CURRENT PEDIATRIC DIAGNOSIS & TREATMENT

2ND EDITION

current
PEDIATRIC
DIAGNOSIS
& TREATMENT

By

C. HENRY KEMPE, MD

Professor of Pediatrics and
Chairman, Department of Pediatrics
University of Colorado School of Medicine
Denver, Colorado

HENRY K. SILVER, MD

Professor of Pediatrics
University of Colorado School of Medicine
Denver, Colorado

DONOUGH O'BRIEN, MD, FRCP

Professor of Pediatrics
University of Colorado School of Medicine
Denver, Colorado

And Associate Authors

Lange Medical Publications

LOS ALTOS, CALIFORNIA

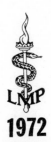

1972

A Concise Medical Library for Practitioner and Student

Current Pediatric Diagnosis & Treatment, 2nd ed. $12.00

Current Diagnosis & Treatment (11th annual revision). Edited by M.A. Krupp and M.J. Chatton. 962 pp.	1972
Review of Physiological Chemistry, 13th ed. H.A. Harper. 529 pp, *illus.*	1971
Review of Medical Physiology, 5th ed. W.F. Ganong. 573 pp, *illus.*	1971
Review of Medical Microbiology, 10th ed. E. Jawetz, J.L. Melnick, and E.A. Adelberg. 518 pp, *illus.*	1972
Review of Medical Pharmacology, 3rd ed. F.H. Meyers, E. Jawetz, and A. Goldfien. 688 pp, *illus.*	1972
General Urology, 7th ed. D.R. Smith. 436 pp, *illus.*	1972
General Ophthalmology, 6th ed. D. Vaughan, T. Asbury, and R. Cook. 316 pp, *illus.*	1971
Correlative Neuroanatomy & Functional Neurology, 14th ed. J.G. Chusid. 453 pp, *illus.*	1970
Principles of Clinical Electrocardiography, 7th ed. M.J. Goldman. 400 pp, *illus.*	1970
Handbook of Psychiatry, 2nd ed. Edited by P. Solomon and V.D. Patch. 648 pp.	1971
Handbook of Surgery, 5th ed. Edited by J.L. Wilson. About 780 pp, *illus.*	1972
Handbook of Obstetrics & Gynecology, 4th ed. R.C. Benson. 774 pp, *illus.*	1971
Physician's Handbook, 16th ed. M.A. Krupp, N.J. Sweet, E. Jawetz, and E.G. Biglieri. 660 pp, *illus.*	1970
Handbook of Medical Treatment, 13th ed. Edited by M.J. Chatton. About 640 pp.	1972
Handbook of Pediatrics, 9th ed. H.K. Silver, C.H. Kempe, and H.B. Bruyn. 713 pp, *illus.*	1971
Handbook of Poisoning: Diagnosis & Treatment, 7th ed. R.H. Dreisbach. 515 pp.	1971

Lithographed in USA

To

Robert J. Glaser, MD

*in recognition of his contribution to the growth of the
Department of Pediatrics of the University of Colorado School of Medicine
and in gratitude for his support and encouragement during his years
as Dean of the School of Medicine (1957–1963).*

Table of Contents

Preface

Rapid advances are being made in almost all areas of child health, and the chief problem in writing a pediatric text is how to be useful without being encyclopedic. We have tried to strike some balances: to emphasize what is more common and more important, but to include also what is uncommon though still important; to pass on to the student and younger pediatrician the practical bedside tips that are his due from foregoing generations of pediatricians who often worked with little else, but to emphasize also the modern aspects of sophisticated procedure; and to balance our desire to leave nothing pertinent unsaid against the necessity of getting the book done and of a size and at a price with which everyone can be satisfied.

As in the First Edition, our attempt is to focus on principles of essential diagnosis and treatment and on current important up-to-date references. The Second Edition contains a new chapter on Ambulatory Pediatrics, a chapter on Teeth, and extensive revisions based on suggestions made by our readers, for which we are most grateful.

Let us stress that the popular *Handbook of Pediatrics* (Silver, Kempe, & Bruyn) continues to be revised and reissued on alternate years. That book is now in its Ninth Edition and serves an entirely different purpose.

The authors and editors have been careful to recommend those drug dosages that are in agreement with current official pharmacologic standards and responsible medical literature, but the dosage recommendations should still be regarded only as estimates in most cases. Since there may be considerable variation in available preparations and dosages of particular drugs offered by individual manufacturers, all clinicians are strongly advised to refer to the drug manufacturer's product information (eg, package inserts), especially in the case of new or infrequently prescribed medications.

–CHK

Denver, Colorado
July, 1972

The Authors

Charles S. August, MD
Disorders of Immune Mechanisms
Assistant Professor of Pediatrics, University of Colorado Medical Center.

Joseph V Brazie, MD
The Newborn & Premature Infant
Director, Section of Newborn Medicine, Presbyterian–St. Luke's Hospital, Chicago; formerly Assistant Professor of Pediatrics, University of Colorado Medical Center.

John D. Burrington, MD
Emergencies & Accidents
Associate Professor of Surgery, University of Colorado Medical Center; Surgeon in Chief, Children's Hospital, Denver.

Winona G. Campbell, MD
Allergic Disorders
Associate Clinical Professor of Pediatrics, University of Colorado Medical Center.

H. Peter Chase, MD
Disorders of Nutrition
Associate Professor of Pediatrics, University of Colorado Medical Center.

Henry E. Cooper, Jr., MD
Adolescence
Associate Professor of Pediatrics and Director of Adolescent Clinic, University of Colorado Medical Center.

Ernest K. Cotton, MD
Respiratory Tract & Mediastinum
Associate Professor of Pediatrics, University of Colorado Medical Center.

Frank J. Cozzetto, MD
Gastrointestinal Tract
Associate Professor of Pediatrics and Director of Clinical Services, University of Colorado Medical Center.

Janice M. Dodds, MS
Normal Nutrition
Education Director, Cook County General Hospital, Chicago.

Marion P. Downs, MA
Ear, Nose, & Throat
Assistant Professor of Surgery (Otolaryngology), University of Colorado Medical Center.

Reuben S. Dubois, MD
Gastrointestinal Tract; Liver & Pancreas
Assistant Professor of Pediatrics, University of Colorado Medical Center.

Burris R. Duncan, MD
Ambulatory Pediatrics
Assistant Professor of Pediatrics, University of Colorado Medical Center.

Jerry J. Eller, MD
Infections: Bacterial & Spirochetal
Assistant Professor of Pediatrics, University of Texas Medical School at San Antonio; formerly Assistant Clinical Professor of Pediatrics, University of Colorado Medical Center.

Elliot F. Ellis, MD
Disorders of Immune Mechanisms
Associate Professor of Pediatrics, University of Colorado Medical Center; Chief of Pediatrics, National Jewish Hospital, Denver.

Philip P. Ellis, MD
Eye
Professor of Surgery and Head, Division of Ophthalmology, University of Colorado Medical Center.

Vincent A. Fulginiti, MD
Immunization; Infections: Viral & Rickettsial; Infections: Mycotic
Professor and Head, Department of Pediatrics, University of Arizona College of Medicine, Tucson; formerly Associate Professor of Pediatrics, University of Colorado Medical Center.

John H. Githens, MD
Hematologic Disorders
Professor of Pediatrics and Associate Dean, Office of Student Affairs, University of Colorado Medical Center.

Ronald W. Gotlin, MD
Endocrine Disorders; Diagnostic & Therapeutic Procedures
Assistant Professor of Pediatrics, University of Colorado Medical Center.

William Hathaway, MD
Hematologic Disorders
Associate Professor of Pediatrics, University of Colorado Medical Center.

Charlene P. Holton, MD
Neoplastic Diseases
Assistant Clinical Professor of Pediatrics, Department of Pediatrics, University of Colorado Medical Center; Director of Clinical Oncology, Children's Hospital, Denver.

Olof H. Jacobson, DDS
Teeth
Clinical Instructor of Surgery, Department of Surgery, University of Colorado Medical Center; Chief of Dental Services, Colorado State Home and Training School, Wheatridge, Colorado.

Jacob T. John, MD
Infections: Parasitic
Chief, Enterovirus Laboratory, Christian Medical College and Hospital, Vellore, South India; formerly Fellow in Pediatric Infectious Diseases, University of Colorado Medical Center.

Leslie L. Kelminson, MD
Heart & Great Vessels
Assistant Clinical Professor of Pediatrics, University of Colorado Medical Center.

C. Henry Kempe, MD
Anti-infective Chemotherapeutic Agents & Antibiotic Drugs
Professor and Chairman, Department of Pediatrics, University of Colorado Medical Center.

Anthony J. Kisley, MD
Psychosocial Aspects of Pediatrics & Psychiatric Disorders
Assistant Clinical Professor of Psychiatry, University of Colorado Medical Center.

Lula O. Lubchenco, MD
The Newborn & Premature Infant
Professor of Pediatrics, University of Colorado Medical Center.

Joan Parker MacReynolds, MS
Normal Nutrition
Nutritionist II, Department of Pediatrics, University of Colorado Medical Center.

Harold P. Martin, MD
Developmental Retardation
Assistant Professor of Pediatrics, John F. Kennedy Center, University of Colorado Medical Center.

John H. Meier, PhD
Developmental Retardation
Associate Professor of Clinical Psychology and Associate Professor of Pediatrics, John F. Kennedy Center, University of Colorado Medical Center.

James S. Miles, MD
Bones & Joints
Professor of Surgery and Head, Division of Orthopedics, University of Colorado Medical Center.

John B. Moon, MD
Kidney & Urinary Tract; Fluid & Electrolyte Therapy
Assistant Professor of Pediatrics, University of Colorado Medical Center.

David N. Myers, MBBCh, DA, FFASA
Respiratory Tract & Mediastinum
Assistant Professor, Department of Anesthesiology, University of Colorado Medical Center.

Gerhard Nellhaus, MD
Neuromuscular Disorders
Associate Professor of Pediatrics and Medicine (Neurology), University of Colorado Medical Center.

James J. Nora, MD
Heart & Great Vessels
Associate Professor of Pediatrics and Director of Pediatric Cardiology, University of Colorado Medical Center.

Donough O'Brien, MD, FRCP
Normal Nutrition; Kidney & Urinary Tract; Connective Tissue Diseases; Diabetes Mellitus; Disorders of Nutrition; Inborn Errors of Metabolism; Fluid & Electrolyte Therapy; Interpretation of Biochemical Values
Professor of Pediatrics, University of Colorado Medical Center.

John E. Ott, MD
Poisoning
Assistant Professor of Pediatrics, University of Colorado Medical Center.

William H. Parry, MD
Respiratory Tract & Mediastinum
Clinical Instructor of Pediatrics, University of Colorado Medical Center.

David Pearlman, MD
Allergic Disorders
Associate Professor of Pediatrics, University of Colorado Medical Center.

James A. Philpott, Jr., MD
Skin
Associate Clinical Professor of Medicine (Dermatology), University of Colorado Medical Center.

Osgoode S. Philpott, Jr., MD
Skin
Assistant Clinical Professor of Medicine (Dermatology), University of Colorado Medical Center.

Dane G. Prugh, MD
Psychosocial Aspects of Pediatrics & Psychiatric Disorders
Professor of Psychiatry and Pediatrics, University of Colorado Medical Center.

Conrad M. Riley, MD
Ambulatory Pediatrics
Professor of Pediatrics and Preventive Medicine, University of Colorado Medical Center.

Arthur Robinson, MD
Genetic & Chromosomal Disorders
Professor of Pediatrics and of Biophysics and Genetics, University of Colorado Medical Center.

Denis O. Rodgerson, PhD
Interpretation of Biochemical Values
Assistant Professor of Pediatrics, University of Colorado Medical Center.

Claude Roy, MD
Gastrointestinal Tract; Liver & Pancreas
Professor of Pediatrics, Hospital Ste. Justin, Montreal; formerly Associate Professor of Pediatrics, University of Colorado Medical Center.

Barton D. Schmitt, MD
Ambulatory Pediatrics
Assistant Professor of Pediatrics, University of Colorado Medical Center.

Henry K. Silver, MD
History & Physical Examination; Growth & Development; Endocrine Disorders; Diagnostic & Therapeutic Procedures; Drug Therapy
Professor of Pediatrics, University of Colorado Medical Center.

Arnold Silverman, MD
Gastrointestinal Tract; Liver & Pancreas
Assistant Clinical Professor of Pediatrics, University of Colorado Medical Center, and Director, Graduate Education, Children's Hospital, Denver.

Clive C. Solomons, PhD
Bones & Joints
Associate Professor of Pediatrics, University of Colorado Medical Center.

Marlin Weaver, MD
Ear, Nose, & Throat
Assistant Clinical Professor of Surgery (Otorhinolaryngology), University of Colorado Medical Center.

Anne S. Yeager, MD
Anti-infective Chemotherapeutic Agents & Antibiotic Drugs
Assistant Professor of Pediatrics, University of Colorado Medical Center.

METRIC SYSTEM PREFIXES
(Small Measurement)

In keeping with the decision of several scientific societies to employ a uniform system of metric nomenclature, the following prefixes have been used in this text:

k	kilo	10^3
c	centi	10^{-2}
m	milli	10^{-3}
μ	micro	10^{-6}
n	nano	10^{-9}
	(formerly	
	millimicro, $m\mu$)	
p	pico	10^{-12}
	(formerly	
	micromicro, $\mu\mu$)	
f	femto	10^{-15}

1...

History & Physical Examination

Henry K. Silver, MD

HISTORY

General Considerations in Taking the History

For many pediatric problems, the history is the most important single factor in arriving at a correct diagnosis.

A. Interpretation of History: The presenting complaint as given by the informant may be a minor part of the problem. One should be prepared to go on, if necessary, to a more productive phase of the interview, which may have little or no apparent relationship to the complaint as originally presented.

B. Source of History: The history should be obtained from the mother or from whoever is responsible for the care of the child. Much valuable information can be obtained also from the child himself.

C. Direction of Questioning: Allow the informant to present the problem as she sees it; then fill in with necessary past and family history and other pertinent information. The record should also include whatever may be disclosed concerning the parents' temperaments, attitudes, and methods of rearing children.

Questions should not be prying, especially about subjects likely to be associated with feelings of guilt or shame; however, the informant should be allowed to volunteer information of this nature when she is prepared to do so.

D. Recorded History: The history should be a detailed, clear, and chronologic record of significant information. It should include the parents' interpretation of the present difficulty, and should indicate the results they expect from consultation.

E. Psychotherapeutic Effects: In many cases the interview and history-taking is the first stage in the psychotherapeutic management of the patient and his parents.

HISTORY OUTLINE: GENERAL

The following outline should be modified and adapted as appropriate for the age of the child and the condition for which he is brought to the physician:

Name, address, home phone number, sex, date and place of birth, race, religion, nationality, referred by, father's and mother's names, father's and mother's occupations, business telephone numbers.

Date: _____ Hospital or case number: _____

Previous entries: Dates, diagnoses, therapy, other data.

Summary of correspondence or other information from physicians, schools, etc.

Presenting Complaint (PC)

Patient's or parent's own brief account of the complaint and its duration.

Present Illness (PI) (or Interval History)

When was the patient last entirely well?

How and when did the disturbance start?

Health immediately before the illness.

Progress of disease; order and date of onset of new symptoms.

Specific symptoms and physical signs that may have developed.

Pertinent negative data obtained by direct questioning.

Aggravating and alleviating factors.

Significant medical attention and medications given and over what period.

In acute infections, statement of type and degree of exposure and interval since exposure.

For the well child, determine factors of significance and general condition since last visit.

Examiner's opinion about the reliability of the informant.

Previous Health

A. Antenatal: Health of mother during pregnancy. Medical supervision, diet, infections such as rubella, etc, other illnesses, vomiting, toxemia, other complications; Rh typing and serology, pelvimetry, medications, x-ray procedure.

B. Natal: Duration of pregnancy, birth weight, kind and duration of labor, type of delivery, sedation and anesthesia (if known), state of infant at birth, resuscitation required, onset of respiration, first cry.

C. Neonatal: Apgar score; color, cyanosis, pallor, jaundice, cry, twitchings, excessive mucus, paralysis, convulsions, fever, hemorrhage, congenital abnormalities, birth injury. Difficulty in sucking, rashes, excessive weight loss, feeding difficulties.

Development

(1) First raised head, rolled over, sat alone, pulled up, walked with help, walked alone, talked (meaningful words; sentences).

(2) Urinary continence during night; during day.

(3) Control of feces.

(4) Comparison of development with that of siblings and parents.

(5) Any period of failure to grow or unusual growth.

(6) School grade, quality of work.

Nutrition

A. Breast or Formula: Type, duration, major formula changes, time of weaning, difficulties.

B. Vitamin Supplements: Type, when started, amount, duration.

C. "Solid" Foods: When introduced, how taken, types.

D. Appetite: Food likes and dislikes, idiosyncrasies or allergies, reaction of child to eating.

Illnesses

A. Infections: Age, types, number, severity.

B. Contagious Diseases: Age, complications following measles, rubella, chickenpox, mumps, pertussis, diphtheria, scarlet fever.

C. Others.

Immunization & Tests

Indicate type, number, reactions, age of child.

A. Inoculations: Diphtheria, tetanus, pertussis, measles, poliomyelitis, typhoid, mumps, others.

B. Oral Immunizations: Poliomyelitis.

C. Percutaneous Vaccination: Smallpox. ("Take" or not? Scar?)

D. Recall immunizations ("boosters").

E. Serum Injections: Passive immunizations.

F. Tests: Tuberculin, Schick, serology, others.

Operations

Type, age, complications; reasons for operations; apparent response of child.

Accidents & Injuries

Nature, severity, sequelae.

Family History

(1) Father and mother (age and condition of health). What sort of people do the parents characterize themselves as being?

(2) Marital relationships. Little information should be sought at first interview; most information will be obtained indirectly.

(3) Siblings. Age, condition of health, significant previous illnesses and problems.

(4) Stillbirths, miscarriages, abortions; age at death and cause of death of immediate members of family.

(5) Tuberculosis, allergy, blood dyscrasias, mental or nervous diseases, diabetes, cardiovascular diseases, kidney disease, rheumatic fever, neoplastic diseases, congenital abnormalities, cancer, convulsive disorders, others.

(6) Health of contacts.

Personality History

A. Relations With Other Children: Independent or clinging to mother; negativistic, shy, submissive; separation from parents; hobbies; easy or difficult to get along with. How does child relate to others? Physical deformities affecting personality.

B. School Progress: Class, grades, nursery school, special aptitudes, reaction to school.

Social History

A. Family: Income; home (size, number of rooms, living conditions, sleeping facilities), type of neighborhood, access to playground. Localities in which patient has lived. Who cares for patient if mother works?

B. School: Public or private, overcrowded, type of students.

C. Insurance: Blue Cross, Blue Shield, or other health insurance?

Habits

A. Eating: Appetite, food dislikes, how fed, attitudes of child and parents to eating.

B. Sleeping: Hours, disturbances, snoring, restlessness, dreaming, nightmares.

C. Exercise and play.

D. Urinary, bowel.

E. Disturbances: Excessive bedwetting, masturbation, thumbsucking, nailbiting, breath-holding, temper tantrums, tics, nervousness, undue thirst, others. Similar disturbances among members of family.

System Review

A. Ears, Nose, and Throat: Frequent colds, sore throat, sneezing, stuffy nose, discharge, postnasal drip, mouth breathing, snoring, otitis, hearing, adenitis.

B. Teeth: Age of eruption of deciduous and permanent; number at 1 year; comparison with siblings.

C. Cardiorespiratory: Frequency and nature of disturbances. Dyspnea, chest pain, cough, sputum, wheeze, expectoration, cyanosis, edema, syncope, tachycardia.

D. Gastrointestinal: Vomiting, diarrhea, constipation, type of stools, abdominal pain or discomfort, jaundice.

E. Genitourinary: Enuresis, dysuria, frequency, polyuria, pyuria, hematuria, character of stream, vaginal discharge, menstrual history, bladder control, abnormalities of penis or testes.

F. Neuromuscular: Headache, nervousness, dizziness, tingling, convulsions, habit spasms, ataxia, muscle or joint pains, postural deformities, exercise tolerance, gait.

G. Endocrine: Disturbances of growth, excessive fluid intake, polyphagia, goiter, thyroid disease.

H. Special senses.

I. General: Unusual weight gain or loss, fatigue, skin color or texture, other abnormalities of skin, temperature sensitivity, mentality. Pattern of growth (record previous heights and weights on appropriate graphs). Time and pattern of pubescence.

The Health Record

Every patient should have a comprehensive medical and health record containing all pertinent information. The parents should be given a summary of this record (including data regarding illnesses, operations, idiosyncrasies, sensitivities, heights, weights, special medications, and immunizations).

PHYSICAL EXAMINATION

Every child should receive a complete systematic examination at regular intervals. One should not restrict the examination to those portions of the body considered to be involved on the basis of the presenting complaint.

Approaching the Child

Adequate time should be spent in becoming acquainted with the child and allowing him to become acquainted with the examiner. The child should be treated as an individual whose feelings and sensibilities are well developed, and the examiner's conduct should be appropriate to the age of the child. A friendly manner, quiet voice, and a slow and easy approach will help to facilitate the examination. If the examiner is not able to establish a friendly relationship but feels that it is important to proceed with the examination, he should do so in an orderly, systematic manner in the hope that the child will then accept the inevitable.

The examiner should wash his hands in warm water before examining the child and should be certain that his hands are warm.

Observation of Patient

Although the very young child may not be able to speak, one still may receive much information from him by being observant and receptive. The total evaluation of the child should include impressions obtained from the time the child first enters until he leaves; it should not be based solely on the period during which the patient is on the examining table. In general, more information is obtained by careful inspection than from any of the other methods of examination.

Holding for Examination

A. Before Age 6 Months: The examining table is usually well tolerated.

B. Age 6 Months to 3–4 Years: Most of the examination may be performed while the child is held in the mother's lap or over her shoulder. Certain parts of the examination can sometimes be done more easily with the child in the prone position or held against the mother so that he cannot see the examiner.

Removal of Clothing

Clothes should be removed gradually to prevent chilling and to avoid the development of resistance in a shy child. In order to save time and to avoid creating unpleasant associations with the doctor in the child's mind, undressing the child and taking his temperature are best performed by the mother. The physician should respect the marked degree of modesty that may be exhibited by some children.

Sequence of Examination

In most cases it is best to begin the examination of the young child with an area that is least likely to be associated with pain or discomfort. The ears and throat should usually be examined last. The examiner should develop a regular sequence of examination that can be adapted as required by special circumstances.

Painful Procedures

Before performing a disagreeable, painful, or upsetting examination, the examiner should tell the child (1) what is likely to happen and how he can assist, (2) that the examination is necessary, and (3) that it will be performed as rapidly and as painlessly as possible.

GENERAL PHYSICAL EXAMINATION
(See also Chapter 2.)

Temperature, pulse rate, and respiratory rate (TPR); blood pressure, weight, and height. The weight should be recorded at each visit; the height should be determined at monthly intervals during the first year, at 3-month intervals in the second year, and twice a year thereafter. The height, weight, and head circumference of the child should be compared with standard charts and the approximate percentiles recorded. Multiple measurements at intervals are of much greater value than single ones since they give information regarding the pattern of growth that cannot be determined by single measurements.

Rectal Temperatures

During the first years of life the temperature should be taken by rectum (except for routine temperatures of the premature infant, where axillary temperatures are sufficiently accurate). The child should be laid face down across the mother's lap and held firmly with her left forearm placed flat across his back; with the left thumb and index finger she can separate the buttocks and insert the lubricated thermometer with the right hand.

Rectal temperature may be 1° F higher than oral temperature. A rectal temperature up to 100° F (37.8° C) may be considered normal in a child.

Apprehension and activity may elevate the temperature.

General Appearance

Does the child appear well or ill? Degree of prostration; degree of cooperation; state of comfort, nutrition, and consciousness; abnormalities; gait, posture, and coordination; estimate of intelligence; reaction to parents, physician, and examination; nature of cry and degree of activity; facies and facial expression.

Skin

Color (cyanosis, jaundice, pallor, erythema), texture, eruptions, hydration, edema, hemorrhagic manifestations, scars, dilated vessels and direction of blood flow, hemangiomas, café-au-lait areas and nevi, Mongolian (blue-black) spots, pigmentation, turgor, elasticity, and subcutaneous nodules. Striae and wrinkling may indicate rapid weight gain or loss. Sensitivity, hair distribution and character, and desquamation.

Practical notes:

(1) Loss of turgor, especially of the calf muscles and skin over the abdomen, is evidence of dehydration.

(2) The soles and palms are often bluish and cold in early infancy; this is of no significance.

(3) The degree of anemia cannot be determined reliably by inspection, since pallor (even in the newborn) may be normal and not due to anemia.

(4) To demonstrate pitting edema in a child it may be necessary to exert prolonged pressure.

(5) A few small pigmented nevi are commonly found, particularly in older children.

(6) Spider nevi occur in about 1/6 of children under 5 years of age and almost 1/2 of older children.

(7) "Mongolian spots" (large, flat black or blue-black areas) are frequently present over the lower back and buttocks; they have no pathologic significance.

(8) Cyanosis will not be evident unless at least 5 gm of reduced hemoglobin are present; therefore, it develops less easily in an anemic child.

(9) Carotenemic pigmentation is usually most prominent over the palms and soles and around the nose, and spares the conjunctivas.

Lymph Nodes

Location, size, sensitivity, mobility, consistency. One should routinely attempt to palpate suboccipital, preauricular, anterior cervical, posterior cervical, submaxillary, sublingual, axillary, epitrochlear, and inguinal lymph nodes.

Practical notes:

(1) Enlargement of the lymph nodes occurs much more readily in children than in adults.

(2) Small inguinal lymph nodes are palpable in almost all healthy young children. Small, mobile, nontender shotty nodes are commonly found as residua of previous infection.

Head

Size, shape, circumference, asymmetry, cephal-hematoma, bosses, craniotabes, control, molding, bruit, fontanel (size, tension, number, abnormally late or early closure), sutures, dilated veins, scalp, hair (texture, distribution, parasites), face, transillumination.

Practical notes:

(1) The head is measured at its greatest circumference; this is usually at the midforehead anteriorly and around to the most prominent portion of the occiput posteriorly. The ratio of head circumference to circumference of the chest or abdomen is usually of little value.

(2) Fontanel tension is best determined with the quiet child in the sitting position.

(3) Slight pulsations over the anterior fontanel may occur in normal infants.

(4) Although bruits may be heard over the temporal areas in normal children, the possibility of an existing abnormality should not be overlooked.

(5) Craniotabes may be found in the normal newborn infant (especially the premature) and for the first 2–4 months.

(6) A positive Macewen's sign ("cracked pot" sound when skull is percussed with one finger) may be present normally as long as the fontanel is open.

(7) Transillumination of the skull can be performed by means of a flashlight with a sponge rubber collar so that it forms a tight fit when held against the head.

Face

Symmetry, paralysis, distance between nose and mouth, depth of nasolabial folds, bridge of nose, distribution of hair, size of mandible, swellings, hypertelorism, Chvostek's sign, tenderness over sinuses.

Eyes

Photophobia, visual acuity, muscular control, nystagmus, Mongolian slant, Brushfield spots, epicanthic folds, lacrimation, discharge, lids, exophthalmos or enophthalmos, conjunctivas; pupillary size, shape, and reaction to light and accommodation; media (corneal opacities, cataracts), fundi, visual fields (in older children).

Practical notes:

(1) The newborn infant usually will open his eyes if he is placed in the prone position, supported with one hand on the abdomen, and lifted over the examiner's head.

(2) Not infrequently, one pupil is normally larger than the other. This sometimes occurs only in bright or in subdued light.

(3) Examination of the fundi should be part of every complete physical examination, regardless of the age of the child; dilatation of pupils may be necessary for adequate visualization.

(4) A mild degree of strabismus may be present during the first 6 months of life but should be considered abnormal after that time.

(5) To test for strabismus in the very young or uncooperative child, note where a distant source of

light is reflected from the surface of the eyes; the reflection should be present on corresponding portions of the two eyes.

(6) Small areas of capillary dilatation are commonly seen on the eyelids of normal newborn infants.

(7) Most infants produce visible tears during the first few days of life.

Nose

Exterior, shape, mucosa, patency, discharge, bleeding, pressure over sinuses, flaring of nostrils, septum.

Mouth

Lips (thinness, downturning, fissures, color, cleft), teeth (number, position, caries, mottling, discoloration, notching, malocclusion or malalignment), mucosa (color, redness of Stensen's duct, enanthems, Bohn's nodules, Epstein's pearls), gums, palate, tongue, uvula, mouth breathing, geographic tongue (usually normal).

Practical note: If the tongue can be extended as far as the alveolar ridge, there will be no interference with nursing or speaking.

Throat

Tonsils (size, inflammation, exudate, crypts, inflammation of the anterior pillars), mucosa, hypertrophic lymphoid tissue, postnasal drip, epiglottis, voice (hoarseness, stridor, grunting, type of cry, speech).

Practical notes:

(1) Before examining a child's throat it is advisable to examine his mouth first. Permit the child to handle the tongue blade, nasal speculum, and flashlight so that he can overcome his fear of the instruments. Then ask the child to stick out his tongue and say "Ah," louder and louder. In some cases this may allow an adequate examination. In others, if the child is cooperative enough, he may be asked to "pant like a puppy"; while he is doing this, the tongue blade is applied firmly to the rear of the tongue. Gagging need not be elicited in order to obtain a satisfactory examination. In still other cases, it may be expedient to examine one side of the tongue at a time, pushing the base of the tongue to one side and then to the other. This may be less unpleasant and is less apt to cause gagging.

(2) Young children may have to be restrained to obtain an adequate examination of the throat. Eliciting a gag reflex may be necessary if the oral pharynx is to be adequately seen.

(3) The small child's head may be restrained satisfactorily by having the mother place her hands at the level of the child's elbows while the arms are held firmly against the sides of his head.

(4) If the child can sit up, the mother is asked to hold him erect in her lap with his back against her chest. She then holds his left hand in her left hand and his right hand in her right hand, and places them against the child's groin or lower thighs to prevent him from slipping down from her lap. If the throat is to be

examined in natural light, the mother faces the light. If artificial light and a head mirror are used, the mother sits with her back to the light. In either case, the physician uses one hand to hold the head in position and the other to manipulate the tongue blade.

(5) Young children seldom complain of sore throat even in the presence of significant infection of the pharynx and tonsils.

Ears

Pinnas (position, size), canals, tympanic membranes (landmarks, mobility, perforation, inflammation, discharge), mastoid tenderness and swelling, hearing.

Practical notes:

(1) A test for hearing is an important part of the physical examination of every infant.

(2) The ears of all sick children should be examined.

(3) Before actually examining the ears, it is often helpful to place the speculum just within the canal, remove it and place it lightly in the other ear, remove it again, and proceed in this way from one ear to the other, gradually going farther and farther, until a satisfactory examination is completed.

(4) In examining the ears, as large a speculum as possible should be used and should be inserted no farther than necessary, both to avoid discomfort and to avoid pushing wax in front of the speculum so that it obscures the field. The otoscope should be held balanced in the hand by holding the handle at the end nearest the speculum. One finger should rest against the head to prevent injury resulting from sudden movement by the child.

(5) The child may be restrained most easily if he is lying on his abdomen.

(6) Low-set ears are present in a number of congenital syndromes, including several that are associated with mental retardation. The ears may be considered low-set if they are below a line drawn from the lateral angle of the eye and the external occipital protuberance.

(7) Congenital anomalies of the urinary tract are frequently associated with abnormalities of the pinnas.

(8) To examine the ears of an infant it is usually necessary to pull the auricle backward and downward; in the older child the external ear is pulled backward and upward.

Neck

Position (torticollis, opisthotonos, inability to support head, mobility), swelling, thyroid (size, contour, bruit, isthmus, nodules, tenderness), lymph nodes, veins, position of trachea, sternocleidomastoid (swelling, shortening), webbing, edema, auscultation, movement, tonic neck reflex.

Practical note: In the older child, the size and shape of the thyroid gland may be more clearly defined if the gland is palpated from behind.

Thorax

Shape and symmetry, veins, retractions and pulsations, beading, Harrison's groove, flaring of ribs, pigeon breast, funnel shape, size and position of nipples, breasts, length of sternum, intercostal and substernal retraction, asymmetry, scapulas, clavicles.

Practical note: At puberty, in normal children, one breast usually begins to develop before the other. In both sexes tenderness of the breasts is relatively common. Gynecomastia is not uncommon in the male.

Lungs

Type of breathing, dyspnea, prolongation of expiration, cough, expansion, fremitus, flatness or dullness to percussion, resonance, breath and voice sounds, rales, wheezing.

Practical notes:

(1) Breath sounds in infants and children normally are more intense and more bronchial, and expiration is more prolonged, than in adults.

(2) Most of the young child's respiratory movement is produced by abdominal movement; there is very little intercostal motion.

(3) If one places the stethoscope over the mouth and subtracts the sounds heard by this route from the sounds heard through the chest wall, the difference usually represents the amount produced intrathoracically.

Heart

Location and intensity of apex beat, precordial bulging, pulsation of vessels, thrills, size, shape, auscultation (rate, rhythm, force, quality of sounds—compare with pulse as to rate and rhythm; friction rub—variation with pressure), murmurs (location, position in cycle, intensity, pitch, effect of change of position, transmission, effect of exercise).

Practical notes:

(1) Many children normally have sinus arrhythmia. The child should be asked to take a deep breath to determine its effect on the rhythm.

(2) Extrasystoles are not uncommon in childhood.

(3) The heart should be examined with the child erect, recumbent, and turned to the left.

Abdomen

Size and contour, visible peristalsis, respiratory movements, veins (distention, direction of flow), umbilicus, hernia, musculature, tenderness and rigidity, tympany, shifting dullness, tenderness, rebound tenderness, pulsation, palpable organs or masses (size, shape, position, mobility), fluid wave, reflexes, femoral pulsations, bowel sounds.

Practical notes:

(1) The abdomen may be examined while the child is lying prone in the mother's lap or held over her shoulder, or seated on the examining table with his back to the doctor. These positions may be particularly helpful where tenderness, rigidity, or a mass must be palpated. In the infant the examination may be aided by having the child suck at a "sugar tip" or nurse at a bottle.

(2) Light palpation, especially for the spleen, often will give more information than deep.

(3) Umbilical hernias are common during the first 2 years of life. They usually disappear spontaneously.

Male Genitalia

Circumcision, meatal opening, hypospadias, phimosis, adherent foreskin, size of testes, cryptorchidism, scrotum, hydrocele, hernia, pubertal changes.

Practical notes:

(1) In examining a suspected case of cryptorchidism, palpation for the testicles should be done before the child has fully undressed or become chilled or had the cremasteric reflex stimulated. In some cases, examination while the child is in a hot bath may be helpful. The boy should also be examined while sitting in a chair holding his knees with his heels on the seat; the increased intra-abdominal pressure may push the testes into the scrotum.

(2) To examine for cryptorchidism, one should start above the inguinal canal and work downward to prevent pushing the testes up into the canal or abdomen.

(3) In the obese boy, the penis may be so obscured by fat as to appear abnormally small. If this fat is pushed back, a penis of normal size is usually found.

Female Genitalia

Vagina (imperforate, discharge, adhesions), hypertrophy of clitoris, pubertal changes.

Practical note: Digital or speculum examination is rarely done until after puberty.

Rectum & Anus

Irritation, fissures, prolapse, imperforate anus. The rectal examination should be performed with the little finger (inserted slowly). Note muscle tone, character of stool, masses, tenderness, sensation. Examine stool on glove finger (gross, microscopic, culture, guaiac), as indicated.

Extremities

A. General: Deformity, hemiatrophy, bowlegs (common in infancy), knock-knees (common after age 2), paralysis, edema, coldness, posture, gait, stance, asymmetry.

B. Joints: Swelling, redness, pain, limitation, tenderness, motion, rheumatic nodules, carrying angle of elbows, tibial torsion.

C. Hands and Feet: Extra digits, clubbing, simian lines, curvature of little finger, deformity of nails, splinter hemorrhages, flat feet (feet commonly appear flat during first 2 years), abnormalities of feet, dermatoglyphics, width of thumbs and big toes, syndactyly, length of various segments, dimpling of dorsa, temperature.

D. Peripheral Vessels: Presence, absence, or diminution of arterial pulses.

Spine & Back

Posture, curvatures, rigidity, webbed neck, spina bifida, pilonidal dimple or cyst, tufts of hair, mobility, Mongolian spot; tenderness over spine, pelvis, or kidneys.

Neurologic Examination (After Vazuka.)

A. Cerebral Function: General behavior, level of consciousness, intelligence, emotional status, memory, orientation, illusions, hallucinations, cortical sensory interpretation, cortical motor integration, ability to understand and communicate, auditory-verbal and visual-verbal comprehension, recognition of visual object, speech, ability to write, performance of skilled motor acts.

B. Cranial Nerves:

1. **I (olfactory)**—Identify odors; disorders of smell.

2. **II (optic)**—Visual acuity, visual fields, ophthalmoscopic examination, retina.

3. **III (oculomotor), IV (trochlear), and VI (abducens)**—Ocular movements, ptosis, dilatation of pupil, nystagmus, pupillary accommodation, and pupillary light reflexes.

4. **V (trigeminal)**—Sensation of face, corneal reflex, masseter and temporal muscles, maxillary reflex (jaw jerk).

5. **VII (facial)**—Wrinkle forehead, frown, smile, raise eyebrows, asymmetry of face, strength of eyelid muscles, taste on anterior portion of tongue.

6. **VIII (acoustic)**—

a. **Cochlear portion**—Hearing, lateralization, air and bone conduction, tinnitus.

b. **Vestibular**—Caloric tests.

7. **IX (glossopharyngeal), X (vagus)**—Pharyngeal gag reflex, ability to swallow and speak clearly; sensation of mucosa of pharynx, soft palate, and tonsils; movement of pharynx, larynx, and soft palate; autonomic functions.

8. **XI (accessory)**—Strength of trapezius and sternocleidomastoid muscles.

9. **XII (hypoglossal)**—Protrusion of tongue, tremor, strength of tongue.

C. Cerebellar Function: Finger to nose; finger to examiner's finger; rapidly alternating pronation and supination of hands; ability to run heel down other shin and to make a requested motion with foot; ability to stand with eyes closed; walk; heel to toe walk; tremor; ataxia; posture; arm swing when walking; nystagmus; abnormalities of muscle tone or speech.

D. Motor System: Muscle size, consistency, and tone; muscle contours and outlines; muscle strength; myotonic contraction; slow relaxation; symmetry of posture; fasciculations; tremor; resistance to passive movement; involuntary movement.

E. Reflexes:

1. **Deep reflexes**— Biceps, brachioradialis, triceps, patellar, Achilles; rapidity and strength of contraction and relaxation.

2. **Superficial reflexes**—Abdominals, cremasteric, plantar, gluteal.

3. **Pathologic reflexes**—Babinski, Chaddock, Oppenheim, Gordon.

●　●　●

General References

Barness LA: *Manual of Pediatric Physical Diagnosis,* 3rd ed. Year Book, 1966.

Frankenburg W, Dodds J: *Denver Developmental Screening Test Manual.* University of Colorado Medical Center & Mead Johnson, 1968.

Judge RD, Zuidema GD (editors): *Physical Diagnosis: A Physiologic Approach to the Clinical Examination,* 2nd ed. Little, Brown, 1968.

Morgan WL, Engel GL: *The Clinical Approach to the Patient.* Saunders, 1969.

Richmond JB, Green M: *Pediatric Diagnosis,* 2nd ed. Saunders, 1962.

2 . . .

Growth & Development*

Henry K. Silver, MD

Body measurements and developmental landmarks provide the best and most practical means of evaluating the health of the individual child, because physical growth and developmental sequence follow a relatively smooth and clearly defined pattern. Growth and development generally progress along expected lines only when the functions of the individual are successfully integrated into a working whole. Failure of the individual to conform to the expected human pattern is completely nonspecific in etiologic terms, since it may equally well result from malnutrition, genetic deficiency, psychologic maladaptation, protracted illness, or a number of other causes. The physician, alerted by disturbances in growth, needs to seek out the specific causes.

Physical or psychologic growth and development generally have a smooth pattern of progression, but some deviation from this pattern is to be expected. The variation between racial groups can be great because of unfavorable factors in some cultures. The standards given here apply to the USA and other Western countries. Standards are derived from the measurement of many individuals and may not be entirely applicable to an individual child.

There is no demonstrated advantage for the child whose height is at the top of the healthy group range over the child whose height falls just within the lower limit of such a range. Gradual change over a period of months or years from one level within the group to another need not be considered as evidence of disease, but marked deviations should be regarded with suspicion. The physician must constantly bear in mind that integration of function occurs within the individual and that disruption of the child's own pattern of growth and development is of greater significance than a deviation from the total population of any one set of measurements.

A knowledge of growth and development is of practical importance in relation to the sick child. Diseases tend to have more impact and to lead to greater permanent impairment when they occur during periods of rapid growth and development than when they occur during intervals of slower and more stable change. For example, loss of growth in the long bones of one leg over a period of several months due to osteomyelitis or prolonged casting in the preadolescent child is of less ultimate significance to the alignment of his spine than it would be if he had been at the height of his adolescent growth.

Development and growth are continuous dynamic processes occurring from conception to maturity and take place in an orderly sequence which is approximately the same for all individuals. At any particular age, however, wide variations are to be found among normal children which reflect the active response of the growing individual to numberless hereditary and environmental factors.

GROWTH

The body as a whole and its various tissues and organs have characteristic growth patterns which are essentially the same in all individuals (Fig 2–1). *Development* signifies maturation of organs and systems, acquisition of skills, ability to adapt more readily to stress, and ability to assume maximum responsibility and to achieve freedom in creative expression. *Growth* refers to a change in size resulting from the multiplication of cells or the enlargement of existing ones.

Rate of growth is generally more important than actual size, and height and weight data must be considered in relation to the variability within a certain age. For more accurate comparisons, data should be recorded both as absolute figures and as percentiles for a particular age.

A number of extrinsic and intrinsic factors influence the rate of total growth and growth of various organ systems. Some of the more important extrinsic factors are nutritional status, climate, season, illness, and activity.

Serial measurements of growth are the best indicators of health. Pertinent measurements should be plotted periodically to determine the pattern of growth and to compare them with normal standards. Graphs designating percentile distribution are particularly useful.

*See also Index and other pertinent chapters.

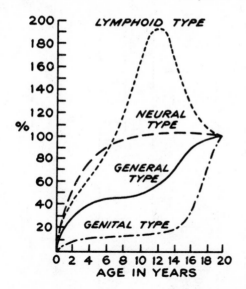

FIG 2-1. Graph showing major types of postnatal growth of various parts and organs of the body. *Lymphoid type:* Thymus, lymph nodes, intestinal lymphoid masses. *Neural type:* Brain and its parts, dura, spinal cord, optic apparatus, many head dimensions. *General type:* Body as a whole, external dimensions (with exception of head and neck), respiratory and digestive organs, kidneys, aorta and pulmonary trunks, spleen, musculature as a whole, skeleton as a whole, blood volume. *Genital type:* Testis, ovary, epididymis, uterine tube, prostate, prostatic urethra, seminal vesicles. (Redrawn and reproduced, with permission, from Holt, McIntosh, & Barnett: *Pediatrics,* 13th ed, Appleton-Century-Crofts, 1962, as redrawn from Harris & others: *Measurement of Man.* University of Minnesota Press, 1930.)

Fetal Growth (See Fig 2-2; Tables 2-1 and 2-2.)

A. Placental Transport:

1. Substances that pass through the placenta by simple diffusion (oxygen, carbon dioxide, water, urea). Some that diffuse are present in lower concentration in the fetus (thyroxine, cholesterol, bilirubin, insulin, progesterone, estrogen), whereas still others are transported actively across the placenta and appear in the fetal blood in higher concentration than in maternal blood (amino acids, glucose, glycerol, fatty acids, minerals).

2. Phosphorus, iodine, and iron are relatively more concentrated on the fetal side of the placenta. Total calcium is present in higher concentration in the blood of the fetus than in the maternal blood, but ionizable calcium is present in equal concentrations in both.

3. Water-soluble vitamins are found in higher concentrations in fetal blood, but fat-soluble vitamins are present in lower concentrations in the fetus.

4. Lipids cross the placenta poorly.

5. The placenta acts as a barrier against thyroid-stimulating hormone, growth hormone, nucleic acids, neutral fats, and many bacteria and viruses.

6. The placenta produces estrogens, progestins, and gonadotropins.

B. Etiology of Fetal Abnormalities: Dietary deficiencies, infections, and numerous other factors in the pregnant woman may cause no manifest symptoms in her while producing significant abnormalities in the offspring; the pregnant woman may fare better than her offspring. Major malformations are present in 1-3.6% of newborn and stillborn infants; minor anomalies have been noted in as many as 15% of newborns.

C. Metabolic Factors:

1. The main source of energy for the growing fetus is carbohydrate.

2. Oxygen saturation in the fetus is lower than that found after birth.

Height (See Figs 2-2 to 2-4, 2-7 to 2-10, and 2-14; Tables 2-1, 2-3, and 2-4.)

A. In Utero:

1. Maximal growth in length occurs during the sixth and seventh months of pregnancy.

2. During fetal life the rate of growth is extremely rapid. During the early months the fetal rate of gain in length is greater than the rate of gain in weight when expressed as percentage of value at birth. By the eighth month the fetus has achieved 80% of his birth length and only 50% of his birth weight. After the second fetal month the greatest relative increase in height is due to an increase in the growth of the extremities.

B. Neonatal:

1. Firstborn infants are usually smaller than later-born infants.

2. At birth, boys are slightly bigger than girls in both height and weight.

3. At birth, the ratio of the lower to the upper segment of the body (as measured from the pubis) is approximately 1:1.7. Subsequently, the legs grow more rapidly than the trunk (Fig 2-5).

C. Childhood: (Figs 2-3, 2-4; Table 2-3.) Height increases at a slowly declining rate until the onset of puberty, when a great spurt in growth occurs. Changes in height are slower in responding to factors that are detrimental to growth than are changes in weight.

1. Birth length is doubled by approximately age 4 and tripled by age 13.

2. The average child grows approximately 20 inches in the 9 months prior to birth, 10 inches in the first year of life, 5 inches in the second, 3-4 inches in the third, and approximately 2-3 inches per year until the growth spurt of puberty appears.

3. At 2 years of age, the midpoint in height is the umbilicus, whereas at adulthood the midpoint is slightly below the symphysis pubis.

4. At 3 years of age, the child is 3 feet tall, and at 4 years, 40 inches tall. At 3½ years the average child weighs 35 pounds.

TABLE 2–1. Fetal and newborn dimensions and weights of the body and its organs.*

Age (Fetal) in Weeks†	Crown-heel (cm)	Crown-rump (cm)	Head Circ. (cm)	Body Wt (gm)	Adrenal (gm)	Brain (gm)	Heart (gm)	Kidney (gm)	Liver (gm)	Lungs (gm)	Pancreas (gm)	Pituitary (gm)	Spleen (gm)	Thymus (gm)	Thyroid (gm)
Prenatal and Newborn															
12	9.0	7.5	7.4	18.6	.087	2.32	.098	.163	.097	.69	.013		.006	.010	.026
16	16.7	12.8	12.6	100	.417	14.4	.662	.962	5.94	3.23	.095	.011	.086	.122	.133
20	24.2	17.7	17.6	310	1.07	43.0	2.08	2.77	16.8	8.18	.314	.024	.410	.553	.352
24	31.1	21.9	22.3	670	2.02	91.0	4.47	5.69	34.5	15.2	.695	.040	1.16	1.53	.684
28	37.1	25.5	26.3	1150	3.16	153	7.70	9.43	57.4	23.7	1.22	.058	2.43	3.14	1.08
30	39.8	27.1	28.1	1400	3.78	189	9.78	11.5	70.3	28.2	1.53	.067	3.26	4.18	1.33
32	42.4	28.5	29.9	1700	4.44	228	11.6	13.8	84.3	33.0	1.88	.076	4.25	5.41	1.54
34	44.8	29.9	31.5	2000	5.11	268	13.7	16.2	100.0	37.8	2.24	.085	5.36	6.77	1.78
36	47.0	31.2	33.1	2450	5.77	309	15.9	18.6	113.0	42.7	2.61	.094	6.55	8.22	2.01
38	49.1	32.4	34.4	2900	6.45	352	18.2	21.0	129.0	47.5	3.01	.103	7.86	9.82	2.26
40	51.0	33.5	35.7	3150	7.10	394	20.6	23.5	143.5	52.5	3.40	.111	9.22	11.5	2.50
Postnatal															
Age (Years)															
1					4	875	43	62	350	160		0.15	30	23	
5					5	1250	90	110	575	305		0.23	55	28	
10					6	1325	145	150	825	450		0.33	77	31	
15					8	1340	245	220	1275	675		0.48	125	27	
Adult‡															
Male					6	1375	300	320	1600	1000			165	14	
Female					6	1280	250	280	1500	750			150	14	

*Adapted from Edith Boyd.
†Time from first day of last menstrual period.
‡Adapted from several sources.

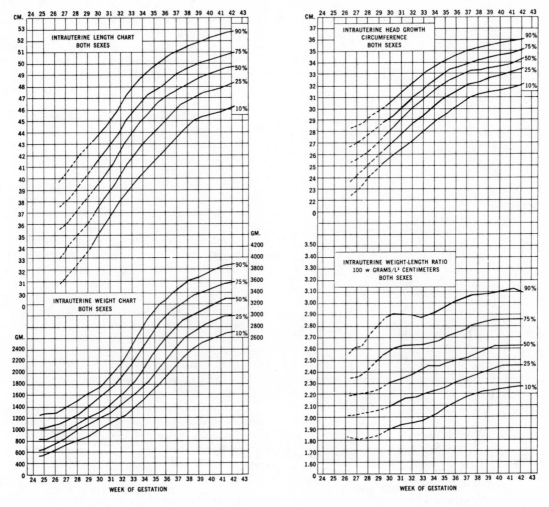

FIG 2–2. **Colorado intrauterine growth charts.** (Reproduced, with permission, from Lubchenco LO & others: Pediatrics 37:403, 1966.)

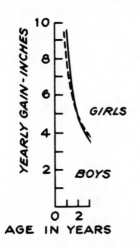

FIG 2–3. Growth rate from birth to age 3 (both sexes).

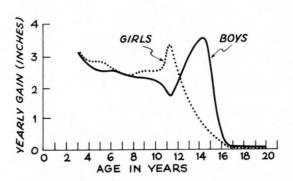

FIG 2–4. Growth rate from age 3–20 (both sexes).

TABLE 2–2. Human fetal development.*

		Fetal Age in Lunar Months
Integument	Three-layered epidermis	3
	Body hair begins	4
	Skin glands form, sweat and sebaceous	4
Mouth	Lip fusion complete	2
	Palate fused completely	3
	Enamel and dentin depositing	5
	Primordia of permanent teeth	6–8
Gastrointestinal	Bile secreted	3
	Rectum patent	3
	Pancreatic islands appear	3
	Fixation of duodenum and colon	4
Respiratory	Definitive shape of lungs	3
	Accessory nasal sinuses developing	4
	Elastic fibers appear in lung	4
Urogenital	Kidney able to secrete	2½
	Vagina regains lumen	5
	Testes descend into scrotum	7–9
Vascular	Definitive shape of heart	1½
	Heart becomes 4-chambered	3½
	Blood formation in marrow begins	3
	Spleen acquires typical structure	7
Nervous	Commissures of brain complete	5
	Myelinization of cord begins	5
	Typical layers of cortex	6
Special senses	Nasal septum complete	3
	Retinal layers complete, light-perceptive	7
	Vascular tunic of lens pronounced	7
	Eyelids open	7–8

*Reproduced, with permission, from Arey LB: *Developmental Anatomy: A Textbook and Laboratory Manual of Embryology*, 5th ed. Saunders, 1947.

5. The legs and feet grow more rapidly than the trunk during childhood. During the first 2–3 years, the feet are flat, and there is an inward bowing of the legs from the knees to the ankles. The feet are often internally rotated ("pigeon-toed") due to internal torsion of the tibia or varus deformity of the medial aspect of the forefoot.

6. During the first year of life, boys grow slightly faster than girls.

7. Between the ages of 1 and 9 years, both boys and girls grow at approximately the same rate.

D. Adolescence:

1. Although children pass through the phase of accelerated growth associated with adolescence at different chronologic ages, the pattern or sequence of adolescent growth tends to be similar in all children.

2. Adolescents undergoing early puberty are taller during early adolescence but have an earlier cessation of growth and shorter stature as adults than adolescents in whom puberty appears later.

3. In the period following the menarche, the average girl grows approximately 5 inches but the range is from less than 1 inch up to 7 inches.

4. The average boy is twice as tall in adult life as he was at age 2.

E. Environmental Factors:

1. Children in this generation are appreciably taller than children in previous generations.

2. Children from high socioeconomic groups are larger than those from lower socioeconomic groups in the same area.

3. Height gains are maximal in the spring and minimal in the fall. The growth of well nourished children is less affected by seasons than is the growth of poorly nourished children. The mechanism in seasonal factors affecting growth is not known.

Weight (See Figs 2–2, 2–6 to 2–10; Table 2–4.)

Body weight is probably the best index of nutrition and growth. Growth responses are noted in changes in weight before they are noted in other aspects of growth. The greatest weight gain occurs in the fall, the least gain in the spring. Obese children are usually taller and exhibit an advanced bone age.

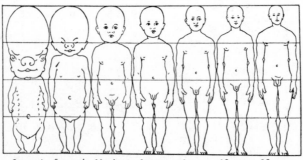

2 months 5 months Newborn 2 years 6 years 12 years 25 years
(fetal)

FIG 2–5. Relative proportions of head, trunk, and extremities at different ages. (From Stratz, modified by Robbins & others: *Growth.* Yale Univ Press, 1928.)

A. Neonatal:

1. The average infant weighs approximately 7 lb 5 oz (3333 gm) at birth.

2. Within the first few days of life, the newborn loses up to 10% of his birth weight. This loss is attributable to loss of meconium, urine, and physiologic edema, and less intake. By 10 days of age, the newborn has generally regained his birth weight.

B. Childhood: (Fig 2–6.)

1. The increment in weight is approximately 1 oz (30 gm)/day during the early months of life.

2. Between the ages of 3 and 12 months, the weight of the child in pounds is equal to his age in months plus 11.

3. Birth weight is doubled between the fourth and fifth months of age, tripled by the end of the first year, and quadrupled by the end of the second year. Between the ages of 2 and 9 years, the annual increment in weight averages about 5 lb per year.

4. At 7 years, the average child weighs 7 times his birth weight.

C. Adolescence: During adolescence, the most rapid gain in weight usually occurs in the year before menarche.

Head & Skull (See Figs 2–5, 2–11, and 2–12.)

Measurements of the head serve as an estimate of brain growth. Growth of the skull as determined by increasing head circumference is a much more accurate index of brain growth than is the presence or size of the fontanel.

A. In Utero: During pregnancy, the head increases in size much more rapidly than the rest of the body.

B. Newborn: At birth, the head is approximately 3/4 its total mature size whereas the rest of the body is only 1/4 its adult size.

C. Childhood:

1. The brain grows very rapidly during infancy and then grows relatively less. At birth, the head makes up 1/4 of the infant's length; by 25 years of age, it measures only 1/8 of the body length.

2. Cranial sutures do not ossify completely until later childhood.

3. While the *averages* of head and chest circumference in the first 4 years of life are approximately equal, during this period the head circumference may normally be from 5 cm larger to 7 cm smaller than the chest.

D. Fontanels:

1. Six fontanels (anterior, posterior, 2 sphenoid, and 2 mastoid) are usually present at birth.

2. The anterior fontanel normally closes between 10 and 14 months of age but may be closed by 3 months or remain open until 18 months.

3. The posterior fontanel usually closes by 2 months but in some children may not be palpable even at birth.

E. Other:

1. The pineal gland may be visualized roentgenographically in 10% of children beyond the tenth year and in 80% of adults of advanced age.

TABLE 2–3. Percent of mature height achieved at each age.

Age in Years	Boys			Girls		
	Average	Accelerated	Retarded	Average	Accelerated	Retarded
Birth	28.6			30.9		
1	42.2	44.5	40.4	44.7	48.0	42.2
2	49.5	51.3	47.0	52.8	54.7	50.0
3	53.8	55.6	51.6	57.0	60.0	55.0
4	58.0	60.0	55.6	61.8	64.9	59.8
5	61.8	64.0	59.7	66.2	69.3	63.8
6	65.2	67.8	63.8	69.3	73.4	67.8
7	69.0	70.5	66.8	74.0	76.0	71.5
8	72.0	73.5	69.8	77.5	79.5	74.5
9	75.0	76.5	73.2	80.7	83.5	77.7
10	78.0	79.7	76.4	84.4	87.9	81.0
11	81.1	83.4	79.5	88.4	92.9	84.9
12	84.2	87.2	82.2	92.9	96.6	88.2
13	87.3	91.3	84.6	96.5	98.2	91.1
14	91.5	95.8	87.6	98.3	99.1	95.2
15	96.1	98.3	91.6	99.1	99.5	97.8
16	98.3	99.4	95.7	99.5	99.5	98.9
16½					100.0	
17	99.3	99.9	98.2	100.0		99.6
17½		100.0				
18	99.8		99.2			100.0
18½	100.0					
19			99.8			
20			100:0			

TABLE 2–4. Percentiles for weight and height: Birth to 5 years and 5–18 years.*

Percentiles (Boys)						Percentiles (Girls)				
3	10	50	90	97		3	10	50	90	97
					Birth					
5.8	6.3	7.5	9.1	10.1	Weight in pounds	5.8	6.2	7.4	8.6	9.4
2.63	2.86	3.4	4.13	4.58	Weight in kg	2.63	2.81	3.36	3.9	4.26
18.2	18.9	19.9	21.0	21.5	Length in inches	18.5	18.8	19.8	20.4	21.1
46.3	48.1	50.6	53.3	54.6	Length in cm	47.1	47.8	50.2	51.9	53.6
					3 Months					
10.6	11.1	12.6	14.5	16.4	Weight in pounds	9.8	10.7	12.4	14.0	14.9
4.81	5.03	5.72	6.58	7.44	Weight in kg	4.45	4.85	5.62	6.35	6.76
22.4	22.8	23.8	24.7	25.1	Length in inches	22.0	22.4	23.4	24.3	24.8
56.8	57.8	60.4	62.8	63.7	Length in cm	55.8	56.9	59.5	61.7	63.1
					6 Months					
14.0	14.8	16.7	19.2	20.8	Weight in pounds	12.7	14.1	16.0	18.6	20.0
6.35	6.71	7.58	8.71	9.43	Weight in kg	5.76	6.4	7.26	8.44	9.07
24.8	25.2	26.1	27.3	27.7	Length in inches	24.0	24.6	25.7	26.7	27.1
63.0	63.9	66.4	69.3	70.4	Length in cm	61.1	62.5	65.2	67.8	68.8
					9 Months					
16.6	17.8	20.0	22.9	24.4	Weight in pounds	15.1	16.6	19.2	22.4	24.2
7.53	8.07	9.07	10.39	11.07	Weight in kg	6.85	7.53	8.71	10.16	10.98
26.6	27.0	28.0	29.2	29.9	Length in inches	25.7	26.4	27.6	28.7	29.2
67.7	68.6	71.2	74.2	75.9	Length in cm	65.4	67.0	70.1	72.9	74.1
					12 Months					
18.5	19.6	22.2	25.4	27.3	Weight in pounds	16.8	18.4	21.5	24.8	27.1
8.39	8.89	10.07	11.52	12.38	Weight in kg	7.62	8.35	9.75	11.25	12.29
28.1	28.5	29.6	30.7	31.6	Length in inches	27.1	27.8	29.2	30.3	31.0
71.3	72.4	75.2	78.1	80.3	Length in cm	68.9	70.6	74.2	77.1	78.8
					15 Months					
19.8	21.0	23.7	27.2	29.4	Weight in pounds	18.1	19.8	23.0	26.6	29.0
8.98	9.53	10.75	12.34	13.33	Weight in kg	8.21	8.98	10.43	12.07	13.15
29.3	29.8	30.9	32.1	33.1	Length in inches	28.3	29.0	30.5	31.8	32.6
74.4	75.6	78.5	81.5	84.2	Length in cm	71.9	73.7	77.6	80.8	82.8
					18 Months					
21.1	22.3	25.2	29.0	31.5	Weight in pounds	19.4	21.2	24.5	28.3	30.9
9.57	10.12	11.43	13.15	14.29	Weight in kg	8.8	9.62	11.11	12.84	14.02
30.5	31.0	32.2	33.5	34.7	Length in inches	29.5	30.2	31.8	33.3	34.1
77.5	78.8	81.8	85.0	88.2	Length in cm	74.9	76.8	80.9	84.5	86.7
					2 Years					
23.3	24.7	27.7	31.9	34.9	Weight in pounds	21.6	23.5	27.1	31.7	34.4
10.57	11.2	12.56	14.47	15.83	Weight in kg	9.8	10.66	12.29	14.38	15.6
32.6	33.1	34.4	35.9	37.2	Length in inches	31.5	32.3	34.1	35.8	36.7
82.7	84.2	87.5	91.1	94.6	Length in cm	80.1	82.0	86.6	91.0	93.3
					2½ Years					
25.2	26.6	30.0	34.5	37.0	Weight in pounds	23.6	25.5	29.6	34.6	38.2
11.43	12.07	13.61	15.65	16.78	Weight in kg	10.7	11.57	13.43	15.69	17.33
34.2	34.8	36.3	37.9	39.2	Length in inches	33.3	34.0	36.0	37.9	38.9
86.9	88.5	92.1	96.2	99.5	Length in cm	84.5	86.3	91.4	96.4	98.7
					3 Years					
27.0	28.7	32.2	36.8	39.2	Weight in pounds	25.6	27.6	31.8	37.4	41.8
12.25	13.02	14.61	16.69	17.78	Weight in kg	11.61	12.52	14.42	16.96	18.96
35.7	36.3	37.9	39.6	40.5	Length in inches	34.8	35.6	37.7	39.8	40.7
90.6	92.3	96.2	100.5	102.8	Length in cm	88.4	90.5	95.7	101.1	103.5
					4 Years					
30.1	32.1	36.4	41.4	44.3	Weight in pounds	29.2	31.2	36.2	43.5	48.2
13.65	14.56	16.51	18.78	20.09	Weight in kg	13.25	14.15	16.42	19.73	21.86
38.4	39.1	40.7	42.7	43.5	Length in inches	37.5	38.4	40.6	43.1	44.2
97.5	99.3	103.4	108.5	110.4	Length in cm	95.2	97.6	103.2	109.6	112.3
					5 Years					
33.6	35.5	40.5	46.7	50.4	Weight in pounds	32.1	34.8	40.5	49.2	52.8
15.24	16.1	18.37	21.18	22.86	Weight in kg	14.56	15.79	18.37	22.32	23.95
40.2	40.8	42.8	45.2	46.1	Length in inches	39.4	40.5	42.9	45.4	46.8
102.0	103.7	108.7	114.7	117.1	Length in cm	100.0	103.0	109.1	115.4	118.8

*The figures for the group from 0–5 years are from Studies of Child Health & Development, Department of Maternal & Child Health, Harvard School of Public Health; those for the group from 5–18 years are from studies by and are reproduced by courtesy of Howard V. Meredith, Iowa Child Welfare Research Station, The State University of Iowa. The figures for 5 years are given twice; their variations are due to the different populations of children used for each group.

TABLE 2—4 (cont'd). Percentiles for weight and height: Birth to 5 years and 5—18 years.

__Percentiles (Boys)__						__Percentiles (Girls)__				
3	10	50	90	97		3	10	50	90	97
					5 Years					
34.5	36.6	42.8	49.7	53.2	Weight in pounds	33.7	36.1	41.4	48.2	51.8
15.65	16.6	19.41	22.54	24.13	Weight in kg	15.29	16.37	18.78	21.86	23.5
40.2	41.5	43.8	45.9	47.0	Height in inches	40.4	41.3	43.2	45.4	46.5
102.1	105.3	111.3	116.7	119.5	Height in cm	102.6	105.0	109.7	115.4	118.0
					6 Years					
38.5	40.9	48.3	56.4	61.1	Weight in pounds	37.2	39.6	46.5	54.2	58.7
17.46	18.55	21.91	25.58	27.71	Weight in kg	16.87	17.96	21.09	24.58	26.63
42.7	43.8	46.3	48.6	49.7	Height in inches	42.5	43.5	45.6	48.1	49.4
108.5	111.2	117.5	123.5	126.2	Height in cm	108.0	110.6	115.9	122.3	125.4
					7 Years					
43.0	45.8	54.1	64.4	69.9	Weight in pounds	41.3	44.5	52.2	61.2	67.3
19.5	20.77	24.54	29.21	31.71	Weight in kg	18.73	20.19	23.68	27.76	30.53
44.9	46.0	48.9	51.4	52.5	Height in inches	44.9	46.0	48.1	50.7	51.9
114.0	116.9	124.1	130.5	133.4	Height in cm	114.0	116.8	122.3	128.9	131.7
					8 Years					
48.0	51.2	60.1	73.0	79.4	Weight in pounds	45.3	48.6	58.1	69.9	78.9
21.77	23.22	27.26	33.11	36.02	Weight in kg	20.55	22.04	26.35	31.71	35.79
47.1	48.5	51.2	54.0	55.2	Height in inches	46.9	48.1	50.4	53.0	54.1
119.6	123.1	130.0	137.3	140.2	Height in cm	119.1	122.1	128.0	134.6	137.4
					9 Years					
52.5	56.3	66.0	81.0	89.8	Weight in pounds	49.1	52.6	63.8	79.1	89.9
23.81	25.54	29.94	36.74	40.73	Weight in kg	22.27	23.86	28.94	35.88	40.78
48.9	50.5	53.3	56.1	57.2	Height in inches	48.7	50.0	52.3	55.3	56.5
124.2	128.3	135.5	142.6	145.3	Height in cm	123.6	127.0	132.9	140.4	143.4
					10 Years					
56.8	61.1	71.9	89.9	100.0	Weight in pounds	53.2	57.1	70.3	89.7	101.9
25.76	27.71	32.61	40.78	45.36	Weight in kg	24.13	25.9	31.89	40.69	46.22
50.7	52.3	55.2	58.1	59.2	Height in inches	50.3	51.8	54.6	57.5	58.8
128.7	132.8	140.3	147.5	150.3	Height in cm	127.7	131.7	138.6	146.0	149.3
					11 Years					
61.8	66.3	77.6	99.3	111.7	Weight in pounds	57.9	62.6	78.8	100.4	112.9
28.03	30.07	35.2	45.04	50.67	Weight in kg	26.26	28.4	35.74	45.54	51.21
52.5	54.0	56.8	59.8	60.8	Height in inches	52.1	53.9	57.0	60.4	62.0
133.4	137.3	144.2	151.8	154.4	Height in cm	132.3	137.0	144.7	153.4	157.4
					12 Years					
67.2	72.0	84.4	109.6	124.2	Weight in pounds	63.6	69.5	87.6	111.5	127.7
30.48	32.66	38.28	49.71	56.34	Weight in kg	28.85	31.52	39.74	50.58	57.92
54.4	56.1	58.9	62.2	63.7	Height in inches	54.3	56.1	59.8	63.2	64.8
138.1	142.4	149.6	157.9	161.9	Height in cm	137.8	142.6	151.9	160.6	164.6
					13 Years					
72.0	77.1	93.0	123.2	138.0	Weight in pounds	72.2	79.9	99.1	124.5	142.3
32.66	34.97	42.18	55.88	62.6	Weight in kg	32.75	36.24	44.95	56.47	64.55
56.0	57.7	61.0	65.1	66.7	Height in inches	56.6	58.7	61.8	64.9	66.3
142.2	146.6	155.0	165.3	169.5	Height in cm	143.7	149.1	157.1	164.8	168.4
					14 Years					
79.8	87.2	107.6	136.9	150.6	Weight in pounds	83.1	91.0	108.4	133.3	150.8
36.2	39.55	48.81	62.1	68.31	Weight in kg	37.69	41.28	49.17	60.46	68.4
57.6	59.9	64.0	67.9	69.7	Height in inches	58.3	60.2	62.8	65.7	67.2
146.4	152.1	162.7	172.4	177.1	Height in cm	148.2	153.0	159.6	167.0	170.7
					15 Years					
91.3	99.4	120.1	147.8	161.6	Weight in pounds	89.0	97.4	113.5	138.1	155.2
41.41	45.09	54.48	67.04	73.3	Weight in kg	40.37	44.18	51.48	62.64	70.4
59.7	62.1	66.1	69.6	71.6	Height in inches	59.1	61.1	63.4	66.2	67.6
151.7	157.8	167.8	176.7	181.8	Height in cm	150.2	155.2	161.1	168.1	171.6

TABLE 2–4 (cont'd). Percentiles for weight and height: Birth to 5 years and 5–18 years.

Percentiles (Boys)						Percentiles (Girls)				
3	10	50	90	97		3	10	50	90	97
					16 Years					
103.4	111.0	129.7	157.3	170.5	Weight in pounds	91.8	100.9	117.0	141.1	157.7
46.9	50.35	58.83	71.35	77.34	Weight in kg	41.64	45.77	53.07	64.0	71.53
61.6	64.1	67.8	70.7	73.1	Height in inches	59.4	61.5	63.9	66.5	67.7
156.5	162.8	171.6	179.7	185.6	Height in cm	150.8	156.1	162.2	169.0	172.0
					17 Years					
110.5	117.5	136.2	164.6	175.6	Weight in pounds	93.9	102.8	119.1	143.3	159.5
50.12	53.3	61.78	74.66	79.65	Weight in kg	42.59	46.63	54.02	65.0	72.35
62.6	65.2	68.4	71.5	73.5	Height in inches	59.4	61.5	64.0	66.7	67.8
159.0	165.5	173.7	181.6	186.6	Height in cm	151.0	156.3	162.5	169.4	172.2
					18 Years					
113.0	120.0	139.0	169.0	179.0	Weight in pounds	94.5	103.5	119.9	144.5	160.7
51.26	54.43	63.05	76.66	81.19	Weight in kg	42.87	46.95	54.39	65.54	72.89
62.8	65.5	68.7	71.8	73.9	Height in inches	59.4	61.5	64.0	66.7	67.8
159.6	166.3	174.5	182.4	187.6	Height in cm	151.0	156.3	162.5	169.4	172.2

2. The eustachian tube is shorter and more horizontal at birth than later.

Nervous System

The CNS makes up 1/4 of the total body weight in the second fetal month, 1/10 at birth, 1/20 at age 5, and only 1/50 of the total weight at full maturity.

A. Myelinization:

1. Myelinization begins by the fourth fetal month and is evident first in the ventral and dorsal spinal routes. The cerebral cortex and thalamus are the last to be myelinated. Myelinization in the cord proceeds in a cephalocaudal direction. At birth, all the cranial nerves, with the exception of the optic and olfactory, are myelinated. At that time, the autonomic nervous system is mature, and some of the segmented spinal nerves are mature, fully myelinated, and functional.

2. The brain stem, those tracts going to the cortex, and some of the finer configurations of the cortex of the brain as well as the nerve tracts connecting the cortex with lower centers are immature and probably incompletely myelinated. Minimal cortical function is present; function is primarily on a subcortical level.

3. Efferent fibers to the voluntary muscles begin to become myelinated soon after birth.

4. Myelinization of the spinal cord, brain stem, and cortex may not be completed for at least 2 years.

B. Reflexes:

1. The cough reflex, Moro reflex, Chvostek's sign, the walking reflex, the patellar reflex, and the grasping reflex are present at birth.

2. The Babinski reflex is seldom elicited in the newborn infant but appears somewhat later and may persist for a year or more.

3. The abdominal and cremasteric reflexes usually cannot be elicited in the neonatal period, nor can the Achilles tendon reflex nor the tonic neck reflex, which is quite inconstant in the newborn but is usually present in the normal 1-month-old infant.

4. By 6 months of age, all the superficial reflexes are present.

C. Blood-Brain Barrier: The blood-brain barrier appears to be more permeable during early infancy than later.

The Respiratory System

A. In Utero:

1. Respiratory movements take place in utero; an exchange of amniotic fluid in the alveoli occurs.

2. The first patterns of respiratory movements become manifest at about the 20th week of pregnancy.

3. The fetus and the newborn can withstand anoxia more effectively than can adults.

B. Newborn:

1. The onset of respiration in the newborn infant is probably dependent on a number of factors, including stimulation of the tactile and thermal receptors on the skin, as well as by hypoxia.

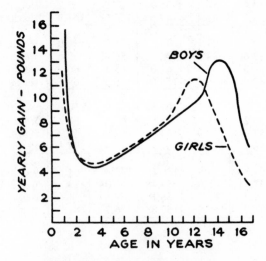

FIG 2–6. **Yearly gain in weight.** (Redrawn and reproduced, with permission, from Barnett: *Pediatrics,* 14th ed. Appleton-Century-Crofts, 1968.)

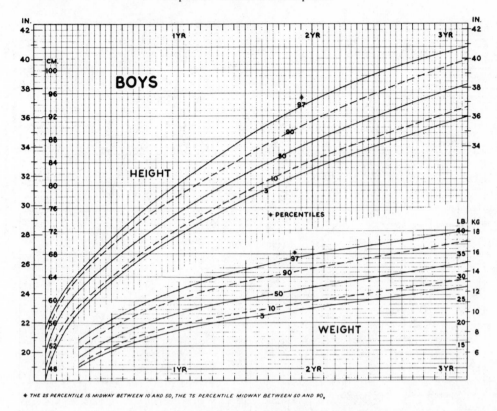

FIG 2−7. Height and weight for boys, age 1−3 years. (Harvard School of Public Health data.)

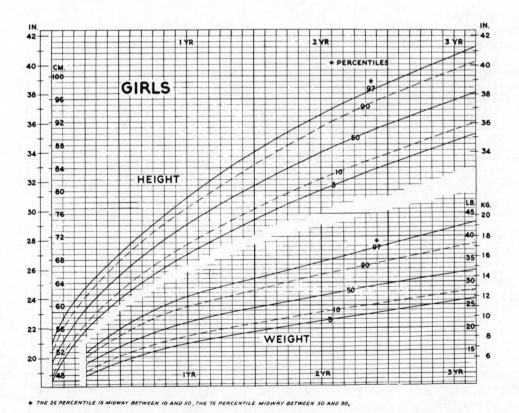

FIG 2−8. Height and weight for girls, age 1−3 years. (Harvard School of Public Health data.)

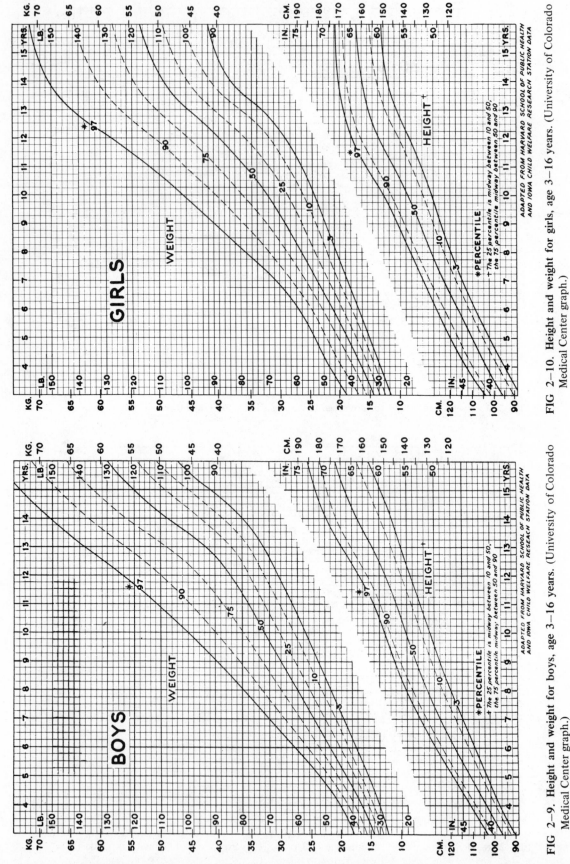

FIG 2–9. **Height and weight for boys, age 3–16 years.** (University of Colorado Medical Center graph.)

FIG 2–10. **Height and weight for girls, age 3–16 years.** (University of Colorado Medical Center graph.)

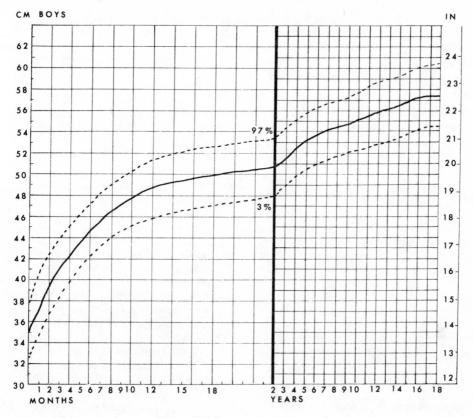

FIG 2–11. Head circumference for boys, birth to 18 years. (Nellhaus: Pediatrics 41:106, 1968.)

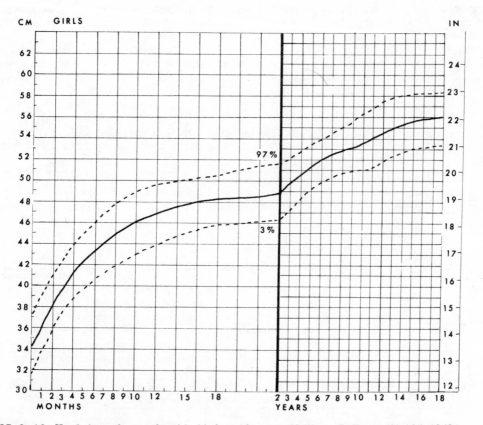

FIG 2–12. Head circumference for girls, birth to 18 years. (Nellhaus: Pediatrics 41:106, 1968.)

TABLE 2−5. Upper limits of the normal P−R interval in children.*

Pulse Rate	Below 70	71−90	91−110	110−130	Above 130
Birth−18 months	0.16	0.15	0.145	0.135	0.125
18 months−6 years	0.17	0.165	0.155	0.145	0.135
6−13 years	0.18	0.17	0.16	0.15	0.14
13−17 years	0.19	0.18	0.17	0.16	0.15

*Reproduced, with permission, from Ashman & Hull: *Essentials of Electrocardiography.* Macmillan, 1941.

2. Respiration in infants is largely diaphragmatic during the first years of life.

C. Childhood:

1. The respiratory rate decreases steadily during childhood, averaging approximately 30/minute during the first year, 25/minute in the second year, 20/minute during the eighth year, and 18/minute by the 15th year.

2. As the child becomes older, the amount of oxygen in the expired air decreases and the amount of CO_2 increases.

D. Adult: Men expel more CO_2 with each breath and have a larger alkali reserve in their blood than women.

Sinuses

A. Newborn: At birth, the mastoid process is only a single cell—the mastoid antrum—and has a relatively wide communication with the middle ear. Its cellular structure appears gradually between birth and age 3. Pneumatization of the tip of the mastoid process becomes demonstrable by the fifth year.

B. Childhood:

1. Maxillary and ethmoid sinuses are present at birth but are usually not aerated and usually cannot be seen by x-ray examination for at least 6 months. The sphenoid sinuses are usually not pneumatized (or visible) until after the third year.

2. Frontal sinuses usually become visible by x-ray between 3 and 9 years of age but seldom before 5.

The Cardiovascular System

A. Heart Rate: The heart rate falls steadily throughout childhood, averaging about 150 beats/minute in utero, 130 beats/minute at birth, 105 beats/minute in the second year of life, 90 beats/minute in the fourth year, 80 beats/minute in the sixth year, and 70 beats/minute in the tenth year.

B. Blood Pressure: (See Table 13−2.)

1. The systolic blood pressure is lower immediately after birth than at any other time during life.

2. The pulmonary and the systemic pressures are approximately equal during the first weeks of life.

C. Heart Sounds:

1. During childhood, the heart sounds have a higher pitch, shorter duration, and greater intensity than later in life. The pulmonary second sound is usually louder than the aortic.

2. Innocent ("functional") murmurs are common during childhood and have been reported to occur in approximately 50% of children at some time during

TABLE 2−6. Changes in the circulatory mechanism at birth. (Adapted from Scammon.)

Structure	Prenatal Function	Postnatal Function
Umbilical vein	Carries oxygenated blood from placenta to liver and heart.	Obliterated to become ligamentum teres (round ligament of liver).
Ductus venosus	Carries oxygenated blood from umbilical vein to inferior vena cava.	Obliterated to become ligamentum venosum.
Inferior vena cava	Carries oxygenated blood from umbilical vein and ductus venosus and mixed blood from body and liver.	Carries only unoxygenated blood from body.
Foramen ovale	Connects right and left atria.	Functional closure by 3 months, although probe patency without symptoms may be retained by some adults.
Pulmonary arteries	Carry some mixed blood to lungs.	Carry unoxygenated blood to lungs.
Ductus arteriosus	Shunts mixed blood from pulmonary artery to aorta.	Generally occluded by 4 months and becomes ligamentum arteriosum.
Aorta	Receives mixed blood from heart and pulmonary arteries.	Carries oxygenated blood from left ventricle.
Umbilical arteries	Carry oxygenated and unoxygenated blood to the placenta.	Obliterated to become the vesical ligaments on the anterior abdominal wall.

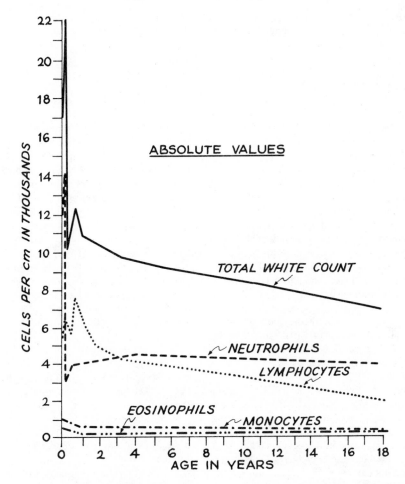

FIG 2–13. **Life patterns of leukocytes.** (Redrawn and reproduced from: *Dynamics of Development: Euthenic Pediatrics,* by D Whipple. Copyright 1966 by McGraw-Hill. Used with permission of McGraw-Hill Book Company.)

childhood, with a peak incidence between the ages of 6 and 9.

3. Less than 10% of murmurs present at birth are the result of a congenital lesion that will persist.

4. A "venous hum" is commonly noted in childhood. It is continuous, located in the parasternal area, usually accentuated in the upright position, and may be either sub- or supraclavicular in location.

D. Heart Volume: Heart volume decreases an average of 25% from birth to the second day as a result of the fluid shift from the vascular compartment and a decreasing flow of blood through the ductus arteriosus.

E. Blood Volume: The total blood volume ranges from 80–110 ml/kg in the newborn infant; averages 115 ml/kg in the premature infant during the first several weeks of life; and is 75–100 ml/kg in the older infant and child and 70–85 ml/kg in the adult.

F. Electrocardiography: (Table 2–5.) During the first months of life there is a tendency to right axis deviation on the ECG.

G. Anatomic Changes Occurring at Birth: (Table 2–6.) The ductus arteriosus and the foramen ovale

close functionally soon after birth; anatomic obliteration of the ductus is complete by the fourth month of postnatal life, whereas anatomic closure of the foramen ovale does not occur until toward the end of the first year.

H. Other:

1. In early childhood, the axis of the heart is more nearly transverse than in later life.

2. Sinus arrhythmia is a normal phenomenon during childhood.

The Blood (See Table 14–1 and Fig 2–13.)

A. In Utero: The first blood-forming centers in the fetus are found in connective tissue (mesenchyme). This later shifts to the liver (most active), spleen, and mesonephros, and finally to the bone marrow. At birth, production of formed elements in the blood occurs primarily in the bone marrow. The liver and spleen retain the ability to make blood cells until early childhood at times of pathologic stress such as excessive hemorrhage.

B. Newborn:

1. If the umbilical cord is not clamped for 2–3 minutes after delivery of the infant, 75–135 ml of blood will be transferred from the placenta to the infant. Late clamping will produce a red blood cell count which is approximately 1 million/cu mm higher, a hemoglobin level approximately 2.5 gm/100 ml higher, and a hematocrit 7% higher than if early clamping were carried out.

2. Nucleated red cells and immature lymphocytes may be present in the newborn but disappear within the first week of life.

3. At birth, 5% of all red blood cells may be reticulocytes; they drop to less than 1% after the second week.

4. Up to 5% of nucleated red blood cells (as a percentage of the total number of nucleated cells) may be present normally for several days after birth.

5. Normally, the number of leukocytes and erythrocytes and the amount of hemoglobin is relatively greater immediately after birth than at any other time in life.

C. Fetal Hemoglobin: Fetal hemoglobin accounts for 80% of total hemoglobin at birth (cord blood), 75% of the total at 2 weeks of age, 55% at 5 weeks, and falls to 5% by 20 weeks of life.

D. White Cells: (Fig 2–13.)

1. The leukocyte count is high at birth, rises slightly during the first 48 hours after birth, falls for the next 2 or 3 weeks, and then rises again. In some children, it reaches its highest level in life sometime before the seventh month; the leukocyte count then falls gradually throughout the remainder of childhood.

2. The lymphocyte count is highest during the first year of life and then falls progressively during the remainder of childhood.

3. The eosinophil count is higher during early infancy than at any other time of life.

4. The basophil count remains essentially unchanged during childhood; at puberty, it falls to adult levels.

E. Sedimentation Rate: Children have an elevated sedimentation rate as contrasted to adults.

The Gastrointestinal Tract

A. Newborn: Gas may be visualized roentgenographically almost immediately after birth in the stomach, within 2 hours in the ileum, and, on the average, in 3 or 4 hours in the rectum.

B. Enzymes:

1. There is a deficiency of the starch-splitting enzyme amylase during early infancy; this prevents optimal handling of long chain polysaccharides. Amylase is present in significant amounts in the pancreatic juice by 3 months of age.

2. Lipase activity is low throughout early childhood. In contrast, trypsin activity is adequate from birth except in the premature infant, in whom low levels are often found.

C. Ketone Bodies: Ketone bodies are not formed as readily by the liver of the young infant as by the older child; acetone is seldom found in the urine at any time during the first 6 months of life.

D. Gastric Acidity: Gastric juice acidity is low during infancy and rises during childhood, with a marked increase during adolescence. Acidity is greater in boys than in girls.

E. Transit Time: Food passes through the stomach more rapidly in the infant than in the older child. Protein digestion is less complete in the stomach of the infant than in the older child.

F. Stomach Capacity: The capacity of the stomach is approximately 30–90 ml at birth, 90–150 ml at 1 month, 210–360 ml at 1 year, approximately 500 ml at 2 years, and averages 750–900 ml in later childhood.

G. Other:

1. Some spitting-up is common in early infancy in almost all children.

2. The abdomen tends to be prominent in infants and toddlers. In the infant, the ascending and descending portions of the colon are short compared with the transverse colon, and the sigmoid extends higher into the abdomen than during later life.

The Urinary System

A. In Utero: The kidney functions during fetal life and contributes some urine to the amniotic fluid, but the fetal kidney probably does not participate in the regulation of electrolyte balance.

B. Newborn:

1. In the kidney of the full-term infant at birth there is a full quota of nephrons, but this may not be the case in the premature infant.

2. The first urine usually has a specific gravity of about 1.015. During the first weeks of life, the urine is scanty and quite dilute (probably as a result of poor response to antidiuretic hormone and immaturity of the renal tubules).

3. During the neonatal period, there is a low clearance of sodium, chloride, and urea, resulting in a hypotonic urine as compared to plasma.

4. The percentage of uric acid is higher in the urine of the neonate than later.

C. Childhood:

1. Renal immaturity probably exists for several months after birth; during the second year of life, the histologic structure of the kidney reaches its mature structure.

2. Glucose and albumin may normally be present in the urine.

D. Urine Volume: The average infant secretes 15–50 ml of urine per 24 hours during the first 2 days of life, 50–300 ml/day during the next week, 250–400 ml/day during the next 2 months, and 400–500 ml/day by the latter 1/2 of the first year. There is subsequently a gradual increase in urinary output; 700–1000 ml are secreted during ages 5–8 and 700–1500 ml between the ages of 8 and 14.

E. Glomerular Filtration: Glomerular filtration rate is low during the first 9 months of life, as are urea clearance, renal plasma flow, and maximal tubular excretory capacity also.

F. Creatine and Creatinine:

1. Creatine is excreted in large amounts by the infant and to a lesser degree by children to the time of puberty; the male adult excretes almost no creatine, whereas female adults excrete very little.

2. Creatinine output increases throughout the growing period, the quantity being directly related to the amount of body musculature.

Fat, Muscle, & Body Water

A. Fat: The body contains equal amounts of fat and protein at or shortly before birth; subsequently, the amount of fat exceeds the amount of protein.

1. Fat is first laid down about the sixth month of pregnancy.

2. The fat of the fetus and newborn infant has a higher degree of saturation, a higher melting point, and contains more palmitic but less stearic and oleic acids than the fat of the older child or adult.

3. There is a gradual decrease in the body stores of fat from the middle of the first year to the age of 6 or 7 years; girls tend to retain more fat than boys, but the differences are slight during childhood. Fat begins to reaccumulate from age 6–7 up to puberty. At that time, the amount of fat decreases in the male but continues to increase in the female.

B. Muscle:

1. At birth, muscle constitutes 20–25% of total body weight as compared with 43% in the adult.

2. During the second trimester of pregnancy, skeletal musculature forms about 1/6 of the body weight; at birth, 1/5 to 1/4; in early adolescence, 1/3; and in early maturity, approximately 2/5.

3. The gain in musculature during childhood equals the growth of all other organs, systems, and tissues combined.

C. Body Water:

1. The water content of the body is approximately 95% by weight in early fetal life; 65–75% at birth; and 55–60% at maturity.

2. The infant ingests and excretes approximately 20% of his total body fluid daily, whereas the adult has a water exchange of only 5% of his total body fluid. For the infant, this represents nearly 50% of his extracellular fluid volume; for the adult, 14% of extracellular fluid volume.

Temperature, BMR, & Steroids (See Table 2–7.)

A. Body Temperature: Body temperature during childhood is on the average 37.3° C (99.1° F) in the first year, 37.5° C (99.4° F) in the fourth year, 37° C (98.6° F) in the fifth year, and 36.7° C (98° F) in the 12th year. During childhood, there is no appreciable difference in the body temperature of boys and girls, but after adolescence women tend to have a higher temperature than men.

B. Basal Metabolic Rate (BMR):

1. Fetal metabolism is lower than that of the newborn.

2. The BMR is highest in the young infant and falls continuously throughout life.

TABLE 2–7. Average body temperatures in well children under basal conditions.*

Age	Temperature and Standard Deviation	
	F	C
3 months	99.4 (0.8)	37.5 (0.4)
6 months	99.5 (0.6)	37.5 (0.3)
1 year	99.7 (0.5)	37.7 (0.2)
3 years	99.0 (0.5)	37.2 (0.2)
5 years	98.6 (0.5)	37.0 (0.2)
7 years	98.3 (0.5)	36.8 (0.2)
9 years	98.1 (0.5)	36.7 (0.2)
11 years	98.0 (0.5)	36.7 (0.2)
13 years	97.8 (0.5)	36.6 (0.2)

*From *Growth and Development of Children,* by Ernest H. Watson, MD. Copyright © 1967. Year Book Medical Publishers, Inc. Used by permission.

3. Boys and girls have comparable metabolic rates, but the rate is higher in men than in women.

C. Steroids:

1. Plasma levels of 17-ketosteroids at birth and for a few days thereafter are 2–5 times higher than in the adult; urinary excretion is higher in the neonatal period than later in infancy.

2. The plasma levels and the urinary excretion of 17-hydroxycorticosteroids are decreased in the newborn infant when compared with the mother's level (which is elevated, particularly during vaginal delivery). Plasma levels remain low for the first 1–2 weeks after birth, gradually rising to adult levels.

Organs of Special Sense

A. Tactile Sensation:

1. At birth the newborn infant has mature sensory receptors for pressure, pain, and temperature from his entire body surface, from his mouth, and from his external genitalia; he also has mature pain receptors in his viscera and proprioceptive receptors in muscles, joints, and tendons.

2. A response to touch is first elicited in the region of the face, particularly the lips.

B. Taste: The ability to taste is present in the newborn infant, and he is capable of distinguishing the 4 basic tastes.

C. Smell: The human infant is born with fully mature receptors for olfaction; the infant may have a stronger sense of smell than the older individual, but this is difficult to test.

D. Hearing:

1. Normal infants can hear almost immediately after birth, but because of a lack of myelinization of cortical auditory pathways they respond to sounds at a subcortical level. Voluntary muscular action in response to sound is present in the average infant by 2 months of age.

2. Although the hearing mechanism in the ear is anatomically mature soon after birth, full maturity of total auditory function may not be present for 5–7 years.

3. The infant can localize a direction of sound by the middle of the first year.

E. Vision: (Table 2—8.) The visual system is relatively immature at birth. The eyeball is less spherical, the cornea is larger, the anterior chamber is more shallow, and the lens more spherical than in the older individual. Because of a lack of myelinization of cerebral neural pathways, the striated muscles which move the eyeballs are not under voluntary control.

TABLE 2—8. Chronology of ophthalmic development.

Age	Level of Development
Birth	Awareness of light and dark. The infant closes his eyelids in bright light.
Neonatal	Rudimentary fixation on near objects (3—30 inches).
2 weeks	Transitory fixation, usually monocular at a distance of roughly 3 feet.
4 weeks	Follows large conspicuously moving objects.
6 weeks	Moving objects evoke binocular fixation briefly.
8 weeks	Follows moving objects with jerky eye movements. Convergence is beginning to appear.
12 weeks	Visual following now a combination of head and eye movements. Convergence is improving. Enjoys light objects and bright colors.
16 weeks	Inspects own hands. Fixates immediately on a 1-inch cube brought within 1—2 feet of eye. Vision 20/300—20/200 (6/100—6/70).
20 weeks	Accommodative convergence reflexes all organizing. Visually pursues lost rattle. Shows interest in stimuli more than 3 feet away.
24 weeks	Retrieves a dropped 1-inch cube. Can maintain voluntary fixation of stationary object even in the presence of competing moving stimulus. Hand-eye coordination is appearing.
26 weeks	Will fixate on a string.
28 weeks	Binocular fixation clearly established.
36 weeks	Depth perception is dawning.
40 weeks	Marked interest in tiny objects. Tilts head backward to gaze up. Vision 20/200 (6/70).
52 weeks	Fusion beginning to appear. Discriminates simple geometric forms, squares and circles. Vision 20/180 (6/60).
12—18 months	Looks at pictures with interest.
18 months	Convergence well established. Localization in distance crude—runs into objects which he sees.
2 years	Accommodation well developed. Vision 20/40 (6/12).
3 years	Convergence smooth. Fusion improving. Vision 20/30 (6/9).
4 years	Vision 20/20 (6/6).

1. Anatomic considerations—

a. The macula begins to differentiate during the first month of life, is well organized by 4 months, and is histologically mature by 8 months.

b. Final development of the macula is reached at about 6 years of age.

c. Tears can be produced during the early weeks of life.

d. The newborn infant is hyperopic; the eyeball grows rapidly for the first 8 years of life, becoming even more hyperopic as a result of changes in the cornea and lens. The eyeball reaches its adult size at about age 8 and then tends to become comparatively myopic. Thus, hyperopia is to be expected in the preschool and early school years.

e. Strabismus normally may be present for the first 6—8 months of life. An infant with an inconstant transient squint need have no treatment until the latter part of the first year. Mature adult function of the eye muscles is usually reached by the end of the first year.

2. Functional considerations—

a. At birth there is an awareness of light and dark, and an infant is capable of rudimentary fixation on near objects.

b. The newborn is capable of peripheral vision, but other visual functions are deficient.

c. The pupillary response is present in late fetal life.

d. The ability to fixate well is usually present by 2—3 months of age.

e. Perception of bright colors is probably present at 3—5 months of age.

f. Depth perception develops at about 9 months of age but does not reach a mature level until age 6.

g. Convergence begins to appear at approximately 8 weeks of age. At 4 months, vision is 20/300—20/200 (6/100—6/70). By 7 months of age, binocular fixation is clearly established. Depth perception becomes apparent at 9 months. At 10 months, vision is 20/200 (6/70). At 1 year, fusion is beginning to appear, and at 18 months convergence is well established. At 2 years, accommodation is well developed; vision is 20/40 (6/12). By 3 years fusion is appearing and vision is 20/30 (6/9). Vision becomes 20/20 (6/6) at age 4.

h. Fusion probably occurs by the sixth year of life.

Immune Mechanisms (See Chapter 15.)

A. In Utero:

1. Antibodies of low molecular weight—the 7S gamma globulins—may appear in higher concentration in fetal than in maternal blood. Antibodies of high molecular weight—the 17S gamma globulins—are usually found in low concentration in the fetus.

2. The placenta permits the transfer of 7S gamma$_1$ globulin to the fetus but selectively withholds the 19S gamma$_1$. Transfer of gamma globulin from the mother to the fetus takes place principally in the last trimester of pregnancy; blood levels of gamma globulin are higher in the full-term infant than in the premature.

3. Gamma globulin is normally not synthesized in utero. The fetus does not synthesize gamma$_2$ globulin. Macroglobulins (19S gamma$_1$) may be synthesized in response to antigenic stimulation.

B. Newborn and Infancy:

1. During the first months of postnatal life, the infant has passive immunity to certain diseases to which the mother was immune, but such immunity is generally limited to those whose antibodies are carried in the 7S gamma$_2$ globulin fraction. Maternal immunity carried solely in macroglobulins is not passed on.

2. In the newborn period, the blood contains a relatively high level of passively transmitted 7S gamma$_2$ globulin and an absence or marked deficiency of 7S and 19S gamma$_1$. The 7S gamma$_2$ globulin which was passively transferred from the mother gradually disappears from the infant's circulation. The lowest level of gamma globulin is reached about the 15th to 80th days.

3. The newborn can manufacture antibody (macroglobulins) as early as the end of the first week of life. By the end of the first year, the child can produce 19S gamma$_1$ globulins as effectively as the adult. However, the newborn is unable to synthesize 7S gamma$_2$ globulin.

C. Childhood: In the normal adult, the presence of 19S gamma$_1$ is followed within a period of 1–2 weeks by the appearance of 7S gamma$_2$, but in the infant relatively little 7S gamma$_2$ appears subsequent to 19S gamma$_1$ formation.

Adolescent Changes (See Tables 2–9 and 2–10.)

A. Both Sexes:

1. The adolescent growth spurt in both sexes is probably due to the production of androgens.

2. Girls mature earlier than boys.

3. Children destined to mature sexually at an early age tend to be tall and have an advanced bone age; late-maturing children are short and show epiphyseal retardation.

4. Sexual maturation is more closely correlated with bone maturation than with chronologic age.

B. Girls: (Table 2–9.)

1. The vaginal mucosa is converted from columnar to squamous type shortly before menarche. This is associated with an increased glycogen content of the mucosa and a lowering of the pH.

2. The maximal yearly increase in height occurs during the year before menarche in most girls.

3. Climate apparently has little effect on sexual development. Nigerian girls and Eskimo girls have their menarche at approximately the same age.

4. If environmental and nutritional factors are similar, girls of different races tend to have their menarche at the same approximate age.

5. During the first 1–2 years following menarche, the menstrual periods of most girls are anovulatory.

6. The first several menses are often irregular, and the interval between periods may be longer or shorter than is characteristic of later life.

7. Girls with early menarche have a more accelerated growth curve than girls with late menarche, but the duration of their growth is shorter.

8. Girls who mature late are taller (on the average) when final stature is attained.

C. Boys: (Table 2–10.) Breast hypertrophy is relatively common in boys at puberty.

"Bone Age" (Epiphyseal Development) (See Table 2–11 and Fig 2–14.)

The ideal method of evaluating bone age would be to x-ray all of the bones. However, this is not practical due to limitations of time, cost, and danger of excessive radiation. At all ages, the most useful areas to evaluate are the wrists and hands; prior to the age of 6 months, x-rays of the feet are also valuable.

The time of appearance and union of various epiphyseal centers follows a specific sequential pattern both during intra- and extrauterine life.

At birth, the average full-term infant has 5 ossification centers demonstrable by x-ray: the distal end of the femur, the proximal end of the tibia, the calcaneus, the talus, and the cuboid.

TABLE 2–9. Time of appearance of sexual characteristics in American girls.*

Pelvis	Female contour assumed and fat deposition begins	8–10 years
Breasts	First hypertrophy or budding	9–11 years
	Further enlargement and pigmentation of nipples	12–13 years
	Histologic maturity	16–18 years
Vagina	Secretion begins and glycogen content of epithelium increases with change in cell type	11–14 years
Pubic hair	Initial appearance	10–12 years
	Abundant and curly	11–15 years
Axillary hair	Initial appearance	12–14 years
Acne	Varies considerably	12–16 years

*From *Growth and Development of Children,* by Ernest H. Watson, MD. Copyright © 1967. Year Book Medical Publishers, Inc. Used by permission.

TABLE 2–10. Time of appearance of sexual characteristics in American boys.*

Breasts	Some hypertrophy, often assuming a firm nodularity	12–14 years
	Disappearance of hypertrophy	14–17 years
Testes and penis	Increase in size begins	10–12 years
	Rapid growth	12–15 years
Pubic hair	Initial appearance	12–14 years
	Abundant and curly	13–16 years
Axillary hair	Initial appearance	13–16 years
Facial and body	Initial appearance	15–17 years
Acne	Varies considerably	14–18 years
Mature sperm	Average range	14–16 years

*From *Growth and Development of Children,* by Ernest H. Watson, MD. Copyright © 1967. Year Book Medical Publishers, Inc. Used by permission.

TABLE 2–11. Time of appearance of epiphyseal ossification centers.*

Hand and Wrist

Age (Year//Month†) Percentile (Boys)			Epiphyseal Centers	Age (Year//Month†) Percentile (Girls)		
5	50‡	95		5	50‡	95
Birth	0 // 2.5	0 // 4	Capitate	< term §	0 // 2.25	0 // 4
Birth	0 // 3.5	0 // 6	Hamate	< term §	0 // 2.5	0 // 5
0 // 8	1 // 0	2 // 0	Distal radius	0 // 6	0 // 10	1 // 6
1 // 0	1 // 6	2 // 0	Proximal third carpal	0 // 9	0 // 11	1 // 3
1 // 0	1 // 6	2 // 0	Proximal second and fourth carpal	0 // 9	0 // 11	1 // 6
1 // 3	1 // 6	2 // 3	Second metacarpal	0 // 9	0 // 11	1 // 6
1 // 0	1 // 6	2 // 3	Distal first carpal	0 // 9	1 // 0	1 // 6
1 // 3	1 // 9	2 // 6	Third metacarpal	0 // 9	1 // 0	1 // 6
1 // 6	2 // 0	2 // 6	Fourth metacarpal	1 // 0	1 // 3	1 // 9
1 // 6	2 // 0	2 // 6	Proximal fifth carpal	1 // 0	1 // 3	2 // 0
1 // 6	2 // 0	2 // 6	Middle third and fourth carpal	1 // 0	1 // 3	2 // 0
1 // 6	2 // 3	3 // 0	Fifth metacarpal	1 // 0	1 // 6	2 // 0
1 // 6	2 // 3	3 // 0	Middle second carpal	1 // 0	1 // 6	2 // 0
1 // 0	2 // 3	4 // 6	Triquetrum	1 // 0	1 // 6	3 // 0
2 // 0	2 // 3	3 // 0	First metacarpal	1 // 6	1 // 6	2 // 6
2 // 6	3 // 0	3 // 6	Proximal first carpal**	1 // 3	1 // 9	2 // 6
2 // 6	3 // 6	5 // 0	Middle fifth carpal**	1 // 6	2 // 0	3 // 3
1 // 6	4 // 0	5 // 6	Lunate**	2 // 6	3 // 0	4 // 0
3 // 6	5 // 3	6 // 6	Greater multangular**	2 // 6	4 // 0	5 // 6
3 // 6	5 // 3	6 // 6	Lesser multangular**	2 // 6	4 // 0	5 // 6
4 // 0	5 // 3	7 // 0	Navicular**	3 // 0	4 // 0	6 // 6
6 // 0	7 // 0	8 // 0	Distal ulna	5 // 0	5 // 6	7 // 0
10 // 0	11 // 0	13 // 0	Pisiform	7 // 6	8 // 0	10 // 6

Extremities
(Excluding Hand and Wrist)

5	50‡	95	Epiphyseal Centers	5	50‡	95
< term §	< term §	2 weeks	Distal femur	< term §	< term §	1 week
< term §	< term §	2 weeks	Proximal tibia	< term §	< term §	1 week
< term §	2 weeks	6 weeks	Tarsal cuboid	< term §	1 week	2 weeks
Birth	3 weeks	0 // 2	Head of humerus	Birth	2 weeks	0 // 1
0 // 3	0 // 4	0 // 9	Distal tibia	0 // 2	0 // 3	0 // 8
0 // 4	0 // 5	0 // 10	Head of femur	0 // 3	0 // 4	0 // 8
0 // 5	0 // 7	1 // 6	Capitellum of humerus	0 // 3	0 // 5	1 // 0
0 // 7	1 // 0	2 // 0	Greater tuberosity of humerus	0 // 4	0 // 8	1 // 6
0 // 8	1 // 0	2 // 0	Distal fibula	0 // 8	0 // 9	1 // 6
2 // 6	3 // 6	4 // 6	Greater trochanter of femur	2 // 0	2 // 6	4 // 0
3 // 0	4 // 0	5 // 6	Proximal fibula	2 // 0	2 // 6	4 // 6
3 // 6	5 // 0	7 // 6	Proximal radius	3 // 0	4 // 0	6 // 0
4 // 6	6 // 0	8 // 0	Medial epicondyle of humerus	3 // 0	3 // 6	6 // 0
7 // 6	10 // 0	12 // 0	Trochlea of humerus	6 // 0	8 // 0	10 // 0
8 // 0	10 // 6	12 // 0	Proximal ulna	6 // 6	8 // 0	9 // 6
10 // 0	12 // 0	13 // 0	Lateral epicondyle of humerus	8 // 0	9 // 6	11 // 0

*Adapted from Marian Maresh. Compiled from data obtained from the Harvard Growth Study, Fels Institute, Brush Foundation, and the University of Colorado Child Research Council.

†Eg, 1 // 3 = 1 year 3 months.

‡50th percentile and mean are approximately the same in most studies.

§< term = before term.

**Centers which are most variable in time and order of appearance.

TABLE 2–12. Dental growth and development.

Primary or Deciduous Teeth

	Calcification		Eruption*		Shedding	
	Begins At	Complete At	Maxillary	Mandibular	Maxillary	Mandibular
Central incisors	4th fetal month	18–24 months	6–10 months (2)	5–8 months (1)	7–8 years	6–7 years
Lateral incisors	5th fetal month	18–24 months	8–12 months (3)	7–10 months (2)	8–9 years	7–8 years
Cuspids	6th fetal month	30–39 months	16–20 months (6)	16–20 months (6a)	11–12 years	9–11 years
First molars	5th fetal month	24–30 months	11–18 months (5)	11–18 months (3)	9–11 years	10–12 years
Second molars	6th fetal month	36 months	20–30 months (7)	20–30 months (7a)	9–12 years	11–13 years

Secondary or Permanent Teeth

	Calcification			Eruption*	
		Begins At	Complete At	Maxillary	Mandibular
Central incisors		3–4 months	9–10 years	7–8 years (3)	6–7 years (2)
Lateral incisors	Maxilla	10–12 months	10–11 years	8–9 years (5)	7–8 years (4)
	Mandible	3–4 months			
Cuspids		4–5 months	12–15 years	11–12 years (11)	9–11 years (6)
First premolars		18–24 months	12–13 years	10–11 years (7)	10–12 years (8)
Second premolars		24–30 months	12–14 years	10–12 years (9)	11–13 years (10)
First molars		Birth	9–10 years	5½–7 years (1)	5½–7 years (1a)
Second molars		30–36 months	14–16 years	12–14 years (12)	12–13 years (12a)
Third molars	Maxilla	7–9 years	18–25 years	17–30 years (13)	17–30 years (13a)
	Mandible	8–10 years			

*Figures in parentheses indicate order of eruption. Many otherwise normal infants do not conform strictly to the stated schedule.

The clavicle is the first bone to calcify in utero, calcification beginning during the fifth fetal week.

Epiphyseal development of girls is consistently ahead of that of boys throughout childhood.

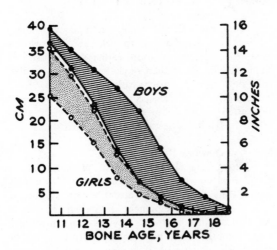

FIG 2–14. **Growth expectancy at bone ages indicated.** (Redrawn and reproduced, with permission, from Holt, McIntosh, & Barnett: *Pediatrics,* 13th ed, Appleton-Century-Crofts, 1962, as redrawn from Harris & others: *Measurement of Man.* University of Minnesota Press, 1930.)

DEVELOPMENT*
(See Table 2–15; Figs 2–15 and 2–16.)

The physician is as responsible for the preservation of health as for the treatment of disease. In order to carry out the former and to identify developmental deviations which may require further assessment, persons responsible for child care must understand the dynamic process involved in what we call development. Development applies to the maturation of organs and systems as well as the acquisition of skills and the ability to adapt to new situations.

*Adapted from Frankenburg WK, Kempe RS, and McCammon R.

Progress of Development

Development is a continuous process that starts with conception and follows an orderly sequential course until death. Children sit before they stand, say single words before they speak phrases and sentences, and draw circles before they can draw squares. Development does not proceed at a constant rate but in bursts of rapid progress interrupted by resting plateaus.

The developmental process takes place in a cephalocaudal direction: control of the head precedes control of the arms, and both precede control of the legs.

Development in the extremities progresses in a proximo-distal direction: control of the arms and legs occurs before control of the wrists and fingers and the feet and toes.

Development proceeds from the massive to the specific. Initially, a young infant seeing a toy moves his entire body; at a later age, he reaches with one hand to grasp it. When an infant learns to say "milk," he may use the word to mean, "Bring me a glass of milk" or "Take the milk"—or the word milk may be used to signify any other drink. Eventually, the word is used to denote what we mean by milk and is combined with other words to form sentences.

Factors Influencing Development

There are "critical periods" of development. At these times, interference with the normal course of development may result in permanent developmental deficits. Just as rubella during the first trimester of pregnancy may result in congenital anomalies, so may untreated cretinism, phenylketonuria, galactosemia, or malnutrition during the first few months after birth result in permanent developmental deficits. On the other hand, rubella, uncontrolled phenylketonuria, hypothyroidism, galactosemia, or malnutrition occurring later in life are usually not associated with permanent significant developmental deficits. Similarly, emotional and psychologic deprivation early in life may produce permanent deficits in personality development.

The pattern of normal development may be influenced by a number of factors, including genetic determinants of rates of development. In certain families, a number of individuals may have a delay in language development. Genetic factors may also determine the intactness of enzyme systems, ie, they may be responsible for inborn errors of metabolism.

Environmental factors may, in turn, influence genetic alternatives. For example, the infant genetically destined to develop cretinism, with its resultant brain damage, may be protected if exogenous thyroid is given. Failure to be appropriately stimulated at critical periods may result in neurologic deficits. Thus, persons deprived of light and auditory stimulation for a prolonged period of time may temporarily develop hallucinations and EEG changes. Environmental influences can either inhibit or enhance the child's motivation and curiosity, and may contain models from which the child learns.

Practice has only a slight influence on normal development; maturation usually plays a much greater role in determining the rate of development.

DEVELOPMENT OF MOTOR SKILLS

The newborn infant can perform a number of motor movements, but these are mainly reflex in character.

Motor development involving the hands tends to proceed along a definite sequential course. First the child looks from his hand to the object. Next, he attempts to grasp objects with 2 hands. Then he learns to grasp with the palm of the hand, first using the ulnar side of the hand and later the radial side. Eventually, he grasps objects with the thumb and index finger.

DEVELOPMENT OF SPEECH & LANGUAGE

The normal development of speech and language requires exposure to language, normal structures of the organs of speech, and the following abilities: hearing in the normal speech frequencies (between 250–4000 cycles/second); comprehending what is heard; recalling what has been heard before; formulating a response; and controlling the muscles of speech. On the average, infants manifest speech and language development as shown in Table 2–13.

Normal Variations in Speech & Language Development

A normal 2-year-old child may have a vocabulary varying from a few words to well over 2000 words. First children tend to speak earlier than subsequent children; twins later than singletons. In some studies, girls developed language earlier than boys. Early development of language is often found in intellectually gifted children, but slow onset of speech is not necessarily an indication of mental deficiency.

Speech & Language Disorders

Though speech and language problems can be detected within the first few years of life, they usually do not come to professional attention until school age.

A. Delayed Development of Speech: If a child does not produce words by 2½ years of age, his speech may be considered to be retarded, but this may not be particularly significant if normal comprehension is present. The principal causes of delayed speech are listed below.

1. Hearing loss or hypoacusis—The effect of hearing loss upon speech and language development varies with the age at which the loss began (more severe in the younger child), the severity of loss, the configura-

TABLE 2–13. Normal speech and language development.

Age	Speech	Language
1 month	Throaty sounds	
2 months	Vowel sounds ("eh"), coos	
2½ months	Squeals	
3 months	Babbles, initial vowels	
4 months	Guttural sounds ("ah," "goo")	
7 months	Imitates speech sounds	
10 months		"Dada" or "Mama" nonspecifically.
12 months		One word other than Mama or Dada.
13 months		Three words.
15–18 months	Jargon (language of his own)	Six words.
21–24 months		Two- to 3-word phrases.
2 years	Vowels uttered correctly	Approximately 270 words; uses pronouns.
3 years	Some degree of hesitancy and uncertainty common	Approximately 900 words; intelligible 4-word phrases.
4 years		Approximately 1540 words; intelligible 5-word phrases or sentences.
6 years		Approximately 2560 words; intelligible 6- or 7-word sentences.
7–8 years	Adult proficiency	

tion of the threshold audiogram, and the efficacy of treatment. (See Chapter 11.) Hypoacusis is frequently associated with incorrect articulation of **b, f,** and **u.** The sounds of **d, y,** and **w** are frequently substituted for **g, l,** and **r,** respectively. The child with a high-frequency hearing loss may react normally to the spoken voice or to sounds of low frequency, clapping of hands, or banging of doors. Hypoacusis, therefore, should only be ruled out by means of a complete audiologic evaluation.

2. Central nervous system dysfunction—The most common type of CNS dysfunction associated with delayed speech development is mental retardation. Neurologic impairments anywhere in the complex speech mechanism may be manifested in delayed speech and language development. Any child with delayed speech development should be evaluated intellectually in terms of his nonverbal as well as his verbal adaptive skills.

3. Maternal deprivation—Children reared without adequate mothering may have delayed speech development. Though other aspects of the child's development may also be delayed, the delay in language is frequently the most prominent. Historically, these children may show a lack of parent-child interaction—diminished affect, decreased motivation, failure to demonstrate stranger anxiety, inability to communicate nonverbally, and a history of an insatiable appetite.

4. Infantile autism—One of the most common manifestations of autism is a delay in speech (see above), probably because of a primary problem in relating to people.

5. Elective mutism—In this condition, children do not talk to certain persons but speak freely at home or elsewhere. Frequently such children are shy. Birth of a sibling may cause a child to stop talking or to talk less and to regress in his development in other ways.

6. Socially disadvantaged background—Since language is learned from other people, deprived environments may fail to provide suitable reinforcement and a sufficient variety of environmental experiences to bring about verbal facility. Children from the lower socioeconomic classes may demonstrate significant deficits in vocabulary, use of adjectives and adverbs, ability to construct complex sentence structures, and a general delay in development of articulation. Their speech and language are similar to normal speech and language of nondisadvantaged children of a younger age.

7. Familial delay—Occasionally, a delay in speech development (possibly due to delayed myelinization) affects several members of a family. The child usually comprehends normally. The delay in speech seldom persists beyond 3 years of age.

8. Histidinemia—In this rare familial aminoaciduria, delayed speech development may occur with mental retardation.

9. Twins—Twins are often late talkers.

10. Bilingualism—Monolingual children are more advanced than bilingual children in language expression but show no differences in the rate of development of language comprehension.

B. Voice Defects (Dysphonia): The loss or impairment of tone and volume is due to excessive loudness and pitch. Though it is generally a functional process, it may evolve into an organic condition with the production of vocal nodules. It may also be due to structural defects (eg, papilloma of the larynx).

C. Articulation Disorders: Articulation errors may be due to omissions, distortions, substitutions, or a combination of these.

1. Causes of articulation disorders—

a. Physiologic and anatomic causes—Defects in the cerebrum and cranial nerves which innervate the muscles of the lips, tongue, and palate may produce

TABLE 2–14. Evaluation of articulation disorders.*

	Age in Years						
	2½–3	3–3½	4–4½	4½–5	5–5½	5½–6	6 and older
Normal number of sounds articulated correctly	7 or more	15 or more	16 or more	18 or more	22 or more	24 or more	25 or more
Normal intelligibility	Understandable half the time or more	Easy to understand					

*Adapted from the Denver Articulation Screening Exam.

articulation defects. Inadequate velopharyngeal closure may also cause articulation disorders, since normal articulation involves movement of the velum between the pendant position to closure against the posterior pharyngeal wall. Inappropriate closure removes the nasality from nasal consonants. Inadequate closure results in resonant properties such as "talking through the nose." Causes of inadequate closure are a cleft palate, a submucous cleft, and velar paresis or disproportion between the soft palate and the posterior pharynx. Since the adenoids sometimes form part of the posterior surface against which the soft palate closes, removal of the adenoids may produce inadequate closure. Children with inadequate closure sometimes present with a history of fluids coming out of the nose during drinking. Failure of fusion of upper lip and hypoplasia of the mandible are other causes of articulation disorders.

b. Environmental factors—Since a child replicates the speech heard in his home, articulation errors may be due to racial, cultural and regional differences or to imitation of articulation errors of the parents. The later a child starts to learn a second language, the more likely he will be to have difficulty in articulating the new language.

2. Evaluation of articulation disorders—The Denver Articulation Screening Exam* is a useful, simple, accurate instrument for determining if a child's articulation is appropriate for his age. The test is designed to detect articulation problems in children age 2½–6 years. To administer the test, one determines the child's ability to correctly articulate each of the 30 italicized sounds found in the following 22 words.

1. *t*able	9. *th*umb	16. wago*n*
2. sh*ir*t	10. too*th*brush	17. *g*u*m*
3. *d*oor	11. *s*ock	18. *h*ouse
4. tru*n*k	12. vacu*um*	19. *p*encil
5. *j*umping	13. *y*arn	20. *f*ish
6. zi*pp*er	14. *m*o*th*er	21. *l*eaf
7. *gr*apes	15. *tw*inkle	22. *c*arro*t*
8. *fl*ag		

The child's articulation is also evaluated for general intelligibility as he puts words together in sentences or phrases (Table 2–14). An abnormal

response either in the articulation of single words or in general intelligibility should be a cause for a diagnostic evaluation by a speech pathologist.

The evaluation should also include a complete neurologic assessment; evaluation of general development or intelligence; assessment of social maturity with a scale such as the Vineland Social Maturity Scale; physical examination of the oropharyngeal cavity; lateral head x-rays during speech production to determine the degree of velopharyngeal closure; and a complete audiologic examination.

D. Dysrhythmia: Three to 4% of children manifest a lack of normal language fluency. In general, lack of fluency is due to interference in the normal control of the respiratory mechanism during speech. Dysrhythmias may be in the form of undue prolongation of word sounds, arrest of speech—mainly at the beginning of a sentence (hesitation)—or repetition of syllables at the beginning of phrases or sentences. Young children between ages 2½–4 years normally manifest breaks in the rhythm of speech, with repetitions being most common.

E. Cluttering: Cluttering is a rapid nervous speech marked by omission of sounds or syllables. The child who clutters may repeat syllables or short words and be unaware of his speech disturbance. Cluttering is due to a dissociation between thinking and speaking. Thus, a child may "get lost" in the middle of a sentence. Individual sounds may be articulated correctly, but the articulation breaks down when the child speaks in longer sentences. Some children who clutter also manifest dysrhythmic handwriting. There is often a family history of cluttering. Occasionally, cluttering may lead to stuttering.

F. Stuttering: Stuttering is a disturbance of rhythm and fluency of speech by an intermittent blocking, convulsive repetition, or prolongation of sounds, syllables, words, or phrases. It is probably caused by many factors. Both organic and psychogenic factors are considered to play a role. Fifty percent of people who stutter begin to do so before age 5, and most begin to stutter before age 11. Between ages 2 and 5, stuttering is usually transient or benign. Stuttering is 2–4 times more frequent in boys. Stuttering causes considerable anxiety in parents, who may then call the child's attention to it in an attempt to make him stop. This, in turn, makes the child more anxious and self-conscious and aggravates the problem. The child may avoid words which are difficult for him to

*Amelia F. Drumwright, University of Colorado Medical Center, 1971.

enunciate, and he may avoid speaking at all. Facial and body movements may be associated with stuttering.

Since one of the factors precipitating or aggravating stuttering is anxiety, it is important to determine the circumstances which led to it. If the stuttering persists or if it has its onset after 11 years of age, the child should be referred to an experienced speech pathologist.

Drumwright A: *Denver Articulation Screening Exam.* University of Colorado Medical Center, 1971.
De Hirsch K: Stuttering and cluttering: Developmental aspects of dysrhythmic speech. J Special Education 2:143, 1969.
Morris HL & others: An articulation test for assessing competency of velopharyngeal closure. J Speech Hearing Dis 1:48, 1961.
Raph JB: Language and speech deficits in culturally disadvantaged children: Implications for the speech clinician. J Speech Hearing Dis 32:203, 1967.

INTELLIGENCE

Intelligence may be defined as the ability to think abstractly and to use abstract symbols for problem solving. It appears to develop when an individual is capable of assimilating (or perceiving) stimuli in the environment and retaining these perceptions in an organized framework.

In general, the development of intelligence occurs in 3 stages. The ages during which these stages take place may vary from one child to another.

First Stage

The first stage involves sensorimotor operations and extends from birth to about 2 years of age.

(1) During the first month of life, the infant responds to stimuli by reflexes.

(2) From 1–4 months, he begins to coordinate reflexes and responses to perform repetitive activities (eg, eye-hand coordination).

(3) From 4–8 months, the child, through memory, may repeat actions to provoke pleasurable responses.

(4) From 8–12 months, he begins to differentiate means from ends, such as the removal of obstacles to obtain a toy.

(5) Starting at 12 months, the child tries new responses to obtain the same goal (experimentation).

Second Stage

The second stage involves concrete operations. It begins at about 18 months or 2 years of age and extends until the child is 11 or 12 years old.

(1) From 2–4 years, he begins to regard stimuli as being representative of other objects (eg, a stick is used as a gun or a wagon as a fire engine).

(2) From 4–7, he begins to form concepts by grouping objects together into classes, such as types of fruit.

(3) From 7–12, he learns about constancy in amounts despite inconstancy of shape (eg, a certain volume of water in a tall narrow glass is the same as that same volume of water in a broad short glass). He also learns that objects can be reversed (eg, 2 and 2 make 4, and 4 can be changed back to 2 and 2).

Third Stage

Stage 3 begins with adolescence. Formal operations are carried out, and the adolescent learns to handle abstract thoughts, to reason, to formulate hypotheses, and to test them in reality and thought.

The development of intelligence is dependent on the brain's capacity to assimilate and accommodate and upon environmental stimuli and models to show how to handle the stimuli. Thus, a child living in a home in which other members are quite vocal will be motivated to develop this skill. When he is tested for verbal ability, he may perform more skillfully than a child with similar intellectual capacity who has not had the same kind of verbal stimulation.

Intelligence Testing

Intelligence tests serve as a relatively accurate assessment of the child's function if such variables as the child's interest, attention span, alertness, motivation, emotional development, and responsiveness are considered in the evaluation of the test.

The tests have a variable degree of accuracy in predicting eventual intelligence but are useful in providing information about a possible organic neurologic abnormality, autism, or emotional deprivation.

DEVELOPMENTAL SCREENING*
(See Fig 2–15.)

There is general agreement that the physician who gives routine pediatric care should have some knowledge of child development and be able to identify abnormal developmental delays.

The Denver Developmental (Frankenburg-Dodds) Screening Test (DDST) is a device for detecting developmental delays in infancy and the preschool years. The test is administered with ease and speed and lends itself to serial evaluations on the same test sheet.

Test Materials

Skein of red wool, box of raisins, rattle with a narrow handle, small aspirin bottle, bell, tennis ball, test form, pencil, 8 one-inch cubical counting blocks.

General Administration Instructions

The mother should be told that this is a developmental screening device to obtain an estimate of the child's level of development and that it is not expected

*From Frankenburg WK: Denver Developmental Screening Test. J Pediat 71:181–191, 1967.

that the child be able to perform each of the test items. This test relies on observations of what the child can do and on report by a parent who knows the child. Direct observation should be used whenever possible. Since the test requires active participation by the child, every effort should be made to put the child at ease. The younger child may be tested while sitting on the mother's lap. This should be done in such a way that he can comfortably reach the test materials on the table. The test should be administered before any frightening or painful procedures. A child will often withdraw if the examiner rushes demands upon the child. One may start by laying out 1 or 2 test materials in front of the child while asking the mother whether he performs some of the personal-social items. It is best to administer the first few test items well below the child's age level in order to assure an initial success-ful experience. To avoid distractions, it is best to remove all test materials from the table except the one that is being administered.

Steps in Administering the Test

(1) Draw a vertical line on the examination sheet through the 4 sectors (gross motor, fine motor adaptive, language, and personal-social) to represent the child's chronologic age. Place the date of the examination at the top of the age line. For premature children, subtract the months premature from the chronologic age.

(2) The items to be administered are those through which the child's chronologic age line passes unless there are obvious deviations. In each sector one should establish the area where the child passes all of the items and the point at which he fails all of the items.

(3) In the event that a child refuses to do some of the items requested by the examiner, it is suggested that the parent administer the item, provided she does so in the prescribed manner.

(4) If a child passes an item, a large letter "P" is written on the bar at the 50% passing point. "F" desig-nates a failure, and "R" designates a refusal.

(5) Failure to perform an item passed by 90% of children of the same age should be considered signifi-cant, although not necessarily abnormal.

(6) Note date and pertinent observations of parent and child behavior (how child feels at time of the evaluation, relation to the examiner, attention span, verbal behavior, self-confidence, etc).

(7) Ask the parent if the child's performance was typical of his performance at other times.

(8) To retest the child on the same form, use a different color pencil for the scoring and age line.

(9) Instructions for administering footnoted items are given below.

Interpretations

The test items are placed into 4 categories: Gross motor, fine motor adaptive, language, and personal-

social. Each of the test items is designated by a bar which is so located under the age scale as to indicate clearly the ages at which 25%, 50%, 75%, and 90% of the standardization population could perform the particular test item. The left end of the bar designates the age at which 25% of the standardization popula-tion could perform the item; the point shown at the top of the bar 50%; the left end of the shaded area 75%; and the right end of the bar the age at which 90% of the standardization population could perform the item.

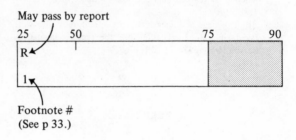

May pass by report

Footnote #
(See p 33.)

Failure to perform an item passed by 90% of chil-dren of the same age should be considered significant. Such a failure may be emphasized by coloring the right end of the bar of the failed item. Several failures in one sector are considered to be developmental delays. These delays may be due to:

(1) The unwillingness of the child to use his abil-ity:

    (a) Due to temporary phenomena, such as fatigue, illness, hospitalization, separation from the parent, fear, etc.

    (b) General unwillingness to do most things that are asked of him; such a condition may be just as detrimental as an inability to perform.

(2) An inability to perform the item due to:

    (a) General retardation.

    (b) Pathologic factors such as deafness or neurologic impairment.

    (c) Familial pattern of slow development in one or more areas.

If unexplained developmental delays are noted and are a valid reflection of a child's abilities, he should be rescreened a month later. If the delays per-sist, he should be further evaluated with more detailed diagnostic studies.

Caution: The DDST is not an intelligence test. It is intended as a screening instrument for use in clinical practice to note whether the development of a particu-lar child is within the normal range.

Directions for Footnoted Items

(1) Try to get child to smile by smiling or by talking or waving to him. Do not touch him.

(2) When child is playing with toy, pull it away from him. Pass if he resists.

(3) Child does not have to be able to tie shoes or button in the back.

(4) Move yarn slowly in an arc from one side to the other, about 6 inches above child's face. Pass if eyes follow 90° to midline. (Past midline, 180°.)

(5) Pass if child grasps rattle when it is touched to the backs or tips of fingers.

(6) Pass if child continues to look where yarn disappeared or tries to see where it went. Yarn should be dropped quickly from sight from tester's hand without arm movement.

(7) Pass if child picks up raisin with any part of thumb and a finger.

(8) Pass if child picks up raisin with the ends of thumb and index finger using an overhand approach.

(9) Copy. Pass any enclosed form. Do not name form. Do not demonstrate.

(10) "Which line is *longer*?" (Not *bigger*.) Turn paper upside down and repeat. (Pass 3 of 3 or 5 of 6.)

(11) Copy. Pass any crossing lines. Do not name form. Do not demonstrate.

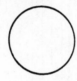

(12) Have child copy first. If he fails, demonstrate. Do not name form.

(13) When scoring symmetrical forms, each pair (2 arms, 2 legs, etc) counts as one part.

(14) Point to picture and have child name it. (No credit is given for sounds only.)

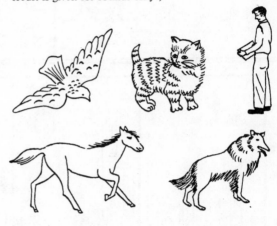

(15) Tell child to, "Give block to Mommie." "Put block on table." "Put block on floor." Pass 2 of 3.

(16) Ask child, "What do you do when you are cold?" "Hungry?" "Tired?" Pass 2 of 3.

(17) Tell child to, "Put block on table." "... under table." "... in front of chair." "... behind chair." Pass 3 of 4. (Do not help child by pointing or by moving head or eyes.)

(18) Ask child, "If fire is hot, ice is –." "Mother is a woman, Dad is a –." "A horse is big, a mouse is –." Pass 2 of 3.

(19) Ask child, "What is a ball?" "... a lake?" "... a desk?" "... a house?" "... a banana?" "... a curtain?" "... a ceiling?" "... a hedge?" "... a pavement?" Pass if defined in terms of use, shape, what it is made of, or general category (eg, banana is *fruit*, not just *yellow*). Pass 6 of 9.

(20) Ask child, "What is a spoon made of?" "... a shoe made of?" "... a door made of?" (No other objects may be substituted.) Pass 3 of 3.

(21) When placed on stomach, child lifts chest off table with support of forearms and/or hands.

(22) When child is on back, grasp his hands and pull him to sitting position. Pass if head does not hang back.

(23) Child may use wall or rail only, not a person. May not crawl.

(24) Child must throw ball overhand 3 feet to within arm's reach of tester.

(25) Child must perform standing broadjump over width of test sheet (8½ inches).

(26) Tell child to walk forward, heel within 1 inch of toe.

(27) Bounce ball to child, who should stand 3 feet away from tester. Child must catch ball with hands, not arms, in 2 out of 3 tries.

(28) Tell child to walk backward, toe within 1 inch of heel. Tester may demonstrate. Child must walk 4 consecutive steps in 2 out of 3 tries.

Date and behavioral observations: (How child feels at time of test, relation to tester, attention span, verbal behavior, self-confidence, etc.)

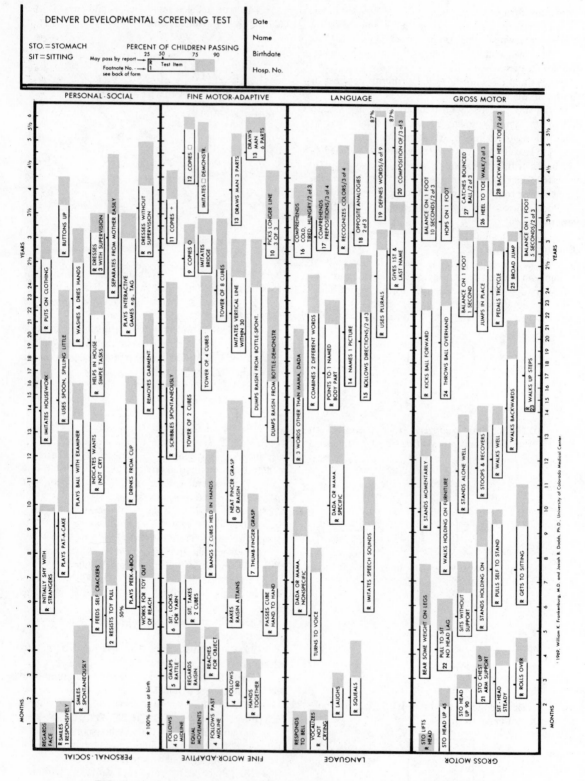

FIG 2–15. Denver Developmental Screening Test. (See p 33 for footnoted items.)

TABLE 2—15. Developmental charts for ages 3–15 years.*

Ages 3–4 Years

Activities to be observed:
Climbs stairs with alternating feet.
Begins to button and unbutton.
"What do you like to do that's fun?" (Answers using plurals, personal pronoun, and verbs.)
Responds to command to place toy *in, on,* or *under* table.
Draws a circle when asked to draw a man (girl, boy).
Knows his sex. ("Are you a boy or a girl?")
Gives full name.
Copies a circle already drawn. ("Can you make one like this?")

Activities related by parent:
Feeds self at mealtime.
Takes off shoes and jacket.

Ages 4–5 Years

Activities to be observed:
Runs and turns without losing balance.
May stand on one leg for at least 10 seconds.
Buttons clothes and laces shoes. (Does not tie.)
Counts to 4 by rote.
"Give me 2 sticks." (Able to do so from pile of 4 tongue depressors.)
Draws a man. (Head, 2 appendages, and possibly 2 eyes. No torso yet.)
"You know the days of the week. What day comes after Tuesday?".
Gives appropriate answers to: "What must you do if you are sleepy? Hungry? Cold?"
Copies + in imitation.

Activities related by parent:
Self care at toilet. (May need help with wiping.)
Plays outside for at least 30 minutes.
Dresses self except for tying.

Ages 5–6 Years

Activities to be observed:
Can catch ball.
Skips smoothly.
Copies a + already drawn.
Tells his age.
Concept of 10 (eg, counts 10 tongue depressors). May recite to higher number by rote.
Knows his right and left hand.
Draws recognizable man with at least 8 details.
Can describe favorite television program in some detail.

Activities related by parent:
Does simple chores at home. (Taking out garbage, drying silverware, etc.)
Goes to school unattended or meets school bus.
Good motor ability but little awareness of dangers.

Ages 6–7 Years

Activities to be observed:
Copies a △.
Defines words by use. ("What is an orange?" "To eat.")
Knows if morning or afternoon.
Draws a man with 12 details.
Reads several one-syllable printed words. (My, dog, see, boy.)
Uses pencil for printing name.

Ages 7–8 Years

Activities to be observed:
Counts by 2s and 5s.
Ties shoes.
Copies a ◇.
Knows what day of the week it is. (Not date or year.)
Reads paragraph #1 Durrell:

Reading:
Muff is a little yellow kitten. She drinks milk. She sleeps on a chair. She does not like to get wet.

Corresponding arithmetic:

$$\begin{array}{cccc} 7 & 6 & 6 & 8 \\ +4 & +7 & -4 & -3 \end{array}$$

No evidence of sound substitution in speech (eg, *fr* for *thr*).
Adds and subtracts one-digit numbers.
Draws a man with 16 details.

Ages 8–9 Years

Activities to be observed:
Defines words better than by use. ("What is an orange?" "A fruit.")
Can give an appropriate answer to the following: "What is the thing for you to do if . . .
—you've broken something that belongs to someone else?"
—a playmate hits you without meaning to do so?"
Reads paragraph #2 Durrell:

Reading:
A little black dog ran away from home. He played with two big dogs. They ran away from him. It began to rain. He went under a tree. He wanted to go home, but he did not know the way. He saw a boy he knew. The boy took him home.

Corresponding arithmetic:

$$\begin{array}{cccc} & 45 & & \\ 67 & 16 & 14 & 84 \\ +4 & +27 & -8 & -36 \end{array}$$

Is learning borrowing and carrying processes in addition and subtraction.

---

*Modified from Leavitt SR, Goodman H, Harvin D: Pediatrics 31:499, 1963. [cont'd]

TABLE 2–15 (cont'd). Developmental charts for ages 3–15 years.

Ages 9–10 Years

Activities to be observed:
Knows the month, day, and year.
Names the months in order. (Fifteen seconds, one error.)
Makes a sentence with these 3 words in it: (One of 2. Can use words orally in proper context.)
1. work .... money .... men
2. boy .... river .... ball
Reads paragraph #3 Durrell:

Reading:
Six boys put up a tent by the side of river. They took things to eat with them. When the sun went down, they went into the tent to sleep. In the night, a cow came and began to eat grass around the tent. The boys were afraid. They thought it was a bear.

Corresponding arithmetic:

$$5204 - 530 \qquad 23 \times 3 \qquad 837 \times 7$$

Should comprehend and answer question: "What was the cow doing?"
Learning simple multiplication.

Ages 10–12 Years

Activities to be observed:
Should read and comprehend paragraph #5 Durrell:

Reading:
In 1807, Robert Fulton took the first long trip in a steamboat. He went one hundred and fifty miles up the Hudson River. The boat went five miles an hour. This was faster than a steamboat had ever gone before. Crowds gathered on both banks of the river to see this new kind of boat. They were afraid that its noise and splashing would drive away all the fish.

Corresponding arithmetic:

$$420 \times 29 \qquad 9\overline{)72} \qquad 31\overline{)62}$$

Answer: "What river was the trip made on?"
Ask to write the sentence: "The fishermen did not like the boat."
Should do multiplication and simple division.

Ages 12–15 Years

Activities to be observed:
Reads paragraph #7 Durrell:

Reading:
Golf originated in Holland as a game played on ice. The game in its present form first appeared in Scotland. It became unusually popular and kings found it so enjoyable that it was known as "the royal game." James IV, however, thought that people neglected their work to indulge in this fascinating sport so that it was forbidden in 1457. James relented when he found how attractive the game was, and it immediately regained its former popularity. Golf spread gradually to other countries, being introduced in America in 1890. It has grown in favor until there is hardly a town that does not boast of a private or public course.

Corresponding arithmetic:

$$536\overline{)4762} \qquad \frac{1}{3} + \frac{1}{3} \qquad 7\frac{1}{6} - \frac{3}{4}$$

Reduce fractions to lowest forms.

Ask to write sentence: "Golf originated in Holland as a game played on ice."
Answers questions:
"Why was golf forbidden by James IV?"
"Why did he change his mind?"
Does long division, adds and subtracts fractions.

PERSONALITY DEVELOPMENT*

Personality development is a dynamic process, and no summary can give a complete picture of what takes place. The goal of the individual, both as a child and as an adult, is to be able to work, to play, to master personal problems, and to love and be loved in a manner that is creative, socially acceptable, and personally gratifying.

The development of personality is a complicated process involving all aspects of the individual and his environment. The process varies from one child to another, but on the whole all children pass through various phases of development of which details differ but of which the broad general outlines are essentially the same.

Each of these successive stages of development is characterized by definite problems which the child must solve if he is to proceed with confidence to the next. The highest degree of functional harmony will be achieved when the problems of each stage are met and solved at an orderly rate and in a normal sequence. On the other hand, it is well to remember that the successive personality gains which the child makes are not rigidly established once and for all but may be reinforced or threatened throughout the life of the individual. Even in adulthood a reasonably healthy personality may be achieved in spite of previous misfortunes and defects in the developmental sequence.

In considering psychologic development it is important to remember that it takes place within a cultural milieu. Not only the form of large social insti-

*Ruth S. Kempe, MD

Smile: In response to an adult or to his voice . . . .

Vocalize: Utters sounds spontaneously or on . . . .
    stimulation
Head control: No head lag when pulled to sitting . . . .
    position from supine
Hand control: Grasps toy with one or both hands . . . .
    when toy is dangled in midline above his chest
Roll over: From back to abdomen . . . .

Sit alone: For several moments . . . .

Crawl: By rolling over and over, pushing along . . . .
    on stomach or back, or any other means
Prehension: Brings together thumb and . . . .
    forefinger to pick up small objects
Pull up: To standing position . . . .

Walk with support: By holding to playpen, ...
    furniture, or an adult
Stand alone: Without any support, for several moments . . . .

Walk alone: Several steps . . . .

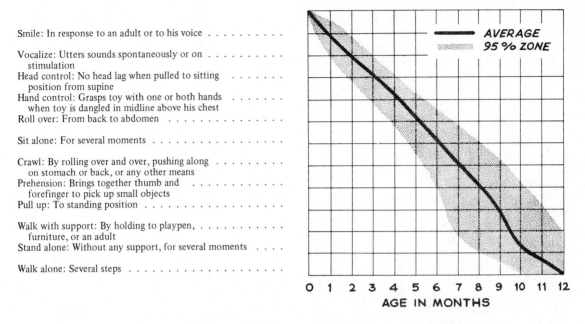

FIG 2—16. Norms of development. (Adapted from Aldrich & Norval: J Pediat 29:304, 1946.)

tutions but the framework of family life, the attitudes of parents, and their practices in child-rearing will be conditioned by the culture of the given period.

Psychologic development in childhood may be roughly divided into 5 stages: infancy (birth to 18 months), early childhood (18 months to 5 years), later childhood (5–12 years), early adolescence (12–16 years), and late adolescence (16 years to maturity).

Infancy

Perhaps the most striking features of the first year are the great physical development which takes place and the infant's growing awareness of himself as an entity separate from his environment.

Much of the psychologic development of the first year is interrelated with physical development, ie, dependent upon the maturation of the body to the extent that the child can discriminate self and nonself. Knowledge of the environment comes with increasing sharpening of the senses (from indiscriminate mouthing to coordinated eye-hand movements). Beginning of mastery over the environment comes with increasingly adept coordination, the development of locomotion, and the beginnings of speech. The realization of himself as an individual in relation to an environment including other individuals is the basis upon which interpersonal relationships are founded.

The newborn infant is at first aware only of his bodily needs—ie, the presence or absence of discomfort (cold, wet, etc). The pleasure of relief from discomfort gradually becomes associated with mothering and later (when perception is sufficient for recognition) with the mother. The child derives a feeling of security when his needs are satisfied and from contact with the mother. The feeding situation provides the first opportunity for

development of this feeling of security, and it is therefore important for the physician to ensure that this is a happy event.

The development of the first emotional relationship, then, comes through this close contact with the mother. It no longer will be just a meeting of the infant's physical needs but a sustained physical contact and emotional interaction with one person. Prolonged absence of this relationship, if no satisfactory substitute is provided, is damaging to the personality. If permanent, it leads to restriction of personality development, even to pseudoretardation in all areas. Such behavior may also occur in a home situation, but it is more striking and more common in infants who remain for long periods of time in the hospital or in other institutions where the nursing personnel is inadequate (either in number or ability) to give sufficient personalized and kindly attention to each child. If the infant is deprived of the security and affection necessary to produce a sense of trust, he may respond with listlessness, immobility, unresponsiveness, indifferent appetite, an appearance of unhappiness, and insomnia. In other cases the continued deprivation of consistent care in infancy may not become apparent until later life, when the individual may feel that he has no reason to trust people; this may result in his feeling no sense of responsibility toward his fellow men.

No particular technics are necessary to develop a baby's feeling of security. The infant is not easily discouraged by an inexperienced mother's mistakes; rather the child seems to respond to the warmth of her feeling and her eagerness to keep trying. The feeling of security derived from satisfactory relationships during the first year is probably the most important single element in the personality. It makes it possible for the child to accept restrictions without fearing that each restriction implies total loss of love.

Toward the end of the first year, other personal relationships also are developing, particularly with the father, who is now recognized as comparable in importance with the mother. Relationships perhaps are also forming with siblings.

Early Childhood

In early childhood the child's horizon continues to widen. Increased body control makes possible the development of many physical skills. The very important development of speech permits extension of the social environment and increasing ability to understand and perfect social relationships.

Perhaps the central problem of early childhood is still, however, the development of control over the instinctive drives, particularly as they arise in relationship to the parents. The acceptance of limitations on the need for bodily love (the realization that complete infantile dependency is not permitted or desirable) and the control of aggressive feelings are prime examples. This control of primitive feelings is largely accomplished through the psychologic process of "identification" with the parents—the desire in the child to be like the parents and to emulate them. With this desire comes the beginnings of conscience, the child's incorporation into his own personality of the moral values of the parents.

The child now begins to have a feeling of autonomy—of self-direction and initiative. The child 18 months to 2½ years of age is actively learning to exercise the power of "yes" and "no." The difficulty the 2-year-old has in making up his mind between the 2 often leads to parental misunderstanding; he may say "no" when he really means "yes," as if he were compelled to exercise this new "will" even against his better judgment.

At this period, parental "discipline" becomes very important. Discipline is an educative means by which the parent teaches the child how to become a self-respecting, likeable, and socially responsible adult. Disciplinary measures have value chiefly as they serve this educative function; if used as an end in themselves, to establish the "authority" of the parent irrespective of the issues at hand, they usually lead only to warfare (open or surreptitious) between parent and child.

The goal is to allow the child to develop the feeling that he is a responsible human being, while at the same time he learns that he is able to use the help and guidance of others in important matters. The favorable result is self-control without loss of self-esteem. As adults, we should allow a child increasingly wide latitude in undergoing experiences which permit him to make the choices he is ready and able to make, and yet we must also teach him to accept restrictions when necessary.

Firmness and consistency in the parent are necessary, for the child must be protected against the potential anarchy of his poorly developed judgment. Perhaps the most constructive rule a parent can follow is to decide which kinds of conformity are really important and then to clearly and consistently require obedience in these areas. Then "discipline" will have the positive goal of making the child socially compatible without making him feel guilty about his basic drives or stifling his need for some expression of independence.

Later Childhood

In this period, the child achieves a rapid intellectual growth and actively begins to establish himself as a member of society. Psychiatrists call this the latency period, because the force of the primitive drives has been fairly successfully controlled, expressed in a socially acceptable way, or repressed. The energy derived from the instinctive drives of which society does not permit direct expression is diverted into the great drive for knowledge—a process of "sublimation." At no time in life does the individual learn more avidly and quickly. Reading and writing (the intellectual skills) and a vast body of information are quickly assimilated. The preoccupation with fantasy gradually subsides, and the child wants to be engaged in real tasks he can carry through to completion. Even in play activities, the emphasis is on developing mental and bodily skills through interest in sports and games.

Late childhood is also a period of conformity to the group. The environment enlarges to include the school and, particularly, other children. Much of the emotional satisfaction previously derived from the parents is now derived from the child's relationships with his peers. His desire to become a member of this larger group of his equals tends to make the qualities of cooperation and obedience to the will of the group (elements of democracy) important. It also paves the way for questioning of the parental values where these differ from those of the group: a direct impact of broader cultural values upon the environment of the home.

Early Adolescence

After the comparative calm of late childhood, early adolescence is a period of upheaval. With the great changes in body size and configuration comes a new confusion about the physical self (the "body image"). Sexual maturation brings with it a resurgence of the strong instinctual drives which have been successfully repressed for several years. In our culture, in contrast to some primitive cultures, the sexual drive is not permitted direct expression in adolescence in spite of physical readiness.

The calm emotional adjustment is disrupted. Again the child has to learn to control strong feelings: love, hate, and aggression. Again the relationship to the parents is disturbed. The former docile acceptance of them as most important, most powerful, is replaced by rebellion. Yet as strongly as the adolescent rebels and insists on independence from his parents, just as strongly does he feel again the old dependence which, although not openly admitted, is revealed in his unwillingness to accept personal responsibility and his tendency to rely on parental care.

Again his position as an individual must be realigned, not in relation to the family circle but in relation to society. Adolescents are constantly preoccupied with how they appear in the eyes of others as compared with their own conceptions of themselves. They find comfort in conformity with their own age group, and fads in clothing and manners reach a peak in early adolescence.

Perhaps most helpful to parents is the ability to "ride" with each swing in adolescent behavior and not assume that each change accurately presages the personality of the future adult. Adolescents are inexperienced in their new roles as potential adults, and their behavior tends to be erratic and extreme. Calm and stability provided by the parents can do much to keep them in equilibrium.

Late Adolescence

By the 16th year most children have again reached comparative equilibrium. Body growth has slowed somewhat, and the adolescent has had time to adapt to his new physique. He has acquired compara- tive mastery over his biologic drives to the extent that they can now be channeled into more constructive patterns, the beginning of heterosexual social activity, which eventually leads to the choice of a marital partner.

The relationship to the parents is now more mature. With the discovery that responsible independence is neither frightening nor overwhelming but a position possible to maintain, the adolescent can cease to rebel and can accept his parents' help in planning constructively for his adulthood.

Again learning is rapid, particularly for the intelligent youth, who can absorb much more than a junior high school education.

Active preparation for adulthood characterizes late adolescence in our culture, although, as in more primitive cultures, some adolescents will have already taken on the responsibilities of job and marriage. Biologically, this is certainly feasible; it is the complexity and competition of our modern culture which so greatly prolongs the emergence into full adulthood.

● ● ●

General References

Watson EH, Lowrey GH: *Growth and Development of Children,* 5th ed. Year Book, 1967.

Whipple DV: *Dynamics of Development: Euthenic Pediatrics.* McGraw-Hill, 1966.

3...

*The Newborn & Premature Infant**

Joseph V Brazie, MD, & Lula O. Lubchenco, MD

The newborn period is usually defined as the interval from birth to age 28 days, though the main clinical emphasis is on the infant's initial nursery stay.

It is obvious that the events leading up to and including birth are vital to the succeeding 28 days, and adequate knowledge of the infant's prenatal and birth history is essential in providing newborn care.

Every newborn infant should be considered a patient in his own right and not a boarder resulting from his mother's admission. Someone must be responsible for the care of the newborn infant from the time of delivery to ensure his satisfactory adjustment to extrauterine life. It is no longer appropriate to organize newborn nurseries only for the care of well newborns, who make these adjustments with minimal difficulty. In order to focus care on the potentially sick infant, the newborn service must have trained personnel available who can anticipate and recognize significant symptoms and signs and institute appropriate diagnostic and therapeutic measures. The specific treatment and general supportive care of the sick newborn infant should be thoroughly understood, and adequate therapeutic facilities must be available.

Certain illnesses can be anticipated before delivery. If the baby is likely to require special care soon after birth, delivery should be planned in or near the hospital where that care is available. Transfer of sick newborns to another hospital for intensive care may result in considerable delay in initiating optimal care, and the transfer itself may introduce additional hazards. Any hospital that assumes the responsibility for delivering newborn infants must provide adequate staff and equipment to manage urgent newborn problems. If the baby's subsequent needs exceed the hospital's capabilities, transfer to a special care newborn center will be necessary.

GROWTH PATTERNS OF NEWBORN INFANTS

Intrauterine growth curves for birth weight, length, and head circumference based on Colorado data are shown in Fig 2–2. A classification of newborn infants based on birth weight, gestational age, and intrauterine growth is given in Fig 3–1.

Birth Weight

In the past, "prematurity"–and, more recently, "low birth weight"–have been defined as a birth weight of 2500 gm or less; in the USA in 1967, the incidence by this criterion was 8.2%. Birth weight is closely related to gestational age, and is a significant factor in morbidity and mortality.

Factors other than gestational age that may influence birth weight include race, sex, socioeconomic status, maternal and paternal height, prenatal care, maternal nutrition and disease, altitude, multiple births, and maternal smoking.

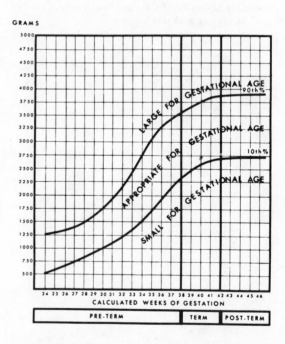

FIG 3–1. Classification of newborn infants by birth weight and gestational age. (University of Colorado Medical Center. Reproduced, with permission, from Battaglia FC, Lubchenco LO: J Pediat 71:160, 1967.)

---

*Special problems of drug treatment in newborn and premature infants are discussed in Chapters 38 and 39.

Gestational Age

Determination of gestational age must be based on careful maternal history correlated with certain findings during the pregnancy, eg, rate of change of uterine height above the symphysis and the time fetal heart sounds and movements were first noted. Determination of gestational age is especially important when elective termination of pregnancy is considered. Obstetric factors may not be known or may be unreliable, so that a clinical estimation of gestational age must also be made from the examination of the infant. This estimation of gestational age is based on physical characteristics and neurologic examination, which change predictably with increasing fetal age (Table 3–3).

Length & Head Size

Most newborns who present with intrauterine growth retardation in weight show relatively less deviation from normal in length and head circumference. Length and head growth appear to be protected to some extent under circumstances of intrauterine undernutrition. However, in severe and prolonged intrauterine undernutrition, such as occurs in the discordant twin, all parameters may be retarded.

Weight-Length Ratio

The weight-length ratio aids in identifying fetal growth abnormalities. It increases with fetal age, ie, the baby becomes heavier for his length as he approaches full term. In intrauterine growth retardation, the weight-length ratio decreases, since the rate of growth in weight is affected more than length. The weight-length ratio is calculated using the following formula:

$$\frac{100 \times \text{Weight in gm}}{(\text{Length in cm})^3}$$

Intrauterine Growth Deviations

Intrauterine growth abnormalities should be looked for in infants who are large or small for gestational age or have disproportionate growth in terms of weight, length, and head circumference. Table 3–1 lists conditions in pregnancy which affect the fetus and are associated with deviations from normal intrauterine growth patterns.

Risk of Mortality or Significant Morbidity

The mortality risk based on gestational age and birth weight is shown in Fig 3–2. In general, infants with an 8% or greater chance of dying, based on these criteria, should be placed in a special newborn nursery. Morbidity risks based on factors other than birth weight and gestational age may dictate special care even though the mortality risk is low. A risk judgment should be made on each pregnancy and newborn.

Additional infant factors affecting risk are discussed in the following sections. Some examples of maternal factors which influence the newborn's outcome are listed below:

Mother's age less than 15 or more than 35 years.
No prenatal care.

Previous fetal or neonatal loss.
Previous preterm delivery.
Preexisting maternal disease: diabetes, hypertensive cardiovascular disease, renal disease.
Prenatal conditions: Rh iso-immunization, toxemia, vaginal bleeding, multiple pregnancy, abnormal presentation, acute infection.
Difficult or surgical delivery.
Fetal distress.
Preterm or postterm delivery.
Premature rupture of membranes.
Polyhydramnios or oligohydramnios.
Apgar score below 5.
Active resuscitation necessary.
Marked pallor or plethora.
Symptoms and signs of significant illness in newborn.

TABLE 3–1. Conditions associated with deviations of intrauterine growth.

	Expected Morbidity
Infants large for gestational age	
Pre-term infants Calculated and clinical estimate of gestational age compatible	Prematurity
More mature clinical estimate of gestational age due to error in calculated gestational age, usually secondary to postconceptual bleeding	Increased risk, cause unknown
Term and post-term infants	Increased risk of birth trauma
Infants of diabetic mothers	Hypoglycemia, respiratory distress, prematurity, birth trauma, fetal death
Infants with transposition of great vessels	Cyanosis, heart failure
Infants small for gestational age	
Intrauterine undernutrition: placental abnormality, discordant twin, multiple birth, hypertensive disease in mother	Short-term undernutrition: decreased growth in weight with normal length and head size Long-term undernutrition: weight, length, and head size diminished. Morbidity: fetal distress, meconium aspiration, feeding problems, hypoglycemia, pulmonary hemorrhage
Infants with congenital anomalies	See text
Infants with chronic intrauterine infection	See text

Battaglia FC, Lubchenco LO: A practical classification of newborn infants by weight and gestational age. J Pediat 71:159, 1967.

Lubchenco LO & others: Intrauterine growth as estimated from liveborn birth-weight data from 24–42 weeks of gestation. Pediatrics 32:793, 1963.

Lubchenco LO, Hansman C, Boyd E: Intrauterine growth in length and head circumference as estimated from live births at gestational ages from 26–42 weeks. Pediatrics 37:403, 1966.

Promoting the Health of Mothers and Children–1970. US Department of Health, Education, and Welfare, 1971. [Available from the Maternal and Child Health Service, Rockville, Maryland 20852.]

OBSERVATION & EXAMINATION OF THE NEWBORN

Because of the rapidly changing physical and behavioral characteristics of the newborn, the physical examination is best described in sequence.

Prior to delivery, the prenatal history, including estimated fetal age and size, is reviewed. The duration, type, and complications of labor and delivery are evaluated. A brief but orderly assessment of the infant and his adnexa is made at birth. These steps allow for more accurate prediction of problems and awareness of significant physical findings.

Behrman RE, Fisher D, Paton JB: In utero disease and the newborn infant. Advances Pediat 17:13–56, 1970.

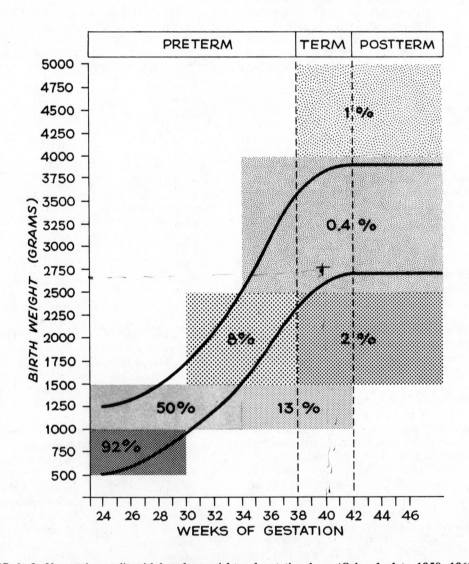

FIG 3–2. Neonatal mortality risk based on weight and gestational age. (Colorado data, 1958–1968.)

Observations During Birth That Indicate Increased Risk

A. Fetal Distress:

1. Tachycardia (> 160 beats/minute).
2. Bradycardia (< 100 beats/minute).
3. Persistent fetal bradycardia at the end of uterine contractions (type II dips).
4. Meconium evacuation from gut.
5. Low pH in fetal scalp blood (< 7.25).

B. Amniotic Membranes and Fluids:

1. Polyhydramnios (2000 ml or more)—Increased incidence of fetal malformations: anencephaly, atresia of the esophagus.
2. Oligohydramnios (300 ml or less)—Associated with renal agenesis, obstruction of the lower urinary tract, premature rupture of membranes.
3. Prolonged rupture of membranes (more than 24 hours)—Increased risk of premature birth and intrauterine infection.
4. Purulent or foul-smelling fluid—Infection.

The Infant Immediately After Birth

A. Apgar Score Evaluation:
Apgar scoring of the infant at 1 and 5 minutes after birth has become a valuable routine procedure (Table 3–2). The newborn in the best condition receives a score of 8–10, is vigorous, pink, and crying. A moderately depressed baby has an Apgar score of 5, 6, or 7. He appears cyanotic, with slow and irregular respirations, but has good muscle tone and reflexes. The severely asphyxiated infant has a score of less than 4 and is limp, pale or blue, apneic, and has a slow heart rate. The 1-minute Apgar score draws attention to the condition of the baby at birth; the 5-minute Apgar score is a useful prognostic indicator.

B. Auscultation of the Lungs:
Auscultation may reveal sticky rales with the first few breaths. In the healthy infant, air exchange is good almost immediately. Respiratory rate ranges from 30–60 for the first few minutes and may be irregular.

C. Temperature:
Body temperature will fall precipitously in a cool environment unless special precautions are taken. With a fall in body temperature, the infant becomes cyanotic—first in the hands and feet, then in the face, and finally over the entire body. He may develop grunting respirations and retractions of the rib cage with respirations if hypothermia persists.

D. Stomach Tube:
Passing a stomach tube confirms patency of the esophagus. Aspiration of more than 25 ml of stomach contents suggests upper intestinal obstruction. The stomach tube should not be passed until the baby has established respirations and is stabilized; otherwise, the tube touching the posterior pharynx may cause laryngospasm and apnea.

E. Other Observations:

1. The sex, amount of vernix, size, and development of the infant are observed and related to the calculated gestational age.
2. The color of the skin, in addition to cyanosis, is evaluated. Pallor, plethora, petechiae, and ecchymoses call for further investigation. Jaundice is a grave sign when present at birth and requires immediate evaluation.
3. Gross malformations or unusual facies or body configuration suggesting "a syndrome" can be seen at a glance and plans for care or treatment can be made.
4. A distended abdomen indicates the need for additional observations for organomegaly, ascites, etc; a scaphoid or "empty" abdomen suggests diaphragmatic hernia.
5. Asymmetric movement of muscle groups or extremities may indicate presence of nerve injury or fracture.

Drage JS, Berendes H: Apgar scores and outcome of the newborn. P Clin North America 13:635, 1966.

The Fetal Adnexa (Placenta, Cord, & Amniotic Membranes)

A. The Umbilical Cord:

1. **Gross appearance**—The diameter of the umbilical cord varies greatly, depending chiefly on the amount of Wharton's jelly present. The cord of term infants with small placentas is likely to be thin and stained yellow. Meconium staining of the umbilical cord indicates prior fetal distress. The cord is usually inserted concentrically on the placenta. When the insertion is velamentous, ie, arising away from the placental margin and supported only by the amnion, there is increased risk of fetal hemorrhage during delivery. Velamentous insertions of the cord occur commonly in multiple births.
2. **Length of umbilical cord**—A very short cord is uncommon but can result in abruptio placentae or rup-

TABLE 3–2. **Infant evaluation at birth.*** One minute and 5 minutes after complete birth of infant (disregarding cord and placenta), the following objective signs should be checked.

Points	0	1	2
1. Heart rate	Absent	Slow (< 100)	> 100
2. Respiratory effort	Absent	Slow, irregular	Good, crying
3. Muscle tone	Limp	Some flexion of extremities	Active motion
4. Response to catheter in nostril (tested after oropharynx is clear)	No response	Grimace	Cough or sneeze
5. Color	Blue or pale	Body pink; extremities blue	Completely pink

*Reproduced, with permission, from Apgar V: JAMA 168:1985, 1958.

ture of the cord. A very long cord (75 cm or more) may loop around the body and neck, resulting in a relatively short cord during delivery. Loops about the neck are rarely a cause of asphyxia.

3. Single umbilical artery—The vessels of the umbilical cord are best observed in a freshly cut section at birth. Normally, 2 arteries and one vein are present. A single artery is present in approximately 1% of births. The incidence rises to 5–6% in twins. The twin with a single umbilical artery is often significantly smaller than the twin with 2 arteries. A single umbilical artery is considered a congenital vascular malformation. Associated congenital abnormalities, especially of the cardiovascular, gastrointestinal, or urinary tracts, should be looked for.

4. Prolapsed cord—If the umbilical cord prolapses and is compressed during labor, acute fetal distress results. This is an obstetric emergency, and prompt treatment is necessary if the life and welfare of the baby are to be preserved. The perinatal mortality rate when an umbilical cord prolapses is about 35%.

B. Placenta: In general, the weight of the placenta is related to the weight of the baby. The average placenta weighs about 500 gm. Small placentas may be due to local disease in the placenta (infarction) or to systemic disease in the mother (severe hypertension or chronic vascular disease). The infant is small and undernourished. Prior to delivery, these infants may have suffered chronic hypoxia. After delivery, they are likely to become hypoglycemic. If the infant is small and the placenta is normal in size, one should suspect congenital anomalies or chronic infection in the infant.

Large placentas occur with large normal babies, with infants of diabetic mothers, in erythroblastosis fetalis, and in chronic intrauterine infection.

Careful examination of placenta and membranes in multiple births can often differentiate single ovum and multiple ovum twinning. In single ovum twins, 2/3 will show one placenta, one chorion, and a double or single amnion distinguishing them as of single ovum origin. The other 1/3 will have 2 placentas (sometimes fused), 2 chorions, and 2 amnions, the same as double ovum twins.

The First Hours After Birth

A. Birth Recovery Period: Desmond has described the physical findings associated with postnatal adjustment in normal newborn infants. The premature infant responds similarly to the full-term infant but more slowly; therefore, each of the periods described below is delayed and prolonged. Infants with low Apgar scores show an initial delay in the first stage but may then recover rapidly. Significant alterations from the basic sequence of events may result from analgesia and anesthesia given the mother (Fig 3–3).

1. First stage—For about 30 minutes after delivery, the infant is active and alert and muscle tone is increased. The heart and respiratory rate are rapid, and transient rales may be heard. Bowel sounds are absent. The infant may drool or vomit mucus. There is usually a fall in body temperature, grunting, flaring of the alae nasi, and costal retractions.

2. Second stage—Between about 30 minutes and 2 hours, there is a decrease in heart and respiratory rates, motor activity declines, and the infant falls asleep.

3. Third stage—After about 2 hours, the infant arouses and the initial findings return. Between 2–6 hours after birth, he again shows an increase in heart rate, vasomotor instability, irregular respirations, and apneic periods. Oral mucus is present, and meconium is passed.

B. Plethora: During the first 4–6 hours after birth, hemoconcentration of the peripheral blood occurs. The hematocrit, determined from heel-stick blood, may rise to as high as 80% at 6 hours. The infant appears red and, with crying, may become purplish red. By 12–24 hours after birth, the hematocrit has returned toward high normal values (60–70%). At the height of hemoconcentration, slight edema may be manifested by a shiny or tight skin.

C. Head: Caput succedaneum (edema of the scalp) is noted over the presenting surface in practically all vertex presentations. The swelling lasts about 24 hours. Cephalhematoma may be difficult to differentiate from caput succedaneum during the first few hours of life but gradually becomes circumscribed by the borders of the individual skull bone. Molding and overriding of the cranial sutures is common. The fontanels may be small as a result of the molding and overriding of the cranial bones.

D. Eyes: The eyes are open and alert during the first 30 minutes after birth and then tend to be closed during the next few hours. Small subconjunctival and retinal hemorrhages may be present.

E. Ears: The amount of cartilage is helpful in estimating maturity (Table 3–3). The eardrums usually cannot be visualized. Abnormal configuration and position of the ears (low-set) are often associated with genitourinary abnormalities.

F. Face: Transient (3 weeks to several months) seventh nerve palsies are not uncommon, and permanent palsy may also occur. With crying, movement of the unaffected side of the face gives a distorted appearance to the mouth. There may be, in addition, inequality in the eyelid openings, the weak side being more open. Facial nerve injury may be caused by forceps trauma, pressure exerted on the face when the head passes over the promontory of the sacrum, or by abnormal position of the infant's shoulder or foot during labor.

G. Mouth: Drooling of mucus is common in the first few hours after birth.

H. Chest:

1. Breasts—Breast tissue is present in full-term infants without intrauterine growth retardation.

2. Lungs—Respiratory movements continue to be irregular. Breath sounds are heard. Overexpansion of the chest (hyperaeration with or without pneumothorax or pneumomediastinum) may occur in premature infants or infants requiring resuscitation. A full chest with increased anteroposterior diameter, increase in respiratory rate, and sometimes distant heart tones are observed.

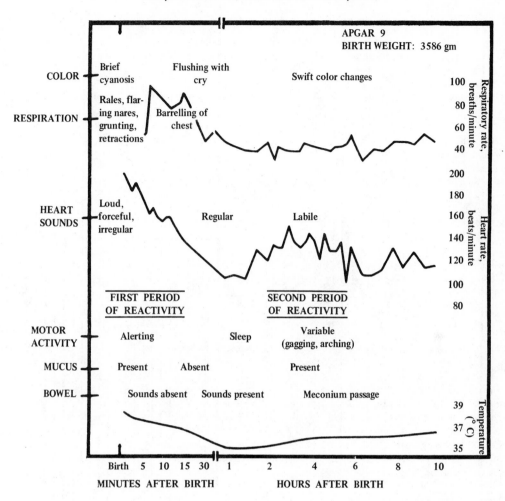

FIG 3–3. Summary of the physical findings noted during the first 10 hours of extrauterine life in a representative high-Apgar-score infant delivered under spinal anesthesia without prior premedication. (Reproduced, with permission, from Desmond MM & others: The transitional care nursery: A mechanism for preventive medicine. P Clin North America 13:656, 1966.)

3. Heart—The heart rate is increased during the first few hours. Sinus arrhythmia is present. Transient murmurs are common, most frequently over the pulmonic area.

I. Abdomen: The abdominal contents are most easily palpated soon after birth, before the bowel becomes filled with gas. Absence of abdominal contents suggests diaphragmatic hernia or dextroversion. The liver edge and the lower poles of both kidneys are palpable. The tip of the spleen may be felt and occasionally is 2–3 cm below the left costal margin.

J. Genitalia: The foreskin is adherent to the glans of the penis. The development of the genitalia is related to gestational age.

K. Anus: Patency should be checked if the infant has not passed meconium.

L. Neurologic Examination: Moro, rooting, and sucking reflexes are present at birth. Absence of these

signs suggests brain damage or marked depression. Other positive pathologic signs indicating CNS damage include a high-pitched cry, hypotonia, hypertonia, unequal tone of the 2 sides of the body, muscular twitching, abnormal eye movements, apneic periods, respiratory distress, pallor, and convulsions.

Desmond MM, Rudolph AJ, Phitaksphraiwan P: The transitional care nursery: A mechansim for preventive medicine. P Clin North America 13:651, 1966.

Clinical Estimate of Gestational Age

The onset of the mother's last menstrual period is still the basic item of information from which the period of gestation is calculated. Because the infant's physical characteristics and neurologic development progress in a predictable fashion with increasing fetal age, it is possible to estimate the gestational age by

TABLE 3–3. Clinical estimation of gestational age: A guide.*

PHYSICAL FINDINGS	EST GA (WEEKS GESTATION) 24 → 44
EXAMINATION FIRST HOURS	
VERNIX	APPEARS (24) — COVERS BODY — DECREASE IN AMOUNT (39–40) — NO VERNIX (43–44)
BREAST TISSUE	
NIPPLES	NONE — BARELY VISIBLE — WELL DEFINED FLAT AREOLA — WELL DEFINED, RAISED AREOLA
SOLE CREASES	NONE — 1, ANTERIOR TRANSVERSE — 2, ANTERIOR TRANSVERSE — ANTERIOR 2/3 SOLE — CREASES INVOLVING HEEL
EAR CARTILAGE	PINNA SOFT, STAYS FOLDED — RETURNS SLOWLY FROM FOLDING — THIN CARTILAGE, SPRINGS BACK — FIRM, REMAINS ERECT FROM HEAD
EAR FORM	FLAT, SHAPELESS — BEGINNING INCURVING OF PERIPHERY — PARTIAL INCURVING ALL OF UPPER PINNA — WELL DEFINED INCURVING ALL OF UPPER PINNA
GENITALIA – TESTES & SCROTUM	UNDESCENDED — TESTES HIGH IN CANAL, FEW RUGAE — TESTES LOWER MORE RUGAE — TESTES DESCENDED, PENDULOUS SCROTUM, RUGAE COMPLETE
LABIA & CLITORIS	LABIA MAJORA WIDELY SEPARATED, PROMINENT CLITORIS — LABIA MAJORA NEARLY COVER LABIA MINORA — LABIA MINORA & CLITORIS COVERED
HAIR (APPEARS ON HEAD @ 20 WKS)	EYEBROWS & LASHES — FINE, WOOLLY HAIR — HAIR SILKY, SINGLE STRANDS
LANUGO (APPEARS @ 20 WKS)	LANUGO OVER ENTIRE BODY — VANISHES FROM FACE — SLIGHT LANUGO OVER SHOULDERS — NO LANUGO
SKIN TEXTURE	THIN — SMOOTH, MEDIUM THICKNESS — DESQUAMATION
SKIN COLOR & OPACITY	TRANSLUCENT, PLETHORIC, NUMEROUS VENULES (ABDOMEN) — PINK, FEW LARGE VESSELS OVERALL — PALE PINK, NO VESSELS SEEN
SKULL FIRMNESS	SOFT TO 1 INCH FROM ANTERIOR FONTANELLE — SPRINGY AT EDGES OF FONTANELLE CENTER FIRM — BONES HARD SUTURES EASILY DISPLACED — BONES HARD, CANNOT BE DISPLACED
POSTURE – RESTING	LATERAL DECUBITUS — HYPOTONIA — SLIGHT INCREASE IN TONE, LOWER EXTREMITY — FROG-LIKE — TOTAL FLEXION
RECOIL	ABSENT — NONE UPPER EXTREMITIES / GOOD LOWER EXTREMITIES — SLOW UPPER EXTREMITIES — GOOD UPPER EXTREMITIES
LATER EXAMINATION	
TONE – HEEL TO EAR	NO RESISTANCE — SLIGHT RESISTANCE — DIFFICULT — ALMOST IMPOSSIBLE — IMPOSSIBLE
SCARF MANEUVER	NO RESISTANCE — MINIMAL RESISTANCE — FAIR RESISTANCE — DIFFICULT
NECK EXTENSORS	ABSENT — SLIGHT — FAIR — GOOD
NECK FLEXORS	ABSENT — MINIMAL — FAIR
REFLEXES – MORO	BARELY APPARENT — COMPLETE, EXHAUSTIBLE — GOOD, COMPLETE — NO ADDUCTION — COMPLETE WITH ADDUCTION
PUPILS TO LIGHT	REACT
GRASP	FEEBLE — FAIR — SOLID, INVOLVES ARMS — MAY PICK INFANT UP
ROOTING	MINIMAL c̄ REINFORCEMENT — GOOD c̄ REINFORCEMENT — GOOD
CROSSED EXTENSION	SLIGHT WITHDRAWAL — WITHDRAWAL — WITHDRAWAL & EXTENSION — WITHDRAWAL, EXTENSION, ADDUCTION
AUTOMATIC WALK	ABSENT — MINIMAL — FAIR, TOES — GOOD, HEELS
TRUNK ELEVATION	ABSENT — SLIGHT — GOOD
GLABELLAR TAP	ABSENT — APPEARS — PRESENT
HEAD TURNS TO LIGHT	ABSENT — APPEARS — PRESENT
CLINICAL ESTIMATE, GA	
CALCULATED GA	24 25 26 27 28 29 30 31 32 33 34 35 36 37 38 39 40 41 42 43 44 WEEKS GESTATION

*Reproduced, with permission, from Lubchenco LO: P Clin North America 17:125–145, 1970.

*Reproduced, with permission, from Lubchenco LO: P Clin North America 17:125–145, 1970. Characteristics which may be altered by intrauterine growth retardation include: (1) Absence of or retardation in growth of breast tissue. (2) Loss of vernix and desquamation of the skin prior to full term. (3) Meconium staining of skin and nails. (4) The decrease in intrauterine growth affects first the weight, then length, and—in severe undernutrition—head circumference. The percentile standings are thus discrepant, with weight being lowest, length next, and head circumference highest.

examining the infant at birth. When the physical signs and the calculated gestational age agree, the information is confirmatory. If the 2 estimates are discrepant, the information derived suggests possible pathologic factors.

Table 3–3 itemizes the clinical criteria used in determining gestational age and outlines the physical and neurologic findings observed at various gestational ages.

Intrauterine growth retardation due to undernutrition of the fetus (rather than due to fetal malformation) alters the physical characteristics associated with gestational age in the following ways:

(1) Absence of or retardation in growth of breast tissue.

(2) Loss of vernix and desquamation of the skin prior to term.

(3) Meconium staining of skin and nails.

(4) Decrease in intrauterine growth affects first the weight, then the length and, in severe undernutrition, the head circumference. Therefore, the percentile standings at birth show the weight to be most affected, the length next most affected, and head circumference the least affected.

(5) Neurologic development is least affected and is appropriate for the gestational age.

Amiel-Tison C: Neurologic evaluation of the maturity of newborn infants. Arch Dis Childhood 43:89, 1968.

Dubowitz LMS & others: Clinical assessment of gestational age in the newborn infant. J Pediat 77:1–10, 1970.

Lubchenco LO: Assessment of gestational age and development at birth. P Clin North America 17:125–146, 1970.

COMPLETE PHYSICAL EXAMINATION

The complete physical examination should be done within 24 hours after the birth recovery period.

A. Prior to Undressing:

1. The resting position of the infant and the character of sleep and spontaneous movements, both normal and abnormal, are observed before the newborn is touched in order to determine the infant's general condition.

2. Respirations are counted at this time. Periodic breathing is often seen in premature infants and occasionally in full-term infants when they are sleeping quietly. It is thought to be associated with some degree of hypoxia.

3. The basal or sleeping heart rate may be observed without disturbing the infant by palpation of the temporal artery.

B. During the Process of Undressing:

1. Evaluation of muscle tone and responsiveness is made at this time. The hypertonic baby is usually jittery and startles easily, his fists are tightly closed, the arms in tight flexion, and the legs stiffly extended. The hypotonic or lethargic infant is "floppy" and has little head control. The extremities fall to the bed loosely when picked up and released. Recoil of arms and legs to flexion when they are extended helps determine tone as well as gestational age.

2. The usual quieting response upon being picked up and held can be demonstrated after the undressing. The tense baby may take longer to calm down or will not stop crying.

General Examination

The general condition of the infant, nutritional status, maturity, and gross deformities are observed.

A. Resting Position: The development of muscle tone determines, to a great extent, the resting position of the infant. The type of presentation prior to delivery may also affect the resting position, eg, an infant delivered as a frank breech remains in a "sitting position" with the thighs flexed on the abdomen and the legs extended at the knees. Asymmetry of the skull, face, jaw, or extremities may result from intrauterine pressures. The infant may be passively "folded" into the position of comfort assumed in utero.

B. Skin and Subcutaneous Tissues: The skin is usually dark red, often bluish-red over the extremities. Cyanosis of the hands and feet occurs frequently. If pallor rather than plethora is present, serious disease such as hemorrhage or hemolytic disease is suspected. Vernix caseosa, a whitish greasy material, normally covers the body of the newborn infant. As term approaches, it decreases in amount and may be present only in the creases. In the postterm infant very little vernix is present.

Dry, cracked, or peeling skin is seen in the postmature infant or the one with intrauterine growth retardation at an earlier gestational age. Edema is abnormal. When present, conditions such as anemia, respiratory distress syndrome, heart failure, etc should be considered. Loss of skin turgor at birth usually is due to loss of subcutaneous fat and indicates inadequate nutrition.

Meconium staining of the skin and umbilical cord is seen in infants who have had fetal distress. Lanugo (fine, downy hair) appears on the entire body at about 20 weeks' gestation. It gradually disappears from the body; the last areas to lose the hair are the face, then the back and shoulders. Milia of the face—tiny pinpoint white papules (distended sebaceous glands)—are commonly present over the bridge of the nose and cheeks.

Mongolian spots—bluish-black areas of pigmentation over the back, buttocks, and, occasionally, the extremities—are seen with greater frequency in dark-skinned races. Capillary hemangiomas are common over the occiput, eyelids, forehead, around the nares, and, occasionally, the lips. As the child grows older, these facial blemishes tend to decrease in intensity.

Petechiae are often seen over the head and face. If unusually numerous or extensive, thrombocytopenia should be considered.

C. Head: Note the size and shape of the head. Molding during the latter part of pregnancy and delivery often results in a shortened anteroposterior diameter. Caput succedaneum is an area of edema over the presenting part. There is overlapping of sutures on the first day, with widening of sutures and fontanels by the second or third days. The size of the anterior fontanel varies but may range from 1–4 cm in any direction. The posterior fontanel barely admits a finger. Occasionally a third fontanel is present between the anterior and posterior fontanel. The third fontanel is a bony defect in the parietal bones.

Rapid enlargement of the head with separation of sutures is found in cerebral edema, intracranial hemorrhage, subdural hematoma, and hydrocephalus. Cephalhematoma can be distinguished from caput succedaneum because the hemorrhage is beneath the periosteum and is limited by the suture lines. Cephalhematoma is more common after difficult or precipitous delivery, and is usually over one or both parietal bones, but it can occur in the occipital area. Linear skull fractures are rarely present at the site of the cephalhematoma.

The hair is fine and silky at term. Transillumination of the head is equal bilaterally, with a circle of light no more than 1.5 cm in diameter being visible. More transillumination of light occurs in premature infants.

Depressed skull fractures are occasionally seen after difficult deliveries, requiring immediate surgical correction.

D. Face: Symmetry of the face and the size and formation of nose, ears, and eyes are observed. Weakness of facial muscles, forceps marks or bruises, rashes or swellings, petechiae and milia, alertness, and frowning or muscle twitchings are determined.

E. Facies: The odd-looking infant may have facial characteristics which indicate various syndromes. Sometimes the conditions are immediately recognized because of gross defects or anomalies; at other times the findings are subtle. Some syndromes with distinctive facies are as follows:

1. Down's syndrome (trisomy 21, mongolism)— The head may be relatively small and short. There is a prominent epicanthal fold, and the lid slits slant upward and outward. The orbits are shallow, giving the face a flat appearance. In the outer edge of the iris are white specks (Brushfield spots). The nose is short and the bridge is flattened. The tongue often protrudes. The pinnas of the ear are small.

2. First arch syndromes—

a. Treacher-Collins syndrome (mandibulofacial dysostosis)—Micrognathia and abnormality of eyes. There is an antimongoloid slant to the fissures, ie, the slant is downward and outward from the midline. The lower lid is notched in the lateral half. Other features may include a high-arched palate, glossoptosis, and large, low-set ears.

b. Pierre Robin syndrome—Micrognathia associated with pseudomacroglossia, glossoptosis, and high-arched or cleft palate.

c. Waardenburg's syndrome—Ocular hypertelorism, heterochromia, and white forelock. In this condition, there is congenital deafness.

d. Other manifestations as single defects—Harelip and cleft palate, ocular hypertelorism, deformities of external and middle ears, mandibular dysostosis, and deafness.

3. Trisomy 13–15—Cleft lip and palate and deformities of eyes and ears.

4. Trisomy 18—Micrognathia, small nose.

5. Turner's syndrome—Micrognathia, prominent pinnas, webbing of neck, and low hairline posteriorly.

6. Birdheaded dwarfism—Micrognathia with beaklike nose and central facial bones. Microcephaly, downslanting eyes, prominent epicanthal folds.

7. Silver's syndrome—Triangular facies with broad forehead, small mandible, downturned mouth.

8. Leprechaunism—Small face with sunken cheeks and pointed chin, wide-set eyes, dark irides, and large, low-set ears (elfin appearance).

9. Cornelia de Lange's syndrome—A thick mop of hair and low hairline on forehead, heavy eyebrows which meet in the midline, long lashes, long upper lip, thin lips, downturned mouth, small nose with upward tilted nares.

F. Eyes: Note size of the eyes and whether they are set close or widely spaced. The presence of epicanthal folds and mongoloid or antimongoloid slant is observed. In the healthy full-term newborn, the eyes will open, especially when the child is picked up, and he will tend to look toward a lighted area. Brief focusing on a face may occur. Occasional uncoordinated movements are not uncommon, but persistent irregular movements would indicate orbital or CNS disorders.

Conjunctival and retinal hemorrhages are occasionally seen. If one has difficulty focusing on the retinal vessels, it is well to dilate the pupils in these cases. Corneal or lens opacities and pupillary size and shape can be observed with an ordinary hand flashlight. Unequal movement of the lids or ptosis may be seen.

G. Nose: The shape and size of the nose and the position of the anterior nares is important in detecting in utero deformities and recognizing syndromes. Nasal discharge, noisy breathing, or complete obstruction to breathing may be present in choanal atresia or other nasal abnormalities. If obstruction is present, the infant may become apneic since he prefers to breathe through his nose. Flaring of the alae nasi occurs with increased respiratory effort.

H. Mouth and Jaws: The color of the lips and mucous membranes of the mouth may indicate pallor. Thinness and downturning are seen in the De Lange syndrome. Note harelip with or without cleft palate.

Epithelial "pearls" or retention cysts are noted on the gum margins and at the junction of the hard and soft palate. They are sometimes mistaken for teeth. Incisors are occasionally present at birth; most often they are soft and deciduous, but occasionally they persist.

Most newborns have relatively small mandibles, usually asymptomatic. When severe, as with Pierre Robin syndrome, obstruction to breathing occurs when the tongue falls back against the nasopharynx, obstructing the airways. If the child sleeps on his abdomen, there is usually less respiratory difficulty. An oral prosthesis is occasionally required to maintain the airway.

I. Throat and Cry: Note the character of the cry. A high-pitched cry often indicates CNS damage. If the cry is hoarse, infection of the pharynx and respiratory tract is suspected. A whining "cat's cry" is a sign of deletion of the short arm of chromosome 5. Expiratory grunting occurs with respiratory distress. Inspiratory stridor occurs in newborns who have soft, collapsible laryngeal or tracheal structures, elongated epiglottides, or other abnormalities resulting in partial obstruction of the upper airway. The tonsils and adenoids are small in newborns.

J. Ears: Malformation of the pinnas and small or low-set ears alert one to the presence of other anomalies, especially of the genitourinary tract. Small, tortuous external canals occur in Down's syndrome. The amount of cartilage in the pinnas is related to gestational age.

Congenital deafness may be detected by standardized hearing tests in the newborn. The response to sound in the newborn is seen as a startle, eye blink, turning of the head toward the sound, or crying.

K. Neck: Webbing of the neck with demonstrable loose skin, sometimes with edema, suggests Turner's syndrome.

Enlargement of the thyroid is occasionally seen. Sinus tracts are also evident in instances of incomplete closure of bronchial clefts. Torticollis, or shortening of the sternomastoid muscle, may occur when there is hemorrhage or fibrosis in the muscle. A persistent tonic neck reflex, assumed spontaneously and maintained by the infant, is seen in brain damage.

L. Thorax: Note shape, symmetry, position, and development of nipples, breasts, and superficial veins. Note the shape of the thorax and its movement with respirations. Absent clavicles permit unusual anterior movement of the shoulders. Fracture of the clavicle is detected by tenderness and crepitus at the fracture site and limited movement of that arm. After a few days, callus is formed and the deformity can be visualized and felt.

"Fullness" of the chest is a frequent finding in overexpansion of the lungs. Note asymmetry in expansion of the 2 sides or retractions during inspiration in the subcostal, intercostal, xiphoid, and suprasternal areas. These signs indicate pulmonary disease or upper airway obstruction.

M. Lungs: Auscultation of the lungs normally reveals bronchial breathing. In the presence of mediastinal emphysema or pneumothorax, the heart sounds may be distant and breath sounds reduced in intensity. The percussion note will be hyperresonant. Retractions, decreased air entry, expiratory grunting with respirations, dilatation of alae nasi, chin lag, and "see-saw" respirations are characteristic findings in the respiratory distress syndrome.

N. Heart: Size and position may be determined by single finger percussion. Dextroposition of the heart may be due to dextrocardia or pulmonary disease, such as pneumothorax on the left side, causing a shift of the mediastinum toward the right.

Murmurs are frequent and transient in the newborn period. The infant may have a serious congenital heart defect without a murmur, or an infant with a normal heart may have an intensely loud murmur as the ductus arteriosus closes.

O. Abdomen: The abdomen will appear scaphoid at birth but will become slightly protuberant as the bowel fills with air. A markedly scaphoid or persistent scaphoid abdomen with respiratory distress suggests the presence of diaphragmatic hernia. Absence of the abdominal musculature occasionally occurs (associated with urinary tract abnormalities), and in rare instances omphalocele is present at birth. Umbilical hernias are common and usually cause no difficulty.

Abdominal distention occurs with gastrointestinal obstruction or may be present in a septic infant who develops paralytic ileus. Palpation of the abdomen for organs or masses should be done with light touch. The spleen is best felt from the patient's right side and is quite far laterally. The liver is usually palpable 1–2 cm below the right costal margin. The kidneys are more likely to be palpated immediately after birth, before the gastrointestinal tract is filled with air or feedings. If bladder distention occurs, the outline of the bladder may be seen above the symphysis, or it may be felt as a ballotable mass in the lower abdomen. Contraction of bladder muscles with voiding often occurs with palpation.

Superficial veins may appear prominent over the abdomen with or without pathologic conditions.

The umbilical cord begins drying within hours after birth, becomes loose from the underlying skin by 4–5 days, and falls off by the seventh to tenth days. Occasionally, a granulating stump remains which heals faster if treated with silver nitrate.

Pulsation of the femoral arteries can be felt immediately after birth. Absent pulsations are significant and require further investigation for conditions such as coarctation of the aorta.

P. Genitalia: Male and female genitalia show findings characteristic of gestational age. In most term male infants the scrotum is pendulous, with rugae completely covering the sac. The testes have completely descended. The size of the scrotum and the penis varies widely in individual normal infants.

In females, the labia majora at term completely cover the labia minora and clitoris. The vagina and hymenal ring may be visible as a protruding tab of tissue. During the first few days after birth, a white mucous discharge issues from the vagina and sometimes contains blood. Occasionally, a septum produced by fusion of the labia minora is present over the vagina. The fusion is easily disrupted with a blunt probe.

Q. Rectum and Anus: Irritation and fissures may occur after the immediate newborn period. Check for patency of the anus. A firm meconium plug as the first stool may occasionally cause symptoms of obstruction.

R. Extremities: Gross abnormalities such as absence of a bone, clubfoot, and fusion or webbing of digits are obvious. Hip dislocation is suspected when there is limitation of abduction of the hips, or a click can be felt when the femur is pressed downward and then abducted. The legs may be unequal in length, and extra skin folds in the affected thigh are seen. Palsies of the extremities are easily recognized, especially when unilateral, and should be suspected whenever there is asymmetric movement of the extremities.

Note the size and shape of the hands and feet. Deformities are frequent with chromosomal abnormalities—eg, in Down's syndrome the little finger is short and incurved and there is a simian crease in the palm.

Neurologic Examination

Some observations are made while the infant is completely undisturbed; some during minimal handling; and some can only be made by observing responses to specific stimuli. The infant should be neither too hungry nor too sleepy. Because a prolonged examination may exhaust the infant or cause irritability, the examination may have to be done in parts.

A. General Observations: Paucity of spontaneous movements may be as important as abnormal movements. Discordant movements of one limb or of one side, hyperactivity, opisthotonos, athetoid movements, and movements ranging from tremors or jerks to frank convulsions may be seen in the infant with CNS damage. Brief seizures may sometimes present as momentary cessation of movements in a crying infant. Continuous chewing or sucking movements, protrusion of the tongue, and frequent yawns are other abnormal movements. The facial expression may be bland, alert, or frowning, or there may be asymmetry of the face and eyes with movement. Facial nerve palsy is suspected if the weakness is unilateral. It is more difficult to diagnose if bilateral (Möbius' syndrome; nuclear agenesis).

B. Tests for Muscle Tone and Strength: Note resting position without disturbing the infant. Test recoil of the extremities. Extend legs and then release; both legs return promptly to the flexed position in the term infant. Extend arms alongside the body; upon release, there is prompt flexion at the elbows in the term infant. The amount of flexion and extension around joints is further tested at the neck, trunk, shoulder, elbow, wrist, hips, knees, and ankles. A general impression of hypotonia or hypertonia can be gained from this testing.

Still another means of testing for tone is by flopping the hand and foot. As the wrist is moved sharply back and forth, the hand flops for a brief period and then the infant resists the movement and holds the hand or wrist firm. Normal term infants show approximately as much flopping as resistance to movement during this maneuver.

C. Response of Infant to Specific Stimuli: Be very gentle with each test.

1. Rooting reflex—The rooting reflex occurs so early in gestation that its absence in a viable baby (26 weeks or more) should cause concern. However, the rooting reflex is strongest when the infant is hungry and may disappear after feeding. The reflex is elicited in 4 areas: at both corners of the mouth and on the upper and lower lips at the midline. The mouth opens or the head turns toward the side of the stimulus.

2. Sucking reflex—The sucking reflex can be obtained by placing a finger in the baby's mouth and noting the vigor of the movements and the amount of suction produced.

3. Traction response, head flexion and extension—The infant's hands and wrists are grasped and he is pulled gently to a sitting position. In the term infant, there is at first a head lag and then active flexion of the neck muscles so that the head and chest are in line when the infant reaches the vertical position. He maintains his head in the upright position for a few seconds, and the head then falls forward. He then spontaneously—or with a slight stimulus, such as stroking the upper lip—will raise his head again.

4. Grasp reflex—

a. Fingers—Stimulate the palm with a finger, and the infant will close the fingers. The grasp should be sufficiently strong in the term infant that he can be lifted from the table by holding onto the examiner's finger.

b. Toes—Pressing the ball of the foot elicits a definite and prompt toe flexion.

5. Biceps, knee jerk, triceps, and ankle jerk reflexes are most often elicited with the finger rather than a percussion hammer. Care must be taken to have the infant relaxed.

6. Ankle clonus is normally present in the newborn; sustained clonus is not usual.

7. Incurvation of the trunk—The infant is lifted up and held over the hand in a prone position. The amount of flexion of head and body is noted for an additional estimate of tone. The incurvation reflex is obtained by stroking or applying intermittent pressure with the finger, first on one side and then the other, parallel to the spine, watching for a movement of the pelvis to the stimulated side.

8. Righting reaction—When the infant is lifted from the table vertically, he will usually flex his legs. If the soles of the feet then touch the table, he will respond with the righting reflex, ie, his legs will extend and then the trunk and then the head.

9. Placing reaction—The baby is held vertically with his back against the examiner and one leg held out of the way. The other leg is moved forward so that the dorsum of the foot touches the edge of the examining table. The baby will flex the knee, bringing his foot up, as though he were trying to step onto the table.

10. Automatic walking—Following the tests for righting the body and placing, the ability to perform automatic walking movements is evaluated. The baby is inclined forward to begin automatic walking. When the sole of one foot touches the table, he tends to right himself with that leg and the other foot flexes. As the next foot touches the table, the reverse action occurs. Term infants will walk on the entire sole of the foot, whereas prematures often walk on their toes.

11. Moro (startle) reflex—In looking for the Moro response, observe the arms, hands, and cry. The arms show abduction at the shoulder and extension of the forearm at the elbow, followed by adduction of the arms in most infants. The hands show a prominent spreading or extension of the fingers. Any abnormality in the character of the movements should be noted, such as jerkiness or tremor, slow response, or asymmetric response. A cry follows the startle, and should be vigorous. The nature of the cry is important, eg, absent, weak, high-pitched, or excessive.

The Moro reflex may be elicited in several ways:

a. Holding the baby's hands, lift his body and neck (but not his head) off the examining table and quickly let go.

b. Holding the infant with one hand supporting his head and the other supporting his body, allow the head to drop a few centimeters rather suddenly.

c. Holding the infant in both hands, lower both hands rapidly a few centimeters so that he experiences a sensation of falling.

d. If the baby is quiet in the bassinet, lift the head of the bassinet a few centimeters and let it drop.

e. A loud noise near the baby's ear or a sharp blow on the table on which he is lying.

Prechtl H, Beintema D: *The Neurological Examination of the Full Term Newborn Infant.* Heinemann, 1964.

Solomon LM, Esterly NB: Neonatal dermatology I: The newborn skin. J Pediat 77:888—894, 1970.

CARE OF THE HEALTHY TERM INFANT

In the Delivery Room

During and immediately after delivery, the nasopharynx is gently suctioned with a bulb syringe or soft rubber catheter to remove mucus or blood and to clear the airway of obstructive debris. The baby should be evaluated immediately after delivery for evidence of life-threatening disease and gross anomalies. During the ensuing minutes, every effort should be made to prevent a fall in body temperature. With increasing use of air conditioning in delivery rooms, maintaining the infant's body temperature has become a major problem. Safe radiant heat devices or early transfer of the baby to the nursery are the best solutions.

Gastric aspiration may be done when the baby is doing well. Observe the cut end of the umbilical cord for the number of arteries. Routine prophylaxis of the eyes against gonorrheal infection must be done; 1% silver nitrate drops (followed by irrigation with isotonic saline solution) or other antimicrobial agent may be used as defined by local health codes. Proper identi-

fication of the infant is done before he is transferred to the nursery. The infant may be shown to the mother, who may wish to hold him, or she may be content for the time being with just a glance.

In the Recovery Area

The infant is weighed and measured immediately upon entering the nursery. He is then placed in an incubator or wrapped in warm, dry blankets and allowed to rest. During the first 4—6 hours he is observed closely for symptoms and signs of illness. (See Birth Recovery Period, p 44.)

A complete review of the history and a brief physical examination, including the estimate of gestational age, are done during this period. The infant is classified by birth weight and gestational age (Fig 3—1) and given a mortality risk grouping (Fig 3—2). After the baby has stabilized, he is bathed and dressed. He is given his first feeding of glucose in water when he shows evidence of hunger. If he is well, he is transferred to the low-risk nursery for care.

In the Low-Risk Nursery

The duration of hospital stay of the mother and baby following an uncomplicated perinatal course is usually only 3—5 days. The short hospitalization period permits the mother and baby to have a relatively earlier "rooming-in" experience in their own home. If there is an understanding adult helper in the home, freeing the mother to care for the baby, the benefits of this early adjustment can be great. However, early discharge is accompanied by a definite risk of delay in detecting problems: breast feeding is not established, the severity of "physiologic" jaundice cannot be evaluated, and subtle symptoms of illness may not be recognized before discharge.

The life situation of the mother and the family is important in their acceptance of the newborn baby. Favorable conditions exist when the mother is married, the child is wanted at this time, there is some financial security, and the parents themselves are emotionally mature. Even when these favorable factors are operative, however, there may be adverse factors which interfere with a satisfactory adjustment. Problems in pregnancy, a difficult delivery, birth of an abnormal or premature infant, and development of maternal or infant illness are a few such factors.

A. Understanding the Mother and Child: The nurse and physician should understand the needs of the mother and child and show their willingness to meet these needs. The following suggestions will help:

1. Become acquainted with the mother and father—prior to delivery, if possible.

2. Show an interest in the total family unit and explore the parents' attitudes about child-rearing.

3. Visit the mother daily while she is in the hospital and pay attention to her expressed anxieties.

4. Institute flexible schedules of feeding, especially for mothers who are breast feeding.

5. Institute flexible schedules for the amount of time the baby spends with the mother.

6. Examine the infant in the mother's room—at time of discharge is usually convenient.

An optimal family-centered program is the rooming-in situation with mother and baby together in the room under the supervision of an understanding and helpful nurse, with free visiting for the father. The mother can get instruction in caring for the baby as she watches her baby being examined, and her questions about the significance of findings can be answered as they arise. Continued help and encouragement from well trained nurses for the mother who is breast feeding is very helpful.

B. Watching for Illness: Watching for illness in the newborn is the joint responsibility of nurses and physicians. Symptoms and signs of illness in newborns are often an accumulation of "insignificant" signs. It is often necessary to employ different methods of detecting illness in newborns from those used in older children.

A list of symptoms and signs which can be observed in newborn infants, given in Table 3–4, provides a guide to "baby watching." Even though many of the signs listed are benign in themselves, the presence of a large number of signs alerts one to the possibility of disease. This will lead to examination of the infant, followed by appropriate diagnostic procedures to clarify the concern about specific illness. A jot sheet based on this list can be used to replace the bulk of nurses' notes in the nursery.

C. Screening for Disease: Since nearly all babies in the USA are born in hospitals, an excellent opportunity exists to screen mothers and newborns for disease that has not become manifest during their stay in the hospital. Some of these tests can be routine:

1. Maternal serologic test for syphilis.

2. Blood group and RH typing and testing for maternal antibodies for blood group iso-immunization.

3. Blood type and Coombs test to verify presence of blood group iso-immunization in baby with incompatibility.

4. Elevated serum phenylalanine and other amino acids.

TABLE 3–4. Check list of significant observations in newborn infants.*

Healthy Findings				Twitching				Cough			
Body temperature				Irritable				Sneeze			
Incubator temperature				Hyperactive				Stuffy nose			
Weight				Tires easily				**Skin Findings**			
Respiratory rate				Less active				Mottled			
Pulse rate				Lethargic				Harlequin syndrome			
Demanding				Weak cry				Jaundice			
Hungry				Shrill cry				Petechiae (specify area)			
Sucks well				Moro reflex poor or absent				Ecchymoses (specify area)			
Gavages well but slowly				**Cardiovascular Findings**				Edema			
Resisted gavage				Pallor				Dehydration			
Weight gain				Plethora				Sclerema			
Good cry				Cyanosis, circumoral				Umbilical redness			
Active				Cyanosis, circumocular				Umbilical oozing			
Color stable				Cyanosis, extremities				Alcohol to cord			
Gastrointestinal Findings				Cyanosis, generalized				Pustular rash			
Gavaged poorly				Bleeding (specify area)				Other rash (specify)			
Sucked poorly				**Respiratory Findings**				Abscess			
Gagged				Oxygen flow (liters/min)				Eye discharge			
Drooled				Oxygen concentration				Skin dry or peeling			
Regurgitated				Shallow respirations				Skin irritated (specify area)			
Hiccups				Labored respirations				**Other**			
Mucus on gavage tube				Deep respirations							
Mucus, other				Irregular respirations							
Abdominal distention				Rest periods, <10 sec							
Abnormal stool				Rest periods, 10–30 sec							
Sore buttocks				Apnea, >30 sec							
Weight loss				Intercostal retractions							
Neurologic Findings				Xiphoid retractions							
Convulsions				See-saw respirations							
Rigid				Dilated alae nasi							
Opisthotonos				Grunting							

*The severity of the sign is indicated by +, ++, or +++. If the symptom is present only ac or pc, these symbols are used. This check list is used by nurses instead of routine nurses' notes, each column used for one period of observation. The signs observed in the infant are checked, the time and date noted, and the column initialed. If situations other than those listed are present, detailed descriptions are written in the regular nurses' notes. A 24-hour summary of nursing observations is given to the physician at morning rounds. This and the physicians' examinations provide the data on which a decision is made concerning illness. (Adapted from Lubchenco LO: P Clin North America 8:471, 1961.)

Other tests may be added as improved testing methods are developed and evaluated, such as screening for hearing, sex chromatin, and galactosemia.

D. Preparation for Discharge of the Well Baby: Preparation for discharge should include the following:

1. Perform a physical examination, preferably with the mother in attendance, and discuss the care of the cord, circumcision, genitalia, etc as the baby is examined.

2. Make sure the mother knows and understands procedures for caring for the baby.

3. Give feeding instructions and a written formula. Careful attention to preparation of the formula is essential, since improperly prepared formula is dangerous to the infant.

4. Give her an appointment to the physician's office or clinic for well baby care or specific problems.

5. Make sure the mother knows whom to call to have questions answered.

6. Check baby's identification.

7. Vitamin A, C, and D supplementation is indicated unless adequate amounts are provided in the formula.

8. Iron supplementation is recommended for the first months of life unless adequate dietary iron is assured. Iron can be provided in iron-fortified formula or given separately if milk low in iron is used (breast milk; whole or evaporated cow's milk).

Lubchenco LO: Watching the newborn for disease. P Clin North America 8:471, 1961.
Standards and Recommendations for Hospital Care of Newborn Infants. American Academy of Pediatrics, 1971.

FEEDING

The Well Baby

An arbitrary fasting period has been imposed on all infants in the majority of hospital nurseries in order to protect the unidentified sick infant. With improved skill in the detection of illness, healthy newborn infants may be fed as soon as they appear hungry. This usually coincides with recovery from birth, at approximately 3–6 hours of age in the normal term infant.

A. What to Feed: The first feeding may be sterile water or 5% glucose in water. As soon as water feedings are taken well, full-strength milk formula (approximately 20 Cal/oz) or breast feedings are given. Diluted or concentrated formulas do not appear to have any special advantages.

Most of the modified cow's milk formulas available commercially are satisfactory during the hospital stay. Those that provide adequate vitamins A, C, and D are recommended.

An evaporated milk formula for use during the first months of life consists of the following: evaporated milk, 13 oz; water, 19 oz; and corn syrup, 2 tbsp. This formula provides about 21 Cal/oz.

B. How Much to Feed: The initial feeding may be a few swallows or several ounces. A healthy term baby will take 2–4 oz per feeding about every 4 hours. He should be allowed to regulate the volume per feeding and the frequency of feedings that will satisfy him and meet his fluid and caloric requirements.

Methods of Feeding the Well or Sick Infant

A. Bottle Feeding: Most commercial bottles and nipples are satisfactory. The nipple may need to have the hole enlarged, and this is easily done with a hot needle. For premature or debilitated babies, a soft nipple with easy flow (cross-cut hole) is required.

B. Breast Feeding: When a mother wants to nurse her infant, success or failure is related to the amount of factual information given her and to the emotional support of physicians and nurses. Physicians and nurses can share the role of listening, giving factual data, and encouraging the mother to continue nursing long enough to overcome whatever problems she may have in establishing lactation. Having a nurse present when the mother first attempts to feed, giving her some explanation of physiologic processes, and making her physically comfortable will assure success.

1. **Increasing milk production**—Failure to satisfy the nursing infant is generally due to inadequate milk production. Adequate diet, fluids, and rest are important for the general welfare of the mother but do not stimulate milk production. Milk production can be increased by complete and frequent emptying of the breasts. In practice, optimum production occurs if the infant nurses when he is hungry (complete emptying) and nurses from both breasts at each feeding. There may be a lag in supply of an adequate quantity of milk for the infant's demand, which will be resolved over the subsequent few days. At times it is necessary to give a milk supplement to the infant. This can be done with minimal risk to continued milk production if the bottle is prepared ahead of time and given immediately after breast feeding as part of the same feeding. If the milk feeding is given in place of nursing, stimulation of milk production will be decreased and the total amount of milk available to the infant will consequently decrease. When lactation is well established, supplementation is rarely necessary.

2. **Breast engorgement**—A variable amount of breast engorgement occurs in mothers on about the third day after delivery. The engorgement may interfere with nursing because the infant is unable to grasp the nipple. A nipple shield may be used to reduce the areolar engorgement and to draw out the nipple. The infant may then nurse directly from the breast. Prolonged use of the nipple shield interferes with complete emptying of the breasts. Nipple soreness may be minimized if the nursing time is kept to approximately 5 minutes during the prelacteal period (ie, until milk flow is established). Only a bland ointment should be used on the nipples.

3. **Variations in hunger**—The mother should be forewarned that her infant will seem to become more hungry about the fourth or fifth day and will want to

nurse more frequently. This behavior lasts only 1—2 days. The baby will then return to a less frequent feeding schedule.

4. Nursing premature and sick infants—Mothers wishing to nurse premature, sick, or debilitated infants may be successful if given some additional suggestions. She must empty her breasts several times a day with a mechanical pump or by manual expression until her infant is able to nurse from the breast. The amount of milk she expresses need not be adequate for the baby, who can be formula fed if necessary, as long as lactation is maintained. The supply will increase in a few days after the infant begins to nurse. If the baby does not empty the breast, milk production can be increased if she pumps the breast after feedings. She may have insufficient milk for a few days, and a supplement immediately after feedings will be necessary until the supply increases.

5. Mothers who work, who are hospitalized in the postpartum period, or who are separated from their infants for other reasons may nurse successfully if the breasts are emptied periodically during the separation period.

C. Gavage Feeding: Intermittent gavage feeding should be used when the baby has a weak sucking and swallowing reflex or tires easily. It can be done safely with minimal handling of the infant. However, in a sick infant with danger of abdominal distention, regurgitation, and aspiration, gavage feeding has the same risk as nipple feeding.

Procedure for gavage feedings: A number 5 or 8 F polyethylene or rubber feeding tube is used.

1. Measure the distance from the xiphoid to the tip of the ear lobe and mark the tube at this length.

2. Pass the tube through the mouth to this mark.

3. Determine that the tip of the tube is in the stomach—

a. Place the free end of the catheter under water to determine that air is not returned with each respiration.

b. Inject a small amount of air with a syringe and listen with a stethoscope over the stomach area for bubbling.

4. Introduce feeding slowly by gravity flow. Do not inject with a syringe under pressure.

5. To remove the tube, pinch it closed as it is withdrawn to avoid dripping fluid into the pharynx.

Indwelling nasogastric tubes have been used for long-term feedings of small premature infants. A small polyethylene (rather than rubber) catheter must be used to minimize local irritation. The location of the end of the tube must be checked before each feeding (see above) to be sure it has remained in the stomach. The presence of the tube in the nose decreases the airway slightly, and this may be a significant problem in some babies. Also, if mucus begins to develop in the nares, the tube should be removed since infection may develop in the nasopharynx or middle ear.

Nipple feedings can be substituted for gavage feedings gradually when the baby shows increased activity before feeding and begins sucking on the gavage tube. The transition should be made slowly, as babies will tire easily with nipple feedings. On nipple feedings, the baby will go from a 3- to a 4-hour schedule, taking larger quantities with each feeding. A rapidly growing premature infant will take 150 Calories and 180 ml/kg/day or more. Demand feeding of prematures is desirable. Intake will vary with different babies, and each will tend to establish his own pattern of intake. Feedings are satisfactory if associated with adequate weight gain.

D. Gastrostomy: This procedure can be done easily and relatively safely in infants when it is indicated. It should be done by an experienced surgeon with careful attention to special problems of the newborn. The main indications are in surgical conditions such as tracheo-esophageal fistula, chest surgery, and some bowel surgery to aid in pre- and postoperative care. Occasionally, a sick or very small premature infant will benefit from the procedure when oral feedings are associated with apnea, abdominal distention, regurgitation, and the danger of aspiration. The danger of distention, regurgitation, and aspiration is minimized because the tube allows increased gastric pressure to be relieved.

E. Intravenous Feeding:

1. Sick infants—Intravenous fluids may be started either via a peripheral vein or an umbilical catheter if the baby is sick and oral foods cannot be tolerated. Use 10% dextrose in water (65—80 ml/kg/day), with maintenance electrolytes added. Do not give potassium until the baby is 24—48 hours old unless serum levels indicate a need for it.

2. Premature infants—Early feedings, even in small premature infants, are preferred over periods of prolonged starvation and dehydration. In babies who are very small or who are sick, intravenous feeding of 10% glucose in water with maintenance electrolytes will fill this need until oral or gavage feedings can be started safely. Babies who are well and will tolerate oral feedings may be fed by nipple or gavage.

3. Termination of intravenous feedings—The first oral feeding should be sterile water. When water is tolerated well, formula feeding is started. A full strength formula containing approximately 20 Calories per ounce is usually satisfactory, avoiding the need for special preparation of more dilute or concentrated formula for premature infants. The volume of the initial feeding depends on the size of the baby and should be adjusted according to how well he tolerated the last feeding. When given by gavage, the first feeding should be about 5 ml in the very small infant. Volumes are then increased by 1—5 ml per feeding every 3 hours as he tolerates more intake. The total 24-hour volume can be adjusted by varying the volume and frequency of ididival feedings. With gavage feedings, gastric emptying can be checked by aspirating the stomach before feedings until a regular feeding pattern has been established. Replace aspirated fluid and add milk to volume desired for that feeding.

Applebaum RM: The modern management of successful breast feeding. P Clin North America 17:203–225, 1970.

Davidson M: Formula feeding of normal term and low birth weight infants. P Clin North America 17:913–928, 1970.

Filer LJ: The case for iron supplements in infant feeding regimens. Hosp Practice 6:79–92, 1971.

THE PREMATURELY BORN INFANT

Babies born prematurely make up a major group of newborns who are at increased risk. For definitions and classification, see the early section of this chapter.

Complications of pregnancy which predispose to premature delivery, either spontaneous or elective, include disease in the mother (eg, diabetes, toxemia, hypertensive cardiovascular disease, heart failure, urinary tract infection), placenta praevia, abruptio placentae, spontaneous rupture of membranes, cervical incompetence, uterine structural anomaly, severe fetal erythroblastosis, and multiple birth.

Most of what appears in the following sections of this chapter on diseases of the newborn applies to the preterm infant as well. In addition, the preterm infant will require certain special considerations discussed here.

Handicaps Due to Prematurity

The increased risk of prematurity is largely due to the functional and anatomic immaturity of various organs. Some of the more important problems include the following:

(1) Weak sucking, swallowing, gag, and cough reflexes, leading to difficult feeding and danger of aspiration.

(2) Pliable thorax and pulmonary immaturity, leading to hypoventilation and hypoxia and respiratory and metabolic acidosis.

(3) Poor control of body temperature.

(4) Decreased ability to excrete solutes in urine.

(5) Increased susceptibility to infection.

(6) Limited iron stores and rapid growth rate, leading to later anemia.

(7) Tendency to develop rickets due to diminished intake of calcium and vitamin D and rapid growth rate.

(8) Nutritional disturbances secondary to feeding difficulties; diminished absorption of fat and fat-soluble vitamins.

(9) Immaturity of some metabolic processes influencing the metabolism of certain nutrients and drugs as well as maintenance of normal homeostasis.

Care of the Premature Infant

A. Delivery Room: As with any other newborn expected to be at increased risk, a physician or well trained nurse should be available in the delivery room who is specifically responsible for care of the infant. This responsibility includes suction of the pharynx and, when necessary, resuscitation to assure that adequate ventilation is established; brief examination of the infant to determine his condition and need for specific procedures; and early placement in an incubator to provide a stable environment during transfer to the nursery.

B. Care in Nursery: In many institutions the sick baby and premature nursery is separate from the normal and full-term nursery. The premature baby is cared for in an incubator designed to provide the following:

1. Maintenance of body temperature—Incubator temperature should be kept high enough to maintain the baby's body temperature at 36–37° C (96.8–98.6° F). The baby is monitored by axillary temperatures or by placing a thermistor on the skin for remote monitoring or control of the incubator heating unit.

2. Atmosphere—To provide clean, warmed, humidified air. Oxygen is added to air as needed to avoid cyanosis when the baby is not sufficiently oxygenated. Humidity is maintained at 50–75%.

3. Isolation—Protect the infant from infection by providing filtered air and a physical barrier from possibly contaminated surroundings. All personnel must wash their hands carefully before and after they care for the baby.

4. Visibility—A most important aspect of care of the small and sick newborn is frequent observation, which implies that the baby can be seen easily and that trained personnel are available to watch him.

C. Transfer From Incubator to Bassinet: When the premature infant is able to maintain his body temperature without added environmental heat, he is placed in an open bassinet. This usually may be done when the infant reaches 1800–2000 gm. His body temperature should be monitored to be sure he continues to maintain normal temperature.

D. Examination: Evaluation and diagnostic procedures are done gently and carefully. The baby may not tolerate excessive handling well, so that the thoroughness of the examination may have to be tempered by a practical limitation of what the baby can tolerate. Careful observation will provide much information, diminishing the amount of handling needed for the physical examination. Diagnostic procedures may have to be spaced to allow the baby to stabilize after periods of handling. Whenever possible, procedures should be done without removing the baby from his incubator and should be done in the nursery, rather than taking him to other parts of the hospital.

E. Feeding: See p 54.

F. Growth of Premature Infant: There will be a period of weight loss, approaching 5–15% of birth weight, during the first days of life. The smaller the baby, the longer it will be until he begins to gain weight. Earlier feedings tend to minimize this period and the degree of weight loss. Plotting weekly weight, length, and head circumference values on an intrauterine growth chart is a useful way to evaluate the infant's growth.

G. Supplements:

1. Vitamins—Vitamins A, C, and D are given as supplements if they are not present in the formula being used. Vitamin K_1 (phytonadione), 1 mg IM, is given on admission to the nursery.

2. Iron—(See p 53.) Infants with birth weights less than 1800 gm have a special need for supplemental iron, since their iron stores at birth are limited, and growth and increase in blood volume are rapid during the first year of life. Intramuscular iron is needed only rarely, when it is known that the infant cannot tolerate oral iron supplementation.

H. Discharge: Discharge should be timed according to how the baby is doing and is usually advised when the infant weighs 2000–2500 gm, he is eating well, and coexistent medical problems have resolved or are sufficiently improved. Persistent medical problems may delay discharge. The parents are encouraged to visit the baby frequently as the time for discharge approaches. The mother may be encouraged to help care for and feed him. A social worker or visiting nurse may be particularly helpful in aiding the mother to care for the baby and in helping to solve special problems.

I. Screening Tests: Should also be done on premature infants. (See p 52.)

J. Follow-Up: Long-term follow-up care is especially important for very premature babies because of the high incidence of significant handicaps occurring later: cerebral palsy, deafness, learning and perceptual problems, and mental retardation. Early recognition of these handicaps and appropriate treatment when indicated will improve outcome.

Schaffer AJ, Avery ME: *Diseases of the Newborn*, 3rd ed. Saunders, 1971.

CARE OF THE SICK NEWBORN

Newborn intensive care nurseries provide facilities for special procedures, nursing technics, and equipment as well as personnel specially trained in sick newborn care.

Transfer to Another Hospital

The newborn intensive care unit may be in another hospital, perhaps some distance away. If the baby's problem can be anticipated prior to delivery, the transfer should be made before the baby is born. If transfer is necessary after the baby is born, it should be done as soon as possible. Telephone consultation about the infant's problem and management facilitates the transfer and allows the staff of the special nursery to be prepared to provide for his specific needs. Adequate clinical information and a tube of the mother's blood, clotted, should accompany the infant to allow efficient evaluation of his status. The mother's blood may be used to evaluate jaundice in the infant or to provide cross-match sera if a transfusion is needed.

General Approach to the Sick Newborn

A careful review of the history, physical findings, and prior treatment is essential. Diagnostic procedures should be done only on clear indications and may have to be spaced, depending on how well the baby tolerates handling. Diagnostic and therapeutic procedures should be done at the incubator or in the intensive care area if possible. Portable x-rays should be used. Exchange transfusion and other procedures can be done in the unit. If the infant must be taken from the ward, a trained person should accompany him.

Fluid and electrolyte therapy and technics of administration of intravenous fluids are discussed elsewhere. Disposable equipment for intravenous fluid administration has been designed to meet the specific needs of newborns.

Kitterman JA, Phibbs RH, Tooley LOH: Catheterization of umbilical vessels in newborn infants. P Clin North America 17:895–912, 1970.

Segal S, Pirie GE: Equipment and personnel for neonatal special care. P Clin North America 17:793–810, 1970.

Sinclair JC & others: Supportive management of the sick neonate: Parenteral calories, water, electrolytes. P Clin North America 17:793–894, 1970.

RESUSCITATION OF THE NEWBORN
(See Fig 3–4 and Table 3–5.)

Someone who is trained in resuscitation of the newborn infant should be in attendance at each delivery. Physicians and nurses working in the delivery area should be able to decide when resuscitation is necessary and be able to give it efficiently.

Gentle suction of the posterior pharynx with a soft rubber bulb or catheter is all that is usually necessary to remove blood and mucus which may have accumulated during delivery. If the baby is in good condition, he will take his first breath and establish normal ventilation rapidly.

Some babies will require more active intervention. Airway obstruction can be recognized when respiratory efforts are accompanied by marked retraction of the chest wall. Additional airway suction will be necessary, sometimes including direct visualization with a laryngoscope. If breathing is not established and a patent airway is assured, assisted ventilation can be given by the mouth-to-mouth or bag and mask technic. An endotracheal tube will occasionally be necessary to maintain a patent airway.

Each baby must be evaluated individually to determine whether assistance is needed to initiate ventilation. In general, babies with 1-minute Apgar scores of 7–10 will be vigorous and initiate breathing with little problem. Infants with 1-minute Apgar scores of 4–6 should be evaluated carefully since they may require help. Severely depressed infants with 1-minute Apgar scores of 3 or less usually require active resuscitative measures. The aim is to establish a patent airway and initiate ventilation with minimal delay.

Occasionally, after ventilation is established, closed chest cardiac massage may be required. Consider this when the heart rate is below 40/minute after ventilation is adequate.

If acidosis is severe, give sodium bicarbonate intravenously as follows: infant < 1000 gm, 2.5 mEq; 1000–2000 gm, 5 mEq; > 2000 gm, 7.5 mEq. (Concentrated sodium bicarbonate solution usually contains about 0.9 mEq $NaHCO_3$ per ml. This should be diluted 1 part bicarbonate solution with 2 parts distilled water, to a final concentration of about 0.3 mEq/ml.)

Technics

A. Tracheal Aspiration: This is best done by direct visualization, using a laryngoscope. The tube should be stiff enough not to collapse when suction is applied and should have a hole at the end as well as one or 2 on the sides. Insert the tube without suction, but remove it while using gentle suction and slow rotation. The tube may have to be removed and reinserted several times to remove large particles, each time maintaining the suction during removal. A DeLee mucus trap works well for this purpose. Mechanical suction machines frequently develop too great a negative pressure.

B. Mouth-to-Mouth Breathing: Resuscitation by this method may be used to assist ventilation when an

TABLE 3–5. Resuscitation equipment.

Emergency resuscitation equipment must be available in all areas where babies are delivered or cared for. Equipment must be of the proper size and in working order. The items of equipment listed below are relatively inexpensive and functional.

Positive pressure breathing bag
Infant and premature masks
Laryngoscope handle (medium)
Laryngoscope blades, premature and newborn
Batteries and bulbs for laryngoscope (extra)
Endotracheal tubes (Cole), sizes 8, 10, 12, and 14 F
Endotracheal tube stilets made from medium weight copper wire, with rounded ends
Endotracheal tube connectors (to fit bag and respirators)
Oral airway
Mucus trap (DeLee) with tracheal catheter
Towel or 4 X 4 inch gauze to wipe face
Drugs:
    Sodium bicarbonate solution, 44.5 mEq/50 ml (approximately 1 mEq/ml)
    Epinephrine, 1:1000 aqueous solution
    Nalorphine (Nalline), 2 mg ampule, or
    Levallorphan (Lorfan), multidose vial, 1 mg/ml
Plastic syringes, 1, 2, 5, and 10 ml
Extra needles, Nos. 23 and 25
Needle, 1 inch, for cardiac injection
Oxygen source and oxygen administration tubes

appropriate bag is not available. Once the airway is patent, mouth-to-mouth ventilation is easily done and should present minimal danger of infection to the baby. The operator's mouth is placed over the baby's mouth and nose. The aim is to expand the lungs and produce an exchange of air. Watch the chest wall for expansion and have someone listen to the lungs for air exchange. Pressure should be delivered between 10–20 cm water, interspersed with occasional ventilation efforts of 20–40 cm water. (The person using mouth-to-mouth resuscitation should practice ahead of time using a pressure gauge to judge how to deliver a safe, adequate pressure to the baby's airway.)

C. Bag and Mask: Several good bag and mask devices are available for use on newborn infants which allow delivery of small volumes and fit snugly over the baby's mouth and nose. The bags fill easily with air or oxygen and can be used over long periods without tiring the operator. Practice with the bag is necessary so that the operator will learn how to deliver the desired pressures. Be sure the airway remains patent. A small plastic or metal oral airway may be helpful.

D. Endotracheal Intubation: (Fig 3–4.) This may be done with appropriate tubes through the mouth under direct visualization. The tip of the tube must extend into the trachea beyond the larynx but must not reach the bifurcation. This distance can be quite short in a small newborn. (If breath sounds are heard only on one side of the chest, the tube is in a main stem bronchus.) Assisted ventilation can be given either by the mouth-to-tube or the bag-to-tube method until the baby has established adequate respiratory effort. Before the tube is removed, suction the pharynx around the tube and apply gentle suction into the tube itself in order to avoid aspiration of pooled secretions.

Kuhns LR, Poznanski AK: Endotracheal tube position in the infant. J Pediat 78:991–996, 1971.

OXYGEN ADMINISTRATION TO NEWBORNS

Supplemental oxygen administration is required in those infants whose arterial oxygen tensions fall below 50–60 mm Hg because of respiratory insufficiency. Generalized cyanosis occurs at oxygen tensions below these levels and can be used as a satisfactory guide for oxygen therapy for short periods; however, cyanosis does not provide a sufficiently accurate indication of arterial oxygen levels as a guide for continued oxygen therapy. The development of retrolental fibroplasia is related to increased arterial oxygen tensions; therefore, careful monitoring of arterial P_{O_2} is required to avoid this added risk yet provide adequate inspiratory oxygen concentrations to maintain arterial P_{O_2} at appropriate levels.

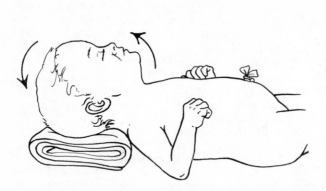

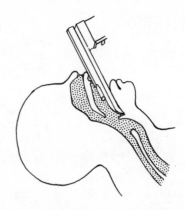

A: A folded towel is placed under the infant's head. With the right hand, the head is rotated into the "sniffing position."

B: A laryngoscope with proper-sized blade is held in the left hand and introduced through the right corner of the infant's mouth. This moves the tongue to the left of the blade. Under direct vision through the slot in the right half of the blade, the tip of the laryngoscope is advanced into the sac at the base of the tongue anterior to the epiglottis.

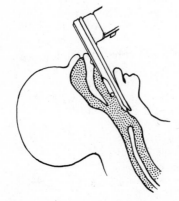

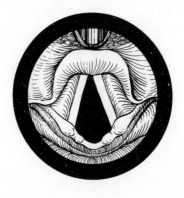

C: The tongue and epiglottis are lifted vertically, bringing the larynx into view. The right hand can now be released, and the infant's jaw is supported with the fifth finger of the left hand. The endotracheal catheter is introduced at the right corner of the mouth and passed into the glottis through the vocal cords. The laryngoscope is then removed.

D: Anterior view of glottis as seen through laryngoscope.

FIG 3–4. Technic of endotracheal intubation.

Methods of Increasing Oxygen Concentration

Warmed (31–34° C) humidified oxygen may be given through the incubator air intake system or by use of a mask or plastic hood. Oxygen concentration at the infant's nose should be monitored frequently.

Indications

(1) During resuscitation for brief hypoxic periods.
(2) Apnea: Needed only if periods of apnea are prolonged and symptomatic (see p 59).
(3) Hypoventilation due to primary lung disease leading to cyanosis.

Recommendations for Administering Oxygen

(1) The aim is to maintain the arterial oxygen tension between 60–80 mm Hg; it should not exceed 100 mm Hg. The inspired oxygen concentration may need to be high to accomplish this; however, use no higher concentrations than needed since oxygen toxicity to other organs, particularly the lungs, may become significant. The inspiratory oxygen concentration must be measured accurately and recorded frequently.
(2) Oxygen added to inspired air should be warmed and humidified; it is administered

through an incubator, funnel, hood, mask, or endotracheal or nasotracheal tube.

(3) Blood for oxygen tension sampling may be drawn from the descending aorta or the temporal or brachial arteries. If blood oxygen tensions cannot be measured, oxygen should be administered in concentrations just high enough to relieve cyanosis. However, the premature infant is at increased risk of developing ocular toxicity and should be transferred to a newborn special care unit where these measurements can be utilized to guide therapy.

(4) As the infant's condition improves, the oxygen concentration should be lowered gradually to determine response, being guided preferably by blood arterial oxygen concentrations.

(5) The eyes of infants who have received oxygen therapy should be examined for evidence of retrolental fibroplasia before discharge and again at 3–6 months of age.

Duc G: Assessment of hypoxia in the newborn. Pediatrics 48:469–481, 1971.

CYANOSIS

When cyanosis occurs, certain groups of diseases should be considered. Some are infrequently encountered but require specific treatment when they occur. Primary pulmonary disease, primary heart disease, and primary brain damage are discussed elsewhere in this text. Peripheral vascular collapse (shock) with poor peripheral circulation usually presents with duskiness or frank cyanosis associated with pallor.

Lees MH: Cyanosis of the newborn infant. J Pediat 77:484–498, 1970.

METHEMOGLOBINEMIA

Oxidation of hemoglobin to methemoglobin may be due to deficiency of erythrocyte nucleotide diaphorase, which is required in the conversion of methemoglobin to hemoglobin, or to the presence of an abnormal hemoglobin M. Toxic causes include ingestion of nitrites or exposure to local anesthetics or aniline dyes.

Methemoglobin does not release oxygen. The baby is cyanotic, although no evidence of lung or heart disease can be found. Distress is minimal unless the degree of methemoglobinemia is severe enough to cause hypoxia. The cyanosis does not improve with oxygen administration. The diagnosis is made when

blood is drawn and the chocolate color of the blood is noted. Confirmation depends on spectroscopic analysis of the hemoglobin.

Treatment consists of the administration of reducing agents which convert methemoglobin back to hemoglobin. Methylene blue or ascorbic acid is usually employed for this purpose. Intravenous administration of methylene blue is fairly dramatic, with resolution of the cyanosis in 15–30 minutes. Every effort must be made to find the agent which has caused the disease so that it may be eliminated from the baby's environment and to prevent the occurrence in other babies.

RESPIRATORY PROBLEMS IN THE NEWBORN PERIOD

APNEA

Apnea is defined as cessation of respiration for 30 seconds or longer and is accompanied by cyanosis and bradycardia. It must be distinguished from **periodic breathing** (see below), in which the apnea is brief (usually less than 10 seconds) and is not accompanied by cyanosis or bradycardia.

Apnea is a symptom of serious significance in the newborn. One episode of apnea demands investigation into the underlying cause, since it so often heralds repeated attacks. Although apnea suggests pulmonary disease, its causes are by no means limited to diseases of the lung. It occurs in association with CNS and metabolic diseases, as well as in a variety of less well defined disorders.

Causes of Apnea

A. Pulmonary Disease: Several diseases of the lungs are characteristically associated with apnea. Although each disease listed below is described in more detail in other sections of this book, the relationship of this important symptom to specific diseases will be stated.

1. Respiratory distress syndrome—Apnea is an ominous symptom of respiratory distress syndrome. It usually indicates severe disease and a poor prognosis. It occurs late, ie, 2–3 days after birth, and sometimes is the terminal event.

2. Pneumothorax—Apnea is frequently a presenting symptom. The association of apnea with or after feeding in cases of pneumothorax has been documented. It is considered to be an indication of pulmonary insufficiency.

3. Pneumonia—Apnea may be the presenting symptom of pneumonia in the newborn or older premature infant. Many continue to have periods of apnea until the disease is controlled. The cause of the apnea is not well understood because the symptom often precedes x-ray evidence of the disease. It is possible that many crib deaths result from this initial apneic episode.

B. Metabolic Derangements:

1. Hypoglycemia—The response of newborns to hypoglycemia may be quite different from that in older children and adults. Rather than irritability, sweating, and convulsions, one may see hunger, cyanosis, pallor, or apnea. Apnea in this instance may be the equivalent of a convulsion.

2. Fluid and electrolyte abnormalities—Small premature infants may have apnea in association with hyponatremia and improve after administration of sodium chloride or sodium bicarbonate. Characteristically, apnea and hyponatremia occur in the very small infant—ie, under 1500 gm—a few days after birth and are often accompanied by other subtle signs of illness. Because intravenous fluids, electrolytes, and glucose are now being given more frequently to small and sick infants, the incidence of apnea due to hyponatremia has decreased. Other factors may also be involved in the etiology of apnea, such as increased bilirubin levels, acidosis, or hyperkalemia.

C. CNS Damage:

1. Kernicterus—Apnea may be a prominent symptom of kernicterus. Decreased respiratory rate and apneic periods may be the major symptoms of kernicterus in the very small premature infant.

2. Idiopathic seizures—Apnea as the equivalent of a seizure has been observed frequently in the high-risk nursery. This symptom usually occurs in babies with a history of perinatal trauma or hypoxia. The onset of periods of apnea may not occur until days or weeks after birth, when the child may be doing well. Signs of acute disease are lacking, and the apnea does not necessarily occur in relation to feeding or other activities. Following the apneic period, the infant again resumes normal vigor, tone, and appetite. The EEG is usually abnormal in this early phase, but the characteristic seizure pattern may not appear until later. When it is a convulsive equivalent, apnea responds to anticonvulsant medication.

D. Other Conditions Associated With Apnea:

1. Choanal atresia—The newborn is reluctant to breathe through his mouth. When the nasal airway is partially or completely obstructed, serious problems may arise. Infants with choanal atresia may become cyanotic, and in some cases apneic. Nursing surveillance in cases of choanal atresia may be lifesaving, and surgery, to produce an airway, becomes an emergency procedure.

2. Pierre Robin syndrome—The combination of micrognathia, harelip, cleft palate, and glossoptosis represents a serious threat to patency of the airway. Unless an airway is established and maintained immediately, the clinical course may be complicated by repeated episodes of apnea.

3. Passage of a stomach tube—Gastric aspiration too soon after birth occasionally results in apnea, probably secondary to reflex stimulation. If nasopharyngeal suction is followed immediately by gastric intubation, the already hypoxic infant may become apneic.

4. Apnea during umbilical vein catheterization—Apnea, as part of a widespread respiratory and circulatory collapse, has been observed in rare instances when an umbilical catheter has been inserted. The mechanisms involved in this reaction are not understood.

Treatment consists of prompt reestablishment of breathing by stimulation or by technics of assisted ventilation described above for active resuscitation. Underlying diseases and metabolic abnormalities, particularly acidosis, must be treated also.

Periodic Breathing

In the small premature infant, a form of Cheyne-Stokes respiration has been described. It characteristically consists of a rhythm of 8–12 respiratory cycles followed by a pause or apneic period of approximately 10 seconds. Periodic breathing is so frequent in premature infants that it scarcely causes concern, and the phrase "rest periods" is often used to describe the breathing pattern. Increasing the concentration of oxygen decreases the rest periods, and the breathing pattern often becomes regular. For this reason, oxygen was used more and more freely for premature infants, and in high concentrations, before the association of high oxygen concentrations with retrolental fibroplasia was appreciated. It is of interest also that the infant with periodic breathing does not become cyanotic; in fact, studies have shown that he is better ventilated than the premature infant with regular respirations.

Periodic breathing is related to altitude as well as to prematurity, since instances of periodic breathing occur in full-term infants in Denver (1 mile above sea level).

Daily WJR, Klaus M, Meyer HBP: Apnea in premature infants: Monitoring, incidence, heart rate changes and an effect of environmental temperature. Pediatrics 43:510, 1969.

Gupta JM, Tizard JPM: The sequence of events in neonatal apnea. Lancet 2:55, 1967.

RESPIRATORY DISTRESS

A number of diseases involving the respiratory and other systems can present with a similar clinical picture of respiratory distress in the newborn. The symptom complex consists of expiratory grunting respirations and retractions of the chest wall, usually involving the lower rib cage and sternum. Depending on the severity of the underlying disease, these findings may be accompanied by varying degrees of cyanosis, increased respiratory rate, and decreased volume of air entry with each respiration. Laboratory studies will show CO_2 retention, hypoxia, and acidosis. Since a variety of different diseases can cause respiratory distress, it is important to give careful consideration in each case to all of the causes. Appropriate diagnostic procedures should be done to determine the diagnosis in a particular patient, including a careful history and physical examination, obtaining cultures, and x-rays. In this way, specific therapy can be instituted when it is needed.

Differential Diagnosis

Hypothermia in the first hours of life, CNS disorders, bleeding, trauma, infection, and abdominal disease may cause respiratory distress.

Respiratory system diseases that cause respiratory distress are as follows:

A. Complete Airway Obstruction: Total obstruction of the airway will be obvious by observing the infant's respiratory effort, with marked retraction but no air exchange. Posterior choanal atresia may also present this picture, since the baby may not open his mouth to breathe and is temporarily supported by means of an oral airway. If obstruction in the upper trachea, larynx, or glottis cannot be removed by suctioning, tracheostomy may be necessary.

B. Partial Airway Obstruction: Vascular rings, laryngeal webs, or other intra- or extraluminal structures may present as respiratory distress and lead to obstructive emphysema, inspiratory or expiratory stridor, or cough.

C. Pulmonary Anomalies: Sequestered lung, congenital cysts, agenesis and hypoplasia of the lung or a portion of lung.

D. Congenital Lobar Emphysema: This occurs when a partial or ball valve type obstruction to the bronchus of one lobe occurs as a result of malformation of the cartilage in the bronchus, partial obstruction of the bronchus due to intra- or extraluminal abnormality, or unknown causes. The symptoms result from the gradually increasing size of that lobe, with secondary compression of the remaining lung on that side of the chest and, if progressive, a shift of the mediastinum with compression of the lung on the opposite side. The clinical course varies, sometimes being rapidly progressive and sometimes stabilizing for long periods. Secondary infection may occur. Surgery is usually indicated and may have to be done urgently as a lifesaving procedure in the child with rapidly developing respiratory insufficiency.

E. Tracheo-esophageal Fistulas With Various Types of Esophageal Atresia: These disorders may present as respiratory distress, although they usually present with findings of excessive mucus from the mouth during the newborn period, cough, and, perhaps, cyanosis.

F. Diaphragmatic Hernias: Diaphragmatic hernias present with varying amounts of respiratory distress depending on the amount of abdominal contents herniated through the defect in the diaphragm. The defect most commonly occurs at the foramen of Bochdalek, at the posterolateral portion of the diaphragm, usually on the left side. The hernia may occur through the esophageal hiatus or in the retrosternal area. The baby has difficulty ventilating in spite of strong respiratory efforts beginning at birth. Asym-

metry of respiration may occur, with the affected side moving less. If the stomach is present in the chest cavity, it may become dilated with air, increasing respiratory distress. This can be treated by passing a tube to decompress the stomach. Bowel sounds may be heard in the chest. The abdomen is typically scaphoid when empty. Diaphragmatic hernia usually constitutes an urgent surgical emergency.

G. Aspiration: Aspirated amniotic fluid probably is not a significant cause of respiratory distress. However, aspirated blood, saliva, stomach contents, and meconium are irritating to the respiratory tract and can cause persistent respiratory symptoms, often with an inordinate amount of cyanosis. The diagnosis is made on the basis of the history and x-ray findings of patchy, coarse infiltrates in the lung fields and the appearance of material obtained by tracheal suction. Treatment consists of oxygen, antibiotics, and careful tracheal toilet if needed to clear the airways.

H. Bacterial Pneumonia: Pneumonia may be congenital or acquired at the time of delivery. It may or may not be associated with a history of prolonged rupture of the membranes and amnionitis. These babies may seem well for several hours and then show symptoms of respiratory tract involvement, when they may deteriorate quite rapidly. X-ray usually aids in making the diagnosis. Bloody sputum may be present.

I. Pulmonary Hemorrhage: This may occur at any time in the newborn period, usually in association with other diseases such as intrauterine growth retardation, respiratory distress syndrome, pneumonia, and sepsis. The baby will develop anemia and signs of respiratory distress, and usually will have bloody mucus coming from the trachea. X-ray often shows a typical picture of symmetrical infiltrates in both lungs. Treatment consists of supportive care, treatment of the underlying condition, and, if possible, correction of the bleeding diathesis.

J. Pneumothorax or Pneumomediastinum: Air may escape from ruptured alveoli, dissect along vascular sheaths to mediastinal tissues, or break through into the pleural space. Pneumothorax may occur with high positive pressure ventilation. The baby develops fairly sudden respiratory distress of varying degree. Mild hypoxia often is manifested as hyperactivity which can be mistaken for hunger. Pneumothorax is occasionally discovered unexpectedly when a chest x-ray has been obtained for another reason. Physical examination may show only an increased anteroposterior diameter of the chest, distant heart tones, and tachypnea. In more severe cases, there may be a bulge of the chest on the side of the pneumothorax and a shift of the cardiac apical pulse. Stomach distention after feedings may compromise ventilation enough to cause cyanosis and apnea. A few cases will progress, and the pneumothorax air will be under tension. Both anteroposterior and lateral chest x-rays are needed to adequately evaluate the extent of free air. Treatment is based on severity of symptoms and progression of the process. When mild, specific treatment may not be needed. Simple needle aspiration of air may relieve moderate symptoms. If progress is rapid or tension develops, aspiration is done, followed by chest tube drainage. In any case, equipment for emergency thoracentesis must be available at the bedside in case sudden increase in respiratory difficulty occurs.

K. Idiopathic Respiratory Distress Syndrome (RDS): See below.

L. Wilson-Mikity Pulmonary Syndrome: See Chapter 12.

Avery ME: *The Lung and Its Disorders in the Newborn Infant,* 2nd ed. Saunders, 1968.

Shaffer AJ, Avery ME: *Disease of the Newborn,* 3rd ed. Saunders, 1971.

Sundell H & others: Studies on infant with type II respiratory distress syndrome. J Pediat 78:754–764, 1971.

IDIOPATHIC RESPIRATORY DISTRESS SYNDROME (RDS) OF THE NEWBORN
(Hyaline Membrane Disease)

Essentials of Diagnosis

- Pre-term birth.
- Onset of grunting and retracting respirations within the first several hours after birth which become progressively more severe by 6 hours of age.
- Poor air entry on auscultation.
- Maternal difficulties at delivery, especially those involving placental perfusion.
- Generalized granularity on x-ray with air bronchograms.

General Considerations

The cause of respiratory distress syndrome is unknown, but it occurs almost exclusively in pre-term infants. It is characterized by increased pulmonary vascular resistance and decreased or absent surface-active substances, resulting in stiff lungs (loss of compliance). Widespread atelectasis of the lung and injury to the pulmonary parenchyma results. Cellular debris and exudate accumulate in the alveolar ducts, forming the membrane seen at autopsy. Vascular engorgement and hemorrhage are frequent. Babies with severe disease who die within the first few hours of life may not show evidence of the membrane although the rest of the pathologic process is consistent with the respiratory syndrome.

Clinical Findings

A. Symptoms and Signs: Retractions and expiratory grunting begin shortly after birth and become progressively more severe. Decreased air exchange, cyanosis, and increased respiratory rate occur as the disease progresses. Symptoms increase in severity until about 24–36 hours of age, when the disease process reaches its peak. The respiratory rate will rise to 70–80/minute. Inspiratory retraction of the sternum and lower costal margin is often associated with abdominal distention. Poor air entry is the main auscultatory finding; rales are not heard in the early stage of the disease. Edema is common, especially in the hands and feet. The limbs are flaccid, and bowel sounds are poor or absent. Progressive ventilatory insufficiency may cause death by 3 days of age.

When recovery ensues, reparative processes result in progressive ventilatory improvement. With supportive care only, babies with the respiratory distress syndrome will have about a 40–50% mortality. However, when given optimal metabolic support with fluid, calories, and electrolytes, in addition to good supportive care, there is an improvement in outcome (a mortality rate of about 25–30%).

B. Laboratory Findings: Blood gas values show the effects of ventilatory insufficiency: acidemia, CO_2 retention, and diminished oxygen tension. In severely affected infants, the arterial oxygen tension is low, with a low arterial blood pH due to metabolic products. P_{CO_2} elevation is a poor prognostic sign. Continued low arterial oxygen tension despite oxygen administration is an unfavorable sign that indicates an increase in right-to-left shunting and bypass of blood to the lungs. Lactate is the main metabolic product causing metabolic acidosis and reflects tissue hypoxia. Serum potassium levels rise as the disease progresses.

C. X-Ray Findings: X-ray of the chest frequently demonstrates the characteristic "ground glass" appearance and an air bronchogram, but is of use mainly to rule out other causes of respiratory distress which need specific therapy.

D. Special Examinations: Pulmonary function studies show stiff, small lungs with a reduced effective pulmonary blood flow.

Differential Diagnosis

Respiratory distress syndrome must be differentiated from cold stress, pneumonia, pneumothorax, pneumomediastinum, lobar emphysema, pulmonary hemorrhage, diaphragmatic hernia, CNS hemorrhage, and occasionally congenital heart disease.

Complications

If the disease is mild, recovery usually is evident by 72 hours of age. Elevation of the arterial CO_2 tension is an unfavorable prognostic sign which indicates that the baby will die unless he receives assisted ventilation. Pulmonary fibrosis and an increased incidence of pulmonary infection are being reported more often in patients receiving certain types of ventilatory assistance. Brain damage usually does not result if the infant survives.

Prevention

The pathophysiology of respiratory distress syndrome is poorly understood, but prematurity is one factor that is clearly involved in its development. Therefore, every effort should be made to prevent preterm births. The mothers at risk (those with diabetes, toxemia, and histories of other premature births or respiratory distress syndrome in other babies) should receive meticulous prenatal care. Transfer to a center where advanced technics are available for caring for the mother and infant should be considered.

Prediction of Respiratory Distress Syndrome

The use of amniocentesis to predict lung maturity by means of the lecithin:sphingomyelin ratio appears promising. As the infant matures, the amount of lecithin increases in relation to the sphingomyelin. A mature lung is associated with a lecithin:sphingomyelin ratio of 2:1 or greater. Severe respiratory distress syndrome can be expected when the ratio is 1:1 or less. Intermediate disease occurs when the ratio is between 1:1 and 2:1.

Treatment of Mild Respiratory Distress Syndrome

Early recognition is important so that the baby can be evaluated and treatment begun as soon as possible. This allows time for transportation to another hospital, if necessary, and for diagnostic procedures to be done while the baby is well enough to tolerate the handling.

The baby is placed in an incubator so that a normal body temperature of 37° C (98.6° F) may be maintained. Humidity should be adequate (70–80%), but mist is not necessary. Oxygen should be added to the atmosphere of the incubator when needed (see p 57). Use of excessive oxygen must be avoided. Intravenous administration of water, glucose, and electrolytes appears to be beneficial: water to maintain adequate hydration and renal output, glucose to provide calories, and electrolytes for maintenance requirements and for specific correction of metabolic derangements. A satisfactory solution is the following: 250 ml of 10% dextrose in distilled water plus 50 ml of concentrated $NaHCO_3$ solution (giving a solution containing 8.3% dextrose and 150 mEq HCO_3/liter), administered at a rate of 65 ml/kg/day by continuous drip.

This solution can be administered safely for 1–2 days as long as the baby's illness does not progress. With improvement, the concentration of bicarbonate is decreased until only maintenance sodium chloride is added to the glucose solution. Potassium is not added during the first 2–3 days unless a specific deficiency is demonstrated. Intravenous fluids are continued until the baby has tolerated several oral or gavage feedings.

Treatment of Severe Respiratory Distress Syndrome

Adequate laboratory support is essential for the management of sicker infants. This emphasizes the need for an early decision to transfer the baby to another hospital for care where these facilities are available.

Some very sick babies may not demonstrate a rising respiratory rate or may not be cyanotic because of peripheral vascular collapse and pallor.

Hypoxia, acidosis, pulmonary vasoconstriction, decreased pulmonary surfactant, and atelectasis play an important role in the pathophysiology of respiratory distress syndrome. Hypovolemia may be present, and the infant will be in shock. Therefore, therapy of the severely affected infant is directed toward correcting hypoxemia and acidosis, improving pulmonary blood flow, expansion of the lung, and correcting blood volume. To this end, inspired oxygen, arterial P_{O_2}, P_{CO_2}, pH, and systemic blood pressure must be monitored. If possible, central venous pressure is also monitored.

Intravenous fluids may be given via a peripheral vein or the umbilical vein. The latter presents some danger to the infant because of the possibility of portal vein thrombosis. Arterial blood is necessary for monitoring oxygen tension, pH, P_{CO_2}, and systemic blood pressure. A satisfactory route for monitoring blood gases and administering fluids is the umbilical artery when fluids are introduced at a constant rate with an infusion pump.

A. Acidosis: Metabolic acidosis as indicated by the calculated base deficit (negative base excess) is corrected with sodium bicarbonate. Standard sodium bicarbonate (0.89 mEq/ml) is diluted with 2 parts of sterile water and infused into the circulation at a rate of 1 mEq/kg/minute or slower. The amount required to correct the metabolic acidosis is calculated from the following formula:

$$\text{mEq of bicarbonate} = \text{body weight in kg} \times \text{the base deficit (negative base excess)} \times 0.3$$

B. Oxygen Therapy: Guidelines from the American Academy of Pediatrics stress the importance of monitoring inspired oxygen concentration as well as arterial oxygen tension. Hypoxemia must be corrected, but too high an arterial oxygen tension may lead to the development of retrolental fibroplasia or pulmonary oxygen toxicity. Therefore, the physician must maintain a balance between the inspired oxygen concentration and arterial oxygen tension so that hypoxemia is corrected with as little inspired oxygen as possible. The goal is to maintain the arterial oxygen tension between 50–80 mm Hg. The oxygen may be given in the incubator up to concentrations of 40%, after which a clear plastic hood is preferred. The oxygen should be warmed and humidified. Flow through the hood should be at least 5 liters/minute to prevent CO_2 rebreathing.

C. Hypovolemia: This condition may be assumed whenever the central venous pressure is less than 2 mm Hg or the mean arterial pressure is less than 25 mm Hg. Volume may be replaced by whole blood or salt-poor albumin (4 gm/100 ml).

D. Temperature: Oxygen expenditure is reduced if the infant remains in a "thermal neutral" state. Moreover, pulmonary blood flow is reduced if the infant is cool. Therefore, the body temperature should be maintained at 37° ± 0.5° C (98.6° ± 1° F) in an incubator or by means of a radiant heater.

E. Fluid and Electrolytes: Intravascular fluids are infused at a rate of 65–100 ml/kg body weight/24 hours. Use 10% dextrose in water with added maintenance electrolytes, or electrolytes required to treat specific needs.

F. Assisted Ventilation: A rising arterial CO_2 tension is a poor prognostic sign. If the arterial oxygen tension cannot be maintained at 50 mm Hg in 100% inspired oxygen, the use of a mechanical respirator must be considered. Because of the time, effort, and laboratory support required, this is best done in centers where an experienced staff is available.

Prognosis

The prognosis depends upon the ability of the nursery staff to give intensive care. The prognosis is good if the infant survives for 72 hours.

Behrman RE: The use of acid-base measurements in the clinical evaluation and treatment of the sick neonate. J Pediat 74:632–637, 1969.

Brumley GW: The critically ill child: XVI. Respiratory distress syndrome of the newborn. Pediatrics 47:758–769, 1971.

Capitanis MA, Kirkpatrick JA Jr: Roentgen examination in the evaluation of the newborn infant with respiratory distress. J Pediat 75:896–908, 1969.

Gluck L & others: Diagnosis of the respiratory distress syndrome by aminocentesis. Am J Obst Gynec 109:440–445, 1971.

Hull D: Lung expansion and ventilation during resuscitation of the asphyxiated newborn. J Pediat 75:47–58, 1969.

Knelson JH & others: Physiologic significance of grunting respirations. Pediatrics 44:393–400, 1969.

Nelson NM: On the etiology of hyaline membrane disease. P Clin North America 17:943–966, 1970.

Reynolds EOR: Indications for mechanical ventilation in infants with hyaline membrane disease. Pediatrics 46:193–202, 1970.

Sundell H & others: Studies on infants with type II respiratory distress syndrome. J Pediat 78:754–764, 1971.

HEART DISEASE IN THE NEWBORN

Signs & Symptoms of Heart Disease in the Newborn Without Heart Failure

A. Physical Examination:

1. Rate and rhythm– Slowed heart rate and arrhythmias may occur with overdigitalization. Tachycardia will occur with early hypoxia, heart failure, and specific cardiac arrhythmias.

2. Heart sounds and murmurs–Considerable information is gained from careful auscultation of the heart for evidence of abnormal heart tones and murmurs. These abnormal findings suggest heart disease and require further diagnostic study. Serious heart disease may exist without a murmur.

3. Cyanosis–Heart disease must be considered whenever cyanosis is present.

4. Peripheral pulses–Absent femoral pulses or bounding pulses suggest heart disease.

B. Electrocardiogram: An ECG should be taken whenever heart disease is suspected. The normal newborn infant has right ventricular dominance due to the relatively large size of the right ventricle at birth. Serial ECG's are helpful when digitalizing a newborn.

C. X-Ray Findings: Chest x-rays show the size and configuration of the heart and pulmonary vasculature, both of which aid in evaluating heart disease in the newborn. Barium swallow is often needed. More specific diagnostic x-ray procedures such as angiocardiography must be done with great care, with special attention to the baby's body temperature and ventilation.

D. Cardiac Catheterization: Cardiac catheterization in newborns is a specialized procedure that requires great care and consideration by expert personnel. The indications for it depend to a large extent on the availability of qualified physicians. The general indications, contraindications, and hazards are discussed in Chapter 13.

Signs & Symptoms of Heart Failure in the Newborn

Heart failure in the newborn infant may be difficult to recognize because the signs and symptoms are not the same as in older infants. The infant in early failure will show only an increased heart and respiratory rate and perhaps irritability. Auscultation of the lungs rarely reveals evidence of pulmonary edema. X-ray examination may show the heart to be enlarged, but in newborn infants minimal cardiac enlargement is difficult to determine, particularly if there is a large thymus shadow. Assessing heart size by physical examination is even more difficult.

Increasing liver size is a most important finding. A significantly enlarged or enlarging liver, in the absence of other disease, is good evidence of heart failure. Liver size should be monitored as a means of evaluating the effectiveness of treatment.

Peripheral edema is present only in severe heart failure.

Congenital Heart Diseases Which Cause Heart Failure in the Newborn

A. Aortic Atresia; Hypoplastic Left Heart Syndrome: The baby usually looks well in the immediate newborn period, with good color and peripheral pulses. Within a few hours, his condition deteriorates, with peripheral vascular collapse, absent pulses, pallor, duskiness, and relentless, progressive heart failure which is unresponsive to therapy. Death occurs in a matter of days.

B. Transposition of Great Vessels: Cyanosis is usually present at birth or soon after. It increases with crying or activity and is not relieved completely by oxygen administration. Murmurs are inconstant. Gallop rhythm is common when failure is present. The cardiac silhouette on x-ray examination has a characteristic "egg shape," although this may not be obvious in the first week of life. There is an increase in pulmonary vascular markings.

C. Coarctation of Aorta: Over half of babies with coarctation become symptomatic in the first year. The postductal type causes symptoms later, with hypertension showing its effect mainly on the left ventricle. In the preductal type, the hypertension affects both ventricles and therefore tends to cause early heart failure even as early as the first week of life. For this reason, peripheral pulses should be routinely evaluated as part of the newborn infant examination. Blood pressures should be taken in the right arm and in one of the lower extremities whenever the diagnosis is considered.

D. Patent Ductus Arteriosus: The ductus arteriosus remains patent for variable periods of time after birth up to a few days or several weeks. A murmur will not develop until the pulmonary artery pressure falls enough to allow a significant flow through the ductus. The murmur in the newborn is usually systolic rather than the typical machinery murmur heard later. The infant is acyanotic; peripheral pulses are bounding; and there is a loud second sound. In the newborn, a simple patent ductus usually does not cause clinical problems, but heart failure does occur in rare instances.

Patent ductus arteriosus is frequently associated with other defects such as coarctation of the aorta, ventricular septal defect, and aortic stenosis. Severe pulmonary hypertension may occur as a complication. X-ray shows pulmonary artery prominence and increased lung vascularity. ECG may show evidence of greater left ventricular predominance than is usually seen in newborns. Congestive heart failure, when it occurs, is treated at first medically and then by surgery, which, if there are no other lesions, will provide a cure.

E. Pulmonary Atresia and Tricuspid Atresia: These defects may occur alone or in association with other heart lesions. The right atrium and left ventricle are enlarged. Other findings include decreased pulmonary vasculature, a harsh systolic murmur along the left lower sternal border, and often severe cyanosis. ECG shows left axis deviation and left ventricular dominance. Heart failure may occur in newborns. The liver may pulsate in tricuspid atresia. Pulmonary valvulotomy may be done for pulmonary atresia. The prognosis for tricuspid atresia is poor.

F. Anomalies of Pulmonary Venous Return: Total anomalous venous return, particularly with infradiaphragmatic insertion of all pulmonary veins, will show marked cyanosis and rapidly developing heart failure in the neonatal period. X-ray examination reveals normal heart size but may show a picture of increased pulmonary vasculature as a result of congestion. Surgery is helpful, and should be done as soon as the condition is diagnosed and the patient can be prepared for the operation.

Acquired Causes of Congestive Heart Failure in the Newborn Period

A. Paroxysmal Atrial Tachycardia: In newborns, symptoms are likely to be dramatic, the baby quickly becoming very ill. He shows restlessness, slight cyanosis, cool skin, rapid respirations, and increasing heart failure as the duration of the attack lengthens. The diagnosis is confirmed by ECG. Digitalis is the treatment of choice.

B. Myocarditis: Myocarditis is usually due to a specific bacterial pathogen (secondary to bacterial septicemia) or to viruses such as those of the Coxsackie B group. Although the clinical picture may vary, the usual picture is that of an infant who shows progressive acute heart failure, often without preceding illness. The heart enlarges and sounds become weak. Treatment is supportive, including digitalization and oxygen. The prognosis is guarded.

C. Pulmonary Disease: Wilson-Mikity syndrome, pulmonary fibrosis, and other pulmonary disorders may cause secondary right heart failure.

D. Other Causes: Severe anemia and arteriovenous fistulas may cause high-output failure. Rapid overexpansion of blood volume secondary to blood, plasma, albumin, or fluid administration may cause heart failure. When severe anemia exists and blood or sedimented red cell transfusion is indicated, the small volume exchange transfusion technic may be necessary to avoid overexpanding the blood volume.

General Management of Heart Disease in Newborn Infants

The goal in management of the newborn infant with congenital heart disease and heart failure is to recognize the presence of the disease early and to decide on timing of definitive diagnostic procedures and specific treatment. Many congenital heart lesions are well tolerated for variable periods and require neither specific diagnosis nor treatment in the newborn period. Careful follow-up is required. Babies who develop clinical evidence of heart failure require treatment of the failure and careful evaluation to decide when further work-up should be done. This may include additional procedures which have some risk, such as cardiac catheterization or angiocardiography. Intervention in surgically correctable lesions should be timed so that the baby is in the best possible condition. If these investigations and definitive treatment can safely be delayed until the baby is older, they will be better tolerated and the outcome may be improved. Each case must be evaluated on its own merits.

The principles of general supportive care are the same as in other sick newborns: minimal handling, adequate ventilation, maintenance of body temperature and adequate fluid, electrolyte, and caloric intake, and treatment of infections when present.

Treatment of Heart Failure in the Newborn

Digitalis is the cornerstone of treatment of heart failure in the newborn just as in any other age group.

The dosage necessary to achieve adequate digitalization in newborn infants may vary widely, and dosage schedules differ from those used in other age groups.

Digoxin is the best preparation to use in the newborn infant. The digitalizing dose in newborns is 0.03–0.05 mg/kg IM or IV; give 1/2 of the dose stat and 1/4 of the dose every 6–8 hours until the baby is digitalized. The maintenance daily dose, usually 1/5–1/10 of the digitalizing dose, must be given in divided doses every 12 hours to maintain an adequate effect throughout the 24-hour period. On once-a-day doses, the baby may have periods of overdigitalization and underdigitalization.

Other measures consist of minimal physical activity, administration of oxygen, and the use of mercurial diuretics if edema is present. Placing the infant in the sitting-up or the cardiac (squatting) position may be very helpful in the newborn with intractable heart failure. Seats are available or can be improvised for this purpose. Be sure that the baby does not slump over.

Morphine will occasionally be needed for sedation in a baby who has acute hypoxic episodes and restlessness.

Lees MH: Heart failure in the newborn infant: Recognition and management. J Pediat 75:139, 1969.

Rowe RD, Mehrizi A: *The Neonate With Congenital Heart Disease.* Saunders, 1968.

Rowe RD: Serious congenital heart disease in the newborn infant: Diagnosis and management. P Clin North America 17:967–982, 1970.

HEMATOLOGIC DISEASES IN THE NEWBORN

Bleeding

A. Clotting Factor Deficiencies:

1. Hemorrhagic disease of the newborn (hypoprothrombinemia)—Vitamin K dependent clotting factors (factors II, VII, IX, X) are normal at birth but the levels decrease within 2–3 days. In vitamin K deficient babies, these levels may be very low, resulting in prolonged bleeding time. Bleeding may occur into the skin or gastrointestinal tract, around the umbilical cord, or at the site of injection of medications or of circumcision. Small amounts of vitamin K are sufficient to correct the clotting factor defects unless liver function is immature in a very sick or premature infant. The preferred drug is phytonadione (vitamin K_1, Aqua-Mephyton), 1–2 mg IM soon after birth. All newborns should receive phytonadione, 1 mg IM, as a routine.

2. Factor VIII (AHF) deficiency (hemophilia)—The X-linked form of clotting factor deficiency accounts for 80% of cases of hemophilia and is likely to be manifest in the newborn period. Bleeding may occur after circumcision or injection. However, some affected infants may show no bleeding in the newborn period. Factor IX and factor XI deficiencies are much less likely to cause bleeding in the newborn period.

B. Thrombocytopenia: Petechiae are frequently seen in newborn infants in the region of the presenting part or over the face and head. The platelet count is normal. When petechiae appear, a blood smear should be done to determine if there is an underlying thrombocytopenia. Frequent causes of thrombocytopenia in newborns are as follows:

1. Chronic intrauterine infection such as rubella syndrome, cytomegalic inclusion disease, and toxoplasmosis.

2. "Consumption coagulopathy" of disseminated intravascular coagulation associated with severe disease.

3. Iso-immunization to platelets can occur in the fetus (analogous to Rh iso-immunization).

4. Mothers with thrombocytopenia may give birth to babies with transient thrombocytopenia.

C. Hypercoagulability: Recent interest in bleeding problems in the newborn period has led to a revaluation of blood clotting factors. The blood of newborn infants clots more rapidly than the blood of normal adults. Sick newborn infants, especially those with respiratory distress syndrome, have even shorter clotting times. They frequently have an elevated hematocrit in the first few hours which increases blood viscosity. Hypercoagulability in the presence of some triggering episode (hypotension, stasis of blood, etc) leads to intravascular clotting and thrombus formation, causing damage to vessel walls and bleeding. The importance of this mechanism in bleeding in the newborn is under study.

D. Hemorrhage Following Prolonged Hypoxia: Hemorrhage associated with prolonged bleeding times is noted in infants delivered after extensive hypoxia.

E. Pulmonary Hemorrhage: Hemoptysis may occur in the sick newborn, particularly in those with intrauterine growth retardation (mechanism unknown) and with congenital pneumonia.

Anemia

Acute blood loss before or during delivery can occur into the maternal circulation, the amniotic sac, a twin, or into the vagina. Acute blood loss after delivery may be external (gastrointestinal, circumcision site, umbilical stump) or internal (a fracture site, cephalhematoma, CNS or pulmonary hemorrhage, soft tissue hematoma, ruptured internal organ). Anemia may be secondary to hemolysis (erythroblastosis, acquired hemolytic disease, red cell metabolic abnormalities, hemoglobinopathies) or to congenital aplastic or hypoplastic anemia.

The clinical findings consist of pallor (to be differentiated from peripheral vascular collapse), tachycardia, decreased hemoglobin and hematocrit, and jaundice (if anemia is due to hemolysis or an enclosed hematoma). Hemoglobin or hematocrit should be determined immediately if the newborn is pale. If it is found to be low, further laboratory and clinical examinations are necessary to determine the cause of the anemia.

If anemia is symptomatic or severe (eg, due to acute blood loss), transfusion of whole blood may be urgently required. If anemia is chronic or due to hemolysis, transfusion may have to be done with sedimented red cells using the small volume exchange transfusion technic. Oral iron supplementation may be needed if the hemoglobin loss has been sufficient to result in later iron deficiency.

Polycythemia

Unusually high hematocrits in newborns may cause symptoms which put the baby at increased risk. A central venous hematocrit over 75% requires careful evaluation.

The cause of polycythemia in the newborn is often not known. Feto-fetal transfusion in twins leaves one twin anemic (and often small for gestational age) and the other plethoric. The clinical findings (due to increased blood viscosity and increased blood volume) include respiratory distress, thrombosis, and jaundice.

Treatment is indicated only for symptomatic infants. Small volume exchange transfusion, removing the high-hematocrit blood and replacing it with plasma or isotonic albumin solution, will reduce the hematocrit to a satisfactory level (60%). Simply removing blood is not adequate since there may be considerable delay before a significant drop in hematocrit occurs.

Hathaway WE: Coagulation problems in the newborn. P Clin North America 17:929–942, 1970.
Hathaway WE, Mull MM, Pechet GS: Disseminated intravascular coagulation in the newborn. Pediatrics 43:233, 1969.
Oski FA, Naiman JL: *Hematologic Problems in the Newborn.* Saunders, 1966.

JAUNDICE OF THE NEWBORN

Jaundice is the most frequent clinical problem occurring in the newborn after he recovers from delivery. The age at onset, the degree of jaundice, and the condition of the baby are important observations in determining the cause and significance of the jaundice.

The outline of the metabolism of bilirubin shown in Fig 3–5 provides a useful basis for considering the differential diagnosis of jaundice. When red blood cells break down, the iron and protein are stored and reused. However, the porphyrin ring must be detoxified and excreted from the body. It is reduced to bilirubin (unconjugated, indirect) in the reticuloendothelial cells and is then transported to the liver via the blood, bound to albumin. In the liver, the bilirubin is conjugated mainly to bilirubin diglucuronide (conjugated, direct) and excreted through the biliary ducts to the gut. The degree of jaundice which develops will depend upon the rate of red cell breakdown (bilirubin load), the rate of conjugation, and the rate of excretion of bilirubin. In normal full-term infants, red blood cells have an average life span of about 100 days; therefore, 1/100 of the cells are removed from the circulation every day. The average capacity of the liver to conjugate bilirubin in the first few days of life approximately equals the bilirubin load, since about ½ of infants will show laboratory evidence of a significant rise in bilirubin levels and about 1/3 show clinical jaundice. Liver conjugation usually improves by the third to fifth day (as late as the seventh day in prematures), so that the peak blood level of bilirubin will occur then. Bilirubin levels should be determined periodically in jaundiced infants because of the special danger of kernicterus in the newborn infant.

Causes of Jaundice of the Newborn

A. Increased Rate of Hemolysis: (Elevated unconjugated bilirubin.)

1. Erythroblastosis fetalis.
2. Bacterial infection.
3. Red cell metabolic defects.
a. Excessive vitamin K administration.
b. Glucose-6-phosphate dehydrogenase deficiency.
c. Pyruvate kinase deficiency.
d. Hereditary spherocytosis.
e. Hemoglobinopathy.
4. Extravascular hemorrhage within the body (eg, cephalhematoma).

B. Decreased Rate of Conjugation: (Elevated unconjugated bilirubin.)

1. Immaturity of glucuronyl transferase system ("physiologic jaundice").
2. Congenital familial nonhemolytic jaundice (inborn errors of metabolism affecting glucuronyl transferase system).
3. Inhibition of glucuronyl transferase maturation (presence of abnormal pregnanediol in breast milk).

C. Abnormalities of Liver Cell Metabolism or Integrity: (Conjugated and unconjugated bilirubin are elevated.

1. Hepatitis—Viral, parasitic, bacterial.
2. Metabolic abnormalities—
a. Galactosemia.
b. Glycogen storage disease.
c. Infant of diabetic mother.

D. Decreased Rate of Excretion: (Conjugated and unconjugated bilirubin are elevated.)

1. Biliary atresia.
2. Choledochal cyst.
3. Obstruction at ampulla of Vater.
4. Fibrocystic disease—Rarely presents with jaundice in newborn because of biliary cirrhosis.

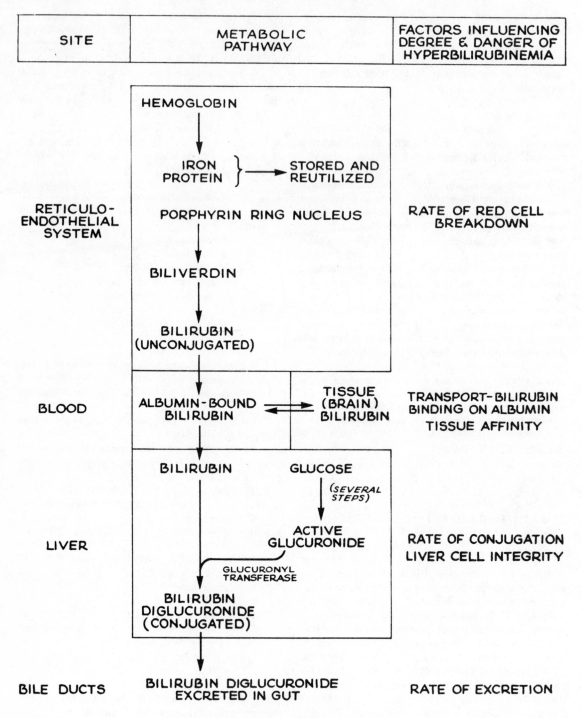

FIG 3–5. Outline of bilirubin metabolism.

ERYTHROBLASTOSIS FETALIS

1. ISO-IMMUNIZATION DUE TO Rh (ANTI-D, E, C, c, or e), KELL (Kk), DUFFY (Fy), LUTHERAN (Lu), KIDD (Jk) FACTORS

The involved red cell antigen is always absent from the mother's red cells; therefore, if fetal red cells containing the involved antigen cross the placenta, the mother will produce antibodies to the "foreign" antigen. These circulating IgG antibodies cross the placenta, enter the fetal circulation, and produce hemolysis of the fetal red cells.

Diagnosis

A. Maternal Past History: Previous infants were jaundiced, anemic, or required exchange transfusion at birth.

B. Current Pregnancy: Blood type and antibody screening should be done on all pregnant women as early as possible. Antibody screening is an easy and inexpensive means of demonstrating the presence or absence of red cell antibody. If antibody is absent in an Rh-negative woman early in pregnancy, it should be repeated at around 34 weeks of gestation to determine if sensitization has occurred during the pregnancy. Significant sensitization to blood groups other than D is unlikely to occur later when no antibody exists in the initial screening. When antibody screening is positive, the specific antibody should be identified and an indirect Coombs titer determined to establish the degree of sensitization. Anti-A and anti-B antibodies are not demonstrated by this test since O cells are used. However, ABO iso-immunization causes little risk to the fetus, and there is ample time to evaluate the infant after delivery.

C. Amniocentesis and Amniotic Fluid Analysis: Amniotic fluid analysis should be done early in the third trimester on all pregnant women with significantly elevated Rh antibody titers to determine if the fetus is affected and to evaluate the severity of the disease. The yellow pigment in the amniotic fluid (unconjugated bilirubin) is quantitated by the method of Liley or Brazie & others. A clinical estimate of severity of disease in the fetus is then made, using the prediction graph based on clinical experience with that method (Fig 3–6 and Table 3–6).

D. Cord Blood Coombs Test: A direct Coombs test is done on cord blood of all infants whose mothers' blood type is Rh-negative and on any infant who shows significant jaundice or anemia in the newborn period (even though the mother is Rh-positive). A positive direct Coombs test in the newborn infant indicates that his cells are coated with antibody and is diagnostic of iso-immunization. A positive indirect Coombs test indicates the presence of antibody in the baby's serum but does not confirm the presence of blood group incompatibility.

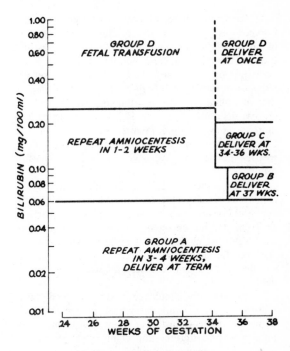

FIG 3–6. Prediction graph for evaluation and management of Rh-sensitized pregnancies based on amniotic fluid examination by chloroform extraction method. See Table 3–6 for description of groups. Location of dashed line at 34 weeks, dividing management of group D patients, is determined by relative risks of premature delivery and intrauterine transfusion. (Redrawn and reproduced, with permission, from Brazie JV & others. Am J Obst Gynec 104:80, 1969.)

Prevention

The passive administration of gamma globulin containing a high titer of anti-D antibody (RhoGAM) to the Rh-negative unsensitized mother has proved successful in preventing sensitization when she has delivered an Rh-positive infant.

After delivery, Rh-negative women must be evaluated and must receive RhoGAM within 72 hours after delivery if it is indicated.

Treatment

Fig 3–6 and Table 3–6 summarize the management of an affected pregnancy and the severity of disease to be expected in the newborn.

Babies born to mothers in groups B, C, and D will have more severe disease. Evaluation of the infant immediately after birth is necessary if infants needing urgent treatment are to be identified. Personnel, equipment, and blood must be available at the time of delivery.

A. Observation and General Care: Observation during the birth recovery period and maintenance of metabolic homeostasis are the same as those required in any sick newborn. Anticipate acidosis and hypoglycemia.

Hemoglobin or hematocrit, blood type, and direct Coombs test results should be determined on cord blood of all infants who may have erythroblastosis. Indirect Coombs titer and bilirubin will help in the evaluation of affected infants. Serial bilirubin levels are required in sensitized infants to follow the degree of hyperbilirubinemia. Serum albumin, blood pH, and glucose determinations will aid in the management of more severely affected infants. Adequate fluid and caloric intake should be maintained in addition to treatment of acidosis, hypoglycemia, and other specific problems.

B. Phototherapy: Light has been demonstrated to enhance degradation of unconjugated bilirubin in the skin into colorless by-products which are apparently nontoxic and are excreted in the urine and bile. Blue light waves are most efficient in detoxifying bilirubin; however, full-spectrum fluorescent bulbs are preferred so that the baby can be observed better under normal light.

Phototherapy should be used only when hyperbilirubinemia is a significant clinical problem. It should be used cautiously—just as any new drug or procedure in a newborn. Certain important routines must be considered whenever phototherapy is used.

1. Phototherapy is used only for unconjugated (indirect) hyperbilirubinemia; it is contraindicated when significant conjugated (direct) hyperbilirubinemia exists ("bronze baby syndrome").

2. The cause of jaundice must always be searched for; phototherapy does not replace any other diagnostic or therapeutic procedures.

3. Serial bilirubin levels must be obtained while the baby is receiving phototherapy. Skin appearance is not a reliable indicator of the degree of jaundice.

4. The indications for exchange transfusion remain unchanged. Although phototherapy clears additional bilirubin from the body, it does not replace the need for exchange transfusion when it is indicated.

5. The effectiveness of phototherapy depends upon the wavelength of light, the intensity of light, and the area of skin exposed. The baby should be undressed and his position should be changed occasionally.

6. The eyes should be protected from intense light by appropriate patching. The patch must be applied carefully and should be removed and the eyes inspected on each nursing shift. Corneal abrasion and conjunctivitis are the main hazards.

7. The baby's temperature must be monitored frequently because of the heat produced by the lights.

C. Exchange Transfusion: The purposes of exchange transfusion are (1) to remove bilirubin from the body when the level is high enough to involve a risk of kernicterus, and (2) to raise the hemoglobin level in severely anemic infants without increasing blood volume. The volume of blood to be exchanged is calculated as twice the infant's blood volume (BV = approximately 85 ml/kg body weight). This amount given by exchange transfusion will result in about 85% exchange of the baby's blood.

TABLE 3–6. Patient groups in erythroblastosis.

Group A: Fetus mildly affected or unaffected. Repeat amniocentesis in 3–4 weeks. Deliver at or near term. Newborn in good condition. If affected, there is time after delivery to evaluate infant.

Group B: Moderate disease; fetus at risk of developing hydrops if pregnancy continued beyond 37 weeks. Repeat amniocentesis in 1–2 weeks. Deliver at 37 weeks. Newborn may be more severely affected. Anticipate immediate evaluation and need for treatment.

Group C: More severe disease; fetus at risk of developing hydrops if pregnancy continues to 37 weeks. Risk of premature delivery less than risk of intrauterine transfusion. Repeat amniocentesis in 1–2 weeks. Deliver at 34–36 weeks. Newborn more severely affected and preterm. Anticipate immediate evaluation and need for treatment.

Group D: Severely affected fetus; hydrops likely prior to 34 weeks. Risk of intrauterine transfusion less than risk of very preterm delivery. Intrauterine transfusions indicated. Deliver at 34 weeks or later, if possible. Newborn condition variable, depending on the efficiency of the fetal transfusions and the degree of prematurity. Anticipate immediate evaluation and need for treatment.

1. **Urgent exchange transfusion**—Done at birth or shortly after.

a. **Purpose**—To treat severe anemia by doing small volume exchange transfusion with sedimented or packed red cells (5–10 ml increments, to a total of 50–100 ml).

b. **Indications**—Exchange transfusion is indicated if the baby is severely anemic at birth (hemoglobin < 8 gm/100 ml); if there is danger of the infant's developing heart failure; or if heart failure is already manifest as frank neonatal hydrops.

c. **Supportive care**—Ensure adequate pulmonary ventilation with oxygen. Treat acidosis. Maintain normal body temperature. Allow the baby to stabilize before exchange transfusion is done.

2. **Early exchange transfusion**—Indicated before hyperbilirubinemia occurs.

a. **Purpose**—To remove sensitized red cells before they hemolyze in order to minimize the bilirubin load presented to babies who are likely to need more than one exchange transfusion.

b. **Indications**—Cord bilirubin over 5 mg/100 ml, cord hemoglobin level below 12 gm/100 ml, rate of bilirubin rise greater than 0.5–1 mg/100 ml/hour in the first 48 hours.

3. **Exchange transfusion for hyperbilirubinemia**—

a. **Purpose**—To clear bilirubin from the body, keeping the serum bilirubin level below 17–23 mg/100 ml.

b. Albumin administration—Exchange transfusion for hyperbilirubinemia can be made more efficient if albumin is used to enhance bilirubin binding in the blood. Salt-poor albumin, 1 gm/kg body weight (4 ml/kg of 25% solution), is given IV 1/2−1 hour before the usual exchange procedure. *Caution:* Albumin solution is hypertonic and will increase blood volume; therefore, never use it in an infant with severe anemia or evidence of early heart failure.

4. If indications are equivocal, do exchange when the following factors are present.

a. Evidence of rapid red cell production and hemolysis—The reticulocyte count is greater than 5% and the nucleated red cell count greater than 10 per white cell, indicating that the bilirubin load will be great.

b. Acidosis—Evidence of other illness in the infant producing acidosis, such as respiratory distress syndrome, infant of diabetic mother, sepsis, or other severe disease.

c. Signs of kernicterus: Absent Moro reflex, severe lethargy, opisthotonos, apnea, high-pitched cry.

5. Blood products to be used—

a. Blood group—Type O, Rh-negative blood is most often used, but type-specific blood may be used if the baby's type is known. Donor blood should be cross-matched with maternal serum.

b. Fresh heparinized whole blood—This is the optimal product. Heparinized blood imposes only a minimal acid load and therefore offers a decided advantage to the infant who is sick, acidotic, premature, etc. Heparinized blood may safely be used for 48 hours after procurement.

c. Acid-citrate-dextrose (ACD) blood less than 5 days old—This blood presents a considerable acid load to the infant; therefore, it should be used with great caution in high-risk newborns. Frequent evaluations of blood pH are necessary. Bicarbonate may be needed to treat acidosis.

d. Buffered blood—Several buffers have been used to minimize the acid load of citrate blood. Tromethamine (THAM) is recommended, adding 10−12 mM/500 ml unit of whole citrated blood, which will bring the donor blood pH toward 7.35 (8−10 ml of a 1.2 M solution or 35−40 ml of an 0.3 M solution). *Caution:* For multiple exchange transfusions, the infant's blood pH should be followed closely. Less THAM may be needed in subsequent units of blood, thus avoiding alkalosis.

D. Special Considerations:

1. Decreased bilirubin binding on albumin—Certain factors affect the albumin binding of bilirubin, thereby increasing the risk of kernicterus at lower serum bilirubin levels.

a. Competition with bilirubin for albumin binding—Sulfonamides, elevated free fatty acids.

b. Decreased absolute binding capacity—Acidosis, hypoalbuminemia.

2. Cardiac arrest—Cardiac arrest (or other catas-trophe) may occur during or shortly after an exchange transfusion. Such accidents are more frequent in sick infants and usually are the result of uncompensated acidosis. The incidence is decreased when fresh heparinized or buffered blood is used. Careful monitoring of heart rate, blood pressure, condition of the infant, etc is important for early recognition. Treatment requires early recognition, adequate pulmonary ventilation, oxygen, closed chest heart massage, intravenous bicarbonate administration (10 mEq by slow push), and other supportive measures as indicated.

3. Babies who have received intrauterine fetal transfusion—The usual indications for exchange transfusion based on cord blood hemoglobin and bilirubin levels need modification. Hemoglobin levels are more stable the higher the percentage of donor cells present. Also, bilirubin levels may rise less rapidly because of the reduced load from red cell breakdown. Therefore, when the baby is stable and the course is in doubt, determine the hemoglobin and bilirubin levels again in 1−2 hours and reevaluate the situation.

4. Later anemia—The baby will continue to have hemolytic anemia until the antibody has decreased to insignificant levels. Therefore, he needs to be followed for several weeks by means of serial hemoglobin or hematocrit determinations until a sustained rise is demonstrated. A single packed red cell transfusion may be needed if the hemoglobin levels fall below 7 gm/100 ml.

2. ISO-IMMUNIZATION DUE TO ABO BLOOD GROUP INCOMPATIBILITY

There is no satisfactory way to predict which full-term infants with ABO sensitization will require exchange transfusion except by following bilirubin levels. Preterm infants are more susceptible. ABO disease requires close observation for several days after birth. They should be kept in the hospital if the bilirubin level continues to rise, or they can be followed closely in outpatient visits.

Blood group combinations that suggest possible incompatibility are as follows:

Mother	Infant
O	A or B (most common clinical problem)
A or B	AB
B	A
A	B

Cord blood typing and Coombs testing can be done whenever potential incompatibility exists. The direct Coombs test is usually mildly positive if done carefully. The indirect Coombs test will be positive in the presence of antibody if type-specific cells are used, although a strongly positive reaction is uncommon. If in doubt about the accuracy of the Coombs test, it is best to assume that sensitization is present whenever maternal-infant major blood group incompatibility exists. Serial bilirubin levels are then obtained.

Hemoglobin levels are normal or nearly so. Mild reticulocytosis may be present. Spherocytes are commonly found on the smear of peripheral blood.

Physical examination is usually normal except for jaundice, which may develop in the first 48 hours. More severe involvement occasionally occurs.

Treatment with supportive care and phototherapy are as indicated with Rh sensitization. Exchange transfusion should be used to keep bilirubin levels below 17–23 mg/100 ml. Cord values or early rates of bilirubin rise are not indications for exchange transfusion in ABO sensitization, since these do not reliably predict eventual bilirubin levels. Pre-exchange administration of albumin is indicated with the same caution as with Rh disease.

For details of volume and products, see above.

Note: Babies who may have both ABO and Rh iso-immunization (eg, mother is type O, Rh-negative; baby type A, Rh-positive) will often be protected from Rh sensitization. However, such a baby with a positive direct Coombs test should have indirect Coombs testing for both antibodies.

Behrman RE, Hsia DY: Summary of a symposium of a phototherapy for hyperbilirubinemia. J Pediat 75:718, 1969.

Brazie JV, Bowes WA Jr, Ibbott FA: An improved, rapid procedure for the determination of amniotic fluid bilirubin and its use in the prediction of the course of Rh sensitized pregnancies. Am J Obst Gynec 104:80, 1969.

Charles AG, Friedman EA: *Rh Isoimmunization and Erythroblastosis Fetalis.* Appleton-Century-Crofts, 1969.

Liley AW: Liquor amnii analysis with management of the pregnancy complicated by rhesus sensitization. Am J Obst Gynec 82:1359, 1961.

Queenan JT: *Modern Management of the Rh Problem.* Harper, 1967.

KERNICTERUS
(Bilirubin Encephalopathy)

Kernicterus refers to the clinical syndrome and pathologic changes in the CNS secondary to deposition of unconjugated bilirubin in certain nuclei of the brain. As a rule, the risk of kernicterus becomes significant at serum bilirubin levels above 17–23 mg/100 ml. However, certain factors predispose to the development of kernicterus at lower serum levels. These factors mainly result in decreased albumin binding capacity for bilirubin (acidosis, low albumin levels, sulfonamide administration, elevated free fatty acid, etc).

The infant with kernicterus has severe hyperbilirubinemia, usually secondary to erythroblastosis but may be associated with jaundice due to other causes. There is a fairly sudden onset of lethargy and poor feedings, a weak or incomplete Moro reflex; a weak, high-pitched cry; and opisthotonos. In premature infants, slowed respiratory rate and apneic periods may be prominent findings. Apnea, respiratory arrest, and convulsions constitute the terminal episode.

Prevention by avoidance of dangerous hyperbilirubinemia is the best treatment. Good supportive care, treatment of acidosis and hypoglycemia, and, in particular, the use of phototherapy and exchange transfusions when indicated will minimize the risk. To what degree brain injury due to bilirubin toxicity is reversible is not known. Surviving infants show varying degrees of athetosis, seizures, deafness, mental deficiency, and other neurologic deficits.

OTHER CAUSES OF JAUNDICE

Infection

Jaundice secondary to bacterial infection is most commonly due to organisms (*Escherichia coli,* staphylococci, and streptococci) which produce hemolysing toxins, increasing the rate of red cell breakdown. The bilirubin is mainly unconjugated. Jaundice may appear shortly after birth or later in the first week, depending on severity and timing of the infection.

Jaundice in infections due to other etiologic agents such as viruses (cytomegalic inclusion disease, hepatitis, herpes simplex, rubella, etc), parasites (toxoplasmosis), and *Treponema pallidum* is associated with elevations of both conjugated and unconjugated bilirubin as a result of liver cell injury and obstruction of biliary canaliculi.

Abnormal Red Cell Metabolism

Two inborn errors of metabolism in the red cells may result in an increased rate of hemolysis: glucose-6-phosphate dehydrogenase (G6PD) deficiency and pyruvate kinase deficiency. The first usually becomes evident only after coincident exposure of the mother or baby to substances such as naphthalene or primaquine. Both are rare. Hereditary spherocytosis may present with a hemolytic crisis in the newborn period, causing jaundice and anemia. By affecting G6PD activity, synthetic vitamin K preparations will cause increased hemolysis of red blood cells if administered in excessive amounts.

Extravascular Hemorrhage

Bleeding within the body, as in cephalhematoma, extensive purpura, or CNS hemorrhage, may result in elevated levels of unconjugated bilirubin because of the increased load of hemoglobin which is broken down to bilirubin.

Immaturity of Glucuronyl Transferase Enzyme System ("Physiologic Jaundice")

The onset of jaundice occurs on the late second or third day in an otherwise well baby, and reaches its peak at 5–7 days. The cause is apparently a delay in maturation of the glucuronyl transferase enzyme to conjugate bilirubin, although other factors may be operative as well. Clinical jaundice is evident in about 1/3 of full-term infants. Serum unconjugated bilirubin is increased, but other laboratory findings are normal. Bilirubin levels rarely exceed 12 mg/100 ml in full-term infants or 15 mg/100 ml in premature infants.

Treatment consists of adequate hydration and caloric intake, phototherapy, and exchange transfusion if the bilirubin level is high.

The prognosis is excellent. Bilirubin levels rarely rise high enough to cause kernicterus. Suspect another diagnosis when jaundice is unusually severe.

Metabolic Defects in the Liver

Galactosemia and glycogen storage disease may cause jaundice in the newborn. In galactosemia, symptoms (which may include hypoglycemia) begin after milk feedings are established. Mild jaundice usually has its onset after the third day and persists into the second week of life.

Obstruction of Biliary Ducts

Bile duct obstruction is manifested principally by an elevation in the level of conjugated bilirubin, but a significant degree of unconjugated bilirubinemia secondary to liver cell injury will also be present. Jaundice may begin on the third day, as with physiologic jaundice, but will persist and become increasingly intense as the conjugated bilirubin levels rise. With persistent jaundice of this type, the skin takes on a greenish yellow hue.

Prolonged & Persistent Jaundice in the Newborn

Most causes of jaundice in the newborn are transient. When jaundice persists into the second week of life, one of the following conditions may be considered.

(1) In small premature infants, jaundice will persist longer due to the delayed maturation of the glucuronyl transferase enzyme system.

(2) Liver disease or anomaly—If there are persistent and increasing levels of conjugated and unconjugated bilirubin, the diagnostic work-up is urgent because irreversible cirrhosis may develop in the presence of a surgically correctable lesion. Therefore, intrahepatic biliary atresia and neonatal hepatitis must be differentiated from extrahepatic atresia, choledochal cysts, or other correctable abnormality. Liver function tests, needle biopsy, and the clinical course may help, but open biopsy and operative cholangiogram are usually necessary to identify the cause of the jaundice.

(3) Choledochal cysts cause obstruction by intermittent filling of the cyst with bile, which causes torsion of the duct. The jaundice is usually intermittent and variable and is often associated with a palpable mass in the upper right quadrant of the abdomen.

(4) An inborn error of metabolism in the mother results in the secretion of an abnormal pregnanediol in breast milk. This substance inhibits the maturation of the glucuronyl transferase enzyme system in the infant and results in prolonged serum elevation of unconjugated bilirubin. When breast milk feedings are omitted for a few days, the enzyme matures quickly and remains functional even though nursing is resumed.

BRAIN & NEUROLOGIC DAMAGE IN THE NEWBORN

Brain damage in the newborn is usually due to birth trauma with hemorrhage and hypoxia, congenital anomaly, or infection. The diagnosis depends on evaluation of the maternal and perinatal history as well as examination of the infant. (Specific neurologic diseases and infections are described in Chapter 21.)

Prolonged & Severe Hypoxia

Intrauterine hypoxia causes brief tachycardia in the fetus and increased fetal movement, followed by depression and bradycardia. Meconium is usually passed into amniotic fluid and may be aspirated.

At delivery, the severely hypoxic infant is hypotonic, cyanotic, and pale and makes little or no respiratory effort. Active resuscitation is indicated, and prolonged assisted ventilation may be necessary. After 1/2–1 hour he may make spontaneous respiratory efforts and gradually establish spontaneous respirations. He will usually have a high-pitched, irritable cry, absent or poor Moro reflex, diminished or absent deep tendon reflexes, decreased muscle tone, and retinal hemorrhages. If the baby dies during the newborn period, the terminal event may be convulsions or apnea with respiratory arrest.

As the infant recovers, reflexes may become hyperactive and muscle tone increases, sometimes asymmetrically. There may be less spontaneous activity and a weak sucking reflex. Spasticity associated with mental and physical retardation, including slow head growth, may be expected. However, some babies recover without any demonstrable handicap.

Trauma Causing Subarachnoid, Intraventricular, or Brain Hemorrhage

There is usually a history of difficult delivery, often precipitous or breech. The baby may appear well after birth, but within a few hours develops clinical findings of irritability, increased muscle tone, high-pitched cry, often respiratory distress, decreased or absent Moro and sucking reflexes, increased or asymmetrical muscle tone, twitching, retinal hemorrhages, and dilated pupils. Convulsions may be a terminal event. Anemia and shock will occur if bleeding has been of sufficient volume. If bleeding is mild and does not recur, symptoms will begin to improve. The degree of permanent neurologic damage will depend on the extent and location of the injury. Long-term follow-up is important.

Congenital Anomaly

Microcephaly, hydrocephaly, and other congenital abnormalities can be identified in the newborn period.

Treatment of the Brain-Damaged Newborn

Except for subdural hematoma, specific treatment is not available for most types of brain trauma in the newborn. Repeated aspiration of subdural fluid or surgical removal of the sac has proved to be effective. The value or danger of lumbar puncture must be considered. Lumbar puncture is probably not indicated in the treatment of CNS hemorrhage. Meningitis may be ruled out by examination and culture of the CSF.

Supportive care includes close observation, with particular attention to the occurrence of apnea and convulsions. Fluid, electrolyte, and caloric needs must be met. Intravenous fluids are usually necessary, since oral feedings may not be tolerated and the risk of regurgitation and aspiration is great.

CONVULSIONS IN THE NEWBORN

Convulsions may occur in a variety of disorders in the newborn period. They are not frequent with intracranial hemorrhage, edema, or hypoxia except as a terminal event. Convulsions in the newborn may take the form of prolonged apneic spells.

Causes of Convulsions in the Newborn

A. Intracranial Disease:

1. Intraventricular, subarachnoid, or brain hemorrhage.

2. Intracranial hypoxia.

3. Cerebral edema (secondary to injury, hypoxia, or infection).

4. Kernicterus.

5. Sinus thrombosis or thrombosis in the great vein of Galen.

6. Arteriovenous fistula or ruptured aneurysm.

7. Infection (meningitis, encephalitis, abscess).

8. Brain malformation.

9. Brain tumor.

B. Generalized Disease:

1. Infection—Sepsis with toxicity.

2. Metabolic—See specific items for discussion.

a. Hypoglycemia—Infant of diabetic mother, intrauterine growth retardation.

b. Hypocalcemia.

c. Hypernatremia.

d. Maple syrup urine disease—Convulsions are rare before 2 weeks of life.

e. Pyridoxine dependency—May have convulsions in first week.

f. Hypomagnesemia.

3. Maternal morphine addiction—Babies show hyperactivity, jerkiness, excessive crying, and extreme hunger. They may have convulsions in the first 2 days.

4. Mepivacaine (Carbocaine) toxicity secondary to its use in paracervical anesthesia.

Treatment of Convulsions in the Newborn

Special attention must be given to maintaining airway and adequate ventilation.

Phenobarbital is an excellent anticonvulsant in the newborn, giving a good anticonvulsive effect at doses which do not cause respiratory depression. Give the first dose intramuscularly or intravenously to control convulsion. The dosage is 8–12 mg/kg/day in 4 doses. Diphenylhydantoin sodium (Dilantin) provides slower initial control but is a good anticonvulsant. The dosage is 3–8 mg/kg/day orally, IM, or IV. Paraldehyde is also an effective anticonvulsant with a wide margin of safety when respiratory depression is a problem. The dose is 0.15 ml/kg every 4–6 hours orally, IM, or rectally.

Towbin A: Cerebral hypoxic damage in the fetus and newborn: Basic patterns and their clinical significance. Arch Neurol 20:35, 1969.

OPHTHALMOLOGIC DISORDERS IN THE NEWBORN

The eyes of each newborn should be examined carefully at least once during his nursery stay, preferably before prophylaxis for ophthalmia neonatorum is given since periorbital edema and conjunctivitis may make examination difficult. This is particularly important when eye disease or trauma is suspected. An ophthalmologist should be readily available for consultation, since loss of sight may result from delay in proper diagnosis and treatment.

Physical examination should include evaluation of the periorbital structures, nerve function, anterior orbital structures, and light reflex. Ophthalmoscopic examination through dilated pupils should be done also. After examination has ruled out the presence of glaucoma or anterior chamber hemorrhage, cyclopentolate (Cyclogyl) or homatropine may be used to dilate the pupils.

Specific eye problems in the newborn period are listed below. (See Chapter 9 for further discussion of specific disorders.)

Strabismus

Many infants show some degree of strabismus in the neonatal period. It is an important finding if it is secondary to peripheral nerve or CNS damage or when there is severe esotropia (turning inward of the eyes).

Congenital Ptosis

Lid ptosis may be unilateral or bilateral and may be due to defective development of or trauma to the superior rectus or palpebral muscles. Ptosis may appear to be present with facial nerve palsy because the infant cannot completely close the lids. Rarely, ptosis accompanies congenital myasthenia gravis.

Nystagmus

Some coarse nystagmus may occur normally because of the infant's inability to fixate. Congenital idiopathic nystagmus without underlying eye disease will persist for life. Cerebellar and other CNS disease may be associated with nystagmus.

Congenital Cataracts

Cataracts may be present at birth or may become apparent within the first few weeks of life. The most common causes are genetic autosomal dominant defects, congenital rubella, and galactosemia.

Congenital Glaucoma

Early detection of congenital glaucoma is critical for preservation of vision. The disease is sometimes transmitted as an autosomal recessive trait. It should be suspected in the presence of unusually large corneas (> 11 mm), unequal size of the corneas, haziness or cloudiness of the corneas (due to edema), blepharospasm, or photophobia. Enlargement of the entire eye is usually a late finding.

Conjunctivitis

Chemical conjunctivitis secondary to instillation of silver nitrate solution should clear in 2–3 days and causes no after-effects. Gonorrheal conjunctivitis, confirmed by smear and culture, should be treated with penicillin systemically and sodium sulfacetamide or neomycin locally. Other causes of neonatal conjunctivitis include *Escherichia coli,* streptococci, staphylococci, pneumococci, and the agent of inclusion conjunctivitis.

Chorioretinitis

May occur with toxoplasmosis, cytomegalic inclusion disease, herpes simplex, and syphilis.

Retro-orbital Abscess & Periorbital Cellulitis

May occur in the newborn period.

Acute Dacryocystitis

Swelling and redness along the course of the lacrimal duct may become apparent in the newborn period.

Dislocated Lens

Diagnosed by noting the presence of a tremulous iris and identifying the lens margin on examination. Lens dislocation occurs in Marfan's syndrome.

Tumors of the Eye & Orbit

Retinoblastoma is transmitted as a dominant characteristic in the offspring of a survivor, but it may also occur sporadically. The diagnosis is considered when the following findings are present: a grayish-yellow light reflection found behind the pupil, strabismus, and one dilated pupil. The differential diagnosis includes retrolental fibroplasia, hyperplastic primary vitreous, inflammatory membranes, and congenital cataract. Other tumors of the orbit occurring in the newborn period include hemangiomas and dermoid cysts. Careful examination of the eye by the ophthalmologist is urgent.

Anterior Chamber Hemorrhage

May occur after difficult delivery, partially filling the anterior chamber with blood. A fluid level will form depending on the baby's position and is best demonstrated with the baby upright. Anterior chamber hemorrhages in the newborn period usually reabsorb completely within a few days, leaving no residual damage. However, careful follow-up examinations are necessary to be sure hemorrhage does not recur and glaucoma does not develop.

Retinal Hemorrhage

Small hemorrhages are found frequently in the retinas of newborn infants. They are secondary to minor trauma and increased pressure in the retinal vessels during delivery. They reabsorb quickly and leave no residual damage. Severe retinal hemorrhages may occur after difficult delivery, particularly when the umbilical cord is tightly wrapped around the neck with shoulder dystocia, with significant CNS trauma (including subdural hematoma), and with bleeding disorders.

Retrolental Fibroplasia

Retrolental fibroplasia develops in the eyes of premature infants who have received prolonged excessive oxygen administration. The retinal vessels become dilated and tortuous. As the severity increases, vessels proliferate into the vitreous, fibrosis occurs, and the retina becomes elevated. Permanent damage will vary in degree from no pathology to complete detachment of the retina and blindness. Glaucoma may occur later in more severe cases. Early mild stages are reversible. Prevention of the disease consists of limiting the duration of high-concentration oxygen administration. Each newborn receiving oxygen administration should have a careful ophthalmoscopic examination before discharge from the nursery. (See also Oxygen Administration to Newborns, p 57.)

Baum JD, Bulpitt CJ: Retinal and conjunctival hemorrhage in newborn infants: Review. Arch Dis Childhood 45:344–349, 1970.

Baum JD, Tizard JP: Retrolental fibroplasia: Management of oxygen therapy. Brit M Bull 26:171–174, 1970.

Hospital for Sick Children, Toronto: *The Eye in Childhood.* Year Book, 1966.

Liebman SD, Gellis SS (editors): *The Pediatrician's Ophthalmology.* Mosby, 1966.

INFECTIONS IN THE NEWBORN*

The newborn is unusually susceptible to generalized, sometimes overwhelming infection. The symptoms may be deceptively mild until the infection is far-advanced, making early recognition and treatment more difficult.

Immunoglobulin G (IgG) is transferred from the mother to the fetus, providing passive protection against some organisms. Antibodies to gram-negative organisms are contained in the IgM fraction, which is not transferred to the fetus. This is one reason why *Escherichia coli* is the commonest etiologic agent in bacterial infection in the newborn period. Other gram-negative organisms, as well as staphylococci, streptococci, and pneumococci, also cause disease. Most of these bacteria produce hemolysin which increase the rate of hemolysis of red blood cells and result in hyperbilirubinemia. Other toxins may be produced which cause systemic symptoms and cellular injury. Bacteria that are usually considered nonpathogenic in older children may cause clinical disease in the newborn. Infection is frequently generalized and manifests itself as septicemia. The frequency of positive blood cultures in newborn infants attests to the ease of invasion of bacteria. Neonatal viral and parasitic infections are also more likely to be generalized, to cause signs and symptoms of multiple organ involvement, and to have a progressive course resulting in multiple sequelae or death. Examples include cytomegalic inclusion disease, toxoplasmosis, rubella, herpes hominis, and echovirus and coxsackievirus infection. They are usually acquired before or during delivery. These infections must be considered in the differential diagnosis of severely ill newborns. Although they involve multiple organs, they frequently have individual characteristics which permit a diagnosis in the newborn period.

Specific diagnosis of newborn infections is based on the characteristic features of the disease and appropriate culture and antibody studies.

Clinical Findings

A. History and Physical Examination: *Note:* The absence of a significant history does not exclude the possibility of congenital infection.

1. Jaundice, lethargy, and poor feeding—usually the earliest findings—strongly suggest the possibility of infection.

2. Delayed gastric emptying with abdominal distention, regurgitation, and aspiration occurs frequently.

3. Localization of infection causes symptoms appropriate to the area involved.

4. Maternal or neonatal history—

a. Active infection in the mother may be transmitted to the infant and requires continued treatment after the baby is born.

b. Prolonged rupture of the membranes, particularly in the presence of fever and toxicity in the mother, is evidence of amnionitis. Under these circumstances, the baby should be considered to have sepsis, particularly if there has been a difficult or premature delivery or severe hypoxia.

B. Laboratory Findings: Cultures are essential in confirming the diagnosis. Blood, stool, urine, and nasopharyngeal cultures should be done whenever infection is suspected and before antibiotic therapy is started. Viral cultures and serial serum samples for antibody titers may be appropriate. CSF examination and culture should be done whenever infection is likely but the focus of infection is not obvious.

Treatment

A. General Measures: Early diagnosis, supportive care, and specific antimicrobial therapy are the ingredients of effective management of bacterial infections in the newborn period. The following categories based on information obtained from the history, physical examination, and careful evaluation of the clinical course will help direct management in an individual case. Frequent reevaluation is essential.

1. Suspected infection—If infection is being considered in the differential diagnosis, obtain cultures and other diagnostic studies and observe carefully.

2. Probable infection—If a presumptive diagnosis of infection is made, based on clinical findings or because the baby is seriously ill and infection may be present, obtain cultures and other diagnostic studies and treat with antibiotics. Do not wait for results of cultures before beginning treatment. Observe carefully.

3. Proved sepsis—If cultures or other diagnostic studies have demonstrated a significant pathogen or definite clinical confirmation of infection, treat with antibiotics.

B. Antimicrobial Therapy: If antibiotics are to be administered to the newborn but a definite etiologic diagnosis has not been made, the drugs should cover both gram-negative and gram-positive bacteria; should be bactericidal rather than bacteriostatic; and should be safe and given in proper dosage for the newborn. Penicillin and kanamycin fit these criteria well in most cases. Ampicillin may replace penicillin when broader coverage is required; methicillin when penicillin-resistant staphylococci are present. Gentamicin may replace kanamycin in the presence of resistant *E coli* organisms. Other antibiotics should be given only on specific indication.

Antibiotic therapy should be continued for 2–3 days beyond the time when the infection appears to

*Syphilis is discussed in Chapter 27.

have cleared and the baby is well. Continued observation is required to make certain the infection does not recur.

Sever JL: *Infectious Agents and Fetal Disease.* McGraw-Hill, 1970.
Symposium on Intrauterine Infections. Birth Defects 4:1–70, Dec 1968.
Williams CPS, Oliver TK: Nursery routines and staphylococcus colonization. Pediatrics 44:640, 1969.

EPIDEMIC DIARRHEA OF THE NEWBORN

Acute diarrhea in infants may be associated with certain types of pathogenic *Escherichia coli.* When it occurs in the nursery, it is potentially quite virulent and communicable. Constant surveillance, quick recognition and treatment, and active measures to avoid epidemic spread are required.

Clinical Findings

The *E coli* strains listed below are not pathogenic for older infants and adults. Because of the virulence of diarrhea and the rapidity of spread among infants in a nursery, emphasis must be placed on early recognition and identification of the etiologic agent. The spread to other infants is chiefly via hand contamination; therefore, hand washing and stool care are the chief measures of control of the epidemic.

A. Symptoms and Signs: Infection with pathogenic *E coli* may be asymptomatic or may cause mild to very severe diarrhea. *E coli* should be suspected particularly when diarrhea occurs in epidemics in infant nurseries. Examination shows dehydration and electrolyte alterations appropriate to the severity of the diarrhea. The amount of fluid lost in the stools is frequently underestimated. Careful physical examination and frequent weighing are most helpful in determining the degree of dehydration.

B. Laboratory Findings: *E coli* obtained from stool cultures is typed by means of agglutination with available type-specific antisera. *E coli* types 026, 055, 0111, 0125, and 0126 are most commonly associated with epidemic diarrhea in infants.

Differential Diagnosis

Other causes of diarrhea include salmonellae, shigellae, and staphylococci. Viruses probably cause diarrhea in the newborn but have been infrequently isolated. Often no etiologic agent can be demonstrated.

Treatment

Fluid and electrolyte losses must be replaced promptly by the intravenous route, followed by oral maintenance of electrolytes and calories. Treatment of shock with blood volume expanders may be needed.

Give neomycin orally or kanamycin systemically (or both) for pathogenic *E coli*, and specific antibiotic therapy if other organisms are identified. Stool cultures should be taken during convalescence to demonstrate the absence of pathogenic *E coli.*

Prognosis

Not all patients will have organisms eliminated from the bowel, although they will become asymptomatic. These infants should be followed closely for recurrence of diarrhea.

Nelson JD: Duration of neomycin therapy for enteropathogenic *Escherichia coli* diarrhea disease: A comparative study of 113 cases. Pediatrics 48:248–258, 1971.
South MA: Enteropathogenic *Escherichia coli* disease: New developments and perspectives. J Pediat 79:1–11, 1971.

PNEUMONIA

Pneumonia may be present at birth or may be acquired after delivery. It is most often due to *E coli* or hemolytic streptococci, but is occasionally caused by staphylococci and rarely by pneumococci or other gram-negative organisms. In addition, several congenital viral infections may present with pneumonia at birth.

The history and physical findings will be those of generalized infection in the newborn, plus evidence of respiratory distress. Percussion and auscultation are of limited aid in diagnosis. Chest x-ray is indispensable.

After cultures have been obtained, antibiotics should include coverage for gram-negative and gram-positive organisms until the specific etiologic agent is identified.

MENINGITIS

Since meningitis results from blood-borne organisms, its presence should be suspected in any infant with septicemia. A lumbar puncture should be done when a diagnosis of meningitis is being considered before antibiotic therapy is started. However, in a very ill baby who may not tolerate a lumbar puncture, the presence of meningitis may have to be assumed and treatment instituted accordingly. A lumbar puncture done after several days of treatment will confirm the original suspicion. The organism involved may grow out of a blood culture.

Irritability in an infant with symptoms of sepsis is a strong reason to suspect meningitis. Localizing physical findings may include a bulging anterior fontanel, meningeal irritation with opisthotonos, and convulsions. Serial head circumference measurements are essential. Newborn infants may respond to CNS infection with little if any localizing findings. *E coli* is a common cause.

General supportive care should include intravenous fluids to avoid vomiting and aspiration of stomach contents. Give specific therapy with antibiotics effective against both gram-positive and gram-negative organisms until the etiologic agent is identified. The drugs should be administered at the highest dosage level safe for newborn infants. Treatment is continued until 2 lumbar punctures show completely normal spinal fluid and negative cultures.

The infant should be observed closely for evidence of recurrence of infection. If infection recurs, an anatomic abnormality of the skull, spinal cord, or vertebral column may be present which allows seeding of organisms to take place—eg, a dermal sinus, fibrin deposits in the base of the brain from the original meningitis, or subdural collections of fluid and small abscesses which have not cleared completely. Localized or generalized brain damage or evidence of developing hydrocephalus should be anticipated.

Greensher J & others: Lumbar puncture in the neonate: A simplified technique. J Pediat 78:1034–1035, 1971.

Overall JC: Neonatal bacterial meningitis. J Pediat 76:499, 1970.

OSTEOMYELITIS

Osteomyelitis is almost always secondary to septicemia in the newborn infant; in rare cases it may be secondary to organisms introduced when a femoral puncture or bone marrow examination is performed. The most common organisms are staphylococci, streptococci, and E coli.

Physical examination will reveal localization of the infection to a bone or joint. There will be tenderness, swelling, redness of the area, and limitation of movement of the extremity involved. The diagnosis is confirmed by aspiration of joint or subperiosteal material for smear and culture. X-ray changes (which may not be present for 1−2 weeks) include periosteal elevation and calcification.

Specific antibiotic therapy should be aimed at the organism most likely to cause the disease. Treatment should be continued until the child is completely well, evidence of local inflammation has completely subsided, and x-rays show that healing is well under way. Follow-up examination and x-rays should be done to make certain that there is no recurrence.

PYELONEPHRITIS

Pyelonephritis in newborns is usually secondary to septicemia rather than contamination via the lower urinary tract. Abnormal fistulous connections between the bowel and the urinary tract, patent urachus, vesicovaginal fistula, or other structural anomaly of the urinary tract associated with obstruction will predispose to urinary tract infection.

Newborn infants with symptoms of infection may have a focus of infection in the urinary tract. This is especially true if the baby is suspected of having a urinary tract anomaly.

Urinalysis and urine culture are essential to a diagnosis of pyelonephritis. A fresh, clean-catch specimen or a specimen taken by means of suprapubic aspiration is desirable for examination and culture. Colony counts above 10,000 organisms/ml of urine in a clean, freshly voided specimen, or any colonies in a suprapubic tap, should be considered evidence of infection. Other diagnostic procedures such as intravenous urography or cystography may be needed to demonstrate congenital anomalies or obstruction of the urinary tract.

Antibiotics should be continued until the urine is normal and cultures negative. Underlying urinary tract pathology may require specific treatment. A baby with documented urinary tract infection must be followed for a long time with repeated urine cultures to be sure that infection does not recur after therapy is discontinued. Underlying urinary tract anomalies and obstruction make recurrence or continued chronic infection more likely.

OMPHALITIS

A normal umbilical cord stump will mummify and separate at the skin level. Saprophytic organisms occasionally cause a small amount of purulent material to form at the base of the cord. Other organisms may colonize and cause infection, especially E coli, streptococci, and staphylococci.

Omphalitis is a potential danger when umbilical vessels are catheterized for administration of intravenous fluids or exchange transfusion. Strict aseptic technic and immediate removal of catheters at the first sign of any complication are important.

Redness and edema of the skin around the umbilicus indicates cellulitis. Serosanguineous or purulent discharge indicates progress of the infection. Systemic reaction occurs as infection becomes more severe. Culture of skin around the cord base and blood cultures should be done.

Appropriate antibiotics for gram-positive and gram-negative organisms are given until the cause is specifically identified, and continued until all evidence of disease has disappeared and blood cultures are negative.

The extent of infection into omphalic vessels determines the prognosis. Septic thrombophlebitis can lead to hepatic abscess, generalized septicemia, and portal vein thrombosis.

SKIN INFECTIONS

The skin is exposed first to *E coli* in the birth canal and then to staphylococci upon contact with nursery personnel and the family. The mere presence of staphylococci on the skin colonization does not indicate pathogenicity, nor does it mean that clinical infection will follow. It is important to watch for evidence of skin infection in babies or their families during their nursery stay and after they have left the nursery. If clinical infection occurs, careful evaluation of nursery babies and personnel must be made to determine which strain of staphylococcus caused the infection and how prevalent it is.

Treatment of babies and personnel may be necessary to rid a nursery of a prevailing virulent organism.

Colonization by organisms other than staphylococci—usually *E coli* or candida—may take place in a newborn infant who is debilitated, has received antibiotic therapy, or has been so well isolated that staphylococcal colonization has not taken place.

Clinical Findings

A. Symptoms and Signs: Infection is manifested by skin pustules with an erythematous base. These may rupture, releasing purulent exudate, and become encrusted. The degree of involvement of the skin may be variable, from a few lesions to extensive coalescing lesions spread over most of the body. **Cellulitis** due to streptococci (less often staphylococci) may spread rapidly. **Ritter's disease** is a grave form of cellulitis caused by staphylococci in which invasion of the skin is extremely rapid, with sloughing of the superficial layers, leaving extensive denuded, weeping areas.

Localized infections may occur around the circumcision site or umbilicus. Breast abscess may occur.

B. Laboratory Findings: Appropriate local cultures and blood cultures should be done. Specific phage typing of staphylococci may be necessary to determine the prevalence of a pathogenic strain in an epidemic.

Treatment

Topical antibiotic ointments are used for limited superficial involvement. Systemic antibiotics are indicated when the lesions are more extensive and progressive, or when septicemia is present.

Melish ME, Clasgow LA: Staphylococcal scalded skin syndrome: The expanded clinical syndrome. J Pediat 78:958–967, 1971.

CYTOMEGALIC INCLUSION DISEASE

The infant infected at birth with cytomegalovirus is often delivered from a mother with a normal pregnancy. The clinical course varies from severely affected infants with fulminating congenital sepsis through intermediate stages with varying degrees of CNS involvement to normal infants.

Clinical Findings

A. Symptoms and Signs: In the severe form, the infant is acutely ill at birth with signs of congenital sepsis, ie, organomegaly, petechiae, and lethargy. He develops jaundice and has feeding problems. He tends to be small for gestational age and have a disproportionately small head circumference when it is compared to length. CNS signs include symptoms of meningitis such as irritability and later development of muscle weakness or spasticity. Chorioretinitis has been observed. Mental retardation accompanies the severe form.

In the intermediate form, the newborn infant shows few signs suggestive of congenital infection. Neonatal jaundice and a few petechiae are common. After a month or longer, symptoms of feeding difficulties, irritability, and development of muscle weakness or spasticity may occur.

Cases of congenital infection with cytomegalic inclusion disease have been documented in which no clinical evidence of disease exists and no late sequelae have been reported.

B. Laboratory Findings: IgM levels in cord blood are elevated, CSF is abnormal, and epithelial cells in the urine show inclusion bodies. Cytomegalovirus may be cultured from urine, saliva, and CSF. An elevated antibody titer in the mother and a rising titer in the infant usually confirm the diagnosis.

C. X-Ray Findings: Skull x-rays may show calcification.

Treatment & Prognosis

Treatment is supportive.

The prognosis has been considered poor, but this opinion may be revised as more subclinical infections are detected.

Burnbaum G & others: Cytomegalovirus infections in the newborn. J Pediat 75:789, 1969.

TOXOPLASMOSIS

Toxoplasmosis and cytomegalic inclusion disease have so many features in common that the preceding discussion applies here just as well. The distinguishing feature between the 2 is the etiologic agent. Toxoplasmosis is due to infection with the intracellular protozoon *Toxoplasma gondii.*

The prenatal course is usually uneventful, and only at birth is the disease suspected. The most severe manifestations at the time of birth include intrauterine growth retardation and micro- or hydrocephalus. Microphthalmia has also been described, as well as

Types	T E	Symptoms and Signs

A

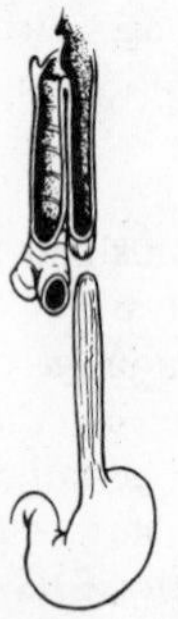

Excessive mucus, aspiration of saliva.
Scaphoid abdomen.
No gas in bowel on x-ray.
Cannot pass catheter into stomach.
Gradually increasing respiratory distress.
Polyhydramnios.

B

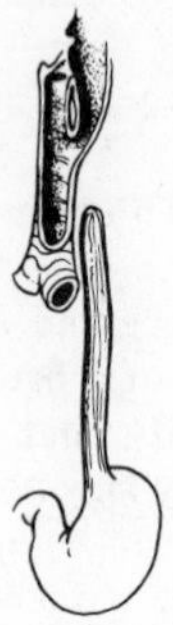

Polyhydramnios.
Coughing, choking, and pneumonia from birth.
Scaphoid abdomen.
No gas in bowel on x-ray.

C

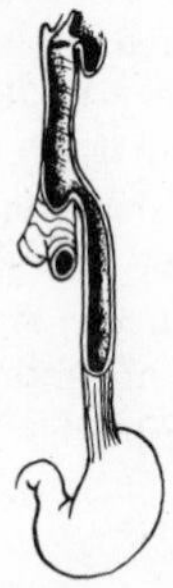

Most common (80% of cases).
Excessive mucus.
Gradually increasing respiratory distress.
Polyhydramnios frequent but not severe.
Gas in bowel on x-ray.

D

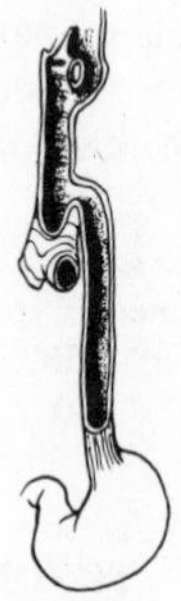

Coughing, choking, and pneumonia from birth.
Gas in bowel on x-ray.

E

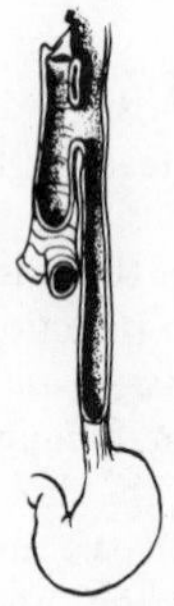

Difficult to diagnose.
Coughing or cyanosis with feeding.
Chronic aspiration pneumonia.

FIG 3−7. Types of tracheo-esophageal fistula and clinical findings.

chorioretinitis and calcifications in the skull x-rays. Hematologic abnormalities may be present. Prolonged jaundice in the neonatal period is common.

Maternal antibody titers to the organism, antibody in the infant which rises on serial determinations, and an elevated IgM in cord blood usually establish the diagnosis. The organism is difficult to grow in tissue culture but is better isolated from intraperitoneal inoculation in mice.

A large number of infants affected at birth die during the neonatal period, and those who survive are usually handicapped. Sequelae include mental retardation, convulsions, neuromuscular disease, poor vision, and micro- or hydrocephalus.

See references on p 727.

RUBELLA

Congenital rubella infection occurs as a result of rubella in the mother primarily during the first trimester of pregnancy. The earlier in pregnancy the disease occurs, the more severely affected the fetus is likely to be. Infection may involve the placenta or fetus (or both) and may persist throughout pregnancy and for a variable period after delivery. A newborn with congenital rubella, therefore, must be considered contagious to those taking care of him, particularly any personnel in the first trimester of pregnancy. Evidence is inconclusive that gamma globulin administered to the mother at the time of exposure or during clinical rubella protects the fetus. Except during an epidemic of rubella, it is essential that the clinical diagnosis of rubella in a pregnant woman be confirmed by hemagglutination inhibition antibody studies of paired sera drawn 10 days apart.

Therapeutic abortion should be offered unless the parents strongly oppose it on religious or other grounds since the incidence of major anomalies, some of which may not be apparent immediately at birth, has been estimated to range from 20–60%, depending on the time of infection in utero. Universal vaccination with attenuated live rubella virus may make intrauterine rubella a disease of the past.

Rubella should be considered in a baby with thrombocytopenia with petechiae or purpura, hepatitis, microcephalus, congenital heart disease (patent ductus arteriosus is the most common lesion), low birth weight for gestational age, cataracts, hepatosplenomegaly, myocarditis, and interstitial pneumonia. X-ray shows characteristic longitudinal radiolucent areas in the distal metaphyses of long bones. Virus isolation and antibody titer rise demonstrated in the mother at the time of infection confirm the clinical diagnosis. Cultures of the baby's nasopharynx, throat secretions, and stool are usually positive, often for several weeks after delivery. Antibody titers, liver function tests, and long bone x-rays are needed. Thrombocytopenia, sometimes only transient, is a consistent finding.

No specific treatment is available. The prognosis is variable, depending on the degree of involvement of various organs. The highest incidence of severe involvement occurs with infection soon after conception.

Krugman S (editor): Rubella symposium. Am J Dis Child 110:345, 1965.

HERPESVIRUS HOMINIS (HERPES SIMPLEX) INFECTION

Congenital or neonatal infection with *Herpesvirus hominis* is becoming a more commonly recognized disease. Infant infection is usually secondary to genital infection (primarily type 2) in the mother. The spectrum of infection in the baby may extend from subclinical with apparent recovery to generalized multiple organ ·involvement and death. Skin vesicles are common and are sometimes present at birth; CNS, eye, and generalized visceral involvement occurs frequently. In those babies who recover, later handicaps are common, particularly when the CNS is affected.

The diagnosis is based on virus culture from maternal and infant lesions and inclusion bodies and positive fluorescent antibody testing in cytologic preparations of cells from the margins of skin lesions. A rising antibody titer in the baby is helpful.

Treatment is supportive. Idoxuridine has been used with variable results. Isolation is necessary to minimize spread to personnel or other infants.

Prevention may be possible by delivering babies by cesarean section when maternal genital lesions are present to avoid fetal contact with the lesions during delivery. This should be done while membranes are intact to minimize the chance of ascending infection.

Nahmias AJ, Alford CA, Korones SB: Infection of the newborn with *Herpesvirus hominis.* Advances Pediat 17:185–226, 1970.

GASTROINTESTINAL DISEASES IN THE NEWBORN

TRACHEO-ESOPHAGEAL FISTULA & ESOPHAGEAL ATRESIA

Determination of abnormal anatomy is usually made on clinical grounds (Fig 3–7). X-ray demonstration of the upper pouch should be done by instilling no more than 1–2 ml of contrast medium if a plain film with a radiopaque catheter in place is not adequate.

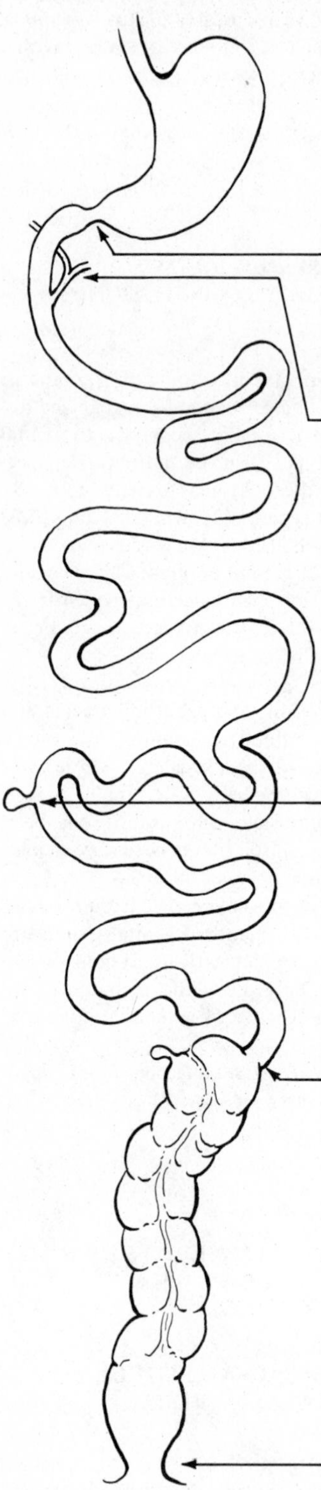

Region of Obstruction	Level	Signs and Symptoms	
		Newborn Period	**Pregnancy and Delivery**
Stomach ... **Pylorus**	A	Early part of feeding tolerated. Stomach distension with gastric waves. Vomiting soon, not bile-stained. X-ray shows gas to level of obstruction.	Polyhydramnios present. Usually over 30 ml stomach content at delivery.
Proximal duodenum ... **Ampulla of Vater**	B	Above plus additional distention and gas-filled first part of duodenum.	As above.
Distal duodenum & jejunum ... **Meckel's diverticulum**	C	Feeding tolerated. Stomach and upper small bowel distention. Vomiting after feeding, bile-stained. X-ray shows gas in upper small bowel.	Degree of polyhydramnios decreases as lesion descends gastrointestinal tract. Stomach contents at birth bile-stained.
Ileum ... **Ileocecal valve**	D	Several feedings tolerated. Gradually increasing distention. Less stomach distention. Vomiting after several feedings, bile-stained.	No polyhydramnios. No increased stomach contents at birth.
Colon	E	More feedings tolerated. More gradual, generalized abdominal distention. Vomiting later, gradually increasing in amount, bile-stained.	As above.
Rectum & anus	F	Above symptoms and signs still more delayed. Physical examination confirms diagnosis.	As above.

FIG 3–8. Sites of intestinal obstruction and clinical findings.

When fistula is present alone, the diagnosis may be difficult to confirm. Careful evaluation must be done in any baby who has respiratory symptoms, particularly coughing, choking, and cyanosis associated with feeding. The differential diagnosis includes pharyngeal muscle weakness, vascular rings, and esophageal diverticula.

Treatment varies depending upon the type of lesion and the degree of abnormality present. Frequent or continuous gentle suctioning of the upper pouch and pharynx will minimize tracheal aspiration of saliva. Gastrostomy may be done early to allow the stomach to be suctioned, minimizing the amount of mucus regurgitated through the fistula into the trachea and allowing early feeding when appropriate.

When the lungs are clear enough to permit surgery, the fistula is closed and, if the 2 ends of the esophagus are close enough, primary anastomosis may be done. However, if this cannot be done easily, closing the fistula and exteriorizing the upper pouch onto the neck is a satisfactory interim measure until final repair is done later.

Careful attention to fluid, electrolyte, and caloric requirements, as well as infection, is important during preparation for surgery and in the postoperative period. Associated congenital anomalies, particularly cardiac and other gastrointestinal abnormalities, may coexist. Evaluation for these should be made prior to surgery.

INTESTINAL OBSTRUCTION

A newborn infant with abdominal distention and vomiting must be suspected of having intestinal obstruction. Fig 3–8 lists the symptoms at various levels of obstruction.

The level of intestinal obstruction can usually be determined and the decision whether or not to undertake surgery can usually be made by careful review of the history and physical examination. A plain film of the abdomen is frequently all that is needed to confirm the clinical impression.

Additional work-up should be done only when needed to clarify the diagnosis or to aid in planning surgery. Unnecessary studies put the baby through needless procedures and delay definitive treatment. The baby may tolerate surgery better soon after birth than he will later. Needless delay must be avoided when vascular supply to the bowel may be compromised. Again, careful attention to the baby's needs in preparation for surgery and during the postoperative period is important.

Surgery may consist of definitive repair of the abnormality or may be palliative, ie, decompression of the bowel followed later by repair of the primary lesion.

Lesions Causing Intestinal Obstruction (Fig 3–8)

A. Atresia and Stenosis: (Levels A, B, C, D, E.) Intestine is narrowed below the level of obstruction.

B. Meconium Ileus: (Level D.) A common presenting clinical picture of cystic fibrosis in the newborn. Small bowel obstruction with very palpable doughy loops of gut. Meconium contains protein. Sweat chloride test may be abnormal.

C. Hypertrophic Pyloric Stenosis: (Level A.) Symptoms begin after 2–3 weeks. Gradually increasing vomiting after feedings, not bile-stained, associated with gastric distention and peristaltic waves. May occur in premature infant while still in the nursery.

D. Meconium Plug: (Levels D, E.) Usually cured by diagnostic barium enema. Check bowel movement carefully during or following barium enema for evidence of typical meconium plug followed by normal meconium.

E. Malrotation With or Without Midgut Volvulus: (Levels C, D.) Urgent because of vascular insufficiency if associated with volvulus.

F. Volvulus: (Levels C, D.) Urgent because of vascular insufficiency.

G. Congenital Peritoneal Bands: (Levels C, D.) May occur alone or in association with malrotation.

H. Incarcerated Hernia, Internal or External: (Levels A, C, D.) Always check the inguinal area when bowel obstruction is present. Acquired intra-abdominal hernia follows surgery or adhesions, or may occur through the diaphragm.

I. Annular Pancreas: (Levels B, C.) X-ray may show abnormality.

J. Duplication and Enteric Cysts: (Levels A, B, C, D, E.) Anywhere along gut; may have associated anomalies (hemivertebrae, neurologic).

K. Intussusception: (Level D.) Usually lower small bowel, crampy, intermittent symptoms, blood in stool which may have a currant jelly appearance. Careful barium enema may reduce the intussusception. If not, surgery is required.

L. Peritoneal Adhesions: (Levels C, D.) Follows bowel perforation, peritonitis, or abdominal surgery.

M. Aganglionosis (Hirschsprung's Disease): (Levels D, E.) Often presents as lower bowel obstruction in newborn. Barium enema with a small amount of barium may demonstrate typical constricted lesion. Rectal biopsy is diagnostic.

N. Paralytic Ileus: (Secondary to sepsis, respiratory distress syndrome, CNS damage, etc.) Generalized distention, decreased bowel sounds, associated with other serious disease.

O. Anal and Lower Rectal Stenosis or Atresia: (Level F.) Can be recognized by careful examination of the perineum at the initial physical examination. The abnormal anatomy may consist of stenosis of the anal opening, an imperforate membrane covering the anal opening, an unformed anus, an unformed anus and terminal rectum, or atresia of the rectum. Fistulas may exist between the terminal rectum and the perineum or vagina or urinary tract. Their presence should be carefully searched for in each case because of the complications, particularly contamination and infection of the urinary tract.

Capitanio MA, Kirkpatrick JA: Roentgenographic evaluation of intestinal obstruction in the newborn infant. P Clin North America 17:983–1001, 1970.

OTHER ABDOMINAL SURGICAL CONDITIONS

Appendicitis & Meckel's Diverticulum

These disorders may occur in the newborn period and may present difficult diagnostic problems. The infant will show general symptoms of illness and may have abdominal distention, decreased bowel sounds, and constipation. Fever and leukocytosis may not be present. Careful examination of the abdomen will usually show localizing findings of peritonitis. The appendix is often ruptured at the time of diagnosis. Meckel's diverticulum may present with sudden bowel bleeding.

Omphalocele

Omphalocele will be present at birth and requires early surgical consultation. Care is needed to keep the sac from rupturing before surgery.

Ruptured Abdominal Viscera

A ruptured abdominal viscus will present with peritonitis and pneumoperitoneum if the stomach or bowel is perforated. Rupture of a solid viscus presents with hemoperitoneum, anemia, and shock.

BLOOD IN VOMITUS OR STOOL

Swallowing maternal blood during delivery is not uncommon. If enough has been ingested, the baby may vomit bright red or dark blood or may pass a stool containing dark or bright red, fresh-appearing blood. He will show no clinical evidence of acute blood loss but may show a transient rise in BUN. If blood in vomitus or stool is of fetal origin, the baby will show evidence of blood loss and anemia, tachycardia, and shock.

Red blood of maternal origin may be differentiated from infant blood since fetal hemoglobin is resistant to alkali denaturation by the following technic: A small amount of red bloody stool or vomitus is mixed with 5–10 ml of water and centrifuged. To 5 parts of pink supernatant, add 1 part 0.25 N sodium hydroxide. If fetal hemoglobin is present, the solution stays pink; if adult hemoglobin is present, the solution becomes brown.

Bowel bleeding in the newborn may be due to any of the following conditions: nasal bleeding, usually secondary to trauma; peptic ulcer, duplication of

bowel, Meckel's diverticulum, intussusception, volvulus, hemangioma or telangiectasia of the bowel, polyp, rectal prolapse, anal fissure (a common cause of small amounts of blood in the stool in infants), infection (salmonellae, shigellae); systemic bleeding disorders, particularly hemorrhagic disease of the newborn; and tumors.

If blood is of maternal origin, no treatment is needed. If bleeding is of fetal origin, treat as for acute blood loss with blood transfusions and supportive care and then proceed with diagnosis and treatment of the underlying disease. If blood loss has been significant but transfusion is not necessary, iron supplementation may be required during the first few months.

Mustard WT & others (editors): *Pediatric Surgery,* 2nd ed. Year Book, 1969.

Swenson O: *Pediatric Surgery,* 3rd ed. Appleton-Century-Crofts, 1969.

CONGENITAL GENITOURINARY TRACT ANOMALIES IN THE NEWBORN

The genitourinary tract is one of the most common sites of congenital anomalies. They should be considered whenever other congenital anomalies are present. Whenever urinary tract infection is diagnosed in the newborn, an underlying congenital anomaly, usually associated with obstruction to urine flow in some part of the urinary tract, should be considered.

Urinary Tract Anomalies

Common congenital anomalies of the urinary tract which may be found in the newborn are as follows: bilateral renal agenesis, cystic disease of the kidney, horseshoe kidney, urinary tract atresia, anomalies of the collecting system, hydronephrosis, urachus anomalies, bladder neck obstruction, with varying degrees of hydronephrosis; exstrophy of the bladder, and fistulas from the urinary tract to other organs or to the perineum.

Anomalies of the External Genitalia

These include hypospadias, meatal stenosis, clitoral enlargement secondary to adrenogenital syndrome, undescended testes, hydrocele, hernia, and many others. When abnormalities of the external genitalia occur in male infants, circumcision should be deferred until the abnormality is evaluated in case the foreskin is required for surgical repair. Hypertrophy of the clitoris should suggest adrenogenital syndrome or ingestion of androgens by the mother during pregnancy.

METABOLIC DISEASES IN THE NEWBORN

HYPOGLYCEMIA IN THE NEWBORN

In normal infants at birth, the blood sugar levels are the same as or slightly lower than those of the mother. During the first hours after delivery, the blood sugar level decreases (rarely below 30—40 mg/100 ml), and by 6—12 hours it stabilizes between 50—80 mg/100 ml. The clinical significance of hypoglycemia in the newborn period (less than 30 mg/100 ml) is not clear because of the frequent observation of low blood sugar levels in a newborn infant who has little or no evidence of symptoms. Babies sick with other diseases may also have hypoglycemia. Severe and prolonged hypoglycemia will cause progressive irreparable brain damage. The effect of less severe hypoglycemia is not known.

Etiology
A. Intrauterine Growth Retardation: Presumably due to lack of available source of glucose.

B. Hyperinsulinism: Infant of diabetic mother, Beckwith's syndrome, erythroblastosis fetalis, islet cell tumor, leucine sensitivity.

C. After Milk Feeds Are Established: Glycogen storage disease, glucose-6-phosphatase deficiency, leucine sensitivity, fructose intolerance (if milk contains sucrose), galactosemia.

D. Other Causes: Idiopathic neonatal hypoglycemia, adrenogenital syndrome, growth hormone deficiency, glycogen synthetase deficiency.

Clinical Findings
A. Symptoms and Signs: Manifestations of hypoglycemia in newborns may be mild and nonspecific: lethargy, poor feeding, regurgitation, apnea, and twitching. As symptoms become more severe, the baby will develop pallor, sweating, cool extremities, and prolonged apnea and convulsions. If these symptoms are due to low blood sugar, they should respond dramatically when the level is raised.

B. Laboratory Findings: Blood sugar levels should be determined on all infants of diabetic mothers (see below) during the first 1—2 hours after delivery, and on infants who are small for gestational age during the first several days. Any sick infant in whom hypoglycemia is suspected should be tested. A careful search for the cause is important but may have to be delayed until the baby is not acutely ill.

Blood collected for glucose determination should be kept cold and tested quickly because of the rapid fall that occurs in whole blood. Glucose oxidase methods should be used, so that actual glucose is determined rather than reducing substances. Simple microchemical technics are available and are easily done with usual laboratory equipment.

Treatment
The lower the blood sugar level and the more symptomatic the infant, the earlier must treatment be given in order to avoid brain damage.

A. Mild Hypoglycemia: Early oral or gavage feeding of milk mixtures may be adequate for transient, mild hypoglycemia. The baby must be watched closely and glucose determinations repeated.

B. Severe Hypoglycemia: The initial treatment of the hypoglycemic infant (< 20 mg/100 ml) is intravenous administration of 10% glucose in water (at a rate of about 65—85 ml/kg/day) with appropriate maintenance electrolytes added. This can be continued until the baby is asymptomatic and able to take oral feedings. If hypoglycemia persists, glucagon, 100—300 μg/kg/dose IM at 1—2 hour intervals for several doses, may be used. Hydrocortisone or prednisone may be needed temporarily to maintain the blood sugar level above 20 mg/100 ml. As soon as feedings are tolerated, the infusion may be decreased and later discontinued. Never allow an intravenous glucose solution to be stopped abruptly in infants with hypoglycemia because of the possibility of a severe reactive hypoglycemia.

Lubchenco LO, Bard H: Incidence of hypoglycemia in newborn infants classified by birth weight and gestational age. Pediatrics 47:831—838, 1971.

INFANTS OF DIABETIC MOTHERS

Before insulin was available, very few pregnancies occurred or were carried to term in diabetic women. This changed radically with the onset of insulin therapy, but new problems arose. Pregnancy in a diabetic woman under adequate control appears to present no special problems up to about the 28th week. In many cases, the fetus then begins to grow at an excessive rate, developing increased fat and glycogen deposition (not edema) as well as increase in length. This appears to be secondary to a state of hyperinsulinism in the fetus. In addition, the fetus is at increased risk of dying in utero as the pregnancy progresses, particularly during the last several weeks of pregnancy. Delivery should be timed to allow the fetus to become as mature as possible, so that the risk of premature delivery is minimal (36 weeks to term, depending on the severity of the disease in the mother and the condition of the fetus), but to avoid the high stillborn rate that occurs during the last several weeks of gestation. In women who have severe diabetes with vascular involvement, the fetus may not be larger than normal, presumably because of placental insufficiency. Ketoacidosis in the mother increases the risk to the fetus at any stage of the pregnancy. In general, the better the control of the mother's diabetes during the pregnancy, the better the risk for the infant.

Management of the newborn infant of a diabetic mother consists of careful resuscitation and evaluation at the time of delivery, and continued observation for hypoglycemia or respiratory distress.

Special Problems

A. Prematurity: Many babies will be delivered following induced labor or cesarean section at 36–37 weeks. Therefore, they need care as do prematures even though their weight may be well over 2500 gm.

B. Hypoglycemia: The newborn of a diabetic mother is usually in a state of hyperinsulinism. Low blood sugars are to be expected within the first 6 hours after birth. The first determinations should be done at 1–2 hours of age. Some may be remarkably asymptomatic, although it is usually possible to demonstrate some clinical evidence of hypoglycemia. Blood glucose should be checked several times during the first few hours. It usually returns to fairly normal levels by 6–12 hours of age. The hypoglycemia is usually transient and responds well to oral feedings. Intravenous administration of 10% glucose solution is occasionally necessary.

C. Respiratory Distress Syndrome: The incidence of respiratory distress syndrome appears to be higher among infants of diabetic mothers than among other premature infants of equivalent gestational age.

Cornblath M, Schwartz R: *Disorders of Carbohydrate Metabolism in Infancy.* Saunders, 1966.

HYPOCALCEMIA IN THE NEWBORN

Hypocalcemia is defined as serum calcium below 8 mg/100 ml or 4 mEq/liter. It may occur as an isolated finding or in the presence of other diseases. It occurs more frequently following abnormal pregnancies. The mechanism is often unknown.

Serum phosphorus and alkaline phosphatase levels should be determined to aid in interpretation of low serum calcium levels.

Clinical Findings

A. Symptoms and Signs: The infant may be twitchy or tremulous, or have frank convulsions, but many babies with low serum calcium levels are without symptoms. Hypocalcemia rarely causes life-threatening symptoms in the immediate newborn period. Convulsions occur infrequently in the newborn period but later may be the presenting symptom of tetany of the newborn.

B. "Tetany of the Newborn": This disorder occurs in the third or fourth week of life, almost exclusively in infants fed evaporated milk formulas. Cow's milk formulas contain excessive solutes, particularly phosphorus, which are not cleared adequately by the kidney. This leads to elevation of serum phosphorus with a secondary lowering of the serum calcium and clinical tetany. It is not known why only a small number of babies are at risk. Relative hypoparathy-

roidism or immaturity of renal function may play a role.

Treatment

Serum calcium should be determined before therapy is started.

A. Oral Calcium: Oral administration of calcium lactate or gluconate is the preferred method of treatment of most cases of hypocalcemia. Calcium can be given either as a diluted solution or added to formula feedings several times a day, in a dose of 0.5–1 gm/kg/day.

In tetany of the newborn it is advisable to lower the solute and phosphorus loads in the feedings as well as to provide extra calcium. This can be done by giving dilute cow's milk formulas with added sugar and calcium until the blood chemistries are normal, or by using special low-solute formulas.

B. Intravenous Calcium: Intravenous administration of calcium solutions may be necessary for prompt relief of symptoms. The infusion must be given slowly, diluted with an equal amount of glucose in water. The heart rate must be monitored carefully during the infusion and immediately afterward; cardiac slowing and arrest can occur as a result of rapid administration of calcium salts. The response to intravenous calcium is usually only transient. (*Note:* Calcium salts cannot be added to intravenous solutions which contain $NaHCO_3$, since they will precipitate as calcium carbonate.) Calcium gluconate is available as 10% solution. The dose is 1–4 ml IV slowly.

Clarke PCN: Hypocalcemic and hypomagnesemic convulsions. J Pediat 70:806, 1967.
Page LA: Clinical implications of recent advances in the understanding of calcium metabolism. Advances Pediat 17:317–358, 1970.

RENAL TUBULAR ACIDOSIS
(See p 454.)

Renal tubular acidosis may occur in premature infants during the first few weeks of life. Early findings consist of a diminished rate of weight gain in spite of adequate intake and a falling serum total CO_2 content. This form is often transient and responds to treatment with bicarbonate orally. Citrate buffer should not be used in the newborn.

INFANTS OF NARCOTIC ADDICTS

Withdrawal symptoms occur in at least 2/3 of infants born of mothers who are addicted to heroin, methadone, or related drugs. Symptoms consist principally of increased tremors, irritability, and hyperactivity, associated with regurgitation, sneezing, hyper-tonicity, sweating, yawning, excessive hunger activities, excessive salivation, and nasal stuffiness. More severely affected babies may have vomiting, diarrhea, and convulsions. This clinical picture of increased activity (often frantic behavior) is typical enough to suggest the diagnosis even though a history had not been elicited prior to delivery. Many infants are small for gestational age.

The diagnosis is usually based on the development of typical symptoms in a mother with a history of narcotic drug abuse. Confirmation can be obtained by doing a screening test for excretory products of the drug on the urine of the mother or baby.

Treatment

Careful observation is required for onset and progression of symptoms. No specific treatment is indicated until symptoms develop.

With the onset of significant irritability, tremors, and hyperactivity, sedation is required. Phenobarbital, 8–12 mg/kg/day orally in 4 divided doses every 6 hours, is recommended because of its safety and predictability of effect. Continue until symptoms are controlled and then gradually decrease the dose as symptoms subside. In addition to phenobarbital, swaddling the baby and allowing the use of a pacifier may help control the excessive activity and allow the baby to rest.

Narcotics may be required to control symptoms that are more severe and life-threatening—particularly vomiting, diarrhea, and respiratory distress. Morphine sulfate, 0.1 mg/kg subcut or IM stat, may be required for immediate treatment of severe symptoms, with a distinct improvement following soon. Oral paregoric, 5 drops/dose every 4–6 hours, gives satisfactory control. As symptoms improve, the dose of narcotic is usually reduced before phenobarbital is reduced.

Prognosis

The prognosis is good for the health of the baby. Individual evaluation must be made in each case. The baby may well be cared for by the mother, but continued interest and long-term support by the health team and the mother's active involvement with a drug treatment program are essential.

Kahn EJ, Neumann LL, Polk G: The course of the heroin withdrawal syndrome in newborn infants treated with phenobarbital or chlorpromazine. J Pediat 75:495–500, 1969.

Reddy AM, Harper RG, Stern G: Observations on heroin and methadone withdrawal in the newborn. Pediatrics 48:353, 1971.

Zelson C, Rubio E, Wasserman E: Neonatal narcotic addiction: 10 year observation. Pediatrics 48:178–189, 1971.

MULTIPLE BIRTHS

Twinning occurs in about one out of 90 pregnancies. The incidence of twins increases with the mother's age and parity and if there is a familial tendency toward multiple births. Twins may develop from a single ovum (monozygotic, identical) or from 2 ova (dizygotic, fraternal).

About 1/3 of twins are of the single ovum type. About 1/3 of identical twins have a double placenta, amnion, and chorion. However, if the partition between the twins consists of 2 layers of transparent amnion without an intervening chorion, a diagnosis of monozygotic twinning can be made with assurance. It is important to determine if the twins are monozygotic or dizygotic, principally because the information may be of vital importance in later life if a question of organ transplantation is raised.

Intrauterine Growth

The fetal growth pattern of twins (or triplets) differs from that of a single fetus. Each twin grows at the same rate as the singleton until approximately 34 weeks of gestation. The rate of weight gain then decreases, so that by the 40th week of gestation the median weight is at the 10th percentile rather than the 50th percentile. This may be considered late gestational placental insufficiency, undernutrition in utero, or intrauterine growth retardation. A similar decreased rate of growth can be seen in triplet gestation, but deviation from the median occurs earlier and the term weight is below the 10th percentile.

Discordant Twins

When twins are of unequal size, the smaller twin not only weighs less but is also shorter and has a smaller head circumference. Vascular anastomosis may occur between monozygotic twins, so that one twin will lose blood chronically into the other and develop anemia and growth retardation while the other twin becomes plethoric and large. The larger twin is at increased risk in the newborn period if he shows significant symptoms due to the high hematocrit.

Complications of Multiple Births

(1) Preterm delivery: Pregnancy is usually several weeks shorter with twins.

(2) Polyhydramnios: Ten times more common.

(3) Preeclampsia and eclampsia: Three times more common.

(4) Placenta praevia: More common because of increased size of placenta.

(5) Abruptio placentae: May occur with second twin placenta due to reduction in size of uterus following delivery of the first twin.

(6) Presentation: Breech and other complications of presentation are more frequent.

(7) Duration of labor: Usually not much longer, though uterine contractions after delivery may be poor, with subsequent bleeding.

(8) Prolapse of the cord: Seven times more frequent than in single deliveries because of abnormal presentations and rupture of the second twin's membranes when unengaged.

Prognosis

The morbidity and mortality risks in multiple births are greater than with single births. More second-born twins die than firstborn twins.

Follow-up studies of twins for later growth and development suggest that the long-term outlook is not so favorable as for single births. Furthermore, the growth and development of the small discordant twin is significantly poorer than for the larger one. Symptomatic neonatal hypoglycemia has been observed in the smaller twin and may contribute to this poorer outcome.

Benirschke K: Multiple birth: Signal for scrutiny. Hosp Pract 1:25, 1966.

Guttmacher AF, Kohn SG: The fetus of multiple gestations. Obst Gynec 12:528, 1958.

Naeye RL: The fetus and neonatal development of twins. Pediatrics 33:546, 1964.

●   ●   ●

General References

Andrews BF (editor): Symposium: The small for date infant. P Clin North America 17:1–227, 1970.

Barnes AC: *Intrauterine Development.* Lea & Febiger, 1968.

Cross KW, Dawes C (editors): The foetus and the newborn. Brit M Bull 22:1, 1966.

Dawes GS: *Foetal and Neonatal Physiology.* Year Book, 1968.

Dawkins M, MacGregor B (editors): *Gestational Age, Size and Maturity.* Heinemann, 1965..

Falkner F (editor): *Human Development.* Saunders, 1966.

James LS (editor): Newborn. P Clin North America 13:573–942, 943–1301, 1966.

Mustard WT & others (editors): *Pediatric Surgery,* 2nd ed. Year Book, 1969.

Schaffer AJ: *Diseases of the Newborn,* 3rd ed. Saunders, 1971.

Silverman WA: *Dunham's Premature Infants,* 3rd ed. Harper, 1961.

Standards and Recommendations for Hospital Care of Newborn Infants. American Academy of Pediatrics, 1971.

Swenson O: *Pediatric Surgery,* 3rd ed. Appleton-Century-Crofts, 1969.

4...

Normal Nutrition

Janice M. Dodds, MEd, Joan Parker MacReynolds, MS, & Donough O'Brien, MD, FRCP

Sensible feeding practices are important through-out infancy and childhood, not only to assure optimal growth but also because mealtimes are occasions for family interaction; particularly in the small infant, feeding is a major source of satisfaction and an opportunity for important closeness with the mother. Parents and those who care for children in hospitals should bear in mind the social as well as the nutritional values of meals and, within sensible limits, be tolerant of the whims of appetite in young people.

Physicians and other health workers have done much to publicize good standards of nutrition for small infants. In most North American families, children continue to be well nourished principally because of the more than adequate eating habits of the people. There are, indeed, reasons for supposing that overnutrition is common.

Until recently, there has been little information on the specific nutritional status of children in the USA. Data now being accumulated show that undernutrition due to poverty or ignorance is prevalent in certain underprivileged groups.

GENERAL NUTRITIONAL REQUIREMENTS & COMPOSITION OF FOODS

Requirements for various nutrients change during childhood depending on the growth rates of different tissues; they also vary considerably with sex, stage of maturation, physical activity, and body build. Nutrition needs during any growth period will depend on the nutritional status of the child at that time and on whether or not a given nutrient can be stored by the body. Periodic review of requirements is desirable because nutritional knowledge is increasing rapidly. Average values (Table 4–1) may be used as guides for estimating requirements at any age; however, differences in needs should be recognized for each child. The child's general health and conformity to established growth percentiles are the best indices of his particular status.

Calories

Total caloric requirements for children rise with age in a curve parallel to the height and weight curves. Following the neonatal weight gain, caloric needs per unit of body weight begin to decline during early childhood. This pattern is similar to the decline in growth rate observed between 18 and 36 months of age. Appetite is a reliable index of caloric needs in most healthy children. During neonatal life, growth is rapid, appetite tends to be good, and caloric intake rises smoothly. Toward the end of the first year, appetite declines with the decrease in growth rate and with increases in physical mobility, interests, and independence.

Mild caloric excess can be as undesirable as mild caloric deficiency. Important factors in considering the quantity of food an infant will voluntarily consume are the bulk of the food and the energy needs of the child. Intake also depends to some extent on the caloric concentration of the feeding. Normally, an infant receiving a low-calorie formula will not be able to consume enough by volume to satisfy his caloric needs. Conversely, an infant receiving a concentrated formula may ingest a smaller volume but more calories than he needs. Human milk and most commercial formulas average 20 calories per ounce.

The Recommended Dietary Allowances (Table 4–1) were developed as a guide for large groups and are misused if applied strictly to one individual. A specific diet may not meet the recommendations, but one cannot conclude that it is inadequate. Children of the same age and size do not necessarily need the same amounts of food. Calories per unit of height/weight per age is the preferable index for determining need; age alone is a poor index. The combination of large caloric intake and rapid weight gain in the absence of rapid change in height suggests overfeeding and may warrant some reduction in calories. Measures to increase caloric intake include the use of a more concentrated formula and the choice of strained foods high in calories. Early introduction of cereals and strained foods can add extra calories if carefully chosen.

Fat

In recent years it has become fashionable to promote the use of nonfat or low-fat milk in an effort to prevent obesity and to retard or prevent the atherosclerotic process. However, neither is recommended as the sole source of calories. Without the addition of sufficient solid foods to the diet, malnutrition is a risk. Vitamin A, linoleic acid, and caloric requirements cannot be met with nonfat or low-fat milk. A further

TABLE 4–1. Recommended daily dietary allowances of the Food and Nutrition Board, National Academy of Sciences-National Research Council.[1]

Age in Years	Weight (kg)	(lb)	Height (cm)	(in)	Calories	Protein (gm)	Fat-Soluble Vitamins			Water-Soluble Vitamins							Minerals				
							Vitamin A Activity (IU)	Vitamin D Activity (IU)	Vitamin E Activity (IU)	Ascorbic Acid (mg)	Folacin[2] (mg)	Niacin (mg eq[3])	Riboflavin (mg)	Thiamine (mg)	Vitamin B6 (mg)	Vitamin B12 (µg)	Calcium (gm)	Phosphorus (gm)	Iodine (µg)	Iron (mg)	Magnesium (mg)
Infants																					
0–1/6	4	9	55	22	kg × 120	kg × 2.2[4]	1500	400	5	35	0.05	5	0.4	0.2	0.2	1.0	0.4	0.2	25	6	40
1/6–1/2	7	15	63	25	kg × 110	kg × 2.0[4]	1500	400	5	35	0.05	7	0.5	0.4	0.3	1.5	0.5	0.4	40	10	60
1/2–1	9	20	72	28	kg × 100	kg × 1.8[4]	1500	400	5	35	0.1	8	0.6	0.5	0.4	2.0	0.6	0.5	45	15	70
Children																					
1–2	12	26	81	32	1100	25	2000	400	10	40	0.1	8	0.6	0.6	0.5	2.0	0.7	0.7	55	15	100
2–3	14	31	91	36	1250	25	2000	400	10	40	0.2	8	0.7	0.6	0.6	2.5	0.8	0.8	60	15	150
3–4	16	35	100	39	1400	30	2500	400	10	40	0.2	9	0.8	0.7	0.7	3	0.8	0.8	70	10	200
4–6	19	42	110	43	1600	30	2500	400	10	40	0.2	11	0.9	0.8	0.9	4	0.8	0.8	80	10	200
6–8	23	51	121	48	2000	35	3500	400	15	40	0.2	13	1.1	1.0	1.0	4	0.9	0.9	100	10	250
8–10	28	62	131	52	2200	40	3500	400	15	40	0.3	15	1.2	1.1	1.2	5	1.0	1.0	110	10	250
Males																					
10–12	35	77	140	55	2500	45	4500	400	20	40	0.4	17	1.3	1.3	1.4	5	1.2	1.2	125	10	300
12–14	43	95	151	59	2700	50	5000	400	20	45	0.4	18	1.4	1.4	1.6	5	1.4	1.4	135	18	350
14–18	59	130	170	67	3000	60	5000	400	25	55	0.4	20	1.5	1.5	1.8	5	1.4	1.4	150	18	400
18–22	67	147	175	69	2800	60	5000	400	30	60	0.4	18	1.6	1.4	2.0	5	0.8	0.8	140	10	400
Females																					
10–12	35	77	142	56	2250	50	4500	400	20	40	0.4	15	1.3	1.1	1.4	5	1.2	1.2	110	18	300
12–14	44	97	154	61	2300	50	5000	400	20	45	0.4	15	1.4	1.2	1.6	5	1.3	1.3	115	18	350
14–16	52	114	157	62	2400	55	5000	400	25	50	0.4	16	1.4	1.2	1.8	5	1.3	1.3	120	18	350
16–18	54	119	160	63	2300	55	5000	400	25	50	0.4	15	1.5	1.2	2.0	5	1.3	1.3	115	18	350
18–22	58	128	163	64	2000	55	5000	400	25	55	0.4	13	1.5	1.0	2.0	5	0.8	0.8	100	18	350
Pregnancy					+200	65	6000	400	30	60	0.8	15	1.8	+0.1	2.5	8	+0.4	+0.4	125	18	450
Lactation					+1000	75	8000	400	30	60	0.5	20	2.0	+0.5	2.5	6	+0.5	+0.5	150	18	450

[1] The allowance levels are intended to cover individual variations among most normal persons as they live in the USA under usual environmental stresses. The recommended allowances can be attained with a variety of common foods, providing other nutrients for which human requirements have been less well defined.

[2] The folacin allowances refer to dietary sources as determined by Lactobacillus casei assay. Pure forms of folacin may be effective in doses less than 1/4 of the recommended allowances.

[3] Niacin equivalents include dietary sources of the vitamin itself plus 1 mg equivalent for each 60 mg of dietary tryptophan.

[4] Assumes protein equivalent to human milk. For proteins not 100% utilized, factors should be increased proportionately.

consideration is that a diet which contains less than 20% of calories as fat may cause diarrhea; the disaccharide content of the diet could exceed the ability of the disaccharidases to split these sugars. A third consideration must be that the protein content of the diet may become so high that renal solute load is excessive. And finally, fat contributes greatly to the satiety value of a diet. Our understanding of the importance of serum lipid concentrations and fatty streaking of arteries during infancy is so meager that it is simpler and safer to alter caloric intake by means other than greatly reducing fat intake. Practical measures for decreasing caloric intake include substitution of low-calorie strained foods for a portion of the milk intake. Replacing the high-calorie strained foods (eg, high meat dinners and desserts) with lower calorie strained foods such as vegetables and breakfast foods will also lower calories.

Caloric needs may vary in the newborn period due to differences in fat absorption and excretion. Calculated caloric intakes may be misleading in terms of energy actually available to the infant. Differences in digestibility exist between human milk fat and other fats. An infant—particularly an infant of low birth weight—may lose an appreciable amount of fat during the first 2 months of life. After the newborn period, fat absorption generally increases.

Other Nutrients

A. Protein: In technically advanced nations, most infants receive abundant amounts of high-quality protein in their diets. However, new infant formulas continue to appear on the market and should be evaluated for amino acid imbalance. For example, soy products are naturally low in methionine and must be supplemented by the manufacturer with this amino acid to prevent its becoming a limiting factor in growth. Animal proteins have a more complete complement of essential amino acids and are of higher quality than vegetable proteins, which are often low in at least one essential amino acid—eg, lysine in wheat. Greater amounts of vegetable proteins must be consumed in order to meet the physiologic demands of the body. When a variety of foods are eaten in combination at a meal, the required intake of each food becomes less when the amino acids complement each other. Small amounts of animal protein can greatly increase the value of vegetable proteins.

In discussing amino acids it must be mentioned that adult humans can synthesize histidine, but there is strong evidence that histidine is an essential amino acid for infants.

B. Water: The water requirement for an infant is small in relation to the usual intakes. The requirement consists of the amount necessary for maintenance of life and growth plus replacement of that lost through the lungs, urine, and feces. In general, the requirement is about 250 ml/day during the first few weeks of life and 600–700 ml/day at 12 months of age.

C. Carbohydrate: Carbohydrate serves primarily as a source of energy, sparing protein for its nitrogen-

ous value. Small amounts of carbohydrate are required for the formation of connective tissue and some body compounds. No specific carbohydrate requirement has been established, but a dietary intake of 40–50% of total calories is common in the USA.

The relationship between carbohydrates and dental caries is strikingly significant. An extensive and well documented investigation completed at Vipeholm in Sweden is of interest in child feeding. The principal findings were that increased sugar consumption can produce caries. However, the effect of sugar as a cariogen is dependent to a large extent on its manner of administration. Increased amounts of sugar given at mealtime caused no increase in caries. When extra sugar was consumed in solution, little or no increase in caries occurred. The greatest increase occurred when sugar confections were eaten between meals.

D. Vitamins and Minerals: The lists in Table 4–2 show the foods which are highest in selected nutrients. They also show other foods which, although lower in food value, are abundantly available. These foods will meet the needs of a child and should be encouraged if economic or cultural circumstances will not permit daily intake of the higher quality foods. Table 4–2 also provides a reference for quick calculation of the major nutrients of a day's diet. When these nutrients are adequate in the diet, other nutrients such as thiamine, riboflavin, and niacin are also present in adequate amounts. The exception is calories. They should be calculated if muscle and adipose tissue are poorly developed.

1. Iron—Premature infants and infants born of mothers with depleted iron stores caused by multiple pregnancies, bleeding, or poor diet have low iron reserves and are prone to anemia. The premature infant is most often prone to this difficulty as he is born before the end of the third trimester, during which time the bulk of the iron stores are normally provided. In addition, the blood volume and red cell mass must parallel the growth spurt of the first year, and there must be adequate iron to meet these needs. Iron can be toxic, however, and infants receiving commercial formulas containing iron and other vitamins and minerals do not need further iron and vitamin supplementation. Mothers may have the mistaken notion that additional iron and vitamins will make their baby more healthy, grow faster, or have fewer infections. Babies taking commercial formulas with iron, plus vitamins with iron, plus iron-fortified cereals are at risk of developing iron toxicity.

2. Calcium—The advisable intake of calcium in an infant who is not fed human milk is tentatively set at 500–600 mg/day. Absorption of calcium may be quite different with feedings other than human milk. The breast-fed infant receives approximately 270 mg/800 ml of human milk. Cow's milk has nearly 4 times as much calcium as human milk, but this is poorly absorbed by infants unless vitamin D is administered. When no additional vitamin D is given, 10% or less of the calcium is retained.

TABLE 4–2. Guides for "rough" assessment of nutritive value of diets.

PROTEIN

Requirements for children:

3 months	1.8 gm/lb
6 months–3 years	1.6 gm/lb
4–6 years	1.4 gm/lb
7–9 years	1.1 gm/lb
10–12 years	0.9 gm/lb
13–15 years	0.7 gm/lb
15 and over	0.5 gm/lb

7 gm protein in:
1 egg
1 oz meat, fish, or fowl
1 oz cheese (1¼ inch cube American, 2 tbsp
    cottage cheese)
8 oz milk
1/2 cup cooked dried beans
2 tbsp peanut butter

3 gm protein in:
1/2 cup cooked cereal
1 cup dry cereal (1 large shredded wheat biscuit)
2/3 cup ice cream
1/2 cup milk pudding
1 slice bacon

2 gm protein in:
1 slice bread
1 serving cake, pie, or cookies
4 soda crackers
1/2 cup gelatin dessert
1 medium potato

1 gm protein in:
1 serving fruit or vegetable

VITAMIN A

Requirements for children:

3–6 months	1500 IU
1–3 years	2000 IU
4–6 years	2500 IU
7–9 years	3500 IU
10–12 years	4500 IU
13 and over	5000 IU

10,000 IU vitamin A in:
1 oz liver
1/2 cup dark greens
1/2 cup carrots, cooked

3000 IU vitamin A in:
1/2 cup broccoli
1/2 cup cantaloupe
1/2 cup sweet potatoes (1 medium)

1000 IU vitamin A in:
1 medium tomato
1/2 cup canned tomato
1 medium apricot
1/2 cup peaches (1 medium)
1/2 cup pumpkin
1/2 cup yellow squash
1/2 cup leaf lettuce

500 IU vitamin A in:
1 large dark green lettuce leaf
1/2 cup head lettuce
1/2 cup light green vegetable (string beans, peas,
    lima beans)
8 oz milk
1 egg
1 tbsp butter or margarine
2 tbsp cream
1½ oz cheddar cheese

CALCIUM

Requirements for children:

3 months	0.6 gm
6–9 months	0.7 gm
1–9 years	0.8 gm
10–12 years	1.1 gm
13–15 years	1.4 gm

0.3 gm calcium in:
8 oz milk
4 oz evaporated milk
1½ oz American cheese (1¾ inch cube)
1 cup dark greens (except spinach, chard, beet
    greens*)
1½ cup ice cream
0.3 gm calcium in remainder of diet

*Calcium not well utilized in these because of oxalic acid.

TABLE 4–2 (cont'd). Guides for "rough" assessment of nutritive value of diets.

<table>
<tr><td colspan="2" align="center">ASCORBIC ACID</td><td colspan="2" align="center">IRON</td></tr>
</table>

ASCORBIC ACID

Requirements for children:

3–9 months	35 mg
1–12 years	40 mg
13–15 years	45 mg
15 and over	50 mg

50 mg vitamin C in:
- 1 medium orange
- 1/2 cup orange juice
- 1/2 cup grapefruit or juice
- 1/2 cup any other citrus
- 1 cup raw cabbage
- 1 large raw tomato
- 1 cup lightly cooked cabbage, cauliflower, broccoli, spinach, or other greens
- 1 cup cantaloupe (1/2 melon)
- 10 large raw strawberries
- 1/3 medium raw pepper

20 mg vitamin C in:
- 1 medium potato, baked, boiled, fried from raw
- 1/2 cup canned tomato or juice
- 1 small sweet potato, baked

10 mg vitamin C in:
- 1 cup other raw fruit or vegetable

5 mg vitamin C in:
- 1/2 cup other cooked fruit or vegetable
- 2 tbsp ketchup
- 20 pieces potato chips (1½ oz)

IRON

Requirements for children:

3 months	6 mg
6 months	10 mg
9 months–3 years	15 mg
4–6 years	10 mg
7–9 years	12 mg
10–12 years	14 mg
13–15 years	15 mg

3 mg iron in:
- 3 tbsp cooked enriched or quick-cooking Cream of Wheat
- 1/2 cup cooked dried beans
- 1/2 cup dark greens
- 1 oz liver
- 1 tbsp dry baby cereal

1 mg iron in:
- 1 oz meat, fish, fowl
- 1 egg
- 1/2 cup cooked cereal
- 1 tbsp molasses
- 2 dried prunes
- 1 cup broccoli
- 9 brussels sprouts

0.5 mg iron in:
- 2 dried apricot halves
- 1 slice whole grain or enriched bread
- 1 medium potato
- 1 tbsp dried raisins
- 1 serving other fruit or vegetable

---

3. Riboflavin—Riboflavin as well as calcium is likely to be deficient in the child who does not receive adequate milk. An ample supply of both is provided if the child receives 1–1½ pints of milk up to age 10 and 1 quart or equivalent during the adolescent growth spurt.

ASSESSMENT OF NUTRITIONAL STATUS

Conformity to established height and weight percentiles and a simple history of an adequate and well balanced intake are usually sufficient to determine that the child's nutritional status is normal. A clinical diagnosis of specific or generalized malnutrition should be supported by the dietary history and, when possible, by laboratory examinations. Normal and deficient biochemical levels are given in Table 4–3. Laboratory appraisals are of significant value in the detection of specific nutritional defects. In children whose nutri-

tional needs are distorted by inborn errors, by illness, or by deprivation, appraisal by a nutritionist or dietitian may be needed.

Dietary information may be collected by using any of the following methods: food record, 24-hour recall, or dietary history.

Food Record

The 4- to 7-day food record is a helpful aid for teaching adequate nutrition, and conscientious mothers are good reporters. However, if the mother has many responsibilities, valid information is hard to obtain from a food record. In addition, the mother may be ashamed of or may feel threatened by revealing the child's normal eating habits and may "exaggerate" the record or temporarily offer more or better foods if the facts are being recorded. In older children and adolescents who tend to be overweight, recording is a useful exercise which may discourage overeating.

24-Hour Recall

The 24-hour recall is a verbal report of all foods eaten by the patient during the preceding 24 hours.

TABLE 4–3. Laboratory data in the interpretation of nutritional status in infants and young children.

Hematologic Data

Hemoglobin, hematocrit	A concentration of hemoglobin of < 10 gm/100 ml in the ages 1–3 and < 11 gm/100 ml in ages 3–6 is presumptive evidence of iron deficiency anemia. Hematocrit at all ages should be > 33% in children living at or near sea level.
Transferrin	Saturation of iron-binding capacity should be > 16% at all ages.
Serum iron	Should be > 30 μg/100 ml up to age 2; ≥ 40 μg/100 ml at age 2–5; and ≥ 60 μg/100 ml over age 5.
MCHC	Should exceed 30% at all ages.

Biochemical Data

Estimation	Deficient or Low	Minimum Normal*
Serum alkaline phosphatase IU/liter as an index of vitamin D deficiency	> 150	60–150
Serum folacin, ng/ml	< 3.0	6.0
Serum protein, gm/100 ml		
0–12 months	< 3.0	5.0
1–5 years	< 5.5	5.5
6–17 years	< 6.0	6.0
Serum albumin, gm/100 ml		
0–5 years	< 3.0	3.0
6–17 years	< 3.5	3.5
Serum vitamin C, mg/100 ml		
0–12 months	< 0.15	0.3
1 year	< 0.15	0.2
Plasma carotene, μg/100 ml		
0–5 months	< 10	10
6–11 months	< 30	30
1–17 years	< 40	40
Plasma vitamin A, μg/100 ml		
0–5 months	< 10	20
6 months–17 years	< 20	30
Urinary thiamine, μg/gm creatinine		
1–3 years	< 125	176
4–15 years	< 125	121
Urinary riboflavin, μg/gm creatinine		
1–3 years	< 150	500
4–6 years	< 100	300
7–9 years	< 85	270
10–15 years	< 70	200
Urinary iodine, μg/gm creatinine	< 50	70
Blood urea nitrogen, mg/100 ml	< 9	10
Serum amylase, Close-Street units	< 6	6

*See also Chapter 40.

The amounts of foods consumed on a typical day must be reported, including a detailed description (how cooked, what added, etc) and the times of the day. A typical day should be described. This information is then used as representative of normal intake during a given period.

Dietary History

The dietary history includes the questions "how often" and "how much" about all foods, including beverages, snacks, etc. The following questions are typically asked in taking a preliminary history. The answers may suggest the need for more detailed and complete data which can easily be acquired by a dietitian or nutritionist.

A. Formulas: What formula is the child now taking? Frequency of feeding? Amount per feeding? How is the formula mixed and put in the bottle?

B. Table Foods: What is the meal pattern? (Times and kinds of foods eaten throughout the day.) Are there particular likes and dislikes? Does he feed himself or show interest in the food? At what ages did he start cereal? fruit? vegetables? meat? Has the introduction of solid food been a problem?

FACTORS AFFECTING THE KIND OF FOODS A CHILD IS OFFERED

A child's nutritional status or dietary intake cannot be examined or altered without looking at his family. The kind of food served in a family is affected by cultural influences, food economics, and food preferences. From the first day of human life, ingestion of food is culturally structured. Foods eaten by individuals are seldom chosen for their nutritional value. Diet modifications must occur within the cultural framework of the family, and one must consider the psychologic need the particular food may be satisfying. Available money and the amount budgeted for food influence the purchasing power of a family. The food allotment is frequently sacrificed when a financial crisis occurs. Fluctuations in price and demands for increased quantities are more acutely felt in poorer families. Food assistance programs are available from the United States Department of Agriculture to families with limited incomes. Finally, a child's choice of foods is determined by his family experience, but new food habits may be acquired through association with peers and school lunch programs.

BREAST FEEDING

Advantages & Disadvantages

A. Advantages: Apart from considerations of economy and convenience (temperature, asepsis, automatic adjustment in most instances to infant's needs), breast feeding is superior to bottle feeding (with vitamin supplements) mainly for its psychologic advantages and because the composition of breast milk is ideal for most infants. Nursing is of benefit to the mother in the postpartum period because it is associated with vigorous contraction of the uterine musculature and speeds the return of that organ to normal size and position.

B. Disadvantages and Contraindications: Breast feeding is usually not possible for a weak, ill, or premature infant or one with a cleft palate or lip, although in such cases breast milk may be fed in some other way. Bottle feeding must be substituted for breast feeding if the mother's supply continues to be inadequate (less than 50% of child's needs) after 3 weeks of effort; if nipple or breast lesions are severe enough to prevent pumping; or if the mother is either pregnant or severely (physically or mentally) ill. Menstruation is not a contraindication to breast feeding.

Management of Breast Feeding

The success or failure of breast feeding is largely determined by the interrelationships of mother, father, baby, and environment, including the physicians who care for the mother and the baby in the prenatal and postnatal periods. Consideration must be given to the mother's attitude toward nursing, her emotional status, home conditions, breast anatomy, general health, the father's interest, and the baby's maturity, weight, vigor, appetite, and feeding characteristics. Each case must be managed individually, and the details of the procedure outlined below must be varied according to the particular situation.

Technic of Nursing

A. Breast Preparation Before Delivery: The decision to nurse should be made by the parents before the birth of the baby rather than after. Preparation of the nipples beginning a few months prior to birth serves 2 purposes. Psychologically, the mother becomes adept at handling her breasts so that aversions are overcome as familiarity is increased, and the nipple epithelium becomes toughened and maximum protractility assures proper nursing grasp by the infant with a minimum of soreness. Two methods of preparation are the following: Cup one breast from below with the palm of the hand and, with a soft washcloth, rub the nipple for 4 or 5 strokes. Then gently pull the nipple several times. This can be done once or twice daily.

B. Preparation for Nursing:

1. Wash hands with soap and water.

2. Assume a comfortable position, either lying down or sitting in a rocking or upright chair.

3. Cleanse nipples and breasts with fresh water.

C. Nursing the Infant: Each baby nurses differently.

1. Compression of the periareolar area and expression of a small amount of colostrum or breast milk for the baby to taste may stimulate him to start nursing.

2. Do not snap the baby's feet, work his jaw, push his head, or press his cheeks.

3. Place the nipple well back in the baby's mouth, resting against his palate, so he can compress the periareolar area with his jaws.

4. The breast should be held away from his nostrils.

5. Before removing the infant from the breast, gently open his mouth to break the suction.

D. After Nursing: Gently wipe the nipples with water.

Colostrum

Colostrum is an alkaline, yellow breast secretion which may be present in the last few months of pregnancy and for the first 2–4 days after delivery. It has a higher specific gravity (1.040–1.060), a higher protein, vitamin A, and mineral content, and a lower carbohydrate and fat content than breast milk.

TABLE 4–4. Composition and schedule of milk feedings for infants up to 1 year of age.*

Age (months)	0	1	2	3	4	5	6	7	8	9	10	11	12
Calories per day†	130–100/kg (60–45/lb)						110–100/kg (50–45/lb)				100–90/kg (45–40/lb)		
Fluid per day (ml)	130–200/kg (2–3 oz/lb)					130–165/kg (2–2½ oz/lb)					130/kg (2 oz/lb)		
Number of feedings per day‡	6 or 7			4 or 5				3 or 4				3	
Ounces per feeding	2½–4	3½–5	4–6	5–7	6–8		7–9						
Milk Evaporated	65 ml/kg (1 oz/lb) up to a total of 13 oz (1 can) daily												
Whole	130 ml/kg (2 oz/lb) up to a total of 28–32 oz daily												
Sugar per day	1–1½ oz						§	None					

*Reproduced, with permission, from Silver HK, Kempe CH, Bruyn H: *Handbook of Pediatrics,* 9th ed. Lange, 1971.

†The larger amount should be used for the younger infant.

‡Will vary somewhat with individual babies.

§Decrease sugar by ½ oz every 2 weeks.

Colostrum contains antibodies which may play a part in the immune mechanism of the newborn. Colostrum has a normal laxative action and is a natural and ideal starter food.

Transmission of Drugs & Toxins in Breast Milk

A. Drugs Secreted in Small Amounts: Alcohol, nicotine, caffeine, opiates, meperidine (Demerol), quinine, hyoscine, atropine, sulfonamides, penicillin, and laxatives (other than cascara) may be taken in moderation by the nursing mother. Although small amounts may be transmitted to breast milk, they will not be sufficient to be harmful. If the mother takes increased amounts of vitamin C, it will be transmitted to her milk.

B. Drugs Secreted in Large Amounts: Barbiturates, salicylates, iodides, thiouracil derivatives, bromides, ergot, and cascara are transmitted in significant quantities. If the mother's intake is excessive, toxicity may be produced in the child.

Weaning

Between the ages of 4 and 8 months, the infant can usually be weaned directly to the cup for fruit juices. However, many infants seem to require a continuation of the sucking provided by a bottle feeding with milk. By 10–14 months of age, most children can be weaned entirely to the cup.

ARTIFICIAL FEEDING
(See Tables 4–4, 4–5, and 4–6.)

Various artificial feeding formulas are in use. One consists of a standard formula for every baby (eg, 13 oz of evaporated milk, 19 oz of water, and 1–1½ oz of added carbohydrate), allowing the appetite and digestive capacity of the baby to determine the volume and number of feedings that will be taken. Although this method is satisfactory for most infants and is of particular value if the child is on a flexible schedule, the physician should be prepared to write an individual formula for each child which takes into account the infant's needs and desires.

If the formula is adequate in amount and composition and the infant is held while being fed, he will gain the physical or emotional satisfaction that accompanies breast feeding.

Whole milk may be substituted for evaporated milk when sugar is no longer added to the formula, but evaporated milk may be continued indefinitely. Milk formulas are deficient in vitamins C and D, and supplements of these vitamins (50 mg of vitamin C and 400 units of vitamin D daily) should be given. The American Academy of Pediatrics has also recommended the general adoption of iron-fortified formulas. Underweight or overweight infants generally have the same food requirements as do infants of the same age with a normal weight. Undiluted whole milk or formulas

providing equal parts of evaporated milk and water should not be used for young infants since these do not provide enough free water in the event of high environmental or body temperature.

Preparation of the Formula

Many companies which supply baby foods prepare instruction booklets for the mother which give the steps in preparation of the formula. The exact ingredients should be determined by the physician. The emphasis presently is on demand feeding, but the physician should make certain that the formulas are diluted correctly and that caloric needs are being met. An infant generally does not need more than 1 quart of whole milk or 1 large can of evaporated milk per day. One pint of whole milk per day is adequate for the older child who otherwise is eating a reasonable diet.

Sterilization of bottles and formulas is not usually necessary. In most city homes, the opened can is stored in the refrigerator and each bottle is diluted as required, using warm tap water. Bottles and nipples are washed in soap and water, rinsed, and dried. Where the water supply may not be clean, boiled water should be used. In situations where cleanliness is more difficult to maintain, powdered milks should be used and dissolved in boiled water.

Feeding the Baby

The bottle should be held, not propped, for 2 reasons: (1) There is a higher incidence of acute and recurrent otitis media in infants who suck bottles in the horizontal position. The short, wide eustachian tube of infants is at such an angle that mucus from rhinitis or nose allergy fills or obstructs the ducts to the middle ear very readily. Also, the eustachian tube orifice is opened during swallowing. (2) The emotional and physical satisfactions gained from being held are well known.

The nipple holes should be wide enough so that a drop of milk forms on the end of the nipple and drops off with little shaking of the cool bottle when turned upside down.

More water may be added to the formula if the infant consistently finishes each bottle, but be certain caloric intake is adequate.

The infant need not take all of every bottle.

The baby should be burped during and at the end of feeding.

TABLE 4–5. Composition of milk and milk formulas.

Percentage of Calories From	Human Milk	Cow's Milk	Diluted Cow's Milk + 10% CHO	Evap Milk 13 oz Water 19 oz CHO 1½ oz
Protein	8%	20%	10%	15%
Fat	50%	50%	25%	39%
CHO	42%	30%	65%	46%

After feeding, the baby should be placed on the right side or on the abdomen.

Additional fluids (without added sugar) should be offered once or twice a day, especially during very hot weather or when the baby is ill, regardless of whether it is ordinarily taken or not.

Vitamin C

If vitamin C (or vitamin preparations containing vitamin C) is added to the formula, it should be added just before feeding and after the bottle has been warmed. Orange juice may be started at any time during the first year; when orange juice is given in adequate amounts (3 oz or more), supplemental vitamin C is no longer necessary.

Solid Foods

There is no exact time or order which is important in starting solid foods. They should be given in small amounts for several consecutive days to determine the child's reaction and any adverse response. The amount given should be gradually increased if the food is well tolerated. If the baby continues to refuse it, another food may be tried; if that, too, is rejected, discontinue the attempt for a week or so before trying again. Commercially prepared baby foods have no nutritional advantage over those prepared by the mother.

Apart from their nutritional value, the purpose of introducing solid foods is to accustom the infant to an increasing range of taste and texture in food. The transition to more textured foods should take place gradually when the infant starts to make chewing motions. Thus, by 6 months, soft table foods (eg, mashed potatoes and applesauce) can be started as well as more grainy junior foods.

Teething biscuits and crackers follow quickly by 8 months; by 9 months, finger feeding, toast, and sandwiches are begun. By 1 year of age, many soft table foods with form such as canned fruits and vegetables, casseroles, and mashed or chopped foods are also included. A complete transition to table foods is accomplished by 1½ years.

Egg and wheat should not be given to potentially allergic children (eg, family predisposition) until the latter part of the first year.

Permit the infant to feed himself with his fingers or a spoon when he wishes to do so.

A. Common Solid Foods and Suggested Time of Introduction: Solid foods may be added to the diet as follows:

2–4 months: Single grain cereal (preferably rice)
3–4 months: Puréed fruits
4–5 months: Puréed vegetables
5–6 months: Strained meat, egg yolk
7 months: Custard, junket, dry toast, bread, bread substitutes
8 months: Bacon
9 months: Chicken, fish
12 months: Egg white

B. Spoon Feeding: Many infants can learn to take semisolid food from a spoon before the fourth month. If the infant cannot master spoon feeding, postpone the attempt for a few weeks; undesirable behavior reactions can occur which may make spoon feeding difficult for months.

Digestion in Infancy

Protein digestion and absorption are excellent in infancy. Amylase is present only in small quantities. The gastric glands are functionally active at birth and secrete hydrochloric acid (small quantities), pepsin, and rennin. Salivary digestion is relatively unimportant during early infancy.

Breast-fed babies usually empty the stomach by 2–3 hours; bottle-fed babies may require 3–4 hours or longer; newborn babies may empty the stomach even more slowly.

Modified Formulas

A wide variety of commercial formulas adapted for specific needs—eg, milk allergy, fat malabsorption, phenylketonuria, galactosemia—are listed in Table 4–6, with the most common conventional formulas.

DEVELOPMENTAL MILESTONES IN FEEDING HABITS

Because the feeding skill is progressing rapidly by 1 year, it can serve as a selective developmental screening method during the first 12 months. Table 4–7 shows the steps in 4 areas which must be accomplished for normal progression of feeding skills. The areas include oral musculature, body position, hand-to-mouth motions, and social development. Table 4–8 outlines the development of feeding skills from age 1 to age 4–7. The tests for those areas of feeding skill and subsequent treatment are explained in Table 4–9.

COMMON FEEDING PROBLEMS & SUGGESTED SOLUTIONS

Birth to Age 1

Rejects solids.

In some cases, when solids are introduced very early (by 2 or 3 months), the infant refuses them. Wait. Although cereal is generally accepted early, 4–6 months is still the age of acceptance of solid foods for most children.

Wants the spoon but cannot feed himself.

Give him the spoon but get another and continue feeding him. He is learning. A dropcloth or news-

TABLE 4–6. Normal and special infant formulas.

	Manufacturer	CHO Source	Fat Source	Indications for Use	Comments (Nutritional Adequacy)
Milk and milk-based formulas					
Cow's milk Evaporated milk	Several brands	Lactose	Butterfat	Feeding of full-term and premature infants with no special nutritional requirements.	Supplement with iron and vitamins C and D if not fortified.
Commercial infant formulas					
Baker's Bottle ready formula Concentrated liquid	Roerig	Lactose, corn sugar*	Coconut, corn, soy	Feeding of full-term and premature infants with no special nutritional requirements.	Supplementation with iron recommended.
Bremil Ready to feed Concentrated liquid	Syntex	Sucrose	Coconut, soy		Available fortified with 8 mg iron/liter.
Enfamil Ready to use Concentrated liquid Powder	Mead Johnson	Lactose	Coconut, corn, oleo, soy, lecithin	Feeding of full-term and premature infants with no special nutritional requirements.	Available fortified with 12 mg iron/liter.
Modilac Concentrated liquid	Gerber	Lactose, corn sugar*	Corn	Feeding of full-term and premature infants with no special nutritional requirements.	Available fortified with 10 mg iron/liter.
Similac Ready to feed Concentrated liquid Powder	Ross	Lactose	Coconut, corn	Feeding of full-term and premature infants with no special nutritional requirements.	Available fortified with 12 mg iron/liter.
Products for milk protein-sensitive infants ("milk allergy")					
Sobee (powder)	Mead Johnson	Dextrin, soy, sucrose, maltose	Coconut, soy	Milk-sensitive infants.	Soy protein isolate.
Mull-Soy liquid	Syntex	Invert sucrose	Soy		Flour.
Neo-Mull-Soy liquid	Syntex	Sucrose	Soy		Soy protein isolate.
Soyalac liquid or powder	Loma Linda	Corn sugar,* sucrose	Soy		Supplement with calcium. Soy protein isolate.
Prosobee	Mead Johnson	Corn sugar,* sucrose	Soy		Soy protein isolate. Zero band antigen.
Isomil	Ross	Corn sugar,* sucrose, corn starch	Corn, coconut		Soy protein isolate.
Non-soy (milk-free) products for milk-sensitive infants					
Meat base	Gerber	Modified tapioca starch	Sesame		Add carbohydrate to increase calories.
Lambase	Gerber	Corn sugar,* modified tapioca starch	Corn		
Dale's goat milk	Cutter	Lactose	Butterfat		Supplement with iron, vitamins C and D.
Low-sodium formulas					
Lonalac powder	Mead Johnson	Lactose	Coconut	Management of children with congestive cardiac failure.	For long-term management, additional sodium must be given. Supplement with vitamins C and D and iron. Na = 1 mEq/liter.

*Composed of glucose, maltose, and dextrins.

TABLE 4–6 (cont'd). Normal and special infant formulas.

	Manufacturer	CHO Source	Fat Source	Indications for Use	Comments (Nutritional Adequacy)
Low-sodium formulas					
Partially demineralized whey formulas					
SMA S-26 Concentrated liquid or powder	Wyeth	Lactose	Coconut, corn, soy, oleo	Use where a low-salt diet is indicated.	Relatively low solute load. Na = 7 mEq/liter.
Similac PM 60/40 Powder	Ross	Lactose	Coconut, corn	Use where a low-salt diet is indicated.	Relatively low solute load. Na = 7 mEq/liter.
Products for infants with fat malabsorption syndromes					
Probana powder	Mead Johnson	Lactose, banana powder, dextrose	Butterfat	Management of celiac disease, cystic fibrosis, and steatorrhea.	In persistent diarrhea, supplement with vitamins E and K. Low-fat, high-protein, low-lactose, supplement with vitamin C and iron.
Portagen	Mead Johnson	Corn sugar,* sucrose	Medium chain triglyceride (coconut source) and safflower	Management of chyluria, intestinal lymphangiectasia, various steatorrhea, biliary atresia.	Fat in medium chain triglycerides and safflower oil.
Alacta	Mead Johnson	Lactose	Butterfat	Infants with poor fat tolerance or poor fat absorption.	Supplement with vitamins A, D, and C and iron. To increase calories, supplement with carbohydrates. Renal solute load is high if powder only is used to increase calories to 67 Cal/100 ml.
Products for infants with carbohydrate malabsorption syndromes					
Nutramigen	Mead Johnson	Sucrose, tapioca	Corn	Feeding of infants and children intolerant to food proteins. Use in galactosemic patients.	Enzymatic hydrolysate of casein.
Cho-Free	Syntex	None	None	Infants intolerant to carbohydrate.	Carbohydrate-free soy protein isolate. Add carbohydrates to increase calories.
For infants with phenylketonuria					
Lofenalac	Mead Johnson	Corn sugar,* sucrose	Corn	Infants and children with phenylketonuria.	

*Composed of glucose, maltose, and dextrins.

papers under the high chair and a spoon and dish of food when he is hungriest will give him the opportunity to practice his new task. He tires easily and mother will want to finish the feeding.

Excessive caloric intake.

See section on calories and fat. If the mother-child relationship appears to be a problem, psychiatric consultation may be required.

Won't eat.

Children ordinarily will eat when hungry and will play with or refuse food only when partly satisfied or not hungry. Stop meal casually when child won't eat and wants only to play with food. Offer a small snack later if he is hungry. *Caution:* Do not stop meal if child is anxious to handle the food but wishes to continue eating; he is learning, and the mother who does not allow the child to

handle his food and try to put some in his mouth is depriving him of a natural and necessary pleasure. If he is not allowed to feed himself with his fingers, he may be delayed in spoon feeding.

Messy eating habits.

It is hard to learn to eat neatly. Eventually, children imitate older, more accomplished eaters and naturally become more adept.

Failure to thrive.

Is the child developmentally able to eat as expected? (See Table 4–8.) In a young child, check that the formula is properly mixed. Psychiatric consultation may be required if there is a mother-child relationship problem.

TABLE 4–7. Developmental sequence of feeding skills (1–12 months).

Age	Oral	Feeding Skills		Social
		Body Position	Hand-to-Mouth	
1 month	Rooting, sucking, swallowing	Total body response		Fearless hunger cry
2 months		Tonic neck reflex position of head		Looks at mother's face
4 months	Mouth poises for nipple, sucks and swallows. Choking response to solids. Tongue projects after spoon or nipple removed. Ejects food with tongue.	Head erect	Arms activate at sight of food. Toy play.	Ability to wait for food
5–6 months			Brings hand to mouth. Strong hand-to-mouth response after spoon or nipple removed. Pats bottle or breast. Closes in on bottle with both hands.	
6 months	Smacking noises with mouth. Sucks liquid from cup.		Grasps and draws bottle to mouth. Grasps spoon or cup rim.	
7 months	Pulls food off spoon with lips. Keeps lips closed while chewing.	Sits leaning forward	Toys to mouth	Lingers over food. Explores and bites. Vocalizes eagerness.
8 months	Bites, chews toys	Acquiring sitting balance. Reaches toward dish.	Feeds self cracker. Holds feeding bottle.	
9 months	Mouth as sensory organ decreasing. Protrudes tongue voluntarily.	Sits well	Combines 2 utensils. Chooses finger feeding.	
10 months	Drinks from cup. Lateral motion of tongue inside and out. Moves tongue to palate.		Tries to feed self	
11–12 months			Holds cup (spills easily). Tries to use spoon (grasps). Neat pincer grasp.	Choosy about food

TABLE 4–8. Developmental sequence of feeding skills (1 year to 4–7 years).

	Months 14	18	24	Years 3	4–7
Motor cup	Holds and dumps (grasps with both hands). Drinking attempted.	Holds, drinks well with one or 2 hands. Lowers to tray well.	Handles well. Drinks with straw.	Spills little. Pours well from pitcher. Feeds self well, using utensils.	Serves self. Can set table. Cuts with knife.
spoon	Spills, fills poorly, turns at mouth.	Lowers to tray well. Fills, turns on mouth.	No turning. Fills. Overhand grasp.		
Social	Hands utensils to mother. Demands to help feed self. Shakes head "no."	Eats rapidly.	Feeds doll. Verbalizes: "Eat, all gone." Asks for food. Feeds self in part.	Combines eating and talking well.	Choosy about food. Eats rapidly.

Age 2 and 3 Years

Will not accept solids; likes only milk.

If milk intake is over 18 oz to 1 quart, cut intake to 18 oz. Is he feeding himself? His developmental feeding tasks may have to begin back at a 6- or 7-month level and then progress. He may not find learning to feed himself at this age as exciting as earlier. If he is slow developmentally, he may not accept solids until other areas are nearer the 6- or 7-month level of development.

Will not drink milk any more.

The toddler has an increasing sense of self (of "I") and of being a distinct and individual person —apart from his mother. His constant use of "no" is not perverse negativism as much as it is his struggle with his ego needs in conflict with his mother's efforts to control him. He wants to do more and decide more for himself. At this age, children go on food jags, have more intense likes and dislikes, and assert their opinions. Puddings, eggnogs, cottage cheese, and cheese are good milk substitutes. Forcing milk is not necessary. He will probably drink it again if it is offered gently from time to time during the period of refusal. Giving him the nutrients milk provides is necessary. Protein and calcium are important at this age.

Does not eat enough; plays with his food.

He is not growing as fast as he was previously. He is less ravenous for food and is exuberantly interested in new activities like feeling and touching foods, tipping the cup, and squeezing or dropping food on the floor. When the child seriously loses interest in eating the food, it should be removed without anger or punishment. If he immediately whimpers for his food, he should be given another chance. However, if the mother always casually stops the meal when the child loses interest, he will learn to pay attention when he is hungry. If the mother acquires the habit of nagging, begging, or bribing him to eat, he will realize that he can become her master in the feeding situation and win any feeding battle. An adequate and nutritious daily diet for most 2- and 3-year-olds should include 18 oz milk, 2 oz meat (4 large adult bites), 1 cup total various fruits and vegetables throughout the day, 2 slices bread or its equivalent, and small amounts of butter and light desserts such as ice cream and jello. This may be less food than he previously ate. At 1 year of age he needs approximately 1000 calories; by the age of 3 years, he needs only 1300–1500 calories. The mother must know that he needs fewer calories per unit of body weight but more protein and minerals. Offer a variety of foods in small amounts. Refined sweets should be reserved for special occasions. The milk will meet his calcium and phosphorus needs.

Does not eat well at mealtimes; wants between-meal snacks.

Snacks must be nutritious and part of the daily food needs; concentrated sweets and foods empty of nutrients except calories are to be avoided. Snack time may be far more pleasant for the child than mealtime, primarily because the mother may insist the child eat certain foods in specific amounts at regular meals but allows snacks which the child likes to eat and can handle more easily, such as finger foods. If the table is too high or if the spoon and fork are too large or a glass too large and heavy, eating becomes difficult and the child may refuse to eat or dawdle at his food. Large servings of food discourage a child. Small servings encourage asking for more.

Age 3–5 Years

Will not eat vegetables.

Children like raw vegetables better than cooked, and most can be eaten raw. Children prefer single foods rather than mixtures with a sauce. Fruits may be substituted for vegetables during times of lagging appetite. A raw vegetable or fruit selection may have more appeal if cut into bite size finger food pieces.

Will only eat peanut butter.

"Food jags" generally last only until the child is tired of the food and should be of no concern.

Will not eat meat.

Meat should be tender and easy to chew. Ground meat cooked so that it is still soft, chicken, turkey, fish, and any soft tender meat should be offered. Children do not like to chew on tough, fibrous meat. Beans (legumes), cheese, eggs; peanut butter, and cottage cheese can be used as meat substitutes. Milk should be combined with the beans and peanut butter to make high-quality-protein. Eating with other children is helpful. He learns by watching them eat and socializing with them.

Will not eat new foods.

The Head Start experience is that it may take 9 months for a child to finally learn to eat with enthusiasm all of the foods which are strange to him and are not served at home. However, the Head Start children are not forced to eat all the food on their plate. With gentle encouragement, children generally have some curiosity and begin to taste new and different foods. New foods served with old foods are easier to accept. The mother can never make her child like a food; she can only allow him to like it. She must be encouraged to continue offering a new food at weekly or monthly intervals. Children often reject a food for some weeks and then, if never forced, will suddenly accept and eat it with gusto. Children enjoy participating in simple tasks in preparation of the meal. A child may eat more if he is allowed to serve himself some food. Devices such as serving a little girl her food on a doll's tea set may make the food more interesting and appetizing to her.

Which rules should be enforced at the table?

Different families have different mealtime habits. Strict rules for young children about eating may cause large problems, however, and give the child a weapon he can use in winning food arguments. Flexibility is the best rule. Children mimic parents and gradually learn to eat and behave at the table as their parents eat and behave. Mealtime should not be the time for settling distressing issues. It should develop as the time that the family has a chance to sit together and share their experiences of the day. Children who run right in from play are often excited and unable to eat. It is helpful to call small children early and have them watch TV, listen to a story, or sit quietly for a few minutes before the meal begins. Parents set the style in a family, and children learn to follow.

Age 6–12 Years

Has horrible table manners.

A child during this period is learning to get along with others and to function with competence. It is a diffuse period of cliques, gangs, and pensive daydreaming. Constant correction at the table by parents rather than setting the example in their own behavior is harmful to the child in his struggle against feelings of inferiority. When the child rebels to the extent that manners once acquired disappear, the parent can be assured that they will reappear after he has established his independence. Girls show less rebelliousness of this nature than boys. A nagging and bossy attitude is more irritating to him than a matter-of-fact request.

Does not eat enough.

Prior to the adolescent growth spurt, growth is erratic, with declines in the food requirement per unit of body weight. The child will eat more in time. Reserves will be built for the demands of the adolescent period to come. Food dislikes and likes are a product of earlier years, but family attitudes are imitated and the child will often begin to eat foods previously refused, particularly if peers eat them and if parents do not prod.

Does not eat breakfast.

When the child is given sole responsibility for his own breakfast, it may be makeshift or nonexistent. The mother may then complain that he does not eat. She should begin or help with breakfast if possible. A departure from traditional breakfast foods such as soup and a sandwich makes a nourishing and perhaps a more acceptable breakfast to the child.

Overweight.

During this age an appropriate mother-child relationship is necessary for successful weight loss. A child needs the support and help of his family. Later, he may make an effort all on his own, but if the mother appears to sabotage his efforts the most one may hope for is to slow the gain. The child will have only a degree of self-control. Older adolescents have more control. A social evaluation may be helpful. (See Obesity, next section.)

Age 12–18 Years

Obesity.

Childhood or juvenile obesity is a difficult problem because it is usually refractory to treatment and tends to persist into adulthood. Many mothers, in their concern over the child's food habits, unwittingly establish a pattern of overeating when they introduce solid foods at a very early age, equate weight gain with good health, or use food as a reward for good behavior. The problem is further complicated by inactivity.

It is important for the physician to establish a good relationship with the adolescent. He must be made to feel that what he is is more significant to you than his "fatness" and that you are more interested in him than in his problem. Try to like him. Find out about his activities, interests, hopes, worries, and satisfactions. When food is his only satisfaction, help him find others. Food will never be eaten in less quantity until another satisfaction can begin to replace it. Give him support. Praise his efforts and be careful to give him goals which you both feel he can successfully accomplish. He will then be able to slowly build on success, no matter how small. He probably has had many failures in the past. Always consider his physical activity. Decide together upon some form of exercise which is more than he is presently getting but which is reasonable for him to realistically accomplish on a daily basis. He must be an active participant in the solution of his own problem. Ask him for suggestions.

Provide him with the nutrition information needed to improve his diet. Then act as a guide and consultant. Be supportive and reward every success. When he does not lose weight, find some event to reward such as refusing a dessert or second helping. Help him develop insight into why he follows the diet and why he does not. Some simple devices which help with weight reduction:

(1) See him often for weigh-in and encouragement.

(2) Have him keep a food intake record and study it together.

(3) Record weights on a graph which exaggerates loss by a steep slope.

(4) Promote exercise in small degrees; increase later.

(5) Promote activities and a hobby.

(6) Encourage other overweight family members to diet.

(7) Have him put reminder signs on the family bulletin board or refrigerator.

(8) Send encouraging notes in the mail.

(9) If he loses a pound, point out that he did **not** eat 3500 calories and he should be very proud.

(10) Always insist that he take all the credit for his weight losses.

(11) Behavior modification technics are helpful with some adolescents.

(12) The following is a 1500-calorie diet with fruit used as dessert:
Milk (2% fat), 3 cups
Meat, 7 oz
Vegetables, as desired
Fat (butter, mayonnaise, etc), 3 tsp
Bread, 4 slices
Fruit, 3 servings

No time for breakfast.

Request he drink milk or juice before leaving for school. This is fast. Suggest a portable food like a sandwich to eat on the way to school. Explain that studies show that students do better work in the morning after breakfast. Suggest he make arrangements the night before: open soup, pour into pan, and refrigerate. Heat in the morning while dressing.

Not hungry for breakfast.

Begin with a drink of milk or orange juice; add foods slowly. Hunger will appear in 2 weeks or 1 month when he conditions his body to eating breakfast.

Skips school lunch: "School food is horrible." "I'm on a diet." "I use my lunch money for other things."

Nibbling on cheap snacks often offers more calories than a small nutritious lunch. No lunch means extreme hunger and possible overeating after school. Have adolescent pack his own lunch, if possible. Explain that eating some food is easier than skipping meals in weight reduction. Skipping and becoming overly hungry weakens will power.

Losing weight rapidly.

In a physically healthy adolescent, this may indicate drug use or serious medical or psychologic problems.

Fad dieting for quick weight loss.

Starvation studies show that weight lost is water and muscle, with little fat. Adherence to most fad diets for the length of time necessary for appreciable loss is impossible. Give valid nutrition information and explain that weight gain was slow; therefore, weight loss may be slow. There is no magic method.

Diets for athletes.

The United States Army has conducted research for 25 years on food and its relationship to physical fitness. They found that the most effective diet for rigorous physical activity is a balance of fat, protein, and carbohydrate with breakfast providing 1/4 to 1/3 of the whole day's needs. Coaches have stressed high-protein diets in the past, but research indicates that protein is not the fuel for working muscles. During mild exercise, fat is the prime fuel. As physical activity increases, carbohydrate becomes more important. Under extreme muscular effort, all muscle energy comes from carbohydrate.

Maximum dietary preparation several days prior to an athletic event is a normal balance of protein and fat, with high carbohydrate intake. The high carbohydrate intake improves the capacity for prolonged exercise when given in addition to the balanced diet. Food eaten immediately prior to the event must be easily and readily digested. Fat takes a longer period for digestion and should be kept to a minimum. Liquid meals of approximately 1000 calories providing 75% carbohydrate and 25% protein are preferable because they are more readily digested and will not induce vomiting, as a heavy protein and fat meal could.

Restricting water is a common practice during hard exercise. There is documented evidence that limiting the water consumed during an athletic event is less beneficial than allowing the players to drink glucose in water or 0.2% sodium chloride solution throughout the game. Maintaining water balance is important for the athlete. One of the principal manifestations of dehydration is fatigue. This is true in cold weather as well as hot weather. Use of special commercial drinks for athletes has its basis in this fact.

Vegetarian diet.

Many peoples of the world subsist on a diet considered by the more affluent to be a vegetarian diet. However, young people may try the various types of vegetarianism by choice. These diets may be categorized into types: Pure vegetarian or vegan diets which are not supplemented with any

TABLE 4–9. Assessment of development of feeding skills and treatment of specific lags.

Deficit In:	Test	Treatment
Oral Musculature		
Swallow	Give liquid and feel throat or watch carefully for spontaneous reflex.	Stroke the outside of the throat firmly, either toward or away from the chin.
Lip control	Feed baby food, hold spoon in mouth, and wait for him to pull away with lips.	Run an ice cube around the lips quickly for 1 minute and rest. Lips should purse. Hold spoon for child to pull food off with lips. Tap firmly around lips quickly while playing.
Tongue control	Put honey in corners of mouth, then middle of upper and lower lip and watch for tongue to lick.	Put honey or peanut butter on corner of mouth or inside cheeks for tongue to get; press down on tongue when putting spoon in mouth; walk back on tongue from tip in very small steps to avoid gag reflex.
Position		
Head control	Observe whether head held steady on his own.	Steady head when propped or sitting; make head secure by supporting on both sides with rolled towels or pillow.
Sitting	Observe whether sits alone or without support.	Recline seat (chair or high chair) by propping front legs up; pad sides with towels or pillows; make secure and not room for much movement.
Feet	(Children are uncomfortable as adults are without foot support while eating.)	Supported or resting on platform.
Hand-to-Mouth		
General	Put toy in front to see if he puts in mouth.	Wait for development of toy-to-mouth play.
Finger feeding	Place cracker on tray and see if he eats it.	Provide initial foods (soft or absorbent) of a consistency such as that of cheese, crackers, toast, banana, canned fruit, or vegetable. Raw fruit such as apples and raw vegetables such as carrots come later. Provide foods in manageable sizes and shapes, with edges large enough to grasp and ready-made handles such as bread sticks.
Glass	Place in front and see if he picks it up and drinks.	Play with toy first. Use glass with lid and spout; handles come later. Use flat-bottomed glass; stand behind with hands over child's hands to guide.
Spoon	Place spoon in front and see if he picks up, how he fills it, brings it to mouth.	If poor grasp, build up handle (fill bicycle handle with plaster of Paris and insert spoon handle). Use spoon holder that straps onto hand. If rotation is poor, bend spoon bowl to compensate. Use sticky food at first; try swivel spoon. If he misses mouth, it is too early to try. Stand behind and guide hand.
Social	(More time must be spent to ensure that the child with a handicap learns to cope with and enjoy eating.)	Mealtimes are especially important times to give attention and training to the handicapped child.

animal foods, dairy products or eggs; lactovegetarian diets, which are supplemented with milk and cheese; or lacto-ovo-vegetarian diets, which are supplemented with milk, cheese, and eggs. The latter 2 diets can be quite adequate. The former, lacking complete proteins, prevents adequate nutrition eventually, as will any extremely narrow choice of foods.

Many young health food addicts are interested and concerned about nutrition but do not have enough knowledge to plan a balanced diet. If they understand that their diet must contain the 8 essential amino acids in the same meal (plus cystine, which is hard to get in an all-vegetable diet), they can plan diets within their health foods and maintain a balance. Health food stores, though expensive, are a source of various vitamins and foods which are acceptable to them. They must be warned, however, that the fat-soluble vitamins can be taken in toxic amounts since they are stored in the body. Iron can also become toxic. Table 4–1 can be used as a guideline for dosage limitations of these nutrients.

TABLE 4–10. Feeding problems in children with cleft palate.

Problem	Suggestions
Difficulty in nursing	Use soft nipples. Enlarge hole. Use Brecht feeder or medicine dropper (milk should hit inside of cheek, not the throat). Child learns to chew out.
Chokes on liquids	Give small amounts. Swallow slowly. Thicken liquid with rice cereal. Fluid should hit the side of the cheek and throat.
Excessive air	If he starts choking, hold him upright and tilted slightly backward while eating (45°) and while burping.
Irritation of mouth and nose by acid and spicy foods	Avoid these foods.
Food getting into opening (happens rarely)	Use pared foods. Thicken with crackers or wafers. Turn spoon over when in mouth. Eat slowly and small bites.
Long time required	Start child before family meal. Feed before or after family meal, but include at the table. Feed 5 or 6 small meals a day. Patience required.
Respiratory infections	Cleanse opening carefully after meals.
Chewing difficulty	Treat dental caries and provide orthodontic repair of faulty alignment.

Health food stores are more expensive than major chain grocery stores, but many so-called health foods are stocked in chain groceries at cheaper prices than at the health food store. Since most food faddists cannot be persuaded to change their diet completely, it is well to know that most vegetarians who take a variety of fruits, vegetables, unrefined cereals, legumes, seeds, nuts, and dairy products have adequate intakes. It is the narrow diet which is restricted to a few foods and is high in carbohydrates which tends to be inadequate.

Pregnancy.
Neonatal, postnatal, and infant mortality rates are higher for infants born to mothers 17 years and under. Superimposed upon the nutrient needs of the growing girl are the nutrient needs of pregnancy. Babies of less than ideal weight are born more often to biologically immature women than to older women. Nutritionally, adolescents are at a definite disadvantage in pregnancy. In ordinary circumstances, girls must make more judicious food choices than boys. (Boys usually have a better appetite and eat larger amounts, which tend to assure an intake of adequate nutrients.) Social and personal pressures concerning figure control and a comparative lack of physical activity may cause girls to follow unwise diets. They therefore may enter pregnancy with poor stores of nutrients. Standardized diets which are often used in prenatal clinics are not suited to the particular nutritional needs of the adolescent. To sustain and complete her own growth, she requires a diet rich in calories, protein, and calcium. Calorie deprivation and restriction of weight gain to less than 24 pounds is poorly tolerated and unwise considering the significance of the intrauterine environment.

SPECIAL PROBLEMS

Children who have special feeding problems include those with specific motor handicaps and cleft palate (Table 4–10). The brain damage which impairs a child's development in walking skills may also impair his feeding and oral development. If a lag is observed, referral to physical or occupational therapy is indicated. In addition, the technics described in Table 4–9 may be implemented by the mother at home, usually before mealtimes and at least twice a day if they do not upset the child.

Meal management is often a problem because parents are uncertain about what demands to place on a handicapped child. They must be encouraged to maintain mealtime discipline similar to what they expect of their normal children—and sometimes more, since concept formation in handicapped children may be slower to appear and often not to the same depth as in normal children.

Cleft Palate

Much of what has been said about children with motor handicaps applies also to children with cleft palate. Specific suggestions which have been collected from parents of cleft palate children are made in Table 4–10.

• • •

General References

Applebaum RM: Modern management of successful breast feeding. P Clin North America 17:203, 1970.

Beal VA: On the acceptance of solid foods, and other food patterns, of infants and children. Pediatrics 20:448, 1957.

Beauregard WG: Positional otitis media. J Pediat 79:294, 1971.

Bowes AD, Church CF: *Food Values of Portions Commonly Used,* 3rd ed. Lippincott, 1970.

Cheek DB: *Human Growth: Body Composition, Cell Growth, Energy and Intelligence.* Lea & Febiger, 1968.

Consolazio CF: *Nutritional Basis for Optimal Performance.* US Army Medical Research and Nutrition Laboratory, Fitzsimmons General Hospital, Denver, Colorado, 1967.

Duncan RB: Positional otitis media. Arch Otolaryng 72:454, 1960.

Erhard D: Nutrition for the now generation. J Nutr Educ 2:135, 1971.

Fomon SJ: *Infant Nutrition.* Saunders, 1967.

Gustaffson BE: The Vipeholm dental caries study. Acta odontol scandinav 11:207, 1953–54.

Guthrie HA: *Introductory Nutrition,* 2nd ed. Mosby, 1971.

Heald FP: *Adolescent Nutrition and Growth.* Appleton-Century-Crofts, 1969.

Illingworth RS, Lister J: The critical or sensitive period, with special reference to certain feeding problems in infants and children. J Pediat 65:839, 1964.

Maternal and Child Health Service: *Screening Children for Nutritional Status.* US Department of Health, Education, & Welfare, 1971.

Maternal Nutrition and the Course of Pregnancy. National Academy of Sciences, 1970.

O'Neal RM, Johnson OC, Schaeffer AE: Guidelines for classification and interpretation of group blood and urine data collected as part of the national nutrition survey. Pediat Res 4:103, 1970.

National Research Council, Food and Nutrition Board: Recommended Dietary Allowances, 7th ed. National Academy of Sciences, 1968.

Snyderman SE & others: The histidine requirement of the infant. Pediatrics 31:786, 1963.

Williams SR: *Nutrition and Diet Therapy,* 2nd ed. Mosby, 1971.

Ziai M & others: *Textbook of Pediatrics.* Little, Brown, 1969.

5...

Immunization

Vincent A. Fulginiti, MD

All pediatric immunizations are planned to prevent specific infectious diseases or their toxic manifestations. Thus, to achieve maximum effectiveness, the vaccines must be administered to the appropriate populations at the appropriate times in life when the individual is immunologically capable and has not yet been exposed to the natural disease. "Routines" of immunization are designed to simplify ordinary practice and to permit reasonable immunization scheduling. However, exceptions to the routine are dictated by peculiar local epidemiologic circumstances (eg, epidemics or absence of a disease in the community) and by individual differences in immunologic response or susceptibility to the adverse effects of specific products. Each immunization should be viewed as a balance between the risk of that disease in the individual and population and the potential adverse effects of the immunizing procedure. This chapter will attempt to present the "routine" as well as the tempering influences for each product and schedule.

Sources of Information

Recommendations for immunization change as experience accumulates and new products and new indications become available. Several sources of such information are available to the practitioner:

A. The American Academy of Pediatrics' *Red Book.* A useful, comprehensive guide to immunization practices. Distributed free to all Fellows of the Academy and available to others at the nominal cost of $2.00 from the Academy, PO Box 1034, Evanston, Illinois 60204. The *Red Book* is supplemented by special information published as needed in the *Academy Newsletter.*

B. *Morbidity and Mortality Reports.* A weekly publication of the National Communicable Disease Center, Atlanta, Georgia, of the US Department of Health, Education, and Welfare—useful reports of the major notifiable diseases supplemented periodically with specific immunization recommendations of the Surgeon General and USPHS.

C. Local public health agencies—either through periodic publications or by special bulletins—make available immunization information, particularly of a local nature. Specific inquiry about requirements for foreign travel, special immunizations, etc can be handled at these agencies.

D. *Immunization Information for Foreign Travel,* a booklet published by the Department of Health, Education, and Welfare (Publication No. 384), may be purchased from the Superintendent of Documents, Government Printing Office, Washington DC, at 25 cents a copy.

STERILITY & SAFETY OF INJECTABLE VACCINE ADMINISTRATION

Avoidance of Bacterial Infection & Hepatitis

Most of the "sterile" or aseptic precautions are recommended in order to prevent the introduction of unwanted infectious agents. Simple cleanliness and the use of sterilized equipment would suffice to prevent most bacterial infections. However, the more stringent precautions are designed to prevent hardier bacteria and the hepatitis agent from gaining access to the vaccinee. The following steps are recommended:

A. **Single-Unit Dosage:** Where possible, single-unit disposable equipment should be used. Plastic syringes or single-dose vaccine units are most desirable.

B. **Sterilization of Equipment:** If glass syringes are used, adequate sterilization procedures must be employed between individual patient usage. The following procedures are recommended by the American Academy of Pediatrics: (1) Autoclaving at a temperature of 121° C for a period of 15 minutes at 15 lb pressure. (2) Dry heat for 2 hours at 170° C or boiling for 30 minutes are also acceptable, but one must be certain that the time and temperature requirements are met.

C. **Disinfection:** For most procedures, it is sufficient to cleanse the intended injection site and the surface of the immunization container with a solution of 70% alcohol. Some prefer 2% tincture of iodine followed by 70% alcohol. Iodine burns have occurred when the tincture is not removed or is allowed to pool in contact with the skin. Our current feeling is that no skin preparation or, at most, gentle washing with soap and water is preferable preceding smallpox immunization.

Routes & Methods of Immunization

All adjuvant or "depot" antigens which contain alum, aluminum hydroxide or phosphate, mineral oil, etc should be administered **intramuscularly only**. Subcutaneous injection results in considerable irritation and pain and may lead to the so-called sterile abscess.

Intramuscular injections should be given into the anterolateral thigh (vastus lateralis muscle) or into the deltoid or triceps muscle mass (older children and adults). This is to avoid sciatic nerve damage, which may follow intragluteal injections.

One should always aspirate prior to injection to avoid intravascular administration.

Aqueous vaccines can be given intramuscularly, subcutaneously or, on occasion, intracutaneously.

Live vaccines should be given on separate occasions separated by at least 1 month unless an emergency situation dictates otherwise. This will minimize potential interference and additive effects such as fever, malaise, etc, and will clarify the etiology of reactions should they occur. An exception to this practice is the use of *proved* live virus vaccine combinations. These preparations have been shown to be effective and safe, with no additive clinical effects.

The "jet gun" or compressed air injection of vaccines is useful for mass immunization. The advantages are ease of administration, rapidity of multiple injections, and greater acceptance. The units are expensive, and single dose administration units are not yet practical. This method may find greater favor with the development of improved, inexpensive equipment.

Host Factors in Safety of Immunizations

Only healthy children should be immunized. Febrile illnesses, incubation of a childhood exanthem, and any active infection are contraindications to immunization. The child who has a "cold" each time he presents for his routine immunizations poses a problem in completion of his primary series. Two alternatives exist to achieve adequate protection: (1) Have the child return between regularly scheduled visits when he is well. (2) Administer the vaccine. This requires judgment, as the child may have a minimal upper respiratory illness and will tolerate the procedure quite well.

Chronic illnesses in themselves are not necessarily contraindications; indeed, they may make immunizations more desirable or even mandatory. Caution must be exercised if CNS damage exists. In general, infants under 1 year of age with cerebral dysfunction should not receive routine immunization. Most authorities feel that a delay until 1 year of age is justified. In particular, infants with convulsive disorders may experience fever and convulsions with the risk of aggravating their basic disorder.

Chronic open skin diseases such as eczema contraindicate smallpox immunization or contact with a vaccinated individual. Acute dermatitis or injury resulting in weeping surfaces again contraindicates vaccination or contact. If vaccination of a sibling or other contact is desirable, the affected child must be completely removed from the environment until the crust has separated and the vaccinee is free of virus.

Immunologic deficiency states are an absolute contraindication to live virus immunization. Whether congenital or acquired, these deficiency diseases expose the host to the danger of dissemination of the vaccine virus. Malignancies of the lymphatic system are frequently overlooked as predisposing the host to such complications. More and more children are being treated with corticosteroids and immunosuppressive agents. These drugs may induce a state of lowered immunologic reactivity, and live virus immunization at such times may result in generalized and frequently fatal infections.

Allergy to a component of the vaccine preparation is infrequent but often can be anticipated. Antibiotic allergies should be elicited by questioning and the antibiotic composition of various viral vaccines known. Many vaccines are prepared in eggs or in fowl tissues, and patients who are sensitive should not receive such preparations. A rough guide which is frequently advised is that if a child can eat a whole egg without adverse effects he can receive egg or fowl tissue prepared vaccines. Infrequently, patients are sensitive to the preservative included in the vaccine, eg, mercury.

THE IMMUNIZING ANTIGENS

Increasing numbers of vaccines, antisera, and gamma globulin preparations are becoming available. They differ significantly in their composition, form, stability, route of administration, and timing. It is essential that the practitioner carefully assess each preparation before he administers it to any patient. The brochure provided with the preparation is almost invariably complete in its description of the product and its proper use.

"Typical" Composition

The typical vaccine does not exist, but the following categories of components are found. The list is presented to point out the complexities of some vaccines and the difficulty in attributing an unusual reaction to a specific component. Immunization involves administering a complex product to a complex individual, and the result of this administration is complex.

A. The Principal Antigen: May be whole bacteria, bacterial products (toxins, hemolysins, etc), whole viruses or substructures of viruses.

B. Host-Derived Antigens: Protein or other constituents of host tissue which are carried along with or intimately associated with the virus particles.

C. Altered Antigens: Distorted proteins and other substances may become incorporated into vaccines as a result of the complex changes associated with the effects of virus infection on the cells in which it is grown.

D. Preservatives and Stabilizers: A variety of chemical compounds are employed to prevent bacterial growth or to maintain the desired antigen in a stable form. Mercury compounds and glycine are typical examples.

E. Antibiotics: Trace amounts may be found in viral vaccines which must be prepared in antibiotic-containing media. Various antibiotics are employed, and the "same" vaccine prepared by different manufacturers may vary in the specific antibiotics used.

F. Menstruum: All vaccines are solutions or suspensions. The fluid phase may consist simply of saline solution or may be as complex as the tissue culture media employed in viral growth.

G. Unwanted or Unknown Constituents: Despite elaborate precautions in preparing vaccines, viruses or other antigens may be included which are not wanted or not even detectable.

H. Adjuvants: A variety of substances may be used to enhance the antigenic effect of the principal antigen. Such materials as alum, aluminum phosphate, and aluminum hydroxide are currently in use, and others (mineral oil, peanut oil, etc) may be employed in the future. The purpose of these materials is to retain the antigen at the depot site and to release it slowly, thus enhancing the response by prolonging contact.

Properties of Antigens

Antigens vary in their ability to produce the desired immunologic response; some do so weakly, and some strongly. For a given antigen, the response may be variable, with some individuals responding poorly and a few not at all. One should be aware of this phenomenon in assessing the clinical effects of a preparation. Some children who receive optimal immunizations will simply not respond and may contract the disease if exposed naturally. This should not condemn the particular antigen for all children, as it may protect the vast majority of recipients.

Adjuvant Vaccines

In general, depot type vaccines are preferred since they provide more prolonged immunity and greater antigenic stimulation and reduce the systemic effects observed with fluid antigens, which are rapidly absorbed. For example, DTP (diphtheria and tetanus toxoid and pertussis organisms) provides prolonged antitoxic immunity against diphtheria and tetanus. In addition, it enhances the antibody response to pertussis, particularly in early infancy. Fluid or aqueous preparations may achieve earlier immunity and are less likely to produce local reactions at the site of injection.

Gamma Globulin Preparations

A variety of gamma globulins are available for clinical use. Whatever the label, they are all essentially the same. They consist of roughly a 16% solution of a limited spectrum of serum proteins in the gamma range of electrophoretic mobility. They differ in their antibody content to a significant degree. Thus, tetanus immune globulin is a preparation obtained by pooling and concentrating donor plasma from individuals recently stimulated with tetanus toxoid, thus assuring a higher level of antitoxin than is found in other gamma globulins obtained from donors irrespective of their tetanus immunization status. This is true for all of the specifically labeled gamma globulins—they contain a standard level of the specific antibody desired, whereas randomly prepared lots do not.

Gamma globulins are intended only for intramuscular injection and should not be given intravenously since intravenous administration results in predictable anaphylactoid reactions. (An intravenous gamma globulin is now in preparation but as of this writing has not been marketed.)

The dosage of gamma globulin is not uniform but varies for each specific preparation and for the specific clinical circumstances of its use. One must learn these variables in order to use the antibody contained in the preparations effectively.

Intradermal testing with gamma globulin is unnecessary and may be misleading. The intradermal inoculation of gamma globulin may result in a wheal and flare reaction which does not indicate sensitivity to intramuscular administration. Thus, this method is not advised.

Whenever gamma globulin is administered simultaneously with an active immunizing antigen, one must be concerned about decreasing the effect of the antigen. This is due to the combination of the specific antibody in the gamma globulin with the antigen that occurs in the host after injection. It may be wise in some situations to administer additional doses of the antigen subsequently to ensure adequate stimulation. These special circumstances are pointed out in the specific immunization sections that follow.

Horse Serum Sensitivity

A major limiting factor in the use of antibody in the form of horse serum is the existence or development of horse serum sensitivity. This possibility must be considered each time the use of horse serum is contemplated. Appropriate medications to treat anaphylactic shock should be instantly available. The possibility of serum sickness developing later should be borne in mind.

To test for preexistent horse serum sensitivity, the following steps should be taken:

A. Allergic History: Elicit a careful history of prior administration of horse serum products and of any allergic reactions. Allergy in general is an indication for caution in administering horse serum.

B. Sensitivity Tests: Skin or conjunctival tests should be performed, bearing in mind that severe reactions may occur from the testing procedure itself and that the physician must be prepared to intercede.

1. Skin test—Give intradermally 0.1 ml of a 1:100 saline dilution of the serum to be used. In allergic individuals, reduce the dose to 0.05 ml of a 1:1000 dilution. The appearance of a wheal in 10—30 minutes indicates hypersensitivity.

2. Conjunctival test—One drop of a 1:10 dilution in saline is placed in the lower conjunctival sac and 1 drop of saline solution in the other eye as a control. A positive reaction consists of conjunctivitis and tearing in 10—30 minutes.

C. Desensitization: Table 5-1 outlines the subsequent procedure to be followed.

TABLE 5–1. Desensitization procedure in horse serum sensitivity.

History	Sensitivity Test	Procedure
–	–	IM dose can be given. For IV use, give 0.5 ml serum in 10 ml fluid first; if there is no reaction in 30 minutes, give the remainder of the dose as a 1:20 dilution.
+ or –	– or +	If serum use is imperative, give 1 ml of 1:10 dilution subcut; if there is no reaction, proceed with 1 ml undiluted and if still no reaction proceed as above.
+	+	Serum should only be used if there is no alternative and it may be lifesaving. Begin with 0.05 ml of a 1:20 dilution subcut and increase every 15 minutes as follows if there is no reaction: 0.1 ml of 1:10, 0.3 ml of 1:10, 0.1 ml undiluted, 0.2 ml undiluted, 0.5 ml undiluted, and then the remainder of the dose. If an untoward reaction occurs at any stage, reduce the dose by half.

SPECIFIC IMMUNIZATIONS

DIPHTHERIA

Immunity against diphtheria is related to the levels of circulating antitoxin. Immunization may not prevent the carrier state. Occasionally, even well immunized individuals develop the disease, although morbidity is less and mortality rates are lower in such cases than in the nonimmunized. Protection is in excess of 85%. The major significant reservoirs of diphtheria in the USA today are the unimmunized, particularly older individuals whose immunity has waned and underprivileged children who have received no immunizations.

Vaccines Available

A. Combined Diphtheria-Tetanus-Pertussis (DTP): See below.

B. Diphtheria Toxoid: (Not available in 1971.) Recommended only when there is a specific contraindication to the combined preparations. It is usually given in 3 doses of 0.5 ml IM 4–6 weeks apart. A recall dose should be given 1 year later.

C. Diphtheria-Tetanus (DT) (Pediatric): This preparation contains full amounts of both diphtheria and tetanus toxoids and is indicated in those individuals who cannot be given pertussis vaccine. It is usually given in 3 doses of 0.5 ml IM 4–6 weeks apart with a booster 1–2 months later. Do not administer to adults because severe reactions may occur.

D. Diphtheria-Tetanus (Td) (Adult): This preparation contains 1/20 the amount of diphtheria toxoid contained in DPT or in pediatric DT. It is designed for use after the age of pertussis immunization. This amount of diphtheria toxoid elicits a booster response but results in far fewer local reactions.

E. Diphtheria Toxoid (Fluid): An infrequently used preparation which does not contain alum.

F. Diphtheria Toxin for Schick Test: Intradermal inoculation of 0.1 ml will result in 10 mm or more of erythema and induration approximately 4 days after injection. Pseudoreactions reach their peak earlier and fade by the third or fourth day. If a reaction occurs, it means that the individual has too little antibody to neutralize the toxin and is susceptible.

Immunization Schedules

Diphtheria immunization should be initiated in early infancy. Three doses of toxoid, alone or in combination with tetanus and pertussis vaccines, are administered at 2, 4, and 6 months. A booster dose is required at 1½ years, at 4 years, at 14–16 years, and every 10 years thereafter (see Table 5–2). If it is desired to avoid pertussis immunization, then 3 doses of pediatric DT should be administered to children younger than 6 years. Older individuals should receive 3 monthly doses of adult Td. In all cases, a booster dose should be administered 1 year later and at 10-year intervals.

Precautions

Diphtheria toxoid is associated with few side-effects in the pediatric age range. As it is a depot type vaccine, it should never be given by a route other than intramuscularly. In older children and adolescents, a reduced dose of diphtheria toxoid will ensure a low reaction rate and still provide effective immunization.

Antibody Preparations

A. Diphtheria Antitoxin, Equine: This material is prepared by hyperimmunization of horses and is available in vials containing 1000, 10,000, 20,000, and 40,000 units.

B. Antitoxin Schedule: Diphtheria antitoxin should be given as early as possible (1/2 intramuscularly and 1/2 intravenously) in the following clinical situations: Tonsillar, 20 thousand units IM; anterior nares, 10–20 thousand units; larynx, 20–40 thousand units; nasopharynx, 40–75 thousand units (dilute 1:20 in saline and administer slowly).

Always test for horse serum sensitivity. Administer all antitoxin intravenously if symptoms are severe and the disease is life-threatening. The actual dose of antitoxin is less critical than early administration. If the patient has been ill more than 48 hours, increase the dose. *Note:* Never substitute antibiotic therapy for antitoxin therapy.

TABLE 5–2. Schedule for active immunization and tuberculin testing of normal infants and children in the USA. (Approved by the Committee on Infectious Diseases, American Academy of Pediatrics, October 1971.)

2 months	DTP
	TOPV
4 months	DTP
	TOPV
6 months	DTP
	TOPV
1 year	Measles
	Tuberculin test
1–12 years	Rubella
	Mumps
1½ years	DTP
	TOPV
4–6 years	DTP
	TOPV
14–16 years	Td (and every 10 years thereafter)

DTP = diphtheria and tetanus toxoids, alum-precipitated or aluminum hydroxide adsorbed, combined with pertussis bacterial antigen. Suitable for young children. Three doses of 0.5 ml IM at intervals of 4–8 weeks. Fourth injection of 0.5 ml IM given about 1 year later.

TOPV = trivalent oral poliovirus vaccine (types 1, 2, and 3 polioviruses combined). Recommended as indicated in the schedule at 2, 4, 6, and 18 months and at 4–6 years. An alternative method would be to administer the monovalent vaccines containing just one of the types of poliovirus at 2, 4, and 6 months, with administration of trivalent vaccine at 15–18 months and at 6 years. The sequence can be type 1, type 3, and type 2 (recommended by Red Book Committee of the Academy of Pediatrics) or type 2, type 1, and type 3 (recommended by the USPHS Advisory Committee on Immunization Practices).

Measles: May be given at 1 year as measles-rubella or measles-mumps-rubella combined vaccines. Do not mix the individual vaccines or give individual vaccines separately but simultaneously. Live measles virus vaccine may be given alone (0.5 ml IM). When using attenuated (Edmonston) strain, give human gamma globulin, 0.01 ml/lb, injected into the opposite arm at the same time, to lessen the reaction to the vaccine. This is not advised with "further attenuated" (Schwarz) strain vaccine. Inactivated measles vaccine should not be used. (*Caution:* Please note the author's reservations about routine rubella vaccination on p 117.)

Tuberculin test: The frequency of repeated tuberculin tests depends upon the risk of exposure of the child and on the prevalence of tuberculosis in the population group.

Rubella: See Measles (above) and note author's comments on p 117.

Mumps: See Measles (above).

Td: Tetanus toxoid and diphtheria toxoid, adult form: Use only this preparation (Td-adult) in children older than 6 years. It contains less diphtheria toxoid than the pediatric preparation (DT) and thus results in fewer local reactions. Booster doses for Td are required on a routine basis at 10-year intervals.

PERTUSSIS

Potent pertussis vaccines confer immunity upon infants given the full schedule. Attack rates can be reduced from 90% to less than 15%. One major problem is the need for early protection in infants since little or no maternal immunity is transferred. Although schedules in which immunization is started at 6–8 weeks of life result in a lower level of antibody than those beginning after 6 months of age, it is vital to begin immunization early, accepting a somewhat lesser immunologic effect for the earlier protection afforded. Furthermore, booster doses eliminate the difference between the early-immunized and the later-immunized.

At the other end of the age scale, a different problem occurs. Outbreaks of pertussis are now being observed in preteen and teen-age children who received full infant immunization but were not boosted beyond the preschool years. We ordinarily refrain from pertussis immunization in older children because the reaction rate is high. Pertussis immunization must therefore be determined by the epidemiologic circumstances. In communities with high attack rates, one might wish to begin immunization in the newborn period and carry booster programs through the 12th year of age, recognizing that booster doses will be necessary in order to achieve a high level of immunity beyond the first few months of life. Untoward reactions in older children include severe fever, convulsions, and, rarely, encephalopathy. In communities where pertussis occurs rarely or never, ordinary scheduling suffices for adequate immunity. It would be unwise to abandon pertussis immunization completely since the child may move from an area of low incidence to one where the incidence is higher.

The efficacy of pertussis immune globulin is in doubt. Some believe it is only effective in preventing pertussis when given to unimmunized infants after exposure. Others also use it therapeutically. Clear-cut evidence of its effectiveness in either clinical situation is not available.

Vaccines Available

A. **Plain Pertussis Vaccine (Without Alum):** Useful in epidemics for rapid protection. Administer 3 IM doses of 0.5 ml (4 NIH units) each at monthly intervals.

B. **Adjuvant Pertussis Vaccine (With Alum, Aluminum Phosphate, or Aluminum Hydroxide):** Give 3 IM doses of 0.5 ml (4 NIH units) each at monthly intervals for primary immunization. Within 8–12 months following primary immunization, whether with plain or adjuvant pertussis vaccine, a booster dose of adjuvant vaccine should be used.

C. **Diphtheria-Tetanus-Pertussis (DTP):** See next section.

Immunization Schedules

Pertussis immunization is usually started at 6–8 weeks of age with combined diphtheria-tetanus vaccine. Three doses at bimonthly intervals complete primary immunization. Booster doses should be administered 8–12 months after completion of the primary series. Ordinarily, pertussis immunization is maintained by boosters at approximately 18 months and 4 years of life.

In areas of high endemicity, one may wish to start immunization with 0.5 ml of adjuvant pertussis vaccine on the second day of life in a healthy infant, with monthly doses at 1 and 2 months. An initial booster dose at 8–9 months of age and the regular boosters at 18 months and 4 years would complete the series. Additional boosters at 8 and 12 years could also be given. If this method is chosen, DTP could be given instead of adjuvant pertussis vaccine. If it is not, then DT (pediatric) should be administered in doses of 0.5 ml at monthly intervals for 3 doses early in infancy.

Precautions

Since pertussis vaccine is usually a depot antigen, it should only be given intramuscularly. Local and systemic reactions (tenderness, induration, and fever) are common, and many physicians prescribe aspirin routinely for 2–12 hours following immunization. Severe reactions are less common, and those involving the CNS least common. The occurrence of a severe febrile reaction or any CNS symptoms following pertussis immunization is an absolute contraindication to further doses. Pertussis vaccine should be administered to infants with CNS disease only after their first birthday—and then cautiously, in fractional doses.

With moderate reactions to vaccine not accompanied by CNS symptoms, it is desirable to reduce the dose to 0.1–0.3 ml and separate it from other immunizations.

Antibody Preparations

Pertussis immune globulin is human gamma globulin obtained from volunteers immunized with pertussis vaccine. It is supplied in 1.25 ml vials. Give 1.25–2.5 ml IM at the time of exposure in infants and repeat in 7 days if exposure continues. Some recommend 2.5 ml daily or every other day for infants with pertussis to a total dose of 7.15–12.5 ml. The author does not recommend its use.

TETANUS

Tetanus vaccine is one of the best immunizing agents available, conferring almost 100% protection in a fully immunized individual. A prolonged period of adequate immunity follows primary immunization, and booster doses are required only 10 years apart. Military personnel who received primary immunization in the 1940s maintained adequate serum antitoxic levels or were easily "boosted" by a single dose as long as 18 years later.

Vaccines Available

A. **Plain Tetanus Toxoid (Fluid):** This preparation is rapidly absorbed, resulting in more rapid immunization, but it is rarely needed.

B. **Tetanus Toxoid, Aluminum Phosphate Adsorbed:** The usual "booster" toxoid. Administer 0.5 ml IM as a booster; 3 doses spaced at monthly intervals provide primary immunization.

C. **Tetanus-Diphtheria Toxoid (Pediatric and Adult):** See Diphtheria, above.

D. **Diphtheria-Tetanus-Pertussis (DTP):** See next section.

Immunization Schedules

Three doses of 0.5 ml of an adjuvant tetanus toxoid suffice for primary immunization. Booster doses should be given 1 year later and every 10 years thereafter.

Management of injuries requires (1) early treatment, (2) adequate surgical care of the wound, (3) antibiotic therapy, if indicated, and (4) tetanus immunoprophylaxis. With minor injuries, prophylaxis is not necessary, although this may be an opportunity to start tetanus immunization in an unimmunized individual. In the case of injuries involving heavy contamination or extensive tissue destruction or delay in treatment, it is desirable to employ both tetanus immune globulin and recall tetanus vaccine in the previously immunized. With lesser injuries, tetanus immune globulin should not be given, but a booster (0.5 ml) dose of toxoid should be administered if a booster dose has not been given in the past 5 years. In the unimmunized, both tetanus immune globulin and tetanus toxoid should be given. It is imperative that full immunization subsequently be completed in the unimmunized.

Precautions

Tetanus toxoid is one of the safest immunizing antigens in the pediatric age range. Reactions are very infrequent and usually mild when they do occur, consisting only of local erythema and tenderness. More severe local reactions, sometimes accompanied by fever, are encountered in older individuals with repetitive doses of toxoid. Reduction in dosage reduces the risk of such reactions.

Antibody Preparations

A. **Tetanus Immune Globulin, Human (Hyper-Tet):** This is the preparation of choice. It has virtually no side-effects and is not immunologically removed from the circulation, ensuring prolonged antitoxin levels. It is supplied in 250 unit vials. Give 4 units/kg IM as prophylaxis to a maximum of 250 units, which is the adult dose. The exact dose for treatment is not known, but 140 units/kg IM is recommended.

B. **Tetanus Antitoxin, Equine:** This preparation should not be used today because of the dangers of horse serum sensitization. (Whenever possible, human tetanus immune globulin should be used.)

The equine preparation is supplied in 1500, 3000, 20,000, and 40,000 unit vials. For prophylaxis against tetanus, give 5—10 thousand units. For therapy of tetanus, give 50—100 thousand units—preferably 1/2 intravenously and 1/2 intramuscularly (given simultaneously) after testing for horse serum.

C. **Tetanus Antitoxin, Bovine:** This preparation was formerly used for individuals sensitive to horse serum. It is available only from Merck Sharp & Dohme by special contact. It has largely been superseded by human tetanus immune globulin.

COMBINED DIPHTHERIA-TETANUS-PERTUSSIS (DTP) IMMUNIZATION

The most common and most practical method for immunizing infants and young children is the combination of diphtheria and tetanus toxoids with pertussis vaccine (DPT). The combination has the advantages of triple immunization simultaneously and in one injection plus the enhancement of pertussis vaccine potency by the adjuvant effect of the toxoids. It has the disadvantage of confusing the etiology of reactions since all 3 antigens are given at once.

Vaccines Available

A. **Diphtheria and Tetanus Toxoids and Whole Pertussis Vaccine:** This is a combination of the bacterial suspension of pertussis plus the 2 toxoids. It is usually distributed in multiple dose vials. The individual dose is 0.5 ml IM.

B. **Diphtheria and Tetanus Toxoids and Extracted Pertussis Antigen:** This preparation contains the 2 toxoids (as above) with a cell-free extract of pertussis organisms. The claim has been made that it causes fewer local and systemic reactions. However, the results of one study show that the reduced reaction rate is attributable solely to a lower incidence of local reactions and that the incidence of systemic reactions is not affected.

Immunization Schedules

Three 0.5 ml doses of vaccine are administered IM at bimonthly intervals, usually beginning at 2 months of age. A booster dose should be given at 18 months and again at 4—5 years. Thereafter, the pertussis component is eliminated and DT or Td preparations are utilized. (Exceptions are noted under Pertussis, above.)

Precautions

As for the individual components.

POLIOMYELITIS

Poliovaccines afford a high degree of protection to individuals adequately immunized against all 3 types. Both inactivated (killed, Salk) and attenuated (oral, live, Sabin) vaccines produce satisfactory immunity.

The advantages of inactivated vaccine are that it cannot cause polio from the vaccine, the assurance that the vaccinee receives the vaccine, and simplicity of storage. The disadvantages include reduction in antibody titer and, presumably, immunity with the passage of time; the ability of wild poliovirus to grow in the intestinal tract of the vaccinee; and the need for repeated intramuscular injections.

The advantages of attenuated vaccine include ease of administration (oral); prolonged immunity; intestinal immunity, which prevents wild poliovirus multiplication in the intestinal tract; a lesser risk of sensitization to vaccine constituents other than poliovirus; and its ability to limit epidemics by mass application. Its disadvantages include uncertainty of adequate immunization if the vaccinee vomits or if it is given early in life or if the mother is breast-feeding; the potential instability of types 3 and 1, which appear to have reverted to neurovirulence and have produced clinical polio in a few recipients or contacts of recipients; and the need for storage and maintenance at freezing temperatures.

Within the pediatric age range, it would appear that attenuated vaccine in its trivalent form represents the safest, simplest, and most effective immunizing material. Until the issues are completely resolved, primary and so-called "booster" doses of poliovaccine should be the trivalent attenuated type.

In epidemics, monotypic vaccine corresponding to the epidemic type should be administered in a mass, short-term campaign. This method will result in limiting the epidemic but should be followed with efforts to provide protection against the nonepidemic types.

Some pediatricians prefer inactivated vaccine for primary immunization in the early months of life, with attenuated vaccine given subsequently. Their reasons include assurance of immunization coupled with demonstrated effectiveness. The only adverse consideration is the inability of inactivated vaccine to protect against intestinal multiplication and possible spread of wild poliovirus to unimmunized contacts.

The early problems with inactivated vaccine production which permitted live polio or simian viruses to remain in supposedly inactivated vaccine lots are no longer existent. The inactivated vaccines produced today are free of any demonstrable viral agent prior to release.

Vaccines Available

A. Inactivated Poliovaccine: This is a formaldehyde inactivated virus containing all 3 types (1, 2, and 3). The viruses are grown on monkey kidney tissue culture containing minute amounts of penicillin. Neomycin is added during manufacture to ensure sterility. The vaccine does not contain alum or any other adjuvant. The vaccine is supplied in 9 ml vials. The usual dose is 1 ml IM. It has become difficult to obtain this preparation.

B. Monovalent Attenuated Poliovirus Vaccine: This vaccine is supplied as the live attenuated virus, which is grown on monkey kidney tissue culture. The vaccines are monospecific, ie, they will confer protection only against the type administered. They must be stored at less than 0° C for maximum stability. If stored at ordinary refrigerator temperatures (0–4° C), the vaccine must be used within 30 days; once the vial is opened, the period of use is reduced to 7 days. In order to ensure stability, the freezer compartment of most office refrigerators will suffice provided ice can be maintained continuously as a solid. The dose is 200–500 thousand $TCID_{50}$. (Consult manufacturer's brochure for exact dosage.)

C. Trivalent Attenuated Poliovirus Vaccine: This preparation is similar to the monovalent preparation except that it contains all 3 types of poliovirus in a single dose. Each dose contains more types 1 and 3 polioviruses than type 2 in order to prevent inhibition of the others by type 2. Storage and dosage considerations are similar to those outlined above for the monovalent vaccine.

Immunization Schedules

Scheduling of polio immunization has undergone many revisions and a number of alternatives are available to the practitioner. A final and definitive schedule awaits long-term safety and immunity data. For the present, the following regimens are listed in the order of preference:

A. Trivalent Attenuated Vaccine Alone:

1. Infants—Three oral doses of trivalent vaccine are administered concurrently with DTP immunization at 2, 4, and 6 months of age. This regimen is followed by single doses of trivalent attenuated vaccine at 18 months and 4–6 years of age (just before entry into nursery school).

2. Older children—Two oral doses of trivalent attenuated vaccine are administered 6–8 weeks apart. This regimen can be utilized in the unimmunized; in those whose previous immunization is uncertain; in those who have received monovalent attenuated vaccines; or in those previously immunized with inactivated vaccine. An additional dose of trivalent vaccine should be given at entry into school or nursery school if this is 12 months or more following the initial series.

B. Monovalent Attenuated Vaccine:

1. Infants—Oral type 1 vaccine should be given first, followed in 6–8 weeks by type 3 and, in an additional 6–8 weeks, by type 2. This sequence is required to ensure that type 2 does not inhibit immunization with types 1 and 3.* Subsequent doses are given as trivalent vaccine at ages 18 months and 4–5 years.

2. Older children—The schedule is the same as for infants. Trivalent "booster" doses are given at suggested ages only if feasible; if the child is older, give one trivalent dose 12 months after the primary series.

C. Inactivated Vaccine: (Available but not recommended.)

1. Infants—Give three 1 ml doses IM at monthly intervals. The vaccine can be given in combination with DPT if mixed immediately prior to injection. Alternatively, give at a different site as a separate injection. Booster doses are given 12 months later and at approximately 2-year intervals for as long as protection is considered necessary. Some prefer to give trivalent attenuated vaccine after infancy. Conversion to live vaccine by 3 doses, 2 months apart, is advised except in cases with immunologic deficiencies.

2. Older children, adolescents, and adults—If inactivated vaccine is the desired method of immunization, follow the recommendations in ¶ 1, but do not administer attenuated vaccine to individuals over age 18. Immunity may be maintained by 1 ml inactivated vaccine every 2 years.

Precautions

Inactivated poliovaccine causes essentially no side-effects. It is an aqueous product and does not contain alum.

Attenuated poliovaccine is felt by some to be associated with a risk of paralytic polio. This is most apt to occur with type 3, less apt to occur with type 1, and rarely (if ever) occurs with type 2. The risk is 1:1,000,000 doses for type 3; 1:5,000,000 doses for type 1. For this reason, the Surgeon General recommends that attenuated poliovaccine not be administered to adults older than 18. The only exception is during an epidemic, when the risk of natural disease far outweighs any risk from the vaccine.

Antibody Preparations

Although much human gamma globulin is labeled polioimmune globulin, its use in the prevention of this disease is antiquated. Such labeling simply implies standardization of the preparation for its polio antibody content. It is true that polio can be prevented by the prophylactic use of gamma globulin, but there are no indications for its use for this purpose in modern medical practice.

*This is in accord with American Academy of Pediatrics recommendations. The USPHS Advisory Committee on Immunization Practices recommends the sequence 2-1-3.

MEASLES

Attenuated measles vaccine affords 95–100% protection against natural disease. Immunity appears to be long-lived—probably lifetime—but the exact duration will only be determined by continued observation. Each of the attenuated vaccines is associated with a predictable febrile response and, in some instances, a morbilliform rash. The incidence of fever and rash is reduced by concomitant administration of measles immune globulin or by the use of further attenuated measles vaccine instead of the Edmonston attenuated strain (see below).

Inactivated measles vaccines are associated with relatively short-term immunity and a sufficient incidence of serious immunologic effects to warrant discontinuation of their use. Inactivated vaccines have demonstrated an altered reactivity to live measles virus, resulting in unusual local reactions to subsequent live virus administration and in a "new" disease—atypical measles—upon exposure to the wild virus.

Vaccines Available

A. **Attenuated Measles Virus Vaccine, Edmonston Strain (Enders Vaccine):** The Edmonston virus, originally isolated in human cells, has been adapted to chick embryo tissue culture, in which the vaccine is prepared. It is supplied in individual 0.5 ml doses and in multiple dose vials as a freeze-dried (lyophilized) vaccine with accompanying diluent and syringe for administration. Since attenuated measles virus is easily inactivated by trace preservatives and antiseptics, great care must be taken to use acceptable reconstituting fluid and syringes. The surest method is to use the supplied equipment and diluent. Dosage is as detailed by the manufacturer, and the vaccine is administered subcutaneously.

B. **Attenuated Measles Virus Vaccine, Edmonston Strain, Canine Kidney Adapted:** This vaccine is prepared essentially as above except that it has been adapted to grow in dog kidney tissue culture and less is known about this system in human immunization. The manufacturer recommends its use in egg-sensitive individuals who cannot be given the chick embryo tissue culture vaccine.

C. **Further Attenuated Measles Virus Vaccine (Schwarz Vaccine):** This product was prepared from Edmonston strain virus and passaged many additional times in chick embryo tissue culture. The result ·is further attenuation, with a lessened capacity for febrile and exanthematous reactions but apparent preservation of immunologic potency. The advantage of this vaccine is that it does not require simultaneous administration of measles immune globulin.

D. **Inactivated Measles Virus Vaccine:** Two preparations are marketed for use. One is prepared in monkey kidney tissue culture and the other in chick embryo tissue culture. The American Academy of Pediatrics has officially advised that its use be discontinued. For children already immunized, it is suggested that a subsequent dose of attenuated vaccine be used (see Immunization Schedules, below).

E. **Combined Vaccines:** Measles (rubeola) vaccine has been combined with rubella (German measles) virus alone, and also with both rubella and mumps viruses. At the time of this writing, only one commercial preparation of each combination is available. It is expected that many products will be forthcoming.

Immunization Schedules

Attenuated measles vaccine should be administered at age 1. Prior to this time, maternal antibody may interfere with immunization. However, in an epidemic situation it may be best to administer attenuated vaccine to the 6–12 month old child and repeat the dose 6 months later. A second dose administered to a child who has been immunized with attenuated virus vaccine has not been associated with any untoward effect. Children who received live measles virus vaccine in the past prior to 12 months of age should be reimmunized at present regardless of age.

For individuals older than age 1, a single dose of attenuated vaccine is sufficient. If the child has had natural measles but this is not certainly known, attenuated vaccine administration causes no untoward effects. A few susceptible adolescents and adults have been immunized with no greater clinical symptoms than those seen in infants and children.

Attenuated vaccine (Edmonston strain) can be given alone or simultaneously with measles immune globulin. If it is given alone, one can expect 80% of vaccinees to demonstrate some degree of fever 6–10 days after immunization. About 30% will have fever over 39.4° C (103° F), although most will be asymptomatic despite the fever. A very few children will appear ill and may be temporarily incapacitated and require bed rest. If measles immune globulin is administered at the same time but in a different site with a separate syringe, the febrile rate will be halved (15% with temperatures greater than 39.4° C). Similarly, the morbilliform rash that occurs in 50% of Edmonston vaccinees will be sharply reduced (to 5%) with simultaneous gamma globulin administration. Further attenuated vaccine administration results in fewer instances of fever (5–15%) and rash (5%). Thus, no concomitant measles immune globulin need be given.

The choice of attenuated vaccine for routine use is not arbitrary. Longer experience is available for the chick embryo adapted Edmonston strain; antibody persistence and protection upon exposure have been observed for almost 9 years after immunization. The further attenuated vaccine has not been evaluated for as long a period but has afforded protection for almost 6 years. Antibody stimulation is slightly less than for the Edmonston vaccine, but this appears to be of little clinical significance. The major virtue of the further attenuated vaccine is that concomitant measles immune globulin administration is not necessary. Significant fever occurs in only 5–15% of vaccinees, and the single injection required is a definite advantage.

A special use of attenuated measles vaccine is in the just-exposed child. If attenuated vaccine is administered just prior to or on the day of exposure to natural disease in a susceptible child, the disease may be prevented by successful immunization. This is because the incubation period of the vaccine is approximately 7 days, in contrast to a 10-day period for the natural disease. However, if exposure has occurred one or more days previously, it is best to administer a preventive dose of measles immune globulin and to administer live virus vaccine 6–8 weeks later.

Inactivated measles virus vaccine is no longer recommended. A state of altered immunologic reactivity to live virus, attenuated or wild, appears to be induced in some vaccinees. This will result in induration, erythema, and tenderness at the site of subsequent attenuated virus vaccine in 6–50% of previous recipients of inactivated vaccine. Additionally, upon exposure to natural disease months or years after receiving inactivated vaccine, some children develop an atypical measles characterized by pneumonia with or without pleural effusion, a petechial rash, edema, and temperatures of 39.4–40.6° C (103–105° F). Because of the risk of atypical measles, children who have been immunized with inactivated vaccine should be given attenuated vaccine. Although this may result in a local reaction in some cases, the risk is acceptable in the face of potential serious atypical measles.

Combinations of inactivated and attenuated vaccines are not recommended. All recipients of such combinations should be regarded as inactivated vaccine recipients, and a second dose of attenuated vaccine should be administered as above.

Precautions

Inactivated measles vaccine is not recommended. Its side-effects have been commented upon above.

Because attenuated measles vaccine has been associated with febrile convulsions, a history of febrile convulsions is a contraindication to its use. The vaccine has rarely been associated with CNS complications. As with any live vaccine, its administration to pregnant females and to infants and children with acquired or congenital immunologic deficiencies is contraindicated.

Vaccines prepared in chick embryo tissue should not be administered to children who cannot eat a whole egg without allergic symptoms. Similarly, dog dander or hair allergy contradicts the use of the canine kidney product. Egg-sensitive individuals can be given the dog kidney vaccine and dog-sensitive children the chick embryo adapted product.

Antibody Preparations

Measles immune globulin is human gamma globulin in which the measles antibody content is standardized at 4000 measles neutralizing units/ml. The dose for use in attenuated measles virus immunization is 0.01 ml/lb (0.025 ml/kg). In the prophylaxis of measles following natural exposure of a nonimmune individual, the dose is 0.1 ml/lb (0.25 ml/kg). This is the so-called preventive dose. Prevention of measles depends upon administration of an adequate dose early in the incubation period, usually within 6 days of exposure. The author believes the concept of modifying measles by administration of a smaller dose (0.02 ml/lb [0.05 ml/kg]) of gamma globulin following exposure is unwise. In the unimmunized susceptible, it is best to attempt protection with gamma globulin upon exposure and to administer attenuated vaccine 6–8 weeks later.

SMALLPOX

Smallpox immunization confers virtually 100% protection within 6–12 months following successful immunization and gradually diminishing protection against disease thereafter. At 20 years after immunization, protection is virtually nil. However, once successfully immunized, protection against death, if the disease is contracted, is of a very high order. Repeat successful vaccinations at 1–4 year intervals aid in the maintenance of a high level of immunity.

A recent decision of the WHO Expert Committee on Smallpox makes the definition of successful takes easier. Reactions following primary immunization are considered *major* if there is evidence of a take 7 days later–a vesicular lesion at 7–10 days in a primary take, or a vesicle, pustule, or definite induration and congestion surrounding an ulcer or scab following revaccination. All other reactions are *equivocal* and an indication for revaccination. Almost everyone can be vaccinated; the few people in whom successful takes repeatedly fail fall into 2 categories: (1) those who are vaccinated by improper technic or with impotent vaccine, and (2) true nonreactors (rare). The former can be successfully vaccinated by an experienced person. The latter probably have had an active-passive immunization earlier and are truly resistant to reimmunization, although a very rare individual defies explanation.

Vaccines Available

A. Calf Lymph Smallpox Vaccine: This preparation is derived from the dermal pulp of vaccinia virus infected calves. The vaccine contains 100 million pock-forming units of vaccinia virus supplied either as a glycerinated aqueous preparation or freeze-dried (lyophilized). The dose is not a measured one but consists of enough virus to produce a localized skin infection when the skin underlying a drop of vaccine is scratched or multiply punctured.

B. "Avianized" Smallpox Vaccine: This product is derived from an egg-adapted vaccinia virus strain. It is as potent in titer as the calf lymph vaccine but produces milder vaccination reactions. Its use is as described under calf lymph vaccine.

Immunization Schedules

Smallpox vaccination as a routine compulsory immunization is no longer recommended. The World

Health Organization, the USPHS Advisory Committee of Immunization Practices, and the Red Book Committee of the American Academy of Pediatrics are unanimous in this recommendation. It is advised that health care personnel, especially those working in hospitals, maintain immunity against smallpox.

Precautions

See Vaccinia in Chapter 26.

Antibody Preparations

Vaccinia immune globulin (VIG) is human gamma globulin collected from young military recruits following vaccination. Its titer is variable but usually approximates 620 neutralizing antibody units—in comparison with a titer of 64 or less in randomly collected gamma globulin. It is used in complications of vaccination, and the dosage is variable (0.3–0.6 ml or more per kg body weight IM). (See Chapter 26.)

RUBELLA

Rubella is a benign disease of childhood. The major reason for immunization is to prevent rubella infection of pregnant females and subsequent fetal infection. In 1964, more than 20,000 infants died or were permanently handicapped as a result of intrauterine rubella infection.

Immunization is recommended by the various immunization advisory committees for all prepubertal children in the USA. In England and elsewhere, immunization is only recommended among women of childbearing age. The basic premise behind the USA recommendation is that herd immunity would result, ie, the primary reservoir of rubella infection (in young school-age children) would be reduced, thereby protecting susceptible pregnant women. This hypothesis is untried, and recent evidence suggests that it may not be valid. In populations with 85–95% immunes, rubella infection occurred in all remaining susceptibles. On the other hand, immunization of adult females has several hazards; the incidence of arthritis is higher, and the potential for infecting products of conception in an undiagnosed pregnancy has been demonstrated.

The efficacy of rubella immunization is conjectural at present. More than 96% of recipients develop demonstrable serum antibody, and short-term exposure trials have demonstrated protection against disease. However, reinfection with mild rubella virus occurs in individuals previously immunized, and it is not known whether a previously immunized pregnant female who is reinfected will transmit the virus to her fetus. Most virologists do not believe intrauterine infection will occur in the fetuses of previously immunized pregnant women because viremia has not been demonstrated.

Rubella virus is recoverable from the throat in more than 75% of recipients of vaccine. The virus is present in low titers, and except in a few instances transmission to a susceptible contact has not been observed. It thus appears unlikely that a susceptible pregnant woman will contract rubella from an immunized child, although the potential exists.

Arthritis and arthralgia have been observed in recipients of rubella virus vaccine. In children, the frequency is low except when canine kidney-grown virus vaccine is used. In adolescents and adults, over 10–30% of recipients have had this manifestation of immunization, paralleling the incidence in natural disease.

Peripheral neuritis, resulting in prolonged and painful neuromuscular syndromes, has been observed infrequently in children who have received rubella vaccine. Two forms are thus far recognized: one affecting the upper extremities with severe, recurrent pain; and another affecting the lower extremities, resulting in a peculiar crouching posture. The exact significance and extent of these syndromes is not defined at present.

The author feels there is sufficient uncertainty about the effectiveness of mass rubella immunization, sufficient question concerning pharyngeal virus growth in the vaccinee, and sufficient doubt about the significance of side-effects to question the wisdom of utilizing rubella vaccine routinely in childhood. A preferable alternative at present would be to immunize all prepubescent females, to test all women in the childbearing age group for rubella antibody, and to immunize those who are susceptible (approximately 15%). It is necessary to make absolutely certain that pregnancy is avoided for at least 2 months following such immunization.

Vaccines Available

Several different preparations are now commercially available. The reader is advised to consult the manufacturers' brochures concerning specific instructions for administration.

Two recently licensed products with which experience is limited incorporate rubella virus with measles in one preparation and with measles and mumps in the other. There is no loss of antigenicity in these combinations, and they appear to be safe.

Immunization Schedules

At present, all official advisory bodies recommend routine immunization of all prepubertal children. For future application, all children at 12 months should be given the vaccine. Please note the author's reservations as detailed above.

Precautions

The usual precautions concerning live virus vaccines apply to rubella virus vaccine also. (See Measles, above.)

In addition, rubella virus immunization of all females who can become pregnant (regardless of chronologic age) should only be undertaken (1) after susceptibility has been determined by serologic testing (available in most State Health Department laboratories), and (2) with assurance by appropriate contraceptive means that the woman will not become pregnant for at least 2 months following immunization.

Rubella virus immunization may result in arthritic symptomatology or in peripheral neuritis syndromes. These conditions postdate immunization by as much as 70 days, and the association may not be apparent unless sought.

Antibody Preparations

No specific rubella gamma globulin preparation exists. Standard pooled adult gamma globulin has been used in exposed pregnant females in an effort to prevent transplacental virus transmission. Results to date have been unsatisfactory with doses of 20–40 ml IM.

Center for Disease Control: Rubella virus vaccine: Recommendation of the Public Health Service Advisory Committee on Immunization Practices. Ann Int Med 75:757–759, 1971.

MUMPS

Mumps is generally a benign disease which in most children is either asymptomatic or causes only mild to moderate symptoms. Infection may be accompanied by aseptic meningitis, pancreatitis, or orchitis or oophoritis. The gonadal complications are the major reasons for protecting adolescents and adults against mumps. An attenuated vaccine has recently become available which induces antibody in 98% of susceptible vaccinees, and early studies indicate almost complete protection for 1 year and possibly for 2 years. Further data on the duration of immunity will become available with continuing observation of vaccinees.

Inactivated vaccine confers only partial and short-lived immunity; it is not a very good immunizing agent.

Vaccines Available

A. Attenuated Mumps Vaccine, Jeryl-Lynn Strain: This vaccine is a chick embryo adapted mumps virus to which neomycin has been added. It is supplied as a freeze-dried (lyophilized) powder to be reconstituted according to the manufacturer's directions. Its stability is such that reconstituted vaccine must be used within 8 hours, preferably immediately. Storage of the dry powder is at ordinary refrigerator temperatures. The vaccine is light-sensitive and should be protected from sunlight. The dosage is 0.5 ml IM.

B. Inactivated Mumps Vaccine: This is a formalin and ethylene oxide inactivated vaccine prepared in hen's eggs. The dosage is 1 ml subcut or IM.

C. Combined Vaccine: Mumps vaccine has been combined with measles and rubella virus vaccines. In the combined vaccine, it appears to be antigenic and safe.

Immunization Schedules

Routine mumps vaccination in childhood is now recommended by the Committee on Infectious Diseases of the American Academy of Pediatrics. Mumps immunization has a lower priority than any of the others discussed above, but it is especially recommended that the following groups who have not had mumps should receive the vaccine: children approaching puberty; adolescents and adults, particularly males; institutionalized children; and children in large groups where epidemic mumps may disrupt normal routines. Routine use in children should be limited to those over age 1 and only after DTP and poliomyelitis immunizations are complete.

Inactivated mumps vaccine has a very limited usefulness. It is generally recommended as a postexposure (within 2–3 days) immunization. The author is not convinced of its efficacy. It is definitely not recommended for routine use.

The susceptible exposed adolescent or adult poses a difficult problem. It has been estimated that oophoritis occurs in 5% of females with mumps and unilateral orchitis in 20–30% of males. Although sterility is an extremely uncommon result, the gonadal infection is an uncomfortable and incapacitating one. Current methods of prophylaxis are not reliable. Inactivated vaccine is of dubious value, and mumps immune globulin (see below) is said to reduce orchitis by 75% (although adequate studies are lacking). The best course appears to be to administer attenuated mumps vaccine prior to exposure. It has no value at or following exposure because antibody development requires 28 days.

Precautions

As with other live vaccines, mumps vaccine should not be given to pregnant females or to children with congenital or acquired immunologic deficiencies. Egg-sensitive individuals should not receive this product (see Measles above). No untoward reactions have been observed in a small number of adults given the vaccine.

Antibody Preparations

Mumps immune globulin is human gamma globulin obtained from hyperimmunized donors. The mumps antibody content is 20 times that of human mumps immune serum.

Mumps immune globulin is supplied in 1.5 and 4.5 ml vials. The dose is 1.5 ml IM for a child and 3–4.5 ml IM for individuals over age 12.

SPECIFIC IMMUNIZATIONS
FOR SPECIAL CIRCUMSTANCES

RABIES

In the USA, about 50,000 persons receive rabies immunization each year. The vast majority of these immunizations are unnecessary, but the disease is so feared and the circumstances surrounding many animal bites so uncertain that administration of the vaccine seems the safer course to follow. However, there is a predictable morbidity with rabies immunization, and if unnecessary immunizations are given too frequently the risk of complications of the vaccine or antiserum will outweigh the potential benefits. The physician must know the epidemiology of rabies in his area. A bite from a pet beagle is not equivalent to a similar bite from a stray street dog. In the first situation, rabies is exceedingly unlikely, and in the second it is a distinct possibility. The often quoted WHO recommendations will not be repeated here since they are not applicable to most of the world and certainly not to most of the USA. The physician is referred to his state health department and to the USPHS for accurate local information about rabies epidemiology in his area of practice.

Vaccines Available
A. **Inactivated Rabies Vaccine, Animal Nervous Tissue Origin (Semple Vaccine):** This is a sterile suspension of rabies virus in rabbit brain and spinal cord. The vaccine is prepared from animals 6 days after inoculation with fixed virus. The virus is then inactivated by phenol (Semple method) and supplied in individual dose ampules.
B. **Inactivated Rabies Vaccine, Duck Embryo Tissue Origin:** This consists of propiolactone inactivated virus to which various stabilizing agents are added plus thimerosal as a preservative. Antibody develops within 10–15 days after initiation of daily immunization. The vaccine is distributed as single dose vials with diluent in a package containing 14 doses. Follow the manufacturer's recommendations for storage, reconstitution, and dosage.

Vaccine Schedules
A. **Preexposure Immunization:** This is recommended for persons at high risk of exposure—veterinarians, laboratory technicians working with diagnostic specimens or rabies virus, deliverymen and others who are frequently bitten by dogs, spelunkers (cave explorers) exposed to bats in caves, etc. Two effective schedules are employed: (1) three injections of 1 ml subcut at weekly intervals, followed by 1 ml subcut in 5–6 months; (2) two injections of 1 ml subcut 1 month apart and then 1 ml subcut 7 months later. Booster doses of 1 ml are suggested every 1–2 years. Antibody titers must be determined, because protection is not 100% effective.

B. **Postexposure Immunization:** Because the incubation period of rabies is often prolonged, postexposure immunization is feasible. The exact regimen used is empiric and largely based upon Pasteur's original schedule coupled with antibody stimulation data. The usual regimen is to give 14–21 subcutaneous injections of 1 ml each. Injections are usually given over the abdomen, each one in a different site. Severe bites or bites about the head and neck are indications for prolonging the daily injections to 21 days. In individuals who have been bitten by wild animals, it may be desirable to give twice daily doses of vaccine for 7 days and daily doses for 7 more days in an attempt to stimulate early antibody production. If the animal is healthy after 5 days, the injections should be discontinued. All other patients are treated for at least 14 days. If severe systemic reactions or neuroparalytic complications occur, the injections must be discontinued.

The most difficult decision is whom to immunize. The WHO guidelines are not universally applicable, and more harm than good may follow indiscriminate rabies immunization in an area where there is no risk of rabies. The practitioner must be guided by the rabies epidemiologic data in his area. Nevertheless, some general guidelines can be suggested.

1. Wild animal bites, particularly those by skunks and bats, are absolute indications for rabies prophylaxis.

2. Pets seldom become infected unless exposed to a rabid animal. Pets with current rabies immunization are obviously not a risk.

3. Provoked bites in toddlers are seldom an indication for immunization, particularly if the animal is a pet.

4. Stray animals pose a special problem since they frequently cannot be found. The physician must depend upon current epidemiologic information and balance the risks of immunizing against the possibility of rabies.

5. Rodents are seldom infected with rabies.

6. If in doubt and the animal is impounded, begin immunization and discontinue the series after 5 days if the animal remains healthy. The complications of immunization are uncommon before the fifth day, and a rabid animal will not appear healthy 5 days after biting someone. If the animal sickens or dies, it is essential that adequate virologic examination be carried out by the local public health authorities.

Surgical Management & Antiserum
Adequate prophylaxis against rabies must include (1) extensive surgical (possibly chemical) debridement of the bites as quickly as possible after the episode (excisional surgery is best) and (2) concomitant use of rabies antiserum (see below). There is strong evidence that rabies antiserum offers protection to some individuals. It should be used in adequate doses (1000 units/40 lb to a maximum of 6000 units). Some experts suggest infiltration around the bite with part of the serum. This is horse serum, and the usual precautions should be observed.

For maximal benefit, the antiserum should be administered as soon as possible after the bite—ie, within 24 hours if possible and certainly within 72 hours. When rabies antiserum is used, additional doses of rabies vaccine (preferably avian type) should be given 10 and 20 days after completion of the primary series.

Precautions

Approximately 1:6000 rabies immunizations with animal brain tissue result in neurologic sequelae. These consist of 3 clinical types: encephalitic, myelitic, and neuritic. The encephalitis has its onset suddenly 6—54 days following the first dose of vaccine. Chills, fever, headache, vomiting, and changes in mental state are observed. The myelitic and neuritic complications are paralytic, usually consisting of flaccid paralysis of the lower extremities. Its onset is more gradual. The neurologic sequelae are usually not fatal, although as many as 35% result in permanent residual deficits.

Duck embryo vaccine has been associated with 4 cases of neurologic sequelae in 90,000 14-day courses—a very low reaction rate. Much more common is the occurrence of tenderness, erythema, and induration at the site of inoculation. These local reactions tend to occur after the fifth day and may be associated with a flare-up at previous injection sites. Lymph node enlargement and tenderness can also be observed. Rarely, anaphylactic shock has occurred. Great caution should be exercised in persons with known egg allergy.

Antibody Preparations

Rabies antiserum is horse serum containing 1000 units/ml of rabies neutralizing antibody. All of the precautions in administration of horse serum should be observed.

INFLUENZA VACCINE

Although some doubt the efficacy of influenza vaccines, most experts agree that protection in excess of 65—75% can be expected with their use. Non-epidemic influenza is a relatively unimportant cause of serious childhood respiratory infections. Epidemic or pandemic influenza may result in significant morbidity in very young infants and in individuals with chronic cardiac, pulmonary, metabolic, renal, or neurologic disease. Furthermore, institutionalized children may constitute a unique epidemiologic setting, facilitating rapid spread. These groups should be immunized regularly, but especially in epidemic years. Pandemic spread may require more broad-scale immunization of healthy infants and children, particularly when a new antigenic strain appears.

Vaccines Available

Inactivated aqueous influenza virus vaccine (polyvalent or bivalent) is an egg-grown vaccine virus inacti-

vated with formaldehyde. All such vaccines contain 600 CCA (chick cell agglutination) units, the maximum allowable. Polyvalent vaccine contains influenza A, A_1, and A_2 viruses plus influenza B viruses; the bivalent vaccine contains influenza A_1 and A_2 viruses and influenza B viruses, allowing a higher concentration of the currently infective strains. The recommended route for primary immunization is subcutaneous injection; for booster doses, either the subcutaneous or intradermal route can be used. For children 3 months to 5 years of age, the recommended dose is 0.1—0.2 ml; for those 6—12 years of age, 0.5 ml; and for children over 12 years of age, the full adult dose of 1 ml is recommended.

Immunization Schedules

Primary immunization should be started in late summer or early fall and be completed by late fall or early winter, depending upon the current epidemiologic situation. Primary immunization consists of the appropriate dose for age administered in 2 doses 2 months apart. For children under 5 years of age, 2 doses 1—2 weeks apart followed in 2—3 months by a third dose is suggested.

Booster doses should be given yearly or at least within 3 years of primary immunization. The appropriate dose for age is administered subcutaneously or intracutaneously.

Precautions

Local and systemic reactions resembling mild to moderate influenza (fever, chills, malaise, tenderness at injection site) may occur in as many as 50% of children inoculated. Higher doses of vaccine are associated with a greater risk.

Since the vaccine is prepared in eggs, it should not be given to egg-sensitive individuals.

TUBERCULOSIS

BCG (bacille Calmette Guérin) vaccine is an attenuated tuberculosis vaccine which is indicated for children in geographic areas or in social circumstances where the risk of infection is high. A positive tuberculin test renders BCG unnecessary and potentially dangerous. The vaccine should not be given to any child with acquired or congenital immunologic deficiency.

Immunization is accomplished by intracutaneous, superficial injection over the deltoid or triceps muscle. The dosage is 0.05 ml (newborns) or 0.1 ml for all other children.

CHOLERA

For infants and children traveling to or resident in cholera endemic areas, 3 intramuscular or subcutaneous injections at weekly (or longer) intervals are advised. The dosage is as follows. Booster doses appropriate to age must be given as often as every 6 months to maintain immunity.

	6 Months– 4 Years	5–9 Years	10 Years– Adult
First dose	0.1 ml	0.3 ml	0.5 ml
Second dose	0.3 ml	0.5 ml	0.5 ml
Third dose	0.3 ml	0.5 ml	Omit

PLAGUE

Plague immunization may be desirable for infants and children traveling to currently endemic areas (consult authorities). Age-related dosage is the same as for cholera vaccine (see above). Plague vaccine is given subcutaneously. In children under 10 years of age, the doses should be spaced at weekly intervals; for those older than 10 years, they may be spaced 7–28 days apart. Booster doses appropriate to age may be given within 4 years of the last dose, but in endemic areas boosters may be required every 4–6 months.

YELLOW FEVER

Yellow fever vaccine is obtainable only from certain public health facilities. A single injection of 0.5 ml of a 1:10 dilution is given, with a similar booster dose every 6 years. For travel to certain areas, this immunization is mandatory. Consult authorities.

EPIDEMIC TYPHUS

Vaccination against epidemic typhus is recommended for persons traveling to endemic areas even though it is not required. The vaccine is given subcutaneously. The dosage is as follows:

	6 Months– 4 Years	5–9 Years	10 Years– Adult
First dose	0.2 ml	0.5 ml	1 ml
Second dose	0.2 ml	0.5 ml	1 ml
Third dose	0.2 ml	0.5 ml	1 ml

For children under 10 years of age the vaccine is given every 1–3 weeks; for those over age 10, the first 2 doses are separated by 1–3 weeks and the third is given 1 year later. Annual boosters are recommended.

IMMUNOPROPHYLAXIS & THERAPY

INFECTIOUS HEPATITIS

Human gamma globulin can convert icteric hepatitis to anicteric disease if administered prior to or following exposure. The dosage has been the subject of controversy, but the following schedule appears reasonable: (1) Household exposure, 0.02–0.04 ml/kg. (2) Intensive prolonged exposure or travel to high-risk areas, 0.1 ml/kg and repeat in 6 months as necessary.

GAS GANGRENE

Passive antibody therapy or prophylaxis with gas gangrene antitoxin is not recommended since it appears to be of no benefit.

RUBELLA

There is no indication for immune prophylaxis of rubella in children. The data on protection of susceptible pregnant females are contradictory. Some authorities suggest giving 20–40 ml of human gamma globulin IM as soon after exposure as possible. Serologic diagnosis is available and should be utilized to prove the existence of susceptibility and infection. (See Chapter 26.)

VARICELLA-ZOSTER

Large doses of human gamma globulin (0.2–0.6 ml/kg) administered to healthy children can ameliorate but not prevent varicella. However, its use in healthy children is not recommended. One may wish to administer gamma globulin to very young infants and to children suffering from lymphatic malignancies since varicella-zoster infections may result in serious illness or death in such cases.

Limited evidence suggests that massive doses (in excess of 1 ml/kg) of gamma globulin may be beneficial in established varicella-zoster infections.

A new preparation, zoster immune globulin (ZIG), is under study, and preliminary data suggest that it will be useful in preventing infection in individuals who are very susceptible to varicella-zoster infection by virtue of congenital or acquired immunologic deficiency. Convalescent plasma may also be useful, although a risk of transmitting serum hepatitis exists with this material.

BOTULISM

Although firm evidence for its efficacy is lacking, botulism antitoxin (horse serum) is accepted as a therapeutic tool in botulism. The dose is 2–10 thousand units of the appropriate antitoxin if the type of toxin present is known; if not, polyvalent antitoxin should be used. The antitoxin should be given intravenously with appropriate precautions against horse serum sensitivity.

IN BURNS

There is suggestive (but inconclusive) evidence that 1 ml/kg of human gamma globulin administered shortly after a major burn and repeated in 2 days may result in a reduction of pseudomonas sepsis in certain children.

UNPROVED OR UNWARRANTED USES OF HUMAN GAMMA GLOBULIN

There is little or no evidence—and in some cases there is contrary evidence—that human gamma globulin exerts any effect in recurrent colds, nasal allergy, asthma, herpes simplex infection, or bacterial infections in general. Although there are advocates for its use in each of these disorders, the evidence is anecdotal and controlled studies have failed to substantiate the claims.

• • •

General References

Committee on Infectious Diseases: *Report,* 16th ed. American Academy of Pediatrics, 1970.

Parry WH: Recent trends in immunization and vaccination. Abstr World Med 43:545–556, 1969.

Plotkin SA: The future of vaccines against viral diseases. P Clin North America 15:447–472, 1968.

Public Health Service Advisory Committee on Immunization Practices: Collected recommendations of the Public Health Service Advisory Committee on Immunization Practices (supplement). Morbidity & Mortality (US Department of Health, Education, and Welfare) 18:1–31, 1969.

Riley HD Jr: Current concepts in immunization. P Clin North America 13:75–104, 1966.

6...

Ambulatory Pediatrics

Barton D. Schmitt, MD, Burris R. Duncan, MD, & Conrad M. Riley, MD

This chapter offers guidelines for the conduct of 4 specific types of pediatric visit: (1) well child care, (2) acute illness care, (3) chronic disease follow-up, and (4) consultation. Each type of visit requires a specific service that is different in many ways from the others. If the pediatrician and his staff can mentally classify the patients in this way and vary their approach accordingly, the delivery of pediatric care will become more logical and consistent.

This organization of ambulatory care has 3 general advantages: (1) The quality of care improves since the patient benefits from the comprehensiveness of care that only a systematic approach can ensure. (2) The practice of pediatrics becomes more enjoyable because the establishment of clear office guidelines and policies prevents many frustrations and much duplication of effort for the physician. (3) The cost of medical care is reduced by increasing the efficiency of health care delivery.

Samples of forms, flow sheets, etc discussed in this chapter may be found on pp 145–160. No permission is required to reproduce them.—*The Editors.*

WELL CHILD VISITS

OBJECTIVES

The well child visit is a multipurpose, triangular experience which is best conducted in a relaxed setting. It should be a scheduled appointment with sufficient time allotted for adequate communication and examination. The patient, the parent, and the physician must be satisfied with the experience.

The visit is a time for unhurried discussion of the parents' concerns about their child and an opportunity for the pediatrician to help educate the parents about growth and development, to clarify behavior and discipline, to dispel parental anxiety, and to offer anticipatory guidance. One objective is to help the parents and child derive greater pleasure from each other. The examination is calculated to serve as a screen for deviations in perceptual, emotional, intellectual, and physical development.

Unfortunately, many parents and some physicians consider immunizations the most important aspect of the well child visit. Most physicians realize that they have a responsibility not only to protect the child against communicable disease but also to help the parents nurture their children in appropriate ways as they develop from dependent infants to mature adults. The well child visit serves an educational function in helping parents accept their children as individuals and guide their development. The early developmental years are difficult ones; the well child visit should be used to make them easier and better.

As the physician listens to and deals with parental concerns, discusses the child's development, and examines the child, there should develop a growing trust between the parents, the physician, and the child. A secure relationship established early will be of great help in the total therapy of the child when he is sick. Children tend to get sick very quickly, and it is during these times of acute stress that a familiar face and a familiar hand can restore balance to the situation.

CONTENT OF THE WELL CHILD VISIT*

1. PARENTAL CONCERNS

The first part of each well child visit should be directed toward dealing with the current concerns of the parent, usually the mother. Most expectant mothers have many questions which should be discussed with their pediatrician several weeks prior to delivery. The most frequent concerns include the arguments for and against breast feeding, preparation of the breasts if breast feeding is to be used, hospital policies about when the mother can hold her baby and begin his care, separation problems with the other children during the mother's confinement, and ways of

*Growth and development are discussed in Chapter 2.

decreasing sibling jealousy. It has been traditional for the first newborn office visit to take place at 6 weeks, probably because 6 weeks is the traditional time for the mother's first postdelivery obstetric visit. However, most mothers—particularly primaparas—have many questions and concerns well before this traditional interval after birth. A 2-week postpartal office visit is perhaps more logical.

The early weeks and months are characterized by rapid change. The infant doubles his birth weight in the first 5 months and triples it within the first year. His length increases 50% in the first year, but it takes 4½ more years for it to increase another 50%. His head circumference increases 40% in 1 year, whereas in the next 17 years head circumference increases only another 16%. The newborn changes from a totally dependent, passive individual who sleeps 18—20 hours a day into a curious, mobile, independent, negative 2-year-old. This constant confrontation with change often causes anxiety, concern, and frustration in the parents. During the well child visit the physician must encourage the parent to vent those feelings and he must be prepared to deal with them. Questions range from, "How frequently should I hold him?" to "Is it all right to spank children?" to "How old should he be before I should let him cross the street alone?" Many of the questions have no clear-cut answers. Many should not be answered, but all should be discussed.

2. ANTICIPATORY GUIDANCE

The well child visit is an opportunity to prepare the parents for the problems which normal development will probably create between this visit and the next. A list of suggested topics to discuss at particular ages is part of the well child flow sheet (see p 145). These topics can be covered in a variety of ways. Some physicians prefer to discuss all the items with the parents personally; others prefer to delegate the discussion of these issues to an assistant, who might be either a nurse or a nonprofessional assistant; and still others use printed materials which can be supplemented by personal comments as the need arises.

American Academy of Pediatrics: *Standards of Child Health Care.* Council of Pediatric Practice, 1967.

Patterson GR, Gullion ME: *Living with Children.* Research Press, 1968.

Silver HK, Kempe CH, Kempe RS: *Healthy Baby—Happy Parents.* Blakiston, 1960.

Smith JM, Smith DE: *Child Management: A Program for Parents.* Ann Arbor Publishers, 1967.

3. EXAMINATION OF THE PEDIATRIC PATIENT

The content of the physical examination of the well child depends upon the age of the child and the purpose for which the examination is done. The examination done in the delivery room or the first newborn office visit is far different from the preschool physical, and each is quite different from the examination required for participation in high school athletics.

THE NEWBORN EXAMINATION

Growth

A. Weight: An infant should gain 15—30 gm/day during the first 4 or 5 months of life. The newborn will regain his birth weight by age 10 days; at 2 weeks, he should weigh at least 60—120 gm more than his birth weight; and at 6 weeks he should weigh 480—960 gm more than he weighed at birth (a gain of 15—30% for a 3200 gm neonate). This evaluation provides a lot of information about nutritional status, feeding and elimination, and perhaps even about the mother-child relationship.

B. Head Circumference: The head circumference at birth is frequently not accurate as a result of molding, scalp edema, or cephalhematoma, and is more accurate at the time of discharge. By 2 weeks of age, an exact measurement can be obtained as a reference point for further measurements of head circumference. By 6 weeks, the head circumference is in its steepest growth curve and should have increased about 3 cm.

C. Length: The newborn's length increases about 10% in the first 6 weeks of life from a mean of 50 cm to a mean of 56 cm.

Vision

Most newborns have the visual capacity to fix on a moving object as early as the first few minutes of life. Infants who do not follow a face at the first well child visit should be suspected of having a visual problem. Ophthalmoscopic examination should be done on one of the earliest possible visits in order to make the diagnosis of cataract, congenital glaucoma, or retinal abnormality.

Hearing

A procedure for detection of congenital deafness is discussed in Chapter 11. Infants are exposed to a sound centering around 3000 cps at 90 db and their responses recorded. Infants found to have significant hearing loss have been fitted with hearing aids by 1 month of age. An audiologic high-risk registry program is also used at the University of Colorado Medical Center, and infants who are put into that registry and who are subsequently found to have a profound neurosensory hearing loss are so identified by 6 months of age. Infants with profound neurosensory hearing loss who are neither screened as newborns nor evaluated as part of a high-risk registry program are (on the average) not detected until they are 20 months of age. Programs are available to prevent this prolonged lag in detection and subsequent treatment so that children can receive the audiologic input necessary for normal language development. Every physician who is responsible for the care of infants should develop similar screening programs in the hospital nursery or at least check the infant's hearing at the first visit by the use of squeak toys and bells which have as close to pure tone sounds as possible. The newborn will only respond by a flicker of his eyelids or a very minute Moro response.

Congenital Anomalies

Close attention to relatively minor malformations detectable by surface examination will alert the physician to the possibility of major internal malformations. In one important study (see Marden reference, below), 14% of newborns examined were found to have a single minor anomaly but no appreciable increase in the frequency of associated major abnormalities over the general newborn population; 0.8% of babies had 2 minor external defects which carried a 15% frequency of major internal abnormalities; and 0.5% with 3 or more minor anomalies had a 90% incidence of major defects. The minor abnormalities described in this study usually go undetected unless specifically looked for. Examples include lateral displacement of the inner epicanthic folds, downslanting or upslanting palpebral fissures, preauricular cutaneous tags or pits, incomplete helix development, absence of the lobulus of the pinna, low-set ears, simian crease, bridged palmar creases, short and broad nails, hypoplasia of the nails, clinodactyly of the fifth finger, deep dimples at bony promontories (elbows, sacrum), low posterior hairline, body hirsutism, multiple hair whorls, pectus excavatum, and short sternum.

The Mother-Child Relationship

A very important question to ask of each new mother is, "Do you enjoy your baby?" The response is sometimes not congruent with what is observed as she handles her child. Many mothers will frankly admit they do not enjoy caring for the child but then feel guilty about that attitude. They need a listener and someone who can help them find ways to derive pleasure from their offspring. This must be done as early as possible; if it is not, the mother-child relationship may become more disturbed and the child will make life miserable for everyone around him. The situation then "snowballs" and becomes extremely difficult to resolve.

Early discussions should include what the parents expect from their child, whether the expectations are realistic, and how the parents resolve the difficulty when the child fails to meet those expectations.

Some mothers are highly maternal and others treat their newborns in a detached way. Observing an occipital bald spot and poor skin care tends to confirm an early suspicion of some disturbance in the mother-child relationship.

EXAMINATION BEFORE ENTERING SCHOOL

The preschool examination of the 4- or 5-year-old child should be designed to answer the basic question, "Is the child ready for school?" Listening to the child's chest at this examination is probably of far less importance than determining if he has any speech impediments, if his vision and hearing are normal, if his developmental age is commensurate with his chronologic age, and if his parents have adequately prepared him for the separation implied by entering school. This is not to say that these variables are not investigated prior to age 5; however, it is at the preschool examination that they are of greatest significance.

Vision

Five to 10% of preschool children have some kind of visual impairment. The illiterate E chart, Snellen chart, or Allen cards can be used for checking visual acuity, and each eye should be tested separately. The 5-year-old child should have a visual acuity of 20/30 or better in both eyes, and there should be no more than a 2-line difference between the 2 eyes. Amblyopia ex anopsia affects 2—5% of children and must be detected early before permanent loss of vision occurs. Amblyopia is frequently secondary to strabismus, which can be detected by noting the position where light is reflected off both corneas or by using the more refined cover test (see Chapter 9).

Hearing

Hearing deficits occur in approximately 1% of young school children, and in 10% of those children the loss is profound and bilateral. Most children with hearing loss have recurrent chronic otitis media or. serous otitis media. Even children with a single episode of otitis media may have some degree of hearing impairment for 3—6 months after the acute episode. Although the losses are generally not too severe, if they occur at an inopportune time they may be sufficient to prevent an early school-age child from learning phonics; hence, the effect of the loss may be carried on and magnified throughout much of the school years. If such losses are detected before entry into school, some of the learning problems and some of the behavior and discipline problems which occur secondary to poor attention might be averted. Detection of such problems is as much a part of preventive pediatrics as is the immunization routine. Audiologic screening tests can be performed by nonprofessional technicians and should be a part of the preschool examination.

Speech

The child entering school should be able to speak distinctly and clearly without difficulty. He should be able to answer questions and, after a period of getting acquainted, carry on a conversation with the physician about recent events or tell a story about something he has experienced. Poor speech may impair the child's general performance in school. An easily administered articulation test has been developed which can be used as a screening test to identify children who should be referred to a speech pathologist for definitive evaluation (see Templin reference, below).

Emotional Development & Behavior

The assessment of emotional development and behavior is an important part of the preschool examination. In one study (see Stein reference, below), 42 physicians were observed conducting 673 well child clinic visits. On the average, they said fewer than 2 sentences per visit to the mother which were relevant to child behavior. Yet, when given the opportunity to respond to a questionnaire about behavior, 85% of mothers of preschool children (ages 1½–6 years) indicated one or more such concerns (mean of 3.5 concerns per child). A simple self-administered questionnaire is an effective and efficient device which not only indicates to the parent that the physician is interested in discussing behavioral problems and the emotional growth of the child but also helps the physician to concentrate on the areas of guidance which are most relevant to the mother's concerns.

A number of easily administered developmental tests are available. The Denver Developmental Screening Test (see Chapter 2) is extremely helpful in the younger age groups. For a school entrance examination, the Peabody Picture Vocabulary Test and Goodenough's Draw-A-Man Test can be useful; both are easily administered in the physician's office by a nurse or a trained allied health worker. They should not be thought of as more than screening tests, but they can be used to identify children with developmental lags who may have difficulty in the early months of school as well as those who may need to be referred for psychologic evaluation.

Physical, emotional, and developmental maturation proceeds at different rates for different children. Some children are ready for school long before their fifth birthday; others are not nearly ready at that age. Some parents tend to push their children into experiences that are beyond their capacities at a given age. Children should begin their school experiences with successes; the child who starts with failure is often criticized and becomes discouraged and less interested in school, so that a pattern of failure may develop. The child may continue to lag behind and miss the early fundamentals of learning which are the basis for further education. Many children develop behavioral disorders and truancy simply because they cannot read and so are unable to understand what is going on in the classroom. Part of the physician's role is to help parents recognize physical, emotional, and developmental lags early so that corrective measures can be taken to prepare the child for school. If, despite these efforts, the child is not ready for school, the physician must advise the parents appropriately.

THE TEENAGER*

The well child visit for the teenager who wants to participate in athletics or attend summer camp is also designed to elicit data about special concerns. Most such visits emphasize the physical fitness and immunologic status of the patient. The physician may be called upon to do mass examinations which are of little value other than to fulfill a legal requirement that all participating children should have "a physical." Physicians who examine professional athletes are interested in the player's strength, endurance, sensory perception, and judgment under game-simulated conditions. The physical examination for the high school athlete is usually done with the patient relaxed after sitting in the physician's office or standing in line at the school gymnasium. It is apt to consist of a standard inspection of the eyes, ears, and throat; auscultation of the heart and lungs; and palpation of the abdomen and checking for hernia. It would make more sense to examine the teenager's cardiovascular and respiratory systems after a quarter-mile run or its equivalent.

Ideally, the adolescent should be given the opportunity to discuss problems which are of concern to him as an adolescent—rapid changes in sexual development and interest, drugs, ambivalent feelings, and identity problems. He needs an understanding listener as much as he needs a physical examiner.

Bergstrom LB & others: A high risk registry to find congenital deafness. Otol Clin North America 4:369, 1971.

Frankenburg WK & others: Training the indigenous nonprofessional. J Pediat 77:564, 1970.

Goodenough FL: *Measurement of Intelligence by Drawing.* Harcourt Brace, 1926.

Harris DB: *Children's Drawings as Measures of Intellectual Maturity.* Harcourt Brace, 1963.

Marden PM, Smith DW, McDonald MJ: Congenital anomalies in the newborn infant, including minor variations. J Pediat 64:357, 1964.

Smith DW: *Recognizable Patterns of Human Malformation.* Saunders, 1970.

Stein OC: Content and method of health supervision by physicians seen in child health conferences in Baltimore, 1959. Am J Pub Health 52:1858, 1962.

Templin MC: Norms on a screening test of articulation for ages through 8. J Speech Hearing Dis 18:323, 1953.

Vision, Screening and the Schools. [Pamphlet.] National Society for Prevention of Blindness, 1969.

Willoughby JA, Haggerty RJ: A simple behavior questionnaire for preschool children. Pediatrics 34:798, 1964.

4. LABORATORY SCREENING TESTS

A well child flow sheet (see p 145) is a helpful reminder to the nurse and physician that certain proce-

*See also Chapter 7, Adolescence.

dures, laboratory tests, developmental evaluations, and immunizations are due. All of these items can be initiated by the nurse if the physician establishes the routine to be followed.

Blood

Iron deficiency anemia is found more often in lower socioeconomic populations and has its highest incidence in infants between 9 and 24 months of age. A routine hemoglobin or hematocrit is recommended in this age group and is particularly important in the child whose diet is low in iron-containing foods.

Some clinics advocate routine screening of all black children for sickle cell trait or disease and G6PD deficiency. The knowledge thus gained is helpful in evaluating anemia in the black population and might be used for genetic counseling.

Screening for phenylketonuria should be done by blood test in the hospital nursery prior to the infant's discharge, and in many states such a test is required by law. A victim of this condition who for some reason failed to ingest sufficient milk protein may have a negative test in the first few days of life and be positive only after hospital discharge. A reliable dip stick test for urine is available and can be used at the first newborn visit.

Urine

Routine urinalysis has a low yield in the asymptomatic patient. In contrast to the adult population, it is unusual for a child to have asymptomatic diabetes, and proteinuria is a very infrequent presentation for a renal abnormality in an asymptomatic child. Transient orthostatic proteinuria is frequently found, but its significance has not been determined. However, since the cost is low and an occasional abnormality is detected, a yearly urinalysis is suggested.

Urine cultures probably have a greater yield than microscopic examination of urinary sediment. Over 1/2 of children with significant bacteriuria have no pyuria. The more cultures taken, the greater the yield in detection of asymptomatic urinary tract infections.

Significant bacteriuria has been found in 1% of infants 1–4 days of age; in 2% of infants between 4–12 months; and in 1–1.5% of school-age girls (see Allen reference, below). If every girl had numerous urine cultures over a period of several years, up to 5% would be found to have a urinary tract infection. Several inexpensive methods are available to screen for bacteriuria (eg, Testuria). Methods that depend upon bacteria in the urinary tract to decrease the quantity of glucose in the urine are more difficult to use as screening tests, particularly in young children.

Screening for lead poisoning is extremely important in areas where the child has access to lead-based paint or soil contaminated by lead or where earthenware pots are used as containers for even mildly acid drinks.

Allen TD: Pathogenesis of urinary tract infections in children. New England J Med 273:1421, 1965.

Benson P, Chisholm J: A reliable qualitative urine coproporphyrin test for lead intoxication. J Pediat 56:759, 1960.

Kunin CM: Emergence of bacteriuria, proteinuria, and symptomatic urinary tract infections among a population of school girls followed for 7 years. Pediatrics 41:968, 1968.

5. IMMUNIZATIONS

A child's immunization status can be easily monitored on the well child flow sheet (see p 145). A record of the child's immunizations should also be given to the parents and updated by the nurse as additional immunizations are given.

The details of routine immunization of children are presented in Chapter 5.

PARTICIPATION OF PARAMEDICAL PERSONNEL

A number of paramedical personnel (social workers, visiting nurses, nutritionists) as well as volunteer or semiprofessional women have been helping physicians take care of patients for many years. Only large clinics or group practices are able to employ and fully utilize such a variety of health workers. Some smaller pediatric offices have found it helpful to employ a social worker 1/2 day a week to help with the problems of patients with serious emotional and social problems, since such patients would otherwise take up an inordinate amount of the physician's time. In the past few years, many programs have been initiated to train new types of allied health workers and to make the actual work a person does more nearly commensurate with his training. Examples include pediatric nurse practitioners, chronic disease nurses, and community health workers. In addition to these programs, Silver and others are training an entirely new type of health worker, the Child Health Associate. This allied health worker, who has completed a minimum of 2 years of college and 3 years of pediatric training, will be licensed to deliver all well child care and to diagnose and treat (under a physician's supervision) most acute ambulatory illnesses. His only responsibility for hospitalized patients will involve healthy newborns. Help is thus becoming available to the physician in caring for the expanding pediatric population. However, it is up to the doctor to utilize these deliverers of health care in an effective way, for he will always be the one who is ultimately responsible for patient care.

In 1965, Silver introduced the concept of the Pediatric Nurse Practitioner (PNP), and since that time many similar training programs have emerged. The PNP is a graduate nurse who has been given additional training which improves her skills as a nurse and equips her to take a complete history, to perform a physical examination which includes use of an otoscope and stethoscope, and to give well child guidance and counseling. Her role is to help the physician deliver well child care and to distinguish the sick child from the well child and the abnormal finding from the normal one. The PNP is well accepted by parents, is able to answer parent's concerns about normal growth and development, and is accurate in her physical assessments. The time thus saved has allowed the pediatrician to spend more time with sick patients and to increase the total number of patients cared for.

Other ways of helping the physician deliver child health care are to give the clinic nurse additional responsibilities. Paramedical personnel trained in developmental appraisal and parents themselves can be used. Social workers, visiting health nurses, and nutritionists can help with selected patients.

The parent—or, in the case of an older child, the patient himself—fills out a history questionnaire while the child is waiting to be seen. The example shown on p 147 is a revised version of the form suggested by the American Academy of Pediatrics in their *Standards of Child Health Care* booklet. These forms are simple to complete and easy for the physician to scan, as the responses which need further elaboration are all in the right-hand column. The nurse obtains the vital statistics, charts the measurements on the appropriate graphs, and updates the well child flow sheet. She scans the patient's chart to find other problems the child has had and lists these on the progress sheet. The use of the "problem-oriented record" discussed in another portion of this chapter greatly simplifies both the nurse's work and the physician's work. The nurse also notes parent-child interactions and lists all the concerns the parent expresses. Thus, before he even sees the child, the physician has a fairly clear idea not only of the well child's current health needs but also of other concerns the parent has expressed. These are enumerated in a problem-oriented fashion, and the physician deals with each of them as necessary within the limits of the time he can devote to a given patient.

The waiting room in a large clinic may need to be supervised by an "activity coordinator"—a person trained in early childhood development and elementary education who can design a curriculum for a pediatric outpatient setting with daily and weekly lesson plans. Such a curriculum provides a direction for her and her volunteers and continuity for the children who return periodically to the clinic for well child or chronic illness care. Her goal, beyond keeping the child occupied, is to observe the child's behavior and the parent-child interaction. She is in an ideal position to report any unusual behavior in that setting to the physician. She attempts to show parents that their child is a capable and unique individual, with the ultimate goal of trying to help the parent and the child find pleasure in each other.

By making use of personnel with varying special competences, the physician is better able to organize his task of caring for patients. With such an organized and directed team, the quality of care given should greatly improve.

Duncan B, Smith AN, Silver HK: Comparison of the physical assessment of children by pediatric nurse practitioners and pediatricians. Am J Pub Health 61:1170, 1971.

Schiff DW, Fraser CH, Walters HL: The pediatric nurse practitioner in the office of pediatrics in pediatric practice. Pediatrics 44:62, 1969.

Silver HK, Hecker JA: The child health associate. Hospitals (J Am Hosp Ass) 44:47, 1970.

Silver HK, Ford LC, Stearly SC: A program to increase health care for children: The Pediatric Nurse Practitioner program. Pediatrics 39:756, 1967.

Townsend EH: The social worker in pediatric practice. Am J Dis Child 107:77, 1964.

ACUTE ILLNESS VISITS

The episodic office visit for the child with an acute illness places special demands on the physician.

OBJECTIVES

Diagnosis and treatment of the chief complaint is the first priority for the parents, patient, and physician. Extenuating circumstances (eg, a crowded waiting room) rarely justify an incomplete work-up of an acute chief complaint.

Detection of problem patients who have a chronic disease or an undiagnosed chronic complaint is of nearly equal importance to the physician.

PROCEDURE IN ASSESSING ILLNESS

Optimal management of an acute illness mainly includes telephone triaging, office triaging, diagnosis, assessment of the need for hospitalization, home therapy, and a follow-up plan.

The detection of multiple problem patients is best accomplished by using a brief screening questionnaire, which should be completed on any new patient who makes his initial contact for sick care. Some parents have only crisis care available to their families (eg, in rural areas). Other parents have access to comprehensive health care but use only crisis care because their daily lives are beset with too many other problems (eg, urban slums). This situation is usually a byproduct of a disorganized poverty environment rather than a reflection of disinterest in preventive medicine. The screening questionnaire is unnecessary for patients already being followed for well child care. It can be deferred if the patient has a true emergency problem. An example of a useful questionnaire is given on p 153.

The parent can complete this questionnaire while waiting to see the physician. Since it identifies only major problems, an affirmative answer to any of the first 4 questions should cause the physician considerable concern. In these cases, he should strongly recommend a follow-up appointment even if the parent has not requested well child care.

TELEPHONE TRIAGING & ADVICE

Does the Patient Need to Be Seen?

The physician himself is the person best qualified to give medical advice, both in the office and over the phone. However, talking with parents on the phone may take too much of a physician's time, so that delegation of this function to another member of the office team is desirable. Most of the questions are routine ones that require only routine answers. An office nurse is probably the best person to manage such routine medical calls. If the physician delegates this responsibility to her, he must first specifically train her for this role. For a nurse to be successful in giving medical advice, office policies should be standardized. Routine instructions for handling minor infections, minor injuries, reactions to immunizations, infant feeding problems, newborn care, and prescription refills are easy to communicate to parents if they are written down in an office protocol book. The protocol book should also clarify at what point each problem requires an office visit. This decision depends on the duration of the symptom, the age of the patient, whether or not the patient acts "sick," an assessment of the parent's anxiety, etc. (For example, most patients under 1 year of age with diarrhea need to be examined in person.) After telephone data are gathered, the nurse must be able to decide whether the child needs to be seen or not. She should err on the side of giving an appointment. For patients not seen, any pertinent telephone data should be entered in the patient's chart.

It is helpful if parents understand 2 general telephone rules: (1) the nurse will screen all calls from parents except emergency ones, and (2) calls regarding routine questions will only be accepted during office hours. Night calls should be restricted to urgent ones. Most routine calls come from overanxious, insecure mothers who need reassurance and acceptance, not criticism and abruptness. The conversation with the nurse should build the mother's confidence and independence. The mother can be asked what she had considered doing and have her approach strongly endorsed if it is at all reasonable. If parents are educated to be more medically independent, unnecessary visits will diminish, as will medical costs for society in general.

The physician directly accepts some calls: (1) emergency calls from parents, (2) calls from other physicians, (3) calls regarding hospitalized patients, (4) long distance calls, (5) calls from a parent who "demands" to talk to the physician, and (6) calls where the nurse is unclear about what should be done. These exceptions to the rule are obvious. Parents reasonably expect their personal physician or his designated substitute to be readily available for emergencies, even if the "emergency" exists only from their viewpoint. The physician must be especially circumspect about calls after midnight, for they usually relate to psychosocial crises or urgent medical problems.

There are 4 other possible methods of dealing with telephone calls, any of which may serve as an alternative to having an office nurse give telephone advice: (1) The physician can accept calls continuously throughout the day. These interruptions are unacceptable to most physicians and parents. (2) The physician can have a telephone hour at the beginning and end of the day and accept only emergency calls at other times. The disadvantages of this approach are that parents must wait for answers to their questions and the physician wastes his time with many routine calls. (3) The physician may charge for telephone advice. This charge decreases the number of calls, but in the process it discourages important calls and thereby interferes with preventive pediatrics. (4) The physician can allow various nonmedical office personnel to protect him from telephone calls by accepting calls randomly themselves. This approach would result in inconsistent medical advice and could be dangerous.

Strain JE, Miller JD: The preparation, utilization, and evaluation of a registered nurse trained to give telephone advice in a private pediatric office. Pediatrics 47:1051, 1971.

Sturtz GS, Brown RB: Concerning A.G. Bell's invention. Clin Pediat 8:378, 1969.

When Does the Patient Need to Be Seen?

Some patients must be seen immediately (eg, a foreign body in the eye). Others can be seen later the same day (eg, a cough that kept the patient awake much of the preceding night). Other patients can be scheduled 1–2 days later (eg, recurrent epistaxis). The nurse can make these decisions.

Where Should the Patient Be Seen?

Most sick patients can be seen in the physician's office by appointment. The physician can keep the first and last hour of each day plus at least 15 minutes out of each hour open for acute problems. Most of the first-hour appointments will be given to parents who call the physician during the preceding evening.

Another facility where patients can be seen for medical care is the hospital emergency room. This routing applies to patients who are highly likely to be admitted (eg, croup). Some physicians also send patients with poisonings, lacerations, or possible fractures to the nearest emergency room.

A third possibility is a house call. Most physicians consider this disadvantageous to themselves financially and to the patient medically since laboratory services are not available. A rare indication for a house call might be a particularly contagious disease that needs confirmation (eg, varicella). The physician could occasionally see such a patient in his office parking lot.

OFFICE TRIAGING & PROCEDURE

How Sick Is the Patient?

The nurse should screen every sick patient as soon as possible after he arrives at the office. She can think in terms of 3 general groups: emergency, contagious, and minor illness. Most patients have a minor illness (eg, cold, accident, earache) and can be seen at their appointed time. Some patients are contagious until proved otherwise and should quickly be moved from the waiting room to an isolated examining room (eg, febrile illnesses with rashes, possible pertussis). An attempt should be made to keep children with bronchiolitis or croup away from infants. When an office emergency is recognized by the nurse, she should notify the physician immediately. He can take appropriate emergency action, stabilize the patient, and arrange for transfer to the hospital (eg, an acidotic, dehydrated infant). (See Chapter 30.)

Preparation of the Patient for the Physician

The office aide can record the sick patient's temperature, height, and weight. The office nurse can record the chief complaint. Depending upon the symptom, the nurse can initiate the laboratory procedures and symptomatic treatment listed below.

Initial Treatment & Laboratory Work-Up

A. **Cough:** If present over 1 month, begin a tine test.

B. **Diarrhea:** Take sample for stool culture if the stool contains blood or mucus, if the child is less than 1 year of age, or if diarrhea has persisted for more than 1 week at any age. For children under age 2, give 60 ml of 5% dextrose in water and record the naked weight on each visit.

C. **Earache:** Give acetaminophen if in obvious pain. If there is a possibility of mumps, isolate the patient.

D. **Fever Over 38.5° C (101.3° F):** Give acetaminophen in age-appropriate dose. Put the child in an examining room and assist the parent in undressing him. Provide a bag for urine if not toilet-trained and save urine in refrigerator for analysis and culture. If unexplained fever has been present over 24 hours, do a white count and differential.

E. **Fractures:** Notify the doctor immediately, obtain equipment to immobilize the site, and fill out the x-ray request.

F. **Head Injury:** Record vital signs and check the pupils for equal size and reaction to light.

G. **Infectious Hepatitis Exposure:** Record weights on persons who have had close contact with the patient in anticipation of giving gamma globulin, 0.02 ml/lb IM.

H. **Lacerations:** Wash thoroughly with hexachlorophene soap and water (at least 10 minutes). Check date of last tetanus shot and record. (The physician must decide whether tetanus protection is needed.) Shave if necessary (but never shave eyebrows). Have parents sign consent for suturing.

I. **Nasal Discharge (Purulent, or Clear Plus Fever):** Take material for culture.

J. **Nosebleed:** Check blood pressure and draw blood for hematocrit. Compress the bleeding site for 10 minutes.

K. **Painful Urination (Burning or Frequency):** Take sample for urinalysis, urine culture, and a Gram-stained smear of unspun drop.

L. **Pinworms:** Record the approximate weights of all family members if the infection is a recurrent one (for calculation of dosage of medication).

M. **Sore Throat:** Take material for throat culture (contraindicated if the patient has croup).

N. **Streptococcal Sore Throat (Positive Culture):** Inquire about penicillin allergy and record. Arrange for symptomatic contacts to have throat cultures taken. Arrange for follow-up urinalysis and heart examination by the physician 1 week after discontinuing penicillin or 3 weeks after benzathine penicillin G injection.

O. **Stomach Ache:** Take samples for urinalysis and urine culture and test for presence of bile in urine; save stool specimen for occult blood testing.

P. **Vomiting:** Give patient emesis basin and sips of iced cola drink while waiting.

WORKING DIAGNOSIS

The physician makes the final decision about the patient's diagnosis and the severity of the disease. He may detect emergency conditions that were not obvious to his nurse (eg, shock or meningitis). His history-taking can be modified according to the chief complaint. A history of recent exposure to disease is often important. Severity can be partially assessed by inquiries about appetite, energy, ability to sleep, and the mother's feelings about how sick her child is this time compared to other times. If a family of sick children is brought in, the physician should ask the mother which children she considers the sickest. The physical examination should also be mainly directed toward the chief complaint. A patient with a dog bite does not require a complete examination, but a patient with an earache must be checked for mastoid swelling and meningeal signs in addition to otoscopic examination.

Utilizing the conventional technics of history, physical examination, and laboratory tests, the physician will correctly diagnose the majority of acute chief complaints. However, unless he maintains a high index of suspicion and applies his keenest clinical judgment, he will occasionally miss a child with septicemia. Septic children usually present as unexplained fevers, but (unlike children with acute viral fevers) they often won't play or smile even with their parents. They frequently are physically exhausted and too weak to resist the physical examination, constantly irritable and unable to sleep, and respond paradoxically to cuddling by the mother. Irritability usually stems from pain and hypoxia. A less common finding in the toxic child is constant lethargy or sleepiness. This is difficult to assess because most sick children sleep more than normally. A child with suspected septicemia requires an intensive work-up and therapy in a hospital setting. Making this diagnosis requires the greatest vigilance by the pediatrician.

INDICATIONS FOR HOSPITALIZATION

For every acute problem, the physician must decide whether to treat the child at home or in the hospital. Overhospitalization is currently a greater problem in the USA than underhospitalization. Overhospitalization takes 3 general forms: (1) Hospitalization for an acute illness sometimes occurs because the primary physician is uncertain of the diagnosis and prognosis. Reassurance in the face of such insecurity can often be gained by immediate consultation with a colleague. (2) Hospitalization is sometimes arranged for a diagnostic evaluation and tests because the patient has no outpatient insurance. Unless the parents are having serious financial difficulty, this custom is unethical. It is to be hoped that more realistic insurance coverage will make ambulatory studies equally reimbursable (3) Periodic hospitalizations sometimes are ordered for routine reevaluations of a chronic disease. Even if the patient travels a great distance, this reevaluation can be done on an ambulatory basis if it is carefully planned in advance. The combined costs of the special studies plus hotel accommodations will be far less than hospitalization charges.

Unnecessary hospitalization carries 4 main problems or risks, the last one probably being the most serious: (1) Children under 3 years of age can experience separation problems. (2) The parents' confidence in caring for a sick child themselves is undermined. (3) There is a danger of cross-infection to the patient and óthers. (4) Society sustains an endlessly rising cost for medical care.

If it is not clear whether or not an acutely ill child should be hospitalized, he should be observed in the office for several hours. This will allow time for any reassurance given to the mother to take effect and permits the physician to compare the patient at 2 points in time and determine whether he is improving or getting worse. This interval also helps one decide what to do when the mother's history and the physical examinations are conflicting (eg, "recurrent vomiting" without dehydration, "no urination" without bladder distention). If necessary, another physician can be called in for consultation during this period.

A patient should be hospitalized if his problems fit into one of the following 3 groups of indications:

Major Emergencies

Some examples of obvious life-threatening conditions are shock, severe dehydration, coma, meningitis (bacterial or of unknown cause), respiratory distress, congestive heart failure, severe hypertension, acute renal failure, status epilepticus, and surgical emergencies.

Potentially Life-Threatening or Crippling Illnesses

Some patients are not in critical condition when first seen but require hospitalization because their problem may be rapidly progressive during treatment. If deterioration occurs in the hospital, emergency therapy can be rapidly instituted. Most of the entities in this group are caused by infection or trauma. Endogenous diseases rarely change this rapidly. Although absolute rules cannot be formulated for every situation, the following guidelines can be applied to most cases of acute illness. Obviously, these rules will have some exceptions. Also, the list is not complete (eg, chronic diseases are not listed).

These problems are listed according to body systems:

A. **Skin:**
   1. Cellulitis if less than 6 months old, omphalitis if less than 2 months old, erysipelas, toxic epidermal necrolysis, in cavernous sinus drainage area, if underlying osteomyelitis is suspected, or if there is no response after 2 days of therapy.
   2. Suspected thrombophlebitis.
   3. Burns (second or third degree) involving more than 10% of surface area (> 15% if more than 1 year old), burns of perineal area, full thickness burns of hand area, electrical burns.
   4. Purpura with fever, without fever but unexplained, or without fever but progressive.

B. **Eyes:**
   1. Gonococcal conjunctivitis, bacterial keratitis.
   2. Eye injury if visual acuity is decreased.
   3. Papilledema.

C. **Ears, Nose, and Throat:**
   1. Acute otitis media if less than 1 month old.
   2. Mastoiditis.
   3. Sinusitis if overlying redness or edema is present.
   4. Nasal obstruction if less than 6 months old and an apneic episode has occurred.
   5. Epistaxis if uncontrolled, if hypertension is present, if there is bleeding elsewhere, or if anemia is present.
   6. Fluctuant tonsillar abscess.
   7. Retropharyngeal abscess.
   8. Diphtheria (any symptoms at any age).

D. **Respiratory System:**
   1. Epiglottitis (all cases).
   2. Viral laryngitis if there is stridor at rest, dyspnea, or drooling; if it is currently progressive; if there is a history of a previous

bout with rapid progression; or if the patient is less than 1 year old (even if the disease is mild).

3. Pertussis if symptomatic and the patient is less than 1 year old.

4. Bronchiolitis if dyspneic, if it is progressive, if infiltrates are seen on x-ray, if appetite is poor, or if the patient is less than 2 months old (even if the disease is mild).

5. Pneumonia if the patient is less than 6 months old; if there is a history of apnea, cyanosis, or choking spells; with dyspnea (any age); with pleural effusion; if staphylococcal pneumonia is suspected; if appetite is poor; or if there is no response after 2 days of therapy.

6. Suspected foreign body of the airway.

7. Hemoptysis if unexplained, if there is bleeding elsewhere, or if anemia is present.

E. Cardiovascular System:

1. Suspected subacute bacterial endocarditis.

2. Any myocarditis or pericarditis.

3. Mild acute hypertension.

4. Unexplained arrhythmias.

F. Gastrointestinal System:

1. Diarrhea if explosive in character, if there is abdominal distention, associated with Kussmaul respirations, suspected typhoid fever at any age, suspected acute shigella enteritis if less than 1 year old, suspected staphylococcal enterocolitis, moderate dehydration, or mild dehydration but with vomiting or if patient is less than 1 year old.

2. Suspected appendicitis or intussusception.

3. Toxic ileus.

4. Abdominal trauma if penetrating injury has occurred or if damage to the spleen, liver, kidneys, pancreas, or intestines is suspected.

5. Hematemesis.

6. Melena or unexplained bright-red blood mixed in the stools.

G. Urinary System:

1. Pyelonephritis if patient is less than 1 year old, toxic, unimproved after 2 days of therapy, if underlying renal disease is present, or if recurrences have been frequent.

2. Acute edema, oliguria, or azotemia.

3. Hematuria with symptoms listed in (2), renal colic, or after trauma.

4. Acute urinary retention.

H. Genitalia:

1. Vaginitis if associated with salpingitis.

2. Vaginal injury with sharp object.

I. Skeletal System:

1. Possible osteomyelitis.

2. Arthritis if possibly septic or acute rheumatic fever.

3. Wringer injury if above the elbow, if a hematoma or avulsed skin is present, if a fracture or nerve injury is present, or if the peripheral pulse is diminished.

J. Nervous System:

1. Aseptic meningitis if the level of consciousness is depressed or there is a motor deficit.

2. Suspected tetanus.

3. Suspected epidural spinal abscess.

4. Febrile seizures if they continue more than 30 minutes, if there are persistent neurologic signs, or if the level of consciousness is decreased.

5. Head injury if the patient has been unconscious longer than 1 minute, if there are persistent neurologic signs, if the level of consciousness is decreased, if a seizure has occurred, with CSF rhinorrhea or otorrhea, or if there is significant swelling over the middle meningeal artery, retinal hemorrhages, or progressive headaches.

6. Skull fractures—depressed, compound (ie, into air sinuses or overlying scalp laceration), or across the middle meningeal artery or venous sinus.

7. Spinal trauma.

8. Progressive muscle weakness.

9. CNS deterioration.

K. General:

1. Possible septicemia.

2. Poisoning if the patient is symptomatic, if the agent was not recovered by ipecac, if the agent is unknown, or if the agent is very toxic.

3. Suspected lead poisoning.

4. Unexplained mass.

5. Unexplained failure to thrive if the patient is less than 6 months old; failure to thrive at any age if neglect is suspected.

Psychosocial Indications for Hospitalization

Patients with acute psychosocial problems now comprise a larger proportion of hospitalized children than was formerly the case. Until society can provide alternative facilities for these crises, hospitalization will continue to fulfill this need. These indications fall into 3 general groups: parent, child, and disease problems.

A. Parent Problems:

1. Child abuse (eg, battering, failure to thrive secondary to neglect, or incest).

2. Incipient battering (eg, the parent has made a homicidal threat against his child).

3. Absent parents (eg, abandonment, emancipated minors without caretakers, or the parents themselves are hospitalized).

4. Physically exhausted parents (eg, no sleep for 2 nights).

5. Emotionally incapacitated parents (eg, if the parents remain immobilized and extremely anxious after a careful explanation of their child's illness).

6. Neglectful parents who seem disinterested in their child's illness or therapy (eg, neglected eczema). This is a rare situation compared to overly anxious parents.

7. Intellectually incompetent parents (eg, a mentally retarded mother who can't reliably follow verbal or written instructions).

8. Emotionally disturbed parents who need psychiatric hospitalization for their own problems (eg, a floridly psychotic mother).

B. **Child Problems:**

1. Suicide attempt—A short hospital admission allows time for the mental health worker to do his evaluation and the family to look seriously at their problems.

2. A destructive, dangerous child can be held on a pediatric ward pending placement. A dangerous adolescent will require a psychiatric setting.

3. Severe delirium (eg, if the parents cannot control it).

4. An incapacitating emotional symptom (eg, a severe conversion reaction such as paraplegia or blindness).

C. **Disease Problems:**

1. An incapacitating (but not life-threatening) physical disease (eg, severe Sydenham's chorea).

2. Initial diagnosis of a disease with a complex treatment regimen. The parents and patient deserve a careful, unhurried, and organized introduction to the complex home management of some chronic disease (eg, diabetes mellitus).

3. Initial diagnosis of a fatal disease—This gives the family time to work through the impact phase (eg, leukemia).

4. Terminal care if the family does not want the child to die at home.

Lovejoy FH & others: Unnecessary and preventable hospitalizations: Report on an internal audit. J Pediat 79:868, 1971.

TREATMENT OF THE NONHOSPITALIZED PATIENT

Words are as necessary as drugs in the treatment of a sick child. The parents expect to be told their child's diagnosis and its causes, prognosis, and treatment. They also need to have their concerns acknowledged and clarified. If this communication does not take place, the parents will often be dissatisfied and their compliance with regard to medications, advice, and follow-up will probably be less than optimal.

If the child has a mild acute illness (eg, viral nasopharyngitis), the parent would be reassured by the following general types of comment:

Diagnosis

"David has a cold." The diagnosis should be conveyed in plain English, not in medical jargon. If the physician does not precisely mention his diagnosis to the parents, they may assume he was unable to arrive at one. (See also Ambiguous Diagnosis, below.)

Etiology

"It's due to a virus." This means to most parents that the infection is not serious. Some parents need an added statement that there was nothing they could have done to prevent it—eg, "Everyone is coming down with this."

Parents' Concerns

Mothers often do not listen to their physician's instructions until their own main concerns have been commented upon. These concerns are easily elicited by 3 questions: (1) "Why did you bring David to the clinic today?" (2) "What worried you most about him?" (3) "Why did that worry you?" After these concerns are out in the open, the physician is in an excellent position to clarify misconceptions. His reassurance can be specific—eg, "He doesn't have meningitis," or, "It won't turn into leukemia."

Treatment

In self-limited disease, the goal of medication is to keep the patient comfortable. The opportunities to use symptomatic medications far exceed those where specific medications are available. A useful list of common sense approaches to management (sometimes overlooked) is as follows: (1) An antipyretic is useful if the patient's fever causes discomfort. (2) Sedatives (eg, chloral hydrate) should be prescribed more often for the acutely restless child since his mother cannot easily function as a nurse without some sleep. (3) Codeine can be freely used for acute cough that interferes with sleep. (4) Advice about diet, bed rest, isolation, and mood are also appreciated by the parent. The patient can usually be allowed to select his own diet while he is sick. (5) Home bed rest is something each child may decide for himself in most cases. (6) Isolation within the family structure is rarely indicated since exposure has usually preceded the diagnosis. (7) Parents can be reassured about temporary emotional regression during an acute illness. A return to the previous level of maturity need not be encouraged until good health returns.

Prognosis

"David will probably feel better in 2 or 3 days. This is not a serious infection. If something new develops or his fever lasts over 3 days, give me a call." Nothing is gained by mentioning all the possible complications that could occur. Without promoting anxiety, the door to additional medical evaluation is quietly left open for any new problems that might arise.

Closing

"You're doing a fine job with David. Just hold the fort and he will be his old self in a few days." The visit should close on a positive note, even a compliment if possible. If the patient is older, an attempt can be made to boost his morale as well—eg, "This won't keep *you* out of action for long."

The Ambiguous Diagnosis

An unclear diagnosis presents special problems in communication with the parents. The physician must be honest about the inconclusive diagnosis and yet not unduly alarm the parents. "David's illness is not far enough along to be diagnosed exactly. Another day or so will be needed to pinpoint the problem. I can tell you a few things for certain. He is not in any serious trouble. He doesn't have meningitis. I definitely want to see him tomorrow. Call me sooner if there are any new developments."

Symptomatic therapy should also be prescribed.

Korsch B & others: Practical implications of doctor-patient interaction analysis for pediatric practice. Am J Dis Child 121:110, 1971.

FOLLOW-UP OF THE NONHOSPITALIZED PATIENT

Most children with an acute illness do not require follow-up unless their clinical course worsens or is prolonged. However, if the child has an ambiguous diagnosis (eg, high fever of unknown origin) or an unpredictable course (eg, vomiting), daily follow-up is necessary. This protects both the patient and the physician. This follow-up can be accomplished by revisits, telephone calls, or a visiting nurse.

Revisits

Daily office visits are the best approach to the more serious problem. The weight of the infant with diarrhea and the degree of respiratory distress in a child with croup cannot be estimated over the phone. If a scheduled revisit appointment is not kept, the office clerk should immediately notify the physician. A phone call or home visit should be made on that same day. If transportation is a problem for the parent, a community service agency can usually arrange this. If the late results of laboratory tests indicate that an illness is quite serious and other attempts at contact fail, the police can be requested to locate the patient and bring him in (eg, a stool culture that grows salmonella in a 4-month-old infant).

Telephone Calls

A daily telephone call will suffice for milder problems when only historical follow-up data are needed (eg, vomiting or lethargy). Since these calls are essential to proper management, the physician or his nurse should make them. A daily telephone list can be kept and the charts pulled prior to calling. If the follow-up is felt to be important, parents should not be depended upon to initiate these calls since some may not be made. Telephone calls become the realistic choice of follow-up when long distances are a factor.

Visiting Nurse

Home management of wounds and burns is an appropriate role for a visiting nurse. Mothers of large families who have both a babysitter problem and a transportation problem appreciate this type of follow-up. Mothers with several sick children or who are themselves in poor health also benefit from home visits.

MEDICOLEGAL PROBLEMS

The management of acute illness offers the greatest potential for malpractice litigation in pediatrics. The physician is responsible not only for his own errors but for those of his nurse as well. Errors can be made in any of the areas previously discussed. An error in telephone triaging can result in a delay in diagnosis (eg, calling meningococcemia a viral exanthem, or arranging an appointment for the next day for scrotal pain that turns out to be testicular torsion). An error in underhospitalization can lead to death (eg, epiglottitis being treated on an outpatient basis). Errors in therapy may result in sciatic nerve palsy if an injection is given into an inappropriate quadrant of the buttocks, or acute rheumatic fever if penicillin is not given for a streptococcal sore throat because it was not cultured. Errors in follow-up can result in undiagnosed abdominal pain silently progressing to a ruptured appendix.

The physician should obtain parental consent forms for all medical procedures (eg, lumbar puncture, vaginal examination, suturing) unless an emergency exists. Consultation should be sought whenever a physician is uncertain about what is happening with an acutely and possibly seriously ill patient.

The errors listed above are not difficult to prevent if the physician bases all of his medical decisions on what is best for the patient.

CHRONIC DISEASE FOLLOW-UP VISITS

Office visits for a child with known or potential chronic disease present special problems. There are 5 broad types of chronic disease, each being progressively more difficult to manage: (1) Potential chronic disease (eg, the small premature, the newborn who has recovered from hypoglycemia, or the older child who has recovered from meningitis). (2) Reversible chronic disease (eg, tuberculosis, eczema, or idiopathic thrombocytopenic purpura). (3) Static chronic disease (eg, cerebral palsy, deafness, or dwarfism). (4) Progressive chronic disease (eg, diabetes mellitus or sickle cell anemia). (5) Fatal disease (eg, leukemia or muscular dystrophy). These children usually receive excellent care when they are hospitalized. They should also receive the same kind of thoughtful care when they do not occupy a hospital bed or have an interesting complication.

Objectives

There are 2 primary objectives in the management of a chronic disease. The first is to counteract the effects of the disease to the extent possible. This requires the aggressive use of every available therapeutic modality that could be useful for the individual patient's problems. The second objective is to help the patient and his parents make a healthy emotional adjustment to the treatment regimen and to the effects of the disease that cannot be controlled. Except for matters relating to his disease, the child should be reared no differently than his healthy siblings. He should live as nearly normal a life as possible.

Procedures of Management

Chronic disease management is optimal when the following general aspects receive ongoing attention: continuity of care, frequent visits, problem-oriented records, chronic disease flow sheets, personal medical identification documents, a chronic disease patient registry kept in the office, and medical passport.

I. Continuity of Care

The patient with a chronic disease may have multiple problems that are difficult to manage. If anyone deserves continuous medical care from one physician, this person does. Discontinuous care by several physicians often results in a confused and maladjusted patient. When the patient has a progressive or fatal disease, depression can occur. In such a situation, patients depend upon a single sustaining physician to help them maintain their tenuous hope for survival. Fragmented medical care usually accentuates a poor psychologic adjustment. When a physician agrees to care for a patient with a chronic disease, he should give his home phone number and encourage its use even on nights he is not on call. If the physician is unable to see the patient personally, he can coordinate arrangements by telephone for the patient to be seen by another physician who has been fully briefed. If the patient is unable to contact his personal physician, he should be able to turn to a substitute physician who has been designated well in advance.

II. Frequent Visits

The patient with a chronic disease should be contacted frequently. Monitoring the patient's disease and response to therapy is impossible without periodic visits or telephone communications. If his problem is stabilized, he should be seen personally at least every 6 months; 3-month intervals are better for progressive diseases. If the disease is in relapse, the patient may need to be seen daily.

III. Problem-Oriented Records

In addition to a personal physician, comprehensive care of the chronically ill patient depends upon good record-keeping. No physician's memory is absolutely reliable, and in any case the patient must have accurate office records when the physician is away from the city or after he dies. An excellent system of record-keeping has been developed and refined in a practice setting (see references, below). It has 4 components: the initial data base, the active problem sheet, the plan for each problem, and the progress notes which contribute to the continually expanding data base and problem list.

Initial Data Base

The conventional present illness, review of systems, past medical history, family history, psychosocial history, physical examination, and laboratory screening tests comprise the data base. Information from all accessible sources is used. (See Chapter 1.)

Active Problem Sheet

The active problem list is the keystone of this system. It lists all the patient's significant problems, including psychosocial ones. These problems are defined from the data base currently at hand. They can be expressed as an etiologic diagnosis (eg, rheumatic heart disease), a pathophysiologic state (eg, congestive heart failure), or a sign or symptom (eg, edema). When the therapy carries considerable risk, it should be defined as a problem (eg, corticosteroids or tracheostomy). An attempt is made to list the problems in order of priority. Each problem is then assigned a permanent number (see p 155). Thereafter, this number should precede any entry in the chart that concerns this problem. The active problem sheet should be kept in the front of the patient's chart where it serves as a table of contents. The dates should be date of onset or date of resolution. New problems are added as identified, and old problems are transferred to the "resolved or inactive" column when appropriate. Symptom problems should be reidentified as diagnosed problems when the data accumulated justify doing so.

Plan for Each Problem

Each problem as listed in the active problem sheet needs an individual diagnostic, therapeutic, and educational plan. If the plans for all the problems are combined, omissions are likely to occur.

Progress Notes

Progress notes contain newly collected data, an analysis of the data, and a reassessment of the plan. These notes should always pertain to one of the problems on the active problem sheet and be so labeled both by number and by title, eg, as follows:

#2—Seizures

>   History—Two seizures last week, lasting 1 minute and 5 minutes. Occurred at 7:00 a.m. and 10:00 a.m. Last seizure 3 months ago. No headaches or vomiting. Not drowsy from medication.
>
>   Examination—Neurologic examination and fundi normal. No nystagmus. Gingival hyperplasia—mild.
>
>   Impression—Seizures still in poor control.
>
>   Plan—Continue phenobarbital, 30 mg tid; increase Dilantin to 50 mg tid.

Bjorn JC, Cross HD: *Problem-Oriented Practice.* Modern Hospital Press, 1970.

Weed LL: Medical records that guide and teach. New England J Med 278:593—600, 652—657, 1968.

Weed LL: *Medical Records, Medical Education and Patient Care.* Case Univ Press, 1969.

IV. The Chronic Disease Flow Sheet

There are many variables in the management of a chronic disease. The variables can become lost in the substance of the chart and relatively unavailable for comparison and interpretation. For a patient with a chronic disease or multiple problems, critical data from the progress note should be recorded on a chronic disease flow sheet which tabulates variables so that trends and correlations can be accurately determined. The long axis of the flow sheet has time intervals. Inpatient flow sheets maintained on a critically ill child usually monitor vital signs, intake and output, blood gases, and numerous chemical determinations. Outpatient flow sheets often contain none of the above. Although a specific flow sheet is designed for each chronic disease, the following variables are commonly present in the ambulatory management of most chronic diseases. An example of a flow sheet for a patient with diabetes mellitus, grand mal seizures, and school phobia is shown on p 154. Most of the variables discussed below are used in monitoring this patient's course.

Disease Status

One must monitor the activity level of the disease to know whether therapy is being effective or not. Such activity can be evaluated through the history, physical findings, laboratory data, and consultations. Variables so determined can be tabulated on the flow sheet.

A. Symptom Data: The frequency and duration of asthma attacks are the main determinants of the success of asthma therapy. Migraine headaches, seizure episodes, and psychogenic recurrent abdominal pain must also be monitored largely by attack rates.

B. Physical Findings: Childhood nephrosis must be followed by weighing the patient and observing the presence or absence of edema. Splenomegaly is an important variable in leukemia. Motor milestones are important in cerebral palsy.

C. Laboratory Data: Chest films are important for following tuberculosis, EEGs for seizures, liver enzymes for chronic active hepatitis, urine cultures for recurrent urinary tract infection, etc.

D. Consultations: One of the patient's problems may be followed by another specialist. The primary physician should record under the dates of these visits the consultant's name and abbreviated conclusions on the flow sheet. The date will permit easy location of the consultation report in the chart when it is needed.

E. Hospitalizations: All hospitalizations should be recorded under the problem that they were required for. They usually represent a marker of increased activity of the disease.

Disease Complications

The physician must take specific precautions to prevent or to detect any treatable complications.

A. Prevention of Complications: Many chronic diseases have predictable and preventable complications if therapy is instituted in advance. If these are listed in the flow sheet, the physician will be certain to remind the parent of them on each visit. Examples are performing daily range of motion exercises to prevent contractures in rheumatoid arthritis, requesting penicillin prophylaxis before dental procedures to prevent subacute bacterial endocarditis in congenital heart disease, avoidance of altitudes over 10,000 feet to prevent a crisis in sickle cell disease, and carrying an antihypoglycemic food in the pocket at all times in diabetes mellitus.

B. Early Detection of Complications: Other chronic diseases have complications that are not preventable but respond much better to therapy if they are detected early. Warning signs of these complications should be listed on the flow sheet. Examples are head circumference measurements to detect early subdural effusions or hydrocephalus after meningitis, and blood pressure measurements to detect early hypertension in chronic renal disease. Once hypertension is discovered, it is no longer an anticipated complication but an indicator of disease activity.

Disease Treatment

Therapy may or may not be responsible for improvement in the patient's disease status. Examining the temporal relationship of one to the other allows a physician to decide if the treatment has been effective. A chronic disease flow sheet should supply this information.

A. Medications: All medications and dosages should be listed with the dates when started and discontinued and when the dosage is changed. The dosage may be increased because the patient has outgrown it or because his problem is not under optimal control (eg, increasing the dosage of digoxin in persistent congestive heart failure). New drugs should be added when previous drugs have been pushed to tolerance without adequate control (eg, adding alternate day prednisone to daily aminophylline/ephedrine therapy in asthma). Any drug the patient is receiving should have at least one related variable listed under disease status that permits rapid assessment of the efficacy of the drug (eg, bowel movements per day recorded for the patient with ulcerative colitis on Lomotil).

B. Toxicity: If drugs with side-effects are being used, these problems should be anticipated. The bone marrow, kidney, or liver function tests that need monitoring should be recorded on the flow sheet, as well as the required frequency of testing. If the potential toxicity is high, the drug should also be recorded on the problem list. If sudden discontinuance of the drug could lead to a severe adverse reaction, this risk should be frequently discussed with the patient (eg, anticonvulsants).

C. Other Therapy: Other methods of treatment besides drugs should be recorded on the flow sheet so that their effect on the course of the disease can also be estimated. Examples are specific food avoidance in recurrent urticaria or bubble bath avoidance in recurrent urinary tract infection. In static diseases, compensatory devices (eg, braces in cerebral palsy or hearing aids in deafness) should be listed as well as the recommended interval for routine checks of these devices. Reassurance and other forms of supportive psychotherapy will generally be given on every visit and need not be listed here.

Disease Adjustment

Maladjustment to a chronic disease is preventable in many cases. Three aspects in this area can be considered:

A. Disease Education Reviews: Patients may not cooperate with a therapeutic plan until they are intellectually and emotionally committed to it. Unless the family fully understands what they are expected to do, they cannot do it. Unless they understand priorities, they may unknowingly discontinue some critical element, in the treatment program when the treatment program as a whole becomes frustrating. Optimal patient education is reached when the patient and his family know as much about the treatment of the disease as the physician does and when they can make decisions about minor adjustments of treatment independently.

When facts regarding the disease and treatment are reviewed, one should begin with basic information even though it has been covered many times before. After the first session, the subject is reviewed by asking the patient questions. In the early years, the facts are covered with the patient and both parents present. If the father excludes himself from the medical care of his child, serious marital problems will usually develop. In the adolescent years, the review sessions should be done privately with the teenager. The patient's knowledge of his problems should be explored approximately every 6 months. In the period immediately following diagnosis, it should be covered on every visit for a few months.

B. School Notification: Each fall the physician should notify the school nurse about any patient that may have manifestations of his disease at school. This notification will prevent any emotional problems secondary to mishandling of the physical problem by the school. The patient with chronic heart or lung disease may need a gym excuse. He may need modified gym (eg, no gym on days of wheezing, or no rope-climbing in a seizure patient). Both the nurse and the teacher need to know how to respond to a seizure or insulin reaction in the classroom. The physician should have this listed on his flow sheet so that it is never overlooked. The parents of the patient's closest friends should also have this information, as should the babysitters also.

C. Disease Adjustment Screen: Emotional maladjustments are a frequent and often unnecessary side-effect of chronic diseases. The physician can prevent them in many instances by reviewing an emotional problem checklist on *every* visit. Some of the more common but unvoiced maladjustments are unnecessary restrictions, overprotectiveness, favoritism, school phobia, underdiscipline, and teasing by peers. This subject is fully covered in Chapter 23.

V. The Medical Identification Card

The patient with a chronic disease should carry an identification card with his active problem list, his physician's telephone number, and his parents' telephone number recorded on it. If he has a disease that can result in sudden changes in consciousness (eg, insulin reaction in diabetes mellitus) or an allergy that could be fatal if it were violated (eg, penicillin allergy), he should obtain a medical identification bracelet or necklace. These can be ordered from Medic Alert Foundation, Turlock, California 95380.

VI. Chronic Disease Patient Registry

Every effort should be made to keep certain patients from becoming "lost to follow-up." People with chronic diseases (eg, those with rheumatic heart disease receiving prophylactic penicillin) fall into this group. To prevent the disappearance of any of these patients, the physician should keep them listed in a chronic disease patient registry. Their charts should have a special mark placed on the corner of the cover to show that they are special high-risk patients. These patients should be sent a reminder card 1 week prior to appointments. If the parent cancels an appointment and promises to call back and make another one, the patient's name should be placed on a critical phone call list which automatically goes into effect if the appointment is not remade within 2 weeks. If the patient misses an appointment, the physician should be notified that same day and he should call the patient. If the parent has no phone, a letter should be sent. If there is no response to the letter, a visiting nurse referral should be sent. This usually returns the patient to his physician or shows that the family has changed physicians. If the family does not wish further medical care from anyone and the patient's disease is life-threatening but treatable (eg, tuberculosis or chronic pyelonephritis), the physician should report the case to the child protective services in his community. Since this is an example of medical care neglect, a court order will be issued for treatment of the child. The physician should assume the personal responsibility to follow indefinitely and tenaciously any high-risk patient until transfer of care occurs.

VII. The Medical Passport

Every year, 20% of American families move. Some of them have children with chronic diseases. Nothing is more frustrating for a physician than to receive a complicated new patient with no past records. Legally, the records belong to the physician; but morally, the records belong to the patient. When he moves, he should carry with him a copy of his active problem list, chronic disease flow sheet, well child flow sheet, consultation reports, hospital discharge summaries, pertinent x-ray reports, and a covering letter. The original copies should never be sent because they may be lost. The physician should also give the family the names of 2 or 3 pediatricians they might use in the city they are moving to. These may be personal acquaintances or selections he has made from the *Directory of Medical Subspecialists*.

CONSULTATIVE VISITS

The physician must know how to act as a consultant when he is qualified and how to seek consultation when he needs it. The pediatrician in daily practice is still the best consultant for most pediatric problems.

Objectives

The usual purposes of consultation are the evaluation of an undiagnosed problem and recommendations for management. Some referrals are for treatment

only. A secondary goal of consultation in a referred case is to provide the referring physician with a postgraduate educational experience.

THE PEDIATRICIAN IN THE ROLE OF CONSULTANT

Referring Source

A. Self-Referral: Although not technically a consultation, some problems require the same kind of intensive approach that is needed when consulting with a colleague. A problem requiring a careful diagnostic evaluation may be detected during a well child visit or a sick child visit. These "big" problems are often not mentioned by the parent until the end of the visit or may be detected by a screening questionnaire. The physician should reschedule such a patient to himself. These diagnostic evaluations can keep practice stimulating. If the physician is "rusty" about the work-up of a particular problem, he will have time to refresh his memory prior to the appointment.

B. Physician Referral: Family practitioners or other specialists occasionally refer patients to a pediatrician for consultation. Within the pediatric community, some pediatricians refer patients to other physicians who have a subspecialty "hobby" or expertise with a specific disease. This is more common in group practice.

C. Nonphysician Referral: A physician who is well thought of receives referrals from dentists, school officials, psychologists, social workers, nurses, and previous patients. Some of these referred patients will require a consultation type visit.

Appointments

Consultations usually require 1-hour appointments. Some require 2 such visits to complete the evaluation. The average pediatrician will need to have 2–5 of these 1-hour appointments blocked out on his schedule each week. The visit will be considerably more productive if a screening questionnaire is completed in advance (see p 147). This questionnaire delineates the patient's physical, intellectual, and emotional problems and serves as his initial data base. The psychosocial portion is different for each of 4 age groups. The physician will then have a tentative problem list at hand before he sees the patient.

These long appointments are easily arranged when the patient is referred by another professional because a telephone call or letter usually precedes the patient. However, a patient with almost any problem requiring a careful evaluation can walk into a physician's office at any time and the physician must have a logical response to such situations. When a 10-year-old patient who is being seen for acute otitis media mentions that he has had 4 years of encopresis or 6 months of "staring spells" at school, the busy physician may feel under some pressure to make a quick recommendation.

He may be tempted to do a 5-minute work-up, order some laboratory tests, do a piecemeal work-up over several short visits, or hospitalize the patient for a work-up. He may decide to disregard the complaint or minimize its importance. None of these approaches are in the patient's best interests. Long-standing diagnostic dilemmas require a comprehensive assessment which takes at least an hour. Most such evaluations can be done on an ambulatory basis. Shortcuts can lead to tentative conclusions, unconvinced parents, postponement of the indicated work-up, "doctor shopping," secondary gain for the patient, and an unresolved problem.

The first visit can serve a useful purpose. One can tell the parents that their child's problem is complicated and deserves a complete evaluation. A few screening laboratory tests such as a blood count and erythrocyte sedimentation rate may be ordered. The parent can fill out the screening data questionnaire. A release can be signed for hospital discharge summaries, prior consultation reports, laboratory test results (especially any tests that were dangerous, painful, or expensive), school reports, and growth information. These data will make the consultation visit more meaningful and avoid duplication of effort. Unlike hospitalized consultations, an immediate appointment is rarely needed and the patient can be rescheduled for the following week or later if more time is needed to accumulate data.

Extent of Services

When the patient is referred by the parents or a nonphysician, the request is usually for total care. When the patient is referred by a physician, there are 4 possible degrees of service the consulting physician can offer. If the referring physician does not specify precisely what is needed, the consulting physician should either ask him or assume that a type C consultation (see below) is wanted.

A. Evaluation Only: The consultant can do a diagnostic evaluation on a patient and tell the parents nothing except that he will discuss his findings with their primary physician. Parents generally dislike this. They have paid for the consultation, and they want to hear something from the expert personally. Common courtesy would suggest they are correct.

B. Evaluation and Interpretation: After the evaluation is completed, the consultant usually explains his findings regarding diagnosis and etiology to the family. If he mentions recommendations for therapy, it should only be in very general terms and with the clear understanding that the referring physician will be coordinating the therapy. The patient should then be returned to the referring physician, who will make specific therapeutic recommendations to the family. A specific return appointment date with the referring physician should be given. This is the usual type of referral process for a patient with a chronic disease. The consultant will usually be called upon periodically as new therapeutic questions arise.

C. Evaluation and Treatment of an Isolated Problem: Sometimes the referring physician desires the consultant to manage the referred problem completely. This usually happens with curable, self-limited problems that will require 3–6 visits (eg, recurrent headaches, breathholding spells, ringworm, Sydenham's chorea). The consultant should clearly define and support the referring physician's role as the continual provider of well child and acute illness care during this period of time. When the referred problem is resolved, the patient should be returned to the referring physician for complete care. A single follow-up visit to the consultant in approximately 1 year is usually acceptable. Sometimes a letter from the parent will suffice to supply the consultant with the progress report he desires.

D. Total Health Care: Occasionally a physician refers a patient to a consultant for a diagnostic problem plus all future medical care. This usually occurs when a family is having financial problems or has recently moved. When the diagnostic problem is minimal and the psychosocial problems maximal, this is commonly known as a "dump" and does not constitute a true consultation.

Correspondence With the Referring Source

Communication is the key to a satisfactory referral process. The consulting physician is mainly responsible for this aspect of consultations. Good communication with both the referring physician and the parent completes the process of consultation and achieves the objective originally defined. The following suggestions might be considered guidelines to the appropriate format for completing the process diplomatically.

A. Acknowledgment of the Referral: As soon as a referral letter is received, the consulting physician should send the referral source a brief note acknowledging the referral. Additional information can also be requested at this time: "Thank you for your recent referral letter on David Jones. I have sent the parents a screening data questionnaire. As soon as it is returned, I will schedule him for an evaluation. I will notify you of the results as soon as I have had the opportunity to study his problem. Best regards."

B. A Brief Note Regarding the Evaluation: In some settings, the complete evaluation report may take 1 or 2 weeks to be typed. The patient may return to his referring physician in the interim. Therefore, on the day of the evaluation the consulting physician should telephone the referring physician or send him a brief note. The content of this communication should simply be the defined problems and the recommendations for each.

C. The Consultation Report: The content of the final report depends on the referring source. School officials do not want to know medical details; they usually just want to know if the patient is physically healthy or, if not, what their responsibility is. A referring physician expects a full report that will help him treat the patient. Recommendations should therefore be specific (drugs, dosages, other forms of therapy, duration of therapy, specific laboratory tests, the recommended frequency of these tests, etc). A copy of or reference to a recent review article on the subject will also be appreciated. The final recommendation in the evaluation should definitely state that the patient was returned to the referring physician for follow-up care. If the referring physician had tentatively made the correct diagnosis prior to referral, the consultant's corroboration should be made clear in the body of the report.

This evaluation should be typed as a formal consultation report. It should not contain personal comments or resemble a letter. When written in this style, it can serve as an official evaluation report for anyone who might request a copy of it in future years. To make this communication to the referring physician more personal, it should be accompanied by a covering letter: "It was a pleasure to see David Jones today. A complete summary of his evaluation is included. The recommendations may need to be modified in the light of your previous experience with this family. As you well know, the marital situation is very stormy. It would be a privilege to see David again if you feel the need arises."

Fees for Services Rendered

Many pediatricians are reluctant to charge adequately for their time. This seems illogical since an ambulatory consultation can prevent the high cost of an unnecessary hospital work-up. Even if ambulatory insurance does not cover the full cost of such an evaluation, the pediatrician should bill for these evaluations as "office consultations" and charge for the time allotted. His hour is worth the same whether it is spent with one consultation or several well or sick children.

THE PEDIATRICIAN IN THE ROLE OF REFERRING PHYSICIAN

Indications for Referral

There are generally 7 indications for seeking consultation. The last 2 are primarily to help the parents deal with realities.

A. The Pediatrician Is Uncertain of the Diagnosis: Referral for a diagnostic evaluation is a time-honored indication. A diagnostic dilemma should not be allowed to continue unresolved. The ambulatory consultation is preferable to hospitalization.

B. The Treatment Requires Special Technical Expertise: When the physician knows the diagnosis but treatment is outside of his specialty, he should refer (eg, surgery).

C. The Treatment Is Complex: A physician no longer needs to say he doesn't know how to treat a certain disease because he can look up the currently recommended therapy in several textbooks. However, every pediatrician must know his limitations. The treatment of some diseases is so complex that the

physician unfamiliar with it should refer (eg, cystic fibrosis, rheumatoid arthritis, leukemia).

D. The Disease Is Unresponsive to Conventional Therapy: When the patient is not doing as well as expected, 2 heads are better than one. Even with diseases that the physician has successfully treated many times, an atypical problem may arise that requires a fresh opinion.

E. The Problem Is a Medicolegal One: Parents bring in children with injuries for which they are suing a physician or other person. The pediatrician's main task is to decide if the alleged disability or defect is real. If the injury proves to be significant, the physician can help the family find an expert consultant whose testimony will stand up in court (eg, an orthopedist for a hand injury). If the physician feels that the parents are exaggerating the child's disability for financial gain, he should declare the child healthy and suggest that he return to full activity without confronting the family about his suspicions.

F. The Parents Insist on Overtreatment: The pediatrician can help the family accept his recommendations for avoiding aggressive intervention by suggesting consultation. There are honest differences of opinion about the indications for tonsillectomy, "corrective" shoes, hyposensitization, etc. If the pediatrician is certain that the patient's interests will be best served by a supporting opinion from another doctor, he should choose consultants who share his philosophy and communicate in advance that he wishes the consultant to discourage an escalation of therapy. Consultants sometimes assume that the intention of the referring physician is to have them provide special equipment rather than special advice, and they are reluctant not to comply.

G. The Parents Are Thinking About a Consultation: When the parents have to ask for a consultation or obtain one without telling their physician, the pediatrician has waited too long. He should recognize that such an attitude is developing when parents criticize him, question his judgment, or seem angry. The parents' tendency to deny the prognosis can be anticipated with certain diseases (eg, fatal diseases and mental retardation). This denial should be respected if it does not interfere with therapy.

A rare or fatal disease is not intrinsically an indication for referral. Some physicians automatically seek "confirmation" of a diagnosis they already know or "approval" of a treatment regimen they are already familiar with. The physician who is confident of his knowledge about a particular disease does not reassure the family by hiding his competence.

Method of Referral

A. Obtain Permission From the Family: The family will usually agree to a referral if the reason for it is made clear. Patients sometimes feel that a referral means they are being abandoned by their physician. The referring physician must make it clear that he will remain available for primary medical care. The family should also be told in advance that the consultation will cost more than a regular visit but that it will be worth more.

B. Help the Family Choose a Consultant: The physician should maintain a file listing the best consultants in his community and at the nearest medical center. The parents can be given the names of 2 or 3 competent physicians. If one is outstanding, the pediatrician should not be reluctant to state his preference. If the parents suggest someone they have heard of but whom the physician feels is unqualified, the pediatrician should tell them he does not consider the person they mention an expert on their particular problem.

C. Make an Appointment for the Family: After the family has made a selection, the physician can ask his secretary to arrange an appointment for them.

D. Send a Referral Letter: A referral letter should be sent immediately so that it will arrive well in advance of the appointment with the consultant. All pertinent information, such as copies of previous evaluations, hospital discharge summaries, and laboratory results, should be included. The referring physician must also specify the degree of consultative service he desires. The 2 most common types of consultation are an evaluation without treatment or evaluation and treatment of the referred problem.

Williams TF, MacKinney LG: Consultation-referral process. In: *Ambulatory Pediatrics.* Green M, Haggerty RJ (editors). Saunders, 1968.

QUALITY CONTROL OF AMBULATORY PEDIATRIC CARE

At a time when the consumer, third-party payers, and physicians themselves are alarmed at rising health care costs, all concerned should attempt to develop some kind of reliable quality control. In general, "organized medicine" has in the past been incapable of effectively penalizing any but the most flagrant examples of medical incompetence. The medical societies and academies are now attempting to develop a system of "peer review" which will at least ensure the consumer that the services billed for are appropriate and properly priced. This concept of peer review or medical audit can be implemented by a group of physicians for the purposes of self-education and the continual improvement of quality.

In any good hospital with an interested staff—especially where house staff are present—quality control is almost a built-in feature. Frequent reassessment of the inpatient's status by the physician, plus constant review by other medical and paramedical personnel, make "peer review" an ongoing process.

Care of ambulatory patients, on the other hand, usually is not reviewed systematically. The following is

a suggestion for developing a program that will both improve the quality of ambulatory practice and make it more challenging and satisfying.

Physicians can attempt to schedule approximately 1 hour a week for chart review. Several pediatricians should be present to make this a maximal learning experience. In group practice, the participants are already available. The pediatrician in solo practice can meet with the 1 or 2 pediatricians with whom he shares night calls. The group can focus on random charts or on selected charts that cover a specific problem. The latter method requires an office indexing system.

CHART REVIEWS

Well Child Chart Review

The delivery of comprehensive well child care can be easily audited by reviewing the well child flow sheet (see p 145). Since the nursing staff is primarily responsible for filling out these flow sheets, this type of review is largely a check on their ability to comply with office protocol and need not be done very often. The office protocols themselves require periodic review and revision.

Acute Illness Chart Review

Acute illness charts can be audited for completeness in diagnosis and therapy of the chief complaint. The following questions can be asked: (1) Was the diagnosis valid? Validity is substantiated if the chart contains adequate historical, physical, or laboratory data to document the diagnosis. (2) Was the therapy optimal? (3) Was the follow-up plan optimal? Charts of patients with a specific acute illness (eg, acute lymphadenitis, streptococcal pharyngitis, or infectious hepatitis) can be pulled and audited to test the group consensus about therapy and follow-up.

Chronic Disease Chart Review

Examination of the chronic disease flow sheet (see p 154) is an easy way to audit chronic disease management. If no such flow sheet exists, the variables recommended above for monitoring chronic disease can be assessed as one reads the chart completely. This chart review process could then result in the formulation of a chronic disease flow sheet for that patient. Chart review sessions can be more educational if only one chronic disease is considered each time and if an "expert" on that disease is present. The expert can be an actual subspecialist or a member of the group who has reviewed the literature or attended a workshop on this disease.

Diagnostic Problem Chart Review

An easy way to review consultations is to criticize the consultation report. The following questions can be asked: (1) Was the data base adequate? (2) Were all the active problems identified? (3) Was the diagnostic plan for each problem optimal? (4) Were the final diagnoses valid? (5) Was the recommended therapy for each diagnosis optimal? (6) Was the role of the referring physician clarified and honored? If these consultations are concerned with general pediatric problems, an outside consultant will generally not be required.

Bjorn JC, Cross HD: *Problem-Oriented Practice.* Modern Hospital Press, 1970.

Weed LL: *Medical Records, Medical Education and Patient Care.* Case Univ Press, 1969.

THE EFFECTIVENESS OF MEDICAL CARE

Correct diagnoses and optimal therapeutic recommendations can be ensured by the voluntary type of peer review discussed above. An aspect of the quality of care which is not easy to assess by chart review but which needs to be borne in mind is patient compliance. Superb recommendations do not guarantee anything. Medical care does not become effective until the parent accepts the diagnosis and carries out the therapeutic recommendations. These matters could be considered beyond the physician's control, but he has some influence over them. A parent's compliance often reflects her satisfaction with the medical care being given. Until there is a better understanding of missed follow-up appointments, missed referrals, missed laboratory tests, ungiven medications, unfollowed advice, and unkept home records, even the best conceived therapeutic goals will often not be achieved.

Fink D & others: Effective patient care in the pediatric ambulatory setting: A study of the acute care clinic. Pediatrics 43:927, 1969.

PRACTICAL TIPS FOR AMBULATORY CARE

A number of problems arise which may be perplexing both to the patient and to the physician in the daily care of ambulatory patients. Some of these apparently complex problems have rather simple solutions.

FOREIGN BODIES

Foreign Body in the Nose

Asking the child to blow his nose will remove some foreign bodies. A crocodile forceps, a magnet, or a catheter attached to wall suction may remove others. If these technics have failed and there is some space between the object and the side of the nose after vasoconstriction, a lubricated Bardex Foley catheter can be placed. After the catheter's balloon rests behind the object, the balloon can be inflated and used to pull the object out of the nose.

Rees AC: "Tip of the Month" Consultant 10(2):12, 1970.

Metallic Foreign Body in the Soft Tissues

Tape a straight pin with the point over the site where the metallic object entered the skin. Then obtain an x-ray of the area. An exact measurement can then be obtained to locate the foreign body in relation to the straight pin. Located in this manner, the foreign body can be removed with minimal exploration.

Inlow PM: "Tip of the Month" Consultant 7(6):27, 1967.

Splinters Under the Nails

Using a single-edged razor blade or a sharp thin scalpel, the nail can be gently shaved over the distal end of the splinter until the splinter is exposed. The sliver can then be easily pulled out with a pair of fine-pointed tweezers.

Mikelionis J: "Tip of the Month" Consultant 5(2):28, 1965.

Imbedded Fishhook

Fishhooks can be removed (eg, from a finger) without local anesthesia or wirecutters by bringing them back through their point of entry. A piece of fishline is looped around the curve of the fishhook. The 2 strands of the fishline are wrapped tightly about the physician's forefinger about 1 foot from where it is looped around the hook. The patient's finger is held against a firm surface to stabilize it. The free shank of the fishhook is pressed against the patient's finger with the physician's free hand until the barb is disengaged and the barb's long axis is parallel to the line of intended expulsion. With the string in this same axis, a quick yank expels the hook immediately.

Friedenberg S: Removing an imbedded fishhook. Hosp Physician 8:48, 1971.

Feasting Ticks

Most imbedded ticks will withdraw when covered with alcohol, nail polish, mineral oil, or an ointment. Occasionally, a needle can be inserted between the tick's jaws and used to pry loose his grip. If the above methods fail, the following definitive method can be employed. Pick up the body of the tick with a pair of forceps. Apply gentle traction so that the skin is tented up at the site where the tick is imbedded. Then take a number 11 scalpel blade (or a razor blade) and quickly cut away the superficial layer of dermis in which the tick has buried its jaws. Brief pressure will stop the bleeding. This method of extracting the tick is relatively painless and ensures removal of the head.

Ring on a Swollen Finger

Pass a piece of string under the ring and then wind the distal end of the string in close loops tightly from the distal edge of the ring past the knuckle. Exert a slow, firm pull on the proximal end of the string. The edema passes underneath the ring and the ring is slowly pulled distally as the cord unwinds.

If there is a dentist's office nearby, another way the ring might be removed is to have the dentist cut it off with a carborundum disk attached to his drill.

Burgoon EB: "Tip of the Month" Consultant 4(4):8, 1964.

Gum in the Hair

An easy and nontraumatic way to remove gum from children's hair is by rubbing the gum with peanut butter until the hairs are freed from the gum. This technic is far superior to pulling or cutting the gum out of the hair.

Tar on the Skin

Tar can be removed by applying ice to it for 1 or 2 minutes. The ice causes the tar to become quite hard and nonsticky, so that it can be easily peeled from the skin. Hydrocarbon solvents merely soften the tar and smear it around, and they are painful if a wound is present.

Bostrom PD: "Tip of the Month" Consultant 8(1):12, 1968.

LACERATIONS

Wound Cleaning in a Resistant Child

The wound can be bathed in 1–5 ml of 1% lidocaine (Xylocaine) for 2 minutes, which will cause momentary discomfort. The area will then be relatively anesthetized, and vigorous wound cleaning will be tolerated. The subcutaneous injection of additional lidocaine after the wound is cleaned will also be better tolerated.

Laceration Closure in a Frightened Child

Wounds can often be closed without local anesthesia or sutures by using microporous adhesive tape (Steri-Strip). The skin adjacent to the laceration is made tacky with tincture of benzoin. The 1/8-inch strips of tape are applied in either a parallel or crisscross pattern. This microporous tape is a decided improvement over "butterfly" tape.

Abramo A: Recent results with sutureless wound closure in children. Am J Dis Child 110:42, 1965.

Suture Removal

There is a way to avoid having to dig imbedded sutures out of the skin of a struggling child. At the time the laceration is closed, a straight needle threaded with silk can be passed under each suture used for skin closure. The ends of this silk suture can be tied together, leaving a loose loop. At the time of removal, picking up this loose loop will lift up the sutures which have been used to close the wound. The scissors can then be easily slid underneath the sutures for snipping.

Floyd BG, McKnight CA: "Tip of the Month" Consultant 10(4):35, 1970.

Traumatic Amputations

When a patient loses a significant piece of his skin (eg, a fingertip) in an accident, the skin should be placed in cold normal saline solution and sent with the patient to a plastic surgeon.

BLUNT TRAUMA

Subungual Hematomas

The painful pressure secondary to a subungual hematoma can easily be relieved by applying a red-hot paper clip or other thick wire to the nail surface. The paper clip is held by a clamp. A hole is quickly burrowed through the nail and the blood is allowed to escape. This "hot iron" approach can be very frightening for a child. If there is a dentist's office nearby, it is preferable to have the dentist bore a hole quickly through the nail with a high-speed drill.

Traumatic Tooth Avulsion

Reimplantation of a tooth is possible only with the permanent teeth. The physician or parent should attempt to replace the avulsed tooth in its socket prior to going to the dentist. If this proves impossible, the tooth should be placed in cold normal saline solution and sent with the patient to his dentist.

Bernick SM: What the pediatrician should know about children's teeth: Dental emergencies. Clin Pediat 9:487, 1970.

INJECTIONS

Painful Rabies Vaccine Injections

The local pain that occurs with daily rabies vaccine injections can be relieved by adding 1 ml of 2% lidocaine (Xylocaine) to the syringe.

Baehren PF: Pain and rabies vaccine. Clin Pediat 10:298, 1971.

Inadvertent Subcutaneous Injections

When intramuscular agents are given subcutaneously by mistake, complications can result. The location of the needle point can be rapidly assessed by trying to wiggle it prior to injection. If it is in a muscle mass, the needle point will be relatively fixed. If it is in the subcutaneous fatty tissues, it can be felt to move freely.

MISCELLANEOUS PROCEDURES

Genital Labial Adhesions

Labial adhesions can usually be separated by introducing a probe into any opening remaining in the introitus and then tearing the adhesions. This method is acceptable for thin adhesions. An ointment should be applied to the newly separated surfaces for several days to prevent them from resealing. A nontraumatic method for separating thicker labial adhesions is application of estrogen cream to the medial line for 3 or 4 days.

Postcircumcision Skin Tags

Parents occasionally bring their baby in during the first month of life because the foreskin has an irregular skin tag. A clamp can be applied along the desired line of cleavage for 1 minute. After the clamp is removed, an iris scissors can be used to cut along the crushed skin line without causing any significant bleeding.

Umbilical Granulomas

Umbilical granulomas usually respond to alcohol cleansing. If a pinch of table salt is placed in the umbilical area after alcohol cleansing once a day for 3 days, the desiccant effect of the salt will rapidly shrink the granuloma.

University of Colorado Medical Center	Name
WELL CHILD FLOW SHEET	Hosp. No.
Enter Dates	Date

History forms — 0–5 years [ ] 6–12 years [ ] 13–18 years [ ]

Hematocrit (yearly after 9 months) [ ][ ][ ][ ][ ][ ]

Urinalysis [ ][ ][ ][ ][ ][ ]

Urine bacteria screen (yearly, females only) [ ][ ][ ][ ][ ][ ]

Blood pressure (yearly after age 4) [ ][ ][ ][ ][ ][ ]

DDST — 9–12 months [ ] 3 years [ ] 5 years [ ]

Peabody Picture Vocabulary Test [ ] Goodenough Draw-A-Man [ ]

Vision screen (every other year after age 4 if not done at school) [ ][ ][ ][ ][ ][ ]

Audiologic screen (every other year after age 4 if not done at school) [ ][ ][ ][ ][ ][ ]

Immunizations:

DPT [ ][ ][ ][ ][ ]

DT [ ][ ][ ][ ][ ]

Tetanus [ ][ ][ ][ ][ ]

Polio [ ][ ][ ][ ][ ]

Tuberculin test (every other year after 9 months) [ ][ ][ ][ ][ ]

Rubeola [ ]   Rubella [ ]   Mumps [ ]

Other _____

Discussion and Guidance (Enter Date When Discussed)

Prenatal	Feeding (breast or formula)	_____		12 months	Negativism	_____
	Preparation for newcomer:				Frequency of respiratory	
	Home	_____			infections	_____
	Older children	_____			Cruising and investigating	_____
					Weaning from the bottle	_____
2 weeks	Vitamins	_____			Control of drugs, poisons	
	Urination	_____			(syrup of ipecac)	_____
	Stools	_____				
				15 months	Temper tantrums	_____
6 weeks	Colic	_____			Obedience	_____
	Spoiling	_____				
	Solid foods	_____		18 months	Reaction toward strangers	_____
	Immunizations	_____			Speech development	_____
3 months	Accidents—rolling over	_____		21 months	Manners	_____
	Frustrations	_____			Change in appetite	_____
					Toilet training	_____
5 months	Adapting to family schedule	_____				
	Attitude of father	_____		24 months	Need for peer relationships	_____
					Staying with a babysitter	_____
7 months	Night crying	_____			Sharing	_____
	Separation anxiety	_____			Dental care	_____
	Fear of strangers	_____				
9 months	Use of cup	_____				
	Accidents	_____				
	Normal unpleasant behavior	_____				
	Discipline	_____				
	Need for affection	_____				

Further discussions and guidance should be based on specific parental concerns. Self-administered question-naires or direct questioning can be used to identify problem areas.

Age	Specific Parental Concern—Topic	Date
_____	_____	_____
_____	_____	_____
_____	_____	_____
_____	_____	_____
_____	_____	_____
_____	_____	_____
_____	_____	_____
_____	_____	_____
_____	_____	_____
_____	_____	_____
_____	_____	_____

University of Colorado Medical Center	Name
CHILD CARE CLINIC	Hosp. No.
Birth through 5 years	Date
(History form to be filled out by parent)	

The Pediatric Clinic at Colorado General Hospital can provide either short-term emergency care or long-term continuous care. If your child is under the care of a private doctor or a convenient health clinic, we do not want to interfere with or duplicate the care you are receiving there.

My child usually gets his care at _____ and his last physical examination was _____ months or _____ years ago.

I am here for this visit only and my child receives his care elsewhere.   Yes _____ No _____
If your response to the above is Yes, there is no need to go any further with this questionnaire.

If you would like your child cared for in a private doctor's office or a public health facility more convenient to you, please ask to speak with one of the Public Health Nurses.

If your child is not receiving care elsewhere and you want him to receive his care here, you can help us take better care of him by answering the following questions:

If your child is over 3 years old, is he/she too sick today to have his eyes checked?   Yes _____ No _____

Is he/she too sick today or are you too rushed for us to test how he/she is developing?   Yes _____ No _____
  (approximately 15 minutes)

I. Pregnancy and Birth   **Circle One**
   1. Did you have any illnesses during your pregnancy? . . . .   No   Yes
   2. Did you carry him/her for a full 9 months? . . . .   Yes   No
   3. Where was your baby born? _____
   4. How much did he/she weigh at birth?   _____ lb, _____ oz
   5. Did your baby have any trouble starting to breathe? . . . .   No   Yes
   6. Did your baby have any trouble in the hospital? . . . .   No   Yes
   7. Did your baby go home with you when you left the hospital? . . . .   Yes   No
   8. How long did he/she stay in the hospital?   _____ days

II. Feeding and Digestion
   1. Did your baby have severe colic or any unusual feeding problems during
     the first 3 months of life? . . . .   No   Yes
   2. If on vitamins, what kind and how much? _____
   3. If still on formula, which one do you use? _____
   4. Is your child's appetite usually good? . . . .   Yes   No
   5. Do any foods bother him/her? . . . .   No   Yes
   6. Does he/she often have diarrhea or runny bowels? . . . .   No   Yes

III. Baby Shots, Tests, and Development
   Has your child had:
    1. A scar from smallpox vaccination? . . . .   Yes   No   Year_____
    2. All 3 of his/her "DPT" shots? . . . .   Yes   No   Booster_____
    3. All 3 doses of poliovaccine by mouth? . . . .   Yes   No   Booster_____
    4. Measles shot? . . . .   Yes   No
    5. Skin test for tuberculosis? . . . .   Yes   No   When _____
    6. Rubella shot (German measles)? . . . .   Yes   No
    7. Mumps shot? . . . .   Yes   No
    8. Did your child sit alone before 7 months of age? . . . .   Yes   No
    9. Did your child walk alone before 15 months of age? . . . .   Yes   No
   10. Did your child say any words by 1½ years of age? . . . .   Yes   No
   11. Is he/she as quick in learning as your other children? . . . .   Yes   No

IV. Allergies

Has your child had:

1. Eczema or hives? . . . .   No   Yes
2. Wheezing or asthma? . . . .   No   Yes
3. Allergies or reactions to any medicines or injections such as penicillin? .   No   Yes
4. Does he/she have a constant cold, hay fever, or sinus trouble? . . . .   No   Yes

V. Family-Social History

1. Are both parents in good health? . . . .   Yes   No
2. Do any other members of your child's immediate family (brothers, sisters, parents, grandparents, aunts, uncles) have a serious health problem (mental or physical)? . . . .   No   Yes
   List each problem and who has it. _____

   _____
3. How many people live in your home?   Children _____   Adults _____
4. With whom does the child live? (circle one)
   both parents   mother   father   legal guardian   other _____
5. Does anyone help you take care of your child on a regular basis? . . . . .   No   Yes

VI. Infections, Illnesses, and Other Problems

Has your child:

1. Had **more** than 6 colds or throat infections each year? . . . .   No   Yes
2. Had **more** than 3 ear infections? . . . .   No   Yes
3. Had any trouble hearing? . . . .   No   Yes
4. Had his/her hearing tested? . . . .   Yes   No   When _____
5. Had any trouble seeing? . . . .   No   Yes
6. Had his/her eyes tested? . . . .   Yes   No   When _____
7. Had any trouble with his/her teeth? . . . .   No   Yes
8. Seen a dentist recently? . . . .   Yes   No   When _____
9. Had any trouble passing his/her urine? . . . .   No   Yes
10. Ever had a convulsion or fit or fainting spell? . . . .   No   Yes
11. Had any of the following? (circle)   3-day measles   7-day measles
    chickenpox   mumps   whooping cough   pneumonia
12. Had other diseases? _____
13. Had to stay in the hospital overnight? . . . .   No   Yes
    Age _____   Hospital _____
    Reason _____

VII. Accidents

1. Has your child had any serious accidents? . . . .   No   Yes
   burns _____ poisoning _____ cuts needing a doctor _____ broken bones _____
2. Does your child use seat belts in your car? . . . .   Yes   No
3. Do you know how to prevent infant smothering or choking? . . . .   Yes   No
4. Do you have firearms (loaded or unloaded) in your home? . . . .   No   Yes

VIII. Behavior and Discipline

1. Is he/she more difficult to raise than your other children? . . . .   No   Yes
2. What is the most effective way of disciplining your child? (circle)
   spanking   putting to room   taking privileges away   other _____
3. Are you concerned about any of the following? (circle which ones)
   bad temper   won't mind   holds his breath   jealousy   sleep problems
   thumbsucking   nailbiting   speech problems   can't toilet train
   very shy   doesn't pay attention   overactive   slow to learn
   eats dirt or paint

Reviewed by _____

University of Colorado Medical Center	Name
CHILD CARE CLINIC	Hosp. No.
6 through 12 years	Date
(History form to be filled out by parent)	

The Pediatric Clinic at Colorado General Hospital can provide either short-term emergency care or long-term continuous care. If your child is under the care of a private doctor or a convenient health clinic, we do not want to interfere with or duplicate the care you are receiving there.

My child usually gets his care at _____ and his last physical examination was _____ months or _____ years ago.

I am here for this visit only and my child receives his care elsewhere.   Yes _____ No _____
If your response to the above is Yes, there is no need to go any further with this questionnaire.

If you would like your child cared for in a private doctor's office or a public health facility more convenient to you, please ask to speak with one of the Public Health Nurses.

If your child is not receiving care elsewhere and you want him to receive his care here, you can help us take better care of him by answering the following questions:

Is your child too sick today to have his/her vision and hearing checked?   Yes _____ No _____

I. Pregnancy and Birth   Circle One
1. Did you have any illnesses during your pregnancy? . . . .   No   Yes
2. Did you carry him/her for a full 9 months? . . . .   Yes   No
3. Where was your baby born? _____
4. How much did he/she weigh at birth? _____ lb, _____ oz
5. Did your baby have any trouble starting to breathe? . . . .   No   Yes
6. Did your baby have any trouble in the hospital? . . . .   No   Yes
7. Did your baby go home with you when you left the hospital? . . . .   Yes   No
8. How long did he/she stay in the hospital? _____ days

II. Baby Shots, Tests, and Development
Has your child had:
1. A scar from smallpox vaccination? . . . .   Yes   No   Year _____
2. All 3 of his/her "DPT" shots? . . . .   Yes   No   Booster _____
3. All 3 doses of poliovaccine by mouth? . . . .   Yes   No   Booster _____
4. Measles shot? . . . .   Yes   No
5. Skin test for tuberculosis? . . . .   Yes   No   When _____
6. Rubella shot (German measles)? . . . .   Yes   No
7. Mumps shot? . . . .   Yes   No
8. Did your child sit alone before 7 months of age? . . . .   Yes   No
9. Did your child walk alone before 15 months of age? . . . .   Yes   No
10. Did your child say any words by 1½ years of age? . . . .   Yes   No
11. Is he/she as quick in learning as your other children? . . . .   Yes   No

III. Allergies
Has your child had:
1. Eczema or hives? . . . .   No   Yes
2. Wheezing or asthma? . . . .   No   Yes
3. Allergies or reactions to any medicines or injections such as penicillin? . .   No   Yes
4. Does he/she have a constant cold, hay fever, or sinus trouble? . . . .   No   Yes

IV. Accidents
1. Has your child had any serious accidents? . . . .   No   Yes
     burns _____ poisoning _____ cuts needing a doctor _____ broken bones _____
2. Does your child use seat belts in your car? . . . .   Yes   No
3. Does your child know how to swim? . . . .   Yes   No
4. Do you have firearms (loaded or unloaded) in your home? . . . .   No   Yes

V. Family-Social History

1. Are both parents in good health? . . . .   Yes   No
2. Do any other members of your child's immediate family (brothers, sisters, parents, grandparents, aunts, uncles) have a serious health problem (mental or physical)? . . . .   No   Yes

   List each problem and who has it. _____

   _____
3. How many people live in your home?   Children _____   Adults _____
4. With whom does the child live? (circle one)

   both parents   mother   father   legal guardian   other _____
5. Does anyone help you take care of your child on a regular basis? . . . . .   No   Yes

VI. Infections, Illnesses, and Other Problems

Has your child:

1. Had **more** than 6 colds or throat infections each year? . . . .   No   Yes
2. Had **more** than 3 ear infections? . . . .   No   Yes
3. Had any trouble hearing? . . . .   No   Yes
4. Had his/her hearing tested? . . . .   Yes   No   When _____
5. Had any trouble seeing? . . . .   No   Yes
6. Had his/her eyes tested? . . . .   Yes   No   When _____
7. Had any trouble with his/her teeth? . . . .   No   Yes
8. Seen a dentist recently? . . . .   Yes   No   When _____
9. Had any trouble passing his/her urine? . . . .   No   Yes
10. Is your child's appetite usually good? . . . .   Yes   No
11. Do any foods bother him/her? . . . .   No   Yes
12. Does he/she often have diarrhea or runny bowels? . . . .   No   Yes
13. Ever had a convulsion or fit or fainting spell? . . . .   No   Yes
14. Had any of the following? (circle)   3-day measles   7-day measles

    chickenpox   mumps   whooping cough   pneumonia
15. Had other diseases? _____
16. Had to stay in the hospital overnight? . . . .   No   Yes

    Age _____   Hospital _____

    Reason _____

VII. Behavior and Discipline

1. What school does your child attend?   _____   Grade _____
2. Does your child get along well in school? . . . .   Yes   No
3. Have you met with the teacher? . . . .   Yes   No
4. Is the teacher worried about any problems? . . . .   No   Yes
5. Does your child get along well with other children? . . . .   Yes   No
6. What is the most effective way of disciplining your child? (circle)

   spanking   putting to room   taking privileges away   other _____
7. Are you concerned about any of the following? (circle which ones)

   bad temper   won't mind   holds his breath   jealousy   sleep problems

   thumbsucking   nailbiting   speech problems   can't toilet train

   wets bed   very shy   doesn't pay attention   overactive   slow to learn

   eats dirt or paint

Reviewed by _____

University of Colorado Medical Center	Name
CHILD CARE CLINIC	Hosp. No.
13 through 18 years	Date
(History form to be filled out by patient)	

The Pediatric Clinic at Colorado General Hospital can provide either short-term emergency care or long-term continuous care. If you are under the care of a private doctor or a convenient health clinic, we do not want to interfere with or duplicate the care you are receiving there.

I usually get my care at _____ and my last physical examination was _____ months or _____ years ago.

I am here for this visit only and I receive my care elsewhere.   Yes ____   No ____
If your response to the above is Yes, there is no need to go any further with this questionnaire.

If you would like to receive your care in a private doctor's office or a public health facility more convenient to you, please ask to speak with one of the Public Health Nurses.

If you are not receiving your care elsewhere and want to receive your care here, you can help us by answering the following questions:

I am too sick today to have my vision and hearing checked.   Yes ____   No ____

I. Medical   **Circle One**

  A. Immunizations
     Do you have your immunization records with you today? .... No Yes
     (If not, please bring them on your next visit.)
      1. Did you get your "DPT" immunizations as an infant? .... Yes No
      2. Date of last tetanus booster _____
      3. Have you had the oral poliovaccine? .... Yes No
      4. Have you had a tuberculin skin test in the past year? .... Yes No
      5. Do you have a smallpox scar? .... Yes No
      6. Have you had the German measles vaccine (rubella)? .... Yes No
      7. Have you had German measles? .... Yes No
      8. Have you had the measles vaccine (rubeola)? .... Yes No
      9. Have you had measles (7-day)? .... Yes No
     10. Have you had the mumps vaccine? .... Yes No
     11. Have you had mumps? .... Yes No

  B. Past History
      1. Have you ever been hospitalized for illness or operation? .... No Yes
        Age _____   Hospital _____
        Reason _____
      2. Any other prolonged or serious illness? .... No Yes
      3. Do you have any allergy (hives, wheezing, asthma, hay fever)? .... No Yes
      4. Have you ever had a reaction (rash, hives, breathing difficulty) to any medicines or
        injections such as penicillin? .... No Yes
      5. Are you taking any medicines now? .... No Yes
        If so, which ones? _____

  C. Family History
      1. Are both of your parents in good health? ·........................... Yes No
      2. Do any other members of your immediate family (brothers, sisters, parents, grandparents,
        aunts, uncles) have a serious health problem (mental or physical)? .... No Yes
        List each problem and who has it. _____

        _____

      3. How many people live in your home?   Children ____   Adults ____
      4. With whom do you live? (circle one)
        both parents   mother   father   legal guardian   other _____
      5. Do your parents get along well with each other? .... Yes No
      6. Do you feel that your parents understand your problems? .... Yes No
      7. Any long-term separations of the family? .... No Yes
      8. Do you feel your parents (circle one)   are too strict   too old fashioned
        don't care   favor your brothers and sisters over you   are fair
      9. Could things be better at home? .... No Yes

D. Accidents

    1. Have you ever had any serious accidents? . . . . No   Yes

       burns _____ poisoning _____ cuts needing a doctor _____ broken bones _____

    2. Do you use seat belts in your car? . . . . Yes   No

    3. Do you know how to swim? . . . . Yes   No

    4. Are firearms (loaded or unloaded) kept in your home? . . . . No   Yes

E. Review of Systems

    1. Do you have any of the following complaints? (circle which ones)

       headaches   dizzy spells   convulsions   difficulty hearing

       blurred or double vision   sinus trouble   seizures

    2. Do you wear glasses? _____   How long? _____

    3. Last time you had your eyes checked _____

    4. Do you have swollen glands of the neck or under the arms? . . . . No   Yes

    5. Have you had pneumonia more than 2 times? . . . . No   Yes

    6. Do you get short of breath before other members of your class do? . . . . No   Yes

    7. Do you smoke? _____   How many per day? _____

    8. Do you have a chronic cough? . . . . No   Yes

    9. Do you have a heart murmur? . . . . No   Yes

   10. Do you have (circle)   chest pain   abdominal pain   constipation

       diarrhea   frequent vomiting

   11. Have you ever had hepatitis (yellow eyes or skin)? . . . . No   Yes

   12. Have you had joint pains or swelling of joints? . . . . No   Yes

   13. Have you ever had a kidney infection? . . . . No   Yes

   14. Does it burn when you pass your urine? . . . . No   Yes

   15. Do you get up at night to urinate? . . . . No   Yes

   16. Do you ever wet the bed? . . . . No   Yes

   17. Have you had venereal disease? . . . . No   Yes

   18. Do you have any questions about venereal disease? . . . . No   Yes

   19. Have you had recurrent fevers? . . . . No   Yes

   20. Do you have problems with acne? . . . . No   Yes

   21. Do you have problems with your teeth? . . . . No   Yes

   22. Are you tired in the morning when you get up? . . . . No   Yes

II. Individual Patterns

    1. What grade are you in? _____   Are you satisfied with your grades? . . . . Yes   No

    2. Do you miss more than 3 days of school each month? . . . . No   Yes

    3. Is something slowing your progress at school? . . . . No   Yes

    4. Do your teachers pick on you? . . . . No   Yes

    5. Is school (circle)   a drag   means to an end   meaningless   worthwhile

    6. What do you plan to do when you graduate? _____

    _____

    7. Do you make friends easily? . . . . Yes   No

    8. Do you often feel left out? . . . . No   Yes

    9. Do things get on your nerves easily? . . . . No   Yes

   10. Do you feel that you are a nervous person? . . . . No   Yes

   11. Do drugs make you feel better? . . . . No   Yes

       Which ones? _____

   12. Do you take drugs when you are alone? . . . . No   Yes

   13. Would you like to learn more about the prevention of pregnancy? . . . . No   Yes

FOR GIRLS ONLY

    1. Have you had your first period? _____   At what age? _____

    2. Would you like to learn more about periods? . . . . No   Yes

    3. Do you have cramping with your periods? . . . . No   Yes

    4. Are your periods regular? . . . . Yes   No

    5. Are you taking the "pill"? . . . . No   Yes

    6. Would you like more information about the "pill"? . . . . No   Yes

Reviewed by _____

University of Colorado Medical Center	Name
ACUTE ILLNESS CLINIC	Hosp. No.
	Date

Brief Screening Questionnaire for Major Problems in New Patients

We realize you are here because your child is sick. We will concentrate on that problem today. Please answer the following questions to help us decide what **other** medical care your child may need.

Circle One

1. Does your child have any important physical problems? . . . . No   Yes
2. Does your child have any important emotional problems? . . . . No   Yes
3. Does your child have any important school problems? . . . . No   Yes
4. Does your child have any other medical problem you would like evaluated? . . . . No   Yes
If the answer to 1, 2, 3, or 4 is Yes, list the problems below.

5. Has your child ever been hospitalized? . . . . No   Yes
If Yes, list date, hospital, and diagnosis below.

6. Is your child allergic to any medicines? . . . . No   Yes
If Yes, which ones?

7. Would you like future well child care at our office? . . . . No   Yes
8. Does your child receive his well child care elsewhere? . . . . No   Yes
If Yes, where?

University of Colorado Medical Center

CHRONIC DISEASE FLOW SHEET

Name

Hosp. No.

Date

Dates ⟶

Variables									
Diabetes Mellitus									
Hypoglycemic episodes									
Weight									
Ketotic episodes									
Hospitalization									
Carrying glucose food									
Insulin									
Subcutaneous dystrophy									
Disease education									
Note to school									
Emotional adjustment									
Seizures									
Frequency									
Duration									
Neurologic exam									
EEG									
Phenobarb									
Dilantin									
Gum hyperplasia									
Disease education									
School Phobia									
Attendance									

University of Colorado Medical Center **PROBLEM LIST**	Name Hosp. No. Date

Column I			Column II	
Problem Number	**Date of Onset**	**Problem (Active)**	**Date of Resolution**	**Problem (Resolved or Inactive)**
1	1964	Diabetes mellitus		
2	1966	Grand mal seizures		
3	Sept 1969	School phobia		
4	Feb 1970	Recurrent epistaxis	May 1970	Resolved

University of Colorado Medical Center **PEDIATRIC REFERRAL CLINIC**	Name Hosp. No. Date

–1–

Date of Birth _____

Reason for Referral (to be completed by a parent)

Describe your child's current problem (or problems).
Be as brief as possible.
Include approximate dates whenever possible.

University of Colorado Medical Center	Name
PEDIATRIC REFERRAL CLINIC	Hosp. No. Date

–2–

PHYSICAL SCREENING DATA

A. Review of Systems

Circle any of the following symptoms that apply to your child.

1. **General:** poor appetite   excessive appetite   excessive thirst   overweight   underweight   weight loss   too tall   too short   difficulty in sleeping   excessive sleeping   confusion   loss of memory   no energy   excessive energy   fevers

2. **Skin:** rash   acne   unexplained lump   easy bruising   dandruff   itching

3. **Eyes:** eye pain   blurred vision   crossed eyes   wears glasses

4. **Ear-Nose-Throat:** earaches   decreased hearing   sneezing attacks   frequent nosebleeds   bad teeth   mouth breathing   difficulty in swallowing

5. **Respiratory:** hoarseness   cough   wheezing   difficulty in breathing   "shortness of breath" attacks

6. **Cardiovascular:** chest pain   heart murmur   high blood pressure

7. **Gastrointestinal:** abdominal pains   nausea   vomiting   frequent indigestion   diarrhea   constipation   blood in stools   stools in underwear (soiling)

8. **Urinary:** painful urination   frequent urination   weak urine stream   daytime wetting   bedwetting

9. **Skeletal:** bone pain   back pain   limp   swollen joints   frequent accidents

10. **Neuromuscular:** headache   migraine   weakness   paralysis   numbness   clumsiness   loss of balance   dizziness   unexplained movements or jerks   convulsions   staring spells   fainting   breathholding spells   unexplained "attacks"

11. If your daughter has started her menstrual periods, complete the following:
    When did they begin?   Month _____   Year _____
    Circle if any of the following apply:
    painful periods   excessive bleeding   other menstrual problems

12. Do you feel that any of your child's symptoms are caused by stress or worry?   No _____   Yes _____

13. Do you feel that your child is physically delicate?   No _____   Yes _____

(This medical information is confidential.)

–3–

B. Past Medical History

1. Newborn: How much did your baby weigh at birth? _____ lb, _____ oz
   How long did your pregnancy last? _____ (weeks or months)
   Did your baby have any complications at birth or in the first days of life? No _____ Yes _____
2. Hospitalizations: Has your child ever been hospitalized? No _____ Yes _____
   If Yes, list the approximate dates, hospital, and reason for admission.

3. Other illness: Has your child had any important illnesses for which he was **not** hospitalized?
   No _____ Yes _____
   If Yes, list the approximate dates and the type of illness.

4. Allergies: *Circle* any of the following allergies your child has:
   asthma   nose allergy   eye allergy   eczema   hives
   drug allergy   food allergy
5. Medications: Is your child on any daily medication? No _____ Yes _____
   If Yes, list the drug and the amount per day.

University of Colorado Medical Center | Name
                                            | Hosp. No.
PEDIATRIC REFERRAL CLINIC | Date

–4–

C. Family History

1. Are there any inherited diseases that run in your family?   No ____ Yes ____
2. Are there any family problems that might be related to your child's symptoms?   No ____ Yes ____
3. List below the name and age of each person who lives in your house. (If any of the people have a medical problem, mention it.)

_____

_____

_____

_____

_____

_____

_____

_____

_____

D. Past Medical Work-Up

1. *Circle* any of the following people that your child has already seen for his problem. Ask that person to send us a copy of his results.

    family physician   pediatrician   osteopath
    neurologist   psychologist   psychiatrist
    chiropractor   any other specialist

2. Has your child already undergone any expensive tests for his problem?   No ____ Yes ____
   If Yes, please request that copies be sent to us.

University of Colorado Medical Center	Name
	Hosp. No.
PEDIATRIC REFERRAL CLINIC	Date

–5–

DEVELOPMENTAL SCREENING DATA (13 years or older)
(to be completed by a parent)

A. Speech and Self Care

Yes _____ No _____   1. Did he walk alone across the room by 18 months?

Yes _____ No _____   2. Did he speak in sentences by age 3?

Yes _____ No _____   3. Did he tie his shoestrings alone by age 6?

Yes _____ No _____   4. Did he develop as quickly as his brothers and sisters?

No _____ Yes _____   5. Does he have a problem with pronouncing words?

No _____ Yes _____   6. Does he stutter?

No _____ Yes _____   7. Does he refuse to talk to some people?

Yes _____ No _____   8. Does he have a plan for his future?

Yes _____ No _____   9. Has he ever had a summer job?

Yes _____ No _____   10. Is he starting to loosen his ties to his family somewhat?

Yes _____ No _____   11. Does he sometimes challenge your ideas?

B. School

1. Name of School: _____ Grade: _____

   Address: _____

   Telephone Number: _____ Name of Teacher: _____

2. *Circle* any of the following that you have been told apply to your child:

   mentally retarded   slow learner   low normal intelligence   brain damaged

   cerebral palsy   perceptual-motor problems   reading problems

   other learning problems

3. Attendance: About how many days has he missed so far this year? _____

              About how many total days did he miss last year? _____

Yes _____ No _____   4. Does he get along well in school?

No _____ Yes _____   5. Has he ever repeated a grade?

No _____ Yes _____   6. Has he ever been in special classes?

No _____ Yes _____   7. Has he usually had difficulties with schoolwork?

No _____ Yes _____   8. Has he recently had difficulties with schoolwork?

No _____ Yes _____   9. Is he so upset about something that it is interfering with his schoolwork?

Yes _____ No _____   10. Is he doing as well in school as his brothers and sisters?

No _____ Yes _____   11. Does he need pressure to do his homework?

No _____ Yes _____   12. Does he seem to have "given up" in school?

No _____ Yes _____   13. Does he have trouble getting to school?

No _____ Yes _____   14. Does he have a problem with classroom misbehavior?

No _____ Yes _____   15. Has he ever been suspended for a while from school?

Yes _____ No _____   16. Does he take gym?

No _____ Yes _____   17. Does he want to drop out of school?

(This medical information is confidential.)

University of Colorado Medical Center

PEDIATRIC REFERRAL CLINIC

Name
Hosp. No.
Date

–6–

C. Mood

No ____ Yes ____   1. Is he often tense?
No ____ Yes ____   2. Does he worry a lot?
No ____ Yes ____   3. Is he often unhappy?
No ____ Yes ____   4. Is he often angry?
Yes ____ No ____   5. Will he readily tell people when something is bothering him?
No ____ Yes ____   6. Does he ever talk to himself?
Yes ____ No ____   7. Does he sometimes have mood swings?

D. Friends

Yes ____ No ____   1. Does he get along well with children his age?
No ____ Yes ____   2. Does he have trouble keeping his friends?
No ____ Yes ____   3. Does he fight a lot with people in his age group?
No ____ Yes ____   4. Has he ever accidentally hurt anyone?
No ____ Yes ____   5. Does he prefer to play alone?
Yes ____ No ____   6. Does he have a really close friend?
Yes ____ No ____   7. Does he spend a lot of time with other teen-agers?
Yes ____ No ____   8. Is he up on the latest music?
Yes ____ No ____   9. Is he quite conscious of clothes?
Yes ____ No ____   10. Is your teen-ager interested in the opposite sex?
Yes ____ No ____   11. Does your teen-ager date?

E. Discipline

No ____ Yes ____   1. Is he a difficult child to discipline?
No ____ Yes ____   2. Does he often break rules?
No ____ Yes ____   3. Does he often try to bend the rules?
No ____ Yes ____   4. Does he quarrel and fight a lot with his brothers and sisters?
Yes ____ No ____   5. Do you think he has a conscience?

F. Behavior

1. *Circle* any of the following that pertain at all to your child:

hyperactive	very shy	running away	gets teased	tics
homesickness	sexual problems	damages property	firesetting	
eating problem	sleep problem	drug problems	juvenile delinquency	
highly conscientious	suicide attempt	ditches school	depression	
panic attacks				

2. *Circle* any of the following that you are concerned about:

crying	stubbornness	fussiness	wants his way	temper tantrums
thumbsucking	nailbiting	fears	biting	swearing
restlessness	teases animals	lying	stealing	smoking

7 ...

Adolescence

Henry E. Cooper, Jr., MD

Adolescence is the period of growth and development during which the child grows to adulthood. The upper developmental limit of adolescence is unclear since there are no objective physiologic events that can be used to define its termination. Physiologic and psychologic changes during this period prepare the individual for mature adult biologic and emotional functioning.

Chronologically, adolescence extends from about 12–13 years of age to the early 20's, with wide individual and cultural variations. Adolescence tends to begin earlier in girls than in boys, and to end earlier in both in some cultures.

Puberty is a more restricted term for the biologic and physiologic changes associated with physical and sexual maturation. Although the gross observable changes of puberty may not manifest themselves clinically until the second decade, subtle physiologic changes may occur as early as 8 years of age. Pubescence is the time during which the reproductive functions mature; it also includes the appearance of secondary sex characteristics as well as the physiologic maturation of the primary sex organs. In general, puberty is reached when full reproductive maturity has been achieved.

PHYSICAL CHANGES DURING ADOLESCENCE

Because the age at onset of the physical and emotional changes characteristic of adolescence is variable, it is convenient to assess the stage of development of adolescent children in terms of degree of maturation and physiologic changes. A prominent feature of adolescence is accelerated growth rate. The adolescent growth spurt occurs in all developing children but is quite variable in time of onset, duration, and extent. The adolescent spurt begins earlier in girls than in boys, usually between 11 and 14 years; in boys, the growth spurt begins, on the average, between the ages of 12 and 16 years. In boys this growth spurt accounts for a gain in height of 10–30 cm (4–12 inches) and a gain in weight of 7–30 kg (15–65 lb). The age of maximum velocity of growth may be anywhere between the ages of 12 and 17. In girls the growth spurt is usually slower and less extensive, and accounts for a gain of 5–20 cm (2–10 inches) in height and 7–25 kg (15–55 lb) in weight. Every organ system seems to be involved, but all organs do not grow at the same rate. One exception is the brain, which does not seem to change appreciably in size after age 10 although an increase in head diameter does occur. Lymphatic tissue increases in size from birth and begins to decrease during adolescence, usually at about the time of the growth spurt.

The adolescent growth spurt usually proceeds in a fairly orderly sequence. Leg length usually begins to increase first, and the legs are the first to reach adult length. After a few months, there is an increase in hip width and chest breadth. Shoulder width increases a few months later, and this is followed by an increase in the length of the trunk and the depth of the chest. A great part of the change in weight and muscle mass tends to occur after the bone growth spurt. During the early adolescent period—especially in boys—there may be an increase in subcutaneous fat before the height spurt occurs. This fat is usually lost 1–2 years later and returns with the onset of the skeletal growth spurt.

The rate and onset of the adolescent growth spurt may be influenced by many factors, including sex, racial origin, nutrition, and illness. In children who mature early, this spurt may proceed faster than in those who mature late. The most important determinant of the time of onset and rate of growth seems to be the genetic heritage. Over the past 100 years, there has been a spectacular acceleration of statural size and biologic maturation. In both the USA and Western Europe, there has been an increase in the height of adolescents of the same age during the 20th century. Acceleration of biologic maturity is manifested by the decreasing age at menarche in girls that has been observed in many areas of the world.

Along with changes in body size, the adolescent assumes the adult physique of his or her sex. The outstanding features are changes in subcutaneous fat distribution, differences in relative bulk growth of the arms, shoulders, and pelvis, and the appearance of secondary sex characteristics. The hormonal changes that occur in the adolescent bring about an increase, in men, in shoulder breadth, leg length, and arm length, particularly the forearm. In girls there is an increase in the width of the hips and a change in the size of the

161

bony pelvis. Girls have a greater amount of subcutaneous fat before adolescence and during the growth spurt, associated with little spurt in bone diameter. In contrast, males have an increase in muscle mass and bone diameter and a smaller increase in subcutaneous fat. (The approximate pattern of appearance of sex characteristics is shown in Tables 2–9 and 2–10.)

PHYSIOLOGIC CHANGES DURING ADOLESCENCE

Hormonal Changes

Hormones are known to have an important influence on the adolescent growth spurt and the physiologic changes during adolescence. Although the origin of the triggering mechanism of adolescence and puberty is not definitely known, it appears to be a response of the anterior pituitary to a stimulus from the hypothalamus. This hypothalamic stimulus produces an elaboration of gonadotropic hormones by the pituitary, and the characteristic changes of adolescence are produced.

The gonadotropic hormones—follicle-stimulating hormone (FSH) and luteinizing hormone (LH), including luteotropic hormone (LTH)—are the major hormones elaborated.

Urinary gonadotropin levels in early childhood are less than 6 mouse units/day; they rise during adolescence to reach adult levels of 6–52 units/day. Illness, nutritional disturbances, or emotional disorders may cause a decline in the amount of gonadotropin produced.

A. Female Hormones: Estrogens and progesterone are produced by the ovaries, the testes, and the adrenals. In the female, the estrogen originates in the graafian follicles; in the male, in the testes and adrenals. Estrogen produced before pubescence is probably of adrenal origin. In girls, the amount of estrogen produced increases after approximately age 11, but in boys there is no increase during puberty. The secretion of estrogens assumes a cyclic pattern starting approximately 2 years before menarche. The female secondary sex characteristics, stimulated by estrogen production, are enlargement of the uterus and ovaries, development of the breasts, labia minora, and fallopian tubes, increase in vaginal acidity, and cornification of the vaginal epithelial cells. Progesterone is produced in the corpus luteum, adrenal cortex, and testes. It is excreted principally as pregnanediol, seems to act primarily on the female genital tissues, and participates in the development and function of the breasts. There appears to be no change in excretion of pregnanediol with age, nor is there any sex difference save for a premenstrual increase in pregnanediol excretion which is thought to be evidence of ovulation.

B. Male Hormones: In males, androgenic hormones are produced by the adrenal cortex (2/3) and

testes (1/3); in females, androgens are produced only by the adrenal glands. Some of the earliest changes of adolescence are a by-product of androgen stimulation. A sharp increase in urinary 17-ketosteroids is noted at around 7–9 years of age, the increase being maintained until puberty. The prepuberal rise is noted in both boys and girls, but is greater in boys at about 10–12 years of age. The androgens are believed to be responsible for the growth spurt during adolescence and for the increase in muscular development. In girls, androgens are believed to be responsible for the growth of the labia majora and clitoris, the appearance of axillary and pubic hair, and the stimulation of the sebaceous glands, with resultant seborrhea and acne. In boys, androgens stimulate the growth of the penis, scrotum, testes, prostate, and seminal vesicles, and are responsible for the increase in sebaceous secretion, the appearance of pubic, axillary, and facial hair, and the enlargement of the larynx with deepening of the voice. Measuring the urinary 17-ketosteroids is a widely used method of determining androgen production.

C. Other Hormones: Adrenal corticosteroids are excreted in gradually increasing amounts from birth to maturity, and in adults the amount is dependent upon body size and appears to have no relation to age and sex. The 17-hydroxycorticosteroids may show a rise starting at about 15 years of age in both males and females, and this rise may also be accounted for by increase in size.

Thyroid hormone may decline slightly after puberty, reaching its lowest point in the greatest period of sexual maturation. The degradation rate of thyroxine during adolescence does not seem to differ significantly from that of the younger child or adult. Parathyroid hormone may increase slightly during adolescence.

Other Physiologic Changes

(1) By about age 16, adult levels of extracellular water are achieved (25% of total body weight) in both sexes.

(2) Hemoglobin rises slightly in both sexes, but the rise is greater in boys.

(3) Blood pressure rises and heart size increases.

(4) Pulse rate decreases.

(5) Strength, speed, and stamina increase in both sexes.

(6) Blood alkaline phosphatase levels fall rapidly at the end of the height spurt, attaining adult levels after bone growth ceases.

Donovan BT, Van Der Werff Ten Bosch JJ: *Physiology of Puberty.* Arnold, 1965.

Heald FP, Dangela M, Brunschuyler P: Physiology of adolescence. New England J Med 268: 192, 243, 299, 361, 1963.

Rauh J, Knox M, Goldsmith R: Effect on sexual maturity of the serum concentration of hormonal iodine in adolescence. J Pediat 64: 697, 1964.

Tanner JM: *Growth at Adolescence,* 2nd ed. Blackwell, 1962.

Wilkins L: *The Diagnosis and Treatment of Endocrine Disorders in Childhood and Adolescence,* 3rd ed. Thomas, 1965.

PSYCHOLOGIC CHANGES DURING ADOLESCENCE

Cognitive Development

Until age 11–12, the child uses concrete operations in problem solving. At adolescence the ability to think scientifically blossoms. The adolescent begins to form hypotheses and to test them in reality or in thought in solving a problem. By the time he is 15, he is able to use logical operations and formal logic in solving problems just as an adult is able to do.

Ego Development

The combination of accelerated growth, physiologic changes, cultural expectations, and the boy's or girl's own inner drives brings about certain characteristics commonly associated with adolescence. In addition to developing the capacity for scientific and abstract thought, the adolescent faces the task of acquiring appropriate feelings and attitudes toward sex and developing an identity of his own.

The awakening of sexual interest and the increase in body awareness and sexual drive may cause the adolescent and his parents to become confused and anxious. The growing individual may find the prospect of adult responsibility difficult, and there may be marked vacillations between childish and adult behavior. These behavior swings may further puzzle the adolescent and his parents and may lead to physical and behavioral symptoms. The rapidly shifting interests assumed by adolescents are to be regarded as experimental attempts to understand life. There may be great concern about the physical adequacy of the developing body, and anxiety caused by fears of physical imperfection may be too overwhelming to be verbalized. This denial can usually be overcome by an understanding adult, particularly a physician.

Concern about body changes may cause a feeling of strangeness in a child who formerly felt comfortable about his physical self. It may produce many fantasies about both the external and internal functions of the body. This concern may cause the child to complain of symptoms, and he may become a "hypochondriac." However, the physician must beware of assuming that all complaints are of emotional origin; a careful medical examination is always required to rule out disease.

With maturation and the attempt to establish a personal identity, the adolescent strives for independence. Early adolescence is the time for testing parental controls and discipline and renouncing parental standards in preparation for breaking close ties with the parents. The adolescent is vociferous in his attempts to act without the direction of adults, particularly his parents. However, the psychologic changes that are taking place may make independent action even more difficult than in past stages of development, and the boy or girl may appear to be compulsive in his behavior and confused about his goals. During this period he is driven to experiment with new ideas and

experiences free of adult supervision. When he meets challenges or obstacles he finds difficult to cope with, he turns to adults for guidance and support. This return to a state of dependency is usually appropriate to the reality situation. If the parents fail to provide adequate reassurance and comfort during these intervals of necessary dependency, the adolescent may seek relief in earlier patterns of childlike behavior and methods of handling anxiety. With appropriate parental support, he will be able to give up his immature behavior. However, he may regard the regressive episode as a defeat in his attempts to achieve adulthood. He protests the regression but wishes to avoid self-blame and to deny his own weakness. Consequently, he blames his parents or other adults who are aware of his period of regression. This "scapegoat" role is important for the adolescent as he strives for independence.

As the adolescent begins to break away from parental influence, the peer group attains increasing importance and may even dominate the adolescent's thinking and behavior. In the group the adolescent finds a sense of security that is a source of comfort in dealing with conflicts. He achieves status and a sense of productivity or achievement simply by belonging to the group. In return, he must accept group standards of dress and behavior and the group's attitude toward authority, education, etc. Although membership in a particular group is determined partly by age and intellectual ability, emotional empathy is just as important. The group is usually composed of individuals at the same stage of emotional development. As an individual matures emotionally, he may give up one group to join another more in harmony with his changing interests and goals. The peer group may be unacceptable to the parents for political or social reasons, but association with such a group is probably a necessary part of the adolescent's experimentation with alternative styles of life.

The Implications of Adolescence for Medical Practice

The physician can play an important role in encouraging and facilitating adolescent development. He can serve as a source of understanding and interest, and provides the opportunity to express feelings and attitudes and to ask questions without criticism or embarrassment. Ample time should be scheduled so that the adolescent and his parents can express their concerns and ask about anything that is puzzling to them. Visits should also be managed so that the physician can focus separately upon problems presented by the parents and by the child. Parents should be informed of the normal physical and emotional changes that occur during adolescence.

The physical examination should be performed with consideration for the shyness and the need for privacy that is characteristic of this age group. Drapes should be used during the examination, and chaperoning is essential during the examination of girls. Vaginal examination during adolescence should be avoided except upon definite medical indication. A useful technic is to conduct a review of systems during the examination. It is important that the physician carefully discuss with the patient any diagnostic procedures used and that the physical findings be interpreted to the patient.

Overidentification with the adolescent or the parents should be avoided. A sure understanding of the social and cultural influences acting on the parents and on the adolescent is necessary so that the parents can confidently set limits and maintain discipline in the home and the community.

Gallagher JR: *Medical Care of the Adolescent,* 2nd ed. Appleton-Century-Crofts, 1966.

Josselyn IM: *The Adolescent and His World.* New York Family Service Association of America, 1957.

Solnit AJ, Prevence SA (editors): *Modern Perspectives in Child Development.* Internat Univ Press, 1963.

GROWTH PROBLEMS DURING ADOLESCENCE

DELAYED ADOLESCENCE

Essentials of Diagnosis

- Delay in growth spurt and appearance of secondary sex characteristics.
- Absence of endocrinopathies.

General Considerations

Delayed adolescence is more common in boys than in girls.

The timing, extent, and pattern of pubertal changes vary widely with different individuals. In the evaluation of delayed puberty, developmental age is more reliable than chronologic age. Developmental age may be based on x-ray determination of skeletal age and on standards of development of secondary sex characteristics. Determination of sexual maturity may be based on the following.

A. Genital Development in Males:

Stage 1: Preadolescent.

Stage 2: Beginning enlargement of the scrotum and testes; reddening of the scrotum, and changes in its texture.

Stage 3: Penile enlargement with increase in length and further growth of the scrotum and testes.

Stage 4: Further increase in penile size; growth in breadth and development of the glans. Further enlargement of the testes and scrotum and continued darkening of the scrotal skin.

Stage 5: Adult genitalia in size and shape.

B. Pubic Hair Development in Males and Females:

Stage 1: Preadolescence, with the vellus over the pubic area no more profuse than that on the abdomen.

Stage 2: Sparse growth of long, slightly pigmented, downy hair which is straight or only slightly curled, and appearing usually at the base of the penis or along the labia.

Stage 3: Pubic hair is darker, coarser, and more curly, and the hair is spreading sparsely over the pubic area.

Stage 4: Further spread of the pubic hair, still considerably less than in the adult, and no extension of hair bilaterally up to the middle of the thighs.

Stage 5: Adult in amount and type of hair.

C. Breast Development in Girls:

Stage 1: Preadolescent, with coloration of the papilla only.

Stage 2: Breast bud stage; breasts and papillae are elevated above the chest in a small mound, with enlargement of the areolar diameter.

Stage 3: Further elevation and enlargement of the breasts and areolas but no separation of the contours.

Stage 4: The areolas and papillae project from the breast to form a secondary mound.

Stage 5: Adult stage; projection of the papillae only, with recession of the areolas into the general breast contour.

Variations in the pubertal changes occur both within and between the groups, boys and girls. Boys may take 1.8–4.7 years to proceed from stage 2 to stage 5 in genital or pubic hair development. Some boys may move from stage 2 to stage 5 in less time than others go from one stage to the next. The peak height velocity in boys usually occurs 2 years later than in girls and generally occurs in stage 4 genital or pubic hair development. Many girls may have their peak height velocity in stage 2 of breast development. Thus, the short boy within the early stages of development may still have considerable growth to come. This is not true for girls.

Girls may take 1.5–8 years in passing from stage 2 to stage 5 breast development and 1.5–3 years from stage 2 to stage 5 pubic hair development. Some girls may progress to stage 3 or 4 breast development before pubic hair stage 2 is reached. Alternatively, pubic hair may progress to stage 3 or 4 before breast development starts. Most girls have their menarche at stage 3 or 4 breast and pubic hair development. The peak height velocity in girls usually occurs just before the menarche.

Marshall WA, Tanner JM: Variations in the pattern of pubertal changes in boys. Arch Dis Childhood 45:13–23, 1970.

Marshall WA, Tanner JM: Variations in the pattern of pubertal changes in girls. Arch Dis Childhood 44:291–303, 1969.

Clinical Findings

A. Symptoms and Signs: Puberty may be delayed until as late as 18–19 years, but most children reach puberty by 15 or 16 years of age. There may be no symptoms except for psychologic problems caused by teasing, exclusion from athletic and social activities, or just a feeling of difference from others. The psychologic import of delayed adolescence may be manifested as poor school work, delinquent behavior, withdrawal, or paranoid tendencies.

The physical examination shows that there is a lag behind children of the same age in body weight, muscular development, stage of sexual maturity, and psychosocial development. The history may show that growth retardation has been evident throughout childhood or that another family member has exhibited the same pattern of development.

B. Laboratory Findings: Endocrinologic studies are unrevealing. Skeletal age may show a delay of 2–4 years which has existed throughout preadolescence. Urinary 17-ketosteroids or FSH are usually at adolescent levels.

Treatment

Observation at intervals will reveal that somatic growth and sexual maturation do occur, but late. A series of visits should be scheduled so that the physician can give continued interest and reassurance. Signs of poor psychologic adjustment should be observed for and handled appropriately when they occur.

A. Boys: In boys 17 years old or more, if pubertal development is considerably retarded, if no progress toward maturity is evident, and if the physician's efforts to give reassurance and support are to no avail, it is probably wise to start hormone therapy to stimulate growth. Chorionic gonadotropins, 2000–4000 units IM twice a week for 3–6 months, usually produce rapid somatic growth and initiate the development of secondary sex characteristics. After one course of therapy, maturation will often continue to progress. If this does not occur after 3–6 months, a second course of treatment may be given.

B. Girls: There is no completely reliable means of initiating puberty in girls with delayed adolescence. In some cases, pubertal changes will begin after a course of continuous estrogen therapy for 2–3 months followed by cyclic estrogen-progesterone treatment for a few more months. Diethylstilbestrol, 1–2 mg daily orally, is given for 2–3 months, during which time feminization will occur. This is followed by diethylstilbestrol, 1–2 mg orally daily for 21 days, adding medroxyprogesterone, 10 mg orally daily on the 15th through the 21st day, and then withdrawing both. In 3–5 days, vaginal bleeding will occur. The treatment is then resumed starting on the third day of bleeding. This is usually carried out for about 6 months. Chorionic gonadotropin is contraindicated because of the cystic ovarian changes it produces.

Prognosis

In all cases of delayed adolescence due to a slow growth pattern, the patient will eventually undergo pubertal changes. Once started, maturation occurs in a rapid spurt or as a gradual development and average adult height is eventually attained.

Bayley LM, Bayley N: *Growth Diagnosis: Selected Methods for Interpreting and Predicting Physical Development from One Year to Maturity.* Univ of Chicago Press, 1965.

Gallagher JR: *Medical Care of the Adolescent,* 2nd ed. Appleton-Century-Crofts, 1966.

Hubble D: *Pediatric Endocrinology.* Davis, 1969.

Wilkins L: *The Diagnosis and Treatment of Endocrine Disorders in Childhood and Adolescence,* 3rd ed. Thomas, 1965.

OVERGROWTH & INCREASED HEIGHT

In some adolescents, the rate of change in height prior to puberty suggests that they may have excessive height as adults. In girls, this may be a cause of great anxiety and may be a severe social handicap. When the question arises, height prediction tables should be used to estimate the probable adult height. In general, patients with advanced bone development have less growing time and may stop growing before they become too tall. If the probability of excessive adult height is great and hormonal intervention is being considered, thorough interviews are necessary before treatment is started in an attempt to encourage the patient to accept her body. The indications for hormone therapy are a family history of excessive tallness, a skeletal age that by age 10 is less than normal or normal, and a probable adult height of over 6 feet as estimated by reference to prediction tables.

Treatment is instituted about 1 year before the predicted time of menarche and after secondary sex characteristics have become manifest. The more advanced the bone age at the time therapy is started, the less effective the treatment in reducing height gain. When the bone age has reached 15 years, the effectiveness of treatment is nil. Reported reductions from predicted heights started before growth is completed range from 1–4 inches. Conjugated estrogenic substances (Premarin), 12.5 mg orally, or diethylstilbestrol, 2 mg orally, is given for 21 days, with medroxyprogesterone, 10 mg orally, added on days 15 through 21, and both drugs are then withdrawn. The cycle is then repeated on the third day of vaginal bleeding which occurs following withdrawal. Treatment is continued for approximately 1 year, at which time there is usually evidence of considerable advance of bone age or evidence of epiphyseal closure. Menorrhagia occasionally occurs during treatment but may be controlled by increasing the dose of diethylstilbestrol to 3 mg/day during the first 5 days of treatment. Pigmentation may occur, particularly over the breasts, nipples, and labia.

The effectiveness of and need for estrogen therapy in preventing excessive height is not universally agreed upon. Some data suggest that estrogens slow growth but may not significantly influence adult height.

Fraser SD, Smith FG Jr: Effect of estrogens on mature height in tall girls: A controlled study. J Clin Endocrinol 28:416, 1968.

Greenblatt RB & others: Estrogen therapy in inhibition of growth. J Clin Endocrinol 26:1185, 1966.

Wetterhall HNB, Roche AF: Tall girls: Assessment and management. Australian Pediat J 1:210, 1965.

GYNECOMASTIA

Enlargement of one or both breasts in boys occurs frequently during puberty and occasionally in the preadolescent years and may cause great anxiety. It may be differentiated from gynecomastia due to Klinefelter's syndrome, liver disease, severe malnutrition, obesity, and feminizing endocrinopathies, particularly carcinoma of the testis.

The cause of physiologic gynecomastia during adolescence is not known, but it is postulated that testicular or adrenal androgens may be converted to estrogens which stimulate enlargement.

Benign adolescent breast hypertrophy presents as mild to moderate enlargement of one or (usually) both breasts. It is palpable as a firm, sometimes slightly tender mass 1–2 cm in diameter just beneath the areola, and may be associated with hyperesthesia of the nipple. It occurs frequently in boys who have well developed testes and are virilizing rapidly.

Gynecomastia is usually transitory and subsides spontaneously after about 6 months. When enlargement is considerable, it may persist for years.

In a few cases, gynecomastia which is not associated with endocrine disfunction may present as unilateral or bilateral breast enlargement typical of the developing female pattern. The breasts may be diffusely enlarged, but much more so in the subareolar area, with no tenderness, and may become pendulous, with enlargement and hyperpigmentation of the areolas. These boys may have normal male secondary sex characteristics in all other respects. This type of gynecomastia causes great embarrassment and anxiety and may seriously impair psychologic development.

Treatment of both types usually consists of assurance that the "growth" is benign and transitory.

In extensive and pendulous enlargement, plastic surgery is indicated for psychologic and cosmetic reasons. The patient must be reassured about physical integrity and normal masculinity.

In patients who have residual gynecomastia following correction of endocrine disorders, plastic surgery may be indicated for cosmetic reasons.

Ginsburg J: Gynaecomastia. Practitioner 203:166–170, 1969.
Nydick M & others: Gynecomastia in adolescent boys. JAMA 178:449–454, 1961.

OBESITY

Obesity, beyond the temporary prepubertal accumulation of subcutaneous fat in most girls and some boys, is becoming more common in the USA and Western Europe, possibly related to the dynamics of affluence and patterns of overeating. Although endocrine factors were formerly felt to be prominently involved in many cases of obesity, they appear now to be only rarely influential. Most cases result basically from an excess of intake over output of calories as a result of hyperphagia, usually in families with tendencies toward overeating. Psychosocial, genetic, environmental, and metabolic factors, especially hyperinsulinism, are well documented contributing causes. A small number of cases are associated with a variety of organic diseases (Table 7–1).

From the psychosocial point of view, seriously obese children and adolescents fall into 2 major groups: reactive and developmental. The reactive type is characterized by obesity, overeating, and underactivity in response to an emotionally traumatic experience such as the death of a parent or sibling, the break-up of a family through divorce, or school failure. Such children tend to use food for emotional purposes as a substitute for more basic emotional gratifications. Supportive psychotherapeutic or environmental measures, often with the aid of psychiatric consultation, may be fairly helpful in this group, although some children from more disturbed families require intensive psychotherapy to relieve persistent depression or other manifestations.

The developmental type of obesity usually has its origins in strong family tendencies toward obesity and overeating, representing a disturbed way of life (family frame) involving the whole family. The mother usually dominates and overprotects the child, and the father plays a relatively passive role; both parents, however, may unconsciously use one particular child to satisfy

TABLE 7–1. Etiologic classification of obesities.

Genetic Origin
    Laurence-Moon-Biedl syndrome
    Prader-Willi syndrome
    Glycogen storage disease
    Familial hypoglycemosis
Hypothalamic Origin
    Diencephalic
    Panhypopituitarism and narcolepsy
CNS Origin
    Postfrontal lobotomy
    Cortical lesions (frontal lesions in particular)
Endocrine Origin
    Insulin-producing adenoma of islets of Langerhans
    Diabetes
    Chromophobe adenoma of pituitary gland
    Hyperadrenocorticism (Cushing's syndrome; iatrogenic due to corticosteroid administration)
    Klinefelter's syndrome
    Turner's syndrome
    Male hypogonadism
    Castration
Miscellaneous Causes
    Immobilization
    Psychic disturbances
    Social and cultural pressure

their own emotional needs or compensatory tendencies. Often the child is overvalued by the parents, sometimes because of the death of a previous child, and overfeeding may represent an attempt to deal with guilt. The child is often large at birth, soon becomes obese with overfeeding, and continues to be obese from early infancy on. After early demanding behavior, the child usually becomes passive, oversubmissive, overdependent, and immature.

In such children, feelings of helplessness, despair, and a tendency to withdraw from social interaction often becomes associated with a tendency to overeat and patterns of inactivity. Food may be used to ward off depression or feelings of hostility; eating or chewing may acquire unconscious symbolic significance as a conversion symptom, or patterns of "addiction" to food may result. Although obesity is a social handicap, some children or adolescents may hide behind the "wall of weight" and ward off sexual conflicts with the feeling that they are ugly or unattractive. Too rapid reduction in weight may produce a "dieting depression" or even a psychotic picture in some markedly obese and seriously disturbed person.

Clinical Findings

Evaluation of the obese patient must include height and weight histories of parents and siblings, eating habits, quality and timing of appetite and hunger patterns, the duration of the obesity, and, when possible, height and weight plotted longitudinally. In experienced hands, the use of skinfold calipers can give an objective measurement of obesity (Pediatrics 42:538, 1968). The history should also include information about family attitudes, the patient's feelings about himself, previous weight reduction attempts, physical activities engaged in, and the general adjustment pattern of the patient. A careful history and physical examination will help to distinguish between exogenous obesity and other, organic causes of increased subcutaneous tissue such as Cushing's syndrome or hypothyroidism. A common error is failure to realize that children with hypothyroidism may be thin rather than fat, and that the excess weight gain with hypothyroidism is myxedema rather than fat. Many patients with exogenous obesity are inappropriately treated with thyroid medication for this reason.

Treatment

The treatment of obesity must be individualized. Only in very rare cases do psychologic factors preclude attempts at weight reduction. The patient-doctor relationship is of paramount importance because treatment must continue over a long time with repeated interviews. The physician must be able to give the patient a feeling of personal worth and an optimistic outlook for the future.

A. Diet: Dietary control should be attempted. As a rule, it should be introduced and discussed after several visits. The physician's attitude should be one of sympathy rather than criticism of failure to adhere to the diet, and the relationship with the patient must not

be jeopardized by insisting that the patient lose weight "for the doctor." In early adolescence, during the growth spurt, good nutrition must be maintained; the diet should include adequate proteins and calcium and fewer concentrated sweets and fats. Since a marked reduction in food intake may affect linear growth, the recommended minimum daily caloric intake during early adolescence should be 1200 calories for girls and 1400 calories for boys. Older adolescents may be given diets containing as little as 1000 calories/day as long as 20% of it is protein and vitamin and mineral requirements are met.

The caloric intake should be spread over 3 meals a day. Raw carrots, celery, and raw vegetables may have the effect of slowing the course of meals and allowing satiety to occur. Artificial sweeteners may be substituted for sugar in beverages.

B. Anorexigenic Drugs: The anorexigenic drugs (amphetamines and related compounds) are of limited value in the treatment of obesity. There is no indication for their use in the patient who eats too much even when not hungry. They may be helpful for the patient who is too hungry on a low-calorie diet. If there is excessive hunger, small doses of dextroamphetamine (5–10 mg) may be given 30 minutes prior to the estimated peak of hunger. In general, the effective duration of amphetamine treatment is usually 6–8 weeks. The patient must be aware that this is an adjunct to therapy and that the responsibility for correction of obesity cannot be delegated to the drug.

C. Exercise: The obese adolescent must be encouraged to exercise at least 1 hour a day during the week and 2–4 hours a day during weekends and when school is not in session. The type of exercise makes no difference as long as it is done consistently and intensely. The physician may suggest new activities and interests which might not only create an interest in exercise but also gain for the patient recognition, friends, and the satisfaction of accomplishment.

D. Other Measures: A useful adjunct in the management of obese girls is grooming tips and "figure" control advice to promote self-esteem. Obesity clubs and summer camps may be of some help.

Complications

Most of the complications of obesity during adolescence are psychosocial ones. Respiratory difficulties (Pickwickian syndrome), hypertension, and cardiovascular complications may occur, and menstrual disorders in young girls. Many of these difficulties can be relieved by weight reduction. The psychologic concomitants of obesity may represent disturbances in emotional development during early life, a manifestation of the adjustment reaction to obesity, or an interplay of both. Transient or prolonged psychic stress may lead to increased food intake and an increase in subcutaneous fat. Patients with long-standing obesity frequently show extreme passivity, poor self-esteem, fear of social gatherings, and passive-aggressive personality traits. Because of their inability, real or imagined, to compete with peers in physical and social activities, they may withdraw. This makes them more unacceptable to their peers, and the sedentary activities in which they engage may contribute to their obesity.

Prognosis

The prognosis in long-standing severe obesity is poor for weight reduction, but these patients can be helped to lead a more normal life by accepting their obesity. Patients whose subcutaneous fat tissue increases to excessive amounts after 9 years of age are usually less obese; with careful management, about ½ of these can achieve average weight as adults.

Gallagher JR: *Medical Care of the Adolescent,* 2nd ed. Appleton-Century-Crofts, 1966.

Mayer J: Some aspects of the problem of regulation of food intake and obesity. New England J Med 274:610–616, 722, 731, 1966.

Nutrition Committee of the American Academy of Pediatrics: Obesity in childhood. Pediatrics 40:455–467, 1967.

MENSTRUAL DISORDERS DURING ADOLESCENCE

DYSFUNCTIONAL UTERINE BLEEDING (Metropathia Haemorrhagica)

Essentials of Diagnosis

- Irregular and noncyclic uterine bleeding.
- Absence of systemic and pelvic disorders.
- Occurs after menarche and before regular ovulation is established.

General Considerations

This common disorder of adolescence is thought to be due to the continuous and fluctuating stimulation of the endometrium by estrogens and the absence of progesterone production. Irregularity in timing and amount of flow may continue for 1–4 years following menarche. Menstrual flow which persists longer than 7 days should be investigated further. Iron deficiency anemia may be a precipitating cause of menorrhagia.

Clinical Findings

It is important to determine the timing of menorrhagia in relationship to the menarche. In the absence of organic causes of abnormal uterine bleeding, the physical examination is normal and there are no other symptoms; examination of the epithelial cells in a centrifuged urine specimen will show evidence of fluctuating levels of estrogens. An ovulatory type of flow can be verified by determining the urine pregnanediol level once a week for 3 or more successive weeks. Pregnanediol will be absent or diminished and is directly proportionate to the amount of progesterone produced.

Differential Diagnosis

Early manifestations of fundamental disorders of the thyroid, adrenals, ovaries, and pituitary may resemble adolescent noncyclic bleeding and should be considered during the history and physical examinations.

Complications

Irregular and prolonged bleeding may cause considerable discomfort and anxiety. Excessive bleeding may cause anemia.

Treatment

A. General Measures: Simple reassurance is an essential part of the total management of this disorder.

B. Specific Measures: When uterine bleeding persists longer than 7 days and significantly influences psychologic well-being or produces anemia and weakness, cyclic hormonal treatment may be undertaken. The treatment consists of Tristerone (estrone, 6 mg; testosterone, 25 mg; and progesterone, 25 mg), 1 ml IM daily for 3–5 days, or conjugated estrogenic substances (Premarin), 20 mg IV every 3 hours or 2.5 mg every 2 hours until bleeding ceases or abates. This is followed by oral estrogens such as diethylstilbestrol, 3–6 mg/day, continued for the next 20–25 days with progesterone added during the last 2 weeks. In rare cases, surgical dilatation and curettage is the quickest and most effective way of stopping bleeding.

To achieve uterine bleeding at regular intervals, ethisterone (Pranone), the anhydrohydroxy form of progesterone, may be given orally in doses of 20 mg twice a day for 4 days a month in small girls and 5 days a month in large girls. Two to 3 days after administration of the last dose, withdrawal menstrual flow will begin. If no flow occurs within 3 days after the initial course, it probably means that endogenous progesterone is being produced. In such cases, no further cyclic therapy is indicated. Following the initial medical curettage, the progesterone compound is given for 4–5 days at 28-day intervals to establish a periodic cycle. This should be continued for about 6 months or until the cycle has been established as indicated by withdrawal bleeding, which occurs for 5 days following the last dose.

Prognosis

In most cases, a regular rhythm of menstruation will eventually be established and reassurance is all that is necessary. After cyclic hormonal therapy, many patients continue with normal menstruation.

AMENORRHEA

Amenorrhea is present (1) when there is an interval of 12 months or more between periods in the first 2 years following menarche; (2) when menarche has not occurred by age 17; or (3) when more than 3 periods have been missed after menses have become established. It may be due to pregnancy; it may be a manifestation of many disorders of endocrinologic, emotional, systemic or nutritional origin; or it may be due to mechanical defects.

Classification

Primary amenorrhea is a delay in menarche associated with otherwise normal puberty. It may be the result of dysfunction in the hypothalamic-pituitary-ovarian axis, other endocrinopathies, uterovaginal anomalies, nutritional disorders, or emotional disorders.

Secondary amenorrhea is prolonged amenorrhea (6–12 months) that develops after several months or years of normal cycles. It may be due to any of the conditions that cause primary amenorrhea. However, most cases of secondary amenorrhea in adolescents are due to functional and transient disorders. Minor emotional disturbances are the most common cause of secondary amenorrhea.

The causes of amenorrhea during adolescence may be further subdivided as follows:

A. Uterine Amenorrhea: Failure of the uterus to respond to cyclic hormonal changes may be due to genital underdevelopment or absence of the uterus. The patient may have normal pubescent changes and regular monthly pelvic discomfort but no menstrual flow.

B. Ovarian Amenorrhea: Patients with ovarian dysgenesis have a typical appearance. Elevated urinary FSH levels, absence of estrogenic effect in the urinary sediment, and absence of the normal female chromatin sex pattern in a buccal smear confirm the diagnosis. Ovarian amenorrhea may also be secondary to mumps, tuberculosis, salpingitis, ovarian tumors, and poliomyelitis. Other causes are Stein-Leventhal syndrome and polycystic ovaries.

C. Pituitary Amenorrhea: Pituitary amenorrhea may be associated with hypopituitarism and absence of FSH in the urine sample. It may also be associated with neoplasms or infarctions of the pituitary gland.

D. Hypothalamic Amenorrhea: In this type of amenorrhea there is a lack of luteinizing hormone from the pituitary which seems to be under the control of the hypothalamus. Without this hormone, the estrogen seems to be biologically ineffective and incapable of promoting endometrial growth and shedding. It is thought that the effect of emotional stimuli on the hypothalamus causes this kind of amenorrhea. Neoplastic or toxic changes in the area of the hypothalamus may produce similar changes.

E. Systemic Amenorrhea: This group includes obesity and malnutrition, adrenal and thyroid hyper- and hypofunction, diabetes mellitus, chronic illness, and pregnancy.

F. Pseudo-amenorrhea: Imperforate hymen or stenosed hymen may be associated with complaints of amenorrhea of the primary type but with a history of pelvic pain and bulging in the vaginal area.

Etiologic Diagnosis

A useful approach to the determination of the cause of amenorrhea is as follows:

A. Medical Examination: A careful history and physical examination are necessary to rule out pregnancy and genital anomalies and an abnormal chromatin sex pattern. If serious endocrine disorders or systemic disorders are suspected, appropriate tests and examinations should be carried out.

B. Trial of Hormone Therapy: Give progesterone, 50 mg IM in one dose.

1. If withdrawal bleeding occurs, no serious disorders of the pituitary-ovarian-uterine axis are present. This may be verified by observing for estrogenic effects in the epithelial cells of the urinary sediment or by means of pregnanediol excretion studies.

2. If no withdrawal bleeding occurs, there is a disturbance in estrogen production or in endometrial response to estrogen which may be due to pituitary, ovarian, or uterine disease or functional interference. Give estrogen in the form of diethylstilbestrol, 1–2 mg twice a day for 21–25 days. If bleeding does not occur, it indicates a failure of endometrial response and directs attention to the uterovaginal area. If bleeding does occur, urinary FSH excretion studies should be done. Elevated FSH levels suggest ovarian failure; low levels indicate pituitary failure; and normal levels indicate amenorrhea of the hypothalamic type.

Treatment

Treatment is directed at the underlying disorder.

In the absence of a functioning endometrium, menstruation cannot be established. In pseudo-amenorrhea, surgical correction of the imperforate or stenosed hymen is curative.

A. Ovarian Amenorrhea: Ovarian dysgenesis is treated with estrogens to produce secondary sex characteristics and artificial menstrual periods. Cyclic therapy must be continued indefinitely. In Stein-Leventhal syndrome, menses are usually restored following wedge resection of the ovaries.

B. Pituitary Amenorrhea: Until recently, the failure of pituitary production of FSH was treated with ovarian steroids to produce menstrual periods. The isolation of human pituitary FSH and some early successes in the production of normal menstruation and ovulation give promise for effective therapy in primary pituitary amenorrhea. Treatment with this hormone is still experimental, and further trials are necessary before it will be available clinically.

C. Hypothalamic Amenorrhea: Reassurance and attention to psychologic problems are indicated. Adolescent menstrual cycles seem to be more sensitive to emotional stress than is the case during later life.

DYSMENORRHEA

Essentials of Diagnosis

- Discomfort associated with menstruation in the form of cramps in the lower abdomen.

- There may also be headache, backache, pain in the thighs, anorexia, nausea and vomiting, diarrhea, constipation, or fainting.

General Considerations

Many healthy women experience lower abdominal cramps on the first day of menstruation. They tolerate it as a normal event and it causes no disturbance or loss of time from normal activity. In others, the cramps are more severe, persist longer, and may be associated with some of the above-listed symptoms.

Most cases of dysmenorrhea are of the primary type with no organic cause. Secondary dysmenorrhea is menstrual pain associated with salpingitis, uterine tumors, and endometriosis. Since these are not common disorders, only primary dysmenorrhea will be discussed here.

The pain that occurs with menstrual periods has been said to be due to irregular uterine contractions and the passage of secretory endometrium through the cervical os. In some girls, moderate or severe dysmenorrhea may be due to low pain tolerance, an emotional reaction to slight pain, or both. Dysmenorrhea is rare in the first 1–2 years after menarche and occurs most commonly after ovulation begins. The occurrence of ovulation and the resulting rising levels of progesterone cause the uterus to contract in large, irregular waves of varying amplitude, and this causes the pain.

Clinical Findings

The history usually reveals the onset of painful menstruation 1–2 years after menarche. The pain is typically intermittent and cramping, in the lower midline, occurring with the onset of flow. There may be uterine and adnexal pain and tenderness on examination.

Differential Diagnosis

Dysmenorrhea must be distinguished from other intra-abdominal and pelvic sources of pain. Pain localized to one side may be indicative of organic disease.

Treatment

A. Psychologic Management: An effort should be made to relieve tension and manipulate attitudes so that the patient can tolerate minor discomfort. Sympathetic discussion of the nature and cause of dysmenorrhea is always valuable. The patient should be given the opportunity to ask questions.

B. Analgesics and Antispasmodics: Edrisal is a commonly used analgesic consisting of aspirin, amphetamine sulfate, and phenacetin. One to 2 tablets every 3–4 hours may be helpful. Isoxsuprine (Vasodilan), 10–20 mg 3 times a day, is a useful antispasmodic. These drugs are most helpful when started 2 days before the expected period.

C. Hormone Therapy: If the above measures are not effective and dysmenorrhea is seriously disabling, it is helpful to give estrogens to produce anovulatory cycles, using cyclic therapy for a few months. This can be done with diethylstilbestrol, 1 mg daily orally for 25 days, starting on the first day of the cycle. If breakthrough bleeding occurs, the dose may be increased to 2 mg. Withdrawal bleeding occurring 3–5 days after the 25th day of therapy represents surface necrosis of the endometrium. Treatment should not be continued for more than 2–3 months because cumulative hyperplasia of the endometrium will occur.

An alternative form of cyclic therapy is available using progestins, eg, norethindrone and norethynodrel, 5–10 mg/day starting on the 5th day of the cycle and continuing daily to the 25th day. The advantage of the progestins is that they can be given in successive months. However, since they are progestational agents, mild cramps may occur with their use.

D. Surgery: There is no indication during adolescence for presacral neurectomy (interruption of the nerve pathways to the cerebral cortex).

Prognosis

Dysmenorrhea during adolescence is a self-limiting process, and most cases can be controlled with the therapeutic regimen outlined above. After 2–3 months of painless anovulatory cycles, dysmenorrhea often diminishes considerably and subsequent periods are free of pain or are associated with only mild cramping. Continued severe dysmenorrhea in the presence of anovulatory cycles may be an indication of severe emotional difficulties which may require psychiatric care.

PREMENSTRUAL TENSION

Premenstrual tension is manifested by one or more of the following symptoms or signs: a sense of abdominal discomfort or bloating, headache, backache, leg edema, breast engorgement, irritability, depression, insomnia, and dizziness. It may appear several days before the onset of menstruation and is relieved when menstrual flow begins.

The cause is not agreed upon. One widely held theory is that premenstrual tension is due to retention of sodium, chloride, and water. Other writers have suggested that it might result from qualitative and quantitative excesses or deficits of estrogens and progesterones. Still others have proposed that emotional factors are the most important consideration. Premenstrual tension does not seem to occur before ovulatory cycles begin and is not a frequent problem in adolescence.

The patient usually complains of physical, mental, and emotional tension which may be straining her personal and family relationships. Many appear hostile and bitter. In severe cases there may be impaired mental alertness and acuity, fatigue, depression, headache, visual disturbances, breast swelling and tenderness, anorexia, nausea and vomiting, constipation, and functional gastrointestinal and urinary tract symptoms. Urinary 17-ketosteroid excretion is occasionally high. The significance of this is not clear, but rising aldosterone levels may be responsible.

Treatment

Since premenstrual tension is mild during adolescence, simple measures are all that are usually necessary.

A. Diuretics: Chlorothiazide (Diuril), 250 mg orally daily for 7–10 days before the expected period; or ammonium chloride, 1–2 gm orally, 4 times daily for the same period.

B. Salt and Fluid Restriction: Limited salt intake and moderate fluid restriction during the 7–10 day period before menstruation.

C. Sedatives: Meprobamate or a similar drug may be used for a short time to relieve psychologic tension and to help in verifying the role of anxiety in the production of symptoms.

An effort should then be made without medication to help the patient deal with the causes of her anxiety.

Prognosis

Most cases of premenstrual tension in adolescence can be managed satisfactorily with psychologic help and medical control of bloating and edema.

Gallagher JR: *Medical Care of the Adolescent,* 2nd ed. Appleton-Century-Crofts, 1966.

Green TH Jr: *Gynecology.* Little, Brown, 1965.

Lang WR, Kupferberg AB, Chapple RV (editors): Adolescent gynecology. Ann New York Acad Sc 142:547–834, 1967.

Pria SD & others: Current thoughts on the management of dysfunctional uterine bleeding. Am J Obst Gynec 105:1185–1191, 1969.

Southam AL: Disorders of menstruation. Clin Obst Gynec 9:779–787, 1966.

Sturgis SH: Menstruation and the adolescent. M Clin North America 49:405–420, 1965.

Widholm D: Menstrual disorders in adolescence: Observation and comments. Clin Pediat 5:118–122, 1966.

. . .

RESPONSE TO ILLNESS DURING ADOLESCENCE

Any severe illness during adolescence involves the risk of impaired development or emotional disorganization that may interfere with effective functioning in later life. Factors that seem to determine the ability of a boy or girl to cope with his state of illness are as follows: (1) Severity and duration of the illness. (2) Psychosexual, social, and physiologic development of the individual. (3) Adaptive capacity of the individual and his family. (4) Past and present nature of the parent-child relationship. (5) Nature of the illness and the meaning it has for the patient and his family.

Types of reaction to illness during adolescence may range from acceptance of the illness (with a realistic view of symptoms and treatment) to regressive behavior and denial of the existence of illness. The intensity of the reaction may be tempered or increased by the patient's prior experience with a similar illness in his own life or in the lives of meaningful persons within his environment, and by the attitudes of others toward the illness. The ability to adapt to the illness will depend upon biologic factors, intellectual endowment, the abilities of tissues and organs to respond normally, and the psychosocial status of the patient and his family.

The nature of the illness may determine the extent of the reaction. Important in this regard are the following: (1) The organ system involved. Most anxiety is attached to illnesses which involve the organs of the vital functions and the genitalia. (2) Symptomatology. Pain and loss of control of body function may be highly stressful and make adaptation difficult. (3) Type of care involved. The adolescent frequently finds it difficult to submit to the types of body manipulations that are sometimes necessary in treatment. (4) Duration of the illness and the prognosis for life or residual handicap.

The initial impact at onset of illness may elicit an aggressive response with various symptomatic manifestations, unrealistic fear, or denial. There may then be a period of depression, eating disturbances, hostility toward the physician or health care agency, and, later, a period of self-pity related to the handicapping nature of the illness. Adaptation involves acceptance of the situation and the evolution of constructive attitudes which permit planning in mastering stress and overcoming difficulties.

In illnesses which require prolonged care or which threaten temporary or permanent handicaps, a more intense reaction occurs. Diabetes, epilepsy, asthma, or hemophilia may significantly influence personality development, and this may itself interfere with medical care and attempts to plan for vocational, educational, and social adjustment. Chronic illness may elicit a variety of reactions, ranging from overdependence and passivity and an attempt to derive secondary gain to overindependence and aggressive behavior and strong denial of the illness. Some patients have a realistic attitude; others have a great need to deny the complications of their disease and may resist the physician's attempts at treatment.

Paralleling the patient's reactions are those of the parents. Parents may blame the physician for the child's illness and may unconsciously push the child physically and emotionally beyond his capacities for adjustment; or they may reject the patient because of the discrepancy between what he is and what they hoped he would be. The physician should help the parents to adapt and realistically help the child by permitting both an appropriate dependency and continued development within the limits imposed by the illness.

The management of the ill adolescent demands the physician's interest and understanding and the establishment of a therapeutic doctor-patient relationship. By providing a setting where the patient can be heard and accepted and where his concerns about illness can be aired and interpreted, the physician can establish this relationship. In prolonged and handicapping illnesses the physician may need to call upon all possible resources—including educational, social, paramedical, and community agencies—to help the patient and the family adapt.

When hospitalization is required, the reaction to the hospital as well as the illness must be dealt with. The hospital setting must be one in which development can continue to the greatest possible extent, and the patient should be returned to home and school at the earliest possible time.

In his therapeutic relationship with the patient, the physician attempts to provide information and understanding to correct misconceptions and to interpret the handicap and illness. The physician should impart an attitude of optimism for future success and should not hesitate to discuss career goals and vocational possibilities in realistic terms. Since many patients frequently test the doctor-patient relationship by being angry at the physician, not cooperating in treatment programs, and in other ways, the physician should be prepared to respond with understanding and without anger or hostility.

Psychologic and psychiatric examinations may be necessary before medical care can be effectively administered, and collaborative care with a psychiatrist or psychologist may be indicated.

EMOTIONAL PROBLEMS DURING ADOLESCENCE

Adolescents may be brought to or may come to the physician with complaints of emotional or behavioral disorders. The initial complaints may be manifestations of emotional stress. An effort must be made to evaluate the extent of the problem and the type and amount of treatment necessary. Many common emotional problems of adolescence can be handled by the pediatrician who has an appropriate orientation to development during adolescence. In many instances the pediatrician will have the advantage of having known the child and the family for many years.

The evaluation and management of emotional problems during adolescence requires the establishment of a good patient-doctor relationship. The physician should schedule adequate time for visits so that he can show his serious interest in and respect for the adolescent as a developing person. This will permit the adolescent to verbalize his own feelings and attitudes and help him to accept counseling. Initial interviews should be carried out unhurriedly, and the physician must resist the impulse to get to the heart of the problem quickly. The medical history should be designed to gather information (in an unobtrusive manner) about the patient's social and interpersonal interrelationships. The history may also reveal personal habits and dream material that will be valuable in understanding the problem. Some adolescents find it difficult to verbalize their concerns and feelings and have to be drawn out with questions. Frequent reassurance is often needed to solidify the patient-doctor relationship.

If a disorder seems to be predominantly emotional, it is often helpful to point this out and to assure the patient of the physician's willingness to help solve the problem. Excessive prying is to be avoided, but the patient should be permitted to talk while the physician asks appropriate questions and makes comments as the occasion arises. The physician does not need to adhere to the classical 1-hour visit each week; shorter visits at intervals of up to 3 weeks are often sufficient. Psychologic or psychiatric consultation may be necessary for evaluating the problem and determining what treatment is required. It is also helpful if the physician has a psychologic or psychiatric colleague with whom he can discuss special problems. Discussions with school authorities or other community agencies with whom the patient has been related will be valuable in the diagnosis and treatment, but the patient's permission must be obtained before anyone outside the family is approached.

Parents should be seen in separate interviews so that their evaluation of the problem, attitudes, and questions may be heard. Conflicts between the adolescent and his parents can sometimes be resolved in this way.

If the physician feels that psychiatric care is required, appropriate referral is indicated. In doubtful cases, psychiatric evaluation can serve as a basis for continued management by the pediatrician. The decision on whether to refer or not often depends upon such factors as the number of emotional problems carried in the practice, availability of time, and the physician's ability to manipulate forces in the environment when these are playing a prominent role in the patient's problem.

Hollender MH (editor): *The Psychology of Medical Practice.* Saunders, 1958.
Korsch BM: *Psychologic Principles in Pediatric Practice: The Pediatrician and the Sick Child.* Year Book, 1958.

•   •   •

General References

Adolescent Newsletter. Society for Adolescent Medicine. [Semiannual. Current publications in adolescent medicine.]

Chapman AH: *Management of Emotional Problems of Children and Adolescents.* Lippincott, 1965.

Gallagher JR: *Medical Care of the Adolescent,* 2nd ed. Appleton-Century-Crofts, 1966.

Heald FP (editor): *Adolescent Gynecology.* Williams & Wilkins, 1966.

Masterson JF Jr: *The Psychiatric Dilemma of Adolescence.* Little, Brown, 1967.

8 ...

Skin*

James A. Philpott, Jr., MD, & Osgoode S. Philpott, Jr., MD

SKIN PROBLEMS OF INFANTS

Many dermatologic conditions appear in the neonatal period. Some are present at birth; others appear shortly afterward. They may be classified into 2 main groups: transient and permanent.

TRANSIENT INFANTILE SKIN DISORDERS

Erythema Toxicum Neonatorum

Erythema toxicum neonatorum is a papuloerythematous eruption of unknown cause that appears spontaneously within the first 2 days of life and lasts about a week. The lesions are usually confined to the trunk. Individual lesions may measure up to 3 mm in diameter and have an erythematous base with a papular appearance or may have a vesicular or pustular surface. Even though the contents appear pustular, culture from vesicle or pustular fluid is sterile. A stained smear of vesicular fluid usually reveals a predominance of eosinophils. This may suggest an allergic relationship, but none has been demonstrated. Erythema toxicum must be differentiated from staphyloderma and miliaria rubra.

No treatment is necessary.

Taylor WB, Bonderant CP: Erythema neonatorum allergicum: A study of the incidence in two hundred newborn infants and a review of the literature. Arch Dermat 76:591, 1957.

Miliaria Rubra (Prickly Heat, Heat Rash)

Miliaria is caused by mechanical obstruction of the eccrine ducts within the epidermis. The lesions may consist of small clear vesicles or pustules with erythema. The face, trunk, neck, and diaper area are most often affected. Differential diagnosis includes erythema toxicum (no eosinophilia), candidiasis, and impetigo (no bacteria).

Treatment consists of cool baths, reduced environmental temperature, and loose clothing. Bathing the skin with aluminum acetate (Burow's) solution, 1:20, followed by a bland dusting powder (corn starch) is helpful.

Diaper Rash (Intertrigo, Diaper Dermatitis)

Diaper rash is a form of intertrigo plus contact irritation. The skin becomes inflamed as a result of heat, maceration, and the chemical irritant effect of urine and feces. Occasionally, candidiasis complicates the picture. In severe cases the effects of ammonia, split from urea, may produce more severe inflammation and the skin may show actual discrete areas of ulceration.

A satisfactory treatment routine is as follows: Gently cleanse the area with clear water and apply a simple paste such as the following ("1-2-3 ointment"):

R	Burow's solution	10.0
	Hydrous lanolin	20.0
	Zinc oxide ointment	30.0

Change diapers frequently and do not use plastic pants over them. Treat diapers with a quaternary ammonium antiseptic (Diaparene) or sodium borate in wash water. Give Pedameth (DL-methionine), 0.2 gm orally daily (in formula or fruit juice), to reduce the urea content of the urine. Treat candidiasis if present.

Speer R: Diaper rash. Cutis 1:459, 1965.

Fat Necrosis

This uncommon condition presents in the first few weeks of life as an indurated, plaque-like area, usually on the thighs, buttocks, posterior trunk, chest, arms, and feet. The lesions are hard and do not pit on pressure. They may have a deeply erythematous or purplish discoloration and may vary in size from 2–10 cm. The child is otherwise well. A history of trauma may be present. The underlying cause has been postulated to be an alteration in the olein content of newborn fat.

The reaction gradually softens and disappears, and no treatment is indicated.

Edema Neonatorum

This rare disorder is manifested as pitting edema on parts or all of the skin. It is usually associated with prematurity, cachexia, malnutrition, or postdiarrheal states. No other causes are known.

The prognosis is poor, but dietary protein replacement, antibiotics, and corticosteroids may be beneficial.

*Contact dermatitis, atopic dermatitis, and urticaria are discussed in Chapter 33.

Sclerema Neonatorum

In contrast to edema neonatorum, in sclerema there is a generalized (sometimes localized) hardening of the skin, presumably as a result of solidification of subcutaneous fat. It may appear first on the legs, but progress is rapid within 3–4 days. The skin becomes pale and cyanotic and is cold to the touch. Prematurity and cachexia are the most common predisposing causes.

Vigorous treatment with dietary regulation, antibiotics, and corticosteroids is indicated, but the prognosis is poor.

Hughes WE, Hammond ML: Sclerema neonatorum. J Pediat 32:676–692, 1948.

Irgang S: Sclerema neonatorum. Cutis 7:547, 1971.

Kellum RE, Ray TL, Brown GR: Sclerema neonatorum. Arch Dermat 97:372–380, 1968.

Kendall N, Ledis S: Sclerema neonatorum successfully treated with corticotropin (ACTH). Am J Dis Child 83:52–53, 1952.

Impetigo Neonatorum (Pemphigus Neonatorum)

Impetigo neonatorum is a staphylococcal or streptococcal infection of the skin in infants that may present as rapidly spreading vesicular or bullous lesions with erythematous advancing zones. The lesions often appear first in the intertriginous areas. The lesions break and dry, leaving an encrusted surface. Unlike impetigo in older children, the reaction can run rampant. Fever, malaise, and even shock may be present. A gram-stained smear of blister contents shows gram-positive cocci. Culture may be done but should not interfere with antibiotic therapy.

The differential diagnosis includes congenital syphilis, bullous erythema multiforme, and dermatitis medicamentosa. Complications include diarrhea with electrolyte imbalance and transient pyuria.

Treatment with systemic antibiotics (preferably penicillin) should be instituted as soon as possible. Local therapy consists of gentle cleansing and topical antibiotics such as neomycin, bacitracin, or tetracycline. The prognosis is good.

Ritter's Disease (Dermatitis Exfoliativa Neonatorum)

Ritter's disease is a rare disorder that usually begins in the first few days of life. It is manifested as generalized erythema with vesicles, bullae, and pustules. Constitutional symptoms are usually present and include fever, malaise, and dehydration, all of which may be severe. Both clinical appearance and laboratory studies support a bacterial etiology.

Prompt and intensive treatment with fluids and antibiotics (both systemic and topical) is required. Otherwise, the prognosis is guarded.

Syphilis

Congenital syphilis of the newborn is clinically similar to the secondary phases in the adult. The cutaneous lesion may be present at birth or may appear shortly afterward. This is the only example of vesicular or bullous lesions in clinical syphilis. The eruption may be disseminated and maculopapular and is most apt to be present on the palms or soles. Moist papular lesions may be noted in the perianal and perineal areas. Fissured, moist, papular lesions may be seen on the lips. Mucous membrane lesions are present also, and runny nose or "snuffles" may be noted.

Confirmation of the clinical diagnosis depends upon darkfield examination of serous fluid from the surface of moist lesions for *Treponema pallidum* and positive blood serology. It is important to test venous blood and not cord blood.

Treatment is with penicillin. For patients under 2 years of age, give aqueous penicillin, 100,000 units/kg in divided doses over a period of 1 week; or benzathine penicillin G, 50,000 units/kg IM as a single injection. The prognosis is excellent.

Curtis AC, Philpott OS Jr: Prenatal syphilis. M Clin North America 48:707, 1964.

Newcomber VD: Venereal disease among adolescents. Cutis 7:169, 1971.

Syphilis: Modern Diagnosis and Management. Publication No. 743. Public Health Service, Washington, DC.

Vaccinia

Most cases of vaccinia in infants are the result of accidental inoculation. This is becoming more common with the trend toward giving smallpox vaccination to children 1 year of age or older. Accidental inoculation usually occurs by contact with mothers or siblings, and usually on an exposed part. The lesion is a typical vaccinial reaction, and involutes in the same way. In rare instances, vaccinia may become widespread or locally invasive (malignant type). The disseminated lesions are at first vesicular and later pustular. They are multiloculated and umbilicated, resembling single vaccinia lesions. The differential diagnosis includes chickenpox, smallpox, and generalized herpes simplex. The latter in an atopic infant is often referred to as Kaposi's varicelliform eruption, but Kaposi's eruption may also be due to vaccinia. The atopic child is susceptible to both.

Diagnosis depends upon the history, clinical appearance, and viral identification studies. Disseminated vaccinia is usually associated with a primary underlying defect in the immune system, abnormal globulin fractions, leukemic states, or atopic dermatitis.

Treatment consists of specific vaccinia immune globulin (human), control of secondary infection, and, at times, surgery. Surgical treatment consists of the removal, even though it may be extensive, of the area of primary vaccinia inoculation, including the surrounding zone of inflammatory reaction. This may necessitate partial or even total amputation of an extremity.

The prognosis is guarded.

Kempe CH: Studies on smallpox and complications of smallpox vaccinations. Pediatrics 26:176, 1960.

TOXIC EPIDERMAL NECROLYSIS
(Scalded Skin Syndrome, Lyell's Disease)

Toxic epidermal necrolysis is not rare, and involves most of the body surface. The skin becomes acutely inflamed and erythematous. The epidermis becomes rapidly necrotic and strips off easily. There are bullae present which demonstrate a positive Nikolsky sign. The patient appears to have been scalded. The disorder occurs with equal frequency in males and females of all ages, and it frequently involves children.

Most cases occurring in infants and children are associated with infections by phage group II *Staphylococcus aureus,* particularly type 71. Some cases are induced by drugs, most commonly the sulfonamides and butazones. The cases originally thought to be caused by penicillin may have actually been associated with the staphylococcal infection for which the penicillin was prescribed. A third group of cases is idiopathic. All cases seem to represent a hypersensitivity state. Those associated with drugs often resemble severe erythema multiforme of the Stevens-Johnson type.

Clinical Findings

Inflammation of the eyelids, conjunctivas, mouth, and genitalia may appear several days or a week before the generalized erythema and "scalded" look. The skin is very tender to touch. The inguinal area and axillas are usually involved early, and the process spreads from these areas. The scalp is spared. Bullas form and are large, fragile, and filled with clear fluid. The epidermis strips off and leaves the skin oozing and raw. Healing requires several weeks.

Treatment

All patients should be hospitalized where expert nursing care is available. Suspected drugs should be withdrawn. In cases associated with staphylococcal infection, sodium oxacillin should be used systemically. Electrolyte and fluid balance must be maintained. The usefulness of systemic corticosteroids is not firmly established, but their use is recommended in the acute phase. Corticosteroids should not be used locally on the skin or in the eyes. Secondary infection must be controlled.

The paramount factor in successful treatment is good nursing care. A turning frame, as used in burn cases, is sometimes indicated. Consultation with a dermatologist and an ophthalmologist is generally suggested.

Prognosis

The outlook is best in young children with the staphylococcal form. The death rate is 7−10% in these cases. The overall mortality in all cases is 25% or higher. The idiopathic form is the most severe and also the most likely to recur. In children under age 1, the prognosis is grave.

Lowney ED & others: The scalded syndrome in small children. Arch Dermat 95:359, 1967.

Lyell A: Toxic epidermal necrolysis: An eruption resembling scalding of the skin. Brit J Dermat 68:355, 1956.

Lyell A: A review of toxic epidermal necrolysis in Britain. Brit J Dermat 79:662, 1967.

Skipworth GB & others: Toxic epidermal necrolysis. Cutis 6:307, 1970.

PERMANENT OR FIXED INFANTILE SKIN DISORDERS
(Hereditary, Congenital, Nevoid)

Aplasia of the Skin

In rare instances an infant is born with incompletely developed or completely undeveloped areas of skin. These areas may occur anywhere on the body and vary greatly in extent; some may be so large that they are incompatible with life. The underlying structures may be completely exposed or covered with a transparent film of embryonic epithelium.

If the surface area is suitable for grafting, this should be considered. Spontaneous epithelialization seldom occurs.

Congenital Alopecia

Congenital alopecia may be manifested as total scalp alopecia from birth or poorly developed hair with increasing age. The eyebrows and eyelashes are frequently involved also. This is usually a dominant characteristic but is occasionally recessive. It may be associated with webbed fingers and cataracts.

Monilethrix

Monilethrix is an inherited dominant condition of the hair in which there are regular intervals of constriction of the hair shafts, resulting in broken hairs at varying lengths. There is also an associated follicular hyperkeratosis. The microscopic appearance of the hair is characteristic.

There is no satisfactory treatment. Careful management of the hair in terms of gentle washing and minimal brushing and combing is indicated.

Pili Torti

Pili torti is an inherited incomplete dominant trait in which the hair is twisted on itself along its long axis so that the hair breaks at the points of twisting.

Pili Annulari

This anomaly produces hairs that are alternately pigmented and depigmented along the lengths of the shafts. The resulting ringed appearance gives the disorder its name. There is no treatment.

Wooly Hair

Sometimes referred to as "wooly haired nevus," this condition is almost self-explanatory. The hair is short, kinky, and tightly matted. There is no treatment.

Congenital Canities

This consists of scattered areas of depigmented hair. The white lock is most often present at birth, although in some individuals it does not appear until puberty. In most individuals the remaining hair is dark so that the apparent difference in hair color is obvious. The white lock is usually just behind the forehead.

The abnormality is most commonly inherited as a simple autosomal dominant characteristic, affecting males and females equally.

In rare instances, mental deficiency has occurred. In most cases, however, there are no other congenital anomalies.

Albinism

Albinism is the principal pigmentary disturbance seen in children. It consists of total or partial absence of melanin in the skin, hair, and irises. The hair is sparse. The basic defect involves the enzyme systems that stimulate the production of melanin from its precursors in the melanocytes. The ocular reaction results in photophobia, lacrimation, and nystagmus. Complete albinism is a recessive characteristic. Incomplete albinism may be inherited as a recessive or irregular dominant characteristic.

Affected individuals must be extremely careful to protect themselves from sun exposure.

In patients with albinism, the skin may be more dry than normal, and sweating may be meager. Many patients exhibit an excess of lanugo, and the scalp hair may be silky and yellowish white in color. There may be imperfect development of the fovea centralis of the retina. Nystagmus may be marked.

Vitiligo

Vitiligo is an acquired type of leukoderma that may appear at any age and on any area of the skin and may remain localized or become generalized. The skin is normal except for lack of pigment. The cause of the biochemical reaction that interferes with normal melanin synthesis in affected areas of skin is not known. There is no satisfactory treatment. The administration of psoralens—methoxsalen (Oxsoralen) or trioxsalen (Trisoralin)—may be considered, but these preparations have not proved satisfactory. Psoralens should not be prescribed for children under 12 years of age. Protection from sunlight is important. If the cosmetic problem is severe, cosmetics such as Covermark may be used. Dihydroxyacetone solutions (Man-Tan, etc) may also be satisfactory as a means of producing temporary color matching of the surrounding skin.

Kanof NB: Disorders of melanin pigmentation. M Clin North America 49:593, 1965.

Nevi

In this discussion, the term nevus will be restricted to signify those neoplasms that contain the nevus cell. The nevus cell is the clear cell found in the basal layer of the epidermis which is derived from the schwannian sheath of embryonic nerve tissue.

Nevi are rarely present at birth and seldom require removal during the first decade. They vary considerably in their color and conformation. In general, during childhood, nevi are flat or slightly elevated and tend to be hyperpigmented. During this period, practically all contain junctional elements. As the lesion matures, it is apt to become elevated and dome-shaped. Some lesions become verrucous or cerebelliform. As maturation progresses, the majority of nevi lose their junctional elements and become intradermal and, therefore, benign. Exceptions are nevi on the face, palms, soles, and genitalia, which tend to retain their junctional elements and, therefore, their malignant potentialities. For practical purposes, lesions in these areas demand the greatest attention from the clinician.

Prophylactic removal in all cases is not practical, but repeated observation is important. Malignant nevi are rare in children but do occur. Junctional nevi, when removed, should be surgically excised. Other nevi can be removed for cosmetic reasons by a variety of surgical technics, including plastic removal or electrosurgical removal.

Any nevus that is removed should be examined microscopically.

Halo Nevus

In this reaction the zone of skin around a nevus becomes depigmented. This apparently is the result of some obscure immune response, and, in the process, the nevus is apt to disappear spontaneously during the teen years. It has recently been pointed out that malignant changes can occur in halo nevi.

Baer RL, Witten VH: Selected benign pigmented cutaneous lesions. In: *Yearbook of Dermatology and Syphilology.* Year Book 1958–59.
Kopf AW, Morril S, Silberg D: Broad spectrum of leukoderma acquisitum centrifugum. Arch Dermat 92:14, 1965.

Hemangiomas

Hemangiomas are the most common tumors of infancy. In approximately half of cases they are present at birth; the remainder develop within the first weeks of life.

Hemangiomas can be divided into 2 main types: capillary and cavernous. Capillary hemangiomas are most common on the brows, eyelids, and nuchal area. They are usually transient with the exception of those on the nuchal area, which remain (especially in females). No treatment is necessary.

Extensive capillary hemangiomas are often called **port wine marks or stains.** These lesions can be very extensive, but almost all are unilateral. When they involve the distribution of the trigeminal nerve, the condition is referred to as **Sturge-Weber syndrome** and assumes added clinical significance. They may be associated with intracranial hemangiomas, seizures, contralateral spastic paralysis, and ipsilateral ocular disorders (usually glaucoma). Treatment of capillary hemangiomas in general is unsatisfactory.

Cavernous hemangiomas vary considerably in size, number, and shape. They appear as elevated, soft, compressible, strawberry-like growths. They are usually 0.5–8 cm in diameter but may be much larger, eg, may cover one side of the face or an entire extremity. They may be solitary or multiple. There is usually a period of growth followed by a period of inertia. In the great majority of instances, spontaneous involution occurs. Various technics of treatment have been recommended, including freezing, surgical extirpation, radiation, and injection of sclerosing solutions. In the authors' opinions, none of these measures give better results than spontaneous involution, and treatment is rarely necessary. Exceptions to this rule may be lesions near the eye that may invade the orbit and exert pressure on the globe. In such cases, surgical removal is indicated.

Binings L: Spontaneous regression of angiomas in children: 22 years' observation covering 236 cases. J Pediat 45:643, 1954.

Frost JF, Caplan RM: Cutaneous hemangiomas and disappearing bones: With a review of cutaneo-visceral hemangiomatosis. Arch Dermat 92:501, 1965.

Lymphangiomas

Lymphangiomas are much less common than hemangiomas and tend to enlarge. They are often found under the tongue also. They are amenable to surgical removal, but recurrences are not uncommon.

Cystic hygroma is a type of lymphangioma that arises in and invades the fascial planes of the neck. It rarely produces pressure phenomena, but surgery is indicated because of the disfigurement produced.

Congenital Ectodermal Dysplasia

This rare hereditary skin disorder is characterized by underdevelopment of the epidermis and the epidermal adnexa. If eccrine sweat glands are absent or deficient, anhidrosis results. The skin is usually thin and glossy, and the hair is sparse, dry, and breaks easily. The teeth and gums are malformed, the nasal bones are often flattened, and there may be frontal bosses. These changes produce a characteristic facies. The anhidrotic component may present a serious problem of hyperthermia. Elevated environmental temperature and extreme physical exertion must be avoided.

There is no satisfactory treatment.

Pachyonychia Congenita

In this condition the nails are extremely thickened and tend to grow straight up from the nail beds. There may be associated anomalies of the hair and increased keratosis of the palms and soles. Bullous lesions may occur on the hands and feet.

Surgical removal of the nails may be necessary.

Cutis Hyperelastica (Cutis Laxa, Ehlers-Danlos Syndrome)

This syndrome consists of hyperelasticity of the skin. Hyperextensibility results in unstable joints and muscle weakness. The skin heals poorly after lacerations or surgery in spite of the care taken. Microscopically, increased numbers of elastic fibers are noted in the skin.

There is no satisfactory treatment.

Epidermolysis Bullosa

This hereditary skin disorder occurs with varying degrees of severity. **Epidermolysis bullosa simplex** is an irregular dominant disorder manifested by the appearance of bullae on the hands, feet, elbows, and knees in response to minor trauma. It usually appears early in childhood but may not appear until later. Treatment consists of protection from trauma and topical antibiotics.

Epidermolysis bullosa dystrophica is a recessive anomaly usually present at birth. Minor trauma in handling the infant causes large bullous lesions to develop. Similar lesions develop on the mucous membranes. Healing is attended by atrophic scarring, which may be so severe that loss of tissue (even bone) may occur. In severe cases, death usually occurs early in life. These infants require the finest nursing care and should be treated as one would manage a burn case. Corticosteroids have been advocated but in the authors' experience have not proved satisfactory.

Severin GL, Farber EM: The management of epidermolysis bullosa in children. Arch Dermat 95:302–309, 1967.

Incontinentia Pigmenti

This rare congenital anomaly is almost exclusively limited to females. The disorder in the skin consists of an inflammatory phase and a hyperpigmented phase. The inflammatory phase is present shortly after birth and consists of papular, verrucous, or vesicular lesions in linear distribution on the extremities or the trunk. These disappear spontaneously within 6–8 weeks, leaving the skin mottled with hyperpigmentation. The importance of the condition is in the associated anomalies of the eyes, teeth, cardiovascular system, bones, and other structures. A thorough search for these changes should be made at an early age.

The prognosis is good.

Curth HO, Warburton D: The genetics of incontinentia pigmenti. Arch Dermat 92:229, 1965.

Ichthyosis

Ichthyosis is a general term for dry and scaling (fish-like) skin. Various types and degrees of this condition are described in infants.

Ichthyosis congenita (so-called **harlequin fetus**), the most severe (usually lethal) form of the disorder, is inherited as a recessive trait and is manifested at birth. It consists of a thickened, wrinkled, and parchment-like skin. The orifices of the nose and ears may be occluded. Eyelid movement may be impossible.

A similar but unrelated disorder is the so-called **collodion fetus**, in which a retained embryonic periderm is present and sheds in a matter of weeks, after which the child is normal.

Ichthyosis hystrix is a severe but somewhat localized form characterized by scattered areas of extreme hyperkeratosis. The skin in areas of involvement may resemble that of a porcupine, with a spiny, horny skin.

Ichthyosis simplex is a dominant condition characterized by generalized dryness and scaling which may vary with the season, being worse during the cold, dry winter months.

There is no satisfactory treatment for ichthyosis, but palliative measures may afford considerable relief. Hydration of the skin by bathing, followed immediately by the application of an emollient, is the most satisfactory form of treatment. Lubriderm, Nivea Oil, Keri Lotion, cold cream, and white petrolatum are all useful emollients. The addition of 2–3% salicylic acid to any of these preparations may be extremely helpful as a keratolytic agent to help remove hyperkeratotic material.

Keratosis Palmaris et Plantaris

This is an inherited condition in which the keratin of the palms and soles is greatly thickened. It may result in fissuring and discomfort, with limitation of certain types of hand movements. Treatment consists of attempting to remove the thickened areas with keratolytics such as salicylic acid in either emollients or plasters (eg, 40% salicylic acid plaster).

Keratosis Pilaris

This condition represents a variant of ichthyosis in which changes are limited to the pilosebaceous apparatus. Discrete hyperkeratotic, papular lesions are present in the orifices of the follicular openings. The condition is most manifest on the scapular areas, the posterior surfaces of the arms, and the anterior surfaces of the thighs. As with ichthyosis, improvement is noted in the summer.

Local treatment is similar to that of ichthyosis.

Wells RS, Kerr CB: Genetic classification of ichthyosis. Arch Dermat 92:1, 1965.

COMMON SKIN DISORDERS OF CHILDREN

SKIN REACTIONS DUE TO DRUGS
(Dermatitis Medicamentosa)

Drug eruptions must be considered in the evaluation of any cutaneous reaction. Common dermatoses may be simulated, eg, lichen planus, pityriasis rosea, psoriasis, acne, and erythema nodosum. The lesions may be eczematous, urticarial, or erythema multiforme-like without the presence of vesicles or bullae.

These reactions may occur in any age group. The offending drug or chemical agent may be obscure. A detailed history is essential, and one must not overlook obscure chemicals such as food additives and preservatives. In puzzling situations, consistent search may be rewarding. In addition to the above, certain reactions may remain fixed and solitary (fixed drug eruptions); upon reexposure, reactions occur in identical sites of previous involvement.

Onset is abrupt, with a symmetrical and usually generalized eruption. Systemic symptoms (arthralgia, fever, headache) may occur.

In all cases of dermatitis medicamentosa, the possible effects of certain drugs on other systems (liver, kidneys, hematopoietic system) must be considered and evaluated. Blood counts and urinalysis are always indicated, and liver function studies are required in some instances.

Terminate exposure to the offending drug and give symptomatic local therapy. Antihistamines and epinephrine are indicated in urticarial reactions, and corticosteroids in severe reactions of the urticarial and erythema multiforme types and exfoliative reactions (Table 8–1).

Baer RL, Witten VH: Drug eruption. Pages 9–37 in: *Year Book of Dermatology.* Year Book, 1960–61.
Weary EW, Cole JE, Hickam LH: Eruptions from ampicillin in patients with infectious mononucleosis. Arch Dermat 101:86, 1970.

ERYTHEMA MULTIFORME

In the pediatric age group, erythema multiforme may be difficult to differentiate from urticaria. Dermatitis herpetiformis and pemphigus also resemble erythema multiforme but are very uncommon, especially in children. In urticaria, there are no vesicles or bullae and no mucous membrane lesions. Itching is a prominent symptom in both disorders. Erythema multiforme may be associated with constitutional symptoms (see below). The severe and generalized form of erythema multiforme, often referred to as Stevens-Johnson syndrome, may be fatal.

Erythema multiforme may be due to drug sensitivity, bacterial or viral sensitivity, foreign protein sensitivity, or other causes. The relationship between herpes simplex virus and erythema multiforme is well established. It may occur in association with a developing type of lymphoblastoma; as a postirridation reaction, eg, following deep x-ray therapy for lymphoblastoma or other malignancies; or occasionally at the onset of one of the collagen diseases. A significant percentage of cases are due to unknown causes, and these may be recurrent.

TABLE 8–1. Common skin reactions associated with frequently used drugs.

Drug	Common Reactions
Aspirin	Urticaria rarely; purpuric eruptions.
Antibiotics:	
Cephaloridine (Loridine)	Three percent develop pruritus; occasional reports of urticaria or maculopapular erythema.
Erythromycin (Ilosone, Erythrocin)	Urticaria; rarely, jaundice.
Griseofulvin (Fulvicin, Grifulvin)	Exanthematous eruptions; rarely, cold urticaria or photodermatitis.
Lincomycin (Lincocin)	Urticaria or exanthematous eruptions.
Penicillin and synthetic penicillins (Dynapen, Omnipen, Polycillin, Prostaphlin, Tegopen, Veracillin)	Atopic individuals more susceptible. Serum sickness, urticaria, exanthematous eruptions, anaphylactic shock. Ampicillin causes a high incidence of exanthematous eruptions in patients with infectious mononucleosis.
Streptomycin	Exanthematous eruptions, urticaria, stomatitis.
Sulfonamides	Urticaria, exanthematous eruptions, bullous reactions, Stevens-Johnson syndrome, photodermatitis.
Tetracycline	Exanthematous eruptions, urticaria; rarely, bullous eruptions. Demethylchlortetracycline (Declomycin) can cause phototoxic reactions.
Antihistamines	Exanthematous eruptions, urticaria, photodermatitis.
Barbiturates	Maculopapular eruptions, urticaria, erythema multiforme, Stevens-Johnson syndrome, bullous eruptions.
Chlorothiazides	Exanthematous eruptions, urticaria, photodermatitis, hemosiderosis of the lower extremities, leading to the development of petechiae with resultant pigmentation (Schamberg's phenomenon).
Codeine (cough syrups)	Exanthematous eruptions, urticaria.
Cortisone and derivatives	Acneiform drug reactions on trunk—pustular, purpuric eruptions. Urticaria from ACTH.
Diphenylhydantoin (Dilantin)	Exanthematous eruptions usually in first 3 weeks of treatment; gingival hyperplasia, hypertrichosis.
Insulin	Urticaria, erythema at injection site. The antidiabetic drugs related to sulfonamides (tolbutamide, etc) may also cause urticaria or pruritus.
Iodides (cough syrups, anti-asthma preparations)	Acneiform pustules over trunk, granulomatous reaction, erythema multiforme (seen occasionally after x-ray studies using iodides).
Prochlorperazine (Compazine)	Urticaria, pruritus, photosensitive dermatitis.

Clinical Findings

A. Symptoms and Signs: The skin lesions are symmetrical in distribution, usually erythematous to violaceous and polymorphous, ranging from erythematous macular lesions to erythematous lesions topped with vesicles or bullae or to bullous lesions simulating pemphigus. The extensor surfaces of the extremities are most commonly involved. An erythematous, edematous lesion with a central vesicle ("iris" lesion) is commonly seen on the palms and soles. The mucous membranes of the conjunctivas, oral cavity, and genitalia may also be affected. Constitutional symptoms of fever, malaise, prostration, and even shock may be present. Pneumonitis may be present.

B. Laboratory Findings: Laboratory examination is seldom helpful. Blood and urine are not often abnormal. Nose and throat cultures may reveal pathogenic bacteria. Nasal and gastrointestinal studies may be helpful in identifying viral agents.

Differential Diagnosis

Erythema multiforme must be differentiated from urticaria, which causes more edema and no vesiculation. Pemphigus and dermatitis herpetiformis may

be confused with bullous erythema multiforme, but these 2 diseases are rare in children. Certain types of viremia (eg, hand, foot, and mouth disease), drug eruptions of many types (especially those produced by iodides and bromides), congenital syphilis, and secondary syphilis may resemble erythema multiforme.

Treatment

Erythema multiforme is usually a self-limited disease which can be treated symptomatically. Antibiotics (especially tetracyclines) may be helpful. Fluid and electrolyte losses should be corrected. Systemic corticosteroids are required in widespread or severe reactions and may be mandatory and lifesaving in some cases.

ERYTHEMA NODOSUM

Streptococcal sensitivity, rheumatic fever, and drug sensitivity are the most important causes of erythema nodosum in the pediatric age group. In endemic areas, coccidioidomycosis may be an important cause. Primary tuberculosis should always be considered. A thorough search for focal infection, especially in the upper respiratory tract (including nose and throat cultures), should be made.

Clinical Findings

A. Symptoms and Signs: The erythematous nodular lesions are quite tender. Prodromal manifestations include fever, malaise, and arthralgia. Pneumonitis may be present. The lesions vary in size from 1–6 cm (occasionally larger) and are discrete, usually on the pretibial surfaces but rarely on the arms and trunk. The lesions rarely become fluctuant and do not drain. They may appear in crops but regress spontaneously within weeks.

B. Laboratory Findings: Biopsy may be helpful but is usually not necessary. Appropriate skin testing (tuberculin, coccidioidin, histoplasmin) and nose and throat cultures are indicated.

C. X-Ray Findings: Chest films should be taken to rule out pulmonary disease.

Differential Diagnosis

Bruises and contusions must be considered. Sporotrichosis is usually unilateral. Erythema multiforme is usually generalized. Nodular vasculitis is rare.

Treatment

Treatment consists of bed rest with elevation of the affected part, specific treatment of infection, and salicylates for fever and joint pain. Corticosteroids, if not contraindicated, will shorten the course.

Prognosis

Erythema nodosum is generally a self-limited disease. It may be recurrent, depending upon the cause (eg, drugs, streptococcal sensitivity).

NUMMULAR DERMATITIS

This type of eczematous reaction is characterized by the development of multiple, discrete discoid or "coin-like" lesions. The lesions are usually exudative and encrusted. Secondary infection is common. The initial lesions often appear on the extremities, especially the legs.

The most important cause appears to be contact with wool, soaps, detergents, starches, and other substances, usually acting as primary irritants on an ichthyotic or asteatotic skin. Pruritus with excoriation leads to secondary infection.

The lesions are frequently confused with those of tinea corporis and sometimes psoriasis. Direct examination should rule out tinea, and lack of typical scaling (rather than crusting) plus distribution would eliminate psoriasis.

Treatment consists of reduction of bathing and elimination of contact factors. Topical corticosteroids

and antibiotics are indicated. In severe generalized reactions, systemic corticosteroids in courses of 7–10 days are justified.

Scott TFM: Hypersensitivity syndrome, erythema multiforme, erythema nodosum, urticaria. P Clin North America 3:771–871, 1956.
Paulus HE: Erythema nodosum. J-Lancet 85:145, 1965.

PHOTOSENSITIVITY DERMATITIS

Essentials of Diagnosis

- Erythema of exposed skin.
- History of ingestion of photosensitizing drugs.
- Photosensitizing underlying illness.

General Considerations

Photosensitivity is manifested by abnormal skin reactions in areas exposed to ultraviolet light (UVL). These reactions are of 2 types: photoallergic or phototoxic. It is often difficult to distinguish the 2 types. In general, photoallergic reactions require prior exposure to the photosensitizing substance. The reaction occurs after a delay of several hours, when the sensitized person is again exposed to the photosensitizing substance and UVL. Only sensitized individuals react, and the wavelength of UVL may be variable. Phototoxic reactions, on the other hand, are similar to exaggerated sunburns. They do not require sensitization by prior exposure (can result from the initial exposure), and the reaction time is shorter than with photoallergic reactions.

More people are subject to phototoxic than to photoallergic reactions. A comparison of photosensitive skin reactions and contact dermatitis will contribute to an understanding of the 2 types of reactions. Allergic contact dermatitis is in many ways similar to the photoallergic response, whereas the phototoxic response is more similar to primary irritant contact dermatitis, ie, it is not truly allergic in action.

Photosensitivity reactions may appear without known cause or may be associated with drugs or underlying disease. The drugs may be topically or systemically administered. A few examples of topical sensitizers are coal tar, eosin, certain plants, and sulfonamides. Common photosensitizing internal drugs are sulfonamides, tolbutamide, chlorpropamide, chlorothiazide, demethylchlortetracycline, phenothiazines, gold, quinine, griseofulvin, barbiturates, and diphenhydramine.

Examples of acquired photosensitivity due to unknown causes include polymorphic light eruption and solar urticaria.

Photosensitivity reactions associated with inherited disorders are common. They include albinism, keratosis follicularis, xeroderma pigmentosum, Rothmund-Thomson syndrome, Bloom's syndrome,

Cockayne's disease, Hartnup's disease, and porphyria (porphyria erythropoietica, porphyria cutanea tarda, and erythropoietic protoporphyria).

Other internal illnesses associated with photosensitivity may be of the acquired type, eg, pellagra, systemic lupus erythematosus.

Hydroa vacciniforme is a vesicular disorder of childhood seen during summer (early) and triggered by UVL. It affects the exposed skin, and is more common in boys. It begins during the first few years of life and clears spontaneously during puberty. A milder nonscarring form is known as **hydroa aestivale**. Any child with hydroa must be tested to rule out protoporphyria.

Clinical Findings

Phototoxic reactions are characterized by marked erythema of exposed skin. The appearance is that of an exaggerated sunburn (the single most helpful clinical finding). Photoallergic reactions may be polymorphic, and occasionally involve unexposed areas. Other clinical forms include erythematous plaques, eczematous lesions, papular or vesicular lesions, and urticarial reactions. Again, however, the paramount finding is distribution.

Differential Diagnosis

Contact dermatitis of the airborne type usually involves the eyelids and flexural folds. Occupational contact dermatitis should have a related history. Lupus erythematosus, especially with the plaque-like reaction, may resemble photosensitivity dermatitis, but it usually demonstrates atrophy and is characterized by more fixed lesions. Erythema multiforme and atopic dermatitis must also be considered.

Treatment

If the photosensitivity reaction is due to a drug or chemical compound, the initial step is to discontinue its use. Acute dermatitis is treated with cold tap water compresses for ½ hour 4 times a day. This can be followed by the use of a corticosteroid cream (not an ointment). Systemic corticosteroids are rarely indicated.

Some photosensitivity reactions due to underlying disorders will gradually improve spontaneously as the patient becomes older. Examples are Rothmund-Thomson syndrome, Cockayne's disease, and Hartnup's disease. Others fail to improve.

Dietary measures may improve a photodermatosis such as pellagra or Hartnup's disease.

Some idiopathic polymorphous light eruptions can be blocked by the use of oral antimalarial drugs. Discoid lupus erythematosus, which is aggravated by sunlight, is often improved by antimalarials.

Protective creams and lotions are often used in the management of polymorphous light eruptions caused by UVL with wavelengths of 290–310 nm. *p*-Aminobenzoic acid, 10–15% in hydrophilic ointment base, is effective. Other preparations of value include Uval lotion, RVP ointment, and A-Fil preparations. Newer preparations include PABAFILM lotion, Presun lotion, and Maxafil cream.

If the photodermatitis is created by long wave UVL in the range of 400 nm (eg, porphyria), protective creams are of little or no benefit and avoidance of UVL is required.

Willis I: Sunlight and the skin. JAMA 217:1088, 1971.

XERODERMA PIGMENTOSUM

Xeroderma pigmentosum is an inherited recessive skin disorder which will briefly be considered separately because of its potential danger. It appears in the first or second year of life and involves both sexes equally. The skin lesions tend to become malignant, and death usually occurs before age 15.

The disease usually begins with freckle-like pigmentation of the exposed skin. Later, unexposed areas become involved, as well as the lips, tongue, and conjunctivas. In the early stages, the lesions are made worse by UVL. Atrophy and telangiectasia follow, so that the condition may resemble chronic radiodermatitis. Malignant degeneration develops, and the most common tumor is a basal cell epithelioma. Squamous cell carcinoma can also be present, and melanomas are occasionally encountered. The skin changes are secondary to UVL with a wavelength of 290–320 nm—the "sunburn range."

The serum α_2 globulin level is elevated. Serum copper is elevated, and blood glutathione is decreased. Both the copper increase and the glutathione decrease may interfere with protective melanin formation. Aminoaciduria (aspartic and glutamic acid) of the overflow type has been reported.

The most important aspect of treatment is to avoid needless UVL. Protective clothing and topical sunscreen creams are indicated. Topical 5-fluorouracil, 1%, may be used for early actinic damage. The preparation is applied twice daily for varying periods of time depending upon the clinical response. Direct sunlight should be avoided during treatment with topical 5-fluorouracil. Tumors should be treated with surgery or electrocautery as soon as they become apparent. It is essential to avoid x-ray therapy in the treatment of tumors arising in xeroderma pigmentosum.

Butterworth T, Strean LP: Light sensitivity and the genodermatoses. Cutis 1:61, 126, 1965.
Carter VH, Smith KW, Noojin RO: Xeroderma pigmentosum: Treatment with topically applied fluorouracil. Arch Dermat 98:526–527, 1968.

CUTANEOUS MANIFESTATIONS OF COLLAGEN DISEASE

SYSTEMIC LUPUS ERYTHEMATOSUS

Systemic lupus erythematosus (SLE) is a disease of multiple organ systems, and the most important consideration is the total clinical picture. This section will deal with skin lesions only.

Approximately 70% of patients with SLE will develop skin lesions at some time during their clinical course. In about 20–25%, skin changes will be the first sign of SLE. The disease is much more common in females.

The most common sign of SLE is cutaneous erythema, particularly of areas exposed to sunlight (photosensitivity). Erythema of the malar area, the so-called butterfly rash, occurs in 1/3 of cases. Erythema may also be found involving other locations: thenar, hypothenar, periungual, over the dorsal phalanges, etc. Photosensitivity occurs in approximately 1/3 of cases. Raynaud's phenomenon is not an infrequent finding. Evidence of cutaneous bleeding, such as petechiae, purpura, or ecchymoses, is found in 20% of cases. Less frequent cutaneous signs include alopecia, hyperpigmentation, mucous membrane lesions, subcutaneous nodules, leg ulcers, bullae, and gangrene. In 75% of cases, laboratory examination for lupus erythematosus cells is positive.

The treatment of SLE is discussed elsewhere in this text.

Jones HE & others: Skin tests with nuclear factors in systemic lupus erythematosus. Arch Dermat 95:559–564, 1967.
Tuffanelli DL, Dubois EL: Cutaneous manifestations of systemic lupus erythematosus. Arch Dermat 90:377, 1964.
See also Markham reference, below.

DERMATOMYOSITIS

The presenting complaints of dermatomyositis relate to the skin and voluntary muscles. In children, as opposed to adults, the condition is not related to internal malignancy. The diagnosis is assisted by serum transaminase or urinary creatine elevations. Muscle biopsy is of help if an affected muscle is selected. Skin biopsy is of no help.

Muscle weakness is the most striking feature of this disease. Cutaneous lesions are often erythematous, and particularly affect the face and hands. Edema of the face is common, and dysphagia is a frequent complaint. Telangiectasia of the upper eyelids can impart to them a heliotrope hue. Calcinosis occurs in 40% of cases, and is seen about 2 years after the condition begins. Dermatomyositis is more frequent in females.

Periungual telangiectasia may be present, and erythematous changes are common over the dorsal phalanges—particularly over the joints. Poikiloderma is frequently present. The clinical picture is sometimes confused with trichinosis.

Muscle contracture, respiratory failure, cardiac failure, and bronchial pneumonia may occur as complications.

The treatment of choice is corticosteroids, starting with prednisone, 30 mg/day, or its equivalent.

Markham RW, Callaway JL: Cutaneous manifestations of systemic lupus erythematosus and dermatomyositis. Cutis 6:169, 1970.

SCLERODERMA

Systemic scleroderma occurs uncommonly in children. Localized scleroderma (linear bands and morphea) is much more common in children than in adults.

Systemic Scleroderma

Systemic scleroderma may be of 3 types: edematous, sclerotic, or atrophic. The sclerotic form is seen most often. Calcinosis occurs much later than in dermatomyositis—on the average, about 11 years after the onset of illness. Hyperpigmentation and Raynaud's phenomenon are frequent components of the clinical picture. Distribution is often distal, including the hands, feet, and face. Early sclerosis may cause loss of sweating and alopecia. In older children, the dorsal phalanges should be evaluated for hair loss. The fingers often taper, and a claw hand forms secondary to contracture. Ulcerative lesions are not frequent on the fingertips. Internal organ involvement is to be expected.

There is no effective treatment. Physical therapy is essential.

Localized Scleroderma

Morphea consists of localized plaques of circumscribed scleroderma. These areas may be inflammatory early but then progress to ivory-colored plaques in which the skin is firm and thickened. The area feels rigid to palpation. The peripheral margin may be violaceous. Morphea is more common in females. The lesions tend to resolve gradually over several years.

Another localized form of scleroderma is **linear bands**. These occur commonly in females and develop during the first decade of life. They are found on the face, scalp, chest, and, less often, on the extremities. Linear lesions of the scalp and forehead (*coup de sabre* lesions) may be associated with hemiatrophy of the face. Linear lesions of the leg may be associated with underlying osseous malformation or may impede future bone growth.

The treatment of linear lesions is difficult; however, one should apply topical corticosteroids under occlusive dressings at bedtime and leave in place overnight. The stronger and newer preparations are preferred. Increased percutaneous absorption of the corticosteroid may be encouraged by the addition of 1–2% salicylic acid to the preparation.

Tuffanelli DL, Winkelmann RK: Systemic scleroderma. Arch Dermat 84:359, 1961.

BACTERIAL INFECTIONS OF THE SKIN

Two organisms—staphylococci and streptococci—account for the great majority of cutaneous bacterial infections. Pseudomonas, *Escherichia coli,* and proteus organisms are occasional causes of primary skin infection. Identification in these situations depends on culture. Certain atypical acid-fast organisms may also cause cutaneous infection.

IMPETIGO

Impetigo is primarily a vesicular eruption that quickly becomes encrusted. There is very little inflammatory reaction. Pruritus is common. The face, particularly about the nares, is most commonly affected. The extent of the reaction is within the epidermis, so that scarring does not ensue unless the lesions are excoriated. The lesions at times are widespread. Identification of the causative organism by culture is usually not necessary.

Treatment is simple and effective and consists of soap and water cleansing, removal of crusts with wet compresses if necessary, and appropriate systemic antibiotics for a period of 8–10 days. Penicillin is usually the antibiotic of choice. Erythromycin may be used alternatively.

PYODERMA

Pyoderma is essentially a deeper extension of infection into the dermis with a tendency toward pustulation and ulceration. The tissue reaction is more severe than in impetigo, with inflammation and cellulitis. Pyoderma may heal with or without scarring. Fever, lymphangitis, and lymphadenopathy may be present. Transient pyuria may be noted. Culture and sensitivity tests are not routinely necessary but should be done if improvement is not satisfactory within 48 hours. Nose and throat cultures should be done.

Treatment consists of soap and water cleansing, wet compresses (saline solution, Burow's solution 1:20, or potassium permanganate 1:8000) for cleansing and reduction of inflammation, and topical antibiotics (as for impetigo). Systemic antibiotics should also be used (as in impetigo).

FURUNCLES & CARBUNCLES

Furuncle begins within a hair follicle and produces a deep inflammatory reaction with pain and tenderness followed by liquefaction necrosis and spontaneous drainage. A group of adjacent furuncles is referred to as a carbuncle.

These lesions infect principally the hairy parts. Furuncles and carbuncles are almost uniformly due to infections with staphylococci. Furuncles may be single or multiple, and frequently are chronic and recurrent. In the latter situation, diabetes mellitus, renal disease, lymphoma, and focal infection should be looked for but are seldom found. Furuncles may be perpetuated by local contamination or, much less often, hematogenous spread. Chronic recurrent furunculosis demands therapeutic ingenuity and strict adherence to the principles of skin hygiene (including fingernails) and antibiotic administration.

General skin cleanliness is mandatory, with special attention to areas immediately surrounding the infection. Topical antibiotic dressings are helpful for this purpose (neomycin, tetracycline). Hexachlorophene soaps may be beneficial. Benzalkonium chloride (Zephiran), 1:1000 solution, may also be helpful as a skin cleanser. Local heat in the form of moist dressings or a controlled hot water heat pad should be applied for 1–2 hours twice daily. This tends to hasten fluctuance.

Systemic antibiotics are indicated. Penicillin G is the drug of choice. Erythromycin and oxacillin are alternative drugs. Culture and sensitivity tests should be done in all cases of recurring lesions and antibiotic therapy selected appropriately. In the treatment of chronic recurrent furunculosis, intensive antibiotic therapy should be continued for 2–6 weeks.

Incision and drainage should be done when the lesion becomes fluctuant. An incision should be made, the wound drained and irrigated, and either an iodoform pack or some type of suitable drain implanted.

Vaccine therapy may be helpful as an adjunct to antibiotic therapy.

PYOGENIC GRANULOMA

Pyogenic granuloma is common in children. The lesion grows rapidly and protrudes from the skin as a cherry-red lesion that, if encrusted, may look black. It bleeds freely and profusely with minor trauma, and can be alarming to parents. Microscopically, it resembles hemangioma with acute inflammation and many polymorphonuclear cells. The lesion apparently develops in response to minor trauma and bacterial infection, presumably streptococcal or staphylococcal. The most common sites are the face, neck, and fingers.

Treatment consists of electrodesiccation, being certain to fulgurate the base even after initial desiccation and removal of the lesion.

SKIN INFECTIONS DUE TO ATYPICAL ACID-FAST ORGANISMS

Several "atypical" mycobacteria are capable of producing cutaneous infections. These infections are not common, although more cases may occur than are recognized. Improved culture technics have aided in identification of the organisms. If the infection is suspected, a pathologist or bacteriologist should be consulted about how to obtain material for culture.

Swimming Pool Granuloma

Swimming pool granuloma is the most widely recognized (and probably the most common) cutaneous infection caused by an atypical acid-fast organism (*Mycobacterium balnei*). The lesions develop at points of trauma such as the dorsa of the feet, knees, elbows, and knuckles. Most infections have been traced to swimming pools, but contaminated fresh water irrigation canals and sea water have accounted for a few instances. No systemic complications have as yet been noted, and regional lymphadenitis such as that seen in a primary tuberculous complex of the skin does not occur. As a result of cross-sensitivity between *M balnei* and *M tuberculosis,* a positive tuberculin test (PPD) is present in up to 80% of cases. In most cases, the course is self-limited, but some lesions have persisted for as long as 3 years.

There is no specific treatment, although liquid nitrogen freezing, electrodesiccation, and local heat have been reported to be successful. Anti-tuberculosis drugs are not helpful.

Other Atypical Mycobacteria

In the USA, there have been scattered reports of cutaneous infection with other mycobacteria, eg, *M kansasii.* In Africa, large ulcerative lesions are produced by *M ulcerans.*

Markowitz M & others: The bacteriologic findings, streptococcal immune response, and renal complications in children with impetigo. Pediatrics 35:393, 1965.

McCoy KL, Kennedy ER: Autogenous vaccine therapy in staphylococcic infections. JAMA 174:35, 1960.

Philpott JA & others: Swimming pool granuloma: A study of 290 cases. Arch Dermat 88:1598, 1963.

SUPERFICIAL MYCOTIC SKIN INFECTIONS

Mycotic infections are divided into 2 general categories: superficial and deep. The superficial lesions are by far the more frequent. Cutaneous fungal infection is more common in males. Mycotic infections are promoted by moisture.

Superficial infection can occur in the skin, hair, or nails. The region involved usually determines the clinical term to be applied: tinea capitis, tinea corporis, etc. Dermatophyte infections are commonly called ringworm or, in the case of tinea pedis, athlete's foot.

Superficial infection is caused by 3 genera of organisms: trichophyton, microsporum, and epidermophyton. Specific identification is valuable in treatment. Cultures of organisms assist the clinician in treatment because only a few specific species are resistant to systemic medications.

TINEA CAPITIS
(Scalp Ringworm)

Tinea capitis is caused by microsporum or trichophyton organisms. (Epidermophyton never attacks hair.) *M audouini* may cause epidemics in which the infected hairs fluoresce under Wood's light. *M audouini* is spread from child to child. *M canis* is a common human pathogen and is contracted from an animal, usually a young cat or dog. *M canis* infections may or may not fluoresce. The more inflammatory lesions tend not to fluoresce.

The most important trichophyton organism in the USA is *T tonsurans.* Infection with *T tonsurans* may also occur in epidemics. The organism sporulates within the hair shaft (endothrix involvement) and does not fluoresce. The scalp lesions caused by *T tonsurans* do not tend to clear spontaneously at puberty, as is the case with microsporum infections.

Clinical Findings

A. Symptoms and Signs: Several children in one family or group may be involved. The lesions are generally asymptomatic. The areas of infection appear bald, but close inspection reveals that the hairs are broken off. This apparent alopecia is reversible. The involved areas are gray and scaly. Any area of hair loss in a child should be considered fungal until shown otherwise.

B. Laboratory Findings: The diagnosis is established by direct examination of an involved hair under the microscope in 20% potassium hydroxide solution. Fungi in the form of spores are seen inside or outside the hair shaft. Wood's light fluorescence is of value if the infection is caused by an organism that reacts. The hair fluoresces a brilliant green. Care must be exercised to exclude artifacts. When possible, select a hair that fluoresces for the direct examination and culture. Sabouraud's agar is the best general culture medium. Histologic study with special stains is rarely indicated.

Differential Diagnosis

Tinea capitis must be differentiated from alopecia areata, trichotillomania, localized neurodermatitis, monilethrix, seborrheic dermatitis, and psoriasis.

Complications

An acute inflammatory reaction, referred to as a kerion, may occur.

Treatment

Griseofulvin, preferably microcrystalline, 0.5 gm orally daily for 2–4 weeks, will cure most cases. Griseofulvin (not microcrystalline, ie, Fulvicin, Grifulvin), 3 gm orally in one dose, will often cure tinea capitis and can be used for irregular clinic attenders. Absence from school, skull caps, shaving of the scalp, shampooing, etc are unnecessary because of the effectiveness of oral antifungal treatment.

Prognosis

With griseofulvin, the prognosis is good. Wood's light should be used to evaluate the effectiveness of treatment. Relapses and reinfections should be treated with a second course of griseofulvin.

TINEA CORPORIS
(Body Ringworm)

Tinea corporis may be caused by any of the dermatophytes. It is more common in warm, humid areas, and more frequently involves children. The lesions may occur on any unhairy part of the body. Contact with animals is often associated with infection, and the incidence of tinea corporis is higher in rural areas. In temperate zones, the warmer months of the year produce more infections. In the USA, the 2 most frequent etiologic organisms are *Microsporum canis* and *Trichophyton mentagrophytes.*

Clinical Findings

A. Symptoms and Signs: A typical lesion begins as a reddish papule which then spreads peripherally. The lesion becomes annular, with an active margin. The advancing border is scaly and erythematous. Vesicles are occasionally present. The area tends to clear centrally. Secondary bacterial infection may occur. The amount of inflammation varies with the causative organism. Pruritus is often present.

B. Laboratory Findings: Examination by Wood's light is of no value. The diagnosis is established by microscopic examination of a scale taken from the active border. The scale is placed on a microscopic slide and a drop of 20% potassium hydroxide is placed over it. A cover slide is placed over the preparation,

and the slide is very gently heated over an alcohol lamp. Care must be exercised not to allow the preparation to boil. The microscopic identification of mycelia in the material is pathognomonic. Culture on Sabouraud's agar is a less effective method of diagnosis. The identification of species depends upon culture and microscopic examination of culture mounts. This is of value in that certain species, *T rubrum* and *M canis,* have occasionally developed resistance to griseofulvin.

Complications

The worst complication of tinea corporis is overtreatment. Secondary bacterial infection occurs occasionally. Allergic reactions (dermatophytid) occur rarely.

Differential Diagnosis

Tinea corporis must be distinguished from pityriasis rosea, pityriasis alba, nummular dermatitis, granuloma annulare, erythema multiforme, and seborrhea.

Prevention

Prevention consists of identification and treatment of infected animals and human contacts.

Treatment

Isolated lesions may be effectively treated with tolnaftate (Tinactin). Generalized involvement is best treated with oral griseofulvin, 1 gm daily orally for 4–6 weeks. The medication is most advantageously taken after meals. Microcrystalline griseofulvin is reportedly superior.

Prognosis

With adequate treatment, the prognosis is good. Organisms resistant to griseofulvin are occasionally encountered, and in these cases the prognosis is guarded.

TINEA CRURIS
(Ringworm of the Inguinal Area)

Tinea cruris consists of symmetrical, sharply demarcated inguinal lesions with active borders; central clearing is uncommon. Tinea cruris occurs most commonly in males and is encouraged by humidity, perspiration, obesity, and chafing. Tinea pedis is often present also. The most frequent causative organisms are *Trichophyton rubrum, T mentagrophytes,* and *Epidermophyton floccosum.*

Itching is usually severe. The lesions may also extend to involve the upper thighs. Involvement of the scrotum is rare (in contrast to candida infections). The active margins of the lesions are scaly and erythematous. Vesicles are sometimes found. The diagnosis is made by finding mycelia in scales taken from the active margins and examined microscopically in 20% potassium hydroxide. Species identification depends upon culture. Wood's light examination is of no value.

The treatment of choice is griseofulvin (Fulvicin, Grifulvin), 1 gm daily for 4–8 weeks depending upon the clinical response. Microcrystalline products are generally given in 1/2 the dosage of plain griseofulvin.

Tinea cruris is easy to overtreat topically, and overtreatment results in a weeping eczematous dermatitis. Topical treatment should be mild if used at all. Tolnaftate (Tinactin) or iodochlorhydroxyquin (Vioform) creams are suggested. Harsh ointments such as Whitfield's ointment used for tinea pedis are definitely to be avoided.

The prognosis is good. Retreatment is occasionally required.

TINEA PEDIS
(Athlete's Foot, Ringworm of the Hands & Soles)

Tinea pedis is very common among older boys. The organisms most frequently responsible are *Trichophyton rubrum* and *T mentagrophytes.* Perspiration and occlusive footwear are common predisposing factors.

In acute cases, vesicles are found predominantly in the instep area. These are tense and pruritic. Maceration, peeling, and fissures may be observed between the toes. In long-standing cases, hyperkeratosis and scaling may be noted. The lesions are almost always on the plantar aspect of the foot. Pruritus is frequently encountered.

Diagnosis depends upon microscopic examination and culture. Direct mount examination for fungus is performed by placing a scale on a microscopic slide. This is then covered with a drop of 20% potassium hydroxide and a cover slip is placed over it. The slide is then gently heated over an alcohol lamp. Care must be taken not to allow the preparation to boil. After heating, the cover slip should be gently pressed down firmly and the slide then examined under the microscope. It is essential that the light of the microscope be reduced in a manner similar to that for studying urinary sediment. The finding of mycelial elements is pathognomonic of mycotic infection.

Griseofulvin often fails to cure tinea pedis, but it should be tried for a period of 4 weeks in a dosage of 1 gm/day orally. Microcrystalline griseofulvin may be substituted in 1/2 the dosage for 4 weeks.

Topical therapy should be employed in combination with griseofulvin. Five percent sulfur added to Whitfield's ointment may be used twice a day for 4–6 weeks. Tolnaftate (Tinactin), twice a day for 4–6 weeks, can be used also.

Complications include secondary bacterial infection and a greater tendency of the feet to blister with trauma.

The prognosis is guarded. Relapses and reinfections are frequent.

TINEA UNGUIUM
(Ringworm of the Fingernails or Toenails)

Toenails are more often infected than fingernails, and in most cases some nails are not involved at all. Tinea unguium is more common than was previously believed. The most common cause is *Trichophyton rubrum.*

Dystrophy of a nail beginning laterally or at the free margin should be considered mycotic infection until proved otherwise. Both microscopic examination in 20% potassium hydroxide and culture are used for diagnosis. The nail should be sectioned into small pieces and left in the potassium hydroxide solution overnight. The cover glass may be sealed with petrolatum to prevent drying.

Treatment consists of griseofulvin (Fulvicin, Grifulvin), 1 gm orally daily for 4–6 months for fingernails and 12–18 months for toenails. Local measures may make the patient more comfortable. Sandpapering or filing of the nails is sometimes recommended. Surgical avulsion of the nails is seldom indicated.

The prognosis is good for fingernail infection but poor for toenail involvement. The treatment of tinea unguium is long-lasting and expensive.

CANDIDIASIS
(Moniliasis)

Essentials of Diagnosis
- Oral mucous membrane involvement (thrush).
- Diaper rash with satellite lesions.
- Potassium hydroxide examination and culture positive.

General Considerations
Candidiasis can occur at any age and involves both sexes equally. Several organisms are capable of causing clinical disease, but by far the most common is *Candida albicans.* The clinical disorders resulting from pathogenic candida infection constitute a wide spectrum. The infection is most often superficial; however, deep forms of infection do occur. The lesions may range in severity from simple thrush to fatal systemic dissemination involving the heart, lungs, gastrointestinal tract, genitourinary tract, brain, blood stream, etc. Systemic candidiasis generally affects persons with lowered resistance due to lymphomas, blood dyscrasias, corticosteroid or chemotherapeutic drug administration, and other factors. While *C albicans* can be cultured from the skin and mucous membranes of a significant number of the general population, any blood culture positive for *C albicans* indicates severe disease (eg, as might be found in candidal endocarditis following open heart surgery). Candidal granulomas

occur but are not common; they afflict only a few individuals with specific but undefined immunologic defects.

Candidiasis is often associated with one of many predisposing factors, including the following: (1) administration of antibiotics (particularly broad spectrum), systemic corticosteroids, or immunosuppressive agents; (2) lymphomas or blood dyscrasias; (3) diabetes mellitus; (4) vitamin deficiency states; (5) congenital ectodermal defects; (6) hypoparathyroidism; (7) acrodermatitis enteropathica; (8) obesity; (9) excessive environmental moisture; and (10) any severe debilitating disorder (burns, starvation, etc).

Clinical Findings

This discussion will be limited to candidal infections common in the pediatric age group. Oral mucous membrane candidiasis (thrush) is not uncommon among infants. The areas consist of white curd-like lesions on an inflamed mucous membrane. The lesion should be cultured on Sabouraud's glucose agar; within 48 hours, a creamy white mucoid colony with a yeast-like or beery odor appears on the culture plate. In many cases, the infection is transmitted from the mother via the birth canal. Isolation of cases in nurseries does not seem to be required because cross-infection is very slight.

Diaper dermatitis is frequently complicated by *C albicans* infection, and there may be a concurrent oral thrush. The lesions are erythematous and sharply marginated, with a scalloped border. A grayish sheen is often present over the surface of the area, and oozing may occur. The lesions are characteristically associated with satellite lesions: small (match-head size) islands of similar clinical appearance. Culture should be done.

Candidal paronychia is not common among children.

Differential Diagnosis

Candidiasis must be distinguished from seborrheic dermatitis in inguinal and axillary areas, simple intertrigo, and, in the oral cavity, stomatitis due to drugs.

Treatment

Thrush can be treated with topical nystatin (Mycostatin) or amphotericin B (Fungizone). Amphotericin B requires an occlusive dressing, and should be used only for nystatin-resistant strains. Gentian violet, 2% aqueous solution, may also be used. The authors have had success by having the child suck a nystatin vaginal suppository twice a day.

Cutaneous candidiasis responds to topical nystatin or amphotericin B applied 3 times a day. Dryness is essential. An excellent preparation for diaper area candidiasis is Mycolog Cream, which incorporates a topical corticosteroid (triamcinolone) and antibiotics (neomycin, gramicidin) with nystatin.

DEEP MYCOTIC INFECTIONS

Deep mycotic infections are uncommon in the pediatric age group. The infections that are occasionally encountered will be briefly described.

SPOROTRICHOSIS

Sporotrichum schenckii is found all over the world. Males are involved more frequently than females. The most common form is the localized lymphatic form. The fungus gains entry through the skin by direct inoculation. The first lesion may appear at any time from 20 days to 3 months later. The initial finding is a firm, nontender, freely movable nodule. This adheres to the skin, which becomes reddened. The area then breaks down to form the sporotrichotic chancre. After a few days, multiple nodules develop along the course of the draining lymphatic channels. Regional adenopathy may or may not be present. The child is generally afebrile.

The diagnosis is strongly suggested by the clinical picture. The best confirmation is by culture on Sabouraud's glucose agar. Biopsy is seldom helpful.

Potassium iodide is the treatment of choice. It is given as SSKI (saturated solution of potassium iodide) in water or milk. Start with 10 drops 3 times daily; then rapidly increase the dosage. The total dose may be increased 9 drops per day until 30–40 drops are given in each dose or until tolerance is reached. Treatment may have to be continued for 2–4 weeks before results begin to appear. It should be continued for 4 weeks after apparent recovery.

The prognosis is excellent for the lymphatic form treated with potassium iodide.

ACTINOMYCOSIS

A few scattered cases of actinomycosis are seen in children each year. *Actinomyces bovis* enters through the mucous membranes and is found commonly in the mouths of the general population. The infection, then, is endogenous. Cervicofacial actinomycosis is the most common form. Thoracic and abdominal forms also occur.

The infection most commonly involves the lower jaw. A history of recent dental work is often present. The area at the angle of the jaw swells, and the overlying skin becomes dusky red. A wooden hardness follows, and the surface is lumpy. Superficial sinus tracts may form. The general health of the patient is good, and pain is minimal. Regional adenopathy is absent. The organism may be demonstrated by direct biopsy examination or culture. Granules obtained from pus may demonstrate the so-called ray fungus of this disease. The organism cannot be grown on culture without specific media. Anaerobic conditions with and without 10% CO_2 are needed.

Penicillin is the drug of choice. The dosage varies from 1–5 million units/day for several months, depending upon the type and clinical severity.

The outlook for the cervicofacial form of actinomycosis is good.

Moses J: Actinomycosis in childhood. Historical review and case presentation. Clin Pediat 6:221–226, 1964.

Neavell UW Jr & others: Pathogenesis of cutaneous lesions of actinomycosis. South MJ 61:849–851, 1968.

COMMON CUTANEOUS VIRAL INFECTIONS

WARTS
(Verruca Vulgaris)

Warts are most common in children but can be encountered in any age group. They are multiple in 50% of cases. All warts, regardless of type, are thought to be caused by a similar virus. Minor trauma and moisture predispose to infection. Warts are contagious.

Warts are usually well circumscribed, gray or brown, elevated, firm papules with a rough surface. They can occur anywhere, and are referred to as plantar, palmar, periungual, etc according to their location. They may be flat (verruca plana) or filiform. Warts are asymptomatic unless they occur on a pressure area (eg, plantar warts). Warts tend to grow above the skin except on the plantar surface, where pressure tends to make them grow inward.

The many methods of wart treatment are difficult to evaluate because warts tend to disappear spontaneously. If only a few lesions are present, they can be removed surgically or with a caustic. The surgical procedure requires the use of a local anesthetic. The area is then removed by means of sharp curved iris scissors, and the base of the evacuated area is curetted with a small sharp skin curet. A sclerosing agent such as ferric subsulfate (Monsel's solution) can then be used for hemostasis. A second surgical method would be to locally anesthetize the wart and then fulgurate entire lesions with an electrofulguration unit. The lesions may then be removed with sharp scissors and curetted (as above) or may be left alone to slough spontaneously. A good method of treatment for pediatric patients is cryotherapy with liquid nitrogen. The wart itself is frozen firmly with liquid nitrogen, and then allowed to slough spontaneously. A blister generally appears within the first 24–48 hours, and within 2 weeks the process has completed itself. Warts fre-

quently respond to suggestion alone, which accounts for many cures. Extensive involvement and mosaic plantar warts are best treated by a dermatologist.

MOLLUSCUM CONTAGIOSUM

Molluscum contagiosum is a form of contagious wart. The lesion is caused by a specific virus. Multiple lesions are often present. Children are particularly susceptible, and auto-inoculation is a common mode of spread.

The lesions may occur anywhere but are more common on the hands, face, and genitalia. Lesions of the palms and soles are extremely rare. They start as pinhead-sized papules and usually enlarge to become hemispheric waxy papules 1–3 mm in diameter with a central depression. The lesion contains a curdlike substance composed of keratin and epithelial cells. Occasionally, the lesions become impetigonized.

Surgical expression of the molluscum body contained within the papules is the best treatment. A curet can be used for this purpose. Ethyl chloride is a good anesthetic. Multiple lesions can be treated with caustics such as phenol or podophyllum resin. Freezing with liquid nitrogen is also an effective method of treatment.

HERPES SIMPLEX

Herpes simplex virus is capable of producing a wide spectrum of clinical disease ranging from simple recurrent fever blisters to primary systemic generalized disease and death. Once a person is infected with the virus, a carrier state persists for life. Over 90% of people are infected before the age of 5 years, but less than 2% develop significant primary clinical disease.

Clinical Findings

A. Gingivostomatitis: Gingivostomatitis occurs mostly in children. The onset is sudden. Widespread vesicular ulcerative lesions may occur anywhere in the mouth, and inflammation may be striking. There is regional adenopathy, pain, tenderness, and high fever. The condition lasts 1–2 weeks.

B. Vulvovaginitis: Vulvovaginitis is equally violent and produces a similar clinical picture. Diagnosis can be made by viral culture or by inoculation of vesicle fluid onto the scarified cornea of a rabbit. The latter leads to keratitis.

C. Primary Inoculation Herpes Simplex: This form of the infection may also cause severe systemic findings. Young adults (often nurses or medical personnel) are frequently involved. The localized cutaneous lesions are vesicles which convert to hemorrhagic bullae. Severe pain and constitutional symptoms are often present.

D. Kaposi's Varicelliform Eruption: Patients with atopic dermatitis may develop generalized, widespread vesicular lesions of herpes simplex.

E. Recurrent Infection: Recurrent herpes simplex infection occurs most often on the lips and is seen as grouped vesicles. The vesicles rupture and crust over in a day or so and persist for 1–2 weeks. There may be regional lymphadenopathy. Occasionally the eruption is preceded for a day or so by tingling or pain. Such lesions can occur anywhere but are most common on the lips, nose, genitals, and buttocks. They can be precipitated by fever, sunlight, menses, anxiety, or other factors. In general, herpetic lesions heal without scarring.

Differential Diagnosis

Herpes simplex must be differentiated from impetigo, varicella and variola (in disseminated cases), lymphogranuloma venereum, and primary syphilis (in herpes progenitalis).

Prevention

Recurrent herpes simplex may be prevented by avoiding predisposing factors to the extent possible. An example is the use of a sun screen for herpes simplex induced by UVL. Occasionally, a series of vaccinations may be helpful, but the mechanism of defense is not known and it may be simple suggestion. Such a series of vaccinations would employ the use of polyvalent influenza vaccine, 0.1 ml intradermally at weekly intervals for 6–8 injections. About 2 out of 3 people so treated will be benefited.

Treatment

Corticosteroids should be avoided because they make the condition worse. Topical corticosteroids should not be applied to the eye infected with herpes simplex. Ointments should never be used because they favor secondary bacterial infection and spread. Dryness is essential, and a lotion should be used. Absolute alcohol applied frequently will help to dry the vesicles and prevent secondary bacterial infection.

Wheeler CE, Huffines WD: Primary herpes simplex of the newborn. JAMA 191:455, 1965.

HERPES ZOSTER
(Shingles)

Herpes zoster is caused by the same virus that causes varicella. Herpes zoster actually represents a localized recurrent varicella in a patient with partial immunity to varicella. Underlying lymphoma may rarely be found in any patient with herpes zoster.

Neuralgic pain often precedes the eruption. The vesicles are grouped, 2–4 mm in diameter, and appear on an erythematous base. The lesions follow the course of a nerve from the posterior ganglia (dermatome distribution). The vesicles are unilateral and do not cross the midline. After a few days, they become encrusted. Necrosis or gangrene occasionally occurs. Postherpetic neuralgia is rare in children. The most common site of involvement is over the thorax, but the lesions may be found anywhere (including the distribution of the cranial nerves).

Rule out underlying disease or immunosuppressive drugs as contributing factors.

Dryness is essential, and ointments should not be used. A lotion consisting of 3 parts 70% alcohol and 1 part flurandrenolone lotion (Cordran) is beneficial; apply on compresses for 1/2 hour 4 times a day. Gamma globulin, 10 ml IM, followed by 5 ml IM 48 hours later and repeated if needed, may be beneficial.

INFESTATIONS & INSECT BITES

PEDICULOSIS
(Louse Infestation)

Pediculosis is more common in conditions of overcrowding, usually in poorer socioeconomic areas. Lice are transmitted by close personal contact or common use of hats, combs, and toilet seats. The louse is an important vector of typhus fever, relapsing fever, and trench fever. The head louse (*Pediculus humanus capitis*) and the pubic louse (*Phthirus pubis*) are parasitic for man. The body louse (*Pediculus humanus corporis*) only comes out of the clothing to feed from the skin.

Pruritus, excoriation, and secondary infection are common to all forms of pediculosis. Pruritus may be more intense in a warm atmosphere. The scalp frequently becomes pustular or impetigonized. In body louse infestation, the trunk becomes markedly excoriated, but there is little evidence of insect bites. Pubic louse nits on hair shafts and in the pubic area are usually easily demonstrated. In infants, the pubic louse may infest eyebrows and eyelashes. Clinical identification of lice or nits establishes the diagnosis.

Pediculosis must be differentiated from papular urticaria, scabies, and pyoderma.

Eczematous dermatitis may occur as a complication of overtreatment of pediculosis.

Pediculosis capitis may be treated effectively with any of the following (applied once daily for 3 days): gamma benzene hexachloride (Kwell, Gexane), benzyl benzoate, or crotamiton (Eurax). Pediculosis corporis is treated with any of the above plus dusting of affected clothing with 10% chlorophenothane (DDT) powder. All affected members of a family must be treated to prevent reinfestation. In infants, pediculosis of eyelashes and eyebrows demands careful manual removal of nits and adult forms.

The prognosis is excellent.

SCABIES

Sarcoptes scabiei infestation was common 2 decades ago but is now rarely seen in the USA. It is still common in other parts of the world. It is characterized by nocturnal pruritus and vesicular or pustular lesions in "burrows" about the wrists and finger webs and the heels of the palms. In addition to the hands and wrists, scabies is commonly found in the axillary folds and on the buttocks, genitalia, elbows, and nipples in females. Pyoderma is a frequent complication. If there is doubt regarding clinical diagnosis, microscopic identification of mites or ova will establish the diagnosis.

Secondary infection should be treated by application of topical antibiotics. This can be followed by any of the following, applied once daily after a bath or shower for 3 days: gamma benzene hexachloride (Kwell, Gexane) lotion or ointment, crotamiton (Eurax) cream or lotion, or benzyl benzoate (25% emulsion). Retreatment is seldom necessary, and overtreatment should be avoided. All contacts and family members must be treated also.

The prognosis is excellent.

CUTANEOUS LARVA MIGRANS
(Creeping Eruption)

Larva migrans is caused by the larvae of helminths, particularly *Ancylostoma braziliense.* It is common in southeast USA and may be carried to other areas by moving families with infected cats and dogs. The organisms are found on lawns and in sand contaminated by excreta from infected animals. Cutaneous entry follows direct contact, usually with the soles of the feet and the hands. The larvae invade the skin, burrow, and migrate, leaving an elevated, erythematous serpentine lesion of bizarre pattern. The course of migration can usually be easily traced. The patient may complain of itching or burning.

Until recently, treatment was far from satisfactory. The use of thiabendazole (Mintezol) has been found to be effective.

Katz R, Ziegler J, Blank H: The natural course of creeping eruption and treatment with thiabendazole. Arch Dermat 91:420–424, 1965.

TICKS

Aside from transmitting rickettsial disease (Rocky Mountain spotted fever) and viral diseases (Colorado tick fever), tick bites are of little importance. In rare cases, hypersensitization to tick bites results in fever and transient paralysis. These are managed by removal of the tick and administration of antihistamines or corticosteroids (or both). Ticks retain infectious microorganisms within their biting parts and inoculate man when feeding on the skin.

Removal is best accomplished by mechanical means.

MYIASIS

This infestation is always disturbing when noted in wounds, ulcers, and sores. It consists of the deposition of eggs by flies—especially botflies and warble flies—which hatch to larvae. The disease is most common in areas of poor hygiene. Foreign body reactions and delayed healing ensue.

Treatment consists of mechanical removal and thorough lavage.

CHIGGERS
(Red Bugs)

Chiggers are larvae of trombiculid mites that infest grasses and weeds in southern and southeastern USA and other geographic areas of the world. These mites attack man on the legs and around the waist and produce extreme pruritic papules with central "red dots." Prevention consists of wearing tight-fitting clothing in infested areas. Insect repellents offer some protection.

Treatment is symptomatic, and the following may give relief: antipruritic lotions, lidocaine (Xylocaine) spray or lotion, and spraying individual lesions with ethyl chloride or Frigiderm (25% ethyl chloride and 75% Freon).

CIMICOSIS
(Bedbugs)

Cimicosis is a papular or urticarial reaction caused by the common bedbug, *Cimex lectularius.* The bites tend to occur on exposed or accessible parts of the body and are grouped in rows of 2 or 3. Bedbugs may be attracted to one individual in preference to others, so that both persons in the same bed are not necessarily affected. Bedbugs also tend to have a disagreeable odor that is much more evident to some persons than others.

Treatment is symptomatic. Prevention consists of DDT spraying of beds and bedding. Used rugs and recently purchased upholstered furniture are common sources of infestation.

PULICOSIS
(Flea Bites)

The most common flea that attacks humans is *Pulex irritans.* Cat and dog fleas may also bite humans. The bites are urticarial and sometimes hemorrhagic. Insect repellents are of limited value. DDT is preventive. Treatment is symptomatic.

PAPULAR URTICARIA

Some children develop a widespread urticarial reaction of a papular type as a result of hypersensitivity to insect bites or insect products. The reaction may be related to atopy, and affected children are frequently of atopic habitus. The lesions are excoriated and sometimes topped with vesicles. Old atrophic scarring from prior episodes is present. In geographic areas where insects (particularly mosquitoes, fleas, chiggers, and bedbugs) are seasonal, the condition may also be seasonal. The child apparently becomes sensitized in this atopic fashion.

Antihistamines should be given systemically and insect repellents topically. Crotamiton (Eurax) is especially useful for this purpose because it is an antipruritic as well as an insecticide. Treatment of the environment with DDT is indicated, and a thorough search for insects is necessary.

COMMON SKIN DISORDERS OF UNKNOWN ETIOLOGY

PSORIASIS

Psoriasis is thought to be an inherited (autosomal dominant) disorder. The family history is positive in 1/3 of cases. It is not common in the pediatric age group but does occur. Acute eruptions are occasionally precipitated by drugs, most often sulfonamides and antimalarials, and infections, most often streptococcal. In children with guttate psoriasis, the antistreptolysin O titer should be determined and throat culture should be done. If culture is positive, appropriate antibiotic therapy must be given.

Association of psoriasis with arthritis is rare in children.

Clinical Findings

The lesions of psoriasis are often rounded or circumscribed. Occasionally lesions are very small and isolated and are then given the term guttate (drop-

like). These early guttate lesions often look like drops of wax on the skin. The larger plaques are erythematous and may have dry, gray to silver scaling. The most common areas of involvement are the scalp, elbows, and knees, although any site may be affected. (Mucous membrane involvement is rare.) Pitting of the fingernails is a typical psoriatic lesion. Children often develop initial lesions in one of 3 ways: cephalic lesions in the scalp, guttate lesions, or (less often) lesions appearing in a follicular pattern. A common but not pathognomonic finding is the isomorphic response (Koebner phenomenon), ie, the development of psoriatic lesions at the site of trauma due to surgical incisions, burns, UVL, scratches, etc.

Differential Diagnosis

Psoriasis must be differentiated from seborrheic dermatitis (when limited to the scalp or genitocrural area), secondary syphilis, parapsoriasis, drug eruptions (especially due to sulfonamides), localized neurodermatitis, and onychomycosis (when the nails are involved).

Treatment

Local lesions are best treated with topical corticosteroids under occlusive dressings. Systemic corticosteroids should not be used. Occlusive dressings should be applied at bedtime and removed in the morning. Widespread lesions can be treated with coal tar solution, 10%, and salicylic acid, 3%, in hydrophilic ointment applied twice daily. The addition of 5% ammoniated mercury is beneficial if the patient is not sensitive to mercury. (Before adding mercury to the ointment, a mercury patch test should be done.) The antifolic acid drugs (eg, methotrexate) are of value in the treatment of severe psoriasis, but they must be used with caution and only by physicians experienced with their administration and effects.

Prognosis

The prognosis for psoriasis acquired in the early years of life is guarded. As a general rule, the younger the individual at the time of onset of psoriasis, the more grave the prognosis for continued future involvement.

Baer RL, Witten VH: Psoriasis: A discussion of selected aspects. In: *Yearbook of Dermatology.* Year Book, 1961–62.

Farher EM, Harris DR: Hospital treatment of psoriasis. Arch Dermat 101:381, 1970.

SEBORRHEIC DERMATITIS

Seborrheic dermatitis consists of erythematous lesions with yellowish scales or crusts, often beginning on the scalp and spreading to the central face and central chest. The cause is not known. Increased oiliness of the skin is frequently noted. Seborrheic dermatitis can cause a widespread eczematous eruption in infants. Cradle cap is a form of seborrheic dermatitis, as is dandruff in older children. The lesions may spread to involve the eyebrows, nasolabial folds, the skin around the mouth, the axillas, the umbilical area, and the inguinal area. The eruption may become generalized. Pruritus is occasionally present. The use of antiseborrheic shampoos (eg, Selsun) or coal tar (eg, Sebutone) is essential. An ointment containing 1% salicylic acid, 3% sulfur, and 1% hydrocortisone in a water-miscible base is effective. The ointment should be rubbed in well 3 times a day. All oils, creams, and ointments should be withheld.

Seborrheic dermatitis tends to be a recurring problem, and it is not uncommon for patients to have long and chronic courses.

PITYRIASIS ROSEA

Pityriasis rosea is a papulosquamous eruption which is suspected of being a microbial infection of very low contagiousness. Most cases occur in the spring and fall. The initial lesion is a salmon-colored macule ("herald patch") with peripheral scaling. The herald patch may be confused with tinea corporis. Several days later, a widespread shower of oval, salmon pink macular lesions appears over the trunk. They may reach 1–2 cm in diameter. The long axis of the lesion follows lines of cleavage. Less often, lesions occur on the arms and legs (inverse pityriasis rosea). Face lesions are rare. Mild constitutional symptoms are occasionally present at the onset of the eruption, and pruritus may be present. The eruption clears spontaneously in about 6–8 weeks. Second attacks are rare, and involvement of more than one member of a family is rare.

For pruritic lesions, an effective topical preparation is menthol, 0.25%, in equal parts of olive oil and lime water. Bathing should be minimized to lessen the chance of eczematization. UVL is beneficial for widespread involvement but is seldom necessary. If a patient is extremely uncomfortable or has rapidly spreading generalized involvement, gamma globulin may be given, though treatment with gamma globulin is expensive and not always effective. The dosage for older children is 10 ml initially and then 5 ml after 48 hours. Occasionally, a third injection of 5 ml is needed.

PITYRIASIS ALBA

The characteristic lesion of this disorder is a rounded area of hypopigmentation which is more apparent when the skin is tan. Pityriasis alba occurs only in children and teenagers and may be associated with the atopic state. The cause is not known. The lesions are small (a few centimeters in diameter), white or pink, with slight scales. The most common areas of involvement are the face, arms, neck, and shoulders. There may be slight pruritus, but the lesions are usually asymptomatic.

Treatment is not usually required, although erythematous or symptomatic lesions may be treated with topical corticosteroid creams.

Pityriasis alba clears spontaneously, usually before or during puberty.

DYSHIDROSIS

Dyshidrosis, or dyshidrotic eczema, is a poorly understood disorder of unknown cause. It is often seen in atopic children and frequently misdiagnosed as ringworm. It is one of the more common causes of eczema in children, and in many cases the lesions are associated with increased perspiration. The hands and feet are the primary sites of involvement. General spread can but usually does not occur. The lesions begin as pruritic clear vesicles, often on the sides of the fingers or just under the skin of the palms or soles. There is little inflammation, and the vesicles can coalesce to form so-called frog-spawn vesicles. The vesicles rupture, and a scaling, keratolytic eczema results. These areas may become secondarily infected and weep. Direct microscopic examination of scales in 20% potassium hydroxide must be done to rule out tinea. Dyshidrosis is far more common than tinea.

Dryness is essential, and swimming and bathing must be limited. Palmar and plantar perspiration is increased by emotion, and steps to reduce anxiety and tension may be required. Mild sedation with barbiturates or tranquilizers is helpful. The use of topical corticosteroids is mandatory. Some patients definitely benefit from the use of topical corticosteroids under occlusive plastic gloves or dressings. Systemic corticosteroids are reserved for the most severe cases. Antibiotics are employed for secondary infection only. Occasionally, anticholinergic drugs are used to decrease perspiration. In general, the side-effects of the anticholinergic drugs limit their usefulness.

ACNE VULGARIS

Essentials of Diagnosis
- Grade 1: Comedones and papules.
- Grade 2: Comedones, papules, and pustules.
- Grade 3: Comedones, papules, pustules, and cysts.
- Grade 4: Grade 3 plus abscesses and communicating sinus tracts.

General Considerations

Acne is the most common of all skin conditions. It usually becomes manifest at puberty but may begin during the third or fourth decade of life. It does not always clear spontaneously at the end of adolescence but may persist well into adulthood. The exact mechanism is not known, but acne is related to overproduction of oil from the sebaceous glands, which are under hormonal control (predominantly androgenic). Genetic predisposition is an important factor in the development of acne.

Clinical Findings

The face is the most common site of involvement. The neck, upper back, and chest are frequently involved also. The scalp must be carefully inspected for seborrheic dermatitis or excessive oiliness. The lesions are generally asymptomatic, but inflamed areas may be tender. Scarring, when present, may be mild to severe. Neurotic excoriations are occasionally observed. These result from obsessive manipulation of the lesions by the patient.

Differential Diagnosis

Acne vulgaris must be differentiated from acneiform drug reactions (iodides, bromides), corticosteroid-induced acne, contact reaction to chlorinated hydrocarbons (electric wiring, etc), and secondary syphilis.

Complications

Cystic abscess formation occurs frequently. Scarring secondary to active lesions may be deep and disfiguring. Post-acne keloids are sometimes observed. The most severe complication is the psychologic crippling caused by the poor cosmetic appearance.

Treatment

A. General Measures: A well balanced diet and sufficient rest are necessary for successful treatment. Ask the patient to stop using all types of oil and grease on the skin and to avoid using hair lotions and creams, cold creams, hand lotions, petrolatum, lip ice, hair spray, and aerosols. Drugs or foods that contain significant amounts of iodides or bromides should be withheld.

The exact role of diet in acne is poorly understood. Patients should be suspicious of chocolate, nuts, and cola drinks; if these foods consistently aggravate acne, they should be avoided. The diet should be low in dairy products (whole milk, butter, cheese, ice cream).

B. Local Measures:

1. Grade 1 acne—Treat with dryness and keratolytics. Washing with lava or an abrasive soap (Brasivol, Pernox) once a day is beneficial. An antiseborrheic shampoo should be prescribed where indicated. Keratolytic lotions or pastes should be started in weak strengths and increased as tolerated. Pigmented preparations are available when a cover-up medication is desired. The mechanical removal of comedones by the doctor is suggested.

2. Grade 2 acne—Less harsh keratolytic measures should be used because of the more erythematous nature of grade 2 acne. One of the tetracyclines, 250 mg/day, or sulfadimethoxine (Madribon), 500 mg/day, is helpful. Pustular acne responds well to topical sulfur preparations such as Pronac.

3. Grade 3 acne—Treat as for grade 2 acne. In addition, cysts may be injected with 0.1 ml of hydrocortisone (Neo-Cortef) or comparable intralesional steroid.

4. Grade 4 acne—Often causes psychologic problems. A specialist should be consulted about the use of systemic corticosteroids.

C. Other Methods of Treatment: The use of vitamins in acne has been disappointing. X-ray, cryotherapy with dry ice, and cold quartz UVL are occasionally used. The most recent advances in therapy include systemic cyclic hormones, such as mestranol, and the topical use of benzoyl peroxide preparations (Vanoxide, Benoxyl).

Andrews GC: Acne. Arch Dermat 84:711, 1961.

Goltz RW, Kjartarsson S: Oral tetracycline treatment of bacterial flora in acne vulgaris. Arch Dermat 93:92, 1966.

Lowney ED: Management of acne vulgaris. GP 38:101–106, 1968.

Noojin RO: How I treat acne vulgaris. Postgrad MJ 41:A95–96, 1967.

Reisner RM: Rational therapy of acne vulgaris. Cutis 7:175, 1971.

UNCOMMON SKIN DISORDERS OF UNKNOWN ETIOLOGY

DERMATITIS HERPETIFORMIS

Dermatitis herpetiformis is unusual in childhood, and the clinical manifestations may differ from those observed in the adult form of the disease. In adults, the reaction is characterized by grouped papulovesicular lesions, especially on the extensors of the extremities, scalp, scapular areas, and sacrum; intense pruritus with extreme excoriation and subsequent scarring; and a protracted course. In the child, pruritus and chronicity are common, but the lesion may be pustular or bullous and the distribution may lack conformity.

The cutaneous lesions may show a predominance of eosinophils, and there may be eosinophilia in the differential white count.

Treatment is suppressive and not curative and usually consists of giving sulfapyridine, 0.25–1 gm orally daily; or one of the sulfones, eg, sulfoxone (Diasone), under specialized consultation.

LICHEN PLANUS

The primary lesion of lichen planus is a discrete, polygonal, flat, red to violaceous, shiny patch usually found on the flexural surfaces of the wrists and ankles. Pruritus is usually marked. Generalized involvement occasionally occurs. A white reticulated lesion may appear on the buccal mucous membranes, tongue, or lips.

Treatment is with topical corticosteroids and antipruritics, sedatives or tranquilizers such as phenobarbital or hydroxyzine, and, in severe cases, systemic corticosteroids.

The acute episodes can usually be controlled but recurrences are common.

Irgang S: Lichen planus. Cutis 6:887, 1970.

PARAPSORIASIS

Parapsoriasis is a group of poorly understood disorders. The most frequent example in childhood is pityriasis lichenoides varioliformis (Habermann's disease).

This reaction consists of an acute onset of crops of papulovesicular lesions. The initial reaction may suggest varicella, and the lesions may be deep enough to produce scarring (varioliformis). The eruption may be generalized, but otherwise the child is not ill. The cause is not known, although this disease may be considered a form of superficial "toxic arteritis." Instances of mild epidemics have been reported.

Treatment is principally symptomatic, with topical antipruritics and short, intensive courses of corticosteroids. Antimalarial drugs—eg, hydroxychloroquine (Plaquenil), chloroquine (Aralen)—have been helpful when given for periods of 3 weeks.

The reaction may be self-limited over a period of 4–8 weeks. Other forms of parapsoriasis may suggest atypical psoriasis, pityriasis rosea, nummular dermatitis, and other papulosquamous disorders.

PEMPHIGUS

Pemphigus is mentioned only because it sometimes enters into the differential diagnosis of erythema multiforme, bullous drug eruptions (iodides, sulfonamides), or bullous impetigo. It is extremely rare in childhood, and most clinicians have never seen a case in children.

FAMILIAL BENIGN CHRONIC PEMPHIGUS
(Hailey-Hailey Disease)

Hailey-Hailey disease is an inherited skin disorder manifested initially as small vesicles that gradually enlarge to form ruptured encrusted areas that heal without scarring. It involves the areas about the neck and axillas and the anogenital area.

Treatment is unsatisfactory. Some patients respond to antibiotics. Topical corticosteroids—especially flurandrenolone (Cordran) and fluocinolone (Synalar)—under occlusive dressings have been helpful. The course is benign.

ACANTHOSIS NIGRICANS

Acanthosis nigricans is characterized by the development of hyperpigmented papillomatous and verruciform lesions. It is most often seen in the axillas and axillary folds, but the gluteal cleft and inguinal folds may be involved also. In adults, this condition is associated with occult or obvious malignancy, usually in the gastrointestinal tract, ovaries, or lungs. In children, this is not true. In the child, the so-called true form of acanthosis may occur in the absence of malignancy. A "pseudoacanthosis nigricans" seen in obese children is characterized by darkening and thickening of the skin, particularly on the nape of the neck and in the axillary areas.

There is no effective treatment.

Curth JO: Significance of acanthosis nigricans. Arch Dermat 66:80, 1952.
Curth JO, Aschner BM: Genetic studies on acanthosis nigricans. Arch Dermat 79:55, 1959.
Szymanski FJ: Pityriasis lichenoides et varioliformis acuta. Arch Dermat 79:7, 1959.

URTICARIA PIGMENTOSA
(Mast Cell Disease)

The cause of urticaria pigmentosa is not known. About 40–50% of patients have an atopic family history of asthma or hay fever. Urticaria pigmentosa may be divided into 3 groups: (1) solitary lesions (mastocytoma), (2) multiple lesions in early childhood, and (3) multiple lesions in adults. Group 3 may be associated with internal involvement, which is not generally the case in either form of pediatric urticaria pigmentosa.

Solitary lesions (group 1) vary in diameter from several millimeters up to 6 cm (or larger) and may be yellow, tan, brown, red, or varying degrees of these colors. In most cases, the lesions are present at birth or appear shortly thereafter. Vesiculation is to be expected, and persists for about 1 year. Urtication upon rubbing the lesion generally occurs (Darier's sign).

Group 2 (multiple) lesions may be macular or maculopapular and are yellow, tan, brown, or red. The distribution is central; the palms, soles, and head are usually spared. In 80% of cases, the onset is within the first 6 months of life. The size of individual lesions varies from a few millimeters to several centimeters. Vesiculation occurs in a significant number of cases and generally clears in about 2 years. Generalized flushing may occur but is not common. Urtication as a result of mild trauma (Darier's sign) is frequently present. More than half of patients experience some degree of pruritus. Lesions should be stained and examined microscopically for increased tissue mast cells. When a lesion is suspected of being urticaria pigmentosa, it is essential that the surgical specimen be fixed in alcohol rather than formaldehyde to preserve the staining properties of the mast cells.

Pruritus can often be controlled by systemic antihistamines, but this does not shorten the course of the disease. Spontaneous clearing occurs in about 50% of cases by adolescence; in the remainder, asymptomatic macular lesions persist. The use of drugs that may cause histamine release should be avoided. The common ones include aspirin, codeine (particularly in cough syrups), and opiates for diarrhea. Solitary lesions should be surgically excised only if particularly symptomatic. Before undertaking surgery, one may try intralesional injection of corticosteroids to control symptoms.

In pediatric cases, the outlook is very good.

Caplan RM: Urticaria pigmentosa and systemic mastocytosis. JAMA 194:1077, 1965.

Orkin M & others: Bullous mastocytosis. Arch Dermat 101:547, 1970.

● ● ●

General References

Andrews GC, Domonkos AN: *Diseases of the Skin,* 5th ed. Saunders, 1963.

Butterworth T, Strean LP: *Clinical Genodermatology.* Williams & Wilkins, 1962.

Hildick-Smith G, Blank H, Sarkany I: *Fungus Diseases and Their Treatment.* Little, Brown, 1964.

Lewis GM, Wheeler CE: *Practical Dermatology,* 3rd ed. Saunders, 1967.

Pillsbury DM, Shelley WB, Kligman AM: *Dermatology.* Saunders, 1956.

Rook A, Wilkinson DS, Ebling FJG: *Textbook of Dermatology.* Davis, 1968.

9 . . .
Eye

Philip P. Ellis, MD

GENERAL PRINCIPLES OF DIAGNOSIS

A careful history is essential in establishing an accurate diagnosis of an ocular disorder. The history should include time and rate of onset of the presenting symptoms, associated symptoms, past history of eye disorders and treatment, and pertinent family and social history. However, many eye problems, such as poor vision in one eye, are asymptomatic and are discovered only on testing of visual acuity or other objective diagnostic methods.

COMMON NONSPECIFIC SYMPTOMS & SIGNS

Tearing
In infants, tearing is usually due to nasolacrimal duct obstruction. Tearing may also be associated with local inflammatory and allergic and viral diseases, and with glaucoma.

Discharge
Purulent discharge is usually associated with bacterial infections. Mucoid discharge is usually associated with chemical irritations, some viral infections, or allergic conditions; it may be secondary to obstructions of the nasolacrimal duct.

Pain
Pain in or about the eye may be due to foreign bodies in the cornea or conjunctiva, corneal abrasions, acute infections of the lid, orbital cellulitis, acute dacryocystitis, acute iritis, or glaucoma. Refractive errors seldom produce headaches in young children. Large refractive errors or poor convergence may produce headaches in older children, particularly those who read a good deal.

Poor Vision
In infants poor vision is usually due to a serious ophthalmologic or neurologic disorder such as congenital nystagmus, corneal or lenticular opacities, dis-orders of the retina, optic nerve and CNS abnormalities, or very high myopia. In older children, the development of poor vision is often associated with refractive errors.

The approximate visual acuity of a 1-year-old child is 20/100; a 2-year-old has approximately 20/60 vision. By age 4–5 years, a visual acuity of about 20/20 has developed.

Leukocoria
A white spot in the pupil is a serious finding which may be due to congenital cataract, retrolental fibroplasia, retinal dysplasia, intraocular infection, retinoblastoma, or persistence and hyperplasia of primary vitreous.

EXAMINATION

Visual Acuity
Routine testing of visual acuity should be a part of every general physical examination. It is the single most important test of visual function. In children 4 years old or older, satisfactory visual acuity tests can usually be obtained with the use of Snellen test cards or illiterate E charts. In using the latter, the child is asked to point in the direction of the "feet" of the figure E. Because of distractions in the office, children are sometimes unable to perform this test adequately; special illiterate E cards may be sent home so that the parents can test the vision at home under better circumstances. The mother, with her interest, can repeat the test at her leisure, and the final result is usually more accurate than testing done in the office by the pediatrician or his nurse.

Visual acuity is difficult to evaluate in infants. One can observe whether an infant will follow a light or a bright attractive object in different directions of gaze. Each eye is tested separately. If the infant fails to respond to such testing, one can observe the pupillary responses for reaction to direct light stimulus, which depend upon a functioning retina and optic nerve. However, cortical blindness can exist with preservation of pupillary light reflexes. Optokinetic nystagmus (slow pursuit movements in the direction of a moving stimulus and quick saccadic movements in the reverse direction; "railway nystagmus") indicates that there

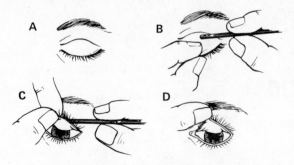

FIG 9–1. Eversion of the upper lid. A. The patient looks downward. **B.** The fingers pull the lid down and a rod is placed on the upper tarsal border. **C.** The lid is pulled up over the rod. **D.** The lid is everted. (Redrawn and reproduced, with permission, from Liebman SD, Gellis DD [editors]: *The Pediatrician's Ophthalmology.* Mosby, 1966.)

are functioning neural receptors in the retina and intact neural pathways. Threat reflexes, such as swiftly bringing an object in the direction of the patient's eyes and observing whether he blinks, are sometimes used to determine if there is a gross deficiency in visual acuity. The difficulty with this test is eliminating the rush of air that can produce corneal sensation and a reflex blink.

Poor visual acuity due to refractive errors in older children can be differentiated from poor vision due to other diseases by a pinhole test. If the reduced visual acuity is due to a refractive error, placement of a pinhole before this eye in line with the pupil will result in improved vision.

External Examination

External examination should include general inspection of the lids and eyeballs, noting their prominence, size, and position as well as any growths, inflammations, discharge, or vascular injection. Forward protrusion (exophthalmos) or retraction (enophthalmos) of the globe should be noted. Unusual size of the globes as indicated by megalocornea or microphthalmos should be noted. The positions of the lids in relation to the globe and the coverage of the lids over the closed eyes should be observed. Normally, with the eyes open, the lower lid margin is at the lower border of the cornea in the forward position of gaze, and the upper lid should cover approximately 2 mm of the cornea. Any drooping of the upper lid (ptosis) or retraction of the eyelids should be noted. The lid margins should be inspected to see if they are against the globes in proper alignment, or whether there is ectropion (turning outward of the lid margins) or entropion (turning inward). The distribution of the lashes and their position should be studied. The lid margins should be inspected for inflammation, crusting, and patency of the lacrimal puncta. If a conjunctival foreign body is suspected, the lids should be everted and the palpebral as well as the bulbar conjunctivas

inspected. The upper lid may be everted by pulling the lid forward (grasping the lashes), placing a small applicator behind the tarsal area, and gently pressing down on the lid (Fig 9–1). The maneuver is facilitated if the patient looks downward. If a corneal abrasion or foreign body is suspected or if there is sudden unexplained pain in the eye, sterile fluorescein solution should be instilled into the conjunctival cul-de-sac and the cornea observed to see if there is any staining. Pupillary light reflexes should be tested for each eye, and both direct and consensual reflexes noted.

Corneal sensitivity may be tested by touching the cornea gently with a fine wisp of cotton. If corneal sensation is intact, a brisk blink reflex will result.

Extraocular Muscles

The position of the eyes should be observed by inspection. As a rule there is little difficulty in telling whether gross strabismus is present. A quick estimation of the alignment of the eyes can be made by the corneal light reflection technic (Hirschberg test). The light reflection should come from corresponding parts of each cornea when a light is shone into the eyes. If there is lateral displacement of the light reflection, esotropia (internal deviation) of the eye is present (Fig 9–2). If the light reflection is displaced nasally, exotropia (outward deviation) is present. A more refined method of judging alignment of the eyes is by means of the cover test. In this test the patient is instructed to look at an object and one eye is then covered. If the uncovered eye has been looking straight forward at the object, there will be no shift in movement of this eye. If, however, the eye has been turned either inward or outward, then a corresponding corrective movement will be made with this eye to align the object in the visual gaze (Fig 9–3). The other eye is then similarly tested. The eye under cover should also be observed to see whether there is inward or outward movement, indicating the presence of a phoria, or a tendency for ocular deviation. If the eye remains in the deviated position after removing the occluder, a tropia (deviation of the eyes not corrected by the fusion mechanism) rather than a phoria (deviation that is corrected by the fusion mechanism) is present.

The cardinal positions of gaze should be checked. An attractive object or light is shown to the infant, and his ability to follow the movement of the object in

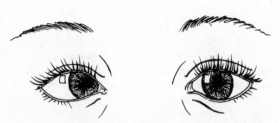

FIG 9–2. Lateral displacement of light reflection showing esotropia (internal deviation) of the left eye. Nasal displacement of the reflection would show exotropia (outward deviation).

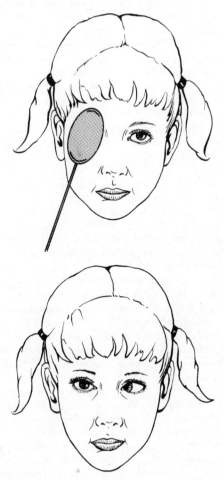

FIG 9–3. Cover test. If the child with an amblyopic eye will fix only when the good eye is covered but does not hold fixation when the cover is removed, vision of the poor eye is usually from 20/100–20/50. (Redrawn and reproduced, with permission, from Havener WH: *Synopsis of Ophthalmology,* 2nd ed. Mosby, 1963.)

different visual directions is tested. If marked strabismus or muscle paralysis is present, there may be limitation of movement in one direction of gaze. To determine whether true paresis of an extraocular muscle is present, the nondeviating eye should be covered ·and the ocular movement of the uncovered eye tested in all directions of gaze.

Nystagmus

If nystagmus is present, its characteristics should be observed and the movements classified, first by rate or variation in rate of movement and then by direction. **Pendular (undulatory) nystagmus** consists of excursions that are equal in each direction of gaze; this type of nystagmus is usually observed in children with poor vision and is usually ocular in origin. **Jerking (rhythmic) nystagmus** is characterized by a slow com-

ponent followed by a quick corrective component; it may be congenital, physiologic (at the extreme positions of gaze), due to inner ear disease, or secondary to CNS disease. **Congenital nystagmus** is a type of jerking nystagmus that is usually not associated with other neurologic disorders. The nystagmus is present in all directions of gaze, but it is usually minimized when the patient turns his eyes lightly to one side or the other.

Nystagmus is further classified according to the direction of movement (horizontal, rotatory, vertical, or mixed). Rotatory and vertical nystagmus result from brain stem disorder. Spasmus nutans is a disorder in which vertical head-nodding is associated with nystagmus; the nystagmus is usually horizontal but may be vertical. The condition occurs in small infants, and usually disappears within the first 2 years of life.

Measurement of Intraocular Tension

The only satisfactory method of measuring ocular tension is with a tonometer. Tactile tension, particularly in infants, is totally unreliable.

If glaucoma is suspected, the intraocular tension should be measured with a tonometer. In infants, general anesthesia is usually required, although in selected cases chloral hydrate sedation and topical corneal anesthesia may be used. In children 6–7 years of age, intraocular tensions can usually be measured with a tonometer after topical anesthesia. Intraocular tensions should be measured in any child with enlarged or hazy corneas or traumatic hyphema (blood in the anterior chamber).

Ophthalmoscopic Examination

Satisfactory ophthalmoscopic examination of the infant eye can be accomplished only after pupillary dilatation. The combined use of 5% homatropine and 2.5% phenylephrine instilled 2–3 times at intervals of 10–15 minutes usually gives satisfactory pupillary dilatation. In children 2 years of age and older, 1% or 2% cyclopentolate (Cyclogyl) instilled twice at 5–10 minute intervals gives good pupillary dilatation.

It is important to study all of the structures in the eye with the ophthalmoscope, including the cornea, lens, and vitreous as well as the optic disk and retina. In the infant eye the optic disk appears paler than in the adult eye. The foveal light reflection is absent. The periphery of the fundus is gray. The peripheral retinal vessels are not well developed.

Refraction

Cycloplegia is necessary to perform satisfactory refractions in infants and small children. The topical instillation of 1% cyclopentolate (Cyclogyl) or 5% homatropine is usually adequate. More complete cycloplegia can be obtained with 0.5–1% atropine instilled into the eyes 2–3 times a day for 3 days, but this is seldom necessary. Retinoscopy is performed with trial lenses. After the child is 7 or 8 years of age, subjective methods of refraction can be used in addition to retinoscopy.

Visual Fields

It is virtually impossible to judge visual fields in infants. One can sometimes estimate gross restriction of peripheral visual fields by covering one eye and directing the infant's gaze to an object. A second attractive object is brought in from the side, and the infant is observed to see when he will first shift his direction of gaze to the new object. Different types of toys and colored lights can be used for the visual test objects.

Perimetry examination of visual fields in children is easier to perform than tangent screen examination. When a child is 6 or 7 years of age, satisfactory perimetric examinations can usually be performed. In this test, attractive toys and large test objects are brought in along the perimetry arm.

Hospital For Sick Children, Toronto: *The Eye in Childhood.* Year Book, 1967.
Liebman SD, Gellis DD (editors): *The Pediatrician's Ophthalmology.* Mosby, 1966.

GENERAL PRINCIPLES OF TREATMENT OF OCULAR DISORDERS

For diseases of the anterior segment of the eye, topical medication is effective. For diseases of the posterior segment of the eye and for diseases of the orbit, systemic medication is necessary. In many instances (eg, severe intraocular infections or uveitis), the combined use of topical and systemic medication is required.

The intraocular penetration of topically applied drugs depends upon their solubility in fat and water. The epithelium of the cornea presents a barrier to medications that are not fat-soluble. The alkaloids, the corticosteroids, and some of the anesthetics penetrate the eye quite easily after topical application to the cornea. Most antibiotics do not penetrate the eye when topically applied.

The degree of intraocular penetration of systemically administered drugs depends upon their ability to pass the blood-aqueous and blood-vitreous barriers. In the normal eye most systemically administered antibiotics do not penetrate the barriers. In the inflamed eye the barriers are broken down, and drugs penetrate in much better concentrations. Systemically administered corticosteroids penetrate the eye quite easily. Certain drugs such as mannitol and glycerol do not cross the blood-aqueous barrier and therefore are valuable in the temporary treatment of acute glaucoma because an osmotic gradient is produced in which the blood is hypertonic to the aqueous and vitreous.

Solutions Versus Ointments

Topical ophthalmic preparations may be administered either as solutions or as ointments. In children, ointments have several advantages over solutions: They are not washed away with the tears; they are quite comfortable upon initial instillation; there is less absorption into the lacrimal passage; and, since the contact time in the eye is much longer, they can be used less frequently. The chief disadvantage of ointments is that they produce a film over the eye and thus interfere with vision. The advantages of solutions are that they do not interfere with vision and cause fewer contact dermatitis reactions than ointments. The chief disadvantage of solutions is that they must be instilled at frequent intervals.

Topical Corticosteroids

The corticosteroids are effective in many eye diseases, including allergic blepharitis and conjunctivitis, vernal conjunctivitis, phlyctenular keratoconjunctivitis, mucocutaneous conjunctival lesions, contact dermatitis of the eyelids and conjunctivas, interstitial keratitis, and many forms of iritis and iridocyclitis. Weaker steroid preparations such as 1% medrysone, 0.5−1.5% hydrocortisone, and 0.125% prednisolone are usually adequate for the management of allergic reactions of the conjunctiva and eyelids.

Many complications follow long and short term administration of topical corticosteroids. Among these are increased incidence or aggravation of herpes simplex keratitis and fungal ulcers of the cornea, decreased healing of corneal abrasions and wounds, glaucoma, and possibly cataract formation. The incidence of complications increases with the use of the more potent corticosteroid preparations such as 0.1% dexamethasone, 1% prednisolone, 0.1% triamcinolone, and 0.1% betamethasone. The use of these agents generally should be reserved for the treatment of severe intraocular inflammation. Any eye disorder severe enough to require prolonged topical corticosteroid therapy should be treated by an ophthalmologist.

Topical Antibiotics & Chemotherapeutic Agents

Ideally, the infecting organism should be identified and its antibiotic sensitivity established before specific antibiotic therapy is started. This is often impractical, however, and topical antibiotics are in most cases instituted empirically. If possible, those antibiotics should be used that are seldom employed systemically in order to decrease the risk of hypersensitivity reactions. For this reason, neomycin, bacitracin, and polymyxin (or mixtures) are frequently used in the treatment of conjunctivitis. Broad spectrum antibiotics and sulfacetamide or sulfisoxazole seldom produce sensitivity. Topical penicillin therapy should be avoided if possible.

In Tables 9−1 and 9−2 are listed the commonly used topical chemotherapeutic and antibiotic ophthalmic agents.

Mydriatics & Cycloplegics

Mydriatics are agents that dilate the pupil without paralyzing the ciliary muscle of accommodation. They are useful for ophthalmoscopic examination and in

TABLE 9–1. Topical chemotherapeutic and antibiotic agents.

Drug	Trade Name	Solution	Ointment
Tetracycline group	Many	5 mg/ml	5–10 mg/gm
Chloramphenicol	Chloromycetin Chloroptic	2.5–5 mg/ml	10 mg/gm
Streptomycin		50 mg/ml	
Neomycin		2.5 mg/ml	5 mg/gm
Polymyxin B	Aerosporin	1 mg/ml	2 mg/gm
Bacitracin		250–1000 units/ml	500 units/gm
Colistin	Coly-Mycin	1.2 mg/ml	
Erythromycin	Many	5 mg/ml	5 mg/gm
Nystatin	Mycostatin	100,000 units/ml	100,000 units/gm
Amphotericin B	Fungizone	2.5–10 mg/ml	
Sulfisoxazole	Gantrisin	40 mg/ml	40 mg/gm
Sulfacetamide sodium	Sulamyd Isopto-Cetamide Bleph 10 Bleph 30	100–300 mg/ml	100 mg/gm
Gentamicin	Garamycin	10 mg/ml	

preventing and breaking posterior synechias (adhesions of the iris to the lens). The commonly used mydriatics are phenylephrine (Neo-Synephrine), 2.5–10%; hydroxyamphetamine (Paredrine), 1%; and eucatropine (Euphthalmine), 5%. The duration of effect of the mydriatics is only a few hours.

Cycloplegic drugs are agents that produce paralysis of accommodation as well as pupillary dilatation. They are used in refraction and in the treatment of acute inflammatory conditions of the iris and ciliary body. The more commonly used cycloplegics are atropine, 0.25–2%; homatropine, 2–5%; scopolamine, 0.2%; cyclopentolate (Cyclogyl), 1–2%; and tropicamide (Mydriacyl), 1%.

Atropine is the most powerful cycloplegic; its effect may last for as long as 14 days. Scopolamine has an effect which lasts 2–5 days, whereas the effects of homatropine are usually gone within 48 hours. Cyclopentolate and tropicamide produce more rapid cycloplegia than the other agents, but their effect is usually

TABLE 9–2. Combinations of anti-infective drugs.

Drugs	Trade Name
Bacitracin and neomycin	Bacimycin
Bacitracin and polymyxin B	Polysporin
Bacitracin, neomycin, and polymyxin B	Mycitracin, Neosporin, Neo-Polycin
Chloramphenicol and polymyxin B	Chloromycetin-Polymyxin B
Oxytetracycline and polymyxin B	Terramycin-Polymyxin B
Neomycin and polymyxin B	Isopto P-N-P, Op-Isophrin-AB, Conjunctin
Neomycin and sulfacetamide	Sulfacidin

gone within 24 hours. It should be pointed out that each drop of 1% atropine contains approximately 0.5 mg of atropine. If 1% atropine drops were instilled into each eye and total absorption occurred, a toxic reaction would occur. When instilling atropine drops into the eyes of infants, it is well to exert pressure over the lacrimal sac to prevent the drop from reaching the nasal mucosa where it could be absorbed; alternatively, the head may be tipped so that the excess of medication will run out of the side of the eye.

Topical Anesthetics

The most commonly used local anesthetics are 0.5% proparacaine (Ophthaine, Ophthetic), 0.4% benoxinate (Dorsacaine), and 0.5% tetracaine (Pontocaine). Other anesthetics such as cocaine and butacaine are seldom used.

Topical anesthetics may be used before the removal of a conjunctival or corneal foreign body. They may be necessary to relieve the blepharospasm induced by a chemical injury before satisfactory irrigation and examination of the eye can be accomplished. Topical anesthetics should never be prescribed for home use since they might mask a serious ocular disorder and since their continued use might result in corneal ulceration.

Sterility of Topical Medication

Any ophthalmic medication may become contaminated. This is particularly true of solutions of fluorescein, which frequently become infected with *Pseudomonas aeruginosa*. It is well to discard all old ophthalmic solutions and any container whose tip has been touched by the examiner's hand or by the patient's eyelids. In the case of fluorescein, fresh solutions should be used for each patient, or strips of filter paper impregnated with fluorescein may be employed.

Ellis PP, Smith DL: *Handbook of Ocular Therapeutics and Pharmacology,* 3rd ed. Mosby, 1969.

OCULAR INJURIES

FOREIGN BODIES

Conjunctival Foreign Body

A conjunctival foreign body can usually be removed with a moist cotton applicator. A common site for foreign bodies is the furrow immediately behind the margin of the upper lid. Eversion of the upper lid, as described above, is necessary to visualize these foreign bodies.

Corneal Foreign Body

Superficial corneal foreign bodies usually can be removed without difficulty. A sterile topical anesthetic should be instilled into the eye and an attempt made to wipe away the foreign body with a moistened cotton applicator. If this is not successful, a blunt spud or small sterile dull hypodermic needle (No. 20) can be used. Care must be taken not to injure the deeper layers of the cornea; if the foreign body is deeply embedded in the stroma, the patient should be referred to an ophthalmologist. All rust rings of foreign bodies should be removed primarily. An antibiotic ointment should be instilled, and the eye should be patched until epithelialization of the cornea has occurred. The patient should be reexamined within 24 hours to make certain that infection has not occurred.

Intraocular Foreign Body

Intraocular foreign bodies are serious injuries which may not be suspected on initial examination. The usual history is that the patient was pounding on a metallic object with a hammer when something flew up into his eye. Examination may show a perforating wound of the cornea, a hole in the iris, and an opaque lens. However, the foreign body may be so small that little evidence of penetration is seen. An x-ray of the eye may be necessary to rule out the possibility of foreign body. If there is any question of a foreign. body, the patient should be referred to an ophthalmologist, since removal of these foreign bodies is extremely difficult. The visual prognosis is poor.

Havener WH, Gloeckner SL: *Diagnostic Techniques and Treatment of Intraocular Foreign Bodies.* Mosby, 1969.
Paton D, Goldberg MF: *Injuries of the Eye, the Lids and the Orbit: Diagnosis and Management.* Saunders, 1968.
Zagora E: *Eye Injuries.* Thomas, 1970.

INJURIES OF THE EYELIDS

Ecchymosis

Severe ecchymosis of the eyelids should be treated first with cold compresses to reduce hemor-rhage and swelling. After 24–48 hours, hot packs will speed absorption of extravasated blood.

Lacerations

Lacerations of the eyelids should be sutured primarily. When the laceration involves the lid margin, particularly the lower lid, it is imperative that the lid margins be sutured as evenly as possible to prevent the development of a notch. Such patients should be referred to an ophthalmologist. Lacerations involving the medial portion of the eyelids should be examined to rule out injury to the lacrimal canaliculi. If the canaliculi are cut, they should be repaired at the time of primary closure of the lid laceration, since delayed attempts to repair lacerated canaliculi are rarely successful.

Tenzel RR: Trauma and burns. Internat Ophth Clinic 10:55–69, 1970.
See Paton & Goldberg and Zagora references, above.

CORNEAL INJURIES

Corneal Abrasions

Corneal abrasions usually produce severe discomfort. The diagnosis is made by instilling fluorescein into the eye and observing the cornea for staining.

Treatment consists of the instillation of a mild cycloplegic such as 5% homatropine or 1% cyclopentolate (Cyclogyl), the application of antibiotic ointments, and firm patching of the eye for 24–48 hours until the epithelium has healed.

Corneal Lacerations

Corneal lacerations should be referred to an ophthalmologist for primary suturing. The patient should be observed for the development of intraocular infection. Systemic antibiotics and tetanus toxoid are indicated if the perforation occurred with a contaminated object.

See Paton & Goldberg and Zagora references, above.

HYPHEMA

Hyphema (blood in the anterior chamber) is a common contusion injury in children. It is a serious injury requiring hospitalization. Secondary bleeding is frequent and occurs usually within 6 days after the primary bleeding. Patients with hyphema should be examined for the development of glaucoma. Ophthalmoscopy should also be attempted to ascertain whether there has been more extensive injury to the posterior part of the eye.

Treatment consists of bed rest, binocular bandages, and sedatives. Binocular bandages are advisable, but if they produce excitement they may be omitted. No pupillary dilating (mydriatic) or pupillary constricting (miotic) drops should be used. If glaucoma develops, the use of carbonic anhydrase inhibitors, intravenous urea or mannitol, or oral glycerol is indicated initially. If this does not control the glaucoma, surgical removal of the blood clot by irrigation with saline or fibrinolysin is indicated.

Another complication of hyphema is blood staining of the cornea. This occurs only if the hemorrhage remains for a long period; it may occur whether or not glaucoma develops.

Coles WH: Traumatic hyphema: An analysis of 235 cases. South MJ 61:813–816, 1968.

Ferguson RHL, Poole LW: Traumatic hyphaema: A preliminary report on 200 cases. Trans Ophth Soc New Zealand 20:54–62, 1968.

BURNS

Burns of the eyelids should be treated in essentially the same way as burns of the skin elsewhere. It is important to protect the eyeballs from infection and exposure. Since burns frequently become contaminated with pseudomonas organisms which can produce severe corneal ulceration, an antibiotic preparation containing either colistin, gentamicin, or polymyxin B should be instilled into the eyes 3–4 times a day. As the burns begin to heal, cicatricial ectropion with corneal exposure may develop. To prevent corneal exposure, ointments should be applied inside the eyelids. Plastic surgery usually is necessary to correct cicatricial ectropion.

Chemical burns of the **cornea and conjunctiva** should be treated initially with thorough irrigation with any clean nonirritating fluid. This may be tap water, saline or boric acid solution, or whatever is available. It may be necessary to instill topical anesthetics into the eye to relieve blepharospasm before irrigation can be accomplished. After irrigation the eye should be inspected for retained chemical particles, which can be removed with a moistened cotton applicator. The extent of the damage is then determined. A weak acid solution such as 0.5% acetic acid may be used to irrigate the eye burned with alkali. In the case of acid burns, 3% sodium bicarbonate may be used for irrigation. In no case should a delay occur while waiting for a certain irrigating solution. If the burn involves the cornea, the eye should be dilated with 1% atropine or 5% homatropine after irrigation. An antibiotic ointment should be instilled, and the eye patched. Any patient who has suffered a severe chemical burn of the eye should be hospitalized and should be seen by an ophthalmologist.

Ultraviolet burns of the cornea usually cause severe pain and tearing. There is a history of exposure to ultraviolet light (eg, a welder's arc, snow on the ski slopes, sunlamp or treatment lamp). Symptoms develop 10–12 hours after exposure. Examination shows superficial corneal edema and pinpoint areas that stain with fluorescein. Treatment consists of the application of a topical anesthetic every 5–10 minutes until the pain is relieved. After pain has subsided, an antibiotic or an antibiotic-corticosteroid ointment is instilled into the eye and the eye is patched. Systemic analgesics and sedatives are then prescribed. Recovery is usually prompt and complete within 48 hours. (*Note:* Topical anesthetics should never be sent home with the patient.)

Retinal burns with permanent loss of vision may occur as a result of exposure to strong infrared light such as from observing an eclipse. If this is suspected, the patient should be referred to an ophthalmologist.

Brown SI, Weller CA: Collagenase inhibitors in prevention of ulcers of alkali-burned cornea. Arch Ophth 83:352–356, 1970.

See Paton & Goldberg reference, above.

FRACTURES OF THE ORBIT

Fractures of the orbit with any degree of displacement of the bones should be surgically reduced. The technics of surgery depend upon the location and extent of the fracture. If the fractures are not satisfactorily reduced, complications occur which include displacement of the globe, enophthalmos, and diplopia. Any injury that is severe enough to cause an orbital fracture may cause further skull fractures and intracranial damage. The patient should be studied for these possibilities.

Bleeker GM, Lyle TK (editors): *Fractures of the Orbit.* Williams & Wilkins, 1970.

Lerman S: Blowout fracture of the orbit. Brit J Ophth 54:90–98, 1970.

Milauskas AT: *Blowout Fractures of the Orbit.* Thomas, 1969.

CONTUSION OF THE GLOBE

In addition to the hyphema mentioned above, contusions of the globe may result in dislocation of the lens, hemorrhage into the vitreous, retinal edema and hemorrhage, retinal detachment, choroidal hemorrhage, choroidal rupture, and rupture of the eyeball. The diagnosis of these conditions is based upon (1) changes in visual acuity and (2) direct observation with the ophthalmoscope and slit lamp. If the fundus can be visualized well and if visual acuity is good, there is little likelihood that any significant damage to the posterior part of the eye has occurred. However, complications such as retinal detachment or dislocation of the lens may appear several weeks after the initial injury.

See Zagora reference, p 202.

REFRACTIVE ERRORS

Myopia (nearsightedness) is easily diagnosed; distant objects are blurred. Near vision is not usually impaired except in very high myopia. Frequently the patient squints his eyes in order to form a physiologic pinhole to improve visual acuity.

The diagnosis of hyperopia or farsightedness in children is more difficult. Children are able to accommodate much more effectively than adults and thus overcome their hyperopia. Sometimes there are associated symptoms of eyestrain or headaches after prolonged periods of close work. Children with severe farsightedness may have internal deviations of the eyes (esotropia).

Astigmatism produces distorted vision. Children will try to overcome the blurry vision by squinting their eyes and forming a pinhole. Children with severe astigmatism may complain of eyestrain and headaches.

Treatment of significant refractive errors consists of the proper fitting of lenses. Small degrees of hyperopia need not be corrected in children. Full correction of myopia is indicated. The use of bifocals in myopic children does not appear to prevent the progressive type of myopia. Other forms of treatment such as the use of cycloplegics, "eye exercises," or certain diets do not appear to influence the progression of myopia.

Contact lenses are seldom indicated in children. The exception is the child with unilateral aphakia (absence of the lens), severe anisometropia (difference of refractive errors in the 2 eyes), corneal scarring producing an irregular astigmatism, or keratoconus. Contact lenses have been purported to reduce the progression of myopia, but there is little evidence for this view.

Duke-Elder S: *The Practice of Refraction,* 8th ed. Mosby, 1969.
Sloane AE: *Manual of Refraction,* 2nd ed. Little, Brown, 1970.

STRABISMUS
(Squint)

Approximately 5% of children have strabismus. The eyes may deviate inward (esotropia), outward (exotropia), upward (hypertropia), or downward (hypotropia). Strabismus is comitant if the same degree of deviation exists in all fields of gaze, and noncomitant if the angle of deviation changes in the various directions of gaze. The terms tropia and phoria are both used to describe abnormal positions of the eye; tropias are manifest deviations, whereas phorias are latent deviations which become manifest only if fusion or binocular vision is broken up.

Strabismus is usually first observed either shortly after birth or at the age of 2–3 years; rarely, the onset is at a later age. Infants do not develop coordinated eye muscle movements until about 4–5 months of age. An occasional infant is observed to have temporary deviation of the eyes, and realignment subsequently occurs. Any child who has a deviation that persists for several months or who develops a deviation after the age of 6 months should be investigated for the cause of the strabismus.

The diagnosis of strabismus is frequently made by simple inspection. If the eyes are deviated considerably, the diagnosis is evident. If there is only a slight deviation or if there is a questionable deviation because of wide epicanthal folds (pseudostrabismus) with more of the white of the eye being exposed temporally than nasally, the diagnosis is established by the corneal light reflection technic (Fig 9–2) or the cover test (Fig 9–3), as described above. Strabismus may also be suspected on the basis of marked reduced visual acuity in one eye. Children with head tilt may have strabismus with very little apparent displacement of the eyes.

During visual development diplopia occurs if alignment of the eyes is such that the object viewed does not fall on corresponding parts of the retina. To avoid diplopia, the child learns to suppress the vision in the deviating eye. If one eye continually deviates, then suppression is always in this eye, with the result that macular vision never develops. The term amblyopia ex anopsia or suppression amblyopia is applied to this condition. Visual screening examination of preschool children is important in diagnosing early suppression amblyopia.

Paralytic or noncomitant strabismus may result from CNS diseases or anatomic maldevelopments of the ocular muscles. The sudden onset of paralytic strabismus in any child should prompt examination for CNS disease.

Treatment

Children do not outgrow strabismus. Early treatment is important and should be given by an ophthalmologist. Treatment is directed toward the development of good visual acuity in each eye, realignment of the eyes in good cosmetic position, and functional cures with the establishment of binocular vision. The following steps are considered in the treatment of strabismus: (1) Careful ophthalmoscopic examination to rule out an organic intraocular cause for the deviation, eg, congenital cataracts, tumors, optic nerve atrophy. (2) Cycloplegic refraction and prescription of lenses. (3) Occlusion of the good eye to develop macular vision in the bad eye. (4) Surgery to align the eyes if glasses are unsuccessful in correcting the deviation.

Early surgery (ages 9–24 months) with alignment of the eyes is more likely to result in a functional cure than surgery performed at age 4–5 years or later.

Orthoptic exercises are of value in establishing binocular vision if the visual axes are nearly aligned. They are also of value in certain forms of intermittent strabismus. **Pleoptics** is a new orthoptic technic of stimulating macular vision in children with suppression amblyopia. These technics are of greatest value for children who do not respond to occlusive therapy. The value of pleoptics is not yet fully established; it appears that some children are able to develop useful macular vision with this form of therapy.

Dyer JA: *Atlas of Extraocular Muscle Surgery.* Saunders, 1970.

Von Noorden GK: Strabismus: Annual review. Arch Ophth 84:103–122, 1970.

Von Noorden GK, Maumenee AE: *Atlas of Strabismus.* Mosby, 1967.

GLAUCOMA

Primary Glaucoma

Primary congenital glaucoma (hydrophthalmos) is due to an abnormal development of the aqueous drainage structures; it may be present at birth or may develop within the first 2 years of life. Diagnosis is based upon (1) enlarged corneas that are frequently edematous and show linear white opacities (breaks in Descemet's membrane), (2) symptoms of photophobia and tearing, and (3) increased intraocular pressure. Since the coats of the eye of an infant are not so rigid as those of an adult, increased intraocular pressure results in stretching of the corneal and scleral tissues.

Early surgical treatment is essential. Medical therapy is of little value. Surgery is successful in controlling intraocular pressure in about 75% of cases. Without treatment, permanent blindness occurs at an early age.

Glaucoma may be associated with other developmental anomalies. These include aniridia, posterior embryotoxon (failure of reabsorption of the mesodermal tissue in the periphery of the iris and drainage angle), Sturge-Weber disease, Lowe's syndrome, Marfan's syndrome, and congenital rubella syndrome.·

Secondary Glaucoma

Secondary glaucoma may be due to many causes. The mechanism of this type of glaucoma is usually an obstruction of the aqueous outflow channels. The various causes include lens dislocation, hemorrhage into the eye, iritis, tumors (including retinoblastoma), retrolental fibroplasia, and xanthogranulomas in the iris. Treatment of these conditions is complicated, and the patient should be referred to an ophthalmologist.

Kolker AE, Hetherington J Jr: *Becker-Shaffer's Diagnosis and Therapy of the Glaucomas,* 3rd ed. Mosby, 1970.

Levene R: Glaucoma: Annual review. Arch Ophth 83:232–253, 1970.

Shaffer RN, Weiss DI: *Congenital and Pediatric Glaucomas.* Mosby, 1970.

CATARACTS

A cataract is an opacity of the lens; it consists of precipitated lens protein. Cataracts may be unilateral or bilateral and partial or complete; considerable variation exists in the extent, position, shape, and density of cataract formation. They may be congenital and associated with other congenital anomalies. They can occur as a result of maternal rubella during the first trimester of pregnancy. Cataracts may be secondary to ocular trauma, or associated with systemic diseases such as diabetes mellitus, galactosemia, atopic dermatitis, Marfan's syndrome, or Down's syndrome. They may also be due to long-term systemic corticosteroid therapy.

The symptoms vary considerably according to location and extent. Vision may be affected very slightly, or considerable reduction in vision can occur. White spots may be observed in the pupil. In a few cases, strabismus or pendular nystagmus is present.

The diagnosis is made by inspection with a flashlight or by examination with an ophthalmoscope or slit lamp. In some cases cataracts can be observed only when the pupils are dilated.

Surgical lens extraction (before age 6 months) is indicated if the cataracts are bilateral and sufficiently dense that vision cannot develop. If cataracts are not dense enough to interfere with visual development, surgery should be deferred since some congenital cataracts do not progress. Surgery is indicated when visual loss is a serious handicap to the child.

Gass JDM: Lens aspiration using a side-opening needle. Arch Ophth 82:87–90, 1969.

Scheie HG, Rubinstein RA, Kent RB: Aspiration of congenital or soft cataracts: Further experience. Am J Ophth 63:3–8, 1967.

Von Noorden GK, Ryan SJ, Maumenee AE: Management of congenital cataracts. Tr Am Acad Ophth 74:352–359, 1970.

DISEASES OF THE EYELIDS

HORDEOLUM

External hordeolum (sty) is a staphylococcal abscess of the sebaceous glands of the lid margin.

Symptoms consist of localized tenderness, redness, and swelling. Internal hordeolum is an acute infection of the meibomian glands that usually points conjunctivally.

Treatment of both types consists of warm moist compresses 3–4 times a day. Instillation of an antibiotic or sulfonamide ophthalmic ointment 4–5 times a day is useful during the acute stage. Treatment should be continued for several days after the lesion has subsided in order to reduce the likelihood of a recurrence.

Spontaneous rupture frequently occurs, but if it does not the lesion should be incised when it becomes large and pointed. The removal of an eyelash will promote drainage of an external hordeolum.

Sexton RR: Eyelids, lacrimal apparatus and conjunctiva: Annual review. Arch Ophth 85:379–396, 1971.

CHALAZION

Chalazion is a granulomatous inflammation of the meibomian glands. The cause is not known. Symptoms consist of slight discomfort in the eyelid and a slight redness and a lump on the conjunctival surface of the lid overlying the involved meibomian gland. Local excision is usually necessary, but chalazions do occasionally disappear after treatment with warm moist compresses.

See Sexton reference, above.

BLEPHARITIS
(Granulated Eyelids)

Chronic inflammation of the lid margins may be seborrheic (nonulcerative), staphylococcal (ulcerative), or a combination of the 2 types. Symptoms are redness, burning, itching, and crusting of the lid margins. In the staphylococcal type the scales are dry; small ulcerative lesions of the skin are observed; the eyelashes may fall out. In the seborrheic type the scales are oily; seborrhea of the scalp is usually present.

Treatment of staphylococcal blepharitis consists of the instillation of antibiotic or sulfonamide ophthalmic ointment into the eye twice a day. Treatment should be continued for a week or so after all symptoms have disappeared. The crusts on the lids should be gently removed with a moist cotton applicator before the ointment is instilled. The treatment of seborrheic blepharitis consists of controlling scalp seborrhea if it exists, removing the scales along the lid margins with a moist cotton applicator, and instilling

sulfacetamide or an antistaphylococcal antibiotic ophthalmic ointment.

Other useful treatments are the careful application of 2.5% ammoniated mercury ointment, 1% silver nitrate solution, or 0.5% selenium sulfide (Selsun) ointment to the lid margins.

Thygeson P: Complications of staphylococcic blepharitis. Am J Ophth 68:446–449, 1969.
See Sexton reference, above.

DISEASES OF THE CONJUNCTIVA

CONJUNCTIVITIS

Conjunctivitis is the most common of all pediatric ocular disorders. It is usually due to bacterial, viral, or fungal infections. Less commonly it may result from an allergic reaction or physical or chemical irritation. Symptoms consist of redness of the conjunctiva, foreign body sensation, a mucoid or purulent discharge, and sticking together of the eyelids in the morning. Vision is not affected. The cornea, anterior chamber, and intraocular pressure are normal.

Bacterial Conjunctivitis

The most common causes of bacterial conjunctivitis are the pneumococcus, *Staphylococcus aureus*, Koch-Weeks bacillus, and hemolytic streptococci. There may be associated bacterial infections elsewhere in the body. Conjunctival membranes (diphtheritic conjunctivitis) or pseudomembranes (streptococcal conjunctivitis) may be present. Discharge, usually a prominent feature of bacterial conjunctivitis, is purulent or mucopurulent in character.

The causative organism should be identified, if possible, by obtaining smears and cultures. Empirical treatment with broad spectrum antibiotics or sulfonamide ophthalmic ointments instilled into the eye 4–5 times a day usually results in improvement within 48–72 hours. If improvement does not occur, it is important to make an etiologic diagnosis if this has not been done earlier. Bacterial conjunctivitis is usually a self-limited disease, but secondary corneal infection and ulceration occur rarely.

Inclusion Conjunctivitis (Swimming Pool Conjunctivitis)

This disease is due to the same organism (TRIC agent; see below) that produces inclusion blennorrhea in the newborn. It is characterized by conjunctival redness, clear or mucoid discharge, and follicles in the lower palpebral conjunctiva. Treatment consists of the local application of sulfonamide or broad spectrum antibiotics 4–5 times a day.

Trachoma

Trachoma is infection of the conjunctiva with TRIC agent, formerly thought to be a large atypical virus but now reclassified as a bacterium of the genus Chlamydia. (TRIC = trachoma-inclusion conjunctivitis.) The disease is usually associated with poor hygiene and poor economic conditions. It is a major cause of blindness in the world, but is rare in the USA except among American Indians.

In the early stages, trachoma is characterized by a catarrhal type of reaction with diffuse redness, mild irritation, and a thin watery discharge. Subsequently the conjunctiva becomes thickened with papillary hypertrophy and formation of follicles, particularly in the tarsal region of the upper lids. Scarring of the conjunctiva develops later, and there is corneal vascularization and opacification.

Local therapy can probably control trachoma adequately, but systemic therapy is usually given also. Systemic sulfonamides are the agents most commonly used, although broad spectrum antibiotics are also effective. The drug of choice is sulfisoxazole (Gantrisin), administered by mouth in a dose of 100 mg/kg body weight daily in 4 divided doses for 1 week, followed by 60 mg/kg body weight for an additional 2 weeks. It is sometimes necessary to repeat this treatment after 1 week without medication. The local treatment of choice is an oil suspension of tetracycline applied 4 times a day for 6 weeks. Since recurrences are common, follow-up evaluation is important.

Viral Conjunctivitis

Viral conjunctivitis is frequently due to infection with one of the adenoviruses. The conjunctivitis may be associated with pharyngitis and preauricular adenopathy. The conjunctiva is quite hyperemic and shows follicular reaction. There is a thin watery discharge. The condition usually lasts 12–14 days.

No treatment is of value. Sulfonamide preparations or broad spectrum antibiotics are instilled locally to prevent secondary infection.

Vaccinial Conjunctivitis

This form of conjunctivitis usually results from auto-inoculation from a recent smallpox vaccination site. Treatment consists of the use of 0.5% idoxuridine (IDU) ophthalmic ointment (Stoxil) instilled into the eye 4 times a day and the intramuscular injection of vaccinia immune globulin (VIG), 0.3 ml/lb body weight. No more than 5 ml of this serum should be given in one site. If no response occurs within 48 hours, VIG treatment should be repeated.

Leptothrix Conjunctivitis

Leptothrix conjunctivitis is characterized by small gray necrotic lesions on the palpebral conjunctiva. There is usually a history of contact with a cat. The course is protracted. Improvement may follow local excision of the necrotic areas. There is no special medical treatment.

Actinomyces Infections

Actinomyces species may produce conjunctivitis. The conjunctivitis is usually on the nasal side of the conjunctiva, and is frequently associated with inflammation of the lacrimal canaliculi. The organisms are susceptible to penicillin and broad spectrum antibiotics. If an infection exists in the canaliculi, this must be cleared before a permanent cure can be effected.

Allergic Conjunctivitis

Allergic conjunctivitis produces symptoms of itching, lacrimation, mild redness, and a stringy mucoid discharge. Eosinophils may be seen on scrapings from the conjunctiva. For acute cases of conjunctivitis, local 1.5% hydrocortisone ophthalmic ointment or its equivalent instilled into the eye 3–4 times a day is quite effective. For chronic forms of allergic conjunctivitis, an attempt should be made to isolate the offending allergen and to eliminate contact with it. Desensitization to the allergen can be carried out if elimination of contact is not possible. Temporary symptomatic relief may be obtained with the use of topical ophthalmic solutions containing vasoconstricting agents and antihistamines.

Phlyctenular Keratoconjunctivitis

Phlyctenular keratoconjunctivitis appears as elevated clear nodules, situated near the limbus, with surrounding hyperemia. The disease has been associated with a hypersensitivity reaction to tuberculin; phlyctenules may also develop as a hypersensitivity reaction to other bacterial products or other antigens.

Treatment consists of the local application of corticosteroids. Systemic tuberculosis should be ruled out.

Vernal Conjunctivitis

This form of conjunctivitis is seen in patients ages 5–20. It tends to be seasonal and becomes less severe with age. Symptoms consist of lacrimation, itching, stringy discharge, and giant "cobblestone" papillary hypertrophy in the tarsal conjunctiva or grayish elevated areas at the limbus. Many eosinophils are seen in the scraping of the lesions.

Treatment consists of the local application of corticosteroid ointment several times a day. Severe cases may require more extensive therapy, but this should be conducted by an ophthalmologist.

Ophthalmia Neonatorum

Ophthalmia neonatorum is inflammation of the conjunctiva of the newborn. It may be due to bacterial infection (gonococcal, staphylococcal, or pneumococcal), viral infection (inclusion blennorrhea), or chemical irritation (silver nitrate). Bacterial conjunctivitis appears 2–5 days after birth; inclusion conjunctivitis appears 5–10 days after birth. Conjunctivitis associated with silver nitrate usually is evident within the first 24–48 hours after birth. A definite diagnosis is established by smears and cultures of the material taken from the conjunctiva. Conjunctivitis due to silver nitrate is sterile, although secondary bacterial infections may occur.

In most states in the USA, chemical (1% silver nitrate) or antibiotic prophylaxis of the newborn eye is required. These laws are highly variable in the different states. Various antibiotics such as penicillin, tetracyclines, or bacitracin are currently used for prophylaxis of gonococcal ophthalmia.

It is most important to treat gonococcal conjunctivitis vigorously, since in untreated or inadequately treated cases corneal ulceration and perforation can occur. The treatment of gonococcal conjunctivitis consists of topical application of either penicillin, erythromycin, or tetracycline drops into the eye every 2 hours and penicillin G, 30,000 units/kg of body weight daily IM, or systemic tetracycline therapy. If one eye is uninvolved, it should be covered with a shield to prevent contamination from the involved eye. The purulent discharge should be irrigated from the conjunctiva with normal saline and allowed to drain toward the outer edge of the eyelids away from the other eye. Cold compresses may be of value in relieving the marked swelling of the eyelids.

Other types of bacterial conjunctivitis of the newborn should be treated by the instillation of appropriate antibiotic ointments 4 times a day. Inclusion blennorrhea is treated by the local instillation of sulfacetamide or tetracycline ointment 4 times a day.

In all cases of conjunctivitis, treatment should be continued for a few days after the symptoms have subsided to prevent early recurrences.

Allen JH: Common external ocular infections. Postgrad Med 45:144–148, 1969.
Thygeson P: Diseases of the conjunctiva. In: *The Eye and Its Diseases,* 2nd ed. Berens C (editor). Saunders, 1950.
Thygeson P, Dawson CR: Trachoma and follicular conjunctivitis in children. Arch Ophth 75:3–12, 1966.
See Sexton reference, p 206.

MUCOCUTANEOUS DISEASES

Conjunctival lesions may be associated with mucocutaneous diseases, including erythema multiforme, Stevens-Johnson syndrome, Reiter's syndrome, and Behcet's syndrome. The conjunctival involvement consists of erythema, vesicular lesions which frequently rupture, membrane formation, and the development of symblepharon (adhesions) between the raw edges of the bulbar and palpebral conjunctivas.

Treatment of the conjunctival lesions associated with these conditions is symptomatic, ie, soothing eye drops and compresses. Topical steroids are helpful in the acute stages in diminishing the intensity and complications of the acute inflammatory phase. Antibiotics are of no benefit except for prevention of secondary infection. Erythema multiforme and Stevens-Johnson

disease may be precipitated by sulfonamide and antibiotic therapy. Topical antibiotic therapy may be used when secondary bacterial infection occurs; care must be taken to choose an antibiotic to which the patient is not sensitive.

Grayson M, Keates RH: *Manual of Diseases of the Cornea.* Little, Brown, 1969.

DISEASES OF THE CORNEA

CORNEAL ULCERS

Corneal ulcers are serious ocular disorders. They may follow corneal injury or conjunctivitis or may be associated with systemic infections. Corneal ulcers are usually diagnosed by simple inspection. There is loss of anterior substance of the cornea with surrounding opaque gray or white necrosis. Corneal ulcers may be peripheral or central. Several ulcers may be present in the same eye. The area of ulceration stains with fluorescein. A serious effort should be made to determine the etiology of any corneal ulcer. Cultures and scrapings should be taken from the ulcer, and if bacterial organisms are found sensitivity tests should be performed.

Bacterial Corneal Ulcers

Central bacterial corneal ulcers are due to infections with pneumococci, hemolytic streptococci, *Pseudomonas aeruginosa,* and, less commonly, gram-positive and gram-negative rods. Marginal corneal ulcers may develop as a result of bacterial sensitivity, most commonly to staphylococcal infections.

Treatment should be started immediately, before sensitivity tests are completed. Subsequently, the antibiotic can be changed if necessary. For mild superficial bacterial ulcers, the topical use of antibiotic drops or ointment at frequent intervals is usually satisfactory. Until the susceptibility of the organism is known, it is well to start the patient on an ophthalmic antibiotic preparation which includes neomycin, bacitracin, and polymyxin B, or else a broad spectrum antibiotic. Cycloplegic drops should be used to relieve the iridocyclitis that accompanies bacterial ulcers. In more severe corneal ulcers which involve the deeper portions of the stroma, more intensive antibiotic therapy should be given. Antibiotics should also be given subconjunctivally and systemically. Corticosteroids should not be given topically, since they interfere with the healing process and might exaggerate an infection that was not susceptible to the treatment being used.

Marginal corneal ulcers respond to topical steroids. If a staphylococcal infection of the conjunctiva or eyelids is present, it should be treated with appropriate antibiotics.

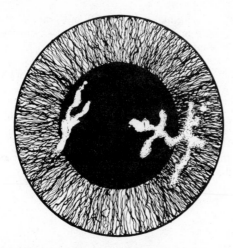

FIG 9–4. Dendritic type of lesion seen in herpes simplex keratitis. (Reproduced, with permission, from Vaughan D, Asbury T, Cook R: *General Ophthalmology*, 6th ed. Lange, 1971.)

Viral Corneal Ulcers

A. Herpes Simplex Ulcer (Dendritic): Herpes simplex keratitis is becoming a more common corneal disease in children. Lesions in the cornea may or may not be associated with herpes labialis. Corneal involvement is frequently precipitated by the topical application of corticosteroids and less commonly with the systemic use of corticosteroids. In the initial infection the lesion has the appearance of a dendrite (Fig 9–4). There are one or more branching vesicular lesions involving the anterior part of the cornea. These vesicles rupture. Subsequently, deeper involvement of the cornea may occur. Iritis may also develop as a complication.

Treatment of acute herpes infections of the cornea consists of the topical application of idoxuridine (IDU) applied as an 0.5% ointment (Stoxil) 4 times a day, or as an 0.1% solution (Herplex, Stoxil) hourly during the day and every 2 hours at night. The eye is usually more comfortable if the pupil is kept dilated with 1% atropine or 5% homatropine. Mechanical denuding of the corneal epithelium is also an effective method of treating fresh cases of superficial herpes simplex keratitis. This should be performed by an ophthalmologist. Deeper involvement of the cornea may represent a hypersensitivity reaction, and the use of topical corticosteroids in conjunction with IDU sometimes improves the condition. However, this type of therapy should be undertaken only by an ophthalmologist, since the use of corticosteroids in an active herpes infection can lead to rapid deterioration of the cornea.

B. Vaccinial Infection: Vaccinial keratitis is usually secondary to auto-inoculation from the site of a recent vaccination. It may also occur as a result of vaccine being splashed into the eye. The treatment of choice is the application of idoxuridine drops or ointments. Drops are employed in 0.1% concentration (Herplex, Stoxil) every hour during the day and every 2 hours at night. Ointment is applied in an 0.5% concentration (Stoxil) 4 times a day.

C. Herpes Zoster Infection: Herpes zoster keratitis is associated with zoster infection of the first branch of the trigeminal nerve. The involvement of the cornea is usually deep. Relief is obtained with the use of topical corticosteroids. Cycloplegic drops should be used for relieving the iridocyclitis which accompanies herpes zoster infection. The physician must be certain of the diagnosis of herpes zoster before employing topical corticosteroids, since other viral diseases of the cornea are aggravated by these agents.

Fungal Corneal Ulcers

Mycotic corneal infections are difficult to diagnose. Usually there is a history of recent trauma or foreign body. Frequently the ulcerated cornea shows surrounding satellite lesions; hypopyon (pus in the anterior chamber) may be present. Fungal corneal ulcers are rare, but their incidence seems to be increasing, possibly from the widespread use of topical corticosteroid and broad spectrum antibiotic medications. Whenever a diagnosis of mycotic corneal ulceration is suspected, cultures and sensitivity tests should be obtained.

Most fungal ulcers of the cornea respond to either nystatin (Mycostatin) or amphotericin B (Fungizone). The nystatin drops are employed in a concentration of 100,000 units/ml; amphotericin B ophthalmic drops are used in a concentration of 4–10 mg/ml. The drops should be used at frequent intervals. Subconjunctival injections of 0.5 ml of amphotericin B or nystatin ophthalmic solutions may also be employed. Cycloplegics should be used to relieve the iridocyclitis.

Kaufman HE, Nesburn AB, Maloney ED: IDU therapy of herpes simplex. Arch Ophth 67:583–591, 1962.

Laibson PR: Cornea and sclera: Annual review. Arch Ophth 85:379–396, 1971.

Polack FM (editor): *Corneal and External Diseases of the Eye.* Thomas, 1970.

ALLERGIC REACTIONS

Allergic reactions in the cornea may involve either the superficial epithelial or deeper stromal layers. Most forms of deep keratitis probably represent hypersensitivity reactions. The allergen may be airborne, or it may enter the cornea by way of the circulation in the limbus. Treatment consists of determining the offending agent, if possible, and then eliminating its contact with the patient. Topical corticosteroids usually give considerable relief.

Interstitial Keratitis

Interstitial keratitis is an acute immune reaction in the cornea usually associated with congenital syphilis. Symptoms consist of intense photophobia, tearing, pain, and decreased vision. On examination the cornea has a diffuse opaque appearance. Fine vessels may be noted in the stroma. There may be aggregates of these vessels which appear as orange-red areas (salmon patches). Other evidence of congenital syphilis may also be present. Serologic tests for syphilis are often negative.

Interstitial keratitis may be associated with other diseases such as tuberculosis and the autoimmune disorders, and any such contributing condition should be ruled out.

Treatment consists of the use of topical steroids and cycloplegics for relief of symptoms. If active syphilis is present, it should be appropriately treated.

Schwartz B (editor): *Syphilis and the Eye.* Williams & Wilkins, 1970.
See Grayson & Keates reference, p 208.

CORNEAL DRYING & EXPOSURE

Keratoconjunctivitis Sicca

This rare condition results from a lacrimal gland insufficiency. The treatment of choice is tear replacement with artificial tears (eg, methylcellulose), 0.5–1% solution as necessary to keep the cornea moist.

Exposure Keratitis

Exposure keratitis may develop after facial nerve palsies or after a period of unconsciousness during which the eyes are exposed. Treatment is similar to that described above.

Neuroparalytic Keratitis

Neuroparalytic keratitis is seen after damage to the ophthalmic division of the trigeminal nerve. It is treated by tear replacement (see Keratoconjunctivitis Sicca, above).

Familial Dysautonomia (Riley-Day Syndrome)

In this condition there is a deficiency of tears, and corneal drying can occur. Tear replacement (see Keratoconjunctivitis Sicca, above) is indicated.

Gasset AR, Kaufman HE: Hydrophilic lens therapy of severe keratoconjunctivitis sicca and conjunctival scarring. Am J Ophth 71:1185–1189, 1971.
Walsh FB, Hoyt WF: *Clinical Neuro-ophthalmology,* 3rd ed. 3 vols. Williams & Wilkins, 1969.

CORNEAL INVOLVEMENT IN OTHER SYSTEMIC DISEASES

The cornea is involved in many systemic diseases. Small calcium deposits may be observed in the corneas of patients with hyperparathyroidism. Cystine crystals are observed in patients with renal rickets (cystinosis). Excessive intake of vitamin D may lead to calcification of the anterior part of the cornea in a band opacity of the exposed portion of the cornea. Deficiency of vitamin A may lead to drying (xerosis) and softening (keratomalacia) of the cornea. Corneal ulceration may occur in patients with severe debilitating diseases such as dysentery. Corneal opacities may occur in children with Hurler's disease (gargoylism).

In all of these conditions it is important to recognize the underlying disease and treat appropriately.

See Grayson & Keates reference, p 208.

UVEITIS

Inflammation of the uveal tract may present anteriorly as iritis or cyclitis (inflammation of the ciliary body), or as posterior inflammations (choroiditis). Uveitis may be associated with other ocular diseases, such as corneal ulceration, keratitis, hypermature cataracts, necrotic intraocular tumors, or optic neuritis.

Uveitis may be classified as exogenous or endogenous. Exogenous uveitis follows the accidental introduction of pathogenic organisms or a foreign substance into the eye. Endogenous uveitis is a result of various systemic processes.

Uveitis may also be classified as suppurative or nonsuppurative according to the type of tissue reaction. Nonsuppurative uveitis, which is the more common form, may further be divided into granulomatous and nongranulomatous types. Nongranulomatous uveitis usually involves the iris and ciliary body and produces symptoms of photophobia, pain, redness, and blurred vision. The pupil is small and often irregular. There is circumcorneal injection. On examination with a slit lamp, cells in the anterior chamber and fine precipitates on the posterior surface of the cornea may be observed. Granulomatous uveitis may involve the iris, ciliary body, or choroid. Pain, redness, and photophobia are not so prominent as in the nongranulomatous form. Vision may be markedly disturbed, particularly if the involvement is in the macular area. On ophthalmoscopy the vitreous may be quite hazy. Active lesions of choroiditis may be seen as swollen, white, indistinct irregular patches. As the choroiditis subsides, pigmentary changes may take place.

Uveitis presents a complex problem. The endogenous nonsuppurative form may be associated with systemic disease. Among the more common associated diseases are toxoplasmosis, histoplasmosis, tuberculosis, sarcoidosis, rheumatoid arthritis and other collagen diseases, bacterial infections of the sinuses or teeth, food and pollen allergies, and viral diseases such as mumps, measles, chickenpox, influenza, herpes simplex, and herpes zoster. The relationship between systemic disease and uveitis may be incidental. There is pathologic evidence that the choroid and retina may be invaded with toxoplasma and *Mycobacterium tuberculosis.* However, aside from these specific instances, causative organisms have not been found to enter the uveal tissue. There is accumulating evidence that most cases of uveitis are due to an immune reaction.

Treatment

If systemic disease is present, it should be appropriately treated. However, successful treatment of systemic disease does not always result in a cure of the uveitis. Nonspecific treatment of uveitis consists of the use of cycloplegics to dilate the pupil and to relieve the ciliary and iris spasm. Atropine, 1–2% solution, or scopolamine, 0.25% solution, should be used 2–3 times daily. In addition, the topical use of 10% phenylephrine hydrochloride is indicated to widely dilate the pupil. Corticosteroids should be used unless they are contraindicated by the presence of a specific bacterial or viral infection. For inflammations of the anterior uveal tract, topical corticosteroids are useful in reducing the inflammation. For posterior uveitis, systemic corticosteroids should be used.

The management of uveitis is difficult. Many complications can occur, including glaucoma, cataract, and retinal detachment. Therefore, these cases should be managed by an ophthalmologist.

Maumenee AE: Clinical studies in "uveitis": An approach to the study of intraocular inflammation. Am J Ophth 69:1–27, 1970.
Schlaegel TF: *Essentials of Uveitis.* Little, Brown, 1969.
Schlaegel TF: The uvea: Annual review. Arch Ophth 85:624–635, 1971.

SYMPATHETIC OPHTHALMIA

Sympathetic ophthalmia is a special form of bilateral granulomatous uveitis. It follows a penetrating ocular injury of the uveal tract. It may occur at any time from 10 days after injury to many years later, but it usually presents within the first 2–4 months after initial injury. The etiology of sympathetic ophthalmia is not understood, but it probably represents a hypersensitivity response to uveal pigment. The diagnosis is based on a history of an injury to one (exciting) eye with the subsequent development of uveitis in the other (sympathizing) eye.

Treatment consists of the use of systemic and topical corticosteroids and topical cycloplegics. Long-term therapy is usually necessary, and maintenance doses of steroids are usually indicated to prevent a flare-up of this condition. The disease can be averted by early enucleation of the exciting eye which has received a severe injury to the ciliary body and which has become visually useless.

See Schlaegel book reference, above.

DISEASES OF THE RETINA

RETINAL DETACHMENT

Detachment of the retina in children is usually associated with severe ocular trauma or with high myopia. In the latter condition there are degenerative changes in the periphery of the retina which lead to subsequent separation of the retina. The diagnosis is established by a history of progressively more severe blurred vision. The visual disturbance may start with the sensation of flashing lights, or the patient may observe a dark cloud coming in from one section of the visual field. On ophthalmoscopy the area of detachment appears elevated and gray. The retinal vessels appear darker, and the retina is seen with increased convex dioptric power in the ophthalmoscope.

The only treatment is surgical repair.

Chisholm L: Retinal detachment in children. Canad J Ophth 6:62–67, 1971.
Tasman W (editor): *Retinal Diseases in Children.* Harper, 1971.

RETINOBLASTOMA

Retinoblastoma is a comparatively rare malignant tumor of children. It usually appears before the third year of life, although rare cases have been reported with onset in adolescence. Retinoblastoma is a hereditary disease due to mutation of an autosomal dominant gene. Patients who have survived retinoblastoma have about a 50% chance of transmitting retinoblastoma to their offspring. Approximately 25% of cases are bilateral.

The presenting symptom is usually a white spot in the pupil. Strabismus may be present. If the tumor becomes very large, glaucoma may occur, with a steamy cornea and red eye. Occasionally retinoblastoma ruptures through the globe and results in a painful red eye. The diagnosis is usually made by ophthalmoscopic examination. To accomplish ophthalmoscopy, wide pupillary dilatation is essential; general anesthesia is often necessary. The tumor appears as a solid yellow or white elevated mass. A small section of the eye may be involved, or the entire eye may be filled with tumor.

Treatment consists of enucleation of the involved eye in unilateral cases. If there is involvement of both eyes, the more severely involved eye should be enucleated and the other eye treated with x-ray therapy together with intravenous or intracarotid injections of triethylenemelamine (TEM).

Some cases of retinoblastoma follow a strong hereditary pattern. If one child is afflicted, the parents should be advised that other children might also suffer from this disease.

Bedford MA, Bedotto C, MacFaul PA: Retinoblastoma: A study of 139 cases. Brit J Ophth 55:19–27, 1971.

Hyman GA & others: Combination therapy in retinoblastoma. Arch Ophth 80:744–746, 1968.

Reese AB: *Tumors of the Eye,* 2nd ed. Hoeber, 1963.

OPTIC NEURITIS

Optic neuritis may involve only the head of the nerve (papillitis) or the orbital portion of the nerve (retrobulbar neuritis). Optic neuritis may occur in association with generalized infectious diseases, demyelinating diseases, blood dyscrasias, or metabolic diseases, or may be due to exposure to toxins or drugs or extension of inflammatory disease such as sinusitis or meningitis. Clinically, there is an acute loss of vision. Involvement may be of one or both eyes; in children the disease is frequently bilateral. Central visual defects are present. There may be some discomfort in the eyes on movement of the globes. On ophthalmoscopic examination, papilledema may be present or the disks may appear normal.

Optic neuritis in children is usually a self-limited disease, and the visual prognosis is generally favorable. If the cause can be determined, it should be treated. Systemic corticosteroid therapy has been advocated for treatment of optic neuritis, but its effectiveness has not been established.

The presence of papilledema may be a sign of increased intracranial pressure. The differentiation between optic neuritis and papilledema secondary to increased intracranial pressure is not always easy. In general, papilledema due to increased intracranial pressure does not produce a severe loss of vision, and there often are associated neurologic signs.

Kennedy C, Carrol FD: Optic neuritis in children. Tr Am Acad Ophth 64:700–712, 1960.

See Walsh & Hoyt reference, p 210.

DISEASES OF THE ORBIT

ORBITAL CELLULITIS

Orbital cellulitis is characterized by proptosis, swelling, redness, and congestion of the eyelids, orbital tissues, and bulbar conjunctiva, discomfort, and frequently fever. In children orbital cellulitis is usually due to bacterial infection. There may be associated infections elsewhere in the body, particularly in the sinuses. Treatment consists of the vigorous use of systemic antibiotics; a favorable response is usually obtained within 48–72 hours.

Howard GM: The orbit: Annual review. Arch Ophth 84:839–854, 1970.

ENDOCRINE EXOPHTHALMOS

This condition is relatively uncommon in children. It may be unilateral or bilateral. Exophthalmos is the principal presenting sign. There may be retraction of the upper lids or swelling of the lids. Injection and swelling of the conjunctiva may be present, and there may also be some extraocular muscle weakness.

Treatment consists of management of the underlying thyroid disturbance. Severe ocular involvement in the form of exposure keratitis, glaucoma, or decreased visual acuity should be treated by an ophthalmologist.

Scheie HG, Grayson MC: Ocular manifestations of systemic disease. Disease-a-Month, pp 1–9, Feb 1971.

See Howard reference, above.

ORBITAL TUMORS

Orbital tumors are rare in children. The most common primary tumors are hemangiomas, neurofibromas, gliomas of the optic nerve, dermoids, rhabdomyosarcomas, and tumors of the lacrimal gland. Neuroblastoma and lymphoma may spread into the orbit. The presenting symptoms are exophthalmos, congestion of the globe and lids, extraocular muscle weakness, and displacement of the globe. Optic nerve gliomas show enlargement of the optic foramen on x-ray examination.

Each case should be carefully evaluated. Treatment includes surgical removal, x-ray therapy, or the use of alkylating agents in certain cases. For certain benign tumors, it is often better not to attempt total removal of the lesion.

Youssefi B: Orbital tumors in children. J Pediat Ophth 6:177–181, 1969.

See Reese and Howard references, above.

DISEASES OF THE LACRIMAL APPARATUS

DACRYOSTENOSIS

In a significant number of babies the nasolacrimal duct fails to completely canalize at the time of birth;

the obstruction is usually at the nasal end of the naso-lacrimal duct. Symptoms consist of persistent tearing and often mucoid discharge in the inner corner of the eye.

Most cases subside without treatment. The obstruction usually opens spontaneously, and relief of symptoms occurs. Massage over the lacrimal sac with expression toward the nose may be helpful in establishing the patency. If a cure does not result within the first few months of life, probing of the nasolacrimal duct should be performed by an ophthalmologist.

Kohler U, Muller W: The treatment of stenoses of the lacrimal passages in infants and children. Ophthalmologica 159:136–141, 1969.
See Sexton reference, p 206.

DACRYOCYSTITIS

Dacryocystitis is usually secondary to obstruction of the nasolacrimal duct. There is resultant stasis of the tears in the sac with secondary bacterial infection. Symptoms consist of tearing and mucopurulent discharge. There may be acute inflammation in the region of the lacrimal sac. Occasionally the sac may rupture to the skin surface.

If possible, cultures should be obtained and the organism identified. For mild cases, expression of the contents of the lacrimal sac followed by instillation of topical antibiotics in the region of the lacrimal puncta may be effective. More severe cases should also be treated with systemic antibiotics. Irrigation of the canaliculi and lacrimal sac with antibiotic solution is a more successful method of delivering adequate concentrations of antibiotics to the area of infection. Once the infection has subsided, an attempt should be made to establish the passage of tears. The nasolacrimal duct should be probed under general anesthesia if the system does not permit passage of fluid irrigated through the canaliculi.

See Kohler reference, above, and Sexton reference, p 206.

DACRYOADENITIS

Inflammation of the lacrimal gland may be associated with systemic disorders such as mumps or sarcoidosis. More rarely, infections of the lacrimal gland may be secondary to tuberculosis and syphilis.

Treatment should be directed toward the specific disease, if present; otherwise, symptomatic treatment should be used. Local applications of heat or cold over the lacrimal gland may give relief. Bed rest and salicylate analgesics are also useful. Systemic corticosteroids may reduce inflammation, but the use of steroids in any viral infection is risky.

See Sexton reference, p 206.

●　　●　　●

General References

Allen JA: *May's Manual of the Diseases of the Eye,* 24th ed. Williams & Wilkins, 1968.
Duke-Elder S: *The Practice of Refraction,* 8th ed. Mosby, 1969.
Ellis PP, Smith DL: *Handbook of Ocular Therapeutics and Pharmacology,* 3rd ed. Mosby, 1969.
Havener WH: *Ocular Pharmacology,* 2nd ed. Mosby, 1970.
Hospital for Sick Children, Toronto: *The Eye in Childhood.* Year Book, 1967.
Hughes WF (editor): *Year Book of Ophthalmology.* Year Book, 1971.
Kaufman HE (editor): *Ocular Anti-inflammatory Therapy.* Thomas, 1970.
Keeney AH: *Ocular Examination: Basis and Technique.* Mosby, 1970.
Liebman SD, Gellis SS (editors): *The Pediatrician's Ophthalmology.* Mosby, 1966.
Moses RA: *Adler's Physiology of the Eye: Clinical Application,* 5th ed. Mosby, 1970.
Newell FW: *Ophthalmology: Principles and Concepts,* 2nd ed. Mosby, 1969.
Scheie HG, Albert DM: *Adler's Textbook of Ophthalmology,* 8th ed. Saunders, 1969.
Sloane AE: *Manual of Refraction,* 2nd ed. Little, Brown, 1970.
Sorsby A: *Ophthalmic Genetics,* 2nd ed. Appleton-Century-Crofts, 1970.
Vaughan D, Asbury T, Cook R: *General Ophthalmology,* 6th ed. Lange, 1971.
Walsh FB, Hoyt WF: *Clinical Neuro-ophthalmology,* 3rd ed. 3 vols. Williams & Wilkins, 1969.

10...

The Teeth

Olof H. Jacobson, DDS

The primary teeth begin to develop by the sixth week of embryonic life; the permanent teeth, by the fourth or fifth month in utero. (Table 2–13 summarizes the sequence of calcification, eruption, and shedding of the teeth.)

ERUPTION OF THE TEETH

Because eruption of teeth is an easily observable part of general growth and development, the progress of tooth eruption may serve as an indicator of the physical condition of a growing individual. Only those cases that are not within the range of normal variation or are clearly not due to a familial tendency should be considered abnormal. Retarded eruption is more frequent than accelerated eruption and may be due to local or systemic causes.

Normal Eruption

As the teeth penetrate the gums, the infant may become irritable and have increased salivation, but "teething" does not cause systemic disturbances. Bacterial invasion through a break in the tissue or under a gingival flap covering the teeth may cause inflammation. Gentle irrigation often helps to relieve inflammation around a gum flap. Gingival incision is rarely indicated. A blunt, firm object or cracked ice wrapped in soft cloth may hasten eruption and relieve pain as the child chews on it.

Abnormal Eruption

Local causes such as premature loss of primary teeth and loss of space by a shift of neighboring teeth may retard eruption or cause impaction of some permanent teeth. Construction of a space maintainer by a dentist is often indicated.

In about 4% of normal individuals, one or more permanent teeth may fail to develop. A family history of similar problems can often be elicited. The third molars are most frequently missing, followed by the upper lateral incisors and the lower second premolars. Congenital absence of teeth in the primary dentition is rare.

Supernumerary teeth appear occasionally, most often in the upper incisor area. Extraction is the treatment of choice, at the discretion of the dentist.

Natal teeth (teeth present at birth or erupting shortly thereafter) may be part of the primary dentition or may be supernumerary teeth. Ordinarily, they should be removed since they present difficulties with nursing and may irritate the infant's lips and tongue.

If a delay in eruption of the entire primary or permanent dentition is observed, hereditary, systemic, and nutritional factors should be evaluated. Hypopituitarism, hypothyroidism, cleidocranial dysostosis, and rickets must be considered. Local causes such as malposition of teeth, supernumerary teeth, cysts, or over-retained teeth may be responsible for failure of eruption of single teeth or small groups of teeth.

Early loss of primary teeth is the most common cause of premature eruption of permanent teeth. If the entire dentition is advanced, an endocrine disorder such as hyperpituitarism must be considered.

Ectopic Eruption

If the jaw size is inadequate or if a permanent tooth is out of position, a tooth may attempt to erupt into the position of its neighbor. This is most common in the upper first permanent molar and occasionally in the lower first permanent molar and the upper permanent cuspid. The molars are tipped mesially, so that they engage the second primary molar. The result is that eruption ceases or pressure resorption causes partial or complete loss of the second primary molar roots. The latter results in premature loss of the primary tooth, which could lead to subsequent impaction of the succedaneous premolar when its time to erupt comes. The dentist can often correct the path of eruption of the permanent tooth and guide it into proper position. If the primary tooth is lost, a space maintainer or space regainer should be placed. Maxillary cuspids frequently tend to erupt in improper position, resulting in pressure resorption of the roots of adjacent teeth or malocclusion. Visits to the pedodontist (at intervals specified by him) and appropriately timed x-ray examination and orthodontic consultation can frequently prevent or minimize problems arising from ectopic eruption.

IMPACTIONS

Impactions are teeth which are so closely lodged in the alveolar bone that they are unable to erupt.

Common usage has applied the term to any tooth which remains within its alveolus and does not erupt. Although there are hereditary patterns leading to impacted teeth, the causative factors of most concern are prolonged retention of primary teeth, localized pathologic lesions, and shortening of the length of the arch.

The teeth most commonly involved are the third molars and maxillary cuspids. Impacted third molars should be removed early, when surgery is less traumatic and healing is more rapid. Because of their anterior position in the mouth, surgery and orthodontics are required both for aesthetic and functional reasons in the case of maxillary cuspids.

The possible formation of dentigerous cysts is the most serious consequence of failure to remove impacted teeth, although pain and malocclusion may also result.

NORMAL OCCLUSION

Normal (class I) occlusion is defined as the circumstance wherein the mesio-buccal cusp of the upper first permanent molar occludes in the buccal groove of the lower first permanent molar. The 3 broad classifications of occlusion are illustrated in Fig 10—1.

Class II occlusion presents a retrognathic posture, whereas class III occlusion causes prognathism. There are several subclassifications, but these are of most interest to the orthodontist. In addition, in normal occlusion, the lower teeth occlude lingually to the uppers.

MALOCCLUSION

Malocclusion may be the result of genetic factors causing abnormal dimensional discrepancies between the jaws and teeth; premature loss of primary or permanent teeth; harmful oral habits such as thumb or finger sucking or tongue thrusting; or "pillowing" (pressure induced by habitually sleeping on the stomach or supporting the head with the hand or fist). If bad habits can be controlled by age 4 or 5 years, physiologic growth may correct malocclusions due to this cause.

Prevention

Speech therapists can sometimes establish normal swallowing habits, eliminating tongue thrust. Thumb or finger sucking is often outgrown. It was once thought that the child was comforted by sucking and that it should be ignored since he might develop more pernicious habits or sustain psychologic trauma if made to stop. Dentists are now beginning to feel that these habits should be stopped early. The trauma to a 5- or 6-year-old child from being deprived of the comfort of sucking is considered to be less than the trauma to a teen-ager wearing orthodontic appliances as he undergoes the changes of puberty—not to mention the cost of orthodontic treatment. Sucking often occurs when the child is bored or tired or has nothing else to do with his hands, as when watching television. The dentist may construct a "crib" to be inserted in the mouth which breaks the suction seal or reminds the child that he is sucking. Mittens or bitter chemicals may be helpful, although eye contamination with chemicals may be dangerous or painful. Constant reminders by siblings or parents or appeals to the child's vanity are often successful.

Habits contributing to malocclusion must be eliminated before orthodontic therapy can be successful.

Treatment

Orthodontic treatment is usually most successful when started at about the time the last primary teeth are shed and before growth ceases, ie, in the early teens. In extreme cases, early consultation—when the permanent incisors and molars are starting to erupt—is advisable.

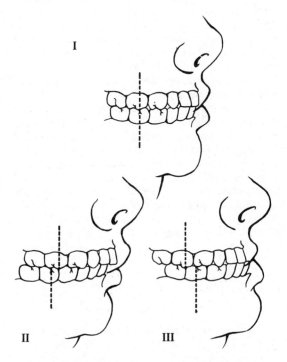

FIG 10—1. Types of occlusions.

DENTAL CARIES

Dental caries is one of the most common chronic diseases of man, occurring in over 50% of 3-year-olds

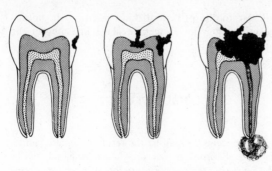

FIG 10–2. Types of caries.

and almost all adults. It has been defined as a disease of the calcified tissues of the teeth which is characterized by destruction beginning on the surface of the tooth in areas of predeliction and progressing inward toward the pulp. The destruction involves (1) decalcification of the inorganic portion and (2) disintegration of the organic substance of the tissue. The decalcification is caused by acids resulting from the action of acidogenic bacteria on refined carbohydrates, particularly sucrose. Three factors are necessary for the development of caries: a tooth, bacteria, and dental plaque.

Three groups of bacteria play a role in producing dental decay: (1) Acidogenic and aciduric organisms, which produce the acids upon the tooth surface necessary to decalcify the hard tissues. *Lactobacillus acidophilus* and certain streptococci are encountered most frequently. (2) Proteolytic organisms which digest the organic matrix after decalcification. (3) Leptotrichia and leptothrix, which form plaques on the smooth surface of the teeth, thus serving to harbor and protect the other organisms; these bacteria are thought to play no primary role in the production of decay.

Two processes are always operating on the enamel surfaces: acid production by bacteria and acid neutralization by the saliva. The rate of acid formation is of importance in caries susceptibility. In some individuals, acid is formed so rapidly that the buffering action of saliva cannot neutralize it. The effectiveness of the buffering action also seems to vary in different individuals.

In certain systemic conditions—and possibly in some emotional states—the quality and quantity of saliva may be altered. This in turn may result in an increase in caries activity. Children and adults suffering from chronic debilitating diseases often show an increase in caries activity. The arrangement of teeth in the arch, their anatomy, and dietary factors may also contribute to the development of caries.

A genetic factor directly related to caries resistance has been established in laboratory animals. In humans, protection from caries seems to be a familial characteristic—as does increased susceptibility also.

Prevention

Dental caries can be controlled in most instances by the following measures:

(1) Frequent observation by a dentist, starting when all of the primary teeth have erupted or at least by age 3. The frequency should be determined by the dentist, depending on the individual child.

(2) Removal of all active decay as soon as detected.

(3) Thorough cleansing of the teeth and rinsing of the mouth after each meal and after between-meal snacks. In the event that brushing is impossible, vigorous rinsing is advisable.

(4) Elimination of all concentrated sugars between meals and keeping the ingestion of sweets at mealtimes to a minimum. Carbohydrates, particularly in forms which cling (taffy, caramels) or have prolonged contact (hard candy, suckers, chewing gum) provide an ideal substrate for the production of tooth-destroying acids by bacteria. Excessive ingestion of sweetened soft drinks and juices can also be harmful. Sugars ingested at mealtimes are less harmful since the acid is buffered by other foods and saliva. The pediatrician should never give candy or gum to his patients as a reward. Inexpensive toys or rings provide a welcome and noncariogenic substitute.

(5) Provision of adequate roughage in the diet for its detergent effect. Such foods as apples, raw carrots, and celery tend to cleanse the surfaces of the teeth as they are masticated. Small children should not be allowed to fall asleep with a bottle of milk or to hold one in the mouth for prolonged periods during the day. A recognizable caries pattern of the primary dentition can often be related to this practice.

(6) Application of topical fluorides, except in areas where fluoride is already present in large amounts (over 3–4 ppm) in the community water supply. Fluoridation of the community water supply is the most effective preventive measure against dental caries, especially from birth to age 10–12. Children born and raised in an area where the water contains 1–1.5 ppm fluoride have 60% less decay than children in areas where the fluoride content is low.

(7) The use of fluoridated toothpastes. The ADA Council on Dental Therapeutics has classified Crest toothpaste (stannous fluoride) and Colgate Dental Cream (monofluorophosphate) in group A, which consists of accepted products which will be listed in Accepted Dental Remedies. Certain other fluoridated toothpastes have been classified in group B, indicating that there is not sufficient evidence to justify present acceptance but that there is reasonable evidence of their usefulness and safety.

PREVENTIVE DENTISTRY

An exciting application of the foregoing is being incorporated into many dental practices today.

Under the supervision of the dentist, trained auxiliary personnel are instructing the patient and the parent in the proper methods of toothbrushing and flossing. Disclosing wafers and solutions containing erythrosine are used to reveal plaque deposits and debris that have been missed by ineffective or non-existent brushing. An explanation of the role of plaque and bacteria in decay and periodontal disease and the importance of oral health to the overall health of the individual is also provided. Cultures of saliva reveal the presence of high bacterial counts which correlate with a high incidence of caries.

Many dentists are also providing nutritional counseling, evaluating the patient's diet and suggesting a more healthy, balanced diet which will improve general health. The use of visual aids and regular return visits are proving that dentistry now has the knowledge to provide a truly preventive service.

The pediatrician can contribute to his patient's oral and general health by (1) recommending early and regular visits to the dentist, (2) acquainting himself with normal and abnormal eruption, occlusion, and tooth form and number, and (3) learning the implications of various soft tissue lesions.

While fewer specific preventive measures are available to the dentist as compared to the physician, increased demand for oral health through education and prepaid dental plans can conceivably lead to a significant reduction in oral disease. Dental research is revealing methods which, with patient cooperation, can achieve this end.

ACCIDENTS TO THE TEETH

Trauma to the teeth may result in fractures of varying degrees of severity. Damaged teeth should be treated by the dentist as soon after the accident as possible to minimize the possibility of loss of tooth vitality and thus avoid the later need for pulpotomy (on primary teeth) or endodontic procedures (on permanent teeth). Loosened teeth will frequently stabilize and survive if they are repositioned and splinted.

Evulsed teeth should be kept moist and handled very carefully until they can be replanted and stabilized. The patient or the parent should be encouraged to replant the tooth as soon as possible, since time is the most important factor in survival. The tooth should be rinsed gently before replantation so as not to remove remnants of the adhering periodontal membrane.

Endodontic therapy is always necessary in the case of an evulsed tooth, and tetanus immunization and antibiotic therapy (penicillin) are usually advisable, especially if the teeth have become contaminated while out of the mouth. The prognosis for replantation of evulsed permanent teeth depends on the time elapsed before replantation and the degree to which closure of the root apex has progressed. If these teeth are retained for 6–8 years (until the growth of the jaws is completed), more effective and aesthetic pros-

thetic devices can be employed. Loss of teeth in the young child adversely affects the development of proper occlusion.

If trauma causes intrusion of the teeth, primary treatment should be directed toward treatment of the soft tissues. Intruded teeth usually reerupt within a month. Most will be retained but will become nonvital, and some will be shed prematurely. Intrusion of primary teeth may cause moderate to severe damage to the developing permanent tooth.

STAINING OF THE TEETH

Hemolytic disease of the newborn may be followed by yellow-green to black staining of enamel and dentin and hypoplasia of the enamel of the primary teeth.

Tetracyclines administered to women in the third trimester of pregnancy, to nursing mothers, or to the infant or child during the period of tooth formation may cause yellow-gray, bright yellow, gray-brown, or dark brown discoloration of teeth forming at the time of exposure to the drug. Under ultraviolet light a yellow to yellow-brown fluorescence is noted, peaking at 340–370 nm.

Mottled enamel is found in persons whose tooth-formative years are spent in an area where the fluoride content of the drinking water is greater than 2 ppm. Mottling varies from small whitish spots to severe brownish discoloration and hypoplasia if the fluoride concentration is greater than 5 ppm.

There are many other varieties of staining, extrinsic and intrinsic, involving a great variety of agents and causes.

DISEASES & DISORDERS OF THE ORAL SOFT TISSUES

Periodontitis

Periodontitis is rare in children. It should alert the clinician to its systemic implications.

Hypophosphatasia, cyclic neutropenia, histiocytosis X, leukemia, scurvy, and vitamin D deficiency should be suspected when periodontal destruction occurs in children.

Children with Down's syndrome are extremely prone to develop periodontitis. Scrupulous home care (brushing) and, occasionally, ascorbic acid therapy (100–300 mg/day) seem to be useful. In spite of all measures, some of these children inevitably lose their teeth to periodontal disease.

Gingivitis

A distressingly high percentage of children exhibit the simple forms of gingivitis which involve the marginal gingivas and interdental papillae. Instruction in good oral hygiene and eating habits will usually eliminate the symptoms in young children and decrease the number of teeth lost to more severe forms of periodontal disease in later life.

Gingival Enlargement

Painless hyperplasia of the entire gingiva, sometimes so extensive that the teeth are entirely covered, may occur after prolonged administration of diphenylhydantoin. The degree of enlargement seems to be related directly to oral hygiene. Therapy should be directed toward improved home care. The tissue may be removed surgically but will almost always recur unless another drug is substituted or scrupulous care of the mouth is maintained.

Necrotizing Ulcerative Gingivitis

This disease goes by many names—NUG, trench mouth, Vincent's infection, fusospirochetal gingivitis, ulcero-membranous gingivitis, etc. It is an acute gingival inflammation characterized by red, swollen gingivas, necrosis beginning in the interdental papilla and extending along the gingival margins, pain, hemorrhage, a necrotic odor, and, often, a pseudomembrane. The tongue may be coated, and salivary flow increases. The mucosa may become involved. It may occur as a response to many factors, including poor mouth hygiene, inadequate diet and sleep, and various other diseases such as mononucleosis, nonspecific viral infections, bacterial infections, oral thrush, blood dyscrasias, and diabetes mellitus. The presence of fusiform and spiral organisms is of no importance as they occur in about 1/3 of clinically normal mouths and are absent in some cases of necrotizing ulcerative gingivitis.

Management depends upon ruling out underlying systemic factors and treating the signs and symptoms as indicated with systemic antibiotics (penicillin), oxygenating mouth rinses, analgesics, rest, and appropriate dietary measures. The patient should be referred to a dentist for gentle, thorough cleansing of the teeth. It is extremely doubtful that the disease is communicable.

Herpetic Infection

Herpetic gingivitis results from infection of the gums with herpes simplex virus. Primary infection usually occurs in childhood. The disease is manifested by red, swollen, tender gingivas and oral mucosa without necrosis of the interdental papillae or gingival margins. The lips are usually swollen and dry. Localized herpetic lesions may be present. The disease is highly infectious and may be mistaken for necrotizing ulcerative gingivitis. The absence of a fetid odor, the lack of gingival necrosis, and the presence of a high temperature in the herpetic infection are the chief differential points. The disease runs its course in about 2 weeks.

Herpetic stomatitis is a vesicular disease of the mouth caused by herpes simplex virus. The term is also used for the secondarily infected ulcerations that follow the vesicles. The lesions have also been called **aphthae**, canker sores, and dyspeptic ulcers. Once a patient has had primary herpetic gingivostomatitis (see above), the virus remains in the cells, apparently without attacking the host. Whenever host resistance is lowered by trauma, infection, menstruation, allergy or sensitivity, psychic factors, or dietary deficiencies, the virus becomes active. The first lesion is the vesicle, but inside the mouth it soon ruptures and becomes secondarily infected. The typical lesion has a yellow, ulcerated center, a bright-red areola, is very painful, and heals in about 10–14 days. Several lesions may coalesce.

Classically, these lesions have been treated by caustics such as phenol, silver nitrate, chromic acid, and alum. These delay healing, although they do cauterize nerve endings and relieve pain. For solitary lesions, tetracycline pastes have proved effective in reducing secondary infection, relieving pain, and hastening healing.

PULPITIS

Pulpitis may be acute or chronic. It may be caused by infection or by physical, thermal, chemical, or electrical trauma. Pulpal invasion by mixed bacteria from the oral cavity is the most common cause. The invading bacteria are usually streptococci or staphylococci, although other forms of bacteria and fungi or viruses may be active causes. When the bacteria enter a tooth from the blood stream after they are attracted to a pulp injured by operative trauma, heat, or other noninfectious causes, the resulting pulpitis is termed anachoretic pulpitis.

Acute Pulpitis

The pulp shows dilatation of blood vessels and cellular infiltration. PMNs predominate and may be in abscess form or diffusely distributed. In its early phases, severe paroxysms of pain occur, often spontaneously and at night. Initially, cold will elicit pain; as the pulpitis passes its earliest phases, heat will cause pain. The tooth responds to the electric pulp tester at lower than average levels early in the disease and to higher levels in later phases. In these earlier phases, the patient can locate the offending tooth. As the pulpitis becomes more severe and extensive, the pain is agonizing, lancinating, and radiating. The application of heat causes excruciating pain which may be partially relieved by tepid or cool water. The pain may be referred to other regions of the face, and the patient cannot locate the tooth and may not even be able to localize the pain to one general region of the jaw. An incisional opening into the pulp may permit the escape of pus and bring immediate relief. Acute pulpitis may cause fever, headache, and malaise.

Acute pulpitis may be resolved if well localized and treated by removing its cause and applying obtundents (eg, eugenol) or, in selected cases by pulpotomy and use of agents such as calcium hydroxide. It may become chronic, or the pulp may become necrotic. In most instances, removal of the pulp or of the tooth is the treatment of choice. Acute pulpitis may lead to periapical inflammation.

Chronic Pulpitis

In chronic pulpitis the pulp shows dilatation of vessels and infiltration by plasma cells and lymphocytes. There are often no symptoms, but at times there may be a dull throbbing pain when the subject lies down or takes hot foods. The tooth usually responds slowly to cold and to electric pulp tests. The application of heat may elicit pain. Pain may be referred. Occasionally, the patient may remember having an acute pain (at the time of acute pulpitis). Chronic pulpitis may progress and necrosis ensue without causing any symptoms. It may act as a source of bacteria or toxins which may spread to remote areas of the body. Any search for possible foci should include tests for chronic as well as for acute pulpitis.

Chronic pulpitis may become acute, or the pulp may become necrotic or calcify. Chronic pulpitis does not usually resolve without treatment, although it could conceivably repair itself with no symptoms ever giving a clue to its presence.

Treatment is by pulp extirpation, apicoectomy, or extraction as determined by local, general, and socioeconomic factors.

PERIAPICAL PATHOSIS

The periapical tissue may become inflamed as a consequence of pulpitis, trauma (a blow, or occlusal or habitual trauma), or injury caused by drugs used in endodontic therapy. Following traumatic or chemical injury, bacteria may become localized from the blood stream by anachoresis. The periapical region may be resorbed or sclerosed with or without inflammation.

Acute Periapical Periodontitis

Also referred to as dento-alveolar abscess, this condition begins when infection from the pulp reaches the periodontal membrane or when the membrane is injured by other means. The severity of the injury (or virulence of the organisms) and the resistance of the tissue will determine whether the inflammation is acute or chronic. A chronic periapical inflammation may become acute, and vice versa. If the inflammation progresses, an abscess forms and the surrounding bone may begin to resorb. The inflammation spreads into the bone marrow. For these reasons, periapical periodontitis is a periostitis, an osteitis, and a focal osteomyelitis.

As a result of edema, the tooth is elevated in its socket. The tooth is sore to percussion, and the patient attempts to limit mastication on the side of the jaw involved. Pain on percussion is the most reliable sign. If the inflammation is due to trauma, relieving the traumatic cause may permit resolution of the inflammation. If infection is present, drainage is essential. Drainage may be accomplished by endodontic therapy, incision, or extraction. If infection is not treated, it may progress to form a distinct dentoperiosteal abscess. At this stage, there is pulsation and severe pain, which is increased on pressure. The patient attempts to keep the teeth out of occlusion. Opening of the pulp canal or extraction of the tooth permits the escape of yellow, creamy pus. The patient feels almost immediate relief, and the condition may resolve or become chronic in a short time.

Fistula

If no treatment is given for infected periapical periodontitis, the infection spreads. In about 3–5 days, the infection will point to as far as the cortical layer of bone, the bone is perforated, and a subperiosteal abscess forms. If the abscess is located subgingivally, it forms a parulis ("gum boil"). These subperiosteal abscesses give rise to a new series of painful symptoms until they rupture and evacuate. One sign of periapical periodontitis is redness, swelling, and tenderness over the root in the labial or buccal region.

When the periosteum and overlying skin or mucosa are penetrated, the abscess evacuates, the patient has relief, and acute symptoms subside. The fistula through which the abscess drained may form at various places opening onto the gingiva (Fig 10–3), the palate, or the skin. Drainage into the mouth is more common than through the skin. In the case of upper posterior teeth, the fistula may occasionally go into the maxillary sinus.

Acute dento-alveolar abscess is often accompanied by cellulitis of the face. If the cause is removed (infected tooth or pulp), the cellulitis usually subsides and the periapical lesion may heal by granulation. The use of local or systemic broad spectrum antibiotics may be necessary to promote healing. Without treatment, the infection may spread, resulting in osteitis or

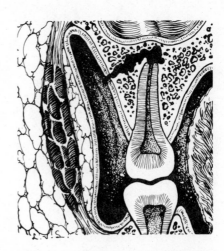

FIG 10–3. Fistula to buccal gingiva.

osteomyelitis, Ludwig's angina, cavernous sinus thrombosis, general toxicity, and possibly death. Infection may become chronic and remain as a potential source of future acute attacks and of toxins and bacteria.

Treatment is directed at removal of the cause, aiding the tissue in its inflammatory response, and minimizing chemical (drug) injury.

•   •   •

General References

Bernier JL, Muhler JC: *Improving Dental Practice Through Preventive Measures,* 2nd ed. Mosby, 1970.

Hirschfeld L, Geiger A: *Minor Tooth Movement in General Practice,* 2nd ed. Mosby, 1966.

Massler M, Schour I: *Atlas of the Mouth and Adjacent Parts in Health and Disease.* American Dental Association, 1958.

Moyer RE: *Handbook of Orthodontics,* 2nd ed. Year Book, 1963.

11...

Ear, Nose, & Throat

Marlin Weaver, MD, & Marion P. Downs, MA

HEARING

PHYSIOLOGY OF HEARING

The special sense of hearing is the result of a series of events beginning with atmospheric radiation and ending with the delivery of nerve impulses to the transverse gyrus of the temporal lobe. Sound energy consists of compressions and rarefactions of an elastic medium, usually air. This force impinges on the tympanic membrane and is relayed by the ossicular chain to the oval window. The tympanic membrane and ossicular chain amplify sound by 2 simple mechanical principles: that of the piston (surface area of the tympanic membrane versus surface area of the stapes footplate) and that of the lever (length of the malleus versus length of the incus). Defects in these structures produce losses in hearing acuity.

The motion of the stapes footplate in the oval window produces motion in the fluid-filled cochlea. Cochlear fluids fill 2 tubular structures: the scala vestibuli and the scala tympani. These parallel scalae are in open communication with each other at the apex of the 2½ turns of the cochlea. When a sound vibration displaces the stapes inward into the scala vestibuli, a simultaneous outward motion occurs in the scala tympani at the round window membrane. For example, when the fundamental frequency of the tone of middle C is sounded, the stapes moves in and out 256 times per second and there is a reciprocal 256 cps motion at the round window.

The vibratory fluid motion is transformed into a nerve impulse by the cochlear neural epithelium acting as a mechanical transducer. The cochlear neural epithelium is composed of approximately 25,000 hair cells arranged in 4 rows and housed in a third fluid-filled duct, the scala media. The scala media is interposed between the scala vestibuli and the scala tympani throughout the 2½ cochlear turns, and its fluid is isolated from that of the other 2 ducts. The hair cells rest on the membranous wall separating the scala media from the scala tympani. The peripheral processes of the cochlear nerve are distributed to the hair cells. The fluid motion in the scala tympani displaces the membrane on which the hair cells rest. This displacement produces torsion of the hair-like processes of the cells, and the torsion stimulates the nerve endings. Thus, the vibratory energy that impinged on the stapes at the oval window is transformed into a nerve impulse.

The peripheral processes of the cochlear nerve carry the nerve impulse to the spiral ganglion cells which are housed in the cone-like center of the cochlea (modiolus). The central processes of these cell bodies leave the base of the modiolus and make up the cochlear portion of the eighth cranial nerve. The cochlear nerve traverses the internal auditory meatus to enter the dorsal surface of the pons in the area of the fourth ventricle. Its fibers are distributed to dorsal and ventral cochlear nuclei. Ascending fibers then reach the inferior colliculus and the medial geniculate body. From these 2 centers, third-order neurons are distributed to the temporal lobe.

MEASUREMENT OF HEARING

Hearing is customarily measured by means of an audiometer—an instrument that produces pure tones of various frequencies and intensities. The individual's threshold for hearing at each frequency is charted on a graph called an audiogram (Figs 11–1 and 11–2). The unit of measurement for determining hearing level is the decibel ("db"), represented on the vertical line, or ordinate, of the audiogram. The top line, or "0 db," represents average normal hearing at all frequencies; 100 db of intensity represents total loss of hearing at all frequencies. The frequencies tested include 250 cps ("middle C") and the octave intervals of 500, 1000, 2000, 4000, and 8000 cps.

Key: Air: Solid line		Bone: Dotted line
R: O——O		R: >--->
L: X——X		L: <---<

Air conduction testing is done by placing an oscillator driven earphone over the external ear. A threshold of response is determined for the various frequencies. This test represents a response of the entire auditory system and thereby reflects the total amount of hearing loss without reference to the site of pathology. A second test, known as bone conduction testing, is done by placing an oscillator on the skull and setting

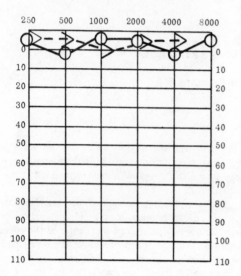

FIG 11−1. Normal audiogram, air and bone conduction, right ear.

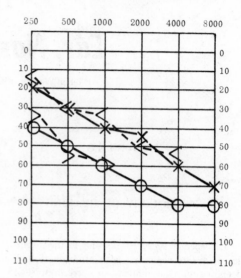

FIG 11−2. Averaging of hearing levels. Average loss, 500−2000. Right: 60 db. Left: 38 db.

it in vibration. The tone in this case stimulates the hair cells directly by the inertial lag of the cochlear fluids, thereby bypassing the middle ear transducers. The threshold in this case reflects the function of the cochlea and the structures central to it.

The important frequency range for hearing speech is the 500−2000 cps range on the audiogram. For this reason, the 3 frequencies 500, 1000, and 2000 cps are commonly averaged to give a single measure of hearing level. An average level of 0−15 db* is considered within normal range for the hearing of speech; beyond 15 db average loss, the individual will begin to have difficulty in understanding speech.

In general, any child with an average hearing level of 15 db or greater should be considered for educational rehabilitation (lip reading, auditory training, speech therapy), preferential seating, or even hearing aid use.

House HP, Linthicum FH Jr, Johnson EW: Current management of hearing loss in children. Am J Dis Child 108:677−696, 1964.

TESTING THE HEARING
OF INFANTS & CHILDREN

With the introduction of sophisticated instrumentation, **hearing losses in children can now be identified and accurately measured at any age.** The younger the child, of course, the more specialized the instrumenta-

*References in this chapter to db levels refer to the American Standards Association, 1951, Reference Level.

tion (and examiner) must be. Gross screening tests may be done in the office or nursery to identify suspected hearing loss; definitive diagnostic follow-up testing is then carried out in the audiology laboratory.

Screening tests for hearing should be done at birth and at all subsequent examinations during the first year so that a hearing loss can be identified before the child is a year old. Ideally, rehabilitation should be begun by 6 months of age so that critical periods for the development of auditory perceptions will not be exceeded. The kinds of tests that can be done in nurseries and in offices to identify hearing losses are outlined below.

Infants at Birth

One method of screening at birth or shortly thereafter utilizes an acoustic signal centering around 3000 cps at 90 db **SPL** (sound pressure level) output. Several instruments have been developed to produce such a signal. The specificity of the signal makes it possible to differentiate from normal hearing those hearing losses that are greater in the high than in the low frequencies. (Figs 11−7, 11−8, and 11−9.)

Normal responses to such signals can easily be observed. They have been categorized as follows: (1) Eye-blink, or auro-palpebral reflex. (2) Moro's reflex, or startle response. (3) Arousal response (eye-opening, limb movements, stirring). (4) Head turn. (5) Sucking activity. (6) Cessation of movement or vocalization.

Observation of these responses can be made not only by physicians and nurses but also by trained volunteer workers or aides. Because a casefinding incidence of only one in 2000 can be expected, this kind of mass screening testing lends itself well to volunteer assistance.

TABLE 11-1. Auditory behavior index up to age 2.*

Age	Acoustic Signal	Mean Signal Strength for Age	Expected Response	Level at Which Subject Listens to or Localizes Measured Speech	Startle to Voice
0-6 weeks	3000 cps	78 db (depending on environment noise). Range: 72-84 db.†	Eye blink, Moro, eye shift or widening, cessation of activity.	...	65 db
	Handclap, horn, "kissing sound"	?	As above		
6 weeks-3¾ months	3000 cps	70 db. Range: 60-80 db.	Eye blink, quieting, rudimentary head turn.	47 db. Range: 45-50 db.	65 db
	Noisemaker, rattle, horn, squeeze toy, bell‡	?	As above		
4-6¾ months	3000 cps	51 db. Range: 40-60 db.	"Listening," head turn on lateral plane and beginning localizing below the ear. §	21 db. Range: 13-29 db.	65 db
	Noisemaker	?	As above		
7-8¾ months	3000 cps	45 db. Range: 30-60 db.	Localization on lateral plane: directly to below ear level, indirectly to above.	15 db. Range: 7.5-22.5 db.	65 db
	Noisemaker	?	As above		
9-12¾ months	3000 cps	38 db. Range: 20-50 db.	Localization directly on lateral and lower plane, and directly above ear level.	8 db. Range: 1-15 db.	65 db
	Noisemaker	?	As above		
13-15¾ months	3000 cps	32 db. Range: 22-42 db.	Direct localization on all planes.	5 db. Range: 0-10 db.	65 db
	Noisemaker	?	As above		
16-20¾ months	3000 cps	25 db. Range: 15-35 db.	Direct localization on all planes.	5 db. Range: 4-6 db.	65 db
	Noisemaker	?	As above		
21-24 months	3000 cps	26 db. Range: 16-36 db.	Direct localization on all planes.	3 db. Range: 1-6 db.	65 db

*These measurements have been made under structured, quiet conditions, not necessarily in soundproof rooms.
†Standard deviations have been used to calculate the range of responses around the mean that can be expected. This means that 66 2/3% of subjects this age can be expected to respond within the range shown.
‡Hardy JB, Dougherty A, Hardy WG: Hearing responses and audiologic screening in infants. J Pediat 55:382-390, 1959.
§Murphy KP: Development of hearing in babies. Child & Family, April, 1962.

If an infant fails to respond to such measurable acoustic signals, follow-up observations and testing should be done. Table 11-1 shows the kinds of responses that can be expected from children at various ages. A variety of noisemakers can be used for testing, but will not differentiate all hearing losses as well as a specific signal.

If an infant persistently fails to respond to acoustic stimuli, clinical testing is required. It is now possible to identify the exact extent of hearing loss in infants through the use of evoked responses of the EEG used in connection with summing computers. Audiology centers which employ this technic are located throughout the USA and are usually found in conjunction with audiologic rehabilitation services.

Bergstrom L, Hemenway WG, Downs M: A high risk registry to find congenital deafness. Otol Clin North America 4:369-399, 1971.
Downs M: Audiological evaluation of the congenitally deaf infant. Otol Clin North America 4:347-358, 1971.

Infants Age 3 Months to 2 Years

By 3 months of age the infant begins to orient to sound by means of a rudimentary searching movement of the head and eyes. In the normal infant this orientation matures rapidly, until by 6 months he is able to turn directly to a soft sound and fix the source with his eyes. The measured acoustic signals described above can be used to stimulate this searching activity. In addition, procedures have been filmed that utilize noisemakers to test the orienting ability of the infant.

Failure to respond in the manner shown on the auditory behavior index (Table 11–1) should arouse a suspicion of hearing loss or of central auditory problems. Referral should be made to an auditory center where facilities and personnel are available to make a differential diagnosis.

Nebraska Educational Television Council for Higher Education: *Auditory Screening of Infants.* 1971. [Film. Available from 1203 Seaton Hall, University of Nebraska, Lincoln.]

Children Age 2 & Older

By the age of 2 years it is possible to elicit voluntary responses from children that will accurately identify the degree of impairment. Audiometric screening can be performed in the office using play conditioning technics with children ages 2–5 and finger raising technics for children age 5 and older.

(1) **Play conditioning procedure:** Place the earphones on the child, telling him that this is a telephone and he is going to hear some telephone bells. Whenever he hears a bell, he is to place a peg in a peg-board, put an animal in a farm, place a block on a block tower, etc. To demonstrate, put the peg or toy in his hand; put his hand up to the earphone; and, when the tone is presented, help him to carry out the instructions. The tone should be loud enough for him to hear (50 db, if no hearing loss seems evident; louder, if a loss is suspected). After a few such conditioning trials, let the child respond to the tone by himself. Once this conditioning has been established, reduce the intensity of the tone to 30 db and then to 10 db, instructing him to listen for a tiny bell this time. If he hears the tone at 10 db, this is sufficient hearing for social and educational purposes. The frequencies 500 cps, 1000 cps, and 2000 cps should be tested, as these constitute the important range of intelligibility for speech. The 10 db level of hearing does not guarantee that no ear pathology is present, and only a careful otoscopic examination will determine the condition of the ear.

If an audiometer is not available, a gross screening test can be given with noisemakers. However, noisemakers do not identify high tone hearing losses; only specific pure tone signals can rule out such losses.

(2) **Finger raising procedure:** For the child age 5 and older, the standard procedure is to ask him to raise his finger whenever he hears the tone. Care should be taken to avoid establishing a rhythm in his responses and to guard against erroneous responses in an effort to please.

If there is any question about the child's hearing level, he should be referred for threshold audiometric testing to an audiology laboratory. There he will be given air conduction and bone conduction tests to determine the presence or absence of an air-bone gap; speech reception tests to determine his ability to hear

and understand speech; and EEG testing if indicated. If the degree of loss is great enough, a specific hearing aid will be recommended. In this case, it is of utmost importance that a course in hearing aid orientation and training be given. The child must be guided in making an adjustment to the aid, and the parents must also be given instructions in home care and use of the aid.

Davis H: The young deaf child: Identification and management. Acta oto-laryng (Suppl) 206:1–258, 1964.

Division of Maternal & Child Health: *Auditory Screening for Infants.* Maryland State Department of Health, 1958.

Downs MP, Sterritt G: Identification audiometry in neonates: A preliminary report. J Audio Res 4:69–80, 1964.

Downs MP, Sterritt G: A guide to newborn testing. Arch Otolaryng 85:15–22, 1967.

McCandless GA, Best L: Summed evoked responses using pure tone stimuli. J Speech Hearing Res 9:266–272, 1966.

Nebraska Educational Television Council for Higher Education: *Auditory Screening of Infants.* 1971. [Film. Available from 1203 Seaton Hall, University of Nebraska, Lincoln.]

TYPES OF HEARING LOSS

Three kinds of hearing losses are identified by audiometric testing: conductive, sensorineural, and mixed.

1. CONDUCTIVE HEARING LOSS

Interference of any sort in the transmission of sound from the external meatus to the inner ear causes a conductive hearing loss. The hair cells of the cochlea are intact, but the sound does not reach them at normal loudness levels. The resulting audiogram is shown in Fig 11–3.

When the conductive impairment is complete, as in atresia, stenosis, complete stapes fixation, and ossicular discontinuity, the audiogram will resemble that shown in Fig 11–4. The greatest possible difference that can occur between air conduction and bone conduction is 60 db.

It should be noted that ear disease may also be present when the air conduction thresholds are normal. Therefore, careful otologic examination is always indicated before ear pathology can be ruled out. For example, chronic serous otitis media is commonly accompanied by normal air conduction thresholds. If bone conduction thresholds are taken, however, a significant air-bone gap (difference between air conduction and bone conduction thresholds) may be shown; young children can be expected to have better than normal thresholds, and the presence of normal hearing by air conduction does not rule out a significant air-bone gap.

In chronic serous otitis media, it is possible to have an audiogram as in Fig 11–5.

2. SENSORINEURAL HEARING LOSS

Dysgenesis, deterioration, or damage to the hair cells results in a sensory impairment; when the dysfunction occurs farther along the eighth nerve pathway, it is a neural impairment. However, the exact location of the lesion is not always known, and any hearing loss that occurs in the cochlea or beyond is therefore called a sensorineural loss. In sensorineural loss the air conduction and bone conduction thresholds are the same. Such a loss is usually greater in the high than in the low frequencies (Fig 11–6).

However, a variety of configurations are found in sensorineural losses (Figs 11–8 and 11–9).

3. MIXED HEARING LOSS

When both a conductive and a sensorineural loss are present, the result is a mixed hearing loss. The resultant audiogram shows the effect of both types of pathology, and the loss is additive. (Sensorineural component plus conductive component = air conduction thresholds.) Any of the lesions responsible for a conductive loss and for a sensorineural loss, when active concurrently, result in a mixed hearing loss.

Jordan RE, Eagles EL: The relation of air conduction audiometry to otological abnormalities. Ann Otol Rhin Laryng 70:819–827, 1961.

DISORDERS ASSOCIATED WITH HEARING LOSS

STENOSIS & ATRESIA OF THE EXTERNAL AUDITORY CANAL

Stenosis of the external auditory canal may occur as a congenital anomaly or may be due to chronic infection. A narrowed canal does not readily eliminate keratin debris and cerumen in the normal way. Periodic aspiration will often suffice to maintain patency; however, surgical enlargement of the canal is sometimes warranted.

Atresia of the external auditory canal may be a congenital malformation or may result from surgical misadventure. In either case, surgical repair is difficult but usually successful, and simultaneous middle ear reconstruction is usually required. In considering whether surgery should be performed, it should be remembered that these children can hear adequately with the help of a bone conduction hearing aid and that no retardation or handicap need ensue if surgery is refused.

OTITIS EXTERNA

Dermatitis of the external ear canal may result from infection with gram-positive and gram-negative organisms (seldom from fungi). A circumstance favorable for infection commonly results from the presence of water deep in the canal against the tympanic membrane. The resultant softening and maceration of the skin provides a suitable environment for bacterial growth. Swelling, pain, and accumulation of cellular debris result. The disease may be further manifested by involvement of the pinna and the regional lymph nodes.

Treatment includes repeated, careful debridement with a suction tip. Burow's solution is applied via a cotton wick placed in the canal to reduce the swelling. After 2–3 days of such treatment, antimicrobial drops may be directly introduced. Satisfactory preparations include various combinations of polymyxin, neomycin, the colistins, and similar topical anti-infective agents. Systemic antibiotics chosen on the basis of culture and sensitivity studies should be used also in cases in which the regional lymph nodes are involved.

Otitis externa. Brit MJ 1:70–71, 1969.

CERUMEN

Cerumen is a combined product of the apocrine and sebaceous glands that protects the ear canal by its adhesive and emollient properties. Massive accumulation causes hearing loss only when it completely occludes the canal or when it has been displaced from the external portion of the canal to press against the tympanic membrane.

Cerumen can be removed with an open head otoscope and a large speculum. The thicker tissue of the posterior and superior portion of the canal will allow the introduction of a curet beyond the mass. For cerumen of softer consistency, an aspirating tip may be more satisfactory. The canal may be irrigated with water if the tympanic membrane is known to be intact. If necessary, glycerite of hydrogen peroxide, detergents, and similar preparations may be used to soften the mass.

FOREIGN BODIES

Foreign bodies in the external auditory canal can usually be removed with an open head otoscope and a large speculum. The child should be immobilized. Grasping forceps should be reserved for handle-like projections or for the extremities of insects. More globular structures should be removed with a curet or a blunt hook (Day hook). If the patient is kept immobile

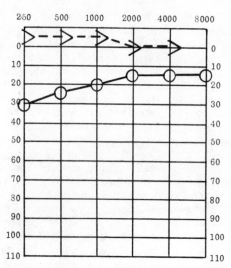

RIGHT EAR
FREQUENCY IN CYCLES PER SECOND

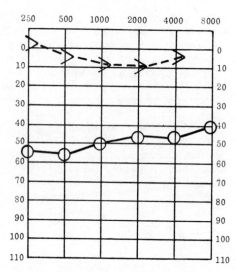

RIGHT EAR
FREQUENCY IN CYCLES PER SECOND

FIG 11−3. Audiogram showing partial impairment of sound transmission in the right ear. The dotted lines >---> represent the hearing of the end organ; the solid lines O——O show the air-conducted hearing level.

FIG 11−4. Audiogram showing complete impairment of sound transmission in the right ear.

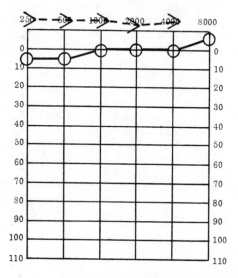

RIGHT EAR
FREQUENCY IN CYCLES PER SECOND

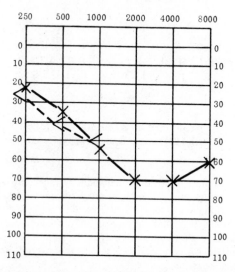

LEFT EAR
FREQUENCY IN CYCLES PER SECOND

FIG 11−5. Audiogram showing normal hearing by air conduction but significant air-bone gap indicating a middle ear problem in the right ear.

FIG 11−6. Audiogram showing typical sensorineural loss in the left ear with large differential between the high and low frequencies.

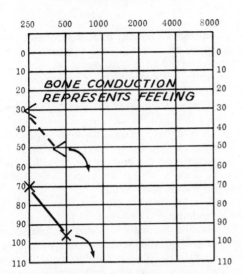

FIG 11—7. Congenital endogenous loss and loss in mumps (left ear).

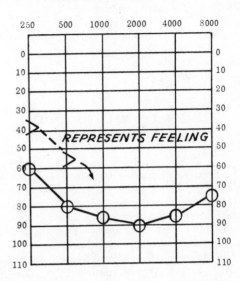

FIG 11—8. Exogenous loss, right ear (rubella and toxicity).

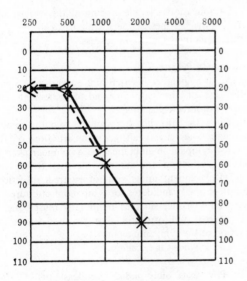

FIG 11—9. Neonatal hypoxia.

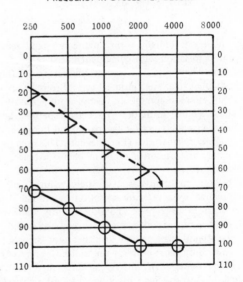

FIG 11—10. Audiogram showing mixed hearing loss.

and a large speculum is used, tympanic membrane trauma can be avoided. Trauma to the canal wall is an evanescent, self-limited problem.

Merkel BM: Foreign bodies in the ear canal. J Iowa Med Soc 47:744–746, 1957.

CONGENITAL MALFORMATIONS OF THE TYMPANIC MEMBRANE

Congenital deformities are usually associated with malformation of the pinna, external auditory canals, and the middle ear. In some cases the tympanic membrane is absent and a bony plate is found in its place; in others, an atrophic tympanic membrane is found when an atretic external auditory canal is opened.

In bilateral cases, treatment consists of the reconstruction of the tympanic membrane in association with repair of the external auditory canal and middle ear to improve hearing. Repair of unilateral defects should probably be deferred until the patient is old enough to understand the hazard of facial nerve injury.

BULLOUS MYRINGITIS

Bullae occasionally form on the tympanic membrane in association with coincident upper respiratory infection. They represent an accumulation of fluid between the squamous epithelial and fibrous layers of the drum, and are commonly mistaken for acute otitis media. A similar formation has been experimentally produced in volunteers by the parenteral injection of *Mycoplasma pneumoniae* (Eaton agent). This organism is probably the causative agent in many instances of bullous myringitis.

Bullous myringitis is exquisitely painful and is accompanied by a pressure sensation in the ear. The pain increases to a peak and subsequently improves with rupture of the bullae.

Treatment may include local heat and anesthetic ear drops. Surgical rupture of the bullae, if employed, should be undertaken with great care since there is danger of introducing infection into an otherwise sterile middle ear. Coincidental otitis media may be identified by noting a marked decrease in the mobility of the tympanic membrane.

The condition is usually self-limited, lasting 1–5 days.

Palmer B: Hemorrhagic bullous myringitis. Eye Ear Nose Throat Month 47:562–565, 1968.
Rifkind D & others: Ear involvement and primary atypical pneumonia following inoculation of volunteers with Eaton agent. Am Rev Resp Dis 479–489, 1962.

PERFORATION OF THE TYMPANIC MEMBRANE

Tympanic membrane perforations result from various forms of trauma (diving, water skiing, a blow to the ear, etc) and acute otitis media.

In acute otitis media the typical perforation is 1–2 mm in diameter. (The tympanic membrane is 8 mm in diameter.) Following the acute infection, such perforation typically will heal spontaneously; however, the hole occasionally persists. In some instances the entire tympanic membrane may slough because of hypersensitivity of the host to the offending microorganism. Such a perforation is not uncommon in severe scarlet fever and rubeola.

Clinical Findings

Conductive hearing loss occurs as a consequence of reduction of vibrating surface of the tympanic membrane. Intermittent painless otorrhea typically occurs with each upper respiratory infection or when the patient gets water in his ear.

On examination the ear canal and middle ear are seen to be filled with mucopurulent exudate. Following aspiration of this debris, the size and position of the perforation may be identified. The middle ear mucosa is typically thick and inflamed.

Complications

Complications include erosion of the ossicles and of the bony confines of the middle ear, causing labyrinthitis, meningitis, or brain abscess.

Treatment & Prognosis

Aural hygiene is essential and consists of keeping water out of the ear, repeated debridement, and topical anti-infective agents.

When the otorrhea has stopped and the middle ear membranes are healthy, reconstruction of the defective tympanic membrane should be undertaken to prevent reinfection and improve hearing. Small children with frequent upper respiratory tract infections are not optimal candidates for tympanoplastic surgery. Autogenous tissue, such as temporalis muscle fascia and external auditory skin, may be used for reconstruction of the tympanic membrane.

The prognosis is excellent.

Beales PH: Acute otitis media. Practitioner 199:752–760, 1967.
Dubow E: Treatment of non-suppurative myringitis and otitis media. Arch Pediat 78:483–489, 1961.

CONGENITAL OSSICULAR DEFORMITY

Malformations of the auditory ossicles are often seen in association with tympanic membrane and external auditory canal deformities. Wide morphologic variations occur, including very rudimentary ossicles and abnormal interossicular fusion and fusion to the surrounding bony structures.

Anomalous ossicular development may also be found in individuals with normal external auditory canals and tympanic membranes, most commonly in association with facial deformities such as mandibulo-facial and craniofacial dysostosis. Fixation of the stapes footplate is commonly associated with these deformities, or may occur in the absence of other abnormalities.

Surgical correction is the procedure of choice. The prognosis is excellent.

Edwards WG: Congenital middle ear deafness and anomalies of the face. J Laryng 78:152–170, 1964.

Wilmot T: Hereditary conductive deafness due to incus-stapes abnormalities and associated with pinna deformity. J Laryng 84:469–479, 1970.

OTOSCLEROSIS

Otosclerosis is a common disease characterized by the growth of abnormal vascular bone at some site in the temporal bone. The usual site is in the oval window, in which case the bony growth reduces the piston-like motion of the stapes and causes hearing loss. It is more common in females, and a positive family history can be elicited in 40% of cases. This process commonly begins in the second decade and becomes manifest by a hearing impairment in the third and fourth decades. Recent clinical experience indicates, however, that children under the age of 10 may have decreased auditory acuity due to otosclerosis.

The defect is surgically correctable.

SEROUS OTITIS MEDIA

The pathophysiology of this disease is not completely understood.

The nasopharyngeal end of the eustachian tube may be blocked by lymphoid tissue, edematous allergic mucosa, a tumor, etc. Under these circumstances the middle ear becomes a closed space and the gases enclosed in it are partially absorbed. The resulting negative atmospheric pressure causes transudation of amber fluid into the middle ear from the mucosal capillary bed, and a hearing impairment results.

Clinical Findings

Conductive hearing loss occurs which commonly goes unnoticed. Pain, when present, is evanescent and minor.

On examination the tympanic membrane is usually retracted. The retraction occurs initially above the lateral process of the malleus in the pars flaccida. As the negative pressure increases, the lower portion of the tympanic membrane also becomes retracted. This process may continue until the tympanic membrane is attached by adhesions to the medial wall of the middle ear.

Complications

Adhesion of the tympanic membrane to the ossicles and the medial wall of the middle ear occurs, with possible erosion of the ossicles.

Treatment

In addition to treatment of the underlying naso-pharyngeal disorder (adenoidectomy, allergic management, etc), the middle ear fluid should be aspirated through a small suction tip following myringotomy. A ventilatory tube is placed in the myringotomy defect to prevent recurrence. Failure to provide adequate treatment may result in irreversible adhesive middle ear disease.

Recalcitrant cases are not uncommon in young children.

Chan JC: Serous otitis media and allergy. Am J Dis Child 114:684–692, 1967.

Everberg G: Conductive lesions in children and young adults. Acta oto-laryng (Suppl) 224:186–194, 1967.

Mawson S & others: Long-term follow-up of 129 glue ears. Proc Roy Soc Med 62:460–464, 1969.

Senturia B: Classification of middle ear effusions. Ann Otol Rhin Laryng 79:358–370, 1970.

Silverstein H & others: Eustachian tube dysfunction as a cause for chronic secretory otitis with children. Laryngoscope 76:259–273, 1966.

Thomas G: Management of chronic middle ear effusion. California Med 110:300–304, 1969.

CHOLESTEATOMA

The continuing maturation process of squamous epithelium produces keratin debris on the surface. When skin finds its way into the middle ear or mastoid following a tympanic membrane perforation, the desquamated keratin accumulates and forms a chole-steatoma. When moisture and bacteria gain access to the accumulated keratin, a foul-smelling otorrhea ensues. This disease process causes erosion of surrounding bone and may produce meningeal complications, eg, extradural abscess, meningitis, or brain abscess.

Cholesteatoma almost invariably requires surgical excision.

Derlacki EL: Congenital cholesteatoma of the middle ear. Laryngoscope 78:1050–1078, 1968.

ACUTE OTITIS MEDIA
& MASTOIDITIS

Essentials of Diagnosis

- Ear pain and pressure sensation, conductive hearing loss.
- Frequently coincident with upper respiratory infection.
- Otorrhea if tympanic membrane ruptures.

General Considerations

The primary defense mechanism of the middle ear is the eustachian tube. This important structure is lined by respiratory (ciliated) epithelium. Protection of the middle ear is afforded by the ciliary propulsion of a "mucous blanket" toward the nasopharynx.

Microorganisms successfully violate this mechanism in 2 ways: (1) by progressive extension of infection along the eustachian tube mucous membrane, or (2) by propulsion of infected droplets from the nasopharynx into the middle ear during moments of high pressure, eg, sneezing and blowing the nose.

Offending organisms include pneumococci, *Hemophilus influenzae,* streptococci, staphylococci, and viruses.

Inflammation of the middle ear is understandably coincident with infection of the mastoid air cell system since these spaces openly communicate with one another.

Clinical Findings

Pain in the ear is of progressive severity, relief occurring with rupture of the tympanic membrane. In contrast, the pain of serous otitis media is typically mild and intermittent, lasting only 10–30 minutes. Another source of pain which may seem to be in the ear is that caused by temporomandibular joint disease. This pain can be quite severe but is related to malocclusion, bruxism, or trauma to the mandible.

The presence of purulent secretion in the middle ear also causes a conductive hearing impairment, a sensation that the patient is "talking in a barrel" and a feeling of pressure in the ear.

On examination, the tympanic membrane is inflamed and thickened. The incus and malleus, which are normally visible, may be obscured from view. With severe pressure behind the tympanic membrane, it may assume a "doughnut-like" appearance with a dimple in the center.

Complications

Acute otitis media and mastoiditis, if unchecked, may spread beyond the confines of the middle ear and mastoid. The disease may extend externally, by perforation of the tympanic membrane, or in any of 4 quadrants: (1) superiorly, through the tegmen tympani (bony plate) into the middle cranial fossa, causing meningitis or abscess; (2) anteriorly, through a bony suture (the petro-tympanic suture), forming a zygomatic abscess; (3) inferiorly, through a bony suture (the tympanomastoid suture), forming an abscess in the neck (Bezold's abscess); or (4) posteriorly, through perforations in the mastoid, forming a postauricular abscess. Superior extension is a life-threatening complication, and a primary goal of treatment of acute otitis media and mastoiditis is the prevention of this complication.

The persistence of inspissated middle ear secretions is a common and frequently unrecognized complication of acute otitis media.

Treatment

Treatment includes (1) topical (warm Auralgan) and systemic (aspirin or Tylenol) analgesics with local heat, (2) selection and application of an appropriate antimicrobial agent, (3) oral and topical decongestants to enhance the patency of the eustachian tube, and (4) in some cases myringotomy or simple mastoidectomy (or both).

Initial antibiotic selection is usually made without the benefit of sensitivity studies. Since *H influenzae* accounts for 20% of otitis media, one should select a drug which will eliminate this organism (eg, ampicillin rather than penicillin).

Cultures of middle ear contents should be made from needle aspiration or from a myringotomy knife. Throat culture results do not correlate precisely with offending middle ear organisms; however, a "pure culture" from the throat of a given organism would be a relevant consideration in selecting a therapeutic agent. Such cultures are valuable in the event that the disease does not respond to the initially chosen antibiotic.

The decision to do a myringotomy must be arrived at after noting the adequacy of medical treatment, the duration of the illness, and the physical characteristics of the tympanic membrane. In most instances of acute ear infection, myringotomy is unnecessary. In the event that appropriate medical treatment has been employed and the tympanic membrane is immobile and bulging but the clinical condition has not improved, myringotomy will be of benefit in preventing serious complications. Myringotomy may be necessary to relieve pain when the tympanic membrane is displaced laterally by elevated middle ear pressure.

Anesthesia for myringotomy varies from no anesthesia for the small child to general anesthesia up to the age of 6 or 7 or regional injection (2 ml of 2% lidocaine with 1:50,000 epinephrine injected in 4 quadrants at the junction of the cartilaginous and bony canal walls) for children over the age of 7.

Care must be taken to make a puncture wound through the layers of the tympanic membrane without dislodging the incus, which is found in the posterior-superior quadrant. The knife blade may pass forward through the drum to the bony middle ear wall with little risk, whereas lateral motion of the knife may cause ossicular damage.

In some instances, incision and drainage of the mastoid air cell system is necessary. This procedure is known as simple mastoidectomy.

Prognosis

With adequate treatment and follow-up, complete recovery can be expected. Hearing tests and pneumatic otoscopy are essential in identifying possible residual middle ear fluid. Continued decongestant (pseudoephedrine) therapy and sometimes myringotomy with aspiration may be required to eliminate persistent fluid.

Brownlee R & others: Otitis media in children. J Pediat 75:636–642, 1969.

Hemenway W & others: Treating acute otitis media. Postgrad Med 47:110–115, 1970.

Hemenway W & others: Treating acute otitis media. Postgrad Med 47:135–138, 1970.

Rubenstein MM: The treatment of acute otitis media in children. Am J Dis Child 109:308–313, 1965.

Towsend EH: Otitis media in pediatric practice. New York J Med 1964:1591–1597, 1964.

Van Dishoeck HE & others: Bacteriology and treatment of acute otitis media in children. Acta oto-laryng 50:250–262, 1959.

Williams S: Acute otitis media of viral origin and other pediatric problems in 1964. MJ Australia 2:235–238, 1965.

CHRONIC OTITIS MEDIA & MASTOIDITIS

Essentials of Diagnosis

- Painless otorrhea, intermittent or persistent.
- Conductive hearing loss.

General Considerations

Chronic otitis media and mastoiditis may result from cholesteatoma or may represent frequent reinfection of an ear with a defect in the tympanic membrane. With perforation of the tympanic membrane, the middle ear and mastoid become infected through 2 routes: the eustachian tube and the external auditory canal. Water is the usual source of infection through the external auditory canal, whereas the eustachian tube allows the transmission of infected droplets of mucus from the nasopharynx during periods of high pressure.

Clinical Findings

Examination shows perforation of the tympanic membrane with mucoid secretions in the middle ear space and the external auditory canal and thickening and inflammation of the middle ear mucosa. With long-standing infection, the mucous membrane of the middle ear may develop granulation tissue which may assume polypoid characteristics.

In the case of a cholesteatoma the defect in the tympanic membrane is usually filled with moist, infected keratin debris which has a foul odor.

The magnitude of the conductive hearing loss is contingent upon the amount of tympanic membrane which has been lost and the extent of damage to the middle ossicles.

Complications

Untreated chronic otitis media may produce extensive development of granulation tissue and polyp formation and subsequent demineralization of surrounding bone. In this way the infection may spread beyond the confines of the middle ear and mastoid, producing labyrinthitis, meningitis, or brain abscess.

Cholesteatomas typically erode surrounding bone, producing the same sort of complications.

Treatment

Treatment is both preventive and therapeutic in nature. The patient is admonished not to blow his nose and to sneeze with his mouth open, thereby avoiding the development of excessive pressure in the nasopharynx. The patient is advised not to swim and to place a small piece of cotton in the ear canal covered with white petrolatum while bathing. Periodic aspiration of the accumulated debris and secretions is required, and topical applications of corticosteroid-containing antibiotic preparations are used twice daily. Virtually all "chronically" infected ears treated carefully in this way will become free of otorrhea, but treatment may have to be continued for 3–6 months. When the middle ear mucosa becomes thin and healthy, a reconstructive surgical procedure may be done. Surgery of this type should be undertaken at an age when the child does not have frequent upper respiratory infections. This usually means 6–9 years of age.

In the case of cholesteatoma, surgery is virtually always necessary to eradicate the disease. Reconstruction may be undertaken only when the surgeon is confident of complete removal of the cholesteatoma.

Armstrong VW: Tympanoplasty in children. Laryngoscope 75:1062–1069, 1965.

Frederickson J: Otitis media and its complications. Arch Oto-laryng 90:387–393, 1969.

CONGENITAL MALFORMATIONS OF THE ORGAN OF CORTI

Congenital lesions of the organ of Corti are divided into 2 groups: an endogenous group due to hereditary transmission and an exogenous group due to misadventures of fetal life.

The typical instance of endogenous congenital deafness is due to the transmission of an autosomal recessive trait. The less common dominant transmission produces deafness in association with renal and other congenital abnormalities. The hearing loss in either case is nearly always bilateral and usually quite severe.

Exogenous congenital hearing loss results from maternal rubella in the first trimester and the administration of ototoxic drugs (dihydrostreptomycin, kanamycin, quinine, etc) to the mother. Other maternal viral illnesses than rubella should probably be incriminated also, but proof of their etiologic role is still forthcoming. Hypoxia and erythroblastosis also cause congenital exogenous hearing loss, but in these cases the pathologic process is in the brain stem.

Individuals with profound bilateral congenital hearing loss constitute what has been known traditionally as the deaf mute population. With early rehabilitative therapy, they can learn to talk. This implies early identification. Too often, congenitally deaf children are not identified until age 2 or 3, which severely compromises the effectiveness of rehabilitation efforts. Routine neonatal auditory screening is not only feasible but essential.

Barr B: Deafness following maternal rubella. Acta oto-laryng 53:413–423, 1961.
Davis H: The young deaf child: Identification and management. Acta oto-laryng (Suppl) 206:1–258, 1964.
Downs MP, Sterritt G: Identification audiometry in neonates: A preliminary report. J Audio Res 4:69–80, 1964.

EFFECT OF DRUGS ON THE ORGAN OF CORTI

The hair cells of the organ of Corti are permanently injured and sometimes totally destroyed by certain antibiotics. Kanamycin and dihydrostreptomycin are the worst offenders. Neomycin, vancomycin, and ristocetin have also been incriminated in this connection. Streptomycin is most often destructive to the vestibular apparatus, but well documented cases of cochlear injury have also been recorded. There is considerable variability in the susceptibilities to these drugs. Impaired renal excretion produces abnormally high blood levels and predictable toxic results from the drugs. Administration of these valuable antibiotics should be undertaken with caution.

Kossowski S: Experimental studies on the ototoxicity of certain antibiotics. Arch Immun Ther Exp 12:402–406, 1964.
Sheehy J: Ototoxic antibiotics. California Med 94:363–365, 1961.

LABYRINTHITIS

The labyrinth consists of the cochlea and the vestibular apparatus. Inflammation of these structures may result from blood-borne deposit of microorganisms in the labyrinth, from extension of middle ear disease or of meningeal infection (via neural sheaths or the cochlear aqueduct), or from surgical accidents. Measles virus is sometimes the causative organism. Vertigo and nausea are usually severe.

Treatment consists of bed rest, motion sickness drugs, adequate hydration, and antibiotics. The disease process may resolve, with complete or partial recovery

of auditory and vestibular function. However, as is often the case in meningitis, an osteitic process may be stimulated, with complete replacement of the labyrinth by solid bone. If that happens, total deafness and absence of vestibular function result.

TRAUMA TO THE ORGAN OF CORTI

Skull fracture lines in the floor of the posterior cranial fossa or in the squamous portion of the temporal bone may extend into the petrous portion of the temporal bone. Since this structure houses the external auditory canal, the middle ear, and the inner ear, one would expect a variety of clinical findings depending upon the site of the injury. Should the fracture cross the external auditory canal, there may be laceration of the skin and bleeding from the external auditory canal with no further damage. A more medial involvement might produce bleeding into the middle ear or damage to the ossicular chain.

The organ of Corti becomes involved when the fracture line passes through the cochlea. Such an injury produces total deafness in the involved ear. In the event of mere concussion without an actual fracture line involving the cochlea, varying degrees of sensorineural hearing impairment result. The loss is permanent and total when a fracture involves the cochlea. In the case of concussion, there may be some recovery.

Ray JW: Bilateral destruction of the internal ear after skull fracture. Ann Otol Rhin Laryng 74:260–263, 1965.
Schuknecht H: Head injury. Arch Otolaryng 63:513–528, 1956.

MUMPS

The effects of mumps virus on various organ systems are well known, and the cochlea is occasionally involved. The hearing loss is permanent, usually severe, and fortunately unilateral in 75% of cases. The other clinical manifestations of mumps need not be severe for deafness to result.

HEARING LOSS DUE TO NOISE

Loud sounds produce destruction of the hair cells, with resultant hearing impairment. The most common exposure in childhood is from explosions, eg, a firecracker exploding close to the ear or in an enclosed space. Sustained exposure to hard rock bands using high amplifications may produce deafness, especially in the performers. Such an injury produces hearing loss of varying severity and pattern. Recovery, if any, is slight. Hearing loss resulting from chronic exposure to loud noises is generally a problem of adult life.

EIGHTH NERVE TUMOR

Tumors arising in the cerebellopontine angle produce a typical auditory phenomenon, ie, unilateral progressive neurosensory hearing loss. Tumors in this area are usually neurilemmomas originating from the vestibular portion of the eighth nerve. Congenital epithelial inclusion cysts (cholesteatomas) and meningiomas occur in this area also. In addition to the auditory findings mentioned above, progressive enlargement of such lesions may produce facial muscle weakness and facial and corneal hypesthesia and anesthesia. The diagnosis is based on the clinical findings, audiometric and vestibular testing, and contrast radiography. Small tumors can be removed through the temporal bone. The morbidity and mortality rate coincident with large tumors is quite high.

House WH: Transtemporal bone microsurgical removal of acoustic neurinomas. Arch Otolaryng 80:599–756, 1964.

DEAFNESS DUE TO ERYTHROBLASTOSIS FETALIS

Kernicterus and resulting neurologic deficits are produced by the deposit of bilirubin in various structures of the CNS. Infants with high bilirubin blood levels resulting from Rh sensitivity may develop kernicterus. This tendency is markedly increased if there is coincident neonatal hypoxia. Kernicterus has been reported in individuals with normal bilirubin levels when neonatal hypoxia occurred. Lowered oxygen tension is thought to make neural tissue more susceptible to bilirubin deposit.

The exogenous congenital deafness of erythroblastosis fetalis is bilateral, permanent, and may be quite severe. Early identification and rehabilitation are essential if these children are to learn to talk.

Hall JG: The cochlea and the cochlear nuclei in neonatal asphyxia. Acta oto-laryng (Suppl) 194:1–93, 1964.

Hall JG: On the neuropathologic changes in the central nervous system following neonatal asphyxia with specific reference to the auditory system in man. Acta oto-laryng (Suppl) 188:331–338, 1964.

Keaster J & others: Hearing problems subsequent to neonatal hemolytic disease or hyperbilirubinemia. Am J Dis Child 117:406–410, 1969.

MISCELLANEOUS BRAIN STEM LESIONS

Demyelinating diseases and lesions responsible for cerebral palsy have no special tendency to involve the auditory system. Hearing impairment frequently does occur, however, and should be taken into account when planning rehabilitation for these unfortunate individuals.

Keats S: *Cerebral Palsy.* Thomas, 1965.

HEARING LOSS DUE TO AGENESIS OR TUMOR OF THE TEMPORAL LOBE CORTEX

Auditory function persists in spite of extensive cortical destruction. Individuals with cortical lesions severe enough to cause deafness are quite disabled due to other defects.

EAR DISORDERS NOT ASSOCIATED WITH HEARING LOSS

CONGENITAL MALFORMATIONS OF THE EXTERNAL EAR

The pinna is formed from 6 mound-like condensations of ectoderm. Congenital deformities include a spectrum of involvement from slight distortion of the free edge of the pinna to complete absence of the external auditory canal and rudimentary remnants of the pinna. These deformities may be either unilateral or bilateral. Surgical repair may be undertaken to improve hearing or cosmetic appearance. Cosmetic repair may be achieved by autogenous implants, plastic implants, or plastic prostheses. Autogenous implants of cartilage require a long series of operations, and the cosmetic result is generally unsatisfactory. Plastic implants generally give a more desirable cosmetic result and require only a series of 3 or 4 operations. With present-day adhesives, plastics, and pigments, a nearly normal appearing prosthetic ear can be constructed and worn satisfactorily.

TRAUMA TO THE EXTERNAL EAR

Lacerations of the pinna should be debrided and closed carefully. In approximating skin edges over cartilage, it is often desirable to resect a small strip of cartilage to facilitate better closure.

Blunt injuries to the pinna which result in hematoma formation are frequently inadequately treated, with a resulting "cauliflower" ear. Such hematomas should be incised and drained to prevent resorption of the cartilage skeleton.

INFECTION OF THE PINNA

Incision and drainage of an infected pinna allows for early resolution of the infection and prevents pressure on the cartilage with subsequent resorption.

FURUNCULOSIS OF THE EXTERNAL EAR CANAL

Furuncles occur in the external portion of the external auditory canal. Treatment consists of incision, drainage, a Burow's solution wick, and systemic antibiotics.

EXOSTOSES OF THE EXTERNAL EAR CANAL

Sessile bony growths in the external auditory canal sometimes favor the development of otitis externa by harboring moisture. Very slight trauma to the overlying skin may produce bleeding. If clinical problems are associated with these lesions, surgical excision is indicated.

NOSE, PARANASAL SINUSES, & PHARYNX

DERMOID CYSTS

Dermoid cysts contain epidermal appendages, ie, hair follicles, sebaceous glands, and sweat glands. They present as a tumor mass on the dorsum of the nose. A sinus tract is often present with an external opening near the nasion. Inflammation and drainage call attention to these otherwise dormant lesions. The intranasal involvement may be quite extensive. Careful excision can be done with minimal cosmetic deformity.

Hoshaw T: Dermoid cysts of the nose. Arch Otolaryng 93:487–491, 1971.
McClean GE: Dermoid cysts of the nose. Am Surgeon 30:203–206, 1964.

MENINGOCELES & ENCEPHALOCELES

Herniation of the cranial contents into the nose begins at birth. Symptoms of nasal obstruction usually present in the first year of life. A smooth, polyp-like mass is seen on anterior rhinoscopy. Excision should be undertaken by a neurosurgeon and a rhinologist.

Jones R: Encephalocele masquerading as a nasal polyp. JAMA 181:640–642, 1962.

CHOANAL ATRESIA

Unrecognized bilateral choanal atresia (closure of the posterior nares) usually results in neonatal death since the newborn may be solely dependent on his nasal airway for respiration. The emergency treatment and initial diagnosis are both accomplished by exerting traction on the tongue or by inserting an oral airway. The diagnosis may be confirmed by attempting to pass a catheter through the nose.

Atresia of the posterior choanae may be membranous or bony. The immediate treatment is designed to provide an airway. In most cases, a nipple with large perforations can be securely fixed in the child's mouth. Satisfactory respiratory exchange takes place through and around the nipple. Mouth breathing is usually learned in 4–6 weeks. Until this time, the infant must be fed by gavage and the airway maintained as described. In some cases, tracheostomy may be necessary. Early perforation of the atretic area is seldom, if ever, indicated. This procedure is hazardous; the resulting airway is tenuous; and definitive repair is more difficult following this maneuver.

When the technic of mouth breathing is acquired, the child progresses well. A definitive transpalatine repair should be undertaken at age 2 or 3.

Diamant H: Congenital choanal atresia: Report of a clinical series. Acta paediat 52:106–110, 1963.
Key F: Bilateral choanal atresia. Obst Gynec 32:58–59, 1968.
Ransome J: Familial incidence of posterior choanal atresia. J Laryng 78:551–554, 1964.
Rowdon RE, Baade EA: Posterior choanal atresia: A practical approach. Eye Ear Nose Throat Month 42:33–37, 1963.

AGENESIS OF SINUSES

At birth the ethmoid sinuses are partially developed; the sphenoid and maxillary sinuses are rudimentary; and the frontal sinuses are absent. The frontal sinuses begin to develop in the second year of life. Any of the paranasal sinuses may fail to develop. Such a finding is usually incidental to x-ray examination for some other purpose and is of no clinical significance.

NASAL SEPTAL DEFORMITY
DUE TO TRAUMA

Newborn infants commonly have obvious nasal deformities, usually a result of subluxation of the nasal septum during childbirth. Gentle manipulation with a cotton-tipped applicator will correct nearly all of these deformities. This should be done at birth or during the first few days of life.

NASAL FRACTURE

Traumatic nasal injury in children may produce deformity and septal hematoma. The diagnosis is made by palpation of the nasal skeleton and by anterior rhinoscopy. X-rays are sometimes helpful in noting the presence or absence of a fracture but are of little benefit assessing the degree of displacement or planning reparative measures. Pre-injury photographs are frequently helpful.

Reduction of the deformity can generally be accomplished within 5 days after the injury. If an operative procedure is necessary, surgical manipulation should be limited to the injured areas only. Extensive surgery should be avoided, since trauma to the nasal growth centers will produce severe deformity as the face and nose develop.

Hematomas of the septum result from bleeding beneath the membrane covering the cartilage. Such a development produces bilateral occlusion of the nasal space by bulging toward the lateral walls. Unless incision and drainage is undertaken, the cartilage may be resorbed as a result of pressure on the cartilage. With loss of this important skeletal support, a severely deformed "saddle" nose may result. Early recognition and treatment of septal hematomas may avoid cosmetic deformity.

Hadley R: Nasal injuries in children. New York J Med 69:281–284, 1969.
Jennes ML: Corrective nasal surgery in children. Arch Otolaryng 79:145–151, 1964.

MAXILLARY FRACTURE

Deceleration injury, blows with club-like objects, and missiles may produce maxillary fractures in children. Acute or latent damage to the CNS should always be the initial consideration in such injuries. When this possibility has been eliminated, one should proceed to evaluation and treatment of the maxillary fracture or fractures.

Several considerations are relevant in detecting the presence of a fracture and determining its extent: (1) pre-injury photographs, (2) visible deformity, (3) palpable deformity, (4) palpable crepitation, (5) malocclusion, (6) limitation of ocular motion, and (7) ocular displacement.

Surgical repair should be conservative. The primary intent should be to correct the deformity with the least possible damage to maxillary growth centers. Special attention must be given to dental and orbital function.

Bailey B & others: Management of mid-facial fractures. Laryngoscope 79:694–713, 1969.
Barclay TL: Some aspects of treatment of traumatic diplopia. Brit J Plast Surg 16:214–220, 1963.
Harrill JA: Midfacial fractures. Am Surgeon 33:931–935, 1967.
Pickering PP: Fractures of the middle third of the face. J Internat Coll Surgeons 40:265–275, 1963.
Woodburn CC: Fractures of the mid-facial skeleton. Arch Otolaryng 78:687–692, 1963.

STENOSIS OF THE ANTERIOR NARES

Trauma to the anterior nares may cause severe deformities. Two types of injury most commonly lead to such misadventures: (1) laceration and (2) corrosive burns. Repair of lacerations about the anterior nares deserves special consideration, particularly in children.

Chemical agents used in the treatment of epistaxis sometimes are inadvertently applied to the anterior nares. The resulting cicatrization may produce stenosis or complete atresia.

NASAL FOREIGN BODY

Foreign bodies within the nose of a child cause unilateral obstruction and rhinorrhea with some bleeding. Immobilization of the child is essential for safe removal and may be achieved by (1) cooperation of the child, (2) physical restraint, or (3) general anesthesia. Nebulizer application of a solution containing 0.5% cocaine and 1% epinephrine gives vasoconstriction and anesthesia. Forceps are of limited value unless the foreign body has a handle-like projection. A hook-like instrument (cerumen curet or Day hook) introduced beyond the foreign body and then withdrawn is usually quite satisfactory. Care must be taken to prevent a nasal foreign body from becoming a bronchial foreign body.

COMMON COLD

This upper respiratory illness is characterized by coryza, sore throat, and occasionally slight fever. In adults it is caused by a group of 30 or more serologically identifiable viruses known as the rhinoviruses. In children a number of additional viruses are probably also responsible.

In children, the identification and treatment of complications are the primary therapeutic aims. Other organ system involvement includes (1) otitis media, (2) sinusitis, (3) aseptic meningitis, (4) croup, (5) bronchitis, or (6) bronchopneumonia.

Dick EC: Epidemiology of infections with rhinovirus. Am J Epidem 86:386–400, 1967.
Douglas R: Pathogenesis of rhinovirus common colds in human volunteers. Ann Otol Rhin Laryng 79:563–571, 1970.
Hilleman MR: Present knowledge of rhinovirus group of viruses. Curr Top Microbiol Immun 41:1–22, 1967.

ACUTE SINUSITIS

Essentials of Diagnosis
- Nasal obstruction with purulent rhinorrhea.
- Facial and dental pain.
- Fever and malaise.

General Considerations
At birth the ethmoid sinuses are partially developed, the sphenoid and maxillary sinuses are rudimentary, and the frontal sinuses are absent. The ethmoid cells reach full development at about age 12. The maxillary sinus begins rapid expansion at age 7 and continues to expand throughout puberty. The frontal sinus is evident on x-ray at age 3 and undergoes significant expansion between ages 7 and 20.

The paranasal sinuses are lined by ciliated respiratory epithelium. An advancing "blanket" of mucus is propelled from the most distal corner of each sinus cavity to the sinus ostium, into the nose, and posteriorly to the nasopharynx. This moving mucus acts as a defense mechanism which under certain circumstances breaks down, allowing the secretions to accumulate and providing a favorable circumstance for infection: The common cold causes thickening of the membranes lining the ostia, thereby occluding them. Nasal allergy produces the same effect. Exposure to cold air immobilizes the cilia. Mechanical obstruction due to polyps, foreign bodies, tumor, etc also produces dysfunction of the defensive system.

The resulting infection is usually due to streptococci, pneumococci, staphylococci, or *Hemophilus influenzae.*

Clinical Findings
Symptoms include facial pain, dental pain, headache, purulent rhinorrhea, and fever. On examination, thick, "boggy" nasal mucous membranes are seen. Purulent secretions are found within the nose, and there is tenderness to percussion of the sinuses. X-rays show opacity of the sinus spaces or an air-fluid level.

Complications
Osteomyelitis of the frontal bone is the most common complication of frontal sinusitis. A frequent historical correlation to this problem is the story of jumping feet first into a chlorinated swimming pool.

A complication of ethmoid sinusitis is the development of an abscess presenting in the area of the inner canthus.

An alarming complication of ethmoid and sphenoid infection is cavernous sinus thrombosis. This complication is fatal in 50% of cases and is characterized by ophthalmoplegia, photophobia, and finally facial anesthesia and blindness. Anticoagulation with heparin should be employed early in this disease. Fibrinolytic agents are applicable in the late stages.

Treatment
The initial treatment of acute sinusitis is aimed at halting bacterial growth with antibiotics selected on the basis of cultures of nasal secretions. Topical and oral decongestants enhance drainage. Antihistamines may be of symptomatic benefit. If the disease worsens in spite of appropriate treatment, lavage of the maxillary sinus or surgical trephine of the frontal sinus may be indicated.

Drettner B: Borderline between acute rhinitis and sinusitis. Acta oto-laryng 64:508–513, 1967.
Klune JP: Septic thrombosis within the cavernous chamber. Am J Ophth 56:33–39, 1963.
McLean D: Sinusitis in children. Clin Pediat 9:342–345, 1970.
Pascarelli E: Diplopia and photophobia as premonitory symptoms of cavernous sinus thrombosis. Ann Otol Rhin Laryng 73:210–217, 1964.

CHRONIC SINUSITIS

Obstructing masses and nasal allergy contribute to the development of chronic sinusitis. Bronchiectasis is commonly associated with sinusitis.

Pneumococci are said to be the most common microorganisms causing sinusitis. Initial treatment is much the same as for acute sinusitis. If repeated irrigation of the maxillary sinus produces purulent secretions, a permanent window should be surgically created in the inferior meatus of the nose.

Axelsson A & others: Treatment of acute maxillary sinusitis. Acta oto-laryng 70:70–76, 1970.
Davison F: Chronic sinusitis and infectious asthma. Arch Oto-laryng 90:202–207, 1969.

FURUNCULOSIS

The veins of the nose and orbit are connected to the cavernous sinus without the protective benefit of valves. For this reason, furuncles and erysipelas in this area deserve special consideration. If cavernous sinus thrombosis is to be prevented, these inflammations deserve early and intensive antibiotic treatment with assiduous observation for developing signs of cavernous sinus involvement.

NASAL ALLERGY & POLYPS

Exposure to antigenic substances capable of producing allergic reactions may occur by inhalation, ingestion, or skin contact. The highly vascular mucosa of the nose and sinuses represents a dramatically reactive shock organ in response to inhaled antigens. Nasal obstruction with thick pallid mucosa is the hallmark of nasal allergy. Chronic exposure with coincident infection may cause nasal polyps.

A more complete discussion of allergic rhinitis is presented in Chapter 33.

A careful clinical history is the most relevant diagnostic tool. The physical characteristics of the mucosa along with eosinophilia in nasal smears are confirmatory. Sinus x-rays commonly show thickened mucosa.

Infections should be treated with systemic antibiotics. Mild symptoms can be controlled with decongestants and antihistamines. Identification of specific allergens and avoidance or desensitization constitute the most direct approach to the problem, but this is not universally successful.

Nasal polyps should be removed after adequate management of the atopic disease is accomplished.

Brown G: Nasal polypsis. Postgrad MJ 45:680–683, 1969.
Rapaport HG: Specific investigation and treatment of allergic diseases in children: A review. Ann Allergy 22:292–302, 1964.

EPISTAXIS

Nasal bleeding in children usually emanates from the anterior portion of the nasal septum. Drying of the mucous membranes, with cracking and fracture of small vessels, is the precipitating circumstance. This type of bleeding can be stopped by compressing the alae against the septum. Twice daily application of an emollient will generally control the problem. Cautery should be avoided, if possible, since destruction of septal tissue may lead to perforation of the septum in adult life.

Posterior bleeding is usually quite severe and commonly reflects defects in the clotting mechanism.

Anterior nasal packing may be required while correction of the systemic disease is accomplished. In some instances a posterior pack or Foley catheter in the nasopharynx will be needed in addition to the anterior packing.

Leukemia victims commonly bleed from "everywhere." Strips of salt pork placed in the nose will have a powerful astringent affect and may be more effective than gauze packing.

Simonton K: The emergency treatment of nosebleed. J Oklahoma MA 62:135–140, 1969.

DISEASES & DISORDERS OF THE MOUTH

CLEFT LIP & PALATE

These deformities are among the most common major congenital malformations. One newborn infant in 600 has either a cleft lip or cleft palate or a combination of both.

The causes of cleft lip and cleft palate are not completely understood. A combination of genetic and nongenetic factors accounts for the deformities. Reports of the percentage of positive family histories range from 12–55%. Maternal factors indicated thus far include (1) viral infections such as rubella, influenza, mumps, and varicella; (2) administration of corticosteroids during pregnancy; (3) anoxia; (4) anemia; and (5) toxemia of pregnancy.

A classification of cleft lip and cleft palate has been proposed by a committee of the American Association for Cleft Palate Rehabilitation. The possible deformities are divided into (1) cleft of the prepalate (including those involving the lip or alveolar process), (2) clefts of the palate, and (3) clefts of the palate and the pre-palate. Laterality, defect size, etc may be noted if a more detailed classification is desired.

Treatment requires the services of several medical and paramedical disciplines. In the presence of a cleft lip, alimentation may be somewhat tedious but is basically quite satisfactory. The cleft lip repair should, therefore, be withheld until the child can best tolerate a major surgical procedure. Cleft lip repair, however, is traditionally done when the child reaches a body weight of 10–12 lb.

The primary consideration in palate repair concerns speech development. Eighteen months is widely accepted as the most appropriate age, since speech begins to develop soon thereafter.

In the formation of many speech sounds it is necessary to approximate the soft palate with the posterior pharyngeal wall, thereby preventing the escape of air into the nose. Deformity and immobility of the repaired palate may prevent satisfactory closure. This problem may be partially compensated for by speech therapy. A permanently constructed flap of tissue from the posterior pharyngeal wall to the soft palate—a pharyngeal flap—may be of benefit. The injection of Teflon granules (50 μm in diameter suspended in glycerine) into the posterior pharyngeal wall may be employed. Satisfactory speech is the result in about 70% of repaired palates.

In the palate repair, the hamulus of the pterygoid plate is usually fractured. This produces redundancy of the soft tissue in the area of the eustachian tube. Occlusion of the eustachian tube orifice results in frequent episodes of secretory and sometimes suppurative otitis media.

Mention should be made of the submucous cleft of the palate. In this circumstance, the mucous membrane of the soft palate is intact, but the muscle which is normally attached in the median raphe is either absent or ineffectively attached in the midline. This deformity may be recognized by palpation and visual observation of the inadequacy of velopalatine closure. Repair of the muscular attachments may suffice; however, a pharyngeal flap or pharyngeal injection of prosthetic material may be necessary.

Cleft palate teams are frequently developed to cope adequately with this multifaceted problem. Plastic surgeons, otolaryngologists, speech therapists, orthodontists, and prosthodontists are all necessary.

Borcbaken C: An analysis of 1000 cases of cleft lip and palate in Turkey. Cleft Palate J 6:210–212, 1969.

Fraser F: The genetics of cleft lip and cleft palate. Am J Human Genet 22:336–352, 1970.

Graham MB: A longitudinal study of ear disease and hearing loss in patients with cleft lip and palate. Tr Am Acad Ophth 67:213–222, 1963.

Harkins CS: A classification of cleft lip and cleft palate. Plast Reconstr Surg 29:31–39, 1962.

Lewin ML: Management of patients with cleft lip and cleft palate. New York J Med 62:2523–2535, 1962.

Oldfield MC: Cleft lip and palate: Some ideas on prevention and treatment. Brit J Plast Surg 17:1–9, 1964.

Schilli W & others: A general description of 315 cleft lip and palate patients. Cleft Palate J 7:573–577, 1970.

PIERRE ROBIN SYNDROME

This malformation is characterized by severe micrognathia and cleft palate. This is a life-threatening problem, since in the supine position the tongue is displaced backward with resulting total occlusion of the pharynx. Within 6–12 months the mandible "catches up" with other skeletal growth and the respiratory problem is solved. Treatment is aimed at preventing asphyxia and providing adequate alimentation until the mandible becomes large enough to accommodate the tongue.

In some instances the child can merely be maintained in a prone position while unattended and fed by gavage. In other cases, surgical intervention is necessary. The Douglas procedure involves placing a large suture through the base of the tongue and anchoring it to the soft tissue in front of the mandible. Tracheostomy is also a satisfactory solution. Selection of the proper management requires careful evaluation of the child's respiratory function. The cleft palate should be repaired at about 18 months of age.

Gunter G & others: Early management of the Pierre Robin syndrome. Cleft Palate J 7:495–501, 1970.

Rankow RM: Micrognathia in the newborn: Pierre Robin syndrome. Plast Reconstr Surg 25:606–614, 1960.

TREACHER-COLLINS SYNDROME
(Mandibulofacial Dysostosis)

This hereditary constellation of deformities reflects genetic abnormalities in the development of the first and second branchial arches. Antimongoloid slant of the eyes; hypoplasia of the malar bones and mandible; notching of the lower eyelid; malformation of the external, middle, and inner ears; and occasional facial clefts may all be included in the "complete" form of this syndrome. Reconstructive surgery for the ear deformities should conform to the principles previously outlined. Other reconstructive surgery should be planned by a qualified plastic surgeon.

Several other rare syndromes involving the facial bone have been described (see references below).

Jervis GA: DeLange syndrome. J Pediat 63:634–645, 1963.

Rogers BO: Berry-Treacher-Collins syndrome. Brit J Plast Surg 17:109–137, 1964.

Russ AL: The oral-facial-digital syndrome: A multiple congenital condition of females with chromosomal abnormalities. Pediatrics 29:985–995, 1962.

TONGUETIE

The frenulum of the tongue is a thin, mobile "web" of oral mucous membrane. Very occasionally this tissue band prevents a child from projecting or elevating the tongue. Very rarely, this may cause abnormalities of speech development. Treatment consists of cutting the frenulum, taking care to avoid injury to the orifices of Wharton's ducts.

FRACTURE OF THE MANDIBLE

Trauma sufficient to fracture the mandible of a child usually occurs as a result of deceleration injury in a fall, automobile accident, or bicycle accident.

Conservative operative treatment to insure normal development and normal epiphyseal growth at the mandibular condyle consists of intermaxillary wiring and interosseous fixation in the case of symphysis fractures. Healing of the condylar fractures is quite satisfactory, with reshaping of the head of the mandible and restoration of normal motion.

Goldberg M & others: The location and occurrence of mandibular fractures. Oral Surg 28:336–341, 1969.
Thomson HG: Condylar neck fractures of the mandible in children. Plast Reconstr Surg 34:452–463, 1964.

LACERATIONS OF THE MOUTH

Lacerations of the lip and buccal mucosa require careful closure. The skin surface should be carefully cleansed and generously debrided. Closure should be done with fine (6–0) sutures. Mucosal surfaces should be closed only loosely, if at all, in order to prevent abscess formation between the skin and mucosa.

Lacerations of the tongue in small children may be a serious problem because of blood loss. Closure should be done with chromic sutures placed in deep mattress fashion. This approach will provide hemostasis and limit subsequent deformity of the tongue.

PUNCTURE INJURIES & HEMATOMAS

Puncture injuries of the tongue, floor of the mouth, and soft palate are common in children. Routine precautions regarding tetanus should be taken. Huge hematomas may develop, and the child should be observed for possible airway obstruction due to hematoma development.

HERPANGINA

A painful vesicular eruption involving the anterior pillars, soft palate, and posterior pharyngeal wall characterizes this viral illness. Coxsackieviruses A are the responsible agents. The disease is brief and self-limited, with little general symptomatic involvement.

HAND, FOOT, & MOUTH DISEASE

This disease is caused by coxsackievirus groups A5 and A16. Its clinical manifestations are vesicular ulcers of the buccal mucosa, tongue, and floor of the mouth. Vesicular lesions are commonly found on the hands and feet, occasionally with a mild generalized rash. Slight fever and malaise may accompany this illness.

Richardson HB: Hand, foot and mouth disease in children: An epidemic associated with Coxsackie A16. J Pediat 67:6–12, 1965.
Whiting D & others: The clinical appearance of hand, foot and mouth disease. South African MJ 43:575–577, 1969.

ORAL HERPES SIMPLEX

This is a common cause of stomatitis in small children. The temperature may reach 40–40.6° C (104–105° F), and malaise and irritability are common. The vesicular eruption involves the gingivas, buccal mucosa, tongue, and soft palate. A yellow-gray membrane forms and later sloughs, leaving a true ulcer. The disease usually lasts 4–9 days.

Cohen L: Chronic oral ulceration. J Oral Med 25:7–11, 1970.
Henle G & others: Observations on childhood infections with the Epstein-Barr virus. J Infect Dis 121:303–309, 1970.
Margoffin RL: Vesicular stomatitis and exanthem. JAMA 175:441–445, 1961.

THRUSH

Candida albicans is a saprophytic inhabitant of the mouth. White, curd-like lesions occur about the gingivas in association with general debility or inadequate diet. Nystatin (Mycostatin) may be applied topically with satisfactory results.

RANULA

These cystic lesions occur in the floor of the mouth, usually to one side of the midline. They are pale blue and contain "stringy" mucoid material. Resection is difficult because of the thinness of the walls and their tendency to interdigitate between the muscle layers of the floor of the mouth. Marsupialization—by removing a portion of the cyst wall and suturing it open—may be employed. A sclerosing agent should not be used.

Olech E: Ranula. Oral Surg 16:1169–1173, 1963.
Redpath T: Congenital ranula. Oral Surg 28:542–544, 1969.

FIBROUS DYSPLASIA

Bone undergoes constant remodeling throughout life, and particularly in childhood. In fibrous dysplasia, the resorbed bone is partially replaced by fibrous tissue. The process commonly involves the mandible but may involve the maxilla or other parts of the skeleton. Extensive facial deformity usually results. Resection of the involved bony tissue may be of some benefit.

Barbary AS: Fibrous dysplasia in the bones of the face. J Laryng 77:593–600, 1963.

MALFORMATIONS OF THE LARYNX & PHARYNX

Congenital laryngeal malformations, with the exception of atresia, are characterized by the development of a weak cry and varying degrees of stridor. The definitive diagnosis in each case is made by direct laryngoscopy. A routine clinical examination should be done prior to this examination. This includes (1) careful history and physical examination, (2) antero-posterior and lateral x-rays of the chest, (3) lateral soft tissue x-rays of the neck, and (4) fluoroscopic examination of the esophagus to·rule out an anomalous aortic arch or subclavian artery.

CONGENITAL LARYNGEAL STRIDOR
(Laryngomalacia)

This clinical entity accounts for 80% of the congenital laryngeal lesions seen by one investigator in a 10-year series (Table 11–2) It consists of an abnormal softness and instability of the epiglottic and arytenoid cartilages. On inspiration, these structures "tumble" into the glottis, causing stridor. An inscrutable aspect of the disease is that stridor is often absent during the first few days of life and appears later.

The diagnosis is made by direct laryngoscopy. In infants, this examination should be done without anesthesia. The child is carefully and firmly restrained while the examiner introduces a No. 8 or No. 9 Jackson laryngoscope. The blade is placed in the vallecula between the epiglottis and the tongue. With forward displacement of the tongue, a satisfactory evaluation of epiglottic and arytenoid movement can be accomplished. The blade can then be placed behind the epiglottis for a more complete view of the larynx and upper trachea. Considerable experience and judgment on the part of the laryngologist are necessary to rule out other congenital lesions and to establish the diagnosis of laryngomalacia.

Other than observation, treatment is seldom needed. Holinger reports that tracheostomy was required in only one out of 305 cases.

LARYNGEAL WEB

Laryngeal web consists of a triangular membrane in the anterior portion of the larynx that limits the respiratory exchange to the posterior glottis. The membrane is usually attached to the superior surface of the true cords. In other instances, an apparent fusion of the anterior part of the true or false cords accounts for the web.

Conservative treatment is usually adequate. Gentle dilatation with triangular laryngeal dilators should be employed. One should be prepared for tracheostomy, although this is seldom necessary.

Simple cutting of the web is inevitably followed by reformation. However, a thin sheet of Teflon or tantalum can be placed within the larynx and between the "leaves" of the divided web. This is attached to the thyroid cartilage and allowed to remain until complete epithelialization has taken place.

LARYNGEAL ATRESIA

Laryngeal atresia is not compatible with life. Several dramatic instances have been recorded of life-saving tracheostomy when this disorder is recognized at birth.

Atresia of the larynx is considered to be quite rare. However, it may be an unrecognized cause of neonatal death.

SUBGLOTTIC STENOSIS

Thickening of the subglottic tissue may account for stridor in the newborn. As the cricoid cartilage increases in size, the stridor disappears. Affected children have a remarkably low tolerance for laryngeal inflammation during the first few months of life.

TABLE 11–2. Congenital laryngeal lesions.
(Holinger, 1954)

Congenital laryngeal stridor	305
Webs	19
Atresia	1
Congenital subglottic stenosis	34
Congenital cysts	5
Laryngoceles	15
	379

LARYNGEAL CYSTS

Congenital cysts of the larynx bulge into the lumen from the laryngeal ventricle. When observed at laryngoscopy they may be resected with the biopsy forceps. More extensive surgery is seldom necessary.

LARYNGOCELE

This congenital lesion is seldom clinically apparent at birth. A defect in the muscular wall of the larynx allows the inflation of an air-filled cyst which presents in the neck when the intralaryngeal pressure is elevated.

HEMANGIOMA

Twenty-one cases of this malformation have been reported, almost all in the subglottic region. If the airway is severely compromised, surgical excision is required. Since the natural history of this lesion is one of progressive atrophy, mildly involved cases should be treated with observation.

Atkins JP: Laryngeal problems of infancy and childhood. P Clin North America 9:1125–1135, 1962.

Cohen S: Unusual lesions of the larynx, trachea, and bronchial tree. Ann Otol Rhin Laryng 78:476–489, 1969.

Davison FW: Inflammatory diseases of the larynx of infants and small children. Ann Otol Rhin Laryng 76:753–761, 1967.

Fox H: Laryngeal atresia. Arch Dis Childhood 39:641–645, 1964.

Holinger P & others: Congenital webs, cysts, laryngoceles and other anomalies of the larynx. Ann Otol Rhin Laryng 76:744–752, 1967.

Imbrie J & others: Laryngotracheoesophageal cleft. Laryngoscope 79:1252–1274, 1969.

Zakraewski A: Subglottic hemangioma of the larynx in an infant, treated surgically. Acta oto-laryng 56:599–602, 1963.

. . .

FRACTURE OF THE LARYNX

Laryngeal fractures and soft tissue injuries in children are commonly the result of the child's being hurled against the dashboard during sudden deceleration in an auto accident. If the larynx is crushed, the airway may be completely blocked and only immediate tracheostomy will save his life. If the child survives the immediate post-injury period, careful observation is necessary during the ensuing 48 hours since edema and expansion of hematomas may compromise the airway.

After attention has been paid to the airway, the important considerations in injuries of this type are debridement and closure of lacerations and treatment of intracranial complications. Then comes the question of what to do with the fractured larynx. The physician is commonly misled at this point by his inclination to be conservative. Expectant treatment is just as inappropriate for the fractured larynx as it is for fracture-dislocation of the tibia. If normal function is to be restored, open reduction of laryngeal fractures is usually necessary.

Fitz-Hugh GS: Injuries of the larynx and cervical trauma. Ann Otol Rhin Laryng 71:419–442, 1962.

Nahum A: Immediate care of acute blunt laryngeal trauma. J Trauma 9:112–125, 1969.

LARYNGEAL FOREIGN BODIES

Laryngeal foreign bodies may completely or partially occlude the larynx. In complete occlusion, immediate extraction (usually with the fingers) or tracheostomy (with any instrument available) is necessary.

Partial obstruction is comparable to bronchial foreign body. Endoscopic removal should be accomplished in an operating theater, with adequate preparation for tracheostomy and bronchoscopy. If possible, the endoscopist should be provided with a duplicate of the foreign body. Extraction of the offending object should be done with little delay, since edema is apt to cause progressive airway obstruction.

ANGIONEUROTIC EDEMA

Extensive edema of the epiglottis of rapid onset causes respiratory obstruction. Edema of the lips or tongue may be present also. Food allergy (see Chapter 33) is commonly believed to be a contributing etiologic factor. Parenteral administration of epinephrine, antihistamines, and corticosteroids has been helpful.

PHARYNGEAL STENOSIS

Pharyngeal surgery such as tonsillo-adenoidectomy may on occasion be complicated by a postoperative inflammatory process and a tendency to develop stenosis. Resection of the stenotic soft tissue only causes recurrent stenosis. This tenacious disease process usually responds to wide excision with immediate placement of a plastic stent which must be kept in place for 6 weeks or more until healing has occurred.

INFLAMMATORY DISORDERS
OF THE LARYNX & PHARYNX

CROUP
(Supraglottitis or Epiglottitis;
Laryngotracheitis)

Essentials of Diagnosis

- Stridor, suprasternal, and intercostal retraction on inspiration.
- Fearfulness and anxiety.
- Laboratory (blood gas) evidence of hypoxia.
- Low-grade fever, leukocytosis.

General Considerations

The term croup has been traditionally applied to inflammatory laryngeal disease causing airway obstruction in children. Recent clinical research clearly divides this disease into 2 separate entities distinguished from each other by etiology, site of involvement, and clinical course.

(1) **Epiglottitis or supraglottitis:** The false cords (ventricular bands), aryepiglottic fold, and epiglottis are involved. The offending organism is usually *Hemophilus influenzae*; however, *Staphylococcus aureus* and beta-hemolytic streptococci may also cause the disease.

(2) **Laryngotracheitis:** Laryngotracheitis is due to parainfluenza viruses types I, II, and III and influenza virus types A_2 and B. The vocal cords, subglottic tissue, and trachea are the sites of infection.

Clinical Findings

There is usually a history of hoarse cough followed by inspiratory stridor, tachycardia, increased respiratory rate, dysphagia, and, ultimately, expiratory stridor. On inspiration there is marked retraction in the supraclavicular and intercostal spaces. The child wears an anxious facial expression, confirming the presence of hypoxia. With prolonged obstruction, the child becomes weary and sleeps fitfully and briefly.

Blood gas studies show decreased oxygen tension and increased CO_2 retention.

Complications

The principal complication of the disease itself is asphyxia. Complications of tracheostomy include bleeding; displacement of the tube into the tissues of the neck, with resultant obstruction of the airway; and stenosis in the trachea at the site of the tracheostomy tube.

Treatment

A. Emergency Treatment:

1. Tracheostomy—The possible need for a tracheostomy must be considered in both of these entities. A clinical decision must be made concerning the tolerable limits of respiratory obstruction. The severity and the duration of the obstruction must be taken into account along with the adequacy of medical treatment and response to treatment.

Several findings characterize the child who needs a tracheostomy. Inspiratory stridor with coincident suprasternal, abdominal, and intercostal retraction are important signs. A state of restless exhaustion is probably the best indicator of approaching asphyxia. Dysphagia is a sign of extensive inflammation and swelling of the larynx and pharynx.

a. Emergency tracheostomy—The emergency tracheostomy is a "feel" operation. The child is positioned with the neck moderately hyperextended. The laryngeal and cricoid cartilages are identified. The trachea, just below the cricoid, is stabilized between the fingers of one hand, while a vertical incision is made with the other hand. This incision extends through the skin, strap muscles, and thyroid isthmus. A cruciate incision is then made in the tracheal wall, allowing the placement of a tracheostomy tube.

b. Elective tracheostomy—The elective tracheostomy should be employed whenever possible. This should be done in an operating suite with adequate light, suction, and instrumentation.

If the tissues of the neck are opened during labored respiration, the negative intrathoracic pressure will allow the entrance of air into the mediastinum and pleural space. For this reason, it is desirable to place a bronchoscope or endotracheal tube through the larynx prior to beginning a tracheostomy. The placement of either of these airway devices should be undertaken with due deliberation, since any manipulation of the larynx under these circumstances is likely to cause complete airway obstruction.

Local anesthesia is adequate, since the child usually goes to sleep following placement of the endotracheal tube or bronchoscope. The diameter of the tracheostomy tube should be approximately 2/3 that of the trachea. The silver tube is probably best for general use. There are different shapes of tubes. The Holinger tube is best for children up to the age of 18 months; the Jackson tube is best in older children.

c. After-care—Constant vigilance is necessary in the care of children with tracheostomies. Well trained, experienced nurses are indispensable. Tracheostomy tubes may become displaced from the trachea into the soft tissues of the neck. This problem must be recognized immediately, and the tube must be replaced.

The necessary equipment and personnel must be at hand if tracheostomy in small children is to successfully reduce the childhood mortality due to upper respiratory problems. Nurses responsible for tracheostomy care should be carefully instructed regarding anatomic considerations.

d. Decannulation—In planning decannulation, the tube should be replaced with progressively smaller sizes and finally blocked for 24 hours. The external fistula closes within several days. Careful and persistent effort is necessary in decannulation of children under 1 year of age.

2. Cricothyroidotomy—An excellent alternative measure is cricothyroidotomy. An incision is made between the cricoid and the thyroid cartilages into the trachea in the subglottic area. A tracheostomy tube or other improvised airway is then introduced. Such a tube placed through the cricothyroid membrane is within a few millimeters of the true vocal cords. Therefore, it must be removed within 24 hours and replaced by an orderly tracheostomy. A well designed instrument for cricothyroidotomy is the cricothyroidotomy scissors.

B. Medical Treatment: Antibiotics are employed for their specific effect on the causative organism in the case of supraglottitis and to prevent secondary bacterial infection in the case of laryngotracheitis. High humidity assists in the removal of secretions and should be provided by a cold mist or ultrasound generator. Intramuscular injections of epinephrine in oil may relieve edema, gaining valuable time for response to antibiotic agents. Corticosteroids may be administered for their anti-inflammatory properties.

Prognosis

A. Viral Croup: This course is often protracted (5–7 days) with gradual improvement or, infrequently, gradual tiring of the patient necessitating elective tracheostomy. The prognosis is generally good.

B. *Hemophilus Influenzae* Croup: Overwhelming and fatal sepsis may occur when antibiotic therapy is not promptly instituted. The course is stormy initially with high fever and toxicity, but with specific antibiotic therapy the prognosis is good.

C. Diphtheritic Croup: (Rare in this country.) Without early antitoxin therapy, the chances of toxic complications of diphtheria are considerable, as is the danger of anoxia from obstruction also.

D. Spasmodic Croup: The disease is self-limited and never fatal. It has a short course. It may clear during the day but show progressively milder exacerbations for a few nights.

E. Foreign Body Croup: Prompt removal of the foreign body results in complete recovery.

Eden AN: Corticosteroid treatment of croup. Pediatrics 33:768–769, 1964.

Fearon B: Acute laryngotracheobronchitis in infancy and childhood. P Clin North America 9:1095–1112, 1962.

McClean DM: Myxoviruses associated with acute laryngotracheobronchitis in Toronto. Canad MAJ 89:1257–1259, 1963.

Strannegard O: Pseudo-croup associated with viral infection. Acta oto-laryng 58:432–440, 1964.

Wulff H: Etiology of respiratory infection: Further studies during infancy and childhood. Pediatrics 33:30–44, 1964.

PHARYNGEAL TONSILLITIS

Pharyngeal lymphoid tissue occurs (1) in the nasopharynx (adenoid), (2) at the base of the tongue (lingual tonsil), (3) between the folds (or "pillars") of the soft palate, and (4) in scattered "islands" on the posterior and lateral pharyngeal walls.

The natural history of this tissue is one of intermittent hypertrophy associated with upper respiratory infection. In children, both the tonsils and the adenoids are commonly involved. However, the tonsils and adenoids have a tendency to atrophy as the child reaches puberty. The lingual tonsil and small pharyngeal deposits are frequently involved in adulthood.

Throat cultures and appropriate antibiotics are the obvious solution to the acute infection. Chronic infection seldom occurs in these tissues. Food particles and epithelial debris are commonly mistaken for purulent material when found in the tonsillar crypts.

The possible merit of tonsillectomy should be considered here. This controversial issue has been examined by pediatricians, otolaryngologists, epidemiologists, and others in many ways.

McCorkle found no difference between the incidence of upper respiratory infections among "tonsillectomized" children as opposed to "nontonsillectomized" children. These subjects were over the age of 3 and were part of a comprehensive family epidemiologic study in Cleveland. Chamovitz investigated military men with proved streptococcal pharyngitis, finding no statistical correlation between the presence of infection and the presence of tonsils and adenoids. Some of his subjects did not receive antibiotics. In this group, the incidence of "suppurative complications" was significantly greater among the nontonsillectomized individuals.

Tonsillectomy should not be recommended unless there is some predictable benefit to the patient. A child who has had a peritonsillar abscess should undergo tonsillectomy. A child with a remarkably small pharyngeal space should have hypertrophied tonsils removed to facilitate swallowing. The child with repeated, well documented tonsillitis should either be treated prophylactically with antibiotics during the winter months or have a tonsillectomy, ie, the treatment is designed to shorten the illness and reduce suppurative complications.

In the tonsillectomized child, vigilance is required to identify subclinical streptococcal infections that may go untreated and lead to rheumatic or renal complications.

ADENOIDITIS

Pharyngeal infection usually involves the nasopharynx, and in prepuberal children causes adenoid hypertrophy. The adenoids may become large enough to occlude the posterior nares and to partially block the orifices of the eustachian tubes. If evidence of such obstruction persists despite adequate treatment for acute infections, adenoidectomy is indicated. It may be necessary to repeat this procedure several times during childhood to prevent serious middle ear disease. The morbidity from this procedure is slight, and the indications are distinctly separate from those for tonsillectomy.

LINGUAL TONSILLITIS

Hypertrophy of the lymphoid tissue at the base of the tongue may become clinically significant in older children and adults. Cultures from this area are seldom helpful except in acute infection. A 10-day course of antibiotics usually produces partial resolution of the hypertrophied tissue.

PERITONSILLAR ABSCESS
(Quinsy)

Tonsillar infection, though usually limited to the lymphoid tissue itself, may sometimes spread to the surrounding muscle and mucosa. Penetration of the infection through the fibrous capsule surrounding the tonsil leads to peritonsillar inflammation and usually to abscess. Clinical findings reflect the expanding mass of the abscess and the inflammatory changes in the muscles of mastication.

The soft palate and uvula are edematous and displaced forward and toward the uninvolved side. Severe trismus and dysphagia are common. The patient expectorates his saliva. Voice quality is severely impaired by the fixation of the soft palate.

Treatment includes culture, sensitivity studies, and appropriate antibiotics. Incision and drainage are done by introducing a needle into the abscess to locate the space and then incising along the needle shaft. Following recovery from the acute infection, tonsillectomy should be done to prevent recurrence.

Chamovitz R: The effect of tonsillectomy on the incidence of streptococcal respiratory disease and its complications. Pediatrics 26:355–367, 1960.

Evans HE: Tonsillectomy and adenoidectomy: Review of published evidence for and against T & A. Clin Pediat 7:71–75, 1968.

Mawson S & others: A controlled study evaluation of adeno-tonsillectomy in children. J Laryng 81:777, 1967.

Mawson S & others: A controlled study evaluation of adeno-tonsillectomy in children. Part 2. J Laryng 82:963–979, 1968.

McCorkle LP: Study of illness in a group of Cleveland families: Relation of tonsillectomy to the incidence of common respiratory diseases in children. New England J Med 252:1066–1069, 1955.

PERIPHARYNGEAL SPACE ABSCESS

The peripharyngeal space is bounded medially by the superior constrictor muscle, laterally by the parotid, anteriorly by the pterygomandibular raphe, and posteriorly by the prevertebral fascia. Abscess formation in children is usually a complication of tonsil infection or dental disease. A tender palpable mass is noted behind the angle of the mandible, and the lateral wall of the oropharynx usually bulges slightly. The prolonged presence of such an abscess may cause erosion into a major vessel.

Drainage is accomplished by an incision in the neck just below the mandible. Exploration of the wound is in a superior direction, and placement of a drain completes the surgical treatment.

Danforth HD: Pharyngeal maxillary space abscess: Changing concepts of etiology. Laryngoscope 73:1344–1350, 1963:

RETROPHARYNGEAL ABSCESS

This potential space is delimited posteriorly by the prevertebral fascia and anteriorly by the pharyngeal mucosa. Lymph nodes present in this area may undergo necrosis in response to infection, with resultant abscess formation. The abscess forms on either side of the midline, since a midline raphe divides the 2 potential spaces. A sessile swelling is seen on the posterior pharyngeal wall or in the nasopharynx, oropharynx, or hypopharynx. Dysphagia and dyspnea may result. Serious hemorrhage has been reported in long-standing cases.

Incision and drainage should be done to prevent extension of the infection and possible hemorrhage. This should be done with the patient in the head-down position to avoid aspiration of purulent material.

Hays H: Retro-pharyngeal hemorrhage: A fatal case. Texas Med 60:904–905, 1964.

LARYNGEAL PAPILLOMATOSIS

This disease is characterized by the development of cauliflower-like squamous papillomas on the mucous membranes of the larynx. The age at onset is usually 2–3 years. Hoarseness and then respiratory obstruction are the chief symptoms. Diagnosis is established by indirect or direct laryngoscopy and biopsy.

The inadequacy of any treatment is reflected in the potpourri of methods currently employed, ie, antibiotics, podophyllin, ultrasound, freezing technics, vaccines, and tracheostomy.

There is significant evidence that the cause is viral, and autogenous and animal vaccines have been employed with some success. Vigilance regarding the upper airway is of paramount importance. A long-standing tracheostomy may be necessary.

Spontaneous remission usually occurs at puberty, but the disease may continue through adulthood.

Boyle W & others: Treatment of papilloma of the larynx in children. Laryngoscope 80:1063–1077, 1970.

Dmochowski L & others: A study of submicroscopic structure and of virus particles in cells of human laryngeal papilloma. Texas Rep Biol Med 22:454–491, 1964.

Holinger P & others: Laryngeal papilloma: Review of etiology and therapy. Laryngoscope 78:1462–1474, 1968.

Klos J & others: A cytopathic agent in laryngeal papilloma of children. Ann Otol Rhin Laryng 75:225–234, 1966.

LARYNGEAL POLYP

This pedunculated cystic lesion usually develops in the anterior part of the larynx and just below the true cords. Hoarseness occurs as the tumor is interposed between the cords on phonation.

Treatment consists of simple excision under direct laryngoscopy.

SINGER'S NODES

This lesion consists of a firm mass of scar occurring along the edge of the true vocal cord. Vocal trauma—shouting or coughing—produces a hemorrhage beneath the epithelium. A nodular scar is subsequently formed which causes hoarseness.

Voice rest will usually allow resolution of the nodule. Since the lesion is on the phonating edge of the cord, excision, if necessary, should be undertaken with extreme care, using the otologic operating microscope, to avoid permanent damage to the vocal cord.

ANGIOFIBROMA

This uncommon tumor of adolescent males originates from the posterior wall of the nasopharynx, and

may extend into the posterior choanae, the maxillary and ethmoid sinuses, the subtemporal fossa, and rarely into the middle cranial fossa. As the name implies, the neoplasm is composed of fibrous and vascular tissue. Presenting symptoms are usually either bleeding or nasal obstruction. The presence of the tumor can be confirmed by anterior rhinoscopy and nasopharyngoscopy.

The primary treatment is surgical excision. The vascularity of the tumor is believed by some to be reduced by giving x-ray treatment and estrogens. Hemorrhage at the time of surgery may be reduced by controlled hypotension with hypothermia or freezing of the tumor with a cryogenic probe.

Fitzpatrick P: The nasopharyngeal angiofibroma. Canad J Surg 13:228–235, 1970.

McGavron M & others: Nasopharyngeal angiofibroma. Arch Otolaryng 90:68–78, 1969.

Patterson CN: Juvenile nasopharyngeal angiofibroma. Arch Otolaryng 81:270–277, 1964.

Pimpinella RJ: The nasopharyngeal angiofibroma in adolescent males. J Pediat 64:260–267, 1964.

MALIGNANT TUMORS OF LARYNX & PHARYNX

Malignancies of the larynx and pharynx are uncommon in children. Rhabdomyosarcoma, lymphoepithelioma, and lymphosarcoma are among the more commonly encountered malignancies found in this area. Adequate physical examination of these areas is essential for early diagnosis.

Rush BF: Cancer of the head and neck in children. Surgery 53:270–284, 1963.

•   •   •

General References

Birrell JF: *The Ear, Nose and Throat Diseases of Children.* Davis, 1960.

Dale DMC: *Applied Audiology for Children,* 2nd ed. Thomas, 1967.

Eagles EL, Wishik SM, Doerfler LG: *Hearing Sensitivity and Ear Disease in Children: A Prospective Study.* Laryngoscope, 1967.

Proctor DF: *The Nose, Paranasal Sinuses and Care in Childhood.* Thomas, 1963.

Valdes M: Sudden and unexpected death in infancy: A review of the world literature. Pediatrics 39:123–138, 1967.

Wilson JG: *Diseases of the Ear, Nose and Throat in Children,* 2nd ed. Grune & Stratton, 1962.

12...

Respiratory Tract & Mediastinum

Ernest K. Cotton, MD, William H. Parry, MD, & David N. Myers, MB

INTRODUCTION

GROWTH OF THE LUNGS

The lungs originate (at 24 days of gestational age) as a ventral outpouching of the primitive gut, which bifurcates into the anlagen of the major bronchi between 26 and 28 days. The subdivision of the endodermal tree continues for the next 12 weeks, by which time the antenatal formation of new bronchi is nearly complete. The endoderm provides the lining cells of the respiratory tract as well as the glandular structures. The surrounding mesenchyme, into which the endoderm insinuates, provides the smooth muscle, cartilage, and connective tissue of the respiratory tree as well as the pulmonary septa and pleura. Cannulization of the airways begins at approximately 20 weeks. Alveoli appear and proliferate from about 26–28 weeks, and during this time the capillary bed proliferates to envelop the developing alveoli.

The airway at birth has little smooth muscle, but by 1 year of age smooth muscle has increased to an amount comparable to that in the young adult. Not all smooth muscle is under nervous system control; in the respiratory unit, smooth muscle is under the control of humoral factors. In contrast, at birth, the smooth muscle of the pulmonary vascular bed is greatly thickened and very reactive. By age 1, the smooth muscle mass of the vascular bed has decreased and is comparable to that of the adult. In newborns, the most reactive portion of the lung is the pulmonary vascular bed; in older children, it is the smooth muscle of the airway.

Postnatal growth of the lungs continues until about 8 years of age. Growth proceeds by increases in the number of generations of branching airways from 17 at birth to 24 by 8 years. Dilatation of major airways occurs, but the ratio between anatomic dead space (internal volume of the airway) and body weight remains constant from birth to adulthood.

PHYSIOLOGIC ASPECTS

Gaseous exchange remains constant with age. Oxygen and CO_2 tensions in the arterial blood of infants do not differ remarkably from those of adults. Chemoreceptor activity likewise is the same in infants, children, and adults. Changes in ventilation and perfusion occur only with alterations of the physiologic state of the individual or changes in the ambient pressures of the inspiratory gases.

All aspects of lung disease relate to alterations in ventilation and perfusion. Since ventilation is dependent upon perfusion and perfusion upon ventilation, it is essential to understand the basic physiologic control of both the airway and the pulmonary vascular bed.

Fig 12–1 summarizes the interaction of ventilation and perfusion as discussed below. This illustration emphasizes acute alterations in normal physiology, but the relationship between changes in oxygen tension and [H⁺] in the arterial blood can also be applied to more chronic states.

Smooth muscle without nervous system control (terminal airway and pulmonary vascular bed) responds to 2 stimuli: hypoxemia and acidemia. The smooth muscle in the airway may actually be constricted by histamine, but this substance is mediated by reduced oxygen tension and increased [H⁺] in the arterial blood. Thus, under conditions of hypoxemia or acidemia due to whatever cause, the pulmonary vascular bed is constricted. Since the pulmonary artery is the major source of nutrients to the respiratory unit, lung metabolism is adversely affected.

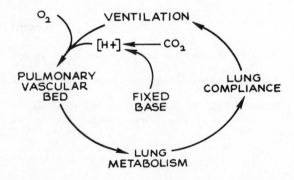

FIG 12–1. Interaction of ventilation and perfusion.

Twelve to 16 metabolic pathways occur within the lung. One of the most important is the production of surfactant by the type 2 pneumocyte located in the alveolus. Surfactant, a lipoprotein lining the alveoli, has the ability to stabilize the lung and prevent atelectasis; therefore, after exhalation, the lung does not start from the degassed state (like the first breath at birth) but as a volume of gas in the alveoli which enables subsequent breaths to take place with little work of breathing. However, with hypoxemia and acidemia leading to constriction of the pulmonary vascular bed and with consequent decrease in alveolar metabolism and decreased production of surfactant, the work of breathing is increased. This is demonstrated by measurement of lung compliance, which is found to be decreased. In other words, the lung is "stiffer," and more work is required to produce comparable ventilation than in a normal lung. Increased work creates greater amounts of organic acids, which further contributes to the acidemia. When the work of breathing increases to the point that the patient cannot maintain ventilation, hypoxemia worsens and hypercapnia still further contributes to the acidemia, completing the cycle and initiating progressive pulmonary disability. The physician who recognizes what is happening may interrupt the process with appropriate therapy at one or several points.

Respiratory smooth muscle with nervous system control (the airway) responds to multiple stimuli. Fig 12–2 outlines the reflex control of the airway. The portion of the respiratory tree distal to the broken line

(the respiratory unit) shows the smooth muscle under humoral control (PO_2 and pH), as described above. The smooth muscle of the airway resides primarily in the bronchiolar area, but enough is present in upper airways to exert a significant influence on airway caliber when cartilaginous support is lacking, as is the case in infants.

Constricting reflexes are (1) irritation of the nose and lower airway, mediated via the CNS, and (2) hypoxemia, mediated via the carotid body. There is one dilating reflex, with afferent fibers localized near the alveoli which are activated with beginning expansion; it results in a widening of the airway far beyond that which can be accomplished by passive means.

The most important laboratory evaluation used in conjunction with the history, physical examination, and radiologic evaluation of a patient with lung disease is measurement of arterial blood gases and pH. Lung volume determinations, airway resistances, flow rates, and diffusion studies are helpful in cooperative patients (usually older than 5 years of age). Arterial blood gas determinations of clinical interest consist of oxygen saturation (SO_2), oxygen tension (PO_2), and CO_2 tension (PCO_2). Included also is the pH and the base excess; the latter is the relationship between the logarithm of the PCO_2 and the pH on a linear scale, which can be helpful in evaluation of metabolic acidosis and alkalosis. Clinical interpretations of physiologic alterations in blood gases and acid-base disorders are discussed in Chapter 37.

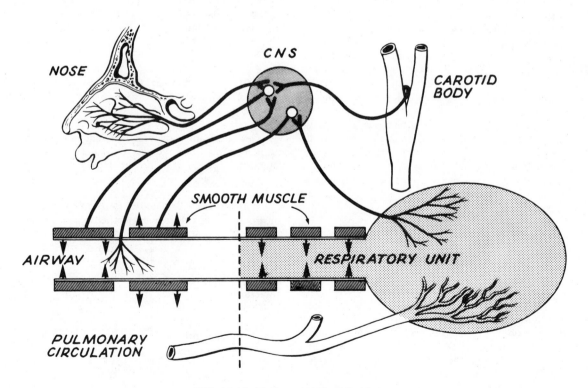

FIG 12–2. Reflex control of the airway.

If the pulmonary bed has become totally constricted, the blood flow from the right heart has 3 possible choices or combinations of choices:

(1) Pooling on the right side, with resultant right-sided failure (cor pulmonale).

(2) Shunting through heart defects such as a patent ductus or foramen ovale, as seen in the newborn with idiopathic respiratory distress syndrome.

(3) Shunting through unventilated portions of the lung with relatively low vascular resistance, as in chronic obstructive airway disease or congenital heart disease with a large bronchial circulation. The degree of right-to-left shunting can be evaluated by giving the patient 100% oxygen to breathe and obtaining an arterial blood gas determination.

PHYSICAL EXAMINATION

Physical findings during examination depend essentially on air entry into and out of the respiratory unit. The most essential evaluation is to determine whether air flow can be heard throughout all portions of the lung.

Chest configuration (retraction, hyperexpansion) gives an indication of the rate of air flow into and out of the airways.

Wheezing, rhonchi, and rales point to specific areas of obstruction of air flow in the bronchiolar area (wheezing), the larger airway (rhonchi), and the respiratory unit (rales).

Physical findings are to a great extent dependent upon age. In infants wheezing often originates in the major airways because of their smaller diameter and nonelastic properties. Furthermore, retractions are more localized to the lower costal area where the diaphragm inserts, since the diaphragm is the major muscle of respiration in infancy.

Cyanosis and clubbing may be a sign of lung disease as well as heart disease. Examination of the fundi may reveal venous engorgement in chronic pulmonary disease. Growth is usually poor in severe lung disease. Headache may be a sign of hypercapnia in an individual with lung disease, and restlessness is a sign of hypoxemia.

PULMONARY FUNCTION TESTS

In older children, the evaluation of lung volumes and flow rates can be helpful in differentiating restrictive and obstructive lung disease. Most of the clinical respiratory problems seen in medicine are obstructive airway problems. In children, these are usually reversible, such as in bronchiolitis and in reactive airway disease. Restrictive lung disease usually is a result of an acute problem such as respiratory distress syndrome.

An example of chronic disease resulting in restrictive pulmonary disease is muscular or connective tissue involvement of the chest wall. Simple pulmonary function studies can be very helpful, and if necessary the child should be referred to a facility where total lung volumes, residual volume, and airway conductance (G) studies can be carried out. These simple studies consist of a vital capacity (VC) measurement and a timed vital capacity measurement. The vital capacity is the maximum volume of air that can be taken in or forced out of the lungs regardless of the time required. The timed vital capacity is the amount of air that can be forced out of the lung from a maximal inspiration (forced expiratory volume; FEV). One-second (FEV_1) and 3-second (FEV_3) intervals are usually evaluated.

Table 12–1 compares the pulmonary function values in obstructive airway disease and restrictive lung disease.

As can be seen, an adequate differentiation between these 2 abnormalities can be made with VC and FEV_1 alone. More complicated pulmonary function studies are necessary for research and evaluation of therapy.

Tidal volume is the amount of air breathed during quiet breathing. This volume multiplied by the respiratory rate is termed the minute volume and is the amount of ventilation necessary or attempted to maintain normal blood gas levels. Whenever a person needs assisted ventilation by artificial means, the tidal volume is set at 10 ml/kg regardless of age, but the accuracy of this value is determined by the resultant blood gas value. In the management of patients who require assisted ventilation, measurement of arterial blood gases is essential.

ANATOMIC & PHYSIOLOGIC DIFFERENCES BETWEEN NEONATES, CHILDREN, & ADULTS

Newborns are nasal breathers, and total airway obstruction may occur unless the nasal passages are patent. (Nonpatency occurs principally in choanal

TABLE 12–1. Pulmonary function tests in obstructive airway disease and restrictive lung disease.

	Obstructive	Restrictive
Vital capacity (VC)	N	↓
Residual volume (RV)	↑	↓
Total lung capacity (TLC)	↑	↓
Timed VC for 1 second (FEV_1)	↓	N
Airway conductance (G)	↓	N
Arterial oxygen tension (P_{O_2})	↓	↓
Arterial CO_2 tension (P_{CO_2})	N or ↑	↓

atresia, Pierre Robin syndrome, and craniofacial dysostosis.)

Because the ribs of newborns are nearly horizontal, the anteroposterior diameter of the thoracic cage cannot increase with inspiration. The diaphragm is displaced upward by the relatively large liver, and ventilation is largely diaphragmatic. The lungs are less efficient ventilating organs, with a respiratory surface per unit weight that is 1/3 that of adults.

The larynx is situated more cephalad, the glottis being situated at the level of the interspace between cervical vertebrae 3 and 4. The laryngeal reflexes are very active, but "bucking" does not occur in the first 3 months. The epiglottis is longer, V or Y shaped, and projects farther posteriorly. The narrowest part of the larynx (and often the entire airway) is at the level of the cricoid cartilage.

Brady JP, Cotton EK, Tooley WH: Chemoreflexes in the newborn infant. J Physiol 172:332–341, 1964.

Chu J & others: Neonatal pulmonary ischemia. Pediatrics 40:709–780, 1967.

Comroe JH & others: *Physiology of Respiration: An Introductory Text.* Year Book, 1965.

Giammonia ST: Evaluation of pulmonary function in children. P Clin North America 18:285–304, 1971.

Widdicombe JG: Regulation of bronchial calibre. Pages 48–82 in: *Advances in Respiratory Physiology.* Caro C (editor). Arnold, 1966.

GENERAL PRINCIPLES IN THE TREATMENT OF LUNG DISEASE

In this chapter, the conventional classification of diseases according to anatomic site of involvement will be used; however, the emerging opinion is that a more appropriate classification would be based on the normal physiology and its alteration by disease. The treatment of these diseases is based on the physiologic alterations that occur—eg, reactive airway disease in bronchiolitis, asthma, and foreign body aspiration. The alterations that occur relate basically to ventilation/perfusion abnormalities. Control of the airway (ventilation) and pulmonary vascular bed (perfusion) have been outlined above. Technics of management will be discussed below, emphasizing physiologic alterations, ie, oxygen is the treatment for hypoxemia.

ARTERIAL BLOOD GASES

Measurement of P_{O_2} and P_{CO_2} is the basis for understanding of the disease process occurring. In most laboratories, arterial blood pH is measured also.

The radial artery is the best site for arterial blood gas sampling as there is no vein nearby. There is little or no place for using "arterialized" capillary blood. The radial artery can be used just as easily in newborns as in older children.

Other potential sites for arterial puncture are the temporal, brachial, and femoral arteries. A 25-gauge needle is used. A complete gas analysis can be done with 0.5 ml of blood. If multiple sampling will be required, percutaneous arterial lines can be placed in older children (5 years and older) or the umbilical artery catheterized in newborns.*

OXYGEN THERAPY

Oxygen therapy is used when arterial blood gases cannot be maintained at a normal gas tension. Enough oxygen should be given by nasal cannula, mask, or hood to maintain an arterial gas tension between 65–85 mm Hg.

Oxygen tents have the disadvantage of not being able to deliver enough oxygen unless they are tightly sealed, which interferes with nursing care.

Nasal prongs are available for children; for infants, a nasal cannula can be constructed from soft rubber or polyvinyl tubing and placed just inside one of the nares. With nasal prongs or a catheter, a 40% concentration of oxygen can be maintained. When nasal obstruction is present or a higher concentration of oxygen is required, a face mask is necessary. The flow through a nasal catheter or prongs should not exceed 3 liters/minute.

High concentrations of oxygen should be avoided. Arterial blood gases at a tension of 120 mm Hg or more can cause eye damage in immature infants. Inspired oxygen concentrations above 240 mm Hg administered for prolonged periods can cause alveolar damage and interstitial fibrosis of the lung. Inspired oxygen concentrations should be set according to the resultant arterial oxygen tension measurement, which should be maintained between 65–85 mm Hg.

HUMIDIFICATION & HYDRATION OF THE AIRWAY

Humidification is definitely indicated in conditions where the large airway is involved. Particles given for large airway conditions should be in the range of 8–10 μm in diameter.

Compressed gases should be bubbled through a humidifier since these gases are dry.

---

*The technic of umbilical artery catheterization is described in Chapter 36.

Ultrasonic nebulizers are available which give a wide range of particle size (Monaghan, 0.5–6 μm) and a 3–6 ml/minute output. There is controversy about whether a tent should be used with these humidifiers for small airway problems. It has been shown (see Wolfsdorf, Swift, & Avery reference, below) that most of the particles rain out in the large airway (nose and pharynx). With deep breathing through the mouth, mist can be delivered to the lower airway. Patients with lower airway problems should be encouraged to breathe the mist deeply from the ultrasonic nebulizer for at least 30 minutes. The number of treatments varies from 2–9 during a 24-hour period.

The most effective way to hydrate the airway is with parenteral fluids. Water is the most effective expectorant, and there is very little evidence that medications such as potassium iodide loosen secretions.

Wolfsdorf J, Swift D, Avery M: Mist therapy reconsidered: An evaluation of the respiratory deposition of labelled water aerosols produced by jet and ultrasonic nebulizers. Pediatrics 43:799–808, 1969.

BRONCHODILATORS

The normal airway is in part supported by normal tissue tone. This tone can be relaxed with bronchodilators (eg, isoproterenol, Bronkosol). A bronchodilator such as Bronkosol (isoetharine, phenylephrine, and thenyldiamine) can be useful in dilating the airway so that medication or humidity can be more effectively breathed. Postural drainage is also more efficient if bronchodilators are used to prevent bronchospasm, which can occur with coughing.

POSTURAL DRAINAGE

Postural drainage is the removal of secretions or foreign matter from the lungs with the aid of gravity. Percussion (with a cupped hand and relaxed arm and wrist) is applied with the patient in the proper position (involved segment upright). These technics help move the secretion into an area where coughing will be effective in its removal. The total time will depend upon area involved; an entire lung can be drained in this way in 15 minutes, or a specific segment in 2–3 minutes.

RESPIRATORY FAILURE

Acute severe respiratory failure is a life-threatening situation and requires immediate therapy.

There is no universally accepted definition of respiratory failure, but it can be presumed to be present when the arterial CO_2 level is elevated or when a moderate to severe degree of hypoxemia exists.

Causes of Respiratory Failure

Respiratory failure may be caused by or secondary to (1) CNS disorders (eg, head injury), (2) neuromuscular diseases (eg, myasthenia gravis, poliomyelitis, Guillain-Barré syndrome), (3) lung diseases (eg, asthma, croup, peripheral lung disease such as respiratory distress syndrome, foreign body aspiration), (4) heart disease (eg, congenital heart disease), or (5) pulmonary vascular bed disorders (eg, pulmonary edema, vasoconstriction).

Principles of Treatment

Treatment is aimed at restoring arterial oxygen and CO_2 tensions to normal. Low arterial oxygen tension can be treated by increasing the concentration of inspired oxygen. In the presence of severe hypercapnia and hypoxia, the predominant respiratory drive may be the hypoxic stimulus; administration of oxygen under these circumstances may result in apnea, but this is a rare occurrence. It should always be borne in mind that lack of oxygen rapidly "wrecks the machinery," and severe hypoxia is not a situation that can be tolerated for very long.*

Increased CO_2 tension is an indication that alveolar ventilation is decreased, and the only way the excess CO_2 can be blown off is by increasing alveolar ventilation. This may require assisted ventilation.

Indications for Assisted or Controlled Ventilation

Assisted ventilation is patient-cycled ventilation augmented by "mechanical means" such as manual resuscitating devices or ventilators. In controlled ventilation, the "mechanical means" controls both the rate and the depth of ventilation.

In general, the indications for assisted or controlled ventilation are as follows:

(1) Arterial oxygen tension which cannot be maintained at or near normal levels by increasing the inspired oxygen concentration.

(2) Elevated CO_2 tension (over 65 mm Hg).

(3) Inability of the patient to perform the necessary work of breathing to maintain normal blood gases. Excessive work of breathing leads to physical exhaustion, and severe respiratory failure may occur suddenly. The oxygen consumption related to excess work of breathing may reach 40% of the total oxygen requirement.

Assisted ventilation may be indicated in the presence of normal blood gas tensions. For example, in Guillain-Barré syndrome, when the vital capacity approaches twice the tidal volume, the patient becomes anxious despite normal blood gases and assisted ventilation is indicated.

---

*See also the discussion of Hypoxic Encephalopathy in Chapter 21.

Application of Assisted Ventilation to the Patient

Some means of connecting the patient to the ventilator is required. This can be achieved by means of an oral or nasal mask, by intubation via either the nasal or oral route, or by tracheostomy. The precise method chosen varies with the specific situation. Some examples are given in the following paragraphs.

In respiratory distress syndrome with an arterial P_{CO_2} of 55 mm Hg and an arterial oxygen tension of 50 mm Hg in 50% inspired oxygen, periodic assisted ventilation with a mask and manual resuscitator is widely used (assisted ventilation for 5 minutes each hour). The CO_2 tension can often be reduced during the period of assisted ventilation, but it rapidly returns to its previously elevated level as soon as ventilatory assistance is discontinued.

Intubation is usually preferred to tracheostomy for diseases of short duration (4–5 days). In the neonate and small infant, nasal intubation is preferable to tracheostomy even if assisted ventilation is continued for long periods.

Tracheostomy is indicated if assisted ventilation will be necessary for a prolonged period (eg, severe Guillain-Barré syndrome).

Tracheostomy in the newborn is a difficult procedure with high morbidity and mortality rates.

A. Ventilators: Ventilators can be broadly classified as volume cycled or pressure cycled. The **volume cycled ventilator** produces a preset volume, the whole volume being transferred to the patient provided no leaks in the ventilator-patient circuit are present. Examples are the Ohio-560 and the Volume Bennett Ventilator (MA1). Volume ventilators may be essential in managing certain respiratory problems where compliance is severely decreased and high pressures are necessary to produce a given volume change (eg, asthma, pulmonary edema).

The **pressure cycled ventilator** produces a certain preset pressure; once this pressure is reached, the ventilator ceases to produce a gas flow. If the compliance of the patient's lungs or chest wall changes, the volume delivered will change. Examples are the Bennett PR2 and the Bird apparatus.

Ventilators can be used to give either assisted or controlled ventilation.

1. Assisted ventilation—The ventilator detects the start of the patient's inspiration (usually by detecting a small negative pressure in the patient's airway at the beginning of inspiration) and transmits its preset volume or pressure to the patient's airway.

2. Controlled ventilation—The ventilator controls both the rate and depth of ventilation. The patient will on occasion breathe out of phase with the ventilator when it is being used as a "controller." The patient's respirations can be brought into phase with the ventilator by hyperventilating the patient for a short time, thus reducing the arterial CO_2 tension and therefore the respiratory drive; by giving narcotics (eg, morphine) to depress the respiratory center; or by giving neuromuscular blocking agents such as curare, 1 mg/5 lb, or gallamine (Flaxedil), 1 mg/lb.

TABLE 12–2. Endotracheal tube sizes.*

Age	Weight (kg)	Internal Diameter (mm)	Length (cm)	
Newborn	2–2.5	3.5	10	uncuffed
Newborn	2.5–3	4	12	
1 month	3–4	4.5	13	
6 months	6	4.5	14	
1 year	10	5	15	
2 years	12	5.5	16	
3 years	14	5.5	16	
4 years	16	6	17	
5 years	18	6	17	cuffed or uncuffed
6 years	22	6.5	18	
8 years	30	6.5	18	
10 years	36	7	20	
12 years	45	7	20	
14 years	50	7.5	24	

*Adapted from Smith RM: Anesthesia for Infants and Children. Mosby, 1968.

B. Endotracheal Tubes: Endotracheal tubes are classified on the basis of the internal diameter of the tube in millimeters. The range of size is 3.5–9.5 mm. The correct tube size is that which comfortably passes through the cords. In general, a tube which will pass through the external nares will pass through the cords.

For an approximate guide to the endotracheal tube sizes appropriate for infants and children, see Table 12–2.

For acute resuscitation (eg, resuscitation of the newborn), oral tubes are generally used. If the tube is to be left in situ for more than a few hours, a nasal tube is indicated since nasal tubes are more easily fixed in place and more comfortable for the patient.

Endotracheal tubes are obtainable with cuffs from size 5 mm upward. The purpose of using a cuffed tube is to provide an airtight seal in the patient-ventilator circuit (may be essential if high inflation pressures are utilized) and to isolate the respiratory tract from the gastrointestinal tract, thus preventing aspiration. If an endotracheal tube is cuffed, the volume of air placed in the cuff should be just enough to produce an air-tight seal* since excess pressure in the cuff may produce tracheal necrosis and stenosis. The cuff should be deflated for 5 minutes each hour to prevent persistent ischemia of the tracheal wall.

All patients in respiratory distress should be intubated by a person experienced in the technic. The intubation is usually done with the patient awake and breathing spontaneously. Preoxygenation is an essential prerequisite of intubation, but in many cases the arterial oxygen tension will not be markedly elevated despite preoxygenation, thus providing only a short time to intubate the patient.

---

*A small leak is permissible.

The equipment necessary for successful intubation is as follows:

1. A suction machine (producing an adequate negative pressure) equipped with a tonsil suction and a wide-bore catheter.

2. A manual resuscitating device capable of producing 100% oxygen.

3. A laryngoscope in good working order. For children under age 2, a straight-bladed laryngoscope should be used.

4. A Magill forceps (utilized in nasal intubation).

5. A cardiac monitor or stethoscope to monitor heart rate and rhythm during intubation.

6. A tube of the correct size (Table 12–2). A tube smaller than the estimated size should be available; if the airway might be obstructed (as in croup), a very small tube should be available.

7. A tracheostomy set.

Tracheostomy

Tracheostomy should always be performed as an elective procedure, preferably in the operating room. All tracheostomies should be done over a previously placed endotracheal tube under controlled conditions. Tracheostomy is occasionally required as an urgent lifesaving procedure.

Manual Resuscitating Devices

Manual resuscitation can be performed with a self-inflating bag (AMBU, Hope, etc), but these bags can only deliver a maximum of approximately 50% oxygen no matter how great the supplementary oxygen inflow is; this is due to the entrainment of room air as the bag fills and severely limits their usefulness.

A simple anesthetic T-piece can also be used (Fig 12–3). A high flow of oxygen (eg, 5–7 liters) is used to prevent rebreathing. This apparatus should be used whenever 100% oxygen is indicated.

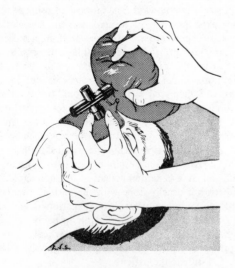

FIG 12–3. Anesthetic T-piece.

Technic of Attaching the Patient to a Ventilator

(1) Set up ventilator, assisting the patient's ventilation with a manual resuscitating device as necessary.

(2) Adjust tidal volume to estimated requirement. An average starting tidal volume is 10 ml/kg. Increase or decrease this on the basis of arterial blood gas determinations.

(3) Adjust rate.

(4) Adjust inspired oxygen tension.

(5) Set humidifier.

(6) Adjust inspiratory flow rate—slower for children, more rapid for larger people.

(7) Make sure warning devices are working.

(8) Observe movement of patient's chest. Auscultate to make sure both lungs are being ventilated.

LOBECTOMY IN CHILDHOOD

Chronically infected lung cysts and those that impair pulmonary function because of airway obstruction are often resected. Lobectomy may also be indicated for sequestered lobes, arteriovenous fistulas, and neoplasms. Persistent bronchiectasis and atelectasis are not indications for surgery and are managed medically.

The operation can usually be performed electively except in the case of emergency resection for lobar emphysema in the neonate. After lobectomy in childhood, the remaining lung has no marked increase in capacity or in the pulmonary capillary bed, although there is minimal hyperplasia.

Cook CD, Bucci G: Studies of respiratory physiology in children. IV. The late effects of lobectomy on pulmonary function. Pediatrics 28:234–242, 1961.

Serg Z & others: Some late sequels of childhood pneumonectomy. Surgery 65:343–351, 1971.

DISEASES OF THE LARYNX, TRACHEA, & BRONCHI*

LARYNGEAL STRIDOR

Common causes of laryngeal stridor are congenital deformity of the epiglottis and supraglottic aperture (most common), epiglottal redundancy, relaxation of the laryngeal wall, congenital absence of the tracheal rings, aortic rings, or other vascular rings, malformation of the vocal cords, a partially occluding laryngeal web, and cysts.

*Drowning is discussed in Chapter 30.

Stridor may also be due to laryngeal infections, tetany, foreign body, neurologic disorders, or anatomic abnormalities (macroglossia, anomalous aortic arch, micrognathia, Pierre Robin syndrome, and some types of congenital heart disease).

Inspiratory stridor, especially pronounced with crying, is present from birth. Congenital laryngeal stridor usually persists for 6–18 months; the child is entirely asymptomatic and without cyanosis. Breathing is noisy (usually on inspiration), and mild intercostal and supraclavicular retraction is evident. Hoarseness, dyspnea, and a laryngeal "crow" may be present. Stridor often disappears when the neck is extended. Direct laryngoscopic examination is helpful in determining the anatomic cause.

Treatment is directed at the underlying cause. Congenital stridor requires no therapy, but special care in feeding is necessary in some cases. Severe stridor due to other causes requires specific etiologic diagnosis and therapy.

Congenital stridor is a self-limited disease with an excellent prognosis. The prognosis of severe stridor due to other causes is that of the specific disease.

Hollinger PH, Johnston KC: The infant with respiratory stridor. P Clin North America 2:403–425, 1955.

Illingsworth RS: Congenital stridor. Clin Pediat 9:94–95, 1970.

CROUP

Croup is a term applied to a symptom complex consisting of a resonant "barking" cough, inspiratory stridor, and variable respiratory distress related to the degree of laryngeal obstruction. Three separate clinical entities are recognized: laryngotracheobronchitis, epiglottitis, and spasmodic laryngotracheitis (Table 12–3).

Croup must be differentiated from aspirated foreign body, allergic diseases (angioneurotic edema), congenital defects such as laryngeal webs, paralysis of the vocal cords, and vascular rings, and diphtheria. Diphtheria can be ruled out by an immunization history. Angioneurotic edema may present as acute respiratory obstruction but is rare in infants and children; epinephrine and antihistamines give prompt relief.

See Table 12–3 for differentiation of other forms of croup.

1. LARYNGOTRACHEOBRONCHITIS
(Viral Croup, Subglottic Croup)

Essentials of Diagnosis
- Gradual onset of symptoms.
- Hoarseness (loss of voice).
- Mild to moderate systemic symptoms.
- White count usually < 15,000/cu mm.

General Considerations

This is the most common form of croup; it usually occurs in children between 6 months and 3 years of age. It is thought to be a viral disease, most commonly due to infection with parainfluenza virus (croup-associated), adenovirus, and respiratory syncytial virus. Measles and influenza viruses have been isolated and have been associated with a prolonged course of croup. The viruses involve mainly the subglottic area (larynx, trachea, and bronchi). Symptoms may vary depending upon which anatomic area is more heavily infected.

Clinical Findings

A. Symptoms and Signs: The onset is usually gradual, with a history of upper respiratory tract symptoms for several days prior to the onset of barking cough and stridor. Fever is generally mild and the child does not appear "sick." If the lower respiratory tract is involved early, wheezing may be present. As the laryngeal obstruction progresses, stridor becomes associated with sternal, intercostal, and abdominal

TABLE 12–3. Differentiating clinical features of laryngotracheobronchitis, epiglottitis, and spasmodic laryngotracheitis.

	Laryngotracheobronchitis	Epiglottitis	Spasmodic Laryngotracheitis
Onset	Gradual	Sudden	Sudden (usually at night)
Voice	Hoarse (loss of voice)	Muffled phonation (quality normal)	Hoarse, sudden loss of voice
WBC	Usually < 15,000/cu mm	Usually > 15,000/cu mm	Normal
Systemic symptoms	Mild to moderate	Marked	None. Usually afebrile.
Other	Dangerous to use O_2 except prior to intubation	Drooling or dysphagia prominent	
Treatment	Varied. Usually humidity, intermittent positive pressure with racemic epinephrine; (?) corticosteroids.	Immediate intubation or tracheostomy	Varied

retractions and the expiratory phase of respiration is prolonged. Auscultation reveals decreased breath sounds. The child becomes anxious and restless as hypoxemia ensues. Cyanosis is a late sign and may herald complete obstruction.

B. Laboratory Findings: The white count seldom rises above 15,000/cu mm. Virus isolation studies have epidemiologic value but are not diagnostically useful.

Complications

The principal complication of viral croup is asphyxia secondary to laryngeal obstruction. Other complications are related to misadventures in attempting to supply an airway in an emergency situation and complications associated with management of a tracheostomy or endotracheal tube after an airway has been provided.

Treatment

A. Medical Measures: Mist is effective in reducing laryngeal edema and relieving respiratory distress. This may be administered in the hospital as cool mist in a "croup tent" or fog room, or at home by means of a cold mist humidifier or by steaming up the bathroom by running the hot water in the bath or shower. Steam vaporizors carry the risk of scalding the child and should not be recommended to parents. Subemetic doses (1–5 ml of syrup of ipecac (**not** ipecac fluidextract) have also been said to be effective; the dose may be repeated in 1 hour if respiratory symptoms persist. Vomiting often gives remarkable relief from symptoms. Antibiotics are not indicated except in case of bacterial superinfection. Sedation is contraindicated since it may depress the respiratory center, promoting hypoventilation and hypoxemia, and may mask the anxiety and restlessness which are the most important signs of hypoxemia. Oxygen as the pressure to generate mist must be used with caution if at all. Hypoxemia is the most useful indication of impending total obstruction of the airway and the need for providing an airway. Administration of oxygen in high concentrations (mask) may delay the onset of clinical hypoxia until the glottis is almost completely obstructed, making a safe intubation much more difficult or the timing of elective tracheostomy much more critical.

The use of corticosteroids is controversial, but many clinicians report good results with dexamethasone (Decadron), 2–4 mg orally every 6 hours.

B. Artificial Airway: If the above measures are not successful in relieving respiratory distress and the patient remains restless and agitated, an airway must be provided. Blood gas analyses are of little value since gas tensions will be normal until a considerable degree of obstruction is present.

Patients who need an artificial airway to relieve airway obstruction require either prolonged nasotracheal intubation or tracheostomy. The important feature of either is to avoid a "crash" intubation or tracheostomy; it is preferred to perform a controlled intubation or tracheostomy under optimal conditions. Once the decision to provide an artificial airway has been made, the child should be given high concentrations of oxygen while arrangements are made. If a nasotracheal tube is employed, it should be small enough to provide a small leak of air around it in order to reduce trauma to the glottis and subglottic area. Tracheostomy should be performed in the operating room over an endotracheal tube or bronchoscopy tube. Postoperative care includes careful suctioning, postural drainage, and pulmonary toilet, including administration of humidified air to the nasotracheal or tracheostomy tube. The patient usually may be extubated or decannulated in 3–5 days.

Prognosis

Most children do not progress beyond the stage of cough, stridor, and mild retractions, and the disease runs its course in 3–7 days with gradual improvement leading to complete recovery.

Eden AN: Corticosteroid treatment of croup. Pediatrics 33:768–769, 1964.

Fearon B: Acute laryngotracheobronchitis in infancy and childhood. P Clin North America 9:1095–1112, 1962.

James JA: Dexamethasone in croup. Am J Dis Child 117:511–516, 1969.

2. EPIGLOTTITIS
(Bacterial Croup, Supraglottic Croup)

This form of croup generally affects children between ages 3–7 years. It has a rapidly progressive, fulminant course. It is most commonly caused by *Hemophilus influenzae* type B, although beta-hemolytic streptococci and pneumonococci have been implicated in rare cases.

See Table 12–3 for differentiations from other forms of croup.

Clinical Findings

A. Symptoms and Signs: The onset of the illness is abrupt. Younger children often present with high fever and respiratory distress; older children complain of difficulty in swallowing and severe sore throat. Because of the dysphagia, pooling of secretions in the pharynx and drooling are prominent signs. Since the site of the pathologic process is the epiglottis and surrounding structures, the larynx is not involved and the patient may not be hoarse. Phonation is muffled, but voice quality is normal. Fever is usually high (> 38.5° C [101.2° F]), and the patient appears "sick" or even shock-like. Blood cultures are frequently positive for *H influenzae* type B. Within hours after onset, the child may be in marked respiratory distress, with stridor and retractions. The pharynx is inflamed (cherry-red), and excessive secretions may be noted. The diagnosis can be made by visualizing the large, swollen, cherry-red epiglottis with a tongue blade. However, this maneuver must be undertaken with great caution because stimulation of the epiglottis has produced abrupt laryngo-spasm and death.

B. Laboratory Findings: Leukocytosis > 15,000/cu mm is usually present.

C. X-Ray Findings: Lateral x-rays of the pharynx may be of value in confirming enlargement of the epiglottis without resorting to direct visualization.

Treatment

When the diagnosis of epiglottitis is suspected, the conservative approach is to provide an artificial airway. Preparations should be made for controlled intubation or tracheostomy. In the operating room, direct visualization of the epiglottis can be performed by the anesthesiologist or someone competent in intubation. If the diagnosis is confirmed, an airway can be immediately provided. Patients may be managed by either nasotracheal tube or tracheostomy. Corticosteroids are of no value. Parenteral (preferably intravenous) antibiotics are indicated; ampicillin is the drug of choice in a dosage of 200–300 mg/kg/day in 6 divided doses for 10 days. In penicillin-sensitive patients, tetracycline or chloramphenicol may be employed.

Prognosis

The disease process usually responds rapidly to antibiotics, and the patient may be extubated or decannulated in 48–72 hours. If an airway is not provided promptly, the mortality rate may be as high as 50%.

Geraci RP: Acute epiglottitis: Prolonged nasotracheal intubation. Pediatrics 41:143–145, 1968.

Rapkin RH: Acute epiglottitis: Pitfalls in diagnosis and management. Clin Pediat 10:312–314, 1971.

3. SPASMODIC CROUP
(Allergic Croup)

This form of croup may affect any age group. There is often a past history or family history of croup. The cause is not known, but the disease may be allergic in nature.

See Table 12–3 for differentiation from other forms of croup.

The onset is abrupt (usually at night), with barking cough and, in some cases, moderate stridor. There are usually no fever or other symptoms.

This disease rarely progresses to airway obstruction, and almost any treatment is effective: change in environmental temperature, enemas, emetics, mist, weather fronts moving through, bronchodilators, and antihistamines have all been reported to be effective. The attack may abate as suddenly as it presented and not recur. More frequently, the symptoms will lessen during the daytime for a few days only to increase at night.

The prognosis is excellent, but recurrences are common.

Dunbar JS: Upper respiratory tract obstruction in infants and children. Am J Roentgenol 109:227–246, 1970.

TRACHEOMALACIA & BRONCHOMALACIA

These congenital disorders are characterized by wheezing, cough, stridor, and dyspnea, which are worse if the child has copious secretions. The basic anatomic abnormality is absence of the tracheal or bronchial cartilages, leading to functional stenosis and obstruction. The chest film shows hyperexpansion of the lungs on an anteroposterior view and tracheal narrowing on a lateral view. Signs are exaggerated, with forced expiration and inspiration such as occur with crying. Bronchomalacia may cause hyperlucent lung or congenital lobar emphysema.

Differentiation from vascular ring, foreign body, and obstructive lesions of the upper airway is by exclusion.

Treatment is directed at control of secretions and infections. Clinical improvement occurs in most cases by age 6 months.

Cox WL, Shaw RR: Congenital chondromalacia of the trachea. J Thoracic Cardiovas Surg 49:1033–1037, 1965.

Lynch JI: Bronchomalacia in children. Clin Pediat 9:279–282, 1970.

MacMahon HE: Congenital segmental bronchomalacia. Am J Dis Child 118:923–926, 1969.

VASCULAR RING

The principal clinical manifestations of vascular ring are noisy respirations at birth, with dyspnea and tachypnea, opisthotonos, increased air trapping, a narrow trachea, and expiratory wheezing. Angiocardiography—either through the venous system or by way of the brachial artery—is diagnostic.

Tracheal obstruction results from one or all of the following: (1) right aortic arch with left ligamentum arteriosum or patent ductus arteriosus, (2) double aortic arch, (3) anomalous innominate or left carotid artery, and (4) aberrant right subclavian artery.

Treatment consists of elective surgical correction. Infections and dehydration should be controlled first.

In experienced hands, the prognosis is good. Cardiac anomalies are usually present and must be corrected also.

Ericsson NO, Söderlund· S: Compression of the trachea by anomalous innominate artery. J Pediat Surg 4:424–431, 1969.

Hallman GL, Cooley DA, Bloodwell RD: Congenital vascular ring. S Clin North America 46:885–892, 1966.

BRONCHITIS

Bronchitis as an isolated clinical entity is uncommon in childhood, but it may be associated with a number of other conditions of the upper and lower respiratory tracts. Viral, bacterial, and fungal infections, allergic disorders, and airborne irritants may initiate symptoms of dry, hacking, and nonproductive cough. Fever, if present, is usually low-grade. Chest pain aggravated by coughing may occur. Within a matter of days, the cough becomes productive, and gagging on the secretions may begin in younger children. After 7–10 days, the mucus thins and the cough gradually disappears.

There is no specific therapy for viral bronchitis. Expectorants may be used but have no proved benefit. Cough suppressants are contraindicated since coughing is necessary to clear secretions. Antihistamines tend to dry secretions, leading to mucous obstruction of bronchi, and should not be employed. Mist or high humidity offers symptomatic relief but does not shorten the course of the disease. Postural drainage and percussion may aid in mobilizing secretions.

Nonviral bronchitis clears with adequate treatment of the underlying cause. Antibiotics are indicated in the rare cases of bacterial or fungal bronchitis; however, in pertussis, antibiotics do not appear to shorten the course of the disease. Chemical aspiration will cause bronchitis similar to that which occurs as a result of smoke inhalation or heat damage (steam inhalation). Noxious chemicals present in urban air pollution are becoming a more prominent cause of chronic bronchitis and repeated lower respiratory tract illness.

Colley JRT, Reed DD: Urban and social origins of childhood bronchitis in England and Wales. Brit MJ 2:213–217, 1970.
Pearlman ME & others: Nitrogen dioxide and lower respiratory illnesses. Pediatrics 47:391, 1971.

BRONCHIOLITIS

Essentials of Diagnosis

- Rhinitis, rales, cough, and wheezing.
- Dyspnea with rapid, shallow respirations.
- Hyperresonance, poor air entry, intermittent cyanosis.
- Increased anteroposterior diameter of the chest.
- Irritability, prostration, low-grade fever.
- Flattened diaphragm and increased radiolucency on chest x-ray.

General Considerations

Respiratory syncytial (RS) virus is the most common viral cause of bronchiolitis, but parainfluenza viruses, adenoviruses, influenza viruses, and *Myco-*

plasma pneumoniae can give the same clinical picture. Recurrent bronchiolitis is frequently followed by childhood asthma. Severe hypoxia with a decline in alveolar oxygen tension (P_{O_2}) is followed by a rise in arterial P_{CO_2}, leading to respiratory acidosis. Hypoxemia may persist for 4–6 weeks after the child has begun to improve clinically.

Clinical Findings

A. Symptoms and Signs: Rhinitis precedes the respiratory disease by several days. Other family members may be ill with a viral respiratory infection. Fever is mild (usually 37.8° C). Tachycardia and tachypnea are prominent findings. Pallor occurs with bronchiolitis of rapid onset, and cyanosis with gradual onset. Retraction with inspiration and overinflation of lungs causes an increase in anteroposterior diameter of the chest and flattening of the diaphragm, with downward displacement of the liver and spleen. Fine crepitation is heard on both inspiration and expiration; however, with marked involvement, air entry is diminished. Expiratory wheezing can be a major finding in some cases but is not essential to the diagnosis.

B. Laboratory Findings: The white blood count is usually normal—an important point in the differentiation from pneumonia and whooping cough. In asthma, nasal and peripheral eosinophilia may be present. Other laboratory findings are noncontributory.

C. X-Ray Findings: Chest x-ray always shows hyperinflation (increased radiolucency), especially on a lateral film, with flattening of the diaphragm. Small areas of collapse are occasionally found.

Differential Diagnosis

In small infants it may be impossible to differentiate bronchiolitis from bronchial pneumonia. Fever is high in bronchial pneumonia, as is the neutrophil leukocyte count.

Whooping cough may be clinically identical with bronchiolitis except that white counts over 15,000/cu mm are unusual in bronchiolitis.

Asthma can occur in infancy, and the differentiation from bronchiolitis may be difficult at first. A positive family history for allergy, repeated attacks, nasal or peripheral eosinophilia, and immediate response to a bronchodilator suggest an allergic etiology.

In severe cases, an erroneous diagnosis of heart failure may be made. Growth retardation, enlarged heart (rare in bronchiolitis), and cardiac murmurs indicate heart disease.

Complications

The principal complication is secondary bacterial infection. Pneumothorax and mediastinal emphysema have been reported. Respiratory failure may occur.

Treatment

Adequate hydration is important since tachypnea increases insensible water loss. In severe cases, hydration must be by the intravenous route since oral intake will be decreased. Forcing oral fluids increases the risk of ... already distressed ... given whether the ... poxemia is invari- ... dministration of ... nd it is hard to ... icosteroids and ... edation should ... gests oxygen ... tics are indi- ... fections. ... rminations ... ry failure. ... mployed ... litis.

... sis is ... % of ... re, ... es ...

Useful clinical and biochemical guidelines for instituting assisted ventilation in severe asthma are as follows: (1) Severe inspiratory retractions. (2) The so-called silent chest (decreased wheezing and breath sounds). (3) $P_{aCO_2} > 65$ mm Hg. (4) Base deficit which cannot be corrected by sodium bicarbonate.

Treatment

Preoxygenation is essential to successful ventilation. Correct acidosis and maintain acid-base balance while the ventilator is being used.

Discontinue isoproterenol or epinephrine until airway responsiveness returns, continue aminophylline therapy (4 mg/kg orally every 4–6 hours) and maintain corticosteroid therapy while on respirator.

Ventilate with a ventilator capable of producing the high pressures required under condition of high airway resistances (see Oxygen Therapy, above, for technic of intubation and ventilation management).

The average time on a ventilator is about 36 hours. Prior to weaning from the ventilator, restart epinephrine or isoproterenol. Assess the patient's ability to maintain normal blood gases by connecting the nasotracheal tube to a T-piece and delivering an oxygen-enriched mixture.

If the blood gases remain satisfactory, remove the tube and observe clinical status and blood gases carefully. A percutaneously placed arterial line (radial artery) greatly facilitates management.

Downes JJ & others: Management of status asthmaticus. Pediatrics 38:286–290, 1966.

Downes JJ & others: Acute respiratory failure in infants with bronchiolitis. Anesthesiology 29:426–434, 1968.

Eisen AH, Bacal HL: The relationship of acute bronchiolitis to bronchial asthma. Pediatrics 31:859–861, 1963.

Leer JA & others: Corticosteroid treatment in bronchiolitis. Am J Dis Child 112:495–584, 1969.

Loda FA & others: Studies on the role of viruses, bacteria, and M pneumoniae as causes of lower respiratory infections in children. J Pediat 72:161–176, 1968.

Wohl MEB & others: Resistance of the total respiratory system in healthy infants and infants with bronchiolitis. Pediatrics 43:495–509, 1969.

Wright FH, Beem MO: Management of acute viral bronchiolitis. Pediatrics 35:334–337, 1965.

BRONCHIECTASIS

Essentials of Diagnosis

- Cough (worse in morning); increased sputum production.
- Consistent physical findings in one lung area.
- Intermittent low-grade fever.
- Clubbing of fingers.

General Considerations

This disease, which essentially results from infection and obstruction or mechanical stress and obstruction, does not necessarily result in permanent damage to the bronchi. It often occurs in children under 5 years of age.

Bronchiectasis occasionally develops after a single episode of pneumonia, pertusis, or measles, but it usually occurs after recurrent infection. Bronchiectasis may be associated with asthma. It is usually present with cystic fibrosis of the lung and is common in children with agammaglobulinemia and its variants. Other causes may include Kartagener's syndrome, foreign body, and tuberculosis.

Some cases are probably congenital in origin and have been postulated to result from an arrest of bron-

MANAGEMENT OF SEVERE ASTHMA
(See also Chapter 33.)

Spasm of smooth muscle of the bronchi and bronchioles results in narrowing of the airway. Edema and retained secretions enhance this effect, and airway resistance increases. Trapping of gas distal to the airway obstruction results in an increase in the functional residual capacity. Work of breathing increases.

Arterial CO_2 tension (P_{aCO_2}) increases. Hypoxemia which has been present since early in the attack increases but can usually be controlled with supplementary oxygen. Metabolic acidosis increases as the severity and duration increase.

The patient becomes fatigued, can no longer perform the work of breathing, and will die unless assisted ventilation is instituted.

The decision whether and when to ventilate becomes a critical one because delay may result in death or the necessity for emergency resuscitation. The advantages of early use of a ventilator must be weighed against the difficulties and complications of the procedure (see Oxygen Therapy, above).

chial development which leads to the formation of cysts which become infected.

Clinical Findings

A. Symptoms and Signs: The clinical manifestations are quite variable. Most children with this disease are healthy in appearance. Cough and sputum production in a child with a history of respiratory infection are the most important symptoms. Cough is much worse in the morning. Sputum varies from whitish to gray and purulent. Bloody sputum is a rare finding. Clubbing of the fingers appears in 25–50% of patients and does not relate to severity. Sinusitis is sometimes present, usually as one component of the triad of sinusitis, situs inversus, and bronchiectasis (Kartagener's syndrome).

Physical findings vary with the amount of retained secretions in the involved area. There may be decreased air entry with dullness to percussion.

B. Laboratory Findings: Sputum culture usually reveals a mixed flora of bacteria, with *Hemophilus influenzae* being the most common.

C. X-Ray Findings: Chest x-rays usually show one or all of the following: increase in pulmonary markings, chronic pneumonia, ring shadows, and displacement of the heart and mediastinum. Normal chest films are occasionally reported. A bronchogram will differentiate the type of involvement (cylindrical or saccular) and the areas of involvement. Bronchography is diagnostic.

Complications

Complications include brain or lung abscess, emphysema, bronchopleural fistula, hemoptysis, cor pulmonale, and amyloidosis.

Prevention

Pneumonia should be treated with appropriate antibiotics in adequate dosages. In cases of pneumonia that are not responding properly, postural drainage should be used in conjunction with a bronchodilator. All children should receive adequate immunizations for pertussis and measles.

Treatment

A. Medical Treatment: Treatment consists of postural drainage exercises, warm moist inhalations, and adequate antibiotics for 10–14 days chosen on the basis of the results of sputum cultures, repeating with each infection.

B. Surgical Treatment: Surgery is restricted to well localized saccular lesions which have not responded to an adequate trial of medical therapy (about 1 year).

Prognosis

Combinations of immunologic deficiency and bronchiectasis have the poorest prognosis. Most children with this disease are well controlled and lead normal lives. It has been repeatedly shown that bronchiectasis is not progressive but remains localized. In some cases, the disease clears entirely by adolescence; in others, repeated upper respiratory infections continue to occur.

Field CE: Bronchiectasis: Third report on a follow-up study of medical and surgical cases from childhood. Arch Dis Child 44:551–561, 1969.

Glauser E, Cook CD, Harris GBC: Bronchiectasis: A review of 187 cases. Acta paediat scandinav 55(Suppl 165):1–16, 1966.

Hartline JV, Zilkowitz PS: Kartagener's syndrome in childhood. Am J Dis Child 121:349–352, 1971.

CYSTIC FIBROSIS

Essentials of Diagnosis

- Elevated sweat chloride.
- Absent or decreased pancreatic exocrine function.
- Recurrent pulmonary infections.
- Characteristic changes in chest x-rays.
- Diarrhea.
- Failure to thrive.

General Considerations

Cystic fibrosis is a genetically transmitted autosomal recessive disease characterized by widespread involvement of the exocrine glands. Approximately 5% of the Caucasian population are carriers of the recessive gene, and one in 2000 births is affected by the disease. Multiple organ systems are involved as well as the lungs, including the gastrointestinal tract, the biliary tree, the sweat glands, and the testes.

The basic pathophysiology in the lung resides mainly in the bronchioles. There is a derangement in the bronchiolar mucous glands which results in an end product which is thick and tenacious. The respiratory cilia, which may also have a disorganized beating pattern, are unable to effectively clear the tenacious mucus. This leads to complete or partial obstruction of the bronchioles and eventually results in air trapping or atelectasis. Secondarily acquired infection occurs and predisposes to destruction of the respiratory epithelium and bronchioles, resulting in bronchiectasis. The disease is progressive and leads to respiratory failure and death. There is wide clinical variability, with some patients severely affected as infants while others remain asymptomatic until adolescence. Any patient with malabsorption problems or repeated pulmonary infections should be suspected of having cystic fibrosis. An elevated sweat chloride (> 70 mEq/liter) is diagnostic.

Clinical Findings

A. Symptoms and Signs: In severe disease, patients have foul-smelling fatty stools, failure to thrive, and repeated pulmonary infection with chronic productive cough. Newborns may present with intestinal obstruction secondary to inspissated meconium (meconium ileus). Mild cases may present symptoms which resemble asthma.

Physical examination may be normal or may reveal signs of pulmonary involvement, including hyperexpansion of the thoracic cage, rales and rhonchi, cyanosis, and clubbing.

Pulmonary function tests reveal obstructive lung disease with increased total lung capacity and residual volumes. Vital capacity may be decreased and the airway resistance increased.

B. Laboratory Findings: Laboratory tests are normal except for the elevated sweat sodium and chloride and increased stool fat excretion.

C. X-Ray Findings: Chest x-ray reveal hyperexpansion with flattening of the diaphragm early in the disease. Later, there are diffuse infiltrates, peribronchial cuffing, and areas of atelectasis.

Differential Diagnosis

Cystic fibrosis must be differentiated from allergic diseases, immunologic deficiency diseases, chronic recurrent pneumonia, and alpha$_1$ antitrypsin deficiency disease.

Complications

Complications include pneumothorax, hemoptysis, empyema, cor pulmonale, respiratory failure, and sepsis.

Treatment

Treatment of the pulmonary component of cystic fibrosis is aimed at relieving the obstruction of the bronchioles by mobilizing the tenacious secretions. Postural drainage and percussion are the mainstays of treatment. Inhalation of mist by mouth through a large-bore tube for 1/2 hour prior to postural drainage aids in loosening secretions. A bronchodilator aerosol is also effective in allowing entrance of air distal to the mucus so that the obstruction may be coughed toward the larger airways. Antibiotics are indicated for infection but should not be used prophylactically since such use favors the emergence of resistant strains. Cor pulmonale may be treated with tolazoline (Priscoline) and oxygen therapy. Constant low-flow oxygen therapy in severely cyanotic patients may add immeasurably to their comfort and productivity at home.

Prognosis

Although recent advances in treatment have prolonged the lives and usefulness of patients with cystic fibrosis, the prognosis remains poor, with most patients dying in their teens or early twenties.

Di Sant'Agnese P: Pathogenesis and physiopathology of cystic fibrosis of the pancreas. New England J Med 271:1287–1295, 1343–1352, 1399–1408, 1967.
Holsclaw DS: Common pulmonary complications in cystic fibrosis. Clin Pediat 9:346–355, 1970.
McCollum AT, Gilson LE: Family adaptation to cystic fibrosis. J Pediat 77:571–578, 1970.

Mellins RB: Site of airway obstruction in cystic fibrosis. Pediatrics 44:315–318, 1970.
Siassi B & others: Cor pulmonale in cystic fibrosis. J Pediat 78:794–805, 1971.
Zapletal A & others: Pulmonary mechanics in asthma and cystic fibrosis. Pediatrics 48:64–72, 1971.

FOREIGN BODY ASPIRATION & ASPIRATION PNEUMONIA

Diagnostic accuracy in these conditions depends upon maintaining a high index of suspicion and proper radiologic examination. Children age 1–3 years are particularly susceptible. The cardinal manifestations are coughing interspersed with symptom-free periods and recurrent pneumonitis in a specific area of the lung. Vomiting when the cough reflex is absent (eg, unconsciousness) leads to aspiration of vomitus. Physical examination discloses absence of air entry in the involved area.

The clinical pattern will vary from immediate death when the trachea is obstructed to unexplained recurrent pneumonia in a specific area of the lung. A detailed history must be taken, questioning the mother about coughing episodes when material such as a peanut or sunflower seed could have been aspirated. Aspiration pneumonia will also occur with ingestion of gasoline, kerosene, or other hydrocarbons. In the infant and small child, wheezing can be an immediate and persistent finding. Hyperexpansion occurs early, followed by atelectasis. Inflammation occurs if obstruction has been incomplete and airway damage has occurred.

Properly performed inspiratory and expiratory x-ray will show air trapping. If cooperation for such a film cannot be obtained, cinefluoroscopy is warranted.

Obstruction of a large airway such as the trachea is an immediate indication for endoscopy.

Postural drainage preceded by isoproterenol aerosol has been successful in removal of a variety of foreign matter, especially when located in a segmental area of the lung.

Antibiotics are of limited value and, if used, should be as specific as possible. Corticosteroids have not been shown to be effective in reducing morbidity or mortality.

Prognosis

The prognosis is excellent after removal and with continued postural drainage until the chest x-ray is normal.

Burrington J, Cotton E: Management of foreign body in the airway of children. J Pediat Surg. In press.
Theander G: Motility of diaphragm in children with bronchial foreign body. Acta radiol 10:113, 1970.

TUMORS OF THE BRONCHI

Papilloma of the trachea is rare and tends to disappear at puberty. It may be asymptomatic or may cause dyspnea and stridor. The diagnosis is based on bronchoscopic examination or bronchography. Treatment consists of surgical removal.

Bronchogenic carcinoma is rare in children. Symptoms depend upon its location (cough, wheezing, etc). None of the reported cases have been resected.

Bronchial adenomas, although rare in children, should be considered in the differential diagnosis of a child with protracted cough and hemoptysis. About 3/4 of these slow-growing tumors are located in primary or secondary bronchi. Two-thirds of patients present with pneumonia and atelectasis distal to the obstructing tumor. Treatment usually requires pulmonary resection; however, if the adenoma is entirely within a main stem bronchus and there is no evidence of local or distant metastasis, wide sleeve resection of the bronchus with end-to-end anastomosis may be curative.

Verska JJ, Connolly JE: Bronchial adenomas in children. J Thoracic Cardiovas Surg 55:411–517, 1968.

BRONCHOGENIC CYST

Congenital bronchogenic cyst occurs in the posterior portion of the mid mediastinum close to or behind the tracheobronchial tree. It usually occurs singly and may be hard to differentiate from acquired lesions. The lining of the respiratory epithelium has a characteristic histologic appearance.

Symptoms of respiratory tract obstruction in infancy are marked when bronchogenic cyst is located in the hilar area. Cysts in other areas lead to chronic respiratory infections and may mimic lung abscess. Pulmonary infiltration and pulmonary abscess formation are present. Asymptomatic bronchogenic cyst may be identified on routine chest x-ray.

The diagnosis is often suggested on fluoroscopic examination when the lesion is observed to ascend on swallowing. Bronchograms are occasionally helpful.

Differentiation must be made from diaphragmatic hernia, tuberculosis, pyogenic lung abscess, sarcoidosis, emphysema, lymphoma, teratoma, hamartoma, mediastinal granuloma, and metastatic lung tumors.

Treatment consists of surgical resection.

Bill AH Jr, Sumner DS: A unified concept of lymphangioma and cystic hygromas. Surg Gynec Obst 120:79–86, 1965.

Griscom NT & others: Fluid filled lung due to airway obstruction in the newborn. Pediatrics 43:383–390, 1969.

Opsahl T, Berman EJ: Bronchogenic mediastinal cysts in infancy: Case report and review of the literature. Pediatrics 30:372–388, 1962.

NONINFECTIOUS DISEASES OF THE LOWER RESPIRATORY TRACT*

IDIOPATHIC DIFFUSE INTERSTITIAL FIBROSIS OF THE LUNG
(Hamman-Rich Syndrome)

Interstitial fibrosis occurs with a variety of conditions such as chronic viral (respiratory syncytial) disease, protozoal (eg, *Pneumocystis carinii*) infections, collagen diseases (eg, rheumatoid arthritis), and sarcoidosis.

Physiologic studies in the past indicated that diffusion was recurrently obstructed at the alveolar level; as our understanding of this disease broadens it has become obvious that ventilation/perfusion abnormalities are the basic abnormality, especially at a regional level.

ALLERGIC ALVEOLITIS (PNEUMOCONIOSIS)
(Farmer's Lung, Pigeon Breeder's Lung, etc)

Organic dust pneumoconiosis is rarely diagnosed in children but may be more common than previously thought. The acute form is characterized by a sudden onset of cough, fever, chills, and weight loss. In the chronic form, cough is progressive and accompanied by dyspnea and pulmonary insufficiency. Chronic exposure or repeated acute episodes can lead to crippling pulmonary fibrosis. Auscultation will generally reveal inspiratory rales. Laboratory studies are noncontributory except for a possible elevation of IgG. Chest films may be normal or may show diffuse infiltrates or streaky densities. Pulmonary function tests show restrictive lung disease.

Numerous organic dusts, moldy hay, bagasse, and fungi in parakeet droppings, pigeon droppings, and mushroom compost can cause the syndrome. Precipitins to specific molds found in the offending organic dust can be found in the patient's serum. Since the pathologic lesion in this acute form is mainly limited to the alveoli, the term allergic alveolitis has been applied to this syndrome. Allergy (hay fever, asthma) is mediated by IgE, whereas allergic alveolitis is thought to be an Arthus reaction in the alveoli mediated by the specific organic dust antigen and an IgG-antibody complex.

Treatment is aimed at avoiding the antigen. Corticosteroids may be of value in decreasing the immunologic response, but the benefit of this method of treatment has not been clearly established.

*Idiopathic respiratory distress syndrome (hyaline membrane disease) is discussed in Chapter 3.

Hughes WF & others: Farmer's lung in an adolescent boy. Am J Dis Child 118:777–780, 1969.

Shannon DC & others: Pigeon breeder's lung and interstitial pulmonary fibrosis. Am J Dis Child 117:504–510, 1969.

PULMONARY ALVEOLAR PROTEINOSIS

This often fatal disease of unknown cause is characterized by progressive dyspnea and productive cough. Fine, soft, diffuse perihilar densities in butterfly distribution are seen on chest x-ray. At autopsy, a laminated structure is found lying close to the alveolar septa; it is thought to be the residual debris of cells rich in protein and lipid. Recent evidence indicates that this disease may be due to an overproduction of surfactant material.

There is no specific therapy. Pulmonary lavage with heparin has been effective in adults.

Colon AR Jr: Childhood pulmonary alveolar proteinosis (PAP). Am J Dis Child 121:481–485, 1971.

Danigelis JA: Pulmonary alveolar proteinosis. Am J Dis Child 118:871–875, 1969.

IDIOPATHIC PULMONARY ALVEOLAR MICROLITHIASIS

This disease of unknown cause (but with a familial tendency) diffusely involves the alveoli with calcium carbonate deposits. There are often no symptoms, and the diagnosis is most often made by chance on the basis of a routine chest x-ray or, rarely, a description of sand in the sputum.

There is no treatment.

Oka S & others: Pulmonary alveolar microlithiasis. Am Rev Resp Dis 93:612–622, 1966.

CONGENITAL PULMONARY LYMPHANGIECTASIS

This uncommon, usually fatal cause of respiratory distress consists of congenital dilatation of the pulmonary lymphatics. The male/female ratio is 2:1. The onset is usually at birth, with severe cases never establishing effective ventilation. A few cases have been reported in which respiratory distress developed days or weeks after birth. X-ray reveals hyperinflation and diffuse infiltrates. The diagnosis is made by lung biopsy. The condition may be associated with generalized (especially intestinal) lymphangiectasia; may be secondary to obstructed pulmonary venous return or

result from a primary developmental defect of pulmonary venous return; or may be due to a primary developmental defect of the pulmonary lymphatics. Prolonged survival is infrequent. The condition should be considered in the differential diagnosis of bilateral obstructive emphysema, cystic fibrosis, asthma, and immunologic deficiency disease.

Treatment is symptomatic.

France NE, Brown RJK: Congenital pulmonary lymphangiectasis. Arch Dis Child 46:528–532, 1971.

Noonan JA & others: Congenital pulmonary lymphangiectasis. Am J Dis Child 120:314–319, 1970.

PULMONARY HEMOSIDEROSIS

Essentials of Diagnosis

- Iron deficiency anemia.
- Cough, hemoptysis, dyspnea, wheezing, rhonchi, cyanosis.
- Episodes of pulmonary bleeding with fever, tachycardia, tachypnea, leukocytosis, elevated sedimentation rate, and abdominal pain.

General Considerations

Pulmonary hemosiderosis can occur either as primary lung involvement with resulting secondary heart or kidney manifestations or as secondary lung involvement associated with primary cardiac or collagen vascular disease. Some cases are related to cow's milk ingestion, but in most instances the cause is not known. Foreign bodies such as grasses and pine needles can mimic this disease.

Clinical Findings

A. Symptoms and Signs: The most helpful findings are iron deficiency anemia associated with chronic pulmonary symptoms: cough, hemoptysis, dyspnea, wheezing, and cyanosis. Hemoptysis is a helpful diagnostic sign, but other causes of hemoptysis must be looked for. Sudden hemoptysis may occur and may be fatal. Fever, tachycardia, and tachypnea accompany episodes of pulmonary hemorrhage. Infection is often wrongly suspected. The physical findings are variable. Besides pallor, all types of airway involvement will be found, such as wheezing, inspiratory rhonchi, and rales. Liver and spleen enlargement may be present.

B. Laboratory Findings: Microcytic hypochromic anemia is present and responds to oral administration of iron salts by elevation of the reticulocyte count. Eosinophilia is present in about 10–25% of cases. The stool guaiac test may be positive. Siderophages are present in the gastric contents and can be found in tracheal washings. Lung biopsy shows alveolar epithelial hyperplasia and degeneration with excessive shedding of cells and large numbers of siderocytes. Biopsy may be necessary in patients where other findings are atypical. Open biopsy is preferred to needle biopsy.

C. X-Ray Findings: These vary from none to mild infiltration to massive parenchymal involvement (atelectasis, emphysema, and adenopathy). The anteroposterior diameter of the chest is increased.

D. Special Examinations: Pulmonary function studies show a reduction of lung volumes, decreased lung compliance, reduced oxygen saturation, and cor pulmonale in severe disease.

Differential Diagnosis

A. Primary Involvement: Differentiate from pulmonary involvement associated with myocarditis, glomerulonephritis (Goodpasture's syndrome), or sensitivity to cow's milk (Heiner's syndrome).

B. Secondary Involvement: Differentiate from chronic increases in pulmonary venous and capillary pressure due to heart disease, diffuse collagen-vascular or purpuric disease, and inhaled foreign body.

Treatment

All associated causative factors must be considered and treated.

Management of acute crises consists of giving blood, oxygen, and corticosteroids. Corticosteroids may suppress the process and must be considered in long-term management.

Patients responding poorly to all agents may respond to deferoxamine (Desferal). Immunosuppressive drugs such as azathioprine (Imuran) have been used with some success.

Prognosis

In minor episodes, recoveries have been reported. Idiopathic disease may disappear.

Gilman PA, Zinkham WH: Severe idiopathic hemosiderosis in the absence of clinical or radiologic evidence of pulmonary disease. Editorial. J Pediat 75:118–121, 1969.

Matsaniotes N & others: Idiopathic pulmonary hemosiderosis in children. Arch Dis Child 43:307–309, 1968.

Soergel KH, Sommers SC: Idiopathic pulmonary hemosiderosis and related syndromes. Am J Med 32:499–511, 1968.

ATELECTASIS

Atelectasis is a condition in which a lung segment, one lobe, or an entire lung fails to expand at birth or collapses after having expanded completely. Microatelectasis is a condition in which atelectasis occurs in many scattered alveoli. The diagnosis depends on the degree of involvement and acuteness of onset. Symptoms include fever, dyspnea, tachypnea, cyanosis, dullness and diminished breath sounds, and mediastinal shift toward the affected side.

In the differential diagnosis one must consider airway obstruction due to any cause, both intrinsic and extrinsic (eg, foreign body, edema, stenosis, tumors, and pericardial effusion), and loss of alveolar lining (eg, pneumonitis).

Pulmonary abscess and bronchiectasis may complicate the condition.

Treatment consists of removal of the underlying cause. Postinfectious atelectasis with mucous obstruction and mucoviscidosis (see Cystic Fibrosis) are best treated with postural drainage assisted by adequate hydration and fine mist atmosphere.

Avery ME: The alveolar lining layer: A review of its role in pulmonary mechanics and in the pathogenesis of atelectasis. Pediatrics 30:324–330, 1962.

Dees SC, Spock A: Right middle lobe syndrome in children. JAMA 197:8–14, 1966.

Lubman WM, St. Geme JW Jr: Management of migratory atelectasis and pneumonitis in Guillain-Barré syndrome. Clin Pediat 9:403–408, 1970.

Qaqundah BY, Taylor WF: Recurrent right middle lobe syndrome in an asthmatic child. Clin Pediat 9:685–687, 1970.

POSTOPERATIVE ATELECTASIS

Following prolonged general anesthesia, parts of the lung occasionally fail to reexpand. Infection often develops in the collapsed areas. Postoperative atelectasis develops most commonly following thoracic surgery, but it may follow any prolonged surgical procedure, particularly when paralytic agents have been given and assisted ventilation used to maintain gas exchange.

Atelectasis develops regularly during anesthesia in experimental animals and man. It can be minimized by intermittent hyperinflation of the lungs. In the nonanesthetized state, this is achieved by periodic sighing. Following surgery, many patients hypoventilate, do not sigh, and thus permit the collapse of the lung to progress.

Clinically, postoperative atelectasis is manifested by sudden development of fever, cyanosis, and varying degrees of respiratory distress. Cough, if present at all, is not marked. Chest x-ray reveals collapse of the lung in the involved areas.

Prevention consists of breathing exercises (use of blow bottles and encouragement of deep breathing), postural drainage to mobilize secretions and to induce coughing, and moderate doses of codeine postoperatively if deep breathing causes pain. Intermittent hyperinflation during surgery and proper hyperinflation with air prior to extubation will help to prevent atelectasis. Unless hypoxemia is present, oxygen inhalation is contraindicated since it accentuates atelectasis.

Antibiotics are indicated, plus isoproterenol inhalation (aerosol) followed by postural drainage at frequent intervals.

Bendixen HH & others: Impaired oxygenation in surgical patients during general anesthesia with controlled ventilation: A concept of atelectasis. New England J Med 269:991–996, 1963.

ADULT RESPIRATORY DISTRESS SYNDROME

Essentials of Diagnosis

- Severe respiratory distress occurring in children or adults.
- Follows a variety of lung insults.
- Resembles respiratory distress syndrome of the newborn.

General Considerations

Adult respiratory distress syndrome can be produced by severe forms of many disorders, eg, aspiration pneumonia, near drowning, shock lung, postperfusion lung (impaired pulmonary function following cardiopulmonary bypass), viral pneumonia, and chest trauma. Factors which may contribute to the syndrome are shock, massive blood transfusion, hypoxemia, and acidemia. Alveolar collapse occurs secondary to loss of surfactant with marked decrease in compliance.

On pathologic examination, the lungs are heavy, noncrepitant, and deep purple in color. Microscopically, there is marked capillary congestion, atelectasis, interstitial edema, and intra-alveolar hemorrhage. A hyaline membrane lining the alveoli can frequently be seen.

Clinical Findings

A. Symptoms and Signs: The syndrome is usually seen 24–48 hours after serious trauma or illness. A history of pulmonary disease is uncommon. The onset is marked by tachypnea, chest retraction, and cyanosis.

B. Laboratory Findings: Blood gas determinations will reveal hypoxemia and acidemia early. As the disease progresses, CO_2 retention occurs.

C. X-Ray Findings: A patchy bilateral infiltrate occurs initially and progresses and coalesces to involve the whole of both lungs.

Treatment

The cyanosis can be corrected initially with small increases in inspired oxygen; as the disease progresses, the concentration of inspired oxygen must be increased to prevent hypoxemia. Corticosteroids should be started early in massive doses—eg, hydrocortisone sodium succinate (Solu-Cortef), 1 gm IV every 6 hours in an adult. This may be of particular value in respiratory distress syndrome associated with pulmonary embolism.

Provide assisted ventilation with a ventilator (usually volume controlled) capable of producing a high inflation pressure to achieve the necessary tidal volume in lungs with markedly decreased compliance.

Constant positive pressure breathing (CPPB) may be lifesaving. CPPB produces a positive airway pressure during expiration which prevents alveolar collapse and reduces congestion and interstitial edema. It may make it possible to reduce the inspired oxygen tension dramatically, thus lessening the hazard of oxygen toxicity.

Fluids should be carefully administered so that a negative fluid balance is maintained and the interstitial fluid compartment in the lung is reduced. Diuretics and salt-free albumin are useful in accomplishing this and should be given as early as possible; 72 hours after insult, collagen may be formed which cannot be transported as fluid.

Prognosis

The prognosis is poor because of the severity of the pulmonary insufficiency and the often severe associated precipitating disease. At postmortem examination, the pathology is that of acute organizing interstitial fibrosis. Skillful use of ventilators, respiratory care, and CPPB may improve the outlook.

Ashbaugh DG & others: Continuous positive pressure breathing (CPPB) in adult respiratory distress syndrome. J Thoracic Cardiovas Surg 57:31–41, 1969.

DESQUAMATIVE INTERSTITIAL PNEUMONITIS

Many reports of this condition in adults and children have appeared since it was first described in 1965. It is one of a host of interstitial lung diseases. Symptoms include dyspnea, tachypnea, cough (usually nonproductive), and cyanosis. There may also be clubbing, chest pain, and weight loss. X-ray reveals a reticular or granular ground-glass interstitial process most marked at the bases—very much like the x-ray findings in hyaline membrane disease. Pulmonary function tests show an increased alveolar-arterial (A–a) oxygen gradient and decreased diffusing capacity. Differential diagnosis must include other interstitial pneumonias such as rheumatoid pneumonia, sarcoidosis, giant cell interstitial pneumonitis, hemosiderosis, and alveolar proteinosis.

The diagnosis is made by lung biopsy. The characteristic findings are proliferation and shedding of the type II granular pneumocyte into the alveolar spaces. The pneumocytes are filled with periodic acid-Schiff (PAS) positive granules.

Treatment with prednisone has produced dramatic improvement in many cases. Combined therapy with corticosteroids and other immunosuppressive agents such as azathioprine (Imuran) have been effective where corticosteroids alone have failed. It is uncertain at present how long treatment should be continued.

Bachta RM & others: Desquamative interstitial pneumonia in a 7-week old infant. Am J Dis Child 120:341–343, 1970.

Rosenow EC III & others: Desquamative interstitial pneumonia in children. Am J Dis Child 120:344–348, 1970.

WILSON-MIKITY PULMONARY SYNDROME

This syndrome is characterized by gradually progressive respiratory distress with ventilatory insufficiency in small premature infants, beginning after several weeks of age. The airway seems to be mainly involved. The cause is not known; it may be viral or due to immaturity of lung. Chest x-ray shows a widespread reticular pattern resembling that of stage III oxygen toxicity (coarser than that of respiratory distress syndrome) with small radiolucent areas (cysts) scattered throughout the lung fields. These changes become more prominent as the disease progresses.

Treatment consists of careful supportive care, oxygen, and ventilatory assistance as needed. Antibiotics have not appeared to influence the course.

Although the course is prolonged and there is extensive lung involvement, only 10–15% of infants with this disorder die of respiratory or right heart failure. The others recover after a few months.

Aherne WA & others: Lung function and pathology in a premature infant with chronic pulmonary insufficiency (Wilson-Mikity syndrome). Pediatrics 40:962–975, 1967.

Krauss AN & others: Physiologic studies on infants with Wilson-Mikity syndrome. J Pediat 77:27–36, 1970.

Hodgman JE & others: Chronic respiratory distress in the premature infant: Wilson-Mikity syndrome. Pediatrics 44:179–195, 1969.

EMPHYSEMA

Essentials of Diagnosis

- Dyspnea.
- Hyperexpansion of lung.
- Cough.
- Biopsy-histology of distention and destruction of alveoli.
- Progressive disease.

General Considerations

Emphysema consists of loss of the elastic properties of the lung with distention or destruction of alveoli, resulting in air trapping. In radiologic terms, emphysema denotes hyperinflation of all or part of the lung. Emphysema may be obstructive or compensatory. Compensatory emphysema occurs when normal lung expands to fill the space of collapsed (atelectasis) or absent (postpneumonectomy) lung.

Localized obstructive emphysema occurs when a bronchus is partially obstructed so that air entry past the obstruction is accomplished more easily than air exit. A whole lung, a lobe of a lung, or a lobule may be involved. The obstruction may be intraluminal, intrabronchial, or extrabronchial. In congenital lobar emphysema, severe respiratory distress may develop in the neonatal period or in early infancy as a result of

compression of normal lung by the emphysematous lobe. In older children with localized emphysema, many conditions involving the airway must be considered, including asthma, foreign body, tumor, vascular ring, local inflammation due to viral or bacterial infection (including tuberculosis), and regional obstructive lung disease.

Generalized obstructive emphysema occurs if there is widespread involvement of bronchioles. It is present in a wide range of clinical conditions, including cystic fibrosis, asthma, bronchiolitis, interstitial pneumonia, and miliary tuberculosis.

Familial emphysema due to alpha$_1$ antitrypsin deficiency is characterized by onset of emphysema at a relatively early age and progressive dyspnea in the absence of clinical bronchitis in the early stages of the disease. The disease is as common in females as males. The pulmonary pathologic picture is that of diffuse panacinar emphysema. The primary pathophysiologic mechanism is not understood, but one theory proposes that the absence of alpha$_1$ antitrypsin allows naturally occurring proteolytic enzymes—as well as proteolytic enzymes released from leukocytes destroyed during infection—to slowly digest the structural protein of normal lung, leading to emphysema.

Alpha$_1$ antitrypsin deficiency is genetically inherited in an autosomal recessive manner. Although some homozygous recessive individuals report no pulmonary symptoms, they are usually symptomatic by the third or fourth decade; isolated cases of adolescents and one girl whose symptoms began at 18 months have been reported. Heterozygous individuals may have an increased incidence of pulmonary disease, but the data are inconclusive. It is estimated that about 5% of the population are carriers of the gene, and one in 2000 births is a homozygous recessive. Alpha$_1$ antitrypsin deficiency has also been associated with a severe form of juvenile hepatic cirrhosis.

The diagnosis may be suspected by the absence of the alpha$_1$ globulin peak in routine protein electrophoresis. Specific assay of antitrypsin activity confirms the diagnosis.

Clinical Findings

A. Symptoms and Signs: The symptoms and signs depend upon the extent of involvement. The cardinal finding is dyspnea. Others are cough, tachypnea, cyanosis, hyperresonant percussion sounds over the involved area, shift of cardiac impulse, and high-pitched wheezing. In localized or lobar involvement, the child may be asymptomatic, but careful examination of the chest will indicate poor air entry to the involved area. In rapid and increasing involvement, progressive respiratory distress will be evident. Increased resonance on percussion, shift of the heart and trachea, wheezing, or absence of breath sounds indicates that the airway involvement is sufficient to cause air trapping.

B. X-Ray Findings: Chest x-ray or fluoroscopic examination in the generalized disease shows increased radiolucency, depressed diaphragms, and horizontal ribs. Chest x-ray is an important diagnostic procedure but does not establish the diagnosis.

Treatment

The treatment of obstructive emphysema is directed toward the underlying cause. In congenital lobar emphysema, therapeutic aspiration bronchoscopy may be successful. If not, lobectomy may be a lifesaving measure in the neonatal period.

Interstitial emphysema, which usually follows resuscitation with intermittent positive pressure breathing, is best treated conservatively. Mediastinal air is seldom of clinical significance, and aspiration is rarely needed.

Browder JA, Billingsley JG: Regional obstructive lung disease in childhood. Am J Dis Child 119:322–325, 1970.

Crawford LV, Stout RH: Obstructive emphysema in preschool children. Ann Allergy 28:17–23, 1970.

DeMuth GR, Sloan H: Congenital lobar emphysema: Long term effects and sequelae in treated cases. Surgery 59:601–607, 1966.

Kruse RL, Lynn HB: Lobar emphysema in infants. Mayo Clin Proc 44:525–534, 1969.

Logan GB, Leonardo E: Obstructive lobe syndrome. J Asthma Res 7:119–125, 1970.

Talamo RC: Symptomatic pulmonary emphysema in childhood associated with hereditary alpha-1-antitrypsin and elastase inhibitor deficiency. J Pediat 79:20–26, 1971.

LUNG CYSTS

A lung cyst is usually thin-walled and contains air or fluid. Most are thought to be acquired through infection, usually with a necrotizing bacterial pathogen, but others are congenital. Pseudocysts (pneumatoceles) following acute bacterial pneumonia may be asymptomatic and tend to regress over a period of several weeks or months. Emergency aspiration is occasionally required when pseudocysts coalesce and impair pulmonary function. Rupture may cause pneumothorax and bronchopleural fistula with empyema.

Surgical removal is reserved for large, nonregressing lesions and those that communicate with a bronchus and are therefore infected.

Brunner S, Poulson P, Vesterdale J: Cysts of the lung in infants and children. Acta paediat scandinav 49:39–49, 1960.

Holder T, Christy M: Cystic adenomatoid malformation of the lung. J Thoracic Cardiovas Surg 7:590–597, 1964.

Merenstein GB: Congenital cystic adenomatoid malformation of the lung. Am J Dis Child 118:772–776, 1969.

Vachier E, Hillman DC: Solitary pulmonary hydatid cyst. Pediatrics 35:699–703, 1965.

ACCESSORY & SEQUESTERED LOBES

An accessory lobe is malformed pulmonary tissue invested with its own pleura. It may communicate with the trachea, major bronchi, or the gut. Its blood supply is aberrant from the aorta, and venous drainage is via the azygous vein. Most accessory lobes have been located on the left, above the diaphragm, occasionally with an infradiaphragmatic portion. Symptoms are rarely present in the newborn period.

Sequestered lung is pulmonary tissue with anomalous nonpulmonary circulation located within a lobe of normal lung (usually the left lower lobe). The sequestered portion is not in communication with the bronchi. Its blood supply is from an aberrant artery of the aorta, and venous drainage is via a pulmonary vein.

Both malformations may undergo cystic degeneration and become infected. Symptoms are uncommon before adolescence. Surgical resection of the malformation is the treatment of choice.

Klein LL: An accessory lobe of the lung in a newborn. Pediatrics 45:118–122, 1970.

Sperling DR, Finck EJ: Intralobar bronchopulmonary sequestration. Am J Dis Child 115:362–367, 1968.

PULMONARY METASTASES

A number of tumors of childhood metastasize to the lungs, often as the first presenting finding. They are Wilms's tumor (kidney), sarcoma (Ewing's, osteogenic, rhabdomyosarcoma), malignant teratoma, neuroblastoma (adrenal, sympathetic chain), and carcinoma (thyroid).

Chemotherapy and irradiation usually precede and follow resection of solitary metastases by wedge resection or lobectomy.

Kilman JW & others: Surgical resection for pulmonary metastasis in children. Arch Surg 99:158–165, 1969.

INFECTIONS OF THE LOWER RESPIRATORY TRACT

BACTERIAL PNEUMONIAS

Essentials of Diagnosis
- History of mild upper airway infection.
- Abrupt rise in temperature to 39.4–40.6° C (103–105° F).
- Cough, dyspnea, abdominal distention, tachypnea.

- Flaring of the nares and rapid, shallow, grunting respirations; splinting of one side on inspiration.
- Auscultation may be normal. Rales are usually not heard early, especially in infancy. In older children, localized signs occur: rales, dullness to percussion, and increased voice transmission.
- Specific etiologic diagnosis depends upon cultures of blood and respiratory secretions.

General Considerations

The characteristic lobar involvement found in adult bacterial pneumonia is rare in children. In infants and children, involvement is more diffuse and the airway is more involved (bronchial pneumonia).

Patients with recurrent pneumonia should be evaluated for immunologic deficiency disease, cystic fibrosis, and foreign body.

Clinical Findings

A. Symptoms and Signs: The onset is usually sudden and follows an upper respiratory infection. Fever and tachypnea are the most important findings, especially in infants, in whom physical examination may be normal. Inspection is often more reliable than auscultation, with the infant splinting the affected side.

Breath sounds are depressed, and inspiratory rales are heard more often in older patients. Other signs are dullness to percussion, tubular breath sounds, and abdominal distention plus increased abdominal tenderness; stiffness of the neck is often present. Older children may complain of chest pain, and rales may not be heard until the disease is resolving. Friction rubs are rare.

B. Laboratory Findings: The white blood count is elevated to 18–40 thousand/cu mm, predominantly PMNs. White counts under 10,000/cu mm with a shift to the left are a poor prognostic sign.

Pneumococci are the most common cause of bacterial pneumonia, but other infective agents must be considered. *Hemophilus influenzae* may cause an identical clinical picture but may not respond to penicillin alone. Streptococcal pneumonia seems to occur most often as a complication of viral infections and is characterized by a more liquid exudate; it also tends to ulcerate the trachea more often than pneumococcal disease, and there may be a higher incidence of empyema. Staphylococcal pneumonia is usually seen in immunologically deficient infants and children; it is more common in hospitals, where debilitated infants are infected by a penicillin-resistant staphylococcus. Staphylococcal infection is more apt to cause abscess formation than other organisms. Tuberculosis should be considered in any case of pneumonia that fails to respond to antibiotic therapy.

C. X-Ray Findings: On chest x-ray the signs of infiltration are patchy (bronchial pneumonia), rarely lobar. Bronchi and interstitial tissues are not involved.

Differential Diagnosis

Bacterial pneumonia may resemble meningitis and acute abdominal disorders. Staphylococcal pneumonia often presents with ileus due to a specific toxin.

Complications

Complications include septicemia, abscess, empyema, bronchiectasis, respiratory failure, pneumothorax, lung hemorrhage, septic shock, pyopneumothorax with shift of the mediastinum, and heart failure. In staphylococcal pneumonia, a fibrinous pleural formation can result.

Treatment

A. Specific Measures: Antibiotics are usually given intramuscularly but in severe cases should be given intravenously. Penicillin is the drug of choice for pneumonia due to pneumococci, streptococci, and penicillin-sensitive staphylococci. Ampicillin should be used in *H influenzae* pneumonia. In resistant staphylococcal infections, the intravenous use of sodium methicillin or nafcillin has been lifesaving.

B. General Measures: Supportive measures such as oxygen, humidity, and intravenous fluids are essential in severe cases.

Prognosis

With adequate therapy, sequelae are rare; however, if staphylococcal, streptococcal, and *H influenzae* pneumonia are not adequately treated, the incidence of lung abscess and empyema is high. Abscess should be resolved by adequate drainage technics.

Barson AJ: Fatal *Pseudomonas aeruginosa* bronchopneumonia in a children's hospital. Arch Dis Child 46:55–60, 1971.

Gourley RH: Staphylococcal pneumonia and empyema in infants. Canad MAJ 87:1101–1105, 1962.

Huxtable KA, Tucker AS, Wedgwood RH: Staphylococcal pneumonia in childhood. Am J Dis Child 108:262–269, 1964.

Jones RS, Owen-Thomas JB, Bouton MJ: Severe bronchopneumonia in the young child. Arch Dis Childhood 43:415–422, 1968.

Nyhan W, Rectanus D, Fausek M: *Hemophilus influenzae* type B pneumonia. Pediatrics 16:31–41, 1955.

Schaedler RW, Choppin RW, Zabriskie JB: Pneumonia caused by tetracycline resistant pneumococci. New England J Med 270:127–129, 1964.

Schreck KM: Observations on the epidemiology of staphylococcal infections. Am J Dis Child 105:646–654, 1963.

Thaler MM: Klebsiella-aerobacter pneumonia in infancy. Pediatrics 30:206–220, 1962.

INTERSTITIAL PLASMA CELL PNEUMONIA
(Pneumocystis Pneumonia)

Pneumocystis carinii is a protozoon that causes pneumonia in premature and debilitated infants and in children with hypo- or dysgammaglobulinemia or those who have been receiving immunosuppressive agents.

The incubation period is about 40 days. The onset usually is in the 6th–16th weeks of life.

The principal findings are failure to thrive, feeding problems, languor and irritability, tachypnea, cyanosis, cough, and radiating bilateral hilar infiltrations on chest x-ray. The chest is usually clear on auscultation, although scattered rales are occasionally heard. The white blood count is usually elevated, with a high eosinophil count. The only way a diagnosis can be made is by lung biopsy.

Differentiation must be made from lipoid pneumonia, primary atypical pneumonia, pulmonary hemosiderosis, alveolar proteinosis, diffuse pulmonary fibrosis, and histiocytic reticuloendotheliosis. Cytomegalic inclusion disease may coexist with this infection.

Treatment is mainly supportive, with humidity, oxygen, and gavage feedings. Pentamidine isethionate (Lomidine) offers specific therapy but may cause reversible megaloblastic bone marrow changes.

Death occurs in a few days in 20–50% of cases.

Bazaz GR & others: *Pneumocystis carinii* pneumonia in three full term siblings. J Pediat 76:767–769, 1970.

Gajdusek DC: *Pneumocystis carinii:* Etiological agent of interstitial plasma cell pneumonia of premature and young infants. Pediatrics 19:543–565, 1957.

Gentry LO & others: *Pneumocystis carinii* pneumonia in siblings. J Pediat 76:769–772, 1970.

Marshall WC, Weston HJ, Bodian M: *Pneumocystis carinii* pneumonia and congenital hypogammaglobulinemia. Arch Dis Childhood 39:18–25, 1964.

Robbins JB & others: Successful treatment of *Pneumocystis carinii* pneumonia in a patient with congenital hypogammaglobulinemia. New England J Med 272:708–713, 1965.

MYCOPLASMA PNEUMONIAE PNEUMONIA
(Eaton Agent Pneumonia;
Primary Atypical Pneumonia)

The symptoms of mycoplasmal pneumonia are similar to those of bacterial and viral pneumonias. There is a dry, hacking cough and substernal pain. Wedge-shaped infiltrations are seen on chest x-ray as well as increased bronchovascular markings and areas of atelectasis. The lower lobes are more frequently involved. Otitis media, serous otitis, pericarditis, and erythema nodosum have been reported as complications.

Mycoplasma pneumoniae may be differentiated from other mycoplasmal species because of its ability to lyse red blood cells.

Serologic tests (cold agglutinins and specific antibody rise) confirm the diagnosis. Culturing the organism ensures definite diagnosis.

Tetracyclines, chloramphenicol, erythromycin, and oleandomycin are all effective in treatment. Illness may be protracted, but recovery is the rule.

Clyde WA Jr, Denny FW Jr: The etiology and therapy of atypical pneumonia. M Clin North America 471:201–218, 1963.

Foy HM & others: *Mycoplasma pneumoniae* in an urban area. JAMA 214:1666–1672, 1970.

Nutu Y & others: Resistance of *Mycoplasma pneumoniae* to erythromycin and other antibiotics. J Pediat 76:438–443, 1970.

VIRAL PNEUMONIA

The symptoms and signs of viral pneumonia are similar to those described for bacterial and mycoplasmal infections. Biphasic illness and a family epidemic of viral upper respiratory disease suggest a viral etiology. Specific diagnosis depends on viral culture and serologic tests and is of benefit only for epidemiologic and research purposes. Radiologically, infiltration tends to be diffuse, ill-defined, and hazy.

Treatment is symptomatic. Antibiotics are of no value.

Avron JM & others: Epidemiology of viral and mycoplasmal agents associated with childhood lower respiratory illness in a civilian population. J Pediat 78:407–414, 1971.

Glezen WP: Epidemiologic patterns of acute lower respiratory disease of children in a pediatric group practice. J Pediat 78:397–406, 1971.

PULMONARY MYCOSES
(Actinomycosis, Nocardiosis, Blastomycosis, Coccidioidomycosis, Cryptococcosis, Histoplasmosis)

Fungal infections of the lung are rare in infants but more common in older children and in those with immunologic defects. Coccidioidomycosis and histoplasmosis (see below) have definite geographic locations.

The symptoms are those of pneumonia or acute lung abscess. Persistent undiagnosed lung disease should suggest fungal infection.

Chest x-ray shows a heavy infiltration or, occasionally, abscess formation. The x-ray often looks worse than the clinical symptoms seem to indicate.

Careful collection and examination of sputum is important for specific diagnosis (culture). Culturing should be done with care since most of these fungi are extremely infectious. Skin tests and complement fixation tests are also of value.

Actinomycosis and coccidioidomycosis cause chronic abscesses. Nocardiosis causes hematogenous dissemination; coccidioidomycosis causes erythema nodosum.

Fungal infections of the lung must be differentiated from pulmonary and miliary tuberculosis, infections with atypical mycobacteria, foreign body, tumors of the airway structures, chronic bacterial infection, and cystic fibrosis.

Amphotericin B (Fungizone) is specific, but it is usually reserved for cases of systemic infection. Most of these diseases are self-limited, and supportive care is usually all that is required.

The prognosis depends on the severity of exposure (dosage of inoculum) and the general physical condition of the patient.

Drips W Jr, Smith CE: Coccidioidomycosis. JAMA 192:1010–1012, 1964.

Seabury JH, Dascomb HE: Results of the treatment of systemic mycoses. JAMA 188:509–513, 1964.

Ziening WH, Rockas HR: Coccidioidomycosis. Am J Dis Child 108:454–459, 1964.

HISTOPLASMOSIS

The most prevalent systemic fungal infection is that due to *Histoplasma capsulatum,* which is endemic on the western Appalachian slopes and along the tributaries of the Ohio, Missouri, and Mississippi rivers. It may be asymptomatic, or there may be fever, weight loss, fatigue, nonproductive cough, diarrhea, and vomiting. Physical examination may be negative. In hematogenous dissemination, persistent fever is present, with hepatomegaly, pallor, regional adenopathy, and purpura.

The blood count is elevated, with a shift to the left; the sedimentation rate is rapid. Skin tests to histoplasmin are positive. Complement fixation tests are positive in comparatively low titer.

Chest x-ray in the active phase reveals an infiltrative lesion suggestive of atypical pneumonia. Lesions are granulomatous, with a caseous necrosis which calcifies readily. X-rays of healed lesions show diffuse calcification.

Pulmonary histoplasmosis must be differentiated from miliary tuberculosis, leukemia, Hodgkin's disease, reticuloendotheliosis, and organic heart disease with emboli.

Complications include ulcerations of the skin and gastrointestinal bleeding resembling ulcerative colitis.

Amphotericin B (Fungizone) is specific, but triple sulfonamides seem to be very effective and less toxic. Corticosteroids are contraindicated. Give supportive measures (blood transfusions, etc) as indicated.

The primary form is benign; the disseminated form almost always fatal. The prognosis is invariably poor in infants because their immunologic defenses have not yet developed.

Christie A: The disease spectrum of human histoplasmosis. Ann Int Med 49:544–555, 1958.

Mager RL & others: Sulfonamides and experimental histoplasmosis. Antibiotics Chemother 6:215–225, 1956.

PSITTACOSIS

Infection with this member of psittacosis-lymphogranuloma venereum group of organisms (recently reclassified as bacteria called chlamydiae) is acquired from infected birds (ornithosis) by persons handling them.

Manifestations range from mild influenza-like symptoms to severe pneumonia. Physical examination shows no characteristic abnormalities. Chest x-rays show diffuse bronchial pneumonia. Only serologic tests are helpful in diagnosis.

Tetracyclines are the most effective drugs.

Dean DJ & others: Psittacosis in man and birds. Pub Health Rep 79:101–106, 1964.

PULMONARY TUBERCULOSIS*

Essentials of Diagnosis

- Family history of tuberculosis or history of recent contact.
- Usually asymptomatic, especially in primary form.
- Miliary and progressive pulmonary disease: fever, anorexia, apathy, weight loss.
- Lymph node involvement (may cause respiratory symptoms if the airway is obstructed).
- Positive tuberculin tests and chest x-ray findings.

General Considerations

Pulmonary tuberculosis should be considered in any child who has been exposed to an adult with the active disease. A recent conversion to a positive tuberculin test indicates active disease in an untreated individual. The mortality rate is higher during infancy and adolescence. Spread is by respiratory droplets, but the disease in children is usually nonprogressive and not contagious.

Clinical Findings

A. Symptoms and Signs: A history of contact with a tuberculous adult is most important. Primary tuberculosis in children is usually asymptomatic. The classical adult syndrome of chronic cough, anorexia, and loss of weight is almost never present in children. Expiratory stridor is rare. Persistent fever of 2 weeks' duration may occur with primary disease. Miliary spread and meningitis are more likely to occur in infants than in older children.

B. Laboratory Findings: Tuberculin testing (tine, Heaf, Mantoux) is the most useful diagnostic tool. The

*See also discussion of tuberculosis in Chapter 27.

tine and Heaf tests are good screening tests, but if the diagnosis is suspected the Mantoux test (intradermal injection of OT or PPD) should be used; it has the basic advantage that the severity of the reaction relates to the severity of the disease. In suspect cases, the test should be read in 48–72 hours by an experienced observer and recorded as millimeters of induration.

Isolation of *Mycobacterium tuberculosis* is best done from gastric contents, and morning washes should be repeated 3 times. When possible, antibiotic sensitivity studies should be done on the organisms recovered.

C. X-Ray Findings: Chest x-ray in primary disease may be read as normal. X-ray will vary with the extent of infection from slight infiltration and hilar node invasion to atelectasis and diffuse involvement, as in miliary spread.

Differential Diagnosis

Pulmonary tuberculosis must be differentiated from atypical pneumonia, bacterial pneumonia, leukemia, malnutrition, tumors, congenital atelectasis, asthma, cystic fibrosis, and Löffler's syndrome.

Complication & Sequelae

Infants and adolescents are more likely to develop complications from pulmonary tuberculosis than people in other age groups. Complications include miliary spread, meningitis, cavitation (adolescents), atelectasis (airway obstruction), lymph node involvement outside of the chest (cervical lymph nodes), epididymitis, renal involvement, osteomyelitis of the spine, retroperitoneal and abdominal involvement, and pleurisy.

Prevention & Treatment

See discussion in Chapter 27.

Prognosis

The prognosis with proper therapy is excellent. If infection is acquired from patients whose organisms are resistant to the antituberculosis drugs, the prognosis is poor.

Anderson SR, Smith MHD: The Heaf multiple puncture tuberculin test. Am J Dis Child 99:764–769, 1960.
Krenﬂig EL Jr, Rogers WL: Tuberculosis in the neonatal period. Am Rev Tuberc 77:418–422, 1958.
Lincoln EM, Sewell EM: *Tuberculosis in Children.* McGraw-Hill, 1963.
Riley RL: Apical localization of pulmonary tuberculosis. Bull Johns Hopkins Hosp 106:232–239, 1960.
Rosenberg M, Gottlieb RP: Current approach to tuberculosis in childhood. P Clin North America 15:513–547, 1968.
Task Force on Tuberculosis Control: *The Future of Tuberculosis Control: A Report to the Surgeon General of the Public Health Service.* US Department of Health, Education, & Welfare. Public Health Service, Communicable Disease Center, Atlanta, Georgia, 1963.
WHO Expert Committee on Tuberculosis: *Eighth Report.* Technical Report Series No. 290. World Health Organization, 1964.

PULMONARY INFILTRATION WITH EOSINOPHILIA
(PIE, Löffler's Syndrome)

Löffler's syndrome consists of transient migratory pulmonary infiltration and eosinophilia (10–60%) which persist 1–6 months or more. Multiple causes include infection with various parasites such as *Toxocara canis* (visceral larva migrans), *Ascaris lumbricoides,* hookworms, etc. The syndrome also occurs in tropical eosinophilia. Symptoms may be very mild or absent. Cough or wheeze and, occasionally, scattered rales, clearing within several days, are the most characteristic findings. Fever is low-grade. Leukocytosis with an eosinophil count of up to 60% is typical.

Löffler's syndrome must be differentiated from pulmonary tuberculosis, asthma, foreign body, primary atypical pneumonia, and polyarteritis nodosa.

Corticosteroids have been reported to shorten the course of the disease. Tuberculosis must be ruled out before corticosteroids are given.

Crofton JW & others: Pulmonary eosinophilia. Thorax 7:1–35, 1952.
Incapuva FP: Pulmonary eosinophilia. Am Rev Resp Dis 84:730–736, 1961.

LUNG ABSCESS

Lung abscess formation is usually the result of foreign body aspiration, necrotizing pneumonitis due to klebsiella, *Staphylococcus aureus,* or *Streptococcus hemolyticus,* or infection of a congenital cyst, atelectatic lung, or tumor.

Treatment depends on the underlying cause, but establishment of postural drainage and eradication of infection with well chosen antibiotics are the conservative course first chosen. Segmental resection and lobectomy are now rarely required.

Moore TC, Battersby JS: Pulmonary abscess in infancy and childhood. Ann Surg 151:496–500, 1960.
Sabisten DC & others: The surgical management of complications of staphylococcus pneumonia in infancy and childhood. J Thoracic Cardiovas Surg 38:421–434, 1959.

DISEASES OF THE PLEURA & CHEST WALL

PLEURISY & EMPYEMA

Pleurisy may be either dry or plastic and serofibrinous or purulent. Dry pleurisy most often occurs with bacterial (pneumococcal) or viral pneumonia, and occasionally with upper respiratory tract disease, tuberculosis, rheumatic fever, subacute bacterial endocarditis, pulmonary embolism, inflammatory lesions of the abdominal wall, subphrenic abscess, and trauma to the chest wall. Serofibrinous pleurisy occurs with infections of the lung and abdomen, metastatic lesions, rheumatic fever, systemic lupus erythematosus, and tuberculosis. Purulent pleurisy (empyema) is usually secondary to bacterial pneumonia and causes an exudate with a specific gravity > 1.015 and a high protein content. It is commonly a complication of staphylococcal, pneumococcal, or *Hemophilus influenzae* pneumonia and is seen in primary tuberculosis.

Clinical Findings

A. Symptoms and Signs: The clinical picture depends upon the amount and type of fluid involvement. In dry pleurisy, a friction rub may be heard and pain is often present with a deep breath or cough. Small effusions may produce no symptoms. Additional findings are related to the amount of fluid present, with decrease in percussion note, absence of breath sounds, and failure to transmit vocal fremitus. Large effusions may cause a shift of the mediastinum and heart. The patient with empyema appears to be sicker, with fever, tachycardia, and tachypnea. Movement of the affected side of the chest may be reduced.

B. X-Ray Findings: Chest x-ray shows a thickened pleural area and occasionally a fluid level. If a thoracentesis has been performed, an air bubble may be present. Lung compression may be marked. The heart and mediastinum may be displaced to the opposite side.

Differential Diagnosis

The presence of a pleural rub in the face of chest pain confirms the diagnosis of pleurisy. Group B coxsackievirus infections may cause the clinical picture of pleurisy (epidemic pleurodynia) in summer outbreaks, but there is no pleural rub and the lungs are clear.

Treatment

Thoracentesis is desirable for diagnosis and treatment in the presence of effusion. Uncomplicated but painful dry pleurisy is treated with analgesics, including ethyl chloride spray or taping of the affected side. Drainage of large pleural effusions (empyema, hydrothorax, hemothorax, or chylothorax) usually brings prompt relief of dyspnea. Fluid should be withdrawn very slowly, in at least 2 or more procedures, through a large (No. 19) needle.

Bacterial empyema is specifically treated with parenteral antibiotic therapy. Pus is best drained by inserting 1–2 adequately sized and properly placed intercostal tubes into the pleural cavity under a negative pressure of 10–15 mm Hg; the tubes must be checked frequently for patency and position.

Injection of antibiotics (penicillin or methicillin) into the pleural space may occasionally be useful. Systemic antibiotics should be chosen on the basis of smear and culture.

Prognosis

Dry pleurisy clears completely since it is usually due to viral infection. In purulent and serofibrinous pleurisy, a residual fibrous formation is present but should not be stripped or decorticated from the lung. The more complete the drainage and control of the instigating lesion, the less the fibrin formation.

Bechamps GJ & others: Empyema in children: A review of Mayo Clinic experience. Mayo Clin Proc 45:43–50, 1970.
Riley H Jr, Bracken E: Empyema due to *Hemophilus influenzae* in infants and children. Am J Dis Child 110:24–28, 1965.
Smith PL & Gerald B: Empyema in childhood followed roengenographically: Decortication seldom needed. Am J Roentgenol 106:114–117, 1969.
Strad WW & others: *Pleural Effusion*. Disease-a-Month, July 1964.

HYDROTHORAX

Hydrothorax is a collection of fluid (transudate) with a specific gravity of 1.015 or less and a protein content of less than 3 gm/100 ml. It is usually caused by cardiac failure (effusion is usually on the right side), acute glomerulonephritis, or nephrotic syndrome or occurs in association with effusions into other serous cavities (peritoneum) in conditions such as atypical measles.

See Chernick reference, below.

HEMOTHORAX

Hemothorax is usually caused by surgical or accidental trauma but may occur in tumors of the pleura and lung. Symptoms are usually related to blood loss.

CHYLOTHORAX

Chylothorax should be suspected in any case of trauma to the chest (accidental or surgical) with injury to the thoracic duct. Obstruction of the thoracic duct may also be caused by tumors or enlarged lymph nodes. Symptoms relate to the amount of accumulated fluid. There is no pain, but tachypnea and dyspnea occur with large accumulations. Chest x-ray shows the fluid. A fat-soluble dye fed to the patient will turn the chylous fluid green. Wasting sometimes occurs. Specific diagnosis is made by obtaining milky fluid from thoracentesis.

Chylothorax must be differentiated from the accumulation of fatty material in serofibrinous pleurisy.

Repeated aspiration may be necessary if respiratory distress occurs. About 1/2 of patients recover completely after repeated aspirations, but there are a few deaths.

Chernick V, Reed MH: Pneumothorax and chylothorax in the neonatal period. J Pediat 76:624–632, 1970.

PNEUMOTHORAX, PNEUMOMEDIASTINUM, & PNEUMOPERICARDIUM

Essentials of Diagnosis

In neonate:
- Irritability and tachypnea.
- Sudden increase in dyspnea.
- Cyanosis and venous engorgement.
- Shock.
- Apex of heart, trachea, and mediastinum displaced to unaffected side.

In older child (additional symptoms; all on affected side):
- Sudden, sharp chest pain.
- Hyperresonance to percussion.
- Reduced breath sounds.

General Considerations

Life-threatening pneumothorax is common in neonates, particularly as a complication of positive pressure resuscitation, difficult deliveries, or cesarean section. In older children, it is a frequent complication of tracheostomy, rupture of pseudocysts, bronchopleural fistula, or staphylococcal pneumonia, or occurs during attacks of asthma. It also occurs following chest trauma (especially with rib fractures) or with rupture of emphysematous blebs. Pneumopericardium and pneumomediastinum are due to the same causes.

Clinical Findings

Seven percent of all infants at birth have some degree of pneumothorax. A small pneumothorax (less than 10% of the hemithorax) may cause few symptoms. Suspicion of the condition should lead to immediate x-ray examination, including, if possible, an expiratory film to show collapsed lung and mediastinal shift optimally. Although pneumopericardium may cause fatal cardiac tamponade, respiratory symptoms (cyanosis, increased respiratory distress) are prominent as well as muffled heart sounds and poor circulation.

Differential Diagnosis

In the neonate, even with an x-ray, diaphragmatic hernia with presence of air-filled bowel in the chest is sometimes mistaken for pneumothorax.

Dyspnea and hypoxia are at times ascribed to primary lung disease, and only x-ray examination reveals the presence of pneumothorax, pneumomediastinum, or pneumopericardium.

Complications

Increasing lung compression and marked mediastinal shift can lead to rapid deterioration and death.

Depending on the underlying cause, pleural effusions, sterile or infected, may follow pneumothorax or its treatment.

Prevention

In the neonate, resuscitation should be gentle. The next most common iatrogenic cause of pneumothorax is tracheostomy. A carefully controlled operation minimizes the risk. Early, effective antibiotic therapy of bacterial pneumonia in childhood lessens the chance of bronchopleural fistula formation and pneumothorax.

Treatment

If pneumothorax is small (less than 20% of the hemithorax) and the patient's general condition is stable, it is best to allow absorption of the loculated air. If symptoms are increasing and the air is under tension, needle aspiration and catheter drainage are required. This is also true in pneumothorax of less than 20% if the underlying lung disease seriously compromises aeration, as is the case in bacterial pneumonia. Pneumopericardium and pneumothorax may resolve spontaneously with no treatment or with breathing 100% oxygen. More often, however, subxiphoid needle aspiration of the pneumopericardium is required to relieve the severe respiratory distress and circulatory collapse. If the condition recurs, constant drainage may be required.

Underwater drainage is obtained through an adequately sized plastic tube inserted through a large (No. 18 or 19) needle, which is then withdrawn. The 7th or 8th intercostal space, just anterior to the margin of the latissimus dorsi, is generally used for emergency needle aspiration and tube placement. (A tube becomes necessary because of recurrence of pneumothorax or a bronchopleural fistula.) If x-ray reveals lung expansion and aspiration bubbles have ceased for 24 hours, the tube is removed.

Needle or tube aspiration may not be feasible in some infants in whom air has dissected through the mediastinum with resulting impairment of cardiovascular function. In these cases, pure oxygen breathing may be lifesaving by hastening absorption of the gas by washing out nitrogen from the blood and tissues. The higher partial pressure of nitrogen in the loculated gas will result in movement to the blood and tissues.

Prognosis

With prompt diagnosis and vigorous therapy, the prognosis is excellent.

Franken EA Jr: Pneumomediastinum in newborn infants with associated dextroposition of the heart. Am J Roentgenol 109:252–260, 1970.

Gershanik JJ: Neonatal pneumopericardium. Am J Dis Child 121:438–439, 1971.

Grosfeld JL & others: Spontaneous pneumopericardium in the newborn infant. J Pediat 76:614–616, 1970.

Lifschitz MI: Pneumothorax as a complication of cystic fibrosis. Am J Dis Child 116:633–640, 1968.

Matthieu JM: Pneumopericardium in the newborn. Pediatrics 46:117–119, 1970.

PHRENIC NERVE PALSY

Essentials of Diagnosis

- Respiratory distress.
- History of obstetric trauma.
- Paradoxic movement of diaphragm.

General Considerations

Paralysis of the diaphragm from phrenic nerve palsy is an uncommon cause of respiratory distress in the neonate. The phrenic nerve arises from the 4th cervical nerve with unconstant secondary branches from the 3rd and 5th cervical nerves. The cause of the palsy is thought to be obstetric trauma. Often there is a history of breech delivery or difficult vertex delivery with traction on the neck. In about 3/4 of reported cases, there is an associated brachial plexus (Erb's) palsy. Approximately 3/4 of cases have been involved on the right side, but this may only mean that the right-sided lesion produces more symptoms.

Clinical Findings

A. Symptoms and Signs: Respiratory distress as evidenced by tachypnea and cyanosis is the most common presentation. This may be present at birth or develop within a few hours. On the other hand, patients may be asymptomatic for weeks or months; and in some cases the diagnosis is made on a routine chest film in a child or adult with no history of symptoms. Asymptomatic congenital eventration of the diaphragm may be a sequel to diaphragmatic paralysis. Other symptoms include feeble cry and poor feeding.

Physical examination reveals cyanosis and tachypnea. Respiratory excursions may be diminished in certain cases; in others, they are exaggerated and accompanied by protrusion of the involved side. More often, there is retraction of the abdomen on the paralyzed side with inspiration. Breath sounds may be diminished on the involved side, and rales may be present.

B. X-Ray Examination: Routine chest film demonstrates an elevated diaphragm on the paralyzed side. The diagnosis is confirmed at fluoroscopy, which reveals paradoxic movement of the involved side.

Differential Diagnosis

The differential diagnosis includes cyanotic congenital heart disease, hyaline membrane disease, aspiration pneumonia, intrauterine pneumonia, intracranial injury with hemorrhage, atelectasis, diaphragmatic hernia, diaphragmatic eventration, sepsis, and various metabolic problems of the newborn, eg, hypoglycemia.

Complications

Complications include atelectasis, pulmonary infection, respiratory failure, poor feeding and regurgitation, hypoxemia, and brain damage.

Treatment

Treatment is aimed at correcting hypoxemia, preventing respiratory failure, and managing the complications that may result from a poorly expanded and poorly ventilated lung. Oxygen administration will correct hypoxemia, bearing in mind that arterial oxygen tensions must be monitored in order to prevent retrolental fibroplasia and to ensure minimum inspired oxygen concentrations to guard against pulmonary oxygen toxicity. Antibiotics should be reserved for pulmonary infection and should not be given prophylactically. Postural drainage is important to remove secretions and to prevent the development of atelectasis and infection. Frequent small feedings (gavage or gastrostomy) may be required if the infant has increased symptoms with feedings.

If arterial CO_2 retention and acidemia develop in spite of the above treatment, the involved side may be mechanically expanded intermittently. This may be accomplished by means of a self-inflating bag and mask if inflation is not required too frequently (eg, 3 times daily); or by prolonged nasotracheal intubation if frequent inflation is required (eg, every hour). The nasotracheal tube allows oral feedings to be continued without danger of inflating the stomach with air and initiating vomiting and aspiration. If the child cannot be maintained by these means, surgical intervention and plication of the paralyzed diaphragm must be considered.

Prognosis

The overall mortality rate is about 20–25%. It is nearly 30% when associated with Erb's palsy and less than 10% when phrenic nerve palsy is an isolated lesion. The first 6 months of life seem most crucial; no deaths have been reported after 6 months of age. If respiratory failure can be prevented, the natural history of the condition is gradual improvement leading often to complete recovery. Recovery of the associated Erb's palsy is considered a good prognostic sign. Thus, if the child can be maintained for the first 6 months of life, surgery probably will not be required.

Bingham JAW: Two cases of unilateral paralysis of the diaphragm in the newborn treated surgically. Thorax 9:248–252, 1954.

France NE: Unilateral diaphragmatic paralysis and Erb's palsy in the newborn. Am J Dis Child 29:357–359, 1954.

Schrifren N: Unilateral paralysis of the diaphragm due to phrenic nerve paralysis with and without associated Erb's palsy. Pediatrics 9:69–76, 1952.

MEDIASTINAL DISEASES

MEDIASTINAL TUMORS

Most mediastinal tumors are asymptomatic and are found on routine chest x-ray. Symptoms develop as a result of pressure on sensitive structures. Respiratory symptoms are more common in children.

Classification

Mediastinal tumors are separated into 4 regions of the mediastinum: superior, anterior, middle, and posterior. Lymph nodes may be enlarged in benign or malignant disease (malignant lymphoma).

A. Primary Mediastinal Cysts: Benign cysts are usually abnormalities of embryologic development. Bronchogenic cyst occurs in the mid mediastinum; esophageal and gastroenteric cysts, in the posterior mediastinum; pericardial coelomic cysts, in the anterior and middle areas; intrathoracic meningoceles (really diverticuli of spinal meninges) lie in the posterior area.

B. Thymus Tumors: The thymus is the most common mediastinal mass in children. A diagnosis of hyperplasia of the thymus should not be made too readily since the size of the gland fluctuates with infections and other influences. Large tumors are rare. Corticosteroids may be employed to "shrink" a normal thymus.

C. Teratoid Tumors: Benign or malignant (teratoma) tumors occur in the anterior mediastinum.

D. Neurogenic Tumors: These are the most common of the posterior mediastinal tumors. Neuroblastoma, neurofibroma, and ganglioneuroma may be present.

Clinical Findings

A. Symptoms and Signs: Respiratory symptoms result from pressure on respiratory tract structures: dry cough, wheezing, and complete obstruction, leading to atelectasis; or incomplete obstruction, causing obstructive emphysema. Infection may be superimposed on incomplete obstruction. Pressure on the recurrent laryngeal nerve will cause hoarseness. Hemoptysis occurs occasionally. Pressure on the esophagus can result in regurgitation. Pain may be pleuritic in type when the intercostal nerves are involved. Dilatation of neck vessels may occur as a result of superior vena caval obstruction. Occasionally, obstruction is so severe that cyanosis of the head can result. Acute obstruction in the newborn period may cause death.

Physical findings are frequently absent except when massive enlargement is present.

B. Laboratory Findings: Definitive diagnosis is made at surgery. Needle aspiration should be reserved for cases in which cystic enlargement has progressed to emergency status or when operation is impossible.

C. X-Ray Findings: Chest x-rays are the main diagnostic tool.

Differential Diagnosis

Mediastinal tumors must be differentiated from asthma, bronchiolitis, cystic fibrosis, hypogammaglobulinemia, endobronchial or endotracheal lesions, foreign body, and widespread neoplasms such as leukemia.

Treatment

Surgical removal is indicated if possible, but deep x-ray therapy can be used in certain situations: hyperplasia of the thymus, Hodgkin's disease, and lymphosarcoma.

Prognosis

The prognosis depends upon the location and type of lesion.

Bratu M: Cystic hygroma of the mediastinum in children. Am J Dis Child 119:348–351, 1970.

Chitale AR: Gastric cyst of the mediastinum. J Pediat 75:104–110, 1969.

Haller JA Jr & others: Diagnosis and management of mediastinal masses in children. J Thoracic Cardiovas Surg 58:385–393, 1969.

Hope JW, Koop CE: Differential diagnosis of mediastinal masses. P Clin North America 6:379–412, 1959.

ACUTE SUPPURATIVE MEDIASTINITIS

Nontraumatic mediastinal infection is rare even as a secondary complication of such likely sources of infection as retropharyngeal abscess, sepsis, pleural empyema, and vertebral or rib osteomyelitis. Early symptoms of mediastinitis are consistent with generalized infection: irritability, fever, and leukocytosis. As the disease process encroaches upon mediastinal structures such as the esophagus, trachea, and vena cava, dysphagia, dyspnea, and venous distention develop. A characteristic respiratory pattern—a spasmodic or "halting" inspiration, sometimes accompanied by grimacing—is thought to result from the pain caused by stretching of the inflamed mediastinal structures during inspiration. Chest x-ray may show mediastinal fluid or widening of the mediastinum.

The disease process is rapidly progressive and requires prompt treatment. Appropriate cultures should be obtained and broad-spectrum antibiotic therapy begun parenterally. Mediastinotomy may be necessary for drainage. Upper airway obstruction is common and requires provision of an artificial airway.

With prompt treatment, the prognosis is good.

Feldman R, Gromisch DS: Acute suppurative mediastinitis. Am J Dis Child 121:79–81, 1971.

•   •   •

General References

Avery ME: *The Lung and Its Disorders in the Newborn Infant,* 2nd ed. Saunders, 1968.

Comroe JH & others: *The Lung: Clinical Physiology and Pulmonary Function Tests.* Year Book, 1962.

Egan DF: *Fundamentals of Inhalation Therapy.* Mosby, 1969.

Filley GF: *Acid-Base and Blood Gas Regulation.* Lea & Febiger, 1971.

Kendig EL: *Disorders of the Respiratory Tract.* Saunders, 1968.

Spencer H: *Pathology of the Lung,* 2nd ed. Saunders, 1968.

13 . . .

Heart & Great Vessels

Leslie L. Kelminson, MD, & James J. Nora, MD

DIAGNOSTIC EVALUATION

SYMPTOMS RELATED TO CARDIOVASCULAR DISEASE

Cyanosis

Cyanosis is gray or bluish discoloration of certain surfaces of the body. Mild cyanosis is limited to the mucous membranes and nail beds; in severe cases, the entire body surface is involved. The presence of cyanosis means that there are at least 5 gm/100 ml of desaturated hemoglobin in the capillary bed (normal: about 2.25 gm/100 ml). This might result either from desaturation of the arterial blood (central cyanosis; right-to-left intracardiac shunt or pulmonary disease) or from unusually great extraction of oxygen from the blood at the capillary level (peripheral cyanosis; low-output congestive heart failure). Central cyanosis secondary to lung disease is markedly improved with the administration of 100% oxygen; in contrast, when cyanosis is due to intracardiac right-to-left shunt, only minimal improvement is noted.

Cyanotic (hypoxic) spells are common in patients with certain cyanotic congenital cardiac defects (primarily tetralogy of Fallot). The spells are characterized by the sudden onset of increased cyanosis, irritability, and marked dyspnea. Unconsciousness, convulsions, and coma may follow if the spell persists.

Squatting

The tendency to squat on exertion and sleep in the knee-chest position is characteristic of tetralogy of Fallot.

Fatigue

Easy fatigability on exertion is common in patients with marked cyanosis, with conditions associated with low systemic cardiac output (eg, heart failure), or with inability to adequately increase systemic cardiac output on exercise (eg, obstruction to ventricular outflow, or large left-to-right shunt). Infants usually manifest easy fatigability by tiring and falling asleep after taking only 2–3 oz of formula.

Tachypnea

A rapid respiratory rate is characteristic of left-sided heart failure or obstruction to flow into the left side of the heart (eg, mitral stenosis). Both of these conditions cause an elevation of pulmonary venous pressure. When this pressure exceeds a critical level (about 25–30 mm Hg), exudation of fluid into the interstitial tissue of the lungs occurs, resulting in a decrease in lung compliance (stiffening of the lungs). Under these circumstances, rapid, shallow breathing is the most efficient means of achieving an adequate minute respiratory volume. In infants, it is of special importance to note the character of breathing during sleep.

Dyspnea

Shortness of breath on exertion, resulting in deep, labored respiration, is common in patients with severe cyanosis or low systemic cardiac output states.

Orthopnea

Shortness of breath in the recumbent position which is helped by sitting up is indicative of pulmonary congestion.

Frequent Respiratory Infections

Patients with large left-to-right shunts often have a history of frequent upper and lower respiratory tract infections.

Anorexia, Vomiting, & Profuse Sweating

These are common in children—and particularly in infants—with inadequate cardiac reserve.

PHYSICAL EXAMINATION

1. CARDIAC EXAMINATION

Inspection & Palpation

Evidence of cardiac enlargement is best obtained by inspection and palpation of the precordium.

Asymmetric prominence of the left anterior chest wall is usually indicative of cardiac enlargement secondary to congenital heart disease.

Right ventricular hypertrophy is characterized by a heaving pulsation at the lower left sternal border or the xiphoid process. Left ventricular hypertrophy is characterized by a thrusting impulse at the apex which is displaced downward and outward. Prominent pulsations both at the apex and at the xiphoid process suggest combined ventricular hypertrophy.

A thrill is a palpable murmur consisting of a high frequency vibration felt by the fingertips. It indicates the presence of a murmur of at least grade IV/VI intensity. Thrills are localized to the area at which the murmur is most intense. The presence of a thrill is characteristic of certain types of congenital and acquired heart disease (aortic stenosis, pulmonary stenosis, ventricular septal defect, etc).

It is at times possible to palpate one or both of the heart sounds. This is frequently referred to as a shock. It is usually an abnormal finding and is often of diagnostic significance (eg, the presence of a palpable second heart sound at the pulmonary area is suggestive of increased pulmonary arterial pressure). However, normal heart sounds may occasionally be palpated through a very thin chest wall.

Percussion

Percussion of the cardiac borders is a gross method of determining heart size but does not differentiate between right or left ventricular hypertrophy. Percussion of the cardiac borders is useful in patients with generalized cardiac dilatation or with pericardial effusion.

Auscultation

A. Heart Sounds:

1. First heart sound (S_1)—The first heart sound is related to closure of the atrioventricular valves. In most cases the first sound seems on auscultation to be single, although there are 4 components which may be detected by phonocardiography.

2. Ejection click—Early ejection clicks are related to dilated great vessels. Early clicks heard at the second left interspace are pulmonary in origin and most often due to pulmonic stenosis. Early clicks which are best localized at the lower left sternal border and apex are frequently aortic and are commonly found in aortic stenosis and truncus arteriosus. Mid- to late-systolic clicks are usually extracardiac when heard at the base and secondary to "mitral dysfunction" when localized at the apex.

3. Second heart sound (S_2)—The second heart sound is due to closure of the semilunar (aortic, pulmonary) valves. The intensity and the manner of splitting of S_2 are extremely important in the diagnosis of heart disease in the pediatric age group. Physiologic splitting consists of widening of the 2 components during inspiration and narrowing (almost complete closure) during expiration. During inspiration, there is a drop in intrathoracic pressure resulting in increased filling of the right side of the heart. This results in a prolonged ejection of blood from the right ventricle and delayed pulmonic closure. The effect of respiration on the filling of the left side of the heart from the pulmonary veins is minimal since both the pulmonary veins and the left atrium are located within the thoracic cavity. Actually, there is a slight decrease in the amount of blood filling the left atrium during inspiration due to dilatation of the pulmonary veins. Accordingly, wide splitting of the second heart sound occurs during inspiration. During expiration, the reverse is true, resulting in narrowing of the 2 components. The presence of the split is detected best at the second intercostal space at the left sternal border in normal patients. The 2 components are usually of equal intensity in the pediatric age group.

4. Third heart sound (S_3)—This is due to the rapid filling of the left ventricle during early diastole. It occurs shortly after (0.12–0.16 seconds) S_2. It is common in infants and children and is best heard at the apex.

5. Fourth heart sound (S_4)— This sound is due to contraction of either atrium; accordingly, if present, it is heard shortly before the first heart sound. It is occasionally audible in patients with congenital heart disease associated with increased pressure within either atrium.

B. Murmurs: The following characteristics of murmurs should be noted: (1) timing in relationship to the cardiac cycle (systolic, diastolic, or continuous); (2) duration; (3) intensity, on a scale of I–VI/VI; (4) quality (blowing, harsh, rough, musical, etc); (5) area of greatest intensity; and (6) transmission (localized, widely transmitted, etc).

Heart murmurs are extremely common, but in the pediatric age group the vast majority are innocent. It is important for all physicians responsible for the care of infants and children to have a clear understanding of the nature and types of innocent heart murmurs. They are usually soft, ie, no more than grade II/VI in intensity, and localized to specific areas of the precordium with poor transmission. They are rarely transmitted to the back. They are systolic, except for venous hum, and usually of short duration, occupying less than ½ of systole and not interfering with the intensity and quality of the heart sounds. Innocent murmurs are usually heard better in the recumbent position, during expiration, and after exercise.

There are 5 types of innocent murmurs:

(1) Still's murmur, vibratory grade I–III/VI systolic murmurs, best heard at the lower left sternal border. This musical, groaning murmur usually disappears with Valsalva's maneuver.

(2) Functional pulmonary ejection murmur. Grade II/VI systolic murmurs may be heard at the pulmonic area in the supine position. They disappear when the patient is upright.

(3) Venous hum. In sitting position, grade II/VI, medium-pitched, slightly humming systolic/diastolic murmur, easily occluded by digital pressure over the jugular veins. The diastolic component disappears in the recumbent position.

(4) Carotid bruit. This ejection murmur originates in a carotid artery and is loudest in that location but may be referred to the base of the heart.

(5) Pericardial pleural "crunch." A very rough grade III–VI/VI systolic and diastolic murmur, best heard at the apex or the lower left sternal border. It varies significantly with respiration and is probably secondary to a pleuro-pericardial adhesion.

2. NONCARDIAC EXAMINATION

Arterial Pulse (Table 13–1)

A. Rate and Rhythm: Cardiac rate and rhythm are usually determined by palpation of the radial or brachial pulse. Throughout infancy and childhood, the rate is subject to great variation. Multiple determinations must be made under properly evaluated conditions before conclusions can be drawn about their significance. This is particularly important in infancy.

Marked variations in heart rate occur with activity; therefore, heart rate should be determined only during sleep. In older children, exercise and emotional factors have a marked effect upon the heart rate. This should be taken into account when examining the child since many children are apprehensive and may react emotionally to the initial phases of the examination.

In the pediatric age group, the rhythm may be regular or there may be a phasic variation in the heart rate (sinus arrhythmia). Occasionally, variations occur without relation to the respiratory cycle. Sinus arrhythmia is a normal finding.

B. Quality and Amplitude of Pulse: Examination of the cardiovascular system should always include a careful examination and comparison of the pulses of the upper and lower extremities. A very wide or bounding (water hammer) pulse is characteristic of aortic regurgitation. Narrow or thready pulses are found in patients with congestive heart failure or severe aortic stenosis.

Examination of the suprasternal notch should always be included. A visible pulsation in the suprasternal notch is usually abnormal, although it may be seen in patients who are emotionally excited. A prominent pulsation is found in aortic insufficiency, patent ductus arteriosus, and coarctation of the aorta. A palpable thrill in the suprasternal notch is charac-

teristic of aortic stenosis, valvular pulmonary stenosis, coarctation of the aorta, and patent ductus arteriosus.

Arterial Blood Pressure (Table 13–2)

A. Procedure: The arterial blood pressure should be determined by the auscultatory technic if possible. In young children, especially premature infants and newborns, the "flush" technic may have to be used. This method enables one to make a gross estimation of the mean arterial pressure. The cuff employed must cover approximately 2/3 of the length of the upper arm or leg. It should be wide enough to cover at least 3/4 of the circumference of the extremity. A cuff that is too narrow or too short will produce an apparent increase in blood pressure. One that is too wide will produce an apparent decrease.

Blood pressures should be obtained in the upper and lower extremities. Systolic pressure in the lower extremities determined by the auscultatory technic is usually higher than that found in the upper extremities in patients older than 1 year of age. In normal infants, the pressure in the arms may be higher. It is also extremely important that the cuff cover the same relative area of the arm and leg; this usually means that a much larger cuff must be used for the leg than for the arm.

B. Pulse Pressure: Pulse pressure is determined by subtracting the diastolic pressure from the systolic pressure. Normally, the pulse pressure is less than 50 mm Hg or less than 1/2 the systolic pressure. A widened pulse pressure (which is associated with a bounding pulse) is present in aortico-pulmonary shunt (eg, patent ductus arteriosus), aortic insufficiency, fever, anemia, and complete heart block. A narrow pulse pressure is seen in congestive heart failure, severe aortic stenosis, and pericardial tamponade.

TABLE 13–2. Normal blood pressures at various ages.*

Ages	Mean Systolic ± 2 SD	Mean Diastolic ± 2 SD
Newborn	80 ± 16	46 ± 16
6–12 months	89 ± 29	60 ± 10
1 year	96 ± 30	66 ± 25
2 years	99 ± 25	64 ± 25
3 years	100 ± 25	67 ± 23
4 years	99 ± 20	65 ± 20
5–6 years	94 ± 14	55 ± 9
6–7 years	100 ± 15	56 ± 9
7–8 years	102 ± 15	56 ± 8
8–9 years	105 ± 16	57 ± 9
9–10 years	107 ± 16	57 ± 9
10–11 years	111 ± 17	58 ± 10
11–12 years	113 ± 18	59 ± 10
12–13 years	115 ± 19	59 ± 10
13–14 years	118 ± 19	60 ± 10

*Reproduced, with permission, from Haggerty RJ, Maroney MW, Nadas AS: Essential hypertension in infancy and childhood. Am J Dis Child 92:535, 1956.

TABLE 13–1. Resting heart rates (per minute) at different ages.

Age	Lower Limits of Normal	Upper Limits of Normal	Average
Newborn	70	160	120
1–12 months	80	140	110
1–5 years	80	110	95
5–10 years	70	100	85
10–15 years	55	90	75

Venous Pressure & Pulse

The level of the distended jugular vein above the suprasternal notch when the patient is at a 45 degree angle is an excellent determinant of venous pressure in older children and adults. Normally, one may observe the level of the transition between collapse and distention of the jugular vein approximately 1–2 cm above the notch. Because of the short, fat neck in infants and young children, this is frequently not too helpful in this age group. In addition to the level of the pulse, the wave pattern should be observed. Two waves can frequently be seen: (1) The "A" wave, due to right atrial contraction, is a rather sharply rising wave and therefore occurs immediately before or with the first heart sound or point of maximum impulse (PMI). (2) The "V" wave, caused by filling of the right atrium during ventricular systole, is a more slowly rising wave and occurs toward the end of ventricular systole. Prominent "A" waves occur with increased right pressure (pulmonary stenosis, tricuspid atresia). Prominent "V" waves occur in tricuspid insufficiency.

If an accurate measurement of the venous pressure is required, direct measurement is recommended. Venous pressure increases slightly with age. Between 3–5 years, a normal venous pressure is about 40 mm water; between ages 5 and 10, about 60 mm water.

Extremities

Cyanosis of the extremities usually indicates congenital heart disease, but severe pulmonary disease must be excluded. Cyanosis is characterized by a bluish discoloration of the nails, but the entire distal portion of the extremity may be involved.

A. Clubbing of Fingers and Toes: Clubbing implies fairly severe cyanotic congenital heart disease. It usually does not appear until approximately age 1, although occasionally, in patients with severe cyanosis, it may occur earlier. The first sign of clubbing is softening of the nail beds. This is followed by rounding of the fingernails and then by thickening and shininess of the terminal phalanx, with loss of creases.

Cyanosis is by far the most common cause, but clubbing occasionally occurs also in patients with subacute bacterial endocarditis, severe liver disease, and pulmonary abscess.

B. Edema: Edema, especially of the lower extremities, is characteristic of right ventricular heart failure in older children and adults. It may be seen in infants and younger children, but in this age group edema fluid usually collects around the periorbital and facial areas before the extremities become involved.

Lungs

Increase in the rate and depth of respiration is seen in cyanotic heart disease and disorders associated with decreased pulmonary blood flow. Shallow, rapid respirations are characteristic of pulmonary venous hypertension (mitral stenosis, cor triatriatum, anomalous pulmonary venous return with obstruction). Pneumonitis is very common with large left-to-right shunts.

Abdomen

Hepatomegaly is one of the cardinal findings in right ventricular heart failure. Presystolic pulsation of the liver may occur with right atrial hypertension, and systolic pulsation with tricuspid insufficiency. Congestive splenomegaly may be present in patients who have had long-standing congestive heart failure. Enlargement of the spleen is one of the characteristic features of subacute bacterial endocarditis. Ascites is occasionally present in right heart failure.

In patients with coarctation of the aorta, attempts should be made to palpate the abdominal aorta. The presence of a pulsating abdominal aorta suggests that the coarctation is in the abdominal portion of the aorta rather than in the descending thoracic aorta.

LABORATORY DATA

Complete Blood Count, Hemoglobin, & Hematocrit

In congenital heart disease, especially the cyanotic types, determinations of hemoglobin, hematocrit, and red blood count should be made. Patients under age 2 with cyanosis are often iron deficient despite the fact that the hematocrit and hemoglobin may be relatively high. It is not infrequent to see a patient with a hemoglobin of 13 gm/100 ml, a hematocrit of 40%, and a red cell count > 7 million. Such results indicate the need for iron therapy. On the other hand, dangerously high hematocrit levels may be encountered. Complete indices should be obtained at regular intervals as a means of following the course of all cyanotic patients.

White blood counts and differentials should be obtained in patients with heart disease if there is evidence of infection.

Urinalysis

Since there is a high incidence of renal disease in patients with various types of congenital heart disease, routine urinalysis is essential. Patients with congestive heart failure frequently have proteinuria. Hematuria is common in subacute bacterial endocarditis.

Erythrocyte Sedimentation Rate (ESR)

The ESR is elevated in subacute bacterial endocarditis and acute rheumatic fever. The combination of rheumatic fever and heart failure causes the sedimentation rate to drop to normal.

Serologic Examination

Acute rheumatic fever is almost always associated with an elevation of the ASO titer. Patients with viral myocarditis occasionally have an elevation of antibodies to a specific virus (eg, coxsackievirus B4). It is necessary to obtain both acute and convalescent serum.

Castle RF, Craige E: Auscultation of the heart in infants and children. Pediatrics 26:511, 1960.

Feinstein AR & others: Glossary of cardiologic terms related to physical diagnosis and history. Parts I–IV. Am J Cardiol 20:206, 1967; 21:273, 1968; 24:444, 1969; 27:708, 1971.

Linde LM, Adams, FH, Rozansky GI: Physical and emotional aspects of CHD in children. Am J Cardiol 27:712, 1971.

Marienfeld CJ & others: A 20-year follow-up study of "innocent" murmurs. Pediatrics 30:42, 1962.

Moss AJ, Adams FH: Flush blood pressure and intraarterial pressure. Am J Dis Child 107:489, 1964.

Park MK, Guntheroth WG: Direct blood pressure measurement in brachial-femoral arteries in children. Circulation 41:231, 1970.

X-RAY OF THE HEART

X-ray examination of the chest for evaluating the cardiovascular system should include views in the postero-anterior, lateral, right anterior oblique, and left anterior oblique projections. Films taken during barium swallow have the advantage that the esophagus is well outlined; with the proper technics, this can be done even in infants. A properly performed cardiac series is invaluable in determining specific chamber enlargement. Each of the 4 different views offers the observer different points of information.

Caffey JP: *Pediatric X-ray Diagnosis,* 5th ed. Year Book, 1967.
Zdansky E: *Roentgen Diagnosis of the Heart and Great Vessels,* 2nd ed. Grune & Stratton, 1965.

THE NORMAL ELECTROCARDIOGRAM

Electrocardiography (ECG) is an essential tool in the diagnosis of congenital and rheumatic heart disease. In addition, it is useful in the diagnosis and management of patients with electrolyte imbalance.

The ECG of the normal child undergoes marked changes during the first several years of life. The stable ECG of the adult does not completely develop until about age 10. The changes in the ECG correlate well with the physiologic changes that take place within the cardiovascular system. At birth, the thickness of the wall and the pressure within the right ventricle are equal to those of the left ventricle. Accordingly, significant electrical forces are directed to the right. Indeed, in the neonatal period, rightward forces predominate. Right ventricular pressure, however, drops rapidly in early life, resulting in a relative decrease in the thickness of the wall. The thickness of the left ventricle, on the other hand, progressively increases. Thus, with increasing age, greater electrical forces are directed to the left and the stable, typical ECG of the adult eventually develops.

In childhood it is essential to obtain not only the usual standard 12 ECG leads but to include right-sided precordial leads (V_{3R} and V_{4R}) as well.

ECG Planes

One way of describing the direction and magnitude (vector) of the electrical forces of the heart is to regard the thorax as a cube and divide it into 3 planes (Fig 13–1). (1) The frontal plane (AB, CD) includes the anterior surface of the thorax in a superior-inferior and right-left direction. (2) The horizontal plane (CD, EG) is a cross-section through the thorax in an anterior-posterior and right-left direction. (3) The sagittal plane (BF, DE) is a sagittal section through the thorax in an anterior-posterior and superior-inferior direction.

P Wave

The P wave results from the conduction of electrical forces through the right and left atria. The normal P wave ranges from 1–2.5 mm in height and 0.04–0.08 mm in duration. The P wave axis in the frontal plane remains at approximately 40–60 degrees throughout childhood without significant change.

The P–R and P–Q Intervals

The P–R interval extends from the beginning of the P wave to the beginning of the R wave; the P–Q interval from the end of the P wave to the beginning of the Q wave.

QRS Complex

The major complex of the ECG is the result of sequential depolarization of the ventricular mass. This sequence is as follows: (1) Ventricular septum from left to right. (2) Anterior and lateral right and left ventricular walls (almost simultaneously). (3) Posterior wall of the left ventricle. (4) Posterior-superior wall of the ventricular septum and, occasionally, the posterior-superior wall of the right ventricle.

The complex that is described in each lead is dependent upon the magnitude and direction of the

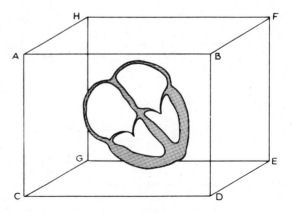

FIG 13–1. Planes of the ECG.

instantaneous electrical forces. Over the right precordial leads, there is an initial R wave followed by an S wave. Occasionally, an r' wave may be present. In the left precordial leads, there is usually a qRs pattern.

The direction of the QRS vector (axis) in the frontal and horizontal planes shifts progressively from the right to the left from birth through adulthood.

Frontal plane:
Neonatal period: +90 to +180 degrees.
1–12 months: +60 to +90 degrees.
Age 1 to adolescence: +40 to +70 degrees.
Adulthood: +40 to +60 degrees.

Horizontal plane:
Neonatal period: Right anterior quadrant.
Age 1 month to adolescence: Progressive shift to the left in the left anterior quadrant.
Adulthood: Left posterior quadrant.

T Wave
The T wave is due to repolarization of the ventricular mass. The axis of the T wave in the frontal plane remains around +60 degrees throughout life. In the right precordial lead, the T wave is normally inverted from 5 days of age to about 5 years. It may be upright or inverted in the right precordial leads from birth through 5 days. After 5 years, it may be either upright or inverted. The T wave in the left precordial leads (V_5 and V_6) is upright throughout life, although it may be inverted normally during the first 24–48 hours.

THE ABNORMAL ELECTROCARDIOGRAM

Right Atrial Hypertrophy
Increase in the height of the P wave (greater than 2.5 mm) with slight narrowing of the wave. This results in a characteristic "peaking," best seen in leads II and V_1.

Left Atrial Hypertrophy
The P wave is prolonged to > 0.08 seconds. A notch usually occurs at a point > 0.05 seconds after the beginning of the wave.

Right Ventricular Hypertrophy
A. Frontal Plane (Limb Leads): Axis > +120 degrees (after age 2); R wave in aVR > 6 mm.
B. Horizontal Plane (Right Precordial Leads): (1) R minus S > 15 mm (under 2 months of age, > 20 mm). (2) R' > 15 mm (under 2 months of age, > 20 mm). (3) q wave in the right precordial leads in the absence of anatomic ventricular inversion (eg, corrected transposition). (4) Presence of upright T waves in the right precordial leads from 5 days to 5 years of life. (5) A combination of tall R waves (with or without a preceding q wave) and deeply inverted T waves

from V_3R through V_3 is indicative of severe right ventricular hypertrophy and "strain."

The appearance of an rsR' pattern in the right precordial leads suggests the type of hypertrophy seen with diastolic or volume overloading of the right ventricle (eg, atrial septal defect). The presence of a very tall R wave, either with upright T waves or deeply inverted T waves, suggests the presence of systolic or pressure overloading of the right ventricle (eg, severe valvular pulmonary stenosis). Although these different patterns may indeed indicate different physiologic states, it is probable that they only represent different degrees of severity of right ventricular hypertrophy.

Left Ventricular Hypertrophy
A. Frontal Plane (Limb Leads): R in lead II + R in lead III > 45 mm; R in aVL or aVF > 25 mm.
B. Precordial Leads (V_5, V_6): (1) R in V_5 + S in V_1 > 60 mm (in children and adolescents). (2) R in V_5 > 40 mm. (3) q > 6 mm associated with tall R and symmetrically peaked T wave (diastolic overload pattern). (4) S in V_1 > 30 mm. (5) Tall R wave associated with depression of the ST segment and inversion of the T wave in V_5 and V_6 suggest severe left ventricular hypertrophy and left ventricular "strain" (systolic overload pattern).

Combined Ventricular Hypertrophy
Combined ventricular hypertrophy may be diagnosed when there is evidence of left ventricular hypertrophy and the following: (1) A dominant R wave in the right precordial leads. (2) Very tall R and very deep S in the mid-precordial leads (R + S > 70 mm). (3) Right axis deviation in the presence of findings of left ventricular hypertrophy.

Effect of Electrolyte Changes on the ECG
A. Hyperkalemia:
1. **Mild (5–7 mEq/liter)**—Tall peaked T waves.
2. **Progressive increase**—Widening of the QRS complex and the P wave and prolongation of the P–R interval.
3. **Severe (> 10 mEq/liter)**—Complete loss of P waves and development of bizarre, wide QRS and T wave complexes.
B. Hypokalemia (> 3 mEq/liter): Widening and lowering of the T waves and appearance of prominent U waves. There is prolongation of the Q–T (Q–U) interval. Occasionally, there may be depression of the S–T segment.
C. Hypercalcemia: May shorten the Q–T interval; produces increased irritability of the heart.
D. Hypocalcemia: Prolongation of the Q–T interval due to prolongation of the S–T segment. (No effect on the T wave.)

Cabrera E, Gaxiola A: A critical re-evaluation of systolic and diastolic overloading patterns. Progr Cardiovas Dis 2:219, 1959.

Hastreiter AR, Abella JB: The ECG in the newborn period. I. The normal infant. J Pediat 78:146, 1971. II. The infant with disease. J Pediat 78:346, 1971.

VECTORCARDIOGRAPHY

During the past several years, technics have been developed to record the instantaneous electrical forces that take place in a 3-dimensional manner. This technic is known as vectorcardiography (VCG). The record that is obtained is in the form of a loop in each of the 3 planes. There are various systems of electrode placement. Loops for the P wave, QRS complex, and T waves are best described in each plane.

This technic has become an important research and diagnostic tool in pediatric cardiology. In future the vectorcardiogram may supplant the conventional ECG in the routine work-up of the cardiac patient.

Hugenholtz PG, Liebman J: The orthogonal vectorcardiogram in 100 normal children (Frank system). Circulation 26:891, 1962.

Liebman J, Nadas AS: An abnormally superior vector (formerly called marked left axis deviation). Am J Cardiol 27:577, 1971.

Namin EP & others: Evolution of the Frank vectorcardiogram in normal infants. Am J Cardiol 13:757, 1964.

CARDIAC CATHETERIZATION; SELECTIVE ANGIOCARDIOGRAPHY & CINEANGIOCARDIOGRAPHY

Cardiac catheterization involves the insertion of a catheter of relatively small caliber into either a peripheral vein or an artery and the manipulation of this catheter into the various chambers of the heart and great vessels. Selective angiocardiography consists of injecting contrast material into a chamber or vessel and following the course of the material (by motion picture or large film x-ray) during several subsequent cardiac cycles. In most laboratories, the cineangiocardiogram is an integral part of the cardiac catheterization procedure. Many laboratories are now equipped with a videotape recorder which permits reevaluation of the cineangiocardiogram immediately following the injection.

In most instances a specific congenital or acquired cardiac lesion can be identified on the basis of clinical information. Therefore, cardiac catheterization and cineangiocardiography are infrequently used for diagnostic purposes alone. Since these technics are potentially dangerous, they should not be performed without sufficient indications, especially in infants and young children.

Indications & Contraindications

A. Indications:

1. To determine the severity of a particular defect in order to assess the need for surgical correction.

2. To confirm a specific clinical diagnosis in an infant in whom the clinical course indicates the need for surgical intervention.

3. For diagnostic purposes in patients whose clinical course indicates a poor prognosis and in whom the diagnosis is in doubt.

4. To rule out the possibility of a surgically correctable condition in patients whose clinical diagnosis is that of a cardiac lesion which is inoperable in the hope that the diagnosis is incorrect.

5. For the postoperative evaluation of patients who have undergone cardiovascular surgery.

6. To gain information concerning the natural history of a particular defect in the course of a well designed and controlled research project.

B. Contraindications: Cardiac catheterization should not be performed for diagnostic purposes in infants who are asymptomatic. In many instances, the diagnosis becomes apparent as one follows the clinical course. If not, cardiac catheterization can be done later when the procedure is less hazardous. These procedures are much more hazardous in infants and young children than in older individuals, in terms of both mortality and morbidity.

Cardiac catheterization is usually not recommended in patients with a clear diagnosis of patent ductus arteriosus and coarctation of the aorta. In some centers, cardiac catheterization is not performed in patients with clear-cut findings of a large ostium secundum atrial septal defect, severe pulmonary stenosis, and aortic stenosis.

Data Obtained in Routine Cardiac Catheterization

A. Oxygen Content and Saturation; Pulmonary and Systemic Blood Flow (Cardiac Output): In most laboratories, evidence of left-to-right shunt is determined by changes of blood oxygen content or saturation during passage of the catheter through the right side of the heart. A significant increase in oxygen content or oxygen saturation from one chamber to another indicates the presence of a left-to-right shunt at the site of the increase. The oxygen saturation of the peripheral arterial blood should always be obtained during the course of cardiac catheterization. The normal arterial oxygen saturation ranges between 94–97%. Any decrease at sea level below 91% is abnormal and indicates the presence of a right-to-left shunt, underventilation, or pulmonary disease.

The size of a left-to-right shunt is usually considered in terms of the ratio of the pulmonary to systemic blood flow. These are determined by application of the Fick principle:

$$\frac{\text{Cardiac output}}{\text{(liters/minute)}} = \frac{\text{Oxygen consumption (ml/minute)}}{\text{Arteriovenous difference (ml/liter)}}$$

B. Pressures: Pressures are obtained in all chambers and vessels entered. Pressures should always be recorded when a catheter is pulled back from a distal chamber or vessel into a more proximal chamber. By this means, gradients across valves may be obtained.

C. Pulmonary and Systemic Vascular Resistance: The vascular resistance is calculated from the following formula:

$$\text{Resistance} = \frac{\text{Pressure}}{\text{Flow}}$$

corrected to the body surface area.

1. Pulmonary vascular resistance = mean pulmonary artery pressure divided by pulmonary blood flow per square meter of body surface area. (Pulmonary blood flow determined from the Fick principle as noted previously.)

2. Systemic vascular resistance = mean systemic arterial pressure divided by systemic blood flow.

The resistance calculated by these formulas is reported in terms of "units." It is also frequently reported in terms of dynes–sec–cm^{-5}–m^2.

Normally, the pulmonary vascular resistance ranges from 2–4 units or 150–300 dynes (at higher altitudes, the upper limit of normal is about 5 units).

D. Special Technics: Special technics are frequently employed during the course of cardiac catheterization. These include the following:

1. The hydrogen electrode catheter–Used to determine the presence of very small left-to-right shunts. This technic enables the operator to detect such shunts even in the absence of any increase in oxygen saturation.

2. Indicator dye dilution curves–This involves injection of an indicator, usually "cardio green," at specific places in the heart and detection of the dye downstream, usually in a peripheral artery. This technic permits the detection of both right-to-left and left-to-right shunts at specific points within the cardiovascular system. Cardiac output is frequently determined by this method.

3. Selective angiocardiography and cineangiocardiography–In this technic, contrast material is injected in a specific chamber or vessel and the course of the contrast material followed by serial large film x-rays (angiocardiography) or by motion pictures (cineangiocardiography).

Agustsson MH, Bicoff JP, Arcilla RA: Hemodynamic studies in fifty-two normal infants and children. Circulation 28:683, 1963.

Brockenbrough EC & others: Left heart catheterization in infants and children. Pediatrics 30:253, 1962.

Simovitch H & others: Percutaneous right and left heart catheterization in children: Experience with 1000 patients. Circulation 16:513, 1970.

Srouji MN, Rashkind WJ: The effect of cardiac catheterization on acid-base status of infants with congenital heart disease. J Pediat 75:943, 1969.

Varghese PJ & others: Cardiac catheterization in the newborn: Experience with 100 cases. Pediatrics 44:24, 1969.

Zimmerman HA (editor): *Intravascular Catheterization,* 2nd ed. Thomas, 1966.

PRENATAL & NEONATAL CIRCULATION

(See Figs 13–2, 13–3, and 13–4.)

Fetal Circulation

In the fetus, the placenta serves as the organ of respiration and for exchange of waste products for nutritive material. Oxygenated blood (80% saturated) passes from the placenta through the umbilical vein to the heart. As it flows toward the heart, it mixes with blood from the inferior vena cava and from the portal vein so that blood entering the right atrium is approximately 65% saturated. A considerable amount of this blood is shunted immediately across the foramen ovale into the left atrium. The venous blood derived from the upper part of the body is much less saturated (approximately 30%), and most of it enters the right ventricle through the tricuspid valve. Thus, the blood in the right ventricle is a mixture of both relatively highly saturated blood from the umbilical vein and desaturated blood from the vena cavae. This mixture results in a blood oxygen saturation of approximately 50% in the right ventricle.

The blood in the left atrium is derived from the blood shunting across the foramen ovale and the blood returning from the pulmonary veins. A great deal of the left ventricular output goes to the head, whereas the lower portion of the body is supplied by blood both from the right ventricle, through the patent ductus arteriosus, and from the left ventricle.

Physiologic Changes at Birth & in the Neonatal Period

At birth, 2 dramatic events occur as far as the cardiovascular-pulmonary system is concerned: (1) The umbilical cord is clamped, removing the placenta from the circulation, and (2) breathing commences. As a result, marked changes in the circulation occur. During fetal life, the placenta offers little resistance to the flow of blood so that the systemic circuit is a low-resistance one. On the other hand, the pulmonary arterioles are markedly constricted and offer marked resistance to the flow of blood into the lung. Clamping the cord causes a sudden increase in resistance to flow in the systemic circuit. As the lung becomes the organ of respiration, the oxygen tension (P_{O_2}) increases in the vicinity of the small pulmonary arterioles, resulting in a release of the constriction and, thus, a significant decrease in the pulmonary arteriolar resistance. Indeed, shortly after birth the pulmonary vascular resistance is less than that of the systemic circuit.

Because of the changes in resistance, the great majority of right ventricular outflow now passes into the lung rather than through the ductus arteriosus into the descending aorta. In fact, functional closure of the ductus arteriosus begins to develop shortly after birth. Recent studies have demonstrated that the ductus

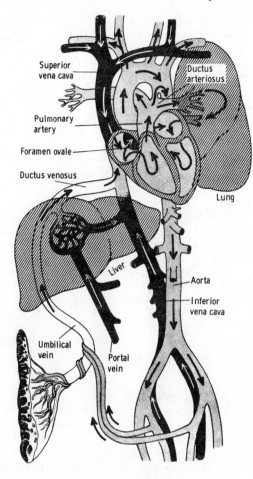

FIG 13-2. Fetal circulation.*

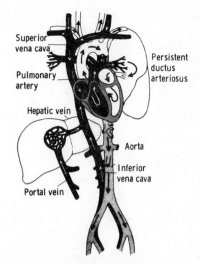

FIG 13-3. Immediate postdelivery circulation.*

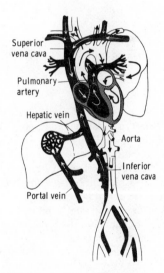

FIG 13-4. Normal circulation.*

*Reproduced, with permission, from Benson RC: *Handbook of Obstetrics & Gynecology,* 4th ed. Lange, 1971.

arteriosus remains patent for a variable period, usually 24-48 hours. During the first hour after birth, there is a small right-to-left shunt (as in the fetus). However, after 1 hour, bidirectional shunting occurs, with the left-to-right direction predominating. In most cases, right-to-left shunting completely disappears by 8 hours. However, in patients with severe hypoxia (in respiratory distress syndrome), the pulmonary vascular resistance remains quite elevated, resulting in a continued right-to-left shunt. The cause of the functional closure of the ductus arteriosus is not completely known. However, recent evidence indicates that the increased PO_2 of the arterial blood causes spasm of the ductus. Anatomically, however, the ductus arteriosus does not close until approximately 3 months of age.

In fetal life, the foramen ovale serves as a one-way valve, permitting shunting of blood from the inferior vena cava through the right atrium into the left atrium.

At birth, because of the changes in the pulmonary and systemic vascular resistance and the increase in the quantity of blood returning from the pulmonary veins to the left atrium, the left atrial pressure rises above that of the right atrium. This functionally closes the flap of the one-way valve, essentially preventing flow of blood across the septum. It has been shown, however, that a small right-to-left shunt does continue for the first week of life. Although the foramen ovale remains functionally closed throughout life, the foramen ovale remains patent in about 25% of patients.

Changes in the First Year of Life

The most significant changes occur at birth and within the neonatal period. However, pulmonary vascular resistance and the pulmonary arterial pressure continue to fall during the first year of life. This results from the involution of the pulmonary arteriole from a relatively thick-walled, small-lumen vessel to a thin-walled, large-lumen vessel. Adult levels of resistance and pressure are usually achieved by 6 months to 1 year of life.

Dawes GS: Changes in the circulation at birth. Brit M Bull 17:148, 1961.

Dawes GS: Physiological changes in the circulation after birth. In: *Circulation of the Blood: Men and Ideas.* Fishman AP, Richards DW (editors). Oxford Univ Press, 1964.

Kaiser IH: Correlation of circulatory changes before birth. In: *The Heart and Circulation in the Newborn and Infant.* Cassels DE (editor). Grune & Stratton, 1966.

Moss AJ, Emmanouilides GC, Duffie ER: Closure of the ductus arteriosus in the newborn infant. Pediatrics 32:25, 1963.

Rowe RD, James LS: The normal pulmonary arterial pressure during the first year of life. J Pediat 51:1, 1957.

Rudolph AM: The changes in the circulation after birth: Their importance in congenital heart disease. Circulation 41:343, 1970.

CONGESTIVE HEART FAILURE

Congestive heart failure is a clinical syndrome in which the heart is not able to supply the oxygen demands of the body. In most cases of heart failure, there is an absolute decrease in the cardiac output (low-output failure). In some instances, cardiac output is actually increased but is still insufficient (high-output failure, eg, hyperthyroidism).

Heart failure is not rare in infants and children. By far the most common cause is congenital heart disease. Less common causes include acute rheumatic fever with pancarditis, viral myocarditis, paroxysmal atrial tachycardia, primary myocardial disease, and chronic renal failure.

Clinical Findings

A. Symptoms and Signs : Most pediatric patients with congestive heart failure present, with findings of combined right and left ventricular failure. Occasionally, signs of pure right heart failure are seen (eg, severe pulmonary stenosis with intact ventricular septum), but pure left ventricular failure is rarely present when the child is seen. The most common signs are as follows: **(1) Tachycardia**: The pulse rate is greater than 140/minute in infants (while asleep) and greater than 100/minute in older children (asleep). It is important to take the pulse during sleep since marked variability can occur while the child is awake and irritable. **(2) Tachypnea**: Respiratory rates of 50–100/minute are not uncommon, and even faster rates are occasionally seen. Tachypnea is an important sign of left heart failure. The increase in left atrial pressure secondary to left heart failure results in an increase in pulmonary venous pressure. This produces transudation of fluid

into the interstitial tissues of the lung. The lungs become stiff and hard to move (ie, lung compliance decreases). Rapid, shallow respirations result since this is the most economical method of producing a satisfactory minute volume. **(3) Hepatomegaly**: Liver enlargement is a characteristic finding of right heart failure. Increase in systemic venous pressure results in accumulation of blood within the liver, and the liver becomes acutely enlarged and often quite tender. Frequently there is a very sharp edge.

These 3 cardinal manifestations of heart failure are found in almost all cases of biventricular failure. Tachypnea, however, does not occur in patients with pure right heart failure.

Other findings include the following: (1) Pulmonary rales. (2) Peripheral edema: When edema occurs in infants and children secondary to congestive heart failure, there is accumulation of fluid in the periorbital area and the face in general. Rarely does one find pretibial edema. (3) Neck vein distention: This is difficult to note in infants because of the short, fat neck. (4) Peripheral cyanosis due to the low cardiac output and the wide arteriovenous oxygen difference in the capillary bed. (5) Fatigue and weakness, the result of the decrease in cardiac output and inability to increase the output with exercise. (6) Weight gain due to the accumulation of fluid.

The peripheral arterial pulses are usually weak in patients with low-output failure. However, they may be quite strong in patients with high-output failure. The mucous membranes and nail beds may be dusky. The heart is generally enlarged and the heart tones poor. Third and fourth heart sounds are frequently heard, producing a gallop effect. Heart murmurs may or may not be present, depending upon the cause of heart failure.

ECG is not helpful in the diagnosis of congestive heart failure.

B. X-Ray Findings: Chest x-rays reveal evidence of diffuse cardiac enlargement and pulmonary venous congestion if there is left heart failure.

Treatment

A. General Measures:

1. Sedation—Children are quite apprehensive and frightened, and infants are very irritable. The drug of choice is morphine, 0.1 mg/kg subcut.

2. Oxygen—Oxygen offers considerable symptomatic relief, increasing the oxygen tension within the pulmonary veins in patients with pulmonary edema and providing the heart with increased oxygen and improving its function.

3. Low-salt diet—This may be difficult to enforce in older children, who will often refuse to eat an extremely low-sodium or low-salt diet. It is advisable, in such cases, to prepare a regular diet but to prohibit added salt.

B. Digitalization: Digitalis is extremely effective in most cases of congestive heart failure. It is probably most beneficial in primary myocardial disease, large left-to-right shunts, and valvular regurgitation. It is not so effective in heart failure secondary to semilunar valve or mitral valve obstruction. High-output failure and cor pulmonale secondary to pulmonary hypertension are usually little affected by the digitalis therapy.

The digitalis product of choice among pediatric cardiologists is digoxin. It has a fairly rapid onset of effect (30 minutes); the maximum effect is achieved in 2–4 hours; and most of the drug disappears from the body within 24–48 hours. Digoxin may be used orally or parenterally; the parenteral dose is ¾ of the oral dose.

The dosage of digoxin required for full digitalization varies from patient to patient, and the following dosage schedule is suggested only as a guide:

Premature and newborn (0–30 days):
>   Digitalizing dose, 0.03–0.05 mg/kg IM
>   Maintenance dose, 1/10–1/5 of digitalizing dose IM

1 month–2 years:
>   Digitalizing dose, 0.06–0.08 mg/kg orally
>   Maintenance dose, 1/5–1/3 of digitalizing dose orally

2–6 years:
>   Digitalizing dose, 0.04–0.06 mg/kg orally
>   Maintenance dose, 1/5–1/3 of digitalizing dose orally

6–12 years:
>   Digitalizing dose, 0.02–0.04 mg/kg orally
>   Maintenance dose, 1/5–1/3 of digitalizing dose orally

It is recommended that ½ the digitalizing dose be given initially, ¼ 8 hours later, and ¼ after another 8 hours.

Digitalization is best done in a hospital with careful monitoring of the pulse. An ECG (rhythm strip) should be done before the last ¼ dose is administered if the heart rate is unduly slow or irregular.

The most common manifestation of digitalis toxicity in childhood is the onset of an arrhythmia or heart block.

C. Diuretics: Since retention of salt and water are major manifestations of congestive heart failure, diuretics play an important role in treatment. This is especially true in infants and children since it is usually very difficult to severely restrict sodium in the diet. Low-sodium formulas and solids are not very palatable and may cause electrolyte disturbances if maintained over a long period of time. It is often necessary to administer diuretics only during the acute phase of congestive heart failure. Continued "maintenance" digitalis therapy is then sufficient to prevent recurrence of heart failure. Occasionally, long-term diuretic therapy is necessary.

The following diuretics have been found to be of clinical value in the pediatric age group:

1. Mercurials—Meralluride (Mercuhydrin) intramuscularly; mercaptomerin (Thiomerin) subcutaneously. These drugs act primarily on the proximal renal tubules to inhibit sodium reabsorption. Chloruresis and diuresis occur as well, since water and chloride ion reabsorption are dependent on sodium reabsorption.

The dosage is as follows: infants, 0.25 ml; small children, 0.5 ml; older children, 1 ml.

Mercurials can be given every other day for several days during the acute treatment phase. If long-term therapy is required, they may be given once or twice weekly.

2. Ethacrynic acid (Edecrin)—This drug is thought to act by inhibiting renal tubular reabsorption of sodium and water. It is a very potent diuretic and causes diuresis extremely rapidly. It is most useful when given intravenously in a dose of 1 mg/kg. Careful determination of serum electrolytes is necessary when the drug is used repeatedly. Nerve deafness has been observed following the use of this drug. This is usually temporary, but permanent deafness has been reported in patients with severe renal disease.

3. Furosemide (Lasix)—This drug is thought to act in a similar fashion to ethacrynic acid. It is given in similar dosage and has an advantage over ethacrynic acid in that it may be given intramuscularly and orally.

4. Thiazides—Chlorothiazide (Diuril) and hydrochlorothiazide (HydroDiuril) are oral diuretics which are used in the treatment of chronic congestive heart failure. These agents seem to have an effect on both the proximal and distal tubules of the nephron. Serum electrolytes must be monitored, since hypokalemia and hyponatremia may occur. The dosage is as follows: chlorothiazide, 25 mg/kg/day in divided doses; hydrochlorothiazide, 2.5 mg/kg/day in divided doses.

Potassium supplements should be provided when these drugs are administered over a prolonged period of time.

5. Spironolactone (Aldactone)—This oral diuretic acts by blocking the sodium-retaining effects of aldosterone on the distal convoluted tubule. It is most useful in combination with a thiazide or with furosemide. The daily dosage for children is 3 mg/kg orally.

Kim KE & others: Ethacrynic acid and furosemide: Diuretic and hemodynamic effect and clinical uses. Am Cardiol 27:407, 1971.

Lees MH: Heart failure in the newborn infant: Recognition and management. J Pediat 75:139, 1970.

Mason DT & others: Current concepts and treatment of digitalis toxicity. Am J Cardiol 27:546. 1971.

Sarnoff SJ, Mitchell JH: The regulation of the performance of the heart. Am J Med 30:747, 1961.

Sparrow AW, Friedberg DZ, Nadas AS: Use of ethacrynic acid in infants and children with congestive heart failure. Pediatrics 42:291, 1968.

Talner NS & others: Congestive heart failure in infancy. 1. Abnormalities in blood gases and acid-base equilibrium. Pediatrics 35:20, 1965.

CONGENITAL HEART DISEASE

I. NONCYANOTIC
HEART DISEASE

ATRIAL SEPTAL DEFECTS

An atrial septal defect is an opening in the atrial septum permitting the shunting of blood between the 2 atria. There are 2 major types: ostium secundum (relatively high) and ostium primum (low). The ostium primum type will be discussed under the endocardial cushion defects.

ATRIAL SEPTAL DEFECT
OF THE OSTIUM SECUNDUM VARIETY

Essential of Diagnosis

- Acyanotic, asymptomatic.
- Right ventricular lift.
- S_2 widely split and fixed.
- Grade I–III/VI ejection systolic murmur at pulmonic area.
- Diastolic flow murmur at the lower left sternal border.

General Considerations

This type of atrial septal defect is relatively common. It occurs in 10–15% of patients with congenital heart disease. The defect occurs in the mid or upper portion of the atrial septum in the area of the foramen ovale. The average size is about 2–3 cm in diameter. In about 10–15% of cases, partial anomalous pulmonary venous drainage is present.

In older infants and in children, the flow across the atrial septal defect is from the left atrium to the right atrium. The flow can be considerable, ranging from 1–20 liters/minute/sq m. The flow is in the left-to-right direction since the resistance to filling of the left ventricle is greater than that of the right ventricle. In the newborn and in the younger infant, the left to-right shunt is usually small because the resistance to filling of the right ventricle is relatively high. As the infant develops, the pressure/volume characteristics of the right ventricle change and resistance to filling of the right ventricle decreases. Accordingly, the left-to-right shunt across the defect increases.

Pulmonary hypertension and increased pulmonary vascular resistance are rare complications in childhood and adolescence but are significant factors after the third decade of life. When increased pulmonary vascular resistance occurs, the left-to-right shunting decreases and right-to-left shunting begins.

Clinical Findings

A. Symptoms and Signs: Children with atrial septal defects are usually small and thin (gracile habitus), but there are usually no cardiovascular symptoms. Some patients remain asymptomatic throughout life; others develop easy fatigability as adults. Cyanosis does not occur until pulmonary hypertension develops. This may never occur; if it does, it is not seen until after the third decade of life. Congestive heart failure is extremely rare until pulmonary hypertension occurs.

The arterial pulses are normal and equal throughout. In the usual case, the heart is hyperactive, with a heaving impulse felt best at the lower left sternal border and over the xiphoid process. A right ventricular outflow thrust at the second intercostal space is palpable. There are no thrills. S_1 at the apex is split with a loud tricuspid (second) component. S_2 at the pulmonary area is widely split and fixed. The pulmonary component is normal in intensity. A grade I–III/VI, somewhat blowing, ejection type systolic murmur is heard best at the left sternal border in the second intercostal space. This murmur radiates well into the interscapular area of the back. An early diastolic murmur can often be heard in the fourth and fifth intercostal spaces at the left sternal border. This murmur is due to increased blood flow across the tricuspid valve during early diastole (tricuspid flow murmur). The presence of this murmur suggests a high flow (pulmonary to systemic blood flow ratio greater than 2:1).

B. X-Ray Findings: Chest x-rays usually demonstrate slight cardiac enlargement. This is due to enlargement of the right atrium and right ventricle. The main pulmonary artery may be dilated. The pulmonary vascular markings are increased as a result of increased pulmonary blood flow.

C. Electrocardiography and Vectorcardiography: The usual ECG shows right axis deviation with a clockwise loop in the frontal plane. In the right precordial leads, there is usually an rsR' pattern. The R' may range from 5–15 mm. Deep S waves can often be identified in the left precordium.

The VCG in the horizontal plane usually shows a terminal vector that is directed rightward and anteriorly.

D. Cardiac Catheterization and Cineangiocardiography: Oximetry reveals evidence of a significant increase in oxygen saturation at the atrial level. The pulmonary artery pressure is usually normal. The right ventricular pressure is occasionally 10–30 mm greater than the pulmonary artery pressure. This is due to "flow," not to organic obstruction. Pulmonary vascular resistance is normal. The pulmonary to systemic blood flow ratio may vary from 1.5:1–4:1. A catheter can easily be passed across the atrial septum into the left atrium if the catheterization is performed through the saphenous vein. Hydrogen electrode curves and dye dilution curves indicate a left-to-right shunt at the atrial level. The systemic arterial saturation is normal.

Cineangiocardiography, with injection of contrast medium into the left atrium, demonstrates a left to right shunt at the atrial level.

Treatment

All ostium secundum atrial septal defects in which the pulmonary to systemic blood flow ratio is greater than 2:1 should be closed. Operation is usually recommended at ages 5–10. The mortality rate for closure is about 1–3%. Once pulmonary hypertension secondary to increased pulmonary vascular resistance occurs, closure of the defect is not recommended.

Course & Prognosis

Patients with atrial septal defects tolerate them very well in the first 2 decades of life. Occasionally patients may live a completely normal life without symptoms. Frequently, however, pulmonary hypertension and reversal of the shunt develops by the third to fourth decade. Heart failure may occur at this time. Subacute bacterial endocarditis is a very rare complication.

Craig RJ, Selzer A: Natural history and prognosis of atrial septal defect. Circulation 37:805, 1968.

Evans JR, Rowe RD, Keith JD: The clinical diagnosis of atrial septal defect in children. Am J Med 30:345, 1961.

Kumar S, Luisada AA: The second heart sound in atrial septal defect. Am J Cardiol 28:168, 1971.

Levin AR & others: Atrial pressure-flow dynamics in atrial septal defects (secundum type). Circulation 37:476, 1968.

McGoon DC, DuShane JW, Kirklin JW: Surgical treatment of atrial septal defect in children. Pediatrics 24:992, 1959.

Nakamura FF, Hauck AJ, Nadas AS: Atrial septal defects in infants. Pediatrics 34:101, 1964.

Nielsen SJ, Fabricius J: Effect of exercise on size of shunt in patients with atrial septal defects. Acta med scandinav 183:91, 1968.

VENTRICULAR SEPTAL DEFECTS

Essentials of Diagnosis

Small- to moderate-sized left-to-right shunt; normal pulmonary arterial pressure.

- Acyanotic, asymptomatic.
- Grade II–IV/VI pansystolic murmur with or without thrill, maximal along the lower left sternal border.
- P_2 not accentuated.

Large left-to-right shunt; pulmonary hypertension:

- Acyanotic.
- Increased respiratory infections.
- Easy fatigability.
- Frequently, congestive heart failure in infancy.
- Hyperactive heart; biventricular enlargement.
- Grade II–VI/VI pansystolic murmur, maximal at lower left sternal border.
- P_2 accentuated.
- Diastolic flow murmur at apex.

Net right-to-left shunt; severe pulmonary hypertension (Eisenmenger's syndrome):

- Cyanosis.
- Quiet precordium with right ventricular lift.
- Palpable P_2.
- Short ejection systolic murmur along left sternal border; single accentuated S_2.
- Systemic arterial oxygen desaturation; pulmonary arterial pressure and systemic arterial pressures are equal; little or no oxygen saturation increase at right ventricular level by catheterization.

General Considerations

Simple ventricular septal defect (ie, without other lesions) is the most common single congenital heart lesion, accounting for about 20% of all cases of congenital heart disease. Defects in the ventricular septum can occur both in the membranous portion of the septum (most common) and in the muscular portion. The size of the defect is more important than its position.

In uncomplicated ventricular septal defect, blood is shunted from the left to the right ventricle. This is because the resistance to filling of the systemic circuit is greater than the resistance to filling of the pulmonary circuit. The amount of blood flow across the ventricular septum is determined not only by the pulmonary vascular resistance but also by the size of the defect. Accordingly, the pulmonary to systemic blood flow ratios may vary from 1.1:1 to greater than 4:1.

Pulmonary hypertension is not uncommon in patients with ventricular septal defect. The increased pressure within the pulmonary circuit may be due to a marked increase in pulmonary blood flow or in pulmonary vascular resistance. (Pressure = flow × resistance.) Pulmonary hypertension rarely develops during infancy and early childhood. If pulmonary hypertension is present in a child with ventricular septal defect, it probably has existed from birth. Furthermore, there is usually very little deterioration of the existing pulmonary hypertension during childhood, ie, development of irreversible changes within the pulmonary vascular bed is rare.

Increased pulmonary vascular resistance in children under 2 is usually the result of muscular constriction of the pulmonary arterioles. This form of increased resistance is reversible by means of pulmonary vasodilators such as oxygen and tolazoline (Priscoline). Following puberty, progressive irreversible changes occur within the pulmonary arteriolar bed, resulting in progressive increase in pulmonary vascular resistance of the "fixed" or irreversible type.

Clinical Findings

A. Symptoms and Signs: Patients with small or moderate left-to-right shunts usually have no cardiovascular symptoms. There may be a history of frequent respiratory infections in infancy and early childhood.

Patients with large left-to-right shunts frequently are sick early in infancy. Such patients have frequent respiratory infections, including bouts of pneumonitis. They grow slowly, with very poor weight gain. Dyspnea, exercise intolerance, and fatigue are quite common. Congestive heart failure may develop between 1–6 months. Patients who survive the first year usually improve, although easy fatigability may persist. With severe pulmonary hypertension (Eisenmenger's syndrome), cyanosis is present.

Arterial pulses are usually normal and equal throughout.

1. Small left-to-right shunt—There are usually no lifts, heaves, thrills, or shocks. The first sound at the apex is normal and the second sound at the pulmonary area is physiologically split. The pulmonary component is normal. A grade II–III/VI, medium to high-pitched, blowing pansystolic murmur is heard best at the left sternal border in the third and fourth intercostal spaces. There is slight radiation over the entire precordium. No diastolic murmurs are heard.

2. Moderate left-to-right shunt—Slight prominence of the precordium is common. There is a moderate left ventricular thrust. A systolic thrill is palpable at the lower left sternal border between the third and fourth intercostal spaces. The first sound is often obliterated by the murmur. The second sound at the pulmonary area is most often split but may be single. A grade IV/VI, harsh pansystolic murmur is heard best at the lower left sternal border in the third and fourth intercostal spaces with radiation well over the xiphoid process to the right lower sternal border. It radiates to the base of the heart and to the apex and the left lung base. A third heart sound and a diastolic flow murmur are often heard. The diastolic flow murmur is due to the increased blood flow across the mitral valve during ventricular diastole. The presence of a flow murmur indicates that the pulmonary blood flow is large and that the pulmonary to systemic blood flow ratio is at least 2:1.

3. Very large ventricular septal defects with pulmonary hypertension—The precordium is prominent and the sternum bulges. A left ventricular thrust and a right ventricular heave are palpable. A shock of the second sound can be felt at the pulmonary area. A thrill may or may not be present at the lower left sternal border. The first heart sound is usually loud. A second heart sound is narrowly split, with accentuation of the pulmonary component. The murmur ranges from grade II–V/VI and is usually harsh and pansystolic. Occasionally, when the defect is very large, very little murmur can be heard. A diastolic flow murmur is heard at the apex.

B. X-Ray Findings: X-rays of the chest vary depending upon the size of the shunt. In patients with small shunts, x-rays may be normal. The heart is normal in size, and the pulmonary vascular markings may be just beyond the upper limits of normal. Patients with large shunts usually show significant cardiac enlargement involving both the left and right ventricles and the left atrium. The aorta is usually small to normal in size, and the main pulmonary artery segment is dilated. The pulmonary vascular markings are significantly increased in patients with large shunts.

C. Electrocardiography and Vectorcardiography: There is some correlation between the ECG and the hemodynamic findings. The ECG is normal in patients with small left-to-right shunts and normal pulmonary arterial pressures. Pure left ventricular hypertrophy with a frontal plane axis to the left of +90 degrees but in the normal quadrant is found in patients with large left-to-right shunts and normal pulmonary vascular resistance. Combined ventricular hypertrophy (both right and left) with a frontal plane axis ranging from −30 degrees to +180 degrees is found in patients with pulmonary hypertension due to increased flow, increased resistance, or both. Pure right ventricular hypertrophy with a frontal plane axis to the right of +150 degrees is found in patients with pulmonary hypertension due to pulmonary vascular obstruction.

D. Cardiac Catheterization and Angiocardiography: Oxygen saturation is increased at the right ventricular level. Pulmonary arterial pressures may vary from normal to that of systemic arterial pressure. Left atrial pressure (pulmonary capillary pressure) may be normal to increased. **Pulmonary vascular resistance** varies from normal to markedly increased. The pulmonary to systemic blood flow ratio may vary from 1.1:1–4:1.

The catheter can frequently be passed across the ventricular septal defect from the right ventricle into the ascending aorta.

Hydrogen electrode curves and dye dilution curves may indicate a shunt at the ventricular level.

Angiocardiographic examination following injection of contrast material into the left ventricle or pulmonary artery reveals a left-to-right shunt at the ventricular level.

Treatment

A. Medical Treatment: Patients who develop congestive heart failure should be treated vigorously with anticongestive measures (see Congestive Heart Failure). If the patient responds well, he should be maintained on digitalis until surgical correction of the defect can be performed. It is often possible to discontinue digitalis after about age 2. If the patient does not respond to vigorous anticongestive measures, surgery is indicated without delay.

B. Surgical Treatment:

1. Pulmonary artery banding—This procedure involves placing a band (frequently umbilical tape) around the main pulmonary artery close to the pulmonary valve. This constriction of the main pulmonary artery increases the resistance to filling of the pulmonary vascular bed. As a result, the left-to-right shunt across the ventricular septal defect is decreased, as is the return of blood back to the left ventricle. This procedure has been employed within the past several years on infants with congestive heart failure who are unresponsive to anticongestive measures and are too small to undergo definitive open heart surgery. The results have been quite successful.

2. Repair of the ventricular septal defect by cardiopulmonary bypass—Repair of the ventricular septal defect is indicated in all patients who have a significant left-to-right shunt and are large enough to undergo open heart surgery. (At some centers, successful open heart surgery has been performed even in children under age 1.) Total repair is recommended in children in whom the pulmonary to systemic blood flow ratio is greater than 1.5:1 and in whom the pulmonary vascular resistance is normal or only slightly increased. Correction of the defect is not recommended in children in whom the pulmonary to systemic blood flow ratio is less than 1.5:1. Repair is contraindicated when there is irreversible pulmonary vascular obstruction and when the net shunt is in the right-to-left direction. Patients with large ventricular septal defects and reactive pulmonary hypertension (increased pulmonary vascular resistance which is reversible with the use of pulmonary vasodilators—tolazoline [Priscoline]—and oxygen) should be operated on earlier (age 3−5) than those with normal pulmonary vascular resistance, for whom surgery is recommended at age 5−10.

Mortality varies depending upon the age of the patient, the degree of pulmonary hypertension, and occasionally on the size and location of the septal defect. Accordingly, the operative mortality rate ranges from less than 5% to 25%. The most serious complication of open heart surgery is the development of complete heart block.

Course & Prognosis

A. Small Ventricular Septal Defects: These patients usually do quite well throughout life and may have a normal life span. They are susceptible, however, to subacute bacterial endocarditis.

B. Moderate Left to Right Shunts: These patients usually do well during infancy and childhood. During or following adolescence, they may develop progressively increasing pulmonary hypertension or congestive heart failure. They are also susceptible to subacute bacterial endocarditis.

C. Large Ventricular Septal Defects: These patients do poorly during infancy, have numerous bouts of pneumonitis, and frequently develop congestive heart failure. If they survive the first year, they often improve symptomatically and do relatively well until adolescence. Following this, however, they develop progressively increasing pulmonary vascular obstruction or congestive heart failure. They are somewhat less susceptible to subacute bacterial endocarditis than patients with smaller ventricular septal defects.

Clarkson PM & others: Prognosis for patients with ventricular septal defect with severe pulmonary vascular obstructive disease. Circulation 38:129, 1968.

Hallidie-Smith KA & others: Effects of surgical closure of ventricular septal defects on pulmonary vascular disease. Brit Heart J,31:246. 1969.

Hoffman JI: Natural history of congenital heart disease: Problems in its assessment with special reference to ventricular septal defect. Circulation 37:97, 1968.

Kirklin JW: Pulmonary artery banding in babies with large ventricular septal defects. Circulation 43:321, 1971.

Lillehei CW & others: Pre- and postoperative cardiac catheterization in 200 patients undergoing closure of ventricular septal defect. Surgery 63:69, 1968.

Rao PS, Sissman NJ: Spontaneous closure of physiologically advantageous ventricular septal defects. Circulation 43:83, 1971.

VENTRICULAR SEPTAL DEFECT IN ASSOCIATION WITH OTHER CARDIAC LESIONS

Ventricular septal defect is often associated with other lesions. The reader is referred to textbooks of pediatric cardiology for a detailed review of these conditions. The more important lesions associated with ventricular septal defects are as follows:

Ventricular septal defect and atrial septal defect
Ventricular septal defect with patent ductus arteriosus
Ventricular septal defect with aortic regurgitation
Ventricular septal defect with absent pulmonary valve
Left ventricular-right atrial shunts
Ventricular septal defect and coarctation of the aorta
Single ventricle

Davachi F, Moller JH: The electrocardiogram and vectorcardiogram in single ventricle. Am J Cardiol 23:19, 1969.

Lev M & others: Single (primitive) ventricle. Circulation 39:577, 1969.

Van Praagh R & others: Diagnosis of the anatomic types of single or common ventricle. Am H Cardiol 15:345, 1965.

ENDOCARDIAL CUSHION DEFECTS

Essentials of Diagnosis

Incomplete form (ostium primum atrial septal defect):

● Acyanotic, asymptomatic.
● Pansystolic murmur of mitral regurgitation at apex.

Complete form (persistent common atrioventricular canal):

● High incidence in Down's syndrome.
● Frequent respiratory infection.
● Congestive heart failure common in infancy.
● Biventricular enlargement.
● Murmurs variable; mitral regurgitation common.
● P_2 accentuated.

General Considerations

An endocardial cushion defect is a congenital cardiac abnormality which results from the incomplete fusion of the embryonic endocardial cushions. The endocardial cushions help to form the lower portion of the atrial septum, the membranous portion of the ventricular septum, and the septal leaflets of the tricuspid and mitral valves. These defects are not very common. They account for about 1–2% of all cases of congenital heart disease. The incidence of this abnormality is increased in patients with Down's syndrome.

Endocardial cushion defects may be divided into incomplete and complete forms. The complete form, also known as a persistent common atrioventricular canal, consists of a high ventricular septal defect, a low atrial septal defect of the ostium primum variety which is continuous with the ventricular septal defect, and a cleft in both the septal leaflet of the tricuspid valve and the anterior leaflet of the mitral valve. In the incomplete form, any one of these components may be present. The most common partial form of endocardial cushion defect is the ostium primum type of atrial septal defect with a cleft in the mitral valve.

The complete form (persistent common atrioventricular canal) results in large left-to-right shunts at both the ventricular and atrial levels, tricuspid and mitral regurgitation, and marked pulmonary hypertension, usually with some increase in pulmonary vascular resistance. When the latter is present, the shunts may be bidirectional. The hemodynamics in the incomplete form are dependent upon the lesions present.

Clinical Findings

A. Symptoms and Signs: The clinical picture varies depending upon the severity of the defect. In the incomplete form, these patients may be indistinguishable from patients with the ostium secundum type of atrial septal defect. They are often completely asymptomatic. On the other hand, patients with an atrioventricular canal usually are severely affected. Congestive heart failure often develops in early infancy; recurrent bouts of pneumonitis are common; and cyanosis may develop in later childhood.

In the complete form, the findings on physical examination vary depending upon the degree of pulmonary vascular obstruction. If the pulmonary vascular resistance is relatively normal, the findings are consistent with a large ventricular septal defect and atrioventricular valve regurgitation. There is no cyanosis; pulses are normal; and the heart is significantly enlarged (both right and left). A pronounced systolic thrill may be palpated at the lower left sternal border. The second heart sound is split, with an accentuated pulmonary component. A loud, harsh pansystolic murmur is heard at the lower left sternal border and transmits over the entire precordium. A pronounced diastolic flow murmur is heard at the apex.

When pulmonary vascular obstruction is present, the findings are quite different. Cyanosis is apparent, and there is evidence of marked right ventricular enlargement and very little left ventricular enlarge-

ment. A shock of the second sound can be palpated at the pulmonary area. No thrill is felt. The second sound is markedly accentuated and single. A nonspecific short systolic murmur is heard at the lower left sternal border. No diastolic flow murmurs are heard.

The physical findings in the incomplete form depend upon the lesions. In the most common variety (ostium primum atrial septal defect with mitral regurgitation), the findings are similar to those of the ostium secundum type of atrial septal defect plus mitral regurgitation (pansystolic murmur at the apex radiating out to the left axilla).

B. X-Ray Findings: Cardiac enlargement is present; the degree depends upon the specific anatomic defect. In the complete (canal) form, there is enlargement of all 4 chambers. The pulmonary vascular markings are increased. In patients with pulmonary vascular obstruction, only the main pulmonary artery segment and its branches are prominent. The peripheral markings are usually decreased.

C. Electrocardiography and Vectorcardiography: In all forms of endocardial cushion defect, left axis deviation with a counterclockwise loop in the frontal plane is present. The mean axis varies from approximately −30 to −90 degrees. Since left axis deviation is present in all patients with this defect, the ECG is a very important diagnostic tool. First degree heart block is present in over 50% of cases. Right, left, or combined ventricular hypertrophy is present, depending upon the particular type of defect and the presence or absence of pulmonary vascular obstruction.

D. Cardiac Catheterization and Cineangiocardiography: The results of cardiac catheterization vary depending upon the type of defect present. When the catheterization is performed from the leg, the catheter is easily passed across the atrial septum in its lowest portion and frequently enters directly into the left ventricle. This is a result of the very low atrial septal defect and the cleft in the mitral valve. Cineangiocardiography is quite helpful in determining the presence or absence of atrioventricular valve regurgitation. Injection of contrast material into the left ventricle in the presence of a cleft mitral valve and atrial septal defect usually results in the passage of contrast from the left ventricle almost directly into the right atrium through the cleft and defect. Tricuspid regurgitation is more difficult to evaluate since the catheter must be positioned in the right ventricle across the tricuspid valve. However, severe degree of tricuspid regurgitation could be determined by an injection into the right ventricle.

The presence of an atrial ventricular communication may be determined by measuring oxygen content and saturation and also by cineangiocardiography. In the complete form, severe pulmonary hypertension is the rule.

Treatment

The treatment of endocardial cushion defects consists of surgical correction. In the incomplete form, surgery is associated with relatively low mortality rate (5–15%). The complete form is associated with a high mortality rate (about 25–50%).

Pulmonary artery banding procedures can be employed in infants with huge left-to-right shunts and congestive heart failure unresponsive to anticongestive measures. The results are not so good as with simple uncomplicated ventricular septal defect.

A frequent complication of correction of an endocardial cushion defect is the development of postoperative complete heart block.

Course & Prognosis

Patients with the complete form of endocardial cushion defect may develop congestive heart failure in early infancy and frequently die in early life. If they survive, pulmonary vascular obstructions develop rapidly. Progressively increasing cyanosis develops.

For a varying period during the development of progressive pulmonary vascular obstruction, the patient seems to improve. After a number of years, however, the course proceeds downhill with marked cyanosis, right ventricular heart failure, pulmonary vascular obstruction, and death. Patients with a partial form may do quite well for long periods.

Patients with the ostium primum atrial septal defect with mitral regurgitation do not do as well as those with the simple type of secundum atrial septal defect, but they can live a relatively normal life into the third or fourth decade.

Lillehei CW & others: Persistent common A–V canal: Recatheterization results in 37 patients following intracardiac repair. J Thoracic Cardiovas Surg 57:83, 1969.

McGoon DC, DuShane JW, Kirklin JW: The surgical treatment of endocardial cushion defects. Surgery 46:185, 1959.

Neufeld HN & others: Isolated ventricular septal defect of the persistent common atrioventricular canal type. Circulation 23:685, 1961.

Rastelli GC & others: Surgical repair of complete form of persistent common atrioventricular canal. J Thoracic Cardiovas Surg 55:299, 1968.

Shah CV, Patel MF, Hastreiter AR: Hemodynamics of complete atrioventricular canal and its evolution with age. Am J Cardiol 29:326, 1969.

PATENT DUCTUS ARTERIOSUS

Essentials of Diagnosis

Typical (left-to-right shunt; normal pulmonary arterial pressure):

- Asymptomatic.
- Continuous machinery murmur, maximal at the pulmonic area.
- Bounding peripheral pulses.
- Widened pulse pressure.

Atypical (large left-to-right shunt; pulmonary hypertension):

- Frequent respiratory infections.
- Congestive heart failure in infancy.

- Murmur variable; rarely continuous in infancy.
- Bounding peripheral pulses.
- Widened pulse pressure.

General Considerations

Patent ductus arteriosus is the persistence in extrauterine life of the normal fetal vessel which joins the pulmonary artery to the aorta. It is a common abnormality, accounting for about 10% of all cases of congenital heart disease. It is very common in children born to mothers who had rubella during the first trimester of pregnancy. There is a higher incidence of patent ductus arteriosus in infants born at high altitudes (over 10,000 feet). It is twice as common in females than in males.

The defect can vary in size from a few mm to over 1 cm in diameter. It joins the main pulmonary artery with the aorta distal to the origin of the left subclavian artery. It usually occurs as an isolated abnormality, but associated lesions are not infrequent (eg, coarctation of the aorta and ventricular septal defect).

In approximately 90% of cases, pulmonary vascular resistance is normal. This results in a left-to-right shunt from the aorta to the pulmonary artery. The size of the left-to-right shunt is related to the pulmonary vascular resistance and the size (diameter) of the ductus itself. In approximately 10% of cases, pulmonary hypertension is present. In such cases, the direction and the degree of shunt is dependent upon the relationship between the pulmonary vascular resistance and the systemic vascular resistance. If the former is greater, the shunt will be predominantly in the right-to-left (pulmonary artery to aorta) direction.

In the neonatal period and during early infancy, the left-to-right shunt in the usual case is relatively small because the pulmonary vascular resistance of the infant is greater than that of the older child and adult. However, within a few months after birth, pulmonary vascular resistance drops to normal and left-to-right shunt progressively increases.

Clinical Findings

A. Symptoms and Signs: Patients with the simple uncomplicated type of patent ductus arteriosus (normal pulmonary arterial pressure) usually have no cardiovascular symptoms throughout infancy, childhood, and adolescence. They are frequently small and thin, but this is probably an associated rather than a related condition. They may have dyspnea on exertion and exercise intolerance when the left-to-right shunt is large. Frequent respiratory infections, including bouts of pneumonitis, may occur.

Patients with pulmonary hypertension are usually quite symptomatic from early infancy. They are usually small, underdeveloped, and poorly nourished and have frequent episodes of pneumonitis. Congestive heart failure is common.

1. Typical patent ductus arteriosus—The pulses are bounding, and pulse pressure is widened (pulse pressure is greater than ½ of the systolic pressure). The first heart sound is normal. The second heart sound is usually narrowly split and very rarely (when the shunt is maximal) paradoxically split. (The second sound closes on inspiration and splits on expiration.) The paradoxic splitting is due to the maximal overload of the left ventricle and the prolonged ejection of blood from this chamber.

The murmur is quite characteristic. It is a very rough "machinery" murmur which is maximal at the second intercostal space at the left sternal border and under the left clavicle. It begins shortly after the first heart sound, rises to a peak at the second heart sound, and passes through the second heart sound into diastole, where it becomes a decrescendo murmur and fades and disappears before the first heart sound. The murmur tends to radiate fairly well over the lung fields anteriorly but relatively poorly over the lung fields posteriorly. A diastolic flow murmur is often heard at the apex. Children under age 1 may have only a systolic murmur.

2. Atypical patent ductus arteriosus (pulmonary hypertension)—The physical findings depend upon the cause of the pulmonary hypertension. If pulmonary hypertension is due primarily to a marked increase in blood flow and only a slight increase in pulmonary vascular resistance, the physical findings are similar to those listed above. The significant difference is the presence of an accentuated pulmonary component of S_2. Bounding pulses and a loud continuous heart murmur are present. In patients with pulmonary hypertension secondary to increased pulmonary vascular resistance and predominant right to left shunt, the findings are quite different. There is usually evidence of generalized cyanosis. Differential cyanosis— involving the left arm and feet but not the head or the right arm—is often present. The second heart sound is single and quite accentuated, and there is no significant heart murmur. The pulses are normal.

B. X-Ray Findings: In simple patent ductus arteriosus, the x-ray appearance depends upon the size of the shunt. If the shunt is relatively small or moderate in size, the heart is not enlarged. If the shunt is large, there is evidence of both left atrial and left ventricular enlargement. In both cases, the aorta is prominent, as is the main pulmonary artery segment also. Occasionally, the shadow of the ductus itself can be seen between the shadow of the descending thoracic aorta and the main pulmonary artery segment. The degree of pulmonary vascular engorgement is dependent upon the degree of left-to-right shunt. In patients with pulmonary hypertension due to increased blood flow and only a mild increase in pulmonary vascular resistance, the findings are similar. The pulmonary artery segment is even more dilated. In those with pulmonary vascular obstruction, the heart is usually small. The main pulmonary artery and its branches are quite prominent, and the distal pulmonary branches are small.

C. Electrocardiography: In simple patent ductus arteriosus, the ECG may be normal or may show a moderate degree of left ventricular hypertrophy. One significant feature which is commonly present is the finding of deep Q waves in the left precordial leads. In patients with pulmonary hypertension due to increased blood flow, there is usually biventricular hypertrophy. In those with pulmonary vascular obstruction, there is pure right ventricular hypertrophy.

D. Catheterization and Angiocardiography: In simple patent ductus arteriosus, there is little justification for cardiac catheterization. If catheterization is performed, there is evidence of increased oxygen content or saturation at the level of the pulmonary artery. Hydrogen electrode curves are positive in the pulmonary artery and negative in the right ventricle. The catheter can often be passed through the ductus from the pulmonary artery into the descending thoracic aorta.

Arteriograms taken following injection of contrast material into the aortic arch show a shunt at the level of the ductus.

Patients with patent ductus arteriosus and pulmonary hypertension due to large left-to-right shunts show a marked increase in oxygen saturation at the pulmonary artery level and normal systemic arterial saturation. Those with marked pulmonary vascular obstruction show no increase in oxygen content at the pulmonary artery and a decrease in systemic arterial saturation. In both cases, a catheter may be passed through the ductus into the descending thoracic aorta.

Treatment

Treatment consists of surgical correction except in patients with pulmonary vascular obstruction. Patients with large left-to-right shunts and pulmonary hypertension should be operated on very early (even under the age of 1 year) to prevent the development of progressive pulmonary vascular obstruction. The optimal age for correction of simple patent ductus arteriosus is between ages 1–5, although the operation may be delayed until a later age without increased mortality.

Patients with irreversible pulmonary vascular obstruction, where the net left-to-right shunt is less than 1.5:1, should not be operated upon. These patients are made worse by closure of the ductus, since the ductus serves as an escape route and limits the degree of pulmonary hypertension.

Course & Prognosis

Patients with simple patent ductus arteriosus and small to moderate shunts usually do quite well. However, in the third or fourth decade of life, symptoms of easy fatigability, dyspnea on exertion, and exercise intolerance appear, usually as a consequence of the development of pulmonary hypertension or congestive heart failure.

Spontaneous closure of a patent ductus arteriosus may occur within the first year of life. This is especially true in infants who were born prematurely. After age 1, spontaneous closure is extremely rare.

Patients with pulmonary hypertension do much less well. Poor growth and development, frequent episodes of pneumonitis, and the development of congestive heart failure are not uncommon in patients with large left-to-right shunts. If these patients do not succumb to congestive heart failure in early infancy, they frequently go on to develop pulmonary vascular obstruction in later childhood or adolescence. Life expectancy is markedly reduced, and these patients often die in their second or third decade. Patients with pulmonary vascular obstruction from very early infancy are actually less symptomatic than those with pulmonary hypertension without obstruction. Their life expectancy is similar to that of patients with large left-to-right shunts (untreated), but the course of their disease throughout life is more uniform. The major symptoms are progressively increasing cyanosis and decreasing exercise tolerance.

Subacute bacterial endocarditis can occur in both varieties.

Campbell M: Natural history of persistent ductus arteriosus. Brit Heart J 30:4, 1968.

Jarmakani MN & others: Effect of site of shunt on left heart volume characteristics in children with ventricular septal defects and patent ductus arteriosus. Circulation 40:411, 1969.

Krovetz LJ, Warden HE: Patent ductus arteriosus: An analysis of 515 surgically proved cases. Dis Chest 42:46, 1962.

Meisner H & others: Surgical correction of aorto-pulmonary septal defects: Review of the literature and report of eight cases. Dis Chest 53:750, 1968.

Rowe RD & others: Cardiovascular disease in the rubella syndrome. In: *The Heart and Circulation in the Newborn and Infant.* Cassels DE (editor). Grune & Stratton, 1966.

Rudolph AM & others: Patent ductus arteriosus: A clinical and hemodynamic study of 23 patients in the first year of life. Pediatrics 22:892, 1958.

MALFORMATIONS ASSOCIATED WITH OBSTRUCTION TO BLOOD FLOW ON THE RIGHT SIDE OF THE HEART

1. VALVULAR PULMONARY STENOSIS WITH INTACT VENTRICULAR SEPTUM

Essentials of Diagnosis

- No symptoms with mild and moderately severe cases.
- Cyanosis and a high incidence of right-sided congestive heart failure in very severe cases.
- Right ventricular lift; intermittent systolic ejection click at the pulmonic area in mild to moderately severe cases.
- No ejection click in severe cases.
- S_2 widely split with soft to inaudible P_2; grade I–VI/VI obstructive systolic murmur, maximal at the pulmonic area.

General Considerations

Obstruction of right ventricular outflow at the pulmonary valve level accounts for about 10% of all cases of congenital heart disease. In the usual case, the cusps of the pulmonary valve are fused to form a membrane or diaphragm with a hole in the middle which varies from 2 mm to 1 cm in diameter. Occasionally, there may be fusion of only 2 cusps, producing a bicuspid pulmonic valve. Very frequently, especially in the more severe cases, there is secondary infundibular stenosis. The pulmonary valve ring is usually small. There is usually moderate to marked poststenotic dilatation of the main pulmonary artery and the left pulmonary artery. There is usually an inverse relationship between the severity of the obstruction and the degree of poststenotic dilation. Patent foramen ovale is fairly common.

Obstruction to blood flow across the pulmonary valve results in an increase in pressure developed by the right ventricle to maintain an adequate output across that valve. Pressures greater than systemic are not unusual, and occasionally may range up to 200 mm Hg. As a consequence of the increased work required of the right ventricle, severe right ventricular hypertrophy and eventual right ventricular failure can occur. This is in contrast to patients with right ventricular outflow obstruction and a large ventricular septal defect (ie, tetralogy of Fallot), in whom—because of the communication between the ventricles—the maximal pressure that the right ventricle may develop is limited (equal to systemic pressure) and heart failure is extremely uncommon.

When the obstruction is severe and the ventricular septum is intact, a right-to-left shunt will often occur at the atrial level through a patent foramen ovale. Accordingly, patients with this condition may have a varying degree of cyanosis. The presence of cyanosis indicates a relatively severe degree of valvular obstruction.

Clinical Findings

A. Symptoms and Signs: The history depends upon the severity of the obstruction. Patients with a mild or even a moderate degree of valvular pulmonary stenosis are completely asymptomatic throughout infancy, childhood, and adolescence. Patients with a more severe type of valve obstruction may develop cyanosis and congestive heart failure very early—even in the neonatal period. In patients with moderately severe but not critical pulmonary stenosis, there may be progressively increasing cyanosis, easy fatigability, and dyspnea on exertion. Cyanotic spells characterized by a sudden onset of marked increase in cyanosis and dyspnea are much less uncommon than in tetralogy of Fallot. Squatting is very uncommon.

Patients with mild to moderate obstruction are acyanotic. Patients with severe or critical stenosis usually show evidence of central cyanosis. These patients are usually well developed and well nourished. They often have a round (moon) face, with high cheek bones and widely spaced eyes. The pulses are normal and equal throughout. Clubbing may occur in severe cases in which cyanosis has persisted for a long time. On examination of the heart, there may be prominence of the precordium. A heaving impulse of the right ventricle can frequently be palpated. A systolic thrill is often palpated in the pulmonic area and frequently in the suprasternal notch. The first heart sound is normal. In patients with mild to moderate stenosis, a prominent pulmonic type of ejection click is heard best at the second left intercostal space. This click varies with respiration. It is much more prominent during expiration than inspiration. In patients with severe stenosis, the click tends to merge with the first heart sound, so that the first heart sound is high-pitched and clicking in quality, but no definite separation between the first sound and the click is heard. The second heart sound also varies with the degree of stenosis. In mild valvular stenosis, the second heart sound is normally split and the pulmonary component is normal in intensity. In moderate degrees of obstruction, the second heart sound is more widely split and the pulmonary component is softer. In severe pulmonary stenosis, the second heart sound is single since the pulmonary component cannot be heard. (On phonocardiography, the pulmonary component of the second heart sound is widely separated from the first heart sound and does not move with respiration.) An ejection type, rough, obstructive systolic murmur is best heard at the second interspace at the left sternal border. It radiates very well over the lung fields anteriorly and over the upper lung fields posteriorly. No diastolic murmurs are audible. In older children, a prominent "A" wave is seen in the jugular venous pulse. If there is congestive heart failure, the liver is enlarged.

B. Electrocardiography: The ECG is usually normal in patients with mild obstruction. Right ventricular hypertrophy is present in patients with moderate to severe valvular obstruction. In cases of severe obstruction, right ventricular hypertrophy and the right ventricular strain pattern (deep inversion of the T wave) is seen in the right precordial leads. In the most severe form, right atrial hypertrophy is also present. Right axis deviation is also seen in the moderate to severe forms. Occasionally the axis is greater than +180 degrees.

C. X-Ray Findings: In the mild form of pulmonary stenosis, the heart may be normal in size. Poststenotic dilatation of the main pulmonary artery segment and the left pulmonary artery is often present. In moderate to severe cases, there may be a slight right ventricular enlargement and there may or may not be poststenotic dilatation of the main pulmonary artery. In patients who are cyanotic, the pulmonary vascular markings are decreased; otherwise they are normal.

D. Cardiac Catheterization and Cineangiocardiography: There is no increase in oxygen saturation or oxygen content in the right side of the heart. In the more severe cases, there is a right-to-left shunt at the atrial level. The pulmonary artery pressure is normal in the milder cases. It is quite low in moderate to severe cases. Right ventricular pressure is always higher than the pulmonary artery pressure. The gradient across the

pulmonary valve varies from 10–200 mm Hg. In severe cases, the right atrial pressure is often elevated, with a predominant "A" wave. Cineangiocardiography with injection of contrast material into the right ventricle shows thickening of the pulmonary valve and the very narrow opening of the pulmonary valve. This produces a "jet" of contrast from the right ventricle into the pulmonary artery. Infundibular hypertrophy may be present. This is seen as a narrowing of the right ventricular outflow track during ventricular systole followed by a widening of this area.

Treatment

Surgery is recommended for all children in whom the right ventricular pressure is greater than 100 mm Hg. In patients with severe obstruction, surgery is usually recommended in early life. Those with cyanosis and congestive heart failure should be operated upon as soon as feasible. Patients who are only mildly or moderately symptomatic should undergo pulmonary valvotomy utilizing cardiopulmonary bypass when they are larger (usually greater than 25 lb). The operative mortality depends upon the age and condition of the patient. It varies from 1–10%.

Course & Prognosis

Patients with mild pulmonary stenosis live a normal life and have a normal life span. Those with stenosis of moderate severity usually show symptoms of easy fatigability and dyspnea on exertion which may be progressive. Those with severe valvular obstruction may develop severe cyanosis and congestive heart failure in early life.

Bassingthwaighte JB & others: The electrocardiographic and hemodynamic findings in pulmonary stenosis with intact ventricular septum. Circulation 28:893, 1963.

Danielson GK & others: Pulmonic stenosis with intact ventricular septum: Surgical considerations and results of operation. J Thoracic Cardiovas Surg 61:228, 1971.

Hultgren HN & others: The ejection click of valvular pulmonary stenosis. Circulation 40:631, 1969.

Koretzky ED & others: Congenital pulmonary stenosis resulting from dysplasia of the valve. Circulation 40:43, 1969.

Leatham A, Weitzman D: Auscultatory and phonographic signs of pulmonary stenosis. Brit Heart J 19:303, 1957.

Mustard WT, Jain S, Trusler GA: Pulmonary stenosis in first year of life. Brit Heart J 30:255, 1968.

2. INFUNDIBULAR PULMONARY STENOSIS WITHOUT VENTRICULAR SEPTAL DEFECT

Pure infundibular pulmonary stenosis is rare. One should suspect infundibular pulmonary stenosis where there is evidence of mild to moderate pulmonary stenosis and intact ventricular septum and (1) no pulmonic ejection click is audible and (2) the murmur is maximal in the third and fourth intercostal space rather than in the second intercostal space. Otherwise, the clinical picture may be identical.

3. DISTAL PULMONARY STENOSIS

Supravalvular Pulmonary Stenosis

This is a relatively rare condition due to coarctation of the body of the main pulmonary artery or of the bifurcation of the main pulmonary artery. The clinical picture may be identical with that of valvular pulmonary stenosis, although the murmur is maximal in the first intercostal space at the left sternal border and in the suprasternal notch. No ejection click is audible. A second heart sound is usually narrowly split, and the pulmonary component is quite loud as a result of closure of the pulmonary valve under high pressure. The murmur radiates extremely well into the neck and over the lung fields.

Supravalvular pulmonary stenosis is a frequent finding in children whose mothers had rubella in the first trimester of pregnancy. The frequent combination of patent ductus arteriosus and supravalvular pulmonary stenosis should make one suspicious of this condition.

Peripheral Pulmonary Stenosis

In this condition there are multiple small coarctations of the branches of the pulmonary artery in the periphery of the lung. They may be unilateral or bilateral. A systolic murmur may be heard over both lung fields both anteriorly and posteriorly. The diagnosis may be established by means of cardiac catheterization, which demonstrates a pressure gradient across the stenotic areas, and by cineangiocardiography.

Absence of a Pulmonary Artery

This condition may exist as an isolated malformation or in association with other congenital heart disease. It is occasionally seen in patients with tetralogy of Fallot.

Coelho E & others: Malformations of the pulmonary artery and its branches, including 2 cases of absence of the right pulmonary artery: Angiographic and hemodynamic study. Am J Cardiol 13:462, 1964.

Delaney T, Nadas AS: Peripheral pulmonary stenosis. Am J Cardiol 13:451, 1964.

Gay BB & others: The roentgenologic features of single and multiple coarctations of the pulmonary artery and branches. Am J Roentgenol 90:599, 1963.

Ross JC & others: Congenital pulmonary artery branch stenosis. Am J Cardiol 24:318, 1969.

Rowe RD: Maternal rubella and pulmonary artery stenosis: Report of 11 cases. Pediatrics 32:180, 1963.

MALFORMATIONS ASSOCIATED WITH OBSTRUCTION TO BLOOD FLOW ON THE LEFT SIDE OF THE HEART

1. COARCTATION OF THE AORTA

Essentials of Diagnosis

Postductal variety:

- No symptoms in most cases.
- Congestive heart failure in infancy in the most severe cases.
- Weak to absent femoral pulses with brachial artery-femoral artery lag.
- Systolic murmur in interscapular area of back.

Preductal variety:

- Cyanosis, occasionally differential cyanosis (head pink, feet blue).
- Congestive heart failure in infancy.
- Weak femoral pulses with right brachial artery-femoral artery lag.
- Nonspecific murmur.

General Considerations

Coarctation is a common cardiac abnormality, accounting for about 5–8% of all cases of congenital heart disease. It is 2–4 times more common in males than in females. In the vast majority of cases, coarctation occurs in the thoracic portion of the descending aorta. The abdominal aorta is very rarely involved. From a pathologic point of view, thoracic coarctations may be divided into the postductal variety, "adult type" (coarctation distal to the entrance of the ligamentum arteriosum), and the preductal variety, "infantile type" (either a long segment of hypoplasia or narrowing of the aorta proximal to the entrance of the ductus arteriosus). Associated congenital cardiac malformations are not uncommon in both types. In the postductal variety, these include patent ductus arteriosus, ventricular septal defect, mitral insufficiency, bicuspid aortic valve (about 40% of cases), and valvular aortic stenosis (about 5% of cases). In the preductal variety, complex intracardiac malformations are usually present.

The presence of a coarctation presents a problem in maintenance of adequate blood flow and pressure to the area of the body distal to the defect. To maintain sufficient flow and pressure, adaptive mechanisms are called into play. These include elevation of the pressure proximal to the coarctation, constriction of the arteriolar bed distal to the coarctation (resulting in an elevation of diastolic pressure), and opening of collateral channels bypassing the area of constriction.

In the preductal type of coarctation, the right arm and the head are supplied by blood derived from the left ventricle. The lower portion of the body distal to the coarctation is supplied by blood from the right ventricle via a patent ductus arteriosus. Accordingly, the blood supplied to the lower portion of the body is desaturated in comparison to the right arm and head. To maintain adequate pressure and flow to the descending aorta, there is persistence of the high pulmonary vascular resistance and pulmonary arterial pressure that is present from birth.

In the postductal type, the blood supplied to the lower extremities as well as the blood supplied to the upper part of the body is derived from the left ventricle. In this case, the pulmonary arteriolar bed resolves in a normal fashion and the pulmonary arterial pressure is normal.

Clinical Findings

A. Postductal Coarctation:

1. Symptoms and signs—Most patients with postductal coarctation have no cardiovascular symptoms throughout infancy, childhood, and adolescence. Symptoms of decreased exercise tolerance and fatigability may appear in early adulthood. The diagnosis is often not made until later childhood or adolescence. In a few cases, however, congestive heart failure develops in early infancy.

In the classical case (asymptomatic older children), there is evidence of better development of the upper than the lower portion of the body. The shoulders are broad, and the mass of muscle in the upper extremities is greater than in the lower extremities. The blood pressure in the upper extremities may be normal or elevated. The blood pressure is frequently normal up to puberty and then increases. The pulses in the upper extremities are strong and usually equal bilaterally. The left subclavian artery is occasionally involved in the coarctation, in which case the left brachial pulse is weak. The pulses in the lower extremities are weak to absent. If femoral pulses are palpable, they are felt later than the brachial pulses (brachial-femoral lag). A visible pulsation is seen in the suprasternal notch. If the coarctation is uncomplicated, the heart sounds are normal. The aortic component of the second heart sound is occasionally increased in intensity. An ejection systolic murmur of grade II/VI intensity is often heard at the aortic area and the lower left sternal border. The pathognomonic murmur of coarctation is heard in the interscapular area of the back, over the area of the coarctation. This murmur is usually systolic in timing. If the coarctation is very severe, the murmur may become continuous. If the coarctation is complicated by other malformations, murmurs associated with these other abnormalities will be audible.

Infants in congestive heart failure will demonstrate the usual findings characteristic of heart failure in infancy and absent femoral pulses. These patients usually have weak pulses in the upper extremities secondary to the congestive heart failure. However, the presence of pulses in the upper extremities and absent pulses in the lower extremities strongly suggests the diagnosis of coarctation of the aorta.

2. X-ray findings—In the older child, the heart may be normal in size, although there is usually some evidence of left ventricular enlargement. The ascending aorta is usually normal in size. On barium swallow, the esophagus has a characteristic **E** shape. The first arc of the **E** is due to dilatation of the aorta just proximal to the coarctation. The second arc is due to poststenotic dilatation of the aorta. The middle line of the **E** is due to the coarctation itself. In older children (usually over age 8), notching or scalloping of the ribs caused by marked enlargement of the intercostal collaterals can be seen.

In infants in congestive heart failure, there is evidence of marked cardiac enlargement and pulmonary venous congestion.

3. Electrocardiography—ECGs may be normal or may show evidence of slight left ventricular hypertrophy. In infants with congestive heart failure, the ECG usually demonstrates right ventricular hypertrophy. According to one group of investigators, pure right ventricular hypertrophy is never present in patients with uncomplicated coarctation after the age of 6 months. Therefore, the presence of right ventricular hypertrophy at this age suggests the presence of associated congenital abnormalities.

4. Cardiac catheterization and cineangiocardiography—In the older patient with uncomplicated coarctation, cardiac catheterization and angiocardiography are unnecessary. If the findings are not classical, however, one might suspect an abdominal coarctation (absent murmur in the interscapular area, absence of the **E** sign on x-rays, and palpable pulsation of the abdominal aorta) and an angiocardiogram should be performed.

In infants with congestive heart failure, cardiac catheterization reveals evidence of pulmonary hypertension and elevation of the pulmonary arterial wedge pressure. The ascending aortic pressure may be normal or elevated; the descending aortic pressure distal to the coarctation is low. There may be arterial unsaturation secondary to the congestive heart failure. This is due to imperfect unsaturation of the pulmonary venous blood and not to a right-to-left intracardiac shunt. The ductus arteriosus is often patent, as shown by an increase in oxygen saturation, a positive hydrogen curve at the pulmonary artery level, and passage of the catheter through the ductus.

B. Preductal Coarctation:

1. Symptoms and signs—Infants with preductal coarctation usually develop left-sided and right-sided heart failure in early infancy, frequently within the first week of life. These children develop generalized cyanosis or, occasionally, differential cyanosis. The total body cyanosis is secondary to congestive heart failure. These patients have a history of very poor feeding from birth, tachypnea and dyspnea, and congestive heart failure. The pulses in the upper extremities are weak but present; the pulses in the lower extremities are absent. If congestive heart failure does not occur, the findings include differential pulses and blood pressures and differential cyanosis.

2. X-ray findings—In preductal coarctation, the heart is enlarged and there is evidence of pulmonary venous congestion. The findings may vary depending upon the intracardiac abnormalities that are usually present.

3. Electrocardiography—There is evidence of severe right ventricular hypertrophy and occasionally a right ventricular strain pattern. The voltage due to left ventricular forces is usually small (hypoplastic left ventricle).

4. Cardiac catheterization and cineangiocardiography—The arterial oxygen saturation in the descending thoracic aorta (or femoral artery) is less than that of the right brachial artery or ascending aorta. There is no increase in oxygen saturation in the right heart. Right ventricular pressure is elevated and equal to the descending aortic pressure. The left ventricular pressure and ascending aortic pressure are usually higher than right ventricular pressure. A pressure gradient may be demonstrated across the coarcted segment. Pulmonary vascular resistance is significantly elevated. The catheter can be passed easily through the ductus from the right ventricle into the descending aorta. Cineangiocardiography following injection of contrast material into the right ventricle or pulmonary artery reveals filling of the descending aorta through the ductus arteriosus.

Treatment

A. Postductal Coarctation: All patients with coarctation of the aorta should undergo surgical correction. The optimal age is 8–15 years. Early operation should be considered when there is significant hypertension, severe symptoms such as easy fatigability and headache, or significant cardiac enlargement. The surgical mortality rate in asymptomatic children is less than 5%.

Infants with postductal coarctation and congestive heart failure should first be treated medically. Vigorous anticongestive measures, including digitalis, diuretics, morphine, and oxygen, often result in dramatic improvement. If they can be maintained without further deterioration, surgery should be deferred until the optimal age. If the response is not adequate within 1–2 days, surgical correction is recommended without further delay. The results, even in this age group, are good.

B. Preductal Coarctation: Congestive heart failure, if present, should be treated vigorously with anticongestive measures. If there is no response, early surgery is recommended. The mortality rate is extremely high because of the young age of the infant and because of the association of this condition with other abnormalities.

Course & Prognosis

A. Postductal Coarctation: Children who survive the neonatal period without developing congestive heart failure do quite well throughout childhood and adolescence. Significant hypertension rarely develops until adolescence. Fatal complications (eg, hypertensive encephalopathy, intracranial bleeding) occur very rarely. Subacute bacterial endocarditis is also rare before adolescence.

Starting in the third decade of life, the patient may develop the onset of easy fatigability, dyspnea on exertion, cardiac enlargement, and left ventricular failure. Only ¼ of these patients may be expected to live through the fourth decade. Death results from subacute bacterial endocarditis or hypertensive cardiovascular disease.

Infants with postductal coarctations who develop congestive heart failure in early infancy usually succumb unless vigorously treated. If they survive this period, they may do very well without surgery and can be operated on at a more optimal age when the surgical risk is less.

B. Preductal Coarctation: The great majority of these infants die within the first 1–2 months of life. Occasionally, however, patients with this defect (if they have no intracardiac abnormality) live even up to the third decade.

Campbell M: Natural history of coarctation of the aorta. Brit Heart J 32:633, 1970.

Sinha SN & others: Coarctation of the aorta in infancy. Circulation 40:385, 1969.

Tawes R & others: Coarctation of the aorta in infants and children: A review of 333 operative cases including 179 infants. Circulation 39(Suppl 1):173, 1969.

Verska JJ & others: Coarctation of the aorta: Abdominal pain syndrome and paradoxical hypertension. J Thoracic Cardiovas Surg 58:746, 1969.

Waterston DJ, Aberdeen E: Preductal coarctation of the aorta. In: *The Heart and Circulation in the Newborn and Infant.* Cassels DE (editor). Grune & Stratton, 1966.

Wielenga G, Dankmeijer J: Coarctation of the aorta. J Path Bact 95:265, 1968.

2. AORTIC STENOSIS

Essentials of Diagnosis

- Usually asymptomatic.
- Occasionally, easy fatigability.
- Congestive heart failure in infancy in most severe cases.
- Left ventricular lift.
- Thrill and murmur along left sternal border.

General Considerations

Aortic stenosis may be defined from the anatomic or physiologic point of view. Anatomically, this indicates an obstruction to the outflow from the left ventricle at or near the aortic valve. Physiologically, aortic stenosis may be defined as a condition in which a systolic pressure gradient of more than 10 mm Hg exists between the left ventricle and the aorta.

Aortic stenosis accounts for approximately 5% of all cases of congenital heart disease.

Anatomically, congenital aortic stenosis may be divided into 4 types:

(1) Valvular aortic stenosis (75%): There is usually a bicuspid aortic valve, with fusion of the right and left coronary cusps. Partial fusion of the commissures of the bicuspid valve results in a smaller than normal orifice during ventricular systole.

(2) Discrete membranous subvalvular aortic stenosis (20%): This consists of a membranous or fibrous ring 5–10 mm below the aortic valve. This membranous ring forms a diaphragm with a hole in the middle and results in obstruction to left ventricular outflow. The aortic valve itself and the anterior leaflet of the mitral valve are often deformed.

(3) Supravalvular aortic stenosis: In this variety there is a constriction of the ascending aorta just above the coronary arteries. This condition is often associated with a family history, abnormal facies, and mental retardation. It is thought to be related to the syndrome of idiopathic hypercalcemia of infancy.

(4) Hypertrophic subaortic stenosis: In this case there is a marked hypertrophy of the entire left ventricle and, predominantly, the ventricular septum. With contraction of the ventricle, the hypertrophic portion of the septum causes a constriction of the left ventricular outflow tract and marked obstruction occurs during mid and late systole. A family history is often present.

Obstruction to outflow from the left ventricle causes the left ventricle to work harder to maintain an adequate pressure and flow in the systemic arterial circuit, resulting in hypertrophy of the left ventricle and increased oxygen requirement. If the stenosis is severe, the oxygen requirements may exceed the capacity of the coronary arteries to supply oxygen, and relative coronary insufficiency may develop. In patients with critical aortic stenosis, left ventricular failure may occur. The left ventricle is usually able to adapt to the increased pressure load for a considerable period of time before developing heart failure or coronary insufficiency.

Clinical Findings

A. Symptoms and Signs: Most patients with aortic stenosis have no cardiovascular symptoms. Except in the most severe cases, the patient may do well up until the third to fifth decade of life, although some patients have mild exercise intolerance and easy fatigability. A small percentage of patients have significant symptoms within the first decade, ie, dizziness and syncope. Sudden death, although uncommon, has occurred in a number of patients with severe or critical stenosis. Congestive heart failure may develop in infancy in the most severe cases.

The physical findings vary somewhat depending upon the anatomic type of lesion:

1. Valvular aortic stenosis—These patients are well developed and well nourished. The pulses are usually normal and equal throughout. If the stenosis is severe and there is a gradient of greater than 100 mm Hg, the pulses are small with a slow upstroke. Examination of the heart reveals a left ventricular thrust at the apex. A systolic thrill is often palpable at the right sternal border in the first and second intercostal spaces. In almost all instances, a thrill can be palpated in the suprasternal notch and along the carotid arteries.

The first heart sound is normal. A prominent aortic type ejection click or ejection sound is best heard at the apex. Very frequently, this click can be heard at the lower left sternal border and at the aortic area. It is separated from the first heart sound by a short but appreciable interval. It does not vary with respiration. The second heart sound at the pulmonary area is physiologically split. The aortic component of the second heart sound is of good intensity. There is a grade III–V/VI, rough, medium- to high-pitched ejection type systolic murmur, maximal at the first and second intercostal spaces, which radiates well into the suprasternal notch and along the carotids. The murmur also radiates fairly well down the lower left sternal border and can be heard at the apex. The murmur transmits to the back but not as well as to the neck. In about 25% of cases, a short early decrescendo diastolic murmur secondary to aortic insufficiency may be heard at the left sternal border in the third intercostal space.

2. Discrete membranous subvalvular aortic stenosis—The findings are essentially the same as those of valvular aortic stenosis. Absence of an aortic ejection click is an important differentiating point, and the thrill and murmur are usually somewhat more intense at the left sternal border in the third and fourth intercostal spaces than at the aortic area. Frequently, however, the murmur is equally intense at both areas. A diastolic murmur of aortic insufficiency is commonly heard after 5 years of age.

3. Supravalvular aortic stenosis—These patients often have abnormal facies and are mentally retarded. The thrill and murmur are characteristically best heard in the suprasternal notch and along the carotids, although they are well transmitted over the aortic area and near the mid left sternal border.

4. Hypertrophic subaortic stenosis—The murmur in this case is heard best at the apex. It is usually mid to late systolic in timing and is grade II–III/VI in intensity. There is often an atrial fourth heart sound and a diastolic murmur. No ejection click is audible. The arterial wave pulse has a rapid upstroke and frequently a bisferiens quality.

B. X-Ray Findings: In most cases, the heart is not enlarged. The left ventricle, however, is slightly prominent. In valvular and discrete subvalvular aortic stenosis, dilatation of the ascending aorta is frequently seen, more commonly in the former. The ascending aorta is usually normal in hypertrophic subaortic stenosis and hypoplastic in supravalvular aortic stenosis.

C. Electrocardiography: There is some correlation between the severity of the obstruction and the ECG. Patients with mild aortic stenosis have normal ECGs. Patients with severe obstruction usually demonstrate evidence of left ventricular hypertrophy and left ventricular strain. However, in about 25% of severe cases the ECG is normal. Progressive increase in left ventricular hypertrophy on serial ECGs indicates a significant degree of obstruction.

D. Cardiac Catheterization and Cineangiocardiography: Left heart catheterization demonstrates the pressure differential between the left ventricle and the aorta and the level at which the gradient exists. From a hemodynamic viewpoint, severe aortic stenosis may be defined as a situation in which there is a peak systolic gradient of more than 65 mm Hg. Since the indications for surgery depend upon the results of cardiac catheterization, the indications for cardiac catheterization include the following: (1) Symptoms such as dizziness or syncope. (2) ECG (or VCG) evidence of significant left ventricular hypertrophy and strain.

Cineangiocardiography is also quite helpful in demonstrating the level of the obstruction.

Treatment

Surgical correction of the obstruction is indicated in all cases of uncomplicated severe aortic stenosis. Operation should be performed under cardiopulmonary bypass. The optimal age ranges from 5 years to adolescence. If syncopal episodes occur, early operation is indicated.

If cardiac catheterization studies reveal only a moderate aortic stenosis (not severe enough to warrant surgery), these patients should refrain from participation in competitive athletics.

Beuren AJ & others: The syndrome of supravalvular aortic stenosis, peripheral pulmonary stenosis, mental retardation and similar facial appearance. Am J Cardiol 13:471, 1964.

Braunwald E & others: Idiopathic hypertrophic subaortic stenosis. I. A description of the disease based upon an analysis of 64 patients. Circulation 30, Suppl 4, 1964.

Fisher RP, Mason DT, Morrow AG: Results of operative treatment in congenital aortic stenosis. J Thoracic Cardiovas Surg 59:218, 1970.

Friedman WF, Modlinger J, Morgan JR: Serial hemodynamic observations in asymptomatic children with valvular aortic stenosis. Circulation 43:91, 1971.

Glew RH & others: Sudden death in congenital aortic stenosis. Am Heart J 78:615, 1969.

Reis RL & others: Congenital fixed subvalvular stenosis: An anatomical classification and correlations with operative results. Circulation 43(Suppl 1):11, 1971.

3. CONGENITAL MITRAL STENOSIS

In this disorder the valve leaflets are thickened and fused to produce a diaphragm-like or funnel-like structure with an opening in the center. The texture of the valve may be described as rubbery. Frequent associated malformations include patent ductus arteriosus, abnormality of the aortic valve, and coarctation. Rarely, a supravalvular diaphragm is present.

Mitral stenosis results in obstruction to blood flow into the left side of the heart, raising the left atrial and pulmonary venous pressures. If the obstruction is very severe, pulmonary edema develops. Other pathologic features include pulmonary arteriolar con-

striction, pulmonary hypertension, and, eventually, right heart failure.

Most patients develop symptoms early in life, though an occasional child may remain asymptomatic throughout childhood. Early symptoms include tachypnea and dyspnea, followed by right heart failure. Physical examination reveals a regular sinus rhythm. The first heart sound is accentuated, and the pulmonic closure sound is loud. No opening snap can be heard. In most cases, a presystolic crescendo murmur is heard at the apex. Occasionally, only a middiastolic murmur can be heard. Rarely, no murmur at all is heard.

ECG shows right axis deviation, biatrial enlargement, and right ventricular hypertrophy. X-ray reveals evidence of left atrial enlargement and frequently pulmonary venous congestion. Cardiac catheterization reveals an elevated pulmonary capillary pressure and wedge pressure and pulmonary hypertension.

Patients with severe disease usually die early in life. Patients with mild disease, however, may live a considerable period of time. If congestive heart failure develops, anticongestive measures should be instituted immediately. If no substantial improvement occurs, operation should be attempted. If the child does improve on medical treatment, he should be observed closely over a number of years and should be subjected to operation at a more optimal.time.

Baker CG & others: Congenital mitral stenosis. Brit Heart J 24:498, 1962.

Castaneda AR & others: Congenital mitral stenosis resulting from anomalous arcade and obstructing papillary muscles: Report of correction by use of ball valve prosthesis. Am J Cardiol 24:231, 1969.

Ferencz C, Johnson AL, Wiglesworth FW: Congenital mitral stenosis. Circulation 9:161, 1954.

Shone JS & others: The developmental complex of "parachute mitral valve," supravalvular ring of left atrium, subaortic stenosis, and coarctation of aorta. Am J Cardiol 11:714, 1963.

4. COR TRIATRIATUM

This is an extremely rare abnormality in which the pulmonary veins enter a separate chamber rather than passing directly into the left atrium. The chamber communicates with the left atrium through an opening of variable size. The physiologic consequences of this condition are very similar to those of mitral stenosis. The clinical findings depend upon the size of the opening. If the opening is extremely small, symptoms develop very early in life. If the opening is large, patients may be asymptomatic for a considerable period of time.

Cardiac catheterization may be diagnostic. Finding a high pulmonary capillary pressure (high pulmonary venous pressure) and a low left atrial pressure (if the catheter can be passed through the foramen ovale into the true left atrial chamber) makes the diagnosis certain. If the catheter cannot be passed into the true left atrial chamber, it is usually impossible to differentiate cor triatriatum from mitral stenosis (elevation of pulmonary wedge pressure in both cases). In this case, diagnosis must be made at surgery.

Surgical repair of cor triatriatum is usually successful only when the patient has reached an adequate size. The surgical mortality rate is very high in young children, but occasional success has been reported.

Van Praagh R, Corsini I: Cor triatriatum. Am Heart J 78:379, 1969.

Wedemeyer AL, Lucas RV, Castaneda AR: Surgical correction in infancy of an unusual form of triatrial heart. J Thoracic Cardiovas Surg 59:685, 1970.

Wolfe RR & others: Cor triatriatum: Total correction in an infant. J Thoracic Cardiovas Surg 56:114, 1968.

OTHER CONGENITAL VALVULAR LESIONS

Congenital Aortic Regurgitation

The most common causes of congenital aortic insufficiency include bicuspid aortic valve, either uncomplicated or with coarctation of the aorta; ventricular septal defect and aortic insufficiency; and fenestration of the aortic valve cusp (one or more holes in the cusp).

Congenital Mitral Regurgitation

This is a relatively rare abnormality which is usually associated with other congenital heart lesions, including corrected transposition of the great vessels, endocardial cushion defect, and endocardial fibroelastosis. Uncomplicated congenital mitral regurgitation is very rare. It is sometimes present in patients with Marfan's syndrome. Occasionally, there is a congenital dilatation of the valve ring with an otherwise normal valve. In other cases the chordae tendineae are congenitally short, resulting in mitral regurgitation.

Absence of the Pulmonary Valve

This rare abnormality is usually associated with ventricular septal defect. In about 50% of cases, severe infundibular pulmonary stenosis is present (tetralogy of Fallot).

Ebstein's Malformation of the Tricuspid Valve

This abnormality is uncommon but not rare. It consists of downward displacement of the tricuspid valve such that the greater portion of the valve is attached to the ventricular wall rather than to the fibrous ring. As a result, the upper portion of the right ventricle is within the right atrium. The portion of the ventricle below the apex of the tricuspid valve is very small and represents the true functioning right ventricle.

Clinically, there is a wide spectrum of abnormalities ranging from relative absence of symptoms to death in early infancy. The severity depends upon the degree of malattachment of the valve.

Flege JB, Vlad P, Ehrenhaft JL: Congenital mitral incompetence. J Thoracic Cardiovas Surg 53:138, 1967.

Hardy KL, Roe BB: Ebstein's anomaly: Further experience with definitive repair. J Thoracic Cardiovas Surg 59:553, 1969.

Saigusa M & others: Tricuspid valve replacement with a preserved aortic valve homograft for Ebstein's malformation. J Thoracic Cardiovas Surg 62:55, 1971.

Schiebler GL & others: Clinical study of 23 cases of Ebstein's anomaly of the tricuspid valve. Circulation 19:165, 1959.

Vlad P: Mitral valve anomalies in children. Circulation 43:465, 1971.

PRIMARY MYOCARDIAL DISEASES

This group of diseases is characterized by significant cardiac enlargement. Murmurs may or may not be present. ECG changes include left ventricular hypertrophy, ST depression, and T wave inversion.

1. GLYCOGEN STORAGE DISEASE OF THE HEART

At least 6 types of glycogen storage disease are recognized. The type that primarily involves the heart is known as Pompe's disease, or type II glycogenosis. In this disease there is a complete absence of 1,4-glucosidase activity at pH 4.0. This enzyme (acid maltase) is necessary for the hydrolysis of the outer branches of glycogen, and its absence results in marked deposition of glycogen within the myocardium. Cardiac glycogenosis is a rare heritable (possibly sex-linked) disorder.

Affected infants are usually normal at birth, but onset usually begins by the sixth month of life. The findings usually include marked cardiac enlargement, a very large tongue, which causes feeding problems, and marked generalized muscular weakness. The liver is usually not enlarged unless there is congestive heart failure. These children usually have a history of retardation of growth and development, feeding problems, poor weight gain, and then the findings of heart failure. Physical examination reveals generalized muscular weakness, a large tongue, cardiomegaly, no significant heart murmurs, and occasionally evidence of congestive heart failure. Chest x-rays reveal marked cardiomegaly, with or without pulmonary venous congestion. ECG shows left ventricular hypertrophy and, usually, ST depression and T wave inversion over the left precordial leads.

Children with this disease usually die within the first year of life. Death may be sudden or due to progressive congestive heart failure.

Hernandez A Jr & others: Cardiac glycogenosis. J Pediat 68:400, 1966.

Hohn AR & others: Cardiac problems in the glycogenoses with special reference to Pompe's disease. Pediatrics 35:313, 1965.

Lauer RM & others: Administration of a mixture of fungal glucosidases to a patient with type II glycogenosis (Pompe's disease). Pediatrics 42:672, 1968.

2. ANOMALOUS ORIGIN OF THE LEFT CORONARY ARTERY

Essentials of Diagnosis

- Colicky pain with pallor from 2–6 months.
- Congestive heart failure.
- Enlarged heart.
- Poor heart tones.
- Frequently, a murmur of mitral regurgitation.
- ECG shows a pattern of myocardial infarction.

General Considerations

In this condition, the left coronary artery arises from the pulmonary artery rather than from the aorta. In the neonatal period, while the pulmonary arterial pressure is relatively high, blood is supplied to the left ventricle from the pulmonary artery. Accordingly, during this period the child is asymptomatic and does well. However, within the first 2 months of life, the pulmonary arterial pressure decreases to normal. This results in a marked decrease of flow to the left coronary artery. Infarction of the heart usually occurs. If the patient survives, collateral channels appear which join the peripheral branches of the right with the branches of the left coronary artery. As a result, the direction of blood flow in the left coronary artery changes. Whereas previously there was some flow from the pulmonary artery into the myocardium through the left coronary, flow now occurs from the right coronary artery through the collateral into the left coronary artery and then into the pulmonary artery. In essence, then, an arteriovenous fistula is formed which further removes blood from the myocardium. This results in further myocardial infarction and fibrosis. Death occurs eventually as a result of marked dilatation of the heart and congestive heart failure. At autopsy, the left ventricle is found to be markedly fibrosed and thin.

Clinical Findings

A. Symptoms and Signs: These patients appear to be normal at birth. Growth and development are relatively normal for a few months, although detailed questioning of the parents often discloses a history of intermittent episodes of severe abdominal pain, pallor, and sweating, especially during or after feeding. These episodes are thought to be secondary to "colic" and attacks are similar to anginal attacks in adults.

On physical examination, the patients are usually well developed and well nourished. They show no evidence of congestive heart failure until terminally. The pulses are usually weak but equal throughout. The heart is enlarged but not very active. A murmur of mitral regurgitation is frequently present, although no murmur may be heard.

B. X-Ray Findings: Chest x-rays show significant cardiac enlargement with or without pulmonary venous congestion.

C. Electrocardiography: The ECG is usually diagnostic. There are T wave inversions in leads I and aVL. The precordial leads show T wave inversions from V_4-V_7. Deep, wide Q waves are often seen in leads I, aVL, and V_4-V_6. These findings are very similar to those of myocardial infarction in adults.

D. Cardiac Catheterization and Cineangiocardiography: The diagnosis depends upon cardiac catheterization and cineangiocardiography. A small left-to-right shunt can often be detected at the pulmonary artery level as a result of the flow of blood from the right through the left coronary artery into the pulmonary artery. Frequently, however, the shunt is very small and can be detected only by the most sensitive technics such as the hydrogen electrode catheter. Cineangiocardiography following injection of contrast material into the root of the aorta shows absence of origin of the left coronary artery from the aorta. A huge right coronary artery fills directly from the aorta, and one can follow the contrast material through the right coronary system into the left coronary arteries. Occasionally, one can actually see the blood flowing into the pulmonary artery.

Treatment & Prognosis

Surgical transplantation of the coronary artery has been highly successful in some hands. Medical management until 4 years of age followed by vein graft anastomosis of the left coronary artery to the aorta gives the patient the security of a 2 coronary artery system. Other workers prefer ligation of the left coronary artery where it enters the pulmonary artery. The rationale for this procedure is that obstructing the flow from the left coronary artery into the pulmonary artery would drive coronary artery blood flow into the myocardium, thus improving myocardial oxygenation.

Edwards JE: The direction of blood flow in coronary arteries arising from the pulmonary trunk. Circulation 29:163, 1964.

Gasior RM & others: Anomalous origin of the left coronary artery from the pulmonary artery: Treatment by aorto-left coronary saphenous venous bypass. Am J Cardiol 27:215, 1971.

Nadas AS, Gamboa R, Hugenholtz PG: Anomalous left coronary artery originating from the pulmonary artery: Report of two surgically treated cases with a proposal of hemodynamic and therapeutic classification. Circulation 24:167, 1964.

Nora JJ & others: Medical and surgical management of anomalous origin of left coronary artery from pulmonary artery. Pediatrics 42:405, 1968.

Perry LW, Scott LP: Anomalous left coronary artery from pulmonary artery: Report of 11 cases; review of indications for and results of surgery. Circulation 41:1043, 1970.

Sabiston DC & others: Surgical management of congenital lesions of the coronary circulation. Ann Surg 157:908, 1963.

3. ENDOCARDIAL FIBROELASTOSIS

Essentials of Diagnosis

- Congestive heart failure in infancy in vast majority.
- Cardiac enlargement.
- No significant murmurs.

General Considerations

This is a fairly common type of "congenital" primary myocardial disease. The cause is not known, though it has been suggested that it might be due to intrauterine infection with mumps virus.

Pathologically, there is a marked milky white thickening of the endocardium and subendocardial layers of the left ventricle and usually the left atrium. The mitral valve is frequently involved also. The myocardial fibers themselves are thickened, but there is no evidence of significant inflammation.

Clinical Findings

A. Symptoms and Signs: These patients appear normal at birth, and growth and development during early infancy are normal. About 50% develop symptoms within the first 5 months of life, and almost all are symptomatic by age 1. An occasional patient may have no symptoms until age 5.

The symptoms and signs that do develop are associated with left ventricular heart failure. These include dyspnea, easy fatigability, feeding difficulties, and, eventually, findings of left and right heart failure.

On physical examination, these children are often small and undernourished. The heart is usually enlarged, and the heart tones are poor (when there is evidence of decompensation). A murmur of mitral regurgitation is often present.

B. X-Ray Findings: Chest x-rays show generalized cardiac enlargement with or without pulmonary venous congestion.

C. Electrocardiography: The ECG almost always shows evidence of left ventricular hypertrophy and, quite frequently, ST depression and T wave inversion. If there has been pulmonary hypertension secondary to the left heart failure, right ventricular hypertrophy may be present. Right atrial hypertrophy is sometimes present. Complete heart block is occasionally seen.

D. Cardiac Catheterization and Cineangiocardiography: Catheterization reveals the absence of left-to-right shunts. Pulmonary hypertension may be present. Cardiac output is usually decreased. Cineangiocardiography demonstrates the poor stroke output (ineffectual contraction) of the left ventricle.

Treatment & Prognosis

The treatment of this disease is medical. Early and vigorous treatment of cardiac failure is essential. There appears to be a definite correlation between favorable outcome and early onset of treatment. In one series, when treatment was initiated later than 1 month after the onset of symptoms of cardiac decompensation, recovery was never complete. If treatment is started promptly, the prognosis is fairly good. (In one series, the overall mortality was 23%.) Other authors, however, have reported a higher mortality rate.

The most important part of the treatment consists of adequate and prolonged digitalis administration. It is recommended that one start with the usual dose of digoxin. If the response to the usual dose is not satisfactory, the dose should be increased until a satisfactory response is noted or toxicity occurs. Digitalis should be continued for at least 2 years. In addition to digitalization, the other usual anticongestive measures should be instituted. Diuretics (chlorothiazide or furosemide plus spironolactone) are recommended in maintenance doses along with the digoxin over a prolonged period of time.

In some cases, the child appears to improve initially but then develops recurrent bouts of heart failure. Complete recovery in such patients is very infrequent, and most eventually die with intractable congestive heart failure.

Gersony WM, Katz SL, Nadas AS: Endocardial fibroelastosis and the mumps virus. Pediatrics 37:430, 1966.

Hastreiter AR, Miller RA: Management of primary endomyocardial disease: The myocarditis-endocardial fibroelastosis syndrome. P Clin North America 11:401, 1964.

Manning JA & others: The medical management of clinical endocardial fibroelastosis. Circulation 29:60, 1964.

Moller JH & others: Endocardial fibroelastosis: A clinical and anatomic study of 47 patients with emphasis on its relationship to mitral insufficiency. Circulation 30:759, 1964.

II. CYANOTIC HEART DISEASE

TETRALOGY OF FALLOT

Essentials of Diagnosis

- Progressively increasing cyanosis dating from infancy.
- Spells of paroxysmal dyspnea (4 months to 4 years).
- Clubbing.
- Right ventricular lift.
- Loud single S_2 at lower left sternal border.
- Grade I–III/VI ejection systolic murmur, maximal in the third intercostal space at the left sternal border.

General Considerations

In Fallot's tetralogy, there is a ventricular septal defect and severe obstruction to right ventricular outflow such that the intracardiac shunt is predominantly from right to left. It is the most common type of cyanotic heart lesion, accounting for 10–15% of all cases of congenital heart disease. The ventricular defect is usually located in the membranous portion of the septum and is usually quite large. Obstruction to right ventricular outflow may be solely at the infundibular level (50%), solely at the valvular level (20%), or at both levels (30%). The term tetralogy has been used to describe this combination of lesions since there is always associated right ventricular hypertrophy and a varying degree of "overriding of the aorta." The overriding is present because of the position of the ventricular septal defect in relation to a dilated and often dextroposed aorta. These 2 factors (right ventricular hypertrophy and overriding aorta) plus the major lesions make up the tetralogy. A right-sided aortic arch is present in 25% of cases and a patent foramen ovale in 25%.

Severe obstruction to right ventricular outflow plus a large ventricular septal defect results in a right-to-left shunt at the ventricular level and desaturation of the arterial blood. The degree of desaturation and the extent of cyanosis depend upon the size of the shunt. This in turn is dependent upon the resistance to outflow from the right ventricle, the size of the ventricular septal defect, and the systemic vascular resistance. The greater the obstruction, the larger the ventricular septal defect, and the lower the systemic vascular resistance—the greater the right-to-left shunt. Although the patient may be deeply cyanotic, the amount of pressure the right ventricle can develop is limited to that of the systemic (aortic) pressure. In other words, right ventricular pressure cannot exceed left ventricular pressure. The right ventricle is usually quite able to maintain this level of pressure without developing heart failure. This is in contrast to cases in which there is right ventricular outflow obstruction and an intact ventricular septum; in these cases, although the pulmonary blood flow is greater and the patient is usually less cyanotic (if at all), the right ventricle can develop sufficient pressure that heart failure is much more common.

Clinical Findings

A. Symptoms and Signs: The clinical findings vary depending upon the degree of right ventricular outflow obstruction. Patients with a mild degree of obstruction are only minimally cyanotic or acyanotic; those with maximal obstruction are deeply cyanotic from birth. However, few children are asymptomatic, most have cyanosis by 4 months of age, and the cyanosis usually is progressive. Growth and development are retarded, and easy fatigability and dyspnea on exertion are common. Squatting is very common when the children become old enough to walk. Hypoxic spells (cyanotic spells) characterized by the sudden onset of marked deepening of cyanosis, irritability, and severe dyspnea, followed occasionally by unconsciousness and convulsions, are quite common between the ages of 4 months and 4 years. These cyanotic spells vary in frequency and severity in different individuals. It is felt that these spells are related to sudden increase of constriction of the infundibulum of the right ventricle, resulting in a marked increase in the degree of right ventricular obstruction.

Patients with tetralogy are usually small and thin. The degree of cyanosis is variable. The fingers and toes show varying degrees of clubbing depending upon the age of the child and the severity of the cyanosis.

On examination of the heart, a right ventricular lift is palpable. No thrills are present. The first sound is normal; occasionally there is an ejection click at the apex. The second sound is single and best heard at the lower left sternal border between the third and fourth intercostal spaces. The second heart sound at the pulmonary area is soft; however, aortic closure is loud and heard best in the third and fourth intercostal spaces at the left sternal border. There is a grade I–III/VI, rough, ejection type systolic murmur which is maximal at the left sternal border in the third intercostal space. This murmur radiates somewhat over the anterior and posterior lung fields. Diastolic murmurs are not present. (The single second heart sound is due to aortic closure. Pulmonary closure cannot be heard, although it may be seen on a phonocardiogram.) During a cyanotic spell, the murmur may decrease significantly in intensity and may be inaudible. (The diamond-shaped ejection murmur is due to the obstruction to pulmonary blood flow and not to the right-to-left shunt at the ventricular level.)

B. X-Ray Findings: Chest x-rays reveal the overall heart size to be normal. However, the right ventricle is hypertrophied, and this is shown in the posteroanterior projection by an upturning of the apex (boot-shaped heart). The main pulmonary artery segment is usually concave, and the aorta in 25% of cases arches to the right. The pulmonary vascular markings are usually on the lower limits of normal.

C. Electrocardiography: The cardiac axis is to the right, ranging from +90 to +180 degrees. The P waves are usually normal, although there may be evidence of slight right atrial hypertrophy. Right ventricular hypertrophy is always present, but right ventricular strain patterns are rare.

D. Laboratory Findings: Hemoglobin, hematocrit, and red blood count are usually mildly to markedly elevated depending upon the degree of arterial oxygen desaturation. (But see Complications, below.)

E. Cardiac Catheterization and Cineangiocardiography: Cardiac catheterization reveals the absence of a significant left-to-right shunt, although the hydrogen electrode curve may be positive in the right ventricle. There is arterial blood desaturation of varying degree. The right-to-left shunt exists at the ventricular level. The right ventricular pressure is at systemic levels, and the pressure contour in the right ventricle is almost identical with that of the left ventricle. The pulmonary artery pressure is extremely low (mean ranges of 5–10 mm). The gradients and pressure may be noted at the valvular level, the infundibular level, or both. The catheter frequently is passed across the ventricular septal defect from the right ventricle into the ascending aorta.

Cineangiocardiography is diagnostic. Injection of contrast material into the right ventricle reveals the right ventricular outflow obstruction and the right-to-left shunt at the ventricular level.

Complications

A. Cerebral Infarction: Brain infarction is not uncommon. The cause varies somewhat depending upon the age of the child. Within the first 2 years of life, it is thought that the major cause of cerebral infarction is anoxia, which results from the marked arterial blood desaturation and the relative iron deficiency anemia that exists in many of these young infants.

Children with a hematocrit under 55% may be liable to the development of an anemic, anoxic infarction. This is much less common over age 2 years, when iron deficiency is less of a problem. Therefore, all children should be followed with a hemoglobin, hematocrit, and red blood count determination. If there is evidence of significant iron deficiency, these patients should be given oral iron therapy.

In older children, cerebral infarction is usually due to thrombosis. When the hematocrit rises above 75% the viscosity of the blood markedly increases and the possibility of thrombotic infarction develops. In these cases, it may be necessary to perform phlebotomy to keep the hematocrit below 75%.

B. Brain Abscess: Children with tetralogy of Fallot over age 2 who develop CNS symptoms and especially brain damage should be considered to have brain abscess until proved otherwise. Brain abscess is now thought to develop in areas of previous infarction which may be microscopic in size. Because of the presence of the right-to-left shunt, bacteria which usually are filtered out by the lungs can pass into the systemic circulation and hence to the area of infarction in the brain. Common presenting symptoms are those of an expanding intracranial mass. There is usually a history of a respiratory infection 1–2 weeks prior to the onset of neurologic symptoms. The most common organism involved is alpha-hemolytic streptococcus. However, many other organisms have been cultured, and multiple organisms may be involved. Treatment consists of antibiotics and, usually, surgical removal of the abscess.

Treatment

The treatment of tetralogy of Fallot is surgery, either palliative or corrective.

A. Palliative Treatment: Palliative treatment is recommended for very small infants or young children who are markedly symptomatic (severely cyanotic, frequent severe anoxic spells), in whom complete correction would be very difficult if not impossible. It is also recommended for individuals who for other reasons are not candidates for complete correction of the defect. If the child seems to be getting along fairly well, it is recommended that surgery be deferred until the child is large enough to permit total correction.

The earliest procedure employed for this disease (Blalock-Taussig) consisted of an anastomosis between the subclavian artery and the pulmonary artery. It is usually done on the side opposite the aortic arch. Another commonly employed anastomotic technic (Potts procedure) anastomoses the descending thoracic aorta to the left pulmonary artery. It is employed in very young infants, in whom the subclavian artery is too small for a sufficient opening. It should not be used in older infants because too large an anastomosis will result in a very large sudden increase in pulmonary blood flow and left heart failure. Furthermore, it is much more difficult to "take down" a Potts operation, which is necessary before complete correction can be undertaken.

The procedure which is gaining favor is construction of an anastomosis between the ascending aorta and the right pulmonary artery. This procedure permits the formation of a large anastomosis and is relatively easy to take down prior to complete correction. It has the same disadvantage as the Potts procedure, ie, it is possible to create too large an opening with resultant left heart failure.

B. Total Correction: Total correction of tetralogy of Fallot is performed under cardiopulmonary bypass. It involves opening the right ventricle, closing the ventricular septal defect, and removing the obstruction to right ventricular outflow. The surgical mortality varies from 2–15%. There seems to be a definite correlation between the severity of the disease and the mortality rate. Children who survive the operation are markedly improved. There is complete disappearance of cyanosis, and clubbing disappears shortly thereafter. Growth and development improve markedly, and these patients often become asymptomatic within a short period of time.

Course & Prognosis

Those with the most severe form of the disease are usually deeply cyanotic at birth. Anoxic spells may occur within the first 1–2 months. Death may occur during a severe anoxic spell. Many patients who survive the first year of life seem to improve. This may be due to the development of bronchial collateral vessels. Although anoxic spells may decrease in severity, these children remain deeply cyanotic and markedly limited in their activity. They seldom survive the second decade of life without surgical treatment.

Those with moderate obstruction to right ventricular outflow do fairly well. Although cyanosis is present in very early life, it is usually not severe. The cyanosis may progress in severity, and anoxic spells may occur. These patients do fairly well in later childhood, but their condition progressively deteriorates during the second and third decade of life. Death occurs by the third decade due to cerebrovascular accidents, brain abscess, subacute bacterial endocarditis, anoxia, or pulmonary hemorrhage.

Patients with the mildest form of the disease are often thought to have the "acyanotic" variety of tetralogy of Fallot. The degree of obstruction is very mild, and the right-to-left shunt is small. Very frequently, there is a predominant left-to-right shunt. However, as the patient gets older, the degree of obstruction frequently increases. This, combined with the increased activity, results in progressively worsening cyanosis. Many of these patients can live a relatively normal life without severe symptoms. Life expectancy, however, is definitely decreased, and death usually occurs by the third to fourth decade.

Cole RB & others: Long-term results following aorto-pulmonary anastomosis for tetralogy of Fallot: Morbidity and mortality. Circulation 43:263, 1971.

Goldman BS, Mustard WT, Trusler GS: Total correction of tetralogy of Fallot: Review of ten years' experience. Brit Heart J 30:563–568, 1968.

Guntheroth WG & others: Venous return with knee-chest position and squatting in tetralogy of Fallot. Am Heart J 75:313, 1968.

Lev M, Eckner FAO: The pathologic anatomy of tetralogy of Fallot and its variations. Dis Chest 45:251, 1964.

Martelle RR, Linde LM: Cerebrovascular accidents in tetralogy of Fallot. Am J Dis Child 101:206, 1961.

Rudolph AM, Danilowicz D: Treatment of severe spell syndrome in congenital heart disease. Pediatrics 32:141, 1963.

PULMONARY ATRESIA
WITH VENTRICULAR SEPTAL DEFECT

This condition consists of complete atresia of the pulmonary valve in association with ventricular septal defect. Essentially it is an extreme form of tetralogy of Fallot. Since there is no flow out from the right ventricle into the pulmonary artery, the pulmonary blood flow must be derived either from a patent ductus arteriosus or from collateral channels which form during intrauterine life.

The clinical picture depends entirely upon the size of the ductus or the collateral channels (or both). If they are large, patients may do quite well and actually do better than those with severe tetralogy of Fallot. If the collateral channels are small, death occurs secondary to severe anoxia early in life.

Cardiac catheterization and cineangiocardiography are diagnostic.

Infants who are severely hypoxemic require urgent systemic-aortic anastomosis in order to provide sufficient oxygenated blood to the body.

A corrective surgical procedure has been developed recently which has been successful (20% mortality) in patients with adequate-sized pulmonary arteries.

Bernhard WF & others: Ascending aorta-right pulmonary artery shunt in infants and older patients with certain types of cyanotic congenital heart disease. Circulation 43:580, 1971.

Kouchoukos NT & others: Surgical treatment of congenital pulmonary atresia with ventricular septal defects. J Thoracic Cardiovas Surg 61:70, 1971.

Miller WW & others: Congenital pulmonary atresia with ventricular septal defect. Am J Cardiology 21:673, 1968.

Mustard WT, Bedard P, Trusler GA: Cardiovascular surgery in the first year of life. J Thoracic Cardiovas Surg 59:761, 1970.

Starke H, Pugh D, Dunn M: Bronchopulmonary arterial communications in pulmonary atresia with ventricular septal defect. Am J Cardiol 24:570, 1969.

Waldhauer J A & others: Ascending aorta-right pulmonary artery anastomosis: Clinical experience with 35 patients with cyanotic congenital heart disease. Circulation 38:463, 1968.

PULMONARY ATRESIA
WITH INTACT VENTRICULAR SEPTUM

Essentials of Diagnosis

- Severely cyanotic infant with marked dyspnea.
- Enlarged heart.
- Murmur of tricuspid insufficiency may or may not be present.
- S_2 single and soft.

General Considerations

In this relatively rare condition, the pulmonary valve is absent and is replaced by a small diaphragm consisting of the fused cusps. The ventricular septum is intact. The main pulmonary artery segment is somewhat hypoplastic but almost always patent. The tricuspid valve is competent in about 75% of cases (type 1). In the remainder (type 2), malformation of the tricuspid valve results in tricuspid insufficiency. In the type 1 deformity, the cavity volume of the right ventricle is extremely small and the wall is thickened and fibrotic. In type 2, the right ventricle cavity is frequently of normal size.

During intrauterine life, if the tricuspid valve is intact and normal, very little blood enters the right ventricle since there is no outlet for this chamber. Almost all of the blood passes through the foramen ovale directly into the left side of the heart. In the type 2 deformity, there is an outlet for the right ventricle (tricuspid valve insufficiency) and the right ventricle receives a sufficient quantity of blood to permit it to develop in a relatively normal fashion.

Following birth, the pulmonary circulation is maintained primarily by a patent ductus arteriosus. Although a bronchial pulmonary collateral network is present, it is usually insufficient to maintain the pulmonary circulation. Accordingly, whether or not these patients live depends upon the patency of the ductus arteriosus. The ductus usually remains open for only a short period of time. As it closes, hypoxia becomes progressively more severe and death eventually occurs.

Clinical Findings

A. Symptoms and Signs: These patients may be normal at birth, although they are usually cyanotic.

Cyanosis becomes progressively more severe and is associated with severe dyspnea. The pulses are usually bounding (due to the patent ductus arteriosus). A blowing systolic murmur can be heard at the pulmonary area and under the left clavicle. This murmur may be continuous. It is due to the patent ductus arteriosus. In type 2 deformity, a loud pansystolic murmur due to the tricuspid insufficiency is heard at the lower left sternal border. Not infrequently, the liver is pulsating.

B. X-Ray Findings: Chest x-rays show a markedly enlarged heart with marked decrease in pulmonary vascular markings.

C. Electrocardiography: ECG reveals an axis which is usually normal in the frontal plane. There is very low voltage over the right precordial leads in the type 1 deformity. In type 2 deformity, the voltage over the right precordial leads may be normal or increased. The voltage over the left precordial leads is usually much greater than normal, suggesting left ventricular hypertrophy.

D. Cardiac Catheterization and Cineangiocardiography: The diagnosis can be made on cardiac catheterization and cineangiocardiography. Right ventricular pressure is very high (greater than systemic). A cineangiocardiogram following injection of contrast material into the right ventricle reveals absence of filling of the pulmonary artery from the right ventricle. It also demonstrates the size of the right ventricular chamber and the presence or absence of tricuspid regurgitation.

Treatment & Prognosis

Surgery should be undertaken as soon as the diagnosis is made. Following the diagnostic aspect of the cardiac catheterization, a Rashkind atrial septostomy is performed. This opens up the communication across the atrial septum and permits adequate flow in both directions. The patient is then taken to the operating room immediately. The current procedure of choice consists of a transventricular pulmonary valvotomy followed by an ascending aorta to right pulmonary artery anastomosis. The latter procedure is performed to ensure adequate blood flow to the lungs, since right ventricular performance (even in type 2) is poor in the immediate postoperative period.

If the patient survives the surgery, the prognosis is good for patients with type 2 malformations since the right ventricle in this type is of adequate size and can develop in a relatively normal fashion after pulmonary valvotomy. In patients with type 1, the right ventricle usually remains hypoplastic.

Bowman FO & others: Pulmonary atresia with intact ventricular septum. J Thoracic Cardiovas Surg 61:85, 1971.

Davignon AL & others: Congenital pulmonary atresia with intact ventricular septum: Clinicopathologic correlation of two anatomic types. Am Heart J 62:591, 1961.

Dhanavaravibul S, Nora JJ, McNamara DG: Pulmonary valvular atresia with intact ventricular septum: Problems in diagnosis and results of treatment. J Pediat 77:1010, 1970.

Hallman GL, Cooley DA: Cardiovascular surgery in newborn infants: Results in 1050 patients less than one year old. Ann Surg 173:1007, 1971.

Miller WW & others: Congenital pulmonary valve atresia with intact ventricular septum. Am J Cardiol 23:128, 1969.

Trusler GA, Fowler RS: The surgical management of pulmonary atresia with intact ventricular septum and hypoplastic right ventricle. J Thoracic Cardiovas Surg 59:740, 1970.

TRICUSPID ATRESIA

Essentials of Diagnosis

- Marked cyanosis from birth.
- Congestive heart failure in early infancy in most cases.

General Considerations

This relatively rare condition (< 1% of cases of congenital heart disease) is characterized by complete atresia of the tricuspid valve. As a result, no direct communication exists between the right atrium and right ventricle.

Tricuspid atresia may be divided into 2 types depending upon the relationship of the great vessels:

Type 1. Without transposition of the great arteries (70%): (a) No ventricular septal defect. Hypoplasia or atresia of the pulmonary artery. Patent ductus arteriosus. (b) Small ventricular septal defect. Pulmonary stenosis. Hypoplastic pulmonary artery. (c) Large ventricular septal defect and no pulmonary stenosis. Normal-sized pulmonary artery.

Type 2. With transposition of the great arteries (30%): (a) With ventricular septal defect and pulmonary stenosis. (b) With ventricular septal defect but without pulmonary stenosis.

Since there is no direct communication between the right atrium and right ventricle, the entire systemic venous return must flow through the atrial septum (either an atrial septal defect or patent foramen ovale) into the left atrium. Accordingly, the left atrium receives both the systemic venous return and the pulmonary venous return. Complete mixing occurs in the left atrium, resulting in a greater or lesser degree of arterial desaturation.

As a result of the lack of direct communication between the right atrium and right ventricle, the development of the ventricle depends upon the presence of a left-to-right shunt at the ventricular level. Therefore, severe hypoplasia of the right ventricle occurs in those forms in which there is no ventricular septal defect or in which the ventricular septal defect is very small.

Clinical Findings

A. Symptoms and Signs: In the great majority of patients with tricuspid atresia, symptoms develop very early in infancy. Except in cases in which the pulmonary blood flow is great, cyanosis is present at birth. Growth and development are very poor, and there is usually easy fatigability on feeding, tachypnea, dyspnea, anoxic spells, and evidence of right heart failure. Patients with marked increase in pulmonary blood flow (types 1c and 2b) will develop evidence of left heart failure as well.

Clubbing is present if the child is old enough. On examination of the heart, a slight bulge on the right side of the sternum may occasionally be seen. The first heart sound is normal. The second heart sound is most often single (due to aortic closure). A murmur is usually present, although it is variable. It ranges from grade I–III/VI in intensity and usually is a harsh blowing murmur heard best at the lower left sternal border.

B. X-Ray Findings: Chest x-rays are variable. The heart may be slightly to markedly enlarged. The main pulmonary artery segment is usually small or absent. The size of the right atrium varies from huge to only modestly enlarged, depending upon the size of the communication at the atrial level. The pulmonary vascular markings are usually decreased, although in types 1c and 2b they are increased.

C. Electrocardiography: ECG is diagnostic. It invariably shows a left axis deviation with a counterclockwise loop in the frontal plane. The P waves are tall and peaked, indicative of right atrial hypertrophy. The size of the P wave depends upon the right atrial pressure, which in turn depends upon the size of the interatrial communication (the taller the P wave, the smaller the communication). Left ventricular hypertrophy or left ventricular preponderance is found in almost all cases. Voltage over the right precordium is usually low.

D. Cardiac Catheterization and Cineangiocardiography: This reveals the marked right-to-left shunt at the atrial level and desaturation of the left atrial blood. Because of the complete mixing in the left atrial chambers, oxygen saturation in the left ventricle, right ventricle, pulmonary artery, and aorta is identical to that in the left atrium. The right atrial pressure is increased. Left ventricular and systemic pressures are normal. The catheter cannot be passed through the tricuspid valve from the right atrium to the right ventricle. The course of the catheter is always from right atrium into left atrium and from there into left ventricle.

Cineangiocardiography following injection of contrast material into the right atrium is diagnostic. It reveals the lack of communication of the right atrium with the right ventricle and the right-to-left shunt at the atrial level.

Treatment

The treatment of tricuspid atresia is surgical. No corrective procedures are at present available, and surgery is therefore limited to palliation directed toward increasing pulmonary blood flow. Two procedures are commonly employed: (1) systemic arterial to pulmonary arterial anastomosis (Blalock-Taussig or Potts procedure), and (2) anastomosis of the superior vena cava to the right pulmonary artery (Glenn procedure). These procedures should be employed only in patients whose pulmonary blood flow is markedly decreased and in whom cyanosis is severe.

Course & Prognosis

The outcome depends on achieving a balance of pulmonary blood flow which permits adequate oxygenation of the tissues without producing intractable congestive heart failure.

Deverall PP & others: Surgical management of tricuspid atresia. Thorax 24:239, 1969.

Edwards WS, Bargeron LM: Superiority of Glenn operation for tricuspid atresia in infancy and childhood. J Thoracic Cardiovas Surg 55:60, 1968.

Hallman GL, Stasnez R, Cooley DA: Surgical treatment of tricuspid atresia. J Cardiovas Surg 9:154, 1968.

Marcano BA & others: Tricuspid atresia with increased pulmonary blood flow: An analysis of 13 cases. Circulation 40:399, 1969.

Neill CA, Brink AJ: Left axis deviation in tricuspid atresia and single ventricle: The electrocardiogram in 36 autopsied cases. Circulation 12:612, 1955.

Riker WL & others: Tricuspid atresia or stenosis complexes: A surgical and pathologic analysis. J Thoracic Cardiovas Surg 45:423, 1963.

HYPOPLASTIC LEFT HEART SYNDROME

This not uncommon syndrome includes a number of conditions in which there are either valvular or vascular lesions on the left side of the heart, resulting in hypoplasia of the left ventricle. A history of maternal diabetes is often present.

The lesions that make up this syndrome are mitral atresia, aortic atresia, atresia of the aortic arch, and hypoplasia of the aortic arch. In all of these conditions, there is severe obstruction to either filling or emptying of the left ventricle. As a result, during intrauterine life, the quantity of blood filling the left ventricle is extremely small, resulting in hypoplasia of this chamber. Following birth, there is marked impairment of the circulation because of the very small size of the left ventricle and the obstructing lesions. Congestive heart failure develops rapidly, in most cases from several days to 3 months of life.

Patients with aortic atresia develop congestive heart failure very early, usually within the first week. Death occurs earliest in this group. Patients with mitral atresia who have large atrial and ventricular communications may live longer. Some patients have lived beyond the first decade. Patients with involvement of the aortic arch usually die within 1–2 months.

The clinical picture depends upon the type of obstructing lesion. Cyanosis is usually present early in life and is usually generalized. Patients with hypoplasia or atresia of the aortic arch may show differential cyanosis. Murmurs may or may not be present and are usually nondiagnostic. Congestive heart failure develops early. Left-sided failure usually appears first, followed by right-sided failure.

Chest x-rays usually are relatively normal at birth. Rapid and progressive cardiac enlargement then occurs, frequently associated with pulmonary venous congestion. These changes occur earliest in patients with aortic atresia.

ECG almost always demonstrates right axis deviation, right atrial hypertrophy, and right ventricular hypertrophy.

No surgical treatment is available. Medical management consists of treatment of congestive heart failure.

Friedman S, Murphy L, Ash R: Aortic atresia with hypoplasia of the left heart and aortic arch. J Pediat 38:354, 1951.

Krovetz LJ, Rowe D, Shiebler GL: Hemodynamics of aortic valve atresia. Circulation 42:953, 1970.

Nadas AS, Mody MR: Preductal coarctation and hypoplastic left heart complexes, with comments on the premature closure of the foramen ovale. Pages 225–236 in: *The Heart and Circulation in the Newborn and Infant.* Cassels DE (editor). Grune & Stratton, 1966.

Sirak H & others: New operation for repairing aortic arch atresia in infancy: Report of three cases. Circulation 37, 38(Suppl 2):43–50, 1968.

Watson DG & others: Mitral atresia with normal aortic valve: Report of 11 cases and review of the literature. Pediatrics 25:450, 1960.

COMPLETE TRANSPOSITION OF THE GREAT ARTERIES

Essentials of Diagnosis

- Severe cyanosis from birth.
- Congestive heart failure in early infancy in most cases.
- Clubbing.
- Cardiac enlargement.
- Single S_2.
- Murmurs variable, depending upon the specific intracardiac abnormalities.

General Considerations

Complete transposition of the great vessels is the second most common variety of cyanotic congenital heart disease, accounting for about 16% of all cases. The male/female ratio is 4:1. It is due to an embryologic abnormality in the spiral division of the truncus arteriosus.

The aorta is located anterior to the pulmonary artery—directly anterior, or to the left or right. The pulmonary artery usually ascends parallel to the aorta rather than crossing it. In most cases, associated intracardiac abnormalities are present. These include ventricular septal defect, atrial septal defect, pulmonic stenosis, and patent ductus arteriosus. Obstructive changes within the pulmonary arteriolar bed are common in patients past infancy.

Transposition of the great vessels can be classified into the following categories:

Group 1. Transposition with intact ventricular septum: (a) Without pulmonic stenosis and (b) with pulmonic stenosis, subvalvular or valvular (or both).

Group 2. Transposition with ventricular septal defect: (a) with pulmonary stenosis, (b) with pulmonary vascular obstruction, (c) without pulmonary vascular obstruction (normal pulmonary vascular resistance).

Since the aorta arises directly from the right ventricle, life would not be possible unless there were mixing between the systemic and pulmonary circulations; oxygenated blood from the pulmonary veins must in some way reach the systemic arterial circuit. In patients with intact ventricular septum (group 1), mixing occurs at the atrial and also at the ductal level. However, in most cases these communications are small, and the ductus arteriosus often closes shortly after birth. These patients are therefore severely cyanotic, and congestive heart failure occurs rapidly as a result of the marked increase in cardiac output. Patients with a ventricular septal defect show greater or lesser degrees of cyanosis depending upon the ratio of the pulmonary to systemic blood flow. Patients with ventricular septal defect and pulmonary stenosis (group 2b) are usually severely cyanotic because of the limited blood flow to the lungs. Patients with ventricular septal defect and pulmonary vascular obstruction (group 2b) show a moderate degree of cyanosis. Patients with ventricular septal defect and normal pulmonary vascular resistance (group 2c) show the least cyanosis but often develop heart failure very early because of the enormous pulmonary blood flow.

Congestive heart failure develops not only because of the high cardiac output but also because of the poor oxygenation of the myocardium and the presence of systemic pressure in both ventricles.

Clinical Findings

A. Symptoms and Signs: Most of the neonates are quite large, often weighing 4 kg (9 lb) at birth, and most are cyanotic at birth although cyanosis occasionally does not develop until later. (Ninety-five percent of children are cyanotic by age 1.) Patients in groups 1 and 2a are most cyanotic; those in group 2c are least cyanotic. Retardation of growth and development after the neonatal period is common. Congestive heart failure occurs in patients in groups 1 and 2c. Patients in group 2a show no evidence of congestive heart failure but often have severe anoxic spells in early life; if they survive the first year of life, retardation of growth and development is common and cyanosis becomes progressively more severe. However, intellectual development, even in patients with severe cyanosis, may be unaffected.

Although these infants are usually large at birth, growth and development is retarded, so that when they reach age 6 months to 1 year they are usually below the third percentile in both height and weight. Cyanosis is marked. Clubbing is present in children over age 1. The findings on cardiovascular examination depend somewhat upon the intracardiac defects. Group 1a patients have only soft murmurs or none at all. The first heart sound is usually normal. The second heart sound is single and accentuated. Patients in group 1b have loud obstructive systolic murmurs loudest at the second and third intercostal spaces and left sternal border, radiating well to the first and second intercostal spaces. Group 2a patients have a murmur of pulmonary stenosis (obstructive systolic murmur at the base of the heart, best heard to the right of the sternum). Those in group 2c have a systolic murmur along the lower sternal border and a mitral diastolic flow murmur at the apex.

B. X-Ray Findings:

1. Group 1a—The heart has a characteristic appearance, "like an egg on its side." The base of the heart is very narrow. Pulmonary vascular markings are markedly increased.

2. Group 1b—Pulmonary vascular markings may be normal, slightly increased, or slightly decreased. The heart is moderately enlarged.

3. Group 2a—The x-ray appearance is almost identical to that seen in tetralogy of Fallot. There is a concave pulmonary artery segment. The pulmonary vascular markings are either at the lower limits of normal or decreased in size.

4. Group 2b—X-ray shows slight cardiac enlargement with a marked bulge of the pulmonary artery segment. The pulmonary vascular markings are prominent at the hilum and decreased in the periphery.

5. Group 2c—There is marked cardiac enlargement involving all 4 chambers. The pulmonary artery segment might be slightly larger than normal. The pulmonary vascular markings are markedly increased.

C. Electrocardiography: In groups 1 and 2a, there is right axis deviation and right ventricular hypertrophy. In groups 2b and 2c, combined right and left ventricular hypertrophy or pure left ventricular hypertrophy is often present.

D. Cardiac Catheterization and Cineangiocardiography: Both catheterization and cineangiocardiography are usually necessary to identify the exact abnormalities that exist, and this should be done before severe symptoms and signs develop. It is usually easy to manipulate the catheter through the defect in the atrial septum into the left side of the heart, and in most cases 4 chambers can be entered. In patients with ventricular septal defects, it is possible to enter both the ascending aorta and the pulmonary artery.

Occasionally it is difficult to distinguish transposition from other types of cyanotic congenital heart disease (eg, tetralogy of Fallot from transposition group 2a).

Treatment

The treatment depends upon the associated intracardiac abnormalities. Until recently, only palliative surgical treatment was available. However, a procedure (Mustard operation) has been developed which totally corrects the defect in some cases.

A. Palliative Treatment:

1. Group 1a—Patients with transposition benefit from mixing of blood across the atrial septum. Those with high flow require venting of the atrial septum to reduce left atrial pressure. A closed chest procedure (the Rashkind septostomy) is preferred by many cardiologists. This is performed at the time of cardiac catheterization by pulling a dye-inflated balloon across the foramen ovale, tearing the septum primum. An open chest surgical septostomy (Blalock-Hanlon operation) is preferred by others.

2. Group 1b—Subvalvular pulmonary obstruction has been noted to develop in a number of patients several months following the performance of a balloon atrial septostomy. If severe hypoxemia develops and the child is too small to have total correction of the defect, a systemic to pulmonary artery anastomosis is indicated.

3. Group 2a—If severe hypoxemia develops, a systemic arterial to pulmonary anastomosis should be performed in addition to the atrial balloon septostomy performed at diagnostic cardiac catheterization.

4. Group 2b—Venting of the left atrium through an atrial septostomy may provide some improvement in mixing and pressure reduction.

5. Group 2c—If severe congestive heart failure occurs because of marked overload of the pulmonary bed, vigorous anticongestive measures should be instituted. A pulmonary artery banding procedure to decrease pulmonary blood flow may be considered in addition to atrial septostomy.

B. Complete Correction: The best candidates for complete surgical correction are patients who have intact ventricular septums and in whom large atrial septal defects are created in early life. The Mustard operation involves complete removal of the atrial septum and rearrangement of the septum with the use of pericardium so that the systemic veins are directed into the mitral valve and the pulmonary veins are directed into the tricuspid valve. This procedure has been quite successful in patients with intact ventricular septums and relatively normal pulmonary vascular resistance. It has been less successful in patients with other intracardiac abnormalities and in those who have irreversible lesions within the pulmonary vascular bed.

Course & Prognosis

Patients in groups 1a and 2c usually develop congestive heart failure early in life; without treatment, death occurs usually between 1 month and 6 months of age.

Patients in group 2a usually do best. If there is a good balance between the pulmonary stenosis and the ventricular septal defect, they can function similarly to those with tetralogy of Fallot. Some patients have been known to survive until the second or third decade or even later. However, patients with severe pulmonary stenosis and markedly diminished pulmonary blood flow have anoxic spells very early in life and die with severe hypoxia.

Patients in group 2b category usually develop severe pulmonary vascular obstruction in early life (2–3 years) and eventually die of congestive heart failure or pulmonary hemorrhage.

Danielson GK & others: Repair of transposition of the great arteries by transposition of the venous return. J Thoracic Cardiovas Surg 61:96, 1971.

Deverall PB & others: Palliative surgery in children with transposition of the great arteries. J Thoracic Cardiovas Surg 58:721, 1969.

Plauth WH Jr & others: Changing hemodynamics in patients with transposition of the great arteries. Circulation 42:137, 1970.

Rashkind WJ, Miller WW: Transposition of the great arteries: Results of balloon atrio-septostomy in 31 infants. Circulation 38:453, 1968.

Tynan MJ & others: Subvalvular pulmonary obstruction complicating the postoperative course of balloon atrial septostomy in transporition of the great arteries. Circulation 39(Suppl 1):223, 1969.

Waldhausen JA & others: Physiologic correction of transposition of the great arteries. Circulation 43:738, 1971.

Treatment consists of total correction which is moderately risky but can be done if the diagnosis is made prior to surgery.

Gomes MMR & others: Double-outlet right ventricle with pulmonic stenosis: Surgical considerations and results of operation. Circulation 43:889, 1971.

Gomes MMR & others: Double-outlet right ventricle without pulmonic stenosis: Surgical considerations and results of operation. Circulation 43(Suppl 1):31, 1971.

Hightower BM & others: Double-outlet right ventricle with transposition of the great arteries and subpulmonary ventricular septal defect: The Taussig-Bing malformation. Circulation 39(Suppl 1):207, 1969.

Neuufeld HN & others: Origin of both great vessels from the right ventricle. 1. Without pulmonary stenosis. 2. With pulmonary stenosis. Circulation 23:399, 630, 1961.

Neufeld HN & others: Origin of both great vessels from the right ventricle without pulmonary stenosis. Brit Heart J 24:393, 1962.

Patrick DL, McGoon DC: Operation for double-outlet right ventricle with transposition of the great arteries. J Cardiovas Surg 9:537, 1968.

ORIGIN OF BOTH GREAT VESSELS FROM THE RIGHT VENTRICLE

In this rare malformation, the aorta is completely transposed but the pulmonary artery occupies a relatively normal position. Accordingly, both great vessels arise from the right ventricle. Ventricular septal defect is present in all cases and provides the only outlet for the left ventricle.

This malformation may be divided into 2 types depending on the presence or absence of valvular pulmonary stenosis.

With Pulmonary Stenosis

Patients with double outlet right ventricle and valvular pulmonary stenosis function very much like those with severe tetralogy of Fallot. There is marked decrease in pulmonary blood flow and marked desaturation of the systemic arterial blood.

Early palliative treatment involves the construction of a systemic to pulmonary artery anastomosis in order to increase pulmonary blood flow. Definitive surgical correction is now being successfully employed in selected patients.

Without Pulmonary Stenosis

When the pulmonary valve is normal and there is no obstruction to flow into the pulmonary artery, the condition may be very difficult to differentiate from a large ventricular septal defect with normal origin of the great vessels. Because of the marked increase in pulmonary blood flow, arterial blood saturation is usually around 90% and cyanosis is not present. The diagnosis is usually made by cardiac catheterization and cineangiocardiography. In some cases the diagnosis is made at surgery.

TOTAL ANOMALOUS PULMONARY VENOUS RETURN WITH OR WITHOUT INCREASED PULMONARY VASCULAR RESISTANCE

Essentials of Diagnosis

No obstruction to pulmonary venous drainage; normal pulmonary vascular resistance:

- Mild cyanosis from early infancy.
- Hyperactive heart.
- Right ventricular lift; S_2 widely split and fixed.
- Grade II–IV/VI pulmonic ejection murmur with wide radiation.
- Tricuspid diastolic flow murmur at lower left sternal border.

Obstruction to pulmonary venous return or increased pulmonary vascular resistance:

- Severe cyanosis.
- Tachypnea and heart failure, usually in early infancy.
- Small heart.
- P_2 loud and single.
- Insignificant murmur.

General Considerations

This malformation accounts for approximately 2% of all congenital heart lesions. The pulmonary venous blood does not drain into the left atrium but either directly or indirectly (via a systemic venous connection) into the right atrium. Thus, the entire venous drainage of the body drains into the right atrium.

This malformation may be classified according to the site of entry of the pulmonary veins into the right side of the heart.

Type 1 (55%): Entry into the left superior vena cava (persistent anterior cardinal vein) or right superior vena cava.

Type 2: Entry into the right atrium or into the coronary sinus.

Type 3: Entry below the diaphragm (usually into the portal vein).

Type 4: Multiple types of entry.

Since the entire venous drainage from the body drains into the right atrium, a right-to-left shunt is always present at the atrial level. This may take the form either of a large atrial septal defect or a patent foramen ovale. Relatively complete mixing of the systemic and pulmonary venous return occurs in the right atrium so that the left atrial and hence the systemic arterial saturation is approximately equal that of the right atrial saturation.

The degree of saturation of the blood (and thus the degree of cyanosis present) is determined by the ratio of the quantity of pulmonary blood flow to that of the systemic blood flow. If pulmonary vascular resistance is normal, the flow of blood into the pulmonary artery is much greater than that into the left side of the heart. In this case, there is much greater return from the pulmonary than from the systemic venous system, and the saturation within the right atrium is high. These patients function very well, with relatively normal pulmonary artery pressures, and at least physiologically are very similar to patients with very large atrial septal defects and normal pulmonary venous return.

If pulmonary vascular resistance is elevated, the ratio of pulmonary to systemic blood flow is much lower. When the pulmonary vascular resistance equals that of the systemic vascular resistance, equal amounts of blood flow in both directions. When this occurs, marked desaturation of the mixed blood develops and the patient is markedly cyanotic. Such patients do much less well, and eventually develop severe right heart failure.

Clinical Findings

A. With Normal Pulmonary Vascular Resistance: The great majority of these patients have some elevation of the pulmonary artery pressure due to the marked increase in pulmonary blood flow. In most cases, the pressure does not reach systemic levels.

1. Symptoms and signs—These patients may have a history of mild cyanosis in the neonatal period and during early infancy. Thereafter, they do relatively well except for frequent respiratory infections. They are usually rather small and thin, and resemble patients with very large atrial septal defects.

Careful examination discloses duskiness of the nail beds and mucous membranes, but definite cyanosis and clubbing are usually not present. The arterial pulses are normal. The jugular venous pulses usually show a significant V wave. Examination of the heart shows left chest prominence. A right ventricular heaving impulse is palpable. On auscultation, the first heart sound is normal to moderately increased in intensity. The second sound is widely split and fixed. Frequently there is a third or fourth heart sound, producing a quadruple or quintuple rhythm. The pulmonary component of the second sound is usually normal in intensity. A grade II–IV/VI ejection type systolic murmur is heard at the pulmonary area. It radiates very well over the lung fields anteriorly and posteriorly. An early to mid diastolic flow murmur is often heard at the lower left sternal border in the third and fourth intercostal spaces (tricuspid flow murmur).

2. X-ray findings—Chest x-ray reveals evidence of cardiac enlargement primarily involving the right atrium, right ventricle, and pulmonary artery. There is a marked increase in pulmonary vascular markings. There is often a specific contour also. The most characteristic contour is the so-called snowman or figure of 8, which is seen when the anomalous veins drain into a persistent left superior vena cava. This produces marked enlargement of the superior mediastinum and results in the characteristic contour.

3. Electrocardiography—ECG reveals right axis deviation and varying degrees of right atrial and right ventricular hypertrophy. There is often a qR pattern over the right precordial leads.

B. With Increased Pulmonary Vascular Resistance: This group includes those patients in which the pulmonary veins drain into a systemic venous structure below the diaphragm. It also includes a large number of patients in whom the venous drainage is into a systemic vein above the diaphragm.

1. Symptoms and signs—These infants are usually quite sick. Half die within the first 6 months; most are dead by age 1 unless treated surgically. Cyanosis is common at birth and is quite evident by 1 week. Another common early symptom is severe tachypnea. Congestive heart failure develops later.

Cardiac examination discloses a striking right ventricular impulse. A shock of the second sound is palpable. The first heart sound is accentuated. The second heart sound is markedly accentuated and single. A grade I–II/VI ejection type systolic murmur is frequently heard over the pulmonary area with radiation over the lung fields. Diastolic murmurs are uncommon. In many cases no murmur is heard at all.

2. X-ray findings—In the most severe and classic cases, the heart is small and pulmonary venous congestion is marked. In less severe cases, the heart may be slightly enlarged or normal in size, with only slight pulmonary venous congestion.

3. Electrocardiography—ECG shows right axis deviation, right atrial hypertrophy, and right ventricular hypertrophy.

4. Cardiac catheterization and cineangiocardiography—These procedures are diagnostic. Cardiac catheterization demonstrates the presence of total anomalous pulmonary venous return and (usually) the site of entry of the anomalous veins. It also demonstrates the ratio of the pulmonary to systemic blood flow and the degree of pulmonary hypertension and pulmonary vascular resistance.

Cineangiocardiography following injection of contrast material into the right ventricle or pulmonary artery demonstrates the presence of anomalous pulmonary venous return and the site of entry of the anomalous veins.

Treatment

Treatment is surgical. The success of surgery depends upon the degree of pulmonary vascular resistance. Patients with normal pulmonary arterial pressure do best. They can be operated on under cardiopulmonary bypass when they are large emough to withstand the procedure. The type of operation depends upon the site of entry of the pulmonary venous return into the systemic bed.

Infants with severe pulmonary hypertension, heart failure, or hypoxemia require diagnostic evaluation and treatment during early infancy. An atrial balloon septostomy is indicated during cardiac catheterization, since frequently the foramen ovale is very small and prevents adequate right-to-left shunting across the atrial septum. This procedure often causes an immediate reduction in symptoms, but in most cases it must be followed by definitive surgical correction. Until recently, the surgical mortality in this age group was greater than 90%. Within the past few years, however, certain centers have reported excellent results employing either cardiopulmonary bypass or extreme hypothermia (cooling to 20° C).

Course & Prognosis

Patients with normal pulmonary vascular resistance and only modest elevation of pulmonary artery pressures may do quite well through the second or third decade. Eventually, however, progressive increase in pulmonary vascular resistance and pulmonary hypertension does occur.

Patients with increased pulmonary vascular resistance and pulmonary hypertension do poorly, and most die unless treated before age 1.

Barratt-Boyes BG, Simpson M, Neutze JM: Intracardiac surgery in neonates and infants using deep hypothermia with surface cooling and limited cardiopulmonary bypass. Circulation 43(Suppl 1):25, 1971.

Gathman GE, Nadas AS: Total anomalous pulmonary venous connection: Clinical and physiologic observations of 75 pediatric patients. Circulation 42:143, 1970.

Gersony WM & others: Management of total anomalous pulmonary venous drainage in early infancy. Circulation 43(Suppl 1):19, 1971.

Gomes MMR & others: Total anomalous pulmonary venous connection: Surgical considerations and results of operation. J Thoracic Cardiovas Surg 60:116, 1970.

Leachman RD & others: Total anomalous pulmonary venous return. Ann Thoracic Surg 7:5, 1969.

Miller WW & others: Total anomalous pulmonary venous return: Effective palliation of critically ill infants by balloon atrial septostomy. (Abstract.) Circulation 35, 36(Suppl 2):189, 1967.

PERSISTENT TRUNCUS ARTERIOSUS

Essentials of Diagnosis

- Cyanosis from early infancy.
- Heart failure frequent in childhood.
- Systolic thrill at lower left sternal border.
- Loud single S_2.
- Grade II–IV/VI, long systolic murmur at lower left sternal border.
- Diastolic flow murmur at apex frequent.

General Considerations

Persistent truncus arteriosus probably accounts for less than 1% of all congenital heart malformations. Only one (huge) great vessel arises from the heart and supplies both the systemic and pulmonary arterial beds. It develops embryologically as a result of complete lack of formation of the spiral ridges that divide the fetal truncus arteriosus into the aorta and pulmonary artery. A high ventricular septal defect is always present. The number of valve leaflets varies from 2–6.

The classification most commonly employed is into 4 types:

Type 1: One pulmonary artery which arises from the base of the trunk just above the semilunar valve and runs parallel with the ascending aorta (48%).

Type 2: Two pulmonary arteries which arise side by side from the posterior aspect of the truncus (29%).

Type 3: Two pulmonary arteries which arise independently from either side of the trunk (11%).

Type 4: No demonstrable pulmonary artery (12%). Pulmonary circulation is derived from bronchials arising from the descending thoracic aorta. (The existence of this variety of truncus is controversial. Many authorities consider it an extreme form of tetralogy of Fallot with an atretic main pulmonary artery.)

In this condition, blood leaves the heart through a single common exit. Therefore, the saturation of the blood in the pulmonary artery is the same as that in the systemic arteries. The degree of systemic arterial oxygen saturation depends upon the ratio of the pulmonary to systemic blood flow. If pulmonary vascular resistance is normal, the pulmonary blood flow is much greater than the systemic blood flow and the saturation is relatively high. If pulmonary vascular resistance is great, due either to pulmonary vascular obstruction or to very small pulmonary arteries, pulmonary blood flow is reduced and oxygen saturation is low. The systolic pressures in both ventricles are identical to that in the aorta.

Clinical Findings

A. Symptoms and Signs: The clinical picture varies depending upon the degree of pulmonary blood flow.

1. Large pulmonary blood flow—These patients do well and are usually acyanotic, though the nail beds are commonly dusky. They function similarly to patients with large ventricular septal defects and pulmonary hypertension. Examination of the heart reveals a hyperactive impulse, felt both at the apex and over the xiphoid process. A systolic thrill is common at the lower left sternal border. The first heart sound is normal. The second sound is single and accentuated. A grade IV/VI, completely pansystolic murmur is audible at the lower left sternal border. A diastolic flow murmur can often be heard at the apex (mitral flow murmur).

2. **Decreased pulmonary blood flow**—These patients have marked cyanosis early and do very poorly. The most common manifestations include retardation of growth and development, easy fatigability, dyspnea on exertion, and congestive heart failure. The heart is not unduly active. The first and second heart sounds are loud. A systolic grade II–IV/VI murmur is heard at the lower left sternal border. No diastolic flow murmur is heard. A continuous heart murmur is very uncommon except in type 4, in which the continuous murmur is due to the large bronchial collateral vessels.

B. X-Ray Findings: Most commonly there is a boot-shaped heart, absence of the main pulmonary artery segment, and a large aorta which frequently arches to the right. The pulmonary vascular markings vary depending upon the degree of pulmonary blood flow.

C. Electrocardiography: The axis is usually normal, though left axis deviation occurs rarely. Evidence of right ventricular hypertrophy or combined ventricular hypertrophy is commonly present. Left ventricular hypertrophy as an isolated finding is rare.

D. Cineangiocardiography: This procedure is usually diagnostic. Injection of contrast material into the right ventricle demonstrates the presence of a ventricular septal defect and the single vessel arising from the heart. The exact type of truncus, however, may be difficult to determine even from cineangiocardiograms. It may be impossible to differentiate this condition from pulmonary atresia and ventricular septal defect (pseudo-truncus).

Treatment

Anticongestive measures and, in some cases, banding of the pulmonary artery are indicated for patients with high pulmonary blood flow and congestive failure. Aortic homografting for "total correction" of the truncus in selected patients is an exciting new therapeutic development.

Course & Prognosis

The outcome depends to a great extent upon the status of the pulmonary circulation. Patients with a low pulmonary blood flow usually do very poorly and die within 1 year. Those with increased pulmonary blood flow can survive for a variable period. A few cases of survival into the third decade have been reported. Death is usually due to congestive heart failure, hypoxia, subacute bacterial endocarditis, or brain abscess.

Becker AE, Becker MJ, Edwards JE: Pathology of the semilunar valve in persistent truncus arteriosus. J Thoracic Cardiovas Surg 62:16, 1971.

McGoon DC, Rastélli GC, Ongley PA: An operation for the correction of truncus arteriosus. JAMA 205:69, 1968.

Tandon E, Hauck AJ, Nadas AS: Persistent truncus arteriosus: A clinical, hemodynamic, and autopsy study of nineteen cases. Circulation 28:1050, 1963.

Van Praagh R, Van Praagh S: The anatomy of the common aortic-pulmonary trunk (truncus arteriosus communis) and its embryologic implications. Am J Cardiol 16:406, 1965.

Victorica BE & others: Persistent truncus arteriosus in infancy: A study of 14 cases. Am Heart J 77:13, 1969.

Wallace RB & others: Complete repair of truncus arteriosus defects. J Thoracic Cardiovas Surg 57:95, 1969.

DEXTROCARDIA

This lesion consists of right-sided heart with or without reversal of position of other organs (situs inversus). If there is no reversal of other organs, the heart usually has other severe defects. With complete situs inversus, the heart is usually normal.

Apical pulse and sounds are heard on the right side of the chest. X-ray shows the cardiac silhouette on the right side. On ECG, the P waves are usually inverted in lead I; QRS is predominantly down in lead I; lead II resembles normal lead III and vice versa.

With situs inversus and no heart defects, the prognosis is excellent. If severe heart defects are present, definitive diagnosis is imperative since corrective surgery is frequently beneficial.

Arcilla RA, Gasul BM: Congenital dextrocardia: Clinical, angiographic and autopsy studies on 50 patients. J Pediat 58:39, 1961.

Cooley DA, Billig DM: Surgical repair of congenital cardiac lesions in mirror-image dextrocardia with situs inversus totalis. Am J Cardiol 11:518, 1963.

Grant RP: The syndrome of dextroversion of the heart. Circulation 18:25, 1958.

Van Praagh R & others: Anatomic types of congenital dextrocardia: Diagnostic and embryologic implications. Am J Cardiol 13:510, 1964.

Van Praagh R & others: Diagnosis of the anatomic types of congenital dextrocardia. Am J Cardiol 15:234, 1965.

ACQUIRED HEART DISEASE

ACUTE RHEUMATIC FEVER

Although acute rheumatic fever has been declining in incidence during the last few decades, it is still an extremely important cause of heart disease in children and adolescents. Rheumatic fever is thought to be a connective tissue disorder resulting from a hypersensitivity reaction to one or more antigenic components or metabolic products of the beta-hemolytic streptococcus.

Jones Criteria (Revised) for Guidance in the
          Diagnosis of Rheumatic Fever
Major Manifestations
          Carditis.
          Polyarthritis.
          Sydenham's chorea.
          Erythema marginatum.
          Subcutaneous nodules.

Minor Manifestations
          Clinical
                    Previous rheumatic fever or rheumatic
                              heart disease.
                    Polyarthralgia.
                    Fever.
          Laboratory
                    Acute phase reactions: elevated
                              erythrocyte sedimentation rate,
                              C-reactive protein, leukocytosis.
                    Prolonged P–R interval.

Plus

Supporting evidence of preceding streptococcal
infection, ie, increased ASO or other streptococcal antibodies; positive throat culture for group A
streptococcus; recent scarlet fever.

Two major manifestations or one major and 2
minor manifestations are strongly indicative of rheumatic fever if evidence of a preceding streptococcal
infection is present. Without such evidence, the diagnosis is doubtful, except when rheumatic fever is first
discovered after a long latent period (eg, Sydenham's
chorea or low-grade carditis).

Predisposing Factors
    A. Family History: There is evidence that familial
predisposition and heredity play a role in susceptibility
to the development of acute rheumatic fever.
    B. Age: Rheumatic fever most commonly occurs
between the ages of 5 and 15 years. The peak incidence is at about age 8. Rheumatic fever is extremely
uncommon under the age of 2 and rare between the
ages of 2 and 5. Recurrences are more likely to occur
in childhood and are rare after age 20. Recurrences are
most likely within the first year following the initial
attack; the longer the patient can go without a recurrence, the more likely that none will occur.
    C. Economic Status: Rheumatic fever occurs
more commonly in the lower socioeconomic groups,
probably because of crowded living conditions and
poor hygiene.
    D. Season: The peak incidence occurs during late
winter and early spring. This is related to the peak
incidence of beta-hemolytic streptococcal infections.
The lowest incidence occurs in August and September.
    E. Climate: The disease is slightly more common
in the temperate zone than in tropical or subtropical
areas.
    F. Previous Attacks: Recurrences of rheumatic
fever following reinfection with beta-hemolytic strep-

tococci are frequent (30%) in children who have had a
prior episode of acute rheumatic fever. Only a few
cases (0.3–3%) of initial attacks of acute rheumatic
fever occur as a complication of all cases of beta-
hemolytic streptococcal infections.

General Considerations
    Rheumatic fever is not a reportable condition in
the USA, and it is difficult to détermine its incidence
accurately. Where rheumatic fever is reportable, the
incidence varies from 3–30 per 10,000 persons.
    Although the association of acute rheumatic fever
and group A beta-hemolytic streptococcal infection
has been well established, the pathogenesis of the disease is still essentially unknown. Furthermore, a specific diagnostic test has not yet been developed.
Accordingly, the diagnosis of acute rheumatic fever
must be made purely on clinical grounds. The physician who makes this diagnosis today assumes a grave
responsibility in view of the intensive treatment program frequently employed during the acute phase and
the institution of an effective and prolonged prophylactic regimen. To help minimize errors, T. Duckett
Jones in 1944 published criteria for guidance and the
diagnosis of acute rheumatic fever. These criteria, as
subsequently modified, are generally accepted in the
USA and elsewhere. The presence of 2 major criteria or
one major and 2 minor criteria indicates a high possibility of acute rheumatic fever. Certainly, there are
some patients with acute rheumatic fever who do not
meet the criteria. Fortunately, these are few, and the
prognosis is usually excellent even when prophylaxis is
not instituted. In most cases, however, it is recommended that the diagnosis of acute rheumatic fever be
restricted to illnesses which meet the modified Jones
criteria.

Major Manifestations of Rheumatic Fever
    A. Active Carditis:
    1. Significant new murmur–(a) Murmur of aortic
insufficiency, short decrescendo, diastolic murmur at
third intercostal space, left sternal border. (b) Murmur
of mitral insufficiency; holosystolic murmur at the
apex. (c) Mid-diastolic murmur at apex.
    2. Pericarditis–Pericardial friction rub or evidence
of pericardial effusion.
    3. Evidence of congestive heart failure.
    4. Evidence of a progressively enlarging heart.
    B. Polyarthritis: Two or more joints must be in-
volved; involvement of one joint does not meet the
criterion. The joints may be involved simultaneously or
in a migratory fashion. The most commonly involved
joints are the ankles, knees, hips, wrists, elbows, and
shoulders. Heat, redness, swelling, severe pain, and tenderness are usually all present. Arthralgia alone without the other signs of inflammation is not sufficient to
meet the criterion.
    C. Subcutaneous Nodules: These appear usually
in severe cases. They are seen most commonly over the
joints, scalp, and spinal column. They vary from a few
mm to 2 cm in diameter. They are nontender and
freely movable under the skin.

D. Erythema Marginatum: This is a specific and major manifestation of acute rheumatic fever. It usually occurs in the most severe cases. It is a macular erythematous rash with a circinate border appearing primarily on the trunk and extremities. The face is usually not involved.

E. Sydenham's Chorea: There is controversy about whether chorea is a manifestation of acute rheumatic fever. This is because it usually occurs alone, without other findings of acute rheumatic fever and without positive laboratory findings. However, since 50–75% of patients with chorea demonstrate other manifestations of acute rheumatic fever at some time before or after the appearance of the chorea, it is felt by most authorities that this is a major manifestation of acute rheumatic fever. In fact, even though it exists by itself without another major manifestation and without other manifestations, it should probably be considered as an attack of acute rheumatic fever.

Sydenham's chorea occurs most commonly in girls between the ages of 8 and 12. It is characterized by the onset of emotional disturbances followed by the development of emotional instability and involuntary movements. These findings become progressively more severe and are often followed by the development of ataxia and slurring of speech. Muscular weakness becomes apparent following the onset of the involuntary movements.

The individual attack of chorea is self-limiting, although it may last up to 3 months. It is not uncommon to find involvement only on one side (hemichorea).

Minor Manifestations of Rheumatic Fever

A. Fever: Usually the fever is low-grade, although occasionally it reaches 39.4–40° C (103–104° F).

B. Polyarthralgia: Polyarthralgia cannot be considered a minor manifestation if polyarthritis is included under the major manifestations.

C. ECG Changes: These include prolongation of the P–R interval, and prolongation of the Q–T_c interval. These ECG abnormalities represent only minor manifestations and do not indicate active carditis.

D. Abnormal Blood Tests: The sedimentation rate is accelerated. The white count is elevated, showing a variable polymorphonuclear leukocytosis. C-reactive protein and gamma globulin are elevated. The serum mucoprotein tyrosine level is elevated. A mild to moderate degree of anemia (normochromic and normocytic) is usually present.

E. Bacteriologic Study: Presence of beta-hemolytic streptococci on throat culture or elevation of ASO titer (250 Todd units or higher).

F. History: A prior history of acute rheumatic fever or the presence of inactive rheumatic heart disease.

In addition to the findings listed above, associated manifestations are often present. These include erythema multiforme; abdominal, back and precordial pain; nontraumatic epistaxis, vomiting, malaise, and weight loss.

In approximately 50% of cases there is a history of an upper respiratory infection, including fever and sore throat. However, in the other 50%, no specific complaints are noted prior to the onset of the findings of acute rheumatic fever.

Treatment

A. Corticosteroids Versus Salicylates: In 1949, Hench and his associates demonstrated that ACTH and cortisone were of substantial value in the treatment of rheumatoid arthritis and other hypersensitivity states. Since then, there has been considerable controversy concerning the effectiveness of the corticosteroids in the treatment of acute rheumatic fever, especially with regard to the prevention of residual valvular damage. This controversy has been at least partly related to the lack of adequate controls in some of the reports and the grouping together of patients presenting with widely varying manifestations of acute rheumatic fever.

The corticosteroids are of significant value and unequivocally superior to the salicylates in the critically ill patient with congestive heart failure. Such patients respond remarkably well to the institution of corticosteroids, and these drugs are frequently life-saving. Congestive heart failure is usually brought under control within 1–2 days without digitalis and other anticongestive measures. The high fever and the marked malaise and anorexia rapidly disappear. Corticosteroid therapy is strongly recommended in all patients with evidence of congestive heart failure. The dosage is as follows: prednisone, 2–3 mg/kg orally (or cortisone, 10–15 mg/kg orally), for 4–6 weeks. The drug is then withdrawn gradually over the next 2–4 weeks. Aspirin, 100 mg/kg daily orally, may be employed during the last 2 weeks to prevent the "rebound" phenomenon.

When corticosteroids are administered, dietary salt should be restricted and potassium given in the form of orange juice or saturated solution.

The physician should be aware of all the possible complications of corticosteroid therapy. Development of a cushingoid state characterized by "moon" facies cannot be considered a complication since it occurs in almost all patients.

For most patients with rheumatic carditis who are not critically ill, corticosteroids are not superior to salicylates in the prevention of residual cardiac damage. There is still considerable controversy, however, about whether corticosteroids alter the natural history of the disease and prevent residual valvular damage. If corticosteroids are to be employed, they must be started early—within 2 weeks of the development of carditis—and probably should be continued for 6–10 weeks.

For patients with acute rheumatic fever without carditis (except in cases of chorea), there is no justification for the use of corticosteroids. Salicylates have been found to be essentially as effective in suppressing the acute inflammatory reaction within the joints, and no permanent damage to the joints develops as a sequel to acute rheumatic fever. The recommended dosage is 60 mg/lb for the first 4–6 weeks in divided doses. The total dose should not exceed 10 gm/day. Following this period of time, the dosage should be gradually reduced. If evidence of the rebound phenomenon appears, (fever, arthritis, increased sedimentation rate), salicylates should be restarted and continued for another 2–4 weeks.

B. Digitalis Therapy: If congestive heart failure persists despite large doses of corticosteroids, digitalis should be administered under careful ECG and clinical control. Patients with carditis may be very sensitive to digitalis, so that doses smaller than those usually given should be administered. Other anticongestive measures such as diuretics and low-salt diets are useful adjuncts. Since corticosteroids and diuretics cause potassium depletion, potassium should be administered—especially since digitalis intoxication is more likely to develop in patients with low serum and intracellular potassium levels.

C. Antibiotics: Although only ½ of patients with acute rheumatic fever grow out beta-hemolytic streptococci on throat culture, all patients should be treated with a full therapeutic course of penicillin, eg, 0.8–1.2 million units of penicillin G daily orally in divided doses, or one injection of benzathine penicillin, 0.6–1.2 million units.

D. Activity: Until recently, patients with acute rheumatic fever with or without carditis were placed at bed rest for periods ranging from several months to several years. There is no convincing evidence that such treatment was of any value, and the tendency now is to get these patients out of bed much earlier. Patients who are toxic, with painful joints, congestive heart failure, or pericarditis, should be kept in bed. However, these patients improve dramatically with anti-inflammatory drugs.

There is no specific time when activity should be resumed. Patients with active carditis should not be called upon to unnecessarily increase their cardiac output. However, sitting in a chair watching television may be more beneficial than restless confinement in bed. When signs of cardiac involvement have stabilized, progressively increasing activity should be permitted. Patients without carditis should be ambulated much more rapidly.

Prophylactic Treatment

Following the completion of the full therapeutic course of penicillin, all patients should be placed on a prophylactic regimen. This consists of the administration of a single monthly injection of benzathine penicillin, oral penicillin, or an oral sulfonamide drug. Recent studies show that benzathine penicillin is slightly more effective than the other 2 drugs in preventing recurrences of rheumatic fever. However, because of the pain associated with the injection, most pediatricians prefer oral penicillin or an oral sulfonamide.

The recommended dosage schedule is as follows:
>Benzathine penicillin, 0.6–1.2 million units IM.
>
>Oral penicillin, 200–400 thousand units/day.
>
>Oral sulfonamide, 0.5–1 gm/day.

Course & Prognosis

Four different patterns of first attacks of acute rheumatic fever have been described. (See Feinstein & Spagnuolo reference.) The most common pattern was that in which the patient sought help for febrile monarticular or polyarticular arthritis. About 30% of these patients had carditis. In the second pattern, the patients sought help primarily because of polyarthralgia. In these, carditis was likely to be more severe than in those with arthritis. In the third pattern, patients developed chorea. Heart murmurs were rare and joint involvement very uncommon. Laboratory evidence of inflammation was seldom found because the chorea often occurred 2–6 months after the initial infection. In the fourth pattern, which rarely came to medical attention, the patients had carditis without involvement of the joints. It is these patients in which pure mitral stenosis is common. Pure mitral stenosis was found to be rare in those patients who had recognizable symptoms and signs during their acute episode. Recurrent attacks of acute rheumatic fever were more frequent in patients with previous valvular damage. Therefore, cardiac involvement was noted to be more common in recurrences of rheumatic fever than in the first attack. In the patients with no evidence of carditis in their initial attack, recurrences usually were associated with arthritis or chorea. Recurrences usually involve the same area of the body that was affected during the first attack.

The prognosis depends mainly upon the degree of residual cardiac damage following the initial attack and the presence or absence of recurrences of carditis. Patients who show no evidence of carditis in their initial attack and who receive prophylactic treatment should have a normal life span. Patients with residual cardiac damage have a varying course depending upon the severity and type of valvular damage.

Initial attacks of acute rheumatic fever—even those which are severe and associated with congestive heart failure—rarely result in death if corticosteroids are given.

Ad Hoc Committee of the Council on Rheumatic Fever and Congenital Heart Disease: Jones's criteria (revised) for guidance in the diagnosis of rheumatic fever. Circulation 32:664, 1965.

Cooperative Rheumatic Fever Study Group: The natural history of rheumatic fever and rheumatic heart disease: Ten-year report of a cooperative clinical trial of ACTH, cortisone, and aspirin. Circulation 32:457, 1965.

Feinstein AR & others: Prophylaxis of recurrent rheumatic fever: Therapeutic continuous oral penicillin vs monthly injections. JAMA 206:565, 1968.

Markowitz M: Eradication of rheumatic fever: An unfulfilled hope. Circulation 41:1077, 1970.

Rheumatic Fever and Rheumatic Heart Disease Study Group: Prevention of rheumatic fever and rheumatic heart disease. Circulation 41:A–1, 1970.

Spagnuolo M & others: Risk of rheumatic recurrences after streptococcal infections. New England J Med 285:641, 1971.

RHEUMATIC HEART DISEASE

Residual cardiac damage resulting from an episode of acute rheumatic fever is limited to involvement of the valves. Although the myocardium and the pericardium may be involved in the acute phase, there is no significant myocardial fibrosis or constrictive pericarditis following recovery.

Although all valves of the heart may be involved, the mitral and aortic valves are by far the most commonly affected. The tricuspid valve is rarely involved, and the pulmonic valve almost never.

Combined mitral insufficiency and mitral stenosis is the rule in adults with mitral valve involvement. However, one or the other usually predominates.

Mitral Insufficiency

The murmur of mitral insufficiency is a common finding in patients with acute rheumatic fever and carditis. However, even when corticosteroids are not given during the acute episode, evidence of mitral insufficiency disappears within 5 years in about 40% of cases.

In patients with persistent mitral insufficiency, the manifestations vary depending upon the severity of involvement. Children and adolescents usually are asymptomatic or show signs of mild exercise intolerance and fatigability. On cardiac examination there is usually evidence of left ventricular hypertrophy; the point of maximal impulse is located in the fifth or sixth intercostal space between the midclavicular line and the anterior axillary line. The left ventricular impulse is heaving. A systolic thrill may or may not be present at the apex. S_1 is soft or absent in more severe cases; it may be relatively normal in very mild cases. S_2 is physiologically split. There is a grade II–IV/VI, high-pitched, pansystolic murmur, heard best at the apex and radiating to the left axilla and to the midaxillary line in the sixth intercostal space.

Mitral Stenosis

This lesion is extremely uncommon in children in the USA. Although mitral stenosis may develop 2 years after the mitral valvulitis, it usually takes much longer to become clinically manifest.

The heart is usually not enlarged. A right ventricular lift is occasionally palpable. In more severe cases, the first sound may be palpated as a shock at the apex. A diastolic thrill is seldom present in children with mitral stenosis, although it is common in adults. On auscultation, S_1 is quite snapping and accentuated. S_2 is usually narrowly split. The pulmonary component may or may not be accentuated. A high-pitched opening snap is often heard at the apex and lower left sternal border. This occurs within 0.1 second after the pulmonary component of S_2. A rumbling, early mid-diastolic murmur is heard at the apex. This develops into a rough, rumbling, crescendo type presystolic murmur which terminates in the booming first sound.

Aortic Valve Involvement

Aortic regurgitation is common in patients with acute rheumatic carditis. In contrast to mitral valve involvement, however, once aortic insufficiency appears, it usually persists. (The aortic insufficiency murmur disappears in only about 5% of cases.) Aortic stenosis secondary to rheumatic carditis is extremely rare in the pediatric age group. If aortic stenosis (even in association with aortic insufficiency) is present in patients under age 20, rheumatic origin should be seriously questioned; aortic stenosis is congenital in the great majority of patients in this age group.

Aortic insufficiency is usually well tolerated for a long period of time. In childhood and adolescence, most patients are asymptomatic. However, in severe aortic insufficiency, syncope, heart failure, and angina may appear. If any of these symptoms develop, the prognosis is usually very poor unless surgery is performed.

The pulses are usually bounding, with a wide pulse pressure. There is left ventricular enlargement, and the point of maximal impulse is between the mid-clavicular line and anterior axillary line. The left ventricular impulse is heaving. No thrill is palpable. S_1 is normal; S_2 at the aortic area is usually decreased. A systolic murmur is usually present even in the absence of aortic stenosis. It is usually grade I–II/VI ejection quality and best heard at the aortic area and at the left sternal border in the third intercostal space. S_2 is followed by a grade I–II/VI, high-pitched, blowing, decrescendo diastolic murmur which is best heard at the left sternal border in the third intercostal space (Erb's point). This murmur usually radiates fairly well down the left sternal border to the fourth and perhaps fifth intercostal spaces. Occasionally it may be heard at the apex. The diastolic murmur may also occasionally be heard in the aortic area (second intercostal space, right sternal border). Frequently, there is a rumbling mid to late diastolic murmur at the apex (Austin Flint murmur).

Complications

Congestive heart failure as a complication of rheumatic heart disease is rare in the pediatric age group. When it occurs it usually represents a recurrence of acute rheumatic fever. However, in patients with severe (especially multiple) valve involvement, heart failure may occur secondary to the mechanical involvement of the valves.

Medical treatment should include all of the anti-congestive measures discussed in the section on congestive heart failure. Patients with mitral valve involvement may be maintained for some time on medical management alone. Patients with aortic insufficiency and heart failure usually do not fare so well, and early surgical intervention is recommended.

Surgical Treatment

The type of surgery performed depends in large measure upon the pathology found at the time of surgery. Most commonly, the valve or valves must be replaced by a prosthesis, though plastic procedures are sometimes possible.

MYOCARDITIS*

Essentials of Diagnosis

- Upper respiratory infection several weeks prior to onset of cardiac symptoms.
- Rapid onset of congestive heart failure or insidious development of heart failure over a number of weeks.
- Signs of right and left heart failure.
- Weak peripheral arterial pulses.
- Poor, muffled heart sounds.
- Gallop rhythm.
- No murmur.

General Considerations

In the great majority of cases, the etiology of myocarditis is not known. However, a number of viral, bacterial, rickettsial, spirochetal, fungal, and parasitic agents have been identified which can cause myocarditis. Severe myocarditis producing signs and symptoms occurs most commonly in acute rheumatic fever, diphtheria, scrub typhus, and Chagas' disease (*Trypanosoma cruzi* infection). Bacteremia, viral pneumonia and encephalitis, and trichinosis may be associated with myocarditis of varying severity.

Clinical Findings

A. Symptoms and Signs: The clinical picture usually falls into 2 separate patterns. In one, there is the sudden onset of congestive heart failure in a patient who had been in relatively good health 12–24 hours previously. These patients are severely ill, with all the symptoms and signs of both right-sided and left-sided congestive heart failure. In the other group, the onset of cardiac findings is much more gradual. There is usually a history of an upper respiratory infection or gastroenteritis 1 month prior to the development of cardiac findings. Following recovery from the initial infection, there is the gradual and progressive development of easy fatigability, dyspnea on exertion, and malaise.

In both groups, the signs of congestive heart failure are usually quite apparent. The skin is pale and gray, and peripheral cyanosis may be present also. The pulses are rapid, weak, and thready. Edema of the face and extremities may be present. Significant cardiomegaly is present, and the left and right ventricular impulses are weak. On auscultation, the heart sounds are very poor, muffled, and distant. Third and fourth heart sounds are common, resulting in a gallop rhythm. Murmurs are usually absent, though a murmur of tri-

cuspid or mitral insufficiency can occasionally be heard. Moist rales are usually present at both lung bases. The liver is enlarged and frequently tender. The level of the jugular venous pulse is elevated.

B. X-Ray Findings: Generalized cardiomegaly involving all 4 chambers of the heart can be seen on x-ray. On fluoroscopy, the cardiac beat is found to be extremely poor, although one can usually see pulsations at the right and left heart borders. There is evidence of moderate to marked pulmonary venous congestion.

C. Electrocardiography: The ECG is variable. Frequently there is evidence of low voltage of the QRS throughout all frontal and precordial leads and depression of the ST segment and inversion of the T waves in leads I, II, and aVF and in the left precordial leads. Arrhythmias are not uncommon, and atrioventricular and intraventricular conduction disturbances may be present. Left ventricular hypertrophy is very rare.

Treatment

A. Digitalis: All patients with clinical findings of myocarditis should be started immediately on digitalis. Because the inflamed myocardium is markedly sensitive to digitalis, only about 2/3 of the usual total digitalizing dose should be employed. During the initial phase of therapy, frequent ECGs should be taken. If serious arrhythmias or other evidence of digitalis intoxication develop, the drug should be stopped and not reinstituted until all evidence of digitalis toxicity has disappeared.

B. Diuretics: Diuretics should be administered after there is evidence of adequate cardiac output and renal function.

Prognosis

The administration of digitalis is usually followed within 12–24 hours by prompt clinical improvement, ie, slowing of the heart rate, disappearance of pulmonary rales, and a decrease in liver size. Evidence of pulmonary congestion on x-ray usually disappears within 2–3 days. However, cardiomegaly may persist for 6 months to 1 year. The ECG may remain abnormal for a varying period of time but usually returns to normal within 1–2 years.

Although most patients respond well to anticongestive treatment, some develop recurrent episodes of congestive heart failure even though they seem to respond well initially to digitalis therapy. These patients have a very poor prognosis and usually die within 3 months to several years after the onset of symptoms. Death is due to severe congestive heart failure secondary to myocardial fibrosis.

Dominguez P, Leindrum BL, Pick A: False "coronary patterns" in the infant electrocardiogram. Circulation 19:409, 1959.

Fine I, Brainerd H, Sokolow M: Myocarditis in acute infectious diseases: A clinical and electrocardiographic study. Circulation 2:859, 1950.

Javett SW & others: Myocarditis in the newborn infant. J Pediat 48:1, 1956.

---

*This discussion will not include patients with rheumatic myocarditis or myocardial involvement secondary to systemic infection elsewhere.

Saphir O: Nonrheumatic inflammatory diseases of the heart: Myocarditis. Pages 784–835 in: *Pathology of the Heart.* Gould SE (editor). Thomas, 1953.

Woodward TE & others: Viral and rickettsial causes of cardiac disease, including the coxsackievirus etiology of pericarditis and myocarditis. Ann Int Med 53:1130, 1960.

BACTERIAL ENDOCARDITIS

Bacterial infection of the endocardial surface of the heart or the intimal surface of certain arterial vessels (coarcted segment of aorta and ductus arteriosus) is a rare condition that usually occurs when an abnormality of the heart or great vessels exists. It may develop in a normal heart during the course of septicemia (acute bacterial endocarditis).

Essentials of Diagnosis

- Preexisting organic heart murmur.
- Persistent fever.
- Increasing symptoms of heart disease (ranging from easy fatigability to heart failure).
- Splenomegaly (70%).
- Embolic phenomena (50%).
- Leukocytosis, elevated erythrocyte sedimentation rate, positive blood culture.

1. SUBACUTE BACTERIAL ENDOCARDITIS (SBE)

The incidence of SBE in the general population has been declining since the advent of antibiotics and chemotherapy. It is extremely rare in infants and uncommon in young children. The incidence increases during the second decade of life.

In the pediatric age group, 2/3 of cases of SBE develop in patients with congenital heart disease. The other 1/3 occurs in patients with rheumatic valvular disease. The most common congenital heart lesions predisposing to the development of SBE are patent ductus arteriosus, coarctation of the aorta, bicuspid aortic valve with or without aortic stenosis, ventricular septal defect, and tetralogy of Fallot. It is very rare in patients with atrial septal defects. In rheumatic heart disease, the mitral and the aortic valves are involved.

Streptococcus viridans accounts for about 75% of cases of SBE in the pediatric age group. *Streptococcus faecalis* (enterococcus) and staphylococci are responsible for 20% of cases. Other organisms that may be involved include *Escherichia coli,* pneumococci, beta-hemolytic streptococci, and pseudomonas.

Clinical Findings

A. History: Almost all patients have a history of heart disease. There may or may not be a history of infection or a surgical procedure (tooth extraction, tonsillectomy).

B. Symptoms, Signs, and Laboratory Findings: In one large study, the following symptoms, signs, and laboratory findings were reported (in order of decreasing frequency):

1. Murmurs (100%).
2. Fever (91%), ranging between 38.3–39.4° C (101–103° F), with considerable daily fluctuation.
3. Weight loss (83%).
4. Cardiomegaly (83%), which may or may not be associated with congestive heart failure.
5. Anemia (80%). The hemoglobin usually ranges between 8 and 12 gm/100 ml. The anemia is usually normochromic and normocytic.
6. Elevated sedimentation rate (74%).
7. Splenomegaly (70%). The presence of an enlarged spleen is an extremely important diagnostic finding. The spleen is usually quite firm and occasionally tender. Infarction of the spleen is not uncommon.
8. Petechiae (50%). This, too, is an important diagnostic finding. Petechiae are usually widely scattered and are probably due to very small septic emboli. Not infrequently, they are found in the nail beds and retinas.
9. Embolism (50%). Small pieces of vegetation may embolize to various parts of the body, including the brain, spleen, and lungs.
10. Leukocytosis (50%).
11. Other findings include caries, hematuria, signs of congestive heart failure, clubbing, joint pains, and hepatomegaly.

Prevention

The decline in incidence of SBE during the past 2 decades is probably due to the use of prophylactic antibiotics in patients with preexisting heart disease before dental work and other operations. It is therefore recommended that prophylactic penicillin be administered before any type of dental work (tooth extraction, cleaning) or operations within the oropharynx. Febrile infections should be treated with antibiotics for at least 1 week. Continuous antibiotic prophylaxis (as in the treatment of rheumatic fever) is not usually recommended in patients with congenital heart disease.

Treatment

In a patient with known heart disease, the presence of fever of 1 week's duration in combination with either splenomegaly or embolic phenomena justifies a diagnosis of SBE. Several blood cultures should be obtained in the first 24–48 hours. If a positive blood culture is obtained and the organism is identified, specific treatment should be begun immediately. If blood cultures are negative after 48 hours, it is advisable to begin penicillin therapy (unless other diagnostic procedures have ruled out SBE) since most positive cultures are obtained within the first 48 hours. Penicillin is the drug of choice in most cases. Other antibiotics may be added (see Chapter 39). Therapy should be continued for at least 6 weeks.

Course & Prognosis

The prognosis depends upon how early in the course of the infectious process treatment is instituted. Patients treated within 1 month of the onset of symptoms usually do quite well. If the disease is not recognized for 3 months or more, the prognosis is extremely poor. The prognosis is better in patients in whom blood culture is positive. Age is also an important factor; older patients are less likely to recover than younger ones. If congestive heart failure develops, the prognosis is usually poor.

Even though bacteriologic cure of the infectious process is achieved, death may occur as a result of congestive heart failure secondary to severe valvular destruction. Intractable congestive heart failure may occur weeks or months following bacteriologic cure. Embolization may occur following bacteriologic cure when vegetations tear off from the involved area.

2. ACUTE BACTERIAL ENDOCARDITIS (ABE)

Infection of the endocardium in patients without preexisting heart disease may occur during the course of septicemia. A number of cases are occurring in patients who have received recent valve prostheses. Patients with ABE are extremely ill, with evidence of severe sepsis. Involvement of the heart becomes clinically manifest with the development of heart murmurs and cardiomegaly. Involvement of the heart is only part of a total systemic infection. Antibiotic treatment is the same, whether or not there is cardiac involvement.

The mortality rate is very high (approximately 50%). Even if bacteriologic cure is effected, residual cardiac damage is the rule and congestive heart failure and death may result.

American Heart Association: Bacterial endocarditis revisited. Mod Concepts Cardiovas Dis 33:831, 1964.

Committee on Prevention of Rheumatic Fever and Bacterial Endocarditis: Prevention of bacterial endocarditis. Circulation 31:953, 1965.

Cutler JG & others: Bacterial endocarditis in children with heart disease. Pediatrics 22:706, 1958.

Hurley EJ & others: Emergency replacement of valves in endocarditis. Am Heart J 73:798, 1967.

Stasen WR & others: Cardiac surgery in bacterial endocarditis. Circulation 38:514, 1968.

Zakrzewski T, Keith JD: Bacterial endocarditis in infants and children. J Pediat 67:1179, 1965.

PERICARDITIS

Essentials of Diagnosis

- Retrosternal pain made worse by deep inspiration and decreased by leaning forward.
- Fever.
- Shortness of breath and grunting respirations are common.
- Pericardial friction rub.
- Tachycardia.
- Hepatomegaly and distention of the jugular veins.

General Considerations

Involvement of the pericardium rarely occurs as an isolated event. In the great majority of cases, pericardial disease occurs in association with a more generalized process. The most common cause of pericardial involvement in children and adolescents is rheumatic pancarditis. Other important causes include viral pericarditis, purulent pericarditis, rheumatoid arthritis, uremia, and tuberculosis.

In the pediatric age group, pericardial disease usually takes the form of acute pericarditis. In most cases, there is effusion of fluid into the pericardial cavity. The consequences of such effusion depend upon the amount, type, and the speed of fluid accumulation. Under certain circumstances, serious compression of the heart occurs. The direct compression and the body's attempt to correct it result in cardiac tamponade. Unless the pericardial fluid is evacuated, death occurs very rapidly.

Clinical Findings

A. Symptoms and Signs: The symptoms depend to a great extent upon the cause of the pericarditis. Pain is common. It is usually sharp and stabbing, located in the midchest and in the shoulder and neck, made worse by deep inspiration, and considerably decreased by sitting up and leaning forward. Shortness of breath and grunting respirations are common findings in all patients.

The physical findings depend upon whether or not a significant amount of effusion is present: (1) In the absence of significant accumulation of fluid, the pulses are normal and the level of the jugular venous pulse is normal. On examination of the heart, a characteristic scratchy, high-pitched friction rub, may be heard. it is not restricted to any cardiac cycle and is usually located at any point between the apex and the left sternal border. The location and timing vary considerably from time to time. The heart sounds are usually normal, and the heart is not enlarged to percussion. (2) If there is a considerable accumulation of pericardial fluid, the cardiovascular findings are different. The heart is enlarged to percussion but, on inspection of the precordium, seems to be very quiet. Auscultation reveals distant and muffled heart tones. Friction rub is usually not present. In the absence of cardiac tamponade, the peripheral, venous, and arterial pulses are normal.

Cardiac tamponade is characterized by distention of the jugular veins, tachycardia, enlargement of the liver, peripheral edema, and "paradoxic pulse," in which the systolic pressure drops by more than 10 mm Hg during inspiration. The term paradoxic pulse is a misnomer since the drop is only an accentuation of a normal event. (Normally, the systolic pressure drops by no more than 5 mm Hg.) This finding is best determined with the use of a blood pressure cuff. At this point, the patient is critically ill and has all the symptoms and signs suggestive of right-sided congestive heart failure.

Not all patients with marked cardiac compression demonstrate all the findings listed above. If the patient appears critically ill and has evidence of pericarditis and effusion, treatment should be instituted even though all the clinical signs of cardiac tamponade are not present.

B. X-Ray Findings: In pericarditis without effusion, chest x-rays are normal. With pericardial effusion, the cardiac silhouette is enlarged, often in the shape of a water bottle, with blunting of the cardio-diaphragmatic borders. When there is evidence of cardiac tamponade, the lung fields are clear. This is in contrast to patients with myocardial dilatation, who show evidence of pulmonary congestion.

Cardiac fluoroscopy usually demonstrates absence of pulsations of the cardiac borders. This is helpful in differentiating this condition from myocarditis, in which the pulsations, although feeble, are present.

C. Electrocardiography: A number of ECG abnormalities occur in patients with pericarditis. Low voltage is commonly seen in patients with significant pericardial effusion, although the voltage may be normal. The ST segment is commonly elevated during the first week of involvement. The T wave is usually upright during this time. Following this, the ST segment is normal and the T wave becomes flattened. After about 2 weeks, the T wave inverts and remains inverted for several weeks and months. In contrast to patients with myocardial infarction, there is no reciprocal relationship between the findings in lead I and lead III in the frontal plane and the right and left precordial leads.

Treatment

Treatment depends upon the cause of the pericarditis. Cardiac tamponade due to any cause must be treated by evacuation of the fluid. It is usually desirable to perform a wide resection of the pericardium through a surgical incision. However, needle insertion into the pericardial sac may be lifesaving in an emergency situation.

Prognosis

The prognosis depends to a great extent upon the cause of the pericardial disease. Cardiac tamponade due to any cause will result in death unless the fluid is evacuated.

SPECIFIC DISEASES INVOLVING THE PERICARDIUM

Acute Rheumatic Fever

When pericarditis occurs during the course of acute rheumatic fever, it is almost always associated with involvement of the myocardium and endocardium (pancarditis). Thus, heart murmurs are almost always present. The pericarditis is usually of the serofibrinous variety and usually not associated with significant pericardial effusion.

Patients with acute rheumatic fever and pericarditis are usually very ill, with severe cardiac involvement. They respond extremely well to corticosteroid therapy. Pericarditis usually disappears rapidly (1 week) after corticosteroid therapy is started. Constrictive pericarditis almost never occurs secondary to this disease.

Viral Pericarditis

Viral pericarditis is uncommon in children and young adults. The most common cause is the coxsackievirus B4. Influenza virus has also been implicated. There is usually a history of a protracted upper respiratory infection.

The pericardial effusion usually lasts for several weeks. Cardiac tamponade is rare. Recurrences of pericardial effusion are quite common even months or years after the initial episode. Constrictive pericarditis has been reported in this disease.

Purulent Pericarditis

The most common causes of purulent pericarditis are pneumococci, streptococci, staphylococci, *Escherichia coli,* and *Hemophilus influenzae.* This is always secondary to infection elsewhere, although occasionally the primary site is not obvious. In addition to demonstrating signs of cardiac compression, these patients are quite septic and run extremely high fevers. The purulent fluid accumulating within the pericardial sac is usually quite thick and filled with polymorphonuclear leukocytes. Although antibiotics will sterilize the pericardial fluid, pericardial tamponade commonly develops and evacuation of the pericardial sac is usually necessary. Wide resection of the pericardium through a surgical incision performed in the operating room is most desirable. Drainage of the purulent fluid is followed by marked symptomatic improvement.

Bain HW, McLean DM, Walker SJ: Epidemic pleurodynia (Bornholm disease) due to coxsackie B-5 virus: Interrelationship of pleurodynia, benign pericarditis and aseptic meningitis. Pediatrics 27:889, 1961.

Benzing G III, Kaplan S: Purulent pericarditis. Am J Dis Child 106:89, 1963.

Lietman PS, Bywaters EG: Pericarditis in juvenile rheumatoid arthritis. Pediatrics 32:855, 1963.

Nadas AS, Levy JM: Pericarditis in children. Am J Cardiol 7:109, 1961.

Shabetai R & others: The hemodynamics of cardiac tamponade and constrictive pericarditis. Am J Cardiol 26:480, 1970.

Surawicz B, Lasseter KC: Electrocardiograms in pericarditis. Am J Cardiol 26:471. 1970.

DISORDERS OF RATE & RHYTHM

The usual or normal pacemaker of the heart is the sino-atrial (SA) node. It is located in the superior portion of the right atrium. From there the impulse spreads through the atrial fibers to the atrioventricular (AV) node. Conduction through the AV node is relatively slow and accounts for the interval in the ECG from the end of the P wave to the beginning of the Q wave. From there the impulse spreads to the common bundle of His, which divides into a right and left bundle. Impulses finally are conducted through the Purkinje fibers to the myocardium and from the endocardium to the epicardial surface.

Although the SA node is a normal pacemaker of the heart, any tissue within the heart can serve in impulse formation. As a rule, the lower the origin of the pulse, the slower the rate of discharge. However, any focus outside the SA node may take over the pacemaker function (either because of decreased irritability of the sinus node or hyperirritability of the ectopic focus) for 1—2 beats (premature contractions) or for a series of beats (ectopic tachycardia).

SINUS ARRHYTHMIA

This arrhythmia is a normal and common finding in children and adolescents. It consists of a phasic change in heart rate, usually associated with the respiratory cycle. It is characterized by acceleration of the heart rate during inspiration and a slowing of the rate with expiration. Occasionally, there may be no relationship to respirations. The P—R and the QRS intervals are normal.

PREMATURE ATRIAL CONTRACTIONS

These result from the discharge of an ectopic focus located within the atrium. Electrocardiographically, they are characterized by the premature appearance of a P wave which is different in size and shape from the normal sinus P wave. The QRS complex and the T wave are normal. The P—R interval of the premature contraction is usually less than 0.12 seconds.

The next normal sinus beat following the premature beat is slightly delayed, but the compensatory pause is incomplete—in contrast to a premature ventricular contraction. If the ectopic focus if located within the AV node, the P—R interval will be extremely short (upper node) or may appear after the QRS complex (lower node), in which case the P wave will be inverted in lead II.

Premature supraventricular contractions may be a normal finding; they occur not infrequently in patients with organic heart disease and with digitalis intoxication. Patients with organic heart disease will always demonstrate other abnormalities besides the ectopic beats (organic murmurs, abnormal x-ray, other ECG abnormalities, and symptoms referable to the cardiovascular system). Furthermore, exercise usually abolishes the ectopic beats in normal children and increases the frequency of premature contractions in patients with organic heart disease.

In normal children, infrequent supraventricular premature contractions require no treatment. The patient and the parents should be reassured that these are harmless. In patients with organic heart disease, frequent premature supraventricular contractions usually require digitalis therapy or, if this is ineffective, quinidine.

PREMATURE VENTRICULAR CONTRACTIONS

In this condition, the ectopic focus is located within the ventricle. Electrocardiographically, the premature beat is recognized by the appearance of an early, bizarre QRS complex and T wave not preceded by a P wave. There is always a complete compensatory pause (interval between 2 beats, including the premature contraction, is equal to 2 normal cardiac cycles).

Premature ventricular contractions may also occur in normal children. They are less common, however, than premature supraventricular contractions. In the normal individual, premature ventricular contractions usually are unifocal in origin and the coupling interval (interval from the end of the previous normal T wave to the beginning of the premature contraction) is exactly the same. Multifocal premature ventricular contractions and varying coupling intervals are found in patients with organic heart disease or drug intoxication. Premature contractions occasionally develop into ventricular tachycardia. Therefore, if the premature contractions are quite numerous or are associated with varying coupling intervals, treatment should be instituted. This consists primarily of the administration of quinidine.

PAROXYSMAL SUPRAVENTRICULAR TACHYCARDIA

In this condition, a hyperirritable ectopic focus located below the SA node (in the atria or AV node) discharges at a very rapid rate and takes over the function of cardiac pacemaker for a period of time ranging from several seconds to several days.

Clinical Findings

A. **Symptoms and Signs:** The onset is usually sudden. During the early phase, older children complain of a fluttering within the chest and will be quite irritable and fearful. Infants are usually asymptomatic during this period, but if the tachycardia persists for more than 24 hours symptoms and signs indicative of impaired cardiac function will develop. In one study (see Nadas reference, below), congestive heart failure developed in about 50% of patients. Three factors seem to influence the development of congestive heart failure: (1) The rate of the tachycardia: Congestive heart failure did not occur in patients who had a heart rate < 180/minute. The more rapid the rate, the more likely the development of congestive heart failure. (2) The duration of the tachycardia: The longer the tachycardia persisted, the more likely congestive heart failure was to develop. Congestive heart failure was not found in patients with tachycardia of less than 24 hours' duration; 19% had evidence of congestive heart failure after 36 hours; and 50% were in congestive heart failure after 48 hours. (3) The age of the patient: The younger the patient, the more common the incidence of congestive heart failure.

Infants in congestive heart failure secondary to paroxysmal supraventricular tachycardia are usually quite ill. They are ashen-gray and often frankly cyanotic. Pulses are difficult to count because they are very rapid and thready. The extremities are cold and clammy. The heart rate is extremely rapid and the heart tones poor. Rales are present within the lung, and the liver is enlarged.

Older children are usually not so ill when first brought to medical attention, probably because the arrhythmia is recognized early in the course.

B. **X-Ray Findings:** X-rays of the chest are normal during the early course of the arrhythmia. If congestive heart failure is present, the heart is enlarged and there is evidence of pulmonary venous congestion.

C. **Electrocardiography:** ECG is the most important tool in the diagnosis of this condition.

1. The heart rate is very rapid, ranging from 160–320/minute.

2. The rhythm is extremely regular. There is no variation in the R–R interval throughout the entire tracing.

3. P waves may or may not be present. If they are present, there is no variation in the appearance of the P wave or in the P–R interval. P waves may be difficult to find because they are superimposed upon the preceding T wave. Furthermore, if the abnormal focus is located within the AV node, the P waves will not be seen.

4. The QRS complex is usually the same as during normal sinus rhythm. However, the QRS complex is occasionally widened. In this case, the condition may be difficult to differentiate from ventricular tachycar-

dia (supraventricular tachycardia with aberrant ventricular conduction).

5. Termination of the tachycardia is characterized by conversion to normal sinus rhythm. Varying degrees of atrioventricular block do not develop, as is the case in atrial flutter.

Treatment

In almost all instances, paroxysmal supraventricular tachycardia can be successfully treated. However, despite conversion to normal sinus rhythm, infants who have been in severe congestive heart failure for prolonged periods with evidence of cardiovascular collapse may still succumb. This emphasizes the need for giving treatment early in the course of the tachycardia—especially in infants, in whom the onset of the arrhythmia cannot be ascertained.

A. **Digitalis:** Paroxysmal supraventricular tachycardia may be treated in a number of ways. In the pediatric age group, the treatment of choice is with digitalis. Conversion of the arrhythmia can almost always be achieved with this drug. Initially, however, reflex vagal stimulation should be attempted. Occasionally, maneuvers such as pressure over the carotid sinus or over the eyeball may convert tachycardia of short duration. If this is unsuccessful, digitalization should not be delayed. Digoxin is the preparation of choice because of its relatively rapid action. Half the calculated digitalizing dose should be administered initially. The other ½ should be given in 2 divided doses within the following 8–16 hours. If, as often happens, tachycardia is terminated before the total digitalizing dose is given, it is desirable to complete digitalization. Reflex vagal stimulation is often successful in terminating the tachycardia during the process of digitalization.

B. **Other Drugs and Procedures:** If digitalis is not effective, the administration of lidocaine (Xylocaine), procainamide (Pronestyl), or quinidine is recommended. The former drugs can be given intravenously under careful ECG control.

Within recent years, electrical countershock has been successful in terminating this type of arrhythmia.

The use of hypertensive agents such as methoxamine (Vasoxyl) or phenylephrine (Neo-Synephrine), by increasing systemic blood pressure and thus stimulating the carotid sinus, has also been successful in conversion of the arrhythmia.

Course & Prognosis

If paroxysmal supraventricular tachycardia persists without treatment, congestive heart failure, cardiovascular collapse, and death usually ensue. If the tachycardia is treated successfully, the great majority of patients do quite well. Symptoms and signs of heart failure clear up rapidly. Cardiac enlargement on x-ray, however, may persist for several days, and the ECG changes, including abnormalities of the P waves and ST and T wave changes, may also persist for up to 1 week.

Recurrences of paroxysmal supraventricular tachycardia are common, especially within the first year after the first attack. This is especially true in patients with Wolff-Parkinson-White syndrome (pre-excitation syndrome). For this reason, all patients should remain on digitalis for at least 2 months. In case of recurrence, digitalis should be reinstituted and maintained for 6–12 months.

ATRIAL FLUTTER

Although atrial flutter may occur in children with normal hearts, it is most common in patients with organic heart disease. It is characterized by an extremely rapid atrial rate (200–350/minute). In contrast to supraventricular tachycardia, however, varying degrees of atrioventricular block often exist. Whether symptoms and signs will occur or not depends upon the ventricular rate. If there is a rapid ventricular response with a heart rate greater than 200/minute, symptoms and signs of congestive heart failure frequently appear. If the ventricular response is slow (one ventricular beat for every 3–4 atrial beats), the patient's status remains essentially unchanged.

Digitalis should be given, especially if the ventricular response is rapid. Digitalization usually converts the flutter to a normal sinus rhythm, but sometimes it merely increases the AV block. In patients with organic heart disease, this may be all that can be accomplished, ie, it may be impossible to convert to normal sinus rhythm. In such a case, one should aim at maintaining the ventricular response at a relatively slow rate (80–140 beats/minute).

ATRIAL FIBRILLATION

Atrial fibrillation is the most severe atrial arrhythmia. It is extremely rare in children. It is always associated with organic heart disease, probably most commonly in patients with acute rheumatic fever.

Clinically, the rhythm is completely irregular and the heart sounds show a varying intensity. There is a variable pulse deficit when the rate of the heart sounds on auscultation is compared with palpation of the peripheral pulse. The ECG reveals a completely irregular rhythm without demonstrable P waves. The QRS complexes are usually normal.

All patients with atrial fibrillation should be digitalized. If the duration of fibrillation has been short, digitalization will often convert the arrhythmia to normal sinus rhythm and in any case will decrease the ventricular rate significantly. If conversion does not occur, it is desirable to maintain the cardiac rate between 70–100/minute at rest. If the ventricular rate falls below 60, digitalis should be discontinued.

If digitalis is not successful in converting the arrhythmia to normal sinus rhythm, quinidine is indicated. However, quinidine should not be administered before digitalization. If quinidine is successful, it should be continued for at least 3 months after conversion.

In refractory cases, electrical countershock may be employed. The experience in children is limited, and the results in adults have been variable.

FIRST DEGREE HEART BLOCK

This is strictly an ECG abnormality, consisting of prolongation of the P–R interval. On physical examination, first degree block is associated with a soft first heart sound.

Prolongation of the P–R interval does not necessarily indicate past or present heart disease. It may occur in normal children, in which case the block is probably congenital in origin. It commonly occurs in the course of acute rheumatic carditis and in varying types of congenital heart disease, including Ebstein's anomaly of the tricuspid valve, corrected transposition of the great vessels, and endocardial cushion defect. Digitalis intoxication is frequently associated with first degree block.

Except as an indication of drug intoxication, prolongation of the P–R interval has no functional significance and requires no specific treatment.

SECOND DEGREE HEART BLOCK

In second degree heart block, an occasional P wave fails to be conducted to the ventricle. There are 2 major types.

Wenckebach Phenomenon
In this condition there is a progressive prolongation of the P–R interval, eventually terminating in complete block of AV conduction. The "dropped" beat usually persists for 3–5 cardiac cycles. Although this may occur in a normal heart, it is usually associated with organic heart disease. Causative factors are the same as those discussed under first degree heart block. The dropped beat usually has no functional significance. Treatment should be directed only toward the underlying heart disease or drug intoxication.

Intermittent AV Block Without Progressive Prolongation of the P–R Interval
This may occur haphazardly or at regular intervals every 3–4 beats. Etiologic and therapeutic considerations are the same as those of Wenckebach phenomenon.

THIRD DEGREE (COMPLETE) HEART BLOCK

In third degree heart block, no atrial impulses can pass through the AV node; this results in independent contraction of the atria and ventricles. This condition should not be confused with AV dissociation, in which conduction through the AV node is intact but, because of a hyperirritable focus within the ventricle, the ventricles beat more rapidly than the atria, resulting in independent atrial and ventricular contractions. In complete heart block (with rare exceptions), the atria always beat more rapidly than the ventricles.

Complete heart block may be congenital or acquired. Congenital complete heart block may occur in the absence of any other intracardiac abnormalities or (occasionally) in association with corrected transposition of the great vessels, endocardial cushion defects, and endocardial fibroelastosis.

In the pediatric age group, almost the only cause of acquired complete heart block is open heart surgery. Transient complete heart block is not uncommon in patients undergoing correction of tetralogy of Fallot or very large ventricular septal defects. In most cases, conversion to normal sinus rhythm occurs within 1–2 weeks. Occasionally, however, complete heart block persists.

Clinical Findings

A. Symptoms and Signs:

1. Congenital complete heart block–Patients with congenital complete heart block usually do quite well. However, a number of recent reports have described Stokes-Adams attacks in these patients. The heart block is usually picked up on routine physical examination. The heart rate usually varies from 60–80/minute. In contrast to acquired heart block or complete heart block in adults, patients with congenital complete heart block can increase their heart rate 20 beats/minute during exercise. On physical examination, the heart is found to be enlarged, the heart rate slow, and loud ejection murmurs are present over the entire precordium. These murmurs are most commonly due to increased stroke volume through normal semilunar valves.

In patients with congenital heart disease and complete heart block, the history and physical findings depend upon the underlying anatomic abnormality.

2. Acquired complete heart block–Patients with heart block secondary to open heart surgery do much more poorly. The rate is usually slower than in congenital complete heart block, varying at rest from 30–50/minute. These patients cannot increase their heart rate significantly with exercise. Stokes-Adams attacks are not uncommon in this group. The mortality rate is high unless treatment is instituted.

B. Electrocardiography: The ECG is characterized by lack of any relationship between the P wave and the QRS complex. The atrial rate is always faster than the ventricular rate. The ventricular complex is usually broadened, with an abnormal T wave. In contrast to AV dissociation, no captured beats can be found on long strips of the ECG.

Treatment

Patients with congenital complete heart block who are completely asymptomatic and have a heart rate of greater than 40/minute during sleep do not require treatment. However, if at any time the heart rate drops below 40/minute, treatment is recommended. This includes the oral administration of isoproterenol (Isuprel) or ephedrine. These drugs increase the ventricular rate. Chlorothiazide (Diuril), an oral diuretic which induces potassium loss, has been recommended in recent years. Potassium diuresis increases the irritability of the myocardium, resulting in a more rapid ventricular rate. If isoproterenol with or without chlorothiazide does not significantly increase the heart rate or decrease the number of Stokes-Adams attacks, surgical insertion of an artificial pacemaker is recommended.

Treatment (as above) should always be instituted in patients with acquired heart block who have a pulse rate under 40.

Any patient with a history of a number of Stokes-Adams attacks should be started on treatment regardless of the heart rate measured at rest.

Because of the inability to significantly increase heart rate and thus cardiac output, patients with complete heart block should be restricted from participating in strenuous activities, especially competitive athletics. Except for this, they may lead normal active lives.

Glenn WWL & others: Heart block in children. J Thoracic Cardiovas Surg 59:361, 1969.

Griffiths SP: Congenital complete heart block. Circulation 43:615, 1971.

Hunsaker MR, Khoury GH: Management of supraventricular tachycardia by atrial stimulation. J Pediat 77:455, 1970.

Nadas AS & others: Paroxysmal tachycardia in infants: Study of 41 cases. Pediatrics 9:167, 1952.

Paul MH: Cardiac arrhythmias in infants and children. Progr Cardiovas Dis 9:136, 1966.

Zoll PM: Rational use of drugs for cardiac arrest and after cardiac resuscitation. Am J Cardiol 27:645, 1971.

● ● ●

General References

Burch LE, De Pasquale NP: *Electrocardiography in the Diagnosis of Congenital Heart Disease.* Lea & Febiger, 1967.

Cassels DE (editor): *The Heart and Circulation in the Newborn and Infant.* Grune & Stratton, 1966.

Cassels DE, Ziegler RF: *Electrocardiography in Infants and Children.* Grune & Stratton, 1966.

Gasul BM, Arcilla RA, Lev M: *Heart Disease in Children: Diagnosis and Treatment.* Lippincott, 1966.

Keith JD, Rowe RD, Vlad P: *Heart Disease in Infancy and Childhood,* 2nd ed. Macmillan, 1967.

Kjellberg SR & others: *Diagnosis of Congenital Heart Disease.* Year Book, 1955.

Moss AJ, Adams FH: *Heart Disease in Infants, Children, and Adolescents.* Williams & Wilkins, 1968.

Robinson SJ, Abrams HL, Kaplan HS: *Congenital Heart Disease.* McGraw-Hill, 1965.

Rowe RD, Mehrizi A: *The Neonate With Congenital Heart Disease.* Saunders, 1968.

Watson H (editor): *Pediatric Cardiology.* Mosby, 1968.

14 . . .

Hematologic Disorders

John H. Githens, MD, & William Hathaway, MD

Knowledge of the normal ranges is essential in the diagnosis of hematologic disorders of infancy and childhood. The normal values for peripheral blood and bone marrow are shown in Tables 14–1 and 14–2. They vary significantly with age.

The important changes shown in Table 14–1 include polycythemia in the neonatal period followed by physiologic anemia of infancy, which is maximal at 2½–3 months. Subsequently, there is a gradual rise of the hemoglobin, hematocrit, and red cell count through childhood. Adult levels are not reached until after puberty.

The red blood cells of the newborn are macrocytic (8–9 μm in diameter). There is a gradual change to microcytosis at 3 months, with return to normal diameter (7.4 μm) by 8 months.

The white blood count may normally remain higher than in the adult throughout infancy and childhood. The differential white count shows a predominance of lymphocytes, which may normally comprise as much as 80% of the white blood cells through the first 6 years of life.

I. ANEMIAS

Anemia is always a manifestation of disease or nutritional deficiency. The cause should be determined by appropriate clinical and laboratory investigations or, if necessary, by therapeutic trial with specific replacement therapy. "Shotgun" treatment with multiple drugs is never indicated.

The cell index that is most useful is the MCHC (mean corpuscular hemoglobin concentration):

$$\frac{\text{Hemoglobin (gm)}}{\text{Hematocrit (\%)}} \times 100 = \text{MCHC. Normal} = 32\text{–}34\%$$

The primary cause of anemia in infancy is nutritional iron deficiency. Anemias due to causes other than iron deficiency fall into 2 major groups: (1) those due to impaired red cell production, maturation, or release from the marrow; and (2) those due to acute blood loss or destruction (hemolysis). The studies needed to determine the exact cause are different for these 2 groups.

The essential test in differentiating anemias due to defective production from the hemolytic group is the reticulocyte count. This must be done prior to treatment with drugs or transfusion.

Diagnosis of Anemia

The following scheme for diagnosis of anemia is useful:

(1) Careful history: Duration of symptoms, diet, rate of growth, evidence of acute or chronic hemorrhage, jaundice, and a family history of anemia, jaundice, or gallbladder disease.

(2) Determination of hemoglobin, hematocrit, red blood cell count, MCHC, and examination of the smear.

(a) If hypochromia is shown, the cause of iron deficiency should be sought and treated. Additional studies—serum iron and iron-binding capacity, serum proteins, examination of stools for blood, and bone marrow examination—may be indicated.

(b) If normochromia (or hyperchromia) is shown, the reticulocyte count is essential. If the reticulocyte count is low (due to defect in marrow production or release), examine bone marrow; if high (due to hemolytic disease or acute hemorrhage), perform blood smear and Coombs test. If the Coombs is negative, perform red cell saline fragility test, autohemolysis test, hemoglobin electrophoresis, fetal hemoglobin determination, and Heinz body preparation. If spherocytosis or a hemoglobinopathy has not been identified, red cell enzyme studies are indicated.

ANEMIAS DUE TO DEFICIENT PRODUCTION

PHYSIOLOGIC "ANEMIA" OF THE NEWBORN & ANEMIA OF PREMATURITY

Essentials of Diagnosis
- Age 2–3 months.

TABLE 14–1. Normal peripheral blood values at various ages.*

	1st day	2nd day	6th day	2 weeks	1 month	2 months	3 months	6 months	1 year	2 years	5 years	8–12 years	Adults Males	Adults Females
Red blood cells (millions/cu mm)	5.9 (4.1–7.5)	6 (4.0–7.3)	5.4 (3.9–6.8)	5 (4.5–5.5)	4.7 (4.2–5.2)	4.1 (3.6–4.6)	4 (3.5–4.5)	4.5 (4–5)	4.6 (4.1–5.1)	4.7 (4.2–5.2)	4.7 (4.2–5.2)	5 (4.5–5.4)	5.4 (4.6–6.2)	4.8 (4.2–5.4)
Hemoglobin (gm)	19 (14–24)	19 (15–23)	18 (13–23)	16.5 (15–20)	14 (11–17)	12 (11–14)	11 (10–13)	11.5 (10.5–14.5)	12 (11–15)	13 (12–15)	13.5 (12.5–15)	14 (13–15.5)	16 (13–18)	14 (11–16)
White blood cells (per cu mm)	17,000 (8–38)		13,500 (6–17)	12,000 (5–16)	11,500 (5–15)	11,000 (5–15)	10,500 (5–15)	10,500 (5–15)	10,000 (5–15)	9,500 (5–14)	8,000 (5–13)	8,000 (5–12)	7,000 (5–10)	
PMNs† (%)	57	55	50	34	34	33	33	36	39	42	55	60	57–68	
Eosinophils (total) (per cu mm)	20–1000				150–1150		70–550	70–550					100–400	
Lymphocytes† (%)	20	20	37	55	56	56	57	55	53	49	36	31	25–33	
Monocytes†	10	15	9	8	7	7	7	6	6	7	7	7	3–7	
Immature white cells (%)	10	5	0–1	0	0	0	0	0	0	0	0	0		
Platelets† (per cu mm)	350,000		325,000	300,000			260,000			260,000		260,000	260,000	
Nucleated red cells/ 100 white cells‡	0–10		0–0.3	0	0	0	0	0	0	0	0	0	0	
Reticulocytes (%)	3 (2–8)	3 (2–10)	1 (0.5–5)	0.4 (0–2)	0.2 (0–0.5)	0.5 (0.2–2)	2 (0.5–4)	0.8 (0.2–1.5)	1 (0.4–1.8)	1 (0.4–1.8)	1 (0.4–1.8)	1 (0.4–1.8)	1 (0.5–2)	
Mean diameter of red cells (μm)	8.6				8.1		5–7		7.4		7.4		7.5	
MCV§ (fl)	85–125		89–101	94–102	90		80	78	78	80	80	82	82–92	
MCHC§ (%)	36		35	34				33		32	34	34	34	
MCH§ (pg)	35–40		36	31	30		27	26	25	26	27	28	27–31	
Hematocrit (%)	54±10	55	51	50	40		35	35	36	37	38	40	40–54	37–47

*Modified and reproduced, with permission, from Silver HK, Kempe CH, Bruyn H: *Handbook of Pediatrics*, 9th ed. Lange, 1971.

†Usual or average values; considerable individual variation may occur.

‡Total nucleated red cells: first day, <1000.

§MCV = mean corpuscular volume. MCHC = mean corpuscular hemoglobin concentration. MCH = mean corpuscular hemoglobin.

Note: μm = micrometer, 10^{-6} meter (formerly μ, micron)

fl = femtoliter, 10^{-15} liter (formerly cμ, cubic micron)

pg = picogram, 10^{-12} gram (formerly μμg or γγ, micromicrogram)

(See explanation facing p 1.)

- Normochromia or hyperchromia; microcytosis.
- Erythroid hypoplasia of marrow.

General Considerations

Physiologic anemia occurs in all full-term infants and reaches its low point (hemoglobin about 10–11 gm/100 ml) at about age 2½ months. The exact cause is not known, although it is recognized that both erythropoietin release and bone marrow production cannot keep pace with somatic growth. At this age it is not due to iron deficiency. It is associated with the transition from production of fetal hemoglobin to adult hemoglobin but is probably not due to this change. The anemia may be more severe in premature infants, in whom the hemoglobin may drop to levels of 5–6 gm/100 ml.

Clinical Findings

A. Symptoms and Signs: Slight pallor may be noted in full-term infants, but usually no other symptoms occur. If the anemia is severe in the premature infant, decreased activity and fatigue with feeding may occur.

B. Laboratory Findings:

1. Blood–Anemia is normochromic or hyperchromic, with microcytosis. Cell diameter may be as small as 5 μm. No other abnormalities are noted in the blood smear.

2. Bone marrow–The marrow appears relatively normal but shows slight erythroid hypoplasia; morphologic changes are not indicative of decreased production.

Differential Diagnosis

Iron deficiency anemia usually does not manifest itself until after the age of 2–3 months. Congenital hemolytic anemias that are associated with red cell membrane or red cell metabolic abnormalities (such as hereditary spherocytosis, pyruvate kinase deficiency, etc) are present from birth and should be considered. Congenital pure red cell hypoplastic anemia presents within the first few months of life; an extremely low reticulocyte count should suggest this diagnosis. Hemolysis associated with sepsis or following erythroblastosis fetalis should be considered.

Treatment

Treatment should not be instituted unless the anemia is of sufficient severity to produce symptoms. Therefore, therapy is not indicated in the full-term infant. Treatment may be necessary in the premature infant if the hemoglobin drops below 7 or 8 gm/100 ml and symptoms of lethargy and fatigue are noted.

The only effective treatment is blood transfusion, which should be given in the form of packed red cells in doses of 5–10 ml/kg. The anemia will not respond at this age to iron or folic acid or other hematinics.

Prognosis

Spontaneous recovery is apparent by about 12–14 weeks of age in all infants. Anemia that persists beyond 3 months usually has another cause.

Guest GM, Brown EW: Erythrocytes and hemoglobin of the blood in infancy and childhood–factors in variability: Statistical studies. Am J Dis Child 93:486–509, 1957.

Mann DL & others: Erythropoietic stimulating activity during the first ninety days of life. Proc Soc Exper Biol Med 118:212, 1965.

O'Brien RT, Pearson HA: Physiologic anemia of the newborn infant. J Pediat 79:132–138, 1971.

NUTRITIONAL ANEMIAS

Anemia is the most common manifestation of nutritional deficiency in children in the USA; it is even more frequent in other parts of the world. In the USA, iron deficiency is responsible for the majority of these nutritional anemias. Folic acid and vitamin B$_{12}$ deficiencies are seen principally in economically underprivileged children. The need for exogenous iron is greatly increased during the first 2 years of life and again in adolescence because of the rapid growth of the child. Milk alone does not meet the iron requirements for normal growth during the first 2 years, and "solid" foods or iron supplementation is needed to prevent the development of anemia.

1. IRON DEFICIENCY ANEMIA

Essentials of Diagnosis

- Pallor, fatigue.
- Good weight gain, poor muscle tone.
- Delayed motor development.
- Poor dietary intake of iron.
- Age 6 months to 2 years.
- Hypochromic microcytic anemia.

General Considerations

The average diet contains 12–15 mg of iron (of which approximately 10% is absorbed), and the normal daily excretion of iron is less than 1 mg/day.

Iron deficiency on a nutritional basis generally occurs between 6 months and 2 years of age and is an extremely rare cause of anemia after age 3 except in adolescence. As the infant rarely outgrows his iron stores prior to the age of 4 months, iron deficiency is almost never a cause of anemia in the first 3 months of life except with severe iron deficiency in the mother or following blood loss by hemorrhage in the infant. It has been demonstrated that iron deficiency is associated with abnormalities of the intestinal mucosa that allow for loss of serum proteins as well as chronic intestinal

TABLE 14–2. Normal values of cellular elements in
bone marrow in older infants and children.*

	Range (%)	Mean (%)
Myeloblasts	1–5	2
Myelocytes (including pro-myelocytes)	10–25	20
Nonsegmented polymorpho-nuclear cells (including metamyelocytes)	15–30	20
Segmented polymorpho-nuclear cells	5–30	25
Lymphocytes	5–25	13
Nucleated red cells (principally normoblasts)	15–30	20
Megakaryocytes	10–35/cu mm	
Total nucleated cell count	100,000–200,000/cu mm	

*From Smith: *Blood Diseases of Infancy and Childhood,* 2nd
ed. Mosby, 1966.

hemorrhage. In some cases, occult gastrointestinal
blood loss may be a major factor. Thus, the exudative
enteropathy that may occur secondary to dietary iron
deficiency further aggravates the iron depletion in the
body. Other primary conditions (eg, milk allergy) may
cause exudative enteropathy and initiate the iron loss.

Iron deficiency is also seen in association with
chronic hemorrhage or rapid growth. Infestation with
hookworm or *Trichuris trichiura* should be considered
as a primary cause of chronic gastrointestinal blood
loss in endemic areas.

The diagnosis depends largely on a history of a
diet low in iron-containing solid foods with a high
intake of milk (greater than 1 quart/day), and evidence
of early rapid weight gain during the first 1–2 years of
life. Hypochromia with microcytosis, decreased MCHC,
and decreased serum iron with increased iron-binding
capacity are characteristic.

Clinical Findings

A. Symptoms and Signs: Pallor, fatigue, irritability, and delayed motor development are common. The
child is often fat and flabby, with poor muscle tone.
Beeturia (red urine from the pigment of beets) occurs
more frequently in iron-deficient children and may be
a clue to the anemia.

B. Laboratory Findings: The hemoglobin is
depressed and may be as low as 3–4 gm/100 ml. The
red cell count and hematocrit are proportionately
higher, producing a significantly lowered MCHC (less
than 30%). The red cells on smear are microcytic and
hypochromic. The reticulocyte count is normal, but it
may be elevated in severe cases.

Serum iron need not be determined in childhood
if the dietary and growth history readily explain the
cause of the hypochromic anemia. Where there is
doubt regarding the diagnosis or the cause, or if exudative enteropathy is suspected, this determination

should be performed. Serum iron is low—usually below
30 μg/100 ml (normal: 90–150 μg/100 ml). Total
iron-binding capacity is usually elevated to 350–500
μg/100 ml (normal: 250–350 μg/100 ml).

Bone marrow examination is usually not necessary in infants for the diagnosis of iron deficiency.
Even normal children under 2 years of age deposit
little or no iron in the form of hemosiderin in the
marrow. In older children and adolescents, marrow
examination with staining for iron may be helpful,
since stainable iron should be present normally over
the age of 2–3 years and will be absent in iron deficiency anemia.

Differential Diagnosis

Iron deficiency anemia must be differentiated
from several other hypochromic microcytic anemias
caused by defective incorporation of iron into the
hemoglobin molecule.

Thalassemia minor is the disorder that is most
frequently confused with nutritional iron deficiency
anemia, and it should be suspected in the child with an
iron-resistant hypochromic anemia. Hypochromia and
anemia may occur with any hemoglobinopathy involving the thalassemia gene. The serum iron will be elevated in these conditions.

Infection and inflammation interfere with the
incorporation and utilization of iron and produce
hypochromic anemias. Although the serum iron and
total iron-binding capacity are low, bone marrow
hemosiderin will be present in the older child; search
should be made for the presence of severe chronic
infection or inflammatory disease. Other iron-resistant
hypochromic anemias include anemia due to lead poisoning and vitamin B_6 dependent anemia.

Complications

Children with iron deficiency anemia are more
susceptible than others to infection. In severe cases,
heart failure may occur. Motor development is often
delayed because of weakness. Anorexia and irritability
cause additional feeding problems and further malnutrition. Severe iron deficiency interferes with the normal integrity of the gastrointestinal tract; exudative
enteropathy associated with protein and additional
iron loss may occur.

Treatment

A. Oral Iron: The recommended oral dose is
1.5–2 mg/kg elemental iron 3 times daily between
meals (4.5–6 mg/kg/day). Although absorption is better if the medication is given between meals, iron can
be administered with food or even in milk. Various
iron complexes and concentrates are available, but
there is little evidence that any one is preferable to the
others. Ferrous sulfate remains the drug of choice.
Patients should be observed for a reticulocyte rise in
3–5 days and for a hemoglobin increase in 1–2 weeks.

The recommended dose for prophylaxis is
0.8–1.5 mg/kg/day of elemental iron, although 0.5
mg/kg/day is probably adequate.

B. Intramuscular Iron: Iron-dextran complex (Imferon) may be given intramuscularly if oral intolerance or malabsorption is present or if parental supervision is inadequate. The dose can be calculated from the following formula:

$$\text{mg iron} = \frac{\text{desired hemoglobin} - \text{initial hemoglobin}}{100} \times$$

$$80 \times \text{weight in kg} \times 3.4$$

An additional 30% should be given to replace deficient iron stores. Daily doses should be limited to 1 ml (50 mg) in infants and 2 ml (100 mg) in very young children. When administering iron-dextran complex, pull the skin to one side before injecting to prevent leakage to the skin.

C. Ascorbic Acid: Large doses of ascorbic acid increase absorption of iron from food but probably do not affect the efficiency of iron medication.

D. Blood Transfusions: Transfusion therapy is reserved for children with extremely low levels of hemoglobin who are bordering on congestive failure or who have serious acute infections. Packed cells should be used and administered slowly in a dose not to exceed 10 ml/kg. In the severely ill child with impending or frank congestive failure, a partial exchange transfusion (isovolumetric) with packed red cells should be given.

E. Diet: Ultimate management requires improvement in the diet, with reduction of milk intake and an increase in iron-containing foods such as meat, eggs, fortified infant cereals, and green vegetables.

Prognosis

Iron therapy will produce rapid and complete recovery if the anemia is due to nutritional inadequacy. If the anemia persists, other causes must be found and treated.

Githens JH, Hathaway WE: Iron deficiency anemia of infancy. Clin Pediat 2:477–483, 1963.
Guha DK & others: Small bowel changes in iron deficiency anemia of childhood. Arch Dis Childhood 43:239, 1968.
Shumway CN: Management of anemia in childhood. GP 39:107, May 1969.
Tunnessen WW & others: Beeturia: A sign of iron deficiency. Am J Dis Child 117:424, 1969.

2. IRON-RESISTANT, HYPOCHROMIC ANEMIAS (Sideroachrestic or Sideroblastic Anemias)

The sideroblastic anemias comprise a group of abnormalities characterized by being iron-resistant and hypochromic. All patients with this type of anemia have large iron stores and high serum iron levels. The anemias are all due to a disturbance in hemoglobin biosynthesis, resulting in an increased number of sideroblasts—nucleated normoblasts containing iron inclusions. The iron accumulates, since the cell is unable to incorporate iron into the hemoglobin molecule. Sideroblasts occur in low concentrations in normal persons but are markedly increased in this group of iron-refractory anemias. Siderocytes, which are erythrocytes containing iron inclusions, are also markedly increased in number.

The most common cause of iron-resistant, hypochromic anemia in childhood is thalassemia minor. Lead poisoning produces a similar pattern.

Pyridoxine-dependent anemia should always be considered since it responds readily to treatment with large doses of vitamin B_6.

Other cases are familial, and some of them are apparently transmitted as an X-linked recessive disorder. Patients are occasionally anemic in early childhood, but the familial forms are more apt to express themselves fully in adult life.

The anemia is always hypochromic, with anisocytosis and poikilocytosis. It is refractory to parenteral iron therapy. The serum iron is increased, with almost complete saturation of the total iron-binding capacity.

Diagnostic tests (in addition to bone marrow examination) include determination of the A_2 hemoglobin level, studies for iron intoxication, and a therapeutic trial with vitamin B_6.

Frimpter GW & others: Vitamin B_6-dependency syndromes: New horizons in nutrition. Am J Clin Nutr 22:794, 1969.
Mollin DL: A symposium on sideroblastic anemia—introduction: Sideroblasts and sideroblastic anemia. Brit J Haemat 11:41, 1965.
Robinson SH: Heme synthesis and hypochromic anemia. New England J Med 280:615, 1969.

3. MEGALOBLASTIC ANEMIAS

Megaloblastic anemias are characterized by oval macrocytes and hypersegmented PMNs in the peripheral blood and megaloblasts in the bone marrow. They are due primarily to a deficiency of folic acid or vitamin B_{12} or a combination of both. These 2 substances function as coenzymes in the synthesis of nuclear protein.

Folic acid must be converted to folinic acid with the assistance of ascorbic acid. The gastric intrinsic factor is necessary for the absorption of vitamin B_{12}. Megaloblastic anemias develop in the absence of gastric intrinsic factor or as a result of dietary deficiencies of folic acid or, rarely, vitamin B_{12}, or they may appear in the presence of ascorbic acid deficiency if the folic acid intake is low.

Megaloblastic Anemia of Infancy (Folic Acid Deficiency)

Megaloblastic anemia of infancy usually occurs in an acute form within the first few months of life. It is almost always due to folic acid deficiency or the combination of low folic acid intake and ascorbic acid deficiency. Practically all types of milk used for infant feeding provide some folic acid, but goat's milk is poor in vitamin B_{12} and may cause megaloblastic anemia. Folic acid deficient megaloblastic anemia also occurs in older children with severe nutritional deficiency or with serious absorption problems such as celiac disease.

The characteristic findings are weakness, pallor, and anorexia in infancy. Glossitis and a beefy red tongue are occasionally noted, but the neurologic manifestations of pernicious anemia are not seen. The anemia is frequently severe, with hemoglobin levels below 4 gm/100 ml. The red cell count is low, and may be < 1 million/cu mm in severe cases. The blood smear shows macrocytes and significant anisocytosis and poikilocytosis. The red cells are usually normochromic or hypochromic (if iron deficiency is also present). Leukopenia with neutropenia is usually present. The PMNs are enlarged and hypersegmented. The platelets are usually moderately reduced. The reticulocyte count is low. Formiminoglutamic acid (FIGLU) is present in the urine in folic acid deficiency after histidine loading. The Schilling test (see Pernicious Anemia) will differentiate folic acid deficiency from defective vitamin B_{12} absorption. Erythrocyte transketolase activity is normal in folate deficiency but elevated in vitamin B_{12} deficiency.

The marrow examination is diagnostic. The smear is characterized by delayed maturation and the presence of the typical megaloblastic forms of the nucleated red cells. Giant metamyelocytes may be seen, and megakaryocyte nuclei may be hypersegmented.

Megaloblastic anemia may also result from infestation with the fish tapeworm (*Diphyllobothrium latum*), the administration of certain anticonvulsant drugs, and various malabsorption syndromes. Megaloblastic anemia is a possible complication of severe chronic hemolytic anemias.

Megaloblastic anemia due to folic acid deficiency responds rapidly to oral or parenteral administration of folic acid in a daily dosage of 5 mg. Two to 3 weeks of treatment are usually sufficient. A significant rise in the reticulocyte count will occur within a few days after therapy is started. Ascorbic acid in a dosage of about 200 mg/day orally should be given at the same time. In generalized malnutrition, vitamin B_{12} should also be given. Dietary changes should be instituted to prevent the recurrence of megaloblastic anemia.

Complete and permanent recovery will follow the administration of folic acid and ascorbic acid. Relapses will not occur unless dietary deficiencies persist.

Luhby AL: Megaloblastic anemia in infancy: Clinical considerations and analysis. J Pediat 54:617, 1959.
Wells DG & others: Erythrocyte transketolase activity in megaloblastic anemia. Lancet 2:543, 1968.

Megaloblastic Anemia of Malnutrition

Megaloblastic anemia occurs among economically underprivileged children, particularly in tropical and subtropical countries, in association with poverty and poor dietary habits. It results from a low intake of both folic acid and vitamin B_{12}, and often is associated with iron deficiency anemia. The bone marrow and other laboratory findings demonstrate the presence of megaloblastic changes in the marrow and iron deficiency. The peripheral blood usually shows both macrocytosis and hypochromia. The anemia of kwashiorkor, which occurs in severe nutritional deficiency associated with protein inadequacy, is usually normochromic and normocytic or, less commonly, macrocytic or megaloblastic.

Treatment should include folic acid, vitamin B_{12}, and iron, with dietary improvement for future prevention.

Mittal VS & others: Observations on nutritional megaloblastic anemias in early childhood. Indian J Med Res 57:730, 1969.

Congenital Megaloblastic Anemia

Cases of megaloblastic anemia have been reported in infancy in association with a congenital metabolic block in nucleic acid formation. Large quantities of orotic acid appear in the urine because of the inborn error in pyrimidine metabolism. These patients respond well to treatment with nucleotides. Therapy must be continued probably throughout life.

Huguley CM & others: Refractory megaloblastic anemia associated with excretion of orotic acid. Blood 14:615–634, 1959.

Juvenile Pernicious Anemia

True pernicious anemia is rare in childhood. The clinical picture is very similar to that in the adult, with anemia resulting in pallor, fatigue, and the development of anorexia and diarrhea. The presence of a beefy, red, smooth, sore tongue and the development of neurologic manifestations differentiate this anemia from the other megaloblastic anemias of childhood. The CNS involvement includes ataxia, paresthesias of the hands and feet, impaired vibratory perception, a positive Babinski sign, and the absence of tendon reflexes. As in the adult, true juvenile pernicious anemia is caused by a deficiency of vitamin B_{12}, which is due to defective absorption in association with absence of the gastric intrinsic factor.

A related familial syndrome has been described in infants in whom there is selective malabsorption of vitamin B_{12} but intrinsic factor activity is present.

Typical laboratory findings include the presence of a macrocytic anemia with anisocytosis and poikilocytosis. Neutropenia and thrombocytopenia are common, and the PMNs are hypersegmented. Reticulocytes are within the normal range. The bone marrow is hyperplastic and shows characteristic megaloblastic abnormalities with a delay in maturation. Giant metamyelocytes and hypersegmented megakaryocytes are found.

The serum vitamin B_{12} concentration is usually less than 100 pg/ml (normal 300–400 pg/ml).

Treatment consists of the administration of vitamin B_{12} (cyanocobalamin) by parenteral injection. In children, a dosage of 15–30 μg IM given 3–5 times per week for 2–4 weeks (or until blood values return to normal) is usually adequate. In large children or adolescents, the dose may be increased to 100 μg given at the same intervals. A maintenance dose of 100 μg should be administered by injection each month. This therapy usually produces an excellent remission, although it must be continued throughout life. Oral administration of vitamin B_{12}, liver injections, and folic acid therapy are not recommended. Treatment with folic acid alone will allow the neurologic manifestations to progress even though the anemia may be controlled.

Hippe E & others: Hereditary factors in pernicious anemia and their relation to serum immuno-globulin levels and age at diagnosis. Lancet 2:721, 1969.

McIntyre OR & others: Pernicious anemia in childhood. New England J Med 272:981, 1965.

4. NORMOBLASTIC MACROCYTIC ANEMIAS

Macrocytosis of the peripheral blood is observed in a number of conditions in which megaloblastic changes are not seen in the bone marrow. These include aplastic anemia, lymphomas, hypothyroidism, scurvy, and liver disease.

Treatment is directed toward correction of the underlying conditions.

APLASTIC & HYPOPLASTIC ANEMIAS

CONGENITAL PURE RED CELL ANEMIA
(Congenital Aregenerative Anemia, Idiopathic Hypoplastic Anemia, Primary Erythroid Hypoplasia, Blackfan-Diamond Syndrome)

Essentials of Diagnosis

- Pallor, weakness, fatigue.
- Onset in first few months of life.
- Normochromic anemia; very low reticulocyte count.
- Normal white blood cells and platelets.

General Consideration

Congenital pure red cell anemia usually manifests itself in the first 4 months of life—often immediately after birth—and should be suspected in an infant with severe normochromic anemia and a very low reticulocyte count in the presence of normal circulating white cells and platelets. The diagnosis is made by bone marrow examination which is characterized by failure of erythropoiesis without equivalent depression of the white cells or platelets. The disorder appears to be caused by a block in the maturation of the erythroid

series at the stem cell or very immature erythroblastic level. Thymoma is not present in the congenital childhood form, although this is sometimes observed in adults with pure red cell anemia.

Clinical Findings

A. Symptoms and Signs: Pallor, fatigue, and weakness becoming progressively more severe from early infancy are produced by the anemia. Small stature and delayed growth are characteristic (in untreated cases). Occasionally there are other associated anomalies, particularly of the thumb and the kidneys.

B. Laboratory Findings:

1. Blood—The anemia is normocytic and normochromic, and the hemoglobin is often less than 5 gm/100 ml. The reticulocyte count is characteristically very low, and may be zero. The platelet count, white count, and differential count are normal.

2. Bone marrow—The bone marrow is characterized by a striking absence of nucleated red cell precursors without any depression of the granulocytic series or the megakaryocytes. Occasionally, very immature cells of the normoblastic series may be seen.

3. Other tests—No other studies are required for diagnosis. Levels of erythropoietin are markedly elevated, and abnormalities of tryptophan metabolites have been described in the urine following a tryptophan loading test.

Differential Diagnosis

Other conditions occurring in the neonatal period with depressed erythropoiesis in the presence of normal granulocytes and platelets include the anemia of prematurity and the anemia which often follows severe erythroblastosis fetalis. In both of these situations, some reticulocytosis should be present and the past history is suggestive.

Congenital pure red cell anemia may occasionally be confused with hemolytic anemia in the first few months of life when physiologic processes inhibit the normal reticulocyte response to hemolysis.

A variant of pure red cell anemia has recently been described in infants with triphalangeal thumbs and neutropenia.

Complications

The principal complications are associated with therapy. Repeated blood transfusions have resulted in widespread hemosiderosis, at times progressing to hemochromatosis. Therapy with corticosteroids has resulted in marked impairment of physical growth and in osteoporosis.

Treatment

A. Corticosteroids: In the majority of cases the anemia responds dramatically to therapy with corticosteroids, particularly if therapy is begun before age 3. Oral prednisone is the most frequently used drug. The dosage ranges from 15 mg/day in infants up to 60 mg/day in older children. It should be given in divided doses. A significant response of the anemia will usually be seen within 3–4 weeks. Following this, the dosage should be reduced to determine the minimal level with which a remission can be obtained. To produce less interference with growth, the total 48-hour dose of prednisone can be given in a single dose every other day, or treatment may consist of therapy on only 3 or 4 days each week.

Other drugs such as testosterone and cobalt have no effect in this condition.

B. Blood Transfusions: Transfusions must be given in the presence of severe anemia and as a chronic supportive measure in the child who does not respond to corticosteroid therapy. Packed cells are preferred, and, as a rule, the transfusion is not given until the hemoglobin drops to approximately 7 gm/100 ml, at which point clinical symptoms usually appear. Therapy with blood alone usually requires a transfusion every 4–8 weeks. The chances of developing hemosiderosis are greatly increased with this form of therapy.

C. Splenectomy: Splenectomy is occasionally of value but is never curative. Its effect is probably greatest in the child who has developed splenomegaly and has an extracorpuscular hemolytic component which is presumably located in the spleen. This can be confirmed by tagging normal donor red cells with radioactive chromium (^{51}Cr) and noting their shortened survival.

Prognosis

Before the adrenocortical steroids came into use, the course of congenital pure red cell anemia in many patients was one of chronic and progressive anemia with a fatal outcome. Repeated transfusions prolonged life but increased the hazards of hemosiderosis and hemochromatosis.

The results of long-term corticosteroid therapy have not yet been evaluated. Many children have been maintained in remission throughout childhood. Markedly impaired growth appears to be the primary complication of corticosteroid treatment.

Occasionally some children will have a spontaneous remission during later childhood or at adolescence. The milder cases that show a few red cell precursors in the bone marrow are more apt to have remissions.

The acquired form of erythrocytic hypoplasia that occurs in adults (often in association with a thymoma) is rarely seen in childhood.

Aase JM, Smith DW: Congenital anemia and triphalangeal thumbs: A new syndrome. J Pediat 74:471, 1969.

Allen DM, Diamond LK: Congenital (erythroid) hypoplastic anemia: Cortisone treated. Am J Dis Child 102:416–423, 1961.

Minagi H, Steinbach HL: Roentgen appearance of anomalies associated with hypoplastic anemias of childhood. Am J Roentgenol 97:100, 1966.

APLASTIC ANEMIA

Essentials of Diagnosis

- Weakness and pallor.
- Purpuras, petechiae, and bleeding.
- Frequent infections.
- Pancytopenia with empty bone marrow.

General Considerations

Aplastic anemia is characterized by a severe pancytopenia with an acellular marrow and normal-sized spleen.

In childhood, aplastic anemia may be of 3 general types.

(1) Fanconi's congenital pancytopenia: See below.

(2) Idiopathic aplastic anemia: In at least 1/2 of cases in childhood, no etiologic agent or specific congenital cause can be found.

(3) Secondary (acquired) aplastic anemia: Aplastic anemia may occur as a toxic reaction to various chemicals and drugs. Chloramphenicol accounts for the majority of cases in childhood. Other antibiotics, sulfonamides, benzene, phenylbutazone (Butazolidin), mephenytoin (Mesantoin), certain insecticides such as DDT, and heavy metals have all been incriminated. Glue sniffing has produced aplastic anemia and has also initiated aplastic crises in patients with sickle cell anemia. Large amounts of radiation and high doses of cytotoxic drugs such as nitrogen mustards and the folic acid antagonists will also produce severe aplasia. Aplastic anemia has also been observed as a complication of severe hepatitis.

Clinical Findings

A. Symptoms and Signs: Weakness, fatigue, and pallor are the result of the anemia; purpura and bleeding occur because of the thrombocytopenia; and severe generalized or localized infections are frequently due to neutropenia.

B. Laboratory Findings: Severe normochromic anemia is usually present, with some microcytosis. The reticulocyte count is usually very low, but in early cases with partial marrow destruction it may be slightly elevated. The white count is usually less than 2000/cu mm, with a marked neutropenia; and the platelet count is usually below 50,000/cu mm. Thrombocytopenia is often the earliest manifestation.

The bone marrow is practically devoid of normal marrow elements and is replaced with fat. A bone marrow section is indicated for absolute diagnosis.

The fetal hemoglobin level frequently remains elevated in congenitally determined aplastic anemia (Fanconi type) but may be normal in acquired forms.

Differential Diagnosis

Other causes of pancytopenia in childhood include infiltration with leukemia, Hodgkin's disease, Niemann-Pick disease, Gaucher's disease, Letterer-Siwe disease, osteopetrosis, myelofibrosis, and various toxic agents. Most of these conditions are associated with splenomegaly.

Complications

The disease is characteristically complicated by overwhelming infection and severe hemorrhage. With long-term transfusion therapy, problems may develop in association with leukoagglutinins, erythrocyte antibodies, and hemosiderosis.

A significant complication of prolonged testosterone therapy in childhood is the development in the male of early secondary sex characteristics, with enlargement of the penis, growth of pubic hair, muscular development, deepening of the voice, and personality changes; and, in the female, evidence of masculinization and hirsutism. Prolonged testosterone therapy may cause closure of the epiphyses and stunting of growth. The patient should be checked periodically with bone x-rays for epiphyseal maturation, and the dosage regulated accordingly.

Treatment

A. General Measures: Severely ill children should be protected from infection in their environment by being placed in "reverse isolation." Specific and appropriate antibiotics should be used for infection.

Transfusions are usually necessary. If bleeding is not present, packed red cells in a dose of 10–20 ml/kg should be used for treatment of the anemia when symptoms develop. For severe hemorrhage, platelet concentrates should be used, although occasionally fresh whole blood will be effective. Buffy coat concentrate containing high numbers of white cells may be tried for severe antibiotic-resistant infections, although this will probably increase the incidence of future transfusion reactions due to the development of leukoagglutinins.

B. Drug Therapy:

1. Testosterone propionate, 1–2 mg/kg/day orally under the tongue (or oxymetholone, 2.4 mg/kg/day orally), will produce remissions in a small proportion of both secondary and idiopathic cases of aplastic anemia in childhood. A patient who has a few residual marrow cells will respond more frequently than a patient with a totally empty bone marrow. The remission will frequently not occur until 1–2 months after treatment is started. Once a remission has been achieved, the lowest possible maintenance dose should be determined by gradual reduction of dosage. Temporary cessation of therapy may be indicated because of untoward drug side-effects. The congenital or Fanconi type of aplastic anemia is more likely to respond than the idiopathic or acquired form, although these patients usually require continued testosterone treatment and do not have spontaneous remissions. When oral medication cannot be used, give testosterone enanthate, 1 mg/kg IM once a month.

2. Corticosteroid therapy–Prednisone and similar drugs are usually not effective alone in aplastic anemia, but they may enhance the effect of testosterone. Therefore, prednisone, 1–2 mg/kg orally, should be given in addition to testosterone for initial therapy; the dose is decreased if a remission occurs. Prednisone in lower doses also has a nonspecific effect which may decrease the bleeding tendency.

C. Bone Marrow Transplantation: To date very little success has been achieved with the use of homologous bone marrow replacement therapy, and this is not recommended. However, isogenic marrow grafting has been successful when an identical twin with unaffected bone marrow is the donor.

Prognosis

The prognosis in either the secondary (acquired) or the idiopathic form of aplastic anemia is extremely poor when the bone marrow is totally empty and complete pancytopenia is present. In spite of supportive measures, these patients usually die of infection or hemorrhage within a period of a few months. Very few will respond to testosterone therapy. If some marrow elements remain, however, spontaneous remissions occasionally occur, and remissions are much more common in association with testosterone therapy. In the acquired form, a spontaneous remission may eventually occur 1–2 years after initiating treatment with testosterone or testosterone plus prednisone. In the congenital form (Fanconi type) of aplastic anemia, the mortality was at one time almost 100%. With testosterone therapy, these children often survive for many years, although relapse usually occurs when the testosterone is discontinued.

Githens JH: Anemias in childhood resulting from bone marrow deficiencies. Postgrad Med 31:128–132, 1967.

Hughes DW: Aplastic anaemia in childhood: A reappraisal. I. Classification and assessment. MJ Australia 1:1059, 1969.

Nora AH, Fernbach DJ: Acquired aplastic anemia in children. Texas Med 65:38, 1969.

Rukin E & others: Syndrome of hepatitis and aplastic anemia. Am J Med 45:88, 1968.

Silink SJ, Firkin BG: An analysis of hypoplastic anemia with special reference to the use of oxymetholone ("Adroyd"). Australasian Ann Med 17:224, 1968.

CONGENITAL APLASTIC ANEMIA WITH MULTIPLE CONGENITAL ANOMALIES (Fanconi's Anemia)

This is a familial aplastic anemia in which hypoplastic or aplastic bone marrow is associated with a number of other congenital anomalies. Occasionally the pancytopenia may occur in association with a hyperplastic marrow as a result of a delay in maturation. The most common defects are skeletal and include hypoplasia or absence of the thumb and the thenar eminence and absence of the radius. Other skeletal anomalies may include syndactyly, congenital dislocation of the hips, and abnormalities of the long bones. Some of these children may have patchy brown pigmentation of the skin, hypogenitalism, microcephaly, short stature, strabismus, ptosis of the eyelids, nystagmus, anomalies of the ears, and mental retardation. The condition may occur in siblings and is probably transmitted as a recessive trait. The hematologic manifestations rarely are manifested prior to age 1 and may appear at any time between ages 1–12. Thrombocytopenia is usually the first abnormality to be noted, followed later by neutropenia and anemia. Although the bone marrow in the majority of patients is hypoplastic and progresses to aplasia, in rare cases it may be hyperplastic, with a delay in maturation of marrow elements.

The hematologic disorder appears to be slowly progressive, and in most cases severe aplasia will develop. Death due to infection or bleeding will eventually occur if therapy is not instituted.

The clinical manifestations are principally those of the aplastic anemia (see above).

The majority of these patients will respond to testosterone therapy or testosterone plus prednisone, although relapse will occur when drug therapy is discontinued. (See section on aplastic anemia for details of therapy.) Transfusion should be used in the patient who does not respond to either testosterone or a combination of testosterone and prednisone.

The prognosis is much better since testosterone therapy came into use. However, long-term experience is beginning to suggest that many of these patients may eventually become resistant to testosterone therapy and die of the aplastic anemia in early adult life. Spontaneous recovery has occurred in a few cases.

Hathaway WE, Githens JH: Pancytopenia with hyperplastic marrow. Am J Dis Child 102:389–394, 1961.

McDonald R, Mibashan RS: Prolonged remission in Fanconitype anemia. Helv paediat acta 23:566, 1968.

O'Gorman-Hughes DW: Varied pattern of aplastic anemia in childhood. Australian Paediat J 2:228, 1966.

Perkins J & others: Clinical and chromosome studies in Fanconi's aplastic anaemia. JM Genet 6:28, 1969.

CONGENITAL HYPOPLASTIC ANEMIA WITHOUT ASSOCIATED ANOMALIES

Several families have been reported with pancytopenia and hypoplastic or aplastic marrow without associated anomalies. This is probably a recessive hereditary disorder and closely related to Fanconi's anemia. Testosterone therapy may be effective.

Zaivov R & others: Familial aplastic anemia without congenital malformations. Acta paediat scandinav 58:151, 1969.

ANEMIA OF RENAL FAILURE
(Anemia of Uremia)

A severe normochromic anemia occurs in almost all forms of renal disease that have progressed to renal failure. Although white cell production remains normal and platelet production may be normal, the bone marrow shows significant hypoplasia of the erythroid series.

The marrow hypoplasia is due to decreased circulating erythropoietin, which is normally produced principally in the kidney. The only treatment available is blood transfusion, which should be given as packed cells in a dosage of 10–20 mg/kg when the hemoglobin drops below 7 gm/100 ml or when symptoms occur. Drug therapy is not effective.

The anemia of renal disease is frequently complicated by an extracorpuscular hemolytic component which occurs in the presence of significant uremia. A more severe form of hemolytic anemia that occurs occasionally in children in association with renal disease is described under the hemolytic-uremic-thrombocytopenic syndrome.

Erslev AJ: Anemia of chronic renal disease. Arch Int Med 126:774–780, 1970.

ANEMIA OF HYPOTHYROIDISM

Certain patients with hypothyroidism develop fairly severe normochromic anemias. The red cells frequently tend to be macrocytic. The bone marrow shows hypocellularity of the erythroid series, with a normoblastic pattern.

Replacement therapy with thyroid hormone is completely effective in treating the anemia of the hypothyroid patient.

ANEMIA OF INFECTION & INFLAMMATION

Significant anemia usually develops in serious chronic infections or inflammatory diseases such as tuberculosis, chronic osteomyelitis, rheumatic fever, and rheumatoid arthritis. The anemia usually ranges between 8 and 11 gm/100 ml of hemoglobin, and is normochromic or slightly hypochromic. The reticulocyte count is usually normal or low. The exact mechanism is not clearly understood, although decreased availability of iron may be the primary case. The bone marrow appears normal and hemosiderin deposits are present, although the serum iron and the total iron-binding capacity are low. Evidence of the underlying infection or inflammatory disease is usually obvious.

There is no effective treatment except control of the infection and transfusions if the anemia is severe.

Anaemia in rheumatoid arthritis. Brit MJ 1:659, 1969.

ANEMIAS ASSOCIATED WITH MARROW REPLACEMENT (Myelophthisic Anemias)

Anemias resulting from bone marrow invasion or replacement are known as myelophthisic anemias. The most common cause in childhood is invasion with leukemic cells or lymphosarcoma. The differentiation from aplastic anemia in the hypoplastic form of leukemia can only be made by bone marrow examination. Hodgkin's disease in its advanced form may also be associated with severe marrow involvement. Other malignancies (particularly neuroblastoma) may cause diffuse involvement of the marrow. The disseminated acute form of histiocytosis or reticuloendotheliosis (Letterer-Siwe disease) may be associated with a diffuse involvement of the marrow. Certain of the lipid storage diseases such as Gaucher's disease and Niemann-Pick disease gradually invade the marrow. Osteopetrosis (Albers-Schönberg disease) in the acute infantile form is associated with severe encroachment on the marrow space by bone and usually presents initially as a myelophthisic anemia. True myelofibrosis with the development of classical agnogenic myeloid metaplasia is rarely seen in childhood.

All of these forms of myelophthisic anemia are characterized by the development of a normochromic anemia and associated thrombocytopenia. The presence of nucleated red cells and immature white cells with an elevated nucleated cell count in the peripheral blood suggests the existence of a myelophthisic process. Immature white and red cells are not always released, and they are probably related to the degree of extramedullary hematopoiesis. Splenomegaly is present in the majority of these conditions. The diagnosis is dependent upon finding the specific infiltrating process, osteopetrosis, or myelofibrosis in the bone marrow.

ANEMIAS DUE TO FAILURE OF RELEASE FROM THE MARROW

PRIMARY REFRACTORY ANEMIA (Refractory Normoblastic Anemia)

This condition is characterized by a moderate to severe chronic anemia, occasionally associated with neutropenia and thrombocytopenia. The reticulocyte count is low to normal. There are usually no other clinical findings, and the spleen is not enlarged. The marrow is markedly hypercellular, with normoblastic hyperplasia. Megaloblastic changes are usually present. Marrow hemosiderin is greatly increased.

The exact cause of this syndrome is not known, although many patients previously given this diagnosis may have had some type of dyserythropoietic anemia associated with intramedullary hemolysis (see next section). Treatment of the primary refractory anemias has been generally without success, and transfusion is the only known treatment. In rare cases, splenectomy has been of slight value; and occasional congenital cases have responded to testosterone therapy. All of these patients should be given a trial of B vitamins since the findings in pyridoxine (vitamin B_6) dependent and thiamine (vitamin B_2) dependent anemias may be similar.

Vilter RW & others: Refractory anemia with hyperplastic bone marrow. Blood 15:1–29, 1960.

DYSERYTHROPOIETIC ANEMIAS

Several reports from different parts of the world have recently described a group of patients who appear to have anemia associated with various forms of dyserythropoiesis. They have all been characterized by evidence of maturation abnormalities in the bone marrow and by evidence of intramedullary hemolysis. The clinical manifestations include the presence of scleral jaundice in a high percentage of cases. This is frequently intermittent. Splenomegaly usually is present. Anemia may or may not be present. Some patients are well compensated, with hemoglobins and hematocrits within the normal range. The majority have a mild to moderate anemia of about 10 gm/100 ml. Occasional patients show intermittent severe anemia associated with increased jaundice. They are frequently not recognized as having a hemolytic process since the destruction takes place in the marrow and an excessive number of reticulocytes are not released. The reticulocyte count usually ranges from normal to a maximum of about 4%. In most of the reported familial cases, the mode of genetic transmission appears to be autosomal recessive.

Additional laboratory findings of importance include the presence of rather marked anisocytosis and poikilocytosis on the blood smear. There is usually an elevation of the indirect serum bilirubin to approximately 2%. Haptoglobin levels are very helpful in diagnosis, particularly in cases in which the serum bilirubin is normal. The haptoglobin is usually low or absent. Urobilin and urobilinogen are increased in the urine. The bone marrow pattern is extremely helpful and is usually diagnostic. All reported cases have demonstrated significant erythroid hyperplasia, and the majority have shown a characteristic picture with multinucleated erythroblasts. In some patients the red cell shows several separate nuclei, and occasionally there is a chromatin bridge. Other patients show erythroblasts with a clover leaf shaped nucleus.

Additional laboratory findings in most patients include an elevated fetal hemoglobin and increased hemolysis in acidified serum (a positive Ham test) in the presence of a negative sugar water test. A high proportion of cells are agglutinated by anti-I antibody. Osmotic fragility is normal or increased. The autohemolysis test and hemoglobin electrophoresis are normal. Iron stores are increased, and iron kinetics show a rapid plasma clearance.

The exact mechanism of the ineffective erythropoiesis and the intramedullary hemolysis has not been specifically explained.

The differential diagnosis in certain patients is primarily from Gilbert's disease, since in patients with little or no anemia the primary finding is elevated unconjugated (indirect reacting) serum bilirubin and intermittent scleral icterus. In patients with anemia, the differential diagnosis initially appears to be from other forms of normochromic anemia, particularly the primary refractory anemias.

Treatment is symptomatic.

Crookston JH & others: Hereditary erythroblastic multinuclearity associated with a positive acidified serum test: A type of congenital dyserythropoietic anemia. Brit J Haemat 17:11, 1969.

HEMOLYTIC ANEMIAS

The hemolytic anemias of childhood may be classified as hereditary or acquired. The hereditary group are of particular importance since the manifestations usually present in infancy or childhood. They may be divided first into those associated with a defect of the red cell membrane, such as hereditary spherocytosis, and those due to abnormalities in red cell glycolysis. (This includes the majority of the nonspherocytic hemolytic anemias that are associated with specific red cell enzyme defects and the drug-induced hemolytic anemias.) Second, there is the large group of hemoglobinopathies, which includes the anemias with abnormal hemoglobin chains, those with a genetically determined decrease in production of one of the hemoglobin chains, and the unstable hemoglobin. The majority of the acquired hemolytic anemias are on an "autoimmune" basis; are secondary to drug or chemical poisoning; or are associated with sepsis from hemolytic organisms.

DISORDERS OF RED CELL MEMBRANE

1. HEREDITARY SPHEROCYTOSIS
(Congenital Hemolytic Anemia, Congenital Hemolytic Jaundice)

Essentials of Diagnosis
- Anemia.
- Sudden weakness and jaundice.
- Splenomegaly.
- Spherocytosis, increased reticulocytes.

- Increased osmotic fragility, abnormal autohemolysis.
- Negative Coombs test.
- Positive family history of anemia, jaundice, or gallbladder disease.

General Considerations

Hereditary spherocytosis is believed to be due to a defect in the red cell membrane, allowing increased permeability to sodium. Increased glycolysis is necessary to prevent the intracellular accumulation of sodium. Spherocytosis and decreased red cell survival occur when the cell is deprived of sufficient glucose. The cells are sequestered and destroyed in the spleen. Transfused cells from normal donors have a normal survival in the patient with spherocytosis, whereas spherocytic cells transfused into a normal recipient maintain their shortened survival rate. The disease may be mild to severe and is characterized by intermittent crises associated with rapid hemolysis and jaundice. Hypoplastic crises occasionally occur in association with decreased erythroid production in the bone marrow. In most instances, the disease is transmitted as an autosomal dominant, and abnormalities can usually be detected in one of the parents of the child even though they are asymptomatic. Occasional families have been reported in which the abnormality cannot be found in other generations, suggesting that it may sometimes be transmitted as a recessive trait or occur as a mutation. Hereditary spherocytosis may be a cause of neonatal hyperbilirubinemia and may be confused with ABO incompatibility because of the presence of spherocytes in both conditions.

Clinical Findings

A. Symptoms and Signs: Jaundice usually occurs in the newborn period. Splenomegaly without other symptoms characterizes many of the cases in childhood. Chronic fatigue and malaise may be present, and abdominal pain is a frequent complaint. Gallbladder pain may occur in the adolescent.

Hemolytic or aplastic crises may develop and are associated with severe weakness, fatigue, fever, abdominal pain, and jaundice.

B. Laboratory Findings: Mild chronic anemia is characteristic. The hemoglobin usually varies from 9–11 gm/100 ml, although a few cases may have almost normal levels of 12–13 gm/100 ml. The red cells are microcytic and hyperchromic (MCV = 70–80 μm and MCHC = 36–40%). Spherocytes characteristically are seen on the smear but may comprise no more than 10% of the cells prior to splenectomy. A persistently elevated reticulocyte count is characteristic. White cells and platelets are usually normal.

The bone marrow shows typical erythroid hyperplasia of hemolytic anemia (except during the hypoplastic crisis, when there may be marked reduction of erythropoiesis).

Osmotic fragility is increased, particularly after incubation at 37° C for 24 hours. Autohemolysis of blood incubated for 48 hours is greatly increased. Incubation with glucose or ATP will decrease the hemolysis (usually to normal levels). Serum bilirubin may show elevation of the unconjugated portion. Stool urobilinogen is usually elevated. The Coombs test is negative, and hemoglobin electrophoresis reveals a normal pattern.

Complications

Severe jaundice may occur in the newborn period with the development of kernicterus if exchange transfusion is not performed. Splenectomy in the first 2 years of life may be associated with increased susceptibility to overwhelming bacterial infections, although the risk is not great. Gallstones (composed principally of bile pigments) occur in up to 85% of young adults with this disease, and may even develop during later childhood if splenectomy is not performed by the middle childhood years.

Treatment

There is no satisfactory medical treatment for this condition, but splenectomy is effective.

A. Exchange Transfusions: For hyperbilirubinemia in the neonatal period, exchange transfusion should be performed.

B. Surgical Treatment: Splenectomy is the treatment of choice in hereditary spherocytosis. Except in unusually severe cases, the procedure should be postponed until the child is at least 3—4 years of age because of the increased risk of infection prior to this time. The operation is indicated in all older children as soon as the diagnosis is confirmed even though the degree of hemolysis may be mild. Cholecystectomy is rarely indicated in childhood, particularly if splenectomy is performed at an early age.

C. Postoperative Anti-infective Prophylaxis: Prophylactic penicillin is recommended following splenectomy in all children under 2 years of age in whom the procedure is done. It should probably be continued until at least 4—5 years of age. In older children, daily penicillin prophylaxis is recommended for at least 1 year postoperatively.

D. Treatment of Hypoplastic Crisis: The crisis is frequently precipitated by an infectious process, which should be treated with appropriate antibiotic therapy. Transfusion with packed red cells is indicated for both the hemolytic and the aplastic crisis.

Prognosis

Splenectomy will eliminate all signs and symptoms, and the red cell survival usually returns to normal following this procedure. The development of cholelithiasis will also be prevented if splenectomy is performed during childhood. The abnormal red cell morphology, increased osmotic fragility, and the abnormal autohemolysis test persist following splenectomy but are of no clinical significance.

Jandl JH: Hereditary spherocytosis. Pages 209—228 in: *Hereditary Disorders of Erythrocyte Metabolism.* Beutler E. Grune & Stratton, 1968.

Oski FA, Naiman JL: *Hematologic Problems in the Newborn.* Saunders, 1966.

2. OVALOCYTOSIS
(Hereditary Elliptocytosis)

Hereditary elliptocytosis is characterized primarily by the presence of large numbers of oval and elliptical cells in the peripheral blood. It is usually discovered on routine examination, and the majority of patients are asymptomatic. The morphologic abnormality of the peripheral blood is transmitted as an autosomal dominant and occurs in both sexes. Approximately 12% of the heterozygous cases demonstrate evidence of mild hemolytic disease characterized by slight splenomegaly and reticulocytosis. There may be low-grade anemia, but even in these patients the hemoglobin is frequently within normal limits. Occasionally, neonatal jaundice is sufficiently severe to require exchange transfusions.

The nucleated precursors of the elliptical cells in the bone marrow are normal in shape, with the oval appearance occurring first at the reticulocyte stage or later. The mechanism of the abnormality is not known.

A few cases have been reported of children who are homozygous for the disease. These children have severe hemolytic anemia, with splenomegaly and hematologic evidence of hemolysis.

Treatment is not usually indicated except in severe cases, for which splenectomy is usually beneficial.

Greenberg LH & others: Hereditary elliptocytosis with hemolytic anemia: A family study of 5· affected members. California Med 110:389, 1969.

3. STOMATOCYTOSIS

A rare form of hemolytic anemia has been described in which the red blood cells have a characteristic cup-shaped appearance. The anemia is mild, and the disease has the characteristics of a hemolytic process with elevated reticulocyte count. The red cells have increased osmotic fragility, increased autohemolysis, and reduced glutathione.

Splenectomy· results in improvement.

Norman JG: Stomatocytosis in migrants of Mediterranean origin. MJ Australia 1:315, 1969.

DISORDERS OF RED CELL GLYCOLYSIS
(The Hereditary Nonspherocytic Hemolytic Anemias)

Essentials of Diagnosis·
- Moderate to severe anemia.
- Elevated reticulocyte count.
- Normal osmotic fragility test with abnormal autohemolysis.

- Splenomegaly.
- Present from birth, with neonatal jaundice.
- Negative Coombs test.

General Considerations

The hereditary nonspherocytic hemolytic anemias include a number of different specific entities which are gradually being differentiated as more refined methods for study of red cell metabolism become available. A large number of specific enzymes necessary for erythrocyte glycolysis have been proved to be deficient in various forms of nonspherocytic hemolytic anemia.

The specific enzyme deficiencies that have already been described include glucose-6-phosphate dehydrogenase (G6PD), 6-phosphogluconate dehydrogenase, pyruvate kinase, triosephosphate isomerase, hexokinase, hexosephosphate isomerase, phosphoglycerate kinase, adenosinetriphosphatase (ATPase), 2,3-diphosphoglycerate mutase, glutathione reductase, glutathione peroxidase, glutathione synthetase, and hereditary absence of glutathione. The most frequently encountered are those associated with G6PD and pyruvate kinase deficiency. These will be discussed in more detail in succeeding sections.

Two general classes of nonspherocytic hemolytic anemia have been described by Dacie. Type I is characterized by normal red cell fragility and a normal to slightly increased autohemolysis test which is corrected by glucose. Patients with severe deficiency of G6PD fall into this type. The specific underlying abnormality in most of the others is not known.

Type II cases are characterized by normal or slightly increased red cell fragility but a markedly increased autohemolysis that is not corrected (or only partially corrected) by glucose. Pyruvate kinase deficiency is characteristic of this group. The hereditary pattern varies. Deficiency of G6PD is usually transmitted as a sex-linked recessive trait, whereas pyruvate kinase deficiency is an autosomal recessive. Other milder forms may be transmitted as an autosomal dominant.

Clinical Findings

A. Symptoms and Signs: Moderate to severe anemia is usually present and exists from early infancy. Neonatal hyperbilirubinemia is usually marked. In severe cases, symptoms of chronic anemia and jaundice persist. The spleen is enlarged.

B. Laboratory Findings: Anemia is moderate to severe, and the hemoglobin usually ranges from 5–9 gm/100 ml. The red cells are normocytic and normochromic, although occasional microcytes are seen and, in pyruvate kinase deficiency, a few spherocytes. The reticulocyte count is markedly elevated; the white cell and platelet counts are normal. Bone marrow shows marked erythroid hyperplasia.

Red cell osmotic fragility is usually within normal limits, although in type II—and particularly in pyruvate kinase deficiency—it may be slightly increased. The autohemolysis test is usually slightly increased in type I, and partially corrected by glucose and ATP, whereas it is markedly abnormal in type II with very little correction by glucose, but complete correction with ATP. A third type (triosephosphate isomerase deficiency) is corrected by both glucose and ATP. The Coombs test is negative, and hemoglobin electrophoresis is normal.

Studies of red cell glycolysis with assays of specific enzymes are indicated in all cases that fall into this group, since the response to therapy may be dependent on the exact type of disease.

Differential Diagnosis

In the newborn period, hereditary nonspherocytic hemolytic anemia must be differentiated from erythroblastosis fetalis and ABO incompatibility by immunologic studies. It is differentiated from acquired hemolytic anemia by the early onset and the absence of a positive Coombs test. The differentiation from hereditary spherocytosis is based on the absence of spherocytes on the smear, the normal or only slightly increased red cell fragility, and the lack of complete correction with glucose in the autohemolysis test in the nonspherocytic hemolytic anemias.

Complications

The severe chronic anemia is usually associated with growth failure; hemosiderosis may occur in cases that require frequent transfusions. Cholelithiasis and cholecystitis may develop in later childhood.

Treatment

There is no specific therapy for most cases of nonspherocytic hemolytic anemia. Splenectomy is not as effective as in hereditary spherocytosis, and is of no benefit in many cases. However, many patients (including those with pyruvate kinase deficiency) do show significant improvement following splenectomy; although no patients are completely cured and many do not respond at all, the operation is probably worth a trial. The possible value of splenectomy can be estimated by determining the red cell survival of cells from a patient with hereditary nonspherocytic hemolytic anemia after infusion into a normal individual who has undergone splenectomy for some other reason.

Prognosis

In the milder form of this disease, the prognosis is good; the patient can usually live with a mild chronic anemia. Cholelithiasis often develops in early adult life. The prognosis is similar in patients with more severe forms that show improvement following splenectomy.

In the severe types that do not respond to splenectomy, frequent transfusions are required, physical growth is stunted, and hemosiderosis and even hemochromatosis may develop.

Beutler E: *Hereditary Disorders of Erythrocyte Metabolism.* Grune & Stratton, 1968.

Dacie JV: Recent advances in knowledge of the hereditary haemolytic anaemias. Schweiz Med Wschr 98:1624, 1968.

1. PYRUVATE KINASE DEFICIENCY HEMOLYTIC ANEMIA

Although this is a rare disease, it is still one of the more frequently encountered specific entities in the group of nonspherocytic hereditary hemolytic anemias. It is transmitted as an autosomal recessive. It presents as a severe hemolytic anemia in the immediate neonatal period, with low hemoglobin levels even in cord blood. Jaundice in the newborn is a common complication, and exchange transfusion is usually required. Splenomegaly is the only consistent clinical finding.

The anemia is normochromic, and there is a marked elevation of the reticulocyte count. The blood smear shows some microcytes and a few spherocytes. Differentiation from hereditary spherocytosis is not easy because spherocytes may be seen in pyruvate kinase deficiency and red cell osmotic fragility may also be slightly increased; the autohemolysis test is markedly increased, as in spherocytosis. The most useful point of differentiation between the 2 diseases is the fact that the red cell fragility is only slightly increased and the autohemolysis test is only partially corrected by glucose in pyruvate kinase deficiency, whereas the latter is markedly corrected in spherocytosis.

Family studies are also helpful in differentiating the 2 conditions, since pyruvate kinase deficiency is a recessive trait whereas spherocytosis is usually a dominant.

Red cell glycolysis and specific enzyme assays for pyruvate kinase are indicated if this condition is suspected. Recently, patients have been described with a similar disorder who appear to have adequate pyruvate kinase activity by the usual assay but who are found to have a pathologic isoenzyme which can be detected only by assays using low levels of substrate.

Treatment consists of splenectomy. Significant improvement usually follows this procedure, although complete cure is not achieved. Prior to splenectomy, repeated transfusions are usually necessary every few months. No drugs or other methods of management are effective.

The prognosis following splenectomy is fairly good, although the complications of cholelithiasis should'be anticipated.

Oski FA, Diamond LK: Erythrocyte pyruvate kinase deficiency resulting in non-spherocytic hemolytic anemia. New England J Med 269:736, 1963.

Poglia DE: An aberrant inherited molecular lesion of erythrocyte pyruvate kinase: Identification of a kinetically aberrant isoenzyme associated with premature hemolysis. J Clin Invest 47:1929, 1968.

2. GLUCOSE-6-PHOSPHATE DEHYDROGENASE DEFICIENCY
(Drug-Sensitive Hemolytic Anemia, Primaquine-Sensitive Hemolytic Anemia)

Drug-induced hemolytic anemia is most commonly associated with a red cell deficiency of glucose–6-phosphate dehydrogenase (G6PD). Although the more severe forms may be manifested by type I chronic hereditary nonspherocytic hemolytic anemia, most persons with a G6PD defect have episodes of hemolysis only after exposure to certain drugs.

The disease is transmitted as a sex-linked trait and is of intermediate dominance. Full expression occurs in males and in rare homozygous females, whereas intermediate expression occurs in the heterozygous female carrier. About 10% of American black males manifest this enzyme deficiency, whereas only 1–2% of American black females tend to be symptomatic when challenged with drugs. This disease occurs also in the Chinese and in whites (particularly Greeks, Italians, and Sephardic Jews). The exact mechanism of the enzyme defect is not quantitatively nor qualitatively identical in all of these racial groups.

Symptoms usually occur only following drug exposure, although in the neonatal period certain racial groups (Greek, Italian, and Chinese) may show increased hyperbilirubinemia, whereas full-term black babies do not. The most common offenders are the antimalarials, sulfonamides, sulfones, nitrofurans, antipyretics, analgesics, synthetic vitamin K, and uncooked fava beans. The clinical picture is characterized by an acute hemolytic episode following exposure to one of these substances. The anemia is normochromic, and Heinz body formation is characteristic. An elevated reticulocyte count will appear within a few days.

Since only the older red cells are susceptible, the process becomes self-limited as a younger red cell population appears in response to the hemolytic process.

A specific laboratory diagnosis may be made by one of several tests, including the glutathione stability· test, the dye reduction test using cresyl blue, the methemoglobin reduction test, or a commercially available dye reduction spot test.

The only treatment required is discontinuing exposure to the offending agent.

Beutler E: *Hereditary Disorders of Erythrocyte Metabolism.* Grune & Stratton, 1968.

Carson PE, Frischer H: Glucose-6-phosphate dehydrogenase deficiency and related disorders of the pentose phosphate pathway. Am J Med 41:744, 1966.

Kirkman HN: Glucose-6-phosphate dehydrogenase variants and drug induced hemolysis. Ann New York Acad Sc 151:753, 1968.

INFANTILE PYKNOCYTOSIS

A transient hemolytic anemia has been described in newborn infants in association with a high degree of pyknocytosis of their red cells. Pyknocytes bear a close resemblance to bur cells and acanthocytes. They occur in small numbers in all newborn and premature infants but in infants with hemolysis as many as 50% of red cells may be pyknocytes. The exact cause remains unknown. The syndrome is characterized by hemolysis beginning during the first week of life, with jaundice, anemia, reticulocytosis, and splenomegaly. The anemia usually reaches its peak by 3 weeks of age, and recovery is spontaneous.

The diagnosis is based on the presence of large numbers of pyknocytes (> 6%) in association with a Coombs-negative hemolytic anemia. Vitamin E deficiency may present an identical laboratory and clinical picture in the newborn, with hemolysis and an increase in burr cells. It can be differentiated by demonstrating an increased hemolysis in hydrogen peroxide and a response to the administration of parenteral vitamin E.

Exchange transfusion may be necessary for the hyperbilirubinemia of pyknocytosis during the first week. Small transfusions are indicated for increasing anemia after that time.

Ackerman BD: Infantile pyknocytosis in Mexican-American infants. Am J Dis Child 117:417, 1969.

SYNTHETIC VITAMIN K-INDUCED HEMOLYTIC ANEMIA OF THE NEWBORN

Another form of drug-induced hemolytic anemia occurs following the administration of synthetic vitamin K (Synkamin, Synkayvite, Hykinone) in large doses in the newborn period. Although the level of G6PD is not decreased in the newborn infant, the drug-induced hemolysis appears to be related to instability of reduced glutathione in the newborn red cells. This may be due in part to the low blood glucose levels which are characteristic of the neonatal period.

This complication can be prevented by limiting the dose of the synthetic vitamin K product to a total of 1 mg or by the use of vitamin K_1 (Mephyton, Aqua-Mephyton, etc), which does not have the same chemical derivation.

Oski FA, Naiman JL: *Hematologic Problems in the Newborn.* Saunders, 1966.

HEMOGLOBINOPATHIES—QUALITATIVE DEFECTS

1. SICKLE CELL ANEMIA

Essentials of Diagnosis

- Anemia, elevated reticulocyte count, jaundice.
- Positive sickling test, hemoglobin S and F.
- Pains in the legs and abdomen.
- Splenomegaly in early childhood, with later disappearance.
- Hemolytic crises.

General Considerations

Sickle cell anemia occurs in individuals who are homozygous for the sickle cell gene. Sickle hemoglobin is characterized by a single amino acid substitution in the beta chain of adult type (A_1) hemoglobin. The sickling trait is transmitted as a dominant; the carrier shows a combination of hemoglobin A and sickle hemoglobin, whereas the patient with sickle cell anemia has only sickle and fetal hemoglobin. The sickling process is often initiated by low oxygen tension and low pH. The sickle cell moves slowly through capillaries, and thrombi are frequent. Thrombosis probably accounts for the abdominal pain, leg pain, and gradual decrease in the size of the spleen ("autosplenectomy").

Clinical Findings

A. Symptoms and Signs: The anemia is moderately severe, but fatigue and weakness are minimal. Mild scleral jaundice is usually present. Crises are frequent, and are characterized by pain in the bones and joints or the abdomen; severe acute hemolysis often occurs. Abdominal tenderness and rigidity may occur. Fever is usually present. Severe anemia, weakness, and increased jaundice may accompany the crisis. Physical growth is slightly delayed, and children are usually of asthenic build. The older child shows an enlargement of the facial and skull bones and may develop a tower skull.

B. Laboratory Findings: The hemoglobin usually ranges between 7 and 9 gm/100 ml. It may drop to levels as low as 2–3 gm/100 ml at the time of a crisis. The reticulocyte count is markedly elevated. The anemia is normocytic and normochromic, but the smear shows increased numbers of target cells and abnormalities of size and shape. Sickling may be seen on the ordinary blood smear and is common at the time of crisis. The sickling phenomenon can be demonstrated by reducing the oxygen tension in the finger with a small tourniquet prior to obtaining blood, or by ringing the cover slip on a slide with petrolatum over a drop of blood. Fresh sodium metabisulfite, 2%, mixed on the slide with the drop of blood will bring out the sickling in a few minutes. Nucleated red cells are present and may equal the number of white cells. The total nucleated cell count is high. Serum bilirubin usually shows a slight elevation of unconjugated (indirect) bilirubin. The specific gravity of the urine becomes fixed at about 1.010 in later childhood, and both hemosiderinuria and hematuria may be seen.

The bone marrow shows marked erythroid hyperplasia. X-rays of the skull and spine reveal cortical thinning, enlargement of the marrow spaces, and increased trabecular markings.

Hemoglobin electrophoresis reveals sickle hemoglobin and fetal hemoglobin. The fetal component usually varies between 5 and 20%.

Differential Diagnosis

The most important differentiation is from the other chronic hemoglobinopathies that are also common in the black population. The differentiation from thalassemia and hemoglobin C disease is made primarily by hemoglobin electrophoresis, fetal hemoglobin determination, and the sickling test. The hematuria that occurs with sickle cell anemia must be differentiated from renal bleeding due to other causes. In crisis, the primary differentiation is from acute appendicitis in the presence of abdominal pain and tenderness and from rheumatic fever because of the frequent joint and bone pains and the systolic precordial murmur in sickle cell disease.

Hemoglobin D migrates electrophoretically on paper and starch at the same rate as S and is indistinguishable by this method. They can be differentiated by the negative sickling test in hemoglobin D disease. Study of the entire family is often of importance in determining the exact nature of the hemoglobinopathy.

Sickle cell trait associated with iron deficiency anemia can be differentiated by the presence of a low reticulocyte count, high red cell count, and hypochromia.

Complications

The primary complications in childhood are associated with vascular thromboses. Cerebral thrombosis and pulmonary infarcts may occur, particularly in younger children; and leg ulcers and aseptic necrosis of the femoral head are common in older children and adolescents. An increased incidence of salmonella osteomyelitis has been reported. In the adolescent, cardiac enlargement and even heart failure may occur in association with prolonged severe anemia and cardiac ischemia. Cholelithiasis is rarely seen in childhood, but will be an eventual complication. Hypoplastic crises may occur and are associated with the development of a very severe and prolonged anemic state.

Treatment

Treatment is instituted primarily for the crises. There is no known effective method for reducing the rate of chronic hemolysis or preventing crises. Both the hemolytic and hypoplastic crises should be treated with transfusion. Transfusions are also helpful in terminating prolonged "painful" crises. Whole blood is preferred, although packed cells may be used in the severely anemic child. The use of oxygen, maintenance of good hydration, and correction of acidosis are the most important measures for management of the symptoms of crisis. Rest, analgesics, and sedatives may be sufficient in mild cases. Corticosteroids have been reported to be helpful in the management of painful swelling of the hands and feet. Recent clinical trials using testosterone to stimulate marrow production have been associated with an increased incidence of thrombosis. The value of treatment with urea (to reduce sickling) must be established by further controlled studies.

Splenectomy may be of value in the child with a persistently enlarged spleen and a need for frequent transfusions. Since there is a natural tendency for the spleen to shrink in size in this disease, splenectomy is seldom indicated.

Prognosis

Relatively few patients with homozygous sickle cell disease die in childhood, although a fatal outcome is occasionally seen in association with overwhelming infections, cerebrovascular accidents, or cardiac failure. Many patients, however, die in early adult life. Progressive renal damage usually occurs, and death from uremia or heart failure is common.

Freedman ML: Treatment of crises in sickle cell anemia. Am J Med Sc 261:305–308, 1971.

Pearson HA & others: Functional asplenia in sickle-cell anemia. New England J Med 281:923, 1969.

Rako J: Sickle cell disease. J Pediat 75:158, 1969.

Smits HL & others: Hemolytic crisis of sickle cell disease: Role of glucose-6-phosphate dehydrogenase deficiency. J Pediat 74:544, 1969.

2. SICKLE CELL TRAIT

Sickle cell trait occurs in about 12% of blacks in the USA and in as much as 50% of the population in certain areas of Africa. It is generally asymptomatic, and anemia, reticulocytosis, and morphologic red cell changes are usually not observed. Hematuria is the principal complication and occurs in 3–4% of cases. Progressive impairment in the ability of the kidneys to concentrate urine is sometimes noted. Infarcts (particularly in the spleen and lung) may occur in the presence of low oxygen tension at extremely high altitudes—particularly with flying in unpressurized aircraft. Except for these unusual circumstances, the prognosis is excellent. The high incidence of the carrier state in African blacks has been attributed to the increased resistance to malaria in these individuals, which tends to selectively increase their representation in the population.

Knochel JP: Hematuria in sickle cell trait. Arch Int Med 123:160, 1969.

3. HEMOGLOBIN C TRAIT & HEMOGLOBIN C DISEASE

Hemoglobin C trait occurs in about 2% of American blacks. Individuals with the trait are heterozygous for the gene and are essentially asymptomatic; they have a normal life expectancy. The blood smear, however, reveals the presence of large numbers of target cells. Renal hematuria has occasionally been reported.

Hemoglobin C disease is rare and occurs in individuals who are homozygous for the gene. It occurs almost exclusively in blacks. Patients usually demonstrate a mild hemolytic anemia with a persistently elevated reticulocyte count. Red cell morphology is characterized by many target cells, which are usually normocytic and normochromic. Tetragonal crystals of hemoglobin can be found in the erythrocyte. Osmotic fragility is decreased. The diagnosis is made by hemoglobin electrophoresis, which usually reveals 100% hemoglobin C. Fetal hemoglobin is usually not elevated. Moderate to marked splenomegaly is the only significant clinical finding. There are usually no symptoms, although abdominal pain, arthralgia, and jaundice may occur occasionally.

Treatment is usually not required, and transfusions are rarely needed. Splenectomy is occasionally indicated if anemia is severe.

Redetski JE, Bickers JN, Samuels MS: Homozygous hemoglobin C disease: Clinical review of 15 patients. South MJ 61:238, 1968.

4. HEMOGLOBIN S-C DISEASE

Hemoglobin S-C disease is caused by the double autosomal heterozygous state for both hemoglobin S and C. The incidence in the American black population is about 1:1500. Symptoms are similar to those described for homozygous sickle cell disease but are much less marked. Target cells are prominent, and a moderate anemia with persistent reticulocytosis is usually present. The diagnosis is confirmed by hemoglobin electrophoresis and the sickling test, along with evaluation of other members of the family. The complications and treatment are similar to those for sickle cell anemia, although most patients require no therapy. Although the severity of the disease may vary, the prognosis is much better than in homozygous sickle disease, and the life span is usually not seriously affected.

River GL, Robins AB, Schwartz SO: S-C hemoglobin: A clinical study. Blood 18:385–416, 1961.

5. HEMOGLOBIN M DISEASE

The designation M is given to several abnormal hemoglobins which are associated with methemoglobinemia. These patients are heterozygous for the gene, and it is transmitted as an autosomal dominant. A number of different types have been described in which various abnormal amino acids are substituted in the polypeptide chain, producing a hemoglobin molecule in which the iron remains in the ferric instead of the ferrous state and cannot combine with oxygen. The defect may be on either the alpha or the beta chain. Hemoglobin electrophoresis at the usual pH will not always demonstrate the abnormal hemoglobin, and special technics are necessary to detect it by electrophoresis as well as spectroscopically.

The patient has marked and persistent cyanosis but is otherwise usually asymptomatic. Exercise tolerance may be normal, and life expectancy is not affected. When the abnormality is on the beta chain, the infant is unaffected for the first few months of life.

This type of methemoglobinemia does not respond to any form of therapy.

Heller P: Hemoglobin M: An early chapter in the saga of molecular pathology. Ann Int Med 70:1038, 1969.

6. OTHER ABNORMAL HEMOGLOBINS

Other hemoglobins such as D, E, G, and H are rare in the USA but occur with a higher incidence in other parts of the world. Hemoglobin D has been reported particularly from the Punjab area of India and in parts of Turkey and Africa, as well as occasionally in American blacks and American Indians. It is generally asymptomatic unless associated with another abnormal hemoglobin such as S. Hemoglobin E occurs particularly in Thailand and is usually asymptomatic except in association with other hemoglobin disorders such as thalassemia. Hemoglobin G, even in the homozygous form, has not been associated with symptoms but has been described in combination with other abnormal hemoglobins as a cause of mild anemia. Hemoglobin H has been reported primarily from Asia and, in particular, from Thailand. It is composed only of beta chains, and symptomatic disease has been described primarily in combination with alpha thalassemia. The red cells demonstrate characteristic inclusion bodies in the presence of supravital stains such as brilliant cresyl blue.

The majority of the other abnormal hemoglobins that have been described occur only in the heterozygous form and are asymptomatic.

Lehmann H: Hemoglobinopathies: Abnormal hemoglobins and thalassemias. Israel J Med Sc 4:478, 1968.

7. THERMOLABILE (UNSTABLE) HEMOGLOBINS

Since the first report in 1960, a number of families have now been described with a mild form of hemolytic anemia due to a hemoglobinopathy in which the hemoglobin is thermolabile. All of these patients with unstable hemoglobins have had mild anemia and scleral jaundice. They frequently report intermittent exacerbations of hemolysis, and in all cases a dark brown urine has been noted. Mild splenomegaly is usually present. The disorders appear to be transmitted as an autosomal dominant with symptoms occurring in the heterozygous form.

The laboratory findings reveal a typical picture of a hemolytic anemia with a mild to moderate depression of the hemoglobin and hematocrit and a significant elevation of the reticulocyte count. The unconjugated (indirect reacting) serum bilirubin is often slightly elevated and haptoglobin levels are usually zero, confirming the evidence for hemolysis. The blood smear in some patients has demonstrated marked basophilic stippling. The osmotic fragility test may show both increased fragility and increased resistance. The autohemolysis test is normal. Specific diagnostic studies include the presence of Heinz bodies, particularly after incubation at 37° C for 48 hours. Hemoglobin electrophoresis in some families has shown an abnormal hemoglobin on paper electrophoresis at pH 8.5. In all cases in which the abnormal hemoglobin was identified on electrophoresis, it has migrated more slowly than hemoglobin A_1 and frequently has been more readily identified on starch gel or agar gel. The percentage of abnormal hemoglobin identified has usually been low (in the range of 5–10%). The heat stability test is the best method for identification of the thermolabile hemoglobin. All of the reported hemoglobins precipitate with heating to 50° C for 1 hour. The dark pigment in the urine has been identified as mesobilifuscin.

The different unstable hemoglobins that have been identified to date include Scott, Zurich, Köln, Ubi-1, Summersmith, Dacy, Seattle, St. Mary's, Genova Galliera, Sydney, and King's County.

The differential diagnosis includes all of the hereditary hemolytic anemias such as spherocytosis and the nonspherocytic group as well as the other hemoglobinopathies. The autosomal dominant genetic transmission tends to exclude the majority of these except for spherocytosis. The diagnostic test is a demonstration of a thermolabile hemoglobin in the blood and the presence of mesobilifuscin in the urine.

The prognosis in most patients is probably good since the anemia appears to be mild. There is no specific treatment.

Saphiapalan R, Robinson MG: Hereditary hemolytic anemia due to an abnormal hemoglobin (hemoglobin King's County). Brit J Haemat 15:579, 1968.

HEMOGLOBINOPATHIES–QUANTITATIVE DEFECTS
(Thalassemia Syndromes)

1. BETA THALASSEMIA MINOR
(Thalassemia Trait, Cooley's Carrier State)

Essentials of Diagnosis
- Mild hypochromic anemia.
- Unresponsiveness to iron.
- Elevated A_2 hemoglobin.
- Usually Mediterranean, black, or Oriental racial lines.

General Considerations

Thalassemia is now known to be due to a genetic defect in the production of hemoglobin. It can affect both the alpha and the beta chains, but the majority of patients seen in the USA have beta thalassemia. The patient with thalassemia minor is heterozygous for the gene, which is transmitted as an autosomal dominant.

Clinical Findings

A. Symptoms and Signs: There are usually no symptoms, and the only physical sign may be slight enlargement of the spleen.

B. Laboratory Findings: The anemia is usually mild; the hemoglobin is rarely under 9 gm/100 ml, and may be within normal limits. The red count and hematocrit are very slightly reduced. The red cells are small and hypochromic, and the MCHC is low. Target cells are often present, and stippled cells are seen occasionally. Variations in the size and shape of the cells are often noted. The reticulocyte count may be slightly elevated but is frequently within normal limits. Osmotic fragility is markedly decreased.

The diagnosis is confirmed by finding an elevation of the A_2 hemoglobin on electrophoresis; fetal hemoglobin is usually not increased. (In alpha thalassemia—see below—the A_2 hemoglobin is normal.) The serum iron and iron-binding capacity are normal or elevated, and the bone marrow may show excessive iron deposition in the older child.

Differential Diagnosis

The primary differentiation is from other mild hypochromic anemias. In childhood, nutritional iron deficiency presents the greatest problem but is readily differentiated by the finding of low serum iron levels and a response to iron therapy, as well as a normal A_2 hemoglobin level. Lead poisoning and pyridoxine responsive anemia may present with a similar hematologic picture.

Several closely related thalassemia-like diseases such as the Lepore trait have recently been described. An abnormal hemoglobin has been demonstrated in the Lepore trait with the use of starch electrophoresis but not with paper. It comprises approximately 10% of the hemoglobin.

Complications

There are no complications of thalassemia trait in childhood. In late adult life, excess accumulation of iron may lead to hemosiderosis.

Treatment

No therapy is indicated. Iron should definitely not be administered.

Weatherall DJ: *The Thalassemia Syndromes.* Davis, 1965.

2. BETA THALASSEMIA MAJOR
(Cooley's Anemia, Mediterranean Anemia)

Essentials of Diagnosis

- Very severe anemia.
- Marked erythroblastemia.
- Splenomegaly and hepatomegaly.
- Elevated fetal hemoglobin.
- Usually Mediterranean, black, or Oriental racial lines.

General Considerations

Thalassemia major appears in individuals who are homozygous for the thalassemia gene. Family studies show that both parents have thalassemia minor. Thalassemia major is almost invariably of the beta thalassemia type, since homozygous alpha thalassemia is incompatible with life. A few infants have been described with alpha thalassemia, but have usually been stillborn with fetal hydrops. Rarely, combinations of alpha and beta thalassemia may occur in individuals who are heterozygous for the 2 genes. Homozygous beta thalassemia is now believed to be due to a quantitative deficiency in production of beta chains. This produces an intracorpuscular defect which is associated with marked hypochromia and a shortened red cell survival time. Ineffective erythropoiesis and increased intramedullary hemolysis contribute to the anemia. The gene is prevalent in a wide belt of equatorial Europe, Africa, and Asia. It is believed that the selective increase in the gene in this area (which may reach an incidence up to 50% in isolated communities) is due to the fact that the heterozygote has an increased resistance to malaria.

Clinical Findings

A. Symptoms and Signs: Severe anemia usually does not manifest itself clinically until about age 1 because of the protective effect of normal fetal hemoglobin. However, splenomegaly and mild anemia are often noted by 6 months. By age 2, there is usually massive splenomegaly and significant hepatomegaly, which continue until the spleen extends into the pelvis. Physical growth is markedly impaired, and there is increased susceptibility to infections. As the child approaches the school years, the widening of the flat bones of the face and skull in association with marrow hypertrophy give all children with thalassemia major a characteristic facies: prominence of the malar eminences, depression of the bridge of the nose, a slightly oblique appearance of the eyes, and an enlargement of the superior maxilla with upward protrusion of the lip. The anemia is severe, and after age 1 usually requires transfusions at frequent intervals. Jaundice may be present.

B. Laboratory Findings: The blood smear reveals a severe hypochromic microcytic anemia with marked anisocytosis and poikilocytosis. Target cells are prominent. Nucleated red cells are numerous and often exceed the circulating white blood cells. The hemoglobin is low (5–6 gm/100 ml). The reticulocyte count is significantly elevated. Platelet and white cell counts are frequently high. Serum bilirubin is elevated. The diagnosis is confirmed by paper or starch block hemoglobin electrophoresis, which reveals no abnormal hemoglobin but a marked increase in fetal hemoglobin. The exact level of fetal hemoglobin should be determined by the alkali denaturation method. Osmotic fragility is markedly decreased. The bone marrow shows marked erythroid hyperplasia with increased iron deposition.

C. X-Ray Findings: Bone x-rays are very characteristic and reveal an increase in the medullary area with thinning of the cortex. The skull has a "hair-on-end" appearance.

Differential Diagnosis

There is usually no problem in the diagnosis of homozygous thalassemia since essentially no other disease shows the characteristic peripheral blood and hemoglobin electrophoresis findings. The primary clinical differentiation is with the combinations of thalassemia and other abnormal hemoglobins such as thalassemia-hemoglobin S disease, thalassemia-hemoglobin E, etc. These have similar clinical pictures but are usually more mild. They are differentiated by the electrophoretic pattern.

Complications

Patients with thalassemia major have multiple complications. They have an increased susceptibility to infections, particularly following splenectomy. Acute benign nonspecific pericarditis is a common problem. Repeated fractures are associated with the thinning of cortical bone. The multiple transfusions which are required are ultimately associated with transfusion reactions and the development of leukocyte antibodies. Growth is impaired, and adolescent development of secondary sex characteristics is delayed. Cholelithiasis and cholecystitis are almost always present in the adolescent or young adult. The major complication, however, is the development of hemochromatosis secondary to excessive absorption and transfusion of iron in these patients. This results in cirrhosis and in heart failure. Cardiac complications are related primarily to the heavy deposition of iron in the myocardium, and death is usually due to heart failure.

Treatment

There is no specific treatment for thalassemia major. Infections should be treated promptly with antibiotics, and heart failure with digitalis and other appropriate therapy.

A. Transfusion: Blood transfusion is the primary therapeutic measure; packed red cells are indicated (in many cases, every 6—8 weeks). In the past, transfusion was given when symptoms occurred or when the hemoglobin fell below 5—6 gm/100 ml; sufficient blood was administered to raise the hemoglobin to approximately 8 gm/100 ml. Maintenance of the hemoglobin level between 10 and 12 gm/100 ml has been associated with improved vigor and well-being and fewer overall complications. There is no good evidence that more frequent transfusions increase hemochromatosis in thalassemia major. In fact, life expectancy may be greater if the hemoglobin is maintained at the higher level.

B. Chelation: Chelating agents such as deferoxamine (Desferal) are valuable in removing some of the iron and may have the potential for prolonging life expectancy. Deferoxamine is indicated particularly in the younger child who does not yet have massive iron deposits. In the older child, the dosage is 0.5—1 gm IM daily. The urinary excretion of iron should be determined to evaluate the effect and duration of therapy.

C. Folic Acid: A relative folic acid deficiency may develop because of the marked overproduction of bone marrow. Folic acid, 5—10 mg daily orally, is often of value.

D. Splenectomy: Splenectomy is usually of value in the older child and is definitely indicated if the transfusion requirements become progressively greater. It is also indicated for the abdominal discomfort and distention associated with massive enlargement of the organ. Although it does not change the basic rate of homolysis, it will eliminate the hypersplenism which further shortens red cell survival. The hazard of severe and overwhelming infection following splenectomy is much greater in patients with thalassemia major than in any other group, and the use of prophylactic penicillin following this procedure is recommended.

Prognosis

Although the prognosis has improved significantly with the use of antibiotics in the past few decades and may continue to improve with the use of chelating agents to remove iron and prevent hemosiderosis, very few patients survive into adult life although the majority reach adolescence.

Lehmann H: Hemoglobinopathies: Abnormal hemoglobins and thalassemias. Israel J Med Sc 4:478, 1968.

Weatherall DJ: The genetics of the thalassemias. Brit M Bull 25:24, 1969.

Weatherall DJ: *The Thalassemia Syndromes.* Davis, 1965.

3. ALPHA THALASSEMIA

Defective production of alpha chains also results in anemia. Several different forms of alpha thalassemia have been described. The disorder has been recognized primarily in Southwest Asia (especially Thailand) and in blacks. Apparently at least 2 alpha thalassemia genes occur in Thailand, with different degrees of severity being reported.

The alpha thalassemia carriers (who are heterozygous for the gene) may be completely asymptomatic and demonstrate normal blood findings, or they may show mild hypochromia and occasional target cells on blood smear. No abnormal hemoglobin is demonstrated, and there are no compensatory increases in hemoglobin A_2 or fetal hemoglobin.

The homozygous form of the disease may be very severe and may be incompatible with life, resulting in fetal hydrops. These severely anemic and hydropic infants have only Bart's hemoglobin, which is composed of 4 gamma chains, since they are unable to produce alpha hemoglobin chains.

The disorder previously designated as thalassemia-hemoglobin H disease is now recognized to be a milder form of homozygous alpha thalassemia. It has been described primarily in Southeast Asia (Philippines, southern China, and Thailand). The patient demonstrates a chronic microcytic anemia which is refractory to iron therapy and tends to resemble beta thalassemia minor. Hemoglobin electrophoresis at pH 8.5 reveals a fast hemoglobin that migrates more rapidly than A_1. This hemoglobin is composed of 4 beta chains. Characteristic red cell inclusions are demonstrated by the reticulocyte stain upon incubation. There is no satisfactory treatment. Iron should not be administered to patients with any form of alpha thalassemia.

Na-Nakorn S & others: Further evidence for a genetic basis of haemoglobin H disease from newborn offspring of patients. Nature 223:59, 1969.

Weatherall DJ: *The Thalassemia Syndromes.*

4. THALASSEMIA VARIANTS

Double heterozygosity of thalassemia with other hemoglobinopathies such as C, S, and E are fairly common in certain parts of the world and manifest themselves clinically as milder forms of thalassemia major. The diagnosis is made by hemoglobin electrophoresis, which shows a predominance of hemoglobin F and other abnormal hemoglobin. Family studies will reveal one parent to be a thalassemia carrier and the other a carrier of C, S, or E.

5. HEREDITARY PERSISTENCE OF FETAL HEMOGLOBIN

Hereditary persistence of fetal hemoglobin has been reported in both black and Greek families. It is usually found in the heterozygous form and is associated with no symptoms. The blood counts and blood smears are normal. The fetal hemoglobin level is approximately 20%. The homozygous form is also asymptomatic, but in combination with the sickle cell trait mild anemia may be present. The defect appears to be in the genetic mechanism that controls the switch from production of gamma to production of beta hemoglobin chains.

Conley CL & others: Hereditary persistence of fetal hemoglobin. Blood 21:261–281, 1963.

ACQUIRED HEMOLYTIC ANEMIAS

1. AUTOIMMUNE HEMOLYTIC ANEMIA

Essentials of Diagnosis
- Sudden pallor, fatigue, and jaundice.
- Splenomegaly.
- Positive Coombs test.
- Reticulocytosis and spherocytosis.

General Considerations
Acquired autoimmune hemolytic anemia is rare during the first 4 months of life but is one of the more common causes of acutely acquired anemia after the first year. It is caused by antibodies which coat the red cells and are responsible for the positive direct Coombs test. Circulating antibodies are demonstrated by the indirect Coombs test. The "primary" (or idiopathic) cases may be associated with an unrecognized preceding infection. The possible importance of cytomegalovirus infection has recently been emphasized. The disease may be "symptomatic" and may occur in association with a known infection such as hepatitis, viral pneumonia, or infectious mononucleosis; or it may occur as a manifestation of a generalized autoimmune disease such as disseminated lupus erythematosus or with a malignancy such as Hodgkin's disease or leukemia.

Clinical Findings
A. Symptoms and Signs: The disease usually has an acute onset and is associated with weakness, pallor, and fatigue. Hemoglobinuria may be present. Jaundice and splenomegaly are often present. Occasional cases are chronic and insidious in onset. Clinical evidence of the underlying disease such as infection or lupus erythematosus may be present.

B. Laboratory Findings: The anemia is normochromic and normocytic and may be very severe, with hemoglobin levels as low as 3–4 gm/100 ml. Occasionally, the secondary form of acquired hemolytic anemia may be very mild and may present with evidence of a positive Coombs test but with compensated anemia. Spherocytes are usually present, and within 24 hours nucleated red cells and reticulocytes are present in the peripheral blood. There is usually a significant leukocytosis, and the platelet count may be elevated. Bone marrow shows a marked erythroid hyperplasia. Both the direct and indirect Coombs tests are usually positive. Autoagglutination may be present, and because of this the patient may be incorrectly typed as AB, Rh-positive. The indirect serum bilirubin may be elevated, and the stool and urine urobilinogen are increased.

Differential Diagnosis
The principal condition to be differentiated in childhood is hereditary spherocytic anemia in crisis, since both diseases present with acute hemolysis and spherocytosis. The Coombs test differentiates the 2 anemias since it is negative in hereditary spherocytosis. The Coombs test likewise differentiates autoimmune hemolytic anemia from essentially all other anemias except erythroblastosis.

Complications
The anemia may be severe and acute and result in shock, requiring emergency management. Thrombocytopenia may occur as an associated autoimmune condition. The complications of the underlying disease such as disseminated lupus erythematosus or lymphoma may be present in the symptomatic form.

Treatment
Medical management of the underlying disease is important in symptomatic cases.

A. Transfusion: Transfusion is necessary in the acute disease and may be an emergency procedure. Difficulty in cross-matching will usually be encountered. A search should be made for blood that will provide the best major cross-match. Packed, washed cells are often more compatible. Transfusion occasionally must be given in spite of agglutination or a positive Coombs test in the major cross-match. Donor cells may be destroyed at a rapid rate, particularly if compatible blood cannot be found. Donor cells may be tagged with ^{51}Cr to determine their rate of survival in severe cases.

B. Immunosuppressive Therapy: Medical treatment to block the immune process is indicated. Corticosteroid therapy in the form of hydrocortisone intravenously in large doses or prednisone, 2 mg/kg/day orally, should be tried initially. If a response is observed, the dose is decreased at weekly intervals until the lowest level that will maintain the patient in remission is reached. Other immunosuppressive drugs such as nitrogen mustards, mercaptopurine, or azathioprine may be tried alone or in conjunction with corticosteroid therapy.

C. Splenectomy: Splenectomy may be beneficial in cases in which all forms of medical treatment have failed. About 50% of cases may be expected to respond to this procedure.

Prognosis

In childhood the disease is self-limited in the majority of idiopathic cases, although hemolysis does not usually cease completely for months to years; the Coombs test often remains weakly positive for years. The majority of cases will show a response to corticosteroid therapy, and about 50% will improve with splenectomy. The majority of chronic cases have a basic underlying disease or immunologic disorder.

Hitzig WH, Massimo L: Treatment of autoimmune hemolytic anemia in children with azathioprine (Imuran). Blood 28:840, 1966.

Zuelzer WW & others: Autoimmune hemolytic anemia: Natural history and viral immunologic interactions in childhood. Am J Med 49:80, 1970.

2. ACUTE ACQUIRED HEMOLYTIC ANEMIA
(Lederer's Anemia)

Severe episodes of hemolytic anemia that are not associated with a positive Coombs test are occasionally seen in children. The onset is acute and the duration short, with spontaneous recovery in a few weeks. As in autoimmune hemolytic anemia, the episode is often precipitated by an infectious process such as a urinary tract infection, but in most cases there is no evidence for red cell antibodies. The term Lederer's anemia is currently reserved for this group.

Transfusion is the treatment of choice; there is usually no problem with cross-matching the donor blood.

The prognosis is good since all cases are self-limited.

Wallerstein RO, Aggeler PM: Acute hemolytic anemia. Am J Med 37:92–104, 1964.

3. MISCELLANEOUS ACQUIRED (NONIMMUNE) HEMOLYTIC ANEMIAS

A wide variety of extracorpuscular mechanisms may also produce hemolysis of a nonimmune type. The role of certain drugs (eg, antimalarials, sulfonamides) and fava beans is discussed elsewhere, since hemolysis in association with this particular group of substances occurs primarily in individuals with a deficiency of G6PD. Certain other chemicals and drugs such as arsenic and benzene may produce hemolysis by their direct effect. Exposure to physical agents such as extreme heat or cold may cause hemolysis. Hemolytic anemia is a common complication of severe burns.

Many bacterial infections with hemolytic organisms such as *Bartonella bacilliformis* and *Clostridium perfringens* produce hemolysis. In the neonatal period, hemolytic anemia may be a complication of almost any infection, but it is seen most commonly with hemolytic staphylococcal and *Escherichia coli* infections. Parasites such as malaria are characteristically associated with hemolysis. The venom of most poisonous snakes (in particular, the pit vipers of North America) contains a hemolysin, as do the venoms of certain spiders also. The management of the majority of the acquired toxic hemolytic anemias is dependent upon the removal of the offending agent or treatment of the toxic disorder. Transfusion may be important in the more severe cases.

Hemolysis in heart disease or after open heart surgery has been reported. This has usually occurred in situations in which a jet of blood was driven against a Teflon prosthesis as well as in certain congenital valvular defects and with prosthetic valve replacement. The hemolysis is on a mechanical basis.

Rodgers BM & others: Hemolytic anemia following prosthetic valve replacement. Circulation (Suppl) 39:155, 1969.

II. POLYCYTHEMIA & METHEMOGLOBINEMIA

PRIMARY ERYTHROCYTOSIS
(Benign Familial Polycythemia)

This is the most common type of primary polycythemia of childhood. It differs from polycythemia vera in that it affects only the erythroid series; the white cell count and platelet count are normal. It frequently occurs on a familial basis, and there are usually no physical findings except for plethora and splenomegaly. The hemoglobin may be as high as 27 gm/100 ml, with a hematocrit of 80% and a red cell count of 10 million/cu mm. There are usually no symptoms other than headache and lethargy.

Treatment is not indicated unless symptoms are marked. Phlebotomy is the treatment of choice.

Geary CG & others: Benign familial polycythaemia. J Clin Path 20:158, 1967.

SECONDARY POLYCYTHEMIA
(Compensatory Polycythemia)

Secondary polycythemia occurs in response to hypoxia in any condition that results in a lowered oxygen saturation of the blood. The most common cause of secondary polycythemia is cyanotic congenital heart disease. It also occurs in chronic pulmonary disease such as cystic fibrosis and in pulmonary arteriovenous shunts. Persons living at extremely high altitudes, as well as those with methemoglobinemia and sulfhemoglobinemia, develop polycythemia. It has on rare occasions been described without hypoxia in association with renal tumors, brain tumors, Cushing's disease, hydronephrosis, and in association with cobalt therapy.

Polycythemia occurs normally in the neonatal period; it is particularly exaggerated in premature infants, in whom it is frequently associated with other symptoms. It has recently been described as a manifestation of Down's syndrome in the newborn and as a complication of congenital adrenal hyperplasia.

Multiple coagulation and bleeding abnormalities have been described in severely polycythemic cardiac patients. These include thrombocytopenia, mild consumption coagulopathy, and increased anticoagulants and elevated fibrinolytic activity. Bleeding at surgery may be severe.

The ideal treatment of secondary polycythemia is correction of the underlying disorder. When this cannot be done, phlebotomy is often necessary to control the symptoms. Adequate hydration of the patient and phlebotomy with plasma replacement are indicated prior to major surgical procedures to prevent the complications of thrombosis and hemorrhage. Isovolumetric exchange transfusion is the treatment of choice in severe cases.

Humbert JR & others: Polycythemia in small for gestational age infants. J Pediat 75:812, 1969.

Smith CH: *Blood Diseases of Infancy and Childhood,* 2nd ed. Mosby, 1966.

METHEMOGLOBINEMIA

Methemoglobin is formed when hemoglobin in a deoxygenated state is oxidized to the ferric form. Methemoglobin is being formed continuously in the red cells and is simultaneously reduced to hemoglobin by enzymes in the erythrocyte. Methemoglobin becomes unavailable for transport of oxygen and causes a shift in the dissociation curve of the residual oxyhemoglobin. Cyanosis is produced with methemoglobin levels of approximately 15% or greater. There are several mechanisms for the production of methemoglobinemia.

Congenital Methemoglobinemia Associated With Hemoglobin M

Congenital and familial methemoglobinemia associated with an abnormal hemoglobin molecule (hemoglobin M) is discussed under the hemoglobinopathies. These patients are cyanotic but asymptomatic. They do not respond to any form of treatment.

Congenital Methemoglobinemia Due to Enzyme Deficiencies

Congenital methemoglobinemia is most frequently caused by congenital absence of a reducing factor in the erythrocyte which is responsible for the conversion of methemoglobin to hemoglobin in normal red cells. The majority of patients with this disease suffer from a deficiency of diaphorase I (coenzyme factor I). It is transmitted as an autosomal recessive trait. These patients may have as high as 40% methemoglobin but usually have no symptoms, although a mild compensatory polycythemia may be present.

Patients with methemoglobinemia associated with a deficiency of diaphorase I respond readily to treatment with ascorbic acid and with methylene blue (see below). However, treatment is not usually indicated.

Drug-Induced Methemoglobinemia

A number of compounds activate the oxidation of hemoglobin from the ferrous to the ferric state, forming methemoglobin. These include the nitrites and nitrates, chlorates, and quinones. Common drugs in this group are the aniline dyes, sulfonamides, acetanilid, phenacetin, bismuth subnitrate, and potassium chlorate. Poisoning with a drug or chemical containing one of these substances should be suspected in any infant or child who presents with sudden cyanosis. Methemoglobin levels in cases of poisoning may be extremely high and can produce severe anoxia and dyspnea with unconsciousness, circulatory failure, and death. Young infants and newborns are more susceptible to poisoning because their red cells have difficulty reducing hemoglobin, probably on the basis of a transient deficiency of DPNH-dependent hemoglobin reductase.

Patients with the acquired form of the disease respond dramatically to methylene blue in a dosage of 2 mg/kg body weight IV. For older children, a dose of 1–1.5 mg/kg is recommended. Ascorbic acid orally or intravenously also reduces methemoglobin, but acts more slowly.

Jaffé ER & others: Hereditary methemoglobinemia, toxic methemoglobinemia and the reduction of methemoglobin. Ann New York Acad Sc 151:795, 1968.

III. DISORDERS OF LEUKOCYTES

LEUKOPENIA & AGRANULOCYTOSIS

Essentials of Diagnosis
- Increased incidence of infections.
- Ulceration of the oral mucosa and throat.
- Neutropenia.
- Normal red cells and platelets.

General Considerations

The neutropenias and agranulocytosis include a wide variety of syndromes which probably have different causes. In the majority of cases the mechanism is not well understood. Many are probably secondary to exposure to drugs and chemicals, and this possibility should be investigated in all cases. In childhood, the more common drug-induced neutropenias occur with anticonvulsants, antimicrobial agents (chloramphenicol), antithyroid drugs (thiouracil), tranquilizers, antihistamines, aminopyrine, phenylbutazone, and the sulfonamides. Neutropenia is a common complication of exposure to large doses of x-ray and to cytotoxic drugs such as the antimetabolites and nitrogen mustards. There is increasing evidence that leukocyte antibodies may produce granulocytopenia on an immunologic basis. This most frequently occurs in association with repeated blood transfusions or as a result of isoagglutinins that develop during pregnancy. Autoagglutinins have also been described, particularly in association with infectious mononucleosis, lymphomas, and autoimmune diseases such as disseminated lupus erythematosus.

Viral infections characteristically produce neutropenia. Bacterial infections, particularly sepsis, are frequently associated with transient neutropenia in the newborn infant, and overwhelming bacterial infections at all ages may be indicated by neutropenia.

Classifications

A number of specific leukopenias have been described in infancy and childhood:

A. Neonatal Agranulocytosis: This term has been applied to the occurrence of agranulocytosis in the neonatal period in repeated siblings. It is usually explained by transplacental iso-immunization of the mother to the leukocytes of her infant in a manner analogous to Rh immunization of the newborn. The granulocytopenia in these cases is accompanied by infection, but it is temporary and improves within 4 weeks.

B. Infantile Genetic Agranulocytosis: Several families have been described in which agranulocytosis occurred from infancy in several siblings without depression of the other circulating cell elements. It has been associated with either depression of the granulocytic series in the marrow or a delay in maturation. The course has been chronic, with a high mortality rate and no response to therapy.

C. Chronic Benign Granulocytopenia in Childhood: Several series of cases have been described in which persistent granulocytopenia was noted throughout childhood. The bone marrow in these cases has usually shown normal cellularity but abnormal maturation of the granulocytes. In most of these cases, the neutrophils have represented about 10% of the circulating leukocytes, and infection has not been a serious problem. Spontaneous remission may occur.

D. Chronic Hypoplastic Neutropenia: A few cases have been described of chronic neutropenia associated with hypoplasia of granulocytic precursors in the marrow. The cause is not known, and complicating infections have been severe.

E. Leukopenia With Pure Red Cell Hypoplastic Anemia: A number of cases of pure red cell hypoplastic anemia have also been associated with leukopenia. This is usually mild, and an increased incidence of infection has not been observed, although oral ulceration and staphylococcal infections of the skin have been reported in a few cases.

F. Pancreatic Insufficiency and Bone Marrow Dysfunction: Neutropenia, anemia, and thrombocytopenia have been reported in association with pancreatic insufficiency in infancy and childhood. Although diarrhea, failure to thrive, and infections have been a problem, the prognosis is better than in cystic fibrosis.

G. Periodic (Cyclic) Neutropenia: This is a rare condition that may occur at any age but usually begins in infancy and childhood. It is characterized by an extreme granulocytopenia that occurs at approximately 3-week intervals, with recovery between attacks. The peripheral blood changes are reflected by a cyclic maturation arrest of the granulocytic series in the bone marrow. During the leukopenic episode, the white count is usually 2–4 thousand/cu mm, with granulocytes representing only 6–10% of the cells. The agranulocytic periods usually last about 10 days and are associated with the development of ulcers of the oral mucosa, fever, and sore throat. Various other infections may complicate the disease, and staphylococcal skin infections are common. Splenomegaly and lymphadenopathy have also been reported.

H. Neutropenia in Association With Immune Deficiency Syndromes: Neutropenia (constant or cyclic) may occur in agammaglobulinemia. It has also been observed in other forms of the immune deficiencies.

Clinical Findings

A. Symptoms and Signs: The symptoms are those of infection, with chills and fever. Sore throat and ulceration of the oral mucosa are common, and chronic or recurrent staphylococcal infection of the skin is frequent. In most cases, the spleen and liver are not enlarged.

B. Laboratory Findings: Neutrophils are absent or markedly reduced in the peripheral blood. In the purer forms of neutropenia or agranulocytosis, the monocytes and lymphocytes will be normal and the red cells and platelets not affected. The bone marrow usually shows a normal erythroid series, with adequate megakaryocytes but a marked reduction in the myeloid cells or a significant delay in maturation of this series.

Differential Diagnosis

The isolated neutropenias should be differentiated from the pancytopenias such as aplastic anemia and the hypoplastic (aleukemic) form of childhood leukemia by bone marrow examination.

Complications

The complications are essentially those of infection, with septicemia and pneumonia being the most serious. Chronic infection with antibiotic-resistant organisms such as staphylococci and pseudomonas are frequent in severe cases.

Treatment

Removal of the toxic agent is essential if one can be identified. Otherwise, treatment consists of administering appropriate antibiotics. Prophylactic antimicrobial therapy is not indicated, and the patient should be managed with specific therapy directed toward the infecting organism.

Marrow stimulation with testosterone or with testosterone plus one of the corticosteroids (see Aplastic Anemia) may be tried in chronic cases, but there is little evidence that it is effective.

Prognosis

The prognosis varies greatly with the underlying cause and the severity of the neutropenia. In severe cases with persistent agranulocytosis, the prognosis is very poor in spite of antibiotic therapy; in mild or cyclic forms of neutropenia, symptoms may be minimal and the prognosis for normal life expectancy is excellent.

Burke V & others: Association of pancreatic insufficiency and chronic neutropenia in childhood. Arch Dis Childhood 42:147, 1967.
Kauder E, Mauer AM: Neutropenias of childhood. J Pediat 69:147, 1966.
Lang JE, Cutter HO: Infantile genetic agranulocytosis. Pediatrics 35:596–600, 1965.

PHYSIOLOGIC NEUTROPENIA

All infants and young children after the first few weeks of life have a neutropenia in comparison with adult levels. The normal white count of the infant and child may be as low as 5–6 thousand/cu mm, and the percentage of neutrophils may normally be as low as 18–20% during the first 3–4 years of life. A diagnosis of neutropenia should be considered in early infancy and childhood only if the absolute neutrophil count is below 1000/cu mm.

See Table 14–1 for normal values of leukocytes at various ages.

ACUTE INFECTIOUS LYMPHOCYTOSIS

Acute infectious lymphocytosis is a specific entity characterized hematologically by marked lymphocytosis that may range between 15–200 thousand cells/cu mm. The predominant cell is a small mature lymphocyte. The disease is apparently infectious and tends to occur in epidemic form in institutions and families. The specific agent has not been

determined, although a virus is suspected. Recent studies suggest that an enterovirus similar to coxsackievirus A may be the cause.

In the majority of cases the condition is asymptomatic, and the diagnosis is made on the basis of a routine blood count. Epidemics have been reported in which symptoms were noted, including fever, upper respiratory manifestations, skin rashes, abdominal pain, diarrhea, and meningoencephalitis. Lymphadenopathy and splenomegaly are not present.

The bone marrow is normal except for a slight increase in mature lymphocytes. The disease can be readily differentiated from leukemia since the lymphocytes of the peripheral blood are all mature and since chronic lymphatic leukemia does not occur in the pediatric age group. Further differentiation is made by bone marrow examination, which is essentially normal. The blood smear is similar to that of pertussis.

There is no specific treatment, and even symptomatic therapy is usually not needed.

The disease is self-limited, and the blood count usually returns to normal within a few weeks.

Horwitz MS, Moore GT: Acute infectious lymphocytosis: Etiology and epidemiologic study of outbreak. New England J Med 279:399, 1968.

CHRONIC NONSPECIFIC INFECTIOUS LYMPHOCYTOSIS

This syndrome is characterized by moderate leukocytosis with a predominance of lymphocytes, low-grade fever, anorexia, pallor, irritability, increased fatigability, and abdominal pain. The peripheral blood usually shows a significant lymphocytosis, with total counts reaching 25,000/cu mm with as many as 80% lymphocytes. Most of the lymphocytes are of the small, mature type, although occasional larger cells may be seen. The cause is not known, but viral infection is suspected.

The symptoms and elevated lymphocyte count often persist for several months, and therapy is not helpful. Antibiotic therapy and restriction of physical activity are not indicated.

Smith CH: Infectious lymphocytosis. Am J Dis Child 62:231–235, 1941.

MYELOID METAPLASIA
(Myelofibrosis, Myelosclerosis, Agnogenic Myeloid Metaplasia)

Myeloid metaplasia is a myeloproliferative condition associated with splenomegaly and a granulocytic leukemoid picture. In childhood it occurs most frequently in the secondary form and is associated with replacement of the bone marrow by tumor, storage cells, or osteosclerosis (osteopetrosis, marble bone disease). The primary form, which is associated with idiopathic myelofibrosis (agnogenic myeloid metaplasia), is extremely rare in childhood.

The peripheral blood in this condition shows not only a marked increase in granulocytes, with many immature forms at all levels of maturation, but also a significant number of nucleated red cells and large immature platelets. The presence of immature hematopoietic cells in the peripheral blood is explained by the marked extramedullary hematopoiesis that occurs in the spleen and liver in this condition.

Treatment should be directed toward the primary disease if possible. The use of testosterone (see Aplastic Anemia) may be helpful in stimulating hematopoiesis in the bone marrow.

Say B, Berkel I: Idiopathic myelofibrosis in an infant. J Pediat 64:580–585, 1964.

CHRONIC GRANULOMATOUS DISEASE

The primary defect in this disorder appears to be inability to kill bacteria despite normal phagocytosis, resulting in persistent infections, frequently with bacteria of low virulence. Onset before age 1 and death before 8 years is the usual course of events. There is a marked defect in degranulation and a marked decrease in the oxidative metabolism normally associated with phagocytosis. The precise relationship of the metabolic abnormalities to the lack of bactericidal activity of the leukocyte is unclear.

The earliest manifestation is an eczematoid dermatosis occurring near a body orifice. This is followed by recurrent lymphadenopathy, suppuration, and draining granulomatous lesions. The lung parenchyma is usually involved, with enlargement of the hilar nodes on x-ray and a distinctive "encapsulating pneumonia" in some cases. Hepatosplenomegaly is characteristic but not uniformly present. Osteomyelitis occurs in about 1/3 of cases. Typical bacteria involved have been staphylococci (including species usually considered nonpathogenic) and enterobacteria such as aerobacter and serratia. The course of the disease is characterized by remissions and exacerbations. Remissions have lasted up to several years. Death usually results from sepsis, pulmonary infections, meningitis, and extensive visceral suppuration.

Humoral- and cell-mediated immunity is normal. Hyperimmunoglobulinemia is present, presumably because of the massive antigenic stimulation of the chronic infection. The inflammatory cycle and complement system are normal, as is the peripheral polymorphonuclear response to bacterial infection. Defective killing of intracellular bacteria is demonstrable in in vitro phagocytic systems by failure to reduce nitroblue tetrazolium to blue formazan.

Treatment is directed toward management of the infections and includes prompt antibiotic therapy with antibiotics that penetrate cell membranes well (eg, chloramphenicol), surgical drainage of suppurative lesions, and general supportive therapy.

Baehner RL, Nathan DG: Quantitative nitroblue tetrazolium test in chronic granulomatous disease. New England J Med 278:971, 1968.

Good RA & others: Fatal (chronic) granulomatous disease of childhood: A hereditary defect of leukocyte function. Seminars Hemat 5:215, 1968.

Quie PG: Chronic granulomatous disease of childhood. Advances Pediat 16:287, 1969.

Quie PG & others: In vitro bactericidal capacity of human polymorphonuclear leukocytes. J Clin Invest 46:668, 1967.

CHEDIAK-HIGASHI SYNDROME

This is a rare familial disorder that is apparently transmitted as an autosomal recessive trait. It is characterized by semialbinism, photophobia, nystagmus, excessive sweating, pale optic fundi, hepatosplenomegaly, generalized lymphadenopathy, and eventually by the development of neurologic signs and symptoms. Hematologically, there is a progressive anemia and granulocytopenia, and typical diagnostic anomalies of the leukocytes. Large granules ranging in size from 2–5 μm in diameter, which may be azurophilic or slate green, occur in the cytoplasm of the neutrophils. Extremely large red granules may also be seen in the eosinophils and are particularly prominent in the myelocytic cells of the marrow.

There is no known treatment.

The course is progressively downhill, with death occurring in childhood.

White JG: The Chediak-Higashi syndrome: A possible lysosomal disease. Blood 28:143–156, 1966.

IV. BLEEDING DISORDERS

Bleeding disorders may be classified as (1) defects in small vessel hemostasis, which include (a) quantitative and qualitative abnormalities of platelets (thrombocytopenia, thrombasthenia, thrombopathia, and thrombocythemia) and (b) the vascular disorders; and (2) intravascular disorders (defects in blood coagulation).

The initial laboratory work-up for screening patients with bleeding disorders should include a careful history and physical examination and the following laboratory investigations:

(1) Bleeding time: To test small vessel integrity and platelet function.

(2) Tourniquet test: To test small vessel integrity and platelet function.

(3) Platelet count or estimation of platelet number on blood smear.

(4) Partial thromboplastin time (PTT) or, if PTT is not available, the less sensitive whole blood coagulation time or plasma recalcification time as a measure of the integrity of the entire coagulation system.

(5) One-stage prothrombin time (PT) to screen the tissue thromboplastin system of coagulation (particularly the prothrombin complex).

(6) Thrombin time to measure antithrombin effect of fibrin split products or heparin as well as fibrinogen level (if very low).

With this battery of screening tests, it is usually possible to determine the general area of the defect and proceed with more specific tests in order to make an exact diagnosis.

ABNORMALITIES OF PLATELET NUMBER OR FUNCTION

IDIOPATHIC THROMBOCYTOPENIC PURPURA (ITP)
(Werlhof's Disease, Purpura Hemorrhagica)

Essentials of Diagnosis

- Petechiae, ecchymoses.
- Other bleeding manifestations.
- Decreased platelet count.
- Prolonged bleeding time, abnormal clot retraction.
- Normal PTT and PT.
- No splenomegaly.

General Considerations

Acute ITP is the most common bleeding disorder of childhood. It most frequently follows infections and is particularly common after certain of the common contagious diseases (rubella, varicella, and rubeola). As a rule it is self-limited; this is particularly true of the postinfectious type, the majority of which cases recover spontaneously within a few months and approximately 90% within a year after onset. Chronic ITP is rare in childhood.

Most cases of ITP are felt to be an immunologic disorder, although platelet antibodies cannot always be demonstrated. The spleen apparently plays a major role by sequestering damaged platelets, by forming antibodies, and perhaps by controlling platelet formation and release in the marrow through a humoral substance.

Clinical Findings

A. Symptoms and Signs: The onset is usually acute, with the appearance of multiple ecchymoses, particularly over the tibias. Petechiae are often present, and epistaxis is common. There are no other physical findings, and the spleen is not palpable.

B. Laboratory Findings:

1. Blood—The platelet count is markedly reduced (usually less than 50,000/cu mm), and platelets are decreased on peripheral blood smear. The white blood count and differential count are normal. Anemia is not present unless hemorrhage has occurred.

2. Bone marrow—The bone marrow usually shows increased numbers of immature megakaryocytes, with little or no evidence of platelet formation. Eosinophils may be increased in the marrow.

3. Other laboratory tests—The bleeding time is prolonged, the tourniquet test is positive, and clot retraction is abnormal. PTT and PT are normal, although prothrombin consumption is decreased.

Differential Diagnosis

The presence of a low platelet count immediately differentiates ITP from all other bleeding disorders except those associated with thrombocytopenia. A normal white blood count and normal granulocytes in the bone marrow differentiate ITP from leukemia and aplastic anemia. The bone marrow is important in making the differential diagnosis.

Complications

Severe exsanguinating hemorrhage and bleeding into vital organs are the primary complications of ITP. Intracranial hemorrhage is the most serious. Complications of treatment include those associated with prolonged corticosteroid therapy. Splenectomy, particularly in children under age 2, may be associated with increased incidence of infection.

Treatment

A. General Measures: Avoidance of trauma is important, and in mild postinfectious cases no other therapy may be required. In the presence of hemorrhage, blood transfusions may be necessary; fresh blood is preferred even though a significant rise in platelet count cannot be expected from whole blood transfusions. Platelet transfusion may be lifesaving if hemorrhage does not respond to medical therapy. The platelets (platelet concentrate or platelet pack) from 1 unit of blood per 5–10 lb of body weight are usually required to produce an observable rise in platelet count.

B. Corticosteroids: Corticosteroids are the treatment of choice in acute ITP if there is a significant hemorrhagic tendency. The initial dose should be high. Prednisone in full therapeutic doses (2 mg/kg orally in divided doses daily) is given initially and continued until the platelet count rises and purpura disappears. A few days to 2 weeks may be required to obtain a remission. Even in the absence of a remission, high doses should not be continued for more than 4 weeks. The dosage is then gradually reduced to the smallest amount that will maintain a remission. If relapse occurs, the patient may be maintained on the lowest dose that previously produced a remission.

In chronic cases, the dosage of prednisone required to maintain elevation of platelets will frequently cause significant hyperadrenocorticism. In this event, low dosage (5–10 mg/day) will often control symptoms due to the "nonspecific" vascular effect of corticosteroids even though an observable rise in platelets does not occur.

C. **Plasma Transfusions:** In chronic thrombocytopenic purpura, a therapeutic trial with small doses of fresh frozen plasma (10–20 ml/kg) is indicated to rule out thrombocytopenia due to a congenital deficiency of the thrombopoietic factors.

Larger doses of fresh frozen plasma (20–30 ml/kg) may occasionally produce remissions in acute ITP because of the presence of this platelet-stimulating plasma factor. This form of therapy may be tried in place of corticosteroids or when corticosteroids fail.

D. **Splenectomy:** Splenectomy produces permanent remission in the majority of cases of ITP; however, it is now usually reserved for children who have shown no evidence of spontaneous remission over a period of 6 months to 1 year, since about 90% of children with ITP will recover without surgical intervention within 1 year after onset. If symptoms are not controlled by medical management, splenectomy may be done prior to this time, and in most cases splenectomy is advised if symptoms persist beyond 1 year after onset. Fifty to 75% of chronic cases in childhood respond to the procedure, although the patient who shows a rise in platelet count with large doses of corticosteroids is most likely to have a satisfactory result.

Bleeding is rarely a complication of splenectomy, but platelet concentrates should be available during surgery. If the patient has been on corticosteroid therapy prior to surgery, the dose should be increased to the full therapeutic level during and after surgery.

Anticoagulant therapy is probably not indicated postoperatively even though the platelets may rise to levels of approximately 1 million.

The risk of overwhelming infection is minimal in the older child undergoing splenectomy. It does represent a significant risk in the child under 2 years of age, and the procedure should be postponed if possible until the child is older. Prophylactic penicillin for at least a year following splenectomy is indicated and is strongly recommended in the very young child.

Prognosis

Spontaneous remission with permanent recovery occurs in almost 90% of cases of ITP in childhood. (The incidence of spontaneous remission is much lower in adults.)

Baldini M: Idiopathic thrombocytopenic purpura. New England J Med 274:1245–1251, 1966.
Choi SI, McClure PD: Idiopathic thrombocytopenic purpura in childhood. Canad MAJ 97:562, 1967.
Karpatkin S: Autoimmune thrombocytopenic purpura. Am J Med Sc 261:126–138, 1971.

THROMBOCYTOPENIA IN THE NEWBORN

Thrombocytopenia is one of the most common causes of purpura in the newborn and should be considered and investigated in any infant with petechiae or a significant bleeding tendency. A number of specific entities may be responsible. The most common are discussed below.

Thrombocytopenia Associated With Platelet Iso-immunization

The most common cause of thrombocytopenia in the neonatal period is platelet iso-immunization, which is similar to the mechanism responsible for Rh blood group iso-immunization. Iso-immunization occurs when the platelet type of the infant differs from that of the mother and when a significant number of platelets cross from the fetal to the maternal circulation. Platelet antibodies can usually be demonstrated by agglutination or Coombs consumption technics. Petechiae are usually present shortly after birth, and a male may bleed from circumcision. The bone marrow usually shows normal to increased megakaryocytes. The disease is self-limited, and severe hemorrhage usually does not occur unless surgery is performed. Platelets show a spontaneous rise within 2 weeks, with complete recovery by 4–6 weeks.

Platelet transfusions may be used in an emergency. In very severe cases, exchange transfusions with fresh whole blood collected in plastic bags is very effective both in removing antibody and in replacing platelets.

Thrombocytopenia Associated With ITP in the Mother

Infants born to mothers with ITP develop thrombocytopenia as a result of passive transfer of antibody from the mother to the infant. Evaluation of the maternal platelet count is indicated in any baby with thrombocytopenia. The persistence of antibodies in the infant's circulation is temporary, and spontaneous recovery the rule.

Congenital Amegakaryocytic Thrombocytopenia

Congenital absence of megakaryocytes is associated with severe chronic refractory thrombocytopenia beginning in the newborn period. It is frequently associated with other congenital abnormalities, particularly absence of the radius. It may be familial. This disease is considered to be the neonatal equivalent of Fanconi's syndrome, which does not usually appear in its classical form until later in childhood.

Treatment is not usually effective, although testosterone with or without corticosteroids may be tried in severe cases.

If the platelet count is extremely low, the prognosis is poor.

Thrombocytopenia Associated With Hemolytic Disease of the Newborn

Thrombocytopenia is a complication of severe erythroblastosis and may represent combined platelet and red cell iso-immunization. In these cases, blood that is rich in platelets is indicated for the exchange transfusion.

Neonatal Thrombocytopenia Associated With Infections

Thrombocytopenia is commonly associated with severe generalized infections of the newborn period, and particularly with those that develop in utero. It may be a major complication of the rubella syndrome in the newborn, and in these instances is usually associated with other malformations, eg, cataracts, congenital heart disease, and skeletal defects. Megakaryocytes are decreased and immature, and splenomegaly is usually present. Other intrauterine infections such as syphilis, toxoplasmosis, and cytomegalic inclusion disease are almost invariably associated with thrombocytopenia, and thrombocytopenia is frequently present with bacterial sepsis and generalized infection with herpes simplex virus. The thrombocytopenia may also be associated with consumption coagulopathy (disseminated intravascular coagulation, DIC) in severe forms of these disorders.

In addition to specific treatment for the underlying disease if available, platelet transfusions in severe cases or heparin for DIC (or both) may be indicated.

Thrombocytopenia Associated With Giant Hemangiomas

A rare but important cause of thrombocytopenic purpura in the newborn is giant hemangioma. Platelet sequestration in the tumor results in peripheral depletion of platelets. The bone marrow usually shows marked hyperplasia of megakaryocytes. In the presence of massive hemangiomas, the thrombocytopenia may be associated with disseminated intravascular coagulation (DIC) and result in fatal hemorrhage.

X-ray treatment of hemangiomas may be indicated. Heparinization is indicated if there is evidence of DIC. Surgery is usually contraindicated because of the risk of hemorrhage.

Hillman RS, Phillips LL: Clotting-fibrinolysis in a cavernous hemangioma. Am J Dis Child 113:649, 1967.

THROMBOCYTOPENIA ASSOCIATED WITH APLASTIC ANEMIA

Thrombocytopenia is frequently the first manifestation of aplastic anemia and may be present before neutropenia and anemia develop. The child who presents with amegakaryocytic thrombocytopenia in the first few years of life—particularly if there are associated skeletal anomalies—should be considered as a possible case of congenital pancytopenia of the Fanconi type.

THROMBOCYTOPENIA IN LEUKEMIA

Thrombocytopenia is almost invariably a major finding in acute leukemia of childhood. This is discussed in Chapter 32.

THROMBOCYTOPENIA DUE TO DEFICIENCY OF THROMBOCYTOPOIETIC FACTOR

Chronic thrombocytopenia may rarely occur in association with a congenital deficiency of thrombopoietin, a plasma factor which apparently is responsible for megakaryocyte maturation and platelet production. The clinical and hematologic picture is similar to that of chronic ITP. The 2 disorders may be differentiated by the administration of fresh or freshly frozen plasma in doses of approximately 10 ml/kg; in thrombocytopoietin deficiency, this produces a dramatic and prolonged response, whereas the patient with classical ITP will respond temporarily only to large doses of plasma (about 30 ml/kg).

Patients with congenital deficiency of the thrombocytopoietic factor may be maintained in good remission with administration of freshly frozen plasma every few months.

Schulman I & others: A factor in normal human plasma required for platelet production; chronic thrombocytopenia due to its deficiency. Blood 16:943–957, 1960.

DRUG-INDUCED THROMBOCYTOPENIA

Drug-induced thrombocytopenia may be either amegakaryocytic or megakaryocytic. The myelosuppressive drugs and chemical toxins, as well as irradiation, tend to affect all marrow elements, including megakaryocytes. Thrombocytopenia thus is a primary presenting complication of the aplastic or hypoplastic anemias produced by these agents. They are discussed in detail in the section on aplastic anemia.

Megakaryocytic thrombocytopenia is an immune reaction resulting from sensitization of the patient by prior administration of drugs such as quinidine, quinine, and allylisopropylacetylcarbamide (Sedormid).

Once the cause of the purpura is understood, prevention is readily effected by removal of the sensitizing drug.

Steinkamp R & others: Thrombocytopenic purpura caused by hypersensitivity to quinine. J Lab Clin Med 45:18–25, 1955.

ECZEMA, THROMBOCYTOPENIA, & RECURRENT INFECTIONS
(Wiskott-Aldrich Syndrome)

The triad of thrombocytopenic purpura, eczema, and recurrent infection occurs as an X-linked familial disorder. The syndrome is fatal, with death occurring as a result of overwhelming infection or hemorrhage. The bone marrow is normal, with adequate megakaryocytes; platelet survival may be greatly decreased. The exact cause is not completely understood, but there is probably a failure to respond to polysaccharide antigens. Isohemagglutinins are low or absent; IgG is quantitatively normal, whereas IgA and IgM may be decreased. Delayed hypersensitivity as measured by appropriate skin testing and lymphocyte blastoid transformation in tissue culture is usually partially impaired. Children with this syndrome may develop a malignant process similar to the Letterer-Siwe type of reticuloendotheliosis, or may have autoimmune complications. There is no specific treatment. Antibiotic therapy is useful in prolonging life, and platelet transfusions (platelet concentrates, 1 unit/5–10 lb) may be indicated in the presence of severe hemorrhage. Bone marrow transplant (although still experimental) or the use of "transfer factor" should be considered since recent success has been reported with these approaches to immunologic reconstitution.

The outcome is usually fatal in spite of all supportive measures.

Aldrich RA & others: Pedigree demonstrating a sex-linked recessive condition characterized by draining ears, eczematoid dermatitis and bloody diarrhea. Pediatrics 13:133–139, 1954.
Cooper MD & others: Wiskott-Aldrich syndrome: Immunologic deficiency disease involving afferent limb of immunity. Am J Med 44:499, 1968.

SECONDARY HYPERSPLENISM

Thrombocytopenia is one of the earliest hematologic manifestations of secondary hypersplenism. This is discussed on p 368.

THROMBOTIC THROMBOCYTOPENIA
(Thrombohemolytic Thrombocytopenic Purpura)

Thrombotic thrombocytopenic purpura is a hemorrhagic disorder characterized by thrombocytopenia, severe purpura, fever, hemolytic anemia, transitory focal neurologic signs, and hepatic involvement. Hemolysis often precedes clinical purpura. The Coombs test may be positive (rarely), and the red blood cells show bizarre forms and fragmentation similar to that seen in the hemolytic uremic syndrome. Other clinical signs and symptoms may occur in association with widespread intracapillary and intra-arteriolar thrombi which may affect not only the brain but also the kidneys, heart, and spleen. It is believed this entity may represent a hypersensitivity syndrome closely related to diseases such as lupus erythematosus and polyarteritis nodosa. Recent evidence suggests that patients with thrombotic thrombocytopenic purpura may be undergoing disseminated intravascular coagulation and that the disease may be related to purpura fulminans.

The course is usually rapidly progressive and terminates fatally within a few weeks, although chronic cases have been described.

Treatment has not been effective, though corticosteroids and splenectomy have both been reported to be of benefit. Heparin given early in the course may be of value in preventing further development of thrombi. Trials of low molecular weight dextran may be indicated.

MacWhinney JB & others: Thrombotic thrombocytopenic purpura in childhood. Blood 19:181, 1962.
Thrombotic thrombocytopenic purpura: Clinico-pathologic conference. Am J Med 27:115–124, 1960.

PLATELET FUNCTIONAL DEFECTS

The terms thrombasthenia, thrombopathia, and thrombocytopathy have been used to describe a variety of conditions characterized by abnormal platelet function in the presence of normal platelet counts. The tests for platelet function include clot retraction test, tourniquet test, bleeding time, platelet adhesiveness, aggregations to collagen, ADP, and thrombin, and estimation of platelet factor 3 content.

Thrombasthenia (Glanzmann's disease) is usually familial and associated with defective function of platelets with abnormal clot retraction; a defect in platelet adhesiveness and aggregation; and inability to release platelet factor 3. The bleeding time is prolonged. Thrombasthenia has been reported both as a recessive and as a dominant, and may be either mild or severe. It should be suspected in a patient with a prolonged bleeding time and should be investigated with platelet function studies. In the presence of severe bleeding, treatment with platelet concentrates may be necessary.

Thrombopathia is characterized by an abnormality of platelet function affecting the clotting mechanism. There is a deficiency of the platelet thromboplastic factor (platelet factor 3). This abnormality is usually associated with mild bleeding. The diagnosis may only be made by investigation of platelet function in the thromboplastin generation test or by the prothrombin consumption test. Platelet concentrates are the recommended therapy. Giant platelets are frequently seen on the blood smear.

TABLE 14–3. Findings in hereditary platelet diseases.*

Disease	Platelet Count	Clot Retraction	Platelet Adhesion to Glass	Platelet Aggregations	Platelet Factor 3 Release	Platelet Survival	Platelet Morphology	Genetic Transmission
Glanzmann's thrombasthenia (membrane defect)	N	↓	↓	Decreased to ADP, collagen, thrombin, epinephrine	↓	N	Decreased absorbed fibrinogen	Autosomal recessive
Thrombopathia (ADP release defect)	N	N	↓ (or N)	Decreased to collagen, epinephrine, low molar ADP	↓ (or N)	N or ↑	No abnormality except(?) small size	Variable; (?)autosomal dominant
Thrombocytopathy (platelet factor 3 defect)	N	N	N (or ↓)	N	↓	. . .	Rare increase in platelet size	(?)Autosomal dominant
Von Willebrand's disease (plasma factor defect)	N	N	↓	N	N	N	N	Autosomal dominant (occasionally recessive)
Macrothrombocytic thrombopathy	↓	N	N (or ↓)	N	↓	↓	Giant platelets	Autosomal dominant
Wiskott-Aldrich syndrome	↓	N	↓	Decreased to ADP, collagen, epinephrine	N (or ↓)	↓	Reduced organelles; large number of tubules	X-linked recessive
Thrombocytopenia with intrinsic platelet defect	↓	N	. . .	N to ADP	N	↓	N	Autosomal dominant

*Modified and reproduced, with permission, from Hathaway WE: Bleeding disorders due to platelet dysfunction. Am J Dis Child 121: 127–134, 1971.

Several other hereditary (Table 14–3) and acquired diseases of platelet function have recently been described. Of practical importance are the acquired platelet function defects found in patients with uremia or after aspirin ingestion.

Hathaway WE: Bleeding disorders due to platelet dysfunction. Am J Dis Child 121:127–134, 1971.

Weiss HJ: Platelet aggregation adhesion and adenosine diphosphate release in thrombopathia (platelet factor 3 deficiency): A comparison of Glanzmann's thrombasthenia and von Willebrand's disease. Am J Med 43:570, 1967.

VON WILLEBRAND'S DISEASE
(Pseudohemophilia, Vascular Hemophilia)

Essentials of Diagnosis
- History of easy bruising and epistaxis from early childhood.
- Prolonged bleeding time with normal platelet count.
- Abnormal platelet adhesiveness.
- Reduced levels of AHF (AHG, factor VIII).

General Considerations
Vascular hemophilia is a familial bleeding disorder that is usually transmitted as a dominant and occurs in both sexes. It is associated both with a bleeding time defect and with a reduced level of factor VIII. Although the whole blood coagulation time is usually normal, the partial thromboplastin test is abnormal.

This bleeding disorder was originally believed to be associated with an abnormality of the capillary wall since increased tortuosity of capillaries may be seen on examination of the loops in the nail bed. There is now evidence that the primary bleeding manifestation is due to a platelet functional defect which is characterized by decreased platelet adhesiveness. This in turn appears to be due to deficiency of a plasma factor which is necessary for the maintenance of normal platelet function. In addition, these patients have a deficiency of antihemophilic factor, which is usually 20–40% of normal but may be as low as 3%.

Clinical Findings
A. Symptoms and Signs: There is usually a history of increased bruising and severe prolonged epistaxis. Increased bleeding will also occur with lacerations or at surgery. Excessive menstrual flow is a problem in the adolescent female. Petechiae are usually not observed, and hemarthrosis does not occur.

B. Laboratory Findings: A prolonged bleeding time is always present; the tourniquet test may or may not be positive. Platelet adhesiveness is usually abnormal. Other platelet function tests are normal. Antihemophilic factor levels are decreased.

Treatment
The depressed levels of AHF can be easily corrected with freshly frozen lyophilized plasma or AHF concentrates (cryoprecipitates). The AHF levels

increase both after transfusion of AHF and as a result of endogenous production of AHF stimulated by another plasma factor; therefore, AHF levels remain elevated longer than in classical hemophilia. In some patients, the platelet adhesiveness and bleeding time can be corrected by the use of freshly frozen, platelet-free plasma. Transfusions with fresh diabetic plasma may be more effective than normal plasma in correcting the bleeding time. Dosage equivalents of 10 ml/kg of freshly frozen plasma every 12 hours will correct the AHF deficiency, but more frequent transfusions may be needed to restore the bleeding time to normal.

Dental procedures involving the gums and tooth extractions should be avoided if possible. When extractions are necessary, management consists of systemic correction of bleeding and local pressure.

Prognosis

Patients with mild forms of the disease usually have a normal life expectancy, and bleeding can be controlled with the measures noted above or may cease spontaneously. In severe cases it may be difficult to control hemorrhage, although recent methods of therapy with plasma and concentrates have greatly improved the outlook. Elective surgical procedures should be avoided.

Larrieu MJ & others: Congenital bleeding disorders with long bleeding time and normal platelet count. 2. Von Willebrand's disease. Am J Med 45:354, 1968.

THROMBASTHENIA WITH ACYANOTIC CONGENITAL HEART DISEASE

Several patients have been observed who demonstrate a history of easy bruising and bleeding from cuts or minor surgery and who have associated acyanotic congenital heart disease. Aortic stenosis is particularly apt to be associated with this problem. It is characterized by a prolonged bleeding time and possibly by abnormal platelet function. The bleeding disorder is usually extremely mild, and some of these patients have undergone surgical correction of their heart disease without excessive hemorrhage.

VASCULAR DEFECTS

ANAPHYLACTOID PURPURA
(Schönlein-Henoch Purpura, Allergic Purpura)

Essentials of Diagnosis
- Purpuric cutaneous rash.
- Urticaria.
- Migratory polyarthritis.

- Gastrointestinal pain and hemorrhage.
- Hematuria.

General Considerations

Anaphylactoid purpura is characterized by a typical purpuric skin rash plus (in any combination) migratory arthritis, gastroenteritis, and nephritis. It is believed to be a sensitivity disease closely related to rheumatic fever, rheumatoid arthritis, and lupus erythematosus. It is characterized by involvement of the small vessels, particularly in the skin, the gastrointestinal tract, and the kidneys. The cause of the allergic reaction is frequently not recognized, although in many parts of the world group A beta-hemolytic streptococcal infection precedes the disease in a high proportion of cases. Other inciting factors such as other infections, food allergens, insect bites, and horse serum have been implicated.

Clinical Findings

A. Symptoms and Signs: Migratory polyarthritis very similar to that of rheumatic fever frequently precedes the onset of the skin rash. Gastrointestinal pain, diarrhea, and gastrointestinal bleeding are common. Nephritis occurs in about 50% of cases and is characterized by hematuria. The skin rash is diagnostic in appearance: It is characteristically distributed on the ankles, buttocks, and elbows; purpuric areas a few millimeters in diameter are present and may progress to form larger hemorrhages. Petechial lesions occur, but the majority of skin or mucous membrane hemorrhages are slightly larger. The rash usually begins on the lower extremities, but the entire body may be involved. Erythematous and urticarial skin eruptions (which may become hemorrhagic) often accompany the hemorrhage. In younger children, edema of the feet and ankles is common. Cardiac involvement is rare.

B. Laboratory Findings: The purpuric manifestation is associated with entirely normal laboratory findings. The platelet count, platelet function tests, bleeding time, and tourniquet test are usually negative, although the latter may be the one abnormal finding. Blood coagulation is normal. Urinalysis frequently reveals hematuria and proteinuria, but casts are unusual. Stool tests may be positive for occult blood, even though gross melena is not observed. The ASO titer is frequently elevated or the throat culture positive for group A beta-hemolytic streptococci.

Differential Diagnosis

The hemorrhagic rash of anaphylactoid purpura can be differentiated from thrombocytopenic purpura by the presence of raised skin lesions in the former and by the platelet count. The rash of septicemia (especially meningococcemia) may be very similar, although the distribution tends to be more generalized in sepsis. Blood culture may be necessary for final diagnosis.

Complications

Intussusception of the small bowel occurs in a significant number of patients with intestinal manifestations. Renal involvement with the development of chronic nephritis is the principal long-term complication.

Treatment

There is no satisfactory treatment for anaphylactoid purpura. Corticosteroid therapy may be useful in patients with acute gastrointestinal manifestations. If the culture is positive for group A beta-hemolytic streptococci or if the ASO titer is elevated, give penicillin in full therapeutic doses for 10 days. In cases of proved streptococcal etiology, the use of prophylactic penicillin may be indicated as in rheumatic fever. In general, the disease must be allowed to run its course, and treatment is symptomatic. Aspirin is useful for the arthritis, and sedatives may benefit the patient with gastrointestinal pain.

Prognosis

The prognosis for recovery is good, although symptoms frequently recur over a period of several months. In patients who develop renal manifestations, approximately 50% may have abnormal urinary findings for several years. This occasionally progresses to significant impairment of renal function.

Allen DM & others: Anaphylactoid purpura in children (Schönlein-Henoch syndrome): Review with a follow-up of the renal complications. Am J Dis Child 99:833, 1960.

Wedgewood RJP, Klaus MH: Anaphylactoid purpura (Schönlein-Henoch syndrome); a long term follow-up study with special reference to renal involvement. Pediatrics 16:196–206, 1955.

INTRAVASCULAR DEFECTS; COAGULATION FACTOR DEFICIENCIES

Essentials of Diagnosis

- Generalized bleeding tendency.
- Ecchymoses (not petechiae).
- Congenital (family history) or acquired (systemic illness).
- Abnormal partial thromboplastin time or prothrombin time (or both).

General Considerations

A congenital or acquired deficiency of one or more of the coagulation factors in the blood can result in a generalized bleeding diathesis. The bleeding tendency may be mild (bleeding only at time of severe traumas or surgical procedures), moderate, or severe (frequent spontaneous hemarthroses and ecchymoses) depending on the degree of the coagulation factor deficit. Fig 14–1 depicts the interaction of these factors in producing coagulation of the blood. Hemostasis in man depends upon platelet and vascular factors as well as blood coagulation.

A specific hemorrhagic diathesis has been seen with a deficiency of each of the coagulation factors except Hageman factor (XII) and calcium deficiency. These disease entities are discussed below.

The diagnosis and classification of clinical coagulation factor deficiencies depend upon proper performance and interpretation of specific clotting tests which are briefly reviewed below.

Coagulation Tests

A. Whole Blood Coagulation Time (Lee-White): This test is too insensitive to be of value in diagnosis or treatment of patients with mild to moderate coagulation factor deficiencies. The clotting time is influenced by heparin and can therefore be used as a rough guide to heparinization. Although simple to perform, this procedure is not an adequate screening test and should be abandoned as a "routine" test. At 37° C, the normal clotting time of whole blood in glass test tubes is less than 10 minutes if the tubes are tipped but may be as long as 15 minutes by the Lee-White method (the third tube is tipped only after the first 2 have clotted).

B. One-Stage Prothrombin Time (Quick): This procedure consists of noting the clotting time of citrated or oxalated plasma after addition of calcium and tissue thromboplastin. Normal adult values are between 11–13 seconds (100%). This is an adequate screening test for proconvertin (VII), proaccelerin (V), Stuart-Prower factor (X), prothrombin (II), and fibrinogen deficiencies. It does not measure the factors necessary for the earlier stages of coagulation.

C. Partial Thromboplastin Time (PTT): This test is performed much like the prothrombin time except that a "crude cephalin" is added instead of tissue thromboplastin. In addition, a contact activator substance like kaolin may be added to avert the influence of glass contact. The test is very sensitive, relatively easy to perform, and inexpensive. All coagulation factors except proconvertin are measured; therefore, it is the screening test of choice. Normal adult values are as follows: with kaolin, 37–50 seconds; without contact activator, 70–100 seconds.

D. Prothrombin Consumption Test: This procedure measures all factors prior to conversion of prothrombin to thrombin (except proconvertin). The test is technically difficult to perform properly and is not as sensitive as the partial thromboplastin time.

E. Thromboplastin Generation Test (TGT): This determination is more difficult to perform than the prothrombin consumption test, but it is a reliable and sensitive estimate of plasma thromboplastin formation and is often used to confirm the diagnosis of AHF or PTC deficiency.

F. Thrombin Time: Bovine or human thrombin is added to plasma and the clotting time recorded. The normal adult range is 7–15 seconds or more, depending upon the amount of thrombin added. The test measures the conversion of fibrinogen to fibrin and is dependent upon the concentration of fibrinogen or inhibitors such as fibrin split products, antithrombins, and heparin.

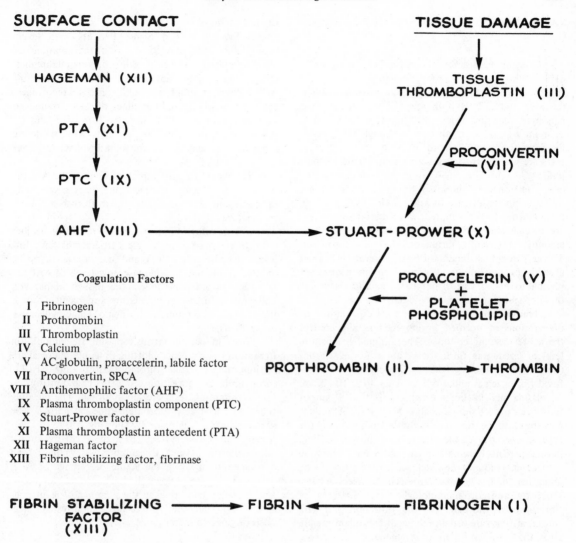

SURFACE CONTACT

HAGEMAN (XII)

PTA (XI)

PTC (IX)

AHF (VIII) ⟶ STUART-PROWER (X)

TISSUE DAMAGE

TISSUE THROMBOPLASTIN (III)

PROCONVERTIN (VII)

PROACCELERIN (V) + PLATELET PHOSPHOLIPID

PROTHROMBIN (II) ⟶ THROMBIN

Coagulation Factors

I	Fibrinogen
II	Prothrombin
III	Thromboplastin
IV	Calcium
V	AC-globulin, proaccelerin, labile factor
VII	Proconvertin, SPCA
VIII	Antihemophilic factor (AHF)
IX	Plasma thromboplastin component (PTC)
X	Stuart-Prower factor
XI	Plasma thromboplastin antecedent (PTA)
XII	Hageman factor
XIII	Fibrin stabilizing factor, fibrinase

FIBRIN STABILIZING FACTOR (XIII) ⟶ FIBRIN ⟵ FIBRINOGEN (I)

FIG 14–1. Blood coagulation scheme and terminology of coagulation factors.

G. Specific Factor Assays: Each of the coagulation factors can be assayed by an indirect clotting method using natural or synthetic factor deficient substrates and compared to the activity of normal plasma (100%). Fibrinogen is the only factor which can be measured directly by a chemical method.

H. Bleeding Time (Ivy): (Hemostasis bleeding time method.) Place a blood pressure cuff on the upper arm and inflate to 40 mm Hg. With an alcohol sponge, clean an area free of visible veins on the flexor surface of the forearm. With a sterile Bard-Parker No. 11 blade, make a puncture wound 5 mm deep and 2 mm wide. Note time of puncture; touch wound gently with sterile filter paper to absorb blood every 30 seconds until bleeding stops. Normal bleeding time is 1–7 minutes.

I. Other Tests: Various other tests, available usually in research laboratories only, such as the thromboelastograph, thrombin generation time, euglobulin fibrinolysin time, and recalcification time are sometimes helpful in identifying unusual circulating anticoagulants or hypercoagulability of the blood.

Macfarlane RG: The basis of the cascade hypothesis of blood clotting. Thromb Diath Haemorrh 15:591–602, 1966.

Owen CA Jr & others: *The Diagnosis and Treatment of Bleeding Disorders.* Little, Brown, 1969.

AFIBRINOGENEMIA & DYSFIBRINOGENEMIA

Congenital absence of fibrinogen produces a definite entity which resembles hemophilia clinically. However, the condition is inherited as an autosomal recessive and affects both sexes. The patients have persistent bleeding from small injuries, hematomas, ecchymoses, and hemarthroses. Although fatal bleeding from the umbilical cord has been reported, most cases are usually much less severe than classical hemophilia.

The principal laboratory finding in afibrinogenemia is complete absence of a fibrin clot by any of the usual clotting tests attempted. Whole blood and plasma are incoagulable even upon the addition of optimal amounts of calcium, thromboplastin, and thrombin. The erythrocyte sedimentation rate is zero. There is an absence of precipitable fibrinogen upon heating of plasma to 56° C for 10 minutes. Specific assays for other coagulation factors are normal.

Transfusion with whole blood, fresh plasma, or preparations of purified fibrinogen generally control the acute bleeding episodes. The minimal hemostatic level of circulating fibrinogen is about 60 mg/100 ml (normal, 250–450 mg/100 ml). The half-life of transfused fibrinogen is about 4 days. Therefore, 10–20 ml of plasma per kg body weight or 0.05–0.1 gm of fibrinogen per kg should achieve hemostasis. This dose may need to be repeated daily depending upon the type and severity of bleeding and the rate of healing. Several patients have been described recently who have a bleeding tendency and delayed clotting due to an abnormal molecule of fibrinogen (congenital dysfibrinogenemia). Immunologic determinations of fibrinogen are normal, but the thrombin and prothrombin times are often prolonged. Treatment is similar to that outlined for afibrinogenemia.

Alexander B & others: Congenital afibrinogenemia: A study of some basic aspects of coagulation. Blood 9:843–860, 1954.

Von Felten A, Frick PG, Straub PW: Studies on fibrin monomer aggregation in congenital dysfibrinogenemia (fibrinogen "Zurich"): Separation of a pathological from a normal fibrin fraction. Brit J Haemat 16:353–361, 1969.

HEMOPHILIA A
(Antihemophilic Factor
[AHF, Factor VIII] Deficiency)

Classical hemophilia (hemophilia A) is a bleeding disorder characterized by decreased amounts of circulating antihemophilic factor (AHF, AHG, or factor VIII). The disease occurs in males and is inherited in an X-linked recessive manner. All degrees of severity of the disease have been reported.

Clinical Findings

A. Symptoms and Signs: Patients with severe hemophilia, characterized by frequent spontaneous bleeding episodes involving skin, mucous membranes, joints, and viscera, apparently have no circulating AHF. However, mild hemophilia is also recognized; these patients bleed only at times of severe trauma or surgical procedures. They have 5–20% AHF activity. An intermediate group of patients with moderate symptoms (usually no severe joint involvement) have 1–5% AHF levels.

The most crippling aspect of hemophilia A is the tendency to develop chronic hemarthroses, especially of knees and elbows, which lead to fibrosis and joint contractures.

B. Laboratory Findings: In about 70% of families with this disease, the female carriers will have low levels of AHF (20–70%) and may occasionally be mildly symptomatic. Otherwise, low levels of AHF are not seen in a female unless the individual has von Willebrand's disease, a circulating anticoagulant, or is the product of the union of a hemophiliac male and a carrier female.

Tests measuring intrinsic plasma thromboplastin formation (whole blood clotting time, plasma recalcification time, partial thromboplastin time [PTT], thromboplastin generation test [TGT], and prothrombin consumption test) are all abnormal. The bleeding time and one-stage prothrombin time are normal. The specific diagnosis is made by showing failure of "correction" in a test system (PTT or TGT) by known AHF-deficient plasma. Coagulation assays have been developed to measure the actual percentage of AHF activity in a given biologic fluid. The whole blood clotting time can be normal in the presence of as little as 1–2% AHF, and, therefore, is not a good test for diagnosis or guide to therapy.

Complications

The principal complication of classical hemophilia is the development of an acquired circulating anticoagulant to AHF. Mild inhibitor or anticoagulant substances specific to AHF not uncommonly can be shown in AHF-deficient patients, but the development of a severe AHF inhibitor is a rare and dreaded complication. When this occurs, the patient is often resistant to all attempts at therapy. The inhibitor has been shown to be an antibody and may be amenable to immunosuppressive therapy.

Another rare complication is the formation of a pseudotumor in the AHF-deficient patient. These are the result of multiple bleeding, fibrosis, serous secretion, and calcium deposition. They should be carefully evaluated and differentiated from bony or soft tissue neoplasms. Crippling due to repeated hemarthroses is the primary long-term complication.

Treatment

The basis of treatment of classical hemophilia is the administration of an AHF-containing substance in order to achieve adequate hemostasis. AHF is temperature and storage labile in biologic fluids.

The in vivo half-life of infused AHF is about 12 hours.

The following substances can be used for therapy: (1) Freshly drawn whole blood, given within 1—3 days. (2) Freshly frozen plasma or cryoprecipitates stored at −30° C for less than 6 months. (3) Lyophilized concentrates of AHF, reconstituted and given immediately.

Dosage and duration of therapy depend upon the type of bleeding seen clinically. "Open" bleeding is that which occurs from lacerations of the skin or mucous membranes, tooth extractions, surgical wounds, or severe traumatic epistaxis. Closed bleeding can be subdivided into (a) joint hemorrhage and non-dissecting hematomas, and (b) dissecting soft tissue hematomas.

A. "Open" Bleeding: Treat in one of the following ways: (1) Freshly frozen plasma or lyophilized plasma, 10 ml/kg body weight immediately and then 5 ml/kg every 6 hours. A level of 20% (in vivo) is achieved by 10 ml/kg. Each dose must be infused as rapidly as the patient can safely tolerate it to ensure peak levels. (2) Cryoprecipitated AHF is prepared from individual blood donors and is usually supplied frozen in 20—30 ml amounts per plastic pack. The units* of AHF activity vary from 75—200 per pack. To achieve a level of 40%, one pack per 5—6 kg of body weight is given. Half of this dose is given every 12 hours to maintain an in vivo level of 20%. (3) AHF concentrates (method 1 or 4, Hyland or Courtland) supplies concentrated AHF in a lyophilized form. The potency of each vial of these products is labeled in units of AHF. Dosage can be calculated as follows:

Units of AHF = weight in kg ×
desired in vivo percentage × 0.5

Treatment must be continued until adequate healing occurs, ie, 2—3 days in case of tooth extractions or epistaxis, but 7—10 days in case of lacerations and surgical wounds. The principle of therapy is to rapidly achieve a hemostatic level of AHF (at least 20%) and to maintain this level until the lesion is adequately healed. For surgical procedures, levels of 30—35% are usually necessary for hemostasis.

B. "Closed" Bleeding: Early closed bleeding in joints or soft tissue areas can often be controlled by a single infusion of freshly frozen plasma, cryoprecipitates, or AHF concentrate to reach a single peak of 20%. If bleeding is severe, this dose should be repeated in 12 hours or a higher level achieved initially (ie, 40%). However, if the lesion is a dissecting hematoma which might threaten nerve function or endanger respiration or vision, a level of 20% should be maintained for at least 48 hours.

Corticosteroids are indicated in cases where a reaction to AHF-fibrinogen might occur or where the presence of an inhibitor is suspected. Patients with renal bleeding have been benefited by corticosteroid therapy. Local hemostatic measures such as pressure or application of Gelfoam soaked in bovine thrombin are often helpful in case of epistaxis.

Prognosis

With prophylaxis against injury, early treatment of bleeding episodes, careful orthopedic care of joint lesions, and attention to emotional, social, and educational adjustment, the prognosis for a useful normal life is good.

Dallman PR, Pool JG: Treatment of hemophilia with factor VIII concentrates. New England J Med 278:199—202, 1968.

Honig GR & others: Administration of single doses of AHF (factor VIII) concentrates in treatment of hemophilic hemarthroses. Pediatrics 43:26—33, 1969.

HEMOPHILIA B
(PTC [Factor IX] Deficiency)

The mode of inheritance and clinical manifestations of hemophilia B (PTC deficiency, factor IX deficiency, Christmas disease) are the same as those of AHF deficiency (hemophilia A). Congenital PTC deficiency is 20—25% as prevalent as AHF deficiency. PTC is made in the liver and is vitamin K dependent; therefore, acquired deficiencies of factor IX are fairly common.

PTC is a storage stable factor which is not consumed during coagulation and is found in the serum. The thromboplastin generation test (TGT) may be used to determine whether the first stage defect is due to PTC (serum) or AHF (plasma) deficiency. Otherwise, the diagnosis is confirmed by failure to "correct" with known PTC-deficient plasma or serum in the PTT or TGT tests. With these exceptions, the laboratory findings are the same as those noted above in the discussion of hemophilia A.

Although factor IX is storage stable and is not consumed during coagulation, the therapy of bleeding episodes is little different from that outlined above for classical hemophilia. The products that can be used include recently outdated blood bank plasma (approximately 3 weeks old) at 4° C, plus freshly frozen plasma, factor IX concentrate, or lyophilized whole plasma. Unlike factor VIII, approximately 1/2 of the administered dose of factor IX diffuses into the extravascular space. Therefore, twice the calculated factor VIII dose (see above) should be given as plasma or factor IX concentrate (Konyne) initially. Subsequently, 1/2 of the initial dose can be given to achieve the desired in vivo level. (Factor IX has a half-life of 20—22 hours in vivo.) Cryoprecipitates and AHF concentrates do not contain sufficient PTC for use in this disease. The prognosis is good if the bleeding episodes are adequately controlled.

*A unit of AHF is the amount contained in 1 ml of fresh plasma at a 100% AHF activity level.

Hoag MS & others: Treatment of hemophilia B with a new clotting factor concentrate. New England J Med 280:581–586, 1969.

Salzman EW, Britten A: Chap 19 in: *Hemorrhage and Thrombosis.* Little, Brown, 1965.

HEMOPHILIA C
(PTA [Factor XI] Deficiency)

PTA (factor XI) deficiency is a bleeding diathesis of mild to moderate severity. Inheritance is by the autosomal recessive mode. Heterozygotes often show a mild bleeding tendency at surgery or following severe trauma. Homozygous patients may have spontaneous hemorrhage (ecchymoses, epistaxis) in addition to bleeding due to trauma. Only rarely do patients with hemophilia C have spontaneous hemarthroses. Hemophilia C has been found mainly in Jews and comprises less than 5% of all hemophilioid diseases.

The defect may be very mild, and a sensitive coagulation test (PTT or TGT) is required to identify the deficiency. Factor XI is a stable factor found in both serum and plasma and shows increased activity on contact with glass or after storage. Therefore, differentiation from PTC deficiency may be difficult unless tests are done with fresh plasma using known PTA-deficient plasma for "correction studies." The prothrombin time and bleeding time (Ivy) are normal in PTA deficiency.

The bleeding defect is mild and requires treatment usually only at times of surgery (eg, tooth extractions) or trauma. PTA is a stable factor, and good levels are found in plasma stored for several weeks at 4° C. Therefore, the principles of treatment outlined for PTC deficiency apply equally well to PTA deficiency.

The prognosis for an average longevity is excellent.

Rapaport SL & others: The mode of inheritance of PTA deficiency: Evidence for the existence of major PTA deficiency and minor PTA deficiency. Blood 18:149–165, 1961.

LIVER-DEPENDENT COAGULATION FACTORS

The following clotting factors are known to be produced in the liver: fibrinogen (I), PTC (IX), prothrombin (II), proconvertin (VII), proaccelerin (V), Stuart-Prower factor (X), PTA (XI), and factor XII. Vitamin K is necessary for the synthesis of II, VII, X, and IX. Hereditary bleeding diseases due to isolated deficiencies of prothrombin, proconvertin, proaccel-erin, or Stuart-Prower factor are exceedingly rare. Congenital deficiencies of fibrinogen and PTC are discussed above.

Hereditary prothrombin deficiency, proconvertin deficiency, Stuart-Prower factor deficiency, and proaccelerin deficiency have been reported in both males and females and have a recessive mode of transmission. Mild to moderately severe bleeding manifestations can occur. The prothrombin time is uniformly prolonged in these disorders; in addition, the PTT is abnormal in all except proconvertin deficiency (formation of intrinsic thromboplastin does not require proconvertin). The diagnosis is suspected when a patient is seen with a history of bleeding manifestations, a prolonged prothrombin time without liver disease, and no response to vitamin K therapy. The diagnosis must be confirmed by specific factor assays.

Treatment consists of transfusion of whole plasma in dosages sufficient to achieve at least 20–30% correction of the prothrombin time. Fresh plasma must be used for proaccelerin (V) deficiency since this is a relatively unstable factor.

Borchgrevink CF & others: A study of a case of congenital hypoprothrombinemia. Brit J Haemat 5:294–310, 1959.

Field JH, Ware AG: Studies in parahemophilia. J Clin Invest 33:923–943, 1954.

Graham JB: Stuart clotting defect and Stuart factor. Thromb Diath Haemorrh 4, Suppl 22, 1960.

Owen CA & others: Congenital deficiency of factor VII. Am J Med 37:71–91, 1964.

HAGEMAN (XII) FACTOR DEFICIENCY

Patients with factor XII deficiency constitute a medical curiosity which consists of a markedly prolonged whole blood and plasma clotting time without clinical bleeding diathesis. This phenomenon cannot be explained at present. The defect is rare and is inherited in an autosomal recessive manner. Hageman factor deficiency becomes of clinical significance in the evaluation of a markedly prolonged coagulation time. These patients have undergone major surgery without excessive bleeding. A newly described coagulation factor defect (tentatively designated "Fletcher factor") has similar laboratory and clinical characteristics.

Hathaway WE, Hathaway HS, Belhasen LP: Evidence for a new plasma thromboplastin factor. 1. Case report, coagulation studies and physicochemical properties. Blood 26:521, 1965.

Ratnoff OD: The biology and pathology of the initial stages of blood coagulation. Progr Hemat 5:204–245, 1966.

FIBRIN STABILIZING FACTOR (XIII) DEFICIENCY

The deficiency of a factor responsible for the stability of the fibrin clot produces a genetically transmitted hemorrhagic disorder called congenital fibrinase (fibrin stabilizing factor, factor XIII) deficiency. Cases reported to date indicate an autosomal recessive inheritance. Affected individuals have a moderately severe bleeding tendency and often present at birth with hemorrhage into the umbilical cord. The usual tests of coagulation such as PTT, prothrombin time, and TGT are all normal. Fibrinogen may be borderline to low, and increased vascular fragility has been reported. The diagnosis is made by demonstrating abnormal stability of the fibrin clot in 5 M urea solution.

Treatment consists of giving plasma transfusions to control the acute bleeding episode.

Britten AFH: Congenital deficiency of factor XIII (fibrin stabilizing factor). Am J Med 43:751–761, 1967.

ACQUIRED COAGULATION FACTOR DEFICIENCIES

1. HEMORRHAGIC DISEASE OF NEWBORN

A generalized bleeding diathesis can occur in newborn infants who are markedly deficient in vitamin K-dependent coagulation factors (PTC, prothrombin, proconvertin, Stuart-Prower factor). This clinical syndrome is called hemorrhagic disease of the newborn. It may be present at birth or may occur any time in the first 3 days of life. All newborn infants show a moderate deficiency of these K-dependent factors at a level of 25–60% of normal adult values. However, when the levels fall below 20% in infants who are vitamin K deficient, a generalized bleeding tendency can ensue. Ecchymoses, gastrointestinal hemorrhage, hematuria, and cerebral hemorrhages may occur on the second to fourth days of life.

The prothrombin time is markedly prolonged to a level below 20% of normal. The PTT is also greatly prolonged. Platelet estimation, bleeding, and clotting times are normal. In this age group, bleeding in association with a greatly prolonged prothrombin time is very suggestive of hemorrhagic disease of the newborn. The diagnosis is confirmed by the response to specific treatment.

By definition, this disorder is due to severe vitamin K deficiency. Therefore, the disease can be prevented and treated adequately by a single intramuscular injection of 1–2 mg of vitamin K_1 (phytonadione). It is also recommended that this dose be given prophylactically to all newborn infants. The prothrombin will become essentially normal within 12–24 hours, and the bleeding will stop within 6–12 hours after treatment with vitamin K. If life-threatening hemorrhage is present, a transfusion of fresh plasma (10 ml/kg) or fresh whole blood (or both) is indicated.

Since the newborn infant can usually ingest, synthesize, and utilize enough vitamin K within a few days after birth to prevent further difficulty, the prognosis is excellent.

Sutherland JM & others: Hemorrhagic disease of newborn: Breast feeding as necessary factor in pathogenesis. Am J Dis Child 113:524–534, 1967.

2. VITAMIN K DEFICIENCY IN OLDER CHILDREN

Older infants and children may develop vitamin K deficiency secondary to chronic diarrhea, malabsorption syndrome, and defective synthesis associated with prolonged antibiotic therapy. The clinical and laboratory manifestations are similar to those seen in hemorrhagic disease of the newborn. Treatment is by administration of vitamin K_1 (phytonadione) in doses of 5–10 mg IV or IM.

3. SECONDARY HEMORRHAGIC DIATHESES OF NEWBORN

Premature and full-term infants frequently develop generalized bleeding tendencies associated with other illness such as respiratory distress syndrome, cyanotic congenital heart disease, cerebral anoxia, and severe sepsis. Factors which are often present and possibly related to this bleeding syndrome are "physiologic" depression of coagulation factors, hypoxia, acidosis, vascular fragility, defective platelet number and function, and increased fibrinolytic activity. Laboratory tests of bleeding and coagulation parameters are usually not very helpful because of the overlap with normal infants. The values for these tests seen in "normal" full-term and premature infants are shown in Table 14–4. The pathophysiologic mechanisms of these secondary bleeding syndromes (cerebral hemorrhage, pulmonary hemorrhage, generalized bleeding tendency) are poorly understood at present.

Occasionally, these infants show the clinical and laboratory signs of disseminated intravascular coagulation (see below). Heparin then becomes an important adjunct to therapy. Otherwise, treatment is symptomatic and is mainly directed at the underlying disease or metabolic disorder. If platelets or coagulation factors are shown to be very low, specific replacement with platelet concentrates or fresh plasma can be given. Vitamin K should always be given to these infants also.

TABLE 14—4. Coagulation factor and test values in normal pregnant women and newborn infants.*

Category	Fibrin-ogen (mg/100 ml)	Factors									Platelet Count (per cu mm)	Euglobulin Lysis Time (minutes)	Partial Thrombo-plastin Time† (seconds)	Pro-thrombin Time (seconds)	Thrombin Time (seconds)
		II (%)	V (%)	VII (%)	VIII (%)	IX (%)	X (%)	XI (%)	XII (%)	XIII (titer)					
Normal adult or child	190–420	100	100	100	100	100	100	100	100	1/16	200,000–450,000	90–300	37–50	12–14	8–10
Term pregnancy	483	92	108	170	196	130	130	69	...	1/16	290,000	278	44	13	8
Premature (1500–2500 gm), cord blood	233	25	67	37	80	↓	29	...	...	1/8	220,000	214	90	17 (12–21)	14 (11–17)
Term infant, cord blood	216	41	92	56	100	27	55	36	...	1/8	190,000	84	71	16 (13–20)	12 (10–16)
Term infant, 48 hours	210	46	105	20	100	↓	45	39	25	...	200,000	105	65	17.5 (12–21)	13 (10–16)

Note: All levels expressed as means or ranges.

*Reproduced, with permission, from Hathaway WE: Coagulation problems in the newborn infant. P Clin North America 17:929–942, 1970.

†Kaolin PTT.

Hathaway WE, Mull MM, Pechet GS: Disseminated intravascular coagulation in the newborn. Pediatrics 43:233, 1969.

4. DISSEMINATED INTRAVASCULAR COAGULATION

Certain diseases occurring in children have been shown to be associated with disseminated intravascular coagulation (DIC) or consumption coagulopathy. These diseases are purpura fulminans, severe overwhelming bacterial sepsis (eg, meningococcemia, *Escherichia coli* infection), viral or rickettsial infections (eg, smallpox, Rocky Mountain spotted fever), severe thermal burns, giant hemangiomas, and the hemolytic-uremic syndrome. DIC can be triggered by a Schwartzman-like phenomenon or release of tissue thromboplastin and leads to widespread fibrin deposition (lungs, kidneys), fibrinolysis, and consumption of coagulation factors which lead to a secondary bleeding tendency.

Laboratory evaluation discloses decreased platelets, fibrinogen, proaccelerin, AHF, and prothrombin (the factors consumed during coagulation). Other factors are usually normal. Fibrinolysins are first increased and later depressed or exhausted. Degradation of fibrin leads to the accumulation of fibrin split products in the blood; these act as an anticoagulant and prolong the thrombin time.

Treatment consists of interrupting intravascular coagulation by the use of heparin in an intravenous dosage of 100–200 units/kg every 4–6 hours until the patient recovers. If marked depletion of consumable clotting factors has occurred, replacement by infusions of freshly frozen plasma or platelets (or both) may be needed.

As shock is often associated with this disorder, early recognition and prompt treatment may be lifesaving.

Abildgaard CF: Recognition and treatment of intravascular coagulation. J Pediat 74:163–176, 1969.

Hathaway WE: Care of the critically ill child: The problem of disseminated intravascular coagulation. Pediatrics 46:767–773, 1970.

5. CIRCULATING ANTICOAGULANTS

Acquired anticoagulants can cause a widespread hemorrhagic diathesis. These inhibitors to coagulation are often associated with "collagen" diseases such as disseminated lupus erythematosus. Also, specific inhibitors to AHF or PTC may occur in hemophilia and may cause a severe intractable bleeding tendency. The anticoagulants appear to be antibodies and are often directed against specific coagulation factors. These inhibitors can be demonstrated using the recalcification time, prothrombin time, and PTT tests. These tests will remain prolonged rather than be corrected by addition of normal plasma in equal quantities. The most effective therapy has been with immunosuppressive agents such as prednisone or azathioprine.

Heparin and bishydroxycoumarin (Dicumarol) are potent anticoagulants when administered as drugs. Heparin affects the whole blood coagulation time or PTT primarily, whereas bishydroxycoumarin affects the prothrombin time by inhibiting the utilization of vitamin K.

Naturally occurring anticoagulants such as heparin, antithromboplastins, and antithrombins are rarely implicated as the cause of a bleeding diathesis, although they can occasionally be demonstrated by special coagulation tests in such disorders as liver disease, malignancies, or disseminated intravascular coagulation. Antithrombins are increased in the normal newborn for unknown reasons.

Bidwell E: Acquired inhibitors of coagulants. Ann Rev Med 20:63–74, 1969.

6. FIBRINOLYSINS

Hemorrhagic tendencies due to hypofibrinogenemia secondary to increased fibrinolysins are rarely seen in children. Circumstances in which increased fibrinolytic activity may be seen include extensive surgery (especially with use of cardiopulmonary bypass procedures), liver disease, carcinomas, leukemia, and disseminated intravascular coagulation (DIC). Increased fibrinolytic activity can be diagnosed by use of the whole blood clot lysis time (normally, a formed clot lyses very slowly–48 hours or more–at 37° C), or the euglobulin lysis time, a more sensitive test. If fibrinolysins are present to a pathologic degree, ie, causing a hemorrhagic tendency, a potent fibrinolysin inhibitor, epsilon-aminocaproic acid (EACA, Amicar) is available. EACA should not be used, however, in DIC, for which heparin is the drug of choice.

Pechet L: Fibrinolysis. New England J Med 273:966–973, 1024–1034, 1965.

V. THE SPLEEN

SPLENOMEGALY

The child with a relatively isolated finding of splenomegaly frequently presents a puzzling diagnostic problem. In the diagnosis of chronic splenomegaly, the following categories of diseases should be considered: congestive splenomegaly, chronic infections, leukemia and lymphomas, hemolytic anemias, reticuloendothelioses, and storage diseases. The clinical findings and diagnostic procedures recommended with each of these entities are summarized in Table 14–5.

DEVELOPMENTAL DEFECTS OF THE SPLEEN

Simultaneous injury, at about the 25th day of embryonic life, of the splenic anlage, atrioventricular cushions of the heart, and mesentery may account for

the triad of situs inversus, congenital lesions of the heart, and asplenia. Fewer than 10% of cases of congenital absence of the spleen occur without serious heart lesions. Most infants with this triad die within a few weeks. The principal evidence of asplenia in these infants consists of erythrocytic inclusions such as Howell-Jolly bodies, nucleated red cells, and Heinz bodies. A mild reticulocytosis and siderocytosis can be found. The discovery of these red cell inclusions in a patient with congenital heart disease is strong presumptive evidence for this syndrome.

No specific therapy is available.

Crosby WH: Hyposplenism: An inquiry into normal functions of the spleen. Ann Rev Med 14:349–370, 1964.

CONGESTIVE SPLENOMEGALY (Banti's Syndrome)

Banti's syndrome consists of an enlarged spleen, pancytopenia, and evidences of hepatic disease such as liver enlargement, decreased liver function as shown by appropriate tests, portal hypertension, and hepatic decompensation. Three separate entities are known to produce this syndrome: (1) vascular anomalies of the splenic and portal venous system; (2) thrombophlebitis of the portal and splenic veins, often secondary to infection following neonatal catheterization of the umbilical vein; and (3) cirrhosis of the liver. The age at onset and the presenting symptoms vary according to the etiology. For further discussion of this disorder, see Chapter 16.

Infections and neoplasms of the spleen are listed in Table 14–5 and discussed elsewhere in the text.

INFECTIONS FOLLOWING SPLENECTOMY

There is good evidence that infants and children who have undergone splenectomy are subsequently more susceptible to severe bacterial infections. These infections are septicemia, meningitis, or pneumonia due to pneumococci, group A streptococci, *Hemophilus influenzae*, and enteric organisms. Children under 2 years of age and those with generalized disorders of the reticuloendothelial system are more frequently affected. The increased susceptibility to infection following splenectomy has not been explained, but it is probably related to the role of the spleen in antibody synthesis and phagocytic function. If possible, splenomegaly should be delayed until after age 2, and prophylactic antibiotic therapy should be used for 1–2 years after splenectomy in susceptible patients.

Ellis E, Smith RT: The role of the spleen in immunity. Pediatrics 37:111–131, 1966.

TABLE 14—5. Causes of chronic splenomegaly in children.

Cause	Associated Clinical Findings	Diagnostic Investigation
Congestive splenomegaly	History of umbilical vein catheter or neonatal omphalitis. Signs of portal hypertension (varices, hemorrhoids, dilated abdominal wall veins); pancytopenia, history of hepatitis or jaundice.	Complete blood count, platelet count, liver function tests, upper gastrointestinal x-rays.
Chronic infections	History of exposure to tuberculosis, histoplasmosis, coccidioidomycosis, other fungal diseases; chronic sepsis (foreign body in blood stream; subacute bacterial endocarditis).	Appropriate cultures and skin tests, ie, blood cultures, PPD, histoplasmin, coccidioidin skin tests; chest film.
Infectious mononucleosis	Fever, fatigue, pharyngitis, rash, adenopathy.	Heterophil antibodies.
Leukemia, lymphoma, Hodgkin's disease	Evidence of systemic involvement with fever, bleeding tendencies, and lymphadenopathy; pancytopenia.	Blood smear, bone marrow examination, spleen biopsy.
Hemolytic anemias	Anemia, jaundice; family history of anemia, jaundice, and gallbladder disease in young adults.	Reticulocyte count, Coombs test, spherocytosis (blood smear, osmotic fragility), autohemolysis test.
Reticuloendothelioses (histiocytosis X)	Chronic otitis media, seborrheic or petechial skin rashes, anemia, infections, lymphadenopathy.	Skeletal x-rays for bone lesions; biopsy of bone, liver, bone marrow, or lymph node.
Storage diseases	Family history of similar disorders, neurologic involvement, evidence of macular degeneration.	Biopsy of rectal mucosa, liver, bone marrow, spleen, or brain in search for storage cells.
Splenic cyst	Evidence of other infections (postinfectious cyst) or congenital anomalies; peculiar shape of spleen.	Aspiration or exploration.

HYPERSPLENISM

An enlarged spleen can produce varying degrees of anemia, leukopenia, or thrombocytopenia regardless of the cause of the enlargement. This pancytopenia is probably due to decreased hemic cell survival due to "trapping" of cells in the splenic pulp, but it may also be due to inhibition of release of cells from the marrow. In such instances of hypersplenism, the bone marrow is usually hyperplastic in appearance.

VI. RETICULOENDOTHELIOSES

The diseases to be discussed under this heading comprise a heterogeneous group of proliferative disorders of the reticuloendothelial system of unknown cause. Eosinophilic granuloma of bone, Hand-Schüller-Christian disease, and Letterer-Siwe disease constitute a complex of diseases of unknown cause, of histiocytic proliferation, and of unpredictable prognosis. Lichtenstein has grouped them under the term histiocytosis X. Although foam cells containing cholesterol are found in these disorders, it is currently believed that the storage cells are not the result of a primary disturbance of lipid metabolism but are secondary either to increased intracellular cholesterol synthesis or to inhibition of cholesterol from necrotic tissue.

Certain patients present primarily with signs and symptoms of lytic lesions limited to the bones—especially the skull, ribs, clavicles, and vertebrae. These lesions are well demarcated and occasionally painful. Biopsy reveals eosinophilic granuloma, which may be the only lesion the patient will develop, although further bone and even visceral lesions may occur.

Another group of patients often present with otitis media, seborrheic skin rash, and evidence of bone lesions, usually in the mastoid or skull area. They frequently also have visceral involvement, which may be indicated by lymphadenopathy and hepatosplenomegaly. This chronic disseminated form is usually known as **Hand-Schüller-Christian disease** and is associated with "foamy histiocytes" on biopsy. The classic triad of Hand-Schüller-Christian disease (bony involvement, exophthalmos, and diabetes insipidus) is rarely seen; however, diabetes insipidus is a common complication.

A third group of patients present early in life primarily with visceral involvement. They often have a petechial or macular skin rash, generalized lymphadenopathy, enlarged liver and spleen, pulmonary involvement, and hematologic abnormalities such as anemia and thrombocytopenia. Bone lesions can occur. This acute visceral form—Letterer-Siwe disease—is often fatal.

In all 3 groups the tissue abnormality is proliferation of histiocytes; aggregations of eosinophils, lymphocytes, and plasma cells; and collection of foam cells.

The principal diseases to be differentiated from histiocytosis X are bone tumors (primary or metastatic), lymphomas or leukemias, granulomatous infections, and storage diseases. The diagnosis is established by biopsy of bone marrow, lymph node, liver, or mastoid or other bone.

Almost any system or area can become involved during the course of the disease. Rarely, these will include the heart (subendocardial infiltrates), bowel, eye, mucous membranes such as vagina or vulva, and dura mater.

Isolated bony lesions are best treated by curettage and local radiotherapy. Multiple bony involvement and visceral involvement often respond well to prednisone, vinblastine (Velban), mechlorethamine (Mustargen), or methotrexate. The current treatment of choice at the authors' institution is prednisone and vinblastine, given in repeated courses or continuously until healing of lesions occurs.

If diabetes insipidus occurs, treatment with vasopressin (Pitressin) gives good control (see Chapter 24).

In idiopathic histiocytosis, the prognosis is often unpredictable. Many patients with considerable bony and visceral involvement have shown apparent complete recovery. In general, however, the younger the patient and the more extensive the visceral involvement, the worse the prognosis.

Lahey ME: Prognosis in reticuloendotheliosis in children. J Pediat 60:664–674, 1962.

Lichtenstein L: Histiocytosis X (eosinophilic granuloma of bone, Letterer-Siwe disease, and Schüller-Christian disease). J Bone Joint Surg 46A:76–90, 1964.

Lieberman PH & others: A reappraisal of eosinophilic granuloma of bone, Hand-Schüller-Christian syndrome and Letterer-Siwe syndrome. Medicine 48:375–400, 1969.

● ● ●

General References

Berry CL & others: Clinico-pathologic study of thymic dysplasia. Arch Dis Child 43:579–584, 1968.

Bostrom PD & others: Splenectomy: An 11-year review. Arch Surg 98:167–170, 1969.

Diamond LK: The concept of functional asplenia. New England J Med 281:958–959, 1969.

Good RA, Gabrielsen AE (editors): *The Thymus in Immunobiology.* Hoeber, 1964.

Kretschmer R & others: Congenital aplasia of the thymus gland (Di George's syndrome). New England J Med 279:1295–1301, 1968.

Levin JM: The thymus gland and immunity. Amer Surg 35:317–321, 1969.

Mauer A: *Pediatric Hematology.* McGraw-Hill, 1969.

Oski FA, Naiman JL: *Hematologic Problems of the Newborn.* Saunders, 1966.

Schwartz E: Therapy for blood disorders in infants and children. P Clin North America 15:473–492, 1968.

Shields TW: The thymus gland. S Clin North America 49:61–70, 1969.

Smith CH: *Blood Diseases of Infancy & Childhood,* 2nd ed. Mosby, 1966.

Wintrobe MM: *Clinical Hematology,* 6th ed. Lea & Febiger, 1967.

Wolman I: *Laboratory Applications in Clinical Pediatrics.* Blakiston, 1957.

15...

Disorders of Immune Mechanisms

Charles S. August, MD, & Elliot F. Ellis, MD

INTRODUCTION

Resistance to infection is a complex phenomenon that depends upon a variety of factors, both non-specific and specific.

NONSPECIFIC FACTORS IN RESISTANCE TO INFECTIONS

Skin & Mucous Membranes

The barrier function provided by intact skin and normal mucous membranes is one of the most important and obvious nonspecific factors in bodily defenses against infection. This function may be compromised in patients with eczema, burns, or cystic fibrosis. In this respect, inhaling irritating substances such as tobacco smoke or other environmental pollutants probably constitutes the most widespread insult to defenses against respiratory infection to which most individuals are exposed.

Phagocytes

Another important defense mechanism against infection resides in the ability of fixed and circulating phagocytic cells to clear the blood stream of infectious agents and to kill or inactivate them. In addition, some phagocytes probably "process" ingested antigens and then deliver them to the lymphoid system to initiate specific immune responses. Patients with granulocytopenia, neutrophil dysfunctions, absent spleens, or "functional asplenia" (as occurs in sickle cell anemia) have diminished phagocytic function, and all are unduly susceptible to infection.

Lysozymes, Complement, & Interferons

The role played by serum lysozymes in resistance to infection is poorly understood. The complement system of serum proteins acts together with specific antibodies to enhance the phagocytosis or killing of certain microorganisms, and this appears now to be its best defined function in the body economy. Interferons—antiviral proteins which are synthesized by almost all virus-infected cells—are thought to play a critical role in the recovery of an organism from a primary viral infection.

Ellis EF, Smith RT: The role of the spleen in immunity. Pediatrics 37:111–131, 1966.

Pearson HA & others: Functional asplenia in sickle-cell anemia. New England J Med 281:923–926, 1969.

Quie PG: Chronic granulomatous disease of childhood. Advances Pediat 16:287, 1969.

Schur PH, Austen KF: Complement in human disease. Ann Rev Med 19:1–24, 1968.

SPECIFIC FACTORS IN RESISTANCE TO INFECTION

Specific immunity is mediated by lymphoid cells: by plasma cells, which synthesize antibodies; and by lymphocytes, which mediate cellular immunity reactions, immunologic memory, and antigen recognition. Both types of cells originate from stem cell precursors which may be found in the bone marrow. Available evidence suggests that such stem cells differentiate to form 2 cell lines: one, dependent on the thymus (so-called T-cells), and another, independent of the thymus (so-called B-cells).

The T-lymphocytes perform a number of functions: (1) Upon antigenic stimulation, they divide to form an expanded population of long-lived "memory" cells. (2) They may be cytotoxic for target cells, eg, graft rejection. (3) They release a number of soluble factors which attract and inhibit the migration of mononuclear phagocytes, increase vascular permeability, and may cause other lymphocytes to divide. (4) They interact and cooperate with B-cells during the immune response to certain antigens. The B-lymphocytes differentiate, proliferate, and mature into plasma cells which synthesize antibody.

The sequence of events that occurs when an antigen—eg, in the form of a bacterium—encounters the normal lymphoid apparatus is illustrated in Fig 15–1. This encounter establishes a population of plasma cells synthesizing specific antibody, a population of small lymphocytes capable of mediating specific delayed hypersensitivity reactions, and a population of long-lived lymphocytes (so-called "memory cells") capable

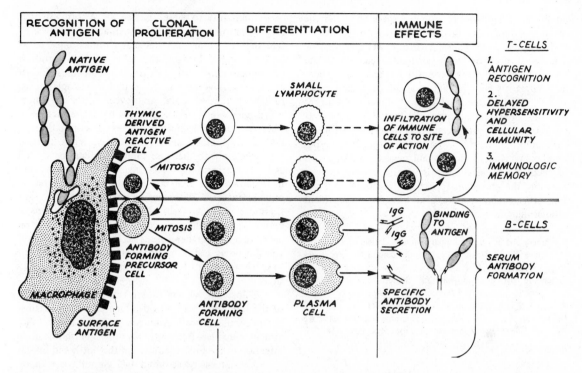

FIG 15–1. A theoretical scheme of cellular and humoral immunity. (Modified and reproduced, with permission, from Meyers FH, Jawetz E, Goldfien A: *Review of Medical Pharmacology,* 3rd ed. Lange, 1972.)

of responding with increased intensity to future challenges with the same antigen.

Since immunologic deficiency diseases may involve defects in humoral or cellular immune mechanisms (or both), it is well to consider these primary mechanisms in greater detail. Immunoglobulins (gamma globulins) are a family of structurally and functionally related glycoprotein molecules with antibody activity composed of 2 different kinds of polypeptide chains known as the H (heavy) and L (light) chains according to their molecular weights. The L chains are of 2 varieties–kappa (κ) and lambda (λ)–

and are antigenically similar in all immunoglobulin molecules. The H chains have regions that are distinctive for each of the immunoglobulin classes. These differences in amino acid sequences are responsible for the distinctive antigenic, physicochemical, and biologic properties of the 5 known members of the immunoglobulin family. The immunoglobulins recognized to date are IgG, IgA, IgM, IgD, and IgE. Some properties of the immunoglobulins are shown in Table 15–1.

Cellular immunity or delayed hypersensitivity is mediated by small lymphocytes (T-cells). Humoral antibodies are not known to play a role in this kind of

TABLE 15–1. Properties of immunoglobulins.

	IgG (γG)	IgA (γA)	IgM (γM)	IgD (γD)	IgE (γE)
Molecular weight	150,000	$(180,000)_n$	900,000	150,000	200,000
Percentage in serum	80	12	7	0.2	0.0016
Serum level (mg/ml)	12	1.8	1.0	0.03	0.00033
Half-life (days)	25	6	5	2.8	. . .
Distribution	ECF	ECF, especially secretions	Blood	. . .	ECF and fixed to target cells
Toxin neutralization	Yes	Yes	No	. . .	. . .
Bactericidal antibody activity	1	. . .	500–1000	. . .	. . .
Placental transfer	Yes	No	No	No	No
Pathologic model	IgG myeloma	IgA myeloma	IgM myeloma	IgD myeloma	IgE myeloma
Subclasses	G1, G2, G3, G4	$A_1\ A_2$	. . .	. . .	. . .
Complement fixation	Yes	No	Yes	No	No

immunity. Histologically, the reactions characteristic of cellular immunity involve infiltration of tissues by lymphocytes and macrophages as well as varying degrees of necrosis. The tuberculin reaction is the prototype of delayed hypersensitivity, and allergic contact dermatitis is a familiar example of disease mediated by this immune mechanism. Cellular immunity is also thought to be the principal factor in homograft rejection and in graft-versus-host reactions. Ultimate containment of certain viral infections such as herpes simplex, vaccinia, varicella, and measles is thought to be mediated by a cellular immunity mechanism. In addition, the granulomatous tissue reactions to fungi and other organisms are also thought to represent cellular immune reactions.

Fudenberg HH & others: Primary immunodeficiencies: Report of a World Health Organization committee. Pediatrics 47:927–946, 1971.

Fudenberg HH: Immunoglobulins: Structure, function, and genetic control. In: *Immunologic Incompetence.* Kagan BM, Stiehm ER (editors). Year Book, 1971.

Robbins JB, Smith RT: The specific immune response. Chap 41 in: *The Biologic Basis of Pediatric Practice.* Cooke RE (editor). McGraw-Hill, 1968.

IMMUNITY IN THE FETUS & NEWBORN

At birth, the fetus emerges from an environment which, if normal, has protected him from antigenic challenge. This lack of antigenic stimulation is reflected in the paucity of lymphoid tissue throughout the body and in a virtual absence of mature plasma cells in the lymph nodes, spleen, and bone marrow.

The serum of the newborn human is deficient in most immunoglobulins. However, IgG is present and is derived from the mother. IgA, IgM, IgD, and IgE are not detected in cord blood in the presence of an intact placenta since these immunoglobulins do not possess the specific structural sites on their heavy chains required for transport across the placenta. IgM antibodies are deficient in the neonatal period, and the fact that they are especially efficient in killing gram-negative bacteria may explain the particular susceptibility of newborn infants to infection with these organisms. The absence in cord blood of IgE antibodies or "reagins" explains the observation that the infant of a mother with ragweed hay fever or other reagin-mediated allergy does not become passively sensitized to substances to which the mother is allergic.

Maternal IgG antibody protects the fetus during the early months of life against diphtheria, tetanus, measles, poliomyelitis, herpes simplex, pneumococcal infections, and group A beta-hemolytic streptococcal infections to the extent that the mother herself possesses immunity to these diseases. Since normally only IgG is transported across the placenta, the low levels of IgM that are sometimes detectable are assumed to be of fetal origin. In fact, the fetus begins to produce immunoglobulins between the second and fourth months of gestation. In syphilis, toxoplasmosis, rubella, herpes simplex, and cytomegalovirus infections, cord blood and serum IgM levels are increased. Therefore, it has been proposed that determinations of IgM in cord blood and subsequently might be used retrospectively to diagnose prenatal infections as well as to detect perinatal infections. However, recent data have shown that IgM concentrations are elevated in only about 50% of proved perinatal infections. Furthermore, in most cases of infection in the neonatal period, signs of illness precede IgM elevation by several days. It appears, therefore, that measurement of IgM will not be as useful for diagnosing perinatal infections as it has proved to be in diagnosing intrauterine infections.

Colostrum, which contains antibodies primarily of the IgA class, may provide some protection against enteric viruses since it is known that attenuated poliovirus is much less frequently able to establish intestinal infection in the breast-fed than in the bottle-fed infant.

As maternally acquired IgG globulin is catabolized with a half-life of 25 days, the IgG levels in the infant fall to a nadir at about 2–3 months of age. Immunoglobulin concentrations then begin to rise as the infant begins to synthesize immunoglobulins as a result of exposure to environmental antigenic stimuli. IgM concentrations reach normal adult levels earliest, followed by IgG and then by IgA. Normal children apparently may have low IgA concentrations until late childhood.

Cell-mediated or delayed hypersensitivity reactions can be elicited during the first weeks of life, and lymphocytes are abundant in the peripheral blood of newborn infants (normal mean = 3400/cu mm). Infants may be regularly sensitized to tuberculin several weeks following BCG immunization at birth. Furthermore, contact sensitization with simple chemicals such as dinitrochlorobenzene (DNCB) can also be accomplished in the neonatal period. Therefore, in contrast to humoral immune mechanisms, cellular immunity seems to be quite fully developed at birth.

Gitlin D: Development and metabolism of the immune globulins. In: *Immunologic Incompetence.* Kagan BM, Stiehm ER (editors). Year Book, 1971.

Smith RT, Robbins JB: Developmental aspects of immunity. Chap 42 in: *The Biologic Basis of Pediatric Practice.* Cooke RE (editor). McGraw-Hill, 1968.

LABORATORY DIAGNOSIS OF IMMUNOLOGIC DEFICIENCY

The laboratory diagnostic approach to a suspected immunologic deficiency state includes the following procedures, some of which are well within the scope of the average hospital laboratory. (See Chapter 40.)

SERUM PROTEIN DETERMINATION

In an individual with immunologic deficiency involving antibodies, the serum protein electrophoresis may reveal diminished or absent gamma globulins. However, the correlation between these results and those obtained by immunochemical methods may not be very close.

IMMUNOELECTROPHORESIS

The technic of immunoelectrophoresis allows the delineation of each of the 3 major immunoglobulins: IgG, IgA, and IgM. IgD and IgE do not ordinarily occur in high enough concentrations in normal serum to allow detection by this technic. The test is semiquantitative at best; however, since a characteristic pattern is seen on immunoelectrophoretic analysis of hypogammaglobulinemic serum, a presumptive diagnosis can be made from the appearance of the precipitin arcs.

QUANTITATIVE DETERMINATION OF IMMUNOGLOBULINS

Quantification of each of the major immunoglobulins is now a standard laboratory procedure. Kits are available from a number of manufacturers for measuring immunoglobulins by the radial diffusion method and are sufficiently reliable for clinical use. Because of the wide range of normal values (Table 15–2), a diagnosis of immunologic deficiency should not be made on the basis of insignificant deviations from the mean.

ISOHEMAGGLUTININ DETERMINATION

Isohemagglutinins are antibodies that react with the blood group antigens A, B, M, N, P, Lewis, and Wright. These blood group substances occur widely in nature, and an individual becomes immunized presumably as a result of exposure to these antigens as they are represented on intestinal bacteria following colonization after birth. Because these antigenic determinants are common both to bacterial and red cell membranes, these antibodies agglutinate the appropriate red blood cells. Isohemagglutinin activity may be detected in cord blood but is usually maternal IgG.

TABLE 15–2. Relation of age to serum immunoglobulin (Ig) levels and isohemagglutinin activity (IHA).

	IgG (mg/100 ml) (Mean ± 1 SD and Range)	IgA (mg/100 ml) (Mean ± 1 SD and Range)	IgM (mg/100 ml) (Mean ± 1 SD and Range)	IHA titer (Mean and Range)
Cord blood	1086 ± 290 (740–1374)	2 ± 2 (0–15)	14 ± 6 (0–22)	0*
1–3 months	512 ± 152 (280–950)	16 ± 10 (4–36)	28 ± 14 (15–86)	1:5 0–1:10†
4–6 months	520 ± 180 (240–884)	22 ± 14 (11–52)	36 ± 18 (21–74)	1:10 0–1:160†
7–12 months	742 ± 226 (281–1280)	54 ± 17 (22–112)	76 ± 27 (36–150)	1:80 0–1:640‡
13–24 months	945 ± 270 (290–1300)	67 ± 19 (9–143)	88 ± 36 (18–210)	1:80 0–1:640‡
25–36 months	1030 ± 152 (546–1562)	89 ± 34 (21–196)	94 ± 23 (43–115)	1:160 1:10–1:640§
3–5 years	1150 ± 244 (546–1760)	126 ± 31 (56–284)	87 ± 24 (26–121)	1:80 1:5–1:640
6–8 years	1187 ± 289 (596–1744)	147 ± 35 (56–330)	108 ± 37 (54–260)	1:80 1:5–1:640
9–11 years	1217 ± 261 (744–1719)	146 ± 38 (44–208)	104 ± 46 (27–215)	1:160 1:20–1:640
12–16 years	1248 ± 221 (796–1647)	168 ± 54 (64–290)	96 ± 31 (60–140)	1:160 1:10–1:320

*IHA is rarely detectable in cord blood.
†50% of normal infants have no isohemagglutinins at age 6 months.
‡10% of normal infants have no isohemagglutinins at age 1.
§Beyond age 2, all normal individuals (except those with blood type AB) have isohemagglutinins.

There is a variable period following birth before the infant begins to produce isohemagglutinins. Therefore, during the first 2 years of life, normal infants may not have detectable isohemagglutinin activity. By the end of the second year, most normal infants have demonstrable isohemagglutinin activity in their serum. These "naturally occurring" isohemagglutinins are primarily IgM but may also be IgG or IgA. Because isohemagglutinins are invariably present in all normal individuals of blood types A, B, or O after the first few years of life, their absence is strong presumptive evidence of an antibody deficiency disorder.

SCHICK TEST

In the Schick test, 0.1 ml of Schick toxin (diphtheria toxin) is injected intradermally. The amount of toxin injected is small (1/50 of the amount necessary to kill a 250 gm guinea pig), but in individuals who have not been immunized against diphtheria or those with immunologic deficiency this amount is sufficient to cause a dermonecrotic reaction at the injection site. The inflammatory reaction begins within a few hours and may be quite severe in the individual totally lacking in diphtheria antitoxin. Therefore, if a positive test is anticipated, the Shick test solution should be diluted 1:5 or 1:10 before injection. Normal individuals who have been well immunized (4 injections of diphtheria toxoid) are uniformly unreactive (Schick-negative). If the test is positive in a well immunized individual, this is strong presumptive evidence of inability to produce antibody. A negative Schick test does not rule out the possibility that an immune deficiency exists since a number of individuals with proved immunologic deficiency states retain the capacity to synthesize small amounts of antibody. Thus, they may produce sufficient diphtheria antitoxin to neutralize the small amount of toxin injected, and a negative Schick test results.

Interpretation of the Schick test reaction is complicated occasionally by the presence of a skin reaction which appears at around 24 hours and reaches its maximum at 48–72 hours. This reaction is thought to be one of delayed hypersensitivity to proteins in the culture from which the toxin is isolated. To avoid this confusion, the use of a Schick control (Schick toxin heated at 60° C for 4 hours to inactivate the toxin) injected simultaneously at another site is required. A positive reaction at the site of the Schick toxin injection and a negative reaction at the control site indicates lack of diphtheria antitoxin in the body.

RESPONSE TO IMMUNIZATION

Since failure to marshal an immune response to an antigenic stimulus is characteristic of the hypo-gammaglobulinemic state, antibody titers should be determined before and after immunization with good immunogens. Immunizing agents used for this purpose should be of potential benefit to the patient. For this reason, only toxoids and vaccines used in conventional immunization regimens should be given. Some that have been successfully used for this purpose include diphtheria toxoid, tetanus toxoid, typhoid vaccine, and influenza vaccine. Administration of live viruses should be avoided in patients suspected of having immunologic deficiency disorders. While low titers of antibody to diphtheria, tetanus, and viral agents are commonly found in the serum of patients with immunologic deficiency disease, immunologically deficient children differ markedly from normals in response to immunization. The normal individual may show a 10-fold greater anamnestic response. The hypogammaglobulinemic individual, on the other hand, even after intensive immunization, will rarely show more than a 1-fold increase in titer and usually shows none at all.

BONE MARROW EXAMINATION FOR PLASMA CELLS

The bone marrow is the most accessible tissue in which to look for the cells which synthesize immunoglobulins. Unfortunately, for developmental reasons, normal children may have very few mature plasma cells in the marrow for the first 2 years of life. After age 2, increasing numbers of plasma cells are seen (Table 15–3).

If a bone marrow biopsy can be obtained, special attention should be paid to the areas around arterioles, which normally are especially rich in plasma cells. Their absence from this location is quite striking in individuals with immunologic deficiency.

TABLE 15–3. Mean values of marrow plasma cells per 5000 nucleated marrow elements of normal and iron-deficient subjects in varying age groups.*

Age	Number of Patients	Mean Value and SD
Newborn	6	0.8 ± 0.2
½–6 months	6	1.2 ± 1.0
6–12 months	5	3.4 ± 2.6
12–24 months	7	5.9 ± 5.2
2–4 years	6	9.2 ± 6.2
4–6 years	5	11.4 ± 3.4
6–12 years	6	17.5 ± 8.3
12–15 years	6	19.3 ± 5.3
Adult	5	19.2 ± 3.6

*Reproduced, with permission, from Steiner MC, Pearson HA: Bone marrow plasmocyte values in childhood. J Pediat 68:562, 1966.

LYMPH NODE BIOPSY

Biopsy of a lymph node draining the site of antigen administration is an extremely useful adjunct to the diagnosis of all of the immunologic deficiency syndromes. Antigen is usually administered intramuscularly into the anterior thigh. Five to 7 days later, the ipsilateral inguinal node is removed. Cortical germinal centers and plasma cells are the morphologic counterpart of the immunoglobulin synthesizing system. The small lymphocytes of the deep cortex (paracortex) are the morphologic counterpart of the thymus-dependent cellular immunity mediating system. Deficiency of either immunologic function will usually be reflected by an abnormality in the appropriate portion of the lymph node.

EVALUATION OF CELLULAR IMMUNITY

Evaluation of the adequacy of cellular immunity or delayed hypersensitivity is considerably more difficult than evaluation of humoral immunity. This is due in part to incomplete understanding of the factors governing cellular immunity. The following tests are used both clinically and investigatively.

Skin Tests

Skin test reagents to detect evidence of delayed hypersensitivity to bacterial, viral, and fungal agents with which the patient has had natural contact include tuberculin, histoplasmin, coccidioidin, candida, mumps, vaccinia, and the group A beta-hemolytic streptococcal enzymes, streptokinase and streptodornase.

For skin testing, the following materials may be injected intradermally:

(1) Tuberculin, 0.1 ml of a 1:10,000 dilution. If negative, repeat at 1:1000. Alternatively, intermediate strength PPD may be injected in the same volume.

(2) Candida, 0.1 ml of 1:10 dilution of stock antigen (infants) or 1:1000 dilution (older children and adults).

(3) Trichophytin, as for candida.

(4) Streptococcal antigens (streptokinase-streptodornase), 0.1 ml at a concentration of 5 units of streptokinase per 0.1 ml. If negative, repeat, using 40 units/0.1 ml.

(5) Mumps antigen, 0.1 ml.

Reactions should be read at 4 hours to assess any Arthus reactions, and at 24 and 48 hours for delayed hypersensitivity. The diameter of redness and induration should be recorded. Only reactions with induration greater than 5 mm in diameter are unequivocally positive.

While a positive delayed hypersensitivity type skin response is consistent with normal cellular immunity, a negative response may indicate only that the patient has had an inadequate sensitizing exposure to the infectious agent from which the skin test material was derived. This is especially true in infants and young children, who by virtue of age have had little opportunity to encounter infectious agents and their products and develop delayed hypersensitivity. For this reason, certain simple chemicals which have the propensity to sensitize human skin have been used to induce delayed hypersensitivity. The agent most commonly used for this purpose is dinitrochlorobenzene (DNCB). This is applied to the skin in a 30% concentration in acetone (10% for infants) applied to the volar surface of the forearm on a piece of filter paper 1 cm in diameter. Two to 3 weeks later, 0.05 ml of the sensitizing agent is reapplied in lower concentration, usually 0.1% or 0.05%. An erythematous indurated reaction appearing at the site of the challenging dose is interpreted to mean that delayed hypersensitivity has been successfully induced and is used as presumptive evidence of normal cellular immunity. Since DNCB is a primary irritant, caution must be exercised in interpreting the results of the challenge in order to be certain that the reaction is truly one of delayed hypersensitivity and not an irritant reaction. This caution is especially pertinent in dealing with infants and small children, whose skin may react in a primary irritant manner to the low concentrations ordinarily used for challenging older children and adults.

Lymphocyte Count, Morphology, & Response to Mitogens

Cellular immunity is mediated by the small lymphocyte. Therefore, an accurate total lymphocyte count should be done and the morphology (number of small lymphocytes) carefully observed. Any child with less than 3000 lymphocytes per cu mm is suspect. Any child with fewer than 1000 lymphocytes per cu mm is definitely lymphopenic. The normal ranges for absolute lymphocyte counts in children of varying ages are given in Table 14–1.

Lymphocyte responsiveness to the nonspecific mitogen phytohemagglutinin (PHA) should be tested. This response is most accurately assessed by methods which measure incorporation by the lymphocyte of an isotopically labeled nucleoside into DNA or RNA. However, if it is not technically feasible to perform the assay by this method, morphologic transformation of the small lymphocyte population into blast forms can be visually estimated. Antigens to which the patient has been sensitized, either naturally or artificially (eg, PPD, candida, diphtheria) also cause blast transformation and nucleoside incorporation, although to a much lesser degree than with PHA.

Bellanti JA, Schlegel RJ: The diagnosis of immune deficiency diseases. P Clin North America 18:49–72, 1971.

Fudenberg HH & others: Primary immunodeficiencies: Report of a World Health Organization committee. Pediatrics 47:927–946, 1971.

Johnston RB, Janeway CA: The child with frequent infections: Diagnostic considerations. Pediatrics 43:596–600, 1969.

TREATMENT OF IMMUNOLOGIC DEFICIENCY DISEASE

The results of treatment of the immunologic deficiency syndromes have been disappointing. Commercial gamma globulin is given in an attempt at replacement therapy in doses of 0.3–0.6 ml/kg IM every 3–4 weeks. It is important to recognize that the available gamma globulin preparations consist largely of IgG, with insignificant amounts of IgA and IgM. Even if preparations rich in IgA and IgM were available, their short biologic half-life would necessitate administration every 5–6 days. While commercial gamma globulin therapy may prevent overwhelming sepsis due to pneumococci in some patients, it does not appear to prevent progression of the otitis media, sinusitis, and bronchiectasis that are seen frequently in older patients.

At this time, gamma globulin cannot be administered intravenously because of the likelihood of producing a severe systemic reaction. Furthermore, even when given by the intramuscular route, gamma globulin administration may not be an entirely innocuous procedure. For this reason, it should only be given to children with proved deficiency of IgG and impaired ability to make specific antibody. Its indiscriminate use is to be condemned.

In selected patients, antibiotic therapy given on a continuous basis seems to be a useful adjunct.

Some patients with severe combined immunodeficiency have been reconstituted immunologically by bone marrow transplantation using cells from a histocompatible sibling.

Githens J: Hematopoietic and immunologic tissue grafting: Current concepts and indications in pediatric patients. Clin Pediat 10:138–147, 1971.

Hitzig WH: Therapy of immunological deficiency diseases. In: *Immunologic Incompetence.* Kagan BM, Stiehm ER (editors). Year Book, 1971.

IMMUNOLOGIC DEFICIENCY DISORDERS

Immunologic deficiency disorders are characterized by increased susceptibility to bacterial infection and, in certain forms, to progressive fungal and viral disease. This may be due to (1) a generalized or selective deficiency in the immunoglobulins; (2) an absent or diminished capacity to form antibodies or to manifest cellular immunity after appropriate antigenic stimulation; and (3) absence of the morphologic components of the normal immunologic apparatus, ie, the mature plasma cell or small lymphocyte.

Children with immunologic deficiency disorders are subject to serious infections such as recurrent bacterial pneumonia, meningitis, sepsis, osteomyelitis, pyoderma, progressive vaccinia, and chronic candidal

TABLE 15–4. Primary immunologic deficiency syndromes.*

	Suggested Cellular Defect		
Type	B-Cells	T-Cells	Stem Cells
Transient hypogammaglobulinemia of infancy†	X		
Infantile X-linked agammaglobulinemia†	X		
Selective immunoglobulin deficiency (dysgammaglobulinemia)†	X (some)		
Thymic hypoplasia (DiGeorge's syndrome)†		X	
Episodic lymphopenia with lymphocytotoxins†		X	
Immunodeficiency with:			
Ataxia-telangiectasia	X	X	
Thrombocytopenia and eczema (Wiskott-Aldrich)	X	X	
Short-limbed dwarfism	X	X	
Severe combined immunodeficiency (thymic alymphoplasia, thymic dysplasia)†			
Autosomal recessive	X	X	X
X-linked	X	X	X
Sporadic	X	X	X
Immunodeficiency with generalized hematopoietic hypoplasia (reticular dysgenesis)†	X	X	X

*Nomenclature of WHO Committee on Primary Immunodeficiencies: Bull World Health Organ 45, 1971 (in press). Modified and reprinted with permission.
†Discussed in the text that follows.

infections. Chronic otitis media, sinusitis, and bronchiectasis are frequently seen. Only rarely does the child with recurrent "colds" turn out to have an immunologic deficiency disease definable by current diagnostic technics. An increased incidence of gastrointestinal dysfunction has recently been recognized, and various hematologic abnormalities, including an increased incidence of lymphoreticular malignancy, are known to occur in certain forms of the disease.

It is now apparent that the immunologic deficiency syndromes include a broad spectrum of entities with enormous variability in clinical and immunologic expression. The best defined of these syndromes are listed in Table 15–4. The nomenclature conforms to recent WHO recommendations. Because most of them are rare, only the more common forms will be described.

TRANSIENT HYPOGAMMAGLOBULINEMIA OF INFANCY

Essentials of Diagnosis

● Recurrent infections of skin, lungs, upper respiratory tract, or meninges, usually with gram-positive bacteria.

● Markedly diminished levels of serum IgG, IgA, and IgM.

- Normal cellular immunity mechanism.
- Lymph node biopsy which reveals absence of mature plasma cells but presence of "plasmacytoid lymphocytes."

General Considerations

Transient hypogammaglobulinemia is a syndrome which occurs in infants in whom there is a prolongation of the low levels of circulating immunoglobulins which normally occur during the first 4–8 weeks of life. If an infant fails to begin synthesizing his own immunoglobulins, the normal catabolism of maternal gamma globulins results in a continuing decline of the infant's immunoglobulin levels. When the level of the infant's passively acquired antibody declines below those that normally protect against pyogenic bacteria and viruses, severe infections begin to appear. These infants usually recover spontaneously between 9 and 15 months of age.

Clinical Findings

A. Symptoms and Signs: Physical signs are related to recurrent infections and the organ systems which may be involved. This particular antibody deficiency syndrome is frequently associated with episodes of bronchitis and wheezing.

B. Laboratory Findings: The principal sign is absence of serum IgG, IgA, and IgM beyond the time when these immunoglobulins normally begin to appear. This varies, of course, with the particular immunoglobulin involved, and Table 15–3 should be consulted in specific instances. Stimulation with specific antigens—eg, diphtheria and tetanus—reveals absent or markedly diminished and delayed responses. Biopsy of the regional lymph nodes carried out 4–7 days after injection of the antigen reveals absence of well formed germinal centers and plasma cells. However, plasmacytoid lymphocytes may be present which help distinguish this condition from infantile X-linked agammaglobulinemia.

Other laboratory findings include normal numbers of circulating small lymphocytes and normal responses of lymphocytes to stimulation in vitro with the mitogen phytohemagglutinin. Cellular immunity mechanisms are normal, as evidenced by positive skin reactions to intradermal injections of candida or streptokinase-streptodornase, and normal ability to become sensitized by dinitrochlorobenzene.

Differential Diagnosis

Differential diagnosis includes virtually all the immunologic deficiency syndromes, which may be excluded by finding (1) normal cellular immune mechanisms, (2) the lymph node biopsy finding as outlined above, and (3) gradual appearance of immunoglobulins.

Treatment

The most effective treatment is a combination of vigorous specific antimicrobial therapy with monthly injections of gamma globulin (see section on Treatment, above).

Prognosis

The infant usually recovers from recurrent infections as he begins to achieve normal immunoglobulin levels. These children probably account for at least some of the instances in which babies with recurrent infections respond to the administration of gamma globulin and later appear to "outgrow" both their infections and the need for therapy.

Janeway CA & others: *The Gamma Globulins.* Little, Brown, 1967.

INFANTILE X-LINKED AGAMMAGLOBULINEMIA
(Congenital Agammaglobulinemia)

Essentials of Diagnosis

- Undue susceptibility to recurrent infections with pyogenic organisms.
- Little or no difficulty with measles, chickenpox, or vaccination.
- Paucity of lymphoid tissues, particularly the tonsils.
- Profound deficiencies of all the major classes of immunoglobulins.
- Absence of cortical germinal centers and plasma cells in lymph node biopsies.

General Considerations

This disease characteristically occurs in male infants and is thought to have an X-linked pattern of inheritance. Undue susceptibility to infection usually becomes evident during the second year of life as these children contract infections with staphylococci, pneumococci, streptococci, and *Hemophilus influenzae*. Purulent sinusitis, pneumonia, sepsis, otitis, meningitis, and furunculosis are common and must be treated vigorously with specific antimicrobial agents or recurrent progressive infections will ensue. Allergic manifestations occur sometimes in a number of children, and some develop a condition similar to rheumatoid arthritis before the diagnosis is established. This puzzling complication usually disappears with treatment.

Clinical Findings

A. Symptoms and Signs: The symptoms and signs of infantile X-linked agammaglobulinemia are those of infection and inflammation in the affected organ systems. In addition, there is an extreme paucity of lymphoid tissue. Tonsils may be absent altogether, and lateral x-rays of the nasopharynx reveal absence of adenoid tissue (Neuhauser's sign).

B. Laboratory Findings: There is marked diminution of all classes of serum immunoglobulins. The serum contains less than 100 mg of IgG per 100 ml, and serum IgA and IgM levels are usually less than 1% of normal adult values. In addition, a failure to synthesize specific antibody may easily be demonstrated by finding absent or markedly low levels of the isohemag-glutinins. A positive Schick test in the presence of a history of DPT immunization is also found. Lymphocyte counts are normal, and cellular immunity mechanisms are intact. Lymph node biopsy 4–7 days after antigenic stimulation is the best means of establishing the diagnosis. Lymphoid tissue from these patients lacks cortical germinal center formation and plasma cells.

Differential Diagnosis

Marked diminution or absence of all classes of immunoglobulins distinguishes this disease from the selected immunoglobulin deficiencies, in which there is a disproportion between the levels of immunoglobulins. The establishment of normal cellular immunity mechanisms serves to distinguish congenital agammaglobulinemia from the immunologic deficiency syndromes relating to abnormalities of the thymus gland. The histology of the lymph nodes and persistence of the syndrome beyond the third or fourth years of life distinguish this from transient hypogammaglobulinemia.

Treatment

These children respond dramatically to monthly injections of gamma globulin. Antibiotics should be used only to treat specific infections. Infections should also be treated with whatever local measures may be indicated.

Prognosis

The prognosis for many children with agammaglobulinemia, if diagnosed early and treated adequately, is quite good. However, some of these patients appear to be unusually susceptible to arthritis, leukemia, and a uniformly fatal syndrome resembling dermatomyositis.

Bruton OC: The discovery of agammaglobulinemia. In: *Immunologic Deficiency Diseases in Man.* Bergsma D (editor). Birth Defects, Original Article Series IV, vol 1. National Foundation (New York), 1968.
Janeway CA & others: *The Gamma Globulins.* Little, Brown, 1967.

SELECTIVE IMMUNOGLOBULIN DEFICIENCY
(Dysgammaglobulinemia)

The ability to measure quantitatively each immunoglobulin class has permitted a more precise definition of situations in which the immunoglobulin deficiency involves only 1 or 2 of the immunoglobulin classes, with the remainder being either normal or elevated. Patients with these disorders may have recurrent infections similar to those suffered by patients with more complete forms of the syndrome. Some have associated abnormalities of cellular immunity,

and for this reason a unified description of all the syndromes is difficult. Patients with dysgammaglobulinemia should be investigated thoroughly in all aspects of their immunologic responses, and a thorough search for underlying disease such as infection, neoplasm, or collagen disease should be made. If the immunoglobulin deficiency involves the IgG fraction, gamma globulin injections may prove therapeutically beneficial.

Ammann AJ, Hong R: Selective IgA deficiency and autoimmunity. Clin Exper Immunol 7:833–838, 1970.
Janeway CA & others: *The Gamma Globulins.* Little, Brown, 1967.
Schur PH & others: Gamma-G globulin deficiencies and recurrent pyogenic infections. New England J Med 283:631–634, 1970.
Stiehm ER & others: Plasma infusions in immunologic deficiency states: Metabolic and therapeutic studies. Blood 28:918–937, 1966.

THYMIC HYPOPLASIA
(Pharyngeal Pouch Syndrome, DiGeorge's Syndrome)

In 1965, DiGeorge described a group of patients with congenital absence of the thymus and parathyroid glands. These patients had hypocalcemic tetany in the neonatal period and then suffered recurrent pyogenic infections. In addition, some had abnormalities of the face, palate, and ears and right-sided aortic arches.

These patients lack cellular immunity mechanisms but retain the ability to synthesize humoral antibodies. They have low normal absolute lymphocyte counts in their peripheral blood and normal levels of serum immunoglobulins. They do not react with delayed hypersensitivity reactions to any of the common skin test antigens. Furthermore, they are unable to be sensitized by dinitrochlorobenzene, and skin allografts undergo markedly delayed rejections. In vitro, their lymphocytes do not undergo blast cell transformation when stimulated with phytohemagglutinin. A partial or less severe form of the syndrome has been described which is thought to be due to hypoplasia of the thymus gland rather than complete aplasia.

It has recently been reported that immunologic function in 2 such patients was markedly improved following implantation of fetal thymus fragments. Beyond experimental transplantation of fetal lymphoid tissue, the treatment of this syndrome is symptomatic. Because all of the patients hitherto described have either died in early infancy or are at this time very young, the natural history and ultimate prognosis remain to be defined.

August CS & others: Establishment of immunological competence in a child with congenital thymic aplasia by a graft of fetal thymus. Lancet 1:1080–1083, 1970.
DiGeorge AM: Congenital absence of the thymus and its immunologic consequences; concurrence with congenital hypoparathyroidism. In: *Immunologic Deficiency Dis-*

eases in Man. Bergsma D (editor). Birth Defects, Original Article Series IV, vol 1. National Foundation (New York), 1968.

Kretschmer R & others: Congenital aplasia of the thymus gland (DiGeorge's syndrome). New England J Med 279:1295–1301, 1968.

EPISODIC LYMPHOPENIA WITH LYMPHOCYTOTOXINS

This condition, also called "immunologic amnesia," is a syndrome of recurrent infections, abnormal small lymphocyte function, and episodic lymphopenia. These children have impaired immunologic memory, ie, poor anamnestic responses to secondary infection of antigens such as diphtheria and tetanus toxoids and defective cellular immunity. In such patients, episodes of lymphopenia are related to the presence of a serum factor which is cytotoxic to lymphocytes. In this respect, the patients resemble experimental animals treated with antilymphocyte serum. These patients are susceptible to recurrent infections with pyogenic bacteria and viruses such as herpes simplex virus. One patient developed an ill-defined lymphoreticular neoplasm which ultimately proved fatal.

Kretschmer R & others: Recurrent infections, episodic lymphopenia and impaired cellular immunity: Further observations on "immunologic amnesia" in two siblings. New England J Med 281:285–290, 1969.

SEVERE COMBINED IMMUNODEFICIENCY
(Thymic Alymphoplasia, Thymic Dysplasia, Swiss Type Agammaglobulinemia)

Essentials of Diagnosis

- Recurrent severe infections with bacteria, viruses, and fungi.
- Chronic skin rashes, diarrhea, and failure to grow.
- Absent immunoglobulins in serum and failure to synthesize specific antibody.
- Lymphopenia and absent cellular immunity mechanisms.
- Absence of thymic shadow on x-ray.
- Marked hypoplasia and disorganization of lymphoid tissue in the thymus, lymph nodes, spleen, nasopharynx, and gastrointestinal tract.

General Considerations

The essential defect in this syndrome is the embryonic failure of the thymus gland to differentiate normally. This appears to be due to absence of the lymphoid stem cell in the bone marrow. Failure of differentiation of both thymus-dependent (T-cell) cellular immunity mechanisms and humoral antibody and B-cell formation is the result. Patients are lymphopenic and totally lack immunologic competence.

Clinical Findings

A. Symptoms and Signs: Infants with combined immunodeficiency become ill in the first few months of life. Persistent candida infection beyond the neonatal period may spread to the pharynx and involve the entire gastrointestinal tract. Infants then usually develop diarrhea and bronchopneumonia. They are unusually susceptible to viral infections; measles, giant cell pneumonia, hemorrhagic varicella, and fatal progressive vaccinia are common. With rare exceptions, these infants die of infection before 3 years of age.

Physical findings relate to the signs of infections in the involved organ systems. In addition, there is marked paucity of lymphoid tissue and absence of a thymic shadow on x-ray.

B. Laboratory Findings: Absence of serum IgG, IgA, and IgM is the rule, although some immunoglobulins are occasionally found. Peripheral blood lymphocyte counts are usually below 1000/cu mm. Isohemagglutinins are usually absent from the peripheral blood, and the Schick test is positive in spite of adequate immunization with DPT. There is no antibody response to any administered antigen. Delayed hypersensitivity reactions are universally absent. Despite chronic candidiasis, patients with this syndrome do not respond to intradermal injections of candida antigen. They cannot be sensitized with simple chemicals such as dinitrochlorobenzene, and skin grafts are accepted indefinitely. Lymphocytes do not respond in vitro to phytohemagglutinin. Lymph node biopsies reveal totally disorganized lymph nodes with absent plasma cells and lymphocytes. At autopsy the thymuses of these patients are found to be tiny epithelial organs containing few, if any, lymphocytes, no corticomedullary differentiation, and no Hassall's corpuscles.

Differential Diagnosis

The differential diagnosis consists of distinguishing this syndrome from thymic hypoplasia (DiGeorge's syndrome) and from infantile X-linked agammaglobulinemia. Patients with the former condition lack cellular immunity but are able to synthesize humoral antibodies and have normal levels of serum immunoglobulins. Patients with the latter are unable to synthesize antibodies, have reduced levels of serum immunoglobulins, but have intact cellular immunity mechanisms. Variants of the thymic dysplasia syndromes exist, and these are usually characterized by the presence in serum of one or all of the immunoglobulins (Nezelof type). In spite of this, it can be demonstrated that antibody synthesis in these patients is not normal, and at autopsy the thymus is identical with that of patients with the complete syndrome.

Treatment

Until recently, no specific treatment existed. However, some centers have recently reported the successful establishment of immunologic function in these patients by transplantation of bone marrow and fetal thymus glands from histocompatible donors. As yet, this mode of therapy is experimental, and patients are best referred to treatment centers with such programs.

The high risk of inducing fatal graft-versus-host reactions in these patients with as few viable leukocytes as are contained in a single unit of transfused blood has been stressed recently. Transfusions, therefore, should be undertaken only upon strong indications and with appropriate preparations for managing complications.

Prognosis

Heretofore, all such patients have died, usually before the end of the third year. Successful transplantation of bone marrow has been achieved too recently for long-term prognosis to be accurately determined.

Githens J: Hematopoietic and immunologic tissue grafting: Current concepts and indications in pediatric patients. Clin Pediat 10:138, 1971.

Hoyer JR & others: Lymphopenic forms of congenital immunologic deficiency diseases. Medicine 47:201–226, 1968.

IMMUNODEFICIENCY WITH GENERALIZED HEMATOPOIETIC HYPOPLASIA (Reticular Dysgenesis)

This is an extremely rare syndrome which consists essentially of the combination of congenital aplastic anemia and severe combined immunodeficiency. The patients are anemic, neutropenic, thrombocytopenic, and lymphopenic. The speculation has been offered that the basic defect is the absence of a common hematopoietic and lymphoid stem cell. The disease is fatal early in the neonatal period.

PRIMARY ACQUIRED AGAMMAGLOBULINEMIA

Acquired agammaglobulinemia is principally a disease of adults but may occur in older children. The sex incidence is equal in males and females. These patients suffer undue susceptibility to pyogenic infection, particularly recurrent sinusitis and pneumonia. Some patients have been found in thoracic clinics with chronic progressive bronchiectasis. More than half of all adults are afflicted with a sprue-like syndrome consisting of diarrhea and steatorrhea. Immunoglobulins in the serum of patients with acquired agammaglobulinemia usually reveal levels of IgG under 500 mg/100 ml, somewhat higher than the level in children with congenital disease. However, striking immunoglobulin deficiency may be seen. IgA and IgM may also be present.

SECONDARY ACQUIRED AGAMMAGLOBULINEMIA

Secondary acquired agammaglobulinemia occurs in patients with protein loss due to any cause or inability to synthesize serum proteins normally. Thus, patients with protein-losing enteropathies, exfoliative dermatitis, and the nephrotic syndrome—or, occasionally, severe malnutrition—may have diminished levels of serum immunoglobulins. Defective synthesis of immunoglobulins not uncommonly accompanies lymphoreticular tumors.

OTHER CONDITIONS ASSOCIATED WITH IMMUNOLOGIC DEFICIENCIES

As mentioned above, the normal newborn is at some risk because of the low levels of serum IgM which he possesses at birth. Transient immunosuppression occurs after certain common viral diseases, the best example being measles. This is self-limited, and immunologic mechanisms usually return to normal within a few weeks. It is also clear that patients being treated with corticosteroids or other immunosuppressive agents such as azathioprine (Imuran) or antilymphocyte globulin have impaired cellular immunity mechanisms. Other syndromes in which impaired cellular immunity has been documented include advanced Hodgkin's disease, sarcoidosis, leprosy, Wiscott-Aldrich syndrome (see Chapter 14), ataxia-telangiectasia (see Chapter 21), and short-limbed dwarfism. Patients with protein-losing enteropathy due to intestinal lymphangiectasia have been found to lose small lymphocytes into their gastrointestinal tracts and suffer an impairment of cellular immunity functions as well as hypogammaglobulinemia.

Aisenberg AC: Immunologic status of Hodgkin's disease. Cancer 19:385–394, 1966.

Waldmann TA: Disorders of immunoglobulin metabolism. New England J Med 281:1170, 1969.

•   •   •

General References

Bellanti JA, Schlegel RJ: The diagnosis of immune deficiency diseases. P Clin North America 18:49, 1971.

Bergsma D (editor): *Immunologic Deficiency Diseases in Man.* Birth Defects, Original Article Series IV, vol 1. National Foundation (New York), 1968.

Cluff LE: Immunological response in infection. Am J Med Sc 256:1, 1968.

Ellis EF, Henney CS: Adverse reactions following administration of human gamma globulin. J Allergy 43:45, 1969.

Fudenberg HH & others: Primary immunodeficiencies: Report of a World Health Organization committee. Pediatrics 47:927, 1971.

Fulginiti V: Immunologic deficiency states. Clin Pediat 8:216, 1969.

Glynn AA: Humoral and cellular aspects of the response to infection. Proc Roy Soc Med 62:285, 1969.

Hoyer JR & others: Lymphopenic forms of congenital immunologic deficiency diseases. Medicine 47:201, 1968.

Janeway CA & others: *The Gamma Globulins.* Little, Brown, 1967.

Janeway CA: Progress in immunology. J Pediat 72:885, 1968.

Kagan BM, Stiehm ER (editors): *Immunologic Incompetence.* Year Book, 1971.

Merler E (editor): *Immunoglobulins: Biologic Aspects and Clinical Uses.* National Academy of Sciences, 1970.

Meischer P, Müller-Eberhard H (editors): *Textbook of Immunopathology.* Grune & Stratton, 1969.

Robbins JB, Smith RT: The specific immune response. Chap 41 in: *The Biologic Basis of Pediatric Practice.* Cooke RE (editor). McGraw-Hill, 1968.

Sever JL: Immunological responses to perinatal infections. J Pediat 75:1111, 1969.

Smith RT, Robbins JB: Developmental aspects of immunity. Chap 42 in: *The Biologic Basis of Pediatric Practice.* Cooke RE (editor). McGraw-Hill, 1968.

Weinstein L, Dalton AC: Host determinants of response to antimicrobial agents. New England J Med 279:467, 524, 581, 1968.

16 ...

Gastrointestinal Tract*

Claude Roy, MD, Arnold Silverman, MD, Frank J. Cozzetto, MD, & Reuben S. Dubois, MB, BS

HIATAL HERNIA & CONGENITALLY SHORT ESOPHAGUS

Hiatal hernias may be classified as follows:

(1) Paraesophageal hernias, where the esophagus is normal up to the esophageal hiatus but the stomach is herniated into the thorax through the hiatus. Regurgitation is not frequent, since the cardia usually maintains its competency.

(2) Sliding hernias, where the esophagogastric junction is located above the esophageal hiatus, is the most common type seen in children. It leads to regurgitation esophagitis and esophageal strictures because of incompetency of the cardiac sphincter. Inflammatory changes secondary to esophagitis lead to shortening of the esophagus and also to metaplastic changes which account for gastric mucosa lining the lower esophagus.

Clinical Findings

Paraesophageal hernias are rare and present with symptoms of complete esophageal obstruction. Symptoms of the sliding type of hiatal hernia may mimic chalasia or "rumination." Dysphagia, failure to thrive, vomiting, aspiration pneumonia, and neck contortions (Sandifer's syndrome) are common features. Pain occurs when esophagitis is present, and bleeding may occur with hematemesis and melena. Stricture formation gives rise to the vomiting of undigested food. Large hiatal hernias often remain completely asymptomatic.

During the first few months of life, the cardiac sphincter is not competent and reflux can be observed. Continuous free reflux observed by cineradiography is abnormal and is almost always associated with the presence of a pouch of stomach above the diaphragm. Considerable skill and patience are needed to demonstrate small hernias. The severity of symptoms may correlate poorly with the size of the hernia. An experienced pediatric radiologist should be responsible for the cine-esophagogram. Esophagoscopy should be performed when medical measures have failed, particularly if there are x-ray changes of esophagitis and pain.

Complications

Gastroesophageal reflux is a well-known cause of disabling esophageal and respiratory complications. Since many severe recurrent respiratory problems of unexplained origin may be the result of gastroesophageal reflux and aspiration, all children with such problems should have the benefit of an esophagogram.

Treatment

In 2/3 of patients, conservative management is efficacious. The most important point is semi-upright positioning of the patient day and night for at least 3 months after all symptoms have ceased. Infants will slip down if just propped with pillows; a special padded frame is helpful. Small thickened feedings and mild sedation combined with antacids and anticholinergics may also be of value.

Failure of medical management and the presence of strictures are indications for surgical treatment. At the time of hernia repair or of esophageal dilatation, pyloroplasty and vagotomy may be indicated—particularly if there is gastric hypersecretion and delayed gastric emptying.

Prognosis

Medical treatment is disappointing, and about 1/3 of patients will develop a stricture requiring bougienage or surgery. However, the condition is not life-threatening.

Lilly JR, LoPresti J, Randolph JG: Hiatal hernia in infants. South MJ 60:545—548, 1967.

McNamara JJ, Paulson DL, Urschel HC Jr: Hiatal hernia and gastroesophageal reflux in children. Pediatrics 43:527—532, 1969.

Sorenson BM: Hiatus hernia in infancy. Acta paediat scandinav 56:513—516, 1967.

ACHALASIA OF THE ESOPHAGUS

Esophageal achalasia is a lesion which has been associated in adults with the absence or degeneration of ganglion cells in Auerbach's plexus. It is characterized by failure of relaxation of the inferior esopha-

---

*Esophageal atresia and tracheo-esophageal fistula are discussed in Chapter 3.

geal sphincter (cardiospasm) and lack of normal peristalsis in the body of the esophagus.

Clinical Findings

A. Symptoms and Signs: Achalasia is occasionally seen in teenage children but is uncommon under the age of 5 years. Psychiatric factors often initiate the presenting symptoms. Typically, the dysphagia is manifested by retrosternal pain and frequent episodes of food "sticking" in the throat or upper chest. The dysphagia is relieved by repeated swallowing movements or by vomiting. Besides dysphagia and vomiting, bouts of coughing and wheezing are reported along with recurrent pneumonitis, anemia, and weight loss.

Dysphagia is a frequent complaint in children born with esophageal atresia (see Chapter 3) even if there is no stenosis of the anastomotic site. Achalasia presents a typical motility pattern. It is now apparent that these motility disturbances are uniformly present in all cases of esophageal atresia, although only a certain percentage of them are symptomatic.

B. X-Ray and Manometric Studies: The barium swallow shows a grossly dilated esophagus except for a narrowing at the distal end. The length of the narrowed segment is usually very short. Cinefluoroscopic examination may show absence of normal peristalsis and failure of relaxation of the gastroesophageal sphincter.

The esophageal motility pattern confirms the abnormal peristalsis and malfunctioning of the lower esophageal sphincter. Injection of a small dose of methacholine (Mecholyl), which does not influence the peristaltic activity of the normal esophagus, increases and further disorganizes the altered motility pattern and is almost pathognomonic.

Differential Diagnosis

Organic stricture of the lower end of the esophagus is the only condition which may cause diagnostic difficulties. Reflux esophagitis secondary to hiatus hernia is the most common cause of organic esophageal stricture in childhood and can be ruled out by esophagoscopy, x-rays, and manometric studies.

Treatment

Special diets and anticholinergic agents have not been successful. Dilatation is of value in a few cases and can be repeated with recurrent symptoms. When the more conservative approach fails, a surgical procedure (Heller's) consisting of longitudinal splitting of all the muscle coats down to the mucosa is advocated.

Prognosis

Because of the shorter duration of the illness in pediatric patients and because of a proximal motility which is less perturbed, the prognosis for return of the esophagus to normal caliber after surgery is very good.

Cloud DT & others: Surgical treatment of esophageal achalasia in children. J Pediat Surg 1:137–144, 1966.

Lind JF, Blanchard RJ, Guyda H: Esophageal motility in tracheo-esophageal fistula and esophageal atresia. Surg Gynec Obst 123:557–564, 1966.

Tachovsky TJ, Lynn HB, Ellis FH: The surgical approach to esophageal achalasia in children. J Pediat Surg 3:226–231, 1968.

CHALASIA

Clinically, 40% of newborn infants have a tendency to regurgitate. On fluoroscopy, regurgitation can be elicited in close to 50% of normal newborns. This is due to immaturity of control over the lower esophageal sphincter.

Vomiting or excessive regurgitation after feedings (chalasia), frequently beginning shortly after birth, is common. Poor weight gain and aspiration pneumonia occasionally occur. Diagnosis is based upon fluoroscopic and film demonstration of retrograde flow of barium from the stomach to the esophagus during respiration and when external pressure is applied over the abdomen.

Gastroesophageal reflux secondary to chalasia may mimic pyloric stenosis, outlet obstruction of the stomach, hiatal hernia, or esophageal stenosis.

Thickened feedings are helpful. The infant should be kept in an erect sitting position for 2–3 hours after each feeding, and it may be necessary to maintain this position 24 hours a day using an "infant seat."

Chalasia is usually a mild transitory condition which usually disappears by 6 months of age. It is compatible with perfectly good health and a normal growth pattern. In rare cases, persistent vomiting, failure to thrive, esophagitis, and repeated bronchopulmonary infections may occur, in which case surgery may be required.

Berenberg W, Neuhauser EBD: Cardioesophageal relaxation (chalasia) as a cause of vomiting in infants. Pediatrics 5:414–420, 1950.

Musslé D, Genton N, Philippe P: Clinical and radiologic course of nonoperated cardio-esophageal incompetence in the infant. Helv paediat acta 24:145–159, 1969.

CAUSTIC BURNS OF THE ESOPHAGUS

Stricture of the esophagus commonly follows ingestion of a caustic alkali, eg, lye, Clorox, Drano, ammonia. Lesions initially are of varying severity. Superficial esophagitis may be the only finding. On the other hand, ulceration and sometimes necrosis may lead to chemical mediastinitis and to peritonitis if the stomach is involved. The extent of burning of the mouth does not correlate well with the presence or the degree of esophageal damage.

Children who have swallowed large amounts of lye may present with oral lesions and shock. The usual clinical picture, however, is that of painful edematous lesions of the lips, mouth, and larynx. Over a period of a few hours or days, the initially extreme dysphagia subsides, and swallowing is resumed. If left untreated, the child remains asymptomatic for a few months until a stricture progressively develops. X-rays usually reveal more severe strictures in the areas of anatomic narrowing, eg, the cervical region and the point at which the left bronchus crosses the esophagus and cardia. Esophagoscopic findings are those of localized escharotic lesions. Later, the entire esophagus is twisted, shortened, and narrowed. Single, dense, fairly localized strictures may occur. Shortening of the esophagus may lead to a hiatal hernia.

The child with a history of alkali ingestion should have a careful examination of his lips and mouth, though esophageal burns are sometimes found in the absence of lip and mouth involvement. Esophagoscopy will demonstrate the lesions but cannot estimate how deeply the esophagus has been burned. Symptoms resulting from strictures may occur within 1 month following the accident, but more commonly the stricture formation does not lead to symptoms for many months or even years. Dysphagia is first manifest for solids and eventually for liquids.

The immediate home care should be familiar to all parents. Vomiting should not be induced. Hospitalization is recommended. Parenteral antibiotics are prescribed along with antacids and sedatives for pain. Intravenous fluids may be necessary. Esophagoscopy should be done within a few hours after ingestion, particularly in the young infant in whom a history of swallowing cannot be obtained. Delay in performing this procedure imposes an increased hazard of perforation. If a burn has been evidenced, corticosteroids and a program of bougienage is started.

Without early treatment, stricture formation is inevitable. Surgical replacement of the esophagus with a segment of colon may be necessary.

Visconi GJ, Beekhuis GJ, Whitten CI: Evaluation of early esophagoscopy and corticosteroid therapy in the management of corrosive injury of the esophagus. J Pediat 59:356–360, 1961.

Weeks RS, Ravitch MM: Esophageal injury by liquid chlorine bleach: Experimental study. J Pediat 74:911–916, 1969.

Yarington CT: Ingestion of caustic: Pediatric problem. J Pediat 67:674–677, 1965.

PYLORIC STENOSIS

Essentials of Diagnosis

- Vomiting, usually projectile.
- Constipation.
- Poor weight gain or weight loss.
- Dehydration.
- Palpable olive-sized tumor in the right upper quadrant.
- "String sign" and evidence of retained gastric contents on x-ray.

General Considerations

Pyloric stenosis is the second most common surgical disorder of the gastrointestinal tract in infancy (after inguinal hernia). The cause of the increase in the size of the circular muscle of the pylorus is not known. There is a coincidence of the disease in twins or fathers and sons. The disease occurs in one out of 500 births, and males are affected 3–4 times more commonly than females. The reported increased incidence in first-borns and in the spring and fall months is controversial.

Clinical Findings

A. Symptoms and Signs: Vomiting usually begins between 2–4 weeks of age and progresses to projectile vomiting after each feeding. In premature infants particularly, the onset of symptoms is often delayed. The vomitus does not contain bile but may be blood-streaked. The infant is hungry and nurses avidly, but there is constipation and failure to gain.

Dehydration, loss of skin turgor, fretfulness, and apathy may be present. The upper abdomen is distended, and gastric peristaltic waves from left to right may be seen. An olive-sized tumor can almost always be felt to the right of the umbilicus and is readily palpable immediately after the infant has vomited.

B. Laboratory Findings: There is metabolic alkalosis with potassium depletion. Hemoconcentration is reflected by elevated hemoglobin and hematocrit values.

C. X-Ray Findings: An upper gastrointestinal series reveals delay in gastric emptying and an elongated narrowed pyloric channel ("string sign"). It is advisable for at least 2 physicians to confirm the presence of the tumor.

Differential Diagnosis

The absence of increased intracranial pressure, virilization, and hyperkalemia rules out intracranial lesions and congenital adrenal hyperplasia with adrenal insufficiency. In achalasia, the food is undigested; in annular pancreas, the vomitus contains bile. Sepsis and urinary tract infections can easily be ruled out. In simple cases of "pylorospasm," there may be a delay in gastric emptying, but the elongated narrow pyloric canal is not seen and no tumor is present.

Treatment

Pyloromyotomy is the treatment of choice and consists of incision down to the mucosa and fully across the pyloric length. Surgery for pyloric stenosis is not an emergency procedure, and the necessary time should be taken to repair dehydration and electrolyte abnormalities and to assuage any gastritis by saline gastric irrigations.

Drug therapy is not widely used or often recommended in the USA but has been used in other countries. Methscopolamine nitrate, 0.1 mg dissolved in water and given orally or subcutaneously 10–15 minutes before each feeding, may be used. It is usually necessary to keep the infant in the hospital for 2–4 weeks while on therapy. It appears that medical management works best in patients whose symptoms begin late (beyond 4 weeks of age) and who suffer little dehydration despite delay in diagnosis.

Prognosis

The outlook is excellent following surgery.

Bell MJ: Infantile pyloric stenosis: Experience with 305 cases at Louisville Children's Hospital. Surgery 64:983–989, 1968.

Day LR: Medical management of pyloric stenosis. JAMA 207:949–950, 1969.

Schärli A, Lieber WK, Keisewetter WB: Hypertrophic pyloric stenosis at the Children's Hospital of Pittsburgh from 1912 to 1967: A critical review of current problems and complications. J Pediat Surg 4:108–114, 1969.

NEONATAL PERFORATIONS OF THE GASTROINTESTINAL TRACT

Sixty percent of neonatal gastrointestinal perforations involve the stomach or the duodenum. The theory of gastric muscular defects or mechanical trauma by catheters has been largely discarded in favor of ischemic necrosis which leads to ulceration and eventually perforation of any segment of the gastrointestinal tract. Stress ulcers and necrotizing enterocolitis of the newborn are other manifestations of ischemic necrosis likely to be seen in asphyxic neonates. A high incidence of colonic perforation has been recently reported in newborn infants after exchange transfusions.

Prematurely born infants are more prone to develop perforation. The syndrome has been observed in identical twins. The affected newborns usually appear normal at birth; the average age at onset of symptoms is the third day of life. Refusal of feedings is followed by vomiting, sometimes bloody. The abdomen becomes rapidly distended; dyspnea and cyanosis frequently ensue and are followed by shock. X-ray findings may reveal free air under the diaphragm. The gastric air bubble is usually absent, especially when the perforation is large.

Fluid and electrolyte balance should be corrected while the abdomen is decompressed by nasogastric suction. The perforation is then repaired.

The prognosis is very poor. The outcome is invariably fatal if surgery is delayed more than 12 hours after onset of symptoms.

Lloyd JR: The etiology of gastrointestinal perforations in the newborn. J Pediat Surg 4:77–84, 1969.

PEPTIC DISEASE

Essentials of Diagnosis

Acute
- Gastrointestinal bleeding is particularly important in the neonatal period and in early infancy.
- Perforation may be the first sign.
- Consider the diagnosis in patients with burns, intracranial lesions, corticosteroid therapy, meningitis, and septicemia.

Chronic
- Atypical symptoms in childhood.
- The cycle of pain relieved by food is more common in the adolescent.
- Not always demonstrated by upper gastrointestinal series.
- Positive family history (20–30%).

General Considerations

The importance of peptic ulceration in pediatric patients is becoming more evident with improvement in diagnostic technics.

The ratio of duodenal to gastric ulcers is about 9:1. Childhood peptic ulcers may occur at any age, but 50% of cases are reported between the ages of 7 and 11. There is a 2:1 ratio of boys to girls.

Peptic ulcers in children occur without obvious cause in most instances.

A recent classification based on symptoms and response to therapy distinguishes 4 types of ulcers.

Type I: An acute primary ulcer presenting usually with hemorrhage or perforation and occurring mainly during the first 2 years of life.

Type II: An acute ulcer that presents with mild to moderate symptoms and responds to medical treatment with complete healing in a few weeks.

Type III: A chronic ulcer syndrome with more typical symptoms. Remissions are followed by exacerbations; resistance to medical management is a problem.

Type IV: An acute and painless ulceration secondary to an accident, surgery, infection, or drug administration (eg, corticosteroids).

Clinical Findings

A. Symptoms and Signs: The typical symptoms observed in adults rarely occur in children. Pain is usually the main symptom, but it conforms to the adult pattern of epigastric location only in older children. In younger patients, periumbilical or generalized abdominal pain without the characteristic relationship to food intake is common. Peptic ulcer disease secondary to known underlying causes occurs more frequently in children under 2 years of age and is manifested at the onset by bleeding or perforation.

B. Gastric Analysis: In children with peptic ulcers, the chief value of gastric fluid analysis is to show that there is no hypersecretion such as would occur with the Zollinger-Ellison syndrome.

C. X-Ray Findings: Radiologic signs of ulceration or a deformity should be present. The frequency with which the radiologic sign of duodenal irritability is found makes the x-ray diagnosis often unreliable. In patients with severe degrees of duodenal irritability, a niche may not be demonstrated since the barium is moved out of the bulb very rapidly.

Complications

Gastric or duodenal perforation or hemorrhage may occur and may be the presenting symptom. Intestinal obstruction occurs rarely.

Treatment

Bed rest is usually unnecessary unless there are signs of duodenal obstruction, active bleeding, or perforation.

With outlet obstruction, gastric suction should be maintained for a few days. Hourly feedings are necessary initially and should be continued until pain has disappeared. Foods that cause pain should be avoided. Beef broth, tea, coffee, spices, and carbonated beverages should be avoided since they enhance gastric secretion. Antacids (15–30 ml) every 1–2 hours and at bedtime are given initially and continued for some time after symptoms have disappeared in both gastric and duodenal ulcers. Anticholinergics are useful only in duodenal ulcers, where gastric hypersecretion can be present.

Surgical management is reserved for the complications, ie, perforation, hemorrhage, and obstruction.

Prognosis

Peptic ulcers of types I, II, and IV in younger children have a natural tendency to heal. About 50% of the type III cases in childhood have a chronic course extending into adulthood. Relapses are associated with a poor prognosis and often require surgery.

Johnston PW, Snyder WH: Vagotomy and pyloroplasty in infancy and childhood. J Pediat Surg 3:238–245, 1968.

Morin C, Davidson M: Pediatric gastroenterology. II. Progress in gastroenterology. Gastroenterology 52:713–726, 1967.

Tudor RB: Peptic ulcerations in childhood. P Clin North America 14:109–139, 1967.

CONGENITAL DIAPHRAGMATIC HERNIA

Between the eighth and tenth weeks of fetal life, the diaphragm is formed and the coelomic cavity divides into its abdominal and thoracic components. During this same stage of morphogenesis, the gastrointestinal tract undergoes its major development, elongating into the umbilical pouch and rotating on its return to the abdominal cavity. Any alteration in these 2 closely interrelated processes leads to a diaphragmatic hernia, which can be secondary to a posterolateral defect in the diaphragm (foramen of Bochdalek) or, more rarely, to a retrosternal defect (foramen of Morgagni).

All degrees of protrusion of the abdominal viscera through the diaphragmatic opening into the thoracic cavity may occur. The extent of herniation determines the severity and the timing of the symptoms. Fewer than 2% of cases are secondary to a retrosternal defect. In the posterolateral variety, more than 80% involve the left diaphragm.

Symptoms of mild to severe respiratory distress and cyanosis are usually present from birth, although some patients remain asymptomatic and the finding of a large diaphragmatic hernia with air-filled coils on x-ray is incidental to an x-ray examination. The abdomen is scaphoid. Breath sounds in the affected hemithorax are absent, with displacement of the point of maximal impulse.

Fatal cases have circulatory problems secondary to the mediastinal shift, giving rise to stretching and kinking of the great vessels. Pulmonary infections also constitute a major cause of death, along with prematurity and a high incidence of associated anomalies, mainly malrotation. The most frequent cause of death, however, is pulmonary insufficiency. The lung on the affected side is compressed and often hypoplastic. The neonate's dependence on diaphragmatic respiration and the right-to-left shunt through a lung incapable of exchanging gases precipitates anoxia and acidosis.

Eventration of the diaphragm is not, strictly speaking, a hernia. A leaf of the diaphragm is ballooned by a diminution of muscular elements, leading to symptoms which are identical though usually much milder.

Baran EM & others: Foramen of Morgagni hernias in children. Surgery 62:1076–1081, 1967.

Johnson DG, Deaner RM, Kooh CE: Diaphragmatic hernia in infancy: Factors affecting the mortality rate. Surgery 62:1082–1091, 1967.

CONGENITAL DUODENAL OBSTRUCTION

Extrinsic duodenal obstruction is usually due to congenital peritoneal bands with or without volvulus associated with midgut malrotation, to annular pancreas, or, more rarely, to an aberrant superior mesenteric artery. An intrinsic type includes atresia, where only the lumen is obliterated by a membrane or where there is a complete gap between the 2 bowel ends. Atresia and stenosis may affect the duodenum proximal or distal to the ampulla of Vater. There is often a history of polyhydramnios.

Clinical Findings

A. Atresia: Vomiting (usually bile stained) begins within a few hours after birth, with epigastric distention. Meconium may be normally passed. The association between duodenal atresia, severe congenital anomalies (30%), prematurity (25–50%), and mongolism (20–30%) is striking.

B. Stenosis: Symptoms of duodenal obstruction appear later and are intermittent, being delayed for weeks, months, or years. Even though a postampullary location of the stenotic area is usual, the vomitus does not always contain bile. X-rays of the abdomen usually show gastric and duodenal gaseous distention proximal to the atretic site ("double bubble"). In cases of protracted vomiting and dehydration, there may be little air in the stomach; it is then advisable to instill 10 ml of air into the stomach to elicit the typical pattern. Total absence of gas in the intestinal tract distal to the obstruction suggests atresia or an extrinsic obstruction severe enough to completely occlude the lumen, while air scattered over the lower abdomen may indicate a partial duodenal obstruction either of the intrinsic or extrinsic variety. A barium enema may be helpful in determining the presence of a concomitant malrotation or of an area of atresia lower in the gastrointestinal tract.

Treatment

Since clinical and radiologic findings cannot do more than indicate either partial or complete duodenal obstruction, thorough exploration is necessary at operation not only to find the cause of the obstruction but to make sure that no additional pathologic anomalies are present lower in the gastrointestinal tract.

Prognosis

The mortality rate (35–40%) is significantly affected by prematurity, mongolism, and associated congenital anomalies.

Aitken J: Congenital intrinsic duodenal obstruction in infancy. J Pediat Surg 1:6, 546–558, 1966.
Fonkalsrud EW, DeLorimier AA, Hays DM: Congenital atresia and stenosis of duodenum. Pediatrics 43:79–83, 1969.
Young DG, Wilkinson AW: Abnormalities associated with neonatal duodenal obstruction. Surgery 63:832–836, 1968.

CONGENITAL JEJUNAL & ILEAL OBSTRUCTION

Bile-stained or fecal vomiting usually begins in the first 48 hours of life, and distention is frequent. Meconium only is passed rectally. Prematurity and severe congenital anomalies may coexist. X-ray features include dilated loops of small bowel and absence of colonic gas. Barium enema will reveal a colon of restricted caliber (microcolon) if the atresia is in the lower small bowel.

The differential diagnosis should include Hirschsprung's disease, paralytic ileus secondary to sepsis, gastroenteritis or pneumonia, midgut volvulus, and meconium ileus. This latter condition, the initial manifestation of cystic fibrosis, can be found in association with intestinal atresia.

Surgery is mandatory. The prognosis remains grave.

Berdon WE & others: Microcolon in newborn infants with intestinal obstruction. Radiology 90:878–885, 1970.
Louw JH: Jejunoileal atresia and stenosis. J Pediat Surg 1:8–23, 1966.

ANNULAR PANCREAS

The pancreas develops from dorsal and ventral endodermal outgrowths which fuse. The ventral pancreatic bud is bilobed; the left bud normally degenerates. If it persists and develops its own pancreatic lobe, it grows around the left side of the duodenum to join the other 2 parts of the pancreas in the dorsal mesentery.

The presence of an annular pancreas is usually associated with failure of segmental duodenal development. The symptoms are those of partial or complete duodenal obstruction. Down's syndrome and severe congenital anomalies of the gastrointestinal tract occur frequently. As with other gastrointestinal obstructive lesions of the neonate, polyhydramnios is commonly found.

Treatment consists of duodenoduodenostomy or duodenojejunostomy without operative dissection or division of the pancreatic annulus.

Elliott GB, Kliman MR, Elliott KA: Pancreatic annulus: A sign or a cause of duodenal obstruction. Canad J Surg 11:357–364, 1968.
Feuchtwanger MM, Weiss Y: Side-to-side duodenoduodenostomy for obstructing annular pancreas in the newborn. J Pediat Surg 3:398–401, 1968.

MIDGUT MALROTATION

Normally, the midgut, which extends from the duodenojejunal junction to the mid-transverse colon and which is supplied by the superior mesenteric artery, returns to the intra-abdominal position during the tenth week of embryonic life while the root of the mesentery rotates in a counterclockwise direction. This causes the colon to cross ventrally; the cecum moves from the left to the right lower quadrant, and the duodenum crosses dorsally to become partly retroperitoneal. When this rotation is incomplete, the posterior fixation of the mesentery is defective so that the bowel from the ligament of Treitz to the mid-transverse colon may twist, causing a volvulus around the pedicle-like mesentery. Duodenal or ileal obstruction may later result through peritoneal bands from the mobile hepatic flexure or cecum. The majority of cases are asymptomatic.

Clinical Findings

A. Symptoms and Signs: Seventy-five percent of symptomatic cases show high intestinal obstruction within the first 3 weeks of life, with bile-stained vomitus, abdominal distention, and visible peristalsis. The first signs may occur later in life, with recurring symptoms of intermittent intestinal obstruction or, more rarely, with celiac syndrome or intermittent profuse watery diarrhea. Acute gastroenteritis may be an early symptom in infants under the age of 6 months. Severe associated congenital anomalies, especially cardiac, are said to occur in over 25% of symptomatic cases.

B. X-Ray Findings: In the newborn period, complete absence of air in the small bowel suggests duodenal atresia. An upper gastrointestinal series may show partial or complete obstruction. The diagnosis of malrotation can be further confirmed by barium enema, which shows a cecum which is mobile and abnormally located.

Treatment & Prognosis

Treatment consists of surgical correction. The prognosis in the newborn period is guarded in view of the incidence of perforation with peritonitis and of extensive intestinal necrosis.

Leslie JWM, Matheson WJ: Failure to thrive in early infancy due to abnormalities of rotation of the midgut. Clin Pediat 4:681–684, 1965.

Rees JR, Redo SF: Anomalies of intestinal rotation and fixation. Am J Surg 116:834–841, 1968.

MAJOR ABDOMINAL WALL DEVELOPMENTAL DEFECTS

Omphalocele

This is a rare condition (1:10,000 births) associated with variable herniation of intra-abdominal viscera into the base of the umbilical cord. There is no defect of the abdominal wall. It is thought to be secondary to an arrest in the intra-abdominal migration of the midgut between the fifth and ninth weeks of gestation. Primary closure of those less than 5 cm in diameter has a good prognosis. Attempts at primary repair of larger ones lead to respiratory failure, necessitating a staged enlargement of the abdominal cavity.

Gastroschisis

This consists of herniation of bowel or other viscus through an extra-umbilical defect in the anterior abdominal wall. There is no covering membrane and the eviscerated bowel loops are dark red, edematous, and adherent. They are encased in a thick matrix of fibrinous material. Gangrene may be present. All patients have associated malrotation and some degree of congenital shortening of the small bowel. Unruptured omphalocele and associated intestinal atresias are

common. Closure is by stages with a prosthetic abdominal wall.

Congenital Deficiency of Abdominal Musculature

This disorder is apparent from the flaccid and wrinkled appearance of the abdominal wall. Almost all of these infants are males with undescended testes; 50% present with club feet. Between 20 and 25% also have cardiac and gastrointestinal anomalies. Urinary tract anomalies consist of urethral and functional bladder neck obstructions associated with a patent urachus. Corseting counteracts the abdominal wall weakness, but 60% die in infancy as a result of renal insufficiency or respiratory failure.

Bourne CW, Cerny JC: Congenital absence of abdominal muscles: Report of 6 cases. J Urol 98:252–259, 1967.

Schuster SR: A new method for the staged repair of large omphaloceles. Surg Gynec Obst 125:837–850, 1967.

Smith RW, Leix F: Omphalocele. Am J Surg 111:450–456, 1966.

MECKEL'S DIVERTICULUM & OMPHALOMESENTERIC DUCT REMNANTS

The remnant of the vitelline duct known as Meckel's diverticulum is present in approximately 1.5% of the population. Complications occur 3 times more frequently in males than in females, and in 50–60% of cases within the first 2 years of life. Heterotopic tissue (gastric mucosa mostly, but also pancreatic tissue and jejunal or colonic mucosa) is 10 times as likely to be present in symptomatic cases.

Clinical Findings

A. Hemorrhage: (40–60% of symptomatic cases.) Massive painless rectal bleeding or dark red stools is characteristic. Shock is common, with hemoglobin levels of 3–4 gm/100 ml. Gastric mucosa and an ulcer of the ileal mucosa are found in the majority of cases presenting with hemorrhage.

B. Intestinal Obstruction: (25% of symptomatic cases.)

1. Intussusception—Ileocolic intussusception with early intestinal infarction. A mass is palpable.

2. Herniation or volvulus—Twisting of the bowel around a fibrous remnant of the vitelline duct extending from the tip of the diverticulum to the abdominal wall may occur with herniation around this cord or strangulation of the diverticulum in an inguinal hernia. In many cases, entrapment of a bowel loop under a band running between the diverticulum and the base of the mesentery has been associated with intestinal obstruction.

C. Diverticulitis: (10–20%.) This condition is clinically indistinguishable from acute appendicitis. Perforation and generalized peritonitis may occur in the young infant.

Treatment

A. Diverticulum: Treatment is surgical. At operation, close inspection of the ileum proximal and distal to the diverticulum may reveal ulcerations and heterotopic tissue adjacent to the neck of the diverticulum.

B. Other Remnants of the Omphalomesenteric Duct: Fecal discharge from the umbilicus is evidence of a patent omphalomesenteric duct. The duct may be completely closed, leading to persistence of a fibrous cord joining ileum and umbilicus and potentially the origin of a volvulus. In other instances, a mucoid discharge may be indicative of a mucocele, which can protrude through the umbilicus and be mistaken for an umbilical granuloma since it is firm and bright red. In all cases, surgical excision of the omphalomesenteric remnant is indicated.

Prognosis

The prognosis for Meckel's diverticulum is good. Marked hemorrhage may occur but is rarely exsanguinating.

Rutherford RB, Akers DR: Meckel's diverticulum. Surgery 59:618–626, 1966.

DUPLICATIONS OF THE GASTROINTESTINAL TRACT

Duplications of the gastrointestinal tract are congenital malformations most often discovered during infancy. Duplications are spherical and tubular structures of various sizes and shapes which may occur anywhere along the gastrointestinal tract from the tongue to the anus. They usually contain fluid and sometimes blood if necrosis has taken place. Although most duplications are not communicating, they are intimately attached to the mesenteric side of the gut and share a common muscular coat. The intestinal epithelium is usually of the same type as that seen in the area of the gastrointestinal tract from which it originates. Some duplications are attached to the spinal cord and are associated with the presence of hemivertebrae (neurenteric cysts). Abdominal duplications are much more common than the thoracic ones, which are usually attached to the esophagus.

Symptoms usually become manifest in infancy and consist of abdominal distention, colicky pain, rectal bleeding, partial or total intestinal obstruction, or an abdominal mass. Physical examination reveals a rounded, smooth, freely movable mass, and x-rays of the abdomen show a noncalcified mass displacing the intestines or compressing the stomach. Involvement of the terminal small bowel can trigger off an intussusception.

Prompt surgical treatment is indicated.

Beardmore HE, Wiggleworth FW: Vertebral anomalies in alimentary duplications. P Clin North America 5:457–474, 1958.

Grosfeld JL, O'Neill JA, Clatworthy HW: Enteric duplications in infancy and childhood. Ann Surg 172:83–90, 1970.

NECROTIZING ENTEROCOLITIS

Although gastric and duodenal perforations are more frequent, a number of reports of small and large bowel perforations in the newborn due to ischemic necrosis have appeared recently. This in turn is due to a perfusion failure resulting from hypoxia or shock.

The syndrome of necrotizing enterocolitis is most commonly found in prematures with a perinatal or postnatal history of asphyxia or in newborns who have had exchange transfusions. Fever in the mother and evidence of amnionitis and early rupture of the membranes are common. Abdominal distention, vomiting, rectal bleeding, and a shock-like picture usually occur in the first week of life. Free air in the peritoneal cavity and intestines is commonly seen. A flat film of the abdomen often shows intramural gas bubbles. Later, air continues to dissociate the intestinal wall and gives rise to the typical picture of pneumatosis intestinalis. Air in the portal vein has been reported. Blood cultures are usually positive for gram-negative organisms. Bland ischemic necrosis is always present, but in 50% of cases there is also a marked inflammatory reaction involving the terminal ileum and the colon.

Surgical closure of the perforations should be attempted.

Orme RLE, Eades SM: Perforation of the bowel in the newborn as a complication of exchange transfusion. Brit MJ 4:349–351, 1968.
Stone HH, Webb HW, Kovalchik MT: Pneumatosis intestinalis of infancy. Surg Gynec Obst 130:806–812, 1970.

PRIMARY PERITONITIS

The incidence of primary peritonitis has decreased remarkably with the advent of antibiotics. Most cases occur below the age of 5. In older children, the disease is 3–5 times more common in girls. The most common infecting organisms are hemolytic streptococci and pneumococci, especially in infants who have undergone splenectomy for conditions such as a hemolytic anemia other than hereditary spherocytosis, a storage disease, or histiocytosis. It also is a potential complication of nephrosis and cirrhosis.

The onset is acute, with severe abdominal pain, fever, nausea, and vomiting. The abdomen is tender, with guarding, involuntary rigidity, and distention. Tenderness is present on rectal examination. The physical signs are identical to those associated with peritonitis secondary to, for example, a perforated appendix. However, the temperature is usually higher and the white count also higher (20,000–50,000/cu mm) than is usual in appendicitis. Diarrhea is not uncommonly seen in primary peritonitis and is much rarer in appendicitis.

Primary peritonitis must be distinguished from secondary peritonitis (see below).

A diagnostic paracentesis should be made and appropriate antibiotic therapy instituted. The prognosis is good.

Fogel BJ, Karpa JN, Luxemberg ER: Primary peritonitis. Clin Pediat 3:578–580, 1967.

SECONDARY PERITONITIS

Secondary peritoneal infection commonly results from an abscessed or ruptured intra-abdominal viscus. usually the appendix. More rarely, peptic ulcer, cholecystitis, pancreatitis, diverticulitis, regional enteritis, ulcerative colitis, midgut volvulus, intussusception, and strangulated hernia can cause secondary peritonitis. Abscesses may form in the pelvic, subhepatic, and subphrenic areas, but localization occurs less commonly in infants and young children than in adults.

Clinical Findings

A. Symptoms and Signs: Signs are often overshadowed by those of the underlying disorder. High fever is common except in newborn or debilitated infants, and shock may be present. Abdominal pain is diffuse and is exacerbated by movement. Vomiting is protracted, and the vomitus is greenish and eventually becomes malodorous. Constipation is marked unless there is localization, when small diarrheal stools may be passed. Restlessness, rapid pulse, and superficial grunting respirations are other common clinical features. Abdominal examination shows diffuse tenderness with muscular resistance and rebound tenderness. Peristalsis is usually absent. Irritation of the pelvic peritoneum is evidenced by pain on rectal examination.

B. Laboratory Findings: A striking polymorphonuclear response is usual; however, as the disease advances, the white blood count often drops to leukopenic levels.

Treatment

Preoperative preparation with hydration, correction of acid-base problems, antimicrobial therapy for *Escherichia coli,* gastric suction, and the relief of pain significantly improve the mortality rate.

The operative management consists of removal or repair of the affected viscus, drainage of the localized abscess, and lavage of the peritoneal cavity with saline and antibiotics.

Prognosis

The mortality rate is probably around 1% in older children and 50% in newborns.

Birch AG, Coran AG, Gross RE: Neonatal peritonitis. Surgery 61:305–313, 1967.

CONGENITAL AGANGLIONIC MEGACOLON
(Hirschsprung's Disease)

Essentials of Diagnosis

- Partial or complete intestinal obstruction in the newborn period.
- Vomiting, diarrhea, abdominal distention, and shock in the newborn period.
- Obstinate constipation, abdominal enlargement, ribbon-like stools, and failure to thrive in infancy or childhood.
- Absence of fecal material on rectal examination.
- Narrowed colonic segment proximal to the anus on x-ray.
- Absence of ganglion cells in the narrowed segment.

General Considerations

Hirschsprung's disease is secondary to congenital absence of parasympathetic ganglion cells in one segment of the colon (a 4–25 cm rectal or rectosigmoid segment in 90% of cases), but it may involve the entire organ. The aperistaltic denervated segment is narrowed, with dilatation of the proximal uninvolved colon. In long-standing cases, the portion proximal to the narrowed segment may become thinned out, and ulcerations of the mucosa occur although perforations are rare. A familial pattern has been described, particularly in total colonic aganglionosis. Hirschsprung's disease is 4 times more common in boys than in girls.

Clinical Findings

A. Symptoms and Signs: Failure to pass meconium in a newborn is rapidly followed by vomiting, abdominal distention, and reluctance to feed. The baby is irritable, and breathing may be rapid and grunting because of the abdominal distention. In other cases, symptoms appear later and are those of partial intestinal obstruction. Stools may be infrequent and loose; vomiting may be bilious initially and fecal later. Abdominal distention is invariably present. Bouts of enterocolitis manifested by fever, explosive liquid diarrhea, and severe prostration are reported in about 50% of newborns with this disease. These episodes are serious and may lead to acute inflammatory and ischemic changes. Perforation and sepsis are not unusual. However, if symptoms during early infancy are not prominent, the child suffers from obstinate constipation, his stools are offensive and ribbon-like, his abdomen enlarged, his veins prominent, peristaltic patterns are readily visible, and fecal masses are easily palpated. Intermittent bouts of intestinal obstruction due to fecal impaction, hypochromic anemia, hypoproteinemia, and failure to thrive are added features.

On digital rectal examination, the anal canal and rectum are devoid of fecal material and may feel narrow. If the involved segment is short, there may be a gush of flatus and of pale, liquid, offensive stool as the finger is withdrawn. The presence of fecal colonic impaction associated with an empty rectum is most suggestive of the disease.

B. Laboratory Findings: The final diagnosis rests on histologic evidence of aganglionosis. Rectal suction biopsies taken at 3, 4, and 5 cm readily establish the diagnosis, although some prefer a full-thickness rectal biopsy in order to have access to the ganglion cells between the muscular layers (Auerbach's flexus).

C. X-Ray Findings: X-ray examination of the abdomen may reveal dilated colonic loops and absence of gas from the pelvic colon on an erect lateral film. A barium enema, introducing a small amount of radiopaque material through a catheter with the tip inserted barely beyond the anal sphincter, will usually demonstrate the narrowed segment. A postevacuation film taken 12−48 hours later will show substantial residual barium. X-ray examination of the urinary tract should be done since an association between megaloureter and Hirschsprung's disease is described.

Differential Diagnosis

Congenital aganglionic megacolon accounts for 15−20% of cases of neonatal intestinal obstruction. Later in life, this disease must be differentiated from psychogenic megacolon. It can also be confused with celiac disease because of the striking abdominal distention and failure to thrive.

A number of disorders are symptomatically similar to Hirschsprung's disease. Hypoganglionosis or immaturity of ganglion cells has been described, as well as some cases of achalasia of the distal rectal segment. Acquired megacolon may be secondary to an anal stricture and is a frequent problem in myxedema and in children with severe mental retardation or deterioration.

Treatment

After preoperative rehydration, a colostomy should be performed in an area of the colon where ganglion cells have been demonstrated by frozen section. If the entire colon is involved, ileostomy is the procedure of choice. If enterocolitis is clinically present and radiologically demonstrated by the typical "saw tooth" appearance, saline irrigations should be started until normal stools return before any surgery is done. Resection of the aganglionic segment is delayed until the infant is at least 6 months of age. In healthy patients, staging is not necessary.

During operation, it is essential to ascertain from biopsies of the bowel that ganglion cells are present in the proximal portion of the resected bowel before the final anastomosis is made. Swenson's abdominoperineal pull-through procedure has been a standard procedure. The Duhamel procedure and Grob's modification of it have been said to reduce the late complications of fecal and urinary incontinence. This may relate to the fact that less pelvic dissection is necessary since the aganglionic rectum is bypassed in both these surgical technics. At present, the technic advocated by Soave is most popular.

Prognosis

In the neonatal period, the mortality rate of Hirschsprung's disease reaches 25−35%. Enterocolitis before or after surgery is an ominous complication, and the mortality rate appears to be higher in infants with a long aganglionic segment.

Bentley JFR, Nixon HH, Ehrenpreis T: Seminar on pseudo Hirschsprung's disease and related disorders. Arch Dis Childhood 41:143−154, 1966.

Campbell PE, Noblet HR: Experience with rectal suction biopsy in the diagnosis of Hirschsprung's disease. J Pediat Surg 4:410−415, 1969.

Fraser GC, Wilkinson AW: Neonatal Hirschsprung's disease. Brit MJ 3:3−10, 1967.

Shim WKT, Swenson O: Treatment of congenital megacolon in 50 infants. Pediatrics 38:185−193, 1966.

THE MECONIUM PLUG SYNDROME

Evidence of low intestinal obstruction becomes apparent on the second day of life. Little or no meconium is passed per rectum, and abdominal distention is usually followed by bile-stained vomiting and dehydration. On rectal examination, the anal canal may be abnormally small. Occasionally, the meconium plug may be passed and large amounts of gas and meconium follow the rectal examination.

In addition to generalized air distention seen on x-ray, fluid levels are observed in half of patients. A barium enema performed under low pressure with a soft-tipped catheter is not only diagnostic, since it reveals a change in the caliber of the colon at the site of obstruction; it can also be therapeutic in dislodging the meconium plug. The finding of a microcolon distal to the plug makes the differentiation from Hirschsprung's disease impossible, especially since the meconium plug syndrome has been reported in Hirschsprung's disease.

Surgical removal is occasionally necessary if the plug is located in the terminal ileum. Ruling out cystic fibrosis by a sweat test and Hirschsprung's disease by a rectal biopsy may be necessary if bowel function is not entirely normal after passage of the meconium.

Ellis DG, Clatworthy HW: The meconium plug syndrome revisited. J Pediat Surg 1:54−61, 1966.

Swischuk LE: Meconium plug syndrome: A cause of neonatal intestinal obstruction. Am J Roentgenol 103:339−346, 1968.

CHYLOUS ASCITES

Congenital chylous ascites may be observed in the newborn before feeding when there is an abnormality in the lymphatic system. If the thoracic duct is involved, chylothorax may be present. Later in life, the cause may be either a congenital lymphatic abnormality or secondary to tumors or peritoneal bands.

Clinical Findings

A. Symptoms and Signs: In both forms, a rapidly enlarging abdomen, diarrhea, and failure to thrive are noted, with a fluid wave and shifting dullness. Unilateral or generalized peripheral lymphedema may be present. In older children, the history is most important in that trauma, infection, tumor, and previous surgery may play an important role.

B. Laboratory Findings: Laboratory findings include hypoalbuminemia, hypogammaglobulinemia, and lymphopenia. Ascitic fluid obtained by paracentesis will have the composition of chyle if the patient has been fed; otherwise, it is indistinguishable from ascites secondary to cirrhosis.

Differential Diagnosis

Chylous ascites must be differentiated from ascites due to liver failure and, in the older child, from constrictive pericarditis and neoplastic or infectious agents causing lymphatic obstruction.

Complications & Sequelae

Severe chylous ascites can be fatal. Chronic loss of albumin and gamma globulin through the gastrointestinal tract may lead to edema and increase the risk of infection. Rapidly accumulating chylous ascites may cause respiratory complications.

Treatment

Specific measures are sometimes helpful when traumatic lesions or secondary obstructive phenomena can be corrected. When a congenital abnormality exists due to hypoplasia, aplasia, or ectasia of the lymphatics, little can be done for the patient. Attempts to relieve the ascites by bringing the saphenous vein into the peritoneal cavity have had partial success. A fat-free diet supplemented with medium chain triglycerides decreases the formation of chylous ascitic fluid.

The congenital form of chylous ascites may spontaneously disappear following paracentesis, exploratory laparotomy, and a medium chain triglyceride diet. Repeated paracentesis is contraindicated. Gamma globulin supplements may be needed if there is hypogammaglobulinemia.

Prognosis

The prognosis is guarded, although spontaneous cures have been reported.

Sanchez RE & others: Chylous ascites in children. Surgery 69:183–188, 1971.

CONGENITAL ANORECTAL ANOMALIES

Anorectal anomalies occur once in every 3000–4000 births and are somewhat more common in males. Inspection of the perianal area is essential in all newborns.

Classification

Five types are now recognized:

A. Anal Stenosis: The anal aperture is very small and filled with a dot of meconium. Defecation is difficult, and there may be ribbon-like stools, fecal impaction, and abdominal distention. This malformation accounts for perhaps 10% of cases of anorectal anomalies. It is readily corrected by digital dilatation.

B. Imperforate Anal Membrane: The infant fails to pass meconium, and a greenish bulging membrane is seen. After excision, bowel and sphincter function are normal.

C. Anal Agenesis: This results from defective development of the anus. The anal dimple is present, and stimulation of the perianal area leads to puckering indicative of the presence of the external sphincter. If there is no associated fistula, intestinal obstruction occurs. Fistulas may be perineal or vulvar in the female and perineal or urethral in the male. A perineal fistula presents as a streak of meconium buried in thickened perineal skin.

D. Rectal Agenesis: Rectal and anal agenesis account for 75% of total anorectal anomalies. Fistulas are almost invariably present. In the female, they may be vestibular or vaginal or may enter a urogenital sinus, which is a common passageway for the urethra and vagina. In the male, fistulas are rectovesical or rectourethral. Associated major congenital malformations are common. Sacral defects, prematurity, and hypoplastic internal and external sphincters significantly influence the prognosis for life and function.

E. Rectal Atresia: A normal anus is seen, but it ends blindly and intestinal obstruction occurs.

X-Ray Findings

X-rays taken with the infant held upside down after the first 24 hours of life and with a radiopaque object held in place at the usual location of the anus will help determine the position of the terminal end of the bowel and ·may help in determining the surgical approach.

Treatment

Colostomy is advocated for all cases of rectal agenesis. In patients with anal agenesis and a visible fistula of sufficient size to pass meconium, treatment can be deferred. The male without a visible fistula may have a urethral fistula; therefore, colostomy is recommended.

Prognosis

The overall mortality rate for anal and rectal agenesis is about 20%. The prognosis is poor in small premature infants and in infants with associated anomalies.

Santulli TV, Schullinger JN, Amoury RA: Malformations of the anus and rectum. S Clin North America 45:1253–1271, 1965.

Stephens FD: Embryologic and functional aspects of "imperforate anus." S Clin North America 50:919–927, 1970.

ACUTE APPENDICITIS

The incidence of acute appendicitis increases with age, and the disease is most frequent between the ages of 15 and 30. Luminal obstruction by fecaliths or parasites is a predisposing factor. The occurrence of appendicitis in association with enteric infections has been described.

Clinical Findings

A. Symptoms and Signs: The triad of persistent localized right lower quadrant pain, localized abdominal tenderness, and slight fever is strongly suggestive of appendicitis. Anorexia, vomiting, and constipation also occur. The clinical picture is often atypical, ie, generalized pain, tenderness around the umbilicus, and no leukocytosis. Diarrhea can substitute for constipation, and a subsiding upper respiratory tract infection may be found. Rectal examination should always be done. Since many infections give rise to symptoms mimicking appendicitis and since physical findings are often inconclusive, it is important to repeat examinations of the abdomen.

B. Laboratory Findings: Leukocytosis, seldom higher than 15,000/cu mm.

C. X-Ray Findings: A radiopaque fecalith can be detected on x-rays and is reportedly present in 2/3 of cases of ruptured appendix.

Differential Diagnosis

Since atypical cases are common, it is better to err on the side of laparotomy after ruling out the presence of intrathoracic infection (eg, pneumonia) or urinary tract infection.

Medical conditions other than pneumonia and urinary tract infections which give rise to an acute abdomen are listed below:

A. Intestinal: Salmonellosis, shigellosis, acute gastroenteritis, regional enteritis, chronic ulcerative colitis, amebiasis, ascariasis, food poisoning, megacolon, incarcerated hernia.

B. Extraintestinal: Rheumatic fever, acute streptococcal infection, infectious lymphocytosis, porphyria, hyperlipidemia, etiocholanolone fever, familial Mediterranean fever, lead poisoning, Henoch-Schönlein purpura, pancreatitis.

Treatment

The only definitive treatment is appendectomy. When surgical facilities are not available, treat as for acute peritonitis.

Prognosis

Even when perforation occurs, the mortality rate is less than 1%.

Liebman WM, St Geme JW Jr: Enteroviral pseudoappendicitis. Am J Dis Child 120:77–78, 1970.

Longino LA, Holder TM, Gross RE: Appendicitis in childhood. Pediatrics 22:238–246, 1958.

FOREIGN BODIES IN THE ALIMENTARY TRACT

Most foreign bodies pass through the esophagus and the rest of the gastrointestinal tract without difficulty, although anything longer than 3–5 cm may have difficulty passing the duodenal loop at the region of the ligament of Treitz. Foreign bodies lodged in the esophagus require immediate attention.

A reasonable rule is that if a foreign body remains distal to the pylorus in one location for longer than 5 days, surgical removal should be considered, especially if symptoms occur. Close observation and, preferably, hospitalization is urged for children who have swallowed open safety pins and long sharp objects.

Esophagoscopy will permit the removal of the majority of foreign bodies lodged in the esophagus.

Erbes J, Babbitt DP: Foreign bodies in the alimentary tract of infants and children. J Lancet 85:247–253, 1965.

TRAUMATIC INJURIES OF THE GASTROINTESTINAL TRACT

Neonatal Period

Severe intra-abdominal injuries are rare in the newborn period. Listlessness, rapid respirations in conjunction with fullness of the abdomen, an abdominal mass, and rapidly developing anemia are characteristic symptoms. The incidence of trauma increases in proportion to the size of the infant and is perhaps higher in breech deliveries. A ruptured spleen usually gives rise to immediate signs. Subcapsular hematomas of the liver secondary to laceration of the liver are quite common, especially if there have been manual attempts at resuscitation. Kidney injuries give rise to retroperitoneal hematomas. Peritoneal taps are helpful in making a diagnosis and deciding whether emergency surgery is indicated. If the peritoneal fluid is bloody, immediate surgery may be required.

Childhood

Abdominal trauma is found in many children brought to the hospital following serious injury. Blunt abdominal trauma gives rise to little external evidence of internal injury, and multiple injuries may distract the examiner from the abdominal injury. Solid organs are more seriously and frequently injured than hollow viscera. Contusion of the pancreas may lead to acute pancreatitis or, later, a pseudocyst. Intramural hematomas in the duodenum or at the duodenojejunal junction are frequently seen in the battered child syndrome.

Eraklis AJ: Abdominal injury from birth trauma. Pediatrics 39:421–424. 1967.

Haller JA: Injuries of the gastrointestinal tract in children. Clin Pediat 4:476–480, 1966.

ANAL FISSURE

Anal fissure consists of a slit-like tear in the anal canal usually secondary to the passage of large, hard, dry fecal masses (scybala). Anal stenosis and trauma can be contributory factors.

The infant or child cries with defecation and will try to hold back his stools, resulting in increasing constipation. Sparse, bright red bleeding usually follows defecation. The fissure can be seen if the patient is held in a knee-chest position and the buttocks spread apart.

When a fissure cannot be identified, it is essential to rule out other causes of rectal bleeding.

Anal fissures should be treated promptly, especially in infancy, to break the constipation-fissure-constipation cycle. Rectal instillation of oil and the introduction of a gloved, lubricated finger twice daily lessens sphincter spasm. Hot sitz baths after defecation may be helpful. In rare cases, silver nitrate cauterization may be necessary. In protracted cases, surgery is indicated.

Arminski TC, MacLean DW: Proctologic problems in children. JAMA 194:1195–1197, 1965.

Duhamel J, Ngo-Binh: Anal fissures in children: Report of 100 cases. Arch franç pédiat 24:1131–1134, 1967.

INTUSSUSCEPTION

Essentials of Diagnosis

- Paroxysmal, episodic abdominal pain and vomiting.
- Sausage-shaped mass in upper abdomen.
- Rectal passage of bloody mucus.
- Barium enema evidence of intussusception.

General Considerations

Intussusception is the most frequent cause of intestinal obstruction in the first 2 years of life. It is 3 times more common in males than in females. In most cases the cause is not apparent, although polyps, Meckel's diverticulum, Henoch-Schönlein purpura, constipation, parasites, and foreign bodies are predisposing factors. Intussusception is relatively common in cystic fibrosis and usually relates to inspissated fecal material in the terminal ileum and in the colon.

In most instances the intussusception starts at a point immediately proximal to the ileocecal valve, so that invagination is usually ileocolic. Other forms include ileo-ileal and colo-colic. Swelling, hemorrhage, incarceration with necrosis, and eventual perforation and peritonitis occur as a result of impairment of venous return.

Clinical Findings

Characteristically, a previously thriving infant between the ages of 3 months and 1 year suddenly develops periodic abdominal pain with screaming and drawing up of the knees. Vomiting occurs soon afterward, and bloody bowel movements with mucus appear within the next 12 hours. Severe prostration and fever supervene, and the abdomen is tender and becomes distended. On palpation, a sausage-shaped tumor may be found in the early stages. In rare cases, diarrhea is an early symptom.

The intussusception can also persist for several days when obstruction is not complete, and such cases may present as separate attacks of enterocolitis. In older children, sudden attacks of abdominal pain may be related to chronic recurrent intussusception with spontaneous reduction.

Treatment

A. Conservative Measures: The use of barium enema in the treatment of intussusception is still controversial. It is a safe procedure if the following recommendations are observed.

1. No attempt should be made at hydrostatic reduction if the onset of the disease was more than 24 hours ago or if there are clinical signs of strangulated bowel, perforation, or severe toxicity.

2. The barium solution should be allowed to drip by gravity through a Foley bag catheter inserted in the rectum from a height not more than 3½ feet above the fluoroscopy table.

3. There should be no manipulation of the abdomen during the hydrostatic reduction under fluoroscopic examination for fear of increasing intraluminal pressure and thus the risk of perforation.

4. Upon reduction, there should be free reflux of barium into the ileum; this is better elicited in a postevacuation film.

B. Surgical Measures: For patients with intussusception who are not suitable for hydrostatic reduction or for those in whom it is unsuccessful (50%), surgery is performed as soon as the patient has been adequately prepared. Surgery has the advantage of demonstrating any lead point (such as Meckel's diverticulum), which occurs in 5% of cases. It may be also that surgical correction is associated with a lower recurrence rate.

Prognosis

Intussusception is almost uniformly fatal if untreated. The prognosis directly relates to the duration of the intussusception before reduction.

Bjarnason G, Pettersson G: The treatment of intussusception: Thirty years' experience at Gottenburg's Children's Hospital. J Pediat Surg 3:19–23. 1968.

Holder TM, Leape LL: The acute surgical abdomen in children. New England J Med 277:921–923, 1967.

INGUINAL HERNIA

A peritoneal sac precedes the testicle as it descends from the genital ridge to the scrotum. The lower portion of this sac envelops the testis to form the tunica vaginalis, and the remainder normally atrophies by the time of birth. Persistence of the processus vaginalis presents as a mass in the inguinal region when an abdominal structure or peritoneal fluid is forced into it. The persistent sac may be very short or may extend into the scrotum. In some cases, peritoneal fluid may become trapped in the tunica vaginalis of the testis (noncommunicating hydrocele). If the processus vaginalis remains open, peritoneal fluid (hydrocele of the spermatic cord, or of the canal of Nuck in the female) or an abdominal structure may be forced into it (indirect inguinal hernia).

Most inguinal hernias are of the indirect type and occur much more frequently in boys than in girls (9:1). Hernias may be present at birth or may appear at any age thereafter.

Clinical Findings

There are no symptoms associated with an empty hernial sac. In most cases, the hernia appears as a painless inguinal swelling which varies in size. There may be a history of inguinal fullness associated with coughing or with long periods in the standing position; or there may be a firm, globular, and tender swelling, sometimes associated with vomiting and abdominal distention.

Spontaneous reduction frequently occurs while sleeping or with mild external pressure. In some instances, a herniated loop of intestine may become partially obstructed, leading to pain, irritability, and incomplete intestinal obstruction. More rarely, the loop of bowel becomes incarcerated, and signs of complete intestinal obstruction are present. In the female, the ovary may prolapse into the hernial sac.

Inspection of the 2 inguinal areas may reveal a characteristic bulging or mass. After crying in the infant or after bearing down in the older child, the patient should be observed for evidence of swelling.

A suggestive history is often the only criterion for diagnosis, along with the "silk glove" feel of the rubbing together of the 2 walls of the empty hernia sac.

Differential Diagnosis

An inguinal mass may represent lymph nodes. They are usually multiple and more discrete. Hydrocele of the cord transilluminates. An undescended testis may be moved along the canal and is associated with absence of the testicle in the scrotum.

Treatment

Surgical treatment is indicated in all cases. There is still some controversy about the advisability of exploration of the opposite side. Herniography is helpful in determining the patency of the processus vaginalis.

Incarcerated inguinal hernias occur most often in the first 6 months of life. Manipulative reduction can be attempted after sedating the child and placing him in the Trendelenburg position with an ice bag on the affected side. This conservative treatment is contraindicated if the incarcerated hernia has been present for more than 12 hours or if bloody stools are noted.

Holcomb GW: Routine bilateral inguinal hernia repair: Evaluation of procedure in infants and children. Am J Dis Child 109:114–120, 1965.

White JJ, Haller JA, Dorst JP: Congenital inguinal hernia and inguinal herniography. S Clin North America 50:823–837, 1970.

UMBILICAL HERNIA

The incidence of umbilical hernia is higher in premature than in full-term infants, in whom the frequency has been estimated to be 20%. This defect is more common in black infants.

Excessive thinning of the skin distended by the hernia and progressive enlargement of the fascial defects are reported very rarely unless there is increased intra-abdominal pressure due to organomegaly or ascites. Incarceration is the only dangerous problem and is limited to smaller hernias.

Most umbilical hernias heal spontaneously if the fascial defect has a diameter of less than 1 cm. Large defects (greater than 2 cm) may still disappear without treatment, but seldom before school age. Large defects and smaller hernias persisting up to school age should be treated surgically. Reducing the hernia and strapping the skin drawn together into a longitudinal fold over the umbilical ring does not accelerate the healing process.

Walker SH: The natural history of umbilical hernias. Clin Pediat 6:29–32, 1967.

TUMORS OF THE
GASTROINTESTINAL TRACT

1. JUVENILE POLYPS

Juvenile polyps are nearly always pedunculated and solitary with a stalk covered by colonic mucosa. The chorion is hyperplastic and inflamed. The glandular portion shows branching, irregular proliferation, and cystic transformation. The polyps are always benign. Eighty percent are within reach of the sigmoidoscope.

Polyps are rare before age 1, but their incidence increases thereafter and reaches a maximum frequency between 4 and 5 years of age. They are uncommon after age 15 because of auto-amputation and self-destruction. Bright red blood in the stools, intermittent melena, and occult painless gastrointestinal bleeding with anemia are the most frequent manifestations. Abdominal pain is infrequent, but a juvenile polyp can be the lead point for an intussusception. Rectal examination, sigmoidoscopy, and barium enema are essential to a full exploration for polyps.

A polyp accessible by sigmoidoscope should be removed for biopsy. If histology confirms that it is a juvenile polyp, nothing further should be done. In the event that 3 or 4 polyps are seen above the rectosigmoid, laparotomy is recommended. Otherwise, treatment is conservative.

The prognosis is excellent, since retention polyps are never malignant and since there is a high incidence of auto-amputation.

Duhamel J, Banche P: Polyps of the colon beyond the reach of the sigmoidoscope. Arch Dis Childhood 40:173–176, 1965.
Shermeta DW & others: Juvenile retention polyps. J Pediat Surg 4:211–215, 1969.

2. FAMILIAL POLYPOSIS

This condition is characterized by the presence in the colon of large numbers of adenomatous polyps varying in size from mucosal excrescences to large stalked polyps. A family history is obtained in roughly 2/3 of cases, and the entity is transmitted genetically as a dominant with reduced penetrance. Carcinoma of the colon usually develops before age 40, or approximately 15 years after onset of symptoms.

The disease has been identified in infants but is more likely to become symptomatic in the late teens. Diarrhea is usually the first symptom. Blood loss, anemia, and abdominal pain usually supervene. The initial symptoms may be those of carcinomatosis.

Sigmoidoscopy reveals great numbers of polyps of various sizes. Barium enema reveals a normal bowel wall but a great number of filling defects.

All members of the family should be carefully examined. Subtotal colectomy has been recommended, but many authors believe that keeping the rectal stump is dangerous since carcinoma may develop despite frequent observation of the stump. Proctocolectomy with an ileostomy is the treatment of choice, since any individual with familial polyposis will eventually develop carcinoma of the colon if untreated.

Abramson DJ: Multiple polyposis in children. Surgery 61:288–301, 1967.

3. PEUTZ-JEGHERS SYNDROME

The polyps in this syndrome are classified as hamartomas. They may occur anywhere between the cardiac sphincter and the anus but occur most often in the small intestine. Mucosal pigmentation is necessary to establish the diagnosis; it usually appears at birth or in infancy and has a tendency to lessen at puberty. The lips and buccal mucosa are usually involved. The syndrome is inherited as an autosomal dominant trait.

Colicky abdominal pain, anemia, and gastrointestinal hemorrhage are common symptoms. Intussusception may occur.

Conservative treatment is advocated. Symptomatic and accessible lesions should be removed surgically. Carcinomatous change has been reported.

4. GARDNER'S SYNDROME

This is a dominantly inherited condition consisting of soft tissue and bone tumors associated with multiple intestinal polyps predisposed to malignant change. The large bowel is the most common site of involvement. Management should be directed at early detection of adenocarcinoma of the bowel. All members of an affected family should be examined periodically.

Duncan BR, Dohner VA, Priest JH: Gardner syndrome: Need for early diagnosis. J Pediat 72:497–505, 19688.

5. CANCER OF THE SMALL &
LARGE INTESTINES

The most common small bowel malignancy in children is lymphosarcoma. Intermittent abdominal pain, an abdominal mass, evidence of intestinal obstruction, or a celiac-like picture may be present. Long-term survivals are reported in patients without lymph node involvement at surgery.

Carcinoid tumors of the small intestine and appendix are usually of low-grade malignancy and rarely show the classical syndrome of diarrhea, asthma, and flushing of the face.

Adenocarcinoma of the colon is rare in the pediatric age group. The transverse colon and rectosigmoid are the 2 most commonly affected sites. The low 5-year survival has to do with the nonspecificity of presenting complaints and the large percentage of undifferentiated types. Children with chronic ulcerative colitis or with familial polyposis are at greater risk but seldom develop cancer before age 20. Cancer of the colon usually develops in a previously intact colon.

Cain AD, Longino LA: Carcinoma of the colon in children. J Pediat Surg 5:527–532, 1970.

Field JL, Adamson LF, Stoeckle HE: Review of carcinoids in children. Pediatrics 29:953–960, 1962.

6. MESENTERIC CYSTS

These tumors are rare in infants and children. They may be small or large, and single or multiloculated. Invariably thin-walled, they contain either serous, chylous, or hemorrhagic fluid. They are commonly located in the mesentery of the small intestine but may also be seen in the mesocolon.

The majority of these cysts are asymptomatic and come to medical attention when the parents note an increase in abdominal girth. However, traction on the mesentery eventually leads to pain in a high percentage of patients. The abdominal discomfort can be mild and recurrent but may present very acutely and lead to vomiting. Volvulus is reported. A rounded mass can occasionally be palpated, and is noted on x-ray to displace adjacent intestine.

Surgical removal is indicated and often includes resection of the adjacent intestine because of a blood supply problem.

Hardin WJ, Hardy JD: Mesenteric cysts. Am J Surg 119:640–645, 1970.

THE IRRITABLE COLON SYNDROME

The typical patient with irritable colon syndrome is a child 1–3 years of age who was a colicky baby and who starts having 3–6 loose mucoid stools per day during the waking hours. The child is active, looks healthy, has a good appetite, and is growing normally. The diarrhea is uninfluenced by diet but may be worse during periods of stress or infection. It clears spontaneously at about 3½ years of age. No organic disease is discoverable. The pathogenesis of the disease remains obscure but may relate to a particularly active gastrocolic reflex. A high familial coincidence of functional bowel disease is observed.

Elimination of chilled fluids and the administration of diiodohydroxyquin (Diodoquin), 100–600 mg orally daily, have been demonstrated to be of value. Toilet training may dramatically cure the nonspecific diarrhea.

Davidson M, Wasserman R: The irritable colon of childhood. J Pediat 69:1027–1038, 1966.

DIARRHEAL DISEASES*

Diarrhea may be defined as water and electrolyte malabsorption leading to accelerated excretion of intestinal contents. What constitutes diarrhea is sometimes difficult to define in terms of number or consistency of stools because there are wide variations in colonic function. Some infants may pass one firm stool every second to third day, whereas others may have 5–8 soft small stools daily. A gradual or sudden increase in the number of stools, a reduction in their consistency coupled with an increase in their fluid content, or a tendency for the stools to be green are more important factors.

Diarrhea may result from the following closely related pathogenetic mechanisms: (1) Interruption of normal cell transport processes. (2) Decrease in the surface area available for absorption by shortening of the bowel or mucosal disease. (3) Increase in intestinal motility. (4) Presence of large amounts of unabsorbable osmotically active molecules. (5) Abnormality of gastric or intestinal permeability, leading to increased secretion of water and electrolytes.

The physiologic consequences of diarrhea vary with its severity and duration, the age of the patient and his state of nutrition prior to onset, and the presence or absence of associated symptoms. Acute diarrhea may lead to dehydration and acid-base disturbances (see Chapter 37). Chronic diarrhea leads to malnutrition.

Causes of Diarrhea Other Than Infectious Gastroenteritis

A. Antibiotic Therapy: Antibiotics such as ampicillin, neomycin, and tetracyclines commonly give rise to diarrhea. They lead to decreased glucose absorption and disaccharidase activity. In a clinical setting where a bacterial infection has been ruled out, they should be stopped and a lactose-free diet administered. At times, antibiotics may give rise to the overgrowth of microorganisms resistant to the antibiotic being given.

*Epidemic diarrhea of the newborn is discussed in Chapter 3; diarrhea due to viral infections, in Chapter 26; diarrhea due to bacterial infections, in Chapter 27; and diarrhea due to parasitic infections, in Chapter 28.

TABLE 16–1. Etiologic classification of diarrhea.*

Type of Disorder	Disease

Infections
  Enteral
    Bacterial
	Pathogenic *Escherichia coli,* shigellosis, salmonellosis, *Staphylococcus aureus, Pseudomonas aeruginosa,* klebsiella, enterobacter, cholera.

Viral	Adenoviruses, enteroviruses.
Parasitic	Amebiasis, giardiasis, ascariasis.
Parenteral	Urinary tract and upper respiratory tract infections.
Inflammatory bowel diseases	Regional enteritis, chronic ulcerative colitis, Whipple's disease, necrotizing enterocolitis of the newborn, nonspecific enterocolitis of infancy.
Anatomic and mechanical causes	Short bowel syndrome, fistula, postgastrectomy, blind loop syndrome, partial duodenal or ileojejunal obstruction, malrotation, Hirschsprung's disease, intestinal lymphangiectasis.
Pancreatic and hepatic disorders	Cirrhosis, hepatitis, biliary atresia, chronic pancreatitis, pancreatic exocrine deficiency, pancreatic hypoplasia.
Biochemical causes	Celiac disease, cystic fibrosis of the pancreas, disaccharidase deficiency, glucose-galactose malabsorption, abetalipoproteinemia, folic acid deficiency, congenital chloridorrhea with alkalosis, acrodermatitis enteropathica.
Neoplastic causes	Carcinoid, ganglioneuroma, Zollinger-Ellison syndrome, polyposis, lymphoma, adenocarcinoma.
Immunity deficiencies	Ataxia, telangiectasia, Wiskott-Aldrich syndrome, agammaglobulinemia, dysgammaglobulinemia, thymic alymphoplasia and dysplasia.
Endocrinopathies	Hyperthyroidism, congenital adrenal hyperplasia.
Malnutrition	Protein malnutrition (kwashiorkor), protein-calorie malnutrition (marasmus).
Dietary factors	Overfeeding, introduction of new foods.
Food allergy	Milk colitis, allergic gastroenteropathy.
Psychogenic or functional disorders	Irritable colon syndrome.
Toxic diarrhea	Ingestion of heavy metals (eg, arsenic, lead).

*Slightly modified and reproduced, with permission, from Silverman A, Roy CC, Cozzetto F: *Pediatric Clinical Gastroenterology.* Mosby, 1971.

B. Parenteral Infections: Infections of the urinary tract and upper respiratory tract (especially otitis media) are at times associated with diarrhea, although the actual mechanism remains obscure. In the opinion of several investigators, a concomitant intestinal infection is likely.

C. Malnutrition: Malnutrition may lead to diarrhea because of an increased occurrence of enteral infections in malnourished children. Decreased disaccharidase activity, altered motility, or changes in the intestinal flora may be other factors.

D. Diet: Dietary causes of diarrhea are numerous. Overfeeding of a colicky infant is a common example. Introduction of new foods such as fruit juices, egg yolk, vegetables, etc can cause diarrhea. Intestinal irritants (spices and foods high in roughage) are also frequent offenders.

E. Allergic Diarrhea: Diarrhea caused by gastrointestinal allergy to dietary proteins is a frequently entertained diagnosis but a poorly documented clinical entity.

Intractable Diarrhea of Early Infancy

A. Symptoms and Signs: The onset is within the first 3 months of life. The benign initial phase is sometimes mistaken for a feeding problem. In most cases,

however, it mimics an infectious diarrhea with loose, greenish stools. The stools are rarely grossly bloody, but microscopic blood is often present. Vomiting and abdominal distention are other features. Dehydration, acidosis, and malnutrition rapidly supervene. After "resting the gastrointestinal tract" by means of intravenous therapy, resumption of oral feedings invariably precipitates a recurrence.

B. Diagnosis: Conditions such as Hirschsprung's disease, enterocolitis, cystic fibrosis, intestinal stenosis, malrotation, blind loop syndrome, short small bowel syndrome, allergic gastroenteropathy, celiac disease, disaccharidase deficiency, immunologic defects, lymphangiectasia, adrenogenital syndrome, sepsis, urinary tract infections, and chloridorrhea may all lead to intractable diarrhea. These diagnoses and infectious gastroenteritis can be verified or ruled out by the following emergency work-up:

(1) Stool cultures (3).

(2) Stool pH.

(3) Tests for fecal blood and reducing substances.

(4) Barium enema, upper gastrointestinal x-ray with small bowel follow-through.

(5) Blood count with small lymphocyte count.

(6) Blood pH and electrolytes.

(7) Sweat chloride test.

(8) Stool chymotrypsin.

(9) Protein electrophoresis and serum immuno-globulins.

(10) Rectosigmoidoscopy and rectal suction biopsy.

If these conditions are ruled out in a young infant who still has diarrhea after 3 weeks and is steadily losing weight, a primary type of intractable diarrhea (nonspecific enterocolitis) becomes the most likely diagnosis.

C. Treatment: Fasting is recommended during the first few days while blood volume, electrolyte, and acid-base disturbances are repaired. A diet free of milk, proteins, and lactose is then recommended. Good success has been achieved with the following formula:

R	Calcium caseinate (Casec) powder	50.0
	Corn oil emulsion (Lipomul-Oral)	58.0
	Medium chain triglyceride oil	10.0
	Fructose	60.0
	Water, qs ad	1200.0

If a favorable response is not obtained, small doses of corticosteroids can be tried—eg, prednisone, 2.5 mg 3 times daily. In most cases, however, parenteral alimentation (see Chapter 4) for a period of 4 weeks appears to be the only solution.

Hyman CJ & others: Parenteral and oral alimentation in the treatment of the nonprotracted diarrheal syndrome of infancy. J Pediat 78:17–29, 1971.

Silverman A, Roy CC, Cozzetto F: Chapter 8 in: *Pediatric Clinical Gastroenterology.* Mosby, 1971.

CONSTIPATION

Constipation is the regular passage of firm or hard stools or of small, hard masses at extremely long intervals (obstipation). In its most severe form, it may be accompanied by fecal soiling or encopresis. Familial, cultural, and social factors influence the genesis, development, and course. Some children with constipation tend to absorb water from the rectum to a greater degree than control subjects. A few babies are constipated in the neonatal period and remain so despite a variety of formula changes. Psychologic factors, toilet training technics, diet (particularly excessive milk intake), overuse of laxatives, and enemas may also influence bowel habits.

Clinical Findings

Many symptoms, such as fever, convulsions, nervousness, school failure, bad breath, and the like have been improperly attributed to constipation.

A. Simple Constipation: The neonate or the infant often appears to be having difficulty passing a stool. His face may turn red, and the legs are drawn up on the abdomen even when the stool passed is quite soft. This pattern may be erroneously considered to be an indication of constipation. Similarly, the infant 6–12 months of age may become flushed, withdraw his legs, and act as though he is having a great deal of difficulty in passing a bowel movement when in fact he may be attempting to withhold a stool. Failure to appreciate this normal developmental pattern may lead to the unwise use of laxatives or enemas. As the child becomes ambulatory, many new and exciting activities interfere with his response to the "call to stool"; he may pass enough stool to relieve the pressure while continuing to play, or may gradually develop an effective capacity to ignore the sensation of rectal fullness. In the older child, school, games, social events, and such aesthetic factors as inadequately cleaned toilets outside the home may all interfere with the development of any pattern of regularity.

B. Constipation With Encopresis: The constant or intermittent involuntary seepage of feces is characteristic of psychogenic constipation, where there is a mass of feces in the rectal ampulla and sigmoid colon. Emotional problems lead to psychogenic constipation and not uncommonly disappear with relief of the constipation.

Differential Diagnosis

Constipation is prevalent among mentally retarded children, particularly those with associated motor deficits. Hypothyroidism is frequently accompanied by constipation, but constipation is usually not the presenting complaint. Stenosis of the anal canal and anal fissure are among the local conditions which must be ruled out.

Distinguishing features from Hirschsprung's disease are summarized in Table 16–2.

Treatment

A. Simple Constipation: High-residue foods such as bran, whole wheat, fruits, and vegetables may be helpful. The use of a barley malt extract such as Maltsupex, 1–2 tsp added to feedings 2 or 3 times daily, is helpful in small infants. Stool softeners such as dioctyl sodium sulfosuccinate (Colace), 5–10 mg/kg/day, prevent excessive drying of the stool and are effective

TABLE 16–2. Differentiation of constipation and Hirschsprung's disease.

	Constipation	Hirschsprung's Disease
Onset	2–3 years	At birth
Abdominal distention	Rarely	Present
Nutritional growth	Normal	Poor
Soiling	Intermittent or constant	Never
Rectal examination	Ampulla full	Ampulla empty

unless there is voluntary stool retention. Cathartics such as senna, 1/2—1 tsp twice daily, can be used for short periods of time.

B. Constipation With Encopresis: Remove the fecal impaction by the administration of hypertonic phosphate enemas (Fleet Enema) after overnight retention of 3—4 oz mineral oil.

Mineral oil in orange juice should be given in amounts sufficient initially (15 ml 3—5 times a day) to lead to incontinence; it should then be reduced so that 4—5 loose stools are passed daily.

The prevention of stool holding and the establishment of a regular soft bowel movement pattern is accomplished by "toileting" the child at regular times each day and by the continued administration of mineral oil over a period of several months in a reduced dosage. Recurrence can be prevented by dietary measures and the occasional use of a laxative. A double dose of water-soluble vitamins is recommended while mineral oil is administered.

Psychiatric consultation may be indicated in cases with recurrent symptoms and in those where there are overt, severe emotional disturbances.

Mercer RD: Constipation. P Clin North America 14:175—185, 1967.

Silber DL: Encopresis: Discussion of etiology and management. Clin Pediat 8:225—231, 1969.

RECTAL BLEEDING

The passage by an infant of bright red or dark blood unrelated to, on the surface of, or mixed with the stool strongly suggests Meckel's diverticulum, intussusception, midgut volvulus, or, more rarely, stress peptic ulcer. Rectal bleeding in children under age 12 is most commonly due to rectal fissure or polyps of the rectum and colon.

TABLE 16—3. Differential diagnosis and treatment of rectal bleeding in infants and children.

Cause	Usual Age Group	Additional Complaints	Amount of Blood	Color of Blood	Blood With Movement	Treatment
Swallowed foreign body	Any age	Usually none	Small	Dark	Yes	Surgery may be necessary.
Systemic bleeding	Any age	Other evidence of bleeding.	Variable	Dark or bright	Yes or no	As indicated.
Hemorrhagic disease of the newborn	Newborn	Other evidence of bleeding.	Variable	Dark or bright	Yes or no	Vitamin K_1, transfusion.
Allergy (milk)	Infants	Colicky abdominal pain.	Moderate to large	Dark or bright	Yes	Eliminate allergen.
Esophageal varices	>4 years	Signs of portal hypertension.	Variable	Usually dark	Yes	Medical initially; sometimes emergency surgery.
Hemangioma or familial telangiectasia	Any age	Often telangiectasia elsewhere.	Variable	Dark or bright	Yes or no	Usually none.
Peptic ulcer	Any age	Abdominal pain.	Usually small; can be massive.	Dark	Yes	Bland diet.
Duplication of bowel	Any age	Variable.	Usually small	Usually dark	Yes	Surgery.
Meckel's diverticulum	Young adult	None or anemia.	Small to large; usually large.	Dark or bright	Yes or no	Surgery.
Volvulus	Infant or young child	Abdominal pain, intestinal obstruction.	Small to large	Dark or bright	Yes or no	Surgery.
Intussusception	<18 months	Abdominal pain, mass.	Small to large	Dark or bright	Yes	Surgery.
Ulcerative colitis	>4 years	Diarrhea, cramps.	Small to large	Usually bright	Yes	Usually medical.
Bacterial enteritis	Any age	Diarrhea, cramps.	Small to large	Usually bright	Yes	Medical.
Polyp	2—8 years	None.	Small to large	Bright	No	Surgery.
Inserted foreign body	Child	Pain.	Small	Bright	No	Removal.
Anal fissure or proctitis	<2 years	Pain.	Small	Bright	No	Soften stool, anal dilatation, habit training.
Swallowed maternal blood	Newborn	None.	Variable	Dark	Yes	None.
Hiatus hernia	Any age	Dysphagia, hematemesis.	Usually small	Dark	Yes	Medical or surgical.

The evaluation of the child who is passing small quantities of blood for several days, weeks, or even months includes a gastrointestinal series, proctosigmoidoscopy, barium enema, and bleeding and clotting studies. Surgery must be considered only if the bleeding is severe and repetitive.

For differential diagnosis and treatment, see Table 16–3.

Brayton D: Gastrointestinal bleeding of unknown origin. Am J Dis Child 107:288–292, 1964.
Shanding B: Laparotomy for rectal bleeding. Pediatrics 35:787–790, 1965.
Spencer R: Gastrointestinal hemorrhage: Review of 473 cases. Surgery 55:718–734, 1964.

RECURRENT ABDOMINAL PAIN

In one survey, one out of 9 unselected school children had experienced at least 3 attacks of recurrent abdominal pain severe enough to affect their activities over a period longer than 3 months. An organic cause can be found in fewer than 10% of cases, and there is usually evidence that the pain is a reaction to emotional stress. The age at onset is usually between 5 and 10 years. The incidence in boys is slightly higher than in girls.

Clinical Findings

A. Symptoms and Signs: Recurrent attacks of umbilical or periumbilical pain last less than 24 hours, usually only about an hour. There may be associated pallor, nausea, vomiting, and slight fever. The pain seldom radiates. An organic cause is suggested by a change in the pattern of the attack, a negative history of colic as a baby, diarrhea, vomiting in infancy, and absence of associated emotional problems or a family history of migraine. The farther the pain is from the umbilicus, the more likely it is that an organic cause will be found. Emotional disturbances are common, with undue fears, enuresis, sleeping problems, food dislikes, and difficulties in school. It is necessary to examine the patient thoroughly both between attacks and during an attack.

The pain bears little relationship with bowel habits and activity. At times, it may occur during meals or before the child leaves for school. A definite precipitating or particularly stressful situation in the child's life at the time the pains began can sometimes be elicited. A history of functional gastrointestinal complaints and migraine headaches is found in the family members of a large number of "little bellyachers."

A thorough physical examination is essential. Abdominal tenderness, if present, is diffuse and mild, although discomfort over the descending colon is common.

B. Laboratory and X-Ray Findings: Complete blood count, sedimentation rate, urinalysis, stool test for occult blood, and tuberculin testing usually suffice. If the syndrome is somewhat atypical, urine cultures, intravenous urography, voiding cystography, barium enema, and upper gastrointestinal x-rays should be done.

Differential Diagnosis

Organic causes relating to the urinary and gastrointestinal tracts, as well as extra-abdominal causes, should be ruled out by appropriate studies if the clinical evidence is suggestive. Oxyuriasis, "mesenteric lymphadenitis," and "chronic appendicitis" are improbable causes of recurrent abdominal pain.

Treatment & Prognosis

Treatment consists of reassurance based on a thorough physical appraisal and a frank and sympathetic explanation of the emotional basis. More specialized therapy for the latter is sometimes required, but drugs should be avoided.

The prognosis is good.

Apley J: *The Child With Abdominal Pain.* Blackwell, 1964.
Stone RT, Barbero GJ: Recurrent abdominal pain in childhood. Pediatrics 45:732–738, 1970.

THE MALABSORPTION SYNDROMES

The majority of diseases causing malabsorption are diseases of the small intestine or conditions which affect its normal function. Not only should the small bowel be of sufficient length, but the mucosal surface area available for absorption must not be decreased beyond a certain minimum. Anatomic abnormalities and impaired motility of the small intestine will not only interfere with normal propulsive movements and mixing of food with pancreatic and biliary secretions; it can also lead to an altered bacterial flora, which may cause malabsorption. Impairment of portal venous return, anoxia, and lymphatic abnormalities are well described causes of malabsorption. Diseases interfering with pancreatic exocrine function and with the production and flow of biliary secretions can have the same effect. Other causes include disaccharidase deficiency, glucose-galactose malabsorption, abetalipoproteinemia, malnutrition, endocrine conditions, immune deficiencies, and emotional factors (maternal deprivation). Many others are listed in the references cited at the end of this section.

Clinical Findings

The chronologic sequence of events is of great importance in determining the onset of malabsorption problems and the relationship between symptoms and the introduction of various nutrients. Gastrointestinal symptoms such as diarrhea, vomiting, anorexia, abdominal pain, and bloating are not always present, and the presenting complaints may not refer to the gastrointestinal tract. Certain physical features such as the pot belly and the wasted buttocks may indicate celiac disease. Personal observation of the stools for abnormal color, consistency, bulkiness, odor, mucus, and blood is important. In general, the investigation of this complex syndrome involves both accurate clinical appraisal and the interpretation of appropriate laboratory data.

The following is a list of the most helpful investigations:

(1) Fat absorption: Seventy-two-hour fecal fat excretion, serum carotene and cholesterol, prothrombin time.

(2) Protein absorption: Serum protein electrophoresis, fecal nitrogen, fecal excretion of chromated Cr 51 serum albumin (Chromalbin).

(3) Carbohydrate absorption: Glucose tolerance test, D-xylose absorption test, disaccharide absorption test, stool pH and reducing substances.

(4) Absorption of folic acid and vitamin B_{12}: Schilling test, serum levels of folic acid and vitamin B_{12}.

(5) Bacteriology: Stool, duodenal juice.

(6) X-ray studies: Upper gastrointestinal series with small bowel follow-through, barium enema.

(7) Sweat test: Chloride determination.

(8) Pancreatic exocrine function: Duodenal aspirate examined for volume, viscosity, pH, bicarbonate, trypsin, lipase, and amylase activity.

(9) Liver function tests: Bilirubin, transaminases, alkaline phosphatase, sulfobromophthalein (BSP) excretion.

(10) Miscellaneous: Peroral small bowel biopsy, rectosigmoidoscopy and rectal biopsy, immunoglobulin levels, lipoprotein electrophoresis, urine catecholamines, endocrine function tests.

Treatment & Prognosis

See specific syndromes—celiac disease, disaccharidase deficiency, etc.

Anderson CM: Intestinal malabsorption in childhood. Arch Dis Childhood 41:571–596, 1966.

Eisenstadt HB: The malabsorption state: A review. Am J Gastroenterol 46:230–237, 1966.

Weser E, Jeffries GH, Sleisenger MH: Malabsorption. Gastroenterology 50:811–828, 1966.

PROTEIN-LOSING ENTEROPATHIES

Excessive loss of plasma proteins into the gastrointestinal tract occurs in association with a number of disorders, some of which are listed below.

Disorders Associated With Protein-Losing Enteropathy

A. Cardiac: Congestive heart failure, constrictive pericarditis, atrial septal defect, primary myocardial disease.

B. Gastric: Giant hypertrophic gastritis (Menetrier's disease).

C. Small Intestine: Celiac disease, intestinal lymphangiectasia, tropical sprue, regional enteritis, Whipple's disease, lymphosarcoma, acute gastrointestinal infection, allergic gastroenteropathy, blind loop syndrome, abetalipoproteinemia, chronic volvulus.

D. Colon: Ulcerative colitis, Hirschsprung's disease.

E. Immunologic deficiency states.

Clinical Findings

The clinical signs and symptoms identified with protein-losing enteropathies are many. These include edema, chylous ascites, poor weight gain, deficiencies of fat-soluble vitamins, hypochromic anemia, or megaloblastic anemia secondary to vitamin B_{12} or folic acid malabsorption. Most patients present with severe and long-standing gastrointestinal symptomatology. Although there is nonselective "bulk loss" of a number of plasma proteins into the enteric lumen, albumin is the most depressed of the plasma proteins and is usually below 2.5 gm/100 ml. A number of methods are available for the detection of increased catabolism of plasma proteins and their quantitation in the gut, but all have certain drawbacks. Normally, the gut probably plays only a minor role in albumin catabolism, and enhanced intestinal losses of protein are solely responsible for the hypoalbuminemia that occurs in a number of conditions leading to protein-losing enteropathies. It is likely, however, that an increased rate of endogenous albumin catabolism or a decreased rate of synthesis may be operative in systemic diseases in which protein-losing enteropathies occur. The simultaneous use of iodinated I 125 serum albumin to measure overall albumin catabolism and chromated Cr 51 serum albumin (Chromalbin) to measure gastrointestinal losses appears to be most informative.

Differential Diagnosis

Malnutrition as a cause of hypoproteinemia must be excluded. Since hypoalbuminemia may be due to either a lowered production or an increased catabolic rate, it is also important to rule out hepatic disease and to make certain that no significant proteinuria is present.

Treatment

Temporary benefits can be derived from plasma or albumin infusions in the presence of severe plasma loss and anasarca. Otherwise, treatment must be directed toward the primary underlying cause.

Kerr RM, Dubois JJ, Holt PR: Use of ^{125}I and ^{51}Cr labeled albumin for the measurement of gastrointestinal and total albumin metabolism. J Clin Invest 46:2064–2082, 1967.

Waldmann TA: Protein-losing enteropathy. Gastroenterology 50:422, 1966.

Wilson JF: Macromolecular aspects of protein absorption and excretion in the mammalian intestine. Report of the 50th Ross Conference on Pediatric Research. Ross Laboratories, 1965.

CELIAC DISEASE
(Gluten Enteropathy)

Essentials of Diagnosis

- Steatorrhea (fecal fat > 5 gm/day).
- Failure to thrive; loss of weight involving mostly the limbs and buttocks.
- Abdominal distention.
- Depressed rate of D-xylose absorption.
- Blunting of the intestinal villi on a small bowel biopsy.
- Improvement on gluten-free diet, and relapse within 2–3 days following reintroduction of gluten (10–30 gm daily) into the diet.
- Normal pancreatic and biliary secretions.

General Considerations

Celiac syndrome denotes the symptom complex resulting from intestinal malabsorption. Celiac disease is a specific disease entity associated with abnormal jejunal mucosa which improves with a strict gluten-free diet.

After cystic fibrosis, celiac disease is the most frequent cause of malabsorption in infants. Most cases present during the second year of life, but the age at onset and the severity are both variable. The disease is more common in Europe than in the USA and is uncommon in Negroes and Orientals. The basic defect is thought to consist of an enzyme deficiency in small bowel mucosal cells leading to incomplete hydrolysis of the water-insoluble protein fraction of wheat, rye, and oats. Experimentally, gliadin, the alcohol-soluble fraction of gluten, has been shown to inhibit peristalsis in vitro and to precipitate symptoms and typical pathologic changes in susceptible individuals. Peptic and tryptic digestion of gliadin does not abolish its harmful effects. The polypeptide products of the peptic and tryptic digestion of gliadin have a molecular weight between 838 and 928 and contain 6 or 7 amino acids, largely proline and glutamine. Since incubation of gliadin with normal intestinal mucosa renders it innocuous to patients with celiac disease, it is suggested that the peptidases responsible for the peptidolysis of the products of tryptic digestion of gliadin are absent. The polypeptides accumulate in the intestinal cells and lead to morphologic changes and alterations in motility patterns. Recently, coproantibodies to gluten have been found in celiac patients, but whether or not they have pathogenetic significance is an unsettled question.

Clinical Findings

A. Symptoms and Signs:

1. Diarrhea—Affected children often present with a history of digestive disturbances starting at 6–12 months of age—corresponding to the age at which wheat, rye, or oat glutens are first fed. Initially, the diarrhea may be intermittent and related to upper respiratory infections. Subsequently, it is continuous, with voluminous, bulky, pale, frothy, greasy, offensive floating stools. During celiac crises, dehydration, shock, and acidosis are commonly seen.

2. Failure to thrive—The onset of diarrhea is usually accompanied by loss of appetite, failure to gain weight, and increased irritability.

3. Wasting and retardation of growth—In established cases, there is a loss of weight which is most marked in the limbs and buttocks. Characteristically, the face remains plump and the abdomen becomes distended secondary to a poor musculature and, more importantly, to accumulation of gas in the hypotonic intestinal tract with altered peristaltic activity.

4. Anemia and vitamin deficiencies—Anemia is usually present; it is often unresponsive to iron and may be megaloblastic. Deficiencies in fat-soluble vitamins are common. Rickets can be seen when growth has not been completely halted by the disease; however, osteomalacia is more common, and pathologic fractures may occur. Hypoprothrombinemia can be severe, and some patients are known to present with severe intestinal hemorrhages.

B. Laboratory Findings:

1. Fat content of stools—A 3-day collection of stools for fat reveals more than 5 gm/day of fecal fat. It is important that a nonabsorbable marker, such as charcoal or brilliant blue, be given for accurate collection. A normal child will absorb 90–98% of ingested fats. The untreated celiac patient, on the other hand, will not absorb more than 65–85% of his daily fat intake.

2. Impaired carbohydrate absorption—A low oral glucose tolerance curve is seen. Absorption of D-xylose is impaired, with a decrease in the 5-hour urine excretion.

3. Hypoproteinemia—Hypoalbuminemia can be severe enough to lead to edema. There is also evidence of increased losses of protein in the gut lumen.

C. X-Ray Findings:

A small bowel series will demonstrate a typical malabsorptive pattern characterized by segmentation and clumping of the barium column. These changes can be accentuated by addition of gluten to the barium meal.

D. Biopsy Findings:

Peroral intestinal biopsy provides the most reliable evidence for the diagnosis of celiac disease. It is a safe and simple procedure even in infants. Hypoprothrombinemia and severe malnutrition, however, are absolute contraindications to this procedure.

A variety of biopsy capsules are available. The Carey capsule is the least likely to cause bleeding and perforation in debilitated infants.

Under the dissecting microscope, the jejunal mucosa presents a "crazy paving" appearance rather than the slender finger-like projections which characterize normal villi. Under the light microscope, the celiac mucosa is readily recognized by amputation of the villi, by lengthening of the crypts of Lieberkühn, and by increased round cell infiltration of the lamina propria. These changes are reversible, and resumption of a normal to nearly normal appearance of the lamina propria can be expected after withdrawl of gluten from the diet.

Differential Diagnosis

The differential diagnosis must include all of the disorders that cause malabsorption. Strict adherence to certain criteria for the diagnosis of gluten enteropathy is helpful (see Essentials of Diagnosis).

Treatment

A. Diet: Treatment consists of dietary gluten restriction for life. However, successful management is not so dependent upon strict adherence to a rigid dietary plan as upon judicious supervision of the diet by a physician who individualizes management according to age, the severity of the illness, and the patient's needs and responses. The diet should provide 25% more calories than calculated for expected weight plus 6–8 gm/kg/day of protein. Lactose is poorly tolerated in the acute stage since the extensive mucosal damage leads to acquired disaccharidase deficiency. Normal amounts of fat are advisable.

In treating a severely affected child, the diet should be tailored to the child's appetite and capacity to absorb. A full gluten-free diet can usually be given after 2–3 weeks. Clinical improvement is usually evident within a week but may take up to 6 months.

B. Corticosteroids: Adrenal corticosteroid therapy can produce dramatic remissions in celiac disease. Corticosteroids are particularly useful in celiac crises and for patients who continue to deteriorate despite the enforcement of a strict gluten-free diet.

Gluten-Free Diet
(All possible sources of wheat, rye, or oats must be eliminated.)

Foods Allowed

Milk and cream	Fruit and fruit juices
Cheese	Cereals: Cornflakes,
Eggs	corn meal, puffed
Meat, fish, and poul-	rice, or precooked
try (unless bread-	gluten-free cereal
ed or creamed)	Soups: All clear soups
Vegetables	Bread: Made from rice,
	corn, or gluten-free
	wheat flour

Foods to Be Avoided

All breads, rolls,	Commercial ice cream
crackers, cakes,	Prepared mixes and
and cookies made	puddings
from wheat or	Postum, Ovaltine,
rye	some instant coffees
All wheat and rye	Beer and ale
cereals, spaghetti,	Commercial candies
macaroni, and	containing cereal
noodles	products
All canned soups ex-	
cept clear broth	

Prognosis

Death due to celiac disease is unusual. Improvement and clinical recovery are the rule. However, disappearance of symptoms can be a protracted, intermittent process. The course may be characterized by periods of rapid improvement and dramatic exacerbations since the potential for the disease always persists. It would appear, however, that the disease tends to partially or completely remit in later childhood even if left untreated.

Hamilton JR, Lynch MJ, Reilly B Jr: Active celiac disease in childhood. Quart J Med 38:135–158, 1969.

Herskovic T & others: Coproantibodies to gluten in celiac disease. JAMA 203:887–888, 1968.

Sheldon W: Prognosis in early adult life of celiac children treated with a gluten-free diet. Brit MJ 2:401–404, 1969.

DISACCHARIDASE DEFICIENCY

Essentials of Diagnosis

- Watery diarrhea, explosive and frothy.
- Stool pH < 5.5.
- Reducing substances present in stools and often in urine.
- Flat glucose tolerance test following disaccharide loading.
- Quantitative decrease or complete absence of disaccharidase activity in intestinal biopsy.

General Considerations

Carbohydrates provide a substantial proportion of the human diet. The polysaccharide starch and the disaccharides sucrose and lactose are quantitatively the most important and require hydrolysis before significant absorption can take place. The accompanying scheme summarizes the digestion sequence of the common polysaccharides and disaccharides.

Disaccharidases are localized in the brush border of the intestinal epithelial cells. Absolute levels are higher in the jejunum and in the proximal ileum than in the distal ileum and in the duodenum. Some substrates can be hydrolyzed by more than one enzyme, and, conversely, some enzymes act on more than one substrate. There are 4 enzymes with maltase activity: IA, IB, II, and III. Maltase IA contributes about 50% of total maltase activity but also has some isomaltase activity. Maltase IB contributes about 25% of total maltase activity but also has some sucrase activity.

Disaccharidase deficiencies are either primary or secondary. In the primary or genetically determined form, the enzyme deficit is isolated, the disaccharide intolerance is likely to persist throughout life, intestinal histology is normal, and a family history is common.

Since disaccharidases are confined to the outer cell layer of the intestinal epithelium, they are very

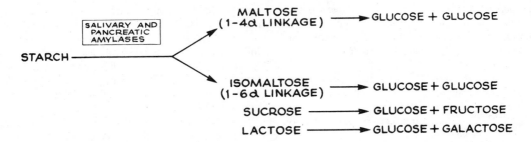

susceptible to mucosal damage. A number of conditions are now known to give rise to the secondary type of disaccharidase deficiency, which is transient and involves a quantitative decrease in all enzymes although lactose intolerance is by far the most common. Histologic examination reveals changes compatible with the underlying disorder. A familial incidence in these cases is uncommon.

Clinical Findings

A. Primary (Congenital):

1. Lactase—Congenital lactase deficiency is a rare condition leading to diarrhea soon after lactose is ingested. A recessive type of inheritance is likely, but this has not been definitely established. Diarrhea is the predominant symptom. The stools are frothy and acid; their pH may fall as low as 4.5 due to a high content of organic acids which stimulate intestinal peristalsis. The osmotic action of unhydrolyzed lactose leads to osmotic catharsis. Vomiting is not uncommon. Severe malnutrition may occur. Reducing substances are usually present in the stools, and lactosuria is a prominent feature. Infants with lactosuria, aminoaciduria, proteinuria, acidosis, and elevated BUN have been described. It is not clear how these other abnormalities are related to lactose intolerance. An oral lactose tolerance test (2 gm/kg) in an infant suspected of the disease and from whose diet lactose has been withdrawn is likely to result in symptoms of intolerance within 8 hours, and the glucose blood levels will show no appreciable rise. If the symptoms are delayed for some time after beginning lactose intake, it is necessary to exclude small intestinal mucosal damage that may cause secondary lactase deficiency; this may be done by means of small bowel biopsy, which also permits direct estimation of the disaccharidase.

Patients respond to the exclusion of lactose from their diet, but over a period of several months most children acquire a tolerance for lactose and eventually show normal lactase levels.

2. Sucrase and isomaltase deficiency—This is a combined defect which is inherited as an autosomal recessive trait. Diarrhea usually occurs only when sucrose is fed. Abdominal distention, failure to thrive, and toilet training difficulties in association with chronic diarrhea may be the presenting symptoms. Since sucrase-isomaltase deficiencies have been found in siblings who had few or no symptoms, it is likely that a number of persons with this trait—particularly adults—remain unrecognized.

In making a diagnosis by estimating reducing substances in the stools, it is important to remember that sucrose is not a reducing sugar. The usual 5 drops of stool and 10 drops of water added to a Clinitest tablet will not give a positive reaction unless 1 N HCl is substituted for the water and the mixture allowed to boil for a few seconds before adding the tablet. A sucrose tolerance test (2 gm/kg) is likely to be flat. As with lactose, a number of gastric and extra-intestinal factors can account for very poor blood glucose rises. It is wise, therefore, to check the stools for the presence of sucrose and to follow the sucrose tolerance test by a glucose tolerance test. Shock may occur due to osmotic water losses in some patients with lactase or sucrase-isomaltase deficiency with a standard dose of the disaccharide for the tolerance test. In sucrase-isomaltase deficiency, exclusion of sucrose is usually sufficient. Starch intolerance is rarely a problem, since the 1–6 linkages of starch hydrolyzed by isomaltase comprise only a small proportion of the whole molecule.

B. Secondary (Acquired):

1. Secondary lactase deficiency—Diarrhea may be produced in normal individuals if a large dose of lactose is ingested. The threshold for lactose tolerance is usually much lower than that for sucrose. Lactose intolerance develops spontaneously in a certain number of children and adults. There is a high prevalence of this form of disease in certain racial groups (70% in American Negroes). Disaccharidase deficiency has been described in association with many different disorders. Neomycin and kanamycin administration have been shown to reduce lactase activity in adults. The list of conditions associated with secondary lactase deficiency includes celiac disease, giardiasis, kwashiorkor, viral or bacterial gastroenteritis, abetalipoproteinemia, cystic fibrosis, immunoglobulin deficiencies, extensive intestinal resections, and regional enteritis.

2. Secondary sucrase deficiency—Intestinal mucosal damage tends to lower the levels of all disaccharidases. Signs of sucrose intolerance are usually masked by the more striking symptoms related to lactose. Infectious diarrhea is the most frequent cause of secondary sucrose intolerance.

Treatment

A. Lactose-Free Diet: Use a proprietary milk formula which does not contain lactose, eg, Nutramigen, meat base, or soybean formulas. Exclude foods containing whey, dry milk solids, and curds. It is important to see if labels indicate any lactose content, particularly with canned puréed baby foods. Cheeses (cottage, cheddar, cream), ice cream, sherbet, and chocolate milk powders should be avoided.

B. Sucrose-Restricted Diet:

1. **Foods allowed**—The diet described here does contain small amounts of sucrose which are usually well tolerated.

> Milk, cream, butter, cheese, salad and cooking oils
> Eggs, meat, fish
> Homemade bread and pastries containing dextrose
> Asparagus, broccoli, brussels sprouts, cucumbers, spinach, tomatoes, lettuce
> Grapes, cherries, strawberries,cranberries, blackberries
> Potatoes
> Homemade ice cream, diet carbonated beverages, diet Kool-Aid, gelatin desserts, unsweetened cocoa, vegetable juices

2. **Foods to be avoided**—

> Fruits and vegetables not included in the above list, especially peas, beans, and lentils
> Kool-Aid, carbonated beverages
> Jam, honey, jelly, candy, molasses, maple syrup
> Commercial ice cream, pies, cookies, cakes
> Breakfast cereals
> Medicines made up in syrup

Prognosis

In the primary type, the enzyme deficiency is theoretically a lifelong defect. However, in both lactase and sucrase deficiencies, tolerance for the offending disaccharide tends to increase with age. The prognosis in the secondary or acquired forms of disaccharidase deficiency is that of the underlying illness. It is important to remember that normal tolerance for lactose may not be regained until many months after an acute mucosal injury, eg, acute gastroenteritis.

Gray GM: Carbohydrate digestion and absorption. Gastroenterology 58:96–107, 1970.
Townley RW: Disaccharidase deficiency in infancy and childhood. Pediatrics 38:127–141, 1966.

GLUCOSE-GALACTOSE MALABSORPTION

Chronic diarrhea indistinguishable from that due to intestinal disaccharide deficiency may be due to a genetic defect in monosaccharide malabsorption. The diarrhea relates to the osmotic effect of the nonabsorbed hexose. A decreased maximal rate of tubular reabsorption of glucose is often associated with the intestinal cell transport defect.

Diarrhea starting within a few days after birth constitutes the cardinal feature. It is usually severe and

can be life-threatening. Small bowel histology is normal. Glycosuria and aminoaciduria may occur. The glucose tolerance test is flat and precipitates symptoms. Fructose is well tolerated. The diarrhea promptly subsides on withdrawal of glucose and galactose from the diet. The stool pH is not so acid as that reported in disaccharidase deficiencies; fecal reducing substances are consistently found.

Initially, total exclusion from the diet of glucose and galactose is mandatory. A satisfactory formula consists of calcium caseinate, corn oil, and fructose.

The prognosis is good if the disease is diagnosed early, since tolerance for glucose and galactose improves with age.

Eggemont E, Loeb H: Glucose-galactose intolerance. Lancet 2:343–344, 1966.
Meeuwisse GW, Melin K: Studies in glucose-galactose malabsorption. Acta paediat scandinav Suppl 188, 1969.

INTESTINAL LYMPHANGIECTASIA

This form of protein-losing enteropathy results from a congenital abnormality of the lymphatic system and is associated with lymphatic aberrations in the extremities. Obstruction to lymphatic drainage of the intestine leads to rupture of intestinal lacteals with leakage of lymph into the lumen of the bowel. Fat loss may be significant and lead to steatorrhea. Chronic loss of lymphocytes and of immunoglobulins is usual and increases the susceptibility to infections.

Clinical Findings

Peripheral edema, diarrhea, abdominal distention, lymphedematous extremities, and repeated infections are common. Laboratory findings are low serum albumin, decreased immunoglobulin levels, lymphocytopenia, and anemia. Serum calcium is frequently depressed, and stool fat may be elevated. Lymphocytes may be seen in large numbers on a stool smear. Albumin turnover studies confirm the gastrointestinal protein loss. X-ray studies reveal an edematous small bowel mucosal pattern, and biopsy reveals dilated lacteals in the villi.

Differential Diagnosis

Other causes of protein-losing enteropathy must be considered, although an associated lymphedematous extremity strongly favors this diagnosis.

Complications & Sequelae

Failure to thrive, tetany, and frequent infections are the common complications of this disease. Extremity lymphedema may be disfiguring since it leads to increased bone growth and hemihypertrophy.

Treatment

Surgery is needed when the lesion is localized to a small area of the bowel or in cases of constrictive pericarditis or obstructing tumors. This may include saphenous vein peritoneal anastomosis in intractable cases.

Medium chain triglycerides as a fat source may reduce the intestinal lymphatic pressure by eliminating long chain fats from the diet. Water-soluble vitamin and calcium supplements and gamma globulin injections may be indicated. Antibiotics are used for specific infections. Corticosteroids should be avoided.

Prognosis

The prognosis at present is not favorable, although dietary manipulations have had dramatic results in some cases.

Herskovic T & others: Hypoproteinemia in intestinal lymphangiectasia. Pediatrics 40:345–353, 1967.
Shimkin PM, Waldmann TA, Krugman RL: Intestinal lymphangiectasia. Am J Roentgenol 110:827–841, 1970.

ALLERGIC GASTROENTEROPATHY
(Milk Allergy)

The gastrointestinal manifestations of milk allergy in infancy are usually mild, consisting of diarrhea and vomiting after milk ingestion, with guaiac-positive stools. Hypoproteinemia is present as a result of the protein-losing enteropathy, and hypochromic anemia secondary to intestinal blood loss. Other manifestations include failure to thrive, chronic fatigue, and low levels of serum albumin and globulin.

A more complete discussion of food allergy is presented in Chapter 33.

Isotope studies show intestinal losses of albumin and red blood cells, but absorption studies of fat, monosaccharides, and disaccharides are normal. X-rays show mucosal edema of the small bowel. Biopsies of the small intestine mucosa reveal either a normal morphology or an eosinophilic infiltrate of the lamina propria which is accompanied by a significant increase in circulating eosinophils.

The majority of patients have eczema, asthma, or allergic rhinitis.

There is a prompt response to removal of milk from the diet. Heat denaturation of the milk proteins may also suppress the fecal red cell losses, and corticosteroids can reverse the abnormal intestinal losses of protein.

The prognosis for the disappearance of the intestinal manifestations of milk allergy is excellent.

Waldman TA & others: Allergic gastroenteropathy. New England J Med 276:761–769, 1967.
Wilson JF, Lahey ME: Unifying concept for pathogenesis of syndrome of iron deficiency anemia, hypocupremia and hypoproteinemia in infants. J Clin Invest 44:11–12, 1965.

IMMUNOLOGIC DEFICIENCY STATES WITH DIARRHEA OR MALABSORPTION

It is now thought that both cellular and humoral immunity serve as a protective mechanism against invasion by pathogenic organisms and also probably prevent mucosal damage which could be caused by the normal intestinal flora.

Intermittent diarrhea is a frequent finding in immunoglobulin deficiency states, but the cause is usually obscure. It is uncommon to find pathogenic bacteria in the stools, but giardiasis is common. Fifty to 60% of idiopathic acquired hypogammaglobulinemics have steatorrhea and histologic changes consistent with the celiac syndrome. Lymphonodular hyperplasia is a common feature in this group of patients. Congenital or Bruton type agammaglobulinemics occasionally have abnormal intestinal morphology. Patients with isolated IgA deficiency have normal intestinal function but may also present with chronic diarrhea, a celiaclike picture, lymphoid nodular hyperplasia, and giardiasis. Patients with isolated cellular immunity defects or combined cellular and humoral immune incompetence all have severe chronic diarrhea leading to malnutrition. The cause of the diarrhea is unknown, and mucosal biopsies are normal. A high incidence of disaccharidase deficiency is associated with immunologic deficits in children.

Treatment must be directed at correction of the immunoglobulin defect. Gluten-free diets have been disappointing in most cases with villous atrophy. Tetracyclines have been effective in a few patients. In patients exhibiting disaccharidase deficiencies, dietary manipulations are helpful.

Bull DM, Tomasi TB: Deficiency of immunoglobulin A in intestinal disease. Gastroenterology 54:313, 1968.
Dubois RS & others: Disaccharidase deficiency in children with immunologic deficits. J Pediat 76:377–385, 1970.

CHRONIC ULCERATIVE COLITIS

Essentials of Diagnosis

- Rectal bleeding, bloody diarrhea, diarrhea with mucus or pus.
- Tenesmus and crampy abdominal pain.
- Extracolonic manifestations, fever, weight loss, retardation of growth, arthralgia, arthritis, mucocutaneous lesions, erythema nodosum, jaundice.
- Ragged mucosa with loss of haustral markings on barium enema.
- Acute inflammatory changes with crypt abscesses on rectal mucosal biopsy.

General Considerations

Ulcerative colitis is an acute or chronic relapsing disease of the mucosa and submucosa of varying lengths of the colon and rectum characterized by bloody stools, irregularly recurring fever, and many local or extracolonic signs and symptoms. It is not a rare disorder in children and has been reported in infants. Twenty percent of cases begin before the age of 20, with a peak between ages 10–19. Impairment of physical growth, delayed appearance of secondary sex characteristics, and the risk of carcinoma make this an important disease.

Rectal involvement is seen in more than 90% of cases. Emotional stress, diet, and infection may provoke relapses. An "autoimmune" basis for this disorder is suggested by the favorable response to local or systemic corticosteroid treatment, especially early in an attack.

Circulating antibodies to colon tissue have been found in about 15% of patients, but it is unlikely that these antibodies play a direct role in the pathogenesis of ulcerative colitis since their attachment to colonic cells cannot be demonstrated in vivo and they are not cytotoxic to colon cells in vitro. However, lymphocytes from patients are toxic to colonic cells obtained from both normal subjects and other patients with ulcerative colitis.

Clinical Findings

The diagnosis of ulcerative colitis is based upon a history of an acute onset of diarrhea or nonspecific gastroenteritis, the passage of bloody stools, abdominal cramping, tenesmus, fever, malaise, and anorexia. The onset may also be insidious, with a change in bowel habits from normal to constipation or continued constipation followed by the passage of blood, mucus, or pus. Less commonly the course is fulminating, with high septic fever, extreme prostration, anorexia, vomiting, and an almost continuous bloody diarrhea. In such cases, the threat of colonic perforation is great and emergency surgery is mandatory.

The extracolonic manifestations may be the presenting symptoms and signs, especially with arthralgia or arthritis (15–20%). This is usually monarticular and involves the major joints. Joint symptoms wax and wane with the remissions and exacerbations of the primary disease. Rarely, they precede the signs of bowel involvement by months or years. Other extracolonic findings are erythema nodosum, pyoderma gangrenosum, and liver disease, either with hepatic enlargement or with abnormalities in liver function studies for which no cause is readily apparent.

The diagnosis of ulcerative colitis is established by sigmoidoscopic examination revealing a hyperemic, friable, bleeding mucosa. Barium enema reveals the serrated edges indicating the location of the ulcers. In active or advanced colitis, there is also a loss of haustral markings and narrowing and shortening of the colon. Biopsy of the rectal mucosa reveals inflammatory cell infiltration and crypt abscesses and is particularly helpful in suggestive cases with negative sigmoidoscopic and radiologic findings.

Differential Diagnosis

Chronic ulcerative colitis must be differentiated from salmonella infections, allergic gastroenteropathy, lupus erythematosus, regional enteritis with colonic involvement (granulomatous ileocolitis), irritable colon syndrome, shigellosis, and amebiasis. The differentiation from shigellosis and amebiasis may be very difficult since these 2 conditions also give rise to crypt abscesses.

Complications

A. Local: With progression of the disease, ulcers within the mucosa may extend to the outer layers, leading to perforations which are occasionally free but which more commonly evolve slowly, resulting in the creation of internal fistulas with other loops of bowel or with an extra-intestinal organ such as the vagina. The chronic course interspersed with acute exacerbations leads to extensive fibrosis and consequently to colonic or rectal stricture. Between areas of fibrosis, mucosa becomes "heaped up" and gives rise to pseudopolyps. Massive hemorrhage is an uncommon complication, and toxic megacolon is very rare in children. Perianal fissures, abscesses, and fistulas occur.

B. Systemic: Arthritis, erythema nodosum, uveitis, and pyoderma gangrenosum may be seen. Retarded growth and chronic invalidism are almost always present. Fatty infiltration of the liver and, rarely, pericholangitis are seen in patients who have had the disease a long time. Sepsis and thromboembolic phenomena also occur.

The risk of carcinoma is about 10% after 10 years of the disease and increases to 25% after 20 years. The mortality rate from carcinoma is very high, so that prophylactic colectomy must always be considered in patients with long-standing disease.

Children with ulcerative colitis demonstrate considerably more disturbance of personality function than children suffering from other chronic diseases of the bowel. Studies have shown them to be emotionally fragile and to have increased dependency needs. Personality strength in affected children is inversely proportionate to the rapidity and severity of onset of the colitis and directly proportionate to the intensity of stress required to precipitate an exacerbation.

Treatment

No method of management has proved uniformly successful. The effectiveness of these measures must be individually determined and will further depend on the kind of relationship the physician has been able to establish with the patient, who is often apprehensive, emotionally immature, hostile, demanding, and depressed.

A. Diet: A high-protein, high-carbohydrate, high-vitamin, normal fat diet is recommended. The main concern should be in serving attractive meals that the child will eat. Restrictive or bland diets are not necessary, although during the first year of the disease, because of a high incidence (40%) of decreased lactase activity, a trial of a milk-free diet is indicated.

B. Antibiotics and Sulfonamides:

1. Antibiotics—Appropriate antibiotics may be indicated during the initial 4−7 days of an exacerbation if stool cultures are positive.

2. Salicylazosulfapyridine (Azulfidine)—This drug is effective acutely and is often useful in long-term therapy. It is relatively nonabsorbable and is said to have a high affinity for the submucosa. The response may be delayed for 1 week. Side-effects include nausea, rash, hemolytic anemia, and agranulocytosis. The dosage is as follows:

a. Children under 10 years of age—Give 0.5−1 gm every 6 hours as acute therapy. The maintenance dosage is 0.5−1 gm 2−3 times daily for 4−8 months.

b. Children over 10 years of age—Give 1−2 gm every 6 hours, followed by a maintenance schedule of 1−2 gm 2−3 times daily for 4−8 months.

C. Corticotropin and Corticosteroids: These drugs are usually restricted to life-threatening situations or to patients in whom salicylazosulfapyridine has not brought about any improvement. Complications of the chronic disease are not reduced by these agents, but emergency surgery is less often required and surgical mortality is therefore reduced.

1. Corticotropin—This drug is said to be superior to corticosteroids in the acute stage of the disease. This may relate to the poor absorption of corticosteroids when the disease is particularly acute. The usual dose of corticotropin is 40 units IV for 7−10 days, overlapping when possible with oral corticosteroids.

2. Corticosteroids—Give prednisone, 1−2 mg/kg orally daily for 2−3 weeks. The maintenance dose of prednisone is 5−20 mg daily. It can also be given on an alternate-day basis in conjunction with salicylazosulfapyridine.

Hydrocortisone retention enemas (Cortenema) are useful when the rectum is severely involved and has been effective also in the treatment of diseased areas in the transverse and descending colon.

D. Symptomatic Therapy: Opiates are useful for pain but should be used with caution because they may contribute to the development of toxic megacolon. Anticholinergic agents are indicated to reduce hypermotility of the bowel. Sedatives and tranquilizers can be used as required.

E. Psychotherapy: The need for a formal psychiatric referral must be individualized. It appears, however, that every patient would benefit from a coordinated psychiatric-pediatric-surgical team approach.

F. Surgical Measures: Emergency surgery is lifesaving in the case of fulminating disease with toxic megacolon. Surgery should also be done on an emergency basis in the presence of severe hemorrhage, perforation, or obstruction. Elective colectomy should be considered in all cases where medical treatment has been unsuccessful, especially in those with 10 years of disease regardless of their degree of incapacitation because of the climbing risk of cancer. This is especially so in patients with total involvement of the colon and in those whose disease has been continuous.

Since most patients undergo total proctocolectomy, the majority have an ileostomy, which is psychologically difficult for children to accept. Also, 25% of ileostomized patients have complications related to their ileostomy.

Prognosis

The overall prognosis for ulcerative colitis is guarded. Sixty percent survival has been reported after 20 years of the disease.

Rarely, the patient may expire during an acute fulminating attack of toxic ulcerative colitis (toxic megacolon).

Many children (30–40%) respond favorably to medical management and psychotherapy, doing well for months or years. These patients may have mild to moderate relapses, but on the whole they are able to lead a fruitful existence.

A group of patients (20–45%) whose symptoms continue despite medical therapy ultimately have one or more surgical procedures.

The patient may die of carcinoma, acute exsanguinating hemorrhage, perforation of the colon, or overwhelming sepsis.

Davidson M: Juvenile ulcerative colitis. New England J Med 277:1408–1410, 1967.

Ehrenpreis T: Surgical treatment of ulcerative colitis in children. Arch Dis Childhood 41:137–142, 1966.

Sadeghi-Nyad A, Senior B: The treatment of ulcerative colitis in children with alternate day corticosteroids. Pediatrics 43:840–845, 1969.

Tumen HJ, Valdes Dapna A, Haddad H: The indication for surgical intervention in ulcerative colitis in children. Am J Dis Child 116:641–651, 1968.

REGIONAL ENTERITIS
(Crohn's Disease)

Essentials of Diagnosis

- Fever, anemia, anorexia, weight loss.
- Crampy abdominal pain, diarrhea.
- Stunting of growth.
- Anal fistulas.
- X-ray evidence of thickened circular folds, cobblestoning, rigidity of the lumen, separation and fixation of loops, "string sign."
- Histologic demonstration of submucosal inflammation with fibrosis and of granulomatous lesions.

General Considerations

The terminal ileum is most commonly involved (80–98%), but any segment or combination of segments of the intestinal tract from stomach to anus may be affected, including the regional lymph nodes. The wall is thickened and rigid, with longitudinal mucosal ulcerations and fissures, submucosal thickening, or cobblestone formation. Sinus tracts and fistulas may be present. Areas of disease may be separated by lengths of normal appearing gut ("skip lesions"). Histologic features consist of a chronic granulomatous inflammatory reaction with edema and fibrosis involving all layers of the intestinal wall. The most useful diagnostic feature is the presence of noncaseating granulomas containing multinucleated giant cells and epithelioid cells. These focal lesions are found in 50% of cases; in another 25%, the inflammatory reaction is more diffuse. In cases where a nonspecific inflammatory process is reported, the diagnosis must be based on other criteria. The frequency of regional enteritis is equal to that of chronic ulcerative colitis in the pediatric age group, and its cause remains unknown. Occurrence of the disease in members of the same family and a significantly higher incidence among Jews suggest a genetic factor. Psychiatric studies of the disease have not disclosed any specific emotional makeup or cause.

Clinical Findings

A. Symptoms and Signs: Teenagers and young adults are most often afflicted. In certain instances, extra-intestinal symptoms such as arthritis, uveitis, stomatitis, erythema nodosum, unexplained fever, or failure to grow may be the presenting symptoms. Anal lesions may antedate the intestinal manifestations by a few years. Crampy abdominal pain, often triggered by food, is usually the predominant symptom. In most instances it is periumbilical, but it may localize in the right lower quadrant. Thus, in 1/3 of patients the symptoms may mimic an attack of acute appendicitis. Diarrhea is the presenting complaint in 1/3 of cases. Bloody diarrhea is less frequent than in ulcerative colitis. Anorexia, weight loss, fever, and anemia are found in the majority of patients and often precede the gastrointestinal complaints.

Sigmoidoscopy may be normal or may show diffuse involvement with lesions indistinguishable from those of ulcerative colitis.

B. Laboratory Findings: Routine laboratory studies contribute little to the diagnosis. Some degree of anemia is usually present. Megaloblastic anemia occurs as a consequence of vitamin B_{12} or folic acid malabsorption. Evidence for a protein-losing enteropathy may be documented by a decreased serum albumin concentration. Stool examination seldom reveals the presence of blood or pus, and cultures for infectious organisms are negative.

C. X-Ray Findings: X-ray examination should include both a small bowel series and a barium enema. When both ileum and colon are involved (granulomatous ileocolitis), the disease may resemble ulcerative colitis with backwash ileitis. However, the differentiation can usually be made on clinical, radiologic, pathologic, and therapeutic grounds.

Complications

Perforation and hemorrhage are rare. Intestinal obstruction, fistulas, and abscess formation and coexistent bowel malignancy have been reported. Malabsorption syndrome may be a serious complication, manifested by protein-losing enteropathy, disaccharidase deficiency, and bile salt induced diarrhea. Systemic complications include perianal disease, pyoderma gangrenosum, arthritis, amyloidosis, and a high incidence of severe growth retardation.

Treatment

Regional enteritis is not surgically remediable. In 33–50% of surgically treated cases, the disease will recur in previously grossly normal bowel. Recurrence at the site of anastomosis is most common; consequently, surgery is reserved for the intestinal complications of the disease such as obstruction, perforation, fistulas, and abscess formation. Recent evidence suggests that when the granulomatous process is limited to the colon (granulomatous colitis), resection may not be followed by involvement of previously intact small bowel.

Evaluation of medical regimens is made difficult by the spontaneous exacerbations and remissions so characteristic of this disease. The medical management is that of a long-term chronic illness, with goals directed toward relieving disability rather than achieving a cure.

A. Diet: Dietary management should center around providing the anorexic patient with a diet high in protein. Supplemental feedings and vitamin and iron supplementation should be encouraged.

B. Symptomatic Treatment: Rest is important when the disease is particularly active. Anxiety, depression, severe diarrhea, and pain can be treated with sedatives, tranquilizers, anticholinergic agents, and opiates or aspirin.

C. Antibiotics: Broad spectrum antibiotics may be helpful if there is evidence that malabsorption is partly due to significant upper small bowel bacterial contamination. Salicylazosulfapyridine is not thought to be as effective in regional enteritis as in ulcerative colitis.

D. Corticosteroids: Both short-term and chronic administration of corticosteroids is useful in control of symptoms, but the response is not so dramatic as in chronic ulcerative colitis. It is doubtful that steroids alter the course of the disease or prevent recurrences in surgically treated patients. In very sick patients, corticotropin may be halpful.

Prognosis

Although the mortality rate is low, the morbidity rate is high. The disease process is progressive in most cases, and its course is interspersed with both acute and chronic complications, leading to variable degrees of invalidism.

Janowitz HD, Present DH: Granulomatous colitis: Pathogenetic concepts. Gastroenterology 51:778–784, 1966.

Law DH: Regional enteritis. Gastroenterology 56:1086–1110, 1969.

Sparberg M, Kirsner, JB: Long term corticosteroid therapy for regional enteritis: An analysis of 58 courses in 54 patients. Am J Digest Dis 11:865–884, 1966.

Winkelman EI: Regional enteritis in adolescence. P Clin North America 14:141–164, 1967.

● ● ●

General References

Bockus HL: *Gastroenterology.* 3 vols. Saunders, 1963, 1964, 1965.

Davidson M: Pediatric gastrointestinal disorders. Chapter 43, pp 1150–1165, in: *Gastroenterologic Medicine.* Paulson M (editor). Lea & Febiger, 1969.

Michener WM (editor): Symposium on gastrointestinal disorders. P Clin North America 14:1–297, 1967.

Morin C, Davidson M: Pediatric gastroenterology. Gastroenterology 52:565, 713, 1967.

Sherlock S: The liver in infancy and childhood. Pages 518–546 in: *Diseases of the Liver and Biliary System.* Davis, 1968.

Silverberg M, Davidson M: Pediatric gastroenterology: A review. Gastroenterology 58:229, 1970.

Silverman A, Roy C, Cozzetto F: *Pediatric Clinical Gastroenterology.* Mosby, 1971.

17...
Liver & Pancreas

Arnold Silverman, MD, Claude Roy, MD, & Reuben S. Dubois, MB, BS

PROLONGED NONHEMOLYTIC NEONATAL JAUNDICE

1. NEONATAL HEPATITIS

Essentials of Diagnosis

- Prolonged neonatal jaundice.
- Hepatosplenomegaly.
- Demonstration of a patent intra- and extrahepatic biliary system.
- Histologic findings on liver biopsy.
- Family history.

General Considerations

Prolonged neonatal obstructive jaundice is most often due to hepatitis, biliary atresia, or sepsis. Hepatitis is the most common cause, accounting for about 50% of cases. However, the clinical and histologic features may be mimicked by a variety of viral, bacterial, protozoal, or metabolic causes.

The isolation of a hepatitis virus from affected newborns has been reported. Previous evidence suggested that the serum hepatitis virus is transplacentally acquired, and genetic factors may be involved in susceptibility and expression of the disease. An increased incidence in males, certain families, and patients with Down's syndrome supports this hypothesis. Measurement of Australia antigen, however, has not confirmed transplacental spread.

Clinical Findings

A. Symptoms and Signs: Jaundice, hepatosplenomegaly, dark urine, and yellow to acholic stools are the most constant physical signs. Lethargy, poor feeding, and failure to thrive accompany the illness.

B. Laboratory Findings: Laboratory tests of liver function usually reflect a combination of hepatocellular injury as shown by elevated SGOT, SGPT, and bilirubin levels and obstructive features with increased serum alkaline phosphatase and acholic stools. Serial rose bengal sodium I 131 tests may be the single most useful laboratory test.

Histologic features on liver biopsy include necrosis, cholestasis (within Kupffer's cells and hepatocytes), multinucleated giant cells, and bile duct proliferation with polymorphonuclear cells, lymphocytes, and eosinophils.

Differential Diagnosis

The major diagnostic difficulty is the differentiation of neonatal hepatitis from biliary atresia on clinical and laboratory grounds without resorting to exploratory laparotomy with liver biopsy and operative cholangiography. A conservative approach may be justified for up to 12 weeks if percutaneous liver biopsy done early in the course of the disease is consistent with hepatocellular injury. If spontaneous resolution of the clinical and laboratory features does not occur within this period, the operative approach becomes mandatory.

Injections and drugs as causes of neonatal jaundice are discussed in the next section.

Genetic metabolic and endocrinologic causes such as galactosemia, tyrosinosis, Wilson's disease, cystic fibrosis, Niemann-Pick disease, hypothyroidism, and the congenital nonhemolytic hyperbilirubinemias must also be considered. Other rare causes include pyloric stenosis, breast milk hyperbilirubinemia, and Lucey-Driscoll syndrome.

Treatment

There is no specific treatment for neonatal hepatitis. Supportive therapy includes a high-caloric formula, preferably one containing medium chain triglycerides (Portagen). Supplementary vitamins A, D, and K in water-soluble form should be given. A hemolytic component may be associated with neonatal hepatitis, and blood transfusions may be needed. Bacterial infections must be treated appropriately.

Corticosteroids are of no proved value in neonatal hepatitis.

Prognosis

About 50% of infants with neonatal hepatitis will recover even after severe and prolonged illness, though most cases show improvement within 2–4 months. The remainder die from hepatic decompensation or go on to cirrhosis.

Danks DM: Prolonged neonatal obstructive jaundice. Clin Pediat 4:499–510, 1965.

Gellis SS, Craig JM, Hsia DY: Prolonged obstructive jaundice in infancy: Neonatal hepatitis. Am J Dis Child 88:285–293, 1954.

Smetena HF, Johnson FB: Neonatal jaundice with giant cell transformation of the hepatic parenchyma. Am J Path 31:747–755, 1955.

2. NEONATAL JAUNDICE SECONDARY TO INFECTIONS & DRUGS

Specific investigative technics should be undertaken to identify the etiologic agent whenever an infectious cause is suspected in prolonged neonatal jaundice.

Bacterial Infections

The jaundice associated with sepsis is often obstructive but may be of the mixed type. Histologic changes attest to the inability of the liver to excrete conjugated bilirubin. Bile stasis predominates, while toxic cellular alterations and giant cell transformation occur less frequently. Cultures from all available body fluids should be obtained. A septic process involving the urinary tract is particularly common.

Viral Infections

Cytomegalovirus infection, rubella, varicella, herpes simplex, coxsackievirus B infection, and adenovirus infection are specific causes of neonatal hepatitis.

Toxoplasmosis

Jaundice and hepatosplenomegaly are common in the congenital variety of this disease. Unless the parasite is demonstrated within the hepatic parenchyma, the liver histopathology is nonspecific. Focal to widespread necrosis, giant cells, and a generalized cellular inflammatory response have been reported.

Syphilis

Syphilis is now a rare cause of neonatal jaundice. Serologic tests for syphilis on the mother and infant and prompt treatment with penicillin in positive cases is important.

Drugs

Vitamin K and the sulfonamides may cause high levels of indirect bilirubin by reducing the available binding sites of albumin or by causing hemolysis in patients with a hereditary deficiency of glucose-6-phosphate dehydrogenase. Novobiocin may impair hepatic bilirubin uptake or conjugation. Tetracyclines, especially when given intravenously, may lead to hepatic necrosis.

3. EXTRAHEPATIC BILIARY ATRESIA

Essentials of Diagnosis

- Prolonged neonatal obstructive jaundice.
- Hepatomegaly (splenomegaly later).
- Acholic stools (persistent).
- Laparotomy and cholangiography.
- Liver histology.

General Considerations

There is no sex or familial tendency for this condition, which has an incidence of 1:8000 to 1:13,000 births. The most common abnormality found is complete atresia of all extrahepatic biliary structures, but a multitude of variations have been reported. The specific cause of biliary atresia is not known, although recent evidence supports an in utero infectious or vascular cause. Extrahepatic biliary atresia has not been found in stillborn infants.

Clinical Findings

A. Symptoms and Signs: Jaundice may be noted in the newborn period but is more often delayed until 2–3 weeks of age. The urine is dark and stains the diaper, and the stools are often acholic. Seepage of bilirubin products across the intestinal mucosa may give some yellow coloration to the stools. Hepatomegaly is common; splenomegaly usually occurs later. Pruritus, digital clubbing, xanthomas, and a rachitic rosary may be noted in slightly older cases. Murmurs reflecting increased cardiovascular output or shunting through bronchial arteries may be heard over the entire precordium.

B. Laboratory Findings: No single laboratory test will consistently differentiate this entity from other causes of obstructive jaundice. Properly performed, serial rose bengal sodium I 131 tests may be the most useful investigation. Persistent elevation of the serum alkaline phosphatase and cholesterol levels, prolongation of the prothrombin time, and elevated leucine aminopeptidase levels suggest biliary atresia, although these findings have also been reported in neonatal hepatitis. These tests will not differentiate the type of atresia (intrahepatic versus extrahepatic) nor indicate which cases are potentially correctable by surgery.

Histologic examination of a liver biopsy specimen obtained either by the percutaneous route or operatively is useful. Although portal tracts may be widened by fibrous tissue and bile duct proliferation, the lobule relationship to the central veins is preserved. Bile duct plugging and bile lakes are common features in extrahepatic atresia, while necrosis is rare. On occasion, giant cells may be seen. In general, biopsy specimens will differentiate neonatal hepatitis from biliary atresia.

Differential Diagnosis

The major diagnostic dilemma is between this entity and neonatal hepatitis. Less commonly, urinary tract infection, intrahepatic atresia, choledochal cyst, intraluminal obstruction, and extrinsic pressure on the ducts by a tumor or lymph nodes may cause prolonged obstructive jaundice.

Surgical exploration is necessary for final diagnosis. Preoperative attention to clotting studies, including partial thromboplastin time as well as prothrombin time, is mandatory. Laparotomy must include biopsy and an operative cholangiogram if a gallbladder is present. The presence of bile in the gallbladder implies patency of the "proximal" extrahepatic duct system.

Radiographic visualization of dye in the duodenum will exclude obstruction to the "distal" extrahepatic ducts. The absence of either gallbladder or bile within its lumen, or failure to visualize the duodenum on cholangiography, dictates thorough exploration of the porta hepatis.

Complications

Failure to thrive, marked pruritus, portal hypertension, hypersplenism, a bleeding diathesis, rickets, ascites, and cyanosis eventually develop.

Treatment

A. Medical Treatment: With the probability that organ transplantation will provide the ultimate treatment for this disorder, medical management during the first 1–2 years is most important. All measures mentioned in the treatment of neonatal hepatitis apply here, with particular emphasis on the use of Portagen, a medium chain fatty acid formula, and water-soluble vitamins. The bile acid binding resin cholestyramine (Questran, Cuemid) is of questionable value in complete atresia. Ascites is best managed by a low-salt diet, spironolactone, and diuretics.

Potassium-depleting diuretics should be avoided. Newer potent diuretics such as triamterene (Dyrenium) and ethacrynic acid (Edecrin) may be used cautiously. Vigorous antibiotic treatment of the frequent bronchial infections will enhance early survival.

B. Surgical Measures: In 80% of cases of complete extrahepatic atresia, liver transplantation offers the most promising solution. In the remainder, surgical correction may be possible, but functional success is achieved in only 5%.

Prognosis

Uncorrected extrahepatic biliary atresia leads to biliary cirrhosis and death within the first 2 years of life in almost all cases.

Danks DM: Prolonged neonatal obstructive jaundice: A survey of modern concepts. Clin Pediat 4:499–510, 1965.

Hays D, Snyder W Jr: Untreated biliary atresia. Surgery 54:373–375, 1965.

Starzl TE & others: The role of organ transplantation in pediatrics. P Clin North America 13:381, 1966.

Thaler MM, Gellis SS: Studies in neonatal hepatitis and biliary atresia. Am J Dis Child 116:257, 262, 271, 280, 1968.

4. INTRAHEPATIC BILIARY ATRESIA

Essentials of Diagnosis

- Obstructive jaundice.
- Absence or hypoplasia of intrahepatic bile ducts.
- Normal extrahepatic biliary system.
- Hepatosplenomegaly.
- Pruritus.
- Xanthomas.

General Considerations

Intrahepatic biliary atresia accounts for 10% of cases of biliary atresia. It may occur sporadically or may be part of a familial syndrome. An in utero inflammatory process (rubella) or a hypoxic episode involving the bile ducts may be involved in the etiology, whereas the familial occurrence suggests a genetic susceptibility. Accumulated bile acids may enhance the cirrhotic process.

Clinical Findings

A. Symptoms and Signs: Features of obstructive jaundice may be present at birth or may appear in the newborn period. Pruritus is usually striking, but the stools are seldom acholic. Hepatomegaly is slight. Splenomegaly and xanthomas are late findings.

B. Laboratory Findings: Serum bilirubin (primarily direct-reacting) is moderately elevated. Serum alkaline phosphatase and cholesterol are moderately elevated. SGOT is normal or slightly elevated. Liver histology reveals a marked reduction in bile duct components of the intrahepatic system. This may involve primarily the major bile ducts, in which case bile plugging of the canaliculi is seen. The smaller ducts and the perilobular or interlobular ducts may be absent or hypoplastic, but large ducts can be seen in the portal triads. The degree of fibrosis may be slight or extensive, with distortion of the architectural pattern. The same variation in bile stasis has been reported.

Differential Diagnosis

Other causes of obstructive jaundice include neonatal hepatitis and extrahepatic biliary atresia. Conditions in which cellular transport of conjugated bilirubin to the canaliculi is impaired must also be considered, eg, Dubin-Johnson syndrome and Rotor's syndrome. The absence of pruritus, acholic stools, steatorrhea, elevated serum alkaline phosphatase, and bile stasis within the liver in these 2 conditions are excluding features.

Three review reports suggest that a clinical spectrum may exist in familial cases: (1) Byler's disease, with marked obstructive jaundice, diminution in intrahepatic bile ducts, and rapid progression of liver disease to an early death has been reported. (2) Survival with obstructive jaundice, pruritus, shortness of stature, peculiar hands, mental retardation, and ataxia were described in 4 out of 7 children in one family. Liver biopsy showed variable degrees of bile stasis, primarily in liver cells, plugging of canaliculi, and a paucity of interlobular bile ducts. (3) Hepatocyte bile stasis, jaundice, pruritus, acholic stools, steatorrhea, and early death in 2 siblings has been reported.

Complications

Slow progressive hepatic fibrosis and biliary cirrhosis occur in most patients. Portal hypertension, hypersplenism, and ascites may develop. Pruritus early and xanthomas late in the disease are common sequelae. Depending upon the degree of obstruction, steatorrhea, failure to thrive, bleeding diathesis, and rickets may occur. Growth failure, mental retardation, ataxia, and early demise would seem to be more common in familial cases.

Treatment

Surgery has little to offer the patient with intrahepatic biliary atresia. Medical management is directed at reducing circulating bile acids by use of the oral bile acid binding resin, cholestyramine (Questran, Cuemid). This relieves the pruritus and lowers the serum cholesterol and bilirubin levels, which theoretically may spare the liver from the injurious effects of the primary and secondary bile acids. Dietary manipulations and water-soluble vitamin supplements are important aspects of the medical therapy.

Prognosis

The prognosis seems better in nonfamilial instances than in the familial cases. In the former, long-term survivors are not uncommonly reported. Large doses of cholestyramine started early in the disease may prolong life.

Carey JB Jr, Williams G: Relief of the pruritus of jaundice with a bile acid sequestering resin. JAMA 176:432—435, 1961.

Gray OP, Saunders RA: Familial intrahepatic cholestatic jaundice in infancy. Arch Dis Childhood 41:328, 1966.

Juberg RC & others: Familial intrahepatic cholestasis with mental and growth retardation. Pediatrics 38:819—836, 1966.

Sharp H, Krivit W, Lowman JT: The diagnosis of extrahepatic obstruction by rose bengal I 131. J Pediat 70:46—53, 1967.

GENETIC, METABOLIC, & ENDOCRINE CAUSES OF NEONATAL JAUNDICE*

1. CYSTIC FIBROSIS

This inherited disorder must be considered in cases of prolonged obstructive jaundice in the newborn period. The findings of bile duct plugging and early fibrosis of the liver have been reported from biopsy.

2. NIEMANN-PICK DISEASE

Prolonged jaundice in the neonatal period may be the earliest manifestation of this disorder of sphingomyelin metabolism. Niemann-Pick cells seen on liver biopsy may be mistaken for the giant cells of neonatal

*Galactosemia and tyrosinosis are discussed in Chapter 35, Inborn Errors of Metabolism.

hepatitis. Other than mild to moderate elevation of bilirubin levels, liver function tests are within normal limits.

Crocker AC, Farber S: Niemann-Pick disease: A review of 18 patients. Medicine 37:1—95, 1958.

3. HYPOTHYROIDISM

Elevation of indirect-reacting bilirubin may be seen in congenital cretinism. The diagnosis should be apparent from other clinical findings.

4. BREAST MILK HYPERBILIRUBINEMIA

Persistent elevation of the indirect bilirubin fraction may be seen in breast-fed infants. The inhibitory action on glucuronyl transferase activity of pregnane-3α,20β-diol in the mother's milk has been shown in vitro. Rapid decline of bilirubin levels may be achieved by temporary discontinuation of breast feeding.

Newman AJ, Gross S: Hyperbilirubinemia in breast-fed infants. Pediatrics 32:995—1001, 1963.

5. LUCEY-DRISCOLL SYNDROME

This is a rare form of transient familial neonatal hyperbilirubinemia developing during the first 48 hours of life. It is due to the presence of an as yet unidentified inhibitor of bilirubin conjugation in both maternal and infant serum.

Lucey JF & others: Transient familial neonatal hyperbilirubinemia. Am J Dis Child 100:787, 1960.

6. FAMILIAL HYPERBILIRUBINEMIA

These entities can be divided into 2 groups depending upon whether unconjugated or conjugated hyperbilirubinemia occurs.

Unconjugated Hyperbilirubinemia

A. Crigler-Najjar Syndrome: Deficiency of the enzyme glucuronyl transferase within liver cells leads to marked elevation of unconjugated bilirubin, serious neurologic defects, and kernicterus in most patients. Occasional instances of this condition without neurologic complications have been found. This disorder appears to be inherited as a recessive trait. Bilirubin excretion in the parents is normal. Liver histology and liver function tests are normal.

B. Gilbert's Disease: The most common form of the congenital hyperbilirubinemias probably represents a syndrome rather than a distinct entity. The common denominator is impaired hepatic uptake of bilirubin. Mild fluctuating jaundice, especially with illness, is the major clinical syndrome. A shortened red cell survival occurs in some patients. Another group has also shown some impairment of glucuronyl transferase activity. Subsidence of hyperbilirubinemia has been achieved in some patients by administration of phenobarbital.

The disease is inherited as an autosomal dominant with incomplete penetrance. Whether another illness (hepatitis) can predispose to Gilbert's disease remains controversial. Liver histology and other liver function tests are normal.

Billing BH, Williams R, Richards TG: Defects in hepatic transport of bilirubin in congenital hyperbilirubinemia: An analysis of plasma bilirubin disappearance curves. Clin Sc 27:245–257, 1964.

Lars W: Congenital non-hemolytic jaundice. Acta paediat scandinav 56:552–556, 1967.

Conjugated Hyperbilirubinemia (Dubin-Johnson Syndrome & Rotor's Syndrome)

These entities are rarely seen in infants, but the elevated levels of conjugated bilirubin may be confused with other causes of obstructive jaundice. Inheritance of both disorders appears to be dominant with incomplete penetrance and variable expression. The basic defect is impaired hepatocyte excretion of conjugated bilirubin, with a variable degree of impairment in uptake and conjugation complicating the picture. The early differentiation of these 2 entities on the basis of the presence or absence of pigment deposition in the liver may have been premature. In Rotor's syndrome, the liver is normal, whereas in Dubin-Johnson syndrome it is darkly pigmented on gross inspection. Microscopic examination reveals numerous dark-brown pigment granules, especially in the centrilobular regions. However, the amount of pigment varies within families, and some jaundiced members may have no demonstrable pigmentation in the liver. Other than retained pigment, the liver is histologically normal. However, excretion of BSP as well as of other dyes is also impaired.

Arias IM: Studies of chronic familial nonhemolytic jaundice with conjugated bilirubin in the serum with and without an unidentified pigment in the liver cells. Am J Med 31:510–518, 1961.

INFECTIOUS HEPATITIS

Essentials of Diagnosis

- Gastrointestinal upset.
- Jaundice.
- Liver tenderness.
- Abnormal liver function tests.
- Positive liver biopsy.
- Local epidemic of the disease.

General Considerations

This disease appears to be caused by a virus or strains of related viruses and tends to occur in both epidemic and sporadic fashion. Transmission by the anal-oral route explains epidemic outbreaks from contaminated food or water supply. Sporadic cases usually result from contact with an affected individual. The overt form of the disease is easily recognized by the clinical manifestations, but a larger number of affected individuals have an anicteric and unrecognized form of the disease. Either form may confer lifelong immunity, although the recurrence rate is slightly higher in anicteric cases. While the great majority of children with infectious hepatitis recover completely, some will develop a fulminating hepatitis, chronic hepatitis, and cirrhosis. Epidemiologic studies suggest that children who die during the initial attack of the disease do so from massive hepatic necrosis secondary to overwhelming viremia, an immunologic deficiency state, or perhaps exposure to a completely different strain of virus.

Clinical Findings

A. History: A history of direct exposure to a previously jaundiced individual or of eating seafood or drinking contaminated water in the recent past should be sought. Following an incubation period of 14–50 days, the initial symptoms of fever, anorexia, and vomiting usually precede the development of obvious jaundice by 5–10 days.

B. Symptoms and Signs: Fever, anorexia, vomiting, headache, and abdominal pain are the usual symptoms. Darkening of the urine, suggesting the presence of bile, precedes jaundice. Jaundice reaches a peak in 1–2 weeks and then begins to subside. The stools may become light or clay-colored during this time. Jaundice and liver tenderness are the most consistent physical findings. Splenomegaly may be present.

C. Laboratory Findings: An elevated serum bilirubin (both direct- and indirect-reacting) is common. The SGOT and SGPT values are elevated, especially early in the course of the disease. The BSP test is of little value initially, as it tends to parallel the bilirubin values. A prolongation of BSP retention following disappearance of jaundice indicates severe residual damage. The cephalin flocculation and thymol turbidity tests are abnormal and indirectly reflect liver damage. Serum proteins are generally normal, but an elevation of the gamma globulin fraction (> 2.5 gm/100 ml) can occur and indicates a worse prognosis. Hypoalbuminemia, hypoglycemia, and marked reduction in prothrombin time are serious prognostic findings. The urine will contain significant amounts of bile and urobilinogen.

If the diagnosis is in doubt, a percutaneous liver biopsy may be safely performed in most children provided the partial thromboplastin time and platelet count are normal, the prothrombin time is greater than 50%, and the serum bilirubin is less than 20 mg/100 ml. The presence of ascites may increase the risk of percutaneous liver biopsy. "Balloon cells" and acidophilic bodies are characteristic histologic findings. Liver cell necrosis may be diffuse or focal, with accompanying infiltration of inflammatory cells containing polymorphonuclear leukocytes, lymphocytes, macrophages, and plasma cells, particularly in portal areas. Some bile duct proliferation may be seen in the perilobular portal areas alongside areas of bile stasis. Regenerative liver cells and proliferation of reticuloendothelial cells are present. Occasionally, massive hepatocyte destruction is seen with scarcely a normal liver cell visible.

Differential Diagnosis

Other diseases with somewhat similar onset include infectious mononucleosis, leptospirosis, drug-induced hepatitis, Wilson's disease, and, most often, serum hepatitis.

Complications

Ninety-five percent of children recover without sequelae. In rare cases of fulminating hepatitis, the patient may die in 5 days or may survive as long as 1–2 months before death ensues. The prognosis is poor if the signs and symptoms of hepatic coma prevail, with deepening of jaundice and development of ascites. Incomplete resolution leads to subacute or chronic active hepatitis, which may have several expressions and clinical patterns. The liver disease may eventually resolve after smoldering for several years or may go on to a chronic hepatitis with cirrhosis. Rare cases of aplastic anemia following acute infectious hepatitis have also been reported.

Some attempt at isolation of the patient is indicated, although maximum exposure has usually occurred by the time of diagnosis. Stool, urine, and blood-contaminated objects should be handled with extreme care for 1 month after the appearance of jaundice.

Prevention

Passive immunization of exposed susceptibles can be achieved. Close contacts may receive 0.06 ml/lb body weight of gamma globulin IM, with casual contacts receiving approximately 1/2 this dose.

Treatment

There are no specific measures. Bed rest during the icteric phase appears to be helpful. Sedatives should be avoided whenever possible.

A. Diet: At the start of the illness, a light diet is preferable. Fruits, vegetables, and plenty of sugars are usually well tolerated. Adequate protein can be supplied by grilled meats or broiled fish with less than normal amounts of fat. B complex vitamins have been used for many years on empiric grounds, but there is no good evidence to show that they alter the course of this disease.

B. Antibiotics: Antibiotics such as neomycin, 20 mg/kg/day orally (or kanamycin in comparable dosage), have been used to decrease the intestinal flora in anticipation of hepatic coma.

Prognosis

See Complications, above.

Conrad ME, Schwartz FD, Young A: Infectious hepatitis—a generalized disease: A study of renal gastrointestinal and hematologic abnormalities. Am J Med 37:789–793, 1964.

Deinhardt F, Holmes AW: Epidemiology and etiology of viral hepatitis. In: *Progress in Liver Diseases.* Vol 2. Popper H, Shaffner F (editors). Grune & Stratton, 1965.

Krugman S, Giles JP, Hammond J: Infectious hepatitis: Evidence for two distinctive clinical epidemiological and immunological types of infection. JAMA 200:365–373, 1967.

Krugman S, Ward R, Giles JP: The natural history of infectious hepatitis. Am J Med 32:717–728, 1962.

Tisdale WA: When to hospitalize the hepatitis patient. Hosp Practice 2:35–41, 1967.

SERUM HEPATITIS

In contrast to infectious hepatitis, serum hepatitis has a slow, insidious onset with an incubation period of 21–135 days. The disease is probably due to a virus, and until recently the parenteral route was the only known means of contracting the disease. The identification of a serum factor (Australia antigen) in 75–100% of patients with serum hepatitis may eventually help in the diagnosis of this entity. The incidence of this disease following blood transfusions varies directly with the number of units received. Recent data suggest that the serum hepatitis agent may be present in 8.7% of blood donors.

Clinical Findings

A. Symptoms and Signs: The symptoms are nonspecific, consisting only of slight fever (which may be absent) and mild gastrointestinal upset. Visible jaundice is usually the first significant finding. It is accompanied by darkening of the urine and pale or clay-colored stools. Hepatomegaly is present.

B. Laboratory Findings: These are similar to those discussed previously for infectious hepatitis (see above). Liver biopsy does not differentiate serum hepatitis from acute infectious hepatitis.

Differential Diagnosis

The differentiation between serum hepatitis and infectious hepatitis is made easier by a history of inoculation and an unusually long period of incubation. The history may indicate a drug-induced hepatitis.

Prevention

The best treatment is prevention. Screening of donors to eliminate individuals who may have had hepatitis is the most dependable way of preventing serum hepatitis. The use of unsterilized hypodermic equipment is a danger that must be considered. Storing plasma at room temperature for 6 months or treating it with ultraviolet rays may decrease the risk of infection. Fibrinogen is just as dangerous as plasma.

Passive immunization of individuals receiving numerous transfusions with gamma globulin has met with variable success. Its specific role in the prevention of serum hepatitis remains uncertain.

Treatment

There are no specific measures. Supportive measures such as bed rest, diet, corticosteroids, and the administration of large doses of gamma globulin have been employed with little success.

Prognosis

The prognosis is good, although fulminating hepatitis and cirrhosis may supervene. The course of the disease is quite variable, but jaundice in children seldom persists for more than 2 weeks. Persistent asymptomatic Australia antigenemia may occur, particularly in children with Down's syndrome or leukemia and those undergoing chronic hemodialysis.

Blumberg BS, Sutnick AI, London WT: Hepatitis and leukemia: Their relation to Australia antigen. Bull New York Acad Med 44:1566–1586, 1968.

Dull HB: Syringe-transmitted hepatitis: A recent epidemic in historical perspective. JAMA 176:413–418, 1961.

Shimizu YO, Tamoto K: The incidence of viral hepatitis after blood transfusions. Gastroenterology 44:740–744, 1963.

FULMINATING HEPATITIS
(Acute Massive Hepatic Necrosis, Acute Yellow Atrophy)

Fulminating hepatitis has a mortality rate close to 100%. Patients with immunologic deficiency diseases are particularly prone to this form of hepatitis.

Clinical Findings

In a number of patients the disease proceeds in a rapidly fulminant course with deepening jaundice, deterioration of laboratory indices, ascites, a rapidly shrinking liver, and progressive coma. Terminally, some laboratory values may improve at the time when the liver is getting smaller (massive necrosis and collapse). Another group of patients start off with a course typical of "benign" hepatitis and then suddenly become ill once again. Fever, anorexia, vomiting, and abdominal pain may be noted, and worsening of liver function tests parallels changes in sensorium or impending coma. A generalized bleeding tendency occurs at this time. Impairment of renal function, manifested by either oliguria or anuria, is an ominous sign. The striking laboratory findings include elevated serum bilirubin levels (usually > 10 mg/100 ml), high SGOT and SGPT (> 500 IU/liter) which may decrease terminally, low serum albumin, hypoglycemia, and prolonged prothrombin time. Blood ammonia levels may be normal, whereas BUN is often very low initially. Hyperpnea is frequent, and a mixed respiratory alkalosis and metabolic acidosis is apparent from serum electrolyte values. A rise in the polymorphonuclear count often presages acute liver failure.

Differential Diagnosis

Other known causes of fulminating hepatitis such as drugs and other poisons may be difficult to exclude. Reye's syndrome is confused with fulminating hepatitis.

Complications

Cirrhosis of the postnecrotic type is the usual sequel in the rare survivor.

Treatment

Many regimens have been tried, but controlled evaluation of therapy remains difficult. Combined exchange transfusion (with fresh heparinized blood) and peritoneal dialysis—sequentially or simultaneously—temporarily repairs both the chemical and hematologic abnormalities. Response may be delayed and repeated exchange transfusions necessary.

Corticosteroids in large doses (100 mg/sq m); sterilization of the colon with antibiotics such as neomycin or kanamycin to decrease ammonia formation; and altering the intestinal flora with *Lactobacillus acidophilus* (Bacid), 2 capsules 2–4 times a day, or with lactulose may have merit. Intravenous arginine and glutamine have been used to decrease blood ammonia levels, but their value is questionable.

Close monitoring of fluid and electrolytes is mandatory. Maintenance of normal blood glucose levels is important. Diuretics, sedatives, and tranquilizers are to be avoided or used sparingly.

Tracheostomy and mechanical support of ventilation in the comatose patient is indicated with respiratory failure. Prophylactic gamma globulin, 0.1 ml/kg IM, should be given to contacts of the patient.

Prognosis

The overall prognosis remains very grave. Exchange transfusions combined with other modes of therapy may improve survival figures, depending on the regenerative capacity of the damaged liver.

Berger RL & others: Exchange transfusion in the treatment of fulminating hepatitis. New England J Med 274:497–499, 1966.

Trey C, Burns DG, Saunders ST: Treatment of hepatic coma by exchange blood transfusion. New England J Med 274:473–481, 1966.

CHRONIC ACTIVE HEPATITIS
(Lupoid Hepatitis, Plasma Cell Hepatitis,
Chronic Hepatitis)

Chronic active hepatitis is most common in teen-age girls, though it does occur at all ages and in either sex. It may follow acute infectious hepatitis or drug-induced hepatitis or may develop in conjunction with such diseases as ulcerative colitis, Sjögren's syndrome, or autoimmune hemolytic anemia. Hepatitis-associated (Australia) antigen has been found in sera of several patients. Positive LE preparations and antinuclear anti-bodies and systemic manifestations, such as arthralgia, acne, and amenorrhea, suggest systemic lupus ery-thematosus with liver involvement. However, the liver histology is consistent with that described for chronic active hepatitis and not that of systemic lupus ery-thematosus.

Clinical Findings
Fever, malaise, recurrent or persistent jaundice, skin rash, arthritis, amenorrhea, gynecomastia, acne, pleurisy, pericarditis, ulcerative colitis, etc may be found in the history of these patients. Cutaneous signs of chronic liver disease may be noted (eg, spider angiomas, liver palms). Digital clubbing and hepato-splenomegaly may be present.

Liver function tests reveal smoldering disease with abnormal values for bilirubin, SGOT, SGPT, BSP reten-tion, and serum alkaline phosphatase. Serum gamma globulin levels are strikingly elevated (in the range 3–6 gm/100 ml), with reports of values as high as 11 gm/100 ml.

Histologic examination of liver biopsy specimens shows "piecemeal" necrosis, with portal fibrosis, an inflammatory reaction in the portal areas as well as perivascularly, and some bile duct and Kupffer cell proliferation and pseudolobule formation.

Differential Diagnosis
Laboratory findings and histology differentiate other types of chronic hepatitis (eg, Wilson's disease, persistent hepatitis, chronic cholangiolitis, subacute hepatitis).

Complications
Continuing disease for months to years eventually results in postnecrotic cirrhosis. Persistent malaise, fatigue, and anorexia follow activity. Bleeding from esophageal varices and development of ascites usually usher in hepatic failure.

Treatment
Corticosteroids and azathioprine (Imuran) are indicated. However, because progressive histopatho-logic changes with normal laboratory indices may occur during treatment, liver biopsy must be under-taken at regular intervals (yearly) to best assess ther-apy.

Supportive and symptomatic therapy is indicated during exacerbations of the disease.

Prognosis
The overall prognosis for chronic active hepatitis is poor, with mean survival rates around 5–8 years. A few patients eventually recover completely.

Bearn AG, Kunkel HG, Slater RJ: The problem of chronic liver disease in young women. Am J Med 21:3–15, 1956.

Kern F Jr & others: The treatment of chronic hepatitis with adrenal cortical hormones. Am J Med 35:310–315, 1963.

MacKay IR: Chronic hepatitis: Effect of prolonged suppressive treatment and comparison of azathioprine with predniso-lone. Quart J Med 37:379–392, 1968.

Mistilis SP, Blackburn SP: Active chronic hepatitis. Am J Med 48:484, 1970.

Page AR, Good RA, & Pollara B: Long-term results of therapy in patients with chronic liver disease associated with hypergammaglobulinemia. Am J Med 47:765, 1969.

POSTNECROTIC CIRRHOSIS

Most cases of postnecrotic cirrhosis occur without a prior episode of known hepatitis, but the disease may occur as a sequel to a chronic active hepatitis, acute viral hepatitis in the preadolescent, or neonatal hepati-tis. The course may be insidious, as in anicteric hepa-titis or Wilson's disease, or the disease may occur as episodes of acute exacerbations of hepatitis.

Clinical Findings
General malaise, loss of appetite, dyspepsia, and nausea and vomiting are frequent complaints. The first indication of underlying liver disease may be ascites or even hepatic coma. There is variable hepatospleno-megaly with spider angiomas and red and warm "liver" palms. Gynecomastia may be noted in males. Digital clubbing may be present. Irregularities of menstruation and amenorrhea in adolescent girls may be early com-plaints.

The most significant laboratory finding is eleva-tion of the BSP retention. Jaundice may or may not be present, and serum protein determinations often reveal a decreased level of albumin and increased level of gamma globulins.

Esophageal varices may be demonstrated by x-ray.

Liver biopsy is necessary for exact confirmation of cirrhosis.

Differential Diagnosis
The most important entity to be considered is Wilson's disease. Others might include glycogen storage disease (especially type IV), galactosemia, fructose intolerance, porphyria, and a_1-antitrypsin deficiency.

Complications
In addition to ascites and hepatic coma, complica-tions manifested by portal hypertension (eg, bleeding esophageal varices, hypersplenism) are frequently found. On the other hand, some individuals with com-

pensated postnecrotic cirrhosis may lead a relatively
normal life.

Treatment

There is no specific treatment for postnecrotic
cirrhosis. If laboratory tests and liver biopsy reveal
ongoing active disease, then corticosteroids, or a
combination of corticosteroids and immunosuppressive
agents, are indicated. Severe hypersplenism may be
treated by splenectomy, and bleeding esophageal
varices by surgical shunting procedures. Ascites may be
treated with a variety of diuretic agents such as chlorothiazide (Diuril) and spironolactone (Aldactone) in
combination with a low-salt diet. Newer and more
potent diuretic agents (eg, ethacrynic acid) must be
used with care because of their tendency to produce
potassium-deficient alkalosis.

Prognosis

The prognosis is guarded since postnecrotic cirrhosis often follows an unpredictable pattern, with
death occurring in the majority of patients within 10
years of diagnosis.

Klatskin G: Subacute hepatic necrotic cirrhosis due to anicteric
    infections with hepatitis virus. Am J Med 25:333–358,
    1958.
Ratnoff OD, Patek AJ Jr: Postnecrotic cirrhosis of liver. J
    Chronic Dis 1:266–291, 1955.
Schaefer JW & others: Progression of acute hepatitis to post-
    necrotic cirrhosis. Am J Med 42:348–358, 1967.
Sharp HL & others: Cirrhosis associated with a_1-antitrypsin
    deficiency: A previously unrecognized inherited disorder.
    J Lab Clin Med 73:934, 1969.

BILIARY CIRRHOSIS

Essentials of Diagnosis

Congenital abnormalities of the bile ducts and
cystic fibrosis account for all but a few cases of biliary
cirrhosis. When the extrahepatic biliary tree is atretic,
the progress of disease is rapid; where intrahepatic
biliary atresia exists, or in cystic fibrosis, progression
to cirrhosis is variable but slow.

The predominating signs and symptoms are those
of persistent jaundice, marked pruritus, hepatosplenomegaly, spider nevi, palmar erythema, xanthomas, and
gynecomastia in males. Failure to thrive (with height
and weight retardation) and steatorrhea are frequent.
Ascites may be present. Laboratory findings show the
typical obstructive pattern of jaundice, with elevations
of blood cholesterol, alkaline phosphatase, and bile
acids. Serum albumin is often reduced, with the
gamma globulin fraction elevated. Esophageal varices
are common in severe biliary cirrhosis secondary to
extrahepatic biliary atresia and cystic fibrosis but
unusual in intrahepatic atresia.

Liver biopsy shows proliferation, dilatation, and
plugging of bile ducts.

Differential Diagnosis

In the neonatal period, extrahepatic or intrahepatic biliary atresia must be considered as the most
likely cause. Stricture or stenosis of the extrahepatic
ducts may also cause biliary cirrhosis. Unrecognized
choledochal cysts and chronic cholelithiasis may lead
to biliary cirrhosis. Cystic fibrosis can be ruled out by
the sweat test. Drug toxicity (Dilantin) should be considered.

TABLE 17–1. Familial hepatic diseases associated with cirrhosis.

	Predominant Hepatic Pathology	Frequency of Hepatic Pathology	Diagnostic Procedure
Wilson's disease	Postnecrotic or macronodular cirrhosis	High	Biopsy, liver copper content, 24-hour urinary copper excretion, copper oxidase levels in serum
Cystic fibrosis	Macronodular biliary cirrhosis	Moderately high	Sweat chloride
Galactosemia	Postnecrotic cirrhosis	High	Galactose-1-phosphate, uridyl transferase levels
Glycogen storage disease (type IV)	Macronodular	High	Amylo-1,4→1,6-transglucosidase (branching enzyme)
Fructose intolerance	Postnecrotic	Rare	Absence of fructose-1-phosphate aldolase
Infantile cirrhosis of India	Postnecrotic	All	Clinical setting
Hepatic porphyrias	Postnecrotic	Rare	Porphyrin excretion, liver biopsy
Rendu-Osler-Weber syndrome	Postnecrotic	Infrequent	Skin lesion, biopsy
Tyrosinosis	Postnecrotic	Frequent	Blood and urine amino acid screening tests
a_1-Antitrypsin deficiency	Postnecrotic	Frequent	Blood a_1-antitrypsin levels

Complications

Progressive deterioration and loss of liver cells with marked disruption of hepatic architecture is the common course. Hepatic decompensation, ascites, and coma eventually supervene. The consequences of portal hypertension, with bleeding esophageal varices and hypersplenism, are life-threatening. Early in the disease, severe pruritus may be disabling.

Treatment

Specific treatment is available only for surgically correctable lesions involving the extrahepatic biliary system. Other cases are treated by supportive measures, including medium chain triglycerides, water-soluble vitamins A, D, and K, and cholestyramine (Cuemid, Questran) in large doses (8–15 gm/day). Antibiotic therapy is indicated in cases where ascending cholangitis or pericholangitis is suspected. Liver transplantation may be of benefit.

Prognosis

The prognosis is good only in surgically corrected lesions. In the remainder, this is a progressive, ultimately fatal disease.

Shier KJ, Horn RI: The pathology of liver cirrhosis in patients with cystic fibrosis of the pancreas. Canad MAJ 89:645–648, 1963.

CHOLECYSTITIS & CHOLELITHIASIS

Gallstones, often related to hemolytic anemias, are more common than cholecystitis in children. Cholecystitis may be seen in association with a systemic disease such as typhoid fever, scarlet fever, measles, etc or secondary to anatomic obstruction, either congenital or acquired. Impairment of bile flow may be a consequence of external pressure from neoplasm, lymph node enlargement in the porta hepatis, pancreatic pseudocyst, or gallstones in the cystic duct, common duct, or ampulla of Vater.

Clinical Findings

A. History: Epigastric or right upper quadrant pain precipitated by eating fatty foods suggests biliary colic. A careful inquiry about hematologic abnormalities may elicit evidence of congenital hemolytic anemia or sickle cell disease.

B. Symptoms and Signs: Recurrent severe, steady upper abdominal pains with tenderness over the right upper quadrant are the most constant physical findings; jaundice and a palpable mass are much less frequent.

C. Laboratory Findings: The white blood count may be normal or elevated. Serum bilirubin and alkaline phosphatase are usually variably elevated. Pancreatic amylase levels are elevated when there is obstruction at the ampulla.

D. X-Ray Findings: X-rays may visualize calculi, and an oral cholecystogram may show impairment or nonfunctioning of the gallbladder with or without calculi. Enlargement of the gallbladder and delayed or incomplete emptying following a fatty meal are definitely abnormal findings in children. Intravenous cholangiography may be necessary if oral cholecystography is nondiagnostic or if better visualization of the common duct is desired.

Differential Diagnosis

The possibilities to be considered for recurrent epigastric and right upper quadrant pain include peptic disease, liver disease, pancreatic pseudocyst, intestinal or colonic inflammatory disease, and kidney disease. The association of abdominal pain in children with hematologic disorders and its postprandial occurrence after fatty foods is most helpful. The triad of pain, jaundice, and a mass should suggest choledochal cyst, but confirmation is best obtained by radiologic studies or even laparotomy.

Complications

The major concern in long-standing cases is biliary cirrhosis. Perforation of the gallbladder is extremely rare in children but does occur in acute cholecystitis. Obstructions at the level of the ampulla can result in pancreatitis.

Treatment

Symptomatic gallbladder disease is best treated by surgical removal of the gallbladder. Common duct patency should be verified by operative cholangiography.

Prognosis

The prognosis in surgically treated patients is good. The postcholecystectomy syndrome is extremely rare in children.

Connelly JP: Clinico-pathological conference. New England J Med 268:731, 1963.

Sorge DV: Cholecystitis and cholelithiasis in children: Report of four cases. Pediatrics 29:46–50, 1962.

LIVER ABSCESS

Pyogenic liver abscesses are usually secondary to pyogenic seeding via the portal vein from infected viscera and occasionally from ascending cholangitis. Unusual causes include omphalitis, subacute bacterial endocarditis, pyelonephritis, and perinephric abscess. Pyogenic liver abscesses are usually multiple, and in the newborn period may be associated with severe sepsis. Amebic hepatic abscesses are rare in children. In adults there is a male preponderance and they are usually solitary.

Clinical Findings

Nonspecific complaints of low-grade to septic fever, chills, malaise, and abdominal pain are frequent. A few patients have shaking chills and jaundice. The dominant complaint is a constant dull pain over an enlarged liver which is tender to palpation. An elevated hemidiaphragm with reduced or absent respiratory excursion may be demonstrated on physical examination and confirmed by fluoroscopy. Laboratory studies show leukocytosis and at times anemia. Liver function tests reveal low-grade bilirubin elevation and an elevated alkaline phosphatase.

A radioisotope liver scan is the most useful diagnostic aid; its overall accuracy is around 80%. Hepatic arteriography or portal venography has had some recent success in demonstrating liver abscesses.

Pyogenic and amebic abscesses can best be differentiated by the indirect hemagglutination test.

Differential Diagnosis

Hepatitis, hepatoma, hydatid cyst, gallbladder disease, or biliary tract infections can mimic liver abscess. Subphrenic abscesses, empyema, and pneumonia may give a similar picture. Inflammatory disease of the intestines or of the biliary system may be complicated by liver abscess.

Complications

Spontaneous rupture of the abscess may occur with extension of infection into the subphrenic space, thorax, peritoneal cavity, and occasionally the pericardium. Metastatic hematogenous spread to the lungs and brain has been reported.

Treatment

When a solitary pyogenic liver abscess is localized, adequate surgical drainage should be performed. Both extraperitoneal and extrapleural drainage are recommended. Cultures are taken and massive specific antibiotic therapy started.

Multiple small abscesses may be impossible to drain surgically, and cultures are needed for specific antimicrobial therapy.

Amebic abscesses should be treated with specific anti-amebiasis therapy. The effect of treatment is best assessed by a liver scan.

Prognosis

An unrecognized and untreated pyogenic liver abscess is universally fatal. The surgical cure rate is about 75%.

Most amebic abscesses are cured with conservative medical management.

Ostermiller CR: Pyogenic liver abscess. Arch Surg 94:353–358, 1967.

Pyrtrek LJ, Bardus SA: Hepatic pyemia. New England J Med 272:551–560, 1965.

EXTRAHEPATIC PORTAL HYPERTENSION

Essentials of Diagnosis

- Splenomegaly.
- Esophageal varices with hematemesis or melena.
- Elevated splenic pulp pressure.
- Normal wedged hepatic vein pressure.
- Abnormal splenoportogram.

General Considerations

Extrahepatic portal hypertension from acquired abnormalities of the portal and splenic veins accounts for 5–8% of cases of gastrointestinal bleeding in children. A history of neonatal omphalitis, sepsis, and umbilical vein catheterization is present in about 50% of cases. Symptoms may occur before 1 year of age, but in most cases the diagnosis is not made until 3–5 years of age. Splenomegaly is often the first symptom. Massive hematemesis or melena occurs within the next few years.

A variety of portal or splenic vein malformations have been described, including valves, cavernous transformation, and atretic segments. The site of the venous obstruction may be anywhere from the hilum of the liver to the hilum of the spleen.

Clinical Findings

A. Symptoms and Signs: Splenomegaly and hematemesis are the most frequent presenting complaints. The presence of extrahepatic portal hypertension is suggested by the following: (1) An episode of severe infection in the newborn period or early infancy—especially omphalitis, sepsis, gastroenteritis, severe dehydration, or prolonged or difficult umbilical vein catheterizations. (2) No previous evidence suggesting liver disease. (3) A feeling of well-being prior to onset or recognition of symptoms.

B. Laboratory and X-Ray Findings: An orderly approach is essential to diagnosis. Most other common causes of splenomegaly may be excluded by proper laboratory tests. Cultures, heterophil titer, blood smear examination, bone marrow, and liver function tests are necessary. Esophagography will reveal varices in over 80% of these patients. In addition to normal liver function tests, confirmation of a normal liver is best obtained directly by liver biopsy or indirectly by measurement of wedged hepatic vein pressure (normal, 3–12 mm Hg). The finding of an elevated splenic pulp pressure (normal, 8–12 mm Hg) and demonstration of the block by simultaneous splenic portography confirms the diagnosis of extrahepatic portal hypertension. Filling of collateral vessels to stomach and esophagus by the dye is frequently demonstrated.

Differential Diagnosis

All causes of splenomegaly must be included in the differential diagnosis, the most common ones being infections, blood dyscrasias, lipidosis, reticuloendotheliosis, cirrhosis of the liver, and cysts or hemangiomas of the spleen. When hematemesis or melena occurs, other causes of gastrointestinal bleeding are possible, ie, esophageal, gastric, or duodenal ulcers, tumors, duplications, ulcerative bowel disease, and suprahepatic or hepatic venous obstructions.

Complications

The major manifestation and complication of this condition is bleeding esophageal varices. Fatal exsanguination appears to be uncommon, but hypovolemic shock or resulting anemia may require prompt treatment. Congestive splenomegaly with granulocytopenia and thrombocytopenia occurs. Rupture of the enlarged spleen due to trauma is always a threat. Leukopenia and thrombocytopenia seldom cause major symptoms. Unexplained fluctuating episodes of ascites may develop, and retroperitoneal edema has been reported.

Treatment

A. Surgical Measures: The surgical treatment of this disease has been disappointing. Portacaval anastomosis would be the most satisfactory procedure, but the portal vein is often involved in the basic disease process, making it unsuitable for anastomosis. Most children have been treated by means of simultaneous splenectomy and splenorenal shunts. Sustained patency of this shunt procedure is unlikely in children under the age of 8–10 years. Thrombosis of the shunt is soon followed by recurrent and often more severe hemorrhage from esophageal varices. Splenectomy perhaps increases the risk to the young child of overwhelming sepsis. More importantly, however, it removes a "safe" group of collateral vessels running from the splenic capsule to the azygos veins, thereby bypassing the esophageal and gastric drainage system.

Other surgical decompression procedures include anastomosis of the superior mesenteric vein to the inferior vena cava. Esophageal and gastric resection of the varices and transthoracic ligation of the varices have been used as more desperate measures.

B. Medical Treatment: Since a few children with this disease will die as a result of esophageal bleeding, every effort should be made to control the disease medically. The chances for successful surgical shunting procedures appear to improve as the child gets older. The patient may even develop his own decompressive shunt which is adequate to prevent major bleeding from the esophageal varices.

Spontaneous cessation of hemorrhage from esophageal varices occurs frequently. Shock must be treated with blood transfusions and anemia with iron. Careful use of a pediatric Sengstaken-Blakemore tube can stop the bleeding. Freezing or cooling the varices is not recommended. A transient reduction of portal venous pressure may be achieved by the use of intravenous vasopressin (Pitressin). Twenty units of vasopressin, diluted in 100 ml of 5% dextrose in water, given IV over a 10-minute period, is suggested. The apparent pharmacologic effect of vasopressin is constriction of the splanchnic and hepatic arterioles and consequent lowering of portal venous pressure.

Antacids, alkalies, anticholinergics, small feedings, and positioning have been suggested to reduce gastric acidity or prevent esophageal reflux. Avoidance of contact sports in the presence of splenomegaly is advisable.

Prognosis

The prognosis depends upon the site of the block and the availability of suitable vessels for shunting procedures. Each unsuccessful surgical procedure worsens the prognosis for life.

The prognosis in patients managed by medical and supportive therapy may be better than in the surgically treated group, especially when surgery is performed at an early age.

Shaldon S, Sherlock S: Obstruction to the extrahepatic portal system in childhood. Lancet 1:63–68, 1962.

Tsakiris A, Haemmerli UP, Buhlmann A: Reduction of portal venous pressure in cirrhotic patients with bleeding from esophageal varices, by administration of phenylalanine-lysine-vasopressin. Am J Med 36:825–839, 1964.

INTRAHEPATIC (NONCIRRHOTIC) PORTAL HYPERTENSION

In the absence of cirrhosis, intrahepatic causes of portal hypertension are rare in the pediatric age group. Two major entities are to be considered:

(1) Hepatic vein occlusion or thrombosis (Budd-Chiari syndrome): In most instances, no cause can be demonstrated. Endothelial injury to hepatic veins by bacterial endotoxins has been shown experimentally. The occasional association of hepatic vein thrombosis in inflammatory bowel disease (ulcerative colitis, regional enteritis, infectious diarrhea) favors the presence of endogenous toxins invading the portal vein and reaching the liver. Allergic vasculitis leading to endophlebitis of the hepatic veins has been occasionally described. In addition, hepatic vein obstruction may be secondary to tumor, hyperthermia, or sepsis.

(2) Jamaican veno-occlusive disease: This entity appears to be the result of ingestion of "bush tea" (*Crotalaria fulva*), a member of the Senecio family. It causes widespread occlusion of the small and medium-sized hepatic veins, with resultant congestion and necrosis of the neighboring parenchymal cells. The acute form of the disease generally follows a nonspecific respiratory illness. The disease may be rapidly fatal, although about 50% of children apparently recover. A subacute and chronic form also exists.

Clinical Findings

Abdominal enlargement due to ascites is the presenting complaint in all but a few cases. Abdominal pain and tender hepatosplenomegaly are frequently found. Jaundice is present in about 25% of cases. Vomiting, hematemesis, and diarrhea are less common.

The presence of distended superficial veins on the anterior abdomen along with dependent edema is usually seen with inferior vena cava obstruction. Absence of the hepatojugular reflex (jugular distention when pressure is applied to the liver) is a helpful clinical sign. Liver function tests are not usually helpful. Localization is difficult. An inferior venacavagram may reveal an intrinsic filling defect from an infiltrating tumor or from extrinsic pressure and obstruction of the inferior vena cava by an adjacent tumor or nodes. Care must be taken in interpreting extrinsic pressure defects of the subdiaphragmatic inferior vena cava in the face of ascites.

Simultaneous wedge hepatic vein pressure and hepatic venography are most useful procedures. Hepatic vein pressure and splenic pulp pressure are elevated. Obstruction to major hepatic vein ostia and smaller vessels may be demonstrated by this procedure. In the absence of obstruction, reflux across the sinusoids into the portal vein branches can be accomplished. In most instances, open liver biopsy should be undertaken. Marked central venous congestion and necrosis without fibrosis is striking. Endothelial thickening of hepatic veins may also be found.

Differential Diagnosis

Cirrhosis of the liver due to any cause must be ruled out. Suprahepatic or infrahepatic (extraprimary) causes of portal hypertension must also be excluded. Although ascites may occur in extrahepatic portal hypertension, it is not common. Cutaneous signs of chronic liver disease are lacking since this entity is usually acute.

Complications

Untreated hepatic vein obstruction will lead to liver failure, coma, and death. A nonportal type of cirrhosis may develop in the chronic form of Jamaican veno-occlusive disease. Hematemesis due to bleeding esophageal varices is frequent in the few survivors.

Treatment

Efforts to correct underlying causes must be promptly undertaken. Surgical removal of the occluding tumor or of the hepatic vein thrombi is possible when the large ostia are involved. Portacaval shunts and right atrial to inferior vena cava grafts have been attempted. Medical management with heparin, corticosteroids, and diuretics has had inconsistent results.

Prognosis

Hepatic vein obstruction carries a very high mortality rate (95%). In veno-occlusive disease, the prognosis is better, with complete recovery possible in 50% of acute forms and 5–10% of subacute forms.

Foster GS: Clinico-pathological conference. New England J Med 273:156–163, 1965.

Parker RGF: Occlusion of the hepatic veins in man. Medicine 38:369, 1959.

HEPATOMAS

Essentials of Diagnosis

- Abdominal enlargement.
- Hepatomegaly.
- Weight loss.
- Anemia.
- Laparotomy and tissue biopsy.

General Considerations

Primary epithelial neoplasms of the liver represent 0.2–5.8% of all malignant conditions in the pediatric age group. There are 2 basic morphologic types with certain clinical and prognostic differences. Hepatoblastoma predominates in male infants and children, with most cases appearing before age 3. The predominance of right-sided lesions has aroused interest since the left lobe is supplied with oxygenated blood from the umbilical vein and the right lobe with portal vein blood, which has a lower oxygen saturation.

Hepatocarcinoma is extremely rare in girls and occurs more frequently after age 5. This type of neoplasm carries a poorer prognosis than hepatoblastoma, and for some reason causes more abdominal discomfort and pain. Hepatocarcinoma has been reported in children with postnecrotic cirrhosis or biliary cirrhosis, but these are the exceptions rather than the rule. An interesting aspect of primary epithelial neoplasms of the liver has been the increased incidence of associated anomalies and unusual conditions found in these children. Virilization has been reported as a consequence of gonadotropin activity of the tumor. Leydig cell hyperplasia without spermatogenesis is found on testicular biopsy. Hemihypertrophy, congenital absence of the kidney, macroglossia, and Meckel's diverticulum have been found in association with hepatocarcinoma.

Clinical Findings

A. History: Noticeable increase in abdominal girth with or without pain is the most constant feature of the history. Constitutional symptoms (anorexia, fatigue, fever, chills, etc) may be present.

B. Symptoms and Signs: Weight loss, pallor, and abdominal pain associated with a large abdomen are common. Physical examination reveals hepatomegaly with or without a definite tumor mass, usually to the right of the midline. Signs of chronic liver disease are usually absent.

C. Laboratory Findings: Normal to slightly distorted liver function tests are the rule. Anemia is frequently seen, especially in cases of hepatoblastoma. Percutaneous liver biopsy can be safely performed, but final tissue diagnosis should be made at laparotomy. Cystathioninuria has been reported. Alpha$_1$ fetoglobulin may be elevated.

D. X-Ray Findings: X-ray is at times helpful in demonstrating the tumor shadow or calcified foci in the neoplasm. It is very helpful in proving the presence or absence of obvious metastases as well as in localizing the lesion to the liver. Specialized technics such as radioactive liver scans and selective celiac axis or umbilical artery angiography may be helpful.

Differential Diagnosis

In the absence of a palpable mass, the differential diagnosis is that of hepatomegaly and anemia. Hematologic and nutritional conditions should be ruled out, as well as less common diseases such as lipid storage diseases, histiocytosis X, glycogen storage disease, hepatic abscess (pyogenic or amebic), cysts, and hemangiomas. Parasitic infections, toxins, and drugs can cause identical symptoms. Veno-occlusive disease and thrombosis of the hepatic veins are also rare possibilities.

Complications

Progressive enlargement of the tumor, abdominal discomfort, ascites, respiratory difficulty, and widespread metastases are the rule. Rupture of the neoplastic liver and intraperitoneal hemorrhage has been reported. Progressive anemia and emaciation predispose to an early septic death. Metastases are most frequently to the lungs and abdominal lymph glands.

Treatment

An energetic surgical approach has brought forth the only long-term survivors. Complete lobectomy appears to be preferred over partial resection. It appears that every isolated lung metastasis should also be surgically resected. Radiotherapy and chemotherapy have been disappointing in the treatment of primary liver neoplasms.

Organ transplantation should be considered when local excision or lobectomy cannot yield the entire tumor.

Prognosis

Survivors are few and occur only following a radical surgical approach. In a recent article, 15 of 37 patients are alive without evidence of metastasis, and 7 patients are reported to have survived more than 5 years following resection.

Alpert ME & others: Alpha$_1$ fetoglobulin in the diagnosis of human hepatoma. New England J Med 278:984, 1968.

Fish JC, McCary RG: Primary cancer of liver in childhood. Arch Surg 93:355–359, 1966.

Ishak KG, Glunz PR: Hepatoblastoma and hepatocarcinoma in infancy and childhood: Report of 47 cases. Cancer 20:396–422, 1967.

WILSON'S DISEASE
(Hepatolenticular Degeneration)

Originally considered to be a molecular defect in ceruloplasmin, Wilson's disease is now thought to involve other copper-containing enzymes, notably those in the respiratory chain. The disease should be considered in all children with evidence of liver pathology or with suggestive neurologic signs. A family history is often present.

Clinical Findings

A. Symptoms and Signs: Hepatic involvement may be acute or may progress to postnecrotic cirrhosis in an insidious manner. Findings include jaundice, Kayser-Fleischer rings, and neurologic manifestations such as tremor, dysarthria, and drooling. The rings can sometimes be detected by unaided visual inspection as a brown band at the junction of the iris and cornea, but slit-lamp examination is usually necessary.

B. Laboratory Findings: Early, liver function tests are consistent with hepatocellular damage. Late in the course, only the BSP may be useful to assess the degree of liver damage.

The laboratory diagnosis of Wilson's disease is sometimes difficult. Serum ceruloplasmin levels are usually < 20 mg/100 ml and are measured as copper oxidase rather than directly. (Normal values are 23–43 mg/100 ml.) Low values, however, are seen normally in infants under 3 months of age, and in 3–5% the levels may be normal. Serum copper levels are low, but the overlap with normal is too great for satisfactory discrimination. Urine copper levels in children over 3 years of age are normally < 30 μg/day; in Wilson's disease, they are > 50 μg/day. Finally, the tissue content of copper from a liver biopsy, normally < 20 μg/gm wet tissue, is > 50 μg/gm wet tissue in Wilson's disease.

Glycosuria and aminoaciduria as well as elevated serum uric acid levels have been reported. Hemolysis and, on rare occasions, bone lesions simulating those of osteochondritis dissecans have been found.

Liver biopsy may distinguish Wilson's disease from other types of hepatitis. Early in the disease, vacuolation of liver cells, fatty degeneration, and lipofuscin granules can be seen, as well as Mallory bodies. The presence of the latter in a child is strongly suggestive of Wilson's disease.

Differential Diagnosis

During the icteric phase, acute viral infectious hepatitis, serum hepatitis, chronic active hepatitis, and drug-induced hepatitis are the usual diagnostic variables. Later, other causes of cirrhosis and portal hypertension need consideration. Laboratory testing for the specific factors listed above will differentiate this disorder from the others.

Complications

Progressive degenerating liver disease and hepatic coma and death are not uncommon. Recovery from the initial episode usually results in a cirrhosis of the postnecrotic type.

Treatment

Penicillamine (Cuprimine), 900–1200 mg/day orally, is the drug of choice in all cases, whether symptomatic or not. Dietary restriction of copper intake is not practical. The dosage of penicillamine may be reduced after urinary copper levels return to normal. Triethylenetetramine dihydrochloride (TETA) or L-dopa may be helpful in cases where penicillamine is unsuccessful. Liver transplantation may be curative.

General treatment measures for acute hepatitis are as outlined for infectious hepatitis.

Prognosis

The prognosis of hepatitis due to Wilson's disease is not favorable.

Barbeau A, Friesen H: Treatment of Wilson's disease with L-dopa after failure of penicillamine. Lancet 1:1180, 1970.

Slovis TL & others: The varied manifestations of Wilson's disease. J Pediat 78:578, 1971.

Sternlieb I, Scheinberg IH: Prevention of Wilson's disease in asymptomatic patients. New England J Med 278:352–359, 1968.

Walshe JM: Management of penicillamine nephropathy in Wilson's disease: A new chelating agent. Lancet 2:1401, 1969.

REYE'S SYNDROME
(Encephalopathy With Fatty Degeneration of the Viscera; White Liver Disease)

Essentials of Diagnosis

- Progressive encephalopathy leading to coma.
- Hepatomegaly.
- Hypoglycemia
- Altered acid-base balance.
- Severe fatty degeneration of liver, kidneys, and brain.

General Considerations

This syndrome is being reported with increasing frequency since its recognition in 1963. Young children seem to be at greater risk. Persistent attempts to implicate a single etiologic factor have failed. Echovirus 2, coxsackievirus A, and rheovirus have been isolated from some patients. Toxic and metabolic causes, particularly salicylates, have also been incriminated. The mode of onset of the disease frequently leads to confusion with other causes of coma, particularly hepatic coma.

The manifestations of Reye's syndrome may be related in part to alterations caused by elevated serum levels of short chain fatty acids.

Clinical Findings

A. Symptoms and Signs: Most cases give a history of minor upper respiratory illness of short duration preceding the development of vomiting, irrational behavior, progressive stupor, and coma. Restlessness and convulsions may also occur. Striking physical findings are hyperpnea, irregular respirations, and hepatomegaly. Jaundice is minimal or absent. Splenomegaly is seldom present. A positive Babinski sign and hyperreflexia in association with decorticate and decerebrate posturing are consistent with severe cerebral edema.

B. Laboratory Findings: CSF is acellular and CSF glucose is often low. The serum glucose is proportionately decreased. Moderate to severe elevations of SGOT, SGPT, and LDH are found. Serum bilirubin and alkaline phosphatase values are normal to slightly elevated. The prothrombin time may be prolonged. A mixed respiratory alkalosis and metabolic acidosis is seen.

The histopathology of Reye's syndrome is most striking in the brain, liver, and kidneys; less commonly, changes in the heart and pancreas may be found. The brain shows gross cerebral edema, occasionally with evidence of herniation.

Histologically, loss of neurons and fatty vacuolation around small vessels have been noted. The liver shows diffuse fatty steatosis with minimal inflammatory changes. Glycogen is virtually absent from the hepatocytes.

The kidney changes consist principally of swelling and fatty degeneration of the proximal lobules.

C. Electroencephalography: The EEG is diffusely abnormal, with marked slow wave activity predominating.

Differential Diagnosis

Differentiation of Reye's syndrome from acute toxic encephalopathy or from hepatic coma or fulminating hepatitis can be made on clinical and laboratory grounds. A negative history for ingestion of poisons and drugs, absence of cells in the CSF, and absence of jaundice are significant. Fulminating hepatitis and hepatic coma in the absence of jaundice have been reported but are extremely rare. Liver biopsy is diagnostic.

Complications

Aspiration pneumonitis and respiratory failure are common, as with any comatose patient. Most patients die of cerebral complications rather than hepatic or renal failure. Herniation of the brain stem due to cerebral edema is the most serious complication.

Treatment

Treatment is empirical and supportive. Tracheostomy and mechanical support of ventilation with increased dead space are recommended to overcome respiratory alkalosis. Maintenance of glycogen stores with a 10% glucose infusion to which insulin is added (1 unit/3 gm of glucose) may be beneficial. Cerebral edema should be treated with minimal maintenance fluids, dexamethasone, and a cooling blanket. In the absence of compromised renal function, mannitol infusion may be tried. Corticosteroids and exchange transfusions have been used without success. Peritoneal dialysis may also be of value.

Prognosis

Less than 1/3 of these patients survive, and severe neurologic residuals may persist in those who recover.

Gellis SS, Jones WA: Varicella in a six-year-old boy with coma and gastrointestinal bleeding: Clinico-pathologic conference. New England J Med 276:47–55, 1967.

Golden GS, Duffell D: Encephalopathy and fatty change in the liver and kidney. Pediatrics 36:67–74, 1965.

Simpson H: Encephalopathy and fatty degeneration of the viscera (acid-base observations). Lancet 2:1274–1277, 1966.

ACUTE PANCREATITIS

Most cases of acute pancreatitis are due to mumps or abdominal trauma. Less common causes resulting in acute obstruction to pancreatic flow include stones in the ampulla of Vater, tumors of the duodenum, and ascariasis. Acute pancreatitis has recently been seen as a consequence of high-dosage corticosteroid therapy.

Clinical Findings

A. Signs and Symptoms: An acute onset of severe upper abdominal pain referred to the back, with vomiting and fever, is the common presenting picture. The abdomen is tender but not rigid, and bowel sounds are diminished. In cases due to trauma, an abdominal mass may be felt that is suggestive of pseudocyst. Ascites may be noted in such cases also.

B. Laboratory Findings: Leukocytosis and an elevated serum amylase and urine diastase should be expected early. Serum calcium may be low and signifies a poor prognosis.

C. X-Ray Findings: An upper gastrointestinal series may demonstrate abnormalities in the duodenum in the case of tumors, stones, pseudocyst, etc and should be ordered in cases where abdominal trauma has occurred. Plain x-rays of the abdomen may show ileus.

Differential Diagnosis

Other causes of acute upper abdominal pain include lesions of the stomach, duodenum, liver, and biliary system, acute gastroenteritis or atypical appendicitis, pneumonia, volvulus, and intussusception.

Complications

Complications include fluid and electrolyte disturbances, ileus, and hypocalcemic tetany. Pseudocyst formation may develop and may be associated with internal fistulas. Chronic pancreatitis and pancreatic lithiasis may occur as sequelae.

Treatment

Medical management includes rest, gastric suction, fluids, electrolyte replacement, and blood or plasma as needed. Pain should be controlled with codeine or meperidine. Atropine may be used intramuscularly.

Surgical treatment is reserved for stones, cysts, and anatomic obstructive lesions.

Prognosis

As most cases are due to mumps, the prognosis is excellent with conservative management. The prognosis following surgical treatment is guarded since the postoperative incidence of pancreatic fistula is high.

Hendren WH, Greep JM, Patton AS: Pancreatitis in childhood: Experience with 15 cases. Arch Dis Childhood 40:132–145, 1965.

Mellinkoff SM: *The Differential Diagnosis of Abdominal Pain.* McGraw-Hill, 1959.

CHRONIC PANCREATITIS

Two general forms of chronic pancreatitis have been reported: chronic fibrosing pancreatitis and hereditary chronic relapsing pancreatitis with a familial tendency.

The causes include stenotic lesions of the ampulla of Vater, strictures of the pancreatic ducts, and parasitic infestations or gallstones in the ampulla. Chronic intermittent disease may rarely follow mumps pancreatitis, and may be a consequence of abdominal trauma with or without pseudocyst formation.

Pancreatitis is rarely symptomatic in cystic fibrosis.

Clinical Findings

The diagnosis of the hereditary form can be made only by a similar history in other family members, aminoaciduria, and sometimes diabetes mellitus and hyperlipidemia. The diagnosis of chronic fibrosing pancreatitis is made by surgical exploration demonstrating a normal duct system and typical histology in the pancreatic biopsy.

A. Symptoms and Signs: There is usually a history of recurrent upper abdominal pain of variable severity but prolonged (1–6 days') duration. Fever and vomiting are not common in the chronic form. Abnormal stools and symptoms of diabetes may develop later in the course of this disease.

B. Laboratory Findings: The serum or urine amylase is usually normal or mildly elevated. Pancreatic insufficiency may be found at duodenal intubation after intravenous administration of pancreozymin (2 units/kg) (available from Professor Jorpes, Karolinska Institute, Stockholm) and secretin (2 units/kg) (available from Boots, Ltd, Nottingham, England). A 3-fold increase of normal serum amylase values is considered a positive test for obstruction.

Blood lipids and urinary amino acids are elevated in familial forms of the disease and should be studied in all cases. Elevated blood sugar levels and glycosuria are frequently found in protracted disease.

C. X-Ray Findings: X-rays of the abdomen may show pancreatic or gallbladder calcifications. Contrast studies may demonstrate other obstructive lesions in the region of the duodenum.

Differential Diagnosis

Other causes of recurrent abdominal pain must be considered. Specific causes such as hyperparathyroidism, infectious disease, and ductal obstruction by tumors, stones, or helminths must be excluded by appropriate tests.

Complications

Disabling abdominal pain, steatorrhea, nutritional deprivation, and diabetes are the most frequent complications.

Treatment

When the hereditary form of chronic pancreatitis is suspected or proved, medical management of acute attacks is indicated (see Acute Pancreatitis, above). If ductal obstruction is strongly suspected, surgical exploration should be undertaken. Pancreatography and cholangiography are usually performed at laparotomy. Sphincterotomy and biopsy are recommended when obvious obstruction is not found. Pseudocysts may be marsupialized to the surface or drained into the stomach or into a loop of jejunum.

Prognosis

In the absence of a correctable lesion, the prognosis is not good. Disabling episodes of pain, pancreatic insufficiency, and diabetes may ensue.

Gross JE: Hereditary pancreatitis: Description of a fifth kindred and summary of clinical features. Am J Med 33:358–364, 1962.

Warwick WJ, Leavitt SR: Chronic relapsing pancreatitis. Am J Dis Child 99:648–652, 1960.

Williams TE, Sherman NJ, Clatworthy HW Jr: Pancreatitis as a cause of abdominal pain. Pediatrics 40:1019–1023, 1967.

ZOLLINGER-ELLISON SYNDROME

This familial syndrome, consisting of non-beta islet cell tumors of the pancreas, marked gastric hypersecretion, and severe intractable peptic ulceration, is most common in males. The youngest patient so far described was 8 years old.

The ulcerogenic, gastrin-like hormone elaborated by these small pancreatic islet cell tumors and their metastases to liver or lymph nodes is responsible for the gastric hypersecretion and the intractable peptic disease. Intractable diarrhea of the secretion type may occur in the absence of peptic disease.

Clinical Findings

Severe, intermittent abdominal pain with vomiting, hematemesis, melena, diarrhea, and steatorrhea are common. X-ray findings of hypertrophied gastric rugae, duodenal dilatation, and edematous small bowel mucosa all suggest gastric hypersecretion. Gastric analysis shows a marked increase in volume and titratable acidity after a 12-hour overnight collection. The histamine test rarely shows more than a 2-fold increase in acid output since these patients are already secreting maximally.

Treatment

Total gastrectomy is the treatment of choice. The hazard of ulcer perforation and the ineffectiveness of medical treatment and of subtotal gastrectomy have been well documented. Primary and metastatic tumor tissue removal should be attempted; however, cures have been reported even when metastases have not been surgically removed and the primary tumor has not been found.

Rosenlund ML: The Zollinger-Ellison syndrome in children. Am J M Sc 140:134–142, 1967.

ISOLATED EXOCRINE PANCREATIC DEFECTS

Trypsinogen Deficiency Disease

In this rare genetic defect, absence of trypsinogen (a pancreatic proenzyme) leads rapidly to severe protein malnutrition and hypoproteinemia.

Trypsinogen is normally converted to trypsin by enterokinase. Once formed, trypsin can replace enterokinase in the activation of the proenzyme. Trypsin is also needed to activate the conversion of chymotrypsinogen to chymotrypsin as well as procarboxypeptidase to carboxypeptidase. Consequently, the absence of trypsinogen results in a complete loss of pancreatic proteolytic enzyme activity. Activation studies with exogenous trypsin have shown that procarboxypeptidase and chymotrypsinogen are present in samples of the patients' pancreatic juice and are qualitatively intact. The sweat chloride test is normal, and the diagnosis is made by duodenal intubation and analysis of pancreatic enzyme activity. Anemia has been associated with this entity but not neutropenia. Enterokinase deficiency must also be excluded.

Treatment consists of feeding a formula containing a casein hydrolysate such as Nutramigen, or by adding pancreatic enzymes to the diet (Cotazym).

Tarlow MJ & others: Intestinal enterokinase deficiency. Arch Dis Childhood 45:651, 1970.

Townes PL, Bryson M, Miller C: Further observations on trypsinogen deficiency disease: Report of a second case. J Pediat 71:220–224, 1967.

Isolated Pancreatic Lipase Deficiency

Deficiencies related to malabsorption of the fat-soluble vitamins are common. Neither pancreatic lipase nor a lipase inhibitor is present, while pancreatic trypsin and amylase activity are normal. The sweat chloride iontophoresis test is normal. Direct assay of pancreatic juice for enzyme activity following stimulation with pancreozymin and secretin, 2 units/kg of each IV, is required for diagnosis.

Improvement in steatorrhea occurs after the addition of pancreatic enzymes to the diet. A low-fat diet or substituting medium chain triglycerides (Portagen) for long chain dietary triglycerides is helpful.

Balzar E: Isolated defect in pancreatic lipase formation. Gastroenterology 5:239–246, 1967.

CYSTIC FIBROSIS
(Fibrocystic Disease, Mucoviscidosis)

Essentials of Diagnosis

- Elevated sweat chloride.
- Absent or decreased pancreatic exocrine function.
- Recurrent pulmonary infections.
- Characteristic changes in chest x-rays.
- Diarrhea.
- Failure to thrive.

General Considerations

The incidence of cystic fibrosis is about 1:1000 live births. It appears to be an autosomal recessive disease with variable expression, prevalent in Caucasians and rare in Negroes and Mongolians. It is a generalized disease affecting all exocrine glands, principally those in the digestive and pulmonary systems. Abnormal mucus glycoproteins, inappropriate water or electrolyte secretion or reabsorption by the ductular epithelial cells, and autonomic nervous system abnormalities are possible causes.

Clinical Findings

A. Symptoms and Signs: The typical patient is easily recognized in the first year of life. Pulmonary involvement is apparent in over 90% of these infants and is manifested by noisy respirations, wheezing, chronic cough (especially at night), and recurrent episodes of bronchitis and bronchopneumonia. Exocrine pancreatic deficiencies show as diarrhea, severe caloric deprivation, and failure to thrive. Appetite seems to be insatiable, but weight gain and growth are strikingly retarded. The stools are frequent, large, greasy, and foul-smelling. The increased fat content makes the stools difficult to remove from the diapers, and repeated toilet flushings are often necessary to dispose of the floating feces. Inanition and chronic pulmonary infection cause a delay in motor development.

As the sweat electrolyte concentration is high, it is not unusual for the mother to find salt deposits in and about the hair and to report that the infant tastes salty when kissed.

The disease may also present in the newborn period, where hyperbilirubinemia, edema with hypo-proteinemia, or intestinal obstruction with or without perforation may be the result of meconium ileus. This complication occurs in about 10–20% of affected newborns. Rectal prolapse may be an early finding and should make one suspect cystic fibrosis. Inability to absorb fat-soluble vitamins may lead to easy bruising and prolonged bleeding episodes. Vitamin D deficiency rickets can occur but is rare, as well as frank episodes of hypocalcemic tetany. At times, nodular biliary cirrhosis and the consequences of portal hypertension can be the major initial findings.

Excessive salt losses via the sweat glands may cause a shock-like state with severe hyponatremia and hypochloremia. Finally, one should suspect cystic fibrosis in a young patient with nasal polyps.

Physical examination usually reveals a thin, tachypneic child with a protuberant abdomen. A mucopurulent rhinitis and nasal polyps may be present. The chest is often emphysematous, and "sticky" rales, rhonchi, or wheezes are frequent auscultatory findings.

B. Laboratory Findings:

1. Sweat test—Quantitative analysis of sweat by pilocarpine iontophoresis for sodium or chloride is a reliable diagnostic test for cystic fibrosis. A sweat chloride measurement above 60 mEq/liter or sweat sodium above 70 mEq/liter is consistent with this diagnosis (data of O'Brien, Ibbott, and Rodgerson). Normal newborns and adults have sweat electrolyte levels higher than those recorded in infancy and childhood, but their levels are rarely in the pathologic range.

2. Gastrointestinal studies—Determination of trypsin content and viscosity of the duodenal fluid is valuable in assaying pancreatic function. However, in approximately 15–20% of patients with this disease, some proteolytic activity may be found in the duodenal fluid.

There is usually no trypsin in the stool, but testing for stool trypsin is of little value in older children, in those receiving antibiotics, or in those with certain other disturbances of the gastrointestinal tract.

C. X-Ray Findings: X-rays of the chest may show no abnormality in early cases, or the changes may be limited to minimal evidence of hyperaeration and increased peribronchial markings. Later, patchy areas of atelectasis and emphysema develop. As the disease progresses, scattered areas of infiltration, more extensive peribronchial markings, and enlargement of the perihilar nodes are noted. Pneumothorax and lung abscess may be seen on occasion.

Differential Diagnosis

Immune deficiency diseases can also present with the combined picture of pulmonary and intestinal disease. Other causes of malabsorption need consideration. If the pulmonary disease predominates, tracheoesophageal fistula, allergy, and dysautonomia should be considered. Other causes of both generalized and isolated exocrine pancreatic insufficiency should be excluded.

Complications

Pulmonary complications due to obstructive secretions include recurrent pneumonitis, atelectasis, abscesses, pneumothorax, progressive fibrosis, pulmonary artery hypertension, and cor pulmonale.

Intestinal complications include meconium ileus in the newborn period, with or without perforation and meconium peritonitis. In older children, symptoms and signs of intestinal obstruction may be due to intussusception, with inspissated stools being the lead point.

Deficiencies of vitamins A, D, K, and E are attended by skin and mucosal lesions, rickets, and hemorrhagic tendencies. Mild focal liver disease is frequent (30–40%), with biliary cirrhosis, portal hypertension, and bleeding esophageal varices seen only rarely in older children. Rectal prolapse and nasal polyps are also frequent complications of cystic fibrosis.

Treatment

A. Surgical Measures:

1. Meconium ileus in the newborn–Meconium ileus in the newborn requires surgery. At laparotomy, atresia or volvulus which requires resection may be found proximal to the meconium ileus. The inspissated meconium may be removed manually or solubilized by luminal perfusions of acetylcysteine (Mucomyst, Respaire). Recently, removal of meconium has also been accomplished by meglumine diatrizoate (Gastrografin) enema.

2. Meconium ileus equivalent in older children– Reduction of suspected intussusception by barium enema and rectal enemas with pancreatic enzymes may be tried. Stool softeners, mineral oil, and liquids should be given by mouth to loosen the inspissated feces. Surgery may be necessary in refractory cases. Careful abdominal palpation for fecal masses in the right lower quadrant should be routine in order to prevent this late intestinal complication. Surgery may occasionally be needed for removal of airway obstruction by nasal polyps and for incarcerated rectal prolapse. Persistent atelectasis, pneumothorax, and empyema may also require surgical attention.

B. Medical Treatment:

1. Pulmonary manifestations–Prevention of progressive pulmonary disease is best achieved by humidification of inspired air combined with vigorous postural drainage. The addition of a mucolytic agent such as acetylcysteine (Mucomyst, Respaire) has been tried with variable results. Bronchodilators such as isoproterenol (Isuprel Mistometer and Duo-Medihaler) are useful adjuncts to postural drainage. Cor pulmonale has been treated with phlebotomy, aminophylline, and tolazoline (Priscoline). Digitalis is probably of little value. Vigorous treatment of pneumonias with antibiotics is essential.

2. Pancreatic insufficiency–A number of commercial products containing lipase, trypsin, and amylase from pork pancreas (eg, Cotazym, Viokase) are available in capsule or tablet form to be taken immediately before meals. The dosage of pancreatic enzyme replacement needs to be individualized, but 1–2 capsules given with each meal, with additional doses for between-meal snacks, will suffice.

Persistence of marked diarrhea in the face of seemingly adequate replacement therapy should make one suspect other causes. Disaccharidase deficiencies and celiac disease have been reported in patients with cystic fibrosis.

The diet should be high in proteins and carbohydrates. A low-fat diet is recommended by some but is not essential. Small infants and even some older children may benefit from diets containing medium chain triglycerides (Portagen). Water-soluble vitamins A, D, and K are given as supplements.

3. Antibiotics for infections–Prophylactic antibiotics even in a rotating schedule have not been shown to decrease mortality or increase survival. A mixed flora is frequently cultured from the tracheal mucosa, with *Hemophilus influenzae*, staphylococci, and *Pseudomonas aeruginosa* predominating.

4. Androgens for growth failure–Variable success has been reported when selected patients have been given androgens. When severe growth and weight retardation cause psychosocial problems, the use of androgens may be reasonable. Improvement in pulmonary status may also be seen with the use of these drugs.

5. Arginine–Buffered L-arginine by mist is of benefit in the pulmonary disease. Oral arginine, 1 gm/kg/day, relieves abdominal pain. It also appears to improve steatorrhea in younger patients.

Prognosis

Twenty-five to 50% of children with cystic fibrosis die by age 5. The severity and progressiveness of the pulmonary damage is the major factor in determining prognosis. There is no connection between sweat electrolyte levels and severity of the disease.

Di Sant'Agnese P, Tolamo RC: Pathogenesis and pathophysiology of cystic fibrosis of the pancreas. New England J Med 177:1287, 1344, 1399, 1967.

Doershuk CF & others: Evaluation of prophylactic and therapeutic program for patients with cystic fibrosis. Pediatrics 36:675–688, 1965.

Schwachman H, Kulczycki LL, Khaw KT: Studies in cystic fibrosis: Report on 65 patients over 17 years of age. Pediatrics 36:689–699, 1965.

Solomons CC, Cotton EK, Dubois RS: The use of buffered L-arginine in the treatment of cystic fibrosis. Pediatrics 47:384, 1971.

PANCREATIC EXOCRINE HYPOPLASIA & CHRONIC NEUTROPENIA

This uncommon disease, characterized by diarrhea and failure to thrive, is due to pancreatic exocrine insufficiency. Pathologically, there is widespread fatty replacement of the gland acinar tissue. There is no fibrosis or inflammation, and the pancreatic ducts appear to be normal. The islet cells are spared. The disease may be confused with cystic fibrosis, but the absence of elevated sweat chlorides distinguishes these entities. The association of bone marrow dysfunction is a curious but fairly constant finding. There is evidence that this entity is genetically determined.

The history of failure to thrive, diarrhea, fatty stools, and, in most cases, freedom from respiratory infections should make one suspect this entity. Important laboratory findings include normal sweat electrolytes but absent or reduced pancreatic lipase, amylase, and trypsin on duodenal intubation. Leukopenia is often present, and the thrombocyte count is sometimes depressed. Small bowel histology is normal, as are studies of absorption not dependent upon pancreatic enzymes. The bone marrow is typically hypocellular, showing a "maturation arrest" of the granulocyte series. Metaphyseal dysostosis and an elevated fetal hemoglobin may occur.

Normal sweat electrolytes and frequent absence of repeated pulmonary infections easily differentiate this disease from cystic fibrosis. Small bowel biopsy supported by absorption tests, particularly with D-xylose, distinguishes the disorder from celiac disease. Cases of isolated lipase, trypsinogen, or enterokinase deficiency may be more difficult to distinguish. Cyclic neutropenia and neutropenia due to other causes must be considered.

The complications and sequelae of deficient pancreatic enzyme secretion are malnutrition, diarrhea, and growth failure. The major sequel seems to be short stature, although long-term follow-up studies are not available. Increased numbers of infections may be the results of chronic neutropenia.

Pancreatic enzyme replacement therapy has been fairly successful, although some patients get along without it. The prognosis appears to be good.

Bodian M, Sheldon W, Lightwood R: Congenital hypoplasia of the exocrine pancreas. Acta paediat 53:282–286, 1964.

Burke V, Colebatch JH, Anderson CM: Association of pancreatic insufficiency and chronic neutropenia in childhood. Arch Dis Childhood 42:147–157, 1967.

•   •   •

General References

Banks PA, Janowitz HD: Some metabolic aspects of exocrine pancreatic disease. Gastroenterology 56:601–617, 1969.

De Reuck AVS, Cameron MP (editors): *CIBA Foundation Symposium on the Exocrine Pancreas: Normal and Abnormal Functions.* Little, Brown, 1962.

Dowdy GS Jr: *The Biliary Tract.* Lea & Febiger, 1969.

Lester R, Troxler RP: Recent advances in biopigment metabolism. Gastroenterology 56:143–169, 1969.

Read AE: Advances in liver disease. Abstr World Med 43:801–820, 1969.

Sherlock S: *Diseases of the Liver and Biliary System,* 4th ed. Davis, 1968.

Silverberg M, Davidson M: Pediatric gastroenterology: A review. Gastroenterology 58:229–252, 1970.

White TT: *Pancreatitis.* Williams & Wilkins, 1966.

18 . . .

Kidney & Urinary Tract

John B. Moon, MD, & Donough O'Brien, MD, FRCP

Renal diseases in infants and children may present in a wide variety of ways. In infants, there may be concomitant physical malformations; in small children, failure to thrive and anorexia are common; in older children, listlessness, headaches, weight loss, and poor school performance may occur. Renal failure often presents in children with a long and indistinct history of headaches, tiredness, and vague abdominal pain. The characteristic findings of dysuria, frequent urination, and fever in urinary tract infections are often not present in children. Such protean manifestations emphasize the need to examine the urine at routine physicals and to consider the possibility of renal or urinary tract disease in any obscure illness.

LABORATORY TESTS OF RENAL FUNCTION

Urinalysis

Urinalysis should be a routine component of any thorough physical examination. The presence of protein, hemoglobin, glucose, acetone, and bilirubin should be investigated. (Convenient test strips—Labstix, Bili-Labstix—are available.) Sediment spun at 3000 rpm for 3 minutes should be examined microscopically using low illumination. Casts and cast inclusions are sought using a low-power objective lens.

Next, tubular epithelial cells and red and white blood cells are studied. These may be easier to distinguish if stained on the slide with 1 drop of 1% eosin, Sternheimer-Malbin stain, or Sedi-Stain. Bacteria, crystals, spores, etc should be searched for using a high-power lens. Polarized light will assist in the identification of fat bodies as evidence of tubular injury.

Fergus EB: Urine sediment: Exploring the body sea with a microscope. Postgrad Med 39:148–155, 1966.
Rutecki GJ & others: Characterization of proteins in urinary casts. New England J Med 284:1049–1052, 1971.

Glomerular Filtration Rate (GFR)

The GFR is a useful index of the total number of functioning glomeruli and is estimated as the clearance of substances such as creatinine, inulin, and iothalamate sodium I 125, which are filtered but not protein-bound, metabolized, secreted, or reabsorbed. GFR = UV ÷ P, where U and P are urine and plasma concentrations, respectively, and V is urine volume in ml/minute. The results are expressed corrected to 1.73 sq m. In the first days of life, GFR averages 40 ml/minute/1.73 sq m, and this value is usually doubled by 2 months of age. Adult values (Table 40–3) of 130 (80–160) ml/minute/1.73 sq m are reached by 2 years of age. Creatinine clearances are highly subject to laboratory and collection error, and in normal circumstances the iothalamate sodium I 125 clearance is preferable. Inulin clearances are reliable but time-consuming tests.

Cohen ML & others: A simple, reliable method of measuring glomerular filtration rate using single, low dose sodium iothalamate [131]I. Pediatrics 43:407–415, 1969.
Kassirer JP: Clinical evaluation of kidney function: Glomerular function. New England J Med 285:385–389, 1971.
Sakai T, Leumann EP, Holliday MA: Single injection clearance in children. Pediatrics 44:905, 1969.

Tests of Renal Tubular Function

A number of renal tubular disorders occur in childhood which lead to impairment of tubular reabsorption of glucose, amino acids, and phosphorus or to the impaired excretion of hydrogen ion.

The urinary excretion of amino acids in generalized tubular disease reflects a quantitative increase rather than a qualitative change. This can be detected by a total urinary amino nitrogen assay, the normal value being 2 mg/kg/24 hours. Glycosuria should not exceed 5 mg/100 ml; one-dimensional paper chromatography is the best test. Phosphaturia is gauged as tubular reabsorption of phosphorus. Normal values should be $\geq 80\%$ calculated as $(1 - C_p/C_{cr}) \times 100$.

The ability of the proximal tubule to reabsorb bicarbonate can only be assessed by the complicated procedure of a bicarbonate infusion test to determine the threshold of HCO_3^- reabsorption. Distal tubular function is estimated by determining hydrogen ion excretion on acid loading.

Net hydrogen ion excretion is expressed as

$$UV_{H^+} = (U_{TA} + U_{NH_4^+} - U_{HCO_3^-})V$$

where U_{TA} titratable acid, $U_{NH_4^+}$ = urine ammonium concentration, $U_{HCO_3^-}$ = urine bicarbonate concentrations, and V = volume of urine (in ml) per minute. Normal values are 45 ± 25 mEq/minute/1.73 sq m during the first year of life and 30 ± 20 mEq/minute/1.73 sq m in later childhood. In the fourth hour, after a single oral ammonium chloride challenge of 130 mEq/24 hours/1.73 sq m, values for both groups rise to 110 ± 30 mEq/minute/1.73 sq m. The hydrogen ion clearance index, H^+ excretion in mEq/minute/1.73 sq m X plasma CO_2 in mEq/liter, is 0.9 ± 0.6 in infancy and 0.6 ± 0.4 in older children. After ammonium chloride loading, this increases in both groups to 2.5 ± 1.4. Values in renal tubular acidosis are usually < 0.7 after ammonium chloride loading.

Kassirer JP: Clinical evaluation of kidney function: Tubular function. New England J Med 285:499–502, 1971.

Tests of the Concentrating Ability of the Distal Tubules & Collecting Ducts

These tests are useful in the differential diagnosis of diabetes insipidus and occasionally in the evaluation of water conservation in chronic renal failure.

Urine osmolality can normally reach 700 mOsm/liter in the first 3 months and 1400 mOsm/liter thereafter on thirsting. More sophisticated ways of expressing this are given in the following tests.

A. Osmolar Clearance:

$$C_{osm} = \frac{U_{osm} \times V}{P_{osm}}$$

Should rise to > 4 ml/sq m/minute in a maximally concentrating situation.

B. Free Water Clearance:

$$C_{H_2O} = V - C_{osm} = V\left[1 - \frac{U_{osm}}{P_{osm}}\right]$$

Should be > 6 ml/sq m/minute during water diuresis.

C. Medullary Water Reabsorption:

$$T^c_{H_2O} = C_{osm} - V = V\left[\frac{U_{osm}}{P_{osm}} - 1\right]$$

Should be > 3 ml/sq m/minute with maximally concentrated urine during solute load.

D. Vasopressin Test for End Organ Sensitivity: Used in the differentiation of psychogenic, pituitary, and renal diabetes insipidus.

RADIOLOGIC TESTS OF RENAL FUNCTION

Intravenous Urography

The bowels should be emptied and the patient thirsted. A scout film should be taken before injection of contrast material to evaluate for stones, calcifications, etc, and a 1–3 minute "early" film should be used to evaluate delayed function on one side, cortical thickness, and renal outline. Interval films at 5, 10, and 15 minutes are primarily used to evaluate the anatomy of the collecting system. An immediate postvoiding film gives an estimate of residual urine.

Combinations of pyelonephritic scarring, obstructive uropathy, and fetal lobulation can coexist and can be difficult to distinguish.

Cystourethrography

A voiding cystourethrogram or scintogram provides visual evidence of bladder trabeculation, residual urine, vesicoureteral reflux, and obstruction distal to the bladder. Voiding cineurethrography is a refinement of the voiding cystourethrogram that may be helpful.

Retrograde Urography

This procedure requires anesthesia and cystoscopy and carries with it a risk of infecting the upper urinary tracts. It therefore should be employed sparingly. It is a useful means of studying the ureters and renal pelves and is often required to evaluate a urinary tract when renal failure prevents visualization by intravenous urography. It is also useful in delimiting obstructive uropathies and for differential renal function studies.

Renogram & Renal Scan

These procedures are of special value in differential renal function studies.

Blaufox MD & others: Radionuclide scintigraphy for detection of vesicoureteral reflux in children. J Pediat 79:239, 1971.

Goldman HS, Freeman LM: Radiographic and radioisotopic methods of evaluation of the kidneys and urinary tract. P Clin North America 18:409–434, 1971.

STRUCTURAL ABNORMALITIES OF THE KIDNEY & URINARY TRACT

Malformations of the kidney and urinary tract are common in children (5–12% of autopsies); fortunately, many of them produce no symptoms or disturbances of function. Anomalous developments of the kidney and urinary tract are of great importance because some lead to obstructive phenomena and, consequently, to infection, calculus formation and eventual renal failure. Furthermore, some of the nonobstructive structural abnormalities involving the kidney may be neoplastic or may directly give rise to renal failure, whereas the nonobstructive anomalies of the lower urinary tract may lead to repeated infections.

Clinical Findings in Urinary Tract Anomalies

A wide spectrum of clinical manifestations is seen. Despite the presence of infection, hydronephrotic atrophy, or renal failure symptoms may be minimal to absent. Signs of infection may be prominent and associated with dysuria, frequency, and urgency. Other symptoms include difficulty in initiating micturition, dribbling, prolonged voiding, or enuresis. A pattern of abdominal pain mimicking peptic disease, gallbladder disease, or appendicitis is not uncommon. Retarded growth, anemia, failure to thrive, "fever of unknown etiology," and hypertension are important clinical manifestations which can reflect an underlying anatomic or functional urologic problem.

A hydronephrotic kidney can sometimes be palpated. A suprapubic abdominal mass is likely to be a distended bladder due to lower urinary tract obstruction such as occurs in posterior urethral valve or due to vesical dysfunction such as in neurogenic bladder. There is a high correlation between external genital malformations and anomalies of the urinary tract. Lumbosacral malformations are commonly associated with bladder dysfunction.

General Management of Urinary Tract Anomalies

Every child with symptoms or physical findings suggestive of a urinary tract anomaly should have a careful urinalysis and urine culture. In addition, GFR should be measured and an intravenous urogram and cystourethrogram performed.

Once the initial investigations have been carried out, the pediatrician may wish to seek the help of the urologist for interpretation of the studies done and a decision about the need for further diagnostic steps such as cystoscopy, cystometrography, and retrograde urography.

Treatment consists of a sustained effort to prevent urinary tract infection in conjunction with any indicated surgical procedure.

OBSTRUCTIVE ANOMALIES OF THE KIDNEY & URINARY TRACT

1. HORSESHOE KIDNEY

The fused renal mass has 2 excretory systems which open laterally but usually empty normally into the bladder. Ureteral compression may result from aberrant vessels or from ureteral overriding of the isthmus joining both kidneys. A mass over the lower lumbar spine is usually palpable.

2. URETEROPELVIC JUNCTION OBSTRUCTION

This lesion is the most common cause of obstructive uropathy. It may be secondary to intrinsic stenosis or compression by a vessel or band, or may be a functional disturbance of the pyelo-ureteral bulb filling or emptying phase. Hydronephrotic atrophy progresses relentlessly and may be compounded by infection, fibrosis, and stone formation. Only a few patients with this malformation remain asymptomatic.

A common variant of this syndrome occurs when a right renal artery compresses the major calyx to the right upper pole. This frequently results in obstruction and infection of the right upper pole and may lead to eventual metastatic infection elsewhere in the urinary tract.

Deckers PJ & others: Vascular obstruction of the superior renal infundibulum in children. Surgery 67:856–862, 1970.

3. DUPLICATION OF THE URETER

This is the most common upper urinary tract anomaly and is usually asymptomatic. In many cases there is a complete division of the pelvic systems. The doubling may be limited to the renal pelvis; may end at any distance from the bladder; or may be complete, leading to separate openings into the bladder. Hydronephrosis may result from obstruction within the duplicated ureters or at the area where they join, or from ureterovesical incompetence. The terminus of one of the double ureters is frequently incompetent, resulting in ureterovesical reflux. (See Ureterocele and Ectopic Ureteral Orifice, below.)

4. URETEROCELE

This is a cystic enlargement of the ureterovesical junction. An intravesical mass resembling an upside down cobra's head may be found on intravenous urography. A large number of ureteroceles are associated with duplicated ureters.

5. ECTOPIC URETERAL ORIFICE

The ectopic ureteral orifice may be found at the base of the bladder, in the bladder neck, in the urethra, or, in females, anywhere from the apex of the vagina to the introitus. The most common location of an ectopic ureteral orifice, however, is just lateral to the trigone of the bladder. When double ureters occur, the upper ureter usually crosses behind the lower and emerges distally and medially to the normally placed orifice of the lower ureter. Ureteral reflux or obstruction often occurs in intravesical ectopia. Any female child over the age of continence who voids normally but is also slightly wet all the time should be suspected of having an ectopic ureteral orifice.

6. CONGENITAL URETERAL STENOSIS

This rare malformation is associated with poor urinary drainage and hydronephrosis.

7. MEGALOURETER

This disorder consists of dilatation and tortuosity of the ureters but no anatomic obstruction to urine flow. It leads to poor drainage since the ureters have little or no peristalsis. Infection is the rule. It has been reported that 3% of patients with Hirschsprung's disease have megaloureters.

8. BLADDER NECK OBSTRUCTION

This condition is much less common than was once thought but it does exist. In the majority of cases, an obstruction such as a posterior urethral valve is found distal to the bladder neck.

9. NEUROGENIC BLADDER

The most common cause of neurogenic bladder in the pediatric age group is spina bifida with or without myelomeningocele. It gives rise to increased or decreased bladder tone, overflow incontinence, residual urine, vesicoureteral reflux, hydronephrosis, repeated infections, renal failure, and calculi.

10. MEGACYSTIS SYNDROME

This anomaly has been identified as a neurogenic bladder dysfunction unassociated with other neurologic abnormalities. An attempt to relate it to Hirschsprung's disease was not successful since there is no diminution in ganglion cells. The bladder capacity is very large, and the walls are thin and smooth. Vesico-

ureteral reflux is usually present; therefore, in most cases, varying degrees of hydroureter, hydronephrosis, and pyelonephritis are present also. Progression to renal failure is common.

11. POSTERIOR URETHRAL VALVES

In this disorder of males, the valves attach at the verumontanum. It may present in the newborn period as absence of voiding, as a urinary tract infection, or even as renal failure since extensive damage has usually taken place by the time of birth.

12. DISTAL URETHRAL STENOSIS

This anomaly is manifested in females by a circle of fibrous tissue at the junction of the meatus with the urethra or at the meatus itself. Meatal stricture in both males and females may be congenital or secondary to local inflammation such as diaper rash. Distal urethral stenosis is much less common than was once thought now that normal urethral variations on cystourethrogram are better appreciated. The history is usually negative, although difficulty starting micturition and voiding a small, thin stream may be described.

Leadbetter GW: Urinary tract infection and obstruction in children. Clin Pediat 5:377–384, 1966.
Schopfner CE: Modern concepts of lower urinary tract obstruction in pediatric patients. Pediatrics 45:194–196, 1970.
Stamey TA: The localization and treatment of urinary tract infections. Medicine 44:1–36, 1965.

NONOBSTRUCTIVE ANOMALIES OF THE KIDNEY AND URINARY TRACT

1. BILATERAL RENAL AGENESIS
(Potter's Syndrome)

Occasionally, neither ureteric bud develops but the fetus continues to grow. It is usually stillborn and premature. Certain facial characteristics are relatively constant and include low-set ears with little cartilage, a receding chin, flattening of the nose, and prominent epicanthal folds forming a wide semicircle on each side of the nose and covering the medial palpebral fissure. Oligohydramnios is present, often causing increased bowing of the extremities.

Rizza J, Downing SR: Bilateral renal agenesis in two female siblings. Am J Dis Child 121:60–63, 1971.

2. EXSTROPHY OF THE BLADDER

Bladder exstrophy represents failure of fusion of the lateral mesodermal and ectodermal somites, allowing the bladder to reach its final development as an open plaque or urothelium on the lower abdominal wall. The trigone and ureteral orifices can be seen, and there is associated complete epispadias in boys, who are twice as commonly affected as girls. Cryptorchidism and inguinal hernias are common; the vagina may be absent in girls. The waddling, duck-like gait of patients affected with this condition relates to a widely spread pubic symphysis.

3. URACHAL REMNANTS

Incomplete obliteration of the urachus will lead to a blind cyst, to a urachal defect leaking mucoid secretions at the umbilicus, or to a tract communicating only with the bladder. More rarely, the entire urachus is patent and there is a constant flow of urine from the umbilical region.

Campbell M: Indications for urologic examination in children. P Clin North America 9:651–666, 1955.

Randolph JG: Congenital abnormalities of the urinary collecting system. P Clin North America 12:381–409, 1965.

URINARY TRACT INFECTIONS

General Considerations

Urinary tract infections are the second most common infections in childhood, exceeded only by infections of the respiratory tract. They vary greatly in their clinical manifestations and range from comparatively mild asymptomatic lower tract infections to life-threatening infections of the renal parenchyma.

The younger the child, the more obscure the symptoms of urinary tract infections. Infants may develop vomiting, poor feeding, lethargy, jaundice, fever, hypothermia, or simply failure to thrive. Toddlers more commonly exhibit signs of abdominal pain, or they may pass foul-smelling urine, void frequently, or scream when they urinate. Not uncommonly, a history of recurrent fevers may be obtained. The older the child, the more apt he is to provide symptoms referable to the urinary tract. Nevertheless, at any age a urinary tract infection may be completely "silent" or may have fever as its only clue.

Note: Examination of the urine is essential in all cases of fever of unknown origin.

Predisposing Factors

A. Age and Sex: Urinary tract infections appear to affect males more frequently than females in infancy, and autopsy reports on very young children show a preponderance of males dying of pyelonephritis. This is due to the higher incidence of serious urinary tract malformations in males.

After early childhood, urinary tract infections are overwhelmingly more common in girls. The short female urethra provides an easy portal of entry for bacteria. Approximately 5% of girls acquire a urinary tract infection at some time during their elementary or high school years.

B. Ureterovesical Reflux: There is still debate about whether ureterovesical reflux, with its concomitant failure of complete bladder emptying, predisposes to urinary tract infection or whether it is simply caused by cystitis and is disclosed by a work-up following urinary tract infection. Lower urinary tract infection in the presence of reflux may be expected to lead to pyelonephritis.

C. Obstructive Uropathy: Obstructive uropathy predisposes to urinary tract infections both by inhibiting the elimination of bacteria and distorting the architecture of the proximal urinary tract. When possible, this should be treated surgically.

D. Other Factors: Additional factors which may predispose to urinary tract infections in females are the existence of pinworms, masturbation, the use of bubble bath, and constipation. It is doubtful that perineal hygiene plays a significant role. Sexual intercourse and pregnancy are well documented correlates of urinary tract infections.

The most common organism which infects the urinary tract is *Escherichia coli:* Over 80% of first infections and over 70% of recurrences are due to this organism. The next most frequent are the klebsiella-enterobacter (aerobacter) group (10–15%). All other microorganisms, including proteus, staphylococcus, and pseudomonas account for 12% or less of all urinary tract infections. The finding of any microorganism other than *E coli* or klebsiella-enterobacter suggests long-standing or recurrent disease and should suggest pyelonephritis rather than lower tract disease.

Clinical Findings

A. Symptoms and Signs:

1. Lower urinary tract infections—Most urinary tract infections are confined to the lower tract. Symptoms in older children, when they occur, usually include dysuria, frequency, urgency, and lower abdominal pain. In uncomplicated lower tract disease, there should be no significant fever, chills, or back pain. Successful treatment usually relieves lower tract symptoms within 24–48 hours.

Symptoms may be absent altogether or may subside spontaneously, precluding reliance on symptomatology as a guide to treatment effectiveness. Recurrences of asymptomatic bacteriuria and cystitis in white females are associated with evidence of caliectasis or reflux (or both) in 15–20% of cases.

2. Pyelonephritis–Pyelonephritis is usually caused by bacteria entering the kidney from the lower urinary tract by way of the ureter. Classically, patients develop costovertebral angle pain and tenderness with fever and chills. Nevertheless, as with lower tract disease, patients with active pyelonephritis may be completely asymptomatic.

Bacteria in the parenchyma localize in the papillae, resulting in the formation of microabscesses. This is a focal process which may occur in only a few areas of an affected kidney. As scar tissue forms, the columns of Bertin and collecting ducts are particularly damaged, with the loss of a significant number of nephrons. This results in calyceal blunting, papillary flattening, and cortical thinning, all of which cause characteristic changes on intravenous urograms.

Examination of the urine may be diagnostic if casts containing polymorphonuclear leukocytes are seen. If the urine is hypo-osmolal, large, swollen polymorphonuclear leukocytes which exhibit brownian movement in their cytoplasm (so-called glitter cells) may also be seen. Occasionally, mild proteinuria will accompany pyelonephritis; heavy proteinuria usually indicates some other process.

The hypertonicity of the renal medulla may favor the persistence of bacteria as L-forms (a special form of many conventional bacteria which lacks a cell wall and thus resists the action of most antibiotics). Some investigators have claimed that reversion from L-form to conventional form accounts for many apparent relapses of pyelonephritis.

B. Laboratory Findings:

1. Bacteriuria–The finding of 100,000 or more organisms per ml in a cleanly voided, promptly cultured midstream urine specimen is presumptive evidence of an active urinary tract infection. However, vulval, vaginal, preputial, and possibly urethral contamination often make interpretation difficult. Unless a cleanly voided midstream urine specimen yields a pure culture of 100,000 *E coli* or klebsiella-enterobacter organisms in the presence of pyuria and symptoms of a urinary tract infection, confirmation should be obtained by suprapubic bladder aspiration. Urine obtained by this means should be sterile. Catheter specimens should generally not be sought.

The finding of one or more organisms per oil immersion field in a gram-stained smear of uncentrifuged urine correlates well with bacterial counts of 100,000 organisms per ml.

2. Hypoglycosuria–A sensitive reagent strip has recently been developed to test for urinary tract infections. Fasting urine normally contains 2–20 mg/100 ml of glucose except in the presence of urinary tract infections. This test has apparent value in mass screening programs and may prove worthwhile in screening

for L-form infections and in follow-up investigations (see above).

3. Urinalysis–A positive test for blood may be seen in hemorrhagic cystitis, and trace or 1+ proteinuria may be observed in pyelonephritis. A consistently alkaline pH may suggest a urea-splitting organism.

Examination of a spun urinary sediment occasionally reveals casts containing white cells–a finding very suggestive of pyelonephritis. Most cellular casts, however, contain only renal tubular epithelial cells. The finding of free white cells is also suggestive (though not diagnostic) of urinary tract infection. The staining of urinary sediment (Sedi-Stain or Sternheimer-Malbin stain) greatly facilitates distinguishing mononuclear renal tubular cells from polymorphonuclear cells.

C. X-Ray Findings: Intravenous urography and voiding cystourethrography are indicated after any first urinary tract infection in a male. Controversy exists about whether these studies should be performed after a first infection in a female. However, the findings of a 20% incidence of reflux and a 16% incidence of caliectasis justify the studies routinely in females. Radiographic evaluation should not be deferred in the case of a female with symptoms, signs, or laboratory findings suggestive of pyelonephritis. This should be carried out before antibiotic therapy is complete in view of the need for catheterization.

Treatment

A. Asymptomatic Bacteriuria: Once significant bacteriuria has been established beyond doubt, treatment should begin with an effective antimicrobial agent such as sulfisoxazole, 120–150 mg/kg/24 hours orally in 4 divided doses, or ampicillin, 100–150 mg/kg/24 hours orally in 4 divided doses. The urine should be recultured 48–72 hours after starting treatment and should be sterile. If it is, treatment should be continued for 10 days to 2 weeks.

If the urine has not been sterilized, the antimicrobial agent should be stopped and a new one selected. Antibiotic sensitivity tests may be used as a guide, but such tests are notoriously unreliable in urinary tract infections. The best guide to the effectiveness of therapy is a reculture 48–72 hours after starting treatment. Other drugs which may be used are nitrofurantoin (Furadantin, Macrodantin), 5–7 mg/kg/day orally in 4 divided doses; cephalexin (Keflex), 100 mg/kg/day orally in 4 divided doses; and nalidixic acid (NegGram), 40–50 mg/kg/day orally in 4 divided doses.

Urinary tract infections commonly recur. Therefore, the urine should be recultured 1 week after stopping treatment, every month for at least 6 months, every 2–3 months for 2 years, and at least every 6 months thereafter.

Patients with asymptomatic bacteriuria during childhood appear to be particularly prone to develop recurrences after beginning sexual activity and after becoming pregnant. They should continue to receive follow-up care throughout adult life.

B. Cystitis (Symptomatic): Treatment for cystitis is the same as for asymptomatic bacteriuria except that therapy is continued for 5–6 weeks.

C. Pyelonephritis: Any evidence of upper urinary tract symptoms (fever, chills, back pain, etc) or upper tract signs (costovertebral angle tenderness, pyelocaliectasis, etc) calls for a diligent attempt to recover the organism followed by treatment with a bactericidal drug (such as ampicillin or cephalexin) instituted with minimal delay. Treatment should be continued for a minimum of 6–8 weeks. Once the infecting organisms have been eradicated, a 3- to 6-month course of treatment with a urinary tract antiseptic may be justified. Appropriate urinary tract antiseptic drugs are nitrofurantoin (Furadantin, Macrodantin), 3–5 mg/kg/day orally in 4 divided doses, or methenamine mandelate (Mandelamine), 50 mg/kg/day orally in 3 divided doses with sufficient ascorbic acid to keep the urine pH below 5.5.

In addition to antimicrobial therapy, patients with pyelonephritis should be treated with water diuresis for several days after beginning antimicrobial therapy. This can best be accomplished by prescribing twice the patient's estimated normal daily water requirements.

D. Management of Recurrent Infections: As a rule, each new infection should be treated as a first infection as outlined above. However, particularly frequent "repeaters" may require one or several protracted (6- to 12-month) courses of urinary tract antiseptic to maintain sterility. Nitrofurantoin, methenamine mandelate plus urinary acidification, and sulfisoxazole are usually the drugs of choice.

Prognosis

As long as urinary tract infections can be confined to the lower urinary tract (bladder and below), the prognosis for life is excellent. Once an infectious process has entered the kidney, the prognosis becomes more guarded. Hence, every diagnostic and therapeutic effort should be made to prevent recurrences.

Forbes PA & others: Initial urinary tract infections. J Pediat 75:187–197, 1969.

Kass EH: Symposium on pyelonephritis. J Infect Dis 120:1–141, 1969.

Kunin CM: Epidemiology and natural history of urinary tract infection in school age children. P Clin North America 18:509–528, 1971.

Matsaniotis N & others: Low urinary glucose concentration: A reliable index of urinary tract infection. J Pediat 78:851–858, 1971.

Whitaker J, Hewstone AS: The bacteriologic differentiation between upper and lower urinary tract infection in children. J Pediat 74:364–369, 1969.

ACUTE GLOMERULONEPHRITIS

Essentials of Diagnosis

- There is usually a history of group A β-hemolytic streptococcal infection 7–14 days previously.
- General malaise, headache, vomiting, fever, loss of appetite, and sometimes abdominal pain.
- Moderate edema, especially of the orbits and the dorsa of the hands and feet.
- Hypertension, usually negligible or moderate, sometimes of rapid onset and capable of causing sudden seizures or cardiac failure.
- Proteinuria and hematuria with hyaline, granular, and red cell casts in the urine. Gross hematuria or "smoky urine" is usually present, but in subclinical cases hematuria may be minimal or absent.
- Occasionally, oliguria or even anuria and acute renal failure can be seen.
- Transient mild to moderate elevation of BUN. ASO titer is commonly elevated. Low C′3 complement level. The erythrocyte sedimentation rate is high.

General Considerations

Acute glomerulonephritis is relatively common in childhood, especially between ages 3 and 10. It is rare before age 2 and affects boys slightly more often than girls. Although several alternative theories have been proposed, the best explanation of the cause of acute glomerulonephritis seems to be that certain cell wall or plasma membrane components of specific strains of streptococci (and possibly other organisms) evoke production of soluble complexes of antigen and antibody which are entrapped by the renal glomerulus as irregular subepithelial deposits. A variety of immune reactions then occur involving, at least in part, the activation of a complement cascade and the fixation of C′3 complement on the subepithelial deposits. The initiation of leukochemotaxis calls forth polymorphonuclear leukocytes which release lysosomal enzymes which damage the glomerular basement membrane, distorting its geometry and making it permeable to serum proteins and to red blood cells.

Grossly, the kidneys are slightly enlarged, with punctate hemorrhages throughout the cortex. Under the light microscope, there is proliferation and swelling of both endothelial and epithelial cells. Blood flow is obstructed. The glomerular tufts become infiltrated with polymorphonuclear leukocytes and monocytes. Epithelial crescent formation and fibrinous adhesions between the glomerular tuft and capsular wall occur rarely.

Clinical Findings

A. Symptoms and Signs: Following an antecedent streptococcal infection and an asymptomatic period of

7–14 days, most patients give a history of passing dark, often "coke"-colored or smoky urine. This is commonly associated with headache, malaise, vague abdominal pains, and a feeling of "heaviness" in the back. Periorbital puffiness is commonly noted in the mornings. Oliguria is common. The stigmas of streptococcal infection (pharyngitis, impetigo, etc) may be present in family members if not in the patient. Occasionally, patients present with seizures or cardiac failure due to hypertension and hypervolemia.

B. Laboratory Findings: Proteinuria is present, but the most important finding in the urine is the massive increase in red cell content, giving it a brown discoloration. Early in the disease, red cell or hemoglobin casts are present, establishing with certainty the renal origin of the bleeding.

BUN and serum creatinine are often mildly elevated. The erythrocyte sedimentation rate is elevated. $C'3$ and $C'5$ serum complement fractions are depressed. The plasma ASO titer is usually above 250 Todd units when there is a history of streptococcal involvement. Only about 80% of group A β-hemolytic streptococci evoke a rise in ASO titer. Hence, it may be necessary to obtain titers to other streptococcal antigens such as streptococcal DNase, M-protein, or hylauronidase. Many patients present at about the time these titers begin to rise. Accordingly, repeat values obtained 2 weeks after onset may reveal a streptococcal illness not otherwise demonstrable. A 2-fold rise in titer indicates that the infection was, in fact, recent and therefore likely to be related to the nephritis. Whenever a group A β-hemoltyic streptococcus is recovered, it should be typed. Types 4, 12, 25, and 49 are commonly nephritogenic.

Complications & Sequelae

Hypertension is occasionally very severe and, if untreated, may lead to cerebrovascular accidents, left-sided failure, convulsions, vomiting, and retinal exudates and hemorrhages. Pulmonary edema is occasionally present, and recent hemodynamic studies have shown that this is not due to systemic hypertension or myocarditis but to increased pulmonary capillary permeability. Very rarely, patients develop acute oliguric renal failure and may require careful fluid and electrolyte management or even peritoneal dialysis or hemodialysis. An occasional patient will be mildly anemic. Blood transfusions in such patients should be diligently avoided, as hypertensive crises are extremely likely to occur.

Treatment

Other than eradication of streptococci, there are no specific therapeutic measures for the acute stage. Corticosteroids are contraindicated.

Bed rest is advisable only during the initial period of illness. Dietary sodium restriction is indicated while edema and hypertension exist. Protein and potassium are ordinarily not restricted unless oliguria is present. All dietary restrictions should be removed once hypertension and oliguria subside. Hypertension is usually

relatively easy to manage with reserpine, 0.03–0.09 mg/kg/dose, and hydralazine, 0.15 mg/kg/dose, both given IM as often as every 4–6 hours as required. Often only 1 or 2 such doses are required.

Prognosis & Follow-up

Well over 95% of children recover completely, although some patients will have hematuria for as long as 2 years and proteinuria for as long as 5 years. Virtually all patients under 7 years of age will go on to complete healing. An occasional patient, usually older, will develop progressive nephritis. Accordingly, patients should receive follow-up care until long after their urinalyses are completely normal. Renal function studies–especially the GFR–should be followed during that time. A falling GFR is cause for alarm.

Lewis EJ, Couse WG: The immunologic basis of human renal disease. P Clin North America 18:467–507, 1971.

Oliver WJ: Acute poststreptococcal glomerulonephritis in children. Hosp Med 6:113–135, 1970.

SUBACUTE & CHRONIC GLOMERULONEPHRITIS

Essentials of Diagnosis

- History of renal disease (sometimes).
- Headaches and fatigue, but often no symptoms at all.
- Hypertension, retinal hemorrhages, edema, pallor, cardiac failure, oliguria, isosmolar urine, proteinuria.
- Progressive renal failure with nitrogen retention, acidosis, hyperphosphatemia, anemia, and, rarely, hyperkalemia.

General Considerations

In progressive glomerulonephritis, the glomerular lesions usually develop insidiously and irreversibly. The lesions may be membranous, proliferative, mixed, or focal.

The end stage of the disease gives rise to small contracted kidneys where hyalinization, crescent formation, and fibrosis lead to the complete obliteration of most of the glomeruli. Extensive tubular changes and interstitial fibrosis are often noted along with prominent vascular damage.

The pathogenesis of progressive glomerulonephritis is rarely known. Some cases undoubtedly occur as a sequel to acute poststreptococcal nephritis or Henoch-Schönlein purpura, or as part of the picture of disseminated lupus erythematosus or Goodpasture's syndrome, but most are unassociated with any defined systemic illness. Most cases are thought to be due to a sustained immunopathy in which accretions of soluble antigen-antibody complexes and subsequent immuno-inflammatory changes damage the glomerular basement membrane or the endothelium and epithelium on either side of it.

The course is variable. Patients with rapidly progressive glomerulonephritis may experience brisk deterioration of renal function and die in uremia a few weeks or months after apparent onset. Others (subacute glomerulonephritis) may progress slowly over 2–3 years, and still others may experience no evident progression over several years.

Clinical Findings

A. Symptoms and Signs: A history of acute infection or renal disease is not always obtained, and defining the onset may not be possible. Exacerbations sometimes appear to follow infections. In general, pediatric patients with progressive glomerulonephritis present either with nephrotic syndrome, with mild to severe signs of glomerular insufficiency along with hematuria, elevated BUN, and hypertension, or with what appears to be an otherwise straightforward acute glomerulonephritis except for the lack of a demonstrable streptococcal component. The clinical picture when the child is first seen can seldom be correlated with the type or severity of the histologic changes.

B. Laboratory Findings: Urine flow may be restricted and is commonly of fixed specific gravity. Variable increases in protein content, as well as of red cells, white cells, and various casts, may be noted. As in any situation where there is proteinuria, it is important to make certain that urinary tract infection is not present. GFR is usually reduced. BUN and serum creatinine are often elevated. Serum albumin is commonly low, and serum globulin levels vary with the magnitude of the renal leak. Heavy (3+ or 4+) proteinuria with nephrotic syndrome, when associated with hypertension, hematuria, and hypogammaglobulinemia, often indicates membranous glomerulonephritis. Serum complement fractions may be variably low or normal. Depending upon the degree of renal failure that exists, acidosis, hyperphosphatemia, anemia, impaired platelet function, and hyperkalemia may be found. Hyperkalemia is an infrequent but ominous sign.

C. Urologic Examinations: An intravenous urogram may produce little or no visualization of the kidneys, owing to their inability to concentrate the contrast material. Isotope scans may show minimal concentrations of radioactivity for the same reason.

D. Renal Biopsy: Renal biopsy may be very informative. Conventional stains such as hematoxylin-eosin and periodic acid-Schiff stain give a good indication of the reversibility of the process and show whether it is primarily membranous, proliferative, mixed, or focal. Methenamine-silver stained sections may reveal basement splitting and even immune deposits. Fluorescence microscopy using anti-IgG, anti-IgM, anti-IgA, anti-C′3 complement, and antifibrin can be extremely valuable by showing whether immune deposition has occurred and, if so, the pattern.

Treatment

Corticosteroids alone are usually ineffective in glomerulonephritis. Evidence is accumulating, however, which suggests that azathioprine (Imuran), 3–5 mg/kg/day orally, in combination with prednisone, 1–2 mg/kg/day orally, may halt or slow the progress of several types of glomerulonephritis, particularly the rapidly progressive forms, those due to systemic lupus erythematosus, Goodpasture's syndrome, and the more fulminant forms of anaphylactoid purpura nephritis.

A recent report has suggested that cyclophosphamide (Cytoxan) may be beneficial in systemic lupus erythematosus nephritis. Heparin may be of value in certain cases where renal fibrin deposition can be demonstrated.

Prognosis

The prognosis in most forms of subacute and chronic nephritis is guarded.

Campbell RA, Jacinto EY: Combined immunosuppressive therapy in steroid-resistant chronic glomerular diseases of childhood. Lancet 2:149–156, 1967.

Herdman RC & others: Anticoagulants in renal disease in children. Am J Dis Child 119:27–35, 1970.

Lewis EJ & others: The immunologic basis of human renal disease. P Clin North America 18:467–507, 1971.

Michael AF & others: Immunosuppressive therapy of chronic renal disease. New England J Med 276:817–828, 1967.

BENIGN RECURRENT HEMATURIA

A significant number of patients present with recurrent gross and microscopic hematuria but completely normal GFRs. Their hematuria is commonly intensified following upper respiratory infections, exposure to allergens, or strenuous exercise. Such patients are often subjected to repeated cystoscopy, urethral dilatations, retrograde studies, etc, and no radiographically discernible lesion is found. Renal biopsy regularly shows either nothing or mild focal glomerular changes. Complement is rarely found with immunofluorescent stains. Noncomplement-fixing IgA is commonly discovered. Benign recurrent hematuria occasionally occurs as a familial trait.

It is important to exclude other obscure causes of painless urinary tract bleeding such as tumor, tuberculosis, and chronic progressive glomerulonephritis. Intravenous urography should be performed. Cystoscopy with retrograde urography while active bleeding is occurring may be very helpful; cystoscopy during periods of microscopic hematuria is seldom helpful owing to the trauma induced by the procedure. Renal biopsy is often diagnostic and should include immunofluorescent studies with anti-IgA.

Treatment is seldom indicated. Many patients have been followed for years with no evident progression of their disease.

Berger J: IgA deposits in renal disease. Transplant Proc 1:939, 1969.

Northway JD: Hematuria in children. J Pediat 78:381–396, 1971.

HEMOLYTIC UREMIC SYNDROME

Essentials of Diagnosis

- Sudden hemolysis, fall in hemoglobin level, and burr cells in peripheral blood.
- Thrombocytopenia.
- Acute renal failure.

General Considerations

Hemolytic uremic syndrome is an uncommon (though not rare) acute disease characterized by thrombocytopenia, the sudden onset of renal failure, and striking hemolysis with fall in hemoglobin and the appearance of burred red cells in the peripheral blood. It is frequently complicated by hypertension, seizures, and extreme oliguria or frank anuria. The disease shows a striking predilection for infants and small children. Its appearance has been correlated with both rickettsial and viral agents and with administration of an investigational interferon-inducing drug. It commonly follows a gastrointestinal or upper respiratory illnesss. The actual pathogenesis of the disease, however, remains obscure.

The disease is regularly associated with fibrin deposition in the renal arterioles. It has been suggested that a consumptive coagulopathy due to a Shwartzman-like phenomenon underlies the fibrin deposition, although numerous studies have failed to provide any convincing evidence in support of this idea. In severe cases, renal cortical necrosis has been demonstrated. It is likely that a variety of insults can set in motion a poorly understood chain of immunologic events which culminate in the hemolytic uremic syndrome.

Clinical Findings

Following an antecedent gastrointestinal or upper respiratory illness, the patient becomes critically ill with pallor, anemia, jaundice, oliguria or anuria, hypertension, convulsions, and stupor. Anemia, thrombocytopenia, burr cells in the peripheral blood, and azotemia usually lead to the diagnosis.

Treatment

The evidence that heparin or corticosteroids, singly or in combination, are beneficial is poor. The only consistently effective therapy is early peritoneal dialysis. In view of the technical problems associated with hemodialysis of small children and the usually reversible nature of the disease, dialysis by the peritoneal route is most often preferable.

In general, peritoneal dialysis should be instituted in any child with hemolytic uremic syndrome who has been anuric for 24 hours or who has oliguria with hypertension and seizures.

The anemia may require transfusion with packed red cells, but the threat of a hypertensive crisis persists throughout the transfusion and for 8–12 hours afterwards. Whole blood exchange transfusion may be safer than merely adding red cells.

An oliguric intravenous fluid regimen (such as described on pp 445 and 927) should be instituted as soon as the oliguria is diagnosed.

Prognosis

Despite the severity of hemolytic uremic syndrome, most patients will survive if vigorous and effective therapy is instituted early and continued long enough. Patients have remained oliguric longer than 3 weeks and survived. Satisfactory return of renal function occurs in most patients. Recurrences have been reported.

Gervis M & others: Immunofluorescent and histologic findings in the hemolytic uremic syndrome. Pediat 47:352–359, 1971.

Kaplan BS & others: An analysis of the results of therapy in 67 cases of the hemolytic-uremic syndrome. J Pediat 78:420–425, 1971.

Katz J & others: Coagulation findings in the hemolytic-uremic syndrome of infancy: Similarity to hyperacute renal allograft rejection. J Pediat 78:426–434, 1971.

Leavitt TJ & others: Hemolytic-uremic-like syndrome following polycarboxylate interferon induction. Am J Dis Child 121:43–47, 1971.

ACUTE HEMORRHAGIC CYSTITIS

Acute hemorrhagic cystitis affects children of any race, age, or sex. It is usually of sudden onset and is characterized by gross total or terminal hematuria, dysuria, frequency, and urgency. It is sometimes associated with suprapubic pain, fever, and enuresis. Examination of urine usually shows only red cells and microscopic pyuria.

In 20–25% of cases, a viral cause can be found; the most common offender thus far identified has been adenovirus 11. As adenovirus carriage is common, it is essential to document rises in viral neutralizing antibody titers as well as to recover the virus if it is desired to establish a viral etiology.

A small proportion of cases appear to be caused by common bacterial pathogens. These should be identified and treated by means of systemic antibiotics.

Most cases are associated with sterile urine and remain idiopathic. Sterile hemorrhatic cystitis is not uncommon in patients receiving cyclophosphamide. Diagnostic studies should exclude other causes of hematuria.

Cases of viral and idiopathic acute hemorrhagic cystitis may be expected to resolve spontaneously in 10–14 days.

Mufson MA & others: Adenovirus infection in acute hemorrhagic cystitis. Am J Dis Child 121:281–285, 1971.

DISEASES OF THE KIDNEYS

RENAL HYPERTENSION

Hypertension in children is most commonly of renal origin (over 90% of diagnosable cases). The renal causes are mainly parenchymal or vascular but may be perinephritic or due to malformations or tumors.

A cause can be identified in 80% of cases of hypertension in children provided a thorough work-up is performed. Failure to diagnose and properly treat significant hypertension in a child may shorten his life expectancy. Therefore, thorough evaluation is mandatory whenever a hypertensive child is found.

Confirmation of the diagnosis depends upon the repeated demonstration of an elevated diastolic blood pressure (2 standard deviations above the mean for age and sex in the presence of a normal pulse rate). Table 18–1 should be consulted whenever a diastolic blood pressure above 70 mm Hg is found in any child. Blood pressure determination should be a routine part of the pediatric physical examination. The blood pressure cuff should be at least 20% wider than the diameter of the arm since too narrow a cuff will cause falsely high readings.

Diagnosis

A. Renoparenchymal Hypertension: A number of children are hypertensive as a result of parenchymal renal disease, which is usually bilateral and chronic. In

TABLE 18–1. Normal blood pressure for various ages (mm Hg).*

Ages	Mean Systolic ± 2 SD	Mean Diastolic ± 2 SD
1 month	80 ± 16	46 ± 16
6 months to 1 year	89 ± 29	60 ± 10†
1 year	96 ± 30	66 ± 25†
2 years	99 ± 25	64 ± 25†
3 years	100 ± 25	67 ± 23†
4 years	99 ± 20	65 ± 20†
5–6 years	94 ± 14	55 ± 9
6–7 years	100 ± 15	56 ± 8
7–8 years	102 ± 15	56 ± 8
8–9 years	105 ± 16	57 ± 9
9–10 years	107 ± 16	57 ± 9
10–11 years	111 ± 17	58 ± 10
11–12 years	113 ± 18	59 ± 10
12–13 years	115 ± 19	59 ± 10
13–14 years	118 ± 19	60 ± 10

*Reproduced, with permission, from Nadas A: *Pediatric Cardiology,* 2nd ed. Saunders, 1963.
†In this study the point of muffling was taken as the diastolic pressure.

sharp contrast to renovascular hypertension, renoparenchymal hypertension is seldom mediated through the renin-angiotensin mechanism, and most patients have normal or low levels of circulating peripheral blood renin. In most cases, the cause is obscure. Recent work has suggested that renal prostaglandin (PGE_2) insufficiency may be causative in at least some cases of renoparenchymal hypertension.

Diagnostic studies should include examination of the urine followed by rapid sequence intravenous urograms and studies of renal function. Renovascular hypertension should be excluded whenever possible. However, the finding of apparent renovascular hypertension in the presence of bilateral renal parenchymal disease should be cause for reevaluation.

Nephrectomy should be avoided unless adequate renal tissue will remain following surgery. Nephrectomy often does not alleviate apparent renovascular hypertension when significant bilateral renoparenchymal disease exists. In particular, patients with chronic bilateral pyelonephritis may exhibit much higher renin levels from one kidney yet remain hypertensive when that kidney is removed.

Patients with renoparenchymal hypertension are often particularly sensitive to sudden expansion of blood volume. A blood transfusion given to a patient with chronic renal disease and mild hypertension may produce dramatic hypertension and often seizures within 12 hours.

B. Renovascular Hypertension: Any hypertensive process mediated through the renin-angiotensin mechanism and caused by interference with the blood supply to or within one kidney is said to be renovascular. Causes include renal artery stenosis, vascular compression by extrinsic masses, and renal arteritis.

Renovascular hypertension is often surgically curable.

Screening tests include rapid sequence intravenous and urea washout urograms and isotope renograms. The most definitive diagnostic tests are renal angiography and bilateral renal vein renin determinations.

If unilateral impairment to blood flow is demonstrated, bilateral renal vein renin levels should be determined. If the renin level from the kidney with impaired flow is 1.5–2 times greater than that of the opposite side, a reasonable likelihood exists that surgical correction of the lesion or unilateral nephrectomy may be curative or beneficial. If any doubt exists regarding the adequacy of the surviving kidney, differential renal function studies should be performed to ascertain how much residual renal function may be anticipated. If anticipated function is marginal or the hypertension is of long duration, open renal biopsy should be performed on the kidney with the lower renal vein renin level to search for hypertensive vascular changes. Failure to correct renovascular hypertension usually results in hypertensive vascular disease in the "good" kidney, and, in time, corrective surgery may become impossible.

C. Miscellaneous Causes of Renal Hypertension: A variety of renal and genitourinary conditions may be associated with hypertension. These include renal malformations, cysts, renal irradiation, Wilms's tumor, renal transplant rejection, hydronephrosis, acute glomerulonephritis, hemolytic uremic syndrome, acute renal failure, and corticosteroid therapy in the presence of renal disease.

Differential Diagnosis

A. Coarctation of the Aorta: One of the most common causes of pediatric hypertension is coarctation of the aorta. Thus, blood pressure recordings in all extremities are mandatory in any child with upper extremity hypertension. This condition is discussed in greater detail in Chapter 13.

B. Adrenal Hypertension: Hypertension may accompany some forms of the adrenogenital syndrome, primary hyperaldosteronism, Cushing's disease, neuroblastoma, and pheochromocytoma. These causes must be excluded in any hypertensive child.

C. Miscellaneous Conditions Associated With Hypertension: A variety of conditions may be associated with hypertension, including burns, increased intracranial pressure, poliomyelitis, Guillain-Barré syndrome, and certain ingestions or overdosages, including reserpine, mercury, and licorice. Recovery from liver transplantation is regularly attended by hypertension.

D. Essential Hypertension: Essential hypertension remains a diagnosis by exclusion. There may be a familial tendency, and blood pressure should be measured in all family members and the results compared carefully with normative tables.

Treatment

A. Hypertensive Emergencies: A hypertensive emergency may be said to exist when CNS signs of hypertension appear, eg, papilledema or seizures. Retinal hemorrhages or exudates also indicate a need for prompt and effective control.

1. One of the most effective drugs for a true hypertensive emergency is diazoxide (Hyperstat), 5 mg/kg by a single, rapid intravenous injection.

2. A combination of intramuscular reserpine and hydralazine is often effective when rapid blood pressure control is desired. This is especially true in acute glomerulonephritis, but less so in long-standing hypertension.

a. Reserpine is given in an initial starting dose of 0.03 mg/kg IM. It may be repeated every 4–6 hours in doubled or tripled doses as necessary. Probably no more than 2–3 mg should be given at one time.

b. Hydralazine (Apresoline), 0.15 mg/kg IM, is given at the same time. The tachycardia caused by hydralazine tends to be counteracted by the bradycardia caused by reserpine.

3. A variety of other drugs are effective in the treatment of hypertensive emergencies. These include methyldopa (Aldomet), sodium nitroprusside, and the still highly-experimental minoxidil.

B. Ambulatory Treatment of Chronic Hypertension: The treatment of renoparenchymal hypertension is usually medical rather than surgical. No hard and fast rules may be laid down regarding the use of antihypertensive drugs or their dosages. In general, treatment is started with a low dose and the dose is raised at intervals (usually every few days) until control of blood pressure is achieved, postural hypotension becomes a problem, or undesirable side-effects occur.

Marked diurnal variations in blood pressure may occur. Hence, it is advisable to teach capable parents how to take and record blood pressures at home. These data should be charted as well as written down. Blood pressure should be taken at least 4 times a day: after arising, at mid-morning if possible, in the afternoon, and during the evening.

Table 18–2 lists the drugs commonly used to treat hypertension on an ambulatory basis. The order and combinations in which these drugs should be used are governed by the potency of the drugs, their freedom from side-effects, and the severity of the hypertension. The mildest drug is probably hydrochlorothiazide used alone, followed by reserpine and hydralazine (often in combination). Methyldopa is particularly valuable in chronic renal failure because of its ability to lower blood pressure while maintaining cardiac output and renal perfusion. Guanethidine is probably the most potent of the "outpatient" antihypertensives, although postural hypotension is a serious side-effect if the dose is increased too rapidly. Acute renal failure may occur when guanethidine is given to patients with

TABLE 18–2. Antihypertensive drugs for ambulatory treatment.

Drug	Oral Dose	Major Side-Effects*
Hydrochloro-thiazide (Esidrix, Hydro-Diuril)	2–4 mg/kg/24 hours as single dose or in 2 divided doses	Potassium depletion, hyperuricemia.
Reserpine (Serpasil, etc)	0.005–0.05 mg/kg/24 hours in 1 or 2 doses	Nasal stuffiness, depression, nausea, bradycardia, sedation.
Hydralazine (Apresoline)	0.75 mg/kg/24 hours in 4–6 divided doses	Lupus-like syndrome, tachycardia, headache.
Methyldopa (Aldomet)	10–40 mg/kg/24 hours in 3 divided doses	False-positive Coombs test, hemolytic anemia, fever, leukopenia, abnormal liver function tests. (Interferes with many laboratory tests.)
Guanethidine (Ismelin)	0.2–1 mg/kg/24 hours as single dose or in 3 divided doses	Postural hypotension, bradycardia; acute renal failure in patients with chronic renal failure.

*Many more side-effects than those listed have been reported.

marginal renal function due to a critically diminished renal perfusion.

Prognosis

The long-term effects of mild hypertension with onset during childhood are not well defined. However, studies by Still & Cottom (see reference, below) indicate that serious hypertension, if not corrected, is associated with a very poor long-term prognosis. Approximately 50% of children with diastolic blood pressures persistently above 120 mm Hg will die within 10 years of diagnosis.

Blaufox MD: Systemic arterial hypertension in pediatric practice. P Clin North America 18:577–593, 1971.

Gruskin AB: Low-renin essential hypertension: Another form of childhood hypertension. J Pediat 78:765–771, 1971.

Leumann E & others: Renovascular hypertension in children. Pediatrics 46:362–370, 1970.

Loggie JMH: Hypertension in children and adolescents. I. Causes and diagnostic studies. J Pediat 74:331–355, 1969.

Loggie JMH: Hypertension in children and adolescents. II. Drug therapy. J Pediat 74:640–654, 1969.

Palmer JM & others: Hypertension, hydronephrosis, and normal plasma renin. New England J Med 283:1032, 1970.

Still JL, Cottom D: Severe hypertension in childhood. Arch Dis Child 42:34–39, 1967.

Strong WB & others: Peripheral and renal vein plasma renin activity in coarctation of the aorta. Pediatrics 45:254–259, 1970.

Zinner SH & others: Familial aggregation of blood pressure in childhood. New England J Med 284:402–404, 1971.

ACUTE RENAL FAILURE

Essentials of Diagnosis

- History of exposure to nephrotoxic agents, sepsis, trauma, surgery, glomerulonephritis, shock, or hemorrhage.
- Severe oliguria or, more rarely, anuria.
- Progressive hyperkalemia, hyponatremia, acidosis, and rising BUN.

General Considerations

Acute renal failure is an important complication of many medical and surgical conditions. It can be defined as the sudden inability to excrete urine of sufficient quantity or adequate composition to maintain normal body fluid homeostasis. It may be due to impaired renal perfusion, as in shock (prerenal), to acute renal disease, or to obstructive uropathy.

Diminished circulating blood volume leads to lowered renal perfusion, and the decreased glomerular filtrate is further diminished by increased tubular reabsorption compounded by excessive amounts of circulating vasopressin (ADH) and aldosterone. Acute renal failure due to hypovolemia usually responds to volume replacement with isotonic saline solution,

plasma, or blood, depending upon the cause of the deficit. If impaired renal perfusion is prolonged, however, renal cortical blood flow ceases, resulting in renal damage which may take days or weeks to resolve.

Occult postrenal obstruction must always be considered since, if the diagnosis is made early enough, urologic treatment will prevent the development of secondary renal failure.

It is useful to consider acute renal failure of renal origin under 2 broad headings: (1) Acute renal failure secondary to exposure of the renal parenchyma to toxic substances or reduced renal perfusion. This type is usually reversible. An initial period of oliguria is generally followed by a high-output phase. (2) Acute renal failure secondary to acute glomerulonephritis, vascular disorders with renal infarction, bilateral cortical necrosis, or necrotizing papillitis.

Clinical Findings

A reliable history of a major infection, trauma (especially crush injury), a surgical procedure, an episode of shock or hemorrhage, or exposure to a potentially nephrotoxic product is helpful in the diagnosis of acute renal failure. The hallmark of the diagnosis is oliguria ($< 200-250$ ml/sq m/day). Frank anuria suggests either obstructive uropathy, bilateral renal infarction, or bilateral renal cortical necrosis. Thus, the physician must be alert to inadequate urine output in any patient at risk of developing acute renal failure.

Complications

Patients with acute renal failure are unable to excrete a water load. Hence, they easily develop hyponatremia and water intoxication. Moreover, they are at great risk of rapidly developing hyperkalemia and acidemia. Hypertension, azotemia, and uremia may supervene after a few hours or days.

Treatment

The objective of treatment is to prevent sustained renal damage and prolonged oliguria, either by averting renal damage altogether or by converting low-output renal failure to high-output renal failure.

A. Acute Management: An indwelling catheter should be inserted and urine output monitored hourly.

1. Prerenal factors—Exclude or rectify any prerenal factors. Oligemia should be corrected with blood, plasma, or isotonic saline solution until the blood pressure is normal. If urine output does not rise above oliguric levels within 30–60 minutes, a central venous pressure line should be inserted and additional blood, plasma, or saline should be infused until the central venous pressure has been restored to 3–6 mm Hg (or 4–8 cm water).

2. Obstructive uropathy—Correct obstructive uropathy or exclude any renal diseases that cannot be expected to respond with immediate diuresis (eg, acute oliguric glomerulonephritis, hemolytic uremic syndrome). Unresponsive renal diseases should be managed by means of an oliguric regimen such as that given on pp 445 and 927.

3. **Other measures**—If diuresis does not occur in response to the above measures, begin a rapid infusion of mannitol, 0.5–1 gm/kg IV over a period of 30 minutes as a 25% solution (up to 25 gm). Also give furosemide (Lasix), 2 mg/kg as an IV push. Allow 2 hours for a response to occur. If the urine output remains low (< 200–250 ml/sq m/24 hours), repeat the dose of furosemide. If no diuresis occurs, go on to the oliguric regimen given below. If diuresis does occur, continue furosemide and mannitol if necessary to sustain it. After several hours, the patient may convert to a phase of high-output renal failure which may last for several days and occasionally requires no further diuretic therapy. When this occurs, manage according to the high-output regimen given below.

4. **Oliguric phase**—Once it has been determined that a prolonged oliguric phase is inevitable, an oliguric renal failure regimen should be instituted without delay. It is essential that close patient monitoring be performed. The patient should be weighed at least daily; strict intake, output, and vital signs records must be kept; and laboratory determinations of hematocrit, serum sodium, potassium, chloride, blood CO_2 content, BUN, and creatinine should be done at least daily.

The principal complications of acute oliguric renal failure are (1) water intoxication and hyponatremia, (2) hyperkalemia, (3) metabolic acidosis, (4) hypertension, and (5) uremia. Therapy is directed against each of these complications.

The tendency to develop water intoxication and hyponatremia requires sharp reductions in fluid intake. This makes it difficult to provide enough calories to minimize tissue catabolism, metabolic acidosis, hyperkalemia, and uremia.

If the patient can retain oral feedings, he may be given carbohydrate and fat-rich supplements provided they are very low in protein, potassium, and sodium (eg, Controlyte). It is usually safer, however, to administer all calories intravenously by augmenting the glucose concentration in the intravenous fluids to 15–20%. Moreover, it is often helpful to place such patients on nasogastric suction so that HCl and NaCl can be removed to be replaced with $NaHCO_3$.

Intravenous fluids are calculated as follows: (1) Give no allotment for urine as long as oliguria persists. (2) Give only about 2/3 of the patient's estimated sensible and insensible water requirements. (The rest will be provided by water of oxidation.) In dry air, such patients usually require about 400 ml/sq m/day. (3) Replace nasogastric fluid losses ml for ml. (4) Replace nasogastric chloride losses with bicarbonate on a mEq for mEq basis.

Hyperkalemia can often be controlled by administration of an ion-exchange resin such as sodium-polystyrene sulfonate (Kayexalate) given as a retention enema every 4 hours made up as an aqueous slurry containing 1 gm of resin/kg body weight.

Severe or persistent hyperkalemia, severe hypertension, congestive failure, severe anemia, or uremic syndrome all justify the use of peritoneal dialysis or, occasionally, hemodialysis.

5. **High-output phase**—Most patients with acute renal failure go through a high-output phase. This phase may follow almost immediately after a renal insult or may be entered by diuretic-induced conversion from a low-output phase or during recovery after a period of prolonged oliguria. In some patients, the high-output phase is mild, lasts only a few days, and is characterized by slightly increased volumes of poorly concentrated urine. Other patients, however, may pass enormous volumes of isosthenuric, sodium-rich urine. Occasionally, this salt wasting state may be accompanied by significant potassium wasting as well.

Management requires the provision of adequate quantities of water, sodium, and potassium to provide for the ongoing losses. Measurement of previous volumes coupled with determinations of urinary electrolytes (Na^+, K^+, Cl^-) provide the best guide to therapy.

B. Dialysis: The indications for dialysis are based on clinical experience. A deteriorating clinical condition, persistent acidosis, a BUN in excess of 150 mg/100 ml, a serum potassium rising above 6 mEq/liter, overhydration, and congestive heart failure are accepted indications. (Intra-abdominal infection, surgery, bowel perforation, severe multiple adhesions, and bleeding are all relative contraindications to dialysis.) Because of recent improvements and simplifications in the technic of peritoneal dialysis, it is now customary to use it when dialysis is required for acute renal failure. At times, however, its effectiveness in removing a dialyzable toxic product or in controlling uremia, hyperkalemia, or severe water and electrolyte derangements is not satisfactory, in which case hemodialysis is recommended.

The technic of peritoneal dialysis is as follows:

1. **Catheter insertion**—

a. Empty the bladder. Scrub the abdomen as for laparotomy. Use strict aseptic technic with surgical scrub, gowns, gloves, etc. (Prophylactic antibiotics are usually not necessary, but strict aseptic technic is essential.)

b. Select a midline site 1/3 of the distance from the umbilicus to the symphysis pubis and infiltrate with local anesthetic (eg, 1% lidocaine). Unless ascites is present, enter the peritoneal cavity with an 18-gauge needle and partially fill the abdomen with 40–50 ml/kg of dialysate fluid (see below) prewarmed to 37° C (99° F). This should be done to reduce the likelihood of perforating a viscus.

c. Insert the peritoneal catheter. (Most commercially available peritoneal catheters come equipped with a stylet to aid in insertion.) Make a 5–10 mm transverse incision through the dermis into the linea alba. Push the stylet through the incision until the resistance of the peritoneum is felt. Apply slow, steady pressure until a "give" occurs as the peritoneal cavity is actually entered.

d. Pass the catheter over the stylet and gently feed it into the peritoneal cavity toward the left pelvic gutter. Unless the catheter is inserted past the last perforation, no siphon effect can be developed and return flow cannot be achieved.

e. Secure the catheter in place with a purse string suture and tie. Apply a sterile dressing.

2. Administration of dialysate—

a. Dialysate (or ascitic fluid) already present in the abdomen should be allowed to drain freely until drainage stops. Hemostats may be used to govern the direction of flow (from dialysate bottle to patient or from patient to reservoir).

b. Fill the peritoneal cavity with 50–80 ml/kg of dialysate. (This usually takes 5–10 minutes.) Allow the dialysate to remain in the abdomen 45–60 minutes and then drain it out to completion (10–15 minutes). Thus, one complete cycle usually takes about 60–85 minutes.

c. It is essential to maintain an accurate running record of volumes in and out. Entries should be made on completion of each infusion or drainage period. Weigh the patient before beginning dialysis and every 6 hours thereafter. Blood pressure, pulse, respiration, and temperature should be recorded hourly.

3. Choosing the proper dialysate—A typical commercial peritoneal dialysate contains approximately 140 mEq/liter Na^+, 100–105 mEq/liter Cl^-, 40–45 mEq/liter lactate$^-$, 3–4 mEq/liter Ca^{++}, and 1–1.5 mEq/liter Mg^{++}. K^+ is usually omitted unless the serum potassium is < 4 mEq/liter. Glucose is also added in varying quantities, usually 15–70 gm/liter depending upon the need to withdraw fluid from the patient. The 15 gm/liter glucose concentration is used to maintain a slight osmotic gradient between the patient's body fluids and the dialysate in order to prevent fluid absorption by the patient. Higher concentrations of glucose may be used to absorb fluid from the patient. When this is done, the volumes recovered after each drainage will exceed the volumes instilled. Unless severe congestive heart failure exists, it is usually unwise to exceed glucose concentrations of 40–45 gm/liter, as excessive water removal can rapidly lead to hypernatremia. Lactate is used instead of HCO_3^- to provide buffer base since HCO_3^- would cause extremely high pH values in the dialysate unless CO_2 were bubbled through it. Five hundred units of heparin should be added to each of the first 4–6 liters of dialysate to prevent clotting in the catheter.

4. Complications of dialysis—The complications include bleeding (rarely major), bowel perforation, failure to obtain return of fluid (usually requiring only repositioning of the patient or the catheter), respiratory distress (usually correctable by using smaller volumes), and infection. Infection is by far the most common and is one of the most serious complications of peritoneal dialysis. Signs of peritonitis should be sought for several days following the procedure.

Disequilibrium syndrome (nausea, vomiting, muscle cramps, heacache, and seizures) may result from too rapid removal of urea. This is a common complication of hemodialysis but is rare with peritoneal dialysis and seldom occurs unless the predialysis BUN is extremely high (> 200 mg/100 ml). It can be corrected by injecting 1–3 ml/kg of 50% glucose solution IV as

needed. Predialysis parenteral administration of diphenylhydantoin, 5 mg/kg, is advisable if peritoneal dialysis is performed on such a patient.

Note: Peritoneal dialysis is much less efficient than hemodialysis and usually requires 20–40 passes over a period of 2 or 3 days. Thus, its use as a long-term therapeutic measure is limited. The catheter should be removed after each dialysis.

Most patients dislike peritoneal dialysis intensely. Anxiety and pain may be relieved with pentazocine (Talwin), 0.3–0.5 mg/kg IV, IM, or subcut every 6–8 hours as necessary.

Course & Prognosis

The period of severe oliguria, if it occurs, usually lasts about 10 days. If oliguria lasts longer than 3 weeks or if there is complete anuria, a diagnosis of acute tubular necrosis is very unlikely and a vascular accident or glomerulonephritis is more probable. The diuretic phase begins with progressive increases in urinary output followed by the passage of large volumes of isosthenuric urine containing 80–150 mEq/liter of sodium. During the recovery phase, signs and symptoms subside rapidly, although polyuria may persist for several days or weeks. Urinary abnormalities usually disappear completely within a few months.

The prognosis is excellent in acute tubular necrosis ($> 90\%$ complete recovery), but poor in other forms of acute renal failure of renal origin such as vascular accident ($< 10\%$ recovery).

Blagg CR: The management of acute reversible intrinsic renal failure. Postgrad MJ 43:290–307, 1967.

Dobrin RS & others: The critically ill child: Acute renal failure. Pediatrics 48:286–291, 1971.

Kaplan SA, Strauss J, Yuceoglu AM: Conservative management of acute renal failure. Pediatrics 25:409–418, 1960.

Luke RG, Kennedy AC: Prevention and early management of acute renal failure. Postgrad MJ 43:280–290, 1967.

CHRONIC RENAL FAILURE

Essentials of Diagnosis

- Usually a history of renal disease.
- Headache, fatigue, anorexia, pallor.
- Hypertension, anemia, acidosis, bone pains, cardiac failure.
- Elevated BUN, proteinuria; red cells and casts in urine.

General Considerations

In renal failure kidney function is reduced to a level at which the kidneys are unable to maintain normal biochemical homeostasis. In acute renal failure, the nephrons are injured, often reversibly; in the chronic form, the nephrons are destroyed progressively, leading to gradually increasing uremia. Many kidney diseases lead to uremia, particularly chronic pyelonephritis and chronic glomerulonephritis. Diabetic nephropathy, renal amyloidosis, systemic lupus erythematosus, cirrhosis, hepatic failure, subacute bacterial endocarditis, hyperparathyroidism, hypercalcemia, renal tubular acidosis, oxalosis, and cystinosis represent some of the conditions which may also lead to uremia. Urinary obstruction is often responsible for uremia, and one should never neglect this possibility since it may be either totally or partially reversible.

The biochemical derangements in chronic renal failure can be summarized as follows:

(1) Water: The kidneys represent the only route of water excretion which can adapt to the metabolic needs of the body since the insensible water losses of lungs and skin are fixed. With a reduction in the number of functioning nephrons, each surviving nephron must handle a larger fraction of the solute load; it therefore passes a larger fraction of its filtrate into the urine without reabsorption, since a urine with a small solute content can be concentrated to a much higher degree than can a urine of large solute load. Consequently, impairment of concentrating capacity relates to the fact that residual nephrons function under conditions of osmotic diuresis. A kidney unable to concentrate urine beyond serum osmolality (285 mOsm/liter) needs about 3 liters of urine to handle a daily solute load of 1000 mOsm. There is usually also a maximum tolerance for water which, when exceeded, leads to edema, hyponatremia, and water intoxication. This ceiling, unfortunately, often is quite close to the minimum tolerance alluded to previously, and water balance can be precarious.

(2) Nitrogenous products: On a normal diet, nitrogen balance can be maintained if an average of 9 mg of urea nitrogen is excreted in the urine per minute. As the filtrate flows down the tubule, 50% of the urea is reabsorbed; therefore, 18 mg of urea nitrogen must be filtered. At a glomerular filtration rate of 100 ml/minute, 18 mg of urea nitrogen will be present in the filtrate if the BUN is 18 mg/100 ml. However, if the filtration rate is 25 ml/minute, a BUN of 72 mg/100 ml is required to filter 18 mg of urea nitrogen. The level of BUN is affected not only by the glomerular filtration rate but also by dietary intake of protein and by urinary flow. Creatinine, on the other hand, is not reabsorbed by the tubules and is not influenced by dietary intake; for these reasons, serum creatinine has several advantages over urea as an index of renal failure.

(3) Sodium and potassium: Sodium loss is enhanced by osmotic diuresis (see above) and by a decreased capacity of the tubules to secrete hydrogen ions in exchange for sodium. For these reasons, sodium retention is rare in chronic renal failure unless there is severe hypertension. Salt wasting can therefore be a serious problem and can be compounded by salt restriction or diuretics. Hyperkalemia is usually a very late problem in chronic renal failure; in actual fact, hypokalemia is often observed.

(4) Phosphorus and calcium: A large percentage (85%) of the filtered phosphorus is normally reab-

sorbed; tubular rejection can therefore compensate for a decrease in glomerular filtration rate. However, retention of phosphorus occurs when the glomerular filtration rate drops below 20 ml/minute. Serum phosphorus levels between 7–10 mg/100 ml are common and, concomitantly, calcium levels drop. This phenomenon relates not only to the fact that the transport of calcium across the bowel wall in uremia is unresponsive to normal amounts of vitamin D but also, perhaps, to the reciprocal relationship of serum phosphorus and serum calcium.

(5) Acid-base balance: Decreased ammonia production and retention of endogenous acid account for the metabolic acidosis seen in chronic renal failure.

Clinical Findings

A. Symptoms and Signs: The lack of correlation between symptoms and chemical abnormalities illustrates the capacity of the patient in chronic renal failure to adapt when changes have taken place slowly. A history of renal disease is not always present. Nocturia for a definable period, headache, fatigue, anorexia, anemia, and loss of weight are common early manifestations, although some patients remain asymptomatic. The skin is commonly sallow, yellow, and dry, and pruritus can be severe.

At a more advanced stage of uremia, the major CNS manifestations include apathy, lethargy, drowsiness, stupor, convulsions, and coma. Kussmaul breathing is not uncommon when severe metabolic acidosis is present.

Anemia is ascribed to decreased erythropoietin, a hemolytic component due to decreased red cell deformability, and toxic suppression of the bone marrow. Hemorrhagic phenomena involving the gastrointestinal tract, the skin, and sometimes the CNS are associated with variable thrombocytopenia and uniformly diminished platelet adhesiveness.

In the cardiovascular system, uremia may cause pericarditis, leading to cardiac enlargement and tamponade. Cardiomyopathy is also described and is partly explained by the cardiac effects of hypertensive disease.

Uremic pneumonitis has the radiologic appearance of pulmonary edema and can become manifest in the absence of left ventricular failure and hypertension.

Congestive heart failure is common. In fact, it is usually impossible to distinguish clearly between congestive heart failure, uremic pneumonitis, and bacterial pneumonia.

Gastrointestinal manifestations are diverse but are dominated by sudden uremic vomiting, which may become intractable and may lead to severe electrolyte disturbances and an increase in the retention of nitrogenous products through protein catabolism.

The skeletal system responds to the biochemical derangements by osteomalacia or by renal rickets.

B. Laboratory Findings: Urinalysis almost always shows proteinuria, red cells, white cells, and various casts. The urine specific gravity is usually

1.008–1.010. The tubular excretion of hydrogen ion and ammonia is low in proportion to the metabolic acidosis which is present, but it correlates well with the residual nephron population. The BUN and serum creatinine are markedly elevated. Serum potassium is normal or low but may rise terminally. Phosphorus retention is usually present. PAH and inulin clearances are proportionately reduced. The anemia is usually normochromic and normocytic. ECG gives valuable information concerning cardiopulmonary manifestations.

C. X-Ray Findings: A plain film of the abdomen may show enlarged or shrunken kidneys. Chest x-ray should be taken to determine whether cardiopulmonary signs are present.

D. Urologic Studies: In the absence of an etiologic diagnosis, a urologic work-up should be done. Intravenous urography is probably worth attempting in patients with BUNs up to 100 mg/100 ml, giving a second dose of the contrast material 30–60 minutes after the first one. Retrograde urography should be done if there are any doubts about the integrity of the urinary tract.

Treatment

The goals of treatment are to prevent further renal damage due to hypertension and infection and to restore maximal homeostasis.

A. Water and Calorie Conservation: Depending upon the degree of renal failure, strict attention must be paid to water conservation. In complete anuria, water should be supplied to replace insensible loss minus water of oxidation (about 400 ml/sq m/24 hours) plus water lost in stools, vomitus, and urine. The amount to be given should be carefully calculated at least daily and checked against body weight and, if possible, urine osmolality.

Diet is difficult to organize for any child with a fickle appetite, and especially so when water must be restricted. However, it is very important to sustain caloric input.

In less severe cases, restriction of protein to 1 gm/kg/24 hours or less may help to lower blood urea, and the so-called Giovanetti diet (Table 18–3) can be made quite palatable for this purpose.

Low-protein (Giovanetti) diet for renal failure: The 37 gm protein diet contains approximately 1600 calories; the 24 gm protein diet contains approximately 1500 calories. This caloric content may be increased and adjusted to the individual patient's needs through the increased emphasis on high-carbohydrate or high-fat foods (or both) in the diet. At both levels of protein restriction, the mineral content of the diet is low: potassium, 1–2 gm; phosphorus, 600–700 mg; sodium, 1 gm.

In cases of severe hypertension or edema, reduction of the sodium intake to 200 mg may be indicated.

Iron, multivitamins, and methionine, 0.5 gm, should be given as supplements. With the exception of methionine, all essential amino acids are provided in adequate amounts.

TABLE 18–3. Low-protein (Giovanetti) diets.*

	37 gm Protein
Milk	2/3 cup daily.
Meat or meat substitute	2 oz meat and 1 egg daily or, when possible, 2 eggs and no meat daily.
Vegetables	2–3 servings daily, ½ cup per serving.
Fruit and fruit juices	As much as possible.
Bread	Low-protein bread ad lib.
Cereal	One serving daily, ½ cup per serving.
Potato or substitute	2 servings daily, ½ cup per serving.
Fats	Use liberally.
Beverages other than milk	Tea, lemonade, Kool-Aid, carbonated beverages, fruit juice.
Soups	Broth containing no meat.
Snacks	Fruit or fruit juice, low-protein bread, desserts made from low-protein flour recipes, hard candy.
Miscellaneous	Jelly, honey, and sugar should be used liberally.
Desserts	Popsicles, hard candy, fruit, desserts made from low-protein flour.

*The 24 gm protein diet is the same as the 37 gm diet with the following changes: *Milk:* 1/3 cup daily. *Meat:* 1 oz meat and 1 egg daily. *Vegetables:* 2 servings daily of ½ cup each. *Potato:* One daily serving of ½ cup.

Newer dietary supplements (eg, Controlyte) can significantly increase caloric intake without adding significant protein, sodium, or potassium.

Salt restriction (ie, no added salt) is advisable in children with hypertension, but low-salt diets are unpalatable and these children have poor appetites.

B. Electrolyte Homeostasis: The principles of fluid and electrolyte therapy are discussed in Chapter 37. Meticulous medical care can often sustain children in renal failure for many weeks without dialysis.

Elevated serum phosphorus can to some extent be controlled by a low-phosphorus diet in conjunction with aluminum hydroxide gel (Amphojel), 1 tbsp 3 times a day. Calcium lactate, 4 gm 3 times a day, usually offsets urinary protein-bound calcium loss, but this is not always effective.

C. Blood Transfusions: Some children with renal failure become severely anemic and transfusions may be essential, but it is remarkable how little they may be affected by hemoglobins as low as 6 gm/100 ml. In general, if there is no cardiac failure and the patient is not overly fatigued, transfusions should be avoided. Since these patients already may have marginally high blood volumes, any increase may precipitate severe hypertension with convulsions or congestive failure. Packed cells should always be used and should be given very slowly and under the closest supervision. If necessary, a total or partial exchange should be used to increase the hematocrit. Vascular accidents are frequent during and immediately after improperly supervised transfusions.

D. Dialysis: Dialysis is indicated for intractable acidosis, hyperkalemia, congestive failure, or clinical uremic syndrome. It may also be essential as an interim sustaining measure when kidney transplant has been decided upon or when an interval between nephrectomy and transplant is required.

Hemodialysis is best carried out by an experienced team. Children should not be given long-term dialysis and (generally) not home dialysis; instead, a decision must be made whether or not to perform a transplant.

E. Management of Acidosis and Osteodystrophy: A low-protein diet will be helpful in decreasing the metabolic acidosis since proteins are the largest contributors of nonvolatile acids. The acidosis can be further alleviated by the administration of an alkalinizing solution. Unless renal failure is very advanced, attempts should be made to relieve bone pain and to improve the osteodystrophy by the administration of vitamin D in doses of 25–50 thousand IU daily or more. Care must be taken to avoid metastatic calcifications. Hyperphosphatemia can be helped by aluminum hydroxide preparations administered after each meal.

F. Management of Hypertension: When hypertension is not controlled on a 0.5–1 gm sodium diet, reserpine and hydralazine (Apresoline) may be helpful. Severe fixed hypertension merits gradually increasing doses of methyldopa (Aldomet), guanethidine (Ismelin) or pentolinium (Ansolysen), singly or in combination. Therapy with ganglion blocking agents must always be started with very small doses because of the risk of cerebral venous thromboses due to postural hypotension. If renal failure is advanced, careful monitoring of glomerular filtration rate should be done since a drastic reduction in blood pressure may provoke a rapid rise in BUN.

G. Control of Infections: Antibiotics should be given at the first sign of infection, keeping in mind that the dosage of certain antibiotics eliminated principally in the urine should be reduced in proportion to the decrease in renal function in order to prevent toxic effects.

H. Renal Transplantation: Renal transplantation is now a realistic and effective means of treating severe renal disease in children. The cost remains high, and for this reason the procedure is usually restricted to specially supported centers. The use of antilymphocyte serum in conjunction with azathioprine (Imuran) and corticosteroids to suppress rejection has led to an immediate survival rate of 80%. This operation should not be undertaken until it is clear that survival depends on it.

Prognosis

Severe chronic renal disease in childhood is all too often progressive and eventually fatal. The rates at which renal diseases progress are quite variable, however, and are hard to predict. Intractable anemia and hypertension are bad signs, as are permanent electrolyte changes and neurologic symptoms. In general, it is best to continue with medical treatment until one of

these unfavorable signs appears before deciding on transplant.

Bricker NS & others: Renal function in chronic renal disease. Medicine 44:263–288, 1965.

Fine RN & others: Hemodialysis in children. Am J Dis Child 119:498–504, 1970.

Holliday MA & others: Treatment of renal failure in children. P Clin North America 18:613–624, 1971.

Lilly JR & others: Renal homotransplantation in pediatric patients. Pediatrics 47:548–557, 1971.

Merrill JP, Hampers CL: Uremia. New England J Med 282:953–961, 1014–1021, 1970.

Potter D & others: The treatment of chronic uremia in childhood. I. Transplantation. II. Hemodialysis. Pediatrics 45:432–443; 46:678–689, 1970.

NEPHROTIC SYNDROME

1. MINIMAL LESION NEPHROTIC SYNDROME

Essentials of Diagnosis

- Sudden onset of generalized edema, with proteinuria, hypoalbuminemia, and often hypercholesterolemia.
- Urine is usually free of red cells unless there is underlying glomerulonephritis.
- Seldom significant hypertension or azotemia.
- Serum protein electrophoretic pattern shows low albumin; high, merged a_2-β peak; and normal or low γ peaks.

General Considerations

Nephrotic syndrome of childhood is usually an idiopathic illness of young children: 65% of patients are under 3 years old at the time of their first attack. It is usually not associated with serious or permenent renal damage, although occasional cases in which nephrotic syndrome is secondary to glomerulonephritis may progress to renal failure. The response to corticosteroid therapy is often dramatic, although recurrences are common. The characteristic findings of nephrotic syndrome (edema, proteinuria, hypoproteinemia, and hypercholesterolemia) are usually present. Most patients demonstrate no significant hypertension, hematuria, or azotemia. Occasionally (2–5%), the disease appears in siblings.

Nephrosis has occasionally been ascribed to exposure to or ingestion of trimethadione, penicillamine, allergens, gold, etc. Congenital forms are reported (see next section). In about 10% of cases, nephrotic syndrome is a complication of a more serious preexisting renal disease such as membranous glomerulonephritis, lupus nephritis, malaria, congenital syphilis, renal vein thrombosis, and amyloid disease. It may occur rarely as a sequel to congestive heart failure, constrictive pericarditis, or tricuspid atresia.

Idiopathic nephrotic syndrome of childhood is usually associated with normal or nearly normal renal biopsy findings on light and immunofluorescence microscopy. Hence, it is commonly called "minimal lesion" nephrosis. Electron microscopy, however, regularly reveals fusion of epithelial cell foot processes which reverts to normal during remissions.

Clinical Findings

A. Symptoms and Signs: Periorbital puffiness in the morning which subsides during the day is usual. Within a few days, the edema worsens and becomes generalized, and ascites and pleural effusions develop.

Striae may develop over the swollen abdomen. The scrotum may become very swollen and pendulous. In long-standing cases, the hair may become coarse and light in color, resembling that seen in kwashiorkor. There may be loss of elasticity of ear cartilage. Anorexia and diarrhea occur as a result of edema of the bowel wall.

B. Laboratory Findings: Heavy proteinuria (> 4–4.5 gm/24 hours) occurs, often in concentrations sufficient to elevate the urinary specific gravity. There should be little or no hematuria. Urinary sediment usually contains numerous hyaline and granular casts and oval fat bodies which show a Maltese cross pattern under polarized light. Serum sodium may be artifactually low if significant hypercholesterolemia is present owing to displacement of serum by fat droplets. Serum albumin is depressed (often to < 1 gm/100 ml), while serum protein electrophoresis shows a strikingly elevated, fused a_2-β peak. Serum gamma globulin may be normal or low. A finding of hematuria, red cell casts, hypogammaglobulinemia, or hypergammaglobulinuria tends to indicate that glomerulonephritis with a serious nonselective protein leak underlies the nephrosis. Minimal lesion nephrosis is usually selective and is seldom associated with heavy globulinuria.

Treatment

A. Corticosteroids: It is useful to define categories on the basis of the response to corticosteroids. Thus, 20–40% of cases are "steroid-sensitive" and are apparently permanently cured with a single course of corticosteroids; 60–80% are "steroid-dependent," responding well to corticosteroids but relapsing at varying intervals after each course; the remainder (5–10%) are at some stage "steroid-resistant," ie, do not respond to corticosteroids.

The usual procedure is to give prednisone, 1.5–2 mg/kg orally daily in 3–4 divided doses. Once diuresis has occurred, the daily dose is increased by 1.5–2 times and given once every 48 hours. Conversion to an alternate-day regimen spares the patient many of the side-effects of corticosteroid therapy. Corticosteroids should be continued for about 3 months, tapered downward over 4–6 weeks, and finally discontinued.

Steroid-dependent and steroid-resistant patients should undergo a renal biopsy to exclude any renal lesion other than "minimal lesion" nephrosis. If another disorder is found, appropriate therapy should be instituted. Steroid-resistant patients and those who are steroid-dependent but require unacceptably high steroid doses may be considered for a course of combined (prednisone-cyclophosphamide) therapy.

B. Combined Therapy: Prednisone and Cyclophosphamide (Cytoxan):

1. Dosage–Cyclophosphamide, 2 mg/kg/day orally, is given as a single dose in the morning with 2 glasses of water. Prednisone, 2–3 mg/kg orally, is given as a single dose every 48 hours. Both drugs are continued for < 2 months; the cyclophosphamide is then abruptly discontinued and the prednisone is tapered to zero by decrements of 5 mg/week. This regimen will usually induce long-term remission.

2. Side-effects–The side-effects of cyclophosphamide are significant. The most common is leukopenia, especially after viral infections or a lowering of the dose of prednisone. Weekly total and differential white counts are essential. The absolute polymorphonuclear leukocyte count should be maintained above 1500–2000/cu mm; if it falls lower than this, the cyclophosphamide should be temporarily withdrawn and reinstituted following a rise in PMN count.

Alopecia may occur but is uncommon in the dosage used. The hair will grow out normally once the cyclophosphamide is discontinued, although a wig may be temporarily necessary. Some hair loosening may be noted during combing.

Sterile hemorrhagic cystitis sometimes occurs. Rare but major bladder hemorrhages have been observed, and severe bladder contractures with fibrosis have been reported. The drug should be discontinued if hematuria occurs; this complication may be preventable by high fluid consumption and frequent voiding.

Fatal varicella has been observed, and some centers reserve cyclophosphamide for patients who have had varicella. Should varicella exposure or eruption occur, the physician should administer commercial gamma globulin, 0.5 ml/kg IM. He is then advised to locate a center where zoster-immune globulin and cytosine or adenine arabinoside may be administered as antiviral chemotherapeutic agents. The cyclophosphamide should be discontinued until the threat has passed, but the prednisone should be continued.

Recent evidence suggests that cyclophosphamide may cause permanent azoospermia and sterility in most if not all males treated for more than 2–3 months. Variable effects on gonadal function have been observed in females. It appears as though cyclophosphamide should not be used unless the patient is willing to pay the price of permanent sterility and the parents are so informed.

C. Diuretics: Hypoproteinemia causes a low circulating plasma volume which, in turn, accelerates renin and eventually aldosterone secretion, thereby causing renal conservation of sodium. Most diuretics are ineffective unless hypoproteinemia is first corrected. If ascites and pleural effusion are causing respiratory difficulty, diuresis should be accomplished. A course of 1–2 gm/kg of salt-poor albumin should be given IV every 6 hours, followed each time by 1–1.5 mg/kg of furosemide IV. Diuresis will usually begin within an hour; if it does not, the dose of albumin should be repeated for a maximum of 3 days.

D. Diet: Unless azotemia occurs, diets should provide generous protein supplementation. Sodium restriction is indicated while edema exists and should be stringent if edema is severe.

E. Antibiotics: Prophylactic antibiotics are not advised. They should be employed readily in patients suspected of having early bacterial infections. Pneumococcal infections, particularly peritonitis, are seen with increased frequency during nephrotic episodes.

Prognosis

Idiopathic nephrotic syndrome of childhood appears to be associated with an excellent prognosis for long-term survival if minimal glomerular lesions are seen on renal biopsy. If the nephrotic syndrome represents a complication of a proliferative, membranoproliferative, or membranous glomerulonephritis, the prognosis is much more guarded and depends on the natural history of the renal disease in question.

Arneil GC: The nephrotic syndrome. P Clin North America 18:547–559, 1971.

Barratt TM, Soothill JF: Controlled trial of cyclophosphamide in steroid-sensitive relapsing nephrotic syndrome of childhood. Lancet 2:479–482, 1970.

Johnson WW, Meadows DC: Urinary bladder fibrosis and telangiectasia after cyclophosphamide therapy. New England J Med 284:290–294, 1971.

Miller DG: Alkylating agents and human spermatogenesis. JAMA 217:1662–1665, 1971.

Saxena KM, Crawford JD: The treatment of nephrosis. New England J Med 272:522–526, 1965.

Tsao YC, Yeung CH: Paired trial of cyclophosphamide and prednisone in children with nephrosis. Arch Dis Child 46:327, 1971.

2. CONGENITAL NEPHROSIS

Congenital nephrosis is a rare congenital, uniformly fatal renal disorder which is often observed in multiple siblings in a single family. Autosomal recessive inheritance is suggested. The kidneys are pale and large and may show microcystic dilatations of the proximal tubules and glomerular changes. The latter consist of proliferation, crescent formation, and thickening of capillary walls.

The pathogenesis is unknown. A fundamental immunologic incompatibility between the mother and the infant is perhaps responsible, since mothers reject skin grafts of their nephrotic infants more rapidly than control mothers reject grafts of normal infants. Evidence of immune injury in the kidneys relates to the finding of gamma globulin and complement components on the glomerular loops.

Low birth weight with an obstetric history of large placenta, wide cranial sutures, delayed ossification, and edema are commonly noted at birth. The edema, however, may be apparent only after the first few weeks or months of life. Anasarca follows, and the abdomen is distended by ascites. Massive proteinuria associated with typical nephrotic serum protein electrophoresis and hyperlipemia is the rule. Hematuria is not uncommon. If the patient lives long enough, progressive renal failure sets in. Most affected infants succumb to infections at the age of a few months.

Treatment has little to offer. Prevention and effective management of urinary tract infection are important. Immunosuppressives and heparin have occasionally appeared to extend renal function for a period.

Hallman N, Norio R, Kouvalainen K: Main features of the congenital nephrotic syndrome. Acta paediat scandinav (Suppl) 172:75–77, 1967.

Kouvalainen K: Immunological features in congenital nephrotic syndrome: Clinical and experimental study. Ann Paediat Fenn (Suppl 22)9:1–137, 1963.

FUNCTIONAL PROTEINURIA

Urine is not normally completely protein-free, but the average output is well below 100 mg/24 hours. Exertional proteinuria is now well recognized and may be accompanied by erythrocytes and casts if the exercise is violent and includes body contact. Orthostatic proteinuria is explained by hemodynamic adjustments leading to renal venous congestion. It has been suggested that lordosis may produce proteinuria by the increased convexity of the aorta compressing the left renal vein. Proteinuria is seen in about 5% of febrile illnesses and is not necessarily due to underlying renal disease.

In spite of these well recognized causes of proteinuria, the physician faced with isolated instances of proteinuria must exercise great care before making such a diagnosis (see below). Asymptomatic nonpostural proteinuria is associated in 50% of cases with histologic kidney changes which may in a small percentage of cases be due to kidney disease.

Diagnosis & Orthostatic Proteinuria

A. Procedure:

1. Have the patient empty his bladder and lie down for 1 hour. Discard urine.

2. Empty the bladder again and lie down for a second hour.

3. Empty the bladder and save the specimen, noting the exact number of minutes since previous voiding.

4. Stand quietly for 1 hour, void, and save urine in a second container, again noting the exact number of minutes since previous voiding.

5. Send both specimens to the laboratory for quantitative protein determinations and measurement of volumes.

B. Normal Values: Supine, < 0.03 mg/minute protein. Standing: < 1 mg/minute in 65%; > 1 mg/minute in 35%.

Note: Patients with true benign orthostatic proteinuria must excrete < 0.03 mg/minute proteinuria. A mere tendency to spill less protein with recumbency is an insufficient criterion.

Hamburger J & others: Page 110 in: *Nephrology.* Vol 1. Saunders, 1968.

Marks MI & others: Proteinuria in children with febrile illnesses. Arch Dis Child 5:250–253, 1970.

McLaine PN, Drummond KN: Benign persistent asymptomatic proteinuria in childhood. Pediatrics 46:548–552, 1970.

Pollak VE & others: Asymptomatic persistent proteinuria: Studies by renal biopsies. Clin Res 6:414–419, 1958.

·   ·   ·

RENAL VEIN THROMBOSIS

Acute blockage of renal venous drainage leads to swelling of the involved kidney, hematuria, and proteinuria. The fate of the kidney depends on the degree and speed of venous occlusion. Hemorrhagic infarction is the usual consequence of an abrupt complete occlusion. More gradual or incomplete impairment of venous drainage leads to nephrotic syndrome or chronic membranous glomerulonephritis.

Most of the cases reported in the pediatric age group are not associated with thromboembolic phenomena elsewhere. In the majority, dehydration, sepsis, or congenital heart disease are the triggering factors.

Primary renal disease (nephrosis) can also lead to renal vein thrombosis. The thrombosis most likely originates in the intrarenal branches of the renal vein; it can involve both kidneys simultaneously or sequentially and may extend to the inferior vena cava.

Renal vein thrombosis is rare; most cases are seen within the first 6 months of life. Cyanotic heart disease, severe congenital anomalies, and difficult deliveries account for a number of cases in the immediate neonatal period. Subsequently, sepsis and gastroenteritis with dehydration are the major initiating factors. Three cases have been found in association with congenital nephrosis.

Acute unilateral renal swelling associated with hematuria and proteinuria is virtually pathognomonic of renal vein thrombosis. Edema of the legs and genitalia coupled with an abdominal superficial circulation suggests inferior vena cava involvement. Shock, oliguria, progressive uremia, hyperkalemia, and hypertension can be helpful diagnostic features. An intravenous urogram may show lack of concentration of the radiopaque material on the affected side; a plain film usually demonstrates an enlarged renal shadow. The contributions of renal scan to the diagnosis relates to a strikingly abnormal vascular phase. In cases of inferior vena cava involvement, cavography can be diagnostic.

Every effort should be made to correct dehydration and control infection. The case for emergency nephrectomy has not been proved. The condition of the patient is rarely improved by this procedure, which is associated with a high mortality rate, and there is no indication that it will prevent the thrombosis from extending to the other kidney. If, following the acute thrombotic episode, the kidney remains enlarged, nephrectomy should probably be done. A second indication for nephrectomy is a scarred kidney with little or no function developing over a period of years.

The prognosis is poor.

Kaufman HF: Renal vein thrombosis. Am J Dis Child 95:377–384, 1958.

Mauer SM & others: Bilateral renal vein thrombosis in infancy: Report of a survivor following surgical intervention. J Pediat 78:509–512, 1971.

McFarland JB: Renal venous thrombosis in children. Quart J Med (NS) 34:269–290, 1965.

Roy CC & others: Congenital nephrosis associated with thrombosis of the inferior vena cava. Canad MAJ 90:786, 789, 1964.

INHERITED OR DEVELOPMENTAL DEFECTS OF THE URINARY TRACT

In recent years there has been a substantial increase in the number of renal or urinary tract diseases which have been discovered to be hereditary or developmental in origin. Many classification schemes have been proposed, although none are entirely adequate. The more important entities are listed below.

Cystic Diseases of Genetic Origin

   A. Polycystic Disease:

      Polycystic disease of early infancy: Neonatal polycystic disease, Meckel's syndrome

      Polycystic disease of childhood: Medullary tubular ectasia, congenital hepatic fibrosis

      Adult polycystic disease

   B. Cortical Cysts:

      Tuberous sclerosis complex

      Lindau's disease (cystic disease in syndromes of multiple malformations):

         Cerebrohepatorenal syndrome of Zellweger

         Autosomal trisomy syndromes D and E

         Lissencephaly and oral-facial-digital syndromes

         Schwartz-Jampel syndrome

Asphyxiating thoracic dystrophy of Jeune
Down's, Turner's, and Ehlers-Danlos syndromes
C. **Medullary Cysts:**
  Medullary sponge kidney
  Medullary cystic disease (nephronophthisis)
D. **Hereditary and Familial Cystic Dysplasia.**

Dysplastic Renal Diseases
Renal aplasia (unilateral, bilateral)
Renal hypoplasia (unilateral, bilateral, total, segmental)
Multicystic renal dysplasia (unilateral, bilateral, multilocular, postobstructive, etc)
Familial and hereditary renal dysplasias
Oligomeganephronia

Hereditary Diseases Associated With Nephritis
Hereditary nephritis with deafness and ocular defects (Alport's syndrome)
Nail-patella syndrome
Familial hyperprolinemia
Hereditary nephrotic syndrome
Hereditary osteolysis with nephropathy
Hereditary nephritis with thoracic asphyxiant dystrophy syndrome

Hereditary Diseases Associated With Intrarenal Deposition of Metabolites
Angiokeratoma corporis diffusum (Fabry's disease)
Familial plasma cholesterol ester deficiency
Heredopathia atactica polyneuritiformis (Refsum's disease)
Various storage diseases (eg, GM_1 monosialogangliosidosis, Hurler's syndrome, Nieman-Pick disease, familial metachromatic leukodystrophy, glycogenosis type I (Von Gierke's disease), glycogenosis type II (Pompe's disease)
Hereditary amyloidosis (familial Mediterranean fever; heredofamilial urticaria with deafness and neuropathy; primary familial amyloidosis with polyneuropathy)

Hereditary Renal Diseases Associated With Tubular Transport Defects
Hartnup's disease
Immunoglycinuria
Fanconi's syndromes
Oculocerebrorenal syndrome of Lowe
Cystinosis (infantile, adolescent, adult types)
Wilson's disease
Galactosemia
Hereditary fructose intolerance
Renal tubular acidosis (many types)
Hereditary tyrosinemia
Renal glycosuria
Vitamin D resistant rickets
Pseudohypoparathyroidism
Vasopressin-resistant diabetes insipidus

Hereditary Diseases Associated With Lithiasis
Hyperoxaluria
L-Glyceric aciduria
Xanthinuria
Lesch-Nyhan syndrome, gout, Lesch-Nyhan disease
Nephropathy due to familial hyperparathyroidism
Cystinuria (types I, II, III)
Glycinuria

Miscellaneous
Hereditary intestinal B_{12} malabsorption.
Total and partial lipodystrophy
Sickle cell anemia
Bartter's syndrome

Bernstein J: Heritable cystic disorders of the kidney: The mythology of polycystic disease. P Clin North America 18:435–444, 1971.

Bernstein J: The morphogenesis of renal parenchymal maldevelopment (renal dysplasia). P Clin North America 18:395–407, 1971.

Carter JE & others: Bilateral renal hypoplasia with oligomeganephronia. Am J Dis Child 120:537–542, 1970.

Crocker JFS & others: Developmental defects of the kidney: A review of renal development and experimental studies of maldevelopment. P Clin North America 18:355–376, 1971.

Milne MD: Genetic aspects of renal disease. Progr Med Genet 7:112–162, 1970.

Pathak IG, Williams DI: Multicystic and cystic dysplastic kidneys. Brit J Urol 36:318–331, 1964.

Perkoff GT: The hereditary renal diseases. New England J Med 277:79–85, 129–138, 1967.

CYSTIC RENAL DISEASES IN CHILDHOOD

Infantile Forms of Polycystic Disease

Polycystic renal diseases constitute a bewildering array of severe, usually fatal hereditary renal diseases in which both kidneys are diffusely involved with gross and microscopic cysts. The cyst lumens communicate with the lumens of nephrons.

It remains uncertain how many forms of infantile polycystic disease actually exist. Virtually all are transmitted by an autosomal recessive mode of inheritance. The course and prognosis tend to be similar in affected siblings. Infants are occasionally born with such massive renal enlargement that dystocia occurs or the infant dies of respiratory failure immediately after birth. In other cases, affected infants may be born with kidneys of nearly normal size which enlarge vastly in the first few days of life. Many infants are stillborn or live only a few days. Others appear able to survive for several months or, rarely, even years. Death due to renal failure is virtually inevitable. The only effective therapy would appear to be homotransplantation, which is still highly experimental in infants.

In some cases, the cystic malformations are confined to the kidneys; in others, the liver, pancreas, lungs, or brain may be involved. The tendency for extrarenal cysts to occur appears to depend upon the particular family pattern of the disease and on time, as protracted survival seems to be associated with the development of more extensive extrarenal cyst formation.

Polycystic Disease (Adult Type)

Adult polycystic disease is a dominantly inherited disorder of gradual onset which seldom becomes manifest before the second decade and is most likely to become symptomatic during the fourth or fifth decades. Its occurrence in pediatric practice is rare though not unknown.

Multiple Renal Cysts

In sharp distinction to the polycystic renal diseases, multiple renal cysts are usually benign asymptomatic lesions with seldom more than 8–12 cysts in either kidney. Rarely, the cysts cause obstructive uropathy or hypertension.

Multicystic Kidney

Multicystic kidneys are severely dysplastic kidneys which usually form no excretable urine, fail to communicate with the bladder, usually present as a unilateral abdominal mass, and are associated with a small noncystic dysplastic kidney on the opposite side about 80% of the time.

Medullary Cystic Disease

Medullary cystic disease is probably the same entity as juvenile nephronophthisis. It is inherited as an autosomal recessive trait, usually causes polyuria with loss of concentrating ability and salt wasting, and results in progressive renal failure with death in the second decade of life. Cysts are usually confined to the renal medulla or corticomedullary junction. The kidneys become small, shrunken, and scarred, with interstitial peritubular and finally periglomerular fibrosis. Round cell infiltrates are usually seen in the interstitium.

Treatment is that of chronic renal failure followed by homotransplantation.

Medullary Sponge Kidney (Renal Tubular Ectasia)

Medullary sponge kidney is a relatively benign, autosomal recessive structural defect involving both kidneys in which the major collecting ducts (of Bellini) become dilated just before they enter the tips of the renal papillae. Most cases are described in adults, although the condition has been demonstrated in children. Patients may be asymptomatic, but not infrequently the ectatic ducts are the sites of small calculi which lead to hematuria and infection.

There is no treatment. The prognosis is good.

Alexander F & others: Familial uremic medullary cystic disease. Pediatrics 45:1024–1028, 1970.

Bernstein J: Heritable cystic disorders of the kidney: The mythology of polycystic disease. P Clin North America 18:435–444, 1971.

Bernstein J: The morphogenesis of renal parenchymal maldevelopment (renal dysplasia). P Clin North America 18:395–407, 1971.

Reilly BJ, Neuhauser EBD: Renal tubular ectasia in cystic disease of the kidneys and liver. Am J Roentgenol 84:546–554, 1960.

DISORDERS OF THE RENAL TUBULES

The proximal renal tubule effects the reabsorption of isotonic salt from the glomerular filtrate as well as of glucose, amino acids, and phosphorus. Both the proximal and the distal renal tubules are concerned with acid-base balance through 2 mechanisms: (1) the exchange of hydrogen ion for intraluminal sodium and (2) the hydrogen ion titration of secreted ammonia into ammonium ion.

Primary tubular disorders in childhood may reflect a defect in a single transport mechanism (eg, renal tubular acidosis) or a defect in all of the major functions (eg, hypophosphatemic vitamin D resistant rickets with aminoaciduria and glycosuria).

Tubular dysfunction may also be secondary to other metabolic disorders such as galactosemia and cystinosis or part of generalized renal failure, as in advanced glomerulonephritis. Tests for these functions are described on p 432.

1. PROXIMAL RENAL TUBULAR ACIDOSIS

Essentials of Diagnosis

- Failure to thrive.
- Hyperchloremic acidosis.
- Low renal threshold for bicarbonate reabsorption.

General Considerations

The renal mechanisms for controlling acid-base equilibrium are illustrated in Fig 18–1. The dominant process in the proximal tubule is the exchange of tubule cell hydrogen ion for intraluminal sodium. Under the influence of surface carbonic anhydrase, CO_2 is then formed, reabsorbed, and rehydrated to HCO_3^- and H^+. About 85–90% of bicarbonate reabsorption is achieved in the proximal tubules. In proximal renal tubular acidosis, the essential lesion is a lowering of the renal bicarbonate threshold, ie, the concentration of bicarbonate in the plasma above which bicarbonate appears in the urine. The exact nature of the lesion is not clear. It does not appear to involve defective function of carbonic anhydrase.

Clinical Findings

The onset is in infancy in males, with failure to thrive and hyperchloremic acidosis but without bone

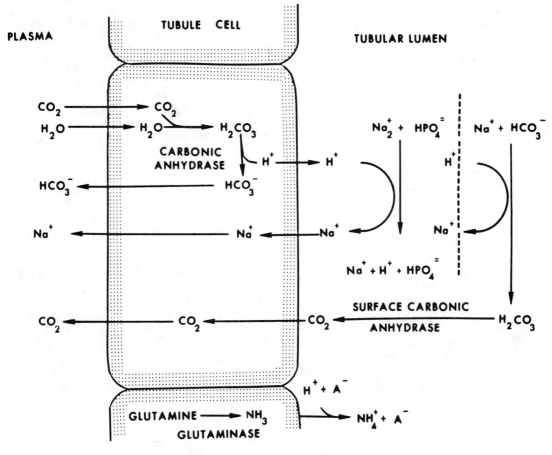

FIG 18–1. Tubular mechanisms for hydrogen ion excretion.

lesions, nephrocalcinosis, or hypokalemia. Secondary forms are seen in association with other tubular disorders, as in Fanconi's syndrome, cystinosis, Lowe's syndrome, Wilson's disease, galactosemia, hereditary fructose intolerance, and tyrosinemia.

Lightwood's syndrome, a condition characterized by failure to thrive, hyperchloremic acidosis, high urine pH, anorexia, vomiting, and constipation starting at around 6 months of age, is probably a special form of this syndrome.

Differential Diagnosis

On bicarbonate loading, these patients may be shown to have a lowered renal threshold for bicarbonate reabsorption. The actual demonstration of lowered HCO_3^- threshold is cumbersome, however, and it may be practical to make an arbitrary differentiation from distal tubular acidosis as follows: A patient who requires > 6 mEq/kg/24 hours of citrate or bicarbonate to sustain a plasma CO_2 of 22 mEq/liter and who under conditions of an acid load can acidify his urine pH below 5.4 may be said to have proximal renal tubular acidosis until proved otherwise.

The possibility that the acidosis is secondary to one of the conditions listed above should be considered.

Treatment

Treatment usually consists of giving sodium bicarbonate, 10 mEq/kg/24 hours in 3 divided doses, or whatever dose is sufficient to maintain a normal plasma HCO_3^- without causing gastrointestinal symptoms. An alternative is to give buffered citrate solution, 50 ml orally 3 times daily:

℞ Sodium citrate	50.0
Potassium citrate	50.0
Citric acid	100.0
Water, qs ad	1000.0

In addition to the above, hydrochlorothiazide (Esidrix, Hydro-Diuril) may be beneficial, although it may require potassium supplementation.

Prognosis

The prognosis appears to be excellent. Alkali therapy can usually be discontinued after several months with no evident recurrence of symptoms or signs.

Donkerwolcke RA & others: Therapy of bicarbonate losing renal tubular acidosis. Arch Dis Child 45:774, 1970.

Edelmann CM & others: Renal bicarbonate reabsorption and hydrogen ion excretion in normal infants. J Clin Invest 46:1309, 1967.

Edelmann CM & others: The renal response of children to acute ammonium chloride acidosis. Pediat Res 1:452, 1967.

Soriano JR: The renal regulation of acid-base balance and the disturbances noted in renal tubular acidosis. P Clin North America 18:529, 1971.

2. DISTAL RENAL TUBULAR ACIDOSIS

Acid-base regulation in the distal tubule is achieved partly by residual bicarbonate reabsorption but also by sodium hydrogen ion exchange against a gradient and by ammonium excretion. The defect in distal renal tubular acidosis appears to be a disability to secrete H^+ against a gradient. It is probably transmitted as an autosomal dominant disorder.

The onset is in later childhood (after age 2) in patients with failure to grow, anorexia, vomiting, and dehydration. There is hyperchloremic acidosis, a urine pH > 6.5, and hypokalemia. Hypercalciuria may lead to rickets, and long-term complications include nephrocalcinosis, nephrolithiasis, and renal failure.

The urinary excretion of titratable acid and ammonium (U_{TA} and U_{NH_4}) is reduced, and the hydrogen ion clearance index (see p 432), which is normally ≥ 1 after an NH_4Cl load, is < 0.7. Urine pH remains above 6.5 even at plasma HCO_3^- concentrations < 13 mEq/liter.

The possibility that the tubular lesion is secondary to malnutrition, hyperparathyroidism, vitamin D intoxication, Fabry's disease, various hypergammaglobulinemic states, amphotericin B intoxication, cirrhosis, and hyperthyroidism should be considered.

In contrast to proximal renal tubular acidosis, the dose of alkali required to achieve normal plasma HCO_3^- concentration and prevent hypercalciuria seldom exceeds 2 mEq/kg/24 hours. Moreover, chlorothiazide may be of particular value in diminishing hypercalciuria.

Distal renal tubular acidosis is a permanent disorder which requires lifelong treatment. The prognosis is good if the diagnosis is made in time to prevent nephrocalcinosis from causing irreversible kidney damage and renal failure.

Edelmann CM Jr: The genetics of primary renal tubular acidosis. Birth Defects 6:25, 1970.

Morris RC Jr: Renal tubular acidosis: Mechanisms, classification and implications. New England J Med 281:1405, 1969.

Pitts RF: The role of ammonia production and excretion in regulation of acid-base balance. New England J Med 284:32, 1971.

Soriano JR: The renal regulation of acid base balance and the disturbances noted in renal tubular acidosis. P Clin North America 18:529, 1971.

CONGENITAL HYPOKALEMIC ALKALOSIS
(Bartter's Syndrome)

This syndrome is characterized by severe hypokalemic, hypochloremic metabolic alkalosis, extremely high levels of circulating renin and aldosterone, and a paradoxical absence of hypertension. The cause and pathogenesis are not known. On renal biopsy, there is striking juxtaglomerular hyperplasia. Most patients present in early infancy with severe failure to thrive. Although the prognosis is very poor, a few patients seem to have less severe forms of the disease that are compatible with longer survival.

There is no effective treatment. Potassium and magnesium supplements may be beneficial in some cases.

Sutherland LE & others: Bartter's syndrome. Acta pediat scandinav Suppl 201, 1970.

Wald MK, Perrin EV, Bolande RP: Bartter's syndrome in early infancy. Physiologic, light and electron microscopic observations. Pediatrics 47:254, 1971.

RENAL GLYCOSURIA

Renal glycosuria is a disorder that apparently involves the proximal convoluted tubule of all nephrons. The basic mechanism does not seem to affect phosphorylation of glucose in the tubule but is assumed to interfere with the sodium and energy dependent steps of incorporation of glucose into the brush border. The degree to which this transport mechanism is interfered with can be quantitated by measuring the maximal tubular reabsorption of glucose (T_mG). Normal values are 260–550 mg/minute/1.73 sq m, whereas in renal glycosuria they range from 80–280 mg/minute/1.73 sq m. The test is carried out in conjunction with an inulin clearance test. The calculation is as follows:

$$T_mG \text{ in mg/minute/1.73 sq m} =$$
$$\text{(Inulin clearance} \times \text{Plasma glucose concentration in mg/ml)} -$$
$$\text{Glucose excretion in mg/minute}$$

Structural alterations of the proximal convoluted tubules have been described; these electronmicroscopic changes are degenerative and correlate well with the functional insufficiency of this area of the nephron.

In most patients the total urinary glucose loss is insufficient to cause any symptoms or metabolic disturbance. Hyperglycemia does not occur. In some affected individuals, polyuria and polydipsia are present. During starvation and occasionally in pregnancy, the obligatory loss of carbohydrates may lead to acidosis.

No treatment is necessary. It is essential to rule out diabetes mellitus and renal tubular disorders, where glycosuria can be associated with aminoaciduria, phosphaturia, and acidification defects.

Horowitz L, Schwarzer S: Renal glycosuria: Occurrence in two siblings and a review of the literature. J Pediat 47:634–639, 1955.

Monasterio G & others: Renal diabetes as a congenital tubular dysplasia. Am J Med 37:44–61, 1964.

Goldman H & others: The use of dithiothreitol to correct cystine storage in cultured cystinotic fibroblasts. Lancet 1:811–812, 1970.

Lietman PS & others: Adult cystinosis: A benign disorder. Am J Med 40:511, 1966.

Mahoney C & others: Renal transplantation for childhood cystinosis. New England J Med 283:397–402, 1970.

Schneider JA & others: Transport and intracellular fate of cysteine-^{35}S in leukocytes from normal subjects and patients with cystinosis. Pediat Res 2:441–450, 1968.

CYSTINOSIS

Three types of cystinosis have been identified: adult, adolescent, and infantile. The adult type is a relatively benign condition characterized by corneal cystine deposition and elevated granulocyte and fibroblast cystine levels but no renal disease. The adolescent type is characterized by cystine deposition in the corneas, granulocytes, and fibroblasts and by the development of mild renal failure with Fanconi's syndrome during adolescence. Growth is normal.

The infantile type is both the most common and the most severe. Characteristically, children present in the first or second year of life with polyuria and on investigation are found to have renal rickets, generalized aminoaciduria, glycosuria, and a variable degree of renal tubular acidosis. The exact biochemical nature of the disease remains obscure. Cystine is stored in cellular lysosomes in virtually all tissues, a finding which has led to the speculation that a lysosomal cystine reductase may be absent or faulty. Eventually, cystine accumulation results in cell damage and cell death, particularly in the renal tubules. Death from renal failure between ages 6 and 12 is the rule. Whenever the diagnosis of cystinosis is suspected, a slit-lamp examination of the corneas should be performed as corneal cystine crystal deposition causes an almost pathognomonic ground-glass "dazzle" appearance. Cystine crystals may also be readily observed in bone marrow aspirates, especially with phase microscopy.

Cystinosis is an autosomal recessive condition which may be diagnosed in utero by obtaining fetal cells by amniocentesis, growing them in tissue culture, and measuring the avidity with which they incorporate ^{35}S-cystine.

A new drug, dithiothreitol, is under investigation for the treatment of cystinosis, but significant side-effects may preclude its use. At present, the management of cystinosis is essentially that of chronic renal failure with particular attention being paid to renal osteodystrophy. Renal homotransplantation shows significant promise in the palliation of cystinosis, although the extent of nonrenal tissue involvement with cystine remains to be defined.

Goldman H & others: Adolescent cystinosis: Comparison with infantile and adult forms. Pediatrics 47:979–988, 1971.

CYSTINURIA

Cystinuria, like Hartnup's disease, is primarily a disorder of amino acid transport across both the enteric and proximal renal tubular epithelium. There appear to be at least 3 biochemical types: (1) The bowel transport of basic amino acids and cystine is impaired but not that of cysteine. In the renal tubule, basic amino acids are again rejected by the tubule but cystine absorption into kidney slices in vitro seems to be normal. The reasons for the cystinuria are, therefore, still obscure. Heterozygotes have no aminoaciduria. (2) The second type is similar except that the heterozygotes excrete excess cystine and lysine in the urine and cystine transport in the bowel is normal. (3) In a third type, only the nephron is involved. The incidence of all types among the institutionalized mentally retarded children is about 0.2%.

The only clinical manifestations relate to stone formation. These include ureteral colic, dysuria, hematuria, proteinuria, and secondary urinary tract infection. The urinary excretion of cystine, lysine, arginine, and ornithine is increased.

The most reliable way to prevent stone formation is to maintain a constant high free water clearance. This involves a water intake of about 400 ml/sq m every 4 hours night and day. If this is not effective, treatment with sodium bicarbonate, 6 gm/sq m/day, should also be given. Such measures will certainly prevent increases in stone formation and very often lead to dissolution.

Operative removal of the stone may occasionally be required. D-Penicillamine (Cuprimine), in doses of 1000–1500 mg/sq m/day, will also decrease cystine excretion and bring about partial or complete dissolution of stones. It is expensive, however, and may give rise to rashes which are just as objectionable as the problem of maintaining a high water intake.

McDonald JE, Henneman PH: Stone dissolution in vivo and control of cystinuria with D-penicillamine. New England J Med 273:578–583, 1965.

Rosenberg LE, Durant JL, Holland JM: Intestinal absorption and renal extraction of cystine and cysteine in cystinuria. New England J Med 273:1239–1245, 1965.

Scriver CR & others: Cystinuria: Increased prevalence in patients with mental disease. New England J Med 283:783–786, 1970.

TABLE 18–4. The renal tubular dystrophies.

N = Normal   ↑ = Elevated   ↓ = Low   + = Defect present   − = No defect present

Disease	Serum Findings					Renal Tubular Transport Defect						Clinical Features
	Ca++	PO₄=	Alk. Ptase	Aci-dosis	Nitrogen Retention	Ca++	TRP	H+	K+	Glu-cose	Amino Acids	
Renal glycosuria	N	N	N	N	N	−	−	−	−	+		Autosomal dominant. Asymptomatic in childhood.
Proximal renal tubular acidosis	N	N	N	↑	N	−	−	+	±	−		Failure to thrive, hyperchloremic acidosis, low HCO₃⁻ threshold.
Distal renal tubular acidosis	N	N	↑	↑	N	+	−	+	+	−		Vomiting, dehydration, failure to thrive, Autosomal dominant. Later, rickets and nephrocalcinosis.
Cystinuria	N	N	N	N	N	−	−	−	−	−	Cystine, lysine, arginine, ornithine	Renal calculi. Variants also have intestinal transport defect.
Hartnup disease[1]	N	N	N	N	N	−	−	−	−	−	Tryptophan and other neutral amino acids	An autosomal recessive with cerebellar ataxia and pellagra-like skin rash. Also, intestinal transport defect.
Glycinuria[2]	N	N	N	N	N	−	−	−	−	±	Glycine	Oxalate renal calculi, usually in females. May occur without calculi in males. Also reported with glycosuria.
Proline oxidase deficiency[3]	N	N	N	↑	↑	−	−	−	−	−	Proline, hydroxyproline, glycine	Associated with congenital renal anomalies and hereditary nephritis.
Iminoaciduria[4]	N	N	N	N	N	−	−	−	−	−	Proline, hydroxyproline, glycine	Asymptomatic, but may be associated with mental retardation and epilepsy. Enteric transport may be similarly affected.
Hydroxyproline oxidase deficiency[5]	N	N	N	N	N	−	−	−	−	−	Proline, hydroxyproline, glycine	Mental retardation.
Simple vitamin D resistant rickets	N	↓	↑	N	N	−	↓	−	−	−		X-linked dominant. Short stature, bowing of legs, enlargement of costochondral junctions, and large joints. May be no bone changes.
Vitamin D resistant rickets with glycinuria	N	↓	↑	↑	N	−	↓	+	−	−	Generalized aminoaciduria	Onset in adolescence with severe bone changes, osteomalacia, and muscle weakness. Responds to vitamin D.

TABLE 18–4 (cont'd). The renal tubular dystrophies.

N = Normal ↑ = Elevated ↓ = Low + = Defect present − = No defect present

Disease	Serum Findings					Renal Tubular Transport Defect					Amino Acids	Clinical Features
	Ca++	PO4=	Alk. Ptase	Acidosis	Nitrogen Retention	Ca++	TRP	H+	K+	Glucose		
Vitamin D resistant rickets with aminoaciduria and acidosis	N or ↓	↓	↑	↑	N or ↑	−	↓	+	±	+	Generalized aminoaciduria	Failure to thrive, bone changes, weakness. Some cases probably confused with tyrosinosis (Fanconi's syndrome).
Lowe's syndrome[6]	N	↓	↑	↑	N	−	↓	+	−	−	Generalized aminoaciduria	X-linked inheritance with physical and intellectual retardation, cataracts, buphthalmos, glaucoma, and rickets.
Cystinosis	N	↓	↑	↑	N or ↑	−	↓	+	+	+	Generalized aminoaciduria	Autosomal recessive with vitamin D resistant rickets and cystine deposits in liver, spleen, kidneys, corneas, etc.
Luder-Sheldon syndrome[7]	N	N	N	N	N	−	−	−	−	+	Generalized aminoaciduria	Autosomal dominant with growth failure.
Ukari syndrome[8]	N	↓	Low	↑	↑	−	+	+	−	+	Generalized aminoaciduria	A temporary tubular nephropathy which lasts a few weeks. Acute onset with acidosis and mild azotemia.
Idiopathic hypercalciuria[9]	N	N	N	N	N	+	−	−	−			Primarily due to excessive transport across the bowel. Urolithiasis. Responds to low calcium intake.
Growth retardation due to cor pulmonale, aminoaciduria[10]	N	N	N	N	N	+	−	−	−	±	Generalized aminoaciduria	Growth retardation, poor muscular development, scanty adipose tissue, recurrent pulmonary infections, right ventricular hypertrophy.
Hypophosphatasia[11]	N or ↑	N	↓	N	N or ↑	−	−	−	−	−	Phosphoethanolamine	Rickets, pseudofractures, premature synostosis of calvarium. Responds to high phosphate load.

[1] Scriver CR: Hartnup disease. New England J Med 273:530–532, 1965.

[2] Wyngaarden JB, Segal S: The hyperglycinurias. Pages 341–352 in: *The Metabolic Basis of Inherited Disease,* 2nd ed. Stanbury JB, Wyngaarden JB, Fredrickson DS (editors). McGraw-Hill, 1966.

[3] Efron ML: Familial hyperprolinemia. New England J Med 272:1243–1254, 1965.

[4] Goodman SI, McIntyre CA, O'Brien CA: Impaired intestinal transport of proline in a patient with familial iminoaciduria. J Pediat 71:246–249, 1967.

[5] Efron ML, Bixby EM, Pryles CV: Hydroxyprolinemia. New England J Med 272:1299–1309, 1965.

[6] Lowe CU, Terry M, MacLachlan EA: Organic aciduria, decreased renal ammonia production, hydrophthalmos, and mental retardation. Am J Dis Child 83:164, 1952.

[7] Luder J, Sheldon W: A familial tubular absorption defect of glucose and amino acids. Arch Dis Child 30:160–164, 1955.

[8] Fellers FX, Kanp J, McKenna J: The Ukari syndrome: A transient tubular nephropathy. Am J Dis Child 100:763–764, 1960.

[9] Dent CE, Watson L: Metabolic studies in a patient with idiopathic hypercalcuria. Brit MJ 2:449–452, 1965.

[10] Rowley PT & others: Familial growth retardation, renal aminoaciduria and cor pulmonale. Am J Med 31:187–204, 1961.

[11] Fraser D: Hypophosphatasia. Am J Med 22:730, 1957.

FAMILIAL HYPERPROLINEMIA

This is a rare hereditary disease in which chronic renal failure with congenital renal malformation is combined with a deficiency of the enzyme that converts proline to Δ^1-pyrroline-5-carboxylic acid. The patients also show deafness, convulsions, and mental retardation. This leads to fasting plasma levels of proline that are over 1 μMol/ml, or about 10 times normal. The overflow prolinuria induces competitive failure to reabsorb hydroxyproline and glycine. The amino acid disorder has been found without renal disease in the siblings of affected cases but not in other family members. Hereditary nephritis was, however, typical on the maternal sides of both observed families.

Efron ML: Familial hyperprolinemia. New England J Med 272:1243–1254, 1965.

PHOSPHATE-LOSING RENAL TUBULAR SYNDROMES & OTHER FORMS OF RICKETS

Recent work on the metabolic products of vitamin D_3 has done much to clarify the causes of various forms of rickets. Those forms due primarily to a lack of available calcium are described elsewhere. They include deficient calcium intake or excessive urinary calcium loss, as in idiopathic hypercalciuria; lack of vitamin D_3 in the diet or from steatorrhea; and vitamin D dependency and azotemic rickets, in which there is (respectively) an inborn or acquired inability to synthesize 1:25-dihydroxycholecalciferol, the calcium transport protein stimulating factor. Treatment consists of giving supplementary calcium or vitamin D in appropriate doses.

Another group of diseases that cause rickets are those in which there is a decreased availability of phosphorus. Excessive use of aluminum hydroxide gels may be responsible, but this is very rare. Most commonly, the defect is an inherited or acquired one of tubular transport defects of amino acids, glucose, potassium, and hydrogen ion. Thus, in Luder-Sheldon syndrome, there is aminoaciduria and glycosuria; in simple vitamin D resistant rickets, phosphaturia only; and in Fanconi's syndrome, aminoaciduria, phosphaturia, glycosuria, and acidosis. Certain generalized metabolic diseases—notably Wilson's disease, galactosemia, and cystinosis—may cause similar tubular damage. Treatment of the primary type is to give extra phosphorus. Treatment of the acquired forms is that of the basic disease. Table 18–4 lists these conditions.

Familial hypophosphatemic vitamin D resistant rickets is an example of a tubular nephropathy in which only phosphorus transport is affected.

Although ordinary rickets is uncommon in patients over 18 months of age, it may manifest itself for the first time in childhood. The majority of cases present during the second year of life, but some have been reported in the first 6 months.

The clinical features are variable. On the one hand the changes may be only biochemical, with a strikingly low serum phosphorus and elevated alkaline phosphatase. Muscular hypotonia may be severe; growth failure, bowing of the legs, and enlargement of wrists, knees, and costochondral junctions are often associated with spinal deformities. Craniosynostosis has been described in infants with this disease. Pathologic fractures may be seen on x-ray, as well as certain unique findings consisting of an irregular mosaic formation of the Haversian system and trabecular "halos" of low-density bone.

In most cases the serum phosphorus is < 2 mg/100 ml. Calcium is very high in stools and can actually exceed dietary intake. Urinary calcium is low, and serum calcium may be normal or slightly low. Aminoaciduria is rare.

Treatment consists of giving 1–3 gm of phosphorus daily as a buffered monosodium and disodium hydrogen phosphate solution at pH 7.4, together with magnesium oxide, 10–15 mg/kg daily by mouth. Supplementary vitamin D (up to 40,000 units daily) should be given if the response to the above is insufficient.

Normal growth is never achieved in patients who chronically maintain abnormally low phosphorus levels despite oral phosphorus supplements and large doses of vitamin D.

Avioli LV & others: Metabolism of vitamin $D_3-{}^3$H in vitamin D resistant rickets and familial hypophosphatemia. J Clin Invest 46:1907–1915, 1967.

Burnett CH & others: Vitamin D resistant rickets: Analysis of twenty-four pedigrees with hereditary and sporadic cases. Am J Med 36:222–232, 1964.

Winters RW & others: A genetic study of familial hypophosphatemia and vitamin D resistant rickets. Medicine 37:97–103, 1958.

HYPOPHOSPHATASIA & PSEUDOHYPOPHOSPHATASIA

The pathogenetic mechanisms proposed for these diseases are largely based on a defective alkaline phosphatase in leukocytes as well as in the spleen, liver, kidneys, and bone. The high plasma level and the urinary excretion of phosphoethanolamine in patients with this condition—and in the majority of their relatives—have suggested to some workers that phosphoethanolamine is the true substrate for bone alkaline phosphatase. However, phosphoethanolamine is not found in the urine of all patients and has been found in one case of ordinary vitamin D deficiency rickets. The disease appears to be familial and is transmitted as an autosomal recessive trait.

Symptoms usually appear within the first weeks of life. Vomiting, anorexia, irritability, seizures, and bouts of cyanosis may be the presenting signs. Spontaneous shedding of deciduous teeth has been noted in infants. Older children may present only with orthopedic deformities and failure to grow.

Serum alkaline phosphatase is low in hypophosphatasia; in pseudohypophosphatasia, it is normal. Serum phosphorus is low and serum calcium elevated.

X-ray evidence of the disease has been detected in utero. The long bones are shorter than expected, and there is poor mineralization throughout. A wide osteoid tissue zone separates the cartilaginous epiphyses from the diaphyses. There are also some focal defects in the metaphyses. Clinically, the signs are those observed in severe rickets; in addition, craniosynostosis has been described along with increased intracranial pressure.

Vitamin D is of no value; there is resistance to its antirachitic properties but not to its toxic manifestations. It also appears that corticosteroids are of no permanent value in the therapy of hypophosphatasia.

In more than 2/3 of cases, death comes within the first year of life.

Fraser D: Hypophosphatasia. Am J Med 22:730–733, 1957.

McCance RA, Morrison AB, Dent CE: The excretion of phosphoethanolamine and hypophosphatasia. Lancet 1:131–132, 1955.

Rosenthal IM & others: Tissue alkaline phosphatase in hypophosphatasia. Am J Dis Child 99:185–192, 1960.

Scriver CR, Cameron D: Pseudohypophosphatasia. New England J Med 281:604, 1969.

RENAL RICKETS

Azotemic osteodystrophy appears in severe renal failure. Failure of the kidney to synthesize 1:25-dihydroxycholecalciferol, the enteric calcium transport protein stimulating factor, is thought to be an important contributing cause.

The clinical picture of uremia is usually present. In the young child, if the growth process has not been completely arrested, signs of rickets are present along with the aches and pains that reflect hyperparathyroidism. Tetany is rare despite a sporadic, strikingly low serum calcium level since systemic acidosis sustains the level of ionized calcium. Tetany, however, may be due to low tissue Mg^{++} levels. Pathologic fractures may occur. Although the renal insufficiency may result from either acute or chronic glomerulonephritis, most cases appear to be caused by obstructive uropathies with superimposed chronic pyelonephritis.

Management ideally should be oriented toward correction of the underlying renal disease. A low-phosphate diet with additional vitamin D is indicated. The specific acquired resistance of the gastrointestinal tract to the action of vitamin D can be overcome by giving doses up to 50,000 IU daily. The danger of nephrocalcinosis, however, necessitates care in the administration of high doses of vitamin D.

In certain cases of renal rickets, the secondary hyperparathyroidism may lead to the formation of a parathyroid adenoma which has autonomous function and is not under the control of calcium levels. Hypercalcemia is usually present, and surgery is indicated.

Merril JP: Management of chronic renal failure. Am J Med 36:736–777, 1964.

Stanbury SW: Azotemic renal osteodystrophy. Brit M Bull 13:57–60, 1957.

HEPATIC & CELIAC RICKETS

A lack of bile salts such as occurs in biliary atresia or hepatocellular disease causes malabsorption of virtually all lipids, including fat-soluble vitamins such as A, D, and K. The emulsifying effect of bile salts is crucial to the surface action of pancreatic lipase and to micelle formation. Severe diffuse diseases of the pancreas, such as in cystic fibrosis, will therefore also lead to malabsorption of vitamin D. Patients with disorders of the small intestine, giving rise to steatorrhea, have large amounts of fecal calcium not only secondary to the washing away of vitamin D but also due to the large amounts of calcium contained in the digestive juices.

The physical stigmas of rickets are present if the underlying hepatic or small bowel disease has not completely arrested growth. Osteomalacia is evident if growth arrest has occurred. Tetany is seldom seen. Jaundice is usually present.

Treatment of the underlying disease should include the prophylactic administration of vitamin D in water-soluble form (2000 IU daily). If rickets has developed despite the regular administration of vitamin D, it will not respond to therapeutic amounts of vitamin D (5000–10,000 IU daily) and will require 25,000–100,000 IU. Cases have been described in which the oral administration of 300,000 IU daily were ineffective and exposure to ultraviolet rays or the parenteral administration of vitamin D proved necessary.

Atkinson M, Nordin BEC, Sherlock S: Malabsorption and bone disease in obstructive jaundice. Quart J Med 25:299–312, 1956.

Coff HD: Calcium and phosphorus metabolism. Am J Med 22:275, 1957.

Gray R & others: Vitamin D metabolism: The role of kidney tissue. Science 172:1232, 1971.

Lumb GA & others: The apparent vitamin D resistance of chronic renal failure: A study of the physiology of vitamin D in man. Am J Med 50:421, 441, 1971.

Stanbury SW, Lumb GA, Nicholson WF: Elective subtotal parathyroidectomy for renal hyperparathyroidism. Lancet 1:793–798, 1960.

THE OCULOCEREBRORENAL SYNDROME
(Lowe's Syndrome)

This condition has been described in males only and is therefore thought to be transmitted as an X-linked recessive gene leading to anomalies involving the eyes, brain, and kidneys. The physical stigmas and the degree of mental retardation are variable. In addition to congenital cataracts and buphthalmos, the typical facies includes prominent epicanthal folds, frontal prominence, and a tendency to scaphocephaly. Muscle hypotonia is a prominent finding. The incidence of hypophosphatemic rickets is variable; it is characterized by low serum phosphorus, low to normal serum calcium, and elevated serum alkaline phosphatase. Some degree of renal tubular acidosis is usually present, characterized by hyperchloremic acidosis, an alkaline urine, and a diminution in both titratable acidity and urinary ammonia in response to an ammonium chloride challenge. Perhaps the most striking urinary abnormality is a type of renal aminoaciduria that affects all the amino acids. In one family, however, the basic amino acids were primarily affected, and ornithine loading permitted the detection of the mother as the genetic carrier. Transport of basic amino acids across the intestinal epithelium also is impaired.

Alkaline therapy should be given to those presenting with tubular acidosis. Vitamin D requirements range from 10,000–20,000 IU daily.

Lowe CU, Terry M, MacLachlan EA: Organic aciduria, decreased renal ammonia production, hydrophthalmos and mental retardation. Am J Dis Child 83:164–169, 1952.

Oetliker O, Rossi E: The influence of extracellular fluid volume on the renal bicarbonate threshold: A study of two children with Lowe's syndrome. Pediat Res 3:140, 1969.

Schwartz R, Hall PW, Gabuzda GJ: Metabolism of ornithine and other amino acids in the cerebro oculorenal syndrome. Am J Med 36:778–786, 1964.

DISORDERS OF THE COLLECTING DUCTS

NEPHROGENIC DIABETES INSIPIDUS

The system of water conservation in the nephron can be described briefly as follows: In the proximal tubule, the water is reabsorbed by osmosis as solutes are being actively and passively reabsorbed. In the descending loop of Henle, water is lost against the osmotic gradient of the papillary countercurrent loop; this is not under the control of vasopressin. In the ascending part of the loop, there is no water exchange, although sodium egress dilutes the urine. Thereafter, reabsorption of water is dependent on ADH-controlled exposure to the countercurrent loop. The exact mechanism of ADH action is not known. The hormone itself is an octapeptide with an intrachain disulfide bridge. It is possible that the molecule is in some way fixed to the tubular membrane and thus alters the geometry to favor water ingress. It is not known whether the defect is in the octapeptide or the membrane acceptor.

Most commonly, the symptoms are limited to polyuria and polydipsia with failure to thrive. In some cases, particularly where the solute intake is unrestricted, some acclimatization to an elevated serum osmolality may develop—so-called diabetes insipidus hyperchloremicus occultus. These children are particularly liable to episodes of dehydration, fever, vomiting, and convulsions.

Clinically, the diagnosis can be made on the basis of a history of polydipsia and polyuria that is not sensitive to the administration of vasopressin or lysine-8 vasopressin. It is wise to confirm this in all cases by performing a vasopressin test. Maximal water restriction, overnight if possible, does not increase the tubular reabsorption of water $(T^C_{H_2O})$ to above 2 ml/minute/sq m. Renal diabetes insipidus will show no increase in urine osmolality with the administration of active vasopressin and only a small change with hypertonic saline. In pituitary insufficiency, there is a normal response to vasopressin but not to hypertonic saline. Theoretically, in psychogenic diabetes insipidus, vasopressin and hypertonic saline increase urine osmolality, but constant water loading seems to diminish renal response to ADH. In a variety of chronic nephropathies, collecting duct function may be diminished; these can be identified by the history, the presence of cells in the urine, and evidence of nitrogen retention or diminished glomerular function.

In infants it is usually best to allow water as demanded and to restrict salt. Serum sodium should be estimated at intervals to ensure against hyperosmolality from inadvertent water restriction. In later childhood, sodium intake should continue to be restricted to 2–2.5 mEq/kg/24 hours. Studies have suggested that chlorothiazide, 60 mg/sq m/24 hours orally, or ethacrynic acid (Edecrin), 120 mg/sq m/24 hours orally, will decrease the C_{H_2O} significantly. When the latter drug is given, potassium chloride, 2–3 mEq/kg/24 hours orally, should also be given to prevent alkalosis due to excessive potassium loss.

Brown DM & others: The use and mode of action of ethacrynic acid in nephrogenic diabetes insipidus. Pediatrics 37:447–455, 1966.

Lant AF, Wilson GM: Long-term therapy of diabetes insipidus with oral benzothiadiazine and phthalimidine diuretics. Clin Sc 40:497–511, 1971.

PRIMARY HYPEROXALURIA

Oxalate production in man is derived from the oxidative deamination of glycine to glyoxylate (about 40%), from the serine-glycolate pathway (about 50%), and from ascorbic acid. At least 2 enzymatic blocks have been described. Type 1 is a 2-oxo-glutarate:glyoxylate carboligase deficiency which inhibits the diversion of glyoxylate to γ-hydroxy-a-ketoglutarate. Type 2 is glyoxylate reductase deficiency.

Excess oxalate combines with calcium to form insoluble deposits in the kidneys, lungs, and other tissues. The onset is in childhood. The joints are occasionally involved, but the main impact is on the kidneys, where progressive oxalate deposition leads to fibrosis and eventual renal failure.

Pyridoxine supplementation and a low-oxalate diet have been tried as therapy, but the overall prognosis is poor and most patients succumb to uremia by early adulthood. Renal transplantation has not so far been successful. Moreover, hemodialysis is associated with severe difficulties in maintaining shunts and preventing ectopic calcification. Calcium carbimide, 1 mg/kg/24 hours, has recently been tried as an inhibitor of the serine-glycolate pathway of oxalate production and was shown to substantially diminish oxalate excretion in type I oxalosis.

Dent CE, Stamp TCB: Treatment of primary hyperoxaluria. Arch Dis Child 45:735–745, 1970.

Solomons CC, Goodman SI, Riley CM: Calcium carbimide in the treatment of primary hyperoxaluria. New England J Med 276:207–210, 1967.

Williams HE, Smith LH: L-Glyceric aciduria: A new genetic variant of primary hyperoxaluria. New England J Med 278:233–239, 1968.

DISEASES OF THE RENAL PELVIS (CALCULI)

Renal calculi in children may occur as a consequence of certain inborn errors of metabolism, eg, cystine in cystinosis, glycine in hyperglycinuria, urates in Lesch-Nyhan syndrome, and oxalates in oxalosis. Stones may occur secondary to hypercalciuria in distal tubular acidosis, and large stones are quite often seen in children with spina bifida with paralyzed lower limbs. Treatment is that of the primary condition if possible. Surgical removal of stones should be considered only for obstruction, intractable severe pain, and chronic infection.

•   •   •

General References

Edelmann CM: Symposium on pediatric nephrology. P Clin North America 18(2), 1971.

Hamburger J: *Nephrology.* Vols 1 & 2. Saunders, 1968.

Heptinstall RH: *Pathology of the Kidney.* Little, Brown, 1966.

James JA: *Renal Disease in Childhood.* Mosby, 1968.

Metcoff J (editor): *Acute Glomerulonephritis.* Little, Brown, 1967.

Pitts RF: *Physiology of the Kidney and Body Fluids.* Year Book, 1963.

Smith DR: *General Urology,* 7th ed. Lange, 1972.

Strauss MB, Welt LG (editors): *Diseases of the Kidney,* 2nd ed. Little, Brown, 1971.

Sunderman F & others: *Laboratory Diagnosis of Kidney Diseases.* W.H. Green, 1970.

Williams DE: *Pediatric Urology,* 2nd ed. Appleton-Century-Crofts, 1969.

19...

Bones & Joints

James S. Miles, MD, & Clive C. Solomons, PhD

In considering orthopedic problems, special attention must be paid to pain, loss of function, and deformity. These should be analyzed in terms of the tissues involved, considering blood vessels, skin, nerves, tendons, joints, bones, and muscles. A conventional history and physical examination remains essential.

The system of classification adopted here is that of the AMA *Standard Nomenclature for Diseases and Operations.* A recent attempt has also been made to standardize nomenclature.

DISTURBANCES OF PRENATAL ORIGIN

CONGENITAL AMPUTATIONS

A wide variety of congenital amputations may occur, secondary to drugs, infections, etc, which may be (1) partial or complete; (2) at the terminal end of the extremity, or intercalary, with the terminal portion of the extremity present but intermediate parts missing; (3) transverse (across the extremity); or (4) paraxial (longitudinal). Amputations may result in complex tissue defects. The child with congenital absence of the sacrum may demonstrate myelodysplasia or complete paraplegia.

Treatment of congenital amputations is reconstructive surgery if feasible. Otherwise, amputation revision is indicated to provide a suitable stump for prosthesis fitting. Recent clinical experience has demonstrated that children may be fitted with lower extremity prostheses by the age of 1 year and with upper extremity prostheses by the age of 18–24 months. These prostheses are entirely functional, and infants readily learn to use them.

Hall CB: Recent concepts in the treatment of the limb-deficient child. Artif Limbs 10:36–51, 1966.

Hall CB, Brooks MB, Dennis JF: Congenital skeletal deficiencies. JAMA 181:590–599, 1962.

DEFORMITIES OF THE EXTREMITIES

1. METATARSUS VARUS OR METATARSUS ADDUCTUS

This disorder is characterized by adduction of the forefoot on the hindfoot. The heel is in normal position. The longitudinal arch may be excessively high on its medial aspect. The lateral border of the foot shows sharp angulation medially at the level of the base of the fifth metatarsal. The deformity may be flexible or rigid. Flexible deformities are postural. The infant usually sleeps in the prone position with his feet curled beneath him and the forefoot adducted.

Treatment of the postural type is by simple manipulations performed by the mother. If the sleeping position contributes to the deformity, a Denis Browne splint may be utilized.

If the deformity is rigid and cannot be corrected by simple passive manipulation, treatment consists of plaster dressings which should be changed weekly until overcorrection is attained.

Shoe wedges have been tried, but in general are ineffective. Corrective shoes with a reversed last and reversal of the shoes (wearing the right shoe on the left foot and vice versa) are usually more soothing to the infant's mother than corrective for the child's feet.

The prognosis is excellent.

Ponseti IV, Becker JR: Congenital metatarsus adductus: The results of treatment. J Bone Joint Surg 48A:702, 1966.

2. CLUBFOOT OR TALIPES EQUINOVARUS

This deformity usually involves equinus (plantar flexion) of the foot at the ankle joint, inversion of the heel, and forefoot adduction. One or another of the 3 deformities may predominate. The incidence of one or the other component is 1:1000 live births. The deformity is usually an isolated one, but similar deformities may be present in arthrogryposis or in myelodysplasia.

Treatment consists of multiple plaster dressings, changed frequently, starting as soon as possible after birth. Wedging of the plaster may be performed in the infant over 3 months of age. The plaster dressings should correct the heel inversion and forefoot adduction first. The equinus is the last deformity to be corrected. Braces may be necessary to maintain correction until the child begins to walk. The deformity may recur during periods of rapid growth. Operations may be needed in childhood or adolescence to correct residual deformity.

The prognosis is guarded.

Hersh A: The role of surgery in the treatment of club feet. J Bone Joint Surg 49A:1684, 1967.
Kite JG: Some suggestions on the treatment of club foot by casts. J Bone Joint Surg 45A:406, 1963.
McCanley JC Jr: Club foot: History of the development of the concepts of pathogenesis and treatment. Clin Orthop 44:51, 1966.
Ponseti IV, Smoley EN: Congenital clubfoot. J Bone Joint Surg 45A:261, 1963.

3. CONGENITAL DYSPLASIA OF THE HIP JOINT
(Congenital Dislocation of the Hip)

This entity consists of a complex deformity of both sides of the hip joint. True dislocation is rarely present at birth but usually develops within the first 3–4 months of life. Excessive anteversion of the femoral neck may be present. Deficiencies of the acetabulum may include shallowness of the weight-bearing quadrant (increased acetabular index) and deficiency of the anterior acetabulum as demonstrated in true lateral x-rays.

Clinical Findings
A. Symptoms and Signs:
1. Prior to dislocation—There may be abnormal muscular splinting of the affected hip, diminished spontaneous movement, flexion of the thigh, limited abduction of the hip, and asymmetry of the gluteal and thigh folds. However, the normal newborn infant may also have asymmetry of skin folds (40%), unilateral extra skin (20%), increased acetabular angle, unequal ability to abduct the legs (4%), apparent shortness of one leg (3%), and inability to abduct a full 90°.
2. Following dislocation—All of the above findings are present, plus marked asymmetry of gluteal, inguinal, and knee folds, external rotation of the leg, shortening of the affected leg, a clicking sound on forced abduction, a bulge of the femoral head, a positive Trendelenburg sign, and delay in learning to walk. With bilateral dislocations, lordosis and waddling gait may be marked.
B. X-Ray Findings: X-ray shows deformity of Shenton's line, delayed appearance or hypoplasia of the femoral epiphyseal center, increased obliquity of the acetabular roof, and dislocation of the femur upward and laterally.

Treatment
Simple dysplasia without subluxation or dislocation requires a splint maintaining the hip in flexion and abduction. Rigid plaster fixation should not be utilized. In most instances, the position can be maintained with a Frejka pillow or very thick and heavy diapers.

Subluxation or dislocation should be treated by closed manipulative reduction without anesthesia. If anesthesia is utilized, too much force may be exerted, damaging the hip. If reduction is obtained by closed means, it should be maintained by well applied plaster. The position chosen for application is the one in which the hip seems most stable, with the hip flexed 90°, abducted 75–90°, and externally rotated maximally. The knee is flexed to 90°, and the ankle is at 90°. The widely abducted and internally rotated position is to be avoided since it has been shown to contribute to the incidence of avascular necrosis of the capital ossification center of the femoral head—not only on the affected side, but also on the sound or normal side. If x-rays show that manipulative reduction is not perfect, open reduction should be performed. An infolded acetabular labrum will usually be found and must be excised.

Acetabular operations have been performed for complex cases at age 2–6.

With skeletal maturity, reconstructive procedures may be necessary if the dislocation is not adequately corrected.

Ponseti IV: Nonsurgical treatment of congenital dislocation of the hip. J Bone Joint Surg 48A:1392, 1966.
Ryder CT: Congenital dislocation of the hip in the older child: Surgical treatment. J Bone Joint Surg 48A:1404, 1966.
Salter RB: *Textbook of Disorders and Injuries of the Musculoskeletal System.* Williams & Wilkins, 1970.

4. TORTICOLLIS

Wryneck deformities may be present in infancy due to sternocleidomastoid muscle injury or disease. The fixed deformity of the neck is rotation of the face to the side opposite the sternocleidomastoid contracture and tilting of the head toward the side of the muscle deformity. The deformity is usually not present at birth but becomes evident in the first 1–2 months of life. A palpable mass may be present in the sternocleidomastoid muscle.

Treatment consists of passive stretching in mild cases and surgical division of the sternocleidomastoid muscle in more severe cases. If left untreated, facial asymmetry may result.

Acute torticollis may follow upper respiratory infections or trauma in older children. X-rays should be taken if there is tenderness or deformity of the cervical spine.

GENERALIZED AFFECTIONS OF THE SKELETON OR OF THE MESODERMAL TISSUES*

1. ARTHROGRYPOSIS MULTIPLEX CONGENITA
(Amyoplasia Congenita)

This congenital syndrome consists of incomplete fibrous ankylosis (usually symmetrical) of many or all of the joints (except those of the spine and jaw). There may be contractures either in flexion or extension. The usual deformities of the upper extremity include normal shoulders, elbows fixed in extension, wrists in palmar flexion, and "club hands" with useless thumbs. In the lower extremities the deformities are similar, with knees fixed in extension and severe club feet. The hips may be dislocated. The joints appear enlarged and cylindrical. The periarticular tissues show contractures and fail to develop normally, and the skin appears thickened. There may be numerous other congenital anomalies in the viscera.

Since muscle power is poor, mobilization of the joints by physical therapy alone is almost useless. If the joints of the upper extremity can be mobilized, dynamic bracing is needed to maintain the joints in a functional position. In the lower extremities, the feet must be corrected to a functional position before bracing and ambulation are possible. The club feet are often most difficult to correct, and surgery is often needed. Heel cord lengthening, posterior capsulotomies of the ankle joint, and medial release operations may be needed to put the stiff foot into a functional position. If the knees are not in full extension, multiple plaster wedgings may be tried to make it possible for the patient to wear long leg braces. Surgical correction of knee flexion contractures may be necessary— posterior capsulotomies, hamstring lengthening, or supracondylar osteotomy. If the hips are dislocated, correction may not be needed. Bilateral dislocation of the hips is not a major obstacle to ambulation in these severely disabled patients.

The prognosis for physical and financial independence is poor.

2. MARFAN'S SYNDROME

This syndrome is associated with abnormal length of fingers, toes, and extremities (arachnodactyly), hypermobility of the joints, subluxation of the lens, other abnormalities of the eyes (cataract, coloboma, megalocornea, strabismus, nystagmus), high palate, defects of the spine and chest (pigeon breast), and congenital cardiovascular disease (particularly weakness of

*Gargoylism is discussed in Chapter 35.

the media of the aorta). Serum mucoproteins may be decreased and urinary excretion of hydroxyproline increased. The condition may be confused with homocystinuria.

Treatment consists only of supportive measures. Rarely do the deformities need bracing or surgical correction. The prognosis for life is poor since most of these patients die from rupture of dissecting aortic aneurysms.

3. CLEIDOCRANIAL DYSOSTOSIS

This syndrome consists of absence of part or all of the clavicle and delay of ossification of the skull. The facial bones may be underdeveloped, the sinuses absent, the palate highly arched, dentition defective, the skull enlarged (especially in the parietal and frontal regions), and other bones defective. Coxa vara deformity of the proximal femur is occasionally present and requires angulation osteotomy to equalize leg length. The clavicular deformity needs no treatment.

4. CRANIOFACIAL DYSOSTOSIS

This syndrome (Crouzon's disease) consists of acrocephaly (tower skull), hypoplastic maxilla, beaked nose, protrusion of the lower lip, exophthalmos, exotropia, and hypertelorism. It may be familial.

No treatment is needed.

5. KLIPPEL-FEIL SYNDROME

This syndrome is characterized by fusion of some or all of the cervical vertebrae or of multiple hemivertebrae into one osseous mass. The neck is short and limited in motion. The hairline is low. Other defects, including scoliosis, cervical rib, spina bifida, torticollis, webbed neck, and congenital high position of the scapula, may be present also.

Treatment is rarely indicated. The scapula may need to be brought down and fixed if the deformity is marked or if function is lost.

6. SPRENGEL'S DEFORMITY

This is a congenital condition in which one or both scapulas are elevated and small. The child cannot raise his arm completely on the affected side, and there may be torticollis. The shoulders are asymmetric.

If the deformity is functionally limiting, the scapula must be surgically relocated lower on the thorax. The scapula is dissected out subperiosteally, moved lower on the rib cage, and anchored there by suture. The operation is an extensive one and should not be performed for cosmetic reasons only.

Woodward J: Congenital elevation of the scapula. J Bone Joint Surg 43A:219, 1961.

7. OSTEOGENESIS IMPERFECTA

Osteogenesis imperfecta is a rare dominantly inherited connective tissue disease which occurs in 2 forms: congenita and tarda. The severe congenita type is characterized by multiple intrauterine or perinatal fractures. These children continue to have fractures and are dwarfed as a result of bony deformities. The shafts of the long bones are slender and reduced in cortical thickness because of defective periosteal bone formation and architecture. Wormian bones are seen in the skull, and immature collagen fibrils are present in bone. Other features include blue scleras, thin skin, hyperextensibility of ligaments, "otosclerosis" with significant hearing loss, and hypoplastic and deformed teeth. Recurrent epistaxis, easy bruisability, mild hyperpyrexia (which may increase significantly during anaesthesia), and excessive diaphoresis are common. In the tarda type, the skeleton appears to be clinically normal at birth but fractures begin to occur at variable times after the perinatal period, resulting in relatively fewer fractures and deformities.

Oral administration of magnesium oxide, 15 mg/kg/day, has decreased fracture rate, diaphoresis, constipation, and fever in the majority of patients treated for 2 years. Magnesium acts by releasing calcitonin, depressing the action of thyroid and parathyroid hormones and increasing calcium and phosphorus balance. The use of sex hormones in prepubertal patients has not been successful. In addition to the usual side-effects of these drugs, an increased fracture rate was seen after withdrawal of the medication. High doses of sodium fluoride, 1 mg/kg (up to a maximum of 20 mg/day), have been given to convert bone mineral to the less soluble fluoroapatite but is not recommended in osteogenesis imperfecta.

Albright JA, Grunt JA: Studies of patients with osteogenesis imperfecta. J Bone Joint Surg 53A:1415–1425, 1971.

Clark I: Effects of magnesium ions on calcium and phosphorus metabolism. Am J Physiol 214:348–356, 1968.

Sofield HA, Millar EA: Fragmentation, realignment, and intramedullary rod fixation of deformities of the long bones in children. J Bone Joint Surg 41A: 1371–1391, 1959.

Solomons CC, Styner J: Osteogenesis imperfecta. Calcif Tissue Res 3:318–326, 1969.

Taves DR: New approach to the treatment of bone disease with fluoride. Fed Proc 29:1185–1187, 1970.

8. IDIOPATHIC JUVENILE OSTEOPOROSIS

This is an acute disease characterized by osteoporosis and unexplained pathologic fractures of the spine and long bones. It affects boys and girls equally in the prepuberal years, and the severity is variable. There is evidence of gross enteric malabsorption of calcium, which may reflect an abnormality of 1:25 dihydroxyergocalciferol synthesis.

9. OSTEOPETROSIS
(Osteitis Condensans Generalisata, Marble Bone Disease, Albers-Schönberg Disease)

The clinical manifestations of this familial and hereditary syndrome are bony deformities due to pathologic fractures, myelophthisic anemia, splenomegaly, visual and auditory disturbances, square head, facial paralysis, pigeon breast, and dwarfing. The findings may appear at any age. On x-ray examination the bones show increased density, transverse bands in the shafts, clubbing of ends, and vertical striations (long bones). There is thickening about the cranial foramens, and there may be heterotopic calcification of soft tissues.

There is no treatment. The prognosis is fair.

10. ACHONDROPLASIA
(Classical Chondrodystrophy)

The clinical manifestations consist of short arms and legs. The upper arms and thighs are proportionately shorter than the forearms and legs. Frequently there is bowing of extremities, waddling gait, limitation of motion of major joints, relaxation of ligaments, short, stubby fingers of almost equal length, a prominent forehead, moderate hydrocephaly, depressed bridge of the nose, and lumbar lordosis. Mentality and sexual function are normal. A family history is often present.

On x-ray the tubular bones are short and thick, the epiphyseal plates generally irregular, and the ends of the bones thick, broad, knob-like, and cupped. The epiphyseal centers may be delayed and small in early childhood. Other x-ray findings include fusion of epiphyses, an enlarged calvarium, and fibulas that are relatively long compared to the tibias.

11. OSTEOCHONDRODYSTROPHY
(Morquio's Disease)

This disorder is characterized by shortening of the spine, kyphosis, scoliosis, moderate shortening of the extremities, protruding sternum, prominent abdomen, hepatosplenomegaly, and a waddling gait due to flexion of the knees and flexion and limitation of motion of the hip joint. The skull is minimally involved. Onset is between 1 and 4 years of age. A family history is often present.

X-ray findings are similar to those of achondroplasia, with wedge-shaped, flattened deformities of the vertebral bodies and irregularity of the epiphyses. The lower extremities tend to be involved more than the upper.

There is no treatment, and the prognosis is fair.

12. CHONDROECTODERMAL DYSPLASIA
(Ellis-Van Creveld Syndrome)

Manifestations include ectodermal dysplasia, congenital heart disease, polydactyly and frequently syndactyly, poorly formed teeth (some or all of the teeth may be absent), and mental retardation.

X-ray examination may show changes of chondrodystrophy, shortening and bowing of the tibias and fibulas, hypoplastic, eccentric proximal tibial epiphyses, and fusion of the carpal bones.

There is no treatment. The prognosis depends on the type of heart disease present.

Rubin P: *Dynamic Classification of Bone Dysplasias.* Year Book, 1964.

GROWTH DISTURBANCES OF THE MUSCULOSKELETAL SYSTEM

IDIOPATHIC SCOLIOSIS

Curvature of the vertebral column in the lateral plane is called scoliosis. The curve is designated by the direction of the convexity of the curve. Accentuation of the normal thoracic curvature in the anteroposterior plane is known as kyphosis; of the normal lumbar curvature, lordosis. Most cases occur in girls 10–14 years of age.

The idiopathic, asymptomatic scoliosis of adolescent girls comprises 80–85% of the total scoliosis problem. In the idiopathic scolioses, girls are affected 7–10 times as frequently as boys. Almost all cases are asymptomatic, but occasionally a traumatic incident may be implicated by parents or child. In these instances, the trauma will merely have precipitated adequate examination. Scoliosis secondary to disorders such as cerebral palsy are relatively uncommon.

Two percent of scolioses may follow muscular problems such as muscular dystrophy. Such curvatures are generally postural, due to gravity, ie, they are present in the upright position and absent when the child is supine or prone. They are long, gentle, single; at first they are quite flexible, but later they may become fixed or rigid.

Five to 7% of scolioses may occur with vertebral anomalies such as hemivertebrae or unilateral vertebral bridges. These curves are fixed and rigid, but quite often will increase with the growth of the child.

A miscellaneous group of curvatures comprises the balance of the cases. Quite often scoliosis is seen in an infant under 1 year of age. These curves are long, gentle, and single, and most of them correct spontaneously.

Not included in the above figures are the postural scolioses which are the result of habit, shortened lower extremities, etc. These secondary curves obviously need treatment of the underlying cause.

Clinical Findings
A. Symptoms and Signs: Scoliosis is asymptomatic. The deformity of the rib cage or prominence of one hip may be quite evident on examination. The curvatures are usually quite limber at first but may become rigid.

B. X-Ray Findings: X-rays should be taken in the standing position. In most cases there is one primary curve, but at times there is a double primary curve each with compensatory curves above and below. If compensatory curves are equal to the primary curve, the scoliosis is "compensated." If the spine is "uncompensated," the head will not be directly over the pelvis. Rotation of the vertebral bodies may be present, with spectacular deformity of the rib cage.

Treatment
Exercise programs may improve postural scoliosis but rarely improve idiopathic scoliosis. The Milwaukee brace, which combines traction with multiple pressure pads, may be effective.

Surgical fusion of the spine may be necessary if the curvature progresses rapidly, if an unsightly curve becomes fixed, or if the rotational element is prominent. Many procedures are available.

Treatment is difficult and prolonged.

Prognosis
Compensated and slowly progressive curves usually have a good cosmetic prognosis. The higher the curve, the worse the prognosis; the greater the rotational deformity, the worse the cosmetic deformity will be. Pelvic obliquity as part of the compensatory curve is a bad prognostic sign. The disorder may continue to progress beyond puberty.

Goldstein LA: Surgical management of scoliosis. J Bone Joint Surg 48A:167, 1966.
James JIP: *Scoliosis.* Williams & Wilkins, 1967.
Risser JC: Treatment of scoliosis during the past 50 years. Clin Orthop 44:109, 1966.
Winter RB, Moe JH, Eilers VE: Congenital scoliosis. In: *Textbook of Disorders of the Musculoskeletal System.* Salter RB. Williams & Wilkins, 1970.

EPIPHYSIOLYSIS
(Slipped Capital Femoral Epiphysis)

Epiphysiolysis is a nontraumatic separation of the femoral head ossification center. It is more common in adolescent boys; in younger overweight boys and girls, and in tall and thin children. Vague symptoms are present, including limitation of motion, limp, pain (which may be referred to the knee), tenderness, shortening of the leg, restriction of internal rotation, and abduction of the hip. X-rays show thickening and irregularity of the epiphyseal cartilage line followed by apparent downward and posterior displacement of the head of the femur.

Treatment consists of immobilization of the femur to prevent separation through additional trauma. Traction may be effective. Internal fixation may be desirable if slipping of the capital femoral epiphysis is marked or is progressing rapidly.

In cases with slight slipping treated early, the prognosis is favorable. Late cases with severe displacement often have permanent disability regardless of the form of therapy. Avascular necrosis of the capital femoral ossification center may result from severe displacement.

Symposium: Slipped capital femoral epiphysis. Clin Orthop 48:7, 1966.

GENU VARUM & GENU VALGUM

Varus (bowleg) and valgus (knock knee) deformities of the knee joints are quite common. They are usually mild, may increase through the first to third years of life, and in most cases correct spontaneously by age 7 or 8.

Treatment is not necessary.

Hugenberger PW: Leg deformities. P Clin North America 14:589, 1967.

TIBIAL TORSION
("Toeing In")

"Toeing in" is a common parental complaint but is usually asymptomatic. The child may stumble, be clumsy, or wear shoes unevenly. Causes include metatarsus adductus (see p 464), internal tibial torsion, and excessive anteversion of the femoral neck.

Treatment is rarely indicated, and the prognosis is good.

COMMON FOOT PROBLEMS

When a child begins to stand and walk, the long arches seem flattened and the feet mildly pronated, the legs and feet turn outward, and the knees show a slight valgum deformity. As the child grows and muscle power develops, more normal relationships develop.

Flatfoot

Flat feet are normal in infants. Muscle power later produces a longitudinal arch. Flatfoot in an older child may represent generalized muscular and ligamentous weakness.

Treatment is rarely indicated. Barefoot exercises are of greatest importance. For persistent or severe cases, a 1/8 inch wedge on the inner heel and sole is prescribed. After age 3, the wedge may be increased to 3/16 inches. Shoes may be either high or low. Arch supports may be necessary later if there is disability or pain, which is rarely the case.

Pronated Foot

This disorder is characterized by lateral rotation of the foot at the talocalcaneonavicular joint, medial inclination of the foot and tibia, and prominence of the medial malleolus. Passive rotation of the foot into a normal position beneath the tibia reveals a good longitudinal arch.

Treatment (indicated only if the deformity is severe or progressive) consists of inner heel wedges as for flatfoot (see above). If the child toes out markedly, use inner heel wedges about 3/16 inches high or a simple Thomas heel. Exercises designed to strengthen the anterior and posterior tibial muscles must be carried out faithfully. These include tiptoe standing and forward knee bends—hands on hips, one foot in front, leaning forward, bending knee and ankle.

The prognosis is good.

Talipes Calcaneovalgus

This disorder is characterized by excessive dorsiflexion at the ankle and eversion of the foot. It is most often present at birth and usually corrects spontaneously. The deformity developing later in life may be due to gastrocnemius paralysis.

If treatment is needed, passive exercises performed by the mother prior to the age of walking are all that is necessary. In older children, scaphoid pads and 1/8 inch or 3/16 inch inner heel and inner sole wedges are used.

Complete correction occurs spontaneously in most cases. If the calcaneovalgus is secondary to muscle paralysis, the prognosis is poor. In such cases, surgical transfer of muscles or foot arthrodeses are the only effective therapy.

Cavus Foot

This disorder may be hereditary or may be due to poliomyelitis, congenital syphilis, or neurologic conditions affecting the posterior and lateral columns of the spinal cord. It is manifested by an excessively high longitudinal arch and overactive long toe extensor tendons, which produce hyperextension at the metatarsophalangeal joint and flexion at the interphalangeal joints.

Early (conservative) treatment consists of metatarsal pads and bars and stretching exercises. Surgical transplantation of the long toe extensor tendons, together with arthrodesis, if indicated, need not be undertaken until later.

Hammer Toe

This is a flexion deformity, usually congenital, of either or both interphalangeal joints. It is most often asymptomatic and requires no treatment except for cosmetic reasons or if a callus forms.

Funk JF Jr: Foot problems in childhood. P Clin North America 14:571, 1967.
Kite JH: Errors and complications in treating foot conditions in children. Clin Orthop 53:31, 1967.

Bunions

These may occur in adolescent girls. Avoidance of pointed shoes is helpful, but bursitis over the head of the first metatarsal may justify a wedge osteotomy of the metatarsal bone.

EPHIPHYSEAL GROWTH DISTURBANCES SECONDARY TO INFECTION OR TRAUMA

Epiphyseal growth disturbances secondary to infection or trauma may necessitate osteotomy or epiphysiodesis. Prevention of epiphyseal damage in patients with pyogenic arthritis or with fractures about the epiphyses is most important; once epiphyseal damage has occurred, reconstructive procedures may be necessary if the deformity is progressive or severe.

METABOLIC DISORDERS OF THE MUSCULOSKELETAL SYSTEM

ORTHOPEDIC ASPECTS OF ENDOCRINE DISEASES

Hormonal problems affecting the skeleton are discussed in Chapter 24. Only a brief orthopedic resume is required here.

Adrenal

Adrenocortical hyperfunction may lead to advanced skeletal age with premature epiphyseal closure.

Osteoporosis and fractures secondary to corticosteroid administration are now rare.

Thyroid

Hyperthyroidism or prolonged thyroid administration may lead to severe osteoporosis with secondary pathologic fracture.

Parathyroid

A. Hyperparathyroidism: Parathormone exerts a direct effect upon bone, producing absorption of bone. Primary hyperparathyroidism is very rare in children. The skeletal effects of hyperparathyroidism may also occur secondarily as a result of parathyroid stimulation by kidney disease. The x-ray findings are of generalized osteoporosis and cortical atrophy, most noticeable in the phalanges and metacarpals, with loss of the normal appearance of the cortices of the diaphyses of these bones. The "brown tumors" of hyperparathyroidism are quite uncommon in childhood.

B. Hypoparathyroidism and Pseudohypoparathyroidism: The symptoms and signs, laboratory findings, and x-ray findings in these 2 disorders are similar, and the distinction between them is difficult. X-rays show club-shaped deformities of bones, particularly prominent in the metacarpals and phalanges. The fourth and fifth metacarpals and metatarsals are usually abnormally short. The epiphyseal ossification centers indent the metaphyses.

C. Pseudopseudohypoparathyroidism: This is a rare syndrome with skeletal deformities similar to those of pseudohypoparathyroidism. Laboratory findings are completely normal. The x-ray features are identical with those of pseudohypoparathyroidism or idiopathic hypoparathyroidism. There is no known treatment.

Gonads

In general, deficiency of gonadal hormones produces osteoporosis with delayed maturation of the skeleton.

DEGENERATIVE PROBLEMS
(Arthritis, Bursitis, & Tenosynovitis)

The degenerative changes include those in joints (degenerative arthritis) or in the bursae and tendons or tendon sheaths (bursitis or tenosynovitis).

Degenerative arthritis may occur in joints which are the seat of severe destructive changes which may follow infection, slipped capital femoral epiphyses, trauma, or hemophilia. Prevention is more important than treatment.

Degenerative changes in the soft tissues of children occur principally in adolescent athletes. Such problems appear about the humeral condyles of boys taught to throw curves in Little League baseball. Treatment is by enforced rest, often with plaster casts. Only rarely is injection of the bursa with corticosteroids justified.

Tenosynovitis is frequently seen about the toes, feet, and ankles of girls taking ballet dancing, particularly toe dancing. The tendon sheaths about the ankle joints can be identified by palpation. Rest is indicated. Only occasionally is corticosteroid injection indicated; if used, it should not be repeated more than once or twice.

TRAUMA

SOFT TISSUE TRAUMA
(Sprains, Strains, & Contusions)

A sprain is the injury that results when a force acts upon a ligament or capsule. A strain is the injury resulting from a force acting upon a tendon or a muscle. Sprains and strains produce some degree of tissue tearing; contusions produce varying degrees of tissue compression, often with vascular damage within the tissue and hematoma formation.

Sprains and strains are classified as mild, moderate, or severe. Mild sprain may be thought of as tearing 5% of the ligament substance; moderate sprain, 50%; and severe sprain 100%.

Mild sprains result from a minor or often ignored injury. The immediate pain of the injury disappears. Function may be normal for 4–12 hours after the injury. Signs and symptoms of pain, point tenderness, swelling, and disability then appear. There is no instability of the joint.

Moderate sprains result from more severe trauma, and symptoms and signs appear sooner. Pain, tenderness, and swelling are greater than in mild sprains. Instability of the joint may be demonstrated by adequate examination, both physically and radiographically.

Severe sprains are the result of major trauma. Deformity of the joint is often evident initially, and both the physician and the patient may make a diagnosis of fracture. The signs and symptoms appear immediately. Disability is immediate, and the patient cannot use the extremity. Instability is grossly evident.

Immediate treatment of sprains is by ice and compression. The ice may be removed in a few hours: Its only function is to produce vasoconstriction and decrease hemorrhage. The compression should be continued for a few days.

In general, mild sprains should be supported by strapping, moderate sprains should be immobilized in plaster, and severe sprains either immobilized in plaster or repaired surgically. Surgical repair is indicated in patients requiring extremes of activity. Strapping should be maintained for 2–3 weeks, followed by a period of graduated exercises to improve muscle power and joint range of motion.

Some specific types of sprains are discussed below.

Ankle Sprains

The history will often indicate whether medial or lateral ligaments are injured. Careful examination for point tenderness will indicate the site and extent of injury. The ankle should be supported or immobilized at a right angle in a functional position. Adhesive elastic strapping should pass from the web of the toes to the tibial tuberosity. Plaster should be similarly extensive. Treatment should be of adequate duration. Inadequate treatment has produced the common statement, "It's too bad you sprained the ankle, for you will always have trouble with it. It would be better if you had broken it." Fractures are more likely to receive adequate treatment.

Knee Sprains

Sprains of the collateral and cruciate ligaments are uncommon in children. Adolescent boys may sustain an injury similar to anterior cruciate rupture in fracture of the anterior tibial spine. Actually, this is an avulsion injury with the anterior cruciate ligament proving stronger than the bone. If the separation of the tibial spine fragment is less than 3 mm, reduction is not necessary, and the knee merely needs to be immobilized in plaster in full extension for 6 weeks. If the separation is greater than that, operation is indicated, and the spine should be sutured in place.

Sprains of the collateral and cruciate ligaments should be treated with support, strapping, or plaster for 6 weeks. This treatment should be followed by an intensive course of physical therapy to build quadriceps muscle strength.

Internal Derangements of the Knee (Meniscus Injuries)

Such injuries are uncommon in children. They may occur in adolescent boys and girls as a result of athletic activities. If the knee is "locked," it should be manipulated in an attempt to "unlock" it. The knee should then be immobilized in plaster for 6 weeks in full extension. Intensive physical therapy is then required. If the knee cannot be unlocked, operative excision of the meniscus is indicated. If locking occurs 3 or 4 times, excision of the meniscus is required.

Back Sprains

Sprains of the ligaments of the back are uncommon in children but may occur in violent trauma such as automobile accidents or athletic injuries. The patient should be placed at bed rest and given heat and sedatives. Complete recovery can be anticipated in 7–10 days. The back may then be strapped with elastic tape, adhesive tape, or elastic bandages and the patient permitted graduated return to full activity.

Contusions

Contusion of muscle with hematoma formation causes the very familiar injury known as "charley horse." Immediate treatment of such injuries is by temporary application of ice and continued compression. Gentle exercises should be started in 5–7 days. Heat should be added then and continued to full recovery.

Myositis Ossificans

Ossification in the muscles is quite common in children. Trauma is always of major degree. The sites most frequently involved are the quadriceps of the thigh and the triceps of the arm. The hematoma of the injury is organized, and ossification begins in the soft tissues adjacent to the bone. The ossification appears 2–3 weeks after the injury. Ossification may reach spectacular proportions and resemble osteosarcoma. Great care must be taken not to diagnose such ossification as sarcoma, resulting in amputation.

Disability of the extremity is great. The part should be immobilized in plaster, and this should be continued until serial roentgenograms demonstrate that the ossification has ceased to progress and has become mature. Gentle active exercises may then be initiated, always staying within the limits of pain. The ossification will then decrease and may entirely disappear. However, a scar remains in the muscle, and it may never return to normal strength and size.

O'Donoghue DH: *Treatment of Injuries to Athletes.* Saunders, 1970.

SUBLUXATIONS & DISLOCATIONS

Such injuries must be considered to be severe sprains because of the ligamentous and capsular damage. In sharp contrast to fracture treatment, which may be delayed with safety, dislocations must be reduced immediately. The reduction can be accomplished in most instances by simple manipulation. No anesthetic is necessary; the parts are usually sufficiently anesthetic as a result of the injury in the first few hours afterward. The part may then be immobilized by splinting and the patient safely transported.

Immobilization should be continued for 3 weeks and the child then urged to perform gentle, graduated, active exercises. Physical therapy is usually not indicated and in fact is contraindicated if the therapist is vigorous. The child should be permitted to perform his own therapy. No stretching should be permitted.

"Pulled Elbow"

Infants frequently sustain subluxation of the radial head as a result of being lifted or pulled by the forearm. The only symptom may be unwillingness to bend the elbow. X-rays are normal. Point tenderness over the radial head is present. The elbow should be placed in full supination and then slowly moved from full flexion to full extension. A click is usually palpable at the radial head as the forearm moves into complete extension, and immediate cure results.

Recurrent Dislocation of the Patella

Recurrent dislocation of the patella is quite common in adolescent girls. The patient states that the knee "gives out" or "jumps out of joint." The patella is always dislocated laterally, the knee flexed, and the patient may notice the patella on the lateral aspect of the knee joint. X-rays will indicate the dislocation. Reduction is performed by extension of the knee and manual pressure on the patella. The knee should be immobilized for 3–4 weeks in full extension. Dislocation is quite apt to recur, and reconstructive surgery on the knee joint capsule should be performed. Exercise to strengthen the quadriceps should then be advised.

EPIPHYSEAL SEPARATIONS

Epiphyseal separations and fractures may be obvious or may be difficult to identify because of the large amount of cartilage present about the ossification centers. Films should be taken of the opposite extremity for comparison. Reduction should be performed as gently as possible in order not to increase the damage already done to epiphyseal cartilage. Imperfect reductions are usually satisfactory because of the tremendous growth potential of the patient. Open reduction is almost never indicated. Simple epiphyseal separations are rarely accompanied by epiphyseal growth disturbance. More traumatic separations or more traumatic reductions may interfere with epiphyseal growth, producing angular deformities which require corrective osteotomies later. Epiphyseal fractures vertically across an ossification center and epiphyseal cartilage are likely to produce growth damage.

TORUS FRACTURES

Torus fractures result from minimal angular trauma. They usually occur in the radius and tibia. On x-ray, one cortex appears to have been folded upon itself, causing minimal angular deformity. Reduction is not necessary. Simple immobilization for 3–5 weeks is sufficient.

GREENSTICK FRACTURES

Greenstick fractures occur in the mid-diaphyseal areas of long bones. It is often said that in greenstick fractures one cortex is fractured and the other not, but this is not true. Nor is it true that the second cortex must be fractured in order to maintain reduction.

Reduction is accomplished simply by manipulation, and immobilization must be in snugly fitting plaster to prevent recurrence of the deformity. The plaster should be changed every 3–4 weeks. These diaphyseal fractures heal more slowly than fractures in the metaphyseal regions, and immobilization must be prolonged (12–14 weeks).

FRACTURES OF THE CLAVICLE

Clavicular fractures are extremely common in infants and children. Reduction is not a problem, and immobilization in a figure-of-8 dressing is all that is necessary.

SUPRACONDYLAR FRACTURES OF THE HUMERUS

These fractures are very common in children 3–6 years old and are dangerous because they are frequently associated with vascular problems. Swelling may be severe, followed by Volkmann's ischemic contracture. Adequate reduction by closed manipulation or by traction is mandatory. If reduction does not restore impaired vascular supply, open exposure of the vessels is necessary. (Stellate ganglion blocks are frequently attempted but are of little value.) Action must be quick and prompt. Supracondylar fractures of the humerus may damage the epiphyseal cartilage with resultant cubitus valgus or varus growth deformity. Extreme cubitus valgus deformity may result in delayed ulnar nerve palsy.

GENERAL COMMENTS ON OTHER FRACTURES IN CHILDREN

Reduction of fractures in children is usually accomplished by simple manipulation or traction. Open reduction is rarely indicated. Remodeling of the fracture callus will produce almost normal appearance of the bone radiographically. Infants will remodel more deformity than will young children or adolescents because of the growth potential still present. Residual displacement and angular deformities may not be so perfectly corrected. Rotational fracture deformities, particularly those in the forearm, must be corrected in reduction.

INFECTIONS OF THE BONES & JOINTS

OSTEOMYELITIS

Osteomyelitis is an inflammatory process which may involve all parts of a bone. It is usually caused by staphylococci, although streptococci, salmonellae (especially in sickle cell anemia), and other organisms may be the causative agents. Hematogenous spread is the usual route of infection, but local extension from an infected focus also occurs. A history of trauma, usually mild, is common in the hematogenous type.

The initial site is usually in the metaphysis of a bone. Pus forms and spreads toward the diaphysis and through the cortex, producing a subperiosteal abscess and elevation of the periosteum and further interference with the blood supply to the shaft. The joint is rarely invaded, but this may occur if the metaphysis lies within the joint capsule. The cortex may undergo necrosis, producing a sequestrum which will be slowly absorbed or extruded through a sinus. Surgical removal of the sequestrum may be necessary. During repair, new bone is laid down beneath the elevated periosteum, forming an envelope of reactive bone about the sequestrum. This reactive bone is called the involucrum. Complete healing takes place only when all dead bone has been reabsorbed, discharged, or excised.

Clinical Findings

A. Symptoms and Signs: Local inflammatory signs may be absent early. Localized erythema, warmth, tenderness, and swelling appear later. Symptoms consist of fever, rapid pulse, severe and constant throbbing pain over the end of the shaft, and limitation of joint motion.

B. Laboratory Findings: Leukocytosis may be marked. Blood cultures are usually positive early in the course. Smears of aspirated pus may show cocci or rods. Cultures (aerobic and anaerobic) of aspirated pus must be performed for sensitivity tests.

C. X-Ray Findings: X-ray shows spotty rarefaction followed shortly by periosteal new bone formation (usually absent during the first 10–14 days of the disease). A considerable portion of bone is usually involved. The bone is at first porotic because of destruction, but subsequent reactive bone formation (the involucrum) produces osteosclerosis.

Treatment

A. Specific Measures: Aspiration of pus (using aseptic technic) provides material for smear and culture and in many cases makes possible immediate bacteriologic diagnosis.

Infection is age related, ie, staphylococcal infections are common in older children and other organisms, especially *Hemophilus influenzae,* in the younger. In suspected cases, methicillin should be given immediately in doses of 250–300 mg/kg/day divided into 6 equal doses until the specific organism has been identified by culture. Then, for penicillin-sensitive staphylococci, pneumococci, or streptococci, give penicillin G, 250,000 units/kg/day in 6 divided doses IV until there is significant amelioration of local signs, whereupon penicillin V should be given orally, 125 mg/kg/day in 4–6 divided doses. For resistant staphylococci, change from methicillin to dicloxacillin, 50 mg/kg/day orally in 4–6 doses and titrate serum killing power level against cultures of the organism.

For *H influenzae* infections, give initially ampicillin, 150–200 mg/kg/day IV in 4–6 doses. Switch to oral penicillin with obvious clinical progress and again titrate the serum.

Treatment should be continued for at least 4–6 weeks in all cases.

B. General Measures: In the early stages, immobilization in a loose-fitting plaster dressing may be helpful in promoting the comfort of the patient. If sequestrum and involucrum formation are marked, limited use of the part will be necessary to prevent fracture.

C. Surgical Measures: Surgical aspiration is of diagnostic value. Surgical debridement is indicated in the following circumstances: (1) rapidly progressive and uncontrolled destruction, (2) evidence of cellulitis not controlled by chemotherapy, (3) abscess formation within the bone, and (4) sequestrum formation when serial x-rays do not show evidence of resorption.

Prognosis

With prompt, sustained, and effective treatment in cases where there is little bone destruction, the prognosis for recovery and restoration of normal bone architecture is excellent. Inappropriate antibiotics, too short a period of therapy, poor drainage, or sequestrum development adversely affect the prognosis.

Waldvogel F & others: Osteomyelitis. New England J Med 282:198–206, 260–266, 316–322, 1970.

PYOGENIC ARTHRITIS

Joint infection occurs by hematogenous spread (most common) or by direct extension of pus-forming organisms. One or more joints may be involved. The most common pathogens are hemolytic streptococci, *Staphylococcus aureus,* gonococci, meningococci, pneumococci, and *Hemophilus influenzae.*

Initially, there is an effusion which rapidly becomes purulent. Destruction of cartilage occurs at areas of joint contact. Bone is not affected in the early stages, but the femoral and humeral heads may undergo septic necrosis, fragmentation, and pathologic dislocation. Epiphyses whose synchondroses are located within the joint capsule are particularly apt to be involved by infection and septic necrosis.

During the chronic phase of the disease and the phase of repair, organization of the exudate occurs in the joint and granulation tissue matures to become fibrous. This may bind the joint surface together with a fibrous ankylosis. When motion is present, the synovial fluid tends to regenerate, but limitation of motion and associated pain generally persist as a result of strong intrasynovial adhesions.

Clinical Findings

A. Symptoms and Signs: The onset of severe systemic findings (fever, malaise, vomiting) may be slow or rapid. Pain may be severe, motion is limited, and the joint is splinted by muscular spasm. In infants, this may produce a pseudoparalysis. Effusion occurs but may not be palpable at first. The overlying tissues become swollen, tender, and warm. Contractures and muscular atrophy may occur late.

B. X-Ray Findings: Distention of the joint capsule is the first radiologic change. Later changes are narrowing of the cartilage space, erosion of subchondral bone, irregularity and fuzziness of the bone surfaces, bone destruction, and diffuse osteoporosis.

Treatment

A. Specific Measures: Aspiration should be done promptly. Surgical drainage may be indicated if symptoms do not subside within 24–30 hours. Appropriate antibiotic therapy in large doses should be administered by parenteral or oral route. Intra-articular administration is indicated if the process does not subside within 24 hours after parenteral administration.

B. General Measures: Immobilization and traction are indicated during the acute phase, and physical therapy when the infectious process has subsided.

Prognosis

With prompt treatment, the prognosis for full recovery of joint function is good.

Clawson DK, Dunn AW: Management of common bacterial infections of bones and joints. J Bone Joint Surg 49A:164, 1967.
Griffin PP: Bone and joint infections in children. P Clin North America 14:533, 1967.

TUBERCULOUS ARTHRITIS

Tuberculosis is less common in the USA than formerly and tends to involve older persons. However, tuberculous arthritis still must be considered in children who demonstrate limited joint motion with pain and swelling around a joint.

Tuberculous infections of the musculoskeletal system almost always involve joint structures. Tuberculous osteomyelitis is rare. Infection begins as a hematogenous extension from tuberculous infection elsewhere. Synovial tissues appear to be involved first, followed by extension into bone, with destruction of the subchondral cortex, and later the formation of a pannus overlying the articular cartilage. Bone destruction is severe. Sequestrum formation is also frequent, particularly in the major joints and in the vertebral bodies. Intervertebral disks are not involved. Adjacent vertebral cortices may be involved, with herniation of the disk into the bodies and narrowing of the disk space on the films.

Clinical Findings

A. Symptoms and Signs: The onset of tuberculous arthritis tends to be more insidious than that of acute pyogenic infections, and local and systemic signs and symptoms are less pronounced. Pain, swelling, and limitation of motion may be the only manifestations. Limp may be present if the infection involves the lower extremity. Deformity may be the only sign if the infection involves the spine. Localized swelling around the joint is attended by very little erythema, warmth, or other evidence of infection. Deformity (gibbus formation) occurs in cases of spine involvement.

B. Laboratory Findings: There is no leukocytosis, and blood cultures are negative. Smears and cultures of joint aspirates may demonstrate acid-fast bacilli.

C. X-Ray Findings: X-ray shows enlargement of the joint capsule, destruction of articular cortices with early preservation of cartilage space, and sequestrum formation. Although intervertebral disks are not involved, the disk space may become narrowed because of destruction of adjacent cortical surfaces of vertebral bodies. The disk then herniates into one or both adjacent vertebral bodies. Gibbus formation may be evident. Very little reactive bone formation occurs.

Treatment

A. Specific Measures: Aspiration or biopsy is necessary to establish a definitive diagnosis. Antituberculosis chemotherapy consists of isoniazid, 8—16 mg/kg orally in divided doses for 18 months; streptomycin, 0.5 gm/day IM for 3 months; and aminosalicylic acid, 10 gm/day orally for 18 months. Isoniazid levels may be determined in the plasma.

B. General Measures: Immobilization and rest in plaster may be desirable. Joints should be maintained in the position of function.

C. Surgical Measures: If destruction of articular surfaces is prominent, arthrodesis may be required even though the joint may be sterilized by appropriate chemotherapeutic procedures. Joint function may be lost as a result of bone destruction and sequestrum formation. Spinal fusion may be necessary to preserve stability of the vertebral column.

Prognosis

Arthritis without joint destruction in primary tuberculosis responds excellently to rest and antituberculous drugs. As noted above, with overt osteitis and cartilage involvement, loss of joint function may occur depending on the severity of the involvement and in spite of chemotherapy.

Kelly PJ, Karlson AG: Musculoskeletal tuberculosis. Proc Mayo Clin 44:73, 1969.

TRANSIENT SYNOVITIS OF THE HIP

This is the commonest cause of painful hip in children in the USA. It is a self-limiting disease of unknown cause, lasting days (usually) to weeks. It affects children between the ages of 3 and 10 years (boys more often than girls). The disease is characterized by a sudden onset of unilateral mild or severe pain in the hip or knee, especially with movement or weight bearing. There is tenderness over the hip joint anteriorly, occasionally palpable swelling, and limp. The hip is usually held in flexion, adduction, and internal rotation, with limitation of motion in extension. X-rays are usually normal.

Treatment is symptomatic. Traction may be necessary in severe cases. Corticotropin and the corticosteroids have been recommended but are seldom indicated since the disease tends to be self-limited. In some patients, Legg-Perthes disease has developed several months after convalescence.

Gladhill HB: Transient gynovitis and Legg-Calvé-Perthes disease. Canad MAJ 100:311, 1969.

Hardinge K: The etiology of transient synovitis of the hip. J Bone Joint Surg 52B:100, 1970.

VASCULAR LESIONS, AVASCULAR NECROSIS, ASEPTIC NECROSIS

EPIPHYSEAL CENTERS

The vascular supply of bone is precarious. When it is interrupted, necrosis of bone results. Unlike other tissues of the body which undergo infarction, bone removes the necrotic tissue and replaces it with living bone in the process known as "creeping substitution." This replacement of necrotic bone may be so complete and so perfect that a completely normal bone results. The adequacy of replacement depends upon a number of physiologic, pathologic, and mechanical factors.

Because of their isolated position, the secondary ossification centers of the epiphyses frequently have their blood supply interrupted. These avascular necrosing lesions of epiphyses were distinguished from tuberculosis and other infections early in the 20th century, and became known by the names of the physicians who originally described the process. The pathologic processes are identical, ie, necrosis of bone followed by replacement by living bone. During replacement, a typical microscopic and radiographic appearance results.

Despite the well known pathologic and radiographic features, the etiology of idiopathic avascular necrosing lesions of the epiphyses is not known. Necrosis of bone may follow such known causes as trauma or infection, but idiopathic lesions usually develop during periods of rapid growth of the epiphysis and its ossification center. Thus, the age incidence of Legg-Perthes disease is from 3–6 years, and Osgood-Schlatter disease of the tibial tuberosity usually begins by the age of 10 or 11.

Clinical Findings

A. Symptoms and Signs: Persistent pain is the most common symptom. Joint dysfunction may be present, with limp and limitation of motion.

B. Laboratory Findings: All laboratory findings, including studies of joint aspirates, are normal.

C. X-Ray Findings: X-ray findings vary depending upon the duration of the replacement process and the extent of the necrosis. Joint effusion is the only early finding. Three to 6 weeks after onset, the surrounding viable tissues will show atrophy due to disability and disuse. The necrotic ossification center will appear more dense than its surrounding viable structures, but this is a relative rather than a true increase in density. In Legg-Perthes disease, the ossification center for the head of the femur will appear to be more dense than the bone of the metaphysis or of the acetabulum.

Subsequent x-rays will demonstrate replacement of the necrotic ossification center. Replacement may take 6–12 months. The necrotic bone is replaced in patchwork fashion, producing apparent "fragmentation" of the ossification center. The living bone is less dense than the preexisting necrotic bone.

The cartilage space may be enlarged, probably due to continued cartilaginous growth without subsequent enchondral ossification and enlargement of the ossification center. The epiphyseal cartilage may be altered. In Legg-Perthes disease, for example, the mediolateral width of the epiphyseal cartilage may be increased. There may also be a large radiolucent lesion in the metaphysis due to infarction of bone there. Widening of the epiphyseal cartilage results in the shortened, thickened, flattened femoral neck (coxa plana) so commonly seen in this process. Varus deformity of the femoral neck also usually results.

Finally, x-rays will demonstrate complete replacement of the necrotic bone of the ossification center with regeneration of a new ossification center. The degree of deformity of the ossification center ranges from minimal to spectacular.

Differential Diagnosis

Differential diagnosis must include inflammatory and infectious lesions of the joints or apophyses. Transient synovitis of the hip joint may be distinguished from Legg-Perthes disease by serial x-rays. Other known causes of necrosing lesions such as trauma and infection must also be excluded.

Treatment

Treatment of these avascular necrosing lesions consists simply of protection. If the lesion is intra-articular and in a weight-bearing joint, the child must not be permitted to bear weight on the extremity. Crutches and various braces are utilized for this purpose. Plaster immobilization may also be utilized, particularly in the uncooperative patient.

If deformity of a weight-bearing epiphysis results, operative treatment may be indicated. Arthroplasty of the femoral head or iliac osteotomy may improve the relationships of the femoral head and the acetabulum.

Prognosis

The prognosis for replacement is excellent. The functional result depends upon the perfection of the replacement or resulting deformity. Some of these secondary ossification centers may be within a joint, and imperfect replacement results in derangement of joint function. Other secondary ossification centers such as those of the tibial tuberosity and the calcaneal tuberosity are outside the joint, and imperfect replacement of the necrotic bone with deformity does not produce disability.

In Legg-Perthes disease, the prognosis depends to some extent upon avoidance of physical damage to the atrophic ossification center of the epiphysis and to damage of the epiphyseal cartilage. In general, patients with metaphyseal defects and those who develop the lesions late in childhood or adolescence have a worse prognosis.

Pappas AM: The osteochondroses. P Clin North America 14:549, 1967.

OSTEOCHONDRITIS DISSECANS

This lesion is a pie-shaped necrosis of bone and cartilage adjacent to the articular surface. The necrotic fragment of bone may be broken off from the host bone and displaced into the joint cavity as a loose body. If it remains attached, the necrotic fragment may be completely replaced by creeping substitution.

The pathologic process is precisely the same as that noted above for avascular necrosing lesions of ossification centers. However, since these lesions are adjacent to articular cortex, the joint damage may be extensive. Deformity of the ossification center usually does not result, and epiphyseal growth disturbance is not apparent.

The most common site of these lesions is the knee joint (lateral aspect of the medial femoral condyle), the elbow joint (the capitellum), and the superior dome of the talus.

Joint pain is the common complaint. However, joint dysfunction may be present—"locking" of the knee, or limp—if the fragment is free within the joint.

TABLE 19–1. The osteochondroses.

Ossification Center	Eponym	Typical Age
Capital femoral	Legg-Calvé-Perthes disease	3–5
Tibial tuberosity	Osgood-Schlatter disease	14
Tarsal navicular	Kohler's disease	6
Metatarsal head, 2	Freiberg's disease	12–14
Vertebral ring	Scheuerman's disease	13–16
Capitellum	Panner's disease	

Laboratory findings, including studies of the joint aspirates, are completely normal. These studies distinguish osteochondritis dissecans from necrosing lesions which develop secondary to infection or tuberculosis.

Treatment consists of protection of the involved area from mechanical damage. This is particularly necessary in weight-bearing joints. If the fragment is free within the joint as a loose body, it must be removed surgically. If adequate replacement does not proceed promptly, surgery is often indicated to speed up replacement.

If large areas of a weight-bearing surface of a joint are involved, secondary degenerative arthritis may result and arthroplasty procedures may be necessary at a later date.

Hatcher CH: *The Fate of Aseptic Necrosis of Bone in Skeletal Diseases and Injuries. The Musculoskeletal System.* Macmillan, 1952.

NEUROLOGIC DISORDERS INVOLVING THE MUSCULOSKELETAL SYSTEM

ORTHOPEDIC ASPECTS OF POLIOMYELITIS

Muscle Recovery

In paralytic poliomyelitis it is impossible to determine how much true anterior horn cell destruction has been sustained, but the pattern of muscle function permits the following generalizations about recovery of muscle function:

(1) "Spotty" paralysis in a number of extremities has a good prognosis.

(2) A completely flail extremity will probably never show a significant functional recovery.

(3) Early muscle recovery is a good prognostic sign, with probable full functional recovery to be expected.

(4) Muscle recovery cannot be expected after 18 months.

(5) Muscle recovery must be steady and continuous. If a "plateau" is reached and maintained for 3 months, no further recovery of that muscle may be anticipated.

(6) Muscle "substitution" may produce functional improvement long after the initial 18 months following the acute infection. Muscle substitution may be functionally beneficial or may be productive of deformity.

Reconstructive Procedures

Reconstructive orthopedic procedures may be directed to the fascia, the muscles, the tendons, the joints, the bones, and extremity length. They are far too numerous to be discussed here. They are the standard reconstructive procedures of tendon transfer, fasciectomy, arthrodesis, and epiphyseodesis.

ORTHOPEDIC ASPECTS OF CEREBRAL PALSY

Physical therapy offers the best hope of improvement for many of these patients. Realistic goals must be established for each patient; if progressive improvement is not apparent, physical therapy should be discontinued.

Bracing and splinting are often of vital importance to prevent or correct deformity. Rigid bracing is more likely to be successful than dynamic or functional bracing. Night splints are often needed.

Reconstructive orthopedic procedures may include tenotomies, muscle and tendon transfers, joint arthrodeses, and denervations. Limb length inequalities are usually not present.

Flexion and adduction deformities of the hip frequently lead to dysplasia of the hip with subluxation or complete dislocation. Prevention of dislocation is extremely important since the treatment is so difficult and unsatisfactory. The principal preventive measure is to maintain the lower extremities in abduction with braces or splints. Night splints alone may suffice.

Athetoid spastics are not good candidates for any reconstructive surgical procedure nor for bracing. Neurosurgical procedures offer the only hope for these individuals.

Orthopedic procedures in patients with cerebral palsy offer less chance of functional improvement than do orthopedic procedures in patients with residuals of poliomyelitis. Spastic paralyses may change with surgical treatment, and deforming muscle actions may be significantly altered by unwise orthopedic operations.

Beals RK: Spastic paraplegia and diplegia: An evaluation of nonsurgical and surgical factors influencing the prognosis for ambulation. J Bone Joint Surg 48A:827, 1966.

Eggers EWN, Evans EB: Surgery in cerebral palsy. J Bone Joint Surg 45A:1275, 1963.

Phelps WM: The cerebral palsies. Clin Orthop 44:83, 1966.

Siffert RS: Children's orthopaedic surgery in the United States: Historical trends. Clin Orthop 44:89, 1966.

Stamp WG: Bracing in cerebral palsy. J Bone Joint Surg 44A:1457, 1962.

ORTHOPEDIC ASPECTS OF MYELODYSPLASIA

Orthopedic reconstructive procedures in patients with myelodysplasia are quite similar to those in patients with traumatic paraplegia or residuals of poliomyelitis. Myelomeningocele should be repaired early, ie, in the first week of life.

Neurotrophic skin problems may require drastic plastic surgical procedures or orthopedic procedures. Prevention of skin problems is far simpler than the correction of severe skin defects. Severe infections may necessitate amputation.

Bracing may be necessary to prevent deformities.

Physical therapy measures are quite similar to those employed in patients with traumatic paraplegia. Realistic functional goals should be established, and physical therapy should not be continued indefinitely if the patient does not improve.

Kilfozel RM: Myelodysplasia. P Clin North America 14:419, 1967.

MISCELLANEOUS DISEASES OF BONE

FIBROUS DYSPLASIA
(Monostotic & Polyostotic Fibrous Dysplasia, Regional Fibrocystic Diseases, Albright's Syndrome)

Dysplastic fibrous tissue replacement of the medullary canal contents of bone is accompanied by the formation of metaplastic bone. Three forms of the disease are recognized: monostotic, polyostotic (most commonly, many long bones of a single extremity), and polyostotic with endocrine disturbance (precocious puberty in females, hyperthyroidism, and hyperadrenalism, ie, Albright's syndrome).

Clinical Findings
A. Symptoms and Signs: The lesion or lesions may be asymptomatic. Café au lait spots may be present on the skin. Pain, if present, is probably due to pathologic fracture. In females, endocrine disturbances may be present in the polyostotic variety.

B. Laboratory Findings: Laboratory findings are normal unless endocrine disturbances are present, in which case the laboratory findings of these disorders (precocious puberty, hyperthyroidism, and hyperadrenalism) will be found.

C. X-Ray Findings: The lesion begins centrally within the medullary canal, usually of a long bone, and expands slowly. Pathologic fracture may occur. If metaplastic bone predominates, the contents of the lesion will be of the density of bone itself. Marked deformity of the bone may result, and limb lengths may be unequal as a result of stimulation of epiphyseal cartilage growth.

Differential Diagnosis
The differential diagnosis must include the fibrous tissue lesions and destructive lesions of bone such as bone cyst, eosinophilic granuloma, aneurysmal bone cyst, nonossifying fibroma, enchondroma, and chondromyxoid fibroma.

Treatment
No treatment is needed if the lesion is asymptomatic. If pathologic fracture occurs, curettage of the lesion may be desirable. Bone grafting may be necessary to fill large defects.

Prognosis
The prognosis is excellent unless the lesions impair epiphyseal cartilage growth and thus cause deformity. The lesions tend to enlarge during childhood and adolescence but not during adult life.

Malignant transformation of the lesion has never been reported.

UNICAMERAL BONE CYST

This lesion appears in the metaphyses of long bones, principally the femurs and humeri. It begins within the medullary canal immediately adjacent to the epiphyseal cartilage. It probably results from some alteration of enchondral ossification. The cyst is "active" as long as it abuts onto the metaphyseal side of the epiphyseal cartilage and "inactive" when a border of normal bone exists between the cyst and the epiphyseal cartilage.

The lesion may be completely asymptomatic. Pain, if present, usually means pathologic fracture. Laboratory findings are normal. On x-ray the cyst begins centrally within the medullary canal. It expands the cortex but is almost never wider than the epiphyseal cartilage. Pathologic fracture may occur.

Treatment consists of curettage of the cyst if it causes pain or has produced pathologic fracture. The lesion is filled with fluid. Curettage should be delayed until the cyst is in an "inactive" phase even if there is pathologic fracture.

The prognosis is excellent. Many cysts will heal following pathologic fracture.

ANEURYSMAL BONE CYST

This lesion is similar to unicameral bone cyst. It usually begins in the long bones in slightly eccentric position, expanding the cortex of the bone, and may produce an extraosseous mass. On x-ray the lesion may appear to be larger than the width of the epiphyseal cartilage, which distinguishes it from unicameral bone cyst.

Aneurysmal bone cyst is filled with large vascular lakes, and the stoma contains fibrous tissue and metaplastic ossification.

Great care must be taken not to overdiagnose this lesion as osteosarcoma or hemangioma. Treatment consists of curettage and bone grafting if necessary. The prognosis is excellent.

INFANTILE CORTICAL HYPEROSTOSIS
(Caffey-Smyth-Roske Syndrome)

This sometimes familial, usually benign disease of unknown cause has its onset before 6 months of age and is characterized by irritability, fever, and non-suppurating, tender, painful swellings. Swellings may involve almost any bone of the body. They are always present in the mandible, in the clavicle in 50% of cases, and in the ulna, humerus, and ribs. The disease is limited to the shafts, does not involve the subcutaneous tissues and joints, and persists for weeks or months. Anemia, leukocytosis, increased sedimentation rate, and elevated serum alkaline phosphatase are usually present. Cortical hyperostosis is demonstrable on x-ray and may be evident on physical examination.

Corticosteroids are effective and should be used, particularly in severe cases.

The prognosis is good, and the disease usually terminates without deformity.

GANGLION

A ganglion is a small, smooth, cystic structure connected by a pedicle to the joint capsule, usually on the dorsum of the wrist. It can be treated by excision if it interferes with function.

BAXTER'S CYST

This is a herniation of the synovium of the knee joint into the popliteal region. It may require excision.

NEOPLASIA OF THE MUSCULO-SKELETAL SYSTEM

Neoplastic diseases of the mesodermal tissues constitute a very serious problem because of the bad prognosis of these malignancies. Few of the benign lesions undergo malignant transformation, and it is important to establish a proper diagnosis and thus avoid undertreatment or overtreatment. The diagnosis

TABLE 19–2. Differentiating features of carcinoma and sarcoma.

	Carcinoma	Sarcoma
Tissue origin	Epithelial	Mesodermal
Age incidence	Middle age	Youth
Metastases	Regional nodes	Lungs
Radiation sensitivity	Sensitive. Some cures.	Resistant
Susceptibility to chemotherapeutic agents	Some specific drug sensitivities	Almost all resistant
Prognosis	Variable	Poor

TABLE 19–3. Benign neoplasms: Osseous.

Disease	Clinical Features	X-Ray Features	Treatment	Prognosis
Osteocartilaginous exostosis (osteochondroma)	Pain-free mass. (Pain, if present, is due to superimposed bursitis.) Single or multiple. Bone mass capped with cartilage. Masses enlarge during childhood and adolescence.	Metaphyseal position. Pedunculated or sessile. Cortex of host bone "turned out" into the lesion. Cartilage cap may be calcified. Long bones predominate.	Surgical excision if symptomatic, if lesion interferes with function, or enlarging mass in adult life.	Excellent. 5–10% of patients may have malignant transformation.
Osteoid osteoma	Pain with point tenderness. Night pain common. Pain often relieved by aspirin.	Radiolucent central nidus (about 1 cm in diameter) surrounded by spectacular osteosclerosis. Sclerosis may obscure nidus.	Surgical excision of nidus.	Excellent. No known malignant transformation.
Osteoblastoma (giant osteoid osteoma)	Pain similar to that of osteoid osteoma.	Nidus larger than 1 cm. Osteolytic phase may predominate.	Surgical excision.	Excellent.

TABLE 19–4. Benign neoplasms: Cartilaginous

Disease	Clinical Features	X-Ray Features	Treatment	Prognosis
Chondroma	Usually silent lesions. Pain may be present. Pathologic fracture may occur.	Radiolucent lesions. Long bones predominate. Most common lesion of phalanges and metacarpals or metatarsals. Calcification may be present centrally. Little or no host reaction.	Surgical excision or curettage.	Excellent. Malignant transformation of chondromas of major bones occurs rarely.
Chondroblastoma (Codman's tumor)	Pain about a joint. Pathologic fracture may occur.	Radiolucent lesion of ossification center of child or adolescent. Occasionally perforates epiphyseal cartilage. Rarely calcification. Little or no reactive bone formation.	Surgical excision or curettage.	Excellent. No known malignant transformation.
Chondromyxofibroma	Usually silent lesion. Mass may be the presenting feature. Pathologic fracture may occur.	Long bones predominate (tibia, fibula, femur, humerus). Radiolucent lesion, may enlarge the host bone. Usually metaphyseal, linearly oriented. Usually well encapsulated.	Surgical excision or curettage.	Excellent.

TABLE 19–5. Benign neoplasms: Fibrous

Disease	Clinical Features	X-Ray Features	Treatment	Prognosis
Nonossifying fibroma (benign cortical defect; benign metaphyseal defect)	Usually silent lesion. Rarely, pathologic fracture.	Radiolucent lesion. Metaphyseal location, linearly oriented. Eccentric position. Thin sclerotic border about lesion. May be multiple lesions.	No treatment needed.	Excellent.
Giant cell tumor	Extremely rare in children.	Radiolucent lesions.	Surgical excision or curettage.	Good. Malignant transformation rare. May undergo change to fibrosarcoma.

depends upon correlation of the clinical, x-ray, and, in many instances, microscopic features.

In general, neoplasms of mesodermal tissues are named according to the tissue produced. However, because of the multiple potentiality of mesodermal cells, several types of tissues may be present within the same tumor. This has resulted in confusion of nomenclature, with some tumors being given a combination of names. It has also resulted in a number of misdiagnoses, since a specimen from a single area may not represent tissue typical of the entire tumor. In addition, some of the tumors are so primitive that they rarely produce any recognizable adult type of tissue.

Biopsy is often necessary. Fears of complications from biopsy are far outweighed by the advantages of correct diagnosis.

Dahlin DC: *Bone Tumors,* 2nd ed. Thomas, 1967.
Ferguson AB Jr: Benign tumors of bone in childhood. P Clin North America 14:683, 1967.
Jaffe HL: *Tumor and Tumorous Conditions of the Bones and Joints.* Lea & Febiger, 1958.
Lichtenstein L: *Bone Tumors.* Mosby, 1952.

TABLE 19–6. Malignant neoplasms.

Disease	Clinical Features	X-Ray Features	Treatment	Prognosis
Osteosarcoma and chondrosarcoma	Pain the most common symptom. Mass, functional loss, limp occasionally present. Pathologic fracture common.	Destructive, expanding, invasive lesion. Minimal host reaction, but, if present, usually is a triangle between tumor, elevated periosteum, and cortex. Usually radiolucent, but lesional tissue may show ossification or calcification. Metaphyseal location common. Femur, tibia, humerus, and other long bones predominate.	Surgical excision or amputation. Radiation resistant. Resistant to presently known chemotherapeutic agents.	Poor. Probably less than 5 or 10% cured. Metastases to lungs, occasionally to other bones.
Fibrosarcoma	Rare lesions in children.	Radiolucent, destructive, expanding, invasive lesion. Little or no host reaction. Long bones predominate.	Surgical excision or amputation.	Poor. Probably 10–15% cured. Metastases to lungs.
Ewing's tumor	Pain very common. Tenderness, fever, and leukocytosis also common. Frequent pathologic fracture. Frequently multicentric.	Radiolucent, destructive lesion, frequently in diaphyseal region of the bone. May be reactive bone formation about the lesion in successive layers—"onion skin" layering.	Radiation sensitive but not curable. Surgical excision usually not desirable because of multiple areas of involvement. Chemotherapy not effective.	Very poor. Metastases to multiple organs.

● ● ●

General References

Banks HH: Symposium on musculoskeletal disorders. P Clin North America 14:299–515, 533–704, 1967.

Bergsma D (editor): *The First Conference on the Clinical Delineation of Birth Defects.* Parts 2, 3, & 4. The National Foundation-March of Dimes, 1969.

Caffey J: *Pediatric X-Ray Diagnosis,* 5th ed. Year Book, 1967.

Fairbank T: *An Area of Generalized Affections of the Skeleton.* Williams & Wilkins, 1951.

Ferguson AB Jr: *Orthopedic Surgery in Infancy and Childhood,* 3rd ed. Williams & Wilkins, 1968.

Salter RB: *Textbook of Disorders and Injuries of the Musculoskeletal System.* Williams and Wilkins, 1970.

20...

Connective Tissue Diseases

Donough O'Brien, MD, FRCP

JUVENILE RHEUMATOID ARTHRITIS
(Still's Disease)

Essentials of Diagnosis

- Nonmigratory monarticular or polyarticular arthropathy, with a tendency to involve large joints or proximal interphalangeal joints.
- Systemic manifestations, with fever, erythematous rashes, nodules, and leucocytosis, and occasionally iridocyclitis, pleuritis, and pericarditis.

General Considerations

Still's disease is a relatively common disorder in the pediatric age group. It may occur at any age after infancy, and is more common in girls. Evidence for a familial tendency is scant and equivocal. Trauma and psychologic stresses are apparently only precipitating factors. Increased collagenase in joint fluid and the presence of antibodies to articular connective tissue may play a role. Recently there has been a return to a belief in the role of infection. Diphtheroids and, more particularly, mycoplasma organisms have been reportedly grown from synovial fluid. Fibroblasts from affected synovial membranes are resistant to infection by rubella, suggesting that they are already colonized.

The idea that an intracellular virus may provoke an altered immune response in certain tissues and thereby permeability changes in the same and other tissues is attractive but still largely unconfirmed.

Clinical Findings

A. Symptoms and Signs: Fever tends to be remittent and irregular rather than sustained. It may occur weeks or months before the onset of joint involvement. Fleeting macular or maculopapular erythematous rashes are common. Joint distribution varies with age at onset. In very small children there may be an acute febrile onset with little joint involvement but widespread systemic changes, including myocarditis, pneumonitis, hepatomegaly, splenomegaly, and lymphadenopathy. In small children also the onset tends to be severe and is more likely to involve many joints, particularly the ankles, the knees, the proximal interphalangeal joints, the wrists, the temporomandibular joints, and the cervical spine. Older children more often have involvement of 1–2 large joints

without systemic manifestations. The proximal interphalangeal joints and wrists are often affected together. The clinical course in older children is much less tempestuous, and the disease tends to abate in the early teen years. Involved joints are not always painful, and rapid loss of movement may take place.

Spondylitis occurs occasionally. Iridocyclitis is commonest in this group.

B. Laboratory Findings: There is no specific diagnostic test for rheumatoid arthritis. The ESR is usually elevated, and the white count may be high or low. Alpha$_2$ globulin and gamma globulins are elevated in 15% of cases. Tests for rheumatoid factor and antinuclear factor are often not positive in children, and if positive are not diagnostic.

C. X-Ray Findings: These are variable. At first there is periarticular soft tissue swelling which later gives rise to atrophy in long-standing cases. With articular destruction, the joint spaces become narrowed. Diminished use then leads to regional osteoporosis. Premature epiphyseal fusion may occur.

Complications

Complications include the occasional severe limitation in daily living from advanced articular involvement and contractures. Chronic iridocyclitis occurs in up to 10% of cases and can progress to blindness from cataracts and keratitis. Renal amyloidosis occurs occasionally in children who have had severe disease from an early age. Cardiac failure from myocarditis occurs but is uncommon.

Differential Diagnosis

Rheumatic fever is now less common than rheumatoid arthritis, and particularly rare in young children. Joint involvement seldom includes the fingers, is migratory, and is usually accompanied by more striking erythema and swelling. Cardiac involvement is more often present in rheumatic fever than in rheumatoid arthritis.

Infectious joint conditions are associated with much more severe joint tenderness and are subject to diagnosis by examination of aspirated joint fluid. Tuberculous arthritis is now rare in the USA. Only one joint is usually involved.

Juvenile rheumatoid arthritis may be mimicked by regional enteritis, chronic active hepatitis, ulcerative colitis, psoriasis, and agammaglobulinemia. Differentiation from systemic lupus erythematosus is at times impossible. Especially in younger children, leukemia and neurofibromatosis may present with symptoms and signs resembling those of rheumatoid arthritis.

Treatment

In most cases, where involvement is predominantly articular, the objective of therapy is to maintain the strength and range of movement of affected joints. This can often be achieved with salicylates. The correct dose is one which alleviates pain, short of toxicity, and does not need to be monitored by blood levels. Home exercises consist of active use of affected joints and passive motion through the maximal range several times a day. Indomethacin is sometimes helpful, but the side-effects (dizziness, rashes, leukopenia) may be severe. Phenylbutazone and gold salts have no place in the treatment of juvenile rheumatoid arthritis.

Corticosteroids may be employed for their analgesic effect during acute flare-ups to permit earlier joint movement. In long-standing cases, small doses may lead to striking improvements. The drug should be given daily and not on alternate days, and should be administered in minimal doses for short periods. Symptoms may increase when the dose is lowered, but will often subside again in a day or two. Corticosteroids on a long-term basis are also given if there is significant pulmonary or cardiac involvement or iridocyclitis. There is increasing evidence that corticosteroids and azathioprine (Imuran), 3 mg/kg/day, or cyclophosphamide (Cytoxan), 2 mg/kg/day, may be helpful in difficult cases. Penicillamine has been helpful in some adult cases. Topical mydriatics should be used for iridocyclitis.

Prognosis

Fatalities sometimes occur in children who are affected at a young age with polyarthritis and systemic involvement, particularly from amyloidosis or carditis. Otherwise, the long-term prognosis depends principally on the degree of irreversible joint involvement. The disease usually remits during the early teen years, although cases presenting in the teen years may presage adult disease.

Calabro JJ: Management of juvenile rheumatoid arthritis. J Pediat 77:355, 1970.
Cytotoxic drugs in rheumatoid arthritis. Lancet 2:1270, 1970.
Denman AM: Rheumatoid arthritis: aetiology. Brit MJ 2:601, 1970.
Ross J & others: Juvenile rheumatoid arthritis persisting into adulthood. Am J Med 45:419, 1968.
Rothfield NF: Diagnosis of lupus erythematosus and rheumatoid arthritis in children. P Clin North America 18:39, 1971.

DISSEMINATED LUPUS ERYTHEMATOSUS

Essentials of Diagnosis

- Fever, joint pains, weakness, weight loss, pallor, emotional problems.
- Malar erythema on face; other skin rashes.
- Tendency to protean involvement, including CNS, kidneys, muscles, lungs, and heart.
- LE cells in blood, hypergammaglobulinemia, especially IgM. Positive fluorescence on skin biopsy, low $C'4$ complement fraction, positive serum antinuclear factors.
- Anemia, leukopenia, thrombocytopenia.

General Considerations

Systemic lupus erythematosus is a disease of connective tissue with vascular and perivascular fibrinoid changes that may involve any organ or system. Onset is most commonly between 9 and 15 years of age. Girls are affected 8 times more commonly than boys. The commonest and most serious complicating lesion is glomerulonephritis. The cause is not known, but the presence in serum of a variety of antinuclear, anti-DNA, and anticytoplasmic antibodies, high levels of Igm, low levels of serum $C'1$, $C'2$, and $C'4$ complement, and, in tissues, of antigen/antibody complexes to native DNA suggests that this is another disease in which the molecular structure of certain tissue proteins has been distorted by superimposed host-generated immune complexes. The possible role of mycoplasma-like structures seen in renal endothelial and lymphoid cells is of great interest but not yet fully understood. Drug sensitivity may also be important, and lupus-like syndromes are evoked by hydralazine, thiazides, procainamide, ethosuximide, heavy metals, sulfonamides, etc.

Clinical Findings

A. Symptoms and Signs: Occasionally in childhood the onset of the disease is fulminating, with fever, loss of weight, hepatosplenomegaly, generalized lymphadenopathy, and malar erythema, together with a variety of indications of system involvement such as renal disease with proteinuria, cardiomegaly, and CNS signs. More often, however, the onset is insidious, with up to 3 years elapsing between the first appearance of symptoms and establishment of a diagnosis. Clinical manifestations are as follows:

1. Joint symptoms are the commonest presenting feature. The larger joints are usually affected. There is pain and swelling and, less often, redness. The joint lesions may come and go irrespective of treatment. Myalgia and myositis are common.

2. Systemic reactions include weakness, anorexia, fever, malaise, and loss of weight.

3. The skin lesions of lupus are less striking in children than in adults. Symmetrical bilateral malar erythema is common but is not always present at the onset. Patchy erythemas occur, and purpura may be present.

4. Lupus glomerulitis may be present in varying degrees of severity. Hematuria and proteinuria occur early. Nephrotic syndrome may be the presenting form of the disease. Chronic renal failure occurs ultimately. Renal involvement, however mild, implies a more serious prognosis.

5. Splenomegaly or hepatomegaly is demonstrable at the time of diagnosis in about 70% of cases. Disseminated intravascular clotting may be a complication.

6. Inguinal, cervical, and axillary lymphadenopathy.

7. Myocarditis with striking cardiomegaly may occur and may initially suggest rheumatic fever. Pericarditis and dysrhythmias are seen. Thrombophlebitis is uncommon, but arteriolitis may affect almost any part of the body.

8. "Lupoid hepatitis"—See Chapter 17.

9. The CNS may be involved, presumably as a result of vasculitis, in a variety of ways manifested as behavioral disturbances, nerve tract lesions, peripheral neuritides, convulsions, and coma.

10. A syndrome very similar to lupus but with skin ulceration, negative LE preparations, and anti-DNA levels has been described. Serum complement levels are < 5% of normal.

B. Laboratory Findings: Leukopenia occurs in 50% of cases and thrombocytopenia in 25%. The sedimentation rate is usually high, and serum gamma globulin levels are frequently in excess of 3 gm/100 ml. In particular, the IgM fraction is elevated and the $C'1$, $C'2$, and $C'4$ fractions of serum complement depressed. Normocytic normochromic anemia is common. Hemolytic anemia may be present with or without a positive Coombs test. Protein, red cells, and white cells in the urine may indicate renal involvement; as this becomes more advanced, both glomerular filtration rate and effective renal plasma flow become diminished, ultimately with nitrogen retention.

The presence in serum of complement-fixing antibodies to DNA or to heat-denatured DNA provides the single most useful diagnostic laboratory test. Simultaneous low serum complement levels suggest an active phase. In particular, complement levels in the presence of complement-fixing antibodies appear to parallel the activity and severity of renal involvement.

A positive LE preparation is found at some time in the course of the disease in over 90% of cases. The LE cell phenomenon reflects the presence of one or more circulating anti-DNA antibodies and consists of a purplish globular inclusion in polymorphonuclear cells exposed to Wright's stain.

An equally reliable diagnostic test is the finding of fluorescent inclusions at the dermal-epidermal border in a skin biopsy using eosin-tagged anti-human complement globulin.

Differential Diagnosis

Disseminated lupus erythematosus is part of a spectrum of autoimmune diseases, and it is sometimes hard to distinguish it from rheumatoid arthritis and related conditions such as polyarteritis and polymyositis. Extensive cardiac involvement may suggest rheumatic fever, and renal involvement may suggest chronic glomerulonephritis or idiopathic nephrosis.

Treatment

A combined regimen of prednisone (or equivalent corticosteroid) and azathioprine (Imuran) should be started as soon as the diagnosis is confirmed. Occasional very mild cases will respond to a 3–6 month course of prednisone given alone in a dose of 1.5–2 mg/kg/day, but sustained remissions are less often achieved in more severe cases. A combination of azathioprine, 3 mg/kg every day, and prednisone, 1–1.5 mg/kg on alternate days, is the treatment of choice. Treatment should be continued for at least 2 years, or even longer if there is any clinical or laboratory evidence of disease beyond that time. Cyclophosphamide (Cytoxan), 2 mg/kg/day, may also be helpful in conjunction with steroids.

Complications of this regimen are uncommon, although all patients receiving azathioprine should have weekly total white counts. Sequential renal clearances may document renal improvement and so justify continued azathioprine therapy in spite of moderate leukopenia. The drug should be discontinued or reduced if the total white count falls below 3000/cu mm or the lymphocytes below 1000/cu mm. Very occasionally, patients will deteriorate rapidly with the institution of azathioprine therapy.

Heparin, 1 mg/kg every 12 hours, is indicated in the occasional case where the disease is complicated by evidence of intravascular clotting associated with thrombocytopenia, low serum proaccelerin (factor V) and AHG (factor VIII), and increased serum fibrin split products. The symptomatic treatment of renal disease is described in Chapter 18.

Dietary and other supportive measures, including analgesics for joint and muscle pain, should be employed, and transfusions ordered as indicated.

Course & Prognosis

Disseminated lupus erythematosus is rarely fulminant in children; characteristically, it progresses over a number of years with episodes of remission. The presence of renal disease is the single most important factor in prognosis. With adequate corticosteroid treatment, about 50% of cases with renal disease will survive 5–6 years; without renal disease, the mean expectation is 11 years. The impact of azathioprine on survival is not yet known.

Cameron JS & others: Treatment of lupus nephritis with cyclophosphamide. Lancet 2:846, 1970.

Meislin AG, Rothfield N: Systemic lupus erythematosus in childhood. Pediatrics 42:37, 1968.

Schur P, Sandson J: Immunologic factors and clinical activity in systemic lupus erythematosus. New England J Med 278:533, 1968.

DERMATOMYOSITIS
(Polymyositis)

Essentials of Diagnosis

- Weak, stiff, tender, and painful muscles, mostly in the limb girdles and extremities, sometimes involving respiratory and swallowing musculature.
- Erythematous, violaceous, and atrophic skin changes, especially on the upper eyelids and knuckles.
- Fever, weakness, irritability, and easy fatigability.
- Edema and lymphadenopathy.
- Prominence of small venules, especially on the eyelids and nail beds.
- Occasional calcium deposits subcutaneously and in muscles.

General Considerations

Dermatomyositis in childhood is primarily a disease of small blood vessels affecting the muscles, skin, connective tissue, fat, peripheral nerves, gastrointestinal tract, and kidneys. The onset is usually between 3 and 8 years of age. There is perivascular cuffing with polymorphonuclear neutrophils, histiocytes, lymphocytes, and plasma cells together with intimal hyperplasia that may lead to vascular occlusion. The final stages of the disease are characterized by widespread evidence of disseminated intravascular clotting. Unlike polymyositis in the adult, vascular changes are common in muscle. There is also endomysial and perimysial inflammation with degeneration, vacuolization, and atrophy of muscle spindles. The condition is rare and begins in childhood. It is more common in boys than in girls. The cause is not known. Various infective and toxic causes have been suggested, but the favorable response to corticosteroids and the clinical and pathologic features which this disease shares with systemic lupus erythematosus suggest that dermatomyositis is one of the "autoimmune" group of diseases.

Clinical Findings

A. Symptoms and Signs: The skin manifestations appear first, with erythema and sometimes edema of the upper eyelids spreading to the periorbital, nasal, malar, and upper lip areas. The extremities are also involved; particularly over the knuckles, knees, and elbows, the erythema may become scaly, atrophic, and violaceous. Especially in the eyelids and nail bases, there is often a prominence of small blood vessels.

Muscular weakness, tenderness, stiffness, and pain usually follow the skin changes. The shoulder muscles are most severely affected, but the muscles of the pelvic girdle are involved also. In general, the proximal limb muscles are more affected than the distal. Flexion contractions occur later. In the later stages, the muscles of chewing, swallowing, respiration, and speech may be involved. Albuminuria, hematuria, and hypertension are sometimes seen. The vasculitis may also lead to permanent retinal damage. Calcium may be deposited in the muscles or subcutaneous tissues, leading to erosion and ulceration of the overlying skin.

Enteric ulcerations may give rise to abdominal pain, gastrointestinal bleeding, and even perforation.

Fever, weakness, irritability, and easy fatigability are common.

B. Laboratory Findings: There are no specific diagnostic laboratory tests. The sedimentation rate and serum IgG levels are elevated, and there is a varying degree of creatinuria reflecting the degree of muscle damage. Serum creatinine, phosphokinase, and LDH muscle enzymes may likewise be elevated. An electromyogram may help to distinguish myositis from wasting due to nerve injury.

Muscle biopsy of an affected area is characterized by perivascular infiltration with polymorphonuclear neutrophils and lymphocytes. These inflammatory changes later involve the media. There is intimal hyperplasia with luminal obstruction and evidence of disseminated intravascular clotting. Infarction of muscle, denervation atrophy, perimysial connective tissue proliferation, and fiber necrosis are seen.

Treatment

Prednisone (or equivalent), 1–1.5 mg/kg/day, should be administered at once and continued in diminishing doses as the disease is controlled and for at least 6 months after all clinical signs have abated. Azathioprine (Imuran), 1.5–2 mg/kg/day, has also been used and appears to be especially successful in the fulminating case. Physical therapy is required to prevent or allay contractures.

Course & Prognosis

Two-thirds of children with this disease recover over a period of 1–3 years. About ½ of survivors have significant resudual muscle weakness. Death is usually due to aspiration pneumonitis secondary to deglutition problems.

Banker BQ, Victor M: Dermatomyositis (systemic angiopathy) of childhood. Medicine 45:261–289, 1966.

Hill RH: Juvenile dermatomyositis. Canad MAJ 103:1152, 1970.

Thompson CE: Polymyositis in children. Clin Pediat 7:24, 1968.

POLYARTERITIS NODOSA

Polyarteritis nodosa is a rare disease which occurs at all ages. About 10% of cases are seen in children under age 15, and a significant proportion of these are infants. In childhood, the sex incidence of the disease is equal. The cause is not known.

The pathologic findings affect primarily the medium-sized arteries, beginning with medial degeneration and leading to an inflammatory response with polymorphonuclear leukocytes, lymphocytes, and plasma cells. Aneurysm and rupture may occur at this stage. There is also intimal proliferation, leading to thrombosis and distal infarction. Healing is accompanied by extensive fibrosis of the vessel wall and surrounding tissues.

Symptomatology involves all tissues, including the heart, lungs, joints, muscles, CNS, gastrointestinal tract, and skin. Cardiac failure, cardiomegaly, myocardial infarction, and pericarditis are seen. Hypertension, edema, proteinuria, hematuria, and ultimately renal failure can occur. Joint and muscle pains are less common, as is gastrointestinal bleeding, though perforations are reported. About 25% of cases show CNS involvement. Fever, skin rashes, and evidence of pulmonary or cardiac involvement are the commonest signs.

Treatment with prednisone, 1–1.5 mg/kg/day, is indicated. If this is unsuccessful, azathioprine (Imuran) should also be used in a dosage of 3 mg/kg/day. Insufficient published experience exists for prognostic accuracy.

Benyo RB, Perrin EV: Polyarteritis nodosa in infancy. Am J Dis Child 116:539, 1968.

Fager DB, Bigler JA, Simonds JP: Polyarteritis nodosa in infancy and childhood. J Pediat 39:65–79, 1951.

DIFFUSE SCLERODERMA

Scleroderma is a rare progressive connective tissue disease. The skin and subcutaneous tissues are principally involved, but multiple internal organs are also affected, including the lungs, heart, and kidneys. The disease is usually slowly progressive, leading ultimately to major respiratory or renal complications. Arrest or quiescence does occur.

This disease is not to be confused with scleredema or localized scleroderma (morphea), both of which are localized benign conditions.

There is no treatment. Corticosteroids and cytotoxic agents are not helpful. Physiotherapy is palliative.

Bradford WD & others: Scleredema of childhood. J Pediat 68:391–399, 1961.

Hanson V & others: Systemic rheumatic disorders in childhood. Bull Rheumat Dis 17:435–441, 1967.

Kass H, Hanson V, Patrick J: Scleroderma in childhood. J Pediat 68:243–256, 1966.

MARFAN'S SYNDROME

First discovered by Marfan in 1896, this syndrome is now considered to be a diffuse abnormality of elastic tissue inherited as an autosomal dominant. The molec-ular defect is unknown, although the high urinary excretion of hydroxyproline indicates an increased rate of turnover of connective tissue fiber. Clinically, the impact of these changes is on the skeletal and cardiovascular systems and the eyes. Patients are characteristically tall and thin, and the upper body segment is proportionately shorter than the lower. In addition to arachnodactyly of the fingers and great toes, bony defects include pectus carinatum and excavatum, a long narrow face and pointed head, high-arched palate, and kyphoscoliosis. The attendant laxity in the ligaments leads to pes planus, winging of the scapulas, genu recurvatum, and subluxation of the patellas, hips, elbows, and other joints. Femoral and diaphragmatic hernias are noted.

Weakening of the aortic media leads to aneurysms, usually of the ascending aorta, which may involve the valve. Lax chordae may lead to mitral as well as aortic incompetence. The pulmonary artery may be dilated. Dislocation of the lens due to weakness of the suspensory ligaments is characteristic but may be confused with homocystinuria. Blue scleras, myopia, retinal detachment, and megalocornea are other abnormalities of the eye, and glaucoma, iridocyclitis, and interstitial keratitis are complications of these disorders.

There is no specific treatment, although surgical correction of the cardiovascular complications may be appropriate. Prognosis is governed by the severity of these cardiovascular lesions.

Monz W: The Marfan's syndrome. Med J Australia 1:571, 1965.

Wong FL & others: Cardiac complications of Marfan's syndrome in a child. Am J Dis Child 107:404, 1966.

EHLERS-DANLOS SYNDROME

This is a rare heritable disorder of collagen which is probably transmitted as an autosomal dominant. Characteristically, the skin is pale, soft, and strikingly hyperextensible without being lax. Subcutaneous nodules develop over pressure points, and the skin in these areas is especially subject to trauma and the formation of shiny, parchment-like, atrophic scars. The joints are hyperextensible, and there is a tendency to dislocation of hips, patellas, elbows, clavicles, and shoulders. Blue scleras, wide epicanthal folds, and dislocation of the lens and other eye signs occur.

A number of other congenital defects have been described in association with this syndrome, notably hiatus hernia, gastrointestinal diverticula, urinary tract anomalies, and aortic aneurysm and insufficiency, the latter being conspicuously difficult to repair because of tissue friability.

There is no specific treatment.

Gellis SS, Feingold M: Picture of the month: Ehlers-Danlos syndrome. Am J Dis Child 118:891, 1969.

Liss SE & others: Ehlers-Danlos syndrome. Med Rec 60:348, 1967.

21...

Neuromuscular Disorders

Gerhard Nellhaus, MD

DISORDERS OF INFANTS & CHILDREN AFFECTING THE NERVOUS SYSTEM

ALTERED STATES OF CONSCIOUSNESS

In the patient who is comatose, stuporous, or drowsy, emergency measures must precede history.

(1) Check respiration, pulse, and color. Ensure an open airway. Consider endotracheal intubation or tracheostomy and administration of oxygen as well as respiratory assistance by mechanical means.

(2) Treat for shock if evident or imminent.

(3) If there is increased intracranial pressure, consider administration of dexamethasone, 1–4 mg IV depending on size of child; mannitol, 2–3 mg/kg of 20% solution IV; or urea, 1 gm/kg IV over a 15–30 minute period.

(4) In known or suspected diabetes, consider insulin reaction and administer glucose intravenously or, if the patient can swallow, orange juice orally.

Causes of Sudden Altered States of Consciousness

(1) **Postictal state.**

(2) **Poisoning:** Common intoxicants in children include salicylates, anticonvulsants, antihistamines, tranquilizers, sedatives, or a mixture of drugs. Ethyl alcohol may cause profound hypoglycemia and coma. Inhalants such as "glue" and carbon monoxide or insecticides must be considered. Heavy metals usually produce an altered state of consciousness over a prolonged period of time.

(3) **Infections:** Bacterial, viral, mycotic, or rickettsial infections causing alterations of consciousness are usually accompanied by signs of meningitis or encephalitis.

(4) **Trauma:** Brain concussion, contusion, and subdural, epidural, or intracerebral hematomas may cause states of altered consciousness. Abdominal trauma resulting in rupture of the spleen or liver may cause massive bleeding with shock and coma.

(5) **Illnesses:** Illnesses to be considered are various intracranial disturbances such as subarachnoid hemorrhage or cerebral infarction; increased intracranial pressure, as may result from obstruction of CSF pathways, tumors, or other space-occupying lesions; and "toxic encephalopathy." Primarily extracranial illnesses causing coma include diabetic coma, hyperinsulinism, liver failure, and uremia.

(6) **Multiple or combined causes:** Keep in mind the possibility that a child may have ingested some drug and then suffered head trauma, or may have been given an overdose of a drug such as salicylates for a febrile illness and phenobarbital for seizures.

Clinical Findings

The degree of alteration of the state of consciousness should be carefully noted and characterized as accurately as possible as coma, semicoma, stupor, drowsiness, or light sleep.

A. Symptoms and Signs:

1. Breathing patterns may give a clue to the underlying cause of the disorder.

a. Slow and deep breathing may be seen in heavy sleep caused by sedatives, following seizures, or in cerebral infections.

b. Slow and often shallow breathing, which may be periodic, is also seen as a result of ingestion of sedatives or narcotics.

c. Periods of hyperpnea alternating with apnea (Cheyne-Stokes breathing) suggest brain stem damage.

d. Deep and rapid (Kussmaul) respirations suggest acidosis.

e. Blowing out of one cheek suggests ipsilateral facial paralysis.

f. The odor of the breath may be helpful, eg, the fruity odor of ketosis, the foul odor of uremia, or the odor of alcohol.

2. Alterations in pulse and in the color of the skin and mucous membranes will vary, as in shock, carbon monoxide poisoning, heat exhaustion, etc.

3. Inspection of the head and body should be done rapidly but carefully for evidence of injury, needle marks, petechiae, and ticks. Particularly in small children, examine the face, mouth, hands, and clothing for evidence of ingestion of toxic substances.

4. Fever may give a clue to acute infection or heat stroke but is also seen in the postictal state and with intracranial bleeding. Hypothermia suggests ingestion of intoxicants (especially barbiturates and alcohol) or shock.

5. Nuchal rigidity suggests meningitis, subarachnoid hemorrhage, or herniation of cerebellar

TABLE 21–1. Characteristics of CSF in the normal child and in some neurologic disorders.

Disease	Initial Pressure (mm H$_2$O)	Appearance	Cells	Protein (mg/100 ml)	Sugar (mg/100 ml)	Other Tests	Comments
Normal	< 180 mm	Clear	0–5 (some accept up to 10) mononuclear cells.	15–35 (lumbar) 5–15 (ventricular)	50–80 (2/3 of blood glucose)	Gamma globulin 8.2% or less of protein. Lactate dehydrogenase (LDH), 2–30 IU/liter.	CSF protein in first month may be up to 150 mg/100 ml; 20–50 red cells in the first days of life.
Bloody tap	Normal or low	Bloody (sometimes with clot)	One white cell for each 700 red cells.	1 mg protein for each 800 erythrocytes above "normal."	Normal		Spin down fluid; supernatant will be clear and colorless.
Acute bacterial meningitis	200–750+	Opalescent to purulent	100 to many thousands, mostly PMNs.	50 to many hundreds.	Decreased; may be none.	Smear and culture mandatory for identification. LDH > 30 IU/liter.	Blood, nose, and throat cultures; very early, sugar may be normal.
Partially treated bacterial meningitis	Usually increased	Clear or opalescent	Usually increased, PMNs usually predominate.	Elevated	Normal or decreased	LDH > 30 IU/liter.	Smear and culture often negative.
Postmeningitic hydrocephalus	Variable	Clear	0–10	Variable; may be low.	Often low	Smear and bacterial cultures negative.	Low CSF glucose may be due to disturbance in transport mechanism.
Tuberculous meningitis	150–750+	Opalescent	250–500. Monocytes predominate.	45–500	Decreased; may be none.	Smear for acid-fast organism; culture and inoculation of CSF.	Very early, PMNs may predominate; tuberculin skin test almost always positive except in fulminant cases; chest x-ray.
Fungal meningitis	Increased	Variable; often clear	10–500; early, mostly PMNs; late, mostly monocytes.	Elevated and increasing	Decreased	India ink preparations, culture, inoculations.	Often superimposed in patients who are debilitated or on immunosuppressive or tumor therapy.
Brain abscess	Normal or increased	Usually clear	5–500 in 80%; mostly PMNs.	Usually slightly increased	Normal; occasionally decreased.		Cell count related to proximity to meninges; findings of purulent meningitis if abscess perforates.
Acute poliomyelitis	Usually normal	Clear or slightly opalescent	10–500+, mostly monocytes; PMNs early.	Normal to 350; often progressive increase.	Normal		Stool virus and serum antibody studies.
Polyneuritis: Early / Late	Normal and occasionally increased	Normal / Xanthochromic if protein high	Normal; occasionally slight increase.	Normal / 45–1500	Normal	Bacterial cultures negative; gamma globulin may be elevated.	Try to find etiology: viral infections, toxins, lupus, infectious mononucleosis, diabetes, etc.
Aseptic meningoencephalitides	Normal or slightly increased	Clear unless cell count is above 300	0 to few hundred, mainly monocytes.	20–125	Normal; may be low in mumps.	CSF, stool, throat wash for viral cultures. LDH < 30 IU/liter.	Acute and convalescent serum antibody studies. Marked pleocytosis (up to 1000 lymphocytes) in mumps.
Neurosyphilis	Normal to 400	Clear unless protein is very high	10–100, mainly monocytes.	25–150: higher in meningitis.	Normal	Positive CSF serology. Gamma globulin may be increased.	Blood serology positive in untreated cases; *Treponema pallidum* immobilization positive.

Parainfectious encephalomyelitis (measles, varicella, vaccinia)	80–450, usually increased	Usually clear	0–50, mainly monocytes.	15–75	Normal	CSF gamma globulin usually normal.	No organisms.
Supratentorial tumors	150–800+, usually increased	Usually clear	Usually normal	Usually normal; increased proximal to obstruction.	Normal	Radiodiagnostic studies	
Brain stem tumors	Usually normal	Clear	Usually normal	Usually normal	Normal	Radiodiagnostic studies	Increase of pressure, cells, or protein occasionally seen in late cases.
Cerebellar and fourth ventricle tumors	150–800+, usually increased	Usually clear	0–150; normal in 80%. Occasionally, cytologic identification of tumor cells.	Normal or slightly elevated	Normal	Tumor cells in CSF occasionally seen on cytologic examination. Contrast studies.	Lumbar tap contraindicated. Ventricular CSF may be normal.
Spinal cord tumors with block	Normal or low; quantitative, manometric studies.	Clear to yellow	0–100, mainly monocytes.	Normal in 15%; 45–3500 in 85%	Normal	Myelography	Color related to amount of protein; very high protein; fluid may clot.
Meningeal carcinomatosis	Often elevated	Clear to opalescent	Cytologic identification of tumor cells.	Often mildly to moderately elevated	Often depressed		Most commonly seen in childhood in leukemia; also in medulloblastoma, meningeal melanosis.
Encephalopathies (lead, anoxic, uremic, toxic)	Increased	Clear to slightly yellow	Normal, occasionally increased; mainly monocytes.	Normal or increased	Normal		Increased lead in blood and urine; increased coproporphyrins in urine; BUN high.
Cerebral concussion	Normal	Clear	Normal	Normal	Usually normal; below 50 in 15%.	Normal	The occasional reduction of sugar is probably related to the presence of blood; protein is increased in relation to admixture.
Cerebral contusion	Increased or normal	Xanthochromic or bloody	Few to several thousand red cells.	Normal		Supernatant fluid xanthochromic	
Subdural hematoma	Increased	Clear in 30%, xanthochromic in 70%	Normal (if fluid is clear).	Often normal in acute subdural hematoma if CSF is not bloody.	Normal	Normal	Blood in CSF due to coexisting other injury.
Epidural hematoma	Above 200 in 2/3 of cases	Clear	See Comments.	See Comments.			Lumbar tap contraindicated if this diagnosis very likely; fluid may be xanthochromic if contusion coexists; cells, protein, and sugar assumed to be normal.
Cerebral hemorrhage	Usually high	Xanthochromic	Amount and type depend on severity of hemorrhage.	Normal to 2000; usually high.	Usually normal; occasionally high or low.	Supernatant fluid xanthochromic	
Subarachnoid hemorrhage	Usually high	Xanthochromic or grossly bloody	Presence of all cellular elements of blood.	Increase related to amount of blood.	Usually high. See Comments.	Supernatant fluid xanthochromic	CSF glucose may be low 7–14 days after initial bleeding.
Demyelinating diseases	Usually high	Clear	0–100, mainly monocytes.	Slightly elevated in 25%	Normal	Gamma globulin usually increased in CSF (ie, > 8.2%).	Schilder's disease, leukodystrophies, neuromyelitis optica, multiple sclerosis, etc.

tonsils. However, nuchal rigidity as a sign of the above may disappear in deep coma.

6. Eyes—(*Caution:* Do not dilate the pupils, as this obliterates critical neurologic signs.)

a. Widely dilated but reactive pupils, sometimes on one side only, are often seen in postictal states.

b. Widely dilated, fixed pupils suggest third nerve paralysis due to tentorial herniation (unless mydriatics have been used).

c. A unilateral fixed pupil usually suggests an expanding lesion on the same side but may be a false localizing sign.

d. Pinpoint pupils are commonly seen with poisonings, eg, with opiates or barbiturates, or in brain stem disorders (hemorrhage, etc).

e. Papilledema indicates increased intracranial pressure. In infants and small children, the presence of subhyaloid hemorrhages is almost always indicative of acute trauma with intracranial bleeding.

f. Visual field examination may be attempted in the lightly comatose or stuporous patient, who may blink in response to threatening movements of the hand coming in from the field of vision to be tested.

g. Check whether eye movements are conjugate or not. Disconjugate movements suggest brain stem lesions. Conjugate deviation of the eyes occurs toward the side of cerebral lesions.

7. Extremities—Asymmetric movements of the limbs or failure to move one side either spontaneously or in response to pain suggests paralysis. A hemiplegic limb will fall uncontrollably.

8. Reflexes—Testing of reflexes may be of limited value.

a. Absence of corneal reflexes usually indicates severe brain damage.

b. A positive Babinski sign may be of value if consistently present, especially if associated with other pyramidal tract signs on the same side. Fluctuating Babinski signs are often observed following seizures or in other states causing stupor.

c. Check for oculomotor paresis by performing the doll's eye maneuver (oculocephalic reflex).

d. The presence of a tonic neck reflex suggests profound brain damage.

B. Laboratory Evaluation: Best guided by the suspected cause:

1. Urinalysis—Urinalysis is generally the most helpful test. It may be necessary to catheterize the patient.

a. Glycosuria is seen with diabetes, salicylism, and sometimes lead poisoning or cerebrovascular accidents.

b. Ketonuria suggests diabetes or starvation state.

c. Proteinuria is seen with renal disease, high fevers, and often lead and other poisonings.

d. A red to purple color on testing the urine with ferric chloride or Phenistix is seen in salicylism and phenothiazine ingestion.

e. Bilirubinuria suggests liver failure.

f. Coproporphyrinuria suggests lead poisoning or other heavy metal intoxication.

2. Blood—

a. Draw blood for typing and cross-matching if transfusion or surgery appears necessary.

b. Blood glucose, urea nitrogen, and pH; serum sodium, chloride, and HCO_3^-.

c. Liver function studies as indicated. High enzyme levels and ammonia, with low bilirubin, are seen in Reye's syndrome.

d. Blood cultures if fever is present.

e. Complete blood count and differential count. Check for "stippling" in small children suspected of having lead poisoning.

f. If possible, set aside blood for toxicologic and viral studies.

3. Gastric contents—Aspirate for diagnostic and therapeutic reasons.

4. Lumbar puncture—Lumbar puncture should be performed immediately **only** when intracranial infection or toxic encephalopathy is suspected. This study can be delayed when intracranial hemorrhage is most likely and is, with rare exceptions, contraindicated in the presence of increased intracranial pressure due to a mass lesion. *Note:* The importance of obtaining CSF opening and closing pressure readings cannot be stressed enough.

C. X-Ray Evaluation: X-rays should be taken when severe head trauma, spinal cord injuries, or abdominal trauma are suspected. Nonessential x-ray studies should be deferred until the patient can cooperate or at least until he is not in an agitated or precarious state.

D. Criteria for "Brain Death": This may be suspected when there is loss of spontaneous respirations, fixed dilated pupils, and nearly total motor and sensory paralysis. Spinal reflexes may be present for a few hours to 2–3 days after "brain death." An isoelectric EEG for 24 hours, except in cases of profound hypothermia and barbiturate poisoning, is confirmatory. More reliable and earlier guides to irreversible brain damage and death, especially when the patient is being considered as an organ donor, are (1) absent cerebral circulation demonstrated by angiography and (2) insignificant drop in oxygen saturation between the arterial and jugular bulb blood.

Treatment

The principle of treatment is to provide specific measures for specific problems. Emergency treatment measures are outlined at the beginning of this section.

(1) Above all, maintain vital functions.

(2) Observe vital signs, the state of the pupils, and levels of consciousness closely.

(3) Turn the patient hourly to prevent hypostatic pneumonia.

(4) Provide fluids by the intravenous route initially and by nasogastric feedings or gastrostomy if coma is prolonged.

(5) Bladder care may require catheterization.

(6) Measures to induce hypothermia may be indicated.

(7) Avoid administration of sedatives but provide anticonvulsants when needed. Diphenylhydantoin is least likely to cloud consciousness. If the patient is very agitated and restlessness threatens to result in injuries, sedate the patient with diphenhydramine, chloral hydrate, or occasionally paraldehyde.

(8) Prophylactic antibiotic therapy is rarely warranted but should be used as for meningitis where a CSF dural leak is present.

(9) Specific therapeutic measures for specific causes.

Prognosis

The prognosis depends on the underlying cause, the severity of the brain damage, and the infections to which the patient with severe depression of consciousness is especially susceptible.

A definition of irreversible coma: Report of the Ad Hoc Committee of the Harvard Medical School to Examine the Definition of Brain Death. JAMA 205:337–340, 1968.

Kunkle EC: *Coma.* Disease-A-Month, Year Book, August 1961.

Nellhaus G: Cerebrospinal fluid immunoglobulin G in childhood. Arch Neurol 24:441–448, 1971.

Pryce JD, Gant PW, Saul KJ: Normal concentrations of lactate, glucose and protein in the cerebrospinal fluid and the diagnostic implications of abnormal concentration. Clin Chem 16:562–565, 1970.

SEIZURE DISORDERS
(Epilepsies)

Essentials of Diagnosis

- Paroxysmal, usually transitory alteration of brain function of sudden onset, frequently recurrent.
- Forced movements, sensory disturbances, autonomic dysfunctions, behavioral changes, alone or in any combination, often accompanied by disturbances of consciousness.
- EEG is frequently abnormal.
- Family history of seizures in 30% of cases.

General Considerations

The causes and modifying conditions of seizures are often unclear, multiple, and additive. In 30% of children with convulsions, others in the family may have a history of epilepsy; migraine is also frequently found. Siblings of epileptic children have a 10% chance of having at least one seizure.

Recognized causes of epilepsy include intrauterine insults, congenital malformations, and perinatal factors. After birth, systemic and CNS infections account for most seizures, with trauma, vascular disorders, metabolic and electrolyte disturbances, toxins,

degenerative diseases, and physical agents responsible for only a few percent. Primary or secondary neoplastic lesions account for less than 1% of "symptomatic" seizures in children, compared with 25% in adults.

Some patients have generalized tonic-clonic or focal motor seizures chiefly during sleep—sometimes just after falling asleep and sometimes in the early morning hours. "Absence" or petit mal, akinetic, and myoclonic spells—often loosely referred to collectively as minor motor seizures—tend to occur in clusters in the morning "after breakfast" and again in the afternoon or around supper time. Marked fatigue, emotional excitement, intercurrent infections, and some drugs may play a "triggering" role. On the other hand, some epileptics who experience difficulty in control at home may do extremely well, with no seizures and on less medication, merely when their situation changes, as when they stay with friends or relatives, go on vacation, or change schools or jobs.

Mixed seizure patterns occur frequently in children. Patterns may also change with maturation, and the treatment of one kind of seizure may unmask another.

Clinical Findings

A. Seizure Types:

1. Generalized convulsions (major motor epilepsy, "grand mal")—Loss of consciousness is usually followed by tonic or clonic movements (or both) and by "the eyes rolling back." The child is usually pale at first and cyanotic later. Auras may occur. Tongue biting, bladder and bowel incontinence, frothing at the mouth, and other visceral disturbances occur in 10–20% of cases. Drowsiness, confusion, fatigue, headache, vomiting, difficulties with speech or movements, and sleep, alone or in any combination, are almost invariably present for a few seconds to hours postictally. The patient is also amnesic for the attack.

While this is the predominant type of childhood epilepsy, over 60% of children with recurrent generalized convulsions exhibit other seizure patterns as well. Partial adversive or abortive attacks are frequently seen. Especially in infants, the generalized seizure may take the form of a "limp" or "stiffening out" spell. In older patients, anticonvulsants may prevent a generalized attack and allow the focal element to emerge.

2. Seizure of localized onset, with or without loss of consciousness—

a. Psychomotor seizures (psychic seizures, "temporal lobe epilepsy")—These seizures are characterized by paroxysmal alteration or clouding of consciousness, usually accompanied by semipurposeful but inappropriate automatic acts which tend to be stereotyped. Young children are often described as seeming suddenly "afraid" or "out in left field." Many children can describe their experience of unpleasant visceral sensations or hallucinations of sight, hearing, taste, or smell, or "forced thoughts." The child may make "mouthing" or "swallowing" movements; he may finger his clothes or other objects; he may run or have inexplicable temper tantrums, or laughing or crying jags. Postictal confusion or giddiness, difficulties with speech, headaches, drowsiness, or sleep generally occur. Many children retain some contact with the environment but feel they have been in a fog, or report that things looked strange or voices were far off. While the child may be amnesic for the attack, some memory of it, particularly of the aura, is often preserved unless the child goes into a generalized convulsion, which occurs at one time or another in over 60% of cases.

This is the predominant seizure type in adults but is reported to begin in childhood in 1/3 of cases, often before the fifth year. One characteristic of "psychomotor seizures" which helps to differentiate them from hysterical attacks is a marked tendency for a particular pattern to repeat itself. Minor variations may occur, and seizures can be modified by the environmental situation. Behavioral and psychic (especially depressive) reactive disturbances are common between episodes. This is even more pronounced around adolescence, when suicidal tendencies may become the most alarming aspect of the problem. Children occasionally "mimic" their attacks for secondary gains. Supportive and sometimes intensive psychiatric therapy, including the judicious use of tranquilizers, may modify the character and frequency of the seizures.

b. Focal seizures—Motor or sensory focal seizures or sensorimotor seizures may be localized in one part of the body, or the seizure may spread in a limited and fixed pattern (jacksonian march). In the focal attack, consciousness is usually preserved. Movements are tonic, clonic, or of mixed type. The attack may become generalized, sometimes so rapidly that it cannot be differentiated from a major motor seizure.

Focal seizures or seizures of focal onset are frequently seen in infants and very young children; however, the "focus" tends to wander and disappear as the child matures. Focal seizures also occur quite commonly in meningitis and encephalitis.

Focal seizures or the focal onset of generalized seizures which repeatedly involve the same locus—especially if associated with lateralizing neurologic deficits—may be due to a specific structural lesion. In many instances, this may be a sclerotic epileptic focus. Further investigation is imperative if the neurologic deficit is progressive or the seizures are difficult to control.

3. Petit mal absence—The term petit mal should be confined to the lapse attacks or absences described below and accompanied by the typical EEG pattern. It should not be used indiscriminately for any seizure that is not grand mal.

Petit mal absence is an attack of "suspended animation," usually lasting 1–2 seconds to 20 seconds. Clusters of a few to 100 attacks may occur, mostly in the midmorning and late afternoon. There is no aura. Awareness is briefly lost, but postural tone is maintained. After the attack, the patient, experiencing no postictal confusion, will usually continue whatever he was doing before. There may be blinking of the eyelids, head nodding, or movements of the lips, hands, or fingers at a rate of about 2–3/second. Petit mal absences are seen predominantly in children age 5–12; they are rare before age 3 and after puberty. When this form of epilepsy occurs by itself, the prognosis is excellent; however, in well over 50% of cases, petit mal absences occur in association with both generalized and minor motor seizures, making the outlook considerably less favorable. Rarely, petit mal may usher in a childhood form of CNS lipidosis.

Petit mal absences may occasionally be accompanied by more complex automatic motor activity, and this makes it difficult to separate them from psychomotor seizures. Here the EEG is of particular help.

4. Minor motor seizures—Three major varieties of epileptic attacks—infantile spasms, myoclonic seizures, and akinetic seizures—are grouped under this term. Lacking the violent tonic-clonic movements of generalized or major convulsions, they are referred to as minor motor seizures. However, the term is misleading in the sense that there is nothing "minor" about the attacks.

These spells share several features. Like petit mal absences, they tend to occur in clusters and are seen during drowsiness or more often in the morning and late afternoon. They may occur for several days in succession and then be absent for days. In contrast to petit mal absences, minor motor seizures often reflect severe and widespread neuronal disturbances, may be exceedingly difficult to control, and are associated with mental retardation at onset or within weeks or months in a high percentage of cases.

a. Infantile spasms—(Massive myoclonic jerks, lightning majors, massive spasms, salaam or "jackknife" seizures.) The typical infantile spasm is a sudden, usually symmetric adduction and flexion of the limbs, with concomitant flexion of the head and trunk; but abduction and extensor movements, simulating an exaggerated Moro reflex, brief tremors, and sudden loss of tone are also seen. Parents may think or be told that the child has "colic."

Infantile spasms arise for the most part in the first year of life and may reflect immature or poorly developed neuronal pathways. Over 1/3 of patients have or will develop generalized seizures. Infantile spasms may cease spontaneously after months or 1–2 years, to be followed after a seizure-free interval by myoclonic, akinetic, or generalized seizures. About 90% of children are or will be retarded, often severely; almost 10% of such patients die by age 3. Prenatal or perinatal brain damage or malformations account for about 1/3 of cases; in another 1/3, various biochemical, infective, traumatic, "fixed," or degenerative brain lesions are implicated; and in about 1/3 no cause can be established. In cases of early onset, pyridoxine dependency, aminoacidurias, and hypoglycemias, including the leucine-sensitive type, should be looked for. Cytomegalovirus infection and toxoplasmosis are among specific infections implicated. Amelanotic spots may be early evidence of tuberous sclerosis. Microcephaly is a common finding.

b. Myoclonic and akinetic seizures—Myoclonic seizures are lightning or shock-like contractions of one or more groups of muscles. The myoclonic jerk may be single or irregularly repetitive, skipping from one part of the body to another.

Akinetic or atonic seizures or "drop attacks" occur when there is a sudden, brief loss of postural control (some describe the child as being "propelled" or flung forward or backward), resulting in a violent drop of the head or fall to the floor.

These 2 types often occur together. The onset is usually at about 2–3 years of age, although the seizures may come on earlier; they diminish progressively after age 6 or 7, but may occasionally still be seen in the second decade. Generalized convulsions are present or will supervene in over 50% of cases. Mental retardation is also evident or will occur in about 50% of cases. Myoclonic and akinetic attacks are not infrequently seen in the CNS degenerative disorders. (See Tables 21–5 and 21–6.) For this reason especially, the cause should be carefully searched for.

These seizures are often difficult to control by medications. To protect the child from head injury, a football helmet with chin padding is advised.

5. "Convulsive equivalents"—("Abdominal epilepsy"; "autonomic," "diencephalic," or "thalamic-hypothalamic" epilepsy; "vegetative" seizures.) These terms are applied to a great variety of episodic visceral or sensory disturbances such as recurrent abdominal pain, cyclic vomiting, headaches, dizzy spells, episodes of profuse sweating, laughing and crying jags, and occasionally incontinence. Brief periods of drowsiness and a fleeting sense of fatigue or "heaviness" may be the only postictal phenomena.

The epileptic nature of these autonomic disorders is often difficult to recognize. The diagnosis depends upon the paroxysmal, repetitive nature of the attacks, the absence of explanatory pathologic findings, and a positive response to therapeutic trials of anticonvulsants, particularly diphenylhydantoin and phenobarbital. A variety of EEG abnormalities are observed in about 70% of cases, but in some cases they are present only during an attack. Older children are most commonly affected (boys twice as often as girls), and 25% or more have or will have other seizures as well as a family history of epilepsy or of migraine.

6. Status epilepticus—Any true seizure lasting an hour or more, or a series of seizures extending over such a period, constitutes status epilepticus. The term is usually applied to a prolonged generalized convulsion or a series of grand mal convulsions occurring in rapid succession without recovery of consciousness between spells. However, patients may also experience focal (motor), "psychomotor," and myoclonic status, as well as petit mal status or "spike-wave stupor" during which consciousness is impaired but not lost.

In treating status epilepticus, vigorous initial therapy is more likely to control seizures than the repeated administration of small doses of various anticonvulsants, whose cumulative effect may produce respiratory depression or marked CNS depression.

7. Neonatal seizures—In the newborn, seizures may not be immediately recognized since they are manifest as twitches or tremors, "jerkiness," eyes rolling upward or staring, cyanotic or apneic spells, or episodes of stiffening or limpness. Focal seizures occur often, but the "focus" changes. Generalized convulsions are frequently violent and terminal.

About 1% of all neonates suffer convulsions (about 1:120–125 in full-term infants; higher in low birth weight infants). Seizures must always be regarded as symptomatic. The diagnosis should be made promptly and specific therapy instituted. Causes include CNS infections, hypocalcemia, hypoglycemia (estimated incidence, 2% of prematures), pyridoxine dependency, hypomagnesemia and other biochemical disorders, and intracranial hemorrhage.

8. Febrile convulsions—Seizures with high fever in children between 6 months and 5 years of age are thought of as "benign": (1) When the fever is due to an intercurrent infection not involving the CNS, eg, tonsillitis, otitis media, or pneumonia. Some pediatricians even include seizures accompanying roseola infantum, though this may be due to an encephalopathy. (2) When the temperature rises rapidly to 40° C (104° F) or higher at the time of the seizures. (3) When the seizures are generalized (although rarely there may be a brief focal onset). (4) When the duration of the convulsion does not exceed 15 minutes. (5) When there are no focal neurologic deficits. (6) When the family history is negative for recurrent nonfebrile seizures (though positive for febrile convulsions in about 40% of cases). (7) When the interictal EEG is normal.

Of the estimated 5% of children 6 months to 5 years of age who have at least one seizure, about 40% will suffer their first convulsion with fever. Boys appear to be twice as susceptible as girls.

The specific cause of the fever should be determined and treated appropriately. A definitely good outcome can be predicted for over 95% of the children whose seizures occur only when fever rises to 40.6° C (105° F), who have no neurologic findings, and who have a normal interictal EEG.

Nevertheless, the chance of recurrence is high. Over 50% will have 2–4 and over 20% more than 4 febrile convulsions. Recurrent nonfebrile seizures develop in 50–75% of children who experience convulsions with lower degrees of fever and those who exhibit focal features or have an abnormal EEG, a family history of epilepsy, or evidence of brain damage.

Febrile convulsions, especially if prolonged and accompanied by significant hypoxemia, may result in brain damage. For these reasons, continuous adequate anticonvulsant therapy (especially phenobarbital or diphenylhydantoin) for 1–2 years significantly reduces the number of recurrences. Exceptions may be made when convulsions have occurred with roseola infantum, salmonella or shigella infections, or fluid and electrolyte disorders provided that no permanent neurologic damage resulted.

9. Breath-holding spells (reflex hypoxic crisis)—
Although not a true epileptic disorder, the typical
breath-holding spell is characterized by violent crying
and breath-holding precipitated by slight injury, anger,
frustration, fear, or the desire for attention in a young
child (usually between 6 months and 4 years of age).
The child becomes hypoxic and cyanotic, loses consciousness, may be opisthotonic, and may have a brief
generalized seizure.

Unless the child sustains a head injury, these
spells are benign. The description usually establishes
the diagnosis. It is helpful to remember that cyanosis—
and rarely pallor—almost always precedes loss of consciousness, whereas in grand mal epilepsy consciousness is lost first. Neurologic examination and EEG are
normal, although reflex slowing produced on the EEG
by ocular compression is diagnostically helpful.

Breath-holding spells almost always disappear
between 4 and 6 years of age. Treatment with phenobarbital usually is of no benefit; in the spells ushered in
by pallor, atropine may be useful.

B. Laboratory Findings: *Note:* The diagnostic
work-up should be guided by the immediate condition
of the child and the demands of the situation.

1. Blood—Glucose, calcium, phosphorus, and
BUN or NPN; when indicated, sodium, magnesium,
and phenylalanine. Check the hemogram specifically
for stippling and sickling of cells. Perform serologic
tests for syphilis and, in infantile spasms, for cytomegalic inclusion disease. Serologic tests for other viral
diseases or for toxoplasmosis may be indicated also.

2. Urine—Reducing substances; ferric chloride or
Phenistix, coproporphyrins and chromatography for
amino acids and organic acids when indicated.

3. Lumbar puncture—Although not a routine
procedure, spinal tap should usually be done in infants
and young children up to about 18 months of age
following the first convulsion, and always if the child is
febrile. *Note:* If meningitis or encephalitis is suspected
as the cause of the seizure, lumbar puncture is mandatory.

Lumbar puncture is not warranted in clear-cut
breath-holding spells, recurrent febrile convulsions
when the cause of the fever is unequivocally extracranial, or when there is a definite risk of brain herniation (as with a posterior fossa mass). Whenever increased intracranial pressure due to a mass is suspected,
skull x-rays should be examined for signs of increased
pressure; if pressure is elevated, the risks of lumbar
puncture should be weighed against its gains, as in
infection or intracranial bleeding.

4. Subdural tap—Subdural tap should always be
considered in an infant with an open anterior fontanel,
particularly if there is any possibility of trauma or
postmeningitic effusion.

C. X-Ray Findings: Skull films should be examined, especially for signs of increased intracranial pressure, calcifications, and lytic lesions. X-rays of long
bones or a skeletal survey should be ordered when
there is a suspicion of lead poisoning, trauma ("battered child"), or occult tumor.

D. Electroencephalography: Almost all children
with gross structural brain disturbances have abnormal
EEGs, which may be enhanced by activating technics
such as light sleep, hyperventilation, and photic stimulation. However, the EEG depends upon the competence of the technician making the recording and the
skill of the physician interpreting the record. Furthermore, about 1/3 of children with a first convulsion
under 4 years of age and about 10% of epileptics later
in life have normal EEGs. In 10–15% of the random
"normal" population and in about 30% of nonpileptic
close relatives of patients with centrencephalic epilepsy, EEG abnormalities may be observed.

1. Diagnostic value—The greatest value of the
EEG in convulsive disorders is in differentiating petit
mal absences and other "minor motor" seizures from
"psychomotor" seizures, and "convulsive equivalents"
from somatic complaints or disorders which are
psychogenic in origin.

The EEG finding of mixed seizure patterns in a
child who clinically demonstrates only grand mal or
petit mal absences may help the physician in choosing
the most appropriate anticonvulsants (Table 21–2).

The EEG may also be useful in localizing a cerebral mass (tumor, abscess, etc). In children who have
persistent seizures despite adequate and prolonged
anticonvulsant therapy, the EEG finding of a constant,
fairly well circumscribed epileptogenic focus may lead
to consideration of surgical excision.

2. Prognostic value—A normal EEG following a
first convulsion suggests (but does not guarantee) a
favorable prognosis. Markedly abnormal EEGs may
become normal (1) immediately following intravenous
injection of 50 mg vitamin B_6 in pyridoxine dependency or deficiency; (2) in infantile spasms (corticotropin or corticosteroids); (3) in petit mal absences
(anticonvulsants); and (4) in petit mal and other minor
motor seizures (ketogenic diet). If so, it is likely that
seizure control will be achieved (although this offers
no clues to the mental status of the patient).

3. Interpretation—The technics of recording and
interpreting the EEG constitute a separate area of
specialization. Examples of the most typical patterns
are the following:

a. Generalized (tonic-clonic) convulsions—
Bilaterally synchronous, symmetrical, multiple high-
voltage spikes, spikes and waves, or mixed patterns.

b. Petit mal absences—Bilaterally synchronous,
symmetrical, high-voltage spikes and waves at a rate of
2–3/second.

c. Minor motor (myoclonic and akinetic) seizures
—Atypical spike and wave patterns, often appearing to
be "petit mal variants," and frequent short bursts of
high-voltage generalized spikes.

d. Infantile spasms—In about 90% of cases, the
EEG shows a rather chaotic pattern ("hypsarhythmia") of very high-voltage slow waves and random
spikes in all leads, and sometimes brief intervals of
electrical silence ("suppression").

e. Psychomotor seizures—A variety of patterns are
seen, including spike and slow wave discharges or 1–4

second bursts of 2–4/second or 4–6/second high-voltage waves, limited to or predominant in the anterior temporal lobe in about 1/3 of cases.

f. The 14 and 6 per second positive spike pattern observed most frequently in adolescents, particularly during light sleep, has been claimed to be associated with convulsive equivalents and dyssocial or asocial behavior; it is now thought to be a normal finding.

E. Special Investigations: Brain scan, pneumoencephalography, cerebral angiography, and ventriculography are usually indicated only when neurosurgical intervention is a distinct possibility, as in the following circumstances: (1) When there is a persistent and progressive neurologic history and findings suggestive of a focal lesion, especially in the presence of markedly localized EEG slowing. (2) When skull films show abnormal calcifications, bony rarefaction, etc, indicative of a lesion amenable to surgery. (3) In the presence of elevated CSF pressure or protein, or persistently depressed CSF sugar, in cases where these findings are not explained by an infectious, toxic, hemorrhagic, or degenerative process. (4) As part of the preoperative evaluation of patients with intractable seizures who may be candidates for cortical excision, anterior temporal lobectomy, or hemispherectomy.

Differential Diagnosis

A. Fainting: In syncope, as cerebral blood flow drops, the patient usually reports that "things went black" before he "sank" to the ground. Convulsive movements do not occur. As blood flow to the brain increases (when the patient lies recumbent or puts his head between his legs), consciousness returns. There are no postictal phenomena, and the patient usually has full memory of fainting.

B. Conversion Hysteria ("Hysteroepilepsy"): The differentiation from epilepsy may be extremely difficult, particularly if the patient has true seizures but also mimics his attacks. This is most often observed in immature adolescents. The character of the attacks (pseudoseizures) may be quite convincing, depending on how much the patient knows about epilepsy and whether he has had the chance to observe generalized or psychomotor seizures. If there is a strong sadomasochistic component to the conversion reaction, the patient may actually injure himself or urinate. In less sophisticated patients, the attacks tend to be "bizarre." During the attack, the patient is often resistive. Even when he mimics postictal stupor, the pupillary dilatation and Babinski responses so often seen immediately after a true seizure are usually not present. The EEG during an attack simply shows muscle artefact, but no preceding "build-up," paroxysmal activity, or postseizure slowing is seen.

C. Narcolepsy: Narcolepsy is uncommon in children. It is characterized by irresistible attacks of sleep, usually of short duration, and is frequently associated with loss of muscle tone (catalepsy) but without sudden loss of consciousness. It is frequently precipitated by acute emotional episodes such as laughing or crying.

Complications

Emotional disturbances—notably anxiety, depression, anger, feelings of guilt and inadequacy—often occur as a reaction to the seizures in the parents of the affected child as well as in the child old enough to understand. The seizures—and particularly the hallucinatory auras and psychomotor attacks—frequently set off in the prepubescent and adolescent youngster fantasies (and sometimes obsessive ruminations) about dying and death which may become so strong as to lead to suicidal behavior and suicidal attempts. The limitations which many school systems place on epileptic children add to the problem. Commonly, the child expresses his feelings by "acting out."

Pseudoretardation may occur in poorly controlled epileptic children because their seizures—or the subclinical paroxysms sustained—may interfere with their ability to concentrate and learn. Anticonvulsants are less likely to "slow the child down," but may do so in toxic amounts.

True mental retardation is most commonly part of the same pathologic process that causes the seizures but may occasionally occur when seizures are frequent, prolonged, and accompanied by hypoxia.

Physical injuries, especially lacerations of the forehead and chin, are frequent in akinetic seizures. In all other seizure disorders in childhood, injuries as a direct result of an attack are impressively rare.

Treatment

The ideal treatment of seizures is the discovery and correction of specific causes. However, even when a biochemical disorder (eg, leucine hypoglycemia) or a tumor is discovered or when septic meningitis is successfully treated, anticonvulsant drugs are often still required.

A. Precautionary Management of Individual Brief Seizures: Position the patient so that he cannot injure himself nor aspirate vomitus. Beyond that, no specific therapy is necessary. The less done to the patient during a relatively brief seizure (up to 10 or 15 minutes), the better. Thrusting a spoon-handle or tongue depressor into the clenched mouth of a convulsing patient or trying to restrain tonic-clonic movements may cause worse injuries than a bitten tongue or bruised limb. Mouth-to-mouth resuscitation is rarely (if ever) necessary.

B. General Management of the Young Epileptic:

1. Education—The patient and his parents must be helped to understand the problem of seizures and their management. Many children—some even as young as 3 years of age—are capable of cooperating with the physician in problems of seizure control.

All bottles containing antiepileptic drugs should bear a contents label. The parents should know the names and dosage of the anticonvulsants being administered.

Pamphlets and books on epilepsy are available from many sources. The local chapter of the Epilepsy Foundation of America and other community and national organizations are eager to be of service and

TABLE 21–2. Guide to anticonvulsant drug therapy.

Seizure Pattern	Drug	Average Total (mg/kg/day)	in	Divided Doses	Toxicity and Precautions	Remarks
All seizures	Phenobarbital	3–5	:	1–3	Irritability and overactivity in many children; sedative effects in others. Mild ataxia, nystagmus, skin rash.	Safest overall drug. Bitter taste.
	Mephobarbital (Mebaral)	4–10	:	1–3	As above.	Tasteless. Twice the quantity of phenobarbital required for comparable effect.
	Primidone (Mysoline)	10–25	:	3–4	Drowsiness, ataxia, vertigo, anorexia, nausea, vomiting, rash.	Start out slowly with 1/4 or 1/3 expected maintenance dose and increase every 2 days until full dose is reached.
	Methsuximide (Celontin)	15–30	:	3–4	Drowsiness, ataxia, headache, diplopia, skin rash.	Effective with phenobarbital in "mixed patterns" where other drugs may be contraindicated.
	Bromides	25–75	:	3–4	Rash, drowsiness, toxic psychosis, mental dullness. Check blood bromide levels regularly.	Rarely used now. Try when usual drugs fail, especially in infantile spasms and "minor motor" seizures.
	Metharbital (Gemonil)	5–15	:	2–3	Drowsiness, irritability, rash.	Not a satisfactory drug. May be useful in seizures due to organic brain damage.
Adjuncts to above	Acetazolamide (Diamox)	5–20	:	3–4	Anorexia; numbness and tingling; increase in urinary frequency.	Supplement to other medications, especially in petit mal and other minor patterns. Also in females 4 days prior to and in the first 2–3 days of menstrual periods.
	Diazepam (Valium)	0.20 ± 0.05	:	3	Somnolence.	Most useful in minor motor seizures and infantile spasms but often ceases to be effective after a few weeks or months.
	Carbamazepine (Tegretol)	Individualize (10–25)	:	2–3 times a day with meals	Bone marrow and liver toxicity.	Experience limited. Useful in psychomotor and generalized seizures. Improved behavior reported.
	Dextroamphetamine (Dexedrine)	0.25–0.75	:	Breakfast and noon	Nervousness, palpitations, anorexia, insomnia.	To counteract sedative effect of other drugs. Narcolepsy. In behavior disorders of younger children.
	Amphetamine (Benzedrine)	0.25–0.75	:	Breakfast and noon	As above.	As above. Less potent, but sometimes better tolerated than Dexedrine.
Any seizures except petit mal absences, akinetic, or myoclonic	Diphenylhydantoin (Dilantin)	5–9	:	1–2	Gum hypertrophy, hirsutism, ataxia, nystagmus, diplopia, rash, anorexia, nausea. Rare: macrocytic anemia, lymph node involvement, exfoliative dermatitis, peripheral neuropathy.	Generally very effective and safe. Will not cause behavior disturbances in children. Good dental hygiene reduces gum hyperplasia. May aggravate petit mal and myoclonic seizures. Severe toxicity may cause pseudodementia and liver damage.

Indication	Drug	Dose	Doses	Side Effects	Comments
	Ethotoin (Peganone)	15–30	2–3	As above.	Not very effective. Worth trying if others fail.
	Mephenytoin (Mesantoin)	4–15	2–3	Mild: Rash, drowsiness, ataxia. *Warning:* Aplastic anemia, agranulocytosis. Obtain at least monthly blood counts.	A good anticonvulsant, but fear of bone marrow depression limits use.
Psychomotor Occasionally primarily akinetic and myoclonic attacks	Phenacemide (Phenurone)	25–50	2–4	Rash, anorexia, nausea. *Warning:* Hepatitis, psychosis, blood dyscrasias. Monthly blood counts, liver function tests.	Especially effective in temporal lobe seizures when all other drugs fail.
Petit mal absences	Ethosuximide (Zarontin)	10–25	3–4	Nausea, gastric discomfort. Take with food. Rare: bone marrow depression.	Drug of choice for petit mal. Occasionally aggravates generalized seizures.
Akinetic and myoclonic attacks	Trimethadione (Tridione)	20–50	3–4	Rash, photophobia, irritability. *Warning:* Leukopenia, agranulocytosis, nephrosis, LE phenomenon. Monthly blood counts and urinalysis.	Useful in petit mal absences if Zarontin fails. May aggravate generalized seizures.
	Paramethadione (Paradione)	20–50	3–4	As above.	As above.
	Phensuximide (Milontin)	20–40	3–4	Drowsiness, headache, slight nephrotoxicity. Monthly urinalysis.	Not very effective, but may be useful when other drugs fail, or in combination.
Status epilepticus, grand mal, focal, psychomotor, and myoclonic	Diazepam (Valium)	0.2 ± 0.05 mg/kg IV initially. Repeat dose 0.1 mg/kg.		Administer slowly IV. Monitor pulse and BP. May cause respiratory depression if given to patient who has already received phenobarbital.	May need to be repeated every 3–4 hours. Follow with phenobarbital or diphenylhydantoin for long-range control.
	Phenobarbital	7–10 mg/kg IV initially. Repeat dose 5 mg/kg IV.		Less if patient has already received barbiturates.	Rule out pyridoxine deficiency, water intoxication.
	Paraldehyde	0.1–0.15 ml/kg IV; 0.2–0.3 ml/kg rectally.		Administer slowly IV mixed in saline; rectal dose in vegetable oil. Avoid in patient with pulmonary disease or in croup.	Avoid IM administration if possible: may cause fat necrosis.
	Lidocaine (Xylocaine)	2 mg/kg IV		Administer slowly.	Useful especially when reluctant to give more barbiturates or paraldehyde. Effect brief.
	General anesthesia if other measures fail.				
Infantile Spasms	Use of corticotropin or corticosteroids and of ketogenic diet discussed in text.				

can be a source of guidance and support as well as an outlet for the anxieties of parents.

2. Privileges and precautions in daily life—Encourage normal daily living within reasonable bounds. The child should engage in physical activities appropriate to his age and social group. After fairly secure seizure control has been established, swimming is generally permissible providing a "buddy system" or adequate lifeguard coverage is maintained. High diving and high climbing should not be permitted. After seizure control is established, physical training and sports in school, camps, community centers, etc are usually to be welcomed rather than restricted. Driving is discussed below.

Excessive fatigue should be avoided.

Emotional disturbances should be treated as indicated.

Prompt attention should be given to infections, and evidence of further neurologic disturbances should be brought to the physician's attention.

Although every effort should be made to control seizures, this must not interfere with a child's ability to function. Sometimes it is better to let a child have an occasional mild seizure than to sedate him so heavily that he cannot function at home, in school, or at play. This often requires much art and fortitude on the part of the physician.

3. Driving—Driving becomes important to most youngsters at age 15 or 16. The restrictions vary from state to state, but in most states a learner's permit or driver's license will be issued if the patient has been under a physician's care and has been free of seizures for at least 2 years, provided the medications or basic neurologic problem do not interfere with the ability to drive.

Epilepsy and the Law, by R.L. Barrow and H.D. Fabing (Hoeber, 2nd ed, 1966), is a helpful guide to this and other legal matters as they pertain to epileptics.

C. Principles of Anticonvulsant Therapy:

1. Treat promptly with the drug most appropriate to the clinical situation as outlined in Table 21–2.

2. Start with one drug—or, in some cases of mixed major and minor motor seizures, with 2—in conventional dosage and increase the dosage until seizures are controlled or to tolerated maximal dosage before adding further drugs or changing medications. The dosages given in Table 21–2 are the usual "guiding" doses, but the actual amount must be individualized.

3. Advise the parents and the patient that the prolonged use of anticonvulsant drugs will not produce "mental slowing" (although the underlying cause of the seizures might) and that prevention of seizures for about 3 years or so substantially reduces the chances of recurrence. Advise them also that anticonvulsants are given to prevent further seizures and that they should be taken as prescribed. Changes in medications or dosages should not be done without the physician's knowledge. Unsupervised sudden withdrawal of anticonvulsant drugs may precipitate severe seizures.

Anticonvulsants must be kept where they cannot be ingested by small children or suicidal patients.

4. Check the patient at intervals, depending on the underlying cause of his seizures, the degree of control, and the toxic properties of the anticonvulsant drug or drugs used. Blood counts, urinalyses, and liver function or other biologic tests must be obtained at frequent intervals in the case of some anticonvulsants as indicated in Table 21–2.

Periodic neurologic reevaluation is important. Repeat skull films may be indicated, eg, if there is a suspicion of a lytic lesion or intracranial calcifications. Repeat EEGs are generally not needed to achieve seizure control and need be obtained in most cases only every 1½–2 years.

5. Continue anticonvulsant treatment until the patient is free of seizures for 2–4 years or, in some cases, through adolescence. A much "improved" or normal EEG (or 2 such tracings 1½–2 years apart) is helpful in determining when anticonvulsant therapy may be discontinued.

6. In general, there is no need to withdraw anticonvulsants before taking an EEG.

7. Discontinue anticonvulsants gradually. If it becomes necessary to withdraw anticonvulsants abruptly, the patient should be under close medical surveillance. If seizures recur during or after withdrawal, anticonvulsant therapy should be reinstituted and again maintained for at least 3–4 years.

D. Side-Effects of Antiepileptic Drugs: (See also Table 21–2.)

1. Serious allergic reactions usually necessitate discontinuance of a drug. However, not every rash in a child receiving diphenylhydantoin, for example, is due to the drug. If a useful antiepileptic drug is discontinued for this reason and the rash disappears, restarting the drug in a smaller dosage is often warranted to see if the allergic reaction recurs.

2. Ataxia and other neurologic signs of drug toxicity will often disappear when the drug is reduced by 25–30% of the last daily dosage.

3. The sedative effect of many of the anticonvulsants is often easily counteracted by the judicious use of dextroamphetamine sulfate (Dexedrine), 2.5–5 mg at breakfast and 2.5 mg at noon.

4. Gingival hyperplasia secondary to diphenylhydantoin is best minimized through good dental hygiene but occasionally requires gingivectomy. This and hypertrichosis usually disappear within 6 months after the drug is discontinued.

E. Guides to Therapy of Specific Seizure Disorders: (See also Table 21–2.)

1. Status epilepticus—Diazepam (Valium) is the drug of choice. In general, 0.2 ± 0.05 mg/kg or 6 mg/sq m administered IV over 1–3 minutes will achieve control; if necessary, 1/2 the initial amount should be given again. Pulse and blood pressure should be monitored during the injection, and if these drop markedly the injection should be temporarily halted until cardiovascular function returns to normal. In recurrent status epilepticus, diazepam may be repeated every 3–4 hours.

Once control is achieved, phenobarbital, 3–5 mg/kg, or diphenylhydantoin, 5–7 mg/kg, should be administered by IV drip, IM, or orally (depending on the particular situation) for long-term seizure control.

Diphenylhydantoin, 10 mg/kg slowly IV, is often useful in major motor and psychomotor status epilepticus, especially where it is desirable to avoid depressing the level of consciousness; lidocaine (Xylocaine) is especially useful to achieve rapid (though short-lived) control of focal motor seizures.

For further details on the use of phenobarbital and paraldehyde in status epilepticus, see Table 21–2.

Note: General anesthesia may have to be used to control status epilepticus if the usual measures fail.

2. Major motor (grand mal) seizures—

a. Phenobarbital—Phenobarbital, 3–5 mg/kg/day orally, is the drug of choice. It may be given once a day, though parents and patients may remember better if the drug is taken with meals, ie, 3 times a day. Phenobarbital can often not be used in young children (particularly those with so-called minimal brain dysfunction syndrome), who may become very hyperactive and irritable when this drug is given; nor in adolescents, in whom the dosage of phenobarbital (if used alone) necessary to control seizures may cause lethargy.

b. Diphenylhydantoin sodium (Dilantin)—Diphenylhydantoin is the drug of choice when phenobarbital cannot be used. It is usually given in addition to phenobarbital if major seizures cannot be controlled even by near-toxic dosages of phenobarbital. Diphenylhydantoin in doses of 5–7 mg/kg/day orally may be given once a day (or in divided doses) to produce a desirable blood level of about 13–17 μg/ml. Some patients conjugate diphenylhydantoin poorly and become toxic on otherwise average doses, whereas other patients tolerate greater amounts. Diphenylhydantoin has a number of undesirable side-effects (Table 21–2) and may aggravate petit mal and possibly other minor motor seizures.

c. Acetazolamide (Diamox)—Give 125 mg/day to 250 mg twice a day orally, depending on the size of the child. This is often an excellent additional drug in any of the seizure groups. It is particularly useful in major motor seizures associated with menstrual periods, when it should be taken for about 4 days prior to and on the first 2–3 days of menses; and in petit mal absences or other minor motor seizures.

d. Mephobarbital (Mebaral)—Some authorities state that children do not become hyperactive on this barbiturate as they do on phenobarbital. This remains open to question. Mephobarbital must be given in twice the dosage of phenobarbital, ie, 6–10 mg/kg/day orally; however, it has the advantages of being tasteless (whereas phenobarbital is bitter) and of being more expensive, so that parents often think it must be better.

e. Less commonly used anticonvulsants—Rarely, mephenytoin (Mesantoin), primidone (Mysoline), or bromides may have to be tried (Table 21–2).

3. Psychomotor seizures—Diphenylhydantoin, 5–7 mg/kg/day orally (as a single dose or in divided doses), is the drug of choice. Primidone (Mysoline) may be added if the seizures continue. The tolerance for primidone is highly variable; in children under 6 years of age, 50 mg orally 3 times daily may suffice; teenagers may tolerate up to 250 mg or more 4 times daily. The patient should build up to the full prescribed dose gradually—eg, 50 mg on day 1, 50 mg twice daily on day 3, 50 mg 3 times daily on day 5—to avoid excessive drowsiness.

Phenobarbital, though related to primidone, is also added when the psychomotor seizures are difficult to control. Acetazolamide and methsuximide (Celontin) have proved effective in some cases.

More recently, carbamazepine (Tegretol) has been used in dosages ranging from 100 mg orally twice a day to 400 mg 3 times a day. Experience with this drug is still limited, but it has been effective in about 50–60% of cases in which other combinations failed to achieve complete control. Blood counts, urinalysis, and liver function tests should be obtained periodically.

In refractory cases, phenacemide (Phenurone) is highly effective. In a limited number of children followed for a long period, no toxic effects on liver or bone marrow have been observed. However, because liver toxicity and blood dyscrasias have been reported, blood counts, urinalyses, and liver function tests should be done monthly at first and later at 3-month intervals. In a few children—each of them with serious preexisting emotional problems—phenacemide triggered psychotic manifestations which promptly disappeared when the drug was discontinued.

In extremely refractory cases, mephenytoin (Mesantoin) might be considered; however, its great tendency to depress bone marrow is a danger to be closely monitored.

4. Focal (motor and sensory) seizures—Phenobarbital is the drug of choice, with primidone or methsuximide and acetazolamide added as necessary.

5. Petit mal absences—Very mild petit mal may respond to phenobarbital, acetazolamide (Diamox), or a combination of the two. In more severe but pure cases of petit mal, the drug of choice is ethosuximide (Zarontin), 250 mg orally daily or twice daily in children up to about 7 years, and up to 500 mg 3 times a day in teenagers. Blood counts should be obtained at 4–6 week intervals. Ethosuximide can precipitate major motor seizures and, in mixed seizures, should be given together with phenobarbital or not used at all.

In mixed petit mal and major motor seizures, the "cocktail" described below under minor motor seizures often works exceedingly well. Occasionally, in severe petit mal, the ketogenic diet is highly effective.

Even though it is highly effective, there is rarely any need to use trimethadione (Tridione), which can cause bone marrow depression, nephrosis, lupus erythematosus, and other serious reactions.

6. Minor motor seizures—In myoclonic and akinetic seizures not due to vitamin B_6 deficiency, start with a combination ("cocktail") of phenobarbital, 3–5 mg/kg/day orally, and methsuximide (Celontin), 15–30 mg/kg/day orally in 3 divided doses. If this does not achieve control in 2–3 days, add acetazolamide.

This "cocktail" is often also very effective in mixed major motor/petit mal epilepsy and even in milder cases of infantile spasm.

In refractory cases, consider the use of corticosteroids and of the ketogenic diet as described below.

F. Corticotropin and Corticosteroids:

1. Indications–These drugs are indicated for infantile spasms not due to causes amenable to specific therapy, and for akinetic and myoclonic seizures which cannot be controlled by anticonvulsant drugs.

The duration of therapy is guided by cessation of clinical seizures and EEG improvement. Corticotropin or the oral corticosteroids are usually continued in full doses for 2–4 weeks and then, if seizures have ceased, are tapered by about 25% every 2 weeks for a total treatment period of about 2 months. If seizures recur, increase the dosage to the last effective level and maintain the patient for up to 6 months on this dosage before again attempting withdrawal.

2. Dosages–

a. Corticotropin gel (Acthar Gel), starting with 4–5 units/kg/day IM in 2 divided doses. Parents can be taught to give the injections.

b. Cortisone, starting with 6–8 mg/kg/day orally in 3 divided doses.

c. Prednisone, starting with 2–4 mg/kg/day orally in 3 divided doses.

d. In akinetic and myoclonic seizures, give phenobarbital and other anticonvulsants also.

3. Precautions–Give additional potassium, guard against infections, and discuss the cushingoid appearance and its disappearance. Do not withdraw oral corticosteroids suddenly.

G. Ketogenic Diet in Treatment of Epilepsy: A ketogenic diet should be recommended in akinetic and myoclonic seizures and petit mal absences not responsive to drug therapy, and occasionally for infantile spasms that do not respond to corticotropin or the corticosteroids. The mechanism for the anticonvulsant action of this diet is not yet understood, although various hypotheses have been put forth. However, it is the ketosis, not the acidosis, which is effective in raising the seizure threshold. It is usually most effective in young children, ie, those under the age of 8 years, but when all other measures fail it should be tried even in adolescents.

As ketosis is achieved, a repeat EEG may be helpful; seizure control by the diet is more likely to occur if the EEG shows improvement.

The ketogenic diet is difficult, expensive, tends to be monotonous, and depends upon the ability of the mother to weigh out the foods as well as absolute adherence to the diet prescribed. Full cooperation of the parents and all other family members is required, including the patient if old enough. However, when seizure control is achieved by this method, the child is alert, often is receiving no anticonvulsants or only

small amounts, and parental and patient satisfaction is most gratifying.

Consult a dietitian and references on ketogenic diet (eg, Keith and Livingston references, below).

Aicardi J, Chevrie JJ: Convulsive status epilepticus in infants and children: A study of 239 cases. Epilepsia 11:187–197, 1970.

Douglas EF, White PT: Abdominal epilepsy: A reappraisal. J Pediat 78:59–67, 1971.

Juul-Jensen P: Frequency of recurrence after discontinuance of anticonvulsant therapy in patients with epileptic seizures. Epilepsia 9:11–161, 1968.

Keith H: *Convulsive Disorders in Children.* Little, Brown, 1963.

Livingston S: *Comprehensive Management of Epilepsy in Infancy, Childhood and Adolescence.* Thomas, 1972.

McInerny TK, Schubert WK: Prognosis of neonatal seizures. Am J Dis Child 117:261–264, 1969.

Niedermeyer E & others: Classical hysterical seizures facilitated by anticonvulsant toxicity. Psychiat Clin 3:71–84, 1970.

Van den Berg BJ, Yerushalmy J: Studies on convulsive disorders in young children. II. Intermittent phenobarbital prophylaxis and recurrence of febrile convulsions. J Pediat 78:1004–1012, 1971.

HEADACHES

Headache is not usually a psychosomatic symptom in very young children, whereas this is more often the case—even in association with vomiting—in older children and adolescents. A careful description of the headaches, associated circumstances, and other neurologic and systemic symptoms should be obtained. The family history and emotional problems should be discussed in detail. Finally, a careful systemic and neurologic examination, including blood pressure, ophthalmoscopic examination, and urinalysis, will help distinguish organic from the more common psychogenic or tension headaches.

EEG, skull and sinus x-rays, ophthalmologic evaluation, and other studies may be indicated as screening tests; even therapeutic trials of diphenylhydantoin, phenobarbital, or ergotamine are occasionally warranted.

If there is evidence of a specific intracranial cause or systemic disorder (eg, renal disease), diagnosis and treatment should be directed at the primary disorder.

Friedman AP, Harms E: *Headaches in Children.* Thomas, 1967.

Tension Headaches

Often described as "dull" or "like a tight band," of slow onset, diffuse or occipital and sometimes nuchal in location, lasting for hours, and rarely disabling, tension headaches are a frequent complaint in school-age and especially adolescent children. Home, school, social, and sexual problems are the usual underlying emotional factors. The history frequently suggests feelings of inadequacy or anxiety in the patient.

Salicylates are often successful in relieving the discomfort. Antianxiety drugs such as chlordiazepoxide (Librium), 5–10 mg 2–3 times daily, are occasionally indicated, along with supportive therapy. Primary attention, however, should be directed at the precipitating and chronic causes of the emotional strain.

Headaches Due to Refractive Error

Although rare in school-age children, more headaches are blamed on eye problems than can be substantiated by ophthalmologic examination. Attention should be directed to underlying emotional disturbances.

Waters WE: Headache and the eye. Lancet 2:1–3, 1970.

Migraine

Migraine attacks are usually paroxysmal, throbbing, pulsating, or pounding in character (initial vasoconstriction of intracranial vessels followed by vasodilatation of extracranial vessels); commonly unilateral; and often preceded by scintillating scotomas, slowly evolving sensory disturbances of the face and arm, and sometimes by psychic disturbances. Less frequent are transient ipsilateral visual disturbances and contralateral hemiplegia. Photophobia, nausea, gastric discomfort, and vomiting are commonly present. The child frequently seeks rest in a dark, quiet room.

Migraine of varying severity may occur in as much as 5% of the population. Onset by age 4 is not uncommon. The family history is often positive for migraine and not infrequently also for epilepsy. The EEG may be slightly abnormal.

Salicylates are often effective in children. The patient should be allowed to remain quiet in a darkened room. In older children, if salicylates are ineffective, and when anxiety and nausea are prominent symptoms, Cafergot P-B,* 1/2–1 tablet at the first sign of an attack and 1/2–1 additional tablet every 30 minutes for a total of 2–4 tablets, is often useful. Cafergot P-B suppositories may have to be used when migraine is severe and vomiting precludes oral medication.

In the prevention of severe, frequent, and disabling migraine, diphenylhydantoin (Dilantin), 5–7 mg/kg/day, may be effective, especially when the EEG is abnormal or there is a family history of epilepsy. In children it is rarely necessary to resort to methysergide maleate (Sansert), 2–6 mg daily with meals in divided doses, depending on age and size. Methysergide is contraindicated in renal disease and vasculitis (eg, "collagen diseases"). It is reported to have caused retroperitoneal fibrosis and vascular complications.

Basser LS: The relation of migraine and epilepsy. Brain 92:285–300, 1969.

Bille B: *Migraine in School Children.* Almquist & Wiksell, Uppsala, 1962.

*Cafergot P-B contains ergotamine tartrate, 1 mg; caffeine, 100 mg; Bellafoline (alkaloids of belladonna, as malates), 0.125 mg; and pentobarbital sodium, 30 mg.

Verret S, Steele JC: Alternating hemiplegia in childhood: A report of eight patients with complicated migraine beginning in infancy. Pediatrics 47:675–680, 1971.

Headache as an Epileptic Phenomenon

Headaches, when associated with epilepsy, may occur as an aura (usually in psychomotor seizures) or in postictal states. Less commonly, they occur as a "convulsive equivalent." (See section on Seizure Disorders.)

Treatment consists of control of seizures. For cyclic headaches not associated with other epileptic phenomena but judged to represent a "convulsive equivalent," a therapeutic trial of an anticonvulsant is warranted. Diphenylhydantoin (Dilantin), 5–7 mg/kg/day orally, is usually more effective than phenobarbital, 3–5 mg/kg/day orally. If effective, treatment should be maintained for 2–3 years of a symptom-free period and then discontinued slowly, with reinstitution of therapy if symptoms recur.

HEAD INJURIES

Initial Evaluation

Check a child brought in because of head trauma rapidly for the following:

A. Respirations: Ensure adequate oxygenation. Hyperventilation is common in excited, irritable children. Deep, rapid, or periodic breathing is seen with brain stem involvement; intermittent gasping often precedes death.

B. State of Consciousness: (See also the section on Altered States of Consciousness.) Alterations of behavior and of consciousness may follow head trauma. In young children, it may be difficult to be certain whether there was a brief loss of consciousness immediately after the injury or whether the child had a breath-holding spell or a seizure. Following a concussion, young children are often extremely irritable.

Immediate stupor or coma suggests severe damage to the diencephalon or brain stem reticular activating system. Initial relative alertness followed by progressively deepening drowsiness, stupor, and coma within minutes, hours, or 3–4 days is observed in more extensive cerebral edema and intracranial bleeding.

C. Pulse: The pulse is often rapid shortly after head trauma. Wide fluctuations in pulse rate or marked slowing accompany direct brain stem damage or increased intracranial pressure.

D. Blood Pressure: Children often look pale and feel clammy after a head injury even though blood pressure is normal. Marked hypotension suggests bleeding into the viscera (consider splenic or hepatic rupture, particularly after an automobile or bicycle accident). Widened blood pressure or marked fluctuations often accompany direct brain stem involvement or increased intracranial pressure.

E. Ocular Signs: Note reactivity of pupils to light and their size. A 1–2 mm inequality with briskly reacting pupils may be due to congenital anisocoria but warrants continued observation. A fixed, dilated pupil in one eye may indicate ipsilateral cerebral damage or hematoma (epidural or subdural) or may be a false lateralizing sign. Bilateral fixed dilated pupils reflect severe brain stem damage, with death often occurring in a few hours. Bilateral fixed constricted pupils may reflect brain stem damage from which the patient may recover but also suggest intoxication, eg, with barbiturates or opiates. Note voluntary and doll's eye movements.

Ophthalmoscopic examination is of paramount importance. Retinal hemorrhages occur in acute head injuries, especially with subdural hematomas. Dilated, nonpulsating retinal veins are the first sign of papilledema, which may develop within a few hours after the onset of increased intracranial pressure.

F. Inspection and Palpation:

1. Skull—Note and record signs of trauma, especially puncture wounds and deep scalp lacerations. Linear fractures, like widely separated sutures, may result in a "cracked pot sound" on percussion of the head; depressed skull fractures may be palpable. The maximum occipitofrontal head circumference should be recorded; the size and tension of the anterior fontanel, if patent, should be noted.

2. Neck—Nuchal rigidity may be due to subarachnoid hemorrhage, but cervical spine injury must be considered. Great caution is urged both in checking the neck and in moving such a patient. Prompt cervical spine films should be taken when there is the least suspicion of cervical spine fracture.

3. Ears—Bleeding from one or both ears or a hematoma over the mastoid region (Battle's sign) suggests basilar skull fracture through the petrous pyramids of the temporal bone; such bleeding may also be due to rupture of the tympanic membrane or the tearing of mucous membranes without perforation of the ear drum, and may occur without skull fracture. Note also leakage of CSF from the ears.

4. Rhinorrhea—A watery nasal discharge strongly positive for glucose (as tested with Dextrostix) suggests CSF leakage as occurs with fracture of the frontal bone and associated dural tearing. However, mucous discharges may also be glucose positive; hence, the discharge must be analyzed chemically and microscopically.

5. Skin and extremities—Rapidly inspect for signs of recent trauma, including fractures. Note also the presence of old scars.

6. Abdomen—Palpate, percuss, and auscultate the abdomen to rule out visceral bleeding, especially from the liver or spleen.

G. Motor, Reflex, and Cerebellar Examination:

1. Motor function may be difficult or impossible to evaluate in a comatose or very irritable child. Spontaneous movements and reflex withdrawal from noxious stimuli should be noted. For a short time after a concussion or convulsion, there may be transient paresis which may alternate from side to side. Consistent paresis is usually due to contusion or laceration of the brain; progressive paralysis occurs with intracranial bleeding and swelling. Paralysis may be on the same side as the injury or hematoma, due to uncal herniation (Kernohan's syndrome).

2. The reflexes (especially the plantar responses) may vary markedly in the immediate posttraumatic period or if there has been a seizure. Pathologic reflexes are of lateralizing value when persistent and associated with motor weakness or spasticity. Transient Babinski signs and absent abdominal reflexes are common with mild head trauma in children.

3. Cerebellar testing requires that the patient be conscious and cooperative. Unsteadiness, mild intention tremor, and generalized clumsiness are common in children after head injuries. Ataxia and nystagmus, especially when associated with vertigo and vomiting, raise a suspicion of posterior fossa hematoma, a potentially curable lesion.

H. Sensory Examination: This is often difficult but should be done, especially where a spinal cord injury is suspected.

I. Temperature: Taking the child's temperature may often be delayed until the end of the examination and until the child is calmed. Never insert a thermometer into the mouth or rectum of a restless or convulsing child. If necessary, axillary temperature may be taken. Mild hypothermia immediately after the injury, followed by mild to moderate fever for 1–2 days, is observed frequently in children. Persistent moderate fever is common with subarachnoid hemorrhage.

Classification & Clinical Findings

Head injuries are usually categorized according to the more prominent clinical and pathologic findings. The clinical status, course, and prognosis of the patient depends on the nature and severity of the cerebral insult rather than on the presence and extent of superficial injuries or of skull fracture.

A. Mild: Disturbance or loss of consciousness, if it occurs at all, is transient, lasting seconds to a few minutes. There are no demonstrable residual neurologic signs. There may be no sequelae, or the posttraumatic period may be characterized by mild headache (easily controlled by salicylates), irritability, drowsiness, and occasionally vomiting in younger children. This picture is usually associated with brain concussion, but it may occur with contusion and even limited subarachnoid bleeding.

B. Moderate: Disturbance or loss of consciousness lasts several minutes to perhaps an hour. Abnormal neurologic signs are frequent (though often transient). The posttraumatic period is characterized by more severe headache, irritability, drowsiness, and confusion. Vomiting for 12–36 hours and mild to moderate fever are common. This state is usually associated with some degree of cerebral edema, contusion, or laceration.

C. Severe: Severe head injuries may result in immediate unconsciousness lasting an hour or more or in sudden or progressive deterioration of the level of consciousness after an initial lucid period. Abnormal neurologic signs may develop and persist for hours or days or may be permanent. If consciousness is preserved, the posttraumatic period may be characterized by severe unremitting headache, mental confusion, marked fluctuations in the level of consciousness, and vomiting. This is usually associated with more extensive cerebral edema, contusion and laceration of the brain, intracranial bleeding, or brain stem damage.

The soft skulls and open cranial sutures in infants and young children may "absorb" some of the force of the head trauma and thus tend to reduce the severity of the injury or result in delayed appearance of neurologic signs.

X-Ray, Laboratory, & Other Methods of Evaluation
A. X-Ray:
1. Skull x-rays—Skull films are indicated in moderate to severe and all open head injuries: (1) to confirm a clinical suspicion of a depressed or basilar fracture; (2) to define the site and extent of bone involvement where neurosurgical intervention is anticipated; and (3) to obtain evidence, where head trauma is suspected but no history of trauma is obtained and no external signs of trauma are found, as may be the case with an abused child. X-rays should be delayed, or bedside portable views obtained, in a very restless, uncooperative child or one in danger of airway obstruction or other serious complication.

Taking skull x-rays routinely has been challenged on both medical and economic grounds. Only about 7% of skull x-rays after head trauma show fractures, but this rarely affects · management. In closed head injuries, there is no correlation between fractures and complications, prognosis, or sequelae.

2. Other plain films—Whenever spinal cord injury is suspected, cervical and other spine films must be obtained (as explained above) as soon as feasible, taking care to move the patient as little as possible. X-rays of the extremities, chest, and abdomen should be taken when injury to these parts is thought likely. One common indication is suspected child abuse.

3. Cerebral angiography—Clinical findings usually indicate the choice of injection site. (Retrograde right brachial angiography is the procedure of choice when there are no clear-cut localizing signs or when a hematoma in the posterior fossa or occipital or posterior parietal region is suspected.) The indications for angiography following head trauma are (1) suspected epidural hematoma, (2) suspected subdural or intracerebral hematoma, (3) suspected thrombosis, (4) rupture of a vascular malformation or aneurysm, and (5) abnormally enlarging head circumference when it is difficult to differentiate clinically between bilateral subdural hematomas and hydrocephalus.

4. Air studies—Ventriculography or lumbar pneumoencephalography may be indicated in children in evaluating posttraumatic hydrocephalus, leptomeningeal or porencephalic cysts, or cerebral atrophy.

In infants and young children with subdural hematomas in whom fluid can be removed by needling the subdural space through the anterior fontanel or an open suture, a small amount of air (10–15 ml) may be injected after removal of an equal amount of fluid; brow-up, brow-down, and right and left lateral skull films will then disclose the extent of the subdural space and of the brain compression or atrophy.

B. Brain Scan: Scanning with radioactive isotopes may be useful, when the patient's status permits, in diagnosing intracranial hematomas or other masses. (Do not use ^{203}Hg in children.)

C. Echoencephalography: This is a rapid, innocuous procedure which is employed in many medical centers today in evaluating patients for possible intracranial hematomas or hydrocephalus.

D. Lumbar Puncture: There are few indications and many contraindications to spinal taps following head injuries. Lumbar puncture is contraindicated by increased intracranial pressure due to a suspected mass lesion, such as in epidural hematoma or intracerebral hemorrhage.

CSF examination is indicated in children when the following are likely: (1) Cerebral infection or toxic encephalopathy. (Many children will become unsteady and fall or suffer a convulsion at the beginning of these processes.) (2) Subarachnoid hemorrhage. Lumbar puncture may help differentiate concussion (CSF pressure normal or slightly elevated but cells, protein, and glucose normal) from contusion and laceration (CSF pressure often increased, with presence of red cells and xanthochromia), but this is of no help in management or prognosis.

E. Subdural Taps: These are often indicated in infants and small children following head trauma (or when there is a strong suspicion of head trauma) when the anterior fontanel is still open or the coronal sutures are sufficiently patent to allow a subdural needle (No. 20 or 22 gauge with short bevel) to pass. Subdural taps are indicated if, following the initial period, the infant continues to do poorly, has convulsions, or develops a fever; if his hemoglobin falls; or if he shows progressive neurologic signs or abnormal enlargement of head circumference. In infants up to about 18 months of age, transillumination of the head will usually be positive in chronic (but not acute) subdural hematomas.

F. Exploratory Bur Holes: Trephination of the skull may be indicated after severe closed head injuries in children whose clinical state is deteriorating rapidly, especially when neurologic signs suggest the presence of extradural or subdural hemorrhage. Bur holes for diagnostic purposes alone are no longer performed in children in whom more definitive studies, such as cerebral angiography or air encephalography, may be safely carried out first.

G. Electroencephalography: EEG is commonly abnormal in the immediate posttraumatic period, with posterior slowing in a high proportion of cases (80% or more). EEG findings are often out of proportion to clinical symptoms and may be of limited prognostic significance. The EEG is indicated in posttraumatic epilepsy. Occasionally it is helpful in the diagnosis of subdural hematoma.

An abnormal posttraumatic EEG does not rule out functional factors and overlay. The EEG is often normal in posttraumatic and compensation neurosis.

Differential Diagnosis

Head trauma, especially when due to an accidental fall, is a common occasion for office or emergency visits. It is important to consider head trauma due to child battering or during an epileptic seizure, falls due to ataxia or other neurologic disorder, loss of consciousness due to hypoglycemia, cerebrovascular accident, intoxication, or other causes discussed in the section on altered states of consciousness (above).

Complications & Sequelae

A. Posttraumatic Seizures: Seizures may be focal or generalized, varying greatly with age and the site and severity of injury. Seizures in the first 24 hours occur in 6–15% of children with head injuries of all types; they are more common in younger children and following brain lacerations.

Chronic posttraumatic epilepsy in children occurs in only about 2% of the total group but in 5–10% of children who suffered brain lacerations or initial unconsciousness of an hour or more. Over 50% of these seizures occur within the first 6 months; over 80% occur within 2 years.

B. Space-Occupying Lesions: (About 1–3% of children with head injuries seen at major hospitals.)

1. Epidural hematoma–The classical picture of a hemispheric extradural (epidural) hematoma is transient disturbance or loss of consciousness followed by a symptom-free ("lucid") interval of a few hours to a day, and then progressive clouding of consciousness and evolution of a dilated fixed pupil and hemiparesis. The usual cause is bleeding from a torn middle meningeal artery or vein.

In children, this classical sequence is rare. A history of unconsciousness or impaired consciousness is frequently lacking. The symptom-free interval is often atypical because of nonspecific irritability, headache, vomiting, and other complaints; in about 1/2 of children, the lucid interval is longer than 48 hours' duration, and the course may be fluctuating rather than progressive, without loss of consciousness. As in adults, the site of injury is usually temporal, but fractures across the middle meningeal artery are often not present and the source of bleeding may be from its smaller branches or from torn diploic veins or bridging vessels. Extradural hematomas of clinical significance are uncommon in children under the age of 4 years.

These differences may be due to the tendency of the softer skull of infants to "give," with no fracture on impact; the escape of epidural blood through widened sutures, the fracture site, or an open fontanel; the less rapid or less massive bleeding that occurs from sources outside the middle meningeal artery; the lower systolic pressures in children, especially after blood loss; and perhaps the fact that the brain is less susceptible to pressure changes in children.

Extradural hematomas of the posterior fossa may be difficult to diagnose clinically in children. The presenting symptoms and signs may relate chiefly to the obstruction of CSF flow and consequent development of increased intracranial pressure. Cerebellar signs and cranial nerve palsies should suggest this diagnosis.

Close observation over several days is necessary to detect early signs of epidural hematoma so that neurosurgical consultation and diagnostic cerebral angiography can be requested early.

2. Subdural hematoma–(About 4–5% of children with a history of head trauma, but the history is often lacking. The male/female incidence is 2:1.) Acute subdural hematoma may occur in association with contusion or laceration. Chronic subdural hematoma is more common. The clinical course is highly variable, depending primarily on the extent of the underlying damage to the cerebral substance and the age of the child. In infants and young children with open fontanels and sutures, there may be considerable delay before symptoms develop. The most common presenting features in children are seizures (about 75% of cases), vomiting (about 60%), drowsiness, irritability, or other personality changes (50%), developmental retardation (20%), and failure to thrive (10%). The presenting signs consist of increased head size and bulging fontanels (80%); retinal hemorrhages (40–65%); anemia (50–70%), extraocular (especially sixth nerve) palsies (40%), hemiparesis (35%), quadriplegia (10%), and fever (10%). There is a high associated incidence of scars and long bone or rib fractures due to "battering."

3. Intracerebral hematoma–(Less than 1% of children with head trauma seen at major hospitals.) Multiple small areas of hemorrhage are more common; larger hematomas may develop beneath a depressed skull fracture. The symptoms and signs vary greatly with the size and location of the hematoma. The frontal and temporal lobes are most frequently involved.

C. Subarachnoid Hemorrhage: In children, traumatic subarachnoid hemorrhage is often relatively asymptomatic and therefore infrequently diagnosed. Nuchal rigidity, disturbance or loss of consciousness, and seizures are usually the outstanding symptoms. (For further details, see Cerebrovascular Disorders.)

D. CSF Rhinorrhea and Otorrhea: (Infrequent in children.) CSF leakage from the nose occurs with fracture of the frontal bone and associated dural and arachnoid tearing. The flow of fluid is increased by erect posture, coughing, and straining. CSF otorrhea with basilar fracture may be of serious prognostic significance.

Infections, particularly meningitis, are a potential threat in CSF leakage. Most CSF leaks heal within 2 weeks in children kept at rest; chronic leaks require surgical repair of the dural tear.

E. Other Acute Paratraumatic Problems:

1. Increased intracranial pressure may be acute or subacute. Manifestations include alterations in consciousness, disturbances of behavior, vomiting, headaches, ataxia, focal weakness, and other neurologic disturbances. Findings are those of a space-occupying lesion, which must be ruled out.

2. Hyponatremia and other electrolyte disturbances are seen most commonly with cerebral edema and CSF rhinorrhea or otorrhea.

3. Infections relate to the nature and severity of the head trauma. There may be pneumonia, often due to aspiration, in children who suffered convulsions or coma. Dural tears may lead to meningitis. Infected skull fractures may result in osteomyelitis.

4. Fever, particularly in younger children, may be due to hypothalamic involvement, dehydration, subdural effusions, resorption of necrotic tissue or subarachnoid blood, and infection.

5. Retrograde amnesia for the events immediately surrounding the head injury is not uncommon, even when there was no seizure.

F. Posttraumatic CNS Structural Complications:

1. Posttraumatic hydrocephalus—The incidence of this complication is not known. It is seen most often in infants and toddlers and is most commonly due to aqueductal gliosis or basilar arachnoiditis. Congenital anomalies of the CSF passageways may play a role.

2. Posttraumatic focal deficits—Cranial nerve palsies (most commonly abducens or facial palsy), optic atrophy, anosmia, motor deficits, diabetes insipidus, or aphasia may occur, depending on the site and nature of the injury.

3. Leptomeningeal cyst—Infants and younger children (usually under age 3) with linear fracture or diastatic suture separation may develop a leptomeningeal cyst—also referred to as cephalhydrocele, spurious cranial meningocele, or "growing skull fracture." This is due to a tear of the dura and arachnoid or entrapment of the arachnoid between the separated bony parts. CSF then accumulates under the scalp, resulting in a fluctuant, often pulsatile swelling which can usually be transilluminated. It should not be aspirated because there is a risk of infection. In some cases, the continued pulsatile effect of the cerebral tissue or loculated fluid causes progressive separation of the bony parts and further damage to the underlying brain. Skull x-rays 2–3 months following the initial trauma usually establish the diagnosis. Early surgical repair of the defect is indicated.

G. Postconcussion Syndrome: The manifestations of the postconcussion syndrome in children vary markedly from those seen in adults. The symptoms also vary with age (preschool, elementary school, older child). The chief complaints usually center around disturbances of behavior (aggressiveness, regression, withdrawal, antisocial acts) and sleep, and may include enuresis, tension phenomena (irritability, emotional lability), phobias (fear of cars, fear of going out alone), and deterioration in school performance. Somatic complaints such as headache, dizziness, tinnitus, and neck pains are relatively uncommon.

Compensation neurosis in children is usually induced by the parents and may cause secondary emotional problems. Repeated questioning by adults concerning somatic symptoms and repeated physical, neurologic, or psychologic examinations may, through suggestion and arousal of anxiety, provoke multiple complaints and behavioral and emotional difficulties in the child.

H. Posttraumatic Mental Retardation: Pseudoretardation (secondary to emotional problems) is not uncommon, but true intellectual loss usually occurs only with very severe injuries. The presence of microcephaly with a head circumference more than 2 SD below the mean for the age at which the accident occurred suggests that mental deficiency antedated the trauma. Psychologic testing may be useful.

Treatment

A. Emergency Measures:

1. Maintain airway and treat shock—See Altered States of Consciousness, above.

2. Anticonvulsants—For status epilepticus, give diazepam (Valium), phenobarbital, or paraldehyde followed by phenobarbital or diphenylhydantoin (Dilantin); the latter is less likely to raise the question of depressing consciousness. (See Seizure Disorders, above.)

B. General Measures:

1. Observation—Careful attention must be paid to level of consciousness, pupillary reactions, and vital signs. Children with severe injuries, loss of consciousness for more than a few minutes, or prolonged and continued seizures must be hospitalized. Most children with mild to moderate concussion need not be hospitalized and can be observed at home if their parents are reliable and live within a reasonable distance from a treatment center. The parents should check the child every few hours, especially to see if the sleeping child can be aroused normally. The parents should maintain telephone contact with the physician, and he should examine the child at least once in the first 24–48 hours after a concussion.

Since the course of epidural hematoma is quite atypical in children, with signs and symptoms often not apparent until more than 24 hours following the head injury, overnight admission of a child lucid on initial examination does not ensure early diagnosis of this serious complication.

Only continued careful observation, maintenance of contact with the parents, and prompt neurologic reevaluation when indicated will ensure early diagnosis of such complications as intracranial hematoma, hydrocephalus, posttraumatic seizures, and leptomeningeal cysts.

2. Restlessness—Diphenhydramine (Benadryl) is often an effective and safe sedative in very young children. Chloral hydrate and paraldehyde may also be used. Do not use opiates or similar compounds such as pentazocine (Talwin).

3. Headache—Give aspirin as necessary in doses appropriate for the size and age of the patient.

4. Fluids—If the child is able to take fluids by mouth, maintain on clear fluids (noncarbonated soft drinks, fruit juices, etc) until it is reasonably certain that vomiting will not occur. Intravenous fluids, if indicated, should be on the low side of maintenance requirements; a slight deficit in the first 3–4 days will counteract cerebral edema and minimize the possibility of water intoxication due to inappropriate ADH secretion.

5. Tetanus prophylaxis—Tetanus toxoid (or tetanus toxoid plus diphtheria toxoid), 0.5 ml, should be given for scalp wounds, particularly if "dirty," and if the child has not had a booster within 4 years.

6. Antibiotics—These are generally best withheld until a specific need arises. With major "dirty" wounds—especially if there is dural tearing, CSF leakage, and extensive cerebral tissue damage—give antibiotics in therapeutic dosages as for purulent meningitis of unknown cause (see Chapter 39).

7. Treatment of cerebral edema—

a. Corticosteroids—The use of methylprednisolone sodium succinate (Solu-Medrol) or dexamethasone-21-phosphate (Decadron phosphate injection) has been advocated to reduce cerebral edema in severe head injuries. Dexamethasone is usually given in a dose of 0.15–0.25 mg/kg IV initially, followed by 0.25 mg/kg/day IM in 3 or 4 doses; it is usually tapered after 72 hours over a 3–4 day period. Methylprednisolone sodium succinate is used in 4–5 times the dose suggested for dexamethasone.

b. Hypertonic solutions—The usefulness of these agents is not clearly established. They have been recommended in the treatment of severe diffuse cerebral edema where no clear-cut structural damage is present. The 2 most widely used agents are urea (1 gm/kg body weight IV every 6–8 hours) and mannitol (1–3 gm/kg body weight IV). The latter may be given repeatedly in smaller doses over several days. Close attention to fluid and electrolyte balance is imperative.

8. Maintenance of normal body temperature—Hypothermia, once favored in the treatment of severe brain injury, is no longer recommended. It is considered safer to maintain normal or nearly normal body temperature. Hyperthermia is often best controlled by covering the child with towels soaked in alcohol and water, using a fan to aid in evaporation.

9. Battering—If clinical and x-ray evidence suggests that the child has been abused, appropriate measures must be taken to ensure social service and psychiatric follow-up (see Chapter 30).

C. Surgical Measures: The chief obligation of the physician caring for the child is early recognition of complications that require prompt diagnostic studies and neurosurgical intervention, eg, extradural hemorrhage, subdural or intracerebral hematoma, posttraumatic hydrocephalus. Many subdural hematomas may be evacuated by "taps" alone.

Note: If there are compelling clinical reasons to suspect epidural hematoma, it is better to relieve pressure surgically immediately than to risk serious delay in treatment by transporting the patient a long distance to a medical center. Major lacerations are best dealt with by the surgeon.

1. Fractures—"Ping-pong ball" skull fractures in very young babies usually correct themselves within a few weeks and require no specific treatment. This is also true of very slightly depressed skull fractures. Depressed fractures involving the inner table of the skull and their accompanying dural and cerebral defects require surgical therapy.

2. Cranioplasty—Repair of major skull defects can often be deferred in young children until the patient is of school age. It is well to remember that the skull attains about 90% of adult growth by 5–6 years of age.

Prognosis

The outlook in children who have suffered head injuries is far better than in adults. Well over 90% of those who sustain concussions and simple linear fractures are free of symptoms after the initial period. Even in severe head trauma, the mortality rate is only about 20%, as compared with 30–35% in adults; similarly, the incidence of neurologic sequelae (including seizures) in such cases is about 20%. Such sequelae are highest in cases of extensive brain laceration (about 40%) and lowest in severe contusions and cerebral edema (about 2–3%). Behavioral and emotional problems constitute the bulk of posttraumatic difficulties in children but normally disappear within a few months or a year.

Bell RS, Loop JW: The utility and futility of radiographic skull examination for trauma. New England J Med 284:236–239, 1971.

Burkinshaw J: Head injuries in children: Observations on their incidence and causes with an enquiry into the value of routine skull x-rays. Arch Dis Child 35:205–214, 1960.

DeVivo DC, Dodge PR: The critically ill child: Diagnosis and management of head injury. Pediatrics 48:129–138, 1971.

Dillon H, Leopold RL: Children and the post-concussion syndrome. JAMA 175:86–92, 1961.

McLaurin RL, Isaacs E, Lewis HP: Results of nonoperative treatment in 15 cases of infantile subdural hematoma. J Neurosurg 34:753–759, 1971.

Mealey JJ: *Pediatric Head Injuries.* Thomas, 1968.

Rabe EF, Flynn RE, Dodge PR: Subdural collections in infants and children. Neurology 18:559–570, 1968.

Shopfner CE, Roberts FF: Skull roentgenograms in children with simple head trauma. Am J Roentgenol. In press.

Silverman D: Electroencephalographic study of acute head injury in children. Neurology 12:273–281, 1962.

Suzuki J, Takaku A: Nonsurgical treatment of chronic subdural hematoma. J Neurosurg 33:548–553, 1970.

PERINATAL HEAD INJURIES

The incidence of head injuries during birth is not known. It has been estimated that such injuries, notably intracranial hemorrhage, account for 3–5 deaths per 1000 live births, or 10–20% of all neonatal deaths. Unlike the violent impact responsible for postnatal head trauma, perinatal injuries are produced by prolonged gradual pressure on the head. A negative pressure gradient as the head goes through the birth canal may play a role. Predisposing or contributing factors include premature birth, cephalopelvic disproportion, shoulder dystocia, breech and precipitate delivery, prolonged labor, and misapplication of forceps or vacuum extractors.

Clinical Findings

A. Symptoms and Signs:

1. Soft tissue injuries—There may be erythema, abrasions, and necrosis of the face and scalp, caput succedaneum, scalpel injuries following cesarian section, or cephalhematoma. The latter usually does not appear until several hours after birth and does not transilluminate; occasionally this subperiosteal hematoma grows so large as to cause symptoms due to hypovolemia.

2. Fractures—Linear skull fractures may be asymptomatic and often are not diagnosed unless accompanied by other findings. About 25% of cephalhematomas are associated with fractures. In occipital fractures with separation of the basal and squamous portions due to undue traction on the hyperextended spine while the head is still fixed in the maternal pelvis during breech delivery, there usually is massive and almost invariably fatal hemorrhage.

3. Intracranial hemorrhage—Tentorial laceration with tearing of the underlying sinuses, rupture of the great vein of Galen, or rupture of veins at the junction of the falx cerebri and tentorium usually results in massive and often fatal hemorrhage.

Rupture of more superiorly placed cerebral veins results in less extensive bleeding, producing subdural hematomas which are more readily diagnosed and treated. Acute subdural hematomas are rare in neonates and result in profound neurologic deficits and depression; subacute and chronic subdural hemorrhages are the rule. Extradural hemorrhage is exceedingly rare during birth.

The clinical manifestations of intracranial bleeding in the newborn are nonspecific, consisting principally of the triad of apneic spells, cyanosis, and convulsions. The neonate may at first be merely listless or floppy, with little spontaneous motor activity; a few hours or a day after delivery, the cry may become shrill ("cerebral cry"), the infant may be jittery or have seizures, muscle tone may become increased, or abnormal postures, including opisthotonos, may be prominent.

The fontanels may be tense and full, the sutures separated widely, the head circumference increased by 1 cm or more (due largely to cerebral edema), and the pupils irregular. Retinal hemorrhages are seen so frequently in infants who do well that no specific conclusions can be drawn from this finding. In neonates, focal neurologic signs are relatively uncommon and usually appear late; these include asymmetry of posture, tone, and reflex responses. The most dependable findings pointing to neurologic damage are persistent asymmetry or absence of the Moro response, marked absence of head control when the infant is pulled gently from the supine into the sitting position (traction response), and poor or absent sucking.

Transillumination is usually negative early since any subdural hematoma is still clotted.

B. Laboratory Findings:

1. Blood—Rapid decreases in the hematocrit or hemoglobin occur with massive bleeding, whether into the subperiosteum or intracranially. Coagulation tests may be abnormal. Hypocalcemia occurs commonly in infants following a traumatic birth, but blood glucose, phosphorus, magnesium, sodium, pH, total CO_2, and P_{CO_2} should also be determined.

2. CSF—Lumbar puncture is imperative. A moderate degree of xanthochromia, 20–50 red cells, and protein up to 150 mg/100 ml are considered by most authorities to be within the limits of normal in neonates; higher values suggest subarachnoid bleeding. A low CSF glucose in the absence of infection is most apt to be due to hypoglycemia, but it occasionally occurs 5–8 days after subarachnoid hemorrhage.

C. Subdural and Ventricular Taps: The subdural tap may yield little or no fluid early, even when there is subdural hematoma, because the blood is clotted. Later, such a tap may not only be diagnostic, but removal of subdural fluid will be therapeutic. Ventricular tap may be indicated when there appears to be intraventricular hemorrhage. It should be performed under experienced supervision.

D. Skull X-Rays: Skull x-rays should be deferred until the infant's condition is stable enough so that adequate views can be obtained; the findings, however, rarely affect management. When depressed skull fractures other than the innocuous "ping-pong ball" type are suspected, tangential views at right angles to the fracture should be obtained to indicate the extent of the depression of bone or bony fragments.

E. Electroencephalography: EEG should be deferred until the infant's condition has stabilized. A "flat" EEG or one with sharply defined paroxysmal activity is a poor prognostic sign. Other abnormalities, such as hemispheric asymmetry or high-amplitude dysrhythmic potentials, are of less prognostic value.

Treatment

Treatment is largely symptomatic. Specific treatment is directed at metabolic and electrolyte disturbances and infections. Anticonvulsants, particularly phenobarbital, 3–5 mg/kg/day IV, should be given for seizures. (See also section on seizure disorders.)

Repeated subdural taps are required in the presence of effusions. Shunting (subdural-peritoneal or subdural-pleural shunts may be necessary) and repeated lumbar punctures (and, rarely, ventricular punctures), particularly when the CSF is grossly bloody, are indicated to relieve irritation or pressure upon vital structures and may improve the infant's status and reduce the frequency and severity of seizures.

Vitamin K_1 (phytonadione), 1 mg IM (if not previously administered to the mother), may be given to the infant with intracranial hemorrhage to reduce the possibility of bleeding associated with vitamin K deficiency.

Significantly depressed skull fractures should be elevated surgically. Most so-called "ping-pong ball" indentations correct themselves as the brain grows.

Prognosis

The prognosis in infants with uncomplicated scalp injuries, linear fractures, "ping-pong ball" depressions, and cephalhematomas is good.

In infants with subacute and chronic subdural hematomas secondary to birth trauma, the prognosis is reasonably good if effusions are evacuated by tapping or by surgical means. However, the incidence of neurologic complications—particularly hydrocephalus, microcephaly, and seizures due to the underlying cortical damage—remains fairly high.

Neonates with major intracranial bleeding who survive frequently have focal neurologic deficits, mental retardation, and seizures. The problem may be compounded by the hypoxia which often initiates or accompanies bleeding.

Focal seizures, especially psychomotor (or "mesial temporal lobe") epilepsy, have been related to the squeezing of the head during the birth process even when there is no significant clinical evidence of trauma at birth. The onset of these seizures may be delayed for many years. Lesser degrees of head trauma may cause minimal cerebral dysfunction.

Gray OP, Ackerman A, Fraser AJ: Intracranial haemorrhage and clotting defects in low-birth-weight infants. Lancet 1:545–548, 1968.

Haller ES, Nesbitt REL, Anderson GW: Clinical and pathologic concepts of gross intracranial hemorrhage in perinatal mortality. Obst Gynec Surv 11:179–204, 1956.

Towbin A: Organic causes of minimal brain dysfunction. JAMA 217: 1207–1214, 1971.

TUMORS OF THE CNS

1. INTRACRANIAL TUMORS

Essentials of Diagnosis

- Focal neurologic deficits, usually slowly progressive.
- Increased intracranial pressure with unremitting headache, vomiting, and papilledema.
- Space-occupying lesion demonstrated by neurodiagnostic studies or at operation.

General Considerations

Malignancies are (after accidents) the second most frequent causes of death in children over age 1, and CNS tumors, usually infratentorial, are second only to the leukemias among neoplasms. For a variety of reasons, specific diagnosis may be delayed for 6 months or more.

The histologic types of brain tumors found in children are as follows:

(1) Gliomas (about 70%–80% of **all** brain tumors in children): (a) astrocytomas, especially of the cerebellum (30% of the total); (b) medulloblastomas (almost 50% of infratentorial tumors of childhood; 20% of gliomas); (c) brain stem gliomas, ependymomas, and malignant gliomas of childhood (variants of the glioblastoma multiforme of adults; each representing nearly 10% of childhood CNS tumors); and (d) gliomas of the optic nerves and chiasm (3–4%).

(2) Craniopharyngiomas (about 10%).

(3) Choroid plexus papillomas (about 3%).

(4) Other tumor types are relatively rare.

Meningiomas, acoustic neurinomas, and pituitary adenomas are rare in children. With the exception of leukemic infiltration, tumors metastatic to the brain are also uncommon; they include neuroblastoma, Wilms's tumor, and Ewing's sarcoma.

Clinical Findings (See Table 21–3.)

A. Symptoms and Signs:

1. Signs of increased intracranial pressure—These include headache, vomiting, abducens palsy, diplopia, papilledema, and, in very young children, a bulging fontanel or greater than normal increase in head circumference. These signs may be due either to obstruction of CSF flow with resulting hydrocephalus or to the tumor mass itself.

2. Focal neurologic signs—Infratentorial (especially cerebellar) tumors most commonly manifest themselves by ataxia, nystagmus, and signs and symptoms of increased intracranial pressure. Supratentorial hemispheric tumors may be manifested by progressive neurologic deficits such as contralateral hemiparesis and spasticity and by seizures; young children rarely are aware of sensory deficits. Visual difficulties, particularly hemianopsias, are rarely reported by young children but may be demonstrated in them by opticokinetic testing or by playing with them, bringing targets into the peripheral field while having the child fix on another object in front. Progressive speech difficulties, particularly when coupled with seizures, point to involvement of the left frontotemporal or parietal lobe. Severe weight loss may occur in diencephalic, cerebellar, brain stem, and intraventricular tumors; marked obesity is sometimes seen in tumors involving the anterior third ventricle and hypothalamus.

Skin lesions may be present, eg, café au lait spots, amelanotic patches, and other stigmas of neurocutaneous dysplasia, in which there is a high incidence of brain tumor of all types.

B. Laboratory Findings: Endocrine status should be assessed if pituitary and hypothalamic involvement is suspected or evident. *Note:* Lumbar puncture for CSF examination is rarely justified—and usually contraindicated—when brain tumor is suspected. CSF obtained at the time of neuroradiologic studies or surgical intervention should be cultured and studied. Cytologic examination of CSF may reveal the presence of tumor cells, as in medulloblastoma, ependymoma, or leptomeningeal sarcoma. CSF protein may be elevated, particularly with malignant gliomas. CSF glucose may be low in the absence of infection when there is extensive meningeal infiltration by tumor, as in leukemia, medulloblastoma, pineal sarcoma, or melanosarcoma.

C. X-Ray Findings:

1. Skull x-rays may show signs of increased intracranial pressure, such as splitting of sutures in younger children and erosion of the posterior clinoids and thinning of sphenoid ridges in older children. Intracranial calcifications are found in the suprasellar region in craniopharyngiomas and also occur, usually asymmetrically, in oligodendrogliomas and other tumors. Enlargement of the optic foramens (> 8 mm) and a strikingly J-, pear-, or banana-shaped sella are seen in optic gliomas. Pineal shifts are rarely encountered on x-rays in children because of the rarity of pineal calcification at this age.

2. Isotopic scanning is becoming increasingly more useful, even in the diagnosis of infratentorial tumors; however, a negative scan does not rule out the presence of tumor.

3. Cerebral angiography via the right brachial, femoral, or carotid artery is often the procedure of choice in the face of increased intracranial pressure and nonspecific or absent focal neurologic findings. For a suspected tumor of a cerebral hemisphere, carotid angiography of the same side should be performed.

4. Ventriculography is most commonly employed, either alone or following angiography, where hydrocephalus is evident and midline tumors, both infra- and supratentorial, are suspected. Contrast medium, such as Pantopaque, is instilled occasionally for better visualization of the posterior third ventricle, the aqueduct, or the fourth ventricle.

5. Pneumoencephalography is of value in lesions not causing increased intracranial pressure, as is usually the case with brain stem glioma, optic glioma, or craniopharyngioma, and for better definition of infratentorial lesions following ventriculography.

Note: Fractional pneumoencephalography, using small amounts of air without removal of fluid and with a surgeon and operating room available, is performed in many centers today even in the presence of increased intracranial pressure.

D. Electroencephalography may show focal slowing and is of localizing value in about 70% of supratentorial tumors. False localization may occur. In infratentorial tumors, the EEG may merely show generalized slowing in the occipital and temporal regions or bifrontal slowing.

E. Echoencephalography may be helpful in rapidly determining the presence of hydrocephalus, third ventricle shift, or the presence of subdural effusions.

Differential Diagnosis

A clinical picture similar to that of brain tumor, with a history of insidious onset and progressive, unremitting course, headache, vomiting, seizures, and focal neurologic deficits, may be produced by any of the following disorders: subdural hematoma, toxic encephalopathies (eg, lead, uremia), "pseudotumor cerebri" of varying causation, brain abscess, tuberculoma or other granuloma, encephalitides (eg, herpes simplex), degenerative CNS diseases, and slowly expanding or "leaking" cerebrovascular malformations. These can usually be differentiated by appropriate diagnostic studies.

Treatment

A. Surgical Treatment: Total extirpation is the procedure of choice if the location and type of tumor permit. Other types of surgical treatment are partial removal or biopsy, surgical decompression, and shunting procedures for relief of CSF obstruction.

B. Radiation Therapy: Radiation therapy is indicated in conjunction with surgery in many tumors. It is of particular importance to give radiation therapy along the entire neuraxis in medulloblastoma after the diagnosis has been confirmed by biopsy. Radiation therapy is given alone for intrinsic tumors of the brain stem and those around the pineal gland and quadrigeminal plate. In the latter instances, shunting for relief of obstructive hydrocephalus may first be necessary.

C. Antitumor Chemotherapy: Methotrexate, 0.5 mg/kg body weight intrathecally, about every fifth day until no cells are seen in the CSF, has been used in medulloblastoma, meningeal sarcoma, and leukemia. Intraventricular perfusion of methotrexate, with removal of perfusant from the lumbar subarachnoid space, is a recently introduced procedure. Other agents, some still in the experimental stage, are being used with increasing frequency.

D. Replacement Hormone Therapy: This is usually required in craniopharyngiomas and pituitary and hypothalamic tumors. Corticosteroids (especially dexamethasone) may be given prior to and for a few days following surgery to reduce cerebral edema. (See sections on altered states of consciousness and head injuries for details.)

E. Anticonvulsants: Anticonvulsants are given as outlined in the section on seizure disorders. In general, phenobarbital, diphenylhydantoin, and primidone (singly or in combination) are the drugs of choice for seizures due to brain tumors.

F. Emergency Medical (Osmotic Diuretic) Treatment for Increased Intracranial Pressure: Give mannitol, 15–20% solution, about 1 gm/kg body weight by push IV; or urea, 1 gm/kg body weight by push IV. The usual duration of effect of these diuretics is about 4–8 hours; the dose may be repeated on indication. Follow osmotic diuretics with dexamethasone.

Prognosis (See Table 21–3.)

The overall operative mortality rate is about 5%. The older the child and the less malignant the tumor, the better the outlook.

A. Benign Tumors: (About 47% of cases.) Total excision is essentially curative. In suprasellar tumors, a normal life span but with neurologic and endocrine

TABLE 21–3. Brain tumors.

Part Affected	Symptoms and Signs	Radiologic Findings	Tumor Type and Characteristics	Treatment and Prognosis
Cerebellum and fourth ventricle	Evidence of increased intracranial pressure.* Cerebellar signs.† Signs due to pressure on adjacent structures.‡ Personality and behavioral changes. Occasionally emaciation.	1. Signs of increased intracranial pressure on skull films.§ 2. Brain scan of posterior fossa may be helpful. 3. Ventriculography (or positive pressure encephalography) may show tumor and hydrocephalus. 4. Brachial angiography often useful in demonstrating hydrocephalus, abnormal vascular patterns, and herniation.	1. Astrocytoma: slow growth, frequently cystic.	Surgical removal. Follow by intensive x-ray therapy if removal is incomplete. Prognosis good if removal complete.
			2. Medulloblastoma: rapid growth, seen most at age 2–6 years, about 75% in boys; seeds along CSF pathways.	Surgical decompression of posterior fossa and x-ray therapy to site, cerebrum, and spinal canal. Chemotherapy. Shunt (ventriculopleural, etc) to relieve CSF obstruction. Prognosis grave: rare 5-year survivors.
			3. Less common: ependymoma, hemangioblastoma, choroid plexus papilloma.	Surgical cure possible with hemangioblastoma and choroid plexus papilloma.
Brain stem	1. Cranial nerve palsies (IX-X, VII, VI, V–chiefly sensory root), pyramidal tract signs (hemiparesis), and cerebellar ataxia. 2. Rarely, signs of increased intracranial pressure or emaciation.	Pneumoencephalographic demonstration of posterior fossa and displacement of aqueduct of Sylvius and fourth ventricle.	Astrocytoma (varying grades; polar spongioblastoma): usually rapid growth and recurrence.	X-ray therapy to site: remission rare for short periods. Prognosis grave: average survival 1 year, particularly when medulla is involved.
Midbrain and third ventricle	1. Personality and behavioral changes, often early. 2. Evidence of increased intracranial pressure.* 3. Pyramidal tract signs and cerebellar signs.† 4. Inability to rotate eyes upward. 5. Sudden loss of consciousness; seizures rare.	1. Signs of increased intracranial pressure on skull films. 2. Brain scan and echoencephalography helpful. 3. Air and contrast ventriculography in third ventricle masses. 4. Pineal rarely calcified in childhood.	Astrocytomas, teratomas including pinealoma (macrogenitosomia praecox in boys), ependymoma.	Shunt procedure (ventriculocisternal, etc) for relief of CSF obstruction and intensive x-ray therapy. Prognosis poor.
			Choroid plexus papilloma and colloid cyst (rare).	With total surgical removal, prognosis good.
Diencephalon	1. Emaciated; good intake. 2. Often very active, euphoric. 3. Few neurologic findings: occasional vertical nystagmus, tremor, ataxia. 4. Pale; without anemia. 5. Frequently: eosinophilia, decreased PBI and pituitary reserve.	Pneumoencephalography shows defect in floor of third ventricle and other midline findings. Echoencephalography may be useful. Brain scan, EEG, and angiography usually nondiagnostic.	Usually astrocytomas; less common, oligodendroglioma, glioma, ependymoma, glioblastoma.	X-ray treatment. CSF shunt for block. Prognosis variable; generally poor.
Suprasellar region	1. Visual disorders (visual field defects, optic atrophy). 2. Hypothalamic disorders (including diabetes insipidus, adiposity). 3. Pituitary disorders (growth arrest, hypothyroidism, delayed sexual maturation). 4. Evidence of increased intracranial pressure.*	1. Skull films: suprasellar calcification in about 90%. Deformity of sella turcica frequent. Enlarged optic foramens in optic gliomas. 2. Pneumoencephalography in absence of increased intracranial pressure; otherwise, ventriculography.	Optic glioma: high incidence of café au lait spots.	X-ray if optic chiasm is involved. Surgical removal if only optic nerve is involved. Prognosis is fair to good. Conservative approach advised.
			Craniopharyngioma: often dormant for years.	Complete excision of craniopharyngioma with hormone replacement is now often feasible; or drainage of cyst and irradiation. Prognosis with complete removal is good.

TABLE 21−3 (cont'd). Brain tumors.

Part Affected	Symptoms and Signs	Radiologic Findings	Tumor Type and Characteristics	Treatment and Prognosis
Cerebral hemispheres and lateral ventricles	1. Evidence of increased intracranial pressure.* 2. Seizures (generalized, psychomotor, focal) in about 40%. 3. Neurologic deficits include hemiparesis (40%), visual field defects, ataxia, personality changes.	1. Signs of increased intracranial pressure. Occasionally calcifications. 2. Angiography preferred where lateralizing signs present. 3. Brain scan may be helpful, as may be echoencephalogram and EEG. 4. Ventriculography, especially for lesions in ventricles. 5. Pneumoencephalography if there is no increased pressure.	Gliomas; primary astrocytomas; glioblastomas in 10%. Meningiomas rare. Leptomeningeal sarcoma.	Surgical biopsy or excision where possible. X-ray treatment. Prognosis varies with tumor type. Chemotherapy gaining in trial and usage.
			Ependymoma and choroid plexus papilloma.	Surgical excision of choroid plexus papilloma; occasionally, hydrocephalus persists and requires shunt procedure.

*Evidence of increased intracranial pressure includes headache, vomiting (often without nausea, and before breakfast), diplopia, blurred vision, papilledema; personality changes, including irritability, apathy, disturbances in sleep and eating patterns, are frequent. Sudden enlargement of the head if head circumferences have been plotted is detectable when sutures are still open or after sutures have split. Alterations of consciousness. Stiff neck with tonsillar herniation.

†Cerebellar signs: ataxia, dysmetria, nystagmus. Truncal ataxia in absence of lateralizing signs most common in vermis tumors.

‡Signs due to pressure on adjacent structures: for posterior fossa, may include head tilting, cranial nerve signs, pyramidal tract signs, suboccipital tenderness, stiff neck.

§X-ray findings of increased intracranial pressure: splitting of sutures, erosion of posterior clinoids and thinning of sphenoid wings. Increased digital markings unreliable.

impairment is common following surgery or irradiation (or both).

B. Malignant Tumors: (About 53% of cases.) Particularly in medulloblastoma, brain stem glioma, and most ependymomas, death within 1−5 years of diagnosis is the usual outcome. Advances in radiation and chemotherapy are improving this outlook.

Matson DD: Neoplasm, cranial and intracranial. Pages 403−642 in: *Neurosurgery of Infancy and Childhood*, 2nd ed. Thomas, 1969.

Panitch HS, Berg BO: Brain stem tumors of childhood and adolescence. Am J Dis Child 119:465−472, 1970.

2. SPINAL CORD TUMORS

The low incidence of spinal cord tumors in children often results in serious delay in diagnosis.

Such tumors may be extra- or intramedullary and include dermoid cysts, teratomas, neuroblastomas, astrocytomas, ependymomas, and other types.

Symptoms and signs usually progress more slowly than in transverse myelitis or other causes of acute flaccid paralysis (Table 21−8) and include disturbances of gait, pain in the back and legs (more common in extramedullary tumors), weakness and disturbances of

sensation in the legs, and urinary incontinence of recent origin.

Neurologic findings—often symmetrical with intramedullary and asymmetrical with extramedullary tumors and varying with their site and extent—include curvature of the spine and localized tenderness; weakness, spasms, sensory deficits, and pathologic reflexes of the lower extremities; and dribbling of urine and loss of anal sphincter tone. Café au lait spots suggest neurofibromatosis. Some forms of spinal dysraphism (see below) may behave like spinal cord tumors.

The diagnosis is made roentgenographically. In 70% of patients, spine films show destructive changes of the vertebra involved; chest x-rays, which should always be obtained, show pulmonary metastases and rib erosion in almost 30% of cases.

Myelography is the procedure of choice for localization of the tumor, but it may have to be performed via a cisternal tap as well as from the usual lumbar site. Where the history extends over only hours or 1−2 days, transverse myelitis is more likely; this may be aggravated by myelography. The CSF may be xanthochromic, with a high protein content, and may contain tumor cells on cytologic examination.

With benign tumors, total excision and cure is often possible. In malignant tumors, decompressive laminectomy, partial excision, irradiation, and chemotherapy are employed, but the prognosis is poor.

TABLE 21–4. Cerebrovascular disorders in childhood.

	Dural Sinus and Cerebral Venous Thrombosis	Arterial Thrombosis	Cerebral Embolism	Intracranial Hemorrhage (Primary Intracerebral and Subarachnoid)
Onset	Usually less sudden and clear-cut than in arterial occlusive disease. Usually unrelated to activity.	Sudden, but prodromal episodes may occur. Unrelated to activity.	Sudden onset; no prodrome. Unrelated to activity.	Sudden onset; severe headache, vomiting, loss of consciousness. Related to activity.
Underlying conditions	Pyogenic infections of leptomeninges and cranial structures (ear, face, sinuses). Marasmic states and severe dehydration. Congenital heart disease. Blood dyscrasias (sickle cell disease, polycythemia, thrombotic thrombocytopenia). Lead and other toxic encephalopathies. Trauma. Metastatic tumor. Sturge-Weber disease.	"Idiopathic" (hemiplegia in infancy). Cyanotic congenital heart disease. Inflammatory disease of arteries: "collagen" diseases, granulomatous (Takayasu's), acute infections, syphilis. Trauma or extrinsic compression. Dissecting aneurysm. Arteriosclerosis (progeria). Thrombotic phenomenon: homocystinuria.	Atrial fibrillation and other "arrhythmias": congenital heart disease (R→L shunt), rheumatic heart disease. Acute or subacute bacterial endocarditis. Air: complications of heart, neck, or chest surgery. Fat: complications of fractures of bone, heart surgery. Septic: pneumonia or lung abscess (especially in congenital heart disease). Newborn: infarcted necrotic placental tissue. Tumor. Coronary.	Trauma: birth (intraventricular), subdural hemorrhage, epidural hemorrhage, cavernous sinus fistula. Vascular malformations: arteriovenous, angiomas, aneurysms. Hemorrhagic disorders (leukemia, aplastic anemia, hemophilia, thrombocytopenic/anaphylactoid purpura, liver disease, vitamin deficiencies [K, C, B$_1$], anticonvulsants). Hypertensive encephalopathy (chronic renal disease, acute glomerulonephritis, pheochromocytoma). Toxic or infectious encephalopathy. Intracranial tumors.
Neurologic findings	Altered state of consciousness. Increased intracranial pressure. Focal neurologic deficits (leg, arm). Seizures, focal and generalized.	Seizures, frequently focal. Focal neurologic deficits. Behavioral and intellectual changes. Rapid improvement at times.	Transient loss of consciousness common. Seizures, often focal. Focal neurologic deficits (sometimes multiple). Rapid improvement at times.	Consciousness commonly lost; may be regained quickly. Marked meningeal signs (not seen in neonate). Focal neurologic deficits. Seizures, generalized and focal.
Special clinical clues	Lateral dural sinus: mastoiditis. Superior sagittal sinus: caput medusae. Cavernous sinus: homolateral exophthalmos, periorbital edema, palsies of cranial nerves III, IV, VI, and V.	Inflammatory disease: multifocal involvement common. Takayasu's: pulseless upper limbs. Somatic constitution (progeria, arachnodactyly). Signs of trauma.	Emboli to other organs (spleen, kidneys, lungs). Air embolism: transient blindness. Fat embolism: respiratory distress, blood-tinged sputum in postoperative period, fat droplets in urine, retinal vessels.	Trauma (hemorrhage, subhyaloid hemorrhages, bruises, fractures on x-rays). Malformations: bruit, heart failure, hydrocephalus, cutaneous stigmas. Previous seizures/neurologic deficit. Coarctation/polycystic kidney. Hemorrhagic diathesis: skin, joints, gastrointestinal tract, newborn. Hypertensive encephalopathy: blood pressure elevated, uremia.
Skull x-rays	Signs of increased intracranial pressure within days or a few weeks, depending on age. Sinus involvement or lytic lesion.	Early: usually normal. Later: hypertrophy of skull on atrophic side of brain. Tumor. Dysplasia. Foreign body.	Normal.	Skull fractures. Characteristic calcifications. Signs of increased intracranial pressure/hydrocephalus. Deep groove in inner table from enlarged vein.
CSF	Findings vary with primary process. Protein often elevated. Sometimes bloody. If PMNs are present, suspect infection.	Early: usually normal. Later: slight monocytic pleocytosis and protein elevation.	Usually normal. Some pleocytosis and protein elevation in bacterial endocarditis.	Bloody CSF all tubes, xanthochromic supernatant. Protein elevated. Sugar may be decreased. Fluid may be clear if hemorrhage is intracerebral only.
Neuroradiologic findings	Angiogram on venous phase or sinogram may show obstruction site. Sinogram may be dangerous.	Angiography early may show occlusion or narrowing. (Later studies usually negative.)	Angiography usually normal as emboli commonly lodge in small peripheral vessels.	Angiography usually able to identify subdural and epidural hematoma, site and type of malformation, intracerebral tumor, clot.
Other studies	Echoencephalography may show midline shift. EEG may show diffuse or focal slowing. Brain scan may show increased uptake. None of these studies are sufficiently specific to obviate the need for other diagnostic—especially angiographic—studies.			

Haft H, Ransohoff J, Carter S: Spinal cord tumors in children. Pediatrics 23:1152–1159, 1959.

CEREBROVASCULAR DISORDERS

General Considerations

About 1–1.5% of all admissions to teaching hospitals (or 5% of pediatric neurologic disorders) are due to cerebrovascular disorders. Intracerebral vascular disease accounts for 17% of pediatric necropsies. About 1/2 of children with leukemia have intracranial bleeding. Homocystinuria is also increasingly recognized as a cause of cerebrovascular accidents.

The deficits in children tend to be more often global or multifocal but also more difficult to demonstrate angiographically than strokes in adults.

Acute hemiplegias in childhood. The special circumstances of this syndrome—often termed acute infantile hemiplegia as if it were a single pathologic entity—require additional description. The essential feature is the relatively rapid acquisition of hemiplegia in a previously neurologically intact child. The syndrome appears most often between 1 month and 6 years of age (usually under 3 years). The onset may be sudden or may evolve over a period of minutes to 1 or 2 days, frequently with an intermittent ("stuttering") progression. Cerebral vasculitis with resultant intravascular thrombosis is considered the principal cause, but it may be difficult to demonstrate angiographically. The syndrome occurs most often in association with infections of the upper respiratory tract and, next most commonly, with head trauma and with blunt injuries to the internal carotid artery or its surrounding tissues. Almost any of the conditions underlying cerebrovascular disorders in childhood (Table 21–4) may be responsible. Frequently, however, no cause can be identified; this has led to the term idiopathic infantile hemiplegia.

Clinical Findings

A. Symptoms and Signs: These are highly variable, depending on the nature, site, and extent of the lesion. Alterations in level of consciousness, disturbances of sensorium, mood, behavior, and of cognitive and perceptual functions, the frequency of seizures, and the more widespread nature of the deficits in younger children may make it difficult to pinpoint the lesions clinically. (See Table 21–4 for a guide to the diagnosis of cerebrovascular disorders in childhood.)

Fever is observed frequently and may be part of an underlying or associated systemic disorder or may be of central origin. Vasomotor disturbances of involved extremities may be observed.

Retinal hemorrhages may occur with sudden increases in intracranial pressure, as in subarachnoid hemorrhage or from subdural hematomas, but should raise the suspicion of head trauma—especially child battering.

Seizures, which may be focal but frequently become generalized, occur in 50% or more of patients. They may precede, accompany, or follow the onset of other neurologic (especially motor) deficits.

In **acute hemiplegia,** the hemiplegia may be flaccid initially. Spasticity usually appears within a few days to 2 weeks. The right side is involved more frequently than the left. Hemianopsia and hemisensory deficits are also often present. The seizures may remain entirely confined to the involved side, resulting in the "hemiplegia-hemiepilepsy" (HHE) syndrome.

B. Laboratory Findings: Blood count, sedimentation rate, urinalysis, and electrolytes are usually normal; when grossly abnormal, they tend to reflect an underlying systemic disease rather than cerebrovascular accident.

Special studies as suggested by clinical indices may include screening for blood dyscrasias, including coagulation and cysteine screening tests, LE cell preparations, or renal function studies. Bacterial, serologic, and virologic studies should be performed in all cases associated with an inflammatory process.

Lumbar puncture should be performed in the presence of fever and meningeal signs to rule out treatable forms of intracranial infections. Except when these findings dominate the clinical picture, lumbar puncture may well be deferred until x-ray studies have shown that tentorial or tonsillar herniation is unlikely. CSF opening and closing pressures should be recorded. The color of the fluid and the distribution of erythrocytes from the initial drops to the last aliquot obtained should be carefully noted. For a differential evaluation of the findings, see Tables 21–1 and 21–4.

C. X-Ray Findings: Skull films are mandatory to rule out evidence of long-standing increased intracranial pressure, calcifications, or fractures. Chest films and a skeletal survey are often indicated—the latter especially in younger children when child abuse is suspected.

Cerebral angiography is the definitive procedure and should be performed as early as possible after the onset of symptoms. It can be done percutaneously even in small infants by those skilled in the procedure. If bilateral involvement is suspected or the possibility of an arteriovenous malformation with multiple feeding vessels exists, retrograde brachial or femoral arteriography may be most informative. In children with congenital heart disease who have had a vascular accident, cerebral angiography may be done at the time of cardiac catheterization by advancing the catheter into the aortic arch and then injecting a bolus of dye. In acute hemiplegia, carotid angiography may demonstrate occlusion of the internal carotid artery or one of the major cerebral vessels—most commonly the middle cerebral artery or one of its branches; or it may show the "beading" typical of arteritis. The pattern may be diagnostic of a space-occupying lesion such as subdural hematoma.

D. Other Neurodiagnostic Studies: EEG is helpful in assessing the effectiveness of anticonvulsant therapy but is of little help in differential diagnosis. (See

Seizure Disorders, above.) Echoencephalography may disclose a shift of midline structures and other intracranial volume changes. Isotopic brain scan may disclose the presence and extent of the lesion or lesions and may be useful in following their resolution.

For subdural and (rarely justifiable) ventricular taps, see Head Injuries (above).

E. Electrocardiography: ECG is indicated where there is clinical evidence of heart disease, hypertension, or an arteriovenous malformation which may be causing a work overload of the heart.

Differential Diagnosis

A. Postictal (Todd's) Paralysis: Focal motor paralysis lasting 2–3 days may follow seizures which are entirely focal or of focal onset.

B. "Cerebral Palsy" with Hemiplegia: Parents sometimes become aware of the presence of hemiplegia or other neurologic deficits only when the child is ill or has his first seizure. The findings of early spasticity—and particularly of atrophy of affected limbs—favor an old deficit, often congenital or of perinatal onset.

C. Other Causes: Focal neurologic deficits, including hemiplegia, may appear suddenly with a variety of inflammatory conditions of the brain, including meningitis, encephalitis, and brain abscess. With CNS tumors, degenerative processes such as Schilder's diffuse sclerosis or multiple sclerosis, or with "slow virus" infections, the deficits are usually slower to evolve than in cerebrovascular disorders but may be apoplectic in onset. In the case of neoplasm, neurologic deficits are usually due to hemorrhage.

Complications

The complications may be those of the underlying disease process. Frequent complications include seizures (particularly generalized status epilepticus), pneumonia, coma, decubiti, contractures, and other injuries of the affected parts, and hydrocephalus.

Treatment

A. General Measures: Careful attention must be paid to airway, fluid and electrolyte balance, and infections. (See Altered States of Consciousness, above.) Anticonvulsant therapy should be administered from the start (even to children who do not present with seizures) because they occur in about 50% or more of cases, especially with acute hemiplegia. The preferred drug is phenobarbital, 3–5. mg/kg/day in 3 divided doses orally, by slow IV drip, or IM. Once seizures (especially status epilepticus) appear, control may be difficult and may require intravenous diazepam (Valium), paraldehyde, and diphenylhydantoin in appropriate doses. If the child has no seizures during the acute phase and none the following year, anticonvulsant therapy may then be gradually discontinued.

Dexamethasone or other corticosteroids should be given to reduce cerebral edema (see Head Injuries, above). Long-term corticosteroid therapy may be indicated in children with arteritis due to lupus erythematosus, polyarteritis nodosa, pulseless disease, and other angiopathies.

Measures to lower systemic hypertension should be employed with caution. Too sudden a drop in arterial pressure may precipitate further cerebral hypoxia.

B. Specific Measures: These depend on the underlying condition and may include heparinization for multiple embolic phenomena or consumption coagulopathies, antibiotics for bacterial infections, and multiple tapping of a subdural hematoma.

C. Neurosurgical Measures: In addition to drainage of subdural hematomas (often performed by pediatricians), specific neurosurgical measures include removal of a large intracerebral clot, endarterectomy of a stenosed carotid artery and removal of thrombus; clipping, trapping, coating, or possibly "embolization" of an aneurysm; extirpation of an accessible arteriovenous malformation; excision or biopsy of a tumor; drainage of a brain abscess; or shunting for hydrocephalus.

D. Long-Term Management: In addition to anticonvulsant treatment, educational, psychologic, physical, and speech therapy are often required.

Corticectomy or hemispherectomy should be considered in children with intractable focal seizures when residual hemiparesis and hemianopsia will not be increased by surgery. In young children, even removal of the left or dominant hemisphere will not cause permanent aphasia; behavioral and functional improvement may also result.

Prognosis

The course may be brief, with complete recovery. Death may occur, depending on the precipitating cause or complications.

Residual motor and sensory deficits are common, especially with hemiplegias which occur at an early age. The upper extremity tends to be more involved than the lower. Visual field and parietal lobe defects—initially not diagnosable in young children—often become apparent later and contribute to the learning disabilities.

Seizures—mostly focal, but also other types—persist in these children.

Impairment of mental abilities roughly parallels the frequency and severity of seizure disorders. In about 3/4 of cases there are learning disabilities, hyperactivity, disturbances of behavior, and other signs of "maturational lag."

Speech is usually least affected permanently. Even when the left hemisphere is involved, the prognosis for normal speech is good in children under age 5 or 6 except as influenced by whatever overall retardation the child may have suffered. In older children, some expressive aphasic difficulties may persist.

Adeloge A & others: Intracranial ventricular haemorrhage as a first presentation of haemophilia. J Neurol Neurosurg Psychiat 32:470–473, 1969.

Banker BQ: Cerebral vascular disease in infancy and childhood. 1. Occlusive vascular disease. J Neuropath Exper Neurol 20:127–140, 1961.

Bax M, Mitchell R: *Acute Hemiplegia in Childhood.* Little Club Clinics In Developmental Medicine, No. 6. Heinemann, 1962.

Hilal SK & others: Primary cerebral arterial occlusive disease in childhood. I: Acute acquired hemiplegia. Radiology 99:71–86; 93–94, 1971.

Taveras JM: Multiple progressive intracranial arterial occlusions: A syndrome of children and young adults. Am J Roentgenol 106:235–268, 1969.

MALFORMATIONS OF THE CNS

1. SPINAL DYSRAPHISM

Essentials of Diagnosis
- Any defect of fusion in the dorsal midline.
- May be cutaneous, vertebral, meningeal, or neural.

General Considerations

Developmental anomalies involving the spinal cord and its coverings are extremely common. Damage to the embryo varies according to when such clefts occur; where they are located; whether they are single or multiple, partial or complete in dividing both the inner and outer limiting neural membranes; whether they are incipient, closed or "healing," or expanding; and how these clefts and their sequelae affect other structures in embryonic life or later.

As a matter of considerable clinical practicality, the various forms of spinal dysraphism can be grouped into (1) noncystic forms, in which there is no hernial protrusion of the meninges of the cord, and (2) cystic forms, with herniation of the meninges through a defect of the neural arch in which the hernial sac contains CSF (meningocele) and often also nervous tissue (meningomyelocele).

The incidence of those forms of neural clefts without meningeal protrusion is not known. Vestigial or primarily superficial manifestations, such as dermal dimples and sinuses, vascular nevi, and abnormal tufts of hair are extremely common. Spina bifida occulta, often an incidental x-ray finding, is estimated to occur in up to 25% of younger children in whom the posterior vertebral arches will eventually fuse, and in about 5% or more of all individuals. Spina bifida cystica occurs in about 2 per 1000 births, with one meningomyelocele per 800 births. Many environmental causes, including viral and irradiation injuries to the embryo, have been implicated epidemiologically and experimentally. Genetic factors may play a role, eg, in spina bifida cystica the family history is positive in about 8% of cases.

Clinical Findings

A. Symptoms and Signs:

1. Cutaneous manifestations—

a. Noncystic—In noncystic forms of spinal dysraphism, these may consist of a skin depression or dermal dimple, which may also mark the outlet of a fistulous or fibrous tract extending to the meninges and representing a dermal sinus. On close inspection, a tiny pore may be seen. There may be chronic or intermittent drainage of a whitish secretion from such a sinus; this may lead to cystic dilatation if the sinus is partially obliterated. Commonly seen also in the midline as evidence of dysraphism are port wine angiomatous nevi; tufts or patches or even tails of hair, which may be long and coarse, sometimes silky, and often dark in blond children; and subcutaneous diffuse, soft lipomatous lesions. Such superficial stigmas may be absent, may appear singly or in close but variable association, or may even "split" on each side of the midline.

b. Cystic—Cystic defects are usually detected on inspection at birth, but occasionally the overlying skin is so thick that detection is delayed. A large vascular nevus, lipoma, or abnormal growth of hair may be associated superficial findings. The differentiation between meningocele and meningomyelocele is usually made by noting the absence (meningocele) or presence of neurologic deficits or the presence of neural elements on transillumination of the sac, or by eliciting reflex responses upon tapping the sac gently; but in some instances a definite diagnosis can only be established by means of surgical exploration. Pressure on the sac may cause the anterior fontanel to bulge. An exception to these statements must be made for the rare neurenteric cysts (see below), in which no superficial lesions are frequently present.

2. Orthopedic manifestations—Plainly visible or palpable anomalies of the spinal column may include scoliosis, those associated with Klippel-Feil syndrome, and occasionally bifid vertebra; in many instances, however, the abnormalities are seen only on x-ray (see below). Deformities of the feet or legs are the most common (and may be the only) evidence of noncystic spinal dysraphism. They may be highly variable in extent and kind and stationary or progressive depending upon the degree of neurologic deficit. There may be a marked difference in size between the 2 legs or feet, inversion (clubfoot) or eversion, and pes cavus or pes cavovarus. Dislocation of the hips may also be present. As would be expected from the low incidence of dysraphism involving primarily the cervical cord, the upper extremities are far less commonly involved.

3. Motor disturbances—The orthopedic manifestations are often accompanied by muscle weakness and reflex disturbances. The nature and extent depend entirely on the lesion in the spinal cord and roots and help to identify the anatomic site. Particularly in such noncystic forms as diastematomyelia (see below)—and in symptomatic spina bifida occulta and "tethering" of the cord—the first signs may appear between 2 and 8 years of age in the form of progressive leg weakness and gait disturbance. In meningomyelocele, the legs may be partially, asymmetrically, or totally paralyzed and areflexic from birth.

4. Urinary and rectal disturbances—Atonic bladder (with dribbling) and poor anal sphincter tone are commonly present at birth in lumbosacral meningo-myeloceles. In noncystic forms of dysraphism, urinary incontinence usually appears after the disturbances of gait and reflects pressure on or traction of the lower cord (or both) by an adherent lipoma or other connective tissue; loss of voluntary control of the anal sphincter in these types is less common but may occur in time. When urinary incontinence is present, intravenous urography may disclose the presence of various upper genitourinary anomalies.

5. Cerebral malformations—Disturbances of brain growth with noncystic forms are relatively infrequent but may occur. With cystic forms, encephalic anomalies are far more common; hydrocephalus occurs in 65% of cases with meningomyelocele, almost invariably in association with some form of Arnold-Chiari malformation, and in 10% of meningoceles. Encephalocele, schizencephaly, cyclopia, and often microcephaly also represent aspects of dysraphism of the neuraxis; indeed, it is not unusual to find a hydrocephalic brain which, after shunting or on postmortem examination, turns out to be microcephalic. A frequent finding in such cases is mental retardation.

6. Sensory deficits—Disturbances of sensation commonly parallel the motor deficits in meningo-myelocele, where the upper level of the defect may be demonstrated by pricking the infant's skin; wrinkling or corrugation denotes an intact dermatome. In noncystic forms of dysraphism, sensory disturbances are much less common; where there is pressure or traction on the cord, there may be loss of pain leading to neurogenic arthropathies (Charcot joints). Trophic disturbances of the skin may also be seen.

B. Laboratory Findings: Abnormal findings relate principally to the 2 major complications of spinal dysraphism: meningitis and urinary tract disease (see below). In meningitis, the infection is frequently mixed, with both skin (*Staphylococcus epidermidis* and others) and gram-negative organisms present. When there is dribbling or other clinical or x-ray evidence of genitourinary tract disturbance, urinalysis, urine cultures, BUN, and creatinine clearance should be obtained and followed.

C. X-Ray Findings:

1. Plain x-rays of the spine—These should be obtained in all cases of symptomatic spinal dysraphism and will usually disclose the extent of the neural arch defect. Plain spine films obtained for other reasons usually establish the diagnosis of spina bifida occulta. In diastematomyelia, a ridge may often be protruding from the body of one or more vertebrae which splits or fixes the spinal cord or cauda equina and which may consist of bone, cartilage, and fibrous tissue; its radiopacity depends on the degree of calcification of this spur; nonvisualization on plain spine films does not rule out this diagnosis.

2. Spine tomograms—These are of particular value in cases of noncystic "tethering" of the cord and with the rarer cases of neurenteric cysts.

3. Myelography—The purpose of this procedure is usually confirmatory, and it should never be under-taken lightly. It should be performed in cases of progressively more symptomatic noncystic forms of dysraphism, particularly where diastematomyelia, tethering of the cord, or a neurenteric cyst—all of which may behave clinically like spinal cord tumors—is a possibility.

4. Skull films—These should be obtained with hydrocephaly, microcephaly, and recurrent bacterial meningitides. In the latter instance, recurrent infection via a dermal sinus must be suspected. Its location may be cephalic, particularly near the midline occipitally or the bridge of the nose. Skull x-rays may disclose a small circular radiolucent area; tomograms may be necessary.

5. Air encephalography—In meningomyelocele, ventriculography to demonstrate hydrocephalus—especially prior to neurosurgical intervention—is frequently required. It should be done shortly after birth to ensure early "shunting." Pneumoencephalography is often also indicated in the work-up of a child with recurrent bacterial meningitis since a congenital dermal sinus must be suspected in such cases.

6. Urologic studies—Cystometrograms and intravenous urograms are indicated in all children with obvious or suspected urinary tract involvement secondary to spinal cord involvement.

Differential Diagnosis

Meningomyelocele usually presents little diagnostic difficulty. Meningocele is not infrequently confused with a subcutaneous lipoma, and indeed the 2 may be associated. The differentiation between meningocele and meningomyelocele is sometimes only made during operation. Because of traction or pressure on the cord (or a combination of both), considerable diagnostic difficulty may be encountered in those forms of dysraphism which give rise to symptoms not unlike those of spinal cord tumors or even syringomyelia. Such may be the case (as the child grows) with fibrolipomas, tethering of the cord or cauda equina by fibrous bands to the bone or skin directly or through meningeal attachment, a tight filum terminale, or a spur which partially or completely bisects the cord (diastematomyelia). Primarily orthopedic findings such as pes cavus or Charcot joints involve consideration of Friedreich's ataxia, diabetes mellitus, congenital insensitivity to pain, familial dysautonomia, and even congenital syphilis. Lastly, the differential diagnosis must include neurenteric cyst, the remnant of an open passage between the yolk sac and neural groove present during the third week of embryonic life, which may be thoracic or lumbosacral in location and may present in infancy or not until the end of the second decade of life. Occasionally, cystic forms of dysraphism are placed anteriorly, causing symptoms of a space-occupying lesion in the thoracic, abdominal, or pelvic cavities, or of a spinal cord tumor. (See also Spinal Cord Tumors, above.)

Complications

Meningitis occurs in nearly 15% of cases of spina bifida cystica if the sac ruptures. It occurs far less frequently with congenital dermal sinus, but when it does it is likely to give rise to recurrent episodes of bacterial meningitis until the sinus is discovered; if it is not readily located in the back or at the nose, shaving the back of the head or air studies may be required. Infections are often due to *Escherichia coli, Pseudomonas aeruginosa,* or *Staphylococcus epidermidis.*

Urinary tract infections, bladder atony, vesicoureteral reflux, hydronephrosis, and eventually renal failure are frequent complications, particularly in spina bifida cystica.

Hydrocephalus is an early and frequent problem with spina bifida.

Skin problems may occur due to breakdown in the saddle area from bladder and bowel incontinence or with trophic disturbances.

Treatment

A. Neurosurgical Considerations:

1. **Noncystic forms of spinal dysraphism**—These may require neurosurgical intervention to relieve pressure or traction on the spinal cord, removal of a diastematomyelic spur, or excision of a dermal fistula and exploration for any connected tumor. It must be emphasized that a dermal sinus should never be probed as this may result in infection, especially of the CNS.

2. **Spina bifida cystica**—Approaches to this complex problem vary radically. Decisions about treatment must be based on the extent of neurologic and systemic involvement, the consequent morbidity, the prognosis for physical and mental function, and the emotional, social, and financial impact on the family.

a. **Meningoceles**—Meningoceles should be repaired early if there is danger of rupture of the sac.

b. **Meningomyeloceles**—The decision about immediate operation or a 3-month delay is controversial.

c. **Hydrocephalus**—A shunt or other measures for the relief of imminent or progressive hydrocephalus may result in collapse of the meningomyelocele, and this may be followed by epithelialization of the sac. Thus, there may be advantages to relief of hydrocephalus as a first procedure.

d. **Contraindications** to neurosurgical intervention include far-advanced hydrocephalus at birth, especially if associated with flaccid paraplegia; the presence of other severely disabling abnormalities; and the presence of a complete spinal cord lesion at about the tenth thoracic level.

B. **Care of the Sac When Neurosurgical Repair Is Delayed:** Application of silver nitrate to the thin membrane covering a sac is advocated by some to encourage epithelialization. A "doughnut" of foam rubber or other spongy material, covered by plastic, wide enough to protect the sac and secured around the abdomen, is a useful protective appliance. It may be roofed by sterile gauze, but contact of the gauze with the sac—whether "dry" or covered with petrolatum—should be avoided.

C. **Orthopedic Considerations:** Surgery and braces are recommended to the extent that these measures will aid ambulation. Correction of foot deformities and dislocation of the hips should not be undertaken if there is little hope that the child will ever walk.

In a child with neurogenic arthropathy, behavioral modification to reduce the frequency of trauma to the joints as well as physically protecting the joints (as by padding) is helpful.

D. **Urologic Considerations:** The renal status should be assessed early and watched closely. Measures for reducing the incidence of pyuria and renal complications include suprapubic manual expression of urine from the bladder, the use of an indwelling catheter, and uretero-ileostomy.

"Prophylactic" antibiotic therapy is not advisable, but specific infections must be treated. Mandelamine (or cranberry juice) to acidify the urine to pH 5.0 or less may reduce the frequency of infections.

E. **Fecal Incontinence:** Constipating foods and drugs may be of help. Colostomy is sometimes advisable for social reasons in older children who are otherwise able to function.

F. **Skin Care:** Skin hygiene should be maintained, particularly around the anus, vulva, and pressure areas, if these are involved.

Prognosis

In noncystic forms of spinal dysraphism, the prognosis for life and function is excellent if proper treatment is carried out. The degree of residual neurologic, orthopedic, and genitourinary deficit is often minimal but depends on the extent of involvement. It is encouraging to realize that with "release" of a tethered cord urinary incontinence and gait disturbances, even when present for several years, may resolve.

In cystic spinal dysraphism, complete cures can be achieved by excision of neurenteric cysts. With meningoceles, the prognosis is that of the complications.

With meningomyeloceles, about 30% of patients can function or be helped to function adequately. About 60% are operable. The overall mortality at present is 15—20%; of these, about 1/2 die within the first 6 weeks of life and another 1/3 within the first year. The most common causes of early deaths are meningitis and hydrocephalus.

Among survivors, 30—45% are mentally normal. Impairment of renal function with uremia is the most serious long-term threat.

Beks JWF, Heybroek G: Le traitement immediate des enfants atteints de spina bifida cystica. Neurochirurgie 15:291—298, 1969.

Ericson NO & others: Factors promoting urinary and anal continence in children with myelomeningocele. Acta paediat scandinav 59:491—496, 1970.

Hoffman EP: The problems of spina bifida and cranium bifidum: A survey of contemporary ideas. Clin Pediat 4:709—716, 1965.

Klump TE: Neurenteric cyst in the cervical spinal canal of a 10-week-old boy. J Neurosurg 35:472—476, 1971.

Lorber J: Neurologic assessment of neonates with spina bifida. Clin Pediat 7:676–679, 1968.

Padget DH: Neuroschisis and human embryonic development. J Neuropath Exper Neurol 29:192–216, 1970.

Talwalker VC, Dastur DK: "Meningoceles" and "meningomyeloceles" (ectopic spinal cord): Clinico-pathological basis of a new classification. J Neurol Neurosurg Psychiat 33:251–262, 1970.

2. HYDROCEPHALUS

Essentials of Diagnosis

- Abnormal enlargement of the cerebral ventricles due to an increased pressure gradient between the intraventricular fluid and the brain.
- In infants and children, hydrocephalus is usually accompanied by macrocephaly.

General Considerations

Most cases of hydrocephalus in infancy and childhood are due to obstruction of CSF flow, the aqueduct between the third and fourth ventricle being the most common site of blockage. Developmental causes include aqueductal stenosis or atresia; absence or atresia of the foramens of Luschka and Magendie (Dandy-Walker syndrome); Arnold-Chiari malformation (3 types are described; myelomeningocele is frequently, but not necessarily, associated); arteriovenous malformation of the great vein of Galen, compressing the aqueduct; and other anomalies, including block of the interventricular foramens (of Monro). Intrauterine and postnatally acquired causes include principally inflammatory states, whether from infection or hemorrhage, with resulting gliosis of the aqueduct, or arachnoiditis ("communicating hydrocephalus"). Intracranial mass lesions such as tumor, abscess, and hematoma also frequently cause obstruction to CSF flow.

A nonobstructive or oversecretion type of hydrocephalus is due to choroid plexus papilloma.

Clinical Findings

A. Symptoms and Signs: Manifestations vary with age at onset, the underlying cause, and the rapidity with which hydrocephalus develops.

In infants with an open anterior fontanel and patent sutures, symptoms of increased intracranial pressure are often delayed or minimal. Instead, the head circumference enlarges too rapidly or exceeds 3 SD above the mean for age and sex as plotted on a standard head circumference graph. The anterior fontanel may be full and tense and the sutures palpably separated; there may be frontal bossing and a "setting sun" sign, in which the eyes appear to be depressed, with more sclera than normal showing above the iris. The head may transilluminate abnormally and percuss like a watermelon.

Abducens palsies with increased intracranial pressure are common in all age groups. When hydrocephalus is due to more acute obstruction, there may be vomiting, irritability and listlessness, and difficulties with vision and gait.

The findings in older infants and children may include Macewen's cracked pot sign of sprung sutures, papilledema or other eye findings, disturbances of muscle tone and reflexes, and incoordination. Cranial bruits are common in children, especially with increased intracranial pressure, but may suggest a vascular malformation.

B. Laboratory Findings: The composition of the ventricular or spinal fluid may offer some clues to the cause of hydrocephalus. Markedly elevated CSF protein is often seen in choroid plexus papilloma and occasionally after a CNS infection or hemorrhage. Low CSF glucose without evidence of current infection is seen in postinfectious hydrocephalus or in meningeal invasion by tumor (eg, leukemia, medulloblastoma). Increased 5-hydroxyindoleacetic acid is found in the CSF in obstructive hydrocephalus. Cytologic examination of CSF may show the presence of tumor cells.

C. X-Ray Findings: X-rays may show the cranium to be disproportionately large with respect to the face; there may be signs of increased intracranial pressure, intracranial calcifications, lytic lesions, or a large, flat occipital shelf suggestive of Dandy-Walker syndrome.

In cases of increased intracranial pressure without focal findings or in children with abnormal head enlargement without other symptoms, right retrograde brachial angiography is recommended to determine the size of the lateral ventricles.

Air encephalography—by the lumbar route if this can be done safely or by the ventricular route (or both)—will usually define the site of CSF block. Sufficient air must be introduced to visualize the entire CSF space, and particularly to rule out a choroid plexus papilloma.

D. Special Examinations: Echoencephalography may show the ventricular dilatation. Isotope scans following the injection of radioiodinated human serum albumin into the lumbar or cisternal subarachnoid space have also been employed.

Differential Diagnosis

In the investigation of a child with a large head (macrocephaly), the following must be considered: (1) nonpathologic megalocephaly, which may be familial; (2) subdural hematoma, usually chronic or subacute and usually bilateral; (3) CNS degenerative diseases (see CNS Degenerative Disorders of Infancy & Childhood); (4) dysplasias, including cerebral gigantism and disorders of bone; (5) hydranencephaly; and (6) brain tumor.

Hydranencephaly consists of replacement of the cerebral hemispheres by a fluid-filled sac, usually due either to profound schizencephaly and bilateral porencephaly or to a massive encephalomalacic process which reduces the cerebral mantle to a thin membrane. The appearance of the neonate may be grossly normal.

The head is usually not enlarged. If the diencephalon and midbrain are intact, as is usually the case, no difficulties occur with feeding, respiration, and other vegetative functions in the first months of life. Diagnosis may be delayed until the parents note slow development or defective vision. Some spasticity and persistence of primitive postural reflexes are usually evident.

Hydranencephaly may be diagnosed by transillumination of the head, air studies, or cerebral angiography.

In cases of increased intracranial pressure without hydrocephalus, the diagnosis of pseudotumor cerebri is one of exclusion. Once this diagnosis is established, its many causes (as discussed in that section) should be investigated.

Complications

In nonoperated cases, continuing increased intracranial pressure leads to neurologic deterioration. Rarely, hydrocephalus may rupture.

In "shunted" cases, complications include (1) sudden rise in intracranial pressure, due either to blockage or other malfunction of the shunt (the site varies with the type of assembly) or to displacement of the shunt mechanism, especially at the distal end as growth proceeds; (2) infections (most frequently due to coagulase-positive *Staphylococcus albus*), including septicemia, meningitis, and ventriculitis, with the shunt itself often the nidus; (3) electrolyte imbalances; and (4) subdural hematoma following abrupt collapse of enlarged ventricles.

Prevention

Early recognition of hydrocephalus is best accomplished by periodic physical and neurologic examinations, which should include head measurements.

Treatment

A. Observations and Evaluation: Careful observation over a short period is required before the decision to operate is made. It is usually best not to operate if the patient is clinically well and the rate of enlargement does not exceed that indicated on a standard head circumference chart or appears to be arresting.

B. Surgical Treatment: The neurosurgical approach is dictated by the underlying condition as well as the surgeon's preference. Associated meningomyelocele or other anomalies must be dealt with also.

1. "Shunting technics" include a variety of ventriculovenous (ventriculojugular or ventriculoatrial) shunts, as well as ventriculoperitoneal or ventriculopleural shunts. Ventriculoureterostomy and ventriculocisternostomy are now performed rarely.

2. "Direct" nonshunting operations consist of third ventriculostomy and choroid plexectomy (imperative in choroid plexus papilloma).

3. Use of the Rickham reservoir and catheter is increasing, at least as a temporary measure.

C. Prophylactic Care of Shunts: Serial head and chest x-rays should be taken to check shunt placement. Other postoperative procedures used to verify the success of surgery are manometric testing of ventricular pressure; ventriculography with CO_2; "isotopic" check with radioiodinated human serum albumin on shunt function; and echoencephalographic estimation of ventricular size.

Prophylactic periodic revision of the shunt is advocated by many neurosurgeons.

Prognosis

In general, if progressive hydrocephalus can be arrested, the prognosis for function is improved. Even if the child is severely retarded and has other handicaps that do not threaten life, "social shunts" are justifiable since the difficulties of caring for the child are markedly eased and the cost of care, by reducing the necessity for institutionalization, is considerably lowered.

The width of the cerebral mantle may not be a reliable prognostic finding.

A. Nonoperated Group: The survival rate at 10 years is about 25%. Of the survivors, about 1/5 can function "competitively" and the remainder require supervision and maintenance. This salvage rate of competitive children is about 5% of the original group.

B. Operated Group: The survival rate at 10 years is about 60%, with over 1/2 of the surviving children able to care for themselves. (About 25% of survivors have normal or higher than normal IQs.)

C. Shunt Dependency: The question of shunt dependency is unsettled. Some data suggest that at some point in ventricular enlargement the ependymal surface may be sufficiently large to absorb the net amount of CSF not handled by the usual pathways. Such "spontaneous arrests" may occur in 40–50% of children surviving the first 1–2 years.

DeLange SA: Ventriculo-atrial shunt in progressive hydrocephalus and shunt dependency. Psychiat Neurol Neurochir 71:65–70, 1968.

Halsey JH, Allen N, Chamberlin HR: The morphogenesis of hydranencephaly. J Neurol Sc 12:187–217, 1971.

Laurence KM: Neurological and intellectual sequelae of hydrocephalus. Arch Neurol 20:73–81, 1969.

Lorber J: Medical and surgical aspects in the treatment of congenital hydrocephalus. Neuropaediatrie 2:239–246, 1971.

Russel DS: *Observations on the Pathology of Hydrocephalus.* Medical Research Council SRS 265, Her Majesty's Stationary Office, 1966.

Shulman K: *Workshop in Hydrocephalus.* University of Pennsylvania, 1966.

3. CRANIOSYNOSTOSIS

Primary craniosynostosis is a developmental disorder of the membranous bones of the skull that results in closure of one or more cranial sutures in utero. Diagnosis at birth is possible by inspection and palpation confirmed by skull x-rays. The ratio of males to females is 3:1. Occasionally there is a genetic basis for the defect. Associated anomalies are found in nearly 1/3 of cases.

Classification

(1) Sagittal sutures only are involved in over 50% of cases, resulting in dolichocephaly (scaphocephaly) with elongation and narrowing of the skull. This deformity may occur as a dominant trait.

(2) Coronal suture involvement accounts for almost 20% of cases. When bilateral, as it is in about 1/2 of these cases, the result is brachycephaly with a broad, shortened skull.

(3) Metopic suture involvement (10%) results in a pointed, ridged forehead or trigonocephaly.

(4) If all of the sutures are involved (about 8%), the result is a "turret" skull (oxycephaly, acrocephaly, turricephaly).

(5) Other combinations occur occasionally, such as fusion of the sagittal and coronal, lambdoidal, or metopic sutures, or of the lambdoidal and squamous sutures.

(6) Allied entities (singly or in combination) are acrocephaly with syndactyly (acrocephalosyndactyly, or Apert's disease), craniofacial dysostosis (Crouzon's disease), and hydrocephalus.

Clinical Findings

In the majority of cases there are no symptoms other than the skull deformity. Signs and symptoms of increased intracranial pressure, strabismus, visual loss, optic atrophy, mental retardation, and occasionally seizures occur with brain compression when multiple sutures are involved, or with hydrocephalus; in the latter case, the head circumference may be abnormally large.

Except where multiple sutures are involved, the normal head circumference and neurologic examination clearly differentiate primary from secondary craniosynostosis, which is usually accompanied by microcephaly.

Skull x-rays will define the suture involvement. The entire suture need not be involved. Decalcification of posterior clinoids and increased digital markings are present when there has been long-standing increased intracranial pressure. Symmetric involvement of sutures plus craniofacial disproportion are seen in microcephaly. Suspicion of hydrocephalus justifies appropriate studies.

Treatment

If multiple sutures are involved, early neurosurgical intervention with excision of sutures in the first weeks of life is recommended. If there is a deformity of the orbits, orbital decompression is required. The principal reason for sagittal synostosis surgery is cosmetic. (See also Hydrocephalus, above.)

About 13% of patients, chiefly those in which both coronal or multiple sutures are involved, require reoperation because of evidence of recurrent increased intracranial pressure or evidence of fusion after craniectomy.

The only fatalities resulting from surgery are due to failure to detect coagulation defects or to provide adequate replacement of blood loss, which is often greater than estimated. Preoperative coagulation screening and close attention to postoperative hemoglobin or hematocrit are therefore mandatory.

Prognosis

Cosmetic improvement occurs in about 75% of patients, with those operated on early and having only one or 2 sutures involved showing the best results, ie, an essentially normal-looking head (about 50% of all operated cases). It is claimed that operation also results in preservation of brain function.

Despite early surgical intervention, however (particularly in trigonocephaly), 3–5% of children with craniosynostosis exhibit varying degrees of mental retardation.

Permanent sequelae of surgical complications are infrequent.

Fishman MA, Hogan GR, Dodge PR: The concurrence of hydrocephalus and craniosynostosis. J Neurosurg 34:621–629, 1971.

Shillito J, Matson DD: Craniosynostosis: A review of 519 surgical patients. Pediatrics 41:829–853, 1968.

NEUROCUTANEOUS DYSPLASIAS

1. RECKLINGHAUSEN'S NEUROFIBROMATOSIS

Recklinghausen's neurofibromatosis is the most common of the neurocutaneous dysplasias, a group of conditions in which nervous and skin tissues, both of ectodermal origin, are chiefly involved. However, tissues arising from meso- and endodermal embryonal layers are often affected as well. Transmitted both as a dominant trait with a highly variable degree of penetrance and as a recessive, Recklinghausen's disease may be expressed by just one of its many features or by any combination of them. Atypical forms are common.

Clinical Findings

    A. Symptoms and Signs:

    1. Dermatologic features—Café au lait spots on skin, freckles under axillas, hemangiomas, lymphangiomas, lipomas, and subcutaneous neurofibromas.

    2. Neurologic features—Neuromas of cranial, peripheral, or autonomic nerves or of the spinal cord; optic nerve gliomas (involving either one nerve or the optic chiasm), not infrequent in childhood; acoustic (eighth nerve) neurinoma, usually bilateral in childhood; intracranial tumors, especially astrocytomas of varying degrees of malignancy; seizures (often indicative of intracranial tumors, but sometimes unrelated);

nonspecifically abnormal EEGs without other neurologic deficit; and CNS malformations, including meningocele and syringomyelia.

3. Mental retardation—Moderate to severe in nearly 10% of individuals with neurofibromatosis.

4. Skeletal involvement—There is a high incidence of kyphoscoliosis, defects of vertebral bodies and of the skull, elephantiasic hypertrophy, and rarefaction and cyst-like destruction of bone. Recklinghausen's disease is occasionally associated with vitamin D resistant rickets.

5. Other systems—Delayed or precocious sex development, diabetes mellitus, thyroid and parathyroid disorders, pheochromocytomas, melanoblastosis, congenital glaucoma, and soft tissue tumors such as retroperitoneal fibrosarcomas.

B. Laboratory, X-Ray, and Other Findings: None are specific. X-rays of the skull, orbits, spine, chest, or long bones, EEGs, brain scans, and other tests such as endocrine studies must be obtained on the basis of suspected involvement.

Differential Diagnosis

The smooth-bordered café au lait spots of Recklinghausen's neurofibromatosis must be distinguished from the jagged-edged "coast of Maine" coffee-hued skin lesions seen in polyostotic fibrous dysplasia (McCune-Albright syndrome).

Treatment

Treatment is directed toward specific problems, eg, neurosurgical removal or radiation therapy for tumors, orthopedic correction of scoliosis. The heritable nature of the disorder should be made clear.

Prognosis

The prognosis depends entirely on the manifestations: excellent where there are only skin or bone lesions, poor with malignant tumors. Most patients live normal lives.

Canale D, Bebin J, Knighton RS: Neurologic manifestations of von Recklinghausen's disease of the nervous system. Confinia neurol 24:359—403, 1964.

2. TUBEROUS SCLEROSIS

Tuberous sclerosis is a neurocutaneous dysplasia, protean in its manifestations, commonly appearing in partial form but accounting for 0.3—0.6% of institutionalized mentally retarded persons.

Clinical Findings

A. Symptoms and Signs:

1. Dermatologic features—Amelanotic spots on the skin and hair (often mistakenly called "vitiligo") may be present at birth or may appear within the first 2 years of life, and may be best demonstrated with Wood's light. Other findings include café au lait spots with smooth borders; Pringle's "adenoma sebaceum" in malar distribution, usually arising in the second to fourth year of life, of 2 types—seed-like, reddish angiofibromatous growths, and yellowish to brown, primarily fibromatous small nodules; angiomas; shagreen spots, which are grayish-green, rough, leathery patches of thickened skin; and subungual fibromas of fingers and toes found at adolescence and chiefly in girls.

2. Neurologic features—Seizures occur in a large number of cases and may be the only manifestation in some family members. About 2—5% of cases of infantile spasms with hypsarhythmia and mental retardation prove eventually to have tuberous sclerosis. Formation of nodules ("tubers") containing atypical large glial cells may result in the finding of cerebral calcifications on skull x-rays or irregularities of the ventricular walls on air encephalograms. The cerebellum, brain stem, and spinal cord are rarely, if ever, involved. Mass lesions include gliomas, gangliogliomas, and cystic lesions. The EEG is often nonspecifically abnormal even in asymptomatic family members.

3. Mental retardation—Mental retardation is frequent, and may be the sole manifestation in a member of an affected family.

4. Ocular involvement—Retinal phakomas or "mulberry lesions" at the edge of the optic disk are found in 7—8% of affected individuals; other eye defects include optic atrophy, nystagmus, and even blindness.

5. Skeletal involvement—Periosteal thickening and central cystic rarefactions of fingers and toes, hyperostosis of cranium, poly- and syndactyly, and vertebral defects.

6. Visceral manifestations—Renal hamartomas, rhabdomyomas of the heart, pulmonary vascular fibrosis, and various mixed tumors of other viscera.

7. Other manifestations—Endocrinopathies, cleft lip and palate, branchial cleft cysts, congenital heart disease, and genital dysplasias are occasionally present.

B. Laboratory Findings: None are specific. Diagnostic tests must be based on clinical judgment.

Differential Diagnosis

The early stages and various atypical forms of tuberous sclerosis may make the diagnosis difficult. The triad of seizures, typical skin lesions (especially of the face), and mental retardation in one individual or when present in any combination in the family supports the diagnosis. The presence of amelanotic skin or hair patches tends to differentiate this entity from Recklinghausen's disease.

Treatment

Treatment is nonspecific except as required for seizures, brain tumors, or visceral lesions. The heritable nature of the disorder should be made clear.

Prognosis

The most severely affected patients have a shortened life span, with death occurring at variable times as a result of status epilepticus, brain or visceral tumors, or intercurrent infections. Mildly affected individuals and those with atypical involvement may have a normal life span.

Lagos JC, Gomez MR: Tuberous sclerosis: Reappraisal of a clinical entity. Mayo Clin Proc 42:26–49, 1967.

Nevin NC, Pearce WG: Diagnostic and genetic aspects of tuberous sclerosis. JM Genet 5:273–380, 1968.

3. ENCEPHALOFACIAL ANGIOMATOSIS
(Sturge-Weber Disease)

Sturge-Weber disease consists of a port wine nevus on the upper part of the face and leptomeningeal angiomatosis of the cerebral cortex on the same side, as indicated by neurologic deficits and skull x-rays. It occurs sporadically. Cutaneous port wine nevi are present at birth, but other manifestations may not become evident for a year or more.

Clinical Findings
A. Symptoms and Signs: A port wine cutaneous nevus covers at least the upper eyelid or supraorbital region of the face and scalp and may involve both sides of the face and other parts of body. Seizures, both focal and generalized, occur in up to 90% of cases, often in the first year of life. Hemiparesis on the side contralateral to the face lesion is found in about 1/3 of cases and is frequently associated with hemiatrophy. Mental retardation of varying degree is present in about 50% of cases.

Buphthalmos (congenital glaucoma) occurs in about 1/3 of cases; hemianopsia is common.

Angiomatous involvement of the oropharynx and viscera and hypertrophy of extremities covered by angiomatous skin may be present.

B. X-Ray Findings: Brain scan may be positive. Diagnostic double-contoured calcifications corresponding to cerebral gyri are seen on skull x-rays usually only after the second year. Skull films may also show bony enlargement with large vascular channels over the involved side. Angiography and pneumoencephalography should be reserved for children in whom complications arise or who are being considered for hemispherectomy.

C. Electroencephalography: The EEG usually shows abnormalities over the involved hemisphere early in the disease, but the findings are nonspecific.

Differential Diagnosis
The diagnosis can usually be made at birth or in the first years of life, especially when seizures and neurologic deficits appropriate to the skin lesion are present. The diagnosis is unmistakable when the typical intracranial calcifications are seen on skull x-rays.

Complications
Intracranial bleeding may occur into the subdural or subarachnoid space, with concomitant worsening of the neurologic status.

Treatment
For the treatment of seizures, see the section on seizure disorders. Physical therapy may be indicated for hemiplegia. Glaucoma should be treated as outlined in Chapter 9. In cases with severe seizures, spastic hemiplegia, and hemianopsia, early hemispherectomy should be given every consideration with a view to preventing further neurologic deterioration.

Prognosis
The prognosis varies with the extent and severity of the leptomeningeal angiomatosis, the occurrence of cerebrovascular accidents, and the severity of the seizure disorder.

Nellhaus G: Sturge-Weber disease with bilateral intracranial calcifications at birth and unusual pathologic findings. Acta neurol scandinav 43:314–347, 1967.

4. VON HIPPEL-LINDAU DISEASE
(Retinal & Cerebellar Angiomatosis)

This unusual, dominantly transmitted disorder is characterized by angiomatosis of the retina and cerebellum. Angiomatosis of the brain stem, spinal cord, and spinal nerve roots, syringomyelia, epithelial cysts, angiomas of the liver, spleen, and kidneys, and other tumors, especially pheochromocytomas, may also be found. Cutaneous hemangiomas occur only rarely. Ocular symptoms and findings include visual difficulties, retinal hemorrhages and exudates, retinal detachment, and glaucoma; cerebellar hemangioblastoma may present as progressive ataxia, increased intracranial pressure, or subarachnoid hemorrhage. Spinal cord symptoms depend on the location and extent of the spinal angiomatosis and whether or not bleeding occurs. Visceral hemangiomas are apt to remain asymptomatic. Polycythemia is frequently present.

The diagnosis may be confirmed by family history, isotope scan of the posterior fossa and cord, and angiography.

Retinal lesions may be dealt with by photo- or diathermy coagulation. Cerebellar and spinal cord hemangioblastomas may require surgical removal.

CNS DEGENERATIVE DISORDERS OF INFANCY & CHILDHOOD

Essentials of Diagnosis
- Arrest of psychomotor development.
- Loss, usually progressive but at highly variable rates, of mental functioning, motor control, and often vision.

- Seizures of varying types are common in some disorders.
- Symptoms and signs vary with age at onset and primary sites of involvement of specific types.

General Considerations

The CNS degenerative disorders of infancy and childhood are fortunately rare. Although they may share many symptoms and signs, a careful history and clinical and laboratory evaluation frequently establish the most likely diagnosis.

Clinical Findings

A. Symptoms:

1. Where white matter is primarily involved, motor disturbances usually appear first. Hypotonia or flaccidity in infants may precede the eventual spasticity, or, if the child has begun to walk, incoordination (ataxia or dystonia) may be noted first, accompanied or followed by derangements of swallowing and of vocalization or speech. Vision is disturbed early. Convulsions usually appear late in the course if at all.

2. Where gray matter is primarily involved, convulsions often precede disturbances of mental and motor functions.

3. Where the disorder is diffuse, the clinical picture may be mixed or may present predominantly with the features of a white or gray matter disturbance.

B. Signs:

1. **Cry**—The cry is irritable and high-pitched in Krabbe's disease, Tay-Sachs disease, and Canavan's disease; diminished, weak, or absent in subacute necrotizing encephalomyelopathy (Leigh's disease); and like that of stridor or laryngospasm in infantile Gaucher's disease.

2. **Head circumference**—Often enlarged early in Canavan's disease and Alexander's disease and in the mucopolysaccharidoses; often enlarged late in metachromatic leukodystrophy and Tay-Sachs disease; and often small in Krabbe's disease and other dysmyelinogenic processes.

3. **Fundi**—"Cherry-red" maculas are seen in Tay-Sachs disease, Niemann-Pick disease, and infantile Gaucher's disease. A "salt and pepper" macula is present in late infantile and juvenile (and adult) forms of neurolipidosis (Batten-Mayou-Bielschowsky disease, Spielmeyer-Vogt disease). Optic atrophy occurs in subacute necrotizing encephalomyelopathy (Leigh's disease), Schilder's disease, and other leukodystrophies. Retinitis pigmentosa is present in abetalipoproteinemia and Refsum's disease.

4. **Hepatomegaly**—In Niemann-Pick disease, infantile Gaucher's disease, Tay-Sachs disease, generalized gangliosidosis, Wilson's disease, mucopolysaccharidoses, glycogen storage diseases, and some organic acidurias.

5. **Muscle tone and reflexes**—These are the least dependable physical clues. However, flaccidity or hypotonia coupled with areflexia may initially occur in white matter disorders in which peripheral nerve involvement is prominent, as in infantile metachromatic leukodystrophy. However, spasticity usually supervenes in time in the degenerative disorders, and deep reflexes may not be obtained because of the flexion contractures which develop.

C. Laboratory Findings: (See also Table 35–7.)

1. **Blood**—Vacuolized lymphocytes are found in many patients with neurolipidosis. Usually 10% or more of the lymphocytes are vacuolated when 300 are counted, but more than one smear may be necessary. The percentage and the size of the vacuoles depend on the duration of the disease. Vacuolized lymphocytes are also often observed in the carriers.

Hypergranulation may be prominent in polymorphonuclear cells, and present but less marked in the mononuclear cells in some of the "storage" diseases. While not present in every patient with such a disorder, they may be observed in a high percentage of close relatives when evident in the patient. Basophilic and more focal granulations are seen in Tay-Sachs disease; azurophilic, dispersed granules are more typical of the late infantile and juvenile forms of familial amaurotic idiocy; and Alder's granulations occur in some of the mucopolysaccharidoses.

Decreased fructose-1-phosphate aldolase is found in Tay-Sachs disease and carriers. SGOT, SGPT, and LDH are often markedly increased in Tay-Sachs disease and Niemann-Pick disease. For enzyme defects in lysosomal disorders, see Chapter 35.

2. **Urine**—A positive screening test is found in mucopolysaccharidosis. Quantitative increases in heparitin and chondroitin sulfate determine the type. Metachromasia of shed epithelial cells and a colorimetric test showing absence of arylsulfatase A help in diagnosis of metachromatic leukodystrophy.

3. **CSF**—Pressure may be elevated in Schilder's diffuse sclerosis. Protein is usually markedly increased in metachromatic and in globoid leukodystrophy. Gamma globulin is increased in Dawson's disease and sometimes in Schilder's sclerosis. Measles antibody titer in CSF is increased in Dawson's disease.

4. **Nerve conduction** is prolonged in metachromatic and globoid leukodystrophy and possibly in other dysmyelinogenic disorders.

D. X-Ray Findings:
Skeletal alterations may suggest Gaucher's disease (thinned cortex, trabeculation) or one of the mucopolysaccharidoses. Gallbladder series shows no uptake of dye in metachromatic leukodystrophy.

E. Biopsies:
The histology of enzyme deficiencies may now be shown in several diseases in the fibroblasts cultured from skin biopsies.

1. **Nerve biopsies**, when indicated by prolonged conduction time, may show typical metachromasia in metachromatic leukodystrophy. In globoid leukodystrophy, nonspecific myelin breakdown is found.

2. **Liver biopsy** is justified when hepatomegaly is present and is most useful in Niemann-Pick disease and in the mucopolysaccharidoses.

3. **Rectal biopsy** involving all muscle layers may show abnormal ganglion cells in the "storage" diseases.

TABLE 21–5. CNS degenerative disorders of infancy.

Disease	Enzyme Defect and Genetics	Onset	Early Manifestations	Vision and Hearing	Somatic Findings	Motor System	Seizures	Laboratory Studies	Biopsy	Course
WHITE MATTER										
Globoid (Krabbe's) leukodystrophy	Recessive. Galactocerebroside-beta-galactosidase deficiency.	First 6 months; rarely later.	Feeding difficulties. Shrill cry. Irritability. Arching of back.	Optic atrophy, mid-course to late. Hyperacusis occasionally.	Head often small. Often underweight.	Early spasticity, occasionally preceded by hypotonia. Prolonged nerve conduction.	Early. Myoclonic and generalized.	Routine blood, urine, and x-rays normal. CSF protein markedly elevated.	Sural nerve: nonspecific myelin breakdown. Brain: globoid cells.	Rapid. Death usually by 1½-2 years.
Metachromatic leukodystrophy	Recessive. Arylsulfatase A deficiency.	Second year. Less often, later in childhood.	Incoordination; especially gait disturbance.	Optic atrophy, usually late. Hearing normal.	Head enlarged late.	Combined upper and lower motor neuron signs. Ataxia. Prolonged nerve conduction.	Infrequent, usually late and generalized.	Metachromatic cells in urine; negative sulfatase A test. CSF protein elevated; occasionally normal early. "Nonfilling" of gallbladder on x-rays.	Sural nerve biopsy: metachromasia.	Moderately slow. Death in infantile form by 3–5 years; in "juvenile" form, by 10–13 years.
Spongy sclerosis (Canavan's)	Recessive. Mostly Jewish. Enzyme defect not known.	First 3 months.	Arrest in development; floppiness.	Optic atrophy, usually early. Hearing normal.	Head enlarged early.	Floppy early, then rapidly very spastic with decerebrate rigidity.	Early; in about 50% of cases.	Blood, urine normal. CSF under increased pressure; protein usually normal. Cranial sutures split.	Brain: (?nonspecific) spongiform degeneration, myelin deficiency.	Rapid. Death usually by 1½-3 years.
Pelizaeus-Merzbacher disease	X-linked recessive; rare female.	(?) Birth to 2 years.	"Eye rolling" often shortly after birth. Head bobbing. Slow loss of intellect.	Slowly developing optic atrophy. Hearing normal.	Head and body normal.	Cerebellar signs early, hyperactive deep reflexes. Spasticity usually only very late.	Usually only late.	Blood, urine, CSF, and x-rays normal.	Brain biopsy rarely helpful; extensive demyelination; small perivascular islands of intact myelin.	Exceedingly slow, often seemingly stationary. Many survive well into adult life.
DIFFUSE, BUT PRIMARILY GRAY MATTER										
Poliodystrophy (Alper's)	Occasionally familial, possibly environmental. (?"Slow virus.")	Infancy to late childhood.	Variable: loss of intellect, seizures, incoordination.	"Cortical blindness and deafness."	Head normal initially; may fail to grow.	Variable: incoordination, spasticity.	Often initial manifestation: myoclonic, akinetic, and generalized.	Blood, urine, and x-rays normal. CSF protein normal or slightly elevated.	Extensive neuronal loss in cortex: may occur very late.	Usually rapid, with death within 1–2 years after onset.

Tay-Sachs disease and variants	93% East European Jewish; often consanguineous. Recessive. Hexoseaminidase A deficiency. In variant forms, non-Jewish.	3–6 months. Under 1 year (hexoseaminidase A and B absent in variant). Over 1 year (partial hexoseaminidase A deficiency).	Variable: shrill cry, loss of vision, infantile spasms, arrest of development.	Cherry-red macula, early blindness. Hyperacusis early.	Head enlarged late. Liver occasionally enlarged.	Initially floppy. Eventual decerebrate rigidity.	Frequent, in mid-course and late. Infantile spasms and generalized.	Blood smears: vacuolated lymphocytes; basophilic hypergranulation. CSF protein normal or slightly elevated. Urine and x-rays normal.	Rectal biopsy: ballooned ganglion cells, often only late.	Moderately rapid. Death usually by 2–3 years.
Niemann-Pick disease and variants	50% Jewish. Higher incidence in girls. Recessive. Sphingomyelinase deficiency. In variants, enzyme defects unknown.	First 6 months. In variants, later onset; often non-Jewish.	Slow development. Protruding belly.	Cherry-red macula in 35–50%. Blindness late. Deafness occasionally.	Head usually normal. Spleen enlarged more than liver. Occasional xanthomas of skin. Emaciation early.	Initially floppy. Eventually spastic. Occasionally extrapyramidal signs.	Rare and late.	Blood: Vacuolated lymphocytes. Increased serum lipids. CSF protein normal or slightly elevated. Urine normal. X-rays: "Mottled" lungs, decalcified bones.	"Foam cells" in bone marrow, spleen, liver, lymph nodes. Rectal biopsy occasionally positive.	Moderately slow. Death usually by 3–5 years.
Gaucher's disease	About 2/3 Jewish. Recessive, rarely dominant. Glucocerebrosidase deficiency.	First 6 months; rarely, late infancy.	Stridor or hoarse cry. Head retraction. Feeding difficulties.	Occasional cherry-red macula. Convergent squint. Deafness occasionally.	Head usually normal. Liver and spleen equally enlarged.	Opisthotonos early, followed rapidly by decerebrate rigidity.	Rare and late.	Peripheral blood findings variable. Increased acid phosphatase. Urine normal. CSF normal. X-rays: Thinned cortex, trabeculation of bones.	"Gaucher cells" in bone marrow, spleen. Positive rectal biopsy.	Very rapid in infantile forms, with death by 1–2 years. Survival for several years in late infantile or juvenile cases.
Generalized gangliosidosis	Recessive. Beta-galactosidase deficiency.	First year; less often, second year.	Arrest of development. Protruding belly.	Occasional "cherry-red spot." Hearing usually normal.	Head enlarged early. Liver enlarged more than spleen.	Initially floppy, eventually spastic.	Usually late.	Blood: Vacuolated lymphocytes. Urine and CSF normal. X-rays: Dorso-lumbar kyphosis, "beaking" of vertebra.	"Foam cells" in bone marrow, spleen. Urine similar to those in Niemann-Pick disease.	Very rapid. Death in 2 years.
Subacute necrotizing encephalomyelopathy (Leigh's)	Recessive. ?Thiamine pyrophosphate-adenosine triphosphate "inhibitor."	Infancy to late childhood.	Difficulties in feeding. Feeble or absent cry. Floppiness.	Optic atrophy, often early. Hearing normal.	Head usually normal; occasionally small.	Flaccid and immobile; may become spastic.	Rare and late.	Increased lactic acid in blood. CSF protein normal or slightly elevated. X-rays normal. Special urine, blood, and CSF studies may demonstrate "inhibitor" factor.	Normal.	Usually rapid in infants, but more slowly progressive, with death after several years in some cases.

TABLE 21–6. CNS degenerative disorders of childhood.*

Disease	Onset	Enzyme Defect and Genetics	Early Manifestations	Vision and Hearing	Motor System	Seizures	Laboratory Studies	Biopsy	Course
Neuroaxonal degeneration (Seitelberger)	1–3 years.	Familial, (?) recessive. Girls more frequent than boys. Defect unknown.	Arrest of development and dementia. Loss of motor functions. Occasionally loss of pain over trunk and legs.	Optic atrophy and blindness, late. Nystagmus frequent. Hearing normal.	Combined upper and lower motor neuron lesions.	Rare.	Electromyography shows partial denervation, elevated serum lactate dehydrogenase and transaminase.	Brain: axonal swellings or "spheroids." Iron deposition in globus pallidus.	Very slowly progressive with death early in second decade.
Cerebromacular degenerations: Late infantile (Bielschowsky)	2–4 years.	Recessive. Defect unknown.	Ataxia. Visual difficulties. Arrested intellectual development.	Pigmentary degeneration of macula. Optic atrophy. Hearing normal.	Ataxia, spasticity progressing to decerebrate rigidity.	Often early: myoclonic and later generalized.	Blood: vacuolated lymphocytes, azurophilic dispersed hypergranulation of polymorphonuclear cells. Electroretinography helpful.	Rectal biopsy: ballooned ganglion cells.	Moderately slow. Death in 3–8 years.
Juvenile (Batten-Mayou, Spielmeyer-Vogt)	5–12 years.	More frequent in Scandinavian and Anglo-Saxon families. Recessive. Relatively common. Defect unknown.	Progressive visual loss. Progressive dementia. Ataxia.	Pigmentary degeneration of macula. Optic atrophy. Hearing normal.	Ataxia, slurred speech, slowly progressive spasticity.	Variable: early to mid-course, "petit mal," myoclonic, generalized.	As in late infantile form.	As in late infantile form.	Slow. Death in 7–15 years after onset.
Adult (Kufs)	15–25 years.	Recessive. Defect unknown.	Psychotic behavior. Dementia. Ataxia.	Normal.	Ataxia.	Myoclonic seizures, usually early.	(?) Normal.	Not known.	Very slow. May live into 60s.
Subacute sclerosing panencephalitis (Dawson's)	3–22 years. Rarely earlier or later.	None. Relatively common. Measles "slow virus" infection.	Impaired intellect, emotional lability, incoordination.	Occasionally chorioretinitis or optic atrophy. Hearing normal.	Ataxia, slurred speech, occasionally involuntary movements, spasticity progressing to decerebrate rigidity.	Myoclonic and akinetic seizures relatively early; later, focal and generalized.	CSF protein normal to moderately elevated. High CSF gamma globulin. Elevated CSF measles antibody titers. Characteristic EEG.	Brain biopsy: inclusion body encephalitis; culturing of measles virus.	Variable, from death in a few months to many years. Remissions and (?)spontaneous cures possible.
Familial sudanophilic leukodystrophy	5–10 years.	Familial. Defect unknown.	Impaired intellect, behavioral problems.	Optic atrophy common. Hearing normal.	Ataxia, spasticity.	Occasionally.	May be associated with hyperpigmentation due to adrenocortical insufficiency.	Brain: sudanophilia, sparing of U fibers.	Fairly rapid, death usually within 2–3 years after onset.

Schilder's diffuse sclerosis and variants†	5–10 years	None. Relatively common. Defect unknown.	Highly variable: may strike mental, motor, or visual systems first, or begin with focal seizures.	Occasionally presents with papilledema. Progressive optic atrophy common. "Psychic deafness."	Ataxia, hemiparesis, or spastic diplegia.	Focal and generalized; variable in onset and frequency.	CSF protein and gamma globulin may be elevated. Occasionally increased CSF pressure.	Leukodystrophy.	Variable: death in months to years after onset.
Neuromyelitis optica (Devic's disease)	Abrupt: late infancy to late childhood. May be preceded by infection.	None. Defect unknown.	Optic neuritis with "painful" blindness or transverse myelitis.	Optic neuritis with loss of vision in one or both eyes. Hearing normal.	Flaccid paraplegia at first, with loss of sphincter control; later, spastic paraplegia.	None.	CSF protein may be elevated; occasionally pleocytosis. CSF gamma globulin may be elevated, usually after several attacks.	None.	Variable: complete remissions possible or recurrent attacks of optic neuritis or transverse myelitis.
Multiple sclerosis	2 years on.	None. Diagnosis difficult in childhood. Defect unknown.	Highly variable: may strike one or more sites of CNS. Paresthesias common.	Optic neuritis; diplopia, nystagmus at some time. Vestibulocochlear nerves occasionally affected.	Motor weakness, spasticity, ataxia, sphincter disturbances, slurred speech, mental difficulties.	Rare: focal or generalized.	CSF may show slight pleocytosis, elevation of protein and gamma globulin.	None.	Variable: complete remissions possible. Recurrent attacks and involvement of multiple sites are prerequisites for diagnosis.

*For late infantile metachromatic leukodystrophy, Pelizaeus-Merzbacher disease, poliodystrophy, Gaucher's disease of later onset, and subacute necrotizing encephalomyelopathy, see Table 21–5.

†This includes the variants Balo's concentric sclerosis and Scholtz's disease as well as transitional sclerosis, which shares features of Schilder's disease and multiple sclerosis.

4. Brain biopsy, if positive, is often definitive and may differentiate an acquired slow viral encephalitis (Dawson's disease) from a biochemically determined degenerative process. In white matter diseases, the biopsy must often be deep to provide proper tissue.

Differential Diagnosis

A period of observation may be necessary before it becomes clear that one is dealing with a degenerative process. Pseudodegeneration may occur as a result of a severe seizure disorder or other illness, or a child may regress because of gross emotional neglect or stress. Retarded children with static brain damage are often thought by their parents to be regressing when in actuality a younger sibling or other child is noted to be outstripping the older one. Thus, the differential diagnosis of CNS degenerative disorders must include "cerebral palsy," seizure disorders, space-occupying lesions (including subdural hematomas or brain tumors), neurocutaneous dysplasias, chromosomal defects, disorders of glucose or protein and amino or organic acid metabolism, and chronic CNS infections.

Tables 21–5 and 21–6 summarize the important differential aspects of the clinical findings and courses of the common CNS degenerative disorders of infancy and childhood.

Complications

Pneumonia, usually due to aspiration, is the most common complication and the usual cause of death.

Prevention

The heritable nature of these disorders should be made clear. Enzymatic technics involving studies of leukocytes, skin fibroblasts, and amniotic cells are being rapidly developed to identify the carriers, affected fetuses, or presymptomatic cases.

Treatment

In most of the CNS degenerative diseases, treatment is purely symptomatic, consisting of control of seizures, maintenance of nutrition, and treatment of infections. In acute attacks of "multiple sclerosis" and optic neuritis or transverse myelitis (neuromyelitis optica, Devic's disease), corticotropin (4 mg/kg/day IM initially, with rapidly decreasing doses if there is a good response) may shorten the duration of the attack but does not alter either the frequency of exacerbations or the ultimate outcome of the disease.

Prognosis

By definition, the CNS degenerative diseases lead to progressive loss of function and premature death within months or a few years, depending on the process.

Brady RO: The sphingolipidoses. New England J Med 275:312–318, 1966.

Desnick RJ & others: Diagnosis of glycosphingolipidoses by urinary-sediment analysis. New England J Med 284:739–744, 1971.

Horta-Barbosa L, Fucillo DA, Sever JL: Chronic viral infections of the CNS. JAMA 218:1185–1188, 1971.

Julius R & others: Diagnostic techniques in metachromatic leukodystrophy. Neurology 25:15–18, 1971.

Menkes JH, Andrews JM, Cancilla PA: The cerebroretinal degenerations. J Pediat 79:183–196, 1971.

O'Brien JS: Ganglioside-storage diseases. New England J Med 284:893–896, 1971.

Poser CM: Myelinoclastic diffuse and transitional sclerosis. Pages 469–484 in: *Handbook of Clinical Neurology.* Vol 9. Vinken PJ, Bruyn GW (editors). North-Holland Publishing Co., 1970.

ATAXIAS OF CHILDHOOD

1. ACUTE CEREBELLAR ATAXIA

Acute cerebellar ataxia occurs most commonly in children 2–6 years of age. The onset is abrupt, and the evolution of symptoms is rapid. In about 1/2 of cases there is a prodromal illness with fever, respiratory or gastrointestinal symptoms, or an exanthem within 3 weeks of onset. Associated viral infections include varicella, rubeola, mumps, rubella, echovirus infections, poliomyelitis, infectious mononucleosis, and influenza. Bacterial infections such as scarlet fever and salmonellosis have also been incriminated.

Clinical Findings

A. Symptoms and Signs: The ataxia of the trunk and extremities may be quite severe, so that the child exhibits a staggering, reeling gait and inability to sit without support or to reach for objects; or there may be only mild unsteadiness. Hypotonia and tremor of the extremities may be present. Abnormal eye movements may include horizontal nystagmus. Speech may be slurred. The child frequently is irritable, and vomiting may occur.

There are no clinical signs of increased intracranial pressure. Sensory and reflex testing usually shows no abnormalities.

B. Laboratory Findings: The CSF is not under increased pressure. CSF protein and glucose are normal, although a slight lymphocytosis (up to about 30%) may be present. Attempts should be made to identify the etiologic viral agent by appropriate studies of CSF, stool, throat washings, and paired sera.

C. X-Ray and Other Findings: Skull films and long bones are normal. EEG may be normal or may show nonspecific slowing.

Differential Diagnosis

Acute cerebellar ataxia must be differentiated from acute cerebellar syndromes due to diphenylhydantoin, phenobarbital, primidone, or lead intoxication. However, with diphenylhydantoin and barbiturate intoxication, the nystagmus is usually fine, rapid, and of equal amplitude, in contrast to the coarser nystagmus of cerebellar disease. The toxic level in serum of diphenylhydantoin is usually above 20 μg/ml. Mean toxic levels of phenobarbital are reported to be above 50 μg/ml; for primidone, above 12 μg/ml. (See section on seizure disorders.) With lead intoxication, papilledema, anemia, basophilic stippling of erythrocytes, proteinuria, typical x-rays, and elevated CSF protein are clinical clues, confirmed by serum, urine, or hair lead levels. (See section on lead poisoning.) The polymyoclonia-opsoclonus syndrome (see below) must also be ruled out.

In rare cases, acute cerebellar ataxia may be mimicked by corticosteroid withdrawal, vasculitides such as in polyarteritis nodosa, trauma, the first attack of ataxia in a metabolic disorder such as Hartnup's disease, or the onset of acute disseminated encephalomyelitis or of multiple sclerosis. The history and physical findings will usually differentiate these disturbances, but appropriate laboratory studies may be necessary, including gas chromatography to identify intoxicants. For ataxias with more chronic onset and course, see the sections on spinocerebellar degeneration (below) and the other degenerative disorders.

Treatment

Treatment is supportive. The use of corticosteroids has no rational justification. Chlorpromazine (Thorazine) may be useful to reduce the irritability and vomiting sometimes seen initially. Reduction of dosage or withdrawal of incriminated drugs will depend on the weight of the indications for them balanced against the severity of the side-effects.

Prognosis

Between 80–90% of children with acute cerebellar ataxia not secondary to drugs recover without sequelae within 6–8 weeks. In the remainder, neurologic disturbances, including disorders of behavior and of learning, ataxia, abnormal eye movements, and speech impairment may persist for months or years, and recovery may remain incomplete.

Weiss S, Carter S: Course and prognosis of acute cerebellar ataxia in children. Neurology 9:711–721, 1959.

2. POLYMYOCLONIA-OPSOCLONUS SYNDROME OF CHILDHOOD
(Infantile Myoclonic Encephalopathy, "Dancing Eyes-Dancing Feet" Syndrome)

Especially at first, the symptoms and signs of this syndrome are similar to those of "acute cerebellar ataxia," and this broad category formerly included cases of the polymyoclonia-opsoclonus syndrome. In addition to severe incoordination of the trunk and extremities, often of relatively sudden onset, there are lightning-like, violent, brief jerking or flinging move-

ments of a group of muscles with the child in constant motion while awake. Extraocular muscle involvement results in sudden jerking, irregular eye movements, or opsoclonus. Irritability and vomiting often accompany these symptoms, but there is no depression of level of consciousness. This syndrome occurs in association with viral infections and in children with tumors of neural crest origin. Immunologic mechanisms have been postulated as responsible. Skull films usually show no evidence of increased intracranial pressure. CSF is not usually under increased pressure and may show normal or mildly increased protein. Special technics are required to show increased CSF plasmacytes and abnormal immunoglobulins. The EEG may be slightly slow, but when performed together with electromyography it shows no evidence of association between cortical discharges and the muscle movements. An assiduous search must be made to rule out tumor of neural crest origin by x-rays of the chest, skeletal survey, and intravenous urography as well as by assays of urinary catecholamine metabolites (VMA, etc) and cystathionine. Urine evaluation should be performed only after proper dietary preparation (omission of foods rich in catecholamines) and should be performed repeatedly if normal since normal results do not rule out the presence of such tumors.

The symptoms respond (often dramatically) to large doses of corticotropin. When a neural crest (or possibly other) tumor is found, surgical excision should be followed by irradiation and chemotherapy. Life span is determined by the biologic behavior of the tumor.

The syndrome is usually self-limited but may be characterized by exacerbations and remissions. However, even after removal of a neural crest tumor and without other evidence of its recurrence, symptoms may reappear. A high incidence of mild mental retardation has also been recorded.

Moe PG, Nellhaus G: Infantile polymyoclonia-opsoclonus syndrome and neural crest tumors. Neurology 20:756–764, 1970.

3. SPINOCEREBELLAR DEGENERATIONS

Essentials of Diagnosis

- Cerebellar and spinal involvement in various combinations.
- Slowly progressive course.
- Family history frequently positive.
- High incidence of associated neurologic or systemic disturbances.

General Considerations

The different heredodegenerative cerebellar ataxias may represent variants of the classical form of Friedreich's ataxia and be indistinguishable from each other in the early stages. Mild and incomplete forms exist. The age at onset and rate of progression may be highly variable, though often similar in the same family or in a given variant of this group of disorders.

Clinical Findings

The following should be looked for carefully, as they appear in various combinations in the entities described briefly below: truncal and extremity ataxia, horizontal or rotatory nystagmus, slurred and staccato speech, hypotonia, kyphosis, scoliosis, high-arched feet with hammer toes, optic atrophy, retinitis pigmentosa, external ophthalmoplegia, cataracts, reflex changes, positive Babinski signs, diminished to absent vibratory and position sense, muscular atrophy, mental retardation, and cardiac disease.

Types of Heredodegenerative Cerebellar Ataxias

A. Friedreich's Spinocerebellar Ataxia: This is not only the commonest form of the hereditary ataxias but also the most variable in its manifestations. Partial forms occur frequently. Affected family members may exhibit only high-arched feet or mild scoliosis. In its complete form, with onset in childhood, findings may eventually include the typical foot deformity (in 75% or more of cases), kyphoscoliosis, ataxia; loss of 2-point discrimination, position sense, and vibratory sensation; loss of knee and ankle jerk reflexes (early) and of arm reflexes (later), positive Babinski signs, horizontal and rotatory nystagmus, staccato speech, muscular hypotonia, and impairment of mental ability. Optic atrophy and cardiac disease may also develop. Variants of peroneal muscular atrophy (Charcot-Marie-Tooth disease) and of progressive muscular dystrophy may occur in association with Friedreich's ataxia.

No specific laboratory findings are helpful. X-rays of the spine may reveal the scoliosis. ECG may show conduction defects with bundle branch block or complete heart block, or changes associated with occlusive coronary disease. Diabetes mellitus should be carefully looked for, as its association with Friedreich's ataxia is not infrequent. Muscle enzyme determinations, electrical studies, and muscle biopsy may establish the presence of muscular atrophy or dystrophy.

B. Roussy-Lévy Syndrome: Beginning usually in early childhood, there is ataxia, pes cavus, diminished or absent knee and ankle jerks, and muscular atrophy of the lower extremities and sometimes of the hands. Dysarthria and nystagmus usually are absent. The course is slowly progressive and often seems to arrest at puberty before symptoms become too severe.

C. Behr's Syndrome: Partial Friedreich's ataxia with spasticity, hyperreflexia, and optic atrophy.

D. Marinesco-Sjögren Syndrome: Partial Friedreich's ataxia with short stature, marked mental retardation, and cataracts.

E. Francheschetti's Syndrome: Partial Friedreich's ataxia combined with external ophthalmoplegia.

F. Hereditary Olivopontocerebellar Atrophy: In the juvenile form, transmitted as a dominant, there may be highly variable involvement of the cranial nerves, pyramidal tract signs, cerebellar disturbances,

and striatal symptoms, including rigidity, tremor, and choreo-athetosis. Mental retardation is variable.

G. Others: Among other entities to be considered are ataxia-telangiectasia of Mme Louis-Bar, abetalipoproteinemia, Refsum's syndrome, and various rare, usually intermittent ataxias associated with disorders of amino acid or ammonia metabolism, such as hyperalaninemia and Hartnup's disease.

Treatment

Supportive care consists of physical therapy, the use of a walker or wheelchair when necessary, and similar measures. Orthopedic surgery may be of value when the disease appears to be only very slowly progressive or is seemingly arrested. Coronary symptoms and cardiac failure may require the use of nitrates (eg, nitroglycerin) and digitalis preparations. Diabetes mellitus should be treated.

Prognosis

In Friedreich's ataxia, many patients are able to walk until the end of their second decade or even longer. Patients usually live for 15–20 years from the date of onset, and death is usually due to heart failure.

Many patients with Roussy-Lévy syndrome live a normal life span. In the rarer forms of spinocerebellar degeneration, the prognosis is highly variable.

Biemond A: Congenital cerebellar ataxia. Psychiat Neurol Neurochir 74:303–314, 1971.

Greenfield JG: *The Spino-cerebellar Degenerations.* Thomas, 1954.

Hariga J, Moutschen J: On the inheritance of the heredoataxias. Human Heredity 19:457–472, 1969.

ATAXIA-TELANGIECTASIA
(Mme Louis-Bar Syndrome)

This heredodegenerative disorder is characterized by ataxia; telangiectasia of the bulbar conjunctivas, external ears, nares, and subsequently other body surfaces; and recurrent respiratory, sinus, and ear infections. The ataxia is usually noted in the second to third years of life; the telangiectatic lesions appear in the third to sixth years. Ocular dyspraxia, slurred speech, choreo-athetosis, hypotonia and areflexia, and psychomotor and growth retardation may be present. In some patients, deficiencies of IgA and IgE exist. There is no treatment other than for the recurrent infections. Several cases of malignancies involving the reticuloendothelial system have been reported.

Terplan KL, Krauss RF: Histopathologic brain changes in association with ataxia-telangiectasia. Neurology 19:446–454, 1969.

THE "EXTRAPYRAMIDAL DISORDERS"

These syndromes are characterized by the presence of one or more of the following features: dyskinesias, especially the choreic syndrome, athetosis and ballismus, tremors, rigidity, and dystonias. (These terms are explained below.)

For the most part, precise pathologic and anatomic localization is not completely understood. In general, motor pathways synapsing in the striatum (putamen and caudate nucleus), globus pallidus, red nucleus, substantia nigra, and the body of Luys are involved; this "system" is markedly influenced by pathways originating in the thalamus, cerebellum, and reticular formation.

Symptoms

A. Chorea: Involuntary, purposeless, sudden jerky, irregular movements involving the face, trunk, and extremities, usually provoked and increased by voluntary activity and tension but decreased by relaxation and disappearing in sleep. Gait, in particular, is markedly disturbed; the legs are flung out or may suddenly flex, and the arms flail about. Hypotonia is frequently present. There is a waxing and waning of the grip ("milkmaid's grip"). The tongue darts in and out. Feeding, writing, and other activities requiring fine muscular coordination are impaired. There is facial grimacing. Speech is irregular and indistinct. The knee jerk may be "hung up," ie, following stimulation, the lower leg may be slow to return to the pre-stimulus position or even the extended position for several seconds. The arm and leg are usually affected equally; however, the 2 sides of the body may be unequally involved, so that only one side may appear to be affected (hemichorea).

B. Athetosis: A recurring series of slow, writhing movements, including vermicular movements in the fingers and waves of grimaces. Muscular hypertonia is frequently evident, and the muscles may become hypertrophied as a result of the constant movements. Speech and swallowing may be severely impaired. Tendon reflexes may be difficult to obtain.

C. Choreo-athetosis: A combination of chorea and athetosis occurs rather frequently.

D. Ballismus: An involuntary movement pattern of violent flinging about of the limbs. The movements are of large amplitude and usually related to contractions of the proximal musculature. This disorder is usually unilateral (hemiballismus), of sudden onset, and may follow transient hemiplegia.

E. Dystonia: Characterized by abnormal postures and disturbed muscle tone, the movements are slow, sustained, and nonpatterned, involving chiefly the muscles of the trunk and neck and the proximal muscles of the extremities. Dystonia is made worse by voluntary activity and emotional tension. The spine is commonly twisted and the feet held in the equinus position and inverted; the hands are less affected. Occasionally, only the neck is involved (spasmodic torticollis). In addition to muscle spasm, hypertonia is common. Tendon reflexes are difficult to elicit. Initially, there are few movements, often confined to one part of the body. Eventually, however, gait and posture become bizarre, and ultimately there may be paucity of movements because of the marked rigidity and contractures.

F. Tremors: These range from fine to coarse, rhythmic oscillatory movements present at rest and often inhibited by voluntary action. Tremors are best demonstrated with the patient's arms outstretched and fingers spread.

G. Rigidity: Increased muscle tone with fairly constant contraction of the flexors and extensors, resulting in increased resistance through the full range of passive motion, and with normal or only slightly increased deep tendon reflexes.

H. "Parkinsonian" Syndrome: A combination of abnormal posture, resting tremor, and rigidity. The "pill-rolling" tremor is increased by emotional tension and inhibited by volitional actions. The rigidity is said to be of the "cogwheel" type because of a regularly jerky "give" in resistance when a flexed extremity is extended passively. Voluntary movements are slow; there is a shuffling gait, and the arms do not swing. There is often a marked paucity of movements. In children, there may be a frozen open-mouthed facies. Speech is slow and monotonous. Coordination and tendon reflexes are usually normal. In many instances, the patient can run much better than he can walk.

1. POSTNATALLY ACQUIRED EXTRAPYRAMIDAL DISORDERS

DRUG-INDUCED EXTRAPYRAMIDAL DISORDERS

Essentials of Diagnosis

- "Parkinsonian" syndrome of acute onset.
- Dystonia, dyskinesia, tetanus-like syndrome, meningismus, myoclonic jerks, or generalized seizures.
- Autonomic disturbances.
- History of administration or ingestion of phenothiazines or "tranquilizers," or presence of such drugs in the home.
- Positive urine test.

General Considerations

The diagnosis may be suspected in children who have received phenothiazine derivatives within the preceding 48 hours. Prochlorperazine (Compazine) is the most common offender. Severe bradykinesia has been reported due to anticonvulsants.

Onset is acute. The clinical picture may be greatly complicated by the signs and symptoms of the illness which led to the administration of a phenothiazine. Phenothiazine intoxication should always be suspected in the presence of extrapyramidal symptoms of acute onset.

Clinical Findings

A. Symptoms and Signs: Frequently seen are cogwheel rigidity, tremors, severe speech and swallowing disturbances, masked facies, dystonias, and dyskinesias. Constant or intermittent spasms of the neck and back muscles, jaws, face, tongue, and limbs, as well as a "sardonic smile," may suggest tetanus. Opisthotonos and spasms of the legs on straight leg raising may suggest meningismus. Oculogyric crisis may occur. Some patients have myoclonic jerks or generalized seizures, including status epilepticus. Bradykinesia may be the chief finding.

Autonomic disturbances such as tachycardia, hypotension, salivation, blurred vision, and paralysis of the bladder may occur.

B. Laboratory Findings: Testing the urine with Phenistix or ferric chloride up to 18–24 hours after the last dose of phenothiazine often gives a reddish-purple reaction. Occasionally—particularly if phenothiazines have been administered over a long period of time—there may be leukopenia and disordered liver function. If antiepileptic drugs are suspected, phenobarbital and (especially) diphenylhydantoin levels should be measured.

The EEG may be normal.

Differential Diagnosis

Common misdiagnoses, as may be suspected from the symptoms, are hysteria, meningitis (especially when there is an underlying febrile illness accompanied by vomiting), tetanus, and Sydenham's chorea.

Treatment

In severe cases, give one of the following: (1) diphenhydramine (Benadryl), 2 mg/kg body weight slowly IV, and repeat cautiously if necessary for a total of 5 mg/kg/day. (2) Caffeine and sodium benzoate, 10 mg/kg IV or IM (may repeat). (3) Promethazine (Phenergan), 0.5 mg/kg IM. (4) Benztropine (Cogentin), 0.5 mg IV, IM, or orally (may repeat). (5) Trihexyphenidyl (Artane), 0.5 mg orally (may repeat). (6) Phenobarbital and atropine have also been used. With bradykinesia due to diphenylhydantoin, that drug should be reduced or withdrawn.

Chien C, Dimascio A: Drug-induced extrapyramidal symptoms and their relations to clinical efficacy. Am J Psychiat 123:1490–1498, 1967.

Prensky AL, DeVivo DC, Palkes H: Severe bradykinesia as a manifestation of toxicity due to antiepileptic medications. J Pediat 78:700–704, 1971.

SYDENHAM'S POST-RHEUMATIC CHOREA

Sydenham's chorea is characterized by an acute onset of choreiform movements and variable degrees of psychologic disturbance. It is frequently associated with endocarditis and arthritis. Although the disorder follows infections with beta-hemolytic streptococci, the interval between infection and chorea may be greatly delayed; throat cultures and ASO titers may therefore be negative. Psychic predisposition may play a role. Chorea has also been associated with hypocalcemia and with vascular (LE), toxic, infectious and parainfectious, and degenerative encephalopathies.

Clinical Findings

A. Symptoms and Signs: See description of chorea in the introduction to this section. In addition to the jerky incoordinate movements, the following are noted: emotional lability, waxing and waning ("milkmaid's") grip, darting tongue, "spooning" of the extended hands and their tendency to pronate, and knee jerks slow to return from the extended to their pre-stimulus position ("hung up").

B. Laboratory Findings: Anemia, leukocytosis, and an increased erythrocyte sedimentation rate may be present. ASO titer may be elevated and C-reactive protein present. Throat culture may occasionally be positive for beta-hemolytic streptococci.

ECG may occasionally show cardiac involvement.

Differential Diagnosis

The diagnosis is usually not difficult. Tics, phenothiazine intoxication, Huntington's chorea, and hepatolenticular degeneration (Wilson's disease) as well as other rare movement disorders can usually be ruled out on historical and clinical grounds.

Treatment

There is no specific treatment. Give sedation with chlorpromazine (Thorazine), 15–25 mg 3 times daily initially and increase slowly until the involuntary movements are markedly reduced or cease or until the patient is overly drowsy; or phenobarbital, 2–3 mg/kg orally 3 times daily—with, if necessary, chloral hydrate, 250–500 mg 2–3 times daily. Meprobamate may be useful in mild cases. In extreme cases, corticotropin or corticosteroids might be considered and occasionally are dramatically effective.

All patients should be given antistreptococcal prophylaxis with penicillin G (200,000 units twice daily) or sulfonamide drugs.

Prognosis

Sydenham's chorea is a self-limiting disease that may last from a few weeks to about 2 years. Two-thirds of patients relapse one or more times, but the ultimate outcome does not appear to be worse in those with recurrences. Valvular heart disease occurs in about 1/3 of patients, particularly if other rheumatic manifestations appear. Psychoneurotic disturbances, if not already present at the onset of illness, occur in a significant percentage of patients.

Aron AM, Freeman JM, Carter S: The natural history of Sydenham's chorea. Am J Med 38:83–95, 1965.

Tierney RC, Kaplan S: Treatment of Sydenham's chorea. Am J Dis Child 109:408–411, 1965.

TICS OR HABIT SPASMS

Tics or habit spasms are quick repetitive movements, often stereotyped, which are alterable at will. Coordination and muscle tone are not affected. A psychogenic basis is usually readily discernible.

Tics usually represent obsessive-compulsive acts, increasing in intensity and becoming more elaborate the more attention they provoke. Unlike the child with an organic movement disorder, the child with tics is little disturbed by their presence. Tics are a common finding in children 9–13 years old.

Facial tics such as grimaces, twitches, and blinking predominate, but the trunk and extremities are often involved as well as twisting or flinging movements. Tourette's disease is a form of tic in which extensive and varied bodily movements are accompanied by guttural or explosive sounds which are choked-off obscenities (coprolalia).

In relatively mild cases, tics are self-limited and, when disregarded, disappear. When attention is paid one tic, it may disappear only to be replaced by another which is often worse. If the tic and its underlying anxiety or compulsive neurosis are severe, psychiatric evaluation and treatment are needed. Drug therapy has little place in the treatment of tics except in Tourette's disease, for which haloperidol (Haldol), 10–15 mg orally daily, has been advocated in conjunction with aversive conditioning.

Moldofsky H: A psychophysiological study of multiple tics. Arch Gen Psychiat 25:79–87, 1971.

Shapiro AK, Shapiro E: Treatment of Gilles de la Tourette's syndrome with haloperidol. Brit J Psychiat 114:345–350, 1968.

Torup E: A follow-up study of children with tics. Acta paediat 51:261, 1962.

2. CONGENITAL CHOREO-ATHETOSIS & RIGIDITY

Congenital chorea, athetosis, and rigidity, in varying combinations and severity, may present in infancy or childhood or may be delayed until adolescence. The symptoms are usually not progressive, and improvement often occurs.

These patients comprise about 20% of all children with cerebral palsy (see below). Patients may be divided into those exhibiting chiefly (1) double chorea, (2) double athetosis, (3) rigidity without movement disorder, (4) atypical movement disorders, (5) transitional types between any of the aforementioned 4 groups (the majority), and (6) those in whom the disorder is complicated by paralysis, spasticity, and other symptoms. The more severe the degree of involvement, the earlier the onset. Other neurologic disorders such as seizures, visual and hearing deficits, and mental retardation may be present.

Laboratory studies often include x-rays of the skull (for microcephaly and calcification) and the hips (for dislocation); EEG, if seizures are evident clinically; amino acid chromatography (aminoacidurias are present in rare cases); tests of vision and hearing; and psychometric evaluation. There is usually little difficulty in establishing the diagnosis because of the early onset and the variety and multiplicity of the neurologic findings.

Treatment is largely asymptomatic. Physical and educational therapy are usually helpful. In selected cases, thalamotomies have been successful. Diazepam (Valium) may reduce the rigidity, but drug therapy to date has generally been of little avail. Levodopa alone or in combination with diazepam has occasionally been effective. Orthopedic correction of deformities is useful in some cases.

Hanson RA, Berenberg W, Byers RK: Changing motor patterns in cerebral palsy. Develop Med Child Neurol 12:309–314, 1970.

3. PROGRESSIVE EXTRAPYRAMIDAL DISORDERS*

HUNTINGTON'S CHOREA

The occurrence of Huntington's chorea in the first decade of life is now being recognized more frequently, although it is still rare. The childhood picture has given rise to the term "striatocortical degeneration." It varies from the adult form in several respects: (1) Dementia occurs early and progresses rapidly. (2) A "striatal" syndrome with rigidity and akinesia predominates over choreo-athetoid features. (3) Cerebellar dysfunctions (tremors and ataxia) are frequent. (4) Seizures occur in over 50% (rare in adults). (5) Average duration of illness after onset is a little over 8 years (compared to over 13 years in adults).

The disease is transmitted in autosomal dominant fashion, but a family history is frequently denied or unobtainable.

*Wilson's disease is discussed in Chapter 17.

Clinical Findings

A. Symptoms and Signs: At onset, Huntington's chorea may present as a behavior disorder. Rigidity, masked facies, slow voluntary movements, and loss of associated movements are almost always present, as well as intention tremor and ataxia. Organic dementia is pronounced. "Pseudo-ophthalmoplegia" with marked abnormalities in coordinated head and eye movements is also a prominent feature.

B. Laboratory and Other Findings: Chromosomal analysis, dermatoglyphics, biochemical studies, and studies of trace metals have not been helpful. Pneumoencephalography frequently shows "butterfly" atrophy in the region of the caudate nucleus and putamen as well as some cortical atrophy. EEG is frequently but nonspecifically abnormal, showing fast, low-voltage activity as well as asymmetry and disorganization.

Differential Diagnosis

Huntington's chorea must be differentiated from the other conditions discussed in this section and from juvenile amaurotic idiocy (Spielmeyer-Vogt disease).

Prognosis & Treatment

There is no treatment, and the disease is fatal within 8 years after onset. Phenothiazines, reserpine, and trihexyphenidyl (Artane) may afford some relief. Genetic counseling to other members of the family is of paramount importance.

Byers RK, Dodge JA: Huntington's chorea in children. Neurology 17:587–596, 1967.

DYSTONIA MUSCULORUM DEFORMANS

This is a rather ill-defined disorder which may be suspected when dystonia is present but encephalitis or toxic encephalopathy, hepatolenticular degeneration, and other extrapyramidal diseases have been ruled out.

Beginning with hypertonia of calf muscles, producing plantar flexion and inversion and adduction of the foot in about 2/3 of cases, it may also start in the wrist and neck. The face, organs of speech, and fingers tend to be spared. The disease soon progresses along the extremity to the trunk, resulting eventually in severe lordosis; slow, powerful, widespread movements, which may succeed each other in waves; and bizarre postures due to spasm of some muscle groups and relaxation of others.

This disorder is inherited (1) as an autosomal recessive, predominantly in Jewish children, with onset between 4 and 16 years of age and a rapid course; and (2) as a dominant, more variable in onset and with a slower course, with no ethnic predilection.

Clinical Findings

A. Symptoms and Signs: These vary with the stage of the disease. The involuntary movements, accentuated by emotional upsets and activity (especially walking or running), are often bizarre and complex. They disappear in sleep. Strength, coordination, and reflexes are intact on examination if proper relaxation can be achieved. Intelligence is not affected, but many emotional problems develop.

B. Laboratory Findings: None are specific. Urinary dopamine levels are increased in some patients.

Differential Diagnosis

This condition must be differentiated from the other progressive extrapyramidal disorders discussed in this section and from hysteria.

Treatment

Pallidectomy and thalamotomy have afforded relief in some patients, at least for several years. Levodopa is being tried. Sedation may be needed for sleep.

Prognosis

The course is usually very slowly progressive, and the disease may be arrested for several years. Children involved earliest have the most rapid course.

Zeman W, Dyken P: Dystonia musculorum deformans. Pages 517–543 in: *Handbook of Clinical Neurology.* Vol 6. Vinken PJ, Bruyn GW (editors). Wiley, 1968.

OTHER PROGRESSIVE EXTRAPYRAMIDAL DISORDERS

Hallervorden-Spatz disease and progressive pallidal degeneration are rare, slowly progressive extrapyramidal disorders whose diagnoses usually depend on the family history or autopsy findings. In familial calcification of the basal ganglia, the diagnosis is made on skull x-rays. Juvenile parkinsonism is a familial disorder due to impaired ability to synthesize dopamine; it may result in clinical symptoms first (or only) when major tranquilizers are used, but it responds to treatment with levodopa. Parkinsonism or dystonia may occur as a consequence of encephalitis.

Martin WE, Resch JA, Baker AB: Juvenile parkinsonism. Arch Neurol 25:494–500, 1971.
Poser CM, Huntley CJ, Polland JD: Para-encephalitic parkinsonism. Acta neurol scandinav 45:199–215, 1969.

INFECTIONS & INFLAMMATIONS OF THE CNS

Infections and infestations of the CNS in children, especially in neonates and infants, present with rather nonspecific symptoms. Early diagnosis depends upon a high index of suspicion, and prompt and appropriate treatment may in many instances prevent or minimize permanent CNS damage.

One of the most significant clinical attributes of any infection or infestation of the CNS is its anatomic distribution, ie, meninges, cerebrum, cerebellum, bulb, or spinal cord. Most CNS infections in infants and young children are meningoencephalitides, although one or the other aspect (meningitis or encephalitis) may be more marked.

Laboratory Findings

A. Cerebrospinal Fluid: The diagnosis usually, though not always, depends on the CSF findings. CSF examination should include total and differential cell count, protein, and glucose with concomitant blood glucose, gamma globulin, lactic dehydrogenase, Gram's stain and cultures (including special studies for acid-fast organisms, viruses, and fungi), and tests for syphilis as indicated. (For characteristics of CSF in various neurologic conditions, see Table 21–1. See comments on lumbar puncture in Chapter 36.

B. Other Means of Identification of Etiologic Agent: The blood, nose, throat, urine, stools, stomach, lungs, and aspirates from petechiae, vesicles, or pus pockets may all provide material for direct isolation of the responsible infective agent. When the child does not clearly have a bacterial infection, serum should be set aside at the time of admission for serologic studies about 3 weeks later with a paired convalescent serum. Heterophil studies, febrile agglutinins, and skin tests (eg, tuberculosis, trichinosis, histoplasmosis) should be performed as indicated.

C. Neurodiagnostic Studies: Special neurodiagnostic studies may occasionally be necessary to differentiate nonsurgical from specifically surgical lesions and infections, eg, encephalitis with marked focal features from brain abscess. Such studies may include echoencephalography, brain scan, EEG, angiography, ventriculography, and lumbar pneumoencephalography.

ACUTE PURULENT MENINGITIS

The symptoms vary greatly with age (see Table 21–7). Nuchal rigidity, especially in the younger age group, may not be present; on the other hand, a stiff neck or meningismus in children is commonly due to other causes—particularly cervical adenopathy.

Clinical Findings

A. Symptoms and Signs: In addition to the symptoms and signs listed in Table 21–7, note the presence of extracranial infections, petechiae, alterations in the state of consciousness, the head circumference in the younger age group, cranial nerve palsies, and other focal neurologic deficits.

TABLE 21–7. Symptoms and signs of purulent meningitis.

Symptoms and Signs	Newborn	Up to 2 Years	Over 2 Years
Irregular respirations/ cyanosis	+		
Fever	+	+	+
Hypothermia	+		
Vomiting	+	+	+
Diarrhea	+		
Jaundice	+		
Drowsiness	+	+	+
Jitteriness	+	+	
Bulging fontanel	+	+	
Convulsions	Early	Early	Late
Stiff neck	Very late	Late	+
Headache			+

B. Laboratory Findings: CSF usually shows pleocytosis, low glucose, variable but often elevated protein, and lactate dehydrogenase values above 30 IU/ liter. Gram's stain and cultures will be positive unless the meningitis has been partially treated.

The most common etiologic agents, in order of frequency, are as follows: (1) In newborns, *Escherichia coli* and other gram-negative organisms; less commonly, *Hemophilus influenzae, Listeria monocytogenes,* hemolytic streptococci, hemolytic staphylococci, and pneumococci. (2) In older infants and children, *H influenzae* (especially in children 2–7 years of age), more prevalent in fall and early winter; pneumococci; and meningococci (epidemics every 8–10 years), more prevalent in early spring.

Complications & Sequelae

A. Seizures: There is a high incidence of convulsions in infants up to about 18 months of age. The prophylactic use of phenobarbital, 3–5 mg/kg/day, is strongly advocated during the acute phase. If a convulsion occurs, even though the child is receiving anticonvulsants, the likelihood of status epilepticus is still greatly reduced and the seizures can usually be brought under control by moderate increases in medication.

Diphenylhydantoin (Dilantin) has been found to be less helpful in the acute stage, partly because, on a maintenance dose of 5–7 mg/kg/day, it takes 7–10 days to build up therapeutic levels. (To build up the blood level of diphenylhydantoin rapidly, 10 mg/kg may be given slowly IV.)

If the patient remains free of seizures during the acute phase, anticonvulsant medication may be gradually withdrawn over a period of several days in the convalescent phase. If the patient had a seizure, it is generally advisable that anticonvulsant medication be maintained for 2–3 years since the recurrence rate of seizures following meningitis is high.

B. Water Intoxication: Cerebral edema may cause inappropriate ADH secretion. Furthermore, if the child is in a croupette, the usual water loss through insensible perspiration does not occur. Hyponatremia is therefore a frequent complication of meningitis. It is best avoided by judicious fluid administration and treated by hypertonic saline or diuretics (mannitol or urea).

C. Subdural Effusions: The incidence of subdural effusion in young infants with meningitis approaches 50%; it is less common after 18 months. Symptoms include prolongation or recurrence of fever, irritability, poor appetite, listlessness, vomiting, and, occasionally, focal or generalized seizures.

Important clues to the presence of a subdural effusion are abnormal increase in head circumference, bulging or tenseness of a previously flat anterior fontanel, positive transillumination in infants up to about 18 months, and widening of sutures on x-ray. The diagnosis is made by finding 2 ml or more of subdural fluid with a high protein content on subdural tap if the fontanel is open, or through a bur hole or suture if the fontanel is closed.

Treatment is by subdural taps, if possible. If significant subdural effusion cannot be "dried up" after 2–3 weeks, neurosurgical intervention may be indicated.

D. Hydrocephalus: Hydrocephalus is most prevalent in neonates and very young infants as a result of inflammatory obstruction of CSF pathways. An important clue to this complication is failure of the CSF glucose to return to normal levels in the face of negative bacterial cultures, most likely due to impairment of the glucose transport mechanism.

E. Other Neurologic Sequelae: Neurologic sequelae of meningitis in childhood occur in 10–20% of survivors, most often in the youngest and in those in whom diagnosis and adequate therapy were delayed. The finding of significant subdural effusions (more than 2 ml) per se has no prognostic significance. Severe seizures, prolonged depression of consciousness, and other evidence of major cerebral injury during the acute phase of meningitis, on the other hand, are the indices of major sequelae. In order of frequency, they are "minimal brain dysfunction" syndrome and mild to severe mental retardation, recurrent seizures, hearing loss, hydrocephalus (see above), and motor deficits, including hemiparesis.

Treatment

Antibiotic and fluid and electrolyte therapy are discussed in separate sections. Corticosteroids are not indicated except possibly when there is massive cerebral edema.

Treatment of complications is discussed above or in the section on tuberculous meningitis.

Prognosis

Purulent meningitis remains, despite potent specific and broad-spectrum antibiotics, a serious threat to life and neurologic competence. Among interacting factors determining outcome—and assuming good medical management once the diagnosis is made—the 3 most important are age, causative agent, and time of diagnosis. In pediatric practice, the highest mortality rate (30–50%) occurs in neonates and young infants with meningitides due to gram-negative organisms or *Staphylococcus aureus* and in those already in coma or near coma at diagnosis.

Platou RV, Rinker A, Derrick J: Acute subdural effusions and late sequelae of meningitis. Pediatrics 23:962–971, 1959.

Swartz MN, Dodge PR: Bacterial meningitis: A review of selected aspects. New England J Med 272:725–731, 779–787, 842–848, 898–902, 954–960, 1003–1010, 1965.

Wehrle PF, Mathies AW, Leedom JM: The critically ill child: Management of acute bacterial meningitis. Pediatrics 44:991–998, 1969.

CIRCUMSCRIBED PYOGENIC INTRACRANIAL INFECTIONS

These infections are usually secondary to a suppurative infection elsewhere; occasionally they are introduced directly, as after a compound skull fracture or penetrating foreign body (eg, pencil points). The source of infection is unknown in 5–15% of cases. Sources of direct extension are chronic otitis media and mastoiditis, the nasal cavity and accessory sinuses (frontal, sphenoid), and meningitis (via venous thrombosis). Metastatic spread occurs from the lungs and pleura or from subacute bacterial endocarditis. *Note:* Brain abscesses occur in nearly 5% of patients with cyanotic congenital heart disease, and are frequent also in patients receiving immunosuppressive agents.

The causative agents are often mixed and tend to be the same organisms responsible for middle ear and sinus infections. In metastatic abscesses, organisms may be even more diversified and include mycotic and parasitic organisms and *Salmonella typhi.*

Clinical Findings

A. Symptoms and Signs: Manifestations often evolve rapidly and include localized severe headache, fever and malaise, drowsiness progressing to confusion and stupor, nausea and vomiting, focal and generalized seizures, and focal motor, sensory, and speech deficits varying with the site and size of the pyogenic collection, the degree of cerebral edema, and the age of the child. (*Note:* Focal neurologic signs may be obscured by depressed level of consciousness and seizures.) Meningismus is seen with meningeal involvement, cerebellar abscess, and tonsillar herniation. Point tenderness to pressure on the cranium over the abscess area may be present. Papilledema may be a late finding.

B. Laboratory Findings:

1. Blood—Leukocytosis with shift to the left and increased sedimentation rate are common.

2. Cerebrospinal fluid—Increased pressure is frequent; pleocytosis is variable, but even one polymorphonuclear cell suggests the possibility of a brain abscess. Protein may be normal to moderately elevated; the glucose is often normal. Cultures are often negative.

C. X-Ray Findings: Skull films may show signs of increased intracranial pressure. Sinus and chest films may show evidence of an inflammatory process. Brain scanning may show increased isotope uptake in the area of an abscess. Cerebral angiography is often the procedure of choice prior to surgical drainage in the localization of a brain abscess.

D. Electroencephalography: EEG may be most helpful. Initially there may be diffuse high-voltage, slow activity. Serial EEGs often show an abscess to be well circumscribed by the evolution of a slow wave focus.

Differential Diagnosis

The differential diagnosis between a cerebral abscess and other intracranial mass lesions may be suspected on clinical grounds but is at times difficult. In extradural abscess, the course may be protracted and relatively benign. There may be no focal findings other than meningeal signs. With subdural empyema, which is commonly a complication of frontal sinusitis and osteomyelitis, the evolution of symptoms is very rapid. The CSF is usually sterile.

Treatment

Antibiotics should be given intravenously in large amounts with broad coverage. Other medical measures include hypothermia and anticonvulsants, especially phenobarbital. Surgical evacuation of pus and excision of the abscess are indicated as soon as feasible to relieve increased intracranial pressure.

Prognosis

The mortality rate is high and is directly related to delay in diagnosis and treatment. With multiple abscesses, mortality is virtually 100%. In about 50% of cases, the duration of illness from first symptoms to death is 5–14 days. Early diagnosis and prompt treatment offer an excellent chance of complete recovery if the underlying disease process is cured.

Raimondi JA, Matsumoto S, Miller RA: Brain abscess in children with congenital heart disease. J Neurosurg 23:588–595, 1965.

Victor M, Banker BQ: Brain abscess. M Clin North America 47:1355–1370, 1963.

SUBACUTE MENINGOENCEPHALITIS

Subacute meningoencephalitis may occur as a complication of primary tuberculosis or may be due to fungal infection or sarcoidosis. These infections involve the meninges of the base of the brain and panarteritis of the pial vessels.

Clinical Findings

A. Symptoms and Signs: Manifestations often evolve gradually and include fever (to 39.4° C [103° F]), malaise, and irritability; headache, vomiting, and photophobia; drowsiness, stupor, and coma; focal and generalized seizures; focal motor deficits, including hemiparesis, paresis of the extraocular muscles, and Bell's palsy; and deafness. Meningeal signs may be absent or minimal, but increased intracranial pressure is common.

B. Laboratory Findings:

1. Blood—The ESR may be elevated. Salt-losing encephalopathy occurs in tuberculosis.

2. Cerebrospinal fluid—(See Table 21–1.) In both tuberculous and mycotic meningitis, cell counts may range from just above 10 to about 500/cu mm, initially mostly polymorphonuclear cells but soon predominantly lymphocytes. CSF protein is mildly to moderately elevated ("pellicle" in tuberculous meningitis). CSF glucose may initially be normal but may fall rapidly. Special stains for tubercle bacilli (acid-fast) and fungi (India ink) and appropriate cultures and inoculations should be obtained.

C. Diagnosis of Specific Types: Disorders with a similar initial clinical course and gross CSF findings include the following:

1. Tuberculous meningitis—Two-thirds of cases occur in the first decade, most between 6 and 24 months of age. A positive tuberculin skin test and chest x-ray strongly favor the diagnosis. Without treatment, the course is unremitting.

2. Mycotic meningitides—The course is usually slowly progressive, but prolonged remissions occur. Definitive diagnosis depends on cultural identification of the etiologic agent. Skin tests are often positive.

a. Cryptococcal meningitis (torulosis) is usually associated with chronic debilitating disorders such as tuberculosis, leukemia, and Hodgkin's disease or occurs in renal or liver transplant recipients.

b. Nocardiosis and aspergillosis are rare, but again are more common in patients who have undergone transplants or are receiving immunosuppressive drugs.

c. Actinomycosis may spread to the CNS from a primary site in the face, neck, or cecum.

d. Mucormycosis may produce systemic infection with orbital cellulitis or thrombosis of the internal carotid artery.

3. Central nervous system sarcoidosis—Recurrent cranial neuropathies are frequent. Eosinophilia is present in about 35% of cases and hypergammaglobulinemia in about 50%. Hypercalcemia with normal serum phosphate levels is common. Lymph node and tongue biopsies and the Kveim test may establish the diagnosis.

D. X-Ray Findings: Skull films should be examined for signs of increased intracranial pressure and calcified tuberculomas (rare). Chest films should be taken for signs of pulmonary tuberculosis or other infections.

Cerebral angiography may be indicated, especially when there is evidence of increased intracranial pressure, to rule out brain abscess or to demonstrate hydrocephalus. Note that narrowed arteries and slow cerebral circulation may be seen in encephalopathies but are particularly frequent with the panarteritis in tuberculous and mycotic meningitides.

Air studies, particularly ventriculography, may be indicated when hydrocephalus is present.

Differential Diagnosis

A. Brain Abscess: This may resemble subacute meningoencephalitis early, but focal headache and neurologic findings usually point to the diagnosis.

B. Meningeal Carcinomatosis: Leukemia, sarcoma, pinealoma, etc. The diagnosis is sometimes made by cytologic studies of the CSF but usually requires demonstration of the tumor by other means.

Treatment

For appropriate antibiotic and anticonvulsant therapy, see under these sections. Observe carefully for signs of toxic reactions to the anti-infective agents used, especially streptomycin, isoniazid, and amphotericin B.

Neurosurgical evacuation of brain abscess may be required (eg, in actinomycosis) as well as neurosurgical relief of hydrocephalus by "shunting."

Prognosis

The prognosis varies with the disease process and its extent and severity. Many fungal infections, especially histoplasmosis, mucormycosis, nocardiosis, and aspergillosis, respond poorly if at all to the best available treatment.

"ASEPTIC" MENINGITIS, ENCEPHALITIS, & MENINGOENCEPHALITIS*

This clinical grouping encompasses those acute and subacute inflammatory conditions of the meninges or encephalon and often, but to a variable extent, both, in which (1) no flaccid paralysis is present, ie, there is no clinical involvement of the spinal cord or peripheral nerves (see below); and (2) no bacterial or fungal organisms are found on smear or cultures of the CSF, which otherwise may show such changes as pleocytosis and increased protein. The diagnosis is often presumptive, and the diagnostic category (and even the specific entity) may be suggested by the patient's history. Clinical differentiation between entities is often difficult, since the presenting signs and symptoms overlap considerably because of the nonspecificity of pathologic involvement. Definitive diagnosis can

---

*For consideration of specific clinical and laboratory features of the individual etiologic syndromes of aseptic meningitis, consult the chapters on viral, bacterial, and fungal diseases. Specific and supportive therapy is discussed in those chapters. Anti-infective therapy is discussed in Chapter 39.

often be established only by laboratory studies, but even this is limited by the laboratory's ability to perform viral cultures or serodiagnostic investigations.

Clues in the Etiologic Differential Diagnosis of Aseptic Meningitis

A. Partially (or Inadequately) Treated Purulent Meningitis: Prior febrile illness and antibiotic therapy.

B. Viral (or Presumably Viral) Meningitis or Encephalitis: Seasonal variation; presence of similar cases in the community; contact of the patient with such cases or with persons having "flu" or "gastrointestinal" symptoms; exposure to mosquitoes, horses, birds, squirrels, cats, or rodents.

1. Viral infections resulting in a predominantly meningitic or meningoencephalitic syndrome—(In approximate order of frequency.)

a. Mumps (winter and early spring). Parotitis, orchitis, oophoritis, and pancreatitis may precede, accompany, or follow the CNS symptoms.

b. Coxsackievirus infections, primarily group B (summer and fall). Herpangina or exanthematous rash suggests coxsackievirus A. Severe chest pain (devil's grip, pleurodynia) suggests coxsackievirus B.

c. Echovirus infections (summer and fall). There may be a petechial rash.

d. Nonparalytic poliomyelitis (summer and early fall).

e. Lymphocytic choriomeningitis (winter and spring).

f. Infectious mononucleosis. Jaundice, lymphadenopathy, petechiae of the soft palate, an exanthematous rash, splenomegaly, hepatomegaly.

g. Cat scratch fever. Lymphadenopathy may be present.

2. Viral infections resulting in a predominantly or often exclusively encephalitic syndrome—

a. Herpes simplex, especially with temporal lobe symptoms.

b. Arthropod-borne viruses (St Louis, eastern and western equine, Japanese, Russian spring-summer, Murray Valley).

c. Cytomegalovirus. Jaundice, splenomegaly, or hepatomegaly may be present.

d. Rabies.

e. Encephalitis lethargica (Von Economo's disease). Oculogyric crisis may occur.

C. Parainfectious and Postvaccinial Encephalitis: Recent infection or vaccination.

1. Exanthematous infections—Measles, varicella, rubella, roseola infantum, scarlet fever.

2. Postvaccinal—Primarily smallpox; also rabies.

D. Rickettsial Infections: Exposure to and bite by ticks (Rocky Mountain spotted fever), louse or flea (typhus), or mite (scrub typhus). There may be an exanthematous rash.

E. Syphilis: The clinical picture is highly variable. There is usually no history of infection. Both congenital and acquired forms are currently on the increase, the latter in adolescents. A history of lesions involving the skin, mucous membranes (rhagades), bones, viscera, and eyes may be obtained. Jaundice and chronic rhinitis in early infancy suggest syphilis.

F. "Chemical" or "Toxic" Meningitis: History of lumbar puncture or other episode (subarachnoid hemorrhage, rupture of a cyst, trauma, neurosurgery), in which an irritative substance (air, oil, blood, etc) was introduced into the subarachnoid space.

G. "Sympathetic" Meningitis: Secondary to a septic, necrotic, or neoplastic focus within the skull or vertebral column.

H. Miscellaneous:

1. Uveo-encephalitic syndrome (Vogt-Koyangi-Harada)–Recurrent uveitis.

2. Behçet's disease–Recurrent mucosal ulcers, uveitis.

3. Mollaret's meningitis–Recurrent acute endothelial lymphocytic meningitis.

4. Eosinophilic meningitis–History of parasitic infestations.

5. Toxoplasmosis–See Chapter 28.

6. Leptospirosis–See Chapter 27.

Lepow ML & others: A clinical, epidemiologic and laboratory investigation of aseptic meningitis during the four-year period 1955–1958. New England J Med 266:1181–1193, 1962.

PYOGENIC SPINAL CORD INFECTIONS

Pyogenic infections of the spinal cord, although relatively uncommon in children, must be considered in the differential diagnosis of cord lesions, as prompt treatment is required. *Staphylococcus aureus* is the most common pathogen. Infection occurs by direct extension or metastasis from a focus of infection such as a skin furuncle, osteomyelitis, empyema, perinephric abscess, infected wound, and other septic processes.

The onset of spinal cord infection, which is more rapid than that of spinal cord tumor, mimics that of noninfectious transverse myelitis. (See Table 21–8.)

Clinical Findings

A. Symptoms and Signs: The principal symptom, sometimes obscured for a while by the underlying illness, is severe localized back pain followed by root pain in the trunk or legs. Flaccid paralysis of the legs, accompanied by sensory loss, develops rapidly. Urinary retention is common. Headache, high fever, a stiff back, and vomiting are present in acute cases but often minimal in chronic ones.

Findings include rigidity of the spine, localized exquisite spine tenderness, lost tendon reflexes, and bilateral plantar extensor signs. Sensory loss, loss of urinary sphincter function, and, less commonly, fecal incontinence may occur.

B. Laboratory Findings:

1. **Blood**–Leukocytocis and elevated ESR are the rule. Blood cultures are often positive.

2. Cerebrospinal fluid–If epidural spinal abscess is suspected, the spinal needle is introduced only into the extradural space at the level of the lesion (region of maximal spine tenderness) to see if pus can be obtained. *Caution:* The utmost care must be exercised not to penetrate the dura and thus introduce infection into the subarachnoid space.

Lumbar puncture should be performed only after spine films have been obtained. CSF manometrics should be performed and dye for myelography instilled while the needle is in place if a CSF block is encountered. CSF xanthochromia and pleocytosis are often present; protein is usually moderately increased; glucose is normal. CSF cultures, however, often are negative.

C. X-Ray Findings: In spinal epidural abscess, evidence of osteomyelitis or an adjacent soft tissue mass is evident on spine x-rays in about 50% of cases.

Myelography is best performed in conjunction with diagnostic lumbar puncture.

Differential Diagnosis

The differential diagnosis involves principally 2 conditions: (1) transverse myelitis (Table 21–8) and other forms of acute flaccid paralysis, and (2) spinal cord tumors (see above).

Treatment

Treatment must be instituted promptly and consists of appropriate antibiotics in massive doses, neurosurgical decompression, and evacuation of the abscess or removal of granuloma.

Prognosis

The prognosis is good if cord compression is relieved early and infection is controlled.

Altrocchi PH: Acute spinal epidural abscess vs acute transverse myelopathy. Arch Neurol 9:17–25, 1963.

SYNDROMES PRESENTING AS ACUTE FLACCID PARALYSIS

Rapidly evolving flaccid paralysis suggests, in the early clinical stages, the following clinical possibilities: paralytic spinal poliomyelitis and encephalomyelitis, Landry-Guillain-Barré syndrome, secondary acute myelopathies and polyneuropathies, tick-bite paralysis, and transverse myelitis. The possibility of spinal cord trauma, tumor, and epidural abscess must be considered; an adequate history will usually tend to make these conditions less likely.

Intercurrent nonspecific infections with predominantly flu-like respiratory and gastrointestinal symptoms are so common in children as to suggest the diagnosis of Landry-Guillain-Barré syndrome ("acute idiopathic polyneuritis") almost too readily, diverting the physician's attention from the search for more specific causes.

TABLE 21–8. Acute flaccid paralyses in children.

	Poliomyelitis (Paralytic, Spinal, and Bulbar), With or Without Encephalitis	Landry-Guillain-Barré Syndrome	Secondary Acute Myelopathies and Polyneuropathies	Tick-Bite Paralysis	Transverse Myelitis and Neuromyelitis Optica
Etiology	Poliovirus types I, II, and III; occasionally mimicked by mumps.	Unknown. An autosensitivity phenomenon has been postulated.	Associated with infections, especially exanthems, diphtheria, etc; vaccination, metabolic and endocrine disturbances, allergic and immune disorders, intoxicants, neoplasms, other miscellaneous conditions.	Probable interference with transmission of nerve impulse caused by toxin in tick saliva.	Unknown.
History	None, or inadequate polio immunization. Upper respiratory or gastrointestinal symptoms followed by brief respite. Bulbar paralysis more frequent after tonsillectomy. Epidemic form more common in late summer and early fall.	Nonspecific respiratory or gastrointestinal symptoms in preceding 5–14 days common. Any season, though slightly lower incidence in summer.	Varies with etiology. Para-infectious paralyses may occur with or after primary illness. Paralyses due to allergic or immune disorders and neoplasms are usually of slow onset.	Exposure to ticks (dog tick in eastern USA; wood ticks). Irritability 12–24 hours before onset of a rapidly progressive ascending paralysis.	Occasionally, symptoms compatible with multiple sclerosis or optic neuritis. Progression from onset to paraplegia very rapid, usually without a history of bacterial infection.
Presenting complaints	Febrile usually. Meningeal signs, muscle tenderness, and spasm. Weakness widespread or segmental (cervical, thoracic, lumbar). Bulbar symptoms early or before extremity weakness. Anxiety. Delirium.	Symmetric weakness of lower extremities, sometimes ascending rapidly to arms, trunk, and face. Muscle tenderness and spinal root pains frequent. Verbal child may complain of paresthesias. Fever uncommon. Facial weakness early.	Symptomatology similar to Landry-Guillain-Barré syndrome, but may be masked by primary disease. In para-infectious and postvaccinal myelitides, initial complaints include low-grade fever, severe back pain, and sensory loss as well as those characteristic of encephalitis.	Rapid onset and progression of ascending flaccid paralysis; often accompanied by pain and paresthesias. Paralysis of upper extremities usually occurs on second day after onset.	Root and back pain in about 1/3–1/2. Sensory loss below level of lesion accompanying rapidly developing paralysis. Sphincter difficulties common.
Findings*	Flaccid weakness, usually asymmetric. Lumbar: legs, lower abdomen. Cervical: shoulder, arm, neck, diaphragm. Thoracic: intercostals, spine, upper abdomen. Bulbar: respiratory, lower cranial, upper cranial nerves. Occasionally papilledema, encephalitic syndrome, ataxia. Fever in first days. Autonomic disturbances common.	Flaccid weakness, symmetric, usually greater proximally, but may be more distal or equal in distribution. Facial diplegia in about 85%, then IX–X, XI, III–VI. Bulbar involvement may occur. Slight distal impairment of position, vibration, touch; difficult to assess in young children.	Findings similar to those in Landry-Guillain-Barré syndrome. Sensory loss may be greater. Level of spinal cord involvement may be better defined. Findings may be masked or distorted by those of the associated primary disorder or encephalitic component.	Flaccid, symmetrical paralysis. Cranial nerve and bulbar (respiratory) paralysis, ataxia, sphincter disturbances, and sensory deficits may occur. Some fever. Diagnosis rests on finding tick.	Paraplegia with areflexia below level of lesion early; later, may have hyperreflexia. Sensory loss below and hyperesthesia or normal sensation above level of lesion. Paralysis of bladder and rectum. Optic atrophy or neuritis may be present.

*Note: In flaccid paralysis, the deep reflexes are depressed or absent.

TABLE 21–8 (cont'd). Acute flaccid paralyses in children.

	Poliomyelitis (Paralytic, Spinal, and Bulbar), With or Without Encephalitis	Landry-Guillain-Barré Syndrome	Secondary Acute Myelopathies and Polyneuropathies	Tick-Bite Paralysis	Transverse Myelitis and Neuromyelitis Optica
CSF	Pleocytosis (about 200 cells) with PMN predominance in first few days, followed by rapid decrease and monocytic preponderance. Glucose normal. Protein frequently elevated (50–200 mg/100 ml).	Cytoalbuminologic dissociation: 10 or fewer cells with high protein after first week. Normal glucose. Gamma globulin may be elevated.	CSF as for Landry-Guillain-Barré syndrome. In parainfectious and postvaccinal cases, mild pleocytosis (15–250 cells, principally monocytes) and mild protein elevation (up to 150 mg/100 ml) common.	Normal.	Usually no manometric block; CSF may show increased protein, pleocytosis with predominantly monocytes, increased gamma globulin.
EMG	Denervation after 10–21 days. Nerve conduction may be slowed slightly.	Denervation after 10–21 days. Nerve conduction velocities markedly decreased.	Denervation after 10–21 days. Nerve conduction slowed only in neuropathies.	Nerve conduction slowed; returns rapidly to normal after removal of tick.	Normal early. Denervation at level of lesion after 10–21 days.
Other studies	Initially, leukocytosis. Virus in stool and throat. Serologic titers.	Rule out specific causes such as infections, intoxications, metabolic or endocrine diseases, allergic phenomena, neoplasms. Lymphocyte transformation demonstrated. *Mycoplasma pneumoniae* implicated.	EEG diffusely slow, with focal or generalized seizure potentials when an encephalitic component is present. Appropriate studies to define associated primary disorder.	Leukocytosis, often with moderate eosinophilia.	Normal spine x-rays speak against spinal epidural abscess. Myelography is often irritative and should be very carefully considered; false positives secondary to swelling of the cord are not unknown.
Course and prognosis	Paralysis usually maximal 3–5 days after onset. Transient bladder paralysis may occur. Outlook varies with extent and severity of involvement. *Note:* Threat greatest from respiratory failure and superinfection. Early muscle atrophy common.	Course progressive over a few days to about 2 weeks. Transient bladder paralysis may occur. *Note:* Threat greatest from respiratory failure and superinfection. Most recover completely; occasional residual weakness.	Course and prognosis vary greatly with underlying disease process, extent of the paralytic and encephalitic involvement, presence of bladder and bowel paralysis, and respiratory complications.	Total removal of tick is followed by rapid improvement and recovery. Otherwise, mortality due to respiratory paralysis is very high.	Large degree of functional recovery possible. Corticosteroids are of benefit in shortening duration of acute attack (especially the first) but not in preventing recurrences or altering the overall course.

While the sensory examination is important in these syndromes, it is often of dubious accuracy and hence of limited usefulness in the younger age group. Diagnosis, outlined in Table 21–8, is based on the clinical features of the illness as well as viral isolation and serologic studies.

Complications

A. Respiratory Paralysis: Early signs of hypoxia are increasing anxiety and a rise in diastolic and systolic blood pressures. Cyanosis is a late sign. The patient's ability to count to 20 on a single breath is a good clinical guide to still adequate vital capacity.

Early and careful attention to oxygenation is essential and may require administration of oxygen, tracheostomy, mechanical respiratory assistance, and careful suctioning of secretions.

B. Infections: Pneumonia is common, especially with respiratory paralysis. Prophylactic antibiotic administration is generally contraindicated. Specific infections are treated with appropriate antibiotics.

Bladder infections are most common when an indwelling catheter is required for bladder paralysis. Prophylactic administration of methenamine mandelate (Mandelamine), 30 mg/kg orally, is recommended, or the use of bladder irrigations with antibiotics. Recovery from myelitis may be delayed by urinary tract infection.

Treatment

There is no specific treatment except removal of ticks in tick-bite paralysis. Recognized associated disorders (eg, endocrine, neoplastic, toxic) should be treated by appropriate means. Patients may require respiratory assistance, fluids, and adequate nutrition, bladder, and bowel care.

Skin breakdown may be prevented by proper nursing care. Give antibiotics and anticonvulsants. Psychiatric support is often needed.

A. Corticosteroids: These agents are believed by some authors to be of benefit in severe and prolonged cases of Landry-Guillain-Barré syndrome, some recurrent polyneuropathies, and "idiopathic" transverse myelitis. *Caution:* They are not advised in parainfectious and postvaccinal encephalopathies.

B. Physical Therapy: Rehabilitative measures are best instituted when acute symptoms have subsided and the patient is stable. The physical therapy regimen will vary from patient to patient.

Prognosis

The prognosis varies greatly with the extent of involvement, duration of the inflammatory process, complications, and other factors. See Table 21—8.

Masucci EF, Kurtzke JF: Diagnostic criteria for the Guillain-Barré syndrome. J Neurol Sc 13:483—501, 1971.

DISORDERS OF CHILDHOOD AFFECTING MUSCLES*

This section is concerned with specific muscle and neuromuscular disorders, including the muscular dystrophies, myasthenia gravis, and miscellaneous congenital neuromuscular disorders.

Certain studies commonly used in the diagnosis of muscle diseases merit special consideration.

Serum Enzymes

The levels of certain enzymes (see normal values, below) may be helpful in establishing the diagnosis and in following the course of some muscle disorders. Blood should be drawn before muscles are traumatized by needle electromyography or muscle biopsy, which may lead to the release of enzymes:

   Creatine phosphokinase (CPK) (most specific): Males, 5—75 IU/liter; females, 6—50 IU/liter.

   Aldolase: Adults, 1.8—4.9 IU/liter; newborn, 4 times adult; children, 2 times adult.

   Glutamic-oxaloacetic transaminase (SGOT): Infants, up to 67 IU/liter; older children, 3—27 IU/liter.

   Lactate dehydrogenase: Infants, 308—1780 IU/ liter; adult males, 98—186 IU/liter; adult females, 87—178 IU/liter.

Electromyography

EMG is often helpful in grossly differentiating "myopathic" from "neurogenic" processes. Fibrilla-

*Polymyositis is discussed in Chapter 20.

tions occur in both. In the myopathies, very slow spikes are more typical and the motor unit action potentials seen during contraction characteristically are of short duration, polyphasic, and increased in number for the strength of the contraction (increased interference pattern).

In myotonic dystrophy, the EMG is characterized by prolonged discharge of electrical activity on movement of the probing needle ("dive bomber" sound), though these discharges may be found to a lesser degree also in other conditions. In myotonic dystrophy during attempted relaxation after a contraction, electrical activity persists parallel with the protracted relaxation of muscle.

Muscle Biopsy

Properly executed, this · is usually most helpful. The introduction of histochemical technics, histogram analysis of muscle fiber types, and electronmicroscopy is offering new insights and hence new classifications of the myopathies. Muscle biopsy findings common to the myopathies include variation in the size and shape of muscle fibers, increase in connective tissue, interstitial infiltration of fatty tissue, degenerative changes in muscle fibers, and central location of nuclei.

Findings more characteristic of certain myopathies include the sarcoplasmic masses and striking chains of central nuclei in myotonic dystrophy; the cysts found in trichinosis or toxoplasmosis; the vacuoles found in the periodic paralyses, thyrotoxicosis, chloroquine myopathy, and lupus erythematosus; the characteristic appearances with special stains of such disorders as central core disease and nemaline myopathy; or the electronmicroscopic findings in giant mitochondrial myopathy.

MUSCULAR DYSTROPHIES

Duchenne's Muscular Dystrophy (Pseudohypertrophic, Juvenile, Infantile)

This is the most common dystrophy in childhood. Onset is usually between 2—5 years; rare cases in infancy have been reported. Inherited as an X-linked recessive, the disease occurs predominantly in males, but 80% of female carriers demonstrate mild clinical, enzyme, and muscle biopsy changes.

Pseudohypertrophy of the gastrocnemius, triceps brachii, and vastus lateralis muscles may occur early. Symmetric weakness of the pelvic girdle results in waddling gait, lumbar lordosis, and difficulties in climbing stairs. The patient often climbs up on his legs in rising from the floor to a standing position. Patients frequently lose patellar reflexes, whereas ankle jerks are preserved. Involvement of the shoulder girdle and sometimes mild articulation difficulties occur later. Contractures develop with lack of exercise; eventually, the patient is confined to a wheelchair. Patients occasionally demonstrate an extensor plantar response which may indicate a relationship to other heredo-familial nervous system disorders. Mild, nonprogressive mental retardation (IQ approximately 85) occurs in many patients. "Barrel chest" and cardiac involvement are seen as the disease progresses in over 50% of cases. A rare subvariety of later onset is more slowly progressive.

Serum enzymes (CPK, aldolase, SGOT) are initially high but gradually decrease to normal as the disease progresses. The EMG and muscle biopsy are myopathic. ECG, chest x-ray, and pulmonary function studies may be indicated.

There is no specific therapy. Testosterone, corticosteroids, and digitalis have been used but are not effective. The patient should be kept ambulatory and receive physical therapy for as long as possible. Special schooling may be indicated. Weight should be kept down. Braces are occasionally of help, but a wheelchair may be necessary within 5–10 years after onset. Infections and cardiac failure must be treated.

Death from pneumonia usually occurs within 10–15 years after recognition of the dystrophic process, with few patients living beyond 20 years of age.

Limb Girdle Type of Muscular Dystrophy (Scapulo-humeral Variety of Erb; Pelvifemoral Type of Leyden-Möbius)

This form of dystrophy is inherited as an autosomal recessive in 60% of cases but also occurs sporadically. Sex distribution is equal. Onset is usually in childhood. The pelvic girdle is involved more than the shoulder girdle; however, some patients first show asymmetrical involvement of the shoulder girdle. The quadriceps and hamstring muscles may be weakest. Spread from the lower to the upper limbs may take 20 years. Many patients show an exaggerated lordosis and winging of the scapulas. Few cases have pseudohypertrophy of calves. The rate of progression is variable.

Serum enzymes are usually normal but may be elevated. EMG and muscle biopsy are myopathic.

There is no specific treatment. Physical therapy may be helpful. The prognosis is usually much better than in Duchenne's dystrophy.

Facioscapulohumeral Type of Muscular Dystrophy

This dystrophy is inherited as an autosomal dominant with equal sex distribution, but sporadic cases are observed. Onset is usually in late childhood and adolescence, but rare instances of onset occur in infancy. The face and scapulohumeral muscles are involved initially, with inability to close the eyes, smile, or whistle. The face may be flat and unlined. Serum enzymes are usually normal. EMG and muscle biopsy are myopathic. The course is slow and may arrest. Survival rates are high, and the disease is consistent with a normal life span.

Myotonic Dystrophy (Steinert's Disease)

This dystrophy is characterized by distal myopathy, with wasting of hand muscles, masseters, and sternocleidomastoids. The myotonic phenomenon consists of prolonged contraction with delay in relaxation of muscles. A "bunching up" of muscle or percussion myotonia may be seen particularly in the tongue, thenar eminence, wrists, and finger extensors after tapping them with a pointed reflex hammer. The disorder is inherited as an autosomal dominant.

The disease may manifest itself at birth with difficulty in nursing because of bilateral facial weakness. Affected infants (in contrast to adults) exhibit proximal muscle weakness. There usually is marked "floppiness," with hyporeflexia and often retarded motor and mental development.

The neostigmine (Prostigmin) test may be useful in differentiating myotonic dystrophy from myasthenia gravis (see below). In the late teens (75% of cases appear after age 15 years), premature frontal baldness, testicular atrophy, and cataracts are fairly constant additional features. Other endocrinopathies may occur. EMG and muscle biopsy show distinctive features. An ECG should be obtained about once a year.

Treatment is with procainamide (Pronestyl), 250 mg 3 times daily orally, increased to tolerance. Diphenylhydantoin (Dilantin), 5–7 mg/kg/day orally, may be useful.

Myotonia Congenita (Thomsen's Disease)

This familial disorder is characterized by myotonia and difficulty in initiating movement after rest. The muscles are often enlarged, giving patients a Herculean appearance. The disability is usually mild, but it may be aggravated by prolonged exposure to cold or emotional excitement.

The EMG shows a myotonic pattern, though less striking than in myotonic dystrophy. Muscle biopsy usually shows no definite structural changes of the muscle fibers.

Treatment is usually not indicated, although the use of diphenylhydantoin (Dilantin), especially during the winter months, occasionally enables a patient to function better.

Distal Myopathy

Two types of this disorder are described: (1) the Gowers type, with early onset and wasting of cranial musculature; and (2) the Welander type, with onset occasionally in adolescence (although more commonly in adulthood), involving the hands and feet, particularly the extensors of the fingers and toes. In this latter type, the muscles of the face and tongue are rarely involved. It is inherited as an autosomal dominant.

The differential diagnosis includes myotonic dystrophy and the neuropathies, and the differentiation may be made by appropriate laboratory studies. The EMG is myopathic, distinguishing this disorder from Charcot-Marie-Tooth disease. Serum enzymes may be mildly elevated, and muscle biopsy shows features common to the myopathies.

There is no specific treatment. The prognosis is good for both function and life span.

Congenital Muscular Dystrophies With Extremely Slow or Nonprogressive Course

These disorders are now diagnosed by special staining technics and electron microscopy. They are inherited as autosomal dominants with nearly equal sex distribution. There usually is proximal muscle weakness, with "floppiness" in infancy and delayed motor development since the muscles of the lower extremities usually are more involved. The bulbar muscles are spared; respiratory involvement is rare. Deep reflexes are usually preserved. Weakness may increase during adolescence.

EMG may be myopathic. Muscle enzymes are usually normal. Muscle biopsy with special histochemical stains and electron microscopy are most important. In central core disease the central areas of the muscle fiber show hyaline changes; these areas are devoid of enzymes and presumably inert. In nemaline myopathy, subsarcolemmal rod-shaped structures are seen; recent evidence suggests that an excess of protein arises from the Z band. Other types, such as giant mitochondrial and myotubular myopathies and new or "mixed" forms, have also been described.

No treatment is usually indicated. Physical therapy is of benefit. The disorders are usually compatible with a normal life span.

Brooke MH, Engel WK: The histographic analysis of human muscle biopsies with regard to fiber types. 4. Children's biopsies. Neurology 19:591, 1969.

Dubowitz V: *Developing and Diseased Muscle.* Heinemann, 1968.

Ocular Myopathy

This disorder often begins in childhood with ptosis and external ophthalmoplegia, which may be asymmetrical. Weakness of the orbicularis oculi muscles and dysphagia occurs in 50% of cases.

Other hereditary neurologic diseases may be found in the patients and their families. Ocular myopathy may be the first manifestation of generalized muscular dystrophy, spinocerebellar degenerative disease, or Refsum's disease. It is sometimes associated with hypogonadism. It must be differentiated from the ophthalmoplegia sometimes seen in demyelinating disorders.

A negative response to edrophonium (Tensilon) and neostigmine (Prostigmin) will differentiate this disorder from myasthenia gravis. Elevation of CSF protein and ECG abnormalities suggest the syndrome of external ophthalmoplegia with conduction block. Serum enzymes are normal. Corticosteroids or corticotropin may be useful. Plastic retraction of the eyelids to correct ptosis may be necessary. The prognosis is good if the disorder is confined to the ocular muscles.

Rosenberg RN & others: Progressive ophthalmoplegia. Arch Neurol 19:362–376, 1968.

THE PERIODIC PARALYSES

Primary Hypokalemic Periodic Paralysis

This condition is inherited as a dominant trait but may occur sporadically. A family history of migraine is often present. The onset is usually about the end of the first decade of life. The proximal muscles are affected first. The muscles innervated by the cranial nerves are spared—eg, the extraocular muscles, the muscles of facial expression, mastication, and swallowing, and the tongue muscles. The diaphragm, which is usually spared, has its embryonic origin in bulbar territory. Attacks of weakness may be precipitated by rest after exercise, exposure to cold, emotional stress, high dietary intake of carbohydrate and sodium, and administration of corticosteroids.

Attacks may last for days but may be aborted by mild exercise. The disease may progress to a chronic form of weakness and atrophy, but in general attacks are less frequent after middle age.

The serum potassium is low during an attack.

Provocative tests which induce weakness and thus confirm the diagnosis include (1) exercise and (2) giving insulin, 0.25 units/kg subcut, simultaneously with glucose, 0.8 gm/kg orally.

Treatment consists of giving potassium chloride, 2–10 gm orally, to terminate an attack, and 2–10 gm at bedtime between attacks. The patient should be encouraged to eat a low-carbohydrate, low-sodium diet. Thiamine may abort the effects of carbohydrates. Unnecessary exposure to cold should be avoided.

The disorder is consistent with a normal life span.

Primary Hyperkalemic Periodic Paralysis (Adynamia Episodica Hereditaria of Gamstorp)

This form of periodic paralysis has its onset in the first decade of life and is usually detected in infancy because of "staring" eyes (myotonic form of lid lag). It is inherited as an autosomal dominant. Pseudohypertrophy of the calves is often present. There is an increased incidence of diabetes mellitus. The attacks are relatively short, lasting 30 minutes to 2 hours, and may be precipitated by rest after exercise, cold, and fatigue. Attacks usually occur in children of school age and then abate.

The serum potassium rises during attacks. The EMG may show myotonia of the external ocular and facial muscles.

Treatment is with hydrochlorothiazide (Hydrodiuril), 50 mg orally daily, or acetazolamide (Diamox), 250 mg orally daily. Dichlorphenamide (Daranide), 50 mg orally daily, has also been recommended. The dose must be adjusted for each case.

The disorder is consistent with a normal life span.

Normokalemic Periodic Paralysis

In this disorder, the onset is in the first decade of life. It is inherited as an autosomal dominant. Attacks come on during rest after exercise, with cold, following ingestion of foods high in potassium (eg, many fruit juices), and following ingestion of alcohol. The attacks may last for days.

In normokalemic paralysis, serum electrolytes do not change during attacks. Muscle biopsy may show vacuolar myopathy.

Treatment consists of increased intake of salt; acetazolamide (Diamox), 250 mg orally daily, with dosage adjusted for each case; and fludrocortisone, 0.1 mg daily orally.

The prognosis is good.

Pearson CM: The periodic paralyses: Differential features and pathological observations in permanent myopathic weakness. Brain 87:341–358, 1969.

MYASTHENIA GRAVIS

Essentials of Diagnosis

- Weakness, chiefly of muscles innervated by the brain stem, usually coming on or increasing with use (fatigue).
- Positive response to neostigmine (Prostigmin) and edrophonium (Tensilon).
- The forms seen in infancy and childhood are often more difficult to distinguish clinically than the adult type.

General Considerations

Myasthenia gravis is characterized by easy fatigability of muscles, particularly the extraocular muscles, muscles of mastication, swallowing, and respiration. However, in the neonatal period or early infancy, the weakness may be constant, so that the physician merely sees another "floppy" infant. Girls are involved more frequently than boys. Siblings may be involved. The age at onset is over 10 years in 75% of cases, often shortly after menarche. If the diagnosis is made in children under age 10, congenital myasthenia should be considered in retrospect. Thyrotoxicosis is found in almost 10% of female patients. The essential abnormality, while associated with altered function of cholinesterase on the acetylcholine released at the neuromuscular junction, is still not defined; altered immunologic responses have recently been demonstrated.

Clinical Findings

A. Symptoms and Signs:

1. Neonatal (transient)—This occurs in infants born of myasthenic mothers, although sometimes the mother is not aware of nor known to have the disease. The condition is due to some substance transmitted from the mother to the infant. Sex distribution is equal. A sibling may have died in the neonatal period with similar symptoms and nondiagnostic autopsy. The infant exhibits hypotonia and a weak Moro reflex, but the knee jerk reflexes are preserved. Most striking are ineffective sucking, difficulty in swallowing, pooling of secretions, and a weak cry despite lack of evidence of other neurologic damage. In contrast to other forms of myasthenia gravis, the eyes are usually wide open, and extraocular muscle palsies are usually not present. There is, however, obvious facial weakness.

2. Congenital (persistent)—In these infants, the mothers rarely have myasthenia gravis but other relatives may. Sex distribution is equal. Extraocular muscle palsies and ptosis are often prominent; there may be a weak cry, fatigue with sucking, and hypotonia. Symptoms are often subtle and not recognized initially. Differential diagnosis includes many other causes of the "floppy infant" syndrome (see below), but particularly ocular myopathy, congenital ptosis, and Möbius' syndrome (facial nuclear aplasia and other anomalies).

3. Juvenile myasthenia gravis—In this form, the symptoms and signs are more similar to those seen in adults. The patient may be first seen by an ENT specialist or psychiatrist. The more prominent signs are difficulty in chewing, dysphagia, a nasal voice, ptosis, and ophthalmoplegia. Pathologic fatigability of limbs, chiefly involving the proximal limb and neck muscles, may be more prominent than the bulbar signs and may lead to an initial diagnosis of conversion hysteria, muscular dystrophy, or polymyositis.

B. Laboratory Findings:

1. Neostigmine test—In neonates and very young infants, the neostigmine (Prostigmin) test is preferable to the edrophonium (Tensilon) test because the longer duration of its response permits better observation, especially of sucking and swallowing movements. The test dose of neostigmine is 0.02 mg/kg subcut, usually given with atropine, 0.01 mg/kg subcut. The physician should be prepared to suction the patient.

2. Edrophonium test—Testing with edrophonium (Tensilon) is used in older children who are capable of cooperating in certain tasks, such as raising and lowering their eyelids and squeezing a sphygmomanometer bulb or the examiner's hands. The test dose is 0.1–1 ml IV, depending on the size of the child. Maximum improvement occurs within 2 minutes.

3. Curare test—This may be done to provoke the myasthenic state but should be performed only if marked diagnostic difficulties are present, under the most controlled conditions, and with an anesthesiologist in attendance.

4. Other laboratory tests—Thyroid function studies and LE cell preparations are indicated in older children. Where available, immunologic studies (eg, for muscle antibodies) may be useful.

C. Electrical Studies of Muscle: Repetitive stimulation of a motor nerve at slow rates (2/sec) with recording over the appropriate muscle reveals a progressive fall in amplitude of the muscle potential in myasthenic patients. A maximal stimulus must be given. At higher rates of stimulation (50/sec), there may be a transient repair of this defect before the progressive decline is seen.

D. X-Ray Findings: Chest x-ray and laminography in older children may disclose thymus enlargement.

E. Electroencephalography: An increased incidence of seizure disorders has been reported in patients with myasthenia gravis.

Treatment

A. General and Supportive Care: In the neonate, or in a child in a myasthenic crisis or cholinergic crisis (see below), suctioning of secretions is essential. Respiratory assistance may be required. Infections should be treated promptly; hospitalization is usually advisable.

The treatment of myasthenia gravis should generally be carried out by physicians with experience and expertise in this disorder. In older children, some of the responsibility for adjustment of the dosage of anticholinesterase drugs may be left to the patient.

B. Anticholinesterase Drug Therapy:

1. Pyridostigmine (Mestinon)—The dose must be adjusted for each patient. A frequent starting dose is 15—30 mg every 6 hours.

2. Neostigmine (Prostigmin)—Fifteen mg are roughly equivalent to 60 mg of pyridostigmine. It often causes gastric hypermobility with diarrhea, but it is the drug of choice in neonates, in whom prompt treatment may be lifesaving.

3. Atropine may be added on a maintenance basis to control mild cholinergic side-effects such as hypersecretion, abdominal cramps, and nausea and vomiting.

4. Patients who become resistant to anticholinesterase drugs may need to be taken off the drugs for a few days and be given respiratory assistance. The use of corticosteroids in such cases is sometimes beneficial.

5. Myasthenic crisis—Relatively sudden difficulties in swallowing and respiration may be observed in myasthenic patients. Edrophonium chloride (Tensilon) will result in dramatic but brief improvement and may be difficult to evaluate in the small child. Suctioning, tracheostomy, respiratory assistance, and fluid and electrolyte maintenance may be required.

6. Cholinergic crises—Cholinergic crisis may result from overdosage of anticholinesterase drugs. The resulting weakness may be similar to that of myasthenia, and the muscarinic effects (diarrhea, sweating, lacrimation, miosis, bradycardia, hypotension) are often absent or difficult to evaluate. The edrophonium (Tensilon) test may help to determine whether the patient is receiving too little of the drug or is manifesting toxic symptoms due to overdosage. Improvement after the drugs are withdrawn suggests cholinergic crisis. Respirator facilities should be available. The patient may require atropine, tracheostomy, and respiratory assistance.

C. Surgical Measures: Thymectomy is beneficial in many patients (especially adolescent girls) who have had the disease for less than 5 years. Some advise irradiation prior to surgery. This requires experienced surgical and postsurgical care.

Prognosis

Neonatal (transient) myasthenia presents a great threat to life, primarily due to aspiration of secretions. With proper treatment, the symptoms usually begin to disappear within a few days to 2—3 weeks, and the child usually requires no further treatment.

In the congenital persistent form, the symptoms may initially be as acute as in the transient variety; more commonly, however, they are relatively benign and constant, with gradual worsening as the child grows older. Life span is not usually affected.

In the juvenile form, a high percentage of patients become resistant or unresponsive to anticholinesterase compounds and require treatment in a hospital where respiratory assistance can be given as needed. Spontaneous remissions in this group are infrequent.

The response to thymectomy after the first few critical days is often most gratifying, with the patient requiring no further drug therapy.

Death in myasthenic or cholinergic crisis may occur unless prompt treatment is given.

Millichap JG, Dodge PR: Diagnosis and treatment of myasthenia gravis in infancy, childhood and adolescence. Neurology 10:1007—1014, 1960.

CONGENITAL ABSENCE OF MUSCLES*

Congenital absence of one or muscles, usually unilateral, and particularly of the pectoralis (sternal portion), trapezius, serratus anterior, quadratus femoris, or omohyoid, is not unusual. Heredofamilial cases have been reported. Other deformities, eg, syndactyly, microdactyly, and muscular dystrophy, may be present. Absence of muscles of the abdominal wall (prune belly) is often associated with urinary tract anomalies (Eagle's syndrome), the latter requiring treatment.

PERIPHERAL NERVE PALSIES

1. THE ASYMMETRIC FACE

Facial asymmetry may be present at birth or develop later, either suddenly or gradually, unilaterally or bilaterally. Nuclear or peripheral involvement of the facial nerves results in sagging or drooping of the mouth and inability to close one or both eyes, particularly with crying in neonates and infants. Inability to wrinkle the forehead may be demonstrated in infants and young children by getting them to follow an

*Arthrogryposis multiplex, or contractures and fixation about multiple joints, is discussed briefly under the section on the floppy infant (below). Clubfoot, Sprengel's deformity, and torticollis are discussed in Chapter 19.

object (light) moved vertically above the forehead. Loss of taste of the anterior 2/3 of the tongue on the involved side may be demonstrated in intelligent, cooperative children by age 4 or 5, though playing with a younger child and the judicious use of a tongue blade may enable the physician to note if the child's face puckers up when something sour, such as lemon juice, is applied with a swab to the anterior tongue. Ability to wrinkle the forehead is preserved, due to bilateral innervation, in supranuclear or central facial paralysis.

Injuries to the facial nerve at birth occur in 0.25–6.5% of consecutive live births. Forceps delivery is the obvious cause in some cases; in others, the side of the face affected may have abutted in utero against the sacral prominence. In many cases, no cause can be established.

Facial weakness in early life may be due to agenesis of the affected muscles, aplasia of the facial nucleus (part of the Möbius syndrome), or may even be familial. Neonatal myasthenia gravis, polyneuritis, and myotonic dystrophy must be considered. Facial asymmetry due to hypoplasia of one side of the cranium associated with contralateral hemiatrophy and spastic hemiparesis (due, in most instances, to an intrauterine cerebrovascular accident affecting one hemisphere) is usually differentiated easily, as is the hemiatrophy of one side of the body seen in Silver's syndrome.

Acquired peripheral facial weakness (Bell's palsy) is common in children. The cause is often not known, but it is important to rule out brain stem gliomas and other posterior fossa tumors, basilar arachnoiditis of whatever cause, and polyradiculoneuropathies (Landry-Guillain-Barré syndrome), which may be parainfectious or related to diabetes mellitus, lupus erythematosus, or polyarteritis nodosa. Malignant hypertension has been reported as a cause. Bell's palsies in children may also be associated with infectious mononucleosis and sarcoidosis.

If there is a history of trauma, skull x-rays, including basilar views, should be obtained to exclude fractures.

In the vast majority of cases of isolated peripheral facial palsy—both those present at birth and those acquired later—improvement begins within 1–2 weeks and near or total recovery of function is observed within 2 months. Methylcellulose drops, 1%, should be instilled into the eyes to protect the cornea during the day, and the eye should be closed with cellophane tape at night. Upward massage of the face for 5–10 minutes 3–4 times a day may help maintain muscle tone. Corticosteroids are sometimes of value.

When little or no improvement occurs in 10–14 days, tests for electrical excitability of the facial nerve and electromyography by specialists are useful diagnostically and prognostically.

In the few children with permanent and cosmetically disfiguring facial weakness, plastic surgical intervention at 6 years of age or older may be of benefit. New procedures, such as attachment of facial muscles to the temporal muscle, are being developed.

Editorial. Bell's palsy and surgery. Brit MJ 4:126–127, 1970.

Lloyd AVC, Jewitt DE, Loyd Still JD: Facial paralysis in children with hypertension. Arch Dis Childhood 41:292–294, 1966.

McHugh H, Sowden KA, Levitt MN: Facial paralysis and muscle agenesis in the newborn. Arch Otolaryng 89:131–143, 1969.

Paine RS: Facial paralysis in children: Review of the differential diagnosis and report of ten cases treated with cortisone. Pediatrics 19:303–313, 1965.

Salam EA, Elyahky WL: Evaluation of prognosis and treatment in Bell's palsy in children. Acta paediat scandinav 57:468–472, 1968.

2. BRACHIAL PLEXUS INJURIES
(Erb's Palsy, Klumpke's Paralysis)

Traction injuries of the brachial plexus are most common in neonates, occurring in 0.1% of spontaneous, 1.2% of breech, 1.3% of forceps, and 0.25% of all deliveries. The complexity of the brachial plexus precludes any absolute classification, but injuries are usually divided into those affecting the upper plexus (Erb's palsy) and those affecting the lower plexus (Klumpke's paralysis).

Erb's palsy, involving chiefly the fifth and sixth cervical roots, is seen in 99% of cases. It is usually associated with difficult breech delivery, forceps delivery (especially in brow and face presentations), or misapplication of the vacuum extractor. The arm is maintained in adduction and internal rotation at the shoulder, with the lower arm pronated, assuming the "waiter's tip" position. Loss of sensation may be difficult to assess in neonates.

In Klumpke's paralysis, involving chiefly the lower brachial plexus (eighth cervical and first thoracic roots), the small muscles of the hand and wrist flexors are affected, causing a "claw hand." Horner's syndrome may also be present. The injury, usually manipulation during delivery, results in hyperabduction of the arm at the shoulder.

Swinging a child by one arm or jerking the arm may also cause lower plexus injuries.

The palsies observed are usually due to avulsion of the plexus with contusion, edema, and some hemorrhage. X-ray studies of the shoulder will rule out fractures of the clavicle or cervical spine, or dislocations.

In most instances, recovery occurs spontaneously within a few days or weeks; however, contractures of the shoulder and especially the elbow joints and atrophy of the affected muscles are not infrequent residuals to which positioning in the so-called Statue of Liberty or airplane wing position, formerly advised, has been said to contribute. Passive range of motion exercises, which can be taught to the parents, are most helpful in preventing contractures. Electromyography can delineate the extent of injury and aid in prognosis. Surgical exploration is justified in the rare instances where residual fibrosis is compressing the roots.

Adler JB, Patterson RL Jr: Erb's palsy: Long-term results of treatment in eighty-eight cases. J Bone Joint Surg 49A: 1052–1064, 1967.

Eng GD: Brachial plexus palsy in newborn infants. Pediatrics 48:18–28, 1971.

3. OTHER PERIPHERAL NERVE INJURIES

Injuries to the radial and ulnar nerves occur with fractures of the humerus; ulnar and median nerve injuries may result from deep wrist lacerations; and fracture of the fibula may cause peroneal palsy. These usually require neurosurgical attention. Femoral nerve palsies occasionally occur with diabetes mellitus in teenage youngsters.

The so-called "shoulder strap" or "pack" paralysis of the long thoracic nerve, resulting in winging of the scapula, occurs in youngsters who carry heavy rucksacks with poorly padded straps. Discontinuing heavy pack carrying results in recovery.

A most unfortunate type of paralysis is that of the sciatic nerve following injections into the buttock. Penicillin and tetracycline injected into neonates or small thin children are the most common offenders. The resulting fibrosis, chiefly around the outer portion of the sciatic nerve, comprising elements making up the common peroneal nerve, causes foot drop and adduction and inversion of the foot. Sensory loss over the outer side of the lower leg and dorsum of the foot may be demonstrated. Electrical studies may delineate the injury.

In most cases, at least partial recovery occurs spontaneously over the course of a few weeks to 6 months. Occasionally, surgical exploration of the buttock with neurolysis is justified. What is most important, however, is to prevent postinjection sciatic neuropathy by giving injections into the anterior lateral aspect of the thigh.

Gilles FH, Matson DD: Sciatic nerve injury following misplaced gluteal injection. J Pediat 76:247–254, 1970.

Watters GV, Barlow CF: Acute and subacute neuropathies. P Clin North America 14:997–1008, 1967.

CHRONIC POLYNEUROPATHY

Polyneuropathy, usually insidious in onset and slowly progressive, occurs in children of any age. The presenting complaints are chiefly disturbances of gait or easy fatigability in walking or running and, slightly less often, weakness or clumsiness of the hands. Pain, tenderness, or paresthesias are infrequently mentioned. Neurologic examination discloses muscular weakness, greatest in the distal portions of the extremities, with steppage gait and depressed or absent deep tendon reflexes. Cranial nerves are sometimes affected. Sensory deficits (difficult to demonstrate in fearful children or those under 5 years of age) cover a stocking-glove distribution. The muscles may be tender, and trophic changes such as a glossy or "parchment" skin and absent sweating may occur. Thickening of the ulnar and peroneal nerves may occasionally be felt. Pure sensory neuropathies show up as chronic trauma.

The cause in children is usually not clear. Known causes include (1) toxins (eg, lead, arsenic, mercurials, vincristine, benzene); (2) metabolic disorders (diabetes mellitus, chronic uremia, recurrent hypoglycemia, porphyria, polyarteritis nodosa, lupus erythematosus); (3) hereditary, often degenerative conditions (eg, Dejerine-Sottas interstitial hypertrophic polyneuritis, some of the leukodystrophies, Refsum's disease, the spinocerebellar degenerations with neurogenic components, especially Charcot-Marie-Tooth disease, abeta-lipoproteinemia, and Recklinghausen's disease); and (4) "inflammatory" states such as "chronic or recurrent Landry-Guillain-Barré syndrome" and neuritis associated with mumps or diphtheria. Causes such as carcinoma, chronic alcoholism, and beriberi and other vitamin deficiencies are not reported in children.

Laboratory diagnosis is made by the marked slowing of nerve conduction. CSF protein is commonly elevated and gamma globulin is sometimes elevated. Electromyography may show a neurogenic polyphasic pattern. Nerve biopsy, with teasing of the fibers as well as staining for metachromasia, is advised to demonstrate loss of myelin and (to a lesser degree) of axons and increased connective tissue or concentric lamellas ("onion skin appearance") around the nerve fiber. Muscle biopsy may show the pattern associated with denervation. Other laboratory studies, directed toward specific causes mentioned above, include screening for heavy metals and for metabolic, renal, or vascular disorders. Chronic lead intoxication, which rarely causes neuropathy in childhood, may escape detection until the child is given calcium disodium edetate (EDTA) and lead levels are determined in timed urines. Three- and 4-fold rises then are diagnostic.

Therapy is directed at specific disorders whenever possible. Occasionally the weakness is profound and involves bulbar nerves, in which case tracheostomy and respiratory assistance are required. In most cases in which the cause is unknown or considered to be due to "chronic inflammation," corticosteroid therapy (as is not the case in acute Landry-Guillain-Barré syndrome) is often of great benefit. Prednisone, 1–2.5 mg/kg/day orally, with tapering to the least effective dose—discontinued if the process seems to be arresting and reinstituted when symptoms recur—is recommended. When treatable, symptoms regress and may disappear altogether over a period of months.

Long-term prognosis varies with the cause and the ability to offer specific therapy. In the "steroid-dependent" group, residual deficits and deaths within a few years are more frequent.

Bradley WG, Aguayo A: Hereditary chronic polyneuropathy. J Neurol Sc 9:131–154, 1969.

Dyck PJ & others: Severe hypomyelination and marked abnormality of conduction in Dejerine-Sottas hypertrophic neuropathy. Mayo Clin Proc 46:432–436, 1971.

Matthews WB, Howell DA, Hughes RC: Relapsing corticosteroid-dependent polyneuritis. J Neurol Neurosurg Psychiat 33:330–337, 1970.

Schoene WC & others: Hereditary sensory neuropathy. J Neurol Sc 11:463–487, 1970.

Tasker W, Chutorian AM: Chronic polyneuritis of childhood. J Pediat 74:699–708, 1969.

MISCELLANEOUS NEUROMUSCULAR DISORDERS

CEREBRAL PALSY

Essentials of Diagnosis

- Impairment of neurologic functions, especially voluntary motor activity.
- Nonprogressive and nonhereditary.
- Present since birth or early infancy.

General Considerations

Cerebral palsy is a term of clinical convenience for disorders of impaired brain and motor functioning with onset before or at birth or during the first year of life, basically nonprogressive, and varying widely in their causes, manifestations, and prognosis. Although the most obvious manifestation is impaired ability of voluntary muscles, the term in its broadest sense has also been applied to the minimal brain dysfunction syndrome (see below). The incidence of cerebral palsy is 1–5/1000 live births.

Classification

Classification is commonly based on the predominant motor deficit.

A. Spastic Forms: About 75% of cases. Often associated with other forms.

1. Tetraplegia—Approximately equal involvement of all 4 extremities. The main lesion is in the cortical gray matter. Cases due to perinatal damage often show symptoms earlier than those due to cortical dysplasias.

2. Hemiplegia—One side involved primarily, the right nearly twice as often as the left. Comprises nearly 40% of all cerebral palsy patients.

3. Diplegia—Legs involved more than arms.

4. Paraplegia—Legs only involved.

5. Monoplegia—One extremity only involved.

6. Triplegia—Three extremities involved.

B. Choreo-athetosis: (See section on extrapyramidal disorders.) Often associated with rigidity or spastic tetraplegia. Comprises about 20% of all cerebral palsy patients.

C. Ataxia: Pure and in combination with other forms. Comprises about 1–2%.

Etiology

The cause is often obscure or multiple. No definite etiologic diagnosis is possible in over 1/3 of cases. The incidence of cerebral palsy is high among infants of low birth weight. Among known causes are intrauterine bleeding, infections, toxins, congenital malformations, birth trauma and hypoxia, neonatal infections, kernicterus, and neonatal hypoglycemia.

Associated Deficits

A. Seizures: Seizures afflict about 60% of children with cerebral palsy (chiefly children with hemi- and tetraplegia) and about 1/3 of children with paraplegia and movement disorders.

B. Mental Retardation: While frequent, it is present primarily in spastic tetraplegics.

C. Sensory and Speech Deficits: Impairment of speech, vision, hearing, and perceptual functions is frequently present in varying degrees and combinations.

Clinical Findings

A. Symptoms and Signs: The typical spastic child exhibits muscular hypertonicity of the clasp-knife type which may eventually end in contractures. Tendon reflexes, if sufficient muscle relaxation can be achieved, are increased; clonus may be present. Plantar responses are often extensor on the involved sides. While voluntary control, especially of fine movements, is decreased, there is spread or overflow of associated movements. In extreme cases, the child may lie with his elbows flexed and fists clenched (straphanger's posture) and his legs crossed or scissored. In early infancy the child may appear floppy, although tendon jerks are abnormally increased (hypotonic, atonic, or prespastic diplegia). Rigidity often accompanies cerebral palsy.

Ataxia may be difficult to delineate due to the simultaneous presence of spasticity or hyperkinetic movements.

Microcephaly (head circumference < 2 SD from mean for age and sex and decreasing) is present in about 25% of spastic tetraplegics.

Partial atrophy of the cranium on the involved side or of involved extremities is observed frequently, but dependable statistics are not available.

A smaller hand or foot, when coupled with mild weakness on muscle testing or hyperreflexia, often justifies a diagnosis of mild cerebral palsy of which the patient or his family may not even have been aware.

B. Laboratory and Other Findings: No routine work-up can be outlined. The clinical findings, the presence or absence of seizures, and the overall outlook for the child—particularly with respect to his ability to carry on activities for daily living and his mental status—determine what studies, if any, should be performed. Hip films in abduction are indicated to rule out dislocations secondary to spasticity. EEG is indicated when seizures are present or suspected.

Pneumoencephalography or cerebral angiography is rarely indicated except when neurosurgical intervention is contemplated, as in hemiplegic children with uncontrolled seizures who may have a porencephalic cyst or may be candidates for hemispherectomy.

Urine screening tests for aminoacidurias and serum uric acid determination, where readily and inexpensively available, are sometimes indicated by the clinical findings.

Children whose motor difficulties, especially incoordination and spasticity, do not begin until the second year of life, should be checked for metachromatic leukodystrophy (Table 21–5).

Differential Diagnosis

The diagnosis is usually not difficult. When there is a suggestion of progressive deterioration, the degenerative and metabolic disorders affecting the nervous system must be considered. In the ataxic form, cerebellar dysgenesis (sometimes familial) and other forms of spinocerebellar degenerations may have to be ruled out; in the former, skull x-rays may show a shallow posterior fossa and a hypoplastic cerebellum on pneumoencephalography.

Treatment

Realistically, a child should be helped to achieve maximum potential rather than "normality." Special educational programming depends on the physical and mental potential of the child. Treat seizures as in other children. The orthopedic aspects of cerebral palsy are discussed in Chapter 19.

Hyperactivity may be controlled to some extent with dextroamphetamine, 2.5–15 mg orally in the morning and at noon, depending on the size and age of the child. Other psychotropic drugs, such as methylphenidate (Ritalin), chlorpromazine (Thorazine), and chlordiazepoxide (Librium), may be useful.

For spasticity, diazepam (Valium), 2–5 mg orally 2–4 times a day, is often of benefit.

Psychologic counseling and support of the child and his family are of paramount importance.

Prognosis

In severely involved cases, especially spastics with profound retardation and seizures which are difficult to control, death due to intercurrent infections during early childhood is not uncommon. Many children with cerebral palsy of average or near-average intelligence lead fairly normal, satisfying, and productive lives.

Bobath K: *The Motor Deficit in Patients With Cerebral Palsy.* Clinics in Developmental Medicine No. 23. Heinemann, 1966.

Christensen E, Melchior J: *Cerebral Palsy: A Clinical and Neuropathological Study.* Clinics in Developmental Medicine No. 25. Heinemann, 1967.

Crothers B, Paines RS: *The Natural History of Cerebral Palsy.* Oxford Univ Press, 1959.

Denhoff E (editor): *Drugs in Cerebral Palsy.* Clinics in Developmental Medicine No. 16. Heinemann, 1964.

Jeubert M & others: Familial agenesis of the cerebellar vermis. Neurology 19:813–825, 1969.

MINIMAL BRAIN DYSFUNCTION SYNDROME

This term is one of many applied to "children of near average, average, or above average general intelligence with certain learning or behavioral disabilities ranging from mild to severe, which are associated with deviations of function of the central nervous system. These deviations may manifest themselves by various combinations of impairment in perception, conceptualization, language, memory, and control of attention, impulse, or motor function."* Certain aspects of this syndrome are discussed briefly in the sections on developmental retardation and chronic brain syndromes. Neurologists are frequently requested to evaluate children whose behavior at home or in school is unacceptable to parents or teachers in order to establish the organic basis of the problem and sometimes in the hope that medical management will provide an easy solution. In terms of daily living, the children, their parents and teachers, and the professionals who become involved find the "dysfunctions" far from "minimal."

Estimates of incidence are imprecise because the syndrome itself is so ill-defined but vary from 4–10% of school-age children. Boys are more frequently affected than girls. Suggested causative factors include virtually any illness or trauma occurring before, during, or after birth and affecting the brain either obviously or by implication. Multiple causes, including psychosocial factors, are usually involved.

Disturbances of feeding and sleeping patterns are often noted in early infancy, with frequent formula changes and delays in sleeping through the night. Motor milestones are usually attained at normal ages, but the child is noted to be clumsy, with troubles learning to dress himself, button his clothes, and tie his shoes. Language development is frequently reported as delayed. When the child attends preschool or school, the chief complaints are "hyperactivity," distractibility, overexcitability, short attention span, and various learning disabilities, particularly in reading and arithmetic.

On neurologic examination, the physician is apt to be less impressed by the child's "hyperactivity" than the parents or teachers. The chief findings are "maladroitness" or nonspecific incoordination; overflow "choreiform" as well as mirror movements or synkinesis (observed best by having the child wiggle the fingers of one outstretched hand and noting extraneous movements of the other hand or the feet); and difficulties in performing rapid rhythmic tasks such as hopping on one foot or clapping the hands in a rhythmic pattern. Disturbances of tone (especially mild spasticity) and hyperreflexia and occasionally Babinski responses are also found. Some clinicians accept even the most minimal of "neurologic soft signs" as evidence of brain damage. Neither eye nor

*Clements SD: Minimal brain dysfunction in children. US Dept of Health, Education, and Welfare, NINDB Monograph No. 3, 1966, pp 9–10.

hand dominance nor "mixed laterality" have proved to be related to the learning problems.

The EEG is mildly and diffusely dysrhythmic in about 40% of cases, but there is no clear correlation between the EEG findings and any of the functional disturbances; indeed, on follow-up studies, children labeled as hyperkinetic who had abnormal EEGs had normal ones later, while those with initially normal studies later had dysrhythmic EEGs.

Far more useful are psychologic tests, including the WISC, Goodenough Draw-A-Man, Bender Gestalt, and Lincoln-Oseretsky Motor Development Scale. These children commonly exhibit a wide scatter on varied subtests, with marked discrepancy between verbal abilities and performances and visual-motor or audio-motor perceptual dysfunctions. Many are also found to be mildly to moderately depressed, compulsive, and anxious because they continually fail to come up to the expectations of others.

The physician's task is not only to rule out severe and possibly progressive neurologic or emotional disorders but also to guide the child and his parents and teachers. He must be as accurate as possible in his diagnosis, keeping in mind that the reported complaints and disabilities, as well as the neurologic, EEG, and even psychometric findings, may be observed in children with different organic, emotional, and social problems, and that these may be present together to a greater or lesser extent. In discussing the problems, the author has often described the child as being "dyssynchronous," ie, "out of phase" in his developmental, behavioral, and educational progression and maturation. Parents quickly appreciate the term "dyssynchronous" when it is explained in terms of such analogies as the automatic shift of an automobile synchronized to changes in speed. Lack of synchronization (or letting the clutch out at the wrong time when using a standard shift) results in grinding the gears or the car's bucking like a bronco. The "dyssynchronous child" may be likened in his effect to an orchestra whose instruments are all playing slightly out of tune and off the beat or whose conductor is not in complete command, so that what is heard is somewhat chaotic and cacophonous. For the more visually oriented parent, the "dyssynchronous child" may be likened to a television image in which the horizontal and vertical alignments are out of focus or where there is a great deal of "snow," offering a recognizable but distorted picture.

The term dyssynchronous may be taken to reflect an imbalance between central excitation and inhibition, the complex feedback mechanisms thought to produce the synchronized discharges essential to the arousal state and attentiveness, fine coordinated movements, and rhythmic electrical brain activity. The term dyssynchronous, while emphasizing the functional aspects of the disorder, also suggests something of its neurophysiologic basis as inferred from clinical findings: a disturbance, possible synaptic in character, of the timing and orderliness of neuronal interplay. This appellation avoids the implication of demonstrable and irreversible anatomic injury contained in u... brain damage; rather, it offers the hope—founded on clinical experience—of adjustment and "synchronization," with maturation aided by education. Thus, this term carries within it the challenge for investigative and therapeutic efforts.

The physician, in his role as an authority figure, can be supportive to parents, teachers, and other professionals. Behavior modification, with emphasis on and rewarding of acceptable behavior, instead of the common tendency to pay greatest attention to the child when he is misbehaving or failing, is of utmost benefit. Parents and siblings, teachers and peers can all be involved in behavior modification programs which may be best outlined by a competent clinical psychologist. Remedial tutoring is best done not by the parents but by an intelligent, calm, patient, and kind high school or college student for 20–30 minute periods several days a week. A wide variety of inexpensive methods to help a child improve his coordination and to overcome any specific learning disabilities may be devised. At present there is little rationale for "patterning" as a form of therapy.

Drug therapy is at times useful, but it is strongly recommended that it be used judiciously, sparingly, and only as an adjunct to behavior modification. Dextroamphetamine (5–20 mg in the morning and 2.5–10 mg at noon) has proved useful in diverting the nondirected "hyperkinetic" behavior into more goal-oriented activity. Methylphenidate (Ritalin) also is used widely in varying dosage, but behavioral and toxic side-effects (the latter in children receiving anticonvulsants) may occur. Diphenhydramine (Benadryl) is recommended for the preschool child. Other psychotropic drugs—particularly chlorpromazine—are also used, singly or in combination.

As he grows older, the restless hyperactive child tends to remain very active but in a more organized and less disturbing fashion. Distractibility continues to be a major handicap, resulting in significantly poorer performance in school or on jobs. Emotional immaturity continues to be characteristic of the child's behavior. Not infrequently, more serious emotional disorders, including delinquency, result from the failures and disapproval experienced by the child.

Obviously, with the large number of children involved, major educational and preventive psychologic efforts are required.

Chalfant JC, Scheffelin MA: *Central Processing Dysfunctions in Children: A Review of Research.* NINDB Monograph No. 9. US Department of Health, Education, and Welfare, 1969.

Clements SD: *Minimal Brain Dysfunction in Children.* NINDB Monograph No. 3. US Department of Health, Education, and Welfare, 1966.

Cohen HJ, Birch HG, Taft LT: Some considerations for evaluating the Doman-Delacato "patterning" method. Pediatrics 45:302–314, 1970.

Kenny TJ & others: Characteristics of children referred because of hyperactivity. J Pediat 79:618–622, 1971.

Lucas AR, Weiss M: Methylphenidate hallucinosis. JAMA 217:1079–1081, 1971.

Millichap JG, Fowler GW: Treatment of "minimal brain dysfunction" syndromes. P Clin North America 14:767–777, 1967.

Pihl RO: Conditioning procedures with hyperactive children. Neurology 17:421–423, 1967.

Touwen BC, Prechtl HFR: *The Neurologic Examination of the Child With Minor Nervous Dysfunction.* Clinics in Developmental Medicine No. 38. Heinemann, 1970.

Weiss G & others: Studies on the hyperactive child: V. The effects of dextroamphetamine and chlorpromazine on behavior and intellectual functioning. J Child Psychol Psychiat 9:145–156, 1968. VII. Five-year follow-up. Arch Gen Psychiat 24:409–414, 1971.

FLOPPY INFANT SYNDROME

Essentials of Diagnosis

- In early infancy, decreased muscular activity, both spontaneous and in response to postural reflex testing and to passive motion.
- In young infants, "frog posture" or other unusual positions at rest.
- In older infants, delay in motor milestones.

General Considerations

In the young infant, ventral suspension, ie, supporting the baby with a hand under the chest, normally results in the baby's holding his head slightly up (45° or less), the back straight or nearly so, the arms flexed at the elbows and slightly abducted, and the knees partly flexed. The floppy infant droops over the hand like an inverted **U**. Even the normal neonate attempts to keep his head in the same plane as his body when pulled up from the supine into the sitting position by his hands ("traction response"). Marked head lag is characteristic of the floppy infant. Hyperextensibility of the joints is not a dependable criterion.

In the older infant, delays in walking, running, or climbing stairs, or difficulties and lack of endurance in motor activities, are the usual reasons for seeking medical evaluation.

Hypotonia or decreased motor activity is a frequent presenting complaint in neuromuscular disorders but may also accompany a variety of systemic conditions or may be due to certain disorders of connective tissue.

Clinical Types

A. Paralytic Group: Significant lack of movement against gravity, such as kicking the legs, holding up arms, or attempting to stand when held or in response to stimuli such as tickling or slight pain.

B. Nonparalytic Group: Floppiness without significant paralysis.

Note: Deep tendon reflexes may be depressed or absent in both groups and thus are of no value in differentiating between them.

1. PARALYTIC GROUP

Hereditary Progressive Spinal Muscular Atrophies

These disorders are inherited as autosomal recessives, but rare instances of dominant transmission occur. Prevention is not possible except for genetic counseling. Treatment is supportive and consists of minimizing respiratory infections, preventing contractures, and enabling those who can do so to use crutches or a wheelchair.

A. Infantile Form (Werdnig-Hoffman Disease): This is the commonest of the paralytic forms of floppy infant syndrome. Onset may be in utero, with loss of fetal movements, or paralysis may appear gradually or fairly abruptly in the early weeks or months of life. The infant usually lies in the frog position, breathing diaphragmatically, exhibiting sternal retraction due to paralysis of intercostal muscles, and moving the legs only slightly if at all. The facies is alert. Cry may be weak, and secretions tend to pool in the pharynx due to bulbar involvement. Fasciculation of the tongue is seen frequently. Tremor of the fingers is less common, especially in younger infants; fasciculations of the muscles of the extremities are usually hidden by baby fat. Deep tendon reflexes are lost early—first in the lower and then in the upper extremities—as the paralysis proceeds cephalad. Sensation is normal.

The diagnosis is based on a "neurogenic" EMG pattern and muscle biopsy, which shows a neuropathic pattern of large bundles of atrophied fibers interspersed with bundles of normal or hypertrophied fibers. Soft tissue x-rays show marked muscle atrophy, and this may help in gauging needed depth for muscle biopsy. Muscle enzymes are usually normal but may be slightly elevated late in the disease.

Pneumonia, often due to aspiration, is the commonest complication, and most of the afflicted infants die within 2–3 years.

B. Variants: Less rapidly progressive forms may represent a continuum of the disorder, but—pending biochemical definition—not specific entities.

1. Weakness appearing late—Muscle weakness, chiefly of the legs, may not be recognized until the time when infants might be expected to sit up by themselves or to be walking; there may be other signs of retarded motor development as well. Intelligence is not affected. Muscles of respiration may be relatively spared, and the upper extremities may be strong enough so that the child can learn to walk with crutches, the legs and lower trunk being braced, or to use a wheelchair. Hence, maximum physical rehabilitation is indicated. In general, the more insidious and the later the onset of weakness and the more limited its extent, the better the prognosis. Some patients may live a normal life span.

2. Juvenile spinal muscular atrophy of Kugelberg-Welander—Onset is between 2 years of age and the late teens. The larger proximal muscles, especially of the pelvic girdle, are affected first; the lower legs and arms are involved relatively late. The muscles of the trunk and those supplied by the cranial nerves are usually spared. Muscle enzymes are usually normal, the EMG is "neurogenic," and muscle biopsy is similar to that seen in Werdnig-Hoffman disease. Progression is usually slow. Males may be affected more severely. Every effort should be made to permit the patient to lead as independent a life as possible.

Myopathies

The congenital, relatively nonprogressive myopathies, muscular dystrophy, myotonic dystrophy, polymyositis, and periodic paralysis are discussed elsewhere. Most cases of congenital or early infantile muscular dystrophy reported in the past probably belong in the group of congenital myopathies.

Glycogenosis With Muscle Involvement

These are described under Glycogen Storage Disease in Chapter 35. Patients with type II (Pompe's disease, due to a deficiency of acid maltase) are most likely to present as floppy infants. The weakness in type III (limit dextrinosis) is less marked than in type II, while the rare instances of type IV (amylopectinosis) are severely hypotonic. Muscle cramps on exertion or easy fatigability, rather than floppiness in infancy, is the presenting complaint in type V (McArdle's phosphorylase deficiency) or the glycogenosis due to phosphofructokinase deficiency or phosphohexose isomerase inhibition.

Myasthenia Gravis

Neonatal transient and congenital persistent myasthenia gravis, presenting as "paralytic" floppy infants, is described elsewhere in this chapter.

Congenital or Early Infantile Idiopathic Polyneuritis

Polyneuritis, which is discussed more fully elsewhere in this chapter, may present at birth or early infancy and may be mistaken for myasthenia gravis or Werdnig-Hoffman disease. Since reliable sensory testing is virtually impossible in this age group, diagnosis rests upon exclusion of myasthenia gravis, in which deep tendon reflexes are present and there is a response to neostigmine; and the demonstration of (1) prolonged nerve conduction time and denervation on EMG examination, (2) elevation of CSF protein, and (3) lack of progressive cerebral involvement, as in the metachromatic and globoid leukodystrophies. Nerve biopsy is often justified. Diagnosis may require a therapeutic trial of corticosteroids, resulting in improvement in the young child, especially in the rare recurrent forms.

Arthrogryposis Multiplex, or Congenital Deformities About Multiple Joints

This symptom complex, sometimes associated with hypotonia, may be of "neurogenic" or "myopathic" origin (or both) and may be associated with a wide variety of other anomalies. Orthopedic aspects are discussed in Chapter 19.

Spinal Cord Lesions

Exceedingly limp newborns, usually the product of breech extraction with stretching or actual tearing of the lower cervical to upper thoracic spinal cord, are still occasionally seen. Klumpke's lower brachial plexus paralysis may be present; the abdomen is usually exceedingly soft, and the lower extremities are flaccid. Urinary retention is present initially, but later the bladder may function autonomously. Spine films are usually not helpful, although myelography may define the lesion. After a few weeks, spasticity of the lower limbs becomes obvious. Treatment is symptomatic, being directed at bladder and skin care, and eventual mobilization on crutches or in a wheelchair. The problem can be prevented by careful obstetric delivery.

2. NONPARALYTIC GROUP

In the "floppy" state without paralysis, tendon reflexes, though depressed, may be elicited. Muscle enzymes and EMG are usually normal. Prolonged nerve conduction velocities point to polyneuritis, metachromatic leukodystrophy, or globoid leukodystrophy. Muscle biopsies, utilizing special staining technics and histographic analysis, often show a remarkable reduction of type II fibers associated with decreased voluntary motor activity.

CNS Lesions (Above Spinal Cord)

Limpness in the neonatal period and early infancy and subsequent delay in achieving motor milestones are the presenting features in a large number of children with a variety of CNS disorders. In many, but not all, the reduction in spontaneous motor activity accompanies mental retardation; in these cases, there may be a history of delayed development or regression suggesting brain damage. Close observation and scoring of motor patterns and adaptive behavior, as by the Denver Developmental Screening Test, usually confirms this. Several categories deserve specific attention.

A. "Prespastic Diplegia": This group includes neonates who have had various forms of pre- or perinatal encephalopathy, eg, encephalopathy due to hypoxia, toxins, and intracranial hemorrhage or infection. Findings include profound limpness at or shortly after birth, depressed or absent deep tendon reflexes initially, other signs of CNS difficulties such as poor sucking and feeding, weak or shrill cry, poor Moro responses, weak or absent grasp responses, and visual and auditory inattention. Tendon reflexes usually become hyperactive within a few weeks. When the infant is held up, supported under the armpits by the examiner's hands, his legs are flexed at the hips and knees and, instead of going limp, the infant exhibits increased tone (Foerster's sign). Because of their floppy state, these infants have been referred to in the past as hypotonic—or even atonic—diplegics; however, most, if not all, eventually exhibit hypertonicity, thus meriting the diagnosis of "prespastic diplegia."

B. Hypotonic, Hypokinetic Forms of "Minimal Brain Dysfunction" Syndrome: Floppiness may occur in children with normal or nearly normal intelligence who eventually exhibit aberrant behavior, maturational lag, and learning disabilities. The diagnosis in early life may be difficult, and close follow-up is indicated.

C. Hypotonia With Various Forms of Mental Deficit: Children with chromosomal defects, particularly trisomy 21, may exhibit floppiness without paralysis. However, in most children with mental retardation who are floppy, presumably because of deficient higher nervous activity, there is no specific diagnosis.

D. Degenerative CNS Disorders: Degenerative diseases of infancy presenting with hypotonia include globoid and metachromatic leukodystrophy, subacute necrotizing encephalomyelopathy, infantile amaurotic idiocy, and generalized gangliosidosis. Though relatively rare, the impact of such a diagnosis on the family, the dire prognosis for the child, and the importance of genetic counseling justify the often exhaustive investigations necessary in these disorders (Table 21–6).

E. Others: Congenital choreo-athetosis, discussed earlier, often presents as hypotonia; involuntary movements of the limbs and facial grimacing are not noted until the second half of the first year or even later. Delays in the attainment of motor milestones are the rule.

Children with congenital cerebellar ataxia and, even more rarely, those with exceedingly early forms of Friedreich's ataxia show hypotonia and subsequent incoordination when they begin to reach, sit, stand, or walk. Pneumoencephalography, sometimes justified by the lack of clear clinical definition and the severity of symptoms, may disclose cerebellar dysplasia.

"Systemic" Causes

Limpness without motor paralysis is a presenting or accompanying feature of many other disorders seen in children. These include the following:

A. Malnutrition: *Examples:* Nutritional deprivation, cystic fibrosis, celiac disease, scurvy, rickets.

B. Debilitating Diseases: *Examples:* Severe infections; congenital heart, lung, and renal diseases.

C. Metabolic Disorders: *Examples:* Infantile hypercalcemia, hypophosphatasia.

D. Endocrinopathies: *Examples:* Hypothyroidism, adrenocortical hyperfunction, gonadal dysgenesis (Turner's syndrome), hypotonia-hypogonadal-obesity (HHO) syndrome of Prader-Willi.

E. Familial dysautonomia of Riley-Day.

Heritable Disorders of Connective Tissue

Children with osteogenesis imperfecta, Marfan's syndrome, Ehlers-Danlos syndrome, and congenital laxity of ligaments, besides being floppy, are often "double-jointed" or "rubber-jointed." The first 3 disorders present characteristic pictures discussed elsewhere. The last condition is entirely benign.

Essential Hypotonia

Floppy infants who do not fall into the previously mentioned categories are often classified as having "essential" or, less properly, "benign congenital" hypotonia. This is, perforce, a diagnosis of exclusion, made less and less frequently as diagnostic acumen and technics improve. In essential hypotonia, the family history is usually negative. The muscles show no atrophy or fasciculations; tendon reflexes may be present, diminished, or absent. Respiratory difficulties are encountered occasionally. "Immaturity" of the motor end plates has been offered as a possible cause of the condition. Muscle biopsy, which should include special stains and electron microscopy, may show either no pathologic features or universally small fibers without histochemical or connective tissue changes. The outlook is for partial to full recovery in well over 50% of children so reported.

Allen JP, Myers GG, Condon VR: Laceration of the spinal cord related to breech delivery. JAMA 208:1019, 1969.

Dubowitz V: *The Floppy Infant.* Clinics in Developmental Medicine No. 31. Heinemann, 1969.

PSEUDOTUMOR CEREBRI
(Benign Intracranial Hypertension, Serous Meningitis, Meningeal Hydrops, Otitic Hydrocephalus, Toxic Hydrocephalus)

Essentials of Diagnosis

- Symptoms and signs of increased intracranial pressure.
- Normal or small ventricular system.

General Considerations

By definition, the diagnosis of pseudotumor cerebri can be made only by excluding intracranial disorders which result in significant distortion, displacement, or enlargement of the ventricular system.

Pseudotumor cerebri, as reflected in its many synonyms, may be due to or associated with any of the following: (1) Inflammatory processes such as mastoiditis and lateral sinus obstruction (more often on the right than the left), poliomyelitis, Landry-Guillain-Barré syndrome, head trauma, Schilder's diffuse sclerosis, and other demyelinating disorders. (2) Encephalopathies such as lead poisoning, hypo- or hypervitaminosis A, or toxicity due to tetracyclines or nalidixic acid, cystic fibrosis and other chronic lung disorders. (3) Endocrinopathies such as hypocalcemia, Addison's disease, functional hyperpituitarism (perhaps); menstrual dysfunctions, including menarche, pregnancy, and galactorrhea. (4) Prolonged corticosteroid therapy, especially with triamcinolone, usually during withdrawal.

Clinical Findings

A. Symptoms and Signs: The presenting symptoms are nonspecific and nonlocalizing: headache, vomiting, blurred vision, photophobia, diplopia, dizziness, tinnitus, incoordination, drowsiness and stupor, and, rarely, convulsions.

On physical examination, signs of the causative or associated disorder may be present. Neurologic findings, in order of frequency, are papilledema, abducens nerve palsies, nystagmus, ataxia, pyramidal tract signs, and central or peripheral facial weakness. Visual acuity and visual fields should be evaluated in any child whose cooperation can be gained and whose intelligence and age (often as early as 3–4 years) permit reliable testing.

B. Laboratory Findings: Studies should be guided by the clinical suspicion of the causes previously mentioned. Lumbar puncture may be performed if the ventricles are normal or small, both to measure and to reduce the elevated CSF pressure. The CSF is acellular, and protein and glucose are normal.

C. X-Ray Findings: X-rays of the mastoid sinuses, chest, and abdomen and a skeletal survey may provide diagnostic information.

D. Neurodiagnostic Studies: As discussed in the section on tumors of the CNS, tests to rule out a space-occupying intracranial lesion include skull x-rays, a brain scan, echoencephalography, and EEG before proceeding to definitive contrast studies. The EEG is normal or slightly slow. In nonlocalized increased intracranial pressure, right retrograde brachial angiography is the procedure of choice to demonstrate the presence or absence of hydrocephalus. Especially when the ventricles are small, as is often the case in pseudotumor cerebri, venticulography may be difficult to perform; hence, if air contrast studies are deemed necessary to supplement angiography, fractional pneumoencephalography is preferred.

Treatment

Specific associated conditions are treated appropriately.

In patients receiving corticosteroids, a temporary increase in dosage may alleviate symptoms, after which very gradual withdrawal may be initiated.

Measures aimed at reducing CSF pressure generally are of transient value. In a child with intractable headache, vomiting, and other somatic complaints, lumbar puncture with removal of sufficient CSF to lower initial pressure by 50% may be of benefit. Acetazolamide and hyperosmolar diuretics have offered no benefit, but glycerol and furosemide have been said to be of value.

Visual acuity should be determined at frequent intervals. If there is loss of acuity or if the disorder is present in a young child (in whom visual acuity is difficult to measure) with long-standing increased intracranial pressure, subtemporal decompression should be considered.

Prognosis

Pseudotumor cerebri is usually a self-limited condition with no residua. Careful follow-up is recommended since some cases recur or a brain tumor eventually becomes manifest.

Greer M: Benign intracranial hypertension (pseudotumor cerebri). P Clin North America 14:819–830, 1967.

HYPOXIC ENCEPHALOPATHY

Essentials of Diagnosis

- Disturbance of neurologic status.
- Any situation resulting in decreased oxygen to brain.

General Considerations

Hypoxic encephalopathy may be due to any one of the 4 types of hypoxia, given here in order of frequency: (1) **hypoxic,** due to reduction in the availability of oxygen to tissues due to a decrease in the partial pressure of oxygen (PO_2) in the arterial blood, as in respiratory difficulties (eg, asphyxiation), interference with gas exchange in the lungs, or arteriovenous shunting; (2) **stagnant,** with reduction of available oxygen due to slowed circulation, as in local brain edema or circulatory failure (cardiac arrest); (3) **anemic,** with reduced oxygen-carrying capacity of the blood, as in anemic hemorrhage or carbon monoxide poisoning; and (4) **histotoxic,** with a reduction of oxygen utilization by tissues due to interference with cellular metabolism, as in certain poisonings (eg, glutethimide [Doriden], propoxyphene [Darvon], or cyanide) or in connection with certain metabolic disorders.

The clinical spectrum of hypoxic encephalopathy and sequelae involves 3 major factors: (1) the nature of the hypoxic process, (2) the neurologic status of the patient prior to the hypoxic episode, and (3) the rapidity of onset, severity, and duration of hypoxia.

Clinical Findings

A. Symptoms and Signs: Mild hypoxia causes headache, troubles in mentation, drowsiness, confusion, listlessness or restlessness, apathy or hyperirritability, and, rarely, delirium.

Moderate hypoxia of gradual onset, allowing cerebral blood flow or the hemoglobin to increase, allows the manifestations just mentioned to be mild and soon to disappear; the symptoms are common when one first moves to a higher altitude.

Severe hypoxia of sudden onset and lasting 1–3 minutes manifests itself by profound disturbance of cerebral function, including loss of consciousness, convulsions, decorticate and decerebrate posturing, often high fever, and rapid evolution of papilledema. If the patient recovers from the immediate episode, he may exhibit true or psychic blindness, aphasia, spasticity, rigidity, choreo-athetotic or pill-rolling movements, and abnormal reflexes such as snouting, sucking, and forced grasp. Seizures are often a continuous problem.

Hypoxia of abrupt onset, marked severity, and lasting 3 or more minutes may result in failure to regain consciousness as well as severe cerebral edema. If the patient survives, he may progress from hypotonic and hyporeflexic to spastic. Such an episode often leads to irreversible brain damage, with medullary compression, and cardiac and respiratory failure.

B. Laboratory Findings: Blood gases and serum electrolytes should be obtained as soon as possible. Blood levels for toxins should be examined as indicated. A chest x-ray and ECG should be obtained as soon as feasible. EEGs can be delayed.

The CSF may be under increased pressure and, with sufficient tissue damage, show an increase in protein and of such enzymes as LDH, GOT and CPK:

Differential Diagnosis

The history of a hypoxic episode establishes the diagnosis. In the absence of such history, hypoglycemic and toxic encephalopathies must be considered. Aspiration of foreign bodies by young children, causing respiratory obstruction, is frequently missed.

Complications

As in any comatose patient, aspiration pneumonitis, infections, electrolyte and fluid imbalances, decubitus ulcers, and contractures may occur. Stress ulcers occur infrequently in children.

Treatment

A. Specific Measures: Prompt reversal of specific causes, eg, removal of a patient from a source of carbon monoxide or extraction of a foreign body, is obviously of urgent importance. Blood gases, fluids, and electrolytes must be monitored closely. Emergency care, treatment of cerebral edema, and antibiotic therapy are discussed in the sections on altered states of consciousness and head trauma.

B. Anticonvulsants: (For treatment of status epilepticus, see Seizure Disorders.) Prophylactic diphenylhydantoin (Dilantin), 10 mg/kg IV, IM, or orally daily, is advised because of the frequency of seizures as a sequel to hypoxic encephalopathy. Seizures may cause further brain damage. If the patient recovers neurologically intact, without seizures and with a normal EEG, anticonvulsant therapy may be gradually discontinued. *Note:* Exercise caution in using paraldehyde in cases of severe pneumopathies. Barbiturates should be avoided because they involve a risk of further depression of the CNS.

Chronic Care: Respiratory toilet, maintenance of nutrition via a nasogastric or gastrostomy tube if necessary, proper skin, bladder, and bowel care, and early physical therapy are often required.

Prognosis

Mild hypoxia usually ends in rapid recovery without sequelae. However, the so-called "minimal brain dysfunction syndrome" has been ascribed to milder hypoxic episodes, especially when these occurred during birth or in early infancy.

Moderately severe hypoxia, particularly if it developed relatively slowly, may result in good recovery, especially in the neonate. The effects of severe hypoxia, however, are often not appreciated in infants for a few weeks or months, after which delayed psychomotor development, microcephaly, spasticity, sometimes choreo-athetosis and ataxia, and frequently seizures become manifest.

Moderately severe hypoxia of acute onset after the neonatal period may be followed by a period of apparent improvement for 1–10 days. The patient may then deteriorate and be permanently impaired mentally and neurologically.

Once there is evidence of medullary compression, with slow irregular respirations, irregular cardiac activity, loss of doll's eye movements and ciliospinal reflexes, fixed pupils, and often flaccidity with absence of deep reflexes but bilateral extensor responses, the prognosis for recovery is extremely poor.

Brierly JB, Meldrun BS (editors): *Brain Hypoxia.* Heinemann, 1971.

CONGENITAL NYSTAGMUS & SPASMUS NUTANS

Two benign types of spontaneous pendular horizontal nystagmus are congenital (familial) nystagmus and spasmus nutans. They occur in about 5% of young infants and are similar initially. Intermittent lateral nodding or tilting of the head is seen in both types; strong light inhibits the nystagmus. Strabismus, neurologic and EEG abnormalities, and a family history of nystagmus, more frequent than in controls, suggest organic causes.

Congenital nystagmus, usually of both eyes, is noted—often as an isolated finding—at or shortly after birth. The family history is often positive, and the disorder may be transmitted as a dominant or an X-linked recessive (hence more common in boys).

Spasmus nutans tends to appear in the third or fourth month as the triad of nystagmus affecting predominantly (or only) one eye (more often the left), head nodding, and head tilting. Sex distribution is equal. Although familial cases are reported, the mode of transmission is not known. Disturbances of the mother-child relationship, nutrition, illumination (room darkness), teething, illness, and trauma are no longer considered to be causative or contributing factors.

The differential diagnosis includes serious causes of nystagmus (often "searching" in type) due to impaired vision as from chorioretinitis, optic atrophy, or optic nerve or cerebellar tumors. Irregular jerking of both eyes may be the principal manifestation of a seizure disorder or part of the polymyoclonia-opsoclonus syndrome.

The passage of time defines congenital nystagmus as permanent. Spasmus nutans is self-limiting, ceasing between the second and fifth year in 3/4 of infants without and in 1/3 of those with associated strabismus or other neurologic abnormalities.

Therapy is directed at any treatable neurologic disorder and correction of strabismus. Congenital nystagmus and spasmus nutans, being benign, require—

in addition to diagnosis—reassurance of the parents. Epileptic nystagmus responds to phenobarbital or diphenylhydantoin.

Jayalakshmi P & others: Infantile nystagmus: A prospective study of spasmus nutans, congenital nystagmus, and unclassified nystagmus of infancy. J Ped 77:177–187, 1970.

Kelly TW: Optic glioma presenting as spasmus nutans. Pediatrics 45:295–296, 1970.

White JC: Epileptic nystagmus. Epilepsia 12:157–164, 1971.

● ● ●

General References

Bray PF: *Neurology in Pediatrics.* Year Book, 1969.

Chusid JG: *Correlative Neuroanatomy & Functional Neurology,* 14th ed. Lange, 1970.

Ford FR: *Diseases of the Nervous System in Infancy, Childhood and Adolescence,* 5th ed. Thomas, 1966.

Gamstorp I: *Pediatric Neurology.* Appleton-Century-Crofts, 1970.

Matson DD: *Neurosurgery of Infancy and Childhood,* 2nd ed. Thomas, 1969.

22...

Developmental Retardation

John H. Meier, PhD, & Harold P. Martin, MD

Developmental retardation can be defined in several ways. This chapter refers to subnormal sensory, motor, perceptual, language, and cognitive functioning. As such the term does not denote a disease or syndrome and is therefore not an adequate diagnosis. Developmental retardation is a symptom of subnormal function of the CNS whether due to damage, altered physiology, environmental deprivation, or abnormally slow maturation. Prevalence figures vary with age group and classification; 1–5% of the population of the USA are considered mentally retarded, and 5–20% of children in regular schools have specific learning disabilities in spite of normal or above normal intelligence.

Verbal development is one of the best indices of developmental rate in human maturation and is a significant factor in the measurement of intelligence. The degree of developmental retardation is usually expressed in a below normal intelligence quotient (IQ). However, there is a growing awareness of the misleading nature of a single quotient, which averages a range of performance. Increasing numbers of children with borderline and above borderline IQs are being classified as having specific learning disabilities instead of general mental retardation. Their development may be retarded in specific language, perceptual, or related functions for which treatment may be available and which have a better prognosis.

When a child is too young to yield an adequate language sample, general physical and social development may be used to predict later placement in tests of mental integrity and power. The resultant developmental quotient (DQ) correlates highly and positively with IQ; however, this is not a cause-effect relationship, as evidenced by well coordinated children who are aphasic or of subnormal intelligence, as well as by congenitally crippled children who are highly articulate and of above average intelligence. Furthermore, the concept that DQs and IQs are stable arises not so much from an individual's static rate of development but more often from the persistence of his environmental conditions.

With present diagnostic sophistication, the exact cause can be determined in only 20–30% of cases of developmental retardation. Furthermore, most organically caused retardation is irreversible. This places the pediatrician in the uncomfortable position of having to admit ignorance about the causes of developmental retardation in specific cases and to have to explain that the symptom is chronic and that there is little chance of totally normal development, ie, the child will probably continue to develop more slowly or less well than his age mates. A comprehensive diagnosis of the developmentally retarded child often requires an interdisciplinary approach in order to fully clarify all of the complex factors affecting the functioning of the child and his family. This requires consultation and cooperation with numerous professionals to determine optimal management. These include psychiatry, neurology, psychology, nursing, social work, nutrition, speech and hearing, and occupational and physical therapy in addition to the pediatrician's care. These additional resources are often available in special clinics and university centers. This chapter presents only certain diagnostic and management considerations in relation to developmental retardation as a symptom.

Diagnostic Objectives

(1) Determine whether or not the slow child is actually developmentally retarded. This includes ruling out neuromuscular disease, gross sensory damage, and emotional disturbance which may result in pseudo-retardation.

(2) Determine the cause if possible, being careful not to overlook those that are treatable, eg, hydrocephalus, cretinism, subdural hematoma, certain inborn errors of metabolism, and malnutrition. Genetically determined disorders are of particular interest for genetic counseling of the parents, who will want to know the probability of subsequent children being similarly affected (chromosomal abnormalities, metabolic errors, tuberous sclerosis, Hunter's syndrome, etc).

(3) Determine the extent and degree of retardation. This also includes looking for associated handicapping conditions such as epilepsy, sensory deficits, congenital anomalies, inappropriate parental nurturing, and cultural differences.

Etiology

Developmental retardation is associated with many diseases and conditions. During the last decade, at least 50 new inborn errors of metabolism have been described. The following classification system is intended only as a broad outline of categories with a few examples listed. It is a modified version of the classification system proposed by the American Association for Mental Deficiency.

A. Infection: Prenatal, eg, rubella, syphilis, toxoplasmosis, cytomegalic inclusion and other viral diseases. Postnatal, eg, meningitis, brain abscess, encephalitis.

B. Intoxication: Eg, toxemia, hyperbilirubinemia, poisoning.

C. Trauma or Physical Agents: Eg, birth injury, postnatal injury, with description as contusion, hemorrhage, vascular occlusion.

D. Metabolism: Eg, galactosemia, phenylketonuria, cerebral lipidosis, lysosomal dystrophies, porphyria, gargoylism, hypoglycemia, malnutrition.

E. Growths: Eg, tuberous sclerosis, neoplasm, neurofibromatosis.

F. Chromosomal Aberrations or Syndromes: Eg, Turner's, Klinefelter's, trisomy 13–15, trisomy 17–18, trisomy 21 (Down's), cri du chat.

G. Unknown Prenatal Influence: Eg, anomalies of brain, craniosynostosis, primary microcephaly, hydrocephalus, intrauterine growth retardation.

H. Associated or Causative Psychologic Problems: Eg, psychosis, neurosis, reactive disorder, deprivation, neglect or abuse, other emotional disturbances.

I. Familial-Cultural: Although cultural or familial patterns, particularly for poverty or minority groups, are often strikingly different and may be deficient relative to majority cultural patterns, polygenic inheritance of low intelligence may also account for many cases in this category. Moreover, consanguinity increases the probability of uncommon recessive traits being inherited by the child.

J. Miscellaneous and Unknown: This and the preceding category account for at least 2/3 of cases of developmental retardation.

Classification of Degree of Retardation

Use commonly accepted standardized test instruments to arrive at an intelligence quotient or a developmental quotient (Table 22–1).

Preliminary Diagnosis

The following procedure serves to alert the pediatrician to the multiplicity of causality, some management recommendations, and the interrelationships between diagnostic and management considerations.

A. Essential Diagnostic Evaluation:

1. Physical examination—Physical examination must emphasize the neurologic function of the child. Head circumference, transillumination of the skull, and

ophthalmoscopic examination through dilated pupils must be included. Subtle signs not historically considered as part of a classical neurologic examination are helpful, eg, grasping patterns, quality of motor performance, and reflex development. Developmental screening in children under age 5 and intelligence screening in the older child are part of the neurologic assessment and can be readily and rapidly administered by trained office personnel. The Denver Developmental Screening Test (see Chapter 2) and the Peabody Picture Vocabulary (IQ) Test are 2 useful examples. Tests to screen visual perception, auditory discrimination, and visual-motor coordination are also available for the pediatrician or office paraprofessionals to administer.

2. History—

a. Past medical history—Attention must be given to the pregnancy, labor, and delivery, including such factors as excessive or minimal weight gain, exposure to radiation, infections, medications, threatened or attempted abortion, toxemia, inadequate prenatal care, excessively rapid or prolonged labor, heavy sedation, and abnormal fetal presentation. A history of the newborn period reveals the baby's sleep pattern, feeding history, and energy level as signs of early CNS system damage as well as any specific neonatal difficulties. Subsequent to the newborn period, a history of unexplained high fevers, trauma, infections, inadequate nutrition, or other medical problem deserves attention.

b. Family history—Any family history of mental retardation or any condition or disease associated with retardation should be ascertained. From a genetic standpoint, it is helpful to know of siblings, uncles, aunts, or cousins of the parents who were stillborn or died in infancy before a diagnosis of retardation could be made. Complete obstetric information about the mother is essential, including questions about previous abortions, relative infertility, and difficulties with previous pregnancies—all of which suggest impaired ability to biologically support a pregnancy.

c. Developmental history—Prior developmental milestones help to clarify the degree of retardation. Regression or changes in the rate of development may indicate the time of a postnatal neurologic insult. It is helpful to see the child's baby book in order to more objectively assess early developmental landmarks such as smiling, reaching, and turning over.

d. Records—Prenatal and nursery records on mother and child often point to etiologic factors not

TABLE 22–1. Classification of mental retardation.*

American Psychiatric Association		World Health Organization		American Association for Mental Deficiency	
IQ	Terminology	IQ	Terminology	IQ	Terminology
70–85	Mild mental deficiency	50–69	Mild subnormality	70–84	Borderline
50–70	Moderate	20–49	Moderate	55–69	Mild
0–50	Severe	0–19	Severe	40–54	Moderate

*Reproduced, with permission, from Solomon P, Patch V (editors): *Handbook of Psychiatry,* 2nd ed. Lange, 1971.

elicited through parental reporting. Apgar scores, length of gestation, newborn head circumference, and nurses' observations of the newborn are important facts parents can rarely recollect. In older children, records from the school should be requested and should include reports of teachers' observations and any testing done by school personnel. Any evaluations by other professionals should be reviewed.

3. Sensory examination—Hearing and vision must be assessed more carefully than in a normally developing child. If there are any doubts, specialist help should be obtained. Auditory disorders often mimic retardation. Associated defects of sensory organs must be diagnosed and treated.

4. Laboratory examination—Laboratory evaluation should include a complete blood count and urinalysis, including a check for galactosuria and phenylketonuria, amino acid and organic acid chromatography, and a copper oxidase screen. If more than one child in the family is retarded, the mother should have a similar biochemical evaluation. Some clinics routinely order bone age films, PBI determinations, serologic tests for syphilis, and an EEG.

5. Family assessment—The physician needs to know how the family views the child, what their questions are, how they perceive retardation, and how the family functions in relation to the child—especially if the family sees the child as completely normal or just lazy. There are many misconceptions about retardation, such as that all retarded children should be institutionalized, that they will sexually act out, will be delinquent, or will cease learning anything at some specific age. Unspoken concerns about inheritance, the part either parent may have played in etiology, and the effect on the siblings are frequent. The physician must answer unspoken questions also and must determine whether the parents need more extensive counseling to assist them in accepting their defective child and planning constructively for his care now and in the future.

B. Other Aspects of Diagnostic Evaluation:

1. Further laboratory evaluation—Electroencephalography, while not diagnostic of mental retardation, is indicated if trauma or a seizure disorder seems likely or localized neurologic findings exist. Skull films are indicated if the child is microcephalic, if prenatal infection seems likely, or if the head is abnormally shaped. Chromosomal analysis is necessary for any retarded child who has a peculiar facies or multiple anomalies or in the child with Down's syndrome born to a mother less than 30 years of age.

When specific diagnoses are associated with developmental retardation, specific laboratory evaluations are indicated, as detailed elsewhere in this book, ie, neuromuscular disorders, cerebral anomalies, errors in metabolism, cerebral palsy, congenital heart disease, etc.

2. Developmental or intelligence testing—If any question remains concerning the child's mental abilities, formal testing by a psychologist or developmental pediatrician is in order. This is particularly germane when adoptability status is being determined, school placement is at issue, development has been erratic or variable, or perceptual handicaps are suspected.

3. Consultation—In abnormal development, many professions have specialized knowledge which the primary physician may profitably use. If the child's behavior seems unusual or bizarre, consultation with a child psychologist or psychiatrist should help determine whether or not a psychic disturbance is the basis for aberrant development. A speech pathologist can clarify the diagnosis of abnormal speech and language. Social workers are particularly helpful in the assessment of complex families in determining etiologic factors as well as providing assistance in treatment. Besides these nonmedical personnel, neurologists, orthopedists, ophthalmologists, psychiatrists, developmental pediatricians, physical and occupational therapists, and public health nurses are but a few of the specialists who can help the primary physician in evaluating and managing the retarded child. Consultation with a mental retardation clinic is sometimes indicated, particularly where multifactorial causation makes it necessary to obtain the help of many professionals. In such cases, efficiency and economy are best served by reference to an interdisciplinary mental retardation clinic. Some families require such a referral for corroboration of the diagnosis and prognosis.

Differential Diagnosis

Several conditions may be confused with mental retardation. Common ones are listed below.

A. Sensory Deficits: Particularly difficult to detect in the office is a high-frequency hearing deficit.

B. Emotional Disturbance: In psychoses or autism, the child may appear retarded but usually manifests other unusual or bizarre behavior. With less serious disturbances such as reactive disorders or neurosis, it is more common for individual functions to be variably normal or retarded. Behavior problems and altered peer or parent-child relationships are usually seen in learning disorders having a primary emotional basis.

C. Minimal Cerebral Dysfunction: This ill-defined syndrome is characterized by various combinations of the following findings: neurologic signs such as poor coordination, associated movements, exaggerated reflexes, tight heel cords, poor eye-tracking, incomplete or mixed brain dominance, drooling, fine tremors, and impaired ability to carry out fine motor tasks. Other findings include wide scatter on subtests of intelligence or psycholinguistic ability, noteworthy learning disabilities in specific school subjects (dyslexia, dysgraphia, dyscalculia, etc), emotional lability, distractibility, hyperactivity, decreased attention span, borderline EEG, perceptual deficit, history of slow language development, and poor sequential memory.

D. Neuromuscular Disorders: Particularly in the first 18 months of life, when the major developmental milestones are motor, the child with altered muscle tone or coordination may appear to be retarded. If retarded, neuromuscular disorders, such as cerebral palsy or hypotonia, make it difficult to assess the degree of retardation.

E. Frequent illness, debilitation, or prolonged hospitalization.

F. Prematurity: Subtract the weeks a child is born prematurely from his chronologic age in determining the age norms.

G. Deprivation: This may take many forms, including neglect, physical abuse, loss of a parent, institutionalization, or more subtle aberrant parent-child interaction. Cultural differences and environmental deprivation are now recognized as a basis for slow development. This can be due to the cultural bias of the intelligence test, which gives higher scores to children with verbal proficiency. Accumulating evidence indicates that deprivation may result in a permanent stunting of the child's mental abilities.

H. Developmental Deviation or Lag: A significant deviation or lag in any one area of development such as language acquisition, motor skills, or social development (from whatever cause) may be misdiagnosed as mental retardation. If some areas of development are within the normal range and the child shows normal ability to learn and solve problems, it can be assumed that his mental capacity is normal.

I. Situational Reaction: Fear, anxiety, or illness may interfere with a child's activity and test performance. Intelligence tests or developmental tests merely sample behavior. When behavior is transiently altered, test results will reflect this. This is most striking during hospitalization, when behavioral regression is typically present. The history taken from the parents or a reassessment of the child at a later time allows a more valid estimate of development.

Prevention

As the causes of various developmental deviations become better understood, specific preventive measures become available. Physical defects due to various prenatal and perinatal CNS damage are explicitly treated in other sections of this book. Several sources of insult to the developing sensory-perceptual-cognitive mechanisms warrant attention here.

A. Genetic Counseling: In addition to the obvious necessity for good prenatal, perinatal, and postnatal care, another promising avenue for prevention of retardation or developmental deviations, whose cause can be traced to chromosomal or genetic aberrations, is genetic counseling. Many hitherto cryptogenic deviations in development have recently been linked to specific chromosomal or genetic anomalies. Thus, the probability of recurrence in the offspring can be communicated to parents contemplating more children. Ideally, all couples who have histories of developmental retardation in their families should obtain genetic counseling and understand the risks involved before conceiving children, or consider the appropriateness of a therapeutic abortion. On the other hand, many of these handicapping conditions are both rare and recessively inherited, so that parents can often be reassured that the chances of giving birth to another handicapped child are relatively slight.

B. Prenatal Care: Although prenatal causes of retardation are multifactorial, early and comprehensive prenatal care should significantly lower the incidence of developmental problems. The goals include adequate maternal nutrition, prevention of prematurity, prompt treatment of maternal infections, expert management of diseases such as diabetes and eclampsia, and avoidance of radiation and rubella. Rubella immunization of all children is critically important in draining the reservoir from which pregnant mothers contract this developmentally crippling fetal disease. The pediatrician or general practitioner who is going to be responsible for the care of the child should see the mother during pregnancy and consult with her obstetrician.

No drug should be given to pregnant women except on urgent medical indication.

C. Perinatal Care: The results of investigations now under way, including a USPHS collaborative study, may help to clarify which perinatal factors most seriously affect subsequent development. Anoxia, hemorrhage, trauma, hyperbilirubinemia, and hypoglycemia have been shown to result in brain damage to animals and humans. Improved obstetric and newborn care can prevent some of these insults. The sensory and maternal deprivation many premature and sick infants experience should be avoided. Sensory and emotional stimulation can often be provided by handling the child, holding him during feedings, and assigning a foster grandmother to infants who must undergo long-term immobilization or isolation.

D. Postnatal Care: Circumstances leading to brain damage or dysfunction must be prevented or promptly treated. Examples include accidents, poisoning, child battering, CNS infections, electrolyte disturbances, inadequate nutrition, and anesthesia.

The President's Panel on Mental Retardation and other epidemiologic studies have shown that 50–75% of retarded children come from the lower socio-economic level and that the developmental problems of a majority of children appear to be related to poverty. Although polygenic inheritance of subnormal mentation remains a possibility, increasing data indicate that the causes of retardation, learning disabilities, and other developmental problems in this large group of children are preventable. It is not the traditional role of physicians to engage in social reform, but their success in recognizing venereal disease and tuberculosis as social problems led to effective intervention and prevention. The pediatrician who takes a similar view of retardation should advocate better nutrition, individualized education, preschool enrichment through improved and more numerous day care centers, family planning, universally available prenatal care, and better medical care for children by whatever means may be required to minimize the incidence of children with damaged or poorly functioning nervous systems and diminished learning ability.

E. Early Infant Stimulation: The vast majority of developmental deviations—especially those manifested by specific perceptual-cognitive deficits—appear to be caused by various forms of environmental deprivation.

Although much of the organism's fundamental equipment is established at birth, optimal growth and development depend upon the environment of the early postnatal years. Animal and human studies lend additional support to the importance of early patterned stimulation of the various sensory modalities in the infant and toddler. The impact of effective stimulation seems to be greatest with the young child and becomes less as the child grows older. Specific patterned stimuli presented to the infant in and out of the crib favor optimal subsequent development of higher cognitive functions such as language, problem solving, abstract thinking, and overall adaptive behavior. The positive feelings about one's self derived from a feeling of basic ability to function effectively among one's peers is a desirable affective side-effect of such sensory-perceptual-cognitive stimulation.

Treatment

A. Specific Pathology: The treatment of specific pathologic conditions causing retardation is discussed in appropriate chapters elsewhere in this book. These conditions include metabolic errors, endocrine dysfunction, cerebral anomalies, and many others. Similarly, specific treatment of associated problems such as seizure control, management of strabismus, and therapy for cerebral palsy is included in other sections of this book.

B. Supportive Care: Prompt treatment of infections, assistance in feeding and diet, medications for hyperactivity, and management of associated medical problems—while they do not constitute specific treatment of developmental retardation—are important in the general care of the child.

C. Parent Counseling: Parents of a retarded child need periodic discussions about their child regarding diagnosis, etiology, prognosis, home management, educational placement, plans for the future, and progress. When the diagnosis is first made, the impact of having a defective child may be overwhelming and the parents may selectively perceive only what they wish to hear, requiring repetition several times. Thereafter, interviews with the physician should be scheduled at regular intervals (eg, every 6–12 months) to discuss the child's current status, problems, and questions which inevitably occur as the child matures. It is important that the parents realize that their physician is interested and willing to talk with them. Occasionally, very difficult parents may require referral to a psychiatrist, psychologist, or social worker. Assistance from a public health nurse or visiting nurse is often helpful; problems stemming from feeding, toileting, and general home management are best handled by means of home visits by such nursing personnel.

D. Parent Organizations: Local chapters of the National Association of Retarded Children or the Association for Children With Learning Disabilities are helpful to many parents. Sharing of common problems, parent education, information about resources and new developments, and a forum for community action to improve services for handicapped children are available through such organizations.

E. School Placement: There is considerable controversy among educators and behavioral scientists regarding the best placement for children whose impaired learning ability reduces their ability to profit from conventional educational programs.

One argument is that the peculiar learning styles and disabilities of these children require placement in a special class with a special teacher who employs special methods and materials. Such special educational provisions are available in most public school systems for children who are functioning intellectually within a range of 50–85% of the capacity of their normal age peers—referred to as "educable mentally retarded" children (IQ 51–80). More severely retarded children (IQ 50 and below) are usually better served in programs for "trainable mentally retarded" children in community centers, cerebral palsy centers, and private schools. Some public schools or communities provide such schooling at no cost to families; financial assistance is available in some communities for parents whose child requires private schooling or care.

The counter-argument is that defective children learn a great deal from their normal peers. When, therefore, children are grouped on the basis of their generalized or specific dysfunctions, they have no opportunity to profit from "peer tutoring." Moreover, as more enlightened school systems move toward instructional programs which are geared to individual differences of learning capacity, speed, and style, segregated special classes are being replaced by special resource centers where individualized learning is offered in a social milieu of mixed abilities and interest. Computer-assisted instruction, flexible scheduling of classes, team teaching, individualized or programmed learning, and other innovations are contributing to the elimination of segregated programs. Some school systems are establishing learning resource centers and training special teachers for children whose general intellectual functioning is not retarded but who have specific perceptual or emotional deficits which make it difficult for them to function satisfactorily in regular classrooms.

When special programs are available to a child with learning disabilities, he should be placed in such a program provided he can be reevaluated within a year to determine his progress. Such reevaluation is especially important for placement in segregated programs, which tend to perpetuate themselves by using a diluted curriculum that prevents a child from catching up with his peers and qualifying for regular class placement.

F. Preschool Experience: Since about 80% of developmental retardation occurs in environmentally deprived backgrounds—and since the majority of intellectual development is completed by school age—preschool intervention is recommended. Nursery school programs which are responsive to individual differences afford opportunities for retarded and deviant children to develop greater self-esteem, independence, sensory and perceptual acuity, and communication and problem-solving abilities.

G. Institutionalization: Placing a retarded child in an institution involves the parents in difficult emotion-laden decisions which may require professional counsel. Retarded children should be kept at home for at least the first 3 years of life because the nondeprived home environment has proved to be more beneficial than an institution for most young retarded children. The decision to institutionalize is typically a last resort for even the severely retarded child in a deprived home environment. When other reasonable options have been exhausted, one should seek placement in an institution where the children are happy, self-sufficient, show intellectual growth, manifest minimal stereotypy (such as rocking), and manifest no excessive need for social reinforcement. Considerable parental counseling is generally required to facilitate the placement and to prevent later resentment and guilt. Some of the bases for institutionalization are as follows: (1) More nursing care is needed than the parents can provide. (2) The family is unable to accept the child in the home.

(3) The community lacks day care educational or training facilities. (4) Disintegrated or negligent family circumstances make it impossible to provide a home for the child.

Prognosis

Specific sensory-perceptual-cognitive deficits or general retardation usually have lifelong implications for management. The chronic nature of these conditions demands a continuity of treatment and follow-up. The pediatrician must be prepared to deal with initial and sometimes accumulating frustration, despair, and even anger on the part of parents who encounter new problems which inevitably arise as the child progresses through various developmental stages.

●　　●　　●

General References

American Association on Mental Deficiency: *Directory of Residential Facilities for the Mentally Retarded.* American Association on Mental Deficiency, 1968.

AMA Conference on Mental Retardation: *Mental Retardation: A Handbook for the Primary Physician.* American Medical Association, 1965.

Directory of Research Centers, University Affiliated Facilities and Community Facilities for Developmentally Disabled Children. In: *Mental Retardation Construction Program.* US Department of Health, Education, & Welfare, 1971.

Dunn L: *Peabody Picture Vocabulary Test.* American Guidance Service, 1959.

Frankenburg W, Dodds J, Fandal A: *The Denver Developmental Screening Test.* Revised. University of Colorado Medical Center, 1970.

Illingworth RS: *The Development of the Infant and Young Child: Normal and Abnormal.* Williams & Wilkins, 1970.

Mussen PH, Conger JJ, Kagan J: *Child Development and Personality.* Harper, 1969.

Poser CM: *Mental Retardation: Diagnosis and Treatment.* Harper, 1969.

Smith DW: Recognizable patterns of human malformation: Genetic, embryologic, and clinical aspects. In: *Major Problems in Clinical Pediatrics.* Vol 7. Saunders, 1970.

Stevenson AC, Davison BCC, Oakes MW: *Genetic Counselling.* Lippincott, 1970.

Tarnopol L (editor): *Learning Disabilities: Introduction to Educational and Medical Management.* Thomas, 1969.

Wortis J: *Mental Retardation: An Annual Review.* 2 vols. Grune & Stratton, 1970, 1971.

23...
Psychosocial Aspects of Pediatrics & Psychiatric Disorders

Dane G. Prugh, MD, & Anthony J. Kisley, MD

GENERAL PRINCIPLES OF PSYCHIATRIC EXAMINATION & TREATMENT

THE APPROACH TO INTERVIEWING

Most physicians find that the traditional question and answer or "check list" method of taking a psychiatric history is not flexible enough to ferret out significant material. The "open-ended question" allows the parent or patient to take the lead and to respond with material that he is most concerned about. The physician should feel comfortable with his own interviewing technics and not attempt to imitate too closely those of someone else.

In addition to what the patient says, the physician can learn much from observation of the patient and from noting how the emotional relationship between himself and the patient is developing. The quality of this relationship will influence both the accuracy of the data obtained and the response to recommended therapeutic measures. A warm, friendly, and nonjudgmental attitude will make it easier for the patient and his parents to talk freely. The doctor's skill in "listening actively" will enable him to discover the multiple determinants in what the patient says. Quick advice should be avoided, as well as premature promises about the success of treatment; both can promote overdependency or lead to disappointment.

Adequate time should be permitted for interviews. A good deal can be learned in 20–30 minutes, and longer interviews can be scheduled if necessary. Appointments should be promptly kept.

Interviewing the Parents

At the initial contact with the family, both parents should be seen together. Valuable impressions can be gained about the marital relationship, attitudes about parenthood, and attitudes toward the child and his illness or adjustment problem.

In most cases, the physician can simply begin by asking what seems to be the matter. The parents should be encouraged to tell the story in their own way, guided as necessary by comments and questions. The ostensible chief complaint may turn out not to be the parents' greatest concern. Considerable patience may be required, and intrusive (or leading) questioning early in the interview only delays the flow of significant material.

Observing the parents' attitudes and feelings will help direct the physician's inquiries to fill in gaps in the history. Repeating an emotion-laden word or phrase may enable a parent who temporarily blocks to continue. A note to oneself about things the parent does not say may give important clues later. The physician should be alert to what the parents' feelings toward him are and what they seem to expect of him. A sympathetic, tolerant, and respectful attitude will help convince them that he is interested in helping them with their problem.

The physician must respect the dignity of the people he deals with in his professional role. He should learn his patients' names and not call all women "mother" to save himself the trouble. If he often encounters "troublesome" parents with whom he cannot seem to get along, he should examine his own attitudes and behavior even to the extent of obtaining psychiatric consultation. Occasionally he may have to suggest that the parents might feel more comfortable with or better served by another physician.

Parental demands for quick advice and easy solutions are usually symptoms of their own anxieties. They soon lose confidence in a physician who jumps to conclusions based on insufficient facts. No parent loses respect for a physician who says he doesn't yet know what is wrong or what to do and that further investigation and thought are necessary.

Certain historical data carry an emotional charge, and some revelations are painful and difficult. This is particularly true of familial or hereditary illnesses and of emotional disturbances in children and parents. For example, parents of children having seizures may at first withhold information about epilepsy in close relatives. Parents also recognize that their feelings about their child may be partly responsible for his behavioral disturbances. In asking questions about behavior problems, it is important not to adopt an approach which the anxious parent may misinterpret as a critical attack. Questions such as, "Did you want this child?" "Does your son masturbate?" "Was she jealous of the new baby?"—all are too frequently doomed, in the initial interview, to provoke conventional and socially acceptable replies or defensive indignation. Such information must be gathered by inference or by the use of indirect questioning. Nonverbal behavior such as blushing, nailbiting, or neuromuscular tension may give important clues.

The history should elicit relevant details about the family's circumstances—eg, their position as members of a minority group, the father's depression about unsatisfying work experiences, the mother's part-time employment which takes her out of the home at the child's bedtime. It is important to determine whether there are or have been family illnesses which may be relevant to the child's problem, but the experienced physician will avoid the monotonous listing of all possible illnesses.

In securing details of the child's birth, growth and development, and past illnesses and of the parent's child-rearing practices, it must be remembered that parents have difficulty in recalling many items with accuracy. Confirmation from other sources may be required.

The most significant emotional data often do not emerge during the first interview. Parents can rarely discuss their deep feelings until a basic sense of trust in their doctor has been allowed to develop. The parents must be allowed to talk at their own pace. The act of talking helps to discharge initial tensions and overcome anxiety. Expectant waiting is vital even if the mother appears to be on the verge of tears. The physician can, with practice, curb his natural impulse to interrupt the expression of strong emotions, and might better encourage crying by a tense and troubled mother. The release of such feeling in a sympathetic atmosphere may be of help to the parent and may strengthen the relationship with the physician.

In terminating the initial interview, it is wise to return to the area of the parents' major concern. The physician can then ask questions prompted by the leads he has gained up to this point. This indicates to the parents that he has fully comprehended their concern and will endeavor to deal constructively with it.

Interviewing the Child

Infants and young children of preschool age are usually seen with the mother. The physician may give the child a toy, tongue depressor, or other object to play with. If the parent talks too freely in the child's presence, the child may play in the waiting room while the pediatrician and the parent talk alone.

The physician may learn a good deal by observing the child at play during the interview. Impressions of the child's level of development can be gained from the degree of complexity and organization of his play, his attention span, and other clues. The child's attitude toward the physician, often reflecting parental anxiety, may also be apparent in his drawings, his play with dolls, and his general demeanor.

With older children and adolescents, the initial interview may be handled in different ways under differing circumstances. If the parents are concerned about what they think is an emotional problem, it may be wise to see them together first without the child so that they can talk freely. If information taken while the appointment is being made reveals a bitter struggle

between an adolescent and his parents, it may be best to see the adolescent first so that he may feel sure he has a chance to tell his story even though he should be told that the doctor cannot take sides. With anxious, suspicious children, it is advisable to see one or both parents and the child together at the first interview since the child may fear that the parent is imparting secret information about him; later, the parents and the child can be seen separately.

At the end of an evaluation, it may help to see the parents and the child together.

At some point, the physician should see the child alone. This is best done in an office rather than an examining room. The parents should tell the child that he is going to see a doctor who is interested in the problems that make boys and girls worried or unhappy.

With an older child, verbal data may be more accurate and voluminous after a positive relationship has been established. At the first contact, school age children or adolescents may be inhibited and withdrawn. The physician should avoid making premature judgments of the child's mental status under these circumstances.

If the physician is unaggressive and friendly and keeps his conversation at the child's level (without talking down to him), he can easily secure the child's cooperation and confidence. He may show the child some toys, suggesting that they talk while he plays. Once engrossed, the child may begin talking spontaneously, or the physician may comment on his activities.

Through observation of the child's play, the physician may learn a great deal about his conflicts or anxieties. The 4-year-old who has a smaller boy doll "beat up" a larger boy doll before "throwing it off a cliff" reveals much about his feelings toward his 6-year-old brother. It is wise not to make immediate interpretations of the child's feelings, however, as he may become too anxious. Later, the physician may bring up the child's feelings about his siblings, referring to the play incident and suggesting that maybe he feels "like that boy." Firm but kindly limits should be set on aggressive or destructive play.

With the child who can talk fairly freely, one can gain impressions of the meaning to him of his symptoms or disability in terms of its effect upon his adjustment at school, within his peer group, and in the home. With frightened or withdrawn children, data of this sort may have to be sought indirectly by asking what they want to do when they grow up. If a school age child cannot offer at least one possibility, it can be inferred that he has some fears about "growing up." The child can be asked to make 3 wishes; a significantly depressed child may not be able to think of one. If an ill child does not include "getting well" as at least one of his wishes, he usually has conflicts about returning to school or other (perhaps unconscious) fears.

A sick child can be asked what he would do if he were well, or a child who cannot talk easily about himself can be asked what a hypothetical child ("Let's pretend we know a boy who . . .") would wish for or do in a particular situation. Most children cannot talk easily at first about their feelings toward their parents. With such an approach, most children from late preschool age onward can be helped to understand their symptoms or behavior as a problem or a worry which can be remedied.

The preadolescent and adolescent child is usually capable of understanding the reason for the interview and, if adequately prepared by the parents, may openly express his desire for help with his problems. If the parents have used the visit to the physician as a threat or punishment, or if the child is present at the recommendation of school or judicial authorities, the physician should quickly clarify the situation with the youngster so that a therapeutic alliance can be established. Authoritarianism, lectures, and unsought advice are detrimental to such a relationship. Frightened adolescents should be put at ease. Hostile or defensive youngsters usually have reasons for their behavior, and a physician who can accept these attitudes nonjudgmentally is likely to discover the reasons. An open and neutral position and an evident desire to help will in time convince even the most resistant adolescent that the physician is sincere.

A formal mental status examination is difficult in children and often insulting to adolescents. Clinical observations, questions about school, and asking the child to write his name or to draw a picture will usually provide sufficiently accurate impressions of his attention span, orientation in time and place, and perceptual and motor functions. School age children, when asked to draw a picture of a person, will usually draw a person of the same sex.

Some estimate of the child's intelligence may be obtained in a rough fashion through similar methods. Pediatricians have demonstrated their capacity, in a controlled study, to make a surprisingly accurate evaluation of the Developmental Quotient of infants and young children. Their main errors lie in underestimating the capacities of physically ill children and in overestimating the abilities of mentally retarded children.

Most available tests of reading ability are complicated and lengthy. The physician should familiarize himself with first, second, and third grade readers and should have one of each available in case a reading problem is suspected. For adequate evaluation in the cognitive area, referral to a clinical psychologist is indicated.

Observation of Child & Parent

From the moment the parent enters the office, valuable clinical impressions are available to the physician or to an alert nurse or secretary. Some parents cannot permit the child to answer a question independently, manifesting a need to dominate the child or the situation. Other parents constantly correct the child or require him to sit impossibly still, disclosing unrealistically high standards of behavior and conformity.

If the father and mother are interviewed together, they may disclose disagreements in child-rearing prac-

tices. Some parents pay little attention to their children, such as the mother who does not stand close to her infant to prevent him from falling off the examining table. Disturbed parents, with unconscious needs to deny the extent or seriousness of the child's obvious illness, may belittle him or urge him to act as if he were well.

The physician should record such observations and test them against later impressions. Observations of this sort are most readily available to the physician who visits the home and enjoys continuity of contact with the parents and child. On a home visit, the standards of parental care and the patterns of family living are often more evident than in the office. Valuable observations of this nature can also be gathered in a clinic waiting room by the receptionist or nurse.

Korsch BM: Practical techniques of observing, interviewing, and advising parents in pediatric practice as demonstrated in an attitude study project. Pediatrics 18:467, 1956.

Korsch BM, Freemon B, Negrete VF: Practical implications of doctor-patient interaction analysis for pediatric practice. Am J Dis Child 121:110, 1971.

THE APPROACH TO PHYSICAL EXAMINATION OF THE CHILD

Preparation for the Examination

The physician can anticipate active participation by the child in the physical examination, but he must be prepared for resigned submission, passive resistance, or even active refusal and violent battle. The degree of rapport already established with the parent and child may determine the diagnostic success of the examination. If the child is seriously ill, the physical examination may be done while the latter portion of the history is being taken to save time and to decrease the suspense of the anxious child and the parent.

Refusal by preschool children to remove certain items of clothing may indicate anxiety over being so completely exposed rather than sexual modesty. This initial apprehension should be respected, and it is soon overcome. Older children may retain their underpants, which can be dropped for genital examination when they are more at ease.

A relaxed and unhurried approach is vital. A few moments spent in conversation, using the child's first name or nickname, may save time and struggle. Some explanation of each step, as in examining the throat or darkening the room for ophthalmoscopic examination, can be given quietly, using terms the child can understand.

Permitting a young child to handle certain instruments such as the stethoscope before they are used (eg, listening to their own heartbeat) may overcome tension. "Blowing out" the light of the otoscope is a time-honored pediatric method of distracting toddlers from their apprehension about the examination.

Variations in Handling of Different Ages

A. Very Young Infants: With the very young infant, little difficulty is encountered if the mother is relaxed and trusting. Pacifiers may be used if the baby is crying or restless. Much of the examination may be performed while the mother holds and feeds the infant, affording the physician an opportunity to observe her feeding approach and the mother a chance to talk about any fears she may have about the infant's physical status or developmental progress.

B. Older Infants Up to Age 1½: In the second half of the first year, stranger or separation anxiety causes most infants to show some fear of the physician even if they have seen him regularly for health examinations. The physician may hand the mother a tongue depressor or similar object to give to the infant while he sits in her lap during the interview, permitting him to appraise the physician from a safe vantage point. If he is crawling or toddling, the infant may later move toward the physician and make friendly overtures.

The infant often resists being examined on his back or on the examining table, and it may be best to examine him on his mother's lap, permitting her to hold his head against her shoulder for examination of the ears and throat. The nurse may be able to obtain a more positive initial response from the older infant than the physician.

C. Ages 1½–3: During the normal period of negativism in the latter part of the second and early part of the third year, the child may refuse to cooperate with some parts of the examination such as opening his mouth to permit examination of the throat. Patience is required. A stubbornly negativistic child, diverted at this point to some other activity, may later abandon his rebellious stand. Physical battles inevitably result in the child's loss of trust in the physician.

D. Preschool Children: The preschool child can usually be examined on a table. Most children at this age are frightened when they are compelled to lie down and feel less anxious when they are in a sitting position.

E. School Age Children: With children of school age, as with older preschool children, much can be learned during the physical examination about the child's attitudes toward his own development; his feelings about himself as a developing individual; his feelings about his body and its adequacy; his fears or misconceptions about parts of his body and how they are working; and his concern about minor blemishes. If the child feels secure with the physician, he may himself bring up his fears or concerns. The parent may verbalize similar concerns during an unhurried examination.

F. Adolescents: With adolescents, feelings of modesty may become apparent during the examination. Such feelings should be respected, and these young people should be handled in the same way as adults. Fears may emerge in boys concerning growth lags or other real or imaginary deviations; in girls, about the onset of menses and the development of secondary sex characteristics. During the examination of girls of this age, a nurse should always be present.

Parent Attendance

Some physicians prefer to exclude an anxious mother from the physical examination, recognizing that the child often submits more passively in her absence. This approach carries with it not only the pain of separation but also the implication of punishment by the physician. The parent may react with feelings of guilt or resentment, surmising that the physician thinks she is a poor parent. It is almost always best to permit the parent to remain with the infant or young child.

An apprehensive parent who asks to leave during the examination should usually be permitted to do so, but it is better that she leave before rather than during the examination. If the mother leaves the room, the child should be told where she will be and when she will return. If restraint is indicated, it should be carried out promptly, with a brief explanation of its need.

Precautions in Examination

The physician's hands and the instruments he uses should be warm, since any coldness to the touch may add to the child's fear or resistance. With younger children, examination of the ears and throat should be done last. Rectal temperatures may be resisted, in which case an axillary temperature reading will suffice. For children beyond infancy, rectal examinations should be performed with great care and gentleness and with adequate explanation. A "blowing" game may aid in securing cooperation during examination of the chest. Time spent in putting the child at ease will provide sufficient relaxation of the abdominal musculature for an accurate examination of the abdomen. Caution should be observed in the vaginal inspection of preadolescent or adolescent girls.

After the examination, the child should be given time to ask questions, if he so desires, about procedures or instruments used or about any other phase of the examination. Plans for preparation of the child for further laboratory procedures, other medical or surgical experiences, or hospitalization should be considered.

The physician should always terminate the interview with a friendly and personal farewell to the child.

SPECIAL TESTS

Psychologic Tests

When properly administered by trained personnel, psychologic tests can be of great diagnostic assistance. Like laboratory tests, they must be interpreted in the light of the clinical findings. A single psychologic test, like a single laboratory test, may not be accurate, especially if the child is tired, sick, or anxious.

Intelligence testing is discussed in Chapter 22.

Electroencephalography

Although the older literature indicates that a large percentage of patients with emotional illnesses have abnormal EEGs, recent investigators have found a strikingly high incidence of so-called abnormal waves in normally developing children. For example, it was once thought that 14- and 6-per-second spikes were associated with behavioral disorders, but these wave patterns have also been found in normal children and adolescents. In one large study, well over ½ of children without symptoms showed these abnormalities, especially children between 4–9 years of age. Many so-called abnormal waves may be better described as transient phenomena occurring during critical periods of integrative development in the CNS.

The EEG should be interpreted only as one of many factors in the clinical evaluation of the patient.

Preparation of the child for EEG testing is important, as the wires and machine may arouse fears of "electricity." The child may also need to be told that the machine cannot read his mind.

Osselton JW, Kiloh LG: *Clinical Electroencephalography.* Butterworth, 1961.
Small JG, Small IF: Fourteen and six per second positive spikes. Arch Gen Psychiat 11:645, 1964.

IMPLEMENTATION OF RESULTS OF THE CLINICAL EXAMINATION

Once the physician has achieved a balanced appraisal of the child and his family, his plan of therapy or his approach to well child care must be communicated effectively to parents and patient. He should be confident and at times authoritative in his recommendations, but humility, patience, and understanding are the most appropriate and useful attitudes. The physician must bear in mind the apprehension with which the parents await his diagnosis and recommendations. He should use simple language and write out detailed or complicated instructions for care.

In discussing with parents a child's emotional problem, the physician should not imply that they have "caused" it. The parents may suspect that the problem is an emotional one. If they initially thought the problem was a physical one, the physician can begin by saying that he is happy to reassure them that there are no serious physical abnormalities. He can add that he feels the symptoms can be caused or aggravated by "emotional tension," and then ask the parents whether they have noticed evidence of any such tension. He can indicate that such problems are "nobody's fault" and can suggest that there are ways of helping the child to oversome his difficulties. He can further indicate that, with help, they might think of things that should be done or things that they might, in hindsight, want to change about their ways of handling the child. Most parents will respond positively, after some initial defensiveness, to such an approach.

The physician should also give the child, in the presence of his parents or alone, a brief explanation of his illness and the plan for treatment, in age-appropriate terms.

INDICATIONS FOR PSYCHIATRIC REFERRAL

The decision about what kind of cases a pediatrician can treat and which he should refer to a child psychiatrist or child guidance clinic depends to a large extent on the pediatrician's interests and training. Of all health professionals, the pediatrician is in the best position to educate parents about the nature of childhood and to help them handle ordinary behavior problems. However, every pediatrician has cases in his practice that he cannot be expected to handle. When doubt exists, consultation with a child psychiatrist is useful.

Criteria for Referral
The following criteria should be considered as guidelines for referral.

A. Home Environment: A severely handicapping home environment or seriously disturbed parents will generally warrant a prolonged relationship with mental health professionals.

B. Age Discrepancy: At certain ages, most children have outgrown particular habits or behavior. If they do not, psychiatric study may be indicated.

C. Intensity or Frequency of Symptoms: Under emotional or physical stress, most children may regress, but persistent regressive behavior may indicate psychologic fixations.

D. Degree of Social Disadvantage or Impairment: Certain modes of behavior tend to be self-perpetuating, eg, the aggressive child who makes many enemies has no choice but to continue to fight.

E. The Child's Inner Suffering: This is frequently overlooked by parents, teachers, and physicians, as with the well behaved student who is not achieving.

F. Intractable Behavior: The persistence of symptoms, despite the efforts of the child and others to change them, is a cardinal clue to intrapsychic conflicts.

Preparation for Referral
When the pediatrician has decided that referral is necessary, his preparation of the child and parents can help to ensure a successful outcome. Parents may be afraid of the word psychiatry; may feel that they have failed as parents; or may fear that they will be lectured or condemned.

The physician must explain to the parents why the child needs help. It is best to discuss the symptoms in terms of the child's discomfort, as indications of "lack of confidence" or of being "mixed up" about himself.

The second step involves dealing with the parents' possible objections to psychiatric aid. Some parents need to be told that normal children can have emotional problems and that they need not fear that the child will be stigmatized. Parents need reassurance about the confidentiality of such matters. A sense of guilt may prevent them from accepting help or recognizing their own involvement. The physician must not argue with the parents and should explain that there are undoubtedly many important reasons for their child's difficulties.

The last step involves conveying a realistic understanding of what psychiatric therapy can accomplish. The physician should not make extravagant promises or concrete predictions but should convince the parents that help is both needed and available.

In talking with the child, openness and honesty are essential. He should be told where he is going and why, and he should know what his basic problem is.

Freud A: Assessment of childhood disturbances. Psychoanal Stud Child 17:149, 1962.

Moskowitz JA: The pediatrician calls for psychiatric referral: Notes on achieving a successful consultation. Clin Pediat 7:733, 1968.

Schwab JJ, Brown J: Uses and abuses of psychiatric consultation. JAMA 205:65, 1968.

PSYCHOTHERAPY

There are several different schools of psychotherapy based on different frames of references, but the aims and methods of treatment tend to be similar in all. In some types of emotional problems, a supportive or directive approach is indicated; in others, exploration of the patient's defenses and life experiences; in still others, the therapeutic effect of allowing the patient to talk about (ventilate) his feelings is of dominant importance. Psychotherapy may also be classified as interpretive, suggestive, persuasive, or educative; or in terms of its depth, duration, and intensity. Isolating a single therapeutic element as a basis for classification is an artificial approach since each of the factors listed is present in some degree in every psychotherapeutic relationship. The dimensions of psychotherapy are best described as a continuum extending from the supportive end, where little uncovering of deeper conflicts occurs, to the insight-promoting end, in which "operative" or interpretative activity is predominant.

Allen FH: *Psychotherapy With Children.* Norton, 1942.

Bowen M: Family psychotherapy. Am J Orthopsychiat 31:40, 1961.

Harrison SI, Carek DJ: *A Guide to Psychotherapy.* Little, Brown, 1966.

Swanson FL: *Psychotherapists and Children: A Procedural Guide.* Pitman, 1970.

PSYCHOPHARMACOLOGIC AGENTS

Psychoactive drugs have achieved a significant place in the treatment of emotional disorders of childhood. They cannot replace the interpersonal relationship which is the main tool of the physician, but they can be effective in reducing anxiety and overactivity. Reduction of impulsiveness and irritability is usually accompanied by less anxiety and improved attention span. On occasion, drug therapy can increase spontaneous activity and responsiveness in states of apathy and depression. The effects upon complex behavior patterns, on the other hand, are much more difficult to predict during drug therapy.

There is no evidence that psychoactive drugs can improve intellectual functioning directly. Although it is possible to modify a child's responses to current experiences with drugs, they cannot undo previously learned behavior or alter neurotic patterns. Much information is still needed on the effects of specific drugs and their mode of action, as our knowledge remains largely empiric.

Principles of Drug Treatment

A. Drug and Diagnosis Must Be Matched: The condition of a disturbed child must be accurately diagnosed if he is to receive the most effective treatment. An appropriate drug—eg, an antipsychotic tranquilizer—can help control behavior even in severe psychoses. With appropriate drug administration, some severely disturbed children may become amenable to psychotherapy. Although neurotic disorders rarely respond lastingly to drugs, some children with intrapsychic conflicts suffering from persistent anxiety, inhibitions, and phobias become more spontaneous and increase their adaptive functioning when given tranquilizing drugs.

Personality disorders and mental retardation are generally not benefited by drugs. Hyperkinesia may benefit from stimulant drugs. Reactive disorders rarely justify drug use except as sedation is necessary for cases of acute anxiety.

B. Benefit Should Exceed Toxicity: The physician who uses drugs should have a thorough knowledge of their pharmacologic properties, including their side-effects and potential toxicity. The severity of the child's disorder and the potential for improvement must justify the possible impact of side-effects and toxicity.

C. Special Precautions in Young Patients: Data cannot always be extrapolated from adult medicine to pediatrics. A child's response to a psychoactive drug may be quite different from that of an adult.

Special clinical testing of drugs potentially valuable for disturbed children is essential, as a drug's action may be other than predicted because of the immature and developing qualities of the child.

Dosage must be individualized for each patient, since undertreatment as well as overtreatment may result from metabolic differences at different ages. Dosage must be carefully regulated so as not to impair a child's intellectual acuity and maturation.

D. Use Familiar Drugs: A well tested and familiar drug should be employed until a newer or unfamiliar one establishes its superiority. Unexpected toxicity from a less well known agent may not become apparent until it has been in general use for a long period.

E. Use Drugs Sparingly: Drugs should not be used any longer than necessary. Lowering the dosage periodically will permit the observation of improvement or worsening of the symptoms being treated.

F. Seek Other Forms of Therapy: Since pharmacotherapy of emotional disorders affects symptoms rather than the underlying disease, the physician must continue his attempts to identify and eliminate the physical, psychologic, and social etiologic factors in the emotional disturbance.

ANTIPSYCHOTIC TRANQUILIZERS

The antipsychotic ("major") tranquilizers have found their greatest usefulness in the treatment of hospitalized, severely disturbed, or psychotic children because they exert a calmative effect on agitated, impulsive, or excited states without causing paradoxical excitement or anesthesia. In addition, they can reduce or eliminate delusions and hallucinations and some schizophrenic ideation and thus make these children more communicative.

The dosage is increased at intervals of several days until a satisfactory response is obtained or until side-effects limit further increases in dosage or force discontinuance of therapy. In acute situations, an initial parenteral dose may be given.

These agents should not be used to alleviate neurotic anxiety.

The antipsychotic tranquilizers can be classified according to their chemical structure or pharmacologic properties.

Phenothiazine Derivatives & Similar Potent Drugs

The tranquilizers most commonly used are phenothiazine derivatives. Chlorprothixene (Taractan) is chemically and pharmacologically similar. Haloperidol (Haldol) is a butyrophenone comparable to the stimulant tranquilizers listed below but is not approved for use in patients under 12.

The phenothiazines can be further classified according to the degree of sedation induced and the likelihood of extrapyramidal side-effects.

A. Sedation Prominent: The only important example is promethazine (Phenergan).

B. Standard Agents: Included are chlorpromazine (Thorazine) and thioridazine (Mellaril).

C. Stimulant Tranquilizers: These agents cause comparatively less sedation for the same therapeutic effect but are also more likely to cause extrapyramidal side-effects. Trifluoperazine (Stelazine) and prochlorperazine (Compazine) are the important drugs in this group. Children are especially susceptible to side-effects and may manifest violent dystonias or choreiform movements as well as tremors, rigidity, and akathisia. Parenteral administration should be avoided.

Other side-effects include atropine-like or anticholinergic responses (constipation, blurred vision, dryness of the mouth, difficult micturition), postural hypotension, and lethargy or drowsiness. Endocrine abnormalities, skin changes (dermatitis, photosensitivity), and lowered body temperature occur less commonly.

Rare cases of aplastic anemia and agranulocytosis have been reported. Cholangiolitic jaundice (intrahepatic obstruction) was once a common side-effect of chlorpromazine administration but is now rare. Convulsions may occur when very high dosages are used or when epilepsy or other predisposition to convulsions is present. The "seizures" that are seen after accidental ingestion of stimulant tranquilizers are usually actually dystonias.

Toxicity or troublesome side-effects can be managed by decreasing the dosage or changing to another drug. Extrapyramidal signs can usually be relieved by antiparkinsonism drugs.

Antihistamines & Other Less Potent Tranquilizers

Diphenhydramine (Benadryl) and other antihistamines and hydroxyzine (Atarax, Vistaril) are tranquilizers of limited potency. The dosage cannot be increased because of atropine-like side-effects.

The antihistamines were used by pediatricians for the induction of sleep even before the concept of tranquilizing drugs was introduced. Children often become excited (disinhibited) when given barbiturates or the antipsychotic tranquilizers. The sedation caused by these agents is not as subjectively unpleasant at bedtime as it is during the day.

Rauwolfia Alkaloids (Reserpine)

Reserpine has been replaced as an antipsychotic tranquilizer by the phenothiazines, and its use is now limited to the treatment of hypertension. In addition to the side-effects mentioned above, it causes nasal congestion, gastric hypersecretion, and diarrhea.

SEDATIVE-HYPNOTICS

In contrast to the antipsychotic tranquilizers, the sedatives are antianxiety agents. They are, of course, also anticonvulsants and used to induce sleep.

The drugs listed below have a number of effects in common. The first 4 properties listed are the stages of anesthesia produced by increasingly larger doses.

(1) Sedation, relief of anxiety, encouragement of normal sleep.

(2) Disinhibition, excitement, drunkenness: Paradoxical excitement is common in children, especially when the continued stimulation of pain, restraint, or anxiety is present.

(3) General anesthesia.

(4) Medullary depression and death.

(5) Anticonvulsant effect.

(6) Habituation and withdrawal: Rare in children, although misuse of secobarbital and other sedatives involves younger age groups each year.

(7) Spinal cord depressant action: These drugs are theoretically but not practically useful as voluntary muscle relaxants.

Classification

The sedatives can be classified according to their chemical structure as barbiturates, piperidinediones (glutethimide [Doriden]), dicarbamates (meprobamate), alcohols (chloral hydrate), ethers (paraldehyde), or benzodiazepines (chlordiazepoxide [Librium]). However, it is more useful to classify them according to their rapidity of action and duration of effect. These properties are correlated—ie, those with a rapid onset of action have short duration of action, and those with a prolonged effect have a longer latent period.

A. Short-Acting: Pentobarbital, secobarbital, chloral hydrate.

B. Intermediate-Acting: Amobarbital, meprobamate, diazepam (Valium).

C. Long-Acting: Phenobarbital, mephobarbital (Mebaral), chlordiazepoxide (Librium), oxazepam (Serax).

STIMULANTS
(Amphetamines)

The amphetamines are effective in the treatment of children who are hyperactive and distractible as a result of brain damage. In such children they often have a paradoxically calming effect, resulting in quieter, better organized behavior and a longer attention span. Prolonged therapy with these agents can be maintained without significant toxicity. Side-effects consist principally of anorexia and insomnia, which can be controlled by lowering the dosage. Overdoses can result in toxic psychosis, and in adolescents there is a risk of habituation.

Treatment for school age children is initiated with 5 mg daily in the morning before breakfast, increasing by 5 mg every several days in divided doses (morning and early afternoon) until improvement occurs or side-effects appear. Doses up to 30 mg/day may be needed to effectively treat a hyperkinetic child. Maintenance doses of about ½ of the above are often effective. If after 2 weeks no noticeable change in symptomatology has occurred, the drug used initially—usually dextroamphetamine (Dexedrine)—should be discontinued and amphetamine (Benzedrine) or methylphenidate (Ritalin) tried.

If effective, these drugs can be continued until puberty, when they are usually no longer necessary and abuse becomes a problem.

ANTIDEPRESSANTS

Whether the antidepressant drugs that closely resemble the tranquilizers will find a place in pediatric practice has not been completely established. The types of depression treated successfully with these drugs in adults do not occur in childhood or adolescence.

The iminodibenzyl derivatives have been said to alleviate enuresis in children. Imipramine (Tofranil), the most commonly used of this class of drugs, appears to be successful for this purpose.

Alexandris A, Lundell F: Effect of thioridazine, amphetamine, and placebo on hyperkinetic syndrome and cognitive area in mentally deficient children. Canad MAJ 98:92-96, 1968.

Conners CK, Eisenberg L, Barcai A: Effect of dextroamphetamine on children: Studies on subjects with learning disabilities and school behavior problems. Arch Gen Psychiat 17:478, 1967.

Costa E, Garattini S (editors): *International Symposium on Amphetamines and Related Compounds.* Raven Press, 1970.

Eisenberg L: The role of drugs in treating disturbed children. Children 11:167, 1964.

Fish B: Drug use in psychiatric disorders of children. Am J Psychiat 124:31, 1968.

Freedman AM: Drug therapy in behavior disorders. P Clin North America 5:573, 1958.

Lasagna L, Epstein LC: The use of amphetamines in the treatment of hyperkinetic children. Page 849 in: *International Symposium on Amphetamines and Related Compounds.* Costa E, Garattini S (editors). Raven Press, 1970.

THE PEDIATRICIAN & OTHER SERVICES IN THE COMMUNITY

The pediatrician can contribute to the early treatment and in some cases prevention of some major social issues facing our communities today. Such social problems as adoption, disturbed families, delinquency, child battering, illegitimate pregnancies, and homicide can be partially solved or prevented by the kind of early intervention the pediatrician is in a position to offer. Physicians responsible for the care of children should be familiar with the mental health, family service, and other agencies in his community and should use them when necessary.

Bender L: Children and adolescents who have killed. Am J Psychiat 116:510, 1959.

Eisenberg E: The sins of the fathers: Urban decay and social pathology. Am J Orthopsychiat 32:5, 1962.

Green M: Pediatrics and the ambulatory patient. Am J Orthopsychiat 32:67, 1962.

Guttmacher AF: Unwanted pregnancy: A challenge to mental health. Ment Hyg 51:514, 1967.

Kempe CH: The battered child and the hospital. Hosp Practice 4:44, 1969.

Matson O & others: Child psychiatric emergencies: Clinical
characteristics and follow-up results. Arch Gen Psychiat
5:591, 1967.

Pettz WL: Sex education programs in schools. Am J Psychiat
125:206, 1968.

Richmond JB: The pediatrician and the individual delinquent.
Pediatrics 26:126, 1960.

Smith DC: Pediatric consultation in adoption practice. Pediatrics 41:519, 1968.

Solnit A, Stark MH: Pediatric management of school learning
problems of under-achievement. New England J Med
261:980, 1959.

PSYCHOTHERAPEUTIC ASPECTS OF THE ROLE OF THE PEDIATRICIAN

Various aspects of the psychotherapeutic role of the pediatrician in dealing with children and their parents include, among others, emotionally supportive contacts during the prenatal period; later, helping the parents to promote the child's healthy personality development; and preparation of the child and parents for potentially stressful experiences such as hospitalization or surgery.

Some aspects of supportive psychotherapy which the pediatrician can use in dealing with parents and with older children and adolescents have already been mentioned. In working with parents of children with mild psychologic disorders or with chronic illnesses or handicaps, he can provide emotional support. He can help them to ventilate their feelings and to develop spontaneous insights by helping to clarify conflicting feelings or by offering gentle confrontation of inconsistencies in their attitudes.

The pediatrician may reflect feelings back to the parents by repeating emotion-laden words, offering them an opportunity to explore conflicts further. At times he can verbalize for them certain feelings or thoughts. He may offer advice or counseling and can help them work through feelings already recognized, particularly in the case of serious illness. By suggestion, persuasion, and other means, he can facilitate constructive changes in the parents' attitudes and behavior.

The use of toys and play interviews can help younger children to clarify their fears, confusion, or conflicts, offering them a chance to discharge tension or master anxieties through "playing out" their feelings.

Verbal discussion and counseling can be helpful for older children and adolescents if they can talk easily, but improvement may often occur on a nonverbal level as a result of the young person's perception of the pediatrician's attitudes toward him and his parents.

Confidentiality of the older child's or adolescent's intimate revelations should be maintained and explained to the parents. Exceptions should be made only with the young person's knowledge and only when obviously necessary, such as a potential suicide attempt or serious delinquency.

Attention should be paid to attitudes or feelings which are transferred from past experiences with key figures onto the pediatrician. Awareness of the origin of these transferences will help the pediatrician to avoid reacting as if the attitudes were directed personally toward him. It may at times be wise to confront the parent or child with the fact that such attitudes or feelings derive from other experiences. If certain types of behavior often make him angry or frustrated, the pediatrician must examine his own responses. Such feelings may be influenced by his own past experiences, representing a type of countertransference which may not be appropriate to the circumstances.

The pediatrician may sometimes employ family interviews, especially if communication between parents and child or adolescent seems blocked. He must take an active, directive approach in such situations, helping the family to maintain control and to avoid explosive releases of hostile feelings. Group discussions, often with the aid of a social worker or other mental health professional, may be of value for parents of chronically ill children or for adolescents with hemophilia, diabetes, or other chronic disorders. They may be employed with groups of parents of well children also in a kind of "child study" approach.

The pediatrician may act as a coordinator of the contributions of other professionals in the health team, as in a comprehensive approach to the management of children in a hospital ward. In the community, he may act as a consultant to nursery schools, public schools, courts, camps, social agencies, or child guidance clinics. He can also use his influence to promote the development of needed mental health resources, which may aid him and other health professionals in preventing emotional disorders and further unhealthy adaptation and personality development.

Bolian GC: Diagnosis and treatment: Psychosocial aspects of
well child care. Pediatrics 39:280, 1967.

Coddington RD: The use of brief psychotherapy in a pediatric
practice. J Pediat 60:259, 1962.

Eisenberg L: Possibilities for a preventive psychiatry. Pediatrics
30:815, 1962.

Green M, Senn MJ: Teaching of comprehensive pediatrics on an
inpatient hospital service. Pediatrics 21:476, 1958.

Korsch B, Fraad L, Barnett HL: Pediatric discussions with
parent groups. J Pediat 44:703, 1954.

Richmond JB: Health supervision of infants and children. J
Pediat 40:634, 1952.

Senn MJE: The psychotherapeutic role of the pediatrician.
Pediatrics 2:147, 1948.

Shulman JL: The management of the irate parent. J Pediat
77:338, 1970.

SPECIFIC CLINICAL DISORDERS

Although the definition of normality in development and behavior has a certain relativity because of individual variations and different cultural settings, an assessment of healthy behavioral responses can be made.

Appropriateness of behavior to the age of the child or stage of development is a basic consideration, and the same is true of the balance of progressive versus regressive forces and the general "smoothness" of development. The latter includes the clinician's assessment of the child's adaptation in the present as well as his mastery of stresses in the past. Such considerations may be modified in accordance with the child's endowment, his current developmental level, the nature of the stresses to which he is subjected in his particular family and social setting, and other factors. The following classification is adapted from that offered by the Committee on Child Psychiatry of the Group for the Advancement of Psychiatry (see reference on p 596).

HEALTHY RESPONSES

1. DEVELOPMENTAL CRISES

Developmental crises are brief and transient upheavals which are definitely related to a particular developmental stage and involve attempts to resolve appropriate psychosocial tasks. The child appears normal except for the manifestations of the developmental crisis.

Examples include "stranger" and "separation" anxieties of the second half of the first year, related to the capacity of the infant to distinguish between the mother and others. Anxiety, oppositional behavior, and other manifestations are most marked when developmental tasks are normally most demanding, as when the young child is first separated from the parent.

Treatment consists of a supportive counseling approach to help the child master the crisis and move on to the next stage of development. Anticipatory counseling of the parents is helpful so that they will not handle the child too permissively or too punitively at such times. Inappropriately handled, a developmental crisis may become a reactive disorder (see below) or may crystallize into a psychoneurotic or personality disorder. If a developmental crisis comes too early or too late, it may represent a developmental deviation.

2. SITUATIONAL CRISES

Situational crises are usually transient and brief and are related to situations in the family or environment which represent acutely stressful circumstances for a particular child. The resulting behavioral problems appear to be normal adaptive responses to crisis situations and not deeply disturbed behavior. The child appears normal on examination except for his behavioral response to the crisis situation.

Examples of situational crises include the death of a parent or other serious family crisis and the mild regression that may occur upon return from the hospital after a tonsillectomy. Depression may be apparent in grief reactions. Depressive equivalents may be manifested by temporary loss of appetite, sleep disturbances, or change in activity level. Regression is often characterized by a transient refusal to speak in infants or loss of bowel and bladder control in toddlers.

Treatment is primarily supportive, since the crises are self-limited. Anticipatory guidance of the parents and preventive measures such as preparation of the child and parents for hospitalization can be vital.

Prolonged stressful circumstances with inadequate parental response can lead to reactive disorders or more structured psychopathology.

Burks HL, Harrison SI: Aggressive behavior as a means of avoiding a depression. Am J Orthopsychiat 32:416, 1962.

Erickson E: Growth and crises of the healthy personality. In: *Symposium on the Healthy Personality.* Supplement II. Josiah Macy Jr Foundation, 1950.

Friedman SB: Management of death in a parent or sibling. In: *Ambulatory Pediatrics.* Green M, Haggerty R (editors). Saunders, 1968.

Sugar M: Children of divorce. Pediatrics 46:588, 1970.

REACTIVE DISORDERS

Pathologic behavior or symptoms may occur in response to disturbing events or situations. They are usually transient but may develop into more severe and chronic psychopathology. Such responses are most common in preschool and early school age children. The child is usually normal on examination but may have had previous adaptive difficulties.

The reactive disorders differ from situational crises in the matter of degree. A disturbing situation arising acutely may have a profound effect. Examples include illness and hospitalization, accidents, loss of a parent, school pressures, and parental behavior problems. The important consideration is not the strength of the stimulus but the intensity of the child's reaction, which is a function of his ego development, his adaptive capacity, his past experience, and his original endowment. Physiologic concomitants such as peptic ulcer or ulcerative colitis may be precipitated in the predisposed youngster. Depression or regressive behavior may include withdrawal, thumbsucking, wetting or soiling, or excessive daydreaming and preoccupation with fantasy.

Treatment is similar to that of situational crisis: supportive counseling for the parents, with anticipatory guidance and clarification of misconceptions, and emotional support for the child. "Replacement" therapy in the hospital, with the use of parent substitutes or liberalized visiting hours, will help to compensate for emotional deprivation. In some cases, a reactive disorder may be superimposed upon a psychoneurosis, a personality disorder, or even a chronic psychosis of moderate severity. A reactive disorder involving temporary arrest in development may evolve into a developmental deviation or psychoneurosis, and formal intensive psychotherapy may be necessary.

Cameron K: Diagnostic categories in child psychiatry. Brit J M Psychol 28:67, 1955.

Spitz RA, Wolf K: Anaclitic depression. Psychoanal Stud Child 2:313, 1946.

DEVELOPMENTAL DEVIATIONS

Developmental deviations become manifest over a period of months or years as characteristics of the child's development. A single parameter of development may be involved (eg, motor or sensory), or the deviation may be characterized by lags, unevenness, or precocities in maturational steps.

Included in this diagnosis are deviations in maturational patterns such as capacity for control or rhythmic integration in such bodily functions as sleeping, eating, speech, or bowel and bladder functions. Specific types of deviations involved are described briefly below.

Types of Developmental Deviations

A. Motor Development: Eg, hyperactivity, hypoactivity, incoordination, and handedness, along with other predominantly motor capacities, where brain damage is not involved.

B. Sensory Development: Difficulty in monitoring stimuli from tactile to social in nature. Such children may overreact or be apathetic to stimuli.

C. Speech Development: Significant delays other than those due to deafness, oppositional behavior, elective mutism, brain damage, or early childhood psychosis. Disorders of articulation, rhythm, or phonation, or an infantile type of speech comprehension, may be evident. Normal word repetition by a healthy child in the preschool phase and stuttering as a conversion symptom are not included in this group.

D. Cognitive Function: Problems of symbolic or abstract thinking such as reading, writing, and arithmetic. "Pseudoretarded" and significantly precocious youngsters are in this category.

E. Social Development: Eg, children with delayed capacities for parental separation, marked shyness, dependence, inhibitions, and immaturely aggressive behavior.

F. Psychosexual Development: Eg, timing of sexual curiosity, persistence of infantile auto-erotic patterns, or markedly precocious or delayed heterosexual interests.

G. Affective (Emotional) Development: Eg, moderate anxiety, emotional lability not appropriate to the child's age, marked overcontrol of emotions, mild depression or apathy, and cyclothymic behavior.

H. Integrative Development: Lack of impulse control or frustration tolerance and the uneven use or overuse of defense mechanisms such as projection or denial.

Treatment

In many cases, no formal treatment is necessary. Explanation to the parents of the nature of the deviation may suffice, and counseling about management of the child is often helpful.

Psychotherapy is necessary in cases involving sweeping lags in maturational patterns or developing personality disturbances.

The amphetamines may be useful for the hyperactive child; speech therapy when there is a lag in speech development; and remedial tutoring for the youngster with a cognitive lag.

Chess S: Individuality in children: Its importance to the pediatrician. J Pediat 69:676, 1966.

PSYCHONEUROTIC DISORDERS

Psychoneurotic disorders are ordinarily chronic and structured in nature, pervading the child's whole personality. They are characterized by psychologic symptoms (free-floating anxiety, obsessive thoughts, and phobias) which can be seriously crippling. They arise from the child's internalized unconscious conflicts, often with apparent reference to current family situations.

Psychoneuroses are not commonly seen in flagrant form before the early school age period. No gross disturbances in reality testing are observed in spite of the apparent irrationality of the child's fears or other symptoms.

Types of Psychoneuroses in the Pediatric Age Group

A. Anxiety Type: The conflict breaks into awareness as an intense and diffuse feeling of apprehension or impending diaster—in contrast to normal apprehensions, conscious fears, or content-specific phobias. The physiologic concomitants of anxiety, in contrast to psychophysiologic disorders, do not lead to structural changes in involved organ systems.

B. Phobic Type: There is unconscious displacement onto an object or situation in the external environment that has symbolic significance for the child. For example, there may be a conscious fear of animals, school, dirt, disease, elevators, etc. Phobias, with their internalized and structured character, should be distinguished from developmental crises involving separation anxiety and the mild fears and transient phobias of the stressful experiences in reactive disorders. School phobias are discussed below.

C. Conversion Type: The original conflict is expressed as a somatic dysfunction of organs supplied by the voluntary portion of the CNS—usually the striated musculature or somatosensory apparatus. Included are disturbances of motor function, as in paralysis or motor tics; alterations in sensory perception, as in cases of blindness or deafness; disturbances in awareness, as in conversion syncope or convulsive-like phenomena; and disturbances in the total body image, as in psychologic invalidism associated with extreme weakness or bizarre paralyses. Dysfunctions of the upper and lower ends of the gastrointestinal tract, as in certain types of vomiting or encopresis; of the voluntary components of respiration, as in hyperventilation and respiration (coughing or barking); and of the genitourinary organs, as in certain types of enuresis or bladder atony may also be conversion expressions. EEG changes are nonspecific, and local structural abnormalities have not been demonstrated except those secondary to long-standing conversions. Personality disorders and borderline psychoses may be associated and may justify multiple diagnoses.

D. Dissociative Type: Includes fugue states, cataplexy, transient catatonic states without underlying psychosis, and conditions with aimless motor discharge or "freezing." Disturbances in consciousness may occur with hypnagogic or hypnopompic or so-called twilight states, marked somnambulism, and pseudodelirious and stuporous states. Depersonalization, dissociated personality, amnesia, Ganser's syndrome (in adolescents), and pseudopsychotic states or "hysterical psychoses" may be present episodically. Although a hysterical personality may be involved, other psychopathologic disorders may be present also. Panic states (usually reactive disorders), acute brain syndromes, psychotic conditions, and epileptic equivalents must be differentiated.

E. Obsessive-Compulsive Type: The countless rituals (eg, excessive orderliness and washing compulsions) with marked anxiety resulting from interference by the parents or others. This disorder must be distinguished from the normal ritualism in early childhood associated with bedtime or toilet training or the pseudocompulsive rituals in the early school age.

F. Depressive Type: Often expressed differently in children than in adults. Symptoms include eating and sleeping disturbances and hyperactivity. Chronic depressive disorders are modified by the child's stage of development and must be distinguished from the more acute reactive disorders, in which depression may be involved (eg, the anaclitic type). Depression may be a component of any clinical problem from developmental crisis to psychosis.

Treatment

Treatment may be minimal, eg, supportive counseling, since some mild psychoneurotic disorders resolve spontaneously. However, intensive psychotherapy for the child and the parents is often required and is generally successful, especially in the anxiety, phobic, conversion, and depressive types. Severe obsessive-compulsive and dissociative types often require child analysis.

Tranquilizing agents are of limited value but may be used to control free-floating anxiety.

Bergman P: Neurotic anxieties in children and their prevention. Nerv Child 5:37, 1946.

Brazelton TB: The pediatrician and hysteria in childhood. Nerv Child 10:306, 1953.

Colin HN: Phobias in children. Psychoanal Rev 46:65, 1959.

Enger NB, Walker PA: Hyperventilation syndrome in childhood. J Pediat 70:521, 1967.

Goodwin DW & others: Follow-up studies in obsessional neurosis. Arch Gen Psychiat 20:182, 1969.

Judd LL: Obsessive-compulsive neurosis in children. Arch Gen Psychiat 12:136, 1965.

Kubie LS: The fundamental nature of the distinction between normality and neurosis. Psychoanal Quart 23:187, 1954.

Langford W.S.: Anxiety states in children. Am J Orthopsychiat 7:40, 1937.

Lapouse R, Monk MA: Fears and worries in a representative sample of children. Am J Orthopsychiat 29:803, 1959.

Proctor JT: Hysteria in childhood. Am J Orthopsychiat 28:394, 1959.

Sandler J, Joffee WG: Notes on childhood depression. Internat J Psychoanal 46:88, 1965.

Toolan JM: Depression in children and adolescents. Am J Orthopsychiat 32:404, 1962.

Weiner H, Braiman A: The Ganser syndrome: A review and consideration of some unusual cases. Am J Psychiat 3:676, 1955.

Ziegler FJ:, Imboden JB: Contemporary conversion reactions. Arch Gen Psychiat 6:259, 1962.

PERSONALITY DISORDERS

Personality disorders in childhood (not commonly seen in flagrant form before late school age) are usually chronic and structured in nature, pervading the child's entire personality. They are manifested as chronic or fixed pathologic behavioral characteristics derived from responses to earlier conflicts which have become ingrained in the personality structure rather than psychologic symptom formation. No gross distortion in reality testing is observed in spite of the apparent irrationality of the child's behavior.

In discussing these disorders, the concept of a continuum is useful. At one end are the relatively well organized personalities with, for example, constructively compulsive traits or somewhat overdependent features, representing mild to moderate exaggerations of healthy personality trends. These may blend into the environment and may almost pass unnoticed unless the interpersonal network of relationships suddenly or radically changes. At the other end are markedly impulsive, sometimes poorly organized personalities which dramatically come into conflict with society as a result of their sexual or social patterns of behavior.

Symptom formation of a psychoneurotic nature is rarely seen, and in most cases the traits are not perceived by the child as a source of anxiety. Premonitory patterns are often seen during infancy and early childhood as fixations in early psychosexual and psychosocial development.

The clinical picture dictates the subcategories, which include compulsive, hysterical, anxious, overly dependent, oppositional, overly inhibited, isolated, mistrustful, tension discharge, sociosyntonic, and sexual deviation.

Treatment & Prognosis

Treatment and prognosis vary according to severity. In its milder forms, the disorder may offer sublimatory outlets (eg, compulsiveness may make for good work habits). More severe forms are more crippling and interfere with effective academic or social functions (eg, delinquency, poor impulse control) or conflict with a new social setting such as the military service when a sociosyntonic personality moves out of his subculture and into the army.

While counseling of children and parents may be sufficient in cases of mild disorders of the obsessive, hysterical, anxious, overly dependent, oppositional, or overly inhibited types, intensive psychotherapy on an outpatient basis is usually necessary for more severe disorders, including the true sexual deviations. Day hospitalization programs with a psychoeducational approach or special classes are indicated if associated learning difficulties are present.

Children with moderate to severe isolated, mistrustful, tension discharge, or impulse ridden personality types generally require intensive treatment on a residential basis. This is particularly the case when delinquency and drug or alcohol problems are involved. A residential setting, whether it be a hospital, cottage type group living setting, group foster home, or treatment-oriented correctional institution, should provide warmth, structure, consistent limits, and positive relationships with a well trained staff who have adequate mental health consultation.

Chodoff P, Lyons H: Hysteria, the hysterical personality, and "hysterical" conversion. Am J Psychiat 114:734, 1958.

Rexford E: A developmental concept of overdependency in young children. Child Develop 25:125–146, 1954.

Zuger B: Effeminate behavior present in boys from early childhood. I. The clinical syndrome and follow-up studies. J Pediat 69:1098, 1966.

PSYCHOTIC DISORDERS

Psychoses may be of sudden or gradual onset in infancy, childhood, or adolescence, with differences in the clinical picture in relation to developmental level. The essential features are failure to develop awareness of or withdrawal from reality, with preoccupation with inner fantasy life; failure to develop emotional relationships with human figures, or retreat from established relationships; inability to express emotions appropriately or to use speech communicatively; and bizarre, stereotyped, or otherwise seriously inappropriate behavior.

Hallucinations and delusions, as well as other classic characteristics of adult psychoses, are rarely encountered until late school age or early adolescence.

Obsessions, compulsions, phobias, and other psychologic or behavioral symptoms may occur in psychotic children. They are markedly intense and tenacious, and the child usually has no awareness of their lack of logic or appropriateness.

Type of Psychoses in the Pediatric Age Group

A. Psychoses of Early Childhood:

1. Early infantile autism—Must be distinguished from autism secondary to brain damage or mental retardation. The onset is within the first year of life, and the child remains aloof from all human contact, being preoccupied with inanimate objects. The child resists any change with outbursts of temper or anxiety when routines are altered. Speech is delayed or absent, and sleep and feeding problems are severe. Intellectual functioning is restricted or uneven, probably related to perceptual and communication problems.

2. Interactional psychotic disorders—These disorders of infancy and early childhood include the so-called "symbiotic psychoses." The problem revolves around the failure of the youngster to master the step of separation and individuation, often because of the mother's inability to allow the child to separate from her. The psychotic disorder is often precipitated in the second to fifth year by some shift in the mother-child relationship such as the birth of a sibling or a family crisis. The overdependent child then shows intense separation anxiety and clinging, with regressive manifestations. The picture is one of gradual withdrawal, emotional aloofness, autistic behavior, and distorted perception of reality.

3. Other psychotic disorders—Other psychoses of early childhood include "atypical" or fragmented ego development in children who exhibit some autistic behavior and emotional aloofness.

B. Psychoses of Later Childhood:
Schizophreniform psychotic disorders occur in the school age period and are characterized by a gradual onset of neurotic symptoms followed by concrete thinking, loose associations, hypochondriacal tendencies, and intense temper outbursts. Later developments may include a breakdown in reality testing, autism, anxiety, and uncontrollable phobias. Bizarre behavior and stereotyped motor patterns, such as whirling, are often observed. Other children may have sudden and wild outbursts of aggressive or self-mutilating behavior, inappropriate mood swings, and suicidal threats or attempts. The range of other psychotic behavior seen in adults may occur, usually in older children. Organic brain syndromes and severe panic states with a temporary thought disorder due to anxiety require careful differential assessment.

C. Psychoses of Adolescence:

1. Acute confusional state—This is a "psychosis" of adolescence with an abrupt onset of acute and intense anxiety, depressive trends, confusion in thinking, and feelings of depersonalization. The crisis of identity is very common, but evidence of a true thought disorder or marked breakdown in reality testing is usually lacking. While rapid recovery is the rule, a deep-seated personality disorder may underlie the psychotic picture. Differential considerations include neurotic panic states and the severe upsets seen in normal adolescents.

2. Adult types of schizophrenia—These occur in late adolescence, with minor differences related to the developmental level. Manifestations include the myriad symptoms seen in adults.

Treatment & Prognosis

Treatment and prognosis vary considerably. The psychotic disorders of early childhood have a more guarded prognosis.

A. Young Children: Patients with early infantile autism have a guarded prognosis and often require long-term hospital care. Interactional psychotic disorders fare somewhat better and may respond to outpatient treatment of the child and the parents. Such treatment can often clarify the child's basic intellectual endowment and help the parents to accept, when necessary, later placement for treatment. In the management of these young children, play therapy as a restitutional experience for emotional deprivation—and simultaneous therapy for the parents—may be usefully combined with the contributions of a therapeutic nursery school. Operant conditioning (positive reinforcement by praise, affection, or reward for healthy behavior) has been helpful in teaching these youngsters speech and socialization. Placement in a nursery school requires preceding treatment to alleviate the separation anxiety of the child and the parents.

Family conjoint therapy and tranquilizing agents have limited value, the latter being useful when the child is very anxious, hyperactive, or destructive.

B. School Age Children: For the school age child with a schizophreniform psychosis, short-term psychiatric hospitalization with several weeks to several months of milieu therapy and individual psychotherapy for the child and parents often assists the youngster with an acute onset to recompensate so that further therapy can be continued on an outpatient basis. This may include family conjoint therapy (wherein the family is treated together and separately). The chronically psychotic child may require long-term residential treatment or long-term placement in small cottage type group living quarters or professional group foster homes.

The psychoactive drugs are useful mainly in controlling outbursts of panic or aggressive behavior.

C. Older Children: The adolescent or postadolescent psychotic disorders often respond well to brief psychiatric hospitalization of only a few days or weeks. This is particularly true of the acute confusional state. Patients with sweeping regressive states may require several months of hospitalization. Very few adolescents, even with adult type schizophrenic

disorders, require long-term hospitalization, and only a small proportion have further episodes or become chronically schizophrenic.

Psychoactive drugs are more effective in adolescents than children and are used adjunctively with psychotherapeutic measures on an outpatient or inpatient basis.

Bender L: Childhood schizophrenia. Am J Orthopsychiat 17:40, 1947.

Eisenberg L: The course of childhood schizophrenia. Arch Neurol Psychiat 78:69, 1957.

Gittelman M, Birch HG: Childhood schizophrenia. Arch Gen Psychiat 17:16, 1967.

Kanner L: Early infantile autism. J Pediat 25:211, 1944.

Mahler MS, Gosliner EJ: On symbiotic child psychosis. Psychoanal Stud Child 10:142, 1955.

Neubauer P, Steinert J: Schizophrenia in adolescence. Nerv Child 10:129, 1954.

PSYCHOPHYSIOLOGIC DISORDERS

The psychophysiologic disorders involve organs or organ systems which are innervated by the autonomic nervous system—in contrast to conversion disorders, which involve the striated musculature and somatosensory apparatus. Biologic predisposing factors appear to be involved, with probable latent biochemical defects. Psychologic and social factors act as additional predisposing, precipitating, and perpetuating influences. More than one organ system may be involved.

Anxiety is not alleviated by these disorders—in contrast to conversion disorders, where anxiety is repressed and "bound" in the symbolic symptom.

No type-specific personality profile, parent-child relationship, or family pattern has as yet been associated with individual psychophysiologic disorders, although some may occur in conjunction with personality disorders.

These disorders may be mild or severe and transient or chronic. A continuum probably exists ranging from cases with milder biologic predisposition and greater psychologic involvement to those which are more heavily "loaded" biologically, requiring less psychologic influence for their appearance and perpetuation.

A brief summary of the various organ systems affected and the clinical manifestations follows. For treatment and prognosis, see p 581.

Skin

Psychophysiologic skin disorders include certain cases of neurodermatitis, seborrheic dermatitis, psoriasis, pruritus, alopecia, eczema, urticaria, angioneurotic edema, and acne. Atopic eczema may persist into childhood or may disappear and recur in late childhood and adolescence, with patches of dermatitis becoming widespread and severe during early adolescence.

Affected children are generally rigid, tense, and at times compulsive, with a tendency to repress strong emotions, particularly toward an overcontrolling mother. Exacerbations during adolescence are usually related to increased conflicts over independence and sexuality. The latter considerations are also involved in urticaria patients, who are often shy, passive, and immature, with feelings of inadequacy, unconscious exhibitionistic trends, and overdependency upon the mother.

Cleveland SE, Fisher S: Psychological factors in neurodermatoses. Psychosom Med 18:209, 1956.

Graham DT: The relations of psoriasis to attitude and to vascular reactions of the human skin. J Invest Dermat 22:379, 1954.

Greenberg SD: Alopecia areata: A psychiatric survey. Arch Dermat 72:454, 1955.

Kaplan H, Reisch M: Universal alopecia: A psychosomatic appraisal. New York J Med 52:1144, 1952.

Kremer MM: Psychological impact of acne in adolescents. J Am Med Wom A 24:309, 1969.

Rosenbaum M: Psychosomatic factors in pruritus. Psychosom Med 7:52, 1945.

Wittkower ED: Acne vulgaris: A psychosomatic study. Brit J Dermat 63:214, 1951.

Musculoskeletal System

Psychophysiologic musculoskeletal disorders include certain cases of low back pain, rheumatoid arthritis, "tension" headaches and other myalgias, muscle cramps, bruxism, and specific types of malocclusion (the latter may involve some conversion components). Children with rheumatoid arthritis often exhibit conflicts over the handling of aggression and dependency, and exacerbations are often related to shifts in family balance.

Blom GE, Nicholls G: Emotional factors in children with rheumatoid arthritis. Am J Orthopsychiat 24:588, 1954.

Cleveland SE, Reitmann EE, Brewer EJ: Psychological factors in juvenile rheumatoid arthritis. Arthritis Rheum 8:1152, 1965.

Respiratory System

Psychophysiologic respiratory disorders may include certain cases of bronchial asthma, allergic rhinitis, chronic sinusitis, hiccup, breathholding spells, and hyperventilation. Psychologic factors contributing to asthmatic attacks include threatened separation and parental marital conflicts.

Enger NB, Walker PA: Hyperventilation syndrome in childhood. J Pediat 70:521, 1967.

Long RT & others: A psychosomatic study of allergic and emotional factors in children with asthma. Am J Psychiat 114:890, 1958.

Purcell K: Distinctions between subgroups of asthmatic children. Pediatrics 31:486, 1963.

Cardiovascular System

Psychophysiologic cardiovascular disorders may overlap with respiratory disorders and include some cases of paroxysmal tachycardia, peripheral vascular spasm (eg, Raynaud's disease and central angiospastic retinopathy), migraine, erythromelalgia, causalgia, vasodepressor syncope, epistaxis, essential hypertension, hypotension, and eclampsia in adolescents. In some children, intense autonomic responses to emotional trauma can trigger paroxysmal tachycardia which may lead to syncope. Children with orthostatic hypotension often appear to be tense, anxious, emotionally restricted, and "not sure where they stand" in their families. Similar characteristics occur in children or adolescents with vasodepressor syncope, often precipitated by sudden fright or pain anticipation. This syncope should be distinguished from conversion syncope which often occurs in hysterical girls who have other conversion phenomena but no vascular changes. Migraine presents during the school age period (headache is rare in preschool children) and is often triggered by emotional crises. The patients tend to be rather rigid, sometimes compulsive individuals in tense families.

Falstein EI, Rosenblum AH: Juvenile paroxysmal supraventricular tachycardia: Psychosomatic and psychodynamic aspects. J Am Acad Child Psychiat 1:246, 1962.

Green M: Fainting. In: *Ambulatory Pediatrics.* Green M, Haggerty R (editors). Saunders, 1968.

Holguin J, Fenichel E: Migraine. J Pediat 70:290, 1967.

Katcher AL: Hypertension in adolescent children. M Clin North America 48:1467, 1964.

Katz J, Friedman AP, Gisolfi A: Psychologic factors of migraine in children. New York J Med 50:2269, 1950.

Gastrointestinal System

The psychophysiologic gastrointestinal disorders comprise a large category of varied clinical disorders. Since the gastrointestinal tract is so responsive to emotional factors, it is unusual to find gastrointestinal disorders which are not affected by the psychic adjustment of the individual. Some of the more common problems include pylorospasm, gastric hyperacidity, pseudo-peptic ulcer syndrome, idiopathic celiac disease, nontropical sprue in adolescents, megacolon (aganglionic type), constipation, diarrhea, and cyclic vomiting in tense, overprotected children in families with these tendencies.

A. Peptic Ulcer: Peptic ulcers in school age children and adolescents are different from those in adults and probably more common. Abdominal pain is not well localized, nausea and vomiting are common, and symptoms are not closely related to meals. Individuals who develop peptic ulcer have high blood pepsinogen levels from infancy, reflecting tendencies toward gastric hypersecretion. In children who have difficulty in handling hostile feelings, are demanding of affection, and are passive and dependent, peptic ulcers are apt to develop in stressful situations.

B. Ulcerative Colitis: Children with ulcerative colitis are often overdependent, passive, inhibited, and compulsive, and frequently manipulate the parents. Precipitation of fulminant cases usually takes place in a situation with actual or threatened loss of emotional support from a key figure. Exacerbations are frequently related to family crises. Other psychologic factors include familial patterns of autonomic response to stress, involving the lower gastrointestinal tract in "bowel oriented" families, conditioning of the defecation reflex to emotional conflict in coercive toilet training, and maternal overprotection and overdominance in early childhood. These factors lead to overdependence associated with resentment on the part of the child.

C. Regional Ileitis: Patients with regional ileitis have psychosocial similarities to those with ulcerative colitis and mucous colitis, the latter being generally less disturbed.

D. Obesity: Obesity results basically from an excess of intake over output of calories as a result of hyperphagia, usually in families with a tendency toward overeating and obesity. From a psychosocial view, there are 2 major groups: the **reactive** type, responding to an emotionally traumatic experience (eg, the death of a parent or a school failure); and the **developmental** type, where the origins are principally in the disturbed family's tendencies toward overeating, with probably some biologic predisposition also involved. The child is often overvalued by the family, sometimes because of the loss of a previous child. He becomes obese as a result of overfeeding and continues to be obese from infancy on. The mother usually dominates and protects the child, and, after an early period of demanding behavior, the child goes on to become passive, overdependent, and immature. In such children, feelings of helplessness, despair, and withdrawal from social interaction are associated with more overeating, and food is used as a solace to ward off depression or feelings of hostility. The "wall of weight" is a way of hiding from social problems and is often used to ward off sexual conflicts with feelings of ugliness or unattractiveness.

E. Anorexia Nervosa: This syndrome occurs in late school age to postadolescence, usually in females. It consists of loss of appetite, denial of physical hunger, aversion to food, severe weight loss, emaciation and pallor, amenorrhea, lowered body temperature, decreased metabolism, pulse rate, and blood pressure, flat or occasionally diabetic blood sugar curves, dry skin, brittle nails, cold intolerance, and, in severe and protracted cases, other symptoms and signs such as gastric hypoacidity and diarrhea. Activity levels remain high even with marked emaciation. Patients are often preoccupied or irritable and have difficulty in verbalizing their feelings. The onset is often related to menarche or traumatic incidents with serious dieting which continues out of control. The parents are frequently in the food business. The mother and daughter often have an ambivalent (hostile-dependent) relationship, and the involvement with the father often has had a seductive quality. During preadolescence, such patients are often overconscientious, energetic, high achievers, but they remain strongly dependent upon the parents. Three main groups of patients are seen: (1) Those with psychoneurotic disorders (mixed hysterical and phobic trends) with sexual implications and symbolic meanings attributed to eating and body weight; (2) those with obsessive-compulsive personality disorders; and (3) schizophrenic or near-psychotic individuals with massive projection tendencies and fears of poisoning. A few show the syndrome as a severe reactive disorder, at times with strongly depressive trends.

F. Recurrent Abdominal Pain: This common syndrome occurs in 10–13% of children, but over 90% show no physical basis for the pain. In most cases, symptoms are epigastric or periumbilical and are usually related to some emotional crisis in tense, apprehensive, timid, and often overly conscientious children who have experienced parental overprotection. Fourteen- and 6-per-second EEG spikes are not diagnostic; they occur in many normal children in the early school age period. School phobia or identification with a family member with abdominal pain is sometimes reported.

Apley J: The child with recurrent abdominal pain. P Clin North America 14:63, 1962.

Bruch H: Obesity. P Clin North America 5:613, 1958.

Chapman AH, Loeb DG, Young JB: A psychosomatic study of five children with duodenal ulcer. J Pediat 48:248, 1956.

Davidson M: The irritable colon of children (chronic non-specific diarrhea syndrome). J Pediat 69:1027, 1966.

Finch SM, Hess JH: Ulcerative colitis in children. Am J Psychiat 118:819, 1962.

Garrard SD, Richmond JB: Psychogenic megacolon manifested by fecal soiling. Pediatrics 10:474, 1952.

Grace WJ: Life stress and regional enteritis. Gastroenterology 23:542, 1953.

Green M: Psychogenic recurrent abdominal pain: Diagnosis and treatment. Pediatrics 40–84, 1967.

Heald F: Obesity in the adolescent. In: *Symposium on Adolescence.* Meiks LT, Green M (editors). Saunders, 1960.

Illingworth RS: Practical observations and reflections. II. Vomiting without organic cause. Clin Pediat 4:685, 1965.

Leiken SJ, Caplan H: Psychogenic polydipsia. Am J Psychiat 123:1563, 1967.

Lesser LI & others: Anorexia nervosa in children. Am J Orthopsychiat 30:572, 1960.

Lowe CU, Coursin DB, Heald FP: Obesity in childhood. Pediatrics 40:455, 1967.

Menking M & others: Rumination: A near-fatal psychiatric disease of infancy. New England J Med 280:802, 1969.

Pinkerton P: Psychogenic megacolon in children: The implication of bowel negativism. Arch Dis Childhood 33:371, 1958.

Prugh DG: Role of emotional factors in idiopathic celiac disease. Psychosom Med 13:220, 1951.

Prugh DG, Jordan K: The management of ulcerative colitis in childhood. In: *Modern Perspectives in International Child Psychiatry.* Howells J (editor). Oliver & Boyd, 1969.

Taboroff LH, Brown WH: A study of personality patterns of children and adolescents with the peptic ulcer syndrome. Am J Orthopsychiat 24:602, 1954.

Genital & Urinary Systems

Psychophysiologic genitourinary disorders include certain cases of menstrual disturbances, functional uterine bleeding, leukorrhea, polyuria and dysuria, vesical paralysis, urethral and vaginal discharges, and persistent glycosuria without diabetes. Disturbances of sexual function (eg, vaginismus, frigidity, frequent erections, dyspareunia, and priapism) are often conversion reactions but may include psychophysiologic components. Menstrual problems are the rule in early adolescence, but they may be intensified or perpetuated by emotional conflicts. Dysmenorrhea has an incidence of up to 12% of high school girls and may be influenced by attitudes of inconvenience or disgust, particularly in middle class girls. Persistence of the symptom indicates difficulty in accepting the feminine role and the responsibilities of womanhood. Premenstrual tension is often intensified by sexual or identity conflicts. Habitual abortion occurs with significant conflicts over sexuality and motherhood. Impotence in adolescent boys is rare, but it may cause problems in teen-age marriages—as may frigidity in girls, which is more common.

Bickers W, Woods M: Premenstrual tension. New England J Med 245:453, 1951.

Heald FP, Masland RP, Sturgis SH: Dysmenorrhea in adolescence. Pediatrics 20:121, 1957.

Heiman M: The role of stress situations and psychological factors in functional uterine bleeding. J Mt Sinai Hosp 23:755, 1956.

Mann EC: Habitual abortion: A report in two parts on 160 patients. Am J Obst Gynec 77:706, 1959.

Endocrine System

Psychophysiologic endocrine disorders include certain cases of hyperinsulinism, growth disturbance, diabetes, hyperthyroidism, and, in adolescents, pseudocyesis and disorders of lactation. Emotional conflicts about "growing up" are related to some cases of delayed puberty or delayed onset of menarche. In pseudocyesis, enlargement of the abdomen is a conversion phenomenon, but the physiologic changes of pregnancy derive from obscure psychologic influences on endocrine function. It usually occurs in hysterical personalities with underlying conflicts over feminine identity and motherhood. In more seriously disturbed adolescents, it may occur after the first experience of kissing or petting. Diabetes is significantly influenced by psychologic mechanisms. It is often precipitated or exacerbated in a setting of increased conflict, most often involving a real or threatened loss of a key relationship. Although most juvenile diabetics show increased symptoms in adolescence, those more disturbed may have an exceptionally "stormy course," with coma precipitated by emotional conflict, rebellious overeating, or inattention to insulin requirements. Children and adolescents with thyrotoxicosis often experience the onset in gradually intensifying stressful situations, particularly those involving emotional relationships.

Bruch H: Physiologic and psychologic interrelationships in diabetes in children. Psychosom Med 11:200, 1949.

Falstein EI, Judas I: Juvenile diabetes and its psychiatric implications. Am J Orthopsychiat 25:330, 1955.

Glaser HH: Physical and psychological development of children with early failure to thrive. J Pediat 73:690, 1968.

Greaves D, Green PE, West LJ: Psychodynamic and psychophysiological aspects of pseudocyesis. Psychosom Med 22:24, 1960.

Ham GC, Alexander F, Carmichael HT: A psychosomatic theory of thyrotoxicosis. Psychosom Med 13:18, 1951.

Hinkle LE, Wolf SG: A summary of experimental evidence relating life stress to diabetes mellitus. J Mt Sinai Hosp 19:537, 1952.

Mandelbrote BM, Wittkower ED: Emotional factors in Graves' disease. Psychosom Med 17:109, 1955.

Portis SA: Life situations, emotions and hyperinsulinism. JAMA 142:1281, 1950.

Romano J, Coon GP: Physiologic and psychologic studies in spontaneous hypoglycemia. Psychosom Med 4:283, 1942.

Silver HK, Finkelstein M: Deprivation dwarfism. J Pediat 70:317, 1967.

Nervous System

Psychophysiologic nervous system disorders include idiopathic epilepsy (grand mal, petit mal, psychomotor epilepsy, and epileptic equivalents), narcolepsy, certain types of sleep disturbance, dizziness, vertigo, hyperactivity, motion sickness, and some recurrent fevers of psychologic origin.

A. Epilepsy: Epilepsy, with its unfortunate stigma, frequently produces psychic trauma, although a personality disorder may antedate its onset. The youngster may have feelings of inferiority, shyness, and feel different from others. Irritability, temper outbursts, or aggressive behavior may be exhibited prior to a seizure. These children tend to experience fears of death before a seizure and may fear they have said or done something "bad" during the interval of postictal amnesia. The parents are understandably anxious about the child and frequently overly restrictive about activity. They often blame themselves for the hereditary factor and often equate the seizures with death or "craziness."

Few children deteriorate, intellectually or otherwise, if adequate seizure control is achieved. Seizures often are more frequent or precipitated initially during periods of emotional conflict or family crises. Some children learn ways of inhibiting or touching off seizures, the latter skill sometimes being used in a manipulative way.

The diagnosis of "epileptic equivalent" on the basis of exaggerated fears, repeated tantrums, aggressive behavior, marked withdrawal, or sleepwalking in association with an abnormal EEG is often inappropriate. Most of the children suspected of such equivalents show disturbances in behavior related to conflicts within the family.

A variety of conditions which were formerly thought to bear some relationship to idiopathic epilepsy include migraine, recurrent abdominal pain, cyclic vomiting, and narcolepsy.

B. Narcolepsy: Narcolepsy is uncommon in childhood and more frequent in boys. It is characterized by paroxysmal and recurrent attacks of irresistible sleep, often precipitated by a sudden alteration in emotional state related to conflictual situations. Attacks may come on suddenly from 1–2 times a day to many times a day. They may be associated with cataplexy and hypnagogic hallucinations. The sleep during attacks is light, and the patient is easily awakened. Nocturnal sleep is usually normal, although an earlier appearance of REM sleep has been reported. The major factors are usually psychopathologic, often related to emotional conflicts over competition or the expression of unacceptable aggressive influences. The EEG is normal between attacks, and there is no significant relationship to epilepsy. Narcolepsy is to be differentiated from the Pickwickian syndrome, in which sudden attacks of somnolence occur in markedly obese children.

C. Motion Sickness: Motion sickness in cars, trains, elevators, swings, etc is more common in children than in adults; seasickness and airplane sickness are less frequent in children. Psychologic factors are involved to varying degrees in different children. Tense, apprehensive, or phobic children are most often affected, and family arguments during driving are frequent precipitating factors. Most children improve markedly by adolescence.

D. Hyperactivity: This picture occurs in many children without signs of brain damage. Anxious children who are active from birth may show this symptom, with impulsiveness and distractibility in response to parental overrestrictiveness or other family tensions.

Barbero GJ: Cyclic vomiting. Pediatrics 25:740, 1960.
Berlin I, Yaeger CL: Correlation of epileptic seizures, electroencephalograms and emotional state. Am J Dis Child 81:664, 1951.
Friedman AP, Harms E: *Headaches in Children.* Thomas, 1967.
Gottschalk LA: Effects of intensive psychotherapy on epileptic children. Arch Neurol Psychiat 70:361, 1953.
Laybourne PC: Psychogenic vomiting in children. Am J Dis Child 86:726, 1953.
Yoss RE, Daly DD: Narcolepsy in children. Pediatrics 25:1025, 1960.

Fever

Fever of psychophysiologic origin may occur in certain children who show excitement or continued emotional tension in the absence of physical overactivity. Chronic low-grade fever may occur in infants with "hospitalism" or in school age children who are anxious or tense. In the latter instance, the mother is often overanxious and continues to take the child's temperature every day long after the subsidence of a mild infection. The fever usually disappears upon discontinuation of the daily measurements. This may be accomplished by discussion of the parents' apprehension related to guilt or other feelings rather than simple reassurance.

Renbourn ET: Body temperature and pulse rate in boys and young men prior to sporting contests: A study of emotional hyperthermia with a review of the literature. J Psychosom Res 4:149, 1960.

White KL, Long WN: The incidence of "psychogenic" fever in a university hospital. J Chronic Dis 8:567, 1958.

Organs of Special Sense

Psychophysiologic disorders of organs of special sense include certain cases of glaucoma, blepharospasm, amblyopia, Ménière's syndrome, and certain types of tinnitus and hyperacusis.

Coleman D: Psychosomatic aspects of diseases of the ear, nose, and throat. Laryngoscope 59:709, 1949.
Fowler EP, Zeckel A: Psychosomatic aspects of Ménière's disease. JAMA 148:1265, 1952.
Ripley HS, Wolff HG: Life situations, emotions, and glaucoma. Psychosom Med 12:215, 1950.

General Principles of Treatment & Prognosis in Pediatric Psychophysiologic Disorders

Treatment and prognosis are related to the multiple interactive factors involved in these disorders. Included are the nature of the biologic predisposition, the degree of personality disturbance and family disruption, the extent of the contribution of psychosocial factors to the perpetuation of the disorder, and the likelihood of its response to psychotherapeutic treatment and medical measures.

The basic approach to treatment should be founded upon an adequate diagnostic evaluation with due consideration to the relative importance of somatic and psychologic factors.

In some disorders, only treatment of the basic emotional deprivation, with "replacement measures" offered by parent substitutes, together with parental treatment, offers any chance of amelioration. In others with mild psychologic components, as in some cases of asthma, medical measures alone will suffice. In some mildly disturbed children—eg, in cases of obesity, menstrual problems, and recurrent abdominal pain—the pediatrician may use a supportive psychotherapeutic approach to the child and parents, with psychiatric consultation initially and as needed. If the patient is hospitalized, seeing him for brief periods at the beginning or end of each day may be more effective than 1–2 hours a week, with the encouragement of an initially dependent relationship upon the pediatrician and, later, gradual "weaning." Long-term follow-up may be indicated, particularly for children with ulcerative colitis (even those treated surgically), who may have later exacerbations at times of emotional trauma.

In more seriously disturbed children with severe conditions of tension headache, asthma, menstrual problems, narcolepsy, quiescent ulcerative colitis, and management problems of diabetes, intensive psychotherapy for the child and parents may have to be carried out by a child psychiatrist or other mental health professional. In most such disorders, supportive psychotherapeutic measures should be undertaken at the beginning, with later use of more intensive measures if necessary. In potentially serious and life-threatening disorders such as acute ulcerative colitis or diabetes, psychotherapeutic treatment should never be undertaken without concomitant medical treatment and follow-up.

In some instances, notably anorexia nervosa, psychiatric hospitalization may be required. Under these circumstances, the psychiatrist may act as a coordinator, drawing upon the contribution of the pediatrician and other consultants regarding the medical or surgical aspects of treatment.

Certain basic principles in the handling of children with psychophysiologic (and many other) illnesses can be listed briefly as follows: *continuity* of the relationship with the child and parents by a single physician (usually the pediatrician); *communication* among professionals, in order to bring about true and respectful *collaboration* among disciplines and *consistency* in management; *consultation* with child psychiatrists and other specialists; and *coordination* of all such activities into a unified plan of therapy with the most appropriate balance of physical, psychologic, and social measures.

Lourie RS: Experience with therapy of psychosomatic problems in infants. In: *Psychopathology of Childhood*. Hoch PH, Zubin J (editors). Grune & Stratton, 1955.

Mirsky IA: Physiologic, psychologic, and social determinants of psychosomatic disorders. Dis Nerv System 21:50, 1960.

See also General References at end of chapter.

BRAIN SYNDROMES

Essentials of Diagnosis

- Impairment of orientation, judgment, discrimination, learning, memory, other cognitive functions; emotional lability.
- Evidence of cerebral dysfunction, including (1) abnormal neurologic findings, (2) definitively abnormal EEG, (3) perceptual-motor disturbances on psychologic testing, and (4) a history of insult to the CNS. (Three out of 4 should be present to establish the diagnosis.)
- Psychologic disturbances, either preexisting or secondary to brain damage. There is no "pure" cerebral dysfunction without accompanying psychologic reactions.

General Considerations

Brain syndromes result from localized or diffuse damage to brain tissue, particularly the cerebral cortex, due to any cause. The severity of the associated psychotic, neurotic, or behavioral disorders is not necessarily proportionate to the degree of brain damage. The psychologic accompaniment of brain damage is determined by predisposing personality patterns, current emotional conflicts, the child's level of development, family interpersonal relationships, and the nature of the brain disorder and its meaning to the child and his parents. As in adults, such associated dis-

orders are often regarded as having been released by the brain disorder or superimposed on or intertwined with it. In infants and young children, however, later personality development may be influenced by such disorders, whose manifestations may be quite different from those in older children and adults. The young child appears to be able to a great extent to compensate for insults to the CNS as he matures. Functions most recently developed may be most vulnerable to such insults, whereas those developed earlier may be less affected. On the other hand, functions not yet developed may be interfered with, particularly those relating to the cognitive aspects of learning and impulse control. It is thus much harder in children than in adults to correlate the severity of cognitive impairment with the severity of the brain pathology.

Children affected by localized rather than diffuse brain lesions may react in various ways depending only in part upon the brain functions which are interfered with.

Brain syndromes of diffuse nature are classified as acute (reversible) or chronic (permanent). The emphasis in the following paragraphs is on the psychologic and social consequences of brain damage in children.

Clinical Findings

A. Acute Brain Syndromes: Acute brain disorders may be due to intracranial infection, systemic infection, drug or poison (including alcohol) intoxication, trauma, circulatory disturbances, certain types of convulsive disorder, metabolic disturbances, and certain disorders of unknown etiology such as multiple sclerosis.

The principal manifestation in children (as in adults) is delirium, a disturbance in awareness resulting from alterations of cerebral metabolism. The clinical picture may be gross and easily identifiable, characterized by wildly agitated or confused behavior and hallucinatory experiences arising from distorted perception or interpretation of stimuli. A subclinical form, however, may present with subtle disturbances in awareness or mildly stuporous states, withdrawn or "difficult" behavior, or irrational fears. In such cases, a rough mental status examination adapted to the child's level of development will often reveal disorientation and misinterpretation of external stimuli. An EEG may aid in diagnosis, revealing large, slow waves and disorganization which disappear upon correction of the disturbance in cerebral metabolism. Perceptual-motor difficulties may persist for some time and may lead to learning difficulties upon return to school even though the brain lesion has completely healed.

Recognition of subclinical forms may be difficult, and the clinician must keep the possibility in mind to avoid overlooking the delirium or to prevent misdiagnosis as psychotic behavior on a psychosocial basis.

Preexisting or underlying psychotic, psychoneurotic, or personality disorders may become more manifest after such insults to the CNS, and reactive disorders or later developmental deviations in cognitive or other areas may result.

B. Chronic Brain Syndromes: These disorders result from relatively permanent, more or less irreversible, diffuse impairment of cerebral tissue function. They may be due to congenital cranial anomalies, cerebral palsy, and other disorders arising from prenatal or perinatal damage to the brain, CNS syphilis, intoxications of various types, brain trauma, convulsive disorders, disturbances of metabolism, growth, or nutrition, intracranial neoplasm, or heredodegenerative factors such as Schilder's encephalopathy, Heller's infantile dementia, etc. Some disturbances in memory, judgment, orientation, comprehension, affect, and learning capacity may persist permanently, accompanied by remarkable compensations at times in individual children during the course of development.

There appears to be no specific type of personality disorder in children with chronic brain syndromes. Many children become overly dependent, with frequent developmental lags in personality organization and other developmental deviations. These psychologic factors appear in varying admixtures with the effects upon behavior of the underlying brain damage, and some of the psychologic features may represent the child's reaction to his perceptions of his own limitations.

One particular syndrome frequently seen in young children with diffuse cerebrocortical damage is frequently but not invariably characterized by hyperactivity, distractibility, impulsiveness, and EEG and EMG abnormalities. Difficulties in perceptual-motor functions, spatial orientation, and cerebral integration lead to problems in employing symbols (eg, reading and writing) and in abstract concept formation. Specific neurologic lesions are rarely demonstrable, and the diagnosis must be based on the history and clinical findings. However, children with significant psychologic disturbances may also exhibit difficulties in impulse control, distractibility, and hyperactivity, together with delayed perceptual-motor development and dysrhythmic EEG patterns. Signs of cerebral dysfunction are not always due to organic lesions alone; therefore, diagnoses of "organicity" or "minimal brain damage" based principally on behavioral manifestations seem open to much question.

Many children with chronic brain syndrome are not significantly retarded in intellectual development. They often show significant learning difficulties, however, due to perceptual-motor handicaps, and may function at a mentally retarded level with psychologic and social factors playing a contributory role. If mental retardation is present, this should be specified by means of appropriate tests. In each instance, the predominant personality picture associated with the brain syndrome should be noted, eg, developmental deviations of affective nature, or personality, psychoneurotic, or psychotic disorders.

Cerebral palsy. (See also Chapter 21.) Children with cerebral palsy exhibit motor disabilities of a predominantly extrapyramidal type characterized by choreiform and athetoid movements and frequent sensory and perceptual defects, all of which predispose to learning difficulties and poor achievement on intelligence tests. Speech problems are often present. The physical defects, combined with the child's inability to discharge tensions through physical activity and play, produce anxiety, emotional conflicts, and feelings of difference from others and a negative self-image. Some parents feel guilty and handle the child overprotectively, whereas others may feel ashamed, resentful, or hopeless. Insufficient stimulation or a pessimistic appraisal of the child's prospects by parents, physicians, and teachers may lead to inadequate education in addition to the inherent learning problems.

Children with cerebral palsy are often emotionally immature, introverted, overly dependent, fearful, irritable, and egocentric. Emotional conflicts are commonly most severe during adolescence, although children with athetosis or ataxia may be surprisingly cheerful and outgoing (often with lack of insight into their limitations).

An important and encouraging characteristic of cerebral palsy is its stationary, nonprogressive course.

Treatment

A. Acute Brain Syndrome: The essential problem in the psychologic management of acute brain syndrome is the control of delirium while the underlying cause is being sought and treated. The child must be helped to deal with misperceptions of stimuli in his environment. He may misinterpret shadows as "witches" or "ghosts," or may see medical instruments as the weapons of "killers"—the doctors and nurses. When his parents are not present, a school age child may fear that they are dead or have abandoned him. Instead of darkening the room to cut down on stimuli, it is important to keep the room adequately lighted, especially at night, when such misperceptions are most severe and frightening. A special nurse, relative, or foster grandmother should be in the room at all times during the day and should be available at night in order to serve as an external "auxiliary ego" who can help the child correct his misperceptions and misinterpretations.

Chloral hydrate is probably the best tolerated sedative in childhood delirium, and large doses may be required. Paraldehyde given orally or rectally is the ideal sedative in adolescents, although the odor may be offensive. Barbiturates tend to cause confusion and should be avoided.

It is essential to maintain the tie with the parents, the only truly familiar figures in the delirious child's confused world, through daily visiting or overnight stay by the mother, even for school age children. If a parent is ill or far away and cannot visit regularly, substitute mothering becomes all the more vital. A familiar blanket or toy from home, or postcards which can be read to the child, will be of some help.

The anxieties and guilt of the parents must also be dealt with, especially in cases involving accidents or poisonings.

B. Chronic Brain Syndrome: Treatment measures, in addition to those directed toward the basic cause of brain dysfunction, include remedial education in small "ungraded" classes from which the child should move to normal classes as soon as possible. Individual tutoring may help to retain the child in his age-appropriate classroom. Special remedial teaching technics using auditory, tactile, and kinesthetic stimuli may be of value.

Children with brain damage and significant emotional problems, including anxiety over performance, problems in impulse control, a negative self-image, and resistance to learning often respond to psychotherapy for themselves and their parents. Such therapy may at first be largely supportive. Educational components, including some tutoring, may be included within the psychotherapeutic approach.

Cerebral palsy. (See also Chapter 19.) Whereas some parents of cerebral palsied children may simply give up, others go to great lengths to push the child toward normality with "gimmicks" or cure-alls such as the Doman-Delacato approach, which involves a great deal of effort and money. This has recently been shown by a controlled study to be of no more value than other training methods, and may cause emotional problems as a result of the pressure it exerts on the child.

In addition to physical therapy, speech therapy, and drug therapy (including tranquilizers) as indicated, special educational measures, sheltered workshops, and group therapy or discussions for the parents of such children may be helpful, as may individual psychotherapy for the more seriously disturbed. There is no substitute for the physician's continuing supportive relationship with the child and his parents, working with representatives of other disciplines. Children with cerebral palsy, many of whom are not inherently retarded, may make surprisingly adequate emotional and vocational adjustments in spite of continuing problems.

Psychoactive drugs may be of some value. Hyperactivity, impulsiveness, and distractibility may be controlled by the judicious use of amphetamines. The phenothiazines may be of help in the control of anxiety or destructive behavior. Residential treatment may be necessary for children with severe emotional disturbances.

Prognosis

A. Acute Brain Syndrome: The prognosis for children with acute brain syndrome depends upon the degree of structural brain damage and upon host resistance factors. With appropriate antibiotic therapy, the various types of bacterial meningitis may resolve with little residual damage. The viral encephalitides cannot be controlled so well, but children who have been in coma even for several months may regain complete function, gradually "relearning" lost skills from walking to reading. In all of these disorders—particularly head trauma—the response of the child is influenced by parental reactions. A minor concussion may provoke overprotective patterns of parental behavior with psychologic difficulties during convalescence in spite of complete recovery.

If the child recovers completely, the possibility of persistence of perceptual-motor deficits for some weeks should be explained to the parents and teachers in order to permit gradual return to optimal academic performance.

B. Chronic Brain Syndrome: Infants and children show a remarkable tendency to compensate for diffuse damage to the cerebral cortex, especially if attention is paid to the psychosocial needs of the child and his parents.

Birch HG (editor): *Brain Damage in Children.* Williams & Wilkins, 1964.

Eisenberg L: Psychiatric implications of brain damage in children. Psychiat Quart 31:72, 1957.

Garrard SD, Richmond JB: Psychological aspects of the management of children with defects or damage of the central nervous system. P Clin North America 15:1033, 1957.

Romano J, Engel GL: Physiologic and psychologic considerations of delirium. M Clin North America 28:629, 1944.

COMMON PROBLEMS IN PEDIATRIC PRACTICE

COLIC

Colic or paroxysmal fussing is a common problem in young infants. It is most common in the evening. It may build up in a crescendo, with the baby drawing his legs up onto the abdomen, and is frequently relieved by the passage of flatus. This period usually begins at age 2–3 weeks and disappears by 10–12 weeks—so-called "3-months colic." The course is not clear, but "developmental colic" may be related to overready response to stimulation, irregular gastrointestinal peristalsis, and other as yet unintegrated autonomic functions characteristic of the first 2–3 months. The evening hours in the home often involve more stimulation from the father, anxiety about the infant's sleep on the part of a tired young mother, and perhaps concerns about the reactions of relatives or neighbors to continued crying.

Clinical observations suggest that prolonged and severe colic, often persisting until the latter part of the first year, occurs most commonly in infants who are overactive and tense from birth (the so-called hypertonic infant, with a "lean and hungry look"). There may be some relationship to greater activity of the infant in utero and higher levels of maternal anxiety during pregnancy. Maternal and family tension, as well as possible allergic tendencies, have also been implicated.

Management of Colic

Anticipatory guidance about avoiding overstimulation (particularly of more active infants) during the first 3 months may be helpful in minimizing developmental colic, and so is the knowledge that it ordinarily disappears by 3 months. A pacifier can be soothing and does no harm unless used too freely by an overly anxious parent to prevent any crying or unless employed as a substitute for tactile, rhythmic, and other forms of soothing. If colic is prolonged and severe, more sucking time during feeding may be required for emotional satisfaction.

Counseling is important, giving the parent an opportunity to "think out loud," with the nonjudgmental help of the physician, about superficial family tensions centering around living arrangements, overstimulation of the infant by the father on his return home in the evening, arguments over handling the infant, criticisms of in-laws in the home, or other matters.

Brazelton TB: Crying in infancy. Pediatrics 29:579, 1962.

Harley LM: Fussing and crying in young infants: Clinical considerations and practical management. Clin Pediat 8:138, 1969.

Paradise JL: Maternal and other factors in the etiology of infantile colic. JAMA 197:191, 1966.

SCHOOL PHOBIA

A special type of inability to attend school called school phobia is a syndrome involving a morbid or irrational dread or fear of some aspect of the school situation. Somatic complaints include abdominal pain, nausea, vomiting, diarrhea, headache, pallor, faintness, feelings of weakness, and low-grade fever. These symptoms appear in the morning before school, usually disappear by the time school is out or before, and do not appear on weekends or school holidays.

The basic fear is not of going to school but of leaving home or of separation from the family. Such fears occur in mild form, often with abdominal pain, in many normal children going off to full day school for the first time. With reassurance and firm support from the parents, they usually disappear within a few days, although they may recur during the first several years of school attendance, after vacations, or during convalescence from illness. Some young school age children with more intense fears are undergoing prolonged separation anxiety or experiencing a developmental crisis.

The classical school phobic picture of psychoneurotic nature usually occurs in an overly dependent, shy, and anxious child who has an overly solicitous or too controlling mother and a passive father. The mother often has a strong need for closeness with the child, fears that he is growing away from her, and communicates her anxiety about his welfare during the process of separation. There is usually a precipitating factor such as an unpleasant experience at school, illness or a new baby at home, or an increase in marital friction. The child's fear of separation is displaced onto the school as a "dangerous" place; his unconscious feelings of resentment over parental domination are projected onto the school as fears of punishment or attack. The mother takes the child's fears too seriously and becomes concerned about his safety.

The child becomes more guilty and socially isolated the longer he is permitted to remain at home and clings more closely to the mother even as she becomes increasingly frustrated and angry at his inability to go to school.

In young children in the early grades, the school phobia syndrome usually involves marked separation anxiety, a developmental crisis, or a mild form of phobic neurosis. In junior and senior high school students, it is usually a manifestation of a more severe personality disorder or occasionally a borderline psychosis.

Management of School Phobia

The pediatrician plays an important role in the management of this pediatric-psychiatric emergency. The emergency situation represents the first phase of treatment, which may be handled by the pediatrician if he understands the background of the difficulty and is willing to work with the parents, the child, and the school authorities.

Early return to school is the immediate goal. The pediatrician should first do a thorough physical appraisal; if abdominal pain or other gastrointestinal symptoms have been present for weeks or months, he should do a barium x-ray series in order to rule out peptic ulcer (often of the acute type), which occasionally coexists with school phobia. If the physical findings are within normal limits, the pediatrician should reassure the parents that no physical abnormalities are present and explain that "emotional tension" can be responsible for all the symptoms. He should further explain, in a noncritical, nonjudgmental way, that the child seems to be easily frightened by "new experiences," of which school is the most typical. Rather than interpreting their role in the problem, he should ask the parents what they feel might be involved.

With this approach, many parents can begin to recognize, without too much defensiveness or guilt, that they have kept the child "too close" to them. The pediatrician can suggest that they "think out loud" with him about ways to help the child become more independent. He should emphasize the importance of the child's early return to school—pointing out, if necessary, that every day at home will only make it harder for the child to have a successful school experience.

The pediatrician should talk with the principal or, with his permission, with the teacher, school social worker, or psychologist in order to learn how they interpret the problem. If the school authorities agree, he should suggest to the mother that she take the child to school and, if necessary, to the classroom, even remaining there briefly. If the mother is too anxious, the father may accompany her or may take the child to school himself. If neither parent feels able to accompany the child, it may be possible for an adult relative, another adult (such as the school nurse), or even an older child to pick up the child and see that he gets to school. Once in the classroom, the younger school age child usually settles in and does well academically. In some cases, it may be necessary to arrange for return to school at first on a part-time basis, to one class only, or even for a change in teachers or schools.

Certain children may be unable to remain for long in the classroom and may ask to go home because of abdominal pain or other symptoms. The teacher should send the child to the school nurse, who can let him lie down briefly and then return him, with reassurance and encouragement, to the classroom. If he is permitted to call his parents, they may not be able to resist his appeals to come and take him home. No matter how worried the parents are, the physician should not give a medical certificate for home teaching since psychologic invalidism and other psychopathology may result.

If these emergency measures are not effective, early referral to a psychiatric clinic is warranted. In a few cases, a threat of legal intervention may be necessary to galvanize helpless parents into action.

Even if early return to school is achieved, referral for psychotherapy is usually indicated to work out underlying conflicts and prevent return of symptoms. If the parents are reluctant to take this step, the pediatrician can take comfort from follow-up studies which show that most such children are able to remain in school and to perform adequately without crippling neurotic symptoms.

With children in junior high or high school, who are usually more severely disturbed, the "first aid" approach should be tried and may be successful. Often it is not, however, and many adolescents with the school phobia syndrome require long-term intensive psychotherapy and even psychiatric hospitalization. With some mildly disturbed adolescents, brief pediatric hospitalization, drawing upon psychiatric consultation, may be all that is required.

Eisenberg L: School phobia: Diagnosis, genesis, and clinical management. P Clin North America 5:645, 1958.
Williams HR, Prugh DG: School phobia. In: *Ambulatory Pediatrics*. Green M, Haggerty R (editors). Saunders, 1968.

ENURESIS & ENCOPRESIS

Two major challenges for the pediatrician are offered by enuresis and encopresis. These symptoms are not necessarily associated with any specific personality picture. Both represent normal patterns until the expected age of training. Thereafter, they may represent a regressive component of a reactive disorder (in late preschool children), a developmental deviation in control mechanisms, a conversion symptom as part of a psychoneurotic disorder, or one of a constellation of symptoms in a chronic personality disorder or psychosis.

1. ENURESIS

Continuing enuresis (beyond about age 4) may be diurnal or nocturnal. Both types are often associated with coercive toilet training in infancy, except for an occasional child whose overpermissive parents have not attempted to train him, the child who has been seriously neglected, or the child with an apparent developmental lag in bladder control mechanisms, without other disturbance, whose parents handle him supportively and continue to pick him up at night. Some family tendencies toward enuresis are seen.

Diurnal enuresis represents constant dribbling during the day beyond the point of occasional accidents caused by anxiety or momentary "forgetting" to empty a full bladder when preoccupied, as often happens in late preschool children. Diurnal enuresis may become a problem if the child enters nursery school, or it may remain mild and relatively unnoticed until the child enters kindergarten. It may or may not be associated with nocturnal enuresis, and is associated with a higher incidence of encopresis.

Diurnal wetting may be influenced by shyness about asking to go to the toilet, fear of strange toilets, negativistic tendencies, or chronic anxiety. In older school age children, it is most often encountered in chronically anxious children, those with personality disorders of the anxiety type, and those with oppositional personality traits. In general, it is more difficult to treat with the usual methods (described below) than the nocturnal type. A supportive relationship with the pediatrician and counseling for the child and the parents may be of help. Psychiatric consultation should usually be obtained, however, and many of these children require referral for intensive psychotherapy.

Children with **nocturnal enuresis** seem to experience greater than normal urgency in response to bladder distention during sleep. Their bladder capacity is not strikingly diminished, however, and, at least as measured by EEG studies, their sleep is not deeper. There appears to be no association with epilepsy (most epileptic children do not have enuresis). Most have no neurologic disorders related to true incontinence or structural abnormalities of the bladder or proximal urethra. The problem seems to be one of external sphincter control, and abnormalities higher in the urinary tract appear to play no significant role.

Diagnostic studies should ordinarily go no further than a urinalysis to rule out cystitis (which might cause urinary urgency) or, at most, an intravenous urogram if abnormalities are suspected. The pediatrician should avoid the use of retrograde cystoscopy in children with normal urine specimens; these can provoke severe anxiety in young school age children, who still have fears of bodily (especially genital) mutilation. If done without general anesthesia in neurotic adolescents, the experience can become paradoxically pleasurable, particularly in girls with hysterical trends and masochistic needs.

Classification of Causes

Children with nocturnal enuresis fall into several groups from a psychosocial point of view, which may account for the conflicting findings in the literature regarding personality pictures and parent-child relationships.

A. Developmental Lag: One group shows a continuing struggle for control with the parents in this area, often arising from an apparent developmental lag in control mechanisms which upsets the parents. These are not usually seriously disturbed children, although they may be timid, somewhat anxious, and show some immature behavior. The symptom is more or less "encapsulated," and may represent a failure to achieve conditioned nighttime control.

B. Psychoneurotic Disorders: Boys with nocturnal enuresis are usually passive, somewhat inhibited, and often overly dependent or with phobic trends. They may identify with a dominant mother or be fearful of a punitive father. The symptoms appear to be of a conversion nature, involving relaxation of the external sphincter in relation to unconscious sexual conflicts, often expressed in terrifying nightmares during which loss of control occurs.

Girls with this symptom seem to be more active, sometimes overly independent, and competitive toward boys, with a tendency toward more masculine identification in an attempt to handle sexual fears. The content of the conversion symptom seems to carry an unconsciously hostile component toward their mothers or toward men who could injure them.

C. Tension Discharge Disorders: Children (usually boys) with tension discharge disorders, frequently of the impulse-ridden type, show problems in control in a number of areas. They often have dysrhythmic EEGs, although these seem to be related to immaturity in CNS development than to other causes. In some children with previously repressed neurotic conflicts, firesetting is encountered, together with dreams of firemen or of firehoses putting out fires. In many cases the fathers have been overly punitive and the mothers unaffectionate. Broken homes are a frequent historical component, and most of these children have experienced considerable emotional deprivation.

D. Other Disorders: A few disturbed children, with much resentment underlying passive-aggressive behavior, demonstrate a "revenge" type of enuresis, ie, their bedwetting represents a conscious, volitional act, usually carried out secretly. Psychotic children may have enuresis because of negativism or as a result of an inability to comprehend the significance of toilet training.

Treatment

Treatment should be related to the type of personality and family picture. For children whose enuresis represents a developmental lag in bladder control

mechanisms, often with a related struggle for control, various methods can be employed successfully, eg, the gold star chart, drugs such as atropine or imipramine (Tofranil), and conditioning approaches such as the Eneurtone apparatus. Probably the most important ingredient in all these approaches is a positive doctor-parent relationship.

In the context of such a relationship, the physician should explain to the parents that the child cannot help the enuresis. They should be assured that the problem is not "their fault" and encouraged to stop pressuring or punishing the child in favor of his prescription, whatever it may be. By developing a positive relationship with the child, the pediatrician can help him with feelings of guilt, shame, or resentment and develop motivation for independent control with the help of the prescribed method. In some instances, control has been achieved during the evaluation process even before the prescription has been written.

Bakwin H: Enuresis in children. J Pediat 58:806, 1961.

Oppel WC, Harper PA, Rider RV: Social, psychological, and neurological factors associated with nocturnal eneuresis. Pediatrics 42:627, 1968.

2. ENCOPRESIS

Children with encopresis fall into 3 different groups. In many cases, the symptom begins as stool withholding in late infancy, and the majority of these children have experienced coercive toilet training.

Classification of Causes

A. Developmental Failure: In one group, failure to develop conditioned control of the external anal sphincter results in continuous soiling from infancy. These children generally have a relaxed anal sphincter. "Paradoxical diarrhea" often occurs, with a flow of mucoid material around a central fecal mass. These children frequently show strong oppositional behavior tendencies, with negativism in response to parental pressure or restrictions. In some cases nonaganglionic megacolon of psychophysiologic origin may be present.

B. Inhibited, Dependent Children: Another group of children with encopresis often exhibit inhibited, dependent, compulsive tendencies and may show much concern about cleanliness in other areas. The symptom, often of regressive onset, seems to be a type of conversion reaction, representing the expression of unconscious hostility and resistance toward the parents—usually a dominating, overcontrolling, compulsive mother with strong unconscious interests in bowel functions and a passive, retiring, uninterested father. Soiling occurs rarely at school but is common on the way home, as the child returns to the area of conflict. "Hiding" the stool, wrapped in underwear, in a bureau drawer where the mother will find it frequently underlines the hostile significance of the soiling. In these children, the stool is often soft and formed, without paradoxical diarrhea.

C. Seriously Disturbed Children: Still another group of children with encopresis are much more seriously disturbed. They may manifest deep personality disorders, of mistrustful or isolated nature, with defects in reality testing of near-psychotic proportions, and some have shown "revenge" encopresis. Some may have been frankly psychotic since infancy, failing to comprehend control, whereas in others encopresis may have developed as one of a group of bizarre symptoms involved in a schizophreniform psychotic disorder. Paradoxical diarrhea may or may not be present. A few children have psychotic parents who have made no attempt to offer training. The parents of most are themselves disturbed, and they may occasionally interfere with treatment because of their fears or suspicions.

Treatment

Treatment should be geared to the personality and family patterns. If fecal impaction is present, hypertonic phosphate or oil retention enemas can be used in the hospital. Later, a mild laxative can be prescribed. Mineral oil is effective, but many children and parents are upset by the "leaking" that occurs. A regular evacuation each day may help reestablish bowel habits.

The support of the pediatrician, helping the parents to understand that the symptom is not their fault nor the child's and encouraging them not to use pressure or punishment in controlling it, is fundamental to any therapeutic approach. The child is usually embarrassed and guilty and can rarely talk about it easily, but he can be encouraged to participate in the reestablishment of bowel routines and control.

The above approach is surprisingly effective in the group who have resisted control by overly rigid parents and to some extent in school age children who develop the regressive type with conversion mechanisms. The doctor can offer the child a "way out," as it were.

Psychiatric consultation may be necessary, and some children and parents may require intensive long-term psychotherapy.

"Cleaning out" procedures and establishment of bowel routines may be resisted by the child or the parents out of fear of harm.

Davidson M: Constipation and fecal incontinence. P Clin North America 5:749, 1958.

Garrard SD, Richmond JB: Psychogenic megacolon manifested by fecal soiling. Pediatrics 10:474, 1952.

Pinkerton P: Psychogenic megacolon in children: The implications of bowel negativism. Arch Dis Childhood 33:371, 1958.

SUICIDAL ATTEMPTS

Depression in adolescents, as in younger children, often takes different forms from depression in adults.

Overt depression, with feelings of worthlessness, psychomotor retardation, and other physical changes, is much less common than in adults. Withdrawal, excessive daydreaming, anorexia, mood swings, sleep disturbances (inability to fall asleep or inability to get up in the morning), hyperactivity or hypoactivity, feelings of helplessness or hopelessness, or even hostility, temper outbursts, or aggressive behavior (warding off a depression) are common depressive equivalents of which the adolescent may not be consciously aware.

Suicidal threats are common in children and often represent attempts to punish the parents. ("You'll be sorry if I die.") Children are unable to comprehend the reality of death until age 9 or 10 years. Suicidal attempts are rare and usually do not reflect serious wishes to die but rather a desire for self-punishment or retaliation against the parents; however, they may accidentally be successful or may be carried out more efficiently than intended. The incidence of attempts rises rapidly after age 14. Although accurate reporting is rare, suicide is the fourth most frequent cause of death in late adolescence and the second most frequent cause in college students of high economic status.

Adolescent suicide rates vary from country to country (highest in Japan, Switzerland, and Finland) and from region to region (highest in the Rocky Mountain and Pacific Coast states in the USA). They appear to be higher in middle class groups and in urban areas, and show some seasonal incidence in temperate countries (highest in the spring) and some variation in relation to historical epochs and social crises. The adolescent suicide rate has increased significantly in the USA in the recent past (from 2.8 per 100,000 in 1954 to 3.8 in 1962, a 36% increase). This increase may be due in part to more honest reporting of suicides previously recorded as accidental. The rate among boys, particularly, may be even higher if automobile accidents are considered, since self-destructive or suicidal motives may be involved in deaths due to vehicle accidents.

In the USA, the suicide rate was formerly higher among adolescent girls than boys. The rate of successful suicide in boys is now at least double that of girls, although girls make more attempts. Boys most commonly employ firearms and explosives, with hanging or strangulation next; girls most frequently have employed poison or drugs, although firearms and explosives have recently become more common.

In addition to social, economic, or historical factors and a greater acceptance of suicide as a method of protest or problem-solving, it may be that child-rearing attitudes related to shame, guilt, or achievement and individual and family or situational factors are involved in most specific suicidal attempts. A small proportion of adolescents who attempt suicide are psychotic, and these episodes may be bizarre attempts at self-mutilation rather than actual suicide. Some have chronic personality disorders (hysterical and others), and their attempts may be clearly manipulative of parents or peers. Immature, sensitive, shy, anxious, emotionally labile adolescents with low self-esteem who come from disorganized or disturbed families are vulnerable to stressful events and may regard suicide as a solution. Others are reasonably healthy adolescents reacting to some specific situation such as chronic illness, pressure for school achievement, or the experience of sudden loss of another person or of self-esteem, as with a broken love affair or a bitter fight with a parent. Depression, feelings of unworthiness, internalized anger at another (with guilt and depression), boredom, attempts to gain affection and esteem or to punish a parent or a boy or girl friend, a desire to join a dead relative, or even the acting out of an unconscious wish of a parent or identification with a parent who has committed suicide may be involved in the attempt, with more than one factor usually involved. Many adolescents do not really wish to die, and the attempt is a "cry for help." Even a true wish to die is more short-lived in adolescents than in adults. The adolescent often tells the parents about the attempt or leaves a note or a bottle where it may easily be found. He may change his mind in the middle of the act (sometimes too late); he may feel backed into a corner by his own threats of suicide if his "bluff is called," and may feel that he has to make the attempt to maintain his integrity.

Many parents are ashamed and guilty when their adolescent son or daughter attempts suicide, and the doctor may unconsciously conspire with them to forget it or "sweep it under the rug." Even suicidal threats should always be taken seriously. If an attempt is made which produces no response from the parents, the adolescent may try again with tragic results.

Signs of depression or depressive equivalents are a serious indication that suicide may be attempted. Although emotional lability is one of the characteristics of adolescence, true depression should never be dealt with by a "pat on the back" or a "buck up" approach. An opportunity to ventilate feelings to an understanding adult may be of great help, or more formal therapy may be necessary.

If an adolescent asks for a chance to talk with a physician or other adult, an interview should be arranged promptly. It is hard enough to encourage teen-agers to talk to adults at most times; if a request for an opportunity to talk is made, granting it may help to prevent impulsive suicidal attempts.

If a suicidal attempt has been made, pediatric hospitalization can provide the time, with the help of a psychiatrist and social worker, to convince the parents of the seriousness of the adolescent's plea for help. Supportive counseling or environmental rearrangement may suffice, or more intensive psychotherapy can be started at once if indicated.

It is unwise to send home from the emergency room an adolescent who has made even a patently superficial and manipulative suicidal attempt such as the ingestion of a small amount of an innocuous drug or a quantity of barbiturates which can easily be dealt with by gastric lavage. The family will often not return for follow-up therapy, and more serious attempts may occur. If the adolescent appears seriously disturbed, emergency psychiatric hospitalization is necessary.

Barter JT, Swaback DO, Todd D: Adolescent suicide attempts. Arch Gen Psychiat 19:523–527, 1968.

Faigel HC: Suicide among young persons: A review of its incidence and causes, and methods. Clin Pediat 5:187, 1966.

Lewis M, Solnit A: The adolescent in a suicidal crisis: Collaborative care on a pediatric ward. In: *Modern Perspectives in Child Development.* Solnit A, Provence S (editors). Internat Univ Press, 1963.

DRUG ABUSE

Drug addiction and the use of drugs by adolescents is one of the most controversial topics of our times. The toxicologic aspects of these subjects are discussed in Chapter 31, and the drugs used are listed in Table 31–6.

LSD & Other Hallucinogens

The biologic effects of LSD and related compounds have been carefully studied; they resemble sympathomimetic agents and produce such changes as increased pulse and heart rate, rise in blood pressure, mydriasis, tremors of extremities, cold sweaty palms, flushing, chills and shivering, increased salivation, nausea, and anorexia. The psychologic effects may last for periods of 1–2 hours to more than a day. The LSD effect usually lasts 4–8 hours.

The effects depend on the person taking the drug, his expectation of what will happen, the setting in which it is taken, the other people in the setting, previous experiences with the drug, the physiologic and psychologic states of the subject, and other variables.

Changes in perception (especially visual) are often experienced by nonpsychotic subjects who take oral doses of LSD as small as 30 μg. They include enhancement of colors, alterations in the perception of one's own body, vivid hallucinations, and synesthesias. Mood changes include depression, euphoria, or lability of mood; anxiety is frequent, sometimes to the point of panic. Feelings of depersonalization and estrangement are often reported. Changes in thinking may include flights of ideas, perseveration, a feeling of insight into universal and transcendental phenomena (the "psychedelic experience"), and intense preoccupation with one's own thought and bodily processes. Other cognitive changes consist of difficulty in concentration on reality-oriented tasks, distractibility, abandonment of logical and causal thinking, and changes in time sense.

Untoward psychologic effects ("bad trips") include the appearance of a serious schizophreniform psychotic illness (usually precipitated by the drug experience in borderline psychotic individuals); prolonged depressive reaction (including a number of reported suicides); continuing anxiety (panic), depersonalization, and recurrent catatonia, with intermittent return ("flashback") of hallucinatory experiences; and serious injury or death in a few cases.

Some reports have indicated that persons who take LSD have an increased number of "breaks" in chromosomes, lasting at least 6 months, and that the offspring of women who have taken LSD early in pregnancy also exhibit such chromosomal alterations (continuing up to 5 years of age). Similar findings have been reported in animals. These results need to be carefully validated, but caution in the use of LSD, especially by pregnant women, seems justified on this basis among others.

Because the manufacture and sale of many of the compounds used as hallucinogens is a federal offense, the extent of their abuse is difficult to determine. Statements regarding large numbers of young people who have experimented with or used these drugs are often exaggerated and inflammatory. Various surveys report that up to 15% of college students in selected colleges have admitted trying LSD. Undoubtedly, a number have tried the experience once only for "kicks" or out of curiosity; some anxious persons with conflicts have continued the practice; and others with "an empty feeling," alienated and isolated (anomie), may continue to seek stimulation of any kind by the use of these drugs. Some report the experience openly as frightening; others describe it in rapturous terms.

Although feelings of universal insight seem to occur in some individuals, there is no evidence that LSD changes personality for the better. In addition, those who experience such insights rarely can describe them clearly to others, and there is little evidence that the experiences have resulted in any personal or social benefit. The use of LSD as an adjunct to psychotherapy in chronic alcoholism and chronic neurosis has been reported, but no carefully controlled studies are available.

LSD is relatively easy to manufacture and easily available from illegal sources, and there is no way to detect its presence in the body. Thus, in spite of realistic concerns about adverse psychologic and biologic effects of LSD (and presumably other psychedelic drugs also), there is no easy way to control its distribution. The largest group of users appears to be teenagers and young adults who characteristically are "looking for answers" and are only too ready to rebel against the established order and break its rules. To make laws against use or possession of these drugs is more likely to encourage experimentation with them than the reverse. Such legislation also means that large numbers of young people who will soon outgrow their rebelliousness in the course of development will be socially hampered by a police record.

At present, the incidence of experimentation with these drugs seems to be decreasing. Young people are aware of the information about chromosomal damage, and appear to respect that type of data even more than rules or laws.

Marihuana

Marihuana is more widely used today than the psychedelic (hallucinogenic, psychotomimetic) drugs, with estimates of up to 20% or more in college students. Its effects are not well studied because of its illegal status; they appear to involve relaxation of inhibitions in some individuals, although most users describe an introspective attitude under the influence of marihuana even in a group setting. The drug does not appear to be significantly involved in episodes of antisocial, destructive, or criminal behavior. It is not addictive and does not predispose to other addictions. The furor among adults over its use seems unjustified, as most young people control its use or eventually give it up.

Heroin

Heroin does seem to have some addictive qualities, although physical dependence on it or other "addictive" drugs (with great desire and increasing tolerance) involves also certain psychologic needs for escape from reality conflicts, fear of withdrawal symptoms, or a conditioning process. Deaths have occurred from overdosage, and tetanus, malaria, hepatitis, syphilis, and other infections have resulted from the use of unsterile needles.

The Hydrocarbons

Inhalation of hydrocarbons (glue or plastic cement, lighter fluid, or gasoline fumes) seems to produce a state somewhat resembling alcoholic intoxication, ie, an initial "jag" with pleasant exhilaration, euphoria, and excitement. Ataxia, slurred speech, and at times diplopia and tinnitus follow, with drowsiness, stupor, and brief coma appearing later. As tolerance develops, large amounts of inhalant become necessary to produce a reaction. Nausea, anorexia, weight loss, irritability, inattentiveness, somnolence, excessive salivation, and fetor oris may result from glue-sniffing, but serious physiologic effects do not occur. Gasoline sniffing, which has been reported in children as young as 18 months of age, has caused occasional accidental deaths.

Although not addictive, the hydrocarbons offer easy habituation. They are used—particularly glue—principally by boys who usually have significant psychosocial problems which lead to the habituation. The same is true of individuals who become habituated to the amphetamines, barbiturates, alcohol, or tobacco in childhood or early adolescence.

Management of Drug Abuse

The approach to the use of drugs should be medical, psychologic, and social rather than restrictive or punitive. This is true of serious addictive problems as well; even alcoholism has been recognized recently by the courts as an illness requiring treatment and not primarily an offense against society. An understanding approach by the parents to guidance and discipline, with some limits but with some flexibility, will prevent many young people from resorting to the habitual use of drugs of any kind.

For those who have experienced "bad trips" or other untoward effects of drug abuse, or those in higher-income families who engage in chronic drug abuse because of emotional disturbance or rebellion, psychiatric treatment is usually indicated. Younger adolescents who have indulged in glue-sniffing because of psychologic problems may often be successfully treated by the pediatrician with the help of psychiatric consultation and therapy for the parents by a social worker or other mental health professional. Other social and economic measures are necessary to deal with the fundamental problems of poverty and discrimination which favor the use of drugs by adolescents in disadvantaged neighborhoods.

Deisher RW & others: Drug abuse in adolescence: The use of harmful drugs—a pediatric concern. Pediatrics 44:131, 1969.

Freedman A, Wilson E: Childhood and adolescent addictive disorders. Pediatrics 34:254, 283, 1964.

Litt IF, Cohen MI: The drug-using adolescent and pediatric patient. J Pediat 77:195, 1970.

MANAGEMENT OF PSYCHOLOGIC ASPECTS OF ILLNESS & INJURY

ACUTE ILLNESS OR INJURY

The child's response to acute illness or injury depends upon the particular organ system affected, his level of psychosocial development, the meaning of the illness to the child and his family, the nature of necessary treatment, and other factors. In general, there are broad patterns of responses characteristic of children at different developmental levels, with variations due to individual differences.

The direct effects of acute illness on behavior may include listlessness, prostration, irritability, or disturbances in sleep and appetite. Restlessness and hyperactivity often complicate the management of milder illnesses, especially in preschool children. In biologically predisposed youngsters, physiologic concomitants of anxiety may appear, including tachycardia, palpitation, hyperventilation, and diarrhea—at times leading to diagnostic confusion with hyperthyroidism, rheumatic fever, etc. Struggles for control between a young child and his parents may cause eating and sleeping problems which may persist long after recovery.

Emotional and behavioral regression in response to illness is common in older infants and young children and occurs to some degree in school age children and adolescents as well. Depression may also occur at times with a return of primitive fears and feelings of helplessness and hopelessness. In more severe reactions, compulsive or ritualized, stereotyped behavior may occur and may subside rapidly or continue as a reactive disorder.

Misinterpretations of the meaning of the illness or accident as punishment are common in preschool children and may occur in school age children as well. Late preschool and early school age children may have fears of bodily mutilation, especially when sensitive areas such as the genitals, eyes, or mouth are involved. In older school age children, conversion and dissociative reactions may be encountered, often associated with subclinical delirium in response to drug administration or high fever or during convalescence.

The potentially deleterious effects of bed rest too strenuously enforced must be borne in mind and balanced against the sometimes doubtful advantages.

CHRONIC ILLNESS & SERIOUS INJURY

Chronic illness or handicapping injuries may have serious consequences for the child's personality development and family functioning. The child's previous adaptive capacity and the parent-child family balance appear to be the most important prognostic factors. These children's personalities appear to fall along a continuum ranging from overdependent, overanxious, and passive or withdrawn to overly independent, with strong tendencies to deny illness. A number of these youngsters become realistically dependent and accept their limitations, developing adequate social roles and methods and sublimating their energies in constructive ways. Parental patterns range from overanxiousness, overprotectiveness, and overindulgence, often with difficulties in setting limits on the child's demands, to refusal to accept the severity of the child's disability, projection of personal guilt onto others (including the doctor), reluctance to cooperate with treatment programs, and, occasionally, rejection or isolation of the child.

Most parents ultimately learn to accept the child's limitations without discomfort, permit an appropriate degree of dependency, and help him explore constructively his capacities and strengths.

Child's Reaction

Many children with chronic illnesses or handicaps have moderate to severe difficulties in maintaining a sound body image. Adolescents especially may show marked reactions to disfigurement or physical handicap.

In reaction to catastrophic illness or injury, school age children and adolescents show a phasic response consisting initially of an *impact phase* involving realistic fears of death, soon followed by marked regression, strong denial of long-term damage, and the use of primitive fantasy (eg, daydreams of being a great athlete). After some days or weeks, the *phase of recoil* is characterized by dawning recognition of the seriousness of the situation and by grief, or "mourning for the loss of the self"; this represents a constructive process, but it may be masked by demanding behavior. Severe depression may be present during this phase. The *phase of restitution* is characterized by the reemergence of premorbid personality traits such as overdependence or unrealistic overindependence. Management must be geared to the patient's progress through these phases.

Parents' Reaction

Parents show a parallel phasic response. A phase of "denial and disbelief" may persist for days, weeks, or months, sometimes accompanied by "shopping" for other opinions. During the succeeding phase of "fear and frustration," the parents may be depressed and guilty and may project blame onto each other or onto other persons. Marital crises may occur during this time. After weeks or months, the parents usually arrive at the phase of "intelligent inquiry and planning," in which they are able to handle their feelings and to live fairly comfortably although with some ambiguity.

Attempts to force either the parents or the child to face the reality of the situation before they are ready only increase the denial. Indeed, some denial—within limits—may be necessary for the maintenance of hope.

Management of Initial Reactions

During the management of chronic illness or handicap, the child and parents can be helped to focus on small, day-to-day steps as well as to ventilate feelings of frustration, anxiety, or guilt. Other supportive measures include suggestions for occupational therapy in the home, encouragement of gradual resumption of activity, and redirecting the child's interests so that he can compensate for activities denied to him by excelling in others. Parents often need to be restrained from overprotecting or overindulging such children.

Home teachers may make it possible for the child to keep up with his schooling. The child should attend school, even on a part-time basis, either in a special class or, ideally, in a regular class. Vocational training compatible with the adolescent's intellectual and physical capacities can be arranged with the help of community resources. For the child who is so seriously handicapped that he cannot leave home, service agencies can often build a social club around him in the home. Group discussions among parents of children with similar problems may be of value in offering emotional support, as may similar approaches with handicapped adolescents.

Paradoxical Responses to Treatment

Children with deep-seated emotional conflicts who have adapted to the role of an invalid in families with unhealthy interpersonal relationships may find it difficult to respond to treatment in a positive way and may instead decompensate or develop a variety of symptomatic reactions. A gradual rehabilitative approach is necessary for such children and parents, and psychiatric consultation or formal psychotherapy is often required.

Prognosis

Emotional factors such as depression over actual or symbolic loss of key figures or lack of motivation to recover may adversely influence the course of serious illnesses such as carcinoma, leukemia, lymphoma, and especially infectious hepatitis, which seems to exert a specific depressive effect upon the psyche. Supportive psychologic measures should be part of the total treatment plan for children and adolescents with many of these disorders. Psychiatric consultation is often helpful and should be sought whenever the physician feels that an emotional component he cannot deal with is menacing his patient's total mental and physical well-being.

Korsch B, Barnett HL: The physician, the child, and the family. J Pediat 58:707, 1961.

Lief HI, Lief VF, Lief NR (editors): *The Psychological Basis of Medical Practice.* Harper, 1963.

Prugh DG: Toward an understanding of psychosomatic concepts in relation to illness in children. In: *Modern Perspectives in Child Development.* Solnit AJ, Provence S (editors). Internat Univ Press, 1963.

Richmond JB: The pediatric patient in illness. In: *The Psychology of Medical Practice.* Saunders, 1958.

Senn MJE: Emotional aspects of convalescence. The Child 10:24, 1945.

HOSPITALIZATION

The management of children before, during, and after hospitalization is an important part of pediatric treatment, since most children have this experience at some time or other (3.5 million a year under age 15). Hospitalization, with its separation from home and the various treatment procedures encountered, may cause a variety of reactions depending upon the child's level of psychosocial development, the family's response, the meaning of the illness and hospitalization, the type of treatment required, and other factors. The older the child, the more he will understand the realistic meaning of this experience and the less likely he will be to misinterpret its significance.

Child's Reaction to Hospitalization

A. Infants Under Age 6 Months: Young infants usually show temporary "global responses" to unfamiliar methods of feeding and handling, which may confuse mothers on return home.

B. Older Infants: Beginning in the second half of the first year, infants experience stranger anxiety and fears of separation, with regression and depression.

C. Young Children: Children up to age 4 appear most vulnerable to separation from the mother. Children of this age often experience a sequence of protest, despair, and detachment, the latter often associated with withdrawal and depression if separation without adequate mother-substitute relationships continues beyond a few days or 1—2 weeks.

D. Age 4 to Early School Age: The child from age 4 through the early school age period, although he may experience separation anxiety, is usually more preoccupied with fears of bodily mutilation.

E. Older School Age Children: Older children are usually able to comprehend the reality of the hospital experience more objectively but may still show signs of mild regression and anxiety over bodily functioning, etc. Fears of genital inadequacy, muscular weakness, and of loss of body control or of helplessness during anesthesia may enhance the feelings of anxiety and inferiority that are characteristic of this stage of development. The same trends may be seen in adolescents but in a muted form. They may have difficulty in accepting the authority of the medical and nursing staff.

Parents' Reaction

Parental reactions to a child's illness may be compounded by hospitalization. Some parents may fear criticism from the hospital staff regarding their role in the illness itself or their effectiveness as parents. Consequently, some may adopt a strongly rival attitude toward nurses or physicians in an attempt to disarm the implied criticism of their own parental abilities. Feeling left out or unwanted is also common among parents. A few parents project their own guilt onto the hospital staff and blame them for the child's difficulties. Some parents with excessive anxiety are themselves unable to separate comfortably from the child; a few, with intense guilt, may be unable to visit.

Preparation for Hospitalization

All children should be told simply and truthfully why they are going to the hospital. They should be given a general impression of what being in a hospital is like and what will be done to make them comfortable. They must be assured that their parents will remain in contact with them. When the physician decides that hospitalization is necessary, he should inform the parents what to tell the child and deal as necessary with their apprehension, guilt feelings, or conflicts. .

Preschool children should not be prepared for elective hospitalization more than a week or so in advance—enough time for questions but not too much for anxiety to build up. In some instances, a group session with the physician, parents, and child may be helpful in order to support anxious parents or to give the child the feeling of being involved in the planning.

Thorough exposition of the medical or surgical implications and procedures is not necessary for most children, although adolescents may wish to know more details. Practical discussions about mealtimes, use of a bedpan, etc may be of value for older preschool children. "Playing out" situations in the hospital with a toy doctor's or nurse's kit may help to prevent anxiety. Visits to the hospital may be useful for school age children. Booklets about "going to the hospital" may be of value if an opportunity for questions is offered, but they should not convey the impression that being in hospital is like "being at a party," with all sorts of entertainment, etc.

Reactions to Painful Procedures

Procedures such as venipunctures, injections, and lumbar punctures are frightening to young children, and very young children cannot be expected to cooperate unassisted. An older child can sometimes be made interested in the doctor's instruments and their purpose, so that he can cooperate to some extent in controlling his response to pain. The doctor should always explain that some pain will occur, without minimizing or exaggerating it. He should tell the child when and where it will hurt and encourage him to cry if he feels like it. Firm but kindly restraint should be used as necessary, with the explanation that it is being done to help the child hold still so that "it won't hurt so much." The main thought to be conveyed is that the young patient, the doctor, and the nurse have an alliance which will help get the task done with as little hurt as possible.

Post-Hospitalization

Most children manifest at least mildly disturbed behavior for a few days or several weeks after returning home. This post-hospitalization reaction may persist if reinforced by parental anxiety or guilt. Anticipatory guidance and support for the parents in gradually "weaning" the child from regressive behavior can be of valuable preventive significance.

During convalescence, some children do not want to relinquish the greater dependency involved in the acute phase of the illness and may dread the imminent return to competitive school responsibilities. Flexibility in matters of bed rest, meals, and treatment routines may be appropriate, eg, rest on the living room couch, in contact with others, may be more therapeutic than in the bedroom, where the relative isolation can lead to further regression.

The child should return to an integrated family life and to school as soon as possible and should resume his responsibilities gradually as his capacities return to normal.

The Child in the Hospital

Hospitalization is not necessarily a traumatic experience for a child, although it should be used as sparingly as possible. Preschool or previously disturbed children are most vulnerable to adverse reactions. In addition to improvement in physical health as a result of hospitalization, some older children benefit from the opportunity to relate to other children and adults outside the home, especially if the family has been disturbed or isolated.

Previously unrecognized psychologic problems in a child with physical illness may become obvious as a result of a comprehensive evaluation in a hospital setting, where one may observe at greater length the behavior of the child and the interaction with his parents.

During hospitalization, the child's "life space" and his ties with reality should be maintained. The teacher is a familiar nonmedical figure, and schooling should be available even during brief periods of hospitalization. Recreational therapists ("play ladies"), social group workers, and occupational therapists can provide valuable emotional support and opportunities for "playing out" feelings about the hospital staff and procedures while at the same time offering age-appropriate recreational outlets.

Early ambulation (in carts if necessary) and family style eating arrangements offer social experiences which may facilitate convalescence and improve appetite.

It is sometimes difficult to coordinate the activities of physicians, consultants, nurses, social workers, teachers, recreational staff, "foster grandmothers," and other persons involved. A weekly or biweekly ward management conference chaired by a senior pediatrician or clinical director will facilitate communication and increase the effectiveness of the total effort.

The most vital mental health need while the child is in the hospital is maintenance of the tie between the child and his family. The "therapeutic alliance" between the parents and the hospital staff is a concept of great importance. Hospital organization should provide a balance between the advantages of the parents' presence and the treatment obligations of the staff, with separate visiting and treatment areas if possible. Flexible daily visiting schedules are directly correlated with less disturbed behavior on the part of the older preschool and school age child, and cross-infection has been shown to be minimal. Some facilities permit unrestricted visiting and overnight stay by parents. For preschool children, who are more anxious over separation and whose understanding is limited, overnight stay or "living in" by the mother is the most effective preventive measure. Individualized planning about visiting is necessary, since some parents will not be able to take advantage of such opportunities for a variety of reasons.

Alternative plans to hospitalization should be considered whenever possible. For example, motel facilities adjacent to a children's hospital have been developed where the parents of a child who is being studied diagnostically may stay. Day care can be planned for children with chronic illnesses or diagnostic problems who do not require hospitalization. Greater use can be made of home care if a "family team" can be organized for this purpose.

Glaser MD: Group discussions with mothers and hospitalized children. Pediatrics 26:132, 1960.

MacKeith R: Children in the hospital: Preparation for operation. Lancet 2:843, 1955.

Mason EA: The hospitalized child: His emotional needs. New England J Med 272:406, 1965.

Plank EM, Coughey PA, Lipson MF: A general hospital child care program to counteract hospitalism. Am J Orthopsychiat 29:94, 1959.

Prugh DG & others: A study of the emotional reactions of children and families to hospitalization and illness. Am J Orthopsychiat 23:70, 1953.

Robertson J: *Young Children in Hospitals.* Basic Books, 1958.

Shore MF (editor): *Red is the Color of Hurting: Planning for Children in the Hospital.* US Department of Health, Education, & Welfare, 1966.

Solnit AJ: Hospitalization: An aid to physical and psychological health in childhood. Am J Dis Child 99:155, 1960.

SURGERY

The child who requires an operation usually needs special preparation if psychologic problems are to be avoided. For school age children, the explanation should be simple and brief, without many details, and the child should be permitted to ask as many questions as he wishes both before and after surgery. Most children can talk more freely and understand more fully if a simple drawing is used to explain the procedure. Even early adolescent boys may fear, for example, that a colectomy for ulcerative colitis may somehow interfere with their capacity for "becoming a man." The pediatrician should make sure that preparation takes place, no matter whether he or the surgeon does it. Preparation of the parents is equally important, as they too may have significant misconceptions. If possible, elective operations should be avoided in children age 4–6 since fears of bodily mutilation are greatest at this time.

Anesthesia

Anesthesia may evoke fears of death or of loss of self-control in school age children. They may have fears they will say or do "something bad" and may also be concerned about what might be done to their bodily organs while they are helpless. Induction and recovery states should be explained in appropriate terms. Some children need to be reassured they will not awaken before the operation is over. Others may mistake the onset of unconsciousness as impending death and need to be told that "forced sleep" is temporary and will be followed by complete awakening and survival. Preliminary "playing out" of the induction process by the anesthetist or other personnel aids in the child's mastery of the situation. If possible, the child should be spared the experience of seeing instruments, the operating room, etc.

Since oral barbiturates may have a stimulant effect on preschool children unless given in large doses, administration of a basal anesthetic (eg, thiopental) in the child's room (with the mother present) may help relax an overly anxious child and prevent resistance on the way to the operating room. When the child awakes, the mother should be there to greet him; this is especially important in young children. School age children can be helped to adjust to the ward setting and staff by being admitted a day in advance of an elective operation. (This is not ordinarily helpful for preschool children.)

Principles of this kind have also been shown to be effective in cutting down on the amount of anesthetic necessary and in reducing the incidence and severity of postoperative reactions.

Mutilating Operations

Special problems may arise in regard to operations with unavoidably mutilating results, such as amputations. If the child misinterprets the procedure as a punishment for a past misdeed, he may become aggressive (in fantasied self-defense) or withdrawn (feeling helpless and hopeless).

Occasionally, persistent denial of loss of a body part, such as a limb, can lead to difficulties in planning for prosthetic devices. Psychiatric consultation should be freely used.

Burns

If a severely burned child is guilty about the accident and fearful of the loss of his parents' love, he may become seriously depressed, respond poorly to surgical procedures, and fail to heal adequately. The presence of a mother substitute such as a foster grandmother may be lifesaving for a regressed and depressed preschool child whose parents cannot hold him because of his burns. Hypnosis may be helpful in stimulating trust and minimizing pain during dressing changes; drugs are not as helpful in children as in adults. Most children with extensive burns have significant emotional problems following even successful surgical treatment. Psychotherapy has been shown to ameliorate or prevent such problems.

Bernstein NR: Observations on the use of hypnosis with burned children on a pediatric ward. Internat J Clin Exper Hypnosis 13:1, 1965.

Fineman L, Blom GE, Waldfogel S: Emotional implications of tonsillectomy and adenoidectomy in children. Psychoanal Study Child 7:126, 1952.

Loomis E: The child's emotions and surgery. In: *Pre- and Post-Operative Care in the Pediatric Surgical Patient.* Kieswelter WB (editor). Year Book, 1956.

TERMINAL ILLNESS

Recent advances in medical and surgical care have brought about a change in the composition of the patient population in many children's hospitals. The pediatric practitioner is spending more and more of his time in caring for children with chronic and sometimes fatal illnesses. The physician must be able to deal constructively with parents and children in these tragic circumstances. The management of dying children is perhaps one of the most difficult tasks the pediatrician faces today.

Explaining a fatal illness is a complicated task often attended by some risk. However, not to interpret the fatal illness at some level is a disservice to the patient and his family. Knowing the individual child and family and understanding the child's concept of death may provide the physician with some guide to individual answers in specific situations.

The Young Child

The young child who is dying expresses mainly his fear of separation from his parents and his wish to avoid pain. When death comes acutely, the child's awareness is often blunted by delirium, stupor, or coma. In a more gradual terminal experience, there is often evidence of depression, withdrawal, fearfulness, and apprehension. Although most children with a fatal illness do not directly ask if they are going to die, this question may be raised by some children over the age of 4 or 5. Parents, physicians, and nurses may have preferences about how to respond. When such questions are raised, the physician can ask why the child thinks he might die and may find that the child is worried about whether he will be alone or whether the doctor will make him feel "all right."

It is better not to tell the child that he might die without first discussing it with the parents and obtaining their permission. They may wish to answer the question themselves or they may wish to have help, either from the physician or from their religious counselors, in answering such questions.

The Older Child

Older children and adolescents have more understanding about impending death than the parents or hospital staff may realize.

Staff members often maintain an unconscious "conspiracy of silence," and may even stay away from the child to avoid the topic. In some cases, everyone involved may feel more comfortable if the topic is brought into the open. The young person can be told that he might die but that everything possible will be done to help him get well. He should be assured that relief from pain will be available and that he will not be left alone if he becomes seriously ill.

When a child dies, other children on the ward inevitably sense that something serious has happened and may need to be reassured that their condition is different.

Reactions of Parents

Parental reactions include the entire continuum from complete withdrawal from the child, through "mourning in advance" and an early detachment, to the extreme of denial and unrealistic expectations accompanied by poor reality testing. The reaction of the parents also depends on the circumstances of the illness or injury, the degree of their guilt, and the nature of the prior family relationship.

The physician must keep in mind the nature of the disease, the age of the child, and the family concept of death. Once he is certain of the diagnosis and prognosis, the parents should be told, frankly but gently, even though they may be overwhelmed and may want to go elsewhere for further medical care. The possibility of a fatal illness should never be mentioned to parents as part of a differential diagnosis, since some disturbed parents may continue to handle the child as if he were going to die even if that possibility is ruled out.

If the parents are able to help care for the child in the hospital during the terminal phase, they should be encouraged to do so. Some parents cannot bring themselves to help, however, and they should not be made to feel guilty if this is so. The physician must be ready to accept whatever feelings the parents display, even permitting them to bring other family members in to mourn with the child or to take the child home to die if that is their cultural tradition. Parents should be allowed to vent their feelings and perhaps even be encouraged to engage in the normal mourning process if there is an obvious lack of expression in an overly inhibited family. In the hospital, parents may gain much emotional support from other parents or social workers. Other community resources may be available also, so that the parents can have someone to whom they can express their feelings outside the hospital. Ministers, other family members, or psychiatric consultants may be helpful in understanding such situations and in working out a plan for some sort of help.

Parents frequently require a continuing supportive relationship with the pediatrician after the child's death. An appointment should be made to see them within several weeks, as their guilt and anxiety may lead them to repeat questions already asked. Such an opportunity for "working through" their feelings may help them to avoid immediately conceiving another child to take the place of the lost one, with obvious difficulties ahead.

Richmond JB, Waisman HA: Psychologic aspects of management of children with malignant diseases. Am J Dis Child 89:42, 1955.

Solnit AJ, Green M: Psychologic considerations in the management of deaths on pediatric hospital services. I. The doctor and the child's family. Pediatrics 24:106, 1959.

Toch R: Management of the child with a fatal disease. Clin Pediat 3:418, 1964.

• • •

General References

Ackerman N: *Treating the Troubled Family.* Basic Books, 1966.

Alt H: *Residential Treatment for the Disturbed Child.* Internat Univ Press, 1960.

Bakwin H, Bakwin RM: *Clinical Management of Behavior Disorders in Children,* rev ed. Saunders, 1967.

Berlin N: *Bibliography of Child Psychiatry: With a Selected List of Films.* American Psychiatric Association, 1963.

Caplan G (editor): *Emotional Problems of Early Childhood.* Basic Books, 1955.

Committee on Child Psychiatry: *The Diagnostic Process in Child Psychiatry.* GAP Report No. 38. Group for the Advancement of Psychiatry, 1957.

Committee on Child Psychiatry: *Psychopathological Disorders in Childhood: Theoretical Considerations and a Proposed Classification.* GAP Report No. 62. Group for the Advancement of Psychiatry, 1968.

Erikson EH: *Childhood and Society.* Norton, 1950.

Finch SM: *Fundamentals of Child Psychiatry.* Norton, 1960.

Freedman AM, Kaplan H: *Comprehensive Textbook of Psychiatry.* Williams & Wilkins, 1967.

Freud A: *Normality and Pathology in Childhood: Assessment of Development.* Internat Univ Press, 1965.

Green M, Haggerty RJ (editors): *Ambulatory Pediatrics.* Saunders, 1968.

Harrison SI, Carek DJ: *A Guide to Psychotherapy.* Little, Brown, 1966.

Helfer RE, Kempe CH: *The Battered Child.* Univ of Chicago Press, 1968.

Hoch P: *Depression.* Grune & Stratton, 1954.

Hoch P, Zubin J (editors): *Psychopathology of Childhood.* Grune & Stratton, 1953.

Hoffman L, Hoffman M (editors): *Review of Child Development Research.* Vol 2. Russell Sage Foundation, 1966.

Hollender M (editor): *The Psychology of Medical Practice.* Saunders, 1958.

Howells JO (editor): *Modern Perspectives in International Child Psychiatry.* Oliver & Boyd, 1969.

Kliman G: *Psychological Emergencies of Childhood.* Grune & Stratton, 1968.

Kanner L: *Child Psychiatry.* Thomas, 1962.

Patton RG, Gardner LI: *Growth Failure and Maternal Deprivation.* Thomas, 1963.

Pearson GHJ (editor): *A Handbook of Child Psychoanalysis.* Basic Books, 1968.

Psychoanalytic Study of the Child. Internat Univ Press, 1945–present. [Annual. Various editors.]

Schulman JL: *Management of Emotional Disorders in Pediatric Practice: With a Focus on Techniques of Interviewing.* Year Book, 1968.

Sex and the College Student. GAP Report No. 60. Group for the Advancement of Psychiatry, 1965.

Shaw CR (editor): *The Psychiatric Disorders of Childhood.* Appleton-Century-Crofts, 1966.

Shirley HF: *Pediatric Psychiatry.* Harvard Univ Press, 1963.

Slavson SR: *Analytic Group Psychotherapy With Children, Adolescents, and Adults.* Columbia Univ Press, 1950.

Solnit AJ, Provence S (editors): *Modern Perspectives in Child Development.* Internat Univ Press, 1963.

Verville E: *Behavior Problems of Children.* Saunders, 1967.

24...

Endocrine Disorders

Henry K. Silver, MD, & Ronald W. Gotlin, MD

Endocrine disorders are relatively frequent in childhood, and a knowledge of the endocrine system is essential in order to differentiate its disorders from congenital malformations and from normal variations in the timing and pattern of development (ie, "constitutional" deviations from average). One should attempt to understand the pathogenesis of endocrine abnormalities so that the physiologic and chemical evidences of specific hormonal dysfunctions can be correlated with structural abnormalities, particularly as they affect growth and development.

DISTURBANCES OF GROWTH & DEVELOPMENT

Disturbances of growth and development are the most common presenting complaints in the pediatric endocrine clinic. It is estimated that over 1 million children in the USA have abnormally short stature and that there are at least 10 million children whose growth is potentially abnormal.

Failure to thrive is a common complaint in infancy and is most often due to undernutrition.

Tall stature is a much less frequent presenting complaint than short stature and is usually a matter of concern only to adolescent girls. The recent trend toward acceptance of tall stature in women has decreased the number of young people evaluated and treated for tall stature.

SHORT STATURE

Abnormally short stature in relation to age is a common finding in childhood. In most instances it is due to a normal variation from the usual pattern of growth. The possible roles of such factors as sex, race, size of parents and other family members, nutrition, pubertal maturation, and emotional status must all be evaluated in the total assessment of the child.

The causes of unusually short stature are listed in Table 24–1. In most instances, the causes can be dif-

ferentiated on the basis of significant findings in the history and physical examination or by laboratory tests.

1. CONSTITUTIONAL SHORT STATURE

Many children have a constitutional delay in growth and skeletal maturation. Puberty is delayed. In all other respects, they appear entirely normal. There is often a history of a similar pattern of growth in one of the parents or other members of the family. Normal puberty eventually occurs, and these children usually reach normal adult height although at a later than average age.

In some children with constitutional short stature, the rate of growth may be decreased in the second year of life. At other times, and throughout childhood in most other children with the condition, the growth curve parallels the third percentile.

No treatment for the short stature is indicated. The child and his parents should be helped to understand the normality of the situation.

2. PITUITARY DWARFISM
(Growth Hormone Deficiency)

Growth hormone (GH) deficiency is an uncommon cause of short stature; approximately 1/2 of cases are idiopathic (rarely familial); the remainder are secondary to pituitary or hypothalamic disease (craniopharyngioma, infections, tuberculosis, sarcoidosis, toxoplasmosis, syphilis, trauma, reticuloendotheliosis, vascular anomalies, and other tumors such as gliomas). GH deficiency may be an isolated defect or may occur in combination with other pituitary hormone deficiencies. Idiopathic growth hormone deficiency affects both sexes equally. The idiopathic form associated with multiple hormone deficiencies is more common in males.

Physical examination may be unremarkable or there may be infantile fat distribution, youthful facial features, small hands and feet, and delayed sexual maturation. Excessive wrinkling of the skin is present

TABLE 24–1. Causes of short stature.

Familial, racial, or genetic

Constitutional retarded growth and delayed adolescence

Endocrine disturbances
Hypopituitarism
Isolated somatotropin deficiency
Somatotropin deficiency with other pituitary hormone deficiencies
Hypothyroidism
Adrenal insufficiency
Cushing's disease and Cushing's syndrome (including iatrogenic causes)
Sexual precocity (androgen or estrogen excess)
Diabetes mellitus (poorly controlled)
Diabetes insipidus
Hyperaldosteronism

Primordial short stature
Intrauterine growth retardation
Placental insufficiency
Intrauterine infection
Primordial dwarfism with premature aging
Progeria (Hutchinson-Gilford syndrome)
Progeroid syndrome
Werner's syndrome
Cachectic (Cockayne's syndrome)
Short stature without associated anomalies
Short stature with associated anomalies (eg, Seckel's bird-headed dwarfism, leprechaunism, Silver's syndrome, Bloom's syndrome, Cornelia de Lange syndrome, Hallerman-Streiff syndrome)

Inborn errors of metabolism
Altered metabolism of calcium or phosphorus (eg, hypophosphatemic rickets, hypophosphatasia, infantile hypercalcemia, pseudohypoparathyroidism)
Storage diseases
Mucopolysaccharidoses (eg, Hurler's syndrome, Hunter's syndrome)
Mucolipidoses (eg, generalized gangliosidosis, fucosidosis, mannosidosis)
Sphingolipidoses (eg, Tay-Sachs disease, Niemann-Pick disease, Gaucher's disease)
Miscellaneous (eg, cystinosis)
Aminoacidemias and aminoacidurias

Epithelial transport disorders (eg, renal tubular acidosis, cystic fibrosis, Bartter's syndrome, vasopressin resistant diabetes insipidus, pseudohypoparathyroidism)
Organic acidemias and acidurias (eg, methylmalonic aciduria, orotic aciduria, maple syrup urine disease, isovaleric acidemia)
Metabolic anemias (eg, sickle cell disease, thalassemia, pyruvate kinase deficiency)
Disorders of mineral metabolism (eg, Wilson's disease, magnesium malabsorption syndrome)
Body defense disorders (eg, Bruton's agammaglobulinemia, thymic aplasia, chronic granulomatous disease)

Constitutional (intrinsic) diseases of bone
Defects of growth of tubular bones or spine (eg, achondroplasia, metatropic dwarfism, diastrophic dwarfism, metaphyseal chondrodysplasia)
Disorganized development of cartilage and fibrous components of the skeleton (eg, multiple cartilaginous exostoses, fibrous dysplasia with skin pigmentation, precocious puberty of McCune-Albright)
Abnormalities of density of cortical diaphyseal structure or metaphyseal modeling (eg, osteogenesis imperfecta congenita, osteopetrosis, tubular stenosis)

Short stature associated with chromosomal defects
Autosomal (eg, Down's syndrome, cri du chat syndrome, trisomy 18)
Sex chromosomal (eg, Turner's syndrome-XO, penta X, XXXY)

Chronic systemic diseases, congenital defects, and malignancies (eg, chronic infection and infestation, inflammatory bowel disease, hepatic disease, cardiovascular disease, hematologic disease, CNS disease, pulmonary disease, renal disease, malnutrition, malignancies, collagen vascular disease)

Psychosocial dwarfism (maternal deprivation)

Miscellaneous syndromes (eg, arthrogryposis multiplex congenita, cerebrohepatorenal syndrome, Noonan's syndrome, Prader-Willi syndrome, Riley-Day syndrome) in older individuals. Dental development and epiphyseal maturation ("bone age") are delayed to a greater degree than height age (median age for patient's height). In cases resulting from CNS disease, headaches, visual field defects, abnormal skull x-rays, and symptoms of posterior pituitary insufficiency (polyuria and polydipsia) may precede or accompany the growth hormone deficiency.

Growth hormone deficiency is associated with low levels of GH in the serum and a failure of GH rise in response to arginine, insulin-induced hypoglycemia, or during normal physiologic sleep. Glucose-6-phosphate dehydrogenase deficiency, spontaneous hypoglycemia, augmented insulin sensitivity, and decreased gonadotropin levels may be present, as well as other pituitary hormone deficiencies.

The ideal treatment is with human pituitary growth hormone, but this agent is not commercially available. Protein anabolic agents (testosterone, fluoxymesterone, oxandrolone, norethandrolone, etc) may be effective in promoting linear growth, but these drugs may cause undue acceleration of epiphyseal closure with resultant limitation of growth potential and short stature in adult life.

3. HYPOTHYROIDISM

Hypothyroidism in childhood (see p 604) is usually associated with poor growth. In occasional cases, short stature may be the principal finding.

4. PRIMORDIAL SHORT STATURE

Primordial short stature may occur in a number of disorders, including craniofacial disproportion (eg, Seckel's bird-headed dwarfism), Silver's syndrome, some cases of progeric and cachectic dwarfism (eg, Hutchinson-Gilford dwarfism), or may occur in individuals with no accompanying significant physical abnormalities. Children with these conditions are small at birth; both birth weight and length are below normal for gestational age. They grow parallel to but below the third percentile. Plasma growth hormone levels are usually normal but may be elevated. In most instances, skeletal maturation ("bone age") corresponds to chronologic age or is only mildly retarded, in contrast to the striking delay often present in children with GH and thyroid deficiency.

There is no satisfactory treatment for primordial short stature, although growth hormone injections have been associated with a growth spurt in a small number of patients.

5. SHORT STATURE DUE TO EMOTIONAL FACTORS

Psychologic deprivation is a recognized cause of short stature and disturbances in motor and personality development. In some instances (deprivation dwarfism), in addition to being small, the child will have increased (often voracious) appetite and a marked delay in skeletal maturation. Plasma growth hormone levels are variable; the normal sleep-related circadian rise may be absent due to restless sleep. Polydipsia and polyuria sometimes occur. These children are of normal size at birth and grow normally for a variable period of time before growth stops. A history of feeding problems in early infancy is common. Emotional disturbances in the family are the rule.

Foster home placement or a significant change in the psychologic and emotional environment at home usually results in significantly improved growth, a decrease of appetite and dietary intake to more normal levels, and personality improvement.

DIFFERENTIAL DIAGNOSIS OF SHORT STATURE

Short stature may accompany or be caused by a large number of conditions (Table 24–1). When the etiologic diagnosis is not apparent from the history and physical examination, the following laboratory studies are useful in detecting the common causes of short stature:

(1) Complete blood count (to detect chronic anemia, infection, malignancies).

(2) Erythrocyte sedimentation rate (elevated in collagen vascular disease, malignancy, chronic infection, inflammatory bowel disease).

(3) Urinalysis and microscopic examination (occult pyelonephritis, glomerulonephritis, renal tubular disease, etc).

(4) Stool examination for occult blood, parasites, and parasite ova (inflammatory bowel disease, overwhelming parasitism).

(5) Serum electrolytes (mild adrenal insufficiency, renal tubular acidosis, etc).

(6) Blood urea nitrogen (occult renal insufficiency).

(7) Buccal smear and karyotyping (should be performed in all short girls with delayed sexual maturation with or without clinical features of Turner's syndrome).

(8) Thyroid function tests: PBI and T_4 (short stature may be the only sign of hypothyroidism).

(9) Growth hormone evaluation. Blood samples for growth hormone determination should be obtained during normal sleep or after administration of one of the conventional provocative agents (arginine, glucagon, Piromen, and insulin-induced hypoglycemia).

Samples obtained during the first 90 minutes of sleep are preferable since they demonstrate both the presence and the physiologic release of growth hormone.

Collipp PJ, Halle JD: Treatment of growth retardation. Pediat Digest, 30–36, March 1970.

Goodman HG, Grumbach MM, Kaplan SL: Growth and growth hormone. 2. A comparison of isolated growth hormone deficiency and multiple pituitary-hormone deficiency in 35 patients with idiopathic hypopituitary dwarfism. New England J Med 278:57–68, 1968.

Gotlin RW, Mace JW, Silver HK: Raised nyctohemeral (night and day) growth-hormone levels in conditions with primordial short stature. Lancet 1:626–627, 1971.

Gotlin RW, Mace JW: Diagnosis and management of short stature in childhood and adolescence. Curr Probl Pediat 2 (4,5), 1972.

Mace JW, Gotlin RW, Beck P: Sleep related human growth hormone release: A test of physiologic growth hormone secretion in children. J Clin Endocrinol 34:339–341, 1972.

Raiti S, Blizzard RM: Human growth hormone: Current knowledge regarding its role in normal and abnormal metabolic states. Advances Pediat 17:99–123, 1970.

Root AW, Bongiovanni AM, Eberlein WR: Diagnosis and management of growth retardation with special reference to the problem of hypopituitarism. Pediatrics 78:737–753, 1971.

Silver HK, Finkelstein M: Deprivation dwarfism. J Pediat 70:317–324, 1967.

Smith DW: Compendium on shortness of stature. J Pediat 70:463–519, 1967.

FAILURE TO THRIVE (FTT)

Failure to thrive is present when there is a perceptible declination of growth from an established pattern or when the patient's height and weight plot consistently below the third percentile. (The term is usually reserved for infants who for various reasons fail to gain weight.) Linear growth and head circumference may also be affected; when this occurs, the underlying condition is generally more severe. There are many reasons for failure to thrive (see below and Table 24–1), although a specific cause often cannot be established.

Classification & Etiologic Diagnosis

The diagnosis of failure to thrive is usually apparent on the basis of the history and physical examination. When it is not, it is helpful to compare the patient's chronologic age with the height age (median age for the patient's height), weight age, and head circumference. On the basis of these measurements, 3 principal patterns can be defined which provide a starting point in the diagnostic approach.

Group 1. (Most common type.) Normal head circumference; weight reduced out of proportion to height: In the majority of cases of failure to thrive, malnutrition is present as a result of either deficient caloric intake or malabsorption.

Group 2. Normal or enlarged head circumference for age; weight only moderately reduced, usually in proportion to height: Structural dystrophies, constitutional dwarfism, endocrinopathies.

Group 3. Subnormal head circumference; weight reduced in proportion to height: Primary CNS deficit; intrauterine growth retardation.

An initial period of observed nutritional rehabilitation, usually in a hospital setting, is often helpful in the diagnosis. The child should be placed on a regular diet for age and his intake and weight carefully plotted for 1–2 weeks. During this period, the presence of lactose intolerance is determined by checking pH and the presence of reducing substances in the stools. If stools are abnormal, the child should be further observed on a lactose-free diet. Caloric intake should be increased if weight gain does not occur but intake is well tolerated. The following 3 patterns are often noted during the rehabilitation period. Pattern 1 is by far the most common.

Pattern 1. (Most common type.) Intake adequate; weight gain satisfactory: Feeding technic at fault. Disturbed infant-mother relationship leading to decreased caloric intake.

Pattern 2. Intake adequate; no weight gain: If weight gain is unsatisfactory after increasing the calories to an adequate level (based on the infant's ideal weight for his height), malabsorption is a likely diagnosis.

If malabsorption is present, it is usually necessary to differentiate pancreatic exocrine insufficiency (cystic fibrosis) from abnormalities of intestinal mucosa (celiac disease). In cystic fibrosis, growth velocity commonly declines from the time of birth and appetite usually is voracious. In celiac disease, growth velocity is usually not reduced until 6–12 months of age and inadequate caloric intake may be a prominent feature.

Pattern 3. Intake inadequate:

(1) Sucking or swallowing difficulties: CNS or neuromuscular disease; esophageal or oropharyngeal malformations.

(2) Inability to eat large amounts is common in patients with cardiopulmonary disease or in anorexic children suffering from chronic infections, inflammatory bowel disease, and endocrine problems (eg, hypothyroidism). Patients with celiac disease often have inadequate caloric intake in addition to malabsorption.

(3) Vomiting: Upper intestinal obstruction (eg, pyloric stenosis), chronic metabolic aberrations and acidosis (eg, renal insufficiency, diabetes mellitus and insipidus, methylmalonic acidemia), increased intracranial pressure.

Laboratory Aids to Diagnosis

The laboratory may provide adjunctive information helpful in the differential.

A. Initial: Initial laboratory investigations at the time of admission might be limited to the following:

1. Blood—Complete blood count, sedimentation rate.

2. Urine—Urinalysis (including microscopic examination of sediment) and culture and colony count.

3. Stool—Culture, pH, reducing substances, and Hematest.

4. Tuberculin test.

5. Other tests as specifically indicated.

B. Definitive: The following laboratory investigations are recommended after the period of nutritional rehabilitation, when the patient has been classified in one of the 3 categories listed above.

1. Pattern 1—No further diagnostic laboratory tests are indicated. Maternal (and family) psychologic evaluation may be indicated.

2. Pattern 2—Evaluation of malabsorption.

a. Stool fat (72-hour specimen) on a diet with normal fat content.

b. Sweat chloride test.

c. Peroral small bowel biopsy with histology, analysis of intestinal disaccharidase activity, duodenal aspiration for pancreatic enzyme activity, culture and examination for *Giardia lamblia.*

d. Liver function tests (eg, serum alkaline phosphatase, serum bilirubin),

3. Pattern 3—

a. With vomiting—

(1) Serum electrolytes, pH, total CO_2, glucose, BUN, serum and urine osmolarities.

(2) Upper gastrointestinal series and cineesophagography.

(3) Skull x-rays for increased intracranial pressure.

b. Without vomiting—

(1) Sigmoidoscopy, rectal biopsy (ulcerative or granulomatous colitis).

(2) Barium enema (ulcerative colitis or Hirschsprung's disease).

(3) Upper gastrointestinal series and follow-through (regional enteritis, malrotations).

(4) Thyroid function test (eg, T_4, PBI).

C. Other Tests: Further evaluation (adrenal function tests, intravenous urograms, etc) may be indicated.

Treatment

Treatment will vary according to the underlying disorder. Most patients will gain weight and thrive on an adequate caloric intake. Maternal counseling and support are often required over a prolonged period. In some cases, foster home placement may be required.

Prognosis

The outcome is dependent on the underlying disorder. In general, infants whose length and, particularly, head circumference are affected along with weight have a less favorable prognosis.

Anderson CM: Intestinal malabsorption in childhood. Arch Dis Childhood 41:571–596, 1966.

Hannaway PJ: Failure to thrive: A study of 100 infants and children. Clin Pediat 9:96–99, 1970.

Kempe CH, Helfer R: *Helping the Battered Child and His Family.* Lippincott, 1972.

Kohler EE, Good TA: The infant who fails to thrive. Hosp Practice 4:54–61, 1969.

TALL STATURE

Tall stature is usually of concern only to adolescent and preadolescent girls. The upper limit of acceptable height of both sexes appears to be increasing, but there are occasions when the patient and her parents desire to influence the pattern of growth.

On the basis of family history, previous pattern of growth, stage of physiologic development, assessment of epiphyseal development ("bone age"), and standard growth data, the physician should make a tentative estimate of the patient's eventual height. Although there are several conditions (Table 24–2) which may produce tall stature, by far the most common cause is a constitutional variation from normal.

Reassurance and counseling should be tried first and are usually the only forms of therapy required. If the predicted height appears to be excessive, hormonal therapy with diethylstilbestrol or, preferably, conjugated estrogenic substances (Premarin), 1.25–5 mg daily orally (continuously or cyclically), may be tried. Estrogens are of little value when the physiologic age (as determined by stage of sexual maturity and epiphyseal development) has reached the 12-year-old level, and some studies indicate that they may be of little

TABLE 24–2. Causes of tall stature.

Constitutional (familial, genetic)

Endocrine causes
    Somatotropin excess (pituitary gigantism)
    Androgen excess (tall as children, short as adults)
        True sexual precocity
        Pseudosexual precocity
    Androgen deficiency (normal height as children, tall as adults)
        Klinefelter's syndrome
        Anorchia (infection, trauma, idiopathic)
    Hyperthyroidism

Genetic causes
    Klinefelter's syndrome
    Syndromes of XYY, XXYY (tall as adults)

Miscellaneous syndromes and entities
    Marfan's syndrome
    Cerebral gigantism (Soto's syndrome)
    Total lipodystrophy
    Diencephalic syndrome (rare)

value even when administered at earlier ages. Estrogens act to accelerate epiphyseal closure and may be continued until fusion occurs.

Because of the unknown long-term effects of hormone administration to children, these agents should be used with great caution.

Frasier SD, Smith FG: Effect of estrogens on mature height in tall girls: A controlled study. J Clin Endocrinol 28:416–419, 1968.

Mace JW, Gotlin RW: Cerebral gigantism: Triad of findings helpful in the diagnosis. Clin Pediat 9:662–667, 1970.

THYROID

FETAL DEVELOPMENT OF THE THYROID

By the seventh week of intrauterine development, the thyroid gland has migrated to its definitive location and the thyroglossal duct has atrophied. Cell differentiation and function progress over the next 7 weeks, and by the 14th week the thyroid is capable of hormone synthesis. At this stage, thyroid-stimulating hormone (TSH; thyrotropin) is detectable in the fetal serum and pituitary gland.

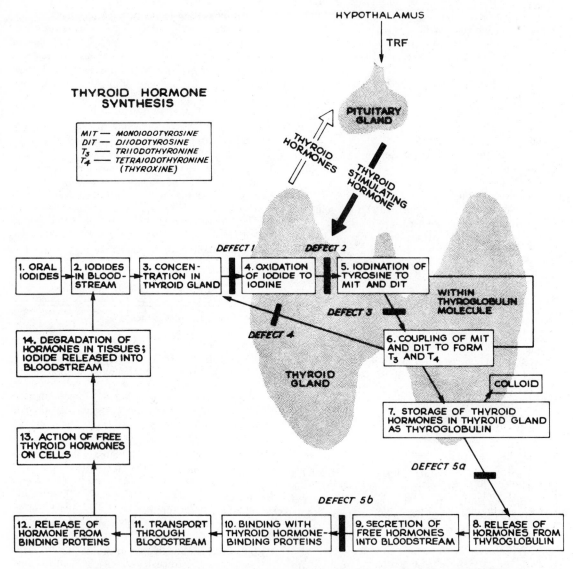

FIG 24–1. Synthesis of thyroxine (T_4) and triiodothyronine (T_3). (Adapted, with permission, from: Current Concepts of Thyroid Disease. [Programmed instruction course in *Spectrum.*] Pfizer Laboratories Division, Chas Pfizer & Co, Inc, 1965.) (See Table 24–3 for causes of defects.)

Under normal conditions, neither TSH nor thyroid hormone crosses the placenta in appreciable amounts, and the fetal pituitary-thyroid axis functions independently of, though in parallel with, the maternal pituitary-thyroid axis.

Trace amounts of free thyroxine (T_4) and triiodothyronine (T_3) are capable of transplacental passage, and administration of the latter in large doses has been recommended in pregnant women when a hypothyroid offspring is anticipated. Antithyroid drugs, including radioactive iodine, freely cross the placenta, and goitrous hypothyroid newborns may be born to hyperthyroid mothers who undergo treatment during pregnancy.

Although maternal TSH does not reach the fetus, pregnant hyperthyroid mothers may transmit long-acting thyroid stimulator (LATS) transplacentally, resulting in thyrotoxic newborns who may exhibit exophthalmos. Since LATS may be present in the serum of "controlled," previously hyperthyroid mothers, the possible transmission of LATS should be considered in all mothers in whom hyperthyroidism is or has been present.

Physiology

Under the stimulation of pituitary TSH, the thyroid gland traps, concentrates, and organifies iodine, synthesizes and couples mono- and diiodotyrosine, and releases active thyroid hormones into the circulation (Fig 24–1).

The quantity released is proportionate to the needs of the organism and is maintained by a negative feedback mechanism involving pituitary TSH and "free" thyroid hormone (Fig 24–2).

Active hormone produced in excess of physiologic needs is stored within the thyroid follicles as colloid. Upon release into the circulation, T_4 and T_3 are bound to thyroxine-binding globulin (TBG), albumin, and prealbumin. The binding affinity of TBG for T_4 is approximately 20 times greater than for T_3. A small percentage ($< 1\%$) of T_3 and T_4 is not bound but is "free" and exists in equilibrium with the "bound" form. The physiologic activity of thyroid hormone depends on the amount of free T_3 and T_4. The level of free hormone is determined by the total amount and binding affinity of the thyroid binding proteins.

Causes of Thyroid Disturbances

Physiologic disturbances of the thyroid gland may be due to the following causes:*

(1) Decreased thyroid tissue: Hypofunction may result from congenital aplasia or hypoplasia, destruction due to inflammatory disease (thyroiditis), neoplasm, antithyroid antibodies, thyroidectomy, or irradiation.

(2) Inborn errors in the synthesis of thyroid hormone: Defects may occur in any of the metabolic steps shown in Fig 24–1 as well as in the binding and release of T_4 and T_3 from thyroglobulin.

(3) Iodine deficiency.

*Adapted from Wilkins.

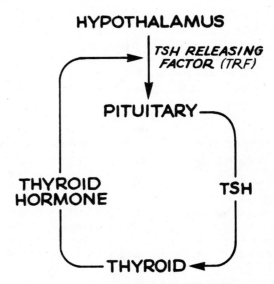

FIG 24–2. Pituitary-thyroid control.

(4) Inhibition of thyroidal iodide uptake and concentration by drugs (eg, thiocyanates, perchlorates, nitrates).

(5) Interference with thyroid enzyme activity by antithyroid compounds. Antithyroid compounds include thiourea, thiouracil and its derivatives, cobalt, large doses of iodides, and certain foods such as cabbage, turnips, and soybeans. Iodides also interfere with the release of thyroid hormone.

(6) Disorders of the hypothalamus and pituitary gland which result in impairment of thyrotropin secretion.

(7) Nervous stresses.

Release of Thyroid Hormone & Its Function

The principal functions of the thyroid gland are to synthesize and store T_4 and T_3 and to release them in response to bodily need. A number of chemical reactions are involved in thyroid hormone formation. The thyroid gland is regulated and stimulated by TSH; LATS is important only in certain disease states. TSH production may be inhibited by either endogenous or exogenous thyroid hormone. At birth, the PBI approximates that of the mother (6–11 μg/100 ml). There is a rapid increase (to 8–13.5 μg/100 ml) during the second to fifth days of life—particularly in the infant who has been allowed to become cool—and then a gradual decrease over several weeks or months.

The T_4 and PBI are low in various forms of hypothyroidism and may be reduced in subacute and chronic thyroiditis, hypopituitarism, nephrosis, cirrhosis, hypoproteinemia, malnutrition, and following therapy with T_3. Prolonged administration of high doses of adrenocorticosteroids as well as sulfonamides, testosterone, diphenylhydantoin (Dilantin), and salicylates may also produce a decrease in the PBI.

The PBI is high in hyperthyroidism and may be elevated in various forms of thyroiditis and hepatitis;

in some types of inborn errors in the synthesis, release, or binding of thyroid hormone; following the administration of estrogens or during pregnancy; and following the administration of various iodine-containing globulins. Individuals receiving T_4 usually have an elevated PBI even though they are maintained in the euthyroid state.

TBG is increased in pregnancy, after estrogen therapy (including oral contraceptives), occasionally as a genetic variation, in certain hepatic disorders, following administration of phenothiazines, and occasionally from unknown cause. TBG is decreased in familial TBG deficiency; following the administration of androgens or anabolic steroids; in nephrotic syndrome with marked hypoproteinemia; in some forms of hepatic disease; in patients receiving diphenylhydantoin; and as an idiopathic finding. T_4 and T_3 are the active components of the thyroid gland, comprising 90% and 10%, respectively, of active thyroid hormone. T_3 acts more rapidly but has a shorter duration of action; there is no marked qualitative difference in its metabolic effect. The thyroid hormones accelerate various oxidative systems, thus increasing the consumption of oxygen.

Editorial: Triiodothyronine. Lancet 1:898, 1971.

Raiti S & others: Evidence for the placental transfer of tri-iodothyronine in human beings. New England J Med 277:456, 1966.

Rall VE: Recent advances in the diagnosis of diseases of the thyroid. Clin chim acta 25:339–344, 1969.

See also General References, p 637, for additional discussions of the subjects in this chapter.

HYPOTHYROIDISM
(Congenital & Acquired [Juvenile] Hypothyroidism)

Essentials of Diagnosis

- Diminished physical activity, sluggish circulation, constipation, thick tongue, poor muscle tone, hoarseness, stunted growth, intellectual retardation.
- Thyroid function studies low (PBI, T_4, and erythrocyte T_3 binding).
- Delayed skeletal maturation. "Stippling" of epiphyses.

General Considerations

Thyroid hormone deficiency may be either congenital (with or without the physical features of cretinism) or acquired (juvenile hypothyroidism) and may be due to many causes.

Various types of enzymatic defects have been described (Table 24–3 and Fig 24–1) which result from inborn errors of metabolism. With the exception of that group associated with congenital nerve deafness (Pendred's syndrome), there are no distinguishing clinical features among the various types. In children who have enzymatic defects, thyroid enlargement may not be present in the newborn period but generally occurs within the first 2 decades of life. In general, enzymatic defects appear to have a familial autosomal recessive inheritance pattern.

In patients with the very rare iodide-trapping defect, the goiter is small and the uptake of radioactive iodine is negligible. In the other types, rapid uptake occurs and reaches peak levels in about 2 hours. Patients with a defect in iodide organification rapidly release labeled iodine from the gland; this release may be significantly and abnormally augmented by the administration of potassium thiocyanate or perchlorate. Comparison of the PBI and T_4 or BEI may be helpful in coupling and deiodinase defects, revealing a greater than normal discrepancy in the blood levels of these substances which reflects impaired thyroglobulin proteolysis, abnormal plasma binding, or the presence of abnormal circulating iodoproteins. Further clarification of the defect generally requires chromatographic fractionation of iodinated compounds in the serum, urine, and thyroid tissue.

A number of drugs and goitrogens taken during pregnancy (eg, cabbage, soybeans, aminosalicylic acid, thiourea derivatives, resorcinol, phenylbutazone, cobalt, and iodides in therapeutic doses for asthma—particularly in individuals who have also received adrenocortical steroids) have been reported to cause goiter and in some instances hypothyroidism also. Since many of these agents cross the placental barrier freely, they should be used with great caution during pregnancy. If taken by the pregnant woman, the goiter and decreased thyroid function that is produced in the newborn are generally transient and seldom a problem.

Many cases of acquired hypothyroidism, particularly in the presence of a history of goiter, appear to be the result of previously unsuspected lymphocytic thyroiditis.

Clinical Findings

The severity of the findings in cases of thyroid deficiency depends on the age at onset and the degree of interference with production of thyroid hormone. Congenital hypothyroidism may be recognized during the first month of life but may be so mild as to go unrecognized for months. Every effort should be made to establish the diagnosis of hypothyroidism as early as possible since untreated hypothyroidism may be associated with irreversible damage to the CNS.

A. Symptoms and Signs:

1. Functional changes—Even with congenital absence of the thyroid gland, the first finding may not appear for several days or weeks. Findings include physical and mental sluggishness; pale, gray, cool or mottled skin; decreased intestinal activity (constipation); large tongue; poor muscle tone, giving rise to a protuberant abdomen, umbilical hernia, and lumbar lordosis; hypothermia; bradycardia; diminished sweating (variable); decreased pulse pressure; hoarse voice or cry; delayed transient deafness; and slow relaxation on

TABLE 24-3. Causes of hypothyroidism.*

A. Congenital (Cretinism):
  1. Aplasia, hypoplasia, or associated with maldescent of thyroid—
    a. Embryonic defect of development.
    b. Autoimmune disease (?).
  2. Familial iodine-induced goiter secondary to metabolic inborn errors—
    a. Iodide transport defect (defect 1).
    b. Organification defect (defect 2)—
      (1) Lack of iodine peroxidase.
      (2) Lack of iodine transferase; Pendred's syndrome associated with congenital nerve deafness.
    c. Coupling defect (defect 3).
    d. Iodotyrosine deiodinase defect (defect 4).
    e. Abnormal iodinated polypeptide (defects 5a and 5b)—
      (1) Resulting from defect in intrathyroidal proteolysis of thyroglobulin.
      (2) Abnormal plasma binding preventing use of T_4 by peripheral cells.
    f. Possible inability of tissues to convert T_4 to T_3.
  3. Maternal ingestion of medications during pregnancy—
    a. Maternal radioiodine.
    b. Goitrogens (propylthiouracil, methimazole).
    c. Iodides.
  4. Iodide deficiency (endemic cretinism).
  5. Idiopathic.

B. Acquired (Juvenile Hypothyroidism):
  1. Thyroidectomy or radioiodine therapy for—
    a. Thyrotoxicosis.
    b. Cancer.
    c. Lingual thyroid.
    d. Isolated midline thyroid.
  2. Destruction by x-ray.
  3. Thyrotropin deficiency—
    a. Isolated.
    b. Associated with other pituitary tropic hormone deficiencies.
  4. TRF deficiency due to hypothalamic injury or disease.
  5. Autoimmune disease (lymphocytic thyroiditis).
  6. Chronic infections.
  7. Medications—
    a. Iodides—
      (1) Prolonged, excessive ingestion.
      (2) Deficiency.
    b. Cobalt.
  8. Idiopathic.

*"Defect 1" etc refers to specific defects in Fig 24-1.

---

eliciting tendon reflexes. Nasal obstruction and discharge and persistent jaundice may be present in the neonatal period.

The skin may be dry, thick, scaly, and coarse, with a yellowish tinge due to excessive deposition of carotene. The hair is dry, coarse, brittle (variable), and may be excessive. Lateral thinning of the eyebrows occurs. The axillary and supraclavicular fat pads may be prominent in infants. Muscular hypertrophy (Debré-Sémélaigne syndrome) occasionally is present.

2. Retardation of growth and development—Findings include shortness of stature, infantile skeletal proportions with relatively short extremities, infantile naso-orbital configuration (bridge of nose flat, broad, and underdeveloped; eyes seem to be widely spaced); delayed osseous development (retarded "bone age"); and retarded dental development. Slowing of mental responsiveness and retardation of development of the brain may occur, and in many cases a coincidental congenital malformation of the brain is present also.

3. Alterations in sexual development (usually retardation, sometimes precocity)—Menometrorrhagia in older girls; galactorrhea occasionally.

B. X-Ray Findings: Epiphyseal development ("bone age") is delayed. Centers of ossification, especially of the hip, may show multiple small centers or a single, stippled, porous or fragmented center (epiphy-seal dysgenesis). The cardiac shadow is increased. Coxa vara and coxa plana may occur.

C. Laboratory Findings: PBI and T_4 are decreased. Radioiodine uptake is below 10% (normal: 10–50%).* (Both may be normal or elevated in goitrous cretinism and in some cases of thyroiditis.) The binding of T_3 by erythrocytes or resin in vitro (T_3 test) is lowered. Serum cholesterol and carotene are usually elevated but often low or normal in infants and rarely low in older children; cessation of therapy in previously treated hypothyroid patients produces a marked rise in serum cholesterol levels in 6–8 weeks. The BMR is low, but the test is difficult to perform and unreliable in children. With primary hypothyroidism, the plasma TSH is elevated. Urinary creatine excretion is decreased and creatinine increased. Serum alkaline phosphatase is occasionally reduced and urinary hydroxyproline is low. Circulating autoantibodies to thyroid constituents are present in about 50% of patients. Erythrocyte glucose-6-phosphate dehydrogenase activity is decreased. Plasma growth hormone may be decreased, with subnormal response to insulin-induced hypoglycemia and arginine stimulation.

*The presence of iodides in bread in recent years has resulted in significant decrease in normal values of radioiodine uptake. The normal levels for any particular area should be ascertained.

Differential Diagnosis

The various causes of primary hypothyroidism due to intrinsic defects of the thyroid gland must be differentiated from pituitary failure with secondary thyroid insufficiency as a result of a deficiency of TSH. PBI and radioactive iodine uptake studies before and after exogenous TSH administration (5–10 units daily for 3 days) are useful in differentiation. Since pituitary insufficiency may be associated with both secondary hypoadrenocorticism as well as secondary hypothyroidism, treatment of the latter alone may precipitate an adrenal crisis.

Down's syndrome, chondrodystrophy, generalized gangliosidosis, I-cell disease, Hurler's and Hunter's syndromes, and certain other causes of short stature as well as macroglossia due to abnormalities of the lymphatics of the tongue can all be readily distinguished by the clinical manifestations and by appropriate laboratory studies. Although other individual findings of the hypothyroid child may suggest exogenous obesity, congenital heart disease, or some type of anemia as the primary diagnosis, a careful appraisal of the entire clinical and laboratory picture should permit establishment of the proper diagnosis.

Treatment

A. Medical Treatment: Desiccated thyroid and L-thyroxine are the drugs of choice. Give desiccated thyroid, 15–30 mg daily, or the equivalent of sodium levothyroxine (60 mg desiccated thyroid = 0.1 mg levothyroxine), for 1–2 weeks. Use the smaller dose for markedly myxedematous infants. Increase dosage by 15 mg every 1–2 weeks to 60 mg daily. Most younger children eventually need 60–150 mg/day; older children will require 90–180 mg daily. Serum T_4 (preferred) or PBI or the T_3 test may be used as a guide to adequate therapy; or the dosage of replacement therapy may be determined by increasing the dose of hormone until toxic manifestations appear and then maintaining the patient on a slightly lower dose.

The hypothyroid patient is quite responsive to thyroid, usually shows improvement 7–21 days after starting therapy, and is very sensitive to slight excesses of thyroid hormone. The normal individual can take comparatively large doses of thyroid with very little effect. If a patient can tolerate significantly more than the usual therapeutic doses of thyroid hormone (> 130 mg in the young child, > 220 mg in the older child), the diagnosis of hypothyroidism should be questioned.

Triiodothyronine (sodium liothyronine, Cytomel) may be employed when a more rapid and short-lived effect is desired (eg, in the TSH suppression test) but probably is not as effective in young children as desiccated thyroid or levothyroxine. If levothyroxine or triiodothyronine is administered, the PBI and T_4 may be difficult to interpret. In the treatment of neonatal goiter with or without hypothyroidism resulting from drugs and goitrogens taken by the pregnant woman, temporary treatment with triiodothyronine or levothyroxine is sufficient to bring about rapid disappearance of the enlargement.

B. Surgical Measures: Rarely, respiratory obstruction may occur, requiring surgical excision of the thyroid isthmus (rather than tracheostomy).

Burke G: Thyroid stimulators and thyroid stimulation. Acta endocrinol 66:558–576, 1971.

Rall VE: Recent advances in the diagnosis of diseases of the thyroid. Clin chim acta 25:339–344, 1969.

Reichlin S, Utiger R: Regulation of the pituitary-thyroid axis in man: Relationship of TSH concentration to concentration of free and total thyroxin in plasma. J Clin Endocrinol 27:251–255, 1967.

HYPERTHYROIDISM

Essentials of Diagnosis

- Nervousness, fatigability, emotional lability, tremor, excessive perspiration, temperature intolerance.
- Exophthalmos, goiter, bruit over thyroid, tachycardia.
- PBI, radioiodine uptake, and other thyroid function studies elevated.

General Considerations

The cause of hyperthyroidism has not been determined, but psychic trauma, psychologic maladjustments, disturbances in pituitary function, infectious disease, heredity, imbalance of the endocrine system, and immunologic disease all have been incriminated. Regardless of the inciting event or agent, the mediation of the disease process is usually by long-acting thyroid stimulator (LATS), an antibody produced by the lymphocytes. Transient congenital hyperthyroidism may occur in infants of thyrotoxic mothers, usually as a consequence of the transplacental passage of LATS. Infantile and early childhood hyperthyroidism may occur, apparently as a familial disease, in the absence of transplacental passage of LATS. Hyperthyroidism may be found with tumors of the thyroid, other tumors producing thyrotropin-like substances, and with exogenous thyroid hormone excess.

Clinical Findings

A. Symptoms and Signs: Hyperthyroidism is much more common in females than in males. The disease is most likely to appear in childhood at 12–14 years, but it may develop at any age and usually progresses rapidly. Findings include weakness, dyspnea, emotional instability, "nervousness" (inability to sit still), marked variability in mood, tremors and movements which may simulate chorea, personality disturbances, warm and moist skin, flushed face, palpitation, tachycardia (even during sleep), systolic hypertension with increased pulse pressure, and dysphagia. Proptosis and exophthalmos are common in hyperthyroid children. Goiter is present in more than 80% of cases and is characteristically diffuse and usually firm. A bruit and thrill may be present. Variable degrees of accelerated growth and development occur, and loss of weight is common in spite of polyphagia. (An occasional adolescent may gain weight.) Amenorrhea is common in adolescent girls. There is an increased incidence of diabetes mellitus in thyrotoxicosis.

B. Laboratory Findings: The T_4 and PBI are elevated;* there is increased binding of radioactive T_3 to shed blood or resin in the T_3 test; radioiodine uptake is above 35–40% at 24 hours and suppressed less than 40% after administration of T_3 (25 μg 3–4 times daily for 7 days). BMR is elevated, but the test is frequently unreliable and is seldom used. Serum cholesterol is low; glycosuria may occur. Agglutinating antibodies to thyroglobulin are found in most patients. Circulating TSH is usually not demonstrable; LATS is often present in plasma (particularly in the newborn infant). Erythrocyte glucose-6-phosphate dehydrogenase activity is increased. Urinary hydroxyproline is increased, and urinary creatine may be elevated.

C. X-Ray Findings: Abnormal skull x-rays are found rarely in some patients with primary pituitary disease. Skeletal maturation may be accelerated; in the newborn it may be associated with subsequent premature closure of the cranial sutures.

Differential Diagnosis

Although the well established case of hyperthyroidism seldom presents a problem in diagnosis, the findings in the early stage of the disease may be confused with chorea, or, more commonly, with the euthyroid child with a goiter (usually an adolescent girl) who is nervous, emotionally labile, and manifests a rapid pulse and increased perspiration. Careful and sometimes repeated clinical and laboratory evaluation may be required before the proper diagnosis can be established. Moreover, it should be recognized that thyrotoxic symptoms may occur with thyroiditis and rarely with thyroid cancer.

Various states with signs of hypermetabolism (severe anemia, leukemia, chronic infections, pheochromocytoma, as well as muscle wasting disease) may occasionally be confused with hyperthyroidism, but differentiation can usually be readily made by the clinical manifestations and by appropriate laboratory studies.

Treatment

The course of hyperthyroidism may exhibit fluctuations of improvement and remission. In some mild cases therapy may not be required.

Both surgical and medical methods are available for treating the manifestations of hyperthyroidism.

A. General Measures: Rest in bed is advisable only in severe cases, in preparation for surgery, or at the

beginning of a medical regimen. The diet should be high in calories, carbohydrates, and vitamins (particularly vitamin B_1).

Fairly large doses of barbiturates or tranquilizers (or both) may be necessary to control symptoms of nervous instability. Sympatholytic drugs, eg, reserpine in combination with one of the barbiturates, may diminish symptoms without altering thyroid function. Propranolol (Inderal), a beta-adrenergic blocking agent, may be helpful in controlling serious cardiac complications.

B. Medical Treatment: With medical treatment, clinical response may be noted in 2–3 weeks and adequate control in 1–3 months. The thyroid frequently increases in size after initiation of treatment but usually will decrease in size within several months.

1. Propylthiouracil—This drug interferes with the binding of iodine to thyroid protein and with hormone synthesis. The correct dose must always be individually assessed. Propylthiouracil may be used in the initial treatment of the patient with hyperthyroidism, but if the T_4 or PBI fails to return to a normal range—or if they rise rapidly with reduction in drug dosage after 18–24 months of therapy—continued or alternative therapy may be necessary. Relapses occur in 10–30% of cases, and severe cases may not respond. Therapy should be continued for at least 2–3 years with the smallest drug dosage that will produce a euthyroid state. The safety of prolonged treatment has not been evaluated.

a. Initial dosage—75–300 mg/day in 3–4 divided doses 6–8 hours apart until tests of thyroid function are normal and all signs and symptoms have subsided. Larger doses may be necessary.

b. Maintenance—50–100 mg/day in 2–3 divided doses. Some authors recommend continuing the drug at higher levels until the euthyroid state is approached or reached and then giving oral thyroid. Thyroid may also be given if the gland enlarges significantly or remains enlarged after 2–3 months with propylthiouracil therapy.

c. Toxicity—Granulocytopenia, fever, and rash may occur. Discontinue the drug and consider giving antibiotics and a short course of one of the adrenocortical steroids.

2. Methimazole (Tapazole)—This drug may be used in 1/10–1/15 the dosage of propylthiouracil. However, toxic reactions may be more common with methimazole than with propylthiouracil.

3. Iodide—Medical treatment with continuous iodide administration alone usually produces a rapid response but is generally not recommended since the effectiveness of iodide is usually short-lived; a progressive increase in dosage is often required for satisfactory control; and toxic reactions to iodide are not uncommon.

C. Surgical Measures: Subtotal thyroidectomy is considered by many to be the treatment of choice, especially when a close follow-up of the patient is difficult or impossible. In childhood, surgery should be employed in patients when medical treatment is impos-

---

*Certain organic iodine compounds, eg, iophenoxic acid (Teridax) may cause prolonged elevation of the PBI. If administered to the mother, they may cross the placenta in significant amounts and will affect the infant's PBI for months to years.

sible or has been unsuccessful. The patient should be prepared first with bed rest, diet, and sedation (as above), and with iodide and propylthiouracil as follows: Propylthiouracil (as above) should be given for 2–4 weeks. Iodide (as saturated solution of potassium iodide) is added 10–21 days before surgery is scheduled. Iodides act by blocking the effect of TSH on the thyroid, with resultant decrease in iodine trapping (with reduction of vascularity), and by inhibiting the release of hormone, thus reducing the possibility of thyroid storm. Give 1–10 drops daily for 10–21 days. Continue the drug for 1 week after surgery.

Progressive exophthalmos following surgery is uncommon in childhood.

D. Radiation Therapy: X-ray and radioactive iodine (^{131}I) generally are not recommended in children because of the possibility of an ultimate increased incidence of cancer, but the significance of this relationship remains to be proved.

E. Congenital (Transient) Hyperthyroidism: Temporary treatment of congenital hyperthyroidism may be necessary, in which case iodides appear to be the drugs of choice. Reserpine or propranolol may be necessary to control cardiac arrhythmias. Transection of an enlarged thyroid isthmus may be of value if respiratory distress is present.

Course & Prognosis

Improvement may occur without therapy in as many as 1/3 of cases, but partial remissions and exacerbations may continue for several years. With medical treatment alone, prolonged remissions may be expected in 1/2–2/3 of cases. Surgical therapy probably yields about the same number of satisfactory results. Postoperative hypothyroidism is not uncommon, and hypoparathyroidism and other complications may occur after surgery. Because of the comparatively high incidence of carcinoma in nodular goiters of childhood, such glands should be removed routinely once the thyrotoxicosis is in remission.

Congenital hyperthyroidism has a significant mortality in the neonatal period, but the eventual prognosis in surviving infants is excellent.

Burke G: The long-acting thyroid stimulation of Graves' disease. Am J Med 45:435–450, 1968.

Hollingsworth DR, Mabry CC, Eckerd JM: Neonatal and early childhood hyperthyroidism: An expression of hereditary Graves' disease. Page 72 in: *Program and Abstracts of the Society for Pediatric Research*, 1971.

Sunshine P, Kusumoto H, Kriss JB: Survival time of circulating long-acting thyroid stimulation in neonatal thyrotoxicosis: Implications for diagnosis and therapy of the disorder. Pediatrics 36:869–876, 1965.

Wilroy RS, Etteldorf JN: Familial hyperthyroidism including 2 siblings with neonatal Graves' disease. J Pediat 78:625–632, 1971.

SIMPLE GOITER

Essentials of Diagnosis

- Enlarged thyroid gland.
- Functional activity of the gland is variable.
- BMR, PBI, serum cholesterol, and radioactive iodine uptake normal, elevated, or decreased.

General Considerations

Goiter or struma is any enlargement of the thyroid gland. It has recently been noted with increasing frequency in children and adolescents. Enlargement of the thyroid may result from inflammation, infiltrative processes, or neoplasms, but in most instances the goiter is produced by the action of a relative excess of TSH or LATS. These may develop autonomously or in response to an increased need for thyroid hormone. When the level of circulating hormone is inadequate, the pituitary usually produces more TSH in an attempt to stimulate the thyroid gland to increased activity.

The enlarged gland may vary greatly in size, shape, and consistency; regardless of these characteristics, the functional activity of the gland may be normal (euthyroid), decreased (hypothyroid), or increased (hyperthyroid). If augmented production is sufficient to produce physiologic quantities of hormone, the individual will be euthyroid; but if maximum stimulation of the thyroid is still associated with deficient production, hypothyroidism results.

Goiters resulting from deficient production of thyroid hormone are seen in children with inborn enzymatic defects, those with both iodine deficiency and excess, and when ingestion of antithyroid drugs or naturally occurring goitrogens has interfered with normal hormonogenesis.

Goiters may also be found in hyperthyroidism, various forms of thyroiditis, tumors, hemorrhage, infiltration with amyloid, and in an idiopathic form, particularly during adolescence. The administration of various drugs (aminosalicylic acid, thiourea derivatives, resorcinol, phenylbutazone, iodides, and cobalt) may be associated with the development of goiter.

Other causes of goiter are discussed above (pp 604–607) and in the following sections.

Classification

A. Neonatal Goiter: Infants whose mothers are deficient in iodine or have been receiving iodides or antithyroid hormones may be born with goiters or may develop them during the first few days of life. The goiter is diffuse and relatively soft but may be large enough to compress the trachea, esophagus, and adjacent blood vessels.

Regression usually occurs in a few weeks. It may be hastened by the administration of small doses of thyroid. If evidence of hyperthyroidism appears, therapy with iodine or thiouracil drugs (or both) for a few weeks may be necessary.

B. Nodular Goiter: Nodular goiter can occur in childhood, and the presence of one or more nodules in the thyroid gland of a child raises the possibility of malignancy. A thyroid nodule is more likely to be malignant in a child than in an adult. Nodules may also occur in chronic thyroiditis or may be the result of cyst formation, hemangiomas, or lymphangiomas.

The likelihood that a nodule is malignant increases when the nodule is single, hard, associated with paratracheal lymph node enlargement, or does not concentrate radioactive iodine. In the absence of these characteristics, nodular goiter in childhood should be treated with full replacement doses of desiccated thyroid or L-thyroxine for a period of 1–2 months. If the nodule fails to decrease in size, it should be removed. Nodules occurring in other conditions (chronic thyroiditis, etc) should also be followed carefully because they too may be associated with an increased risk of malignancy.

C. Goiter With Normal Thyroid Function: Goiter unaccompanied by manifestations of altered thyroid function may occur without apparent cause in non-endemic areas. It is more likely to become evident early in adolescence and is more common in females. In most cases, histologic changes are compatible with chronic lymphocytic thyroiditis (see below).

Clinical Findings

The thyroid is large and soft; bruits and thrills may be present, and occasionally a nodule may be palpable. Usually there is no associated disturbance of function, although in some instances mild hypothyroidism may occur. Symptoms of pressure due to goiter are very uncommon in childhood. Serum T_4 and PBI and radioiodine uptakes are usually normal but may be elevated or reduced.

Prevention

Prevention in endemic areas consists of the use of iodized salt containing 1 mg of iodine per 100 gm of salt, or the administration of an iodide-containing drug. Routine iodinization of the water supply is also a satisfactory preventive measure.

Treatment

Remove or avoid precipitating factors if possible. Desiccated thyroid, 65–195 mg daily orally, is of value when treatment is necessary. Iodine therapy alone is usually not effective.

Surgery is occasionally necessary if significant pressure symptoms persist or for possible malignancy if a nodular lesion fails to regress despite therapy with thyroid hormone.

Course & Prognosis

Simple adolescent goiter usually subsides without treatment, but therapy will hasten shrinking. Iodine is specific for goiters due to iodine deficiency. Recent evidence suggests that many cases of adolescent goiter are the result of chronic lymphocytic thyroiditis.

Silver HK, Gotlin RW: Goiter in infancy and childhood. Postgrad Med 42:133–138, 1967.

ACUTE THYROIDITIS

Acute thyroiditis is uncommon but may occur after various infections, including those of the skin, pharynx, or larynx. At present, acute thyroiditis is apt to be the result of viral infections (mumps, adenovirus, measles, cat scratch fever, etc) or may be caused by bacteria (streptococci, pneumococci, staphylococci). There is usually no associated endocrine disturbance. Specific antibiotic therapy, if available, should be administered. Adrenocortical steroids may be of value.

Gillie RB: Endemic goiter. Sc Am 224:92, 1971.
See also Silver & Gotlin reference, above.

SUBACUTE THYROIDITIS

Subacute thyroiditis (DeQuervain's giant cell thyroiditis, granulomatous thyroiditis, giant cell thyroiditis) is rare in this country. In most cases the cause cannot be identified. Subacute thyroiditis is characterized by an insidious onset, fever, malaise, sore throat, dysphagia, pain in the thyroid gland that may radiate to the ears, and mild and transient manifestations of hypermetabolism. The thyroid gland is firm, and the enlargement may be confined to one lobe. The PBI is elevated and the radioiodine uptake is usually reduced.

The disease is usually self-limited and of short duration, but it may persist for years. Thyroid hormone preparations and adrenocorticosteroids have been employed with variable success in the treatment of serious cases.

Greene JN: Subacute thyroiditis. Am J Med 51:97–108, 1971.
See also Silver & Gotlin reference, above.

CHRONIC LYMPHOCYTIC THYROIDITIS
(Chronic Autoimmune Thyroiditis, Hashimoto's Thyroiditis, Lymphadenoid Goiter)

Essentials of Diagnosis

- Firm, freely movable, and diffusely enlarged goiter.
- PBI relatively higher than T_4 or BEI.
- Antibodies to various thyroid gland fractions.

General Considerations

Chronic lymphocytic thyroiditis is being seen with increasing frequency in all age groups and currently is the most common cause of goiter in childhood. In children and adolescents, it has a peak incidence between the ages of 8–15 years and occurs most commonly in females. The exact cause is not known, but many authors believe chronic thyroiditis to be associated with an "autoimmune phenomenon" since antibodies to various thyroid gland fractions have been reported in many cases. Antibody formation is believed to be stimulated by the release of abnormal thyroid gland proteins which then act as antigens. At present there is no conclusive evidence that antithyroid antibodies actually initiate the changes involving normal thyroid tissue, and the finding of "autoantibodies" has neither been consistent nor unique to chronic thyroiditis.

Clinical Findings

A. Symptoms and Signs: The goiter is characteristically firm, freely movable, nontender, and diffusely enlarged, although it may be asymmetrical, "pebbly," and tender. In long-standing cases, nodules and malignant changes have been described. The onset is usually insidious. Most cases occur without clinical manifestations and are completely painless. The symptoms consist mainly of moderate tracheal compression with a sense of fullness, hoarseness, and dysphagia. There are no local signs of inflammation and no evidence of systemic infection.

B. Laboratory Findings: Laboratory findings may be variable. The PBI may be normal, elevated, or depressed; but there is usually a significantly increased difference between the level of PBI and T_4 or BEI, with the former being higher. Radioactive iodine uptake is usually elevated at 4–6 hours, but the iodine is not bound normally to thyroglobulin and is instead transferred to metabolically inactive pools where it may subsequently be released at an abnormally rapid rate. The enhanced release is reflected by a low 24-hour radioiodine uptake value. The rate of release is increased after the administration of perchlorate or thiocyanate.

Treatment

The treatment of choice for autoimmune thyroiditis is thyroid hormone in full therapeutic doses. Approximately 1/3–1/2 of patients will have a good response. Adrenocorticosteroids have been used and do produce a reduction in the size of the gland, but the gland usually enlarges again when corticosteroids are discontinued. Subtotal thyroidectomy is occasionally necessary when the gland is particularly large and fails to respond adequately to medical therapy. Regardless of the type of treatment employed, hypothyroidism is a common end result.

Greenberg AH & others: Juvenile chronic lymphocytic thyroiditis: Clinical, laboratory and histological correlations. J Clin Endocrinol 30:293–301, 1970.

Humbert JR & others: Lymphocytic (autoimmune Hashimoto's) thyroiditis. Arch Dis Childhood 43:227, 1968.

Ling SM & others: Euthyroid goiters in children: Correlation of needle biopsy with other clinical and laboratory findings in chronic lymphocytic thyroiditis and simple goiter. Pediatrics 44:695–708, 1969.

Silver HK, Gotlin RW: Goiter in infancy and childhood. Postgrad Med 42:133–138, 1967.

RIEDEL'S STRUMA
(Chronic Fibrous Thyroiditis, Woody Thyroiditis, Invasive Thyroiditis)

Riedel's struma is rare in this country, particularly in children. The cause is not known, but the disease may represent a late stage of chronic lymphocytic thyroiditis. The disease is characterized by marked and invasive fibrosis which extends beyond the thyroid gland to involve the trachea, esophagus, blood vessels, nerves, and muscles of the neck, so that the gland becomes fixed to these tissues. Since differentiation from carcinoma of the thyroid is usually impossible by clinical means alone, the diagnosis is usually made by surgical biopsy.

Adrenocorticosteroids may be helpful, but surgery is frequently necessary to relieve fibrotic obstruction or constriction of neighboring structures.

Greene JN: Subacute thyroiditis. Am J Med 51:97–108, 1971.

CARCINOMA OF THE THYROID

Carcinoma of the thyroid is uncommon in childhood, but there is evidence that its incidence is increasing. In a significant number of cases, a history of irradiation, particularly to the neck and chest, can be obtained. The most prominent findings are localized thyroid enlargement, neck discomfort, dysphagia, and voice changes of recent onset. The thyroid gland may be fixed to surrounding tissues. Thyroid function studies are normal.

Papillary carcinoma is the most common form in childhood, and the prognosis with treatment is relatively good, with a survival rate greater than 80% after 10–20 years. Surgical extirpation of the entire gland and removal of all involved lymph nodes is the treatment of choice. Radical neck dissection is seldom necessary. About 1–2 months following surgery, when the patient has become definitely hypothyroid, a diagnostic scan should be carried out with radioactive iodine; if metastases are found, they should be removed or treated with therapeutic doses of radioactive iodine. Replacement therapy with thyroid hormone is initiated and continued for about 6–12 months, at which time thyroid therapy is temporarily withdrawn and the patient rescanned after becoming mildly hypothyroid. Follow-up scanning and skeletal survey by x-ray is recommended at yearly intervals.

Other less common malignant tumors of the thyroid include follicular, medullary, and undifferentiated carcinomas, lymphomas, and sarcoma. The treatment and prognosis depends on the cell type present.

Silver HK, Gotlin RW: Goiter in infancy and childhood. Postgrad Med 42:133–138, 1967.

THE PARATHYROIDS

HYPOPARATHYROIDISM

Essentials of Diagnosis

- Tetany with numbness, tingling, cramps, carpopedal spasm, positive Trousseau and Chvostek signs, loss of consciousness, convulsions.
- Photophobia, candidal infections, defective nails and teeth, cataracts, and calcific bodies in the subcutaneous tissues and basal ganglia.
- Serum calcium low; serum phosphorus high; alkaline phosphatase normal, azotemia absent.

General Considerations

Hypoparathyroidism may be idiopathic (possibly as the result of an autoimmune phenomenon) or may result from parathyroidectomy. Hypoparathyroidism may develop following thyroidectomy, when it may appear acutely (with variable severity of symptoms) or insidiously over several years and may be transient or permanent. Parathyroid deficiency has been reported following x-ray radiation of the neck or the administration of therapeutic doses of radioactive iodine for carcinoma of the thyroid. Transient hypoparathyroidism may occur in the neonate; in the offspring of hyperparathyroid or diabetic mothers; or as a physiologic variation in some infants, particularly those who have received a milk formula with a high phosphate/calcium ratio.

Idiopathic, apparently autoimmune hypoparathyroidism with demonstrable antibodies to parathyroid tissue, is frequently associated with candidal infection, Addison's disease, pernicious anemia, thyroiditis, and steatorrhea. Congenital absence of the parathyroids may occur in association with congenital absence of the thymus (with resultant thymic dependent immunologic deficiency) and cardiovascular, cerebral, and ocular defects (DiGeorge's syndrome).

Clinical Findings

A. Symptoms and Signs: Prolonged hypocalcemia causes tetany (see below), photophobia, blepharo-spasm, diarrhea, chronic conjunctivitis, cataracts, numbness of the extremities, poor dentition, skin rashes, alopecia, ectodermal dysplasias, candidal infections, "idiopathic" epilepsy, or symmetrical punctate calcifications of basal ganglia. In early infancy, respiratory distress may be the presenting finding.

Tetany is manifested by numbness, cramps, and twitchings of the extremities; carpopedal spasm and laryngospasm; positive Chvostek sign (tapping of the face in front of the ear produces spasm of the facial muscles), positive peroneal sign (tapping the fibular side of the leg over the peroneal nerve produces abduction and dorsiflexion of the foot), positive Trousseau sign (prolonged compression of the upper arm produces carpal spasm), and positive Erb sign (use of a galvanic current to determine hyperexcitability); unexplained bizarre behavior, irritability, loss of consciousness, convulsions, and retarded physical and mental development. Headache, vomiting, diarrhea, increased intracranial pressure, papilledema, and pseudopapilledema may occur. The symptoms of hypocalcemic tetany may be confused with respiratory or metabolic alkalosis or primary hyperaldosteronism.

B. Laboratory Findings: (Table 24–5.) Serum calcium is decreased; serum phosphorus increased; serum alkaline phosphatase usually normal. Urinary excretion of calcium and phosphorus is decreased. The Ellsworth-Howard test is positive, ie, there is a markedly increased excretion of urinary phosphorus following a single intravenous injection (2 ml) of parathyroid extract. False-negative results are common. There is a rise in serum calcium, a fall in serum phosphorus, and an increase in urine phosphate following the intramuscular injection of parathyroid extract, 5–10 ml in divided doses daily for 3–4 days. Renal clearance of phosphorus is decreased and the maximum tubular reabsorption of phosphorus is high.

C. X-Ray Findings: Soft tissue and cerebral (basal ganglia) calcification may occur in idiopathic hypoparathyroidism.

Differential Diagnosis

The differential diagnosis of hypoparathyroidism includes pseudohypoparathyroidism (Table 24–4) and the other causes of hypocalcemia listed in Table 24–5. The presence of convulsions may suggest epilepsy and other chronic disorders of the CNS, while the combination of findings referable to the CNS (headache, vomiting, increased intracranial pressure, and convulsions) may make the differentiation from brain tumor difficult.

Other causes of cataracts and basal ganglia calcification as well as chronic diarrhea also enter into the differential diagnosis.

Treatment

The objective of treatment is to increase and maintain the serum calcium at an approximately normal level. A simple, practical method of regulating therapy is with the Sulkowitch urine test, but this test may not always accurately reflect hypercalciuria, particularly in infants.

TABLE 24–4. Differential features of hypoparathyroid states.

	Hypoparathyroidism	Pseudo-hypoparathyroidism	Pseudopseudo-hypoparathyroidism
Genetic features	May be familial.	X-linked dominant "complete"	X-linked dominant "incomplete"
Associated clinical features	Often associated with Addison's disease, candidiasis, and occasionally chronic thyroiditis, pernicious anemia, and diabetes mellitus.	Candidiasis absent	Candidiasis absent
Physical features			
Mental subnormality	Common	Common	Common
Short stature	Occasionally	Common	Common
Hand deformities	Absent	Common	Common
Round face	Rare	Common	Common
Tetany	Common	Common	Absent
Seizures	40–50%	40–50%	Rare
Abnormal calcification			
Intracranial	Common	Common	Uncommon
Subcutaneous	Rare or absent	Common	Rare
Cataracts	Common	Common	Uncommon
Serum			
Calcium	Low	Low	Normal
Phosphorus	Normal to high	Normal to high	Normal
Alkaline phosphatase	Normal to high	Normal to high	Normal to high
Urine			
Calcium	Normal to low	Normal to low	Normal
Phosphorus	Low	Low	Normal to low
Renal response to parathyroid hormone	Responsive (may be hyperresponsive)	Resistant	Slightly responsive

TABLE 24–5. Laboratory findings in hypocalcemia.*†

	Serum Concentration			Urinary Excretion		Bone Pathology
	Ca++	P	Ptase	Ca++	P	
Hypoparathyroidism	↓	↑	N	N or ↓	↓	Usually none
Pseudohypoparathyroidism	↓	↑	N	N or ↓	↓	Tendency to congenital malformations
Renal insufficiency, glomerular	N or ↓	↑	N or ↑	↓	↓	Possible osteitis fibrosis.
Renal insufficiency, tubular	↓	↓	↑	↑	↑	Rickets, osteomalacia
Infantile rickets	N or ↓	↓	↑	↓	↓	Rickets
Tetany of newborn	↓	N or ↑	N	N or ↓	N or ↓	
Steatorrhea	↓	N or ↓	↑	↓	↓	Rickets, osteomalacia
Postacidotic hypocalcemia	↓	↓	N	↓ (?)	↓ (?)	
Hypoproteinemia	Total, ↓ Ionized, N	N	N	N	N	

*Modified and reproduced, with permission, from Silver, Kempe, & Bruyn: *Handbook of Pediatrics,* 9th ed. Lange, 1971.
†Tubular reabsorption of phosphate (TRP) normally is 83–98%; the lower values are associated with higher serum levels of phosphorus. In hypoparathyroidism, TRP varies from 40–70%. Low values for TRP are also found in some forms of inherited renal tubular disease.
(?) = Sometimes occurs.

A. Acute or Severe Tetany: Correct hypocalcemia immediately with calcium intravenously and orally. Dihydrotachysterol may be of value. Parathyroid hormone is seldom employed in the treatment of hypoparathyroidism because of its erratic action, unpredictable potency, and the potential danger of impure parenterally administered commercially available preparations.

Because calcium chloride may cause necrosis and abscess formation at the site of injection, calcium gluconate, 0.1–0.2 gm/kg as a 10% solution injected slowly IV, is generally preferred. Injection should be made slowly, with careful monitoring of the heart. Subsequent control may be obtained with calcium orally, although intravenous calcium may be repeated. For short-term therapy, calcium chloride as a dilute solution orally is useful because it produces systemic acidosis and an increase of ionized calcium; calcium lactate is preferred for prolonged therapy.

B. Maintenance Management of Hypoparathyroidism and Chronic Hypocalcemia:

1. Drugs—Give calciferol (most valuable) or dihydrotachysterol. Calciferol may not reach its peak effect for 3–7 days, but activity persists for weeks or months. Careful control of dosage with frequent determinations of serum calcium is essential to avoid hypercalcemia, with resultant nephrocalcinosis and renal damage.

2. Diet—Give a high-calcium diet, with added calcium gluconate or lactate. The latter is preferable since it appears to possess a vitamin D-like effect at the intestinal level, lowering the dosage requirement of vitamin D. The dose is 300–600 mg of calcium lactate 3 times daily with meals. The diet should be low in phosphorus (omit milk, cheese, and egg yolk).

Course & Prognosis

The initial manifestations of the idiopathic form of hypoparathyroidism may appear in the neonatal period, thus suggesting tetany of the newborn. More often, they appear at a later age in a previously well child. Some of the less dramatic manifestations (unresponsiveness, dullness, unhappiness, irritability, apprehension) may be present for a prolonged period before the presence of convulsions bring the patients to the attention of a physician.

With adequate treatment, many but not all of the findings may be reversed and normal progress expected.

Blizzard RM, Gibbs JH: Candidiasis: Studies pertaining to its association with endocrinopathies and pernicious anemia. Pediatrics 42:231–237, 1968.

Moshkowitz A & others: Congenital hypoparathyroidism simulating epilepsy, with other symptoms and dental signs of intrauterine hypocalcemia. Pediatrics 44:401, 1969.

Parfitt AM: Vitamin D treatment in hypoparathyroidism. Lancet 2:614, 1970.

PSEUDOHYPOPARATHYROIDISM
(Seabright Bantam Syndrome & Pseudopseudohypoparathyroidism)

Pseudohypoparathyroidism is a familial hereditary X-linked disease with a female to male ratio of approximately 2:1 in which there is adequate parathyroid hormone but a failure of response of the end organ, the renal tubule (and perhaps bone), to the hormone. It may have the same symptomatology, physical signs, and chemical findings as idiopathic hypoparathyroidism (Table 24–4). In addition, these patients have round, full faces, irregularly shortened fingers (with the index finger often longer than the middle finger), a short, thick-set body, delayed and defective dentition, and mental retardation. The hair is dry and coarse and nails and skin are thickened, but candidiasis has not been reported. X-rays may show thickness of the long bones with limitation of growth at the metaphyseal ends. There may be chondrodysplastic changes in the bones of the hands, demineralization of the bones, thickening of the cortices, and exostoses. The first, fourth, and fifth metacarpals and metatarsals may be relatively more shortened than the second or third, so that there may be "dimples" in place of some of the knuckles when the hand is clenched into a fist. Ectopic calcification of the basal ganglia and subcutaneous tissues may occur, and corneal and lenticular opacities may be present.

Treatment is the same as for hypoparathyroidism.

Similar clinical findings may be found in **pseudopseudohypoparathyroidism**, which is probably a variant of pseudohypoparathyroidism in which the blood chemistry findings are normal. No treatment is necessary. Lenticular and intracranial calcifications may occur in the presence of normal serum calcium. There may be an unexplained relationship between pseudopseudohypoparathyroidism and Turner's syndrome.

In both pseudo- and pseudopseudohypoparathyroidism, the parathyroid glands are hyperplastic, serum levels of parathyroid hormone are elevated, and abnormal amounts of calcitonin have been noted in the thyroid gland and serum. Thyroidectomy is only temporarily effective in controlling the hypocalcemia of pseudohypoparathyroidism, and the increase in thyroid calcitonin quantities is currently believed to be the consequence rather than the cause of hypocalcemia.

Lee JB & others: Parathyroid hormone and thyrocalcitonin in familial pseudohypoparathyroidism. New England J Med 279:1179–1184, 1968.

Potts JF Jr: Pseudohypoparathyroidism. Chap 52 in: *The Metabolic Basis of Inherited Disease,* 3rd ed. Stanbury JB, Wyngaarden JB, Fredrickson DS (editors). McGraw-Hill, 1972.

Sherwood LM: Parathyroid hormone and thyrocalcitonin in calcium homeostasis. New England J Med 278:663–669, 1968.

HYPERPARATHYROIDISM

Essentials of Diagnosis

- Renal stones, nephrocalcinosis, polyuria, polydipsia, hypertension, uremia, intractable peptic ulcer, constipation.
- Bone pain, cystic lesions, and, rarely, pathologic fractures.
- Serum and urine calcium elevated; urine phosphate high with low to normal serum phosphate; alkaline phosphatase normal to elevated.
- "Band keratopathy" on slit lamp examination of eye.
- X-ray: Subperiosteal resorption, loss of lamina dura of teeth, renal parenchymal calcification or stones, bone cysts.

General Considerations

Hyperparathyroidism may be primary or secondary. The most common causes of primary hyperparathyroidism are adenoma of the gland (rare in childhood) and diffuse parathyroid hyperplasia or hypertrophy. The most common causes of the secondary form are chronic renal disease (glomerulonephritis, pyelonephritis) and congenital anomalies of the genitourinary tract. Rarely, hyperparathyroidism may be found in osteogenesis imperfecta, malignancies with bony metastases, and rickets. Familial hyperparathyroidism may be associated with multiple adenoma of the parathyroid, anterior pituitary, and pancreas, and peptic ulcer in adult life.

Clinical Findings

A. Symptoms and Signs:

1. Due to hypercalcemia—Hypotonicity and weakness of muscles; apathy, nausea, vomiting, and poor tone of the gastrointestinal tract with constipation; loss of weight, hyperextensibility of joints, hypertension, cardiac irregularities, bradycardia, and shortening of the Q–T interval. Calcium deposits may occur in the cornea or conjunctivas. Coma occurs rarely. Intractable peptic ulcer occurs in adults and rarely in children.

2. Due to increased calcium and phosphorus excretion—Loss of renal concentrating ability with resultant polyuria, polydipsia, precipitation of calcium phosphate in the renal parenchyma or as urinary calculi (ie, sand or gravel), and progressive renal damage.

3. Related to changes in the skeleton—Osteitis fibrosa, subperiosteal absorption of phalanges, absence of lamina dura around the teeth, spontaneous fractures, "moth-eaten" appearance of skull, and bone pain. If the patient drinks adequate quantities of milk, renal stones will occur but bone disease will not.

B. Laboratory Findings: See Table 24–6.

C. X-Ray Findings: Bone changes do not occur in children who receive an adequate milk intake; in these children, renal stones may be observed in the urine, and nephrocalcinosis may be observed radiographically. When bone changes occur, one finds a generalized demineralization with a predilection for the subperiosteal cortical bone.

Treatment

Treatment consists of complete removal of the tumor or subtotal removal of hyperplastic parathyroid glands. Preoperatively, fluids should be forced and the intake of milk restricted. The administration of phosphate and sulfate salts has been reported to be successful in reducing the hypercalcemia in primary hyperparathyroidism without renal damage. Adrenocortical steroids are usually ineffective. Postoperatively, observe carefully for evidence of hypocalcemic tetany; this may occur with serum calcium within normal

---

TABLE 24–6. Laboratory findings in hypercalcemia.*

	Serum Concentration			Urinary Excretion		Bone Pathology
	Ca++†	P	Ptase	Ca++	P	
Hyperparathyroidism	↑	↓ or N	N or ↑	N or ↑	↑	Generalized osteitis fibrosa cystica
Hyperparathyroidism with impaired renal function	↑	N or ↑	↑	↑	↑	Generalized osteitis fibrosa cystica
Excessive vitamin D	↑	↑	N or ↑	↑	N or ↑	
Excessive dihydrotachysterol	↑	↓		↑	↑	
Neoplasms of bone	N or ↑	N	N or ↑	↑	N or ↑	Bone destruction
Hyperproteinemia	Total, ↑ Ionized, N	N	N	N	N	
Idiopathic hypercalcemia	↑	N or ↑	N	N or ↑	N	See below.

*Reproduced, with permission, from Silver, Kempe, & Bruyn: *Handbook of Pediatrics,* 9th ed. Lange, 1971.

†Repeated determinations are advisable; serum calcium levels may be within normal limits in some cases of hyperparathyroidism.

limits if a precipitous drop in calcium has occurred. The diet should be high in calcium, phosphorus, and vitamin D.

Treatment of secondary hyperparathyroidism is directed at the underlying disease. Diminish the intake of phosphate with aluminum hydroxide orally and reduce the intake of milk.

Course & Prognosis

Although the condition may recur, the prognosis following subtotal parathyroidectomy or removal of an adenoma is usually good. Renal function may remain abnormal. The prognosis of the secondary forms depends on correcting the underlying defect.

Bjernulf A & others: Primary hyperparathyroidism in children. Acta pediat scandinav 59:249, 1970.

Goldsmith RS: Hyperparathyroidism. New England J Med 281:367, 1969.

Sherwood LM: Parathyroid hormone and thyrocalcitonin in calcium homeostasis. New England J Med 278:663–669, 1968.

OTHER RELATED DISEASES

1. IDIOPATHIC HYPERCALCEMIA

Idiopathic hypercalcemia is an uncommon disorder characterized in its severe form by peculiar ("elfin") facies (receding mandible, depressed bridge of nose, relatively large mouth, prominent lips, hanging jowls, large low-set ears, prominent eyes, occasional esotropia, and hypertelorism), failure to thrive, mental and motor retardation, irritability, purposeless movements, constipation, hypotonia, polyuria, polydipsia, hypertension, and cardiac defects (most often supravalvular aortic stenosis). Generalized osteosclerosis is common, and there may be premature craniosynostosis and nephrocalcinosis with evidence of urinary tract disease. In addition to the hypercalcemia, there may be hypercholesterolemia, azotemia, and elevation of serum vitamin A.

Clinical manifestations may not appear for several months. Severe forms of the disease may terminate fatally. Mild forms may occur without the typical facies and certain other findings and with a good prognosis.

The disease may be due to a defect in the metabolism of, or responsiveness to, vitamin D, abnormal sterol synthesis, or to some as yet unrecognized mechanism.

Treatment is by rigid restriction of dietary calcium and vitamin D and, in severe cases, adrenocorticosteroids, which interfere with calcium absorption from the gastrointestinal tract. The addition of sodium sulfate to the diet and the administration of thyroxine have also been reported to be of value.

Friedman WF, Mills LF: The relationship between vitamin D and the craniofacial and dental anomalies of the supravalvular aortic stenosis syndrome. Pediatrics 43:12, 1969.

2. HYPOPHOSPHATASIA

Hypophosphatasia is an uncommon inherited (autosomal recessive) condition characterized by a specific deficiency of alkaline phosphatase activity in serum, bone, and tissues. Inadequate calcification of bone matrix, with localized areas of radiolucency, are radiographically and histologically similar to the bone lesions of other types of rickets, although in hypophosphatasia the lesions are not limited to sites of rapid growth. The earlier the age at onset, the more severe the condition. Failure to thrive, feeding problems, dwarfing, hyperpyrexia, premature loss of teeth, widening of the sutures, bulging fontanels, convulsions, bony deformities, hyperpigmentation, conjunctival calcification, band keratopathy, and renal lesions have been reported in some cases. Premature closure of cranial sutures may occur. Signs and symptoms may be similar to those of idiopathic hypercalcemia; late features include osteoporosis, pseudofractures, and rachitic deformities. Serum calcium is frequently elevated. The plasma and urine of patients and heterozygote carriers contain phosphoethanolamine in excessive amounts. In some cases, marked metaphyseal irregularities may occur.

No specific treatment is available, but adrenocorticosteroids may be of value. The mortality is high in severe cases, particularly in infancy, but improvement may occur in children who survive early childhood. Adults are usually asymptomatic.

Condon JR: Pathogenesis of rickets and osteomalacia in familial hypophophatemia. Arch Dis Childhood 46:269, 1971.

Danovitch SH, Baer PN, Laster L: Intestinal alkaline phosphatase activity in familial hypophosphatasia. New England J Med 278:1253, 1968.

ADRENAL CORTEX

ADRENOCORTICAL INSUFFICIENCY
(Adrenal Crisis, Addison's Disease)

Essentials of Diagnosis

Acute form (adrenal crisis):

- Vomiting, dehydration, hypotension, circulatory collapse.
- Serum sodium low; serum potassium high.
- Eosinophilia; blood and urine adrenocorticosteroids low.

- A definite precipitating factor usually present (eg, acute illness, trauma).

Chronic form (Addison's disease):

- Weakness, fatigue, pallor; episodes of nausea, vomiting, and diarrhea; increased appetite for salt.
- Increased pigmentation, hypotension; small heart.
- Serum sodium low, serum potassium high; blood and urine adrenocorticosteroids decreased; eosinophilia.

General Considerations

Adrenocortical hypofunction may be due to congenital absence; atrophy (toxic factors, autoimmune phenomena); an enzymatic defect leading to decreased production of cortisol; infection (eg, tuberculosis); destruction of the gland by tumor or hemorrhage (Waterhouse-Friderichsen syndrome) and calcification; or may occur as a consequence of inadequate secretion of corticotropin (ACTH) due to anterior pituitary or hypothalamic disease. In the latter condition, hyperpigmentation does not occur. Any acute illness, surgery, trauma, or exposure to excessive heat may precipitate an adrenal crisis. A temporary salt-losing disorder, possibly due either to mineralocorticoid deficiency or renal tubular insensitivity to mineralocorticoid, may occur during infancy.

Fractional adrenocortical types of insufficiency, including forms with deficiency of glucocorticoid, aldosterone, or other mineral-regulating steroids but normal production of other hormones of the adrenal have been described.

Clinical Findings

A. Symptoms and Signs:

1. Acute form (adrenal crisis)—Manifestations include nausea and vomiting, diarrhea, abdominal pain, dehydration; fever, which may be followed by hypothermia; hypotension, circulatory collapse, and confusion or coma.

2. Chronic form (Addison's disease)—Although tuberculosis of the adrenals was formerly the commonest cause of Addison's disease, congenital adrenocortical atrophy, hereditary enzymatic defects with congenital adrenal hyperplasia, destructive lesions secondary to infection, and neoplasms are more common causes at present. Addison's disease may be familial and has been described in association with hypoparathyroidism, candidiasis, Hashimoto's lymphocytic thyroiditis, hypothyroidism, pernicious anemia, diabetes mellitus, cerebral sclerosis, and spastic paraplegia. The finding of circulating "autoantibodies" to adrenal tissue and other tissues involved in these conditions implies an autoimmune mechanism which remains to be proved.

Signs and symptoms include vomiting, which becomes forceful and sometimes projectile; diarrhea, weakness, fatigue, hypotension, failure to gain or loss of weight, increased appetite for salt, dehydration, and, occasionally, opisthotonos. Diffuse tanning with increased pigmentation over pressure points and mucous membranes, hypotension, and small heart size may be present also.

B. Laboratory Findings:

1. Suggestive of adrenal insufficiency—Serum sodium, chloride, and CO_2 content are decreased, serum potassium and NPN are increased; urinary sodium is elevated and the Na^+/K^+ ratio is high despite low serum sodium. Eosinophilia and moderate neutropenia* are present. The fasting blood glucose level is usually normal but may be low in crisis. The patient is unable to excrete fluid normally ($< 75\%$ in 4 hours following a water load of 20 ml/kg body weight).

2. Confirmatory tests—The following tests measure the functional capacity of the adrenal cortex:

a. Corticotropin (ACTH) stimulation test—See p 964.

b. Plasma 17-hydroxycorticosteroids and cortisol levels are low and fail to rise with ACTH stimulation. Acute allergy will not affect this test.

c. Urinary 17-hydroxycorticosteroid excretion is decreased.

d. Urinary 17-ketosteroid output is decreased except in cases due to congenital hyperplasia or tumor of the cortex. This test is of no value in younger children, who may normally excrete less than 1 mg/day.

e. The metyrapone (Metopirone) test (see p 964) is useful in establishing the competence of the pituitary-adrenal axis and in the diagnosis of adrenal insufficiency secondary to pituitary insufficiency.

f. If there are fewer than 50 eosinophils/cu mm of blood, the diagnosis of primary adrenocortical insufficiency is doubtful.

Differential Diagnosis

Acute adrenal insufficiency must be differentiated from severe acute infections, diabetic coma, various disturbances of the CNS, and acute poisonings. In the neonatal period, adrenal insufficiency associated with severe adrenal hemorrhages may be clinically indistinguishable from respiratory distress or intracranial hemorrhage.

Chronic adrenocortical insufficiency must be differentiated from anorexia nervosa, certain muscular disorders (myasthenia gravis, etc), salt-losing nephritis, chronic debilitating infections (tuberculosis, etc), and recurrent spontaneous hypoglycemia.

Treatment

A. Acute Form (Adrenal Crisis):

1. Replacement therapy—

a. Give hydrocortisone sodium succinate (Solu-Cortef), 1–2 mg/kg diluted in 2–10 ml of water IV over 2–5 minutes. Follow with an infusion of normal saline and 5–10% glucose, 100 ml/kg/24 hours IV, containing 50–250 mg of hydrocortisone sodium

---

*A normal number of eosinophils during stress (eg, the day after operation or in the presence of a severe infection) is also suggestive of insufficiency.

succinate. Cortisone acetate, 1 mg/kg IM, may be used after initial replacement therapy; the onset of action of this preparation given intramuscularly is delayed, and its effect may continue for several days.

b. Repeat intramuscular medication every 24 hours until control is achieved and then reduce gradually.

c. Give deoxycorticosterone acetate, 1–2 mg/day IM, or aldosterone as part of initial therapy and regulate dose depending on state of hydration, electrolyte status, weight, and heart size.

d. Ten percent glucose in saline, 22 ml/kg IV in the first 2 hours, may be of value, particularly in infants with adrenal crisis who have congenital adrenal hyperplasia. Avoid overtreatment.

2. Hypotension—Combat hypotension by one of the following methods:

a. Isoproterenol (Isuprel), 2.5–5 mg in 500 ml of 5% dextrose and 0.45% saline solution infused over a period of 2–8 hours to maintain blood pressure. Plasma or blood transfusion, 22 ml/kg, should be used also as necessary to maintain blood pressure.

b. Levarterenol bitartrate (Levophed), 4 ml (1 mg/ml) added to 1000 ml of electrolyte solution for use by IV drip. Determine response to an initial dose of 0.25–0.5 ml of dilute solution per 10 kg and then stabilize flow at a rate sufficient to maintain blood pressure (usual rate: 0.5–1 ml/minute). This drug is very potent, and great care must be employed in its use.

c. Phenylephrine (Neo-Synephrine)—See Chapter 38 for dosage.

3. Infections—Treat infections with large doses of appropriate antibiotic or chemotherapeutic agents.

4. Waterhouse-Friderichsen syndrome with fulminant infections—The use of adrenal corticosteroids and levarterenol in the treatment or "prophylaxis" of fulminant infections is felt by some not to be justified since it may augment the generalized Shwartzman reaction seen in the renal cortices of fatal cases of meningococcemia. However, corticosteroids probably should be used in the presence of adrenal insufficiency, particularly with hypotension and circulatory collapse.

5. Fluids and electrolytes—Give 10% glucose in saline, 22 ml/kg IV. *Caution:* Avoid overtreatment. Total parenteral fluid in the first 8 hours should not exceed the maintenance fluid requirement of the normal child (see Chapter 37). Fruit juices, ginger ale, milk, and soft foods should be given as soon as possible.

B. Maintenance Therapy of Chronic Form (Addison's Disease): Following initial stabilization, the most effective substitution therapy generally consists of giving hydrocortisone or cortisone together with a high salt intake or supplementary deoxycorticosterone (or both).

Additional deoxycorticosterone, sodium chloride, and cortisone, singly or in combination, may be necessary with acute illness, surgery, trauma, exposure to sudden change in temperature, or other stress reactions.

Supportive adrenocortical therapy should be given whenever surgical operations are performed on patients who have at some time received prolonged therapy with adrenocortical steroids. (See below.)

1. Cortisone or hydrocortisone (or equivalent)—Give 1.25 mg/kg/24 hours IM in 3–4 doses, or 2.5–10 mg IM (infant dose) once or twice daily. Increase to 2–4 times the regular dosage during intercurrent illness or other periods of stress. Prednisone, 0.25 mg/kg/24 hours orally in 3–4 doses, may be equally effective, but more potent corticosteroids should not be used. Either a salt-retaining corticosteroid (eg, aldosterone, deoxycorticosterone acetate, or fludrocortisone; see below) or an increase in dietary salt is almost always necessary when prednisone is employed.

2. Desoxycorticosterone (DCA) and related drugs—The effects of overdosage of DCA are increased blood volume, hypertension, cardiac dilatation, peripheral edema, muscular weakness, and excessive weight gain.

a. Give DCA in oil, 0.5–3 mg/day IM, and increase or decrease gradually to the amount needed to maintain hydration, blood pressure, heart size, and weight. DCA also comes in propylene glycol for sublingual administration and as Linguets or Buccalets.

b. Deoxycorticosterone trimethylacetate (DOCTMA) may be given following prolonged stabilization; 25 mg/ml IM of this long-acting macrocrystalline suspension every 3–4 weeks corresponds to about 1 mg of DCA in oil IM daily. Hypertension (without hypernatremia) may occur following DOCTMA administration and may persist for months following its discontinuation.

c. Pellets of DCA may be implanted. For each 0.5 mg of DCA in oil needed daily, one 125 mg pellet is implanted every 6–9 months.

d. Fludrocortisone (Florinef), 0.05–0.2 mg orally once a day, may be used in place of DCA, in which case the dose of glucocorticoid may usually be reduced.

3. Salt—Give sodium chloride (as enteric-coated salt pills if they can be taken), 1–3 gm/day. Reduce dose if salt retention and edema appear.

C. Corticosteroids in Patients With Adrenocortical Insufficiency Who Undergo Surgery:

1. Preoperatively—Give cortisone acetate IM as follows (single dose):

a. 24 hours before surgery, 100% of maintenance.

b. 12 hours before surgery, 100% of maintenance.

c. 1 hour before surgery, 100% of maintenance.

2. During operation—Give hydrocortisone sodium succinate (Solu-Cortef), 1–2 mg/kg by IV infusion over a 6–12 hour period.

3. Postoperatively—Give cortisone acetate intramuscularly, 100–200% of maintenance daily, for 1–2 days. Begin oral preparation as soon as possible and give full maintenance doses daily. If the maintenance dose is unknown, give 1.25 mg/kg orally, divided as follows: 100% of total at 8 a.m.; 50% of total at 2 p.m. and at 10 p.m. If significant stress occurs postoperatively, give 3–5 times the maintenance dose.

Course & Prognosis

A. Acute: The course of acute adrenal insufficiency is rapid, and death may occur within a few hours unless adequate treatment is given. Spontaneous recovery is unlikely. Newborn infants with severe adrenal hemorrhages seldom respond even to vigorous therapy. Patients who have received treatment with adrenal corticosteroids may exhibit adrenal collapse if they undergo surgery or other acute stress for as long as 6–24 months after corticosteroids are discontinued.

In all forms of acute adrenal insufficiency, once the crisis has passed, the patient should be observed carefully and evaluated with appropriate laboratory tests to assess the degree of permanent adrenal insufficiency.

B. Chronic: Adequately treated chronic adrenocortical insufficiency is consistent with a relatively normal life. Since these patients may become dehydrated quickly during minor infections, they must be observed carefully and receive prompt treatment under such circumstances.

Aceto T, Blizzard RM, Migeon CJ: Adrenocortical insufficiency in infants and children. P Clin North America 9:177–189, 1962.

Bongiovanni AM: Care of the critically ill child: Acute adrenal insufficiency. Pediatrics 44:109–110, 1969.

Moses AM, Millen M: Stimulation and inhibition of ACTH release in patients with pituitary disease. J Clin Endocrinol 27:1581–1588, 1967.

ADRENOCORTICAL HYPERFUNCTION

1. CUSHING'S SYNDROME

Essentials of Diagnosis

- "Truncal type" adiposity with thin extremities, moon face, weakness, plethora, easy bruisability, purplish striae, growth retardation.
- Hypertension, osteoporosis, glycosuria.
- Elevated serum and urine adrenocorticosteroids with loss of normal diurnal variation; low serum potassium; eosinopenia.
- Usually due to adrenal tumor in childhood.

General Considerations

The principal findings in Cushing's syndrome probably result from excessive secretion of the carbohydrate-regulating hormones, with depletion of body protein stores and abnormal carbohydrate and fat metabolism. There may also be lesser degrees of overproduction of the mineralocorticoids and of androgens. It has been suggested that in Cushing's syndrome with bilateral adrenal hyperplasia there is decreased responsiveness of the hypothalamic-pituitary "feedback" mechanism which regulates the release or producton of ACTH. This may then result in a constant but only slightly excessive elevation in the secretion of ACTH or lead to qualitative or quantitative change in the diurnal variation.

Cushing's syndrome is more common in females; in children under 12, it is usually iatrogenic (secondary to therapeutic doses of corticotropin or one of the corticosteroids), but it may rarely be due to an adrenal tumor. In children, it may be associated with a basophilic adenoma of the pituitary gland, adrenocortical hyperplasia (20–30%), or an extrapituitary ACTH-producing tumor.

Clinical Findings

A. Symptoms and Signs:

1. Due to excessive secretion of the glucocorticoid hormones—"Buffalo type" adiposity, most marked on the face, neck, and trunk (a fat pad in the interscapular area is characteristic); easy fatigability and weakness, plethoric facies, purplish striae, easy bruisability, ecchymoses, hirsutism, osteoporosis, hypertension, diabetes mellitus (usually latent), pain in the back, muscle wasting and weakness, and marked retardation of growth.

2. Due to excessive secretion of mineralocorticoids—Edema and hypertension.

3. Due to excessive secretion of androgens (unusual and generally mild)—Hirsutism, acne, and varying degrees of excessive masculinization.

4. Menstrual irregularities occur during puberty in older girls.

B. Laboratory Findings:

1. Blood—

a. Serum cortisol and 17-hydroxycorticosteroid levels are elevated. There is a loss of the normal diurnal variation.

b. Serum chloride and potassium may be lowered.

c. Serum sodium and CO_2 content may be elevated (metabolic alkalosis).

d. Plasma ACTH concentrations are slightly elevated with adrenal hyperplasia; decreased in cases of adrenal tumor; and greatly increased with ACTH-producing pituitary or extrapituitary tumors. Plasma volume is high. The white count shows polymorphonuclear leukocytosis with lymphopenia, and the eosinophil count low (below 50/cu mm). The red cell count may be elevated.

2. Urine—Urinary 17-hydroxycorticosteroid levels are elevated; the normal diurnal variation does not occur. Urinary 17-ketosteroids may be normal, elevated, or low. Glycosuria may be present alone or secondary to hyperglycemia ("diabetic" type of blood glucose curve). Urine volume is increased.

3. Response to corticotropin (ACTH) and corticosteroids—The response to corticotropin (ACTH) stimulation is excessive in patients with adrenal hyperplasia; a poor response is usually found in those with tumor. There is a diminished adrenal response to small doses (0.5 mg) of dexamethasone in the dexamethasone suppression test; larger doses will cause suppression of adrenal activity when the disease is due to adrenal hyperplasia, occasionally when it is due to adenoma, and rarely if it is due to carcinoma.

C. X-Ray Findings: Urograms may be abnormal. Adrenal calcification may be present. Osteoporosis (evident first in the spine and pelvis) with compression fractures may be seen in advanced cases.

Differential Diagnosis

Children with obesity, particularly in the presence of striae and hypertension, are frequently suspected of having Cushing's syndrome. Although the color of the striae (purplish in Cushing's syndrome, pink in obesity), the abnormal growth pattern in Cushing's syndrome, and the distribution of the obesity assist in differentiating the two, the urinary excretion of corticosteroids may not be helpful since they may be elevated in obesity (usually in proportion to the weight and surface area). A loss in the normal diurnal variation of plasma hydrocortisone is helpful in establishing the diagnosis of Cushing's syndrome. In obesity, suppression of corticosteroid production occurs with the oral administration of dexamethasone.

Treatment

Since almost all cases of primary adrenal hyperfunction in childhood are due to tumor, surgical removal, if possible, is indicated. Corticotropin (ACTH) should be given preoperatively and postoperatively to stimulate the nontumorous adrenal cortex, which is generally atrophied. Adrenocortical steroids should be administered for 1–2 days before surgery and continued during and after operation. Supplemental potassium, salt, and mineralocorticoids may be necessary. (See above outline of corticosteroid administration in surgical patients.)

For the treatment of adrenal hyperplasia, total or subtotal adrenalectomy is often necessary although pituitary irradiation, radioactive implantation, electrocoagulation, or ablation have sometimes been of value in adults. Substitution therapy may be necessary.

The use of o,p'DDD (a DDT derivative toxic to the adrenal cortex) has been suggested, but the drug's usefulness in children has not been determined.

Prognosis

If the tumor is malignant, the prognosis is poor; if benign, cure is to be expected following proper preparation and surgery.

Pituitary enlargement has been reported in some cases of Cushing's syndrome following both partial and complete adrenalectomy.

Cushing's syndrome (perhaps due to adrenal hyperplasia) may occasionally undergo spontaneous remission.

Although most of the changes resulting from adrenocorticosteroid excess disappear, hypertension, diabetes mellitus, and osteoporosis may persist.

Loridan L, Senior B: Cushing's syndrome in infancy. J Pediat 75:349–359, 1969.

Orth DN, Liddle GW: Results of treatment in 108 patients with Cushing's syndrome. New England J Med 285:243–247, 1971.

2. ADRENOGENITAL SYNDROME

Essentials of Diagnosis

- Pseudohermaphroditism in females, with urogenital sinus, enlargement of clitoris, and other evidence of virilization.
- Isosexual precocity in males with infantile testes.
- Excessive (isosexual) masculinization in males.
- Excessive growth; early development of sexual hair.
- Urinary 17-ketosteroids elevated; urinary pregnanetriol increased in commonest form.
- May be associated with water and electrolyte disturbances, particularly in the neonatal period.

General Considerations

The congenital familial (autosomal recessive) form of adrenogenital syndrome is due to an inborn error of metabolism with a deficiency of an adrenocortical enzyme. Various types are recognized, including the following:

(1) Deficiency of 21-hydroxylase (most common), resulting in inability to convert 17-hydroxyprogesterone into compound S (11-deoxycortisol). Mild forms result in androgenic changes (virilization) alone, but severe cases are associated with salt loss and electrolyte imbalance.

(2) Deficiency in 11β-hydroxylation and a failure to convert compound S to compound F (cortisol). Associated with virilization and usually with hypertension but no disturbance of electrolytes. Deoxycorticosterone and its metabolites are present.

(3) A defect in 17-hydroxylase, with the enzyme deficiency in both the adrenals and the gonads. Hypertension, virilization, and eunuchoidism may be present. Serum aldosterone levels may be low.

(4) A defect in 3β-hydroxysteroid dehydrogenase activity and a failure to convert Δ5-pregnenolone to progesterone. Associated with incomplete masculinization, with hypospadias and cryptorchidism in the male. Some degree of masculinization may occur in the female. Severe sodium loss occurs, and the infant mortality rate is high.

(5) Cholesterol desmolase deficiency with congenital lipoid adrenal hyperplasia. Clinical features are similar to those of 3β-hydroxysteroid dehydrogenase deficiency (above). Urinary corticosteroid excretion does not occur.

Over 90% of cases manifest a deficiency of either the 21- or 11β-hydroxylase enzyme.

In some forms the infant may appear normal at birth, with onset occurring later. In all forms there is excessive secretion of ACTH, causing adrenal hyperplasia and increased urinary excretion of metabolites of various precursors but decreased production of hydrocortisone. Increased pigmentation, especially of the scrotum, labia majora, and nipples, frequently results from excessive ACTH secretion.

Pseudohermaphroditism in the female may also occur as a result of virilizing maternal tumors or the administration of androgens, synthetic progestins, diethylstilbestrol, and related hormones to the mother during the first trimester of pregnancy. In these cases the condition does not progress after birth, and cortisol deficiency and abnormal steroidogenesis are not present. Pseudohermaphroditism may occur with gonadal dysgenesis.

Adrenogenital syndrome may also result from tumors of the adrenal, ovary (rare in childhood), or testes or from idiopathic adrenal hyperplasia later in life.

Clinical Findings

A. Symptoms and Signs:

1. Adrenogenital syndrome in females—In females with potentially normal ovaries, masculinization occurs and sexual development is along heterosexual lines.

a. Congenital bilateral hyperplasia of the adrenal cortex (pseudohermaphroditism)—Various abnormalities of the external genitalia have been described, including an enlarged clitoris and a common urogenital sinus. Growth in height and skeletal maturation are excessive, and patients become muscular and well developed. Pubic hair appears early (often before the second birthday); acne may be excessive; and the voice may be deep. Excessive pigmentation may develop. Dentition is normal or only slightly advanced for the chronologic age. Similar abnormalities may be present in siblings and cousins. Signs of associated adrenal insufficiency may be present during the first days of life or later.

b. Postnatal adrenogenital syndrome (virilism)—This disorder may be due to adrenal hyperplasia or tumor or to a rrhenoblastoma (extremely rare). Enlargement of the clitoris occurs, but other changes of the genitalia are not found. The family history is negative for similar abnormalities.· If a tumor is present, it may be palpably enlarged. Other findings are similar to those of pseudohermaphroditism.

2. Adrenogenital syndrome in males (macrogenitosomia praecox)—In males, sexual development is along isosexual lines.

a. Congenital bilateral hyperplasia of the adrenal cortex—The infant may appear normal at birth, but during the first few months of life enlargement of the penis will be noted. Spermatogenesis does not occur. There may be increased pigmentation resulting from excessive secretion of ACTH. Other symptoms and signs are similar to those of the congenital form in females. The testes are not enlarged except in an occasional male in whom aberrant adrenal cells may be present in the testes and produce unilateral or bilateral symmetrical or asymmetrical enlargement. Males with the 3β-hydroxysteroid dehydrogenase defect usually show incomplete masculinization with cryptorchidism and hypospadias, whereas females show a mild degree of masculinization. Signs of adrenal glucocorticoid insufficiency may be present.

b. Tumor—The findings may be identical with those of congenital bilateral hyperplasia of the adrenal cortex except that they appear at a later age. The tumor may be palpably enlarged. Rarely, an adrenal tumor in a male may produce feminization with gynecomastia.

B. Laboratory Findings:

1. Urine—

a. 21-Hydroxylase deficiency—17-Ketosteroids, pregnanetriol, and testosterone levels are elevated. (*Note:* During the first 3 weeks of life, normal infants may excrete up to 2.5 mg/day. Urinary pregnanetriol levels are sometimes normal in the neonatal period.) Aldosterone may be reduced, and excessive sodium loss occurs in salt-losing forms.

b. 11β-Hydroxylase deficiency—11-Desoxycortisol (compound S), tetrahydro-compound S, desoxycorticosterone, and 17-ketosteroids and testosterone levels elevated.

c. 17-Hydroxylase deficiency—17-Ketosteroid and aldosterone levels decreased; corticosterone and desoxycorticosterone levels increased.

d. 3β-Hydroxysteroid dehydrogenase deficiency—17-Ketosteroid levels moderately elevated.

e. Cholesterol desmolase deficiency—All steroid excretion is markedly decreased.

f. Tumor—Excretion of dehydroepiandrosterone may be greatly elevated.

g. Urinary excretion of gonadotropins may be elevated.

2. Blood—Plasma renin activity may be elevated with 21-hydroxylase defect and decreased in the hypertensive form of the disease.

3. Dexamethasone suppression test—If the administration of dexamethasone, 2–4 mg/day in 4 doses for 7 days, reduces 17-ketosteroids to normal, hyperplasia rather than adenoma is the probable diagnosis.

4. Buccal smear—In female pseudohermaphrodites, the nuclear chromatin pattern is positive.

C. X-Ray Findings:
Vaginograms using contrast media may indicate the presence of a urogenital sinus. Defects in the urogram, displacement of the kidney, and calcification in the area of the adrenal may be seen on x-rays of patients with tumors. Bone age is advanced with 21- and 11β-hydroxylase defects but may not be evident in the first year. The adrenal may be radiologically enlarged on plain films of the abdomen, but extraperitoneal pneumography *(caution)* may be required to demonstrate the increased size.

Treatment

A. Congenital Hyperplasia of the Cortex:

1. Cortisone acetate, 10–25 mg/day orally to infants and 25–100 mg/day to older children (depending on size), will usually suppress 17-ketosteroid and other adrenal corticosteroid excretions to normal levels within 2–4 weeks. The maintenance dosage is usually about 1.2–1.7 mg/kg/day. The drug may be given orally in divided doses several times a day, or the total 3- to 4-day dose may be given intramuscularly every 3–4 days. The dosage increases with age; older children generally need 37.5–75 mg/day in divided doses. Dosage is regulated by maintaining the urinary level of 17-ketosteroid excretion near normal limits and, in cases due to 21-hydroxylase deficiency, keeping the level of pregnanetriol within normal limits. Concentrated hydrocortisone acetate in 14 times the daily dose of cortisone may be effective when given deeply intramuscularly every 2 weeks. Therapy should be continued throughout life.

2. Clitoridectomy is occasionally indicated in a girl with an abnormally large or sensitive clitoris.

3. In the past, some of these girls have been raised as boys, but with early diagnosis and the effectiveness of control of the disorder with corticosteroids this should no longer be necessary.

4. Other aspects of treatment are as for Addison's disease.

B. Tumor: Because the malignant lesions cannot be distinguished clinically from the benign ones, surgical removal is indicated whenever a tumor has been diagnosed. Preoperative and postoperative treatment is as for Cushing's syndrome due to tumor.

Course & Prognosis

When therapy is started in early infancy, abnormal metabolic effects are not observed and masculinization does not progress.

Unless adequately controlled, uncomplicated congenital adrenal hyperplasia causes sexual precocity and masculinization throughout childhood. They will be tall as children but short as adults. Treatment with the corticosteroids permits normal growth, development, and sexual maturation. If started in females whose somatic development is over 13 or 14 years (as determined by bone age), breast hypertrophy often occurs and menses may appear.

Female pseudohermaphrodites mistakenly raised as males for more than 3 years may have serious psychologic disturbances if their sex is "changed" after that time. If the condition is not recognized for several years and the child is raised as a male, removal of the ovaries and uterus is indicated.

When adrenogenital syndrome is caused by a tumor, progression of signs and symptoms will cease after surgical removal; however, evidences of masculinization, particularly deepening of the voice, may persist.

Bongiovanni AM, Root AW: The adrenogenital syndrome. New England J Med 268:1283–1289, 1342–1351, 1391–1399, 1963.

Federman DD: Disorders of sexual development. New England J Med 277:351–360, 1967.

Kenny FM & others: Virilizing tumors of the adrenal cortex. Am J Dis Child 115:445–451, 1968.

Lovas B, Hasur F, Bertrand J: Exchangeable sodium and aldosterone secretion in children with congenital adrenal hyperplasia due to 21-hydroxylase deficiency. Pediat Res 4:145–156, 1970.

Sternberg WH, Barclay DL: Women with male sex chromosomes: The syndromes of testicular feminization and XY gonadal dysgenesis. J Am Med Wom Ass 22:885–893, 1967.

Summitt RL: Turner's syndrome and Noonan's syndrome. J Pediat 74:155–156, 1969.

Tibbs BS: An approach to the problem of intersex: The role of the general pediatrician. Pediatrics 38:430–435, 1966.

3. PRIMARY HYPERALDOSTERONISM

Primary hyperaldosteronism may be caused by a benign adrenal tumor or by adrenal hyperplasia. It is characterized by paresthesias, tetany, weakness, periodic "paralysis," low serum potassium, elevated serum sodium, hypertension, metabolic alkalosis, and production of a large volume of alkaline urine with elevated protein content and low fixed specific gravity; the latter does not respond to vasopressin (Pitressin). The glucose tolerance test is frequently abnormal. Plasma and urinary aldosterone are elevated, but other steroid levels are variable. Edema is absent. Plasma renin levels are decreased (in contrast to increased levels in secondary hyperaldosteronism, eg, that due to renal vascular disease and Bartter's syndrome). In patients with tumor, the administration of ACTH may further increase the excretion of aldosterone. Marked decrease of aldosterone-induced hypokalemia, alkalosis, hypochloremia, or hypernatremia after the administration of a glucocorticoid or an aldosterone antagonist such as spironolactone (Aldactone), which blocks the action of aldosterone upon the renal tubule, may be of diagnostic value.

Treatment is with glucocorticoid administration, surgical removal of the tumor, or subtotal or total adrenalectomy for hyperplasia.

Giebink GS & others: Familial primary aldosteronism with delayed glucocorticoid responsiveness: A new syndrome? Pediat Res 5:400, 1971.

Goodman AD, Vagnucci AH, Hartroff PM: Pathogenesis of Bartter's syndrome. New England J Med 281:1435–1439, 1969.

New ML, Peterson RE: Disorders of aldosterone secretion in childhood. P Clin North America 13:43, 1966.

· · ·

ADRENOCORTICOSTEROIDS & CORTICOTROPIN (ACTH)

Under the regulation of adrenocorticotropin hormone (ACTH, corticotropin), the intact adrenal elaborates adrenocorticosteroids having glucocorticoid activity and a minimal but significant amount of mineralocorticoid effect. The latter is complemented by adrenocorticosteroids which possess primarily mineralocorticoid activity and are under the regulatory control of vascular compartment volume and electrolyte concentration (ie, sodium). Adrenal androgens are also elaborated, but in the normal subject the quantity is insignificant before puberty.

Numerous synthetic preparations possessing variable ratios of glucocorticoid and mineralocorticoid activity are available (Table 24–7), and are employed widely in a variety of clinical conditions. These agents are not curative and may have many undesirable side-effects. Moreover, prolonged use of these agents orally, parenterally, or topically may result in suppression of ACTH with ultimate adrenal atrophy and insufficiency.

Actions

The adrenocorticosteroids exert an effect on virtually every tissue of the body, but the exact mechanism of their action is not known.

(1) Glyconeogenesis and glycogen synthesis in the liver.

(2) Stimulation of fat synthesis and redistribution of body fat.

(3) Catabolism of protein with an increase in nitrogen and phosphorus excretion.

(4) Decrease in lymphoid and thymic tissue, resulting in a decreased cellular response to inflammation and hypersensitivity.

(5) Alteration of CNS excitation.

(6) Retardation of connective tissue mitosis and migration, decreasing wound healing.

(7) Improved capillary tone and increased vascular compartment volume and pressure.

(8) In the case of mineralocorticoids, control of cation flux across membranes, with sodium retention and potassium excretion.

Uses

The adrenocorticosteroids and corticotropin are commonly employed in the following conditions in childhood:

(1) Adrenogenital syndrome, adrenal insufficiency. (Corticotropin is not effective in these disorders.)

(2) Nephrotic syndrome.

(3) Ulcerative colitis and ileitis.

(4) Allergic disorders: Bronchial asthma (including status asthmaticus), intractable hay fever (pollinosis), urticaria, angioneurotic edema, serum sickness, atopic dermatitis, atopic eczema, exfoliative dermatitis.

(5) Inflammatory eye disease: Uveitis, chorioretinitis, sympathetic ophthalmia, iritis, iridocyclitis, retinitis centralis, herpes zoster (not herpes simplex) ophthalmicus, optic neuritis, retrobulbar neuritis.

(6) Collagen diseases: Rheumatoid arthritis, acute rheumatic fever, disseminated lupus erythematosus, scleroderma, dermatomyositis.

(7) Neoplastic diseases (temporary remission): Pulmonary granulomatosis, lymphoma, Hodgkin's disease, acute leukemia.

(8) Blood dyscrasias: Idiopathic thrombocytopenic purpura, allergic purpura, aplastic anemia, acquired hemolytic anemia.

(9) Miscellaneous conditions: Idiopathic hypoglycemia, infantile cortical hyperostosis, reticuloendotheliosis, thymic enlargement, sarcoidosis, pulmonary fibrosis, transfusion reactions, contact dermatitis (including poison oak), drug reactions, neurodermatitis.

Contraindications

A. Absolute Contraindications: Active, questionably healed or suspected tuberculosis (unless treated concomitantly with specific antituberculosis agents).

B. Relative Contraindications: These drugs should be used with extreme caution in herpes simplex of the eye, osteoporosis, peptic ulcer and other active diseases of the gastrointestinal tract (except ileitis and ulcerative colitis), active infections, marked emotional instability, and thrombophlebitis.

Untoward Reactions of Therapy

With high dosage or prolonged use, adrenocorticosteroids may lead to any or all of the clinical manifestations of Cushing's syndrome. These side-effects may result from either synthetic and exogenous agents (by any route, including topical) or from the use of corticotropin, which stimulates excess production of endogenous adrenocorticosteroids. Use of a large single dose given once every 48 hours (alternate day therapy) may lessen the incidence and severity of side-effects.

A. Endocrine Disorders:

1. Hyperglycemia and glycosuria (of particular significance in early or potential diabetes).

2. Production of Cushing's syndrome.

3. Persistent suppression of pituitary-adrenal responsiveness to stress with danger of hypoadrenocorticism or pituitary insufficiency.

B. Electrolyte and Mineral Disorders:

1. Marked retention of sodium and water, producing edema, increased blood volume, and hypertension.

2. Potassium loss with symptoms of hypokalemia.

3. Hypocalcemia, tetany.

C. Protein and Skeletal Disorders:

1. Negative nitrogen balance, with loss of body protein and bone protein, resulting in osteoporosis and pathologic fractures and aseptic bone necrosis.

2. Suppression of growth, retarded skeletal maturation.

3. Muscular weakness.

D. Effect on Gastrointestinal Tract:

1. Excessive appetite and intake of food.

2. Activation or production of peptic ulcer.

3. Gastrointestinal bleeding from ulceration or from unknown cause (particularly in children with hepatic disease).

4. Fatty liver with embolism, pancreatitis, nodular panniculitis.

E. Lowering of Resistance to Infectious Agents; Silent Infection; Decreased Inflammatory Reaction:

1. Susceptibility to acute pulmonary or disseminated fungal infections; intestinal parasitic infections.

2. Activation of tuberculosis; false-negative tuberculin reaction.

3. Stimulation of activity of herpes simplex virus.

F. Neuropsychiatric Disorders:

1. Euphoria, excitability, psychotic behavior, and status epilepticus with EEG changes.

2. Increased intracranial pressure with "pseudotumor cerebri" syndrome.

G. Hemorrhagic Disorders:

1. Bleeding into the skin as a result of increased capillary fragility.

2. Thrombosis, thrombophlebitis, cerebral hemorrhage.

H. Miscellaneous:

1. Myocarditis, pleuritis, and arteritis following abrupt cessation of therapy.

2. Cardiomegaly.

3. Nephrosclerosis proteinuria.

4. Acne (in older children), hirsutism, amenorrhea.

5. Posterior subcapsular cataracts; glaucoma.

Controls to Minimize Dangers of Corticosteroid Therapy

A. Laboratory Controls: During therapy with corticosteroids the following determinations should be obtained at periodic intervals: Blood pressure, weight, hematocrit and sedimentation rate, urinary glucose, serum potassium and CO_2 content (if prolonged therapy with large doses is necessary), stool examination for occult blood.

B. Other Recommendations:

1. Always reduce the dosage as soon as therapeutic objectives are achieved. Intermittent use may be a preferable and safer method of treatment.

2. Terminate administration gradually. Abrupt withdrawal of corticotropin or the corticosteroids may cause a severe "rebound" of the disease; abrupt withdrawal of corticosteroids may cause symptoms of adrenal insufficiency. When discontinuing therapy, withdraw the evening dose first.

3. When treating less severe disorders, give corticosteroids during the daytime only, since this causes less suppression of endogenous ACTH.

4. When prolonged therapy with adrenocortical steroids is necessary, the short-acting drugs may be preferred since the long-acting corticosteroids may cause pituitary growth hormone suppression.

5. Give therapeutic doses of adrenocortical steroids to any child undergoing surgery, severe infection, or other significant stress who has received therapy with adrenocortical steroids during the past 6 months to 2 years unless adrenal response to corticotropin has been shown to be normal.

6. If a child receiving steroids develops chickenpox, the dosage of the steroid should not be reduced but increased (unless it is already at a high level). Steroid withdrawal in these circumstances may have a fatal outcome.

7. If edema develops, place the patient on a low-sodium diet or administer mercurial or thiazide diuretics.

8. Give potassium in divided doses if prolonged therapy or high dosage is employed.

9. Sodium fluoride has been reported to stimulate calcium retention in some patients with corticosteroid-induced osteoporosis.

10. Liberal intake of protein may decrease the risk of developing osteoporosis.

Dosage

Precise dosage of these drugs in various diseases has not been determined. The recommended dosages listed below may be used as a guide for the therapy of most diseases. (See specific diseases for further guidance.) Maintenance dosage should be adjusted depending upon the clinical response and the effect desired; if possible, it should be no higher than the minimum dosage required for adequate control of the disease (as shown by symptoms, signs, and laboratory evidence of activity).

A great many topical corticosteroids are available in various strengths for the treatment of inflammatory skin conditions. A significant amount of percutaneous absorption of corticosteroids may occur through both intact and inflamed skin.

See Table 24–7 for conversion of other adrenocortical steroids to hydrocortisone equivalents.

A. Corticotropin Gel: 0.5 units/kg or 15 units/sq m IM daily in 2 equal doses 12 hours apart.

B. Hydrocortisone:

1. **Physiologic maintenance**–

a. **IM**–0.44 mg/kg (13 mg/sq m) once daily.

b. **Orally***–0.66 mg/kg (20 mg/sq m) per day.

2. **Early pharmacologic therapy**–

a. **IM**–4.4 mg/kg (130 mg/sq m) once daily.

b. **Orally***–6.6 mg/kg (200 mg/sq m) per day.

3. **Therapeutic maintenance**–

a. **IM**–1.3–2.2 mg/kg (40–66 mg/sq m) once daily.

b. **Orally***–2–3.3 mg/kg (60–100 mg/sq m) per day.

---

*In 4 equal doses 6 hours apart (preferred) or 3 equal doses every 8 hours.

TABLE 24-7. Adrenocorticosteroids.

	Trade Names	Potency/mg Compared to Hydrocortisone* (Glucocorticoid Effect)	Potency/mg Compared to Hydrocortisone (Sodium-Retaining Effect)
Glucocorticoids			
Hydrocortisone (cortisol, compound F)	Cortef, Cortril, Hydrocortone, Solu-Cortef	1	1
Cortisone (compound E)	Cortogen, Cortone	4/5	1
Prednisone	Deltasone, Deltra, Meticorten, Paracort	4-5	2/5
Prednisolone	Delta-Cortef, Hydeltra, Meticortelone, Paracortol, Prednis, Sterane, Sterolone	4-5	2/5
Methylprednisolone†	Medrol	5-6	Minimal effect
Triamcinolone†	Aristocort, Kenacort, Kenalog	5-6	Minimal effect
Paramethasone	Haldrone	10-12	
Fluprednisolone	Alphadrol	13	
Fludrocortisone	Alflorone, F-Cortef, Florinef	15-20	100-200
Dexamethasone	Decadron, Deronil, Dexameth, Gammacorten, Hexadrol	25-30	Minimal effect
Betamethasone†	Celestone	33	
Mineralocorticoids			
Desoxycorticosterone	Percorten	...	15
Desoxycorticosterone pivalate (trimethylacetate)			
Desoxycorticosterone acetate	Doca	... / ...	15 / 15
Aldosterone	Electrocortin	30	500

*To convert hydrocortisone dosage to equivalent dosage in any of the other preparations listed in this table, divide by the potency factors shown.
†There is no indication that these preparations offer any advantage over prednisone and prednisolone.

ADRENAL MEDULLA

PHEOCHROMOCYTOMA
(Chromaffinoma)

Pheochromocytoma is an uncommon tumor which may be located wherever there is any chromaffin tissue (adrenal medulla, sympathetic ganglia, carotid body, etc). It may be multiple, familial (autosomal recessive), recurrent, and sometimes malignant.

Clinical manifestations of pheochromocytoma are due to excessive secretion of epinephrine or norepinephrine. Attacks of anxiety and headaches should arouse suspicion. Other findings are palpitation and tachycardia, dizziness, weakness, nausea and vomiting, diarrhea, dilated pupils with blurring of vision, abdominal and precordial pain, hypertension (usually persis-

tent), discomfort from heat, and vasomotor and sweating episodes. The symptoms may be sustained, producing all of the above findings plus papilledema, retinopathy, and enlargement of the heart. There is an increased incidence of pheochromocytomas in patients and families with the pheochromatoses (eg, neurofibromatosis, etc) and carcinoma of the thyroid. Neuroblastomas, neurogangliomas, and other neural tumors may cause increased secretion of pressor amines and occasionally simulate the findings of a pheochromocytoma. Carcinoid tumors may produce cardiovascular changes similar to those associated with pheochromocytoma.

Laboratory diagnosis is possible in over 90% of cases. Serum catecholamines are elevated, particularly while the patient is symptomatic, and urinary excretion of catecholamines parallels this elevation. (Elevated levels may be limited to the period of a paroxysm.) The 24-hour urine collection shows increased excretion of metanephrines and vanillylmandelic acid

(VMA, 3-methoxy-4-hydroxymandelic acid). Attacks may be provoked by mechanical stimulation of the tumor or by administration of histamine, tyramine, or glucagon. The phentolamine (Regitine) test is abnormal but usually is not necessary for diagnosis. Displacement of the kidney may be shown by routine x-ray or after presacral insufflation of air.

Surgical removal of the tumor is the treatment of choice; this is a dangerous procedure, and may produce sudden paroxysm and death. The oral administration of phentolamine (Regitine) preoperatively has been recommended to prevent the extreme fluctuations of blood pressure which sometimes occur during surgery. Profound hypotension may occur as the tumor is removed; this may be controlled with an infusion of levarterenol, which may have to be continued for 1–2 days.

Complete relief of symptoms is to be expected after recovery from removal of the nonmalignant tumor unless irreversible secondary vascular changes have occurred. If untreated, severe cardiac, renal, and cerebral damage may result.

Saxena KM: Endocrine manifestations of neurofibromatosis in children. Am J Dis Child 120:265, 1970.
Weber AL, Janower ML, Griscom NT: Pheochromocytoma in children. Radiology 88:117, 1967.
Wurtzman RJ: Catecholamines. New England J Med 273:637–645, 693–700, 746–752, 1965.

PITUITARY

DIABETES INSIPIDUS

Essentials of Diagnosis

- Polydipsia (4–40 liters/day); excessive polyuria.
- Urine sp gr < 1.006.
- Inability to concentrate urine on fluid restriction. Hyperosmolality of plasma.
- Responsive to vasopressin.

General Considerations

Diabetes insipidus with inability to elaborate a concentrated urine may result from deficient secretion of vasopressin (ADH), lack of response of the kidney to ADH, or failure of osmoreceptors to respond to elevations of osmolality.

Hypofunction of the hypothalamus or posterior pituitary with deficiency of vasopressin (neurogenic diabetes insipidus) may be idiopathic or may be associated with lesions of the posterior pituitary or hypothalamus (trauma, infections, suprasellar cysts, tumors, reticuloendotheliosis, or some developmental abnormality). Familial ADH deficiency may be transmitted

as an autosomal dominant or X-linked recessive trait. In nephrogenic diabetes insipidus, the renal tubules fail to respond to physiologic or pharmacologic doses of vasopressin, and no lesion of the pituitary or hypothalamus can be demonstrated; this disease is believed to be an X-linked disorder with variable degrees of penetrance, with a milder variant in carrier females. When no specific cause can be determined, the search for an underlying lesion should be continued for many years.

Clinical Findings

The onset is often sudden, with polyuria, intense thirst, constipation, and evidences of dehydration. When the child awakens at night to urinate, he is very thirsty and drinks copiously. In young infants on an ordinary feeding regimen, polyuria may not be obvious and the infant may present with severe dehydration manifested by a high fever, circulatory collapse, and convulsions. In long-standing cases, growth retardation, lack of sexual maturation, and CNS damage may occur. The inability to concentrate urine is reflected by serum osmolalities that may be elevated to 305 mOsm/kg (occasionally higher), but urine osmolality remains below this level. Familial diabetes insipidus may have an insidious onset and a progressive course.

In cases of ADH deficiency and associated damage to the hypothalamic thirst center or hypothalamic-pituitary centers controlling ACTH production, the clinical features may be "masked" and polydipsia may not occur. The administration of corticotropin (ACTH) or adrenocorticosteroids may "unmask" the ADH deficiency by increasing the glomerular filtration rate and distal tubule perfusion, resulting in polyuria.

Differential Diagnosis

Diabetes insipidus may be differentiated from psychogenic polydipsia and polyuria (compulsive water drinking, potomania) by permitting the usual intake of fluid and then withholding water for 7 hours. The test should be terminated if distress is clinically notable and associated with a weight loss exceeding 3% of body weight. Patients with long-standing psychogenic polydipsia may be unable to concentrate urine initially, and the test may have to be repeated on several successive days. Eventually, in these patients, dehydration will increase urine osmolality well above plasma osmolality. With neurogenic and nephrogenic diabetes insipidus, the urine osmolality usually does not increase above 280 (occasionally as high as 305) mOsm/kg (sp gr 1.010) even after the period of dehydration. Normal children and those with psychogenic polydipsia will respond to the dehydration with a urinary osmolality above 450 mOsm/kg (sp gr > 1.020). The vasopressin (Pitressin) and hypertonic saline tests may be employed to distinguish between the various forms of diabetes insipidus. The subcutaneous injection of nicotine, which is a direct stimulus of vasopressin release, may be of value in identifying cases due to primary osmoreceptor failure but has had limited clinical trial in children.

Decreased urinary concentrating ability may also occur in various forms of hypercalcemia, with hypokalemia, and in various forms of renal tubular abnormalities.

Treatment

A. Medical Treatment: Replacement with lypressin (lysine-8-vasopressin, Syntopressin Spray, lysine-8-vasopressin drops [Diapid]), vasopressin tannate (Pitressin Tannate), or posterior pituitary powder for nasal insufflation is of value for cases with a deficiency of pitressin.

The use of one of the thiazide diuretics, ethacrynic acid, or even salt restriction may be of value for short periods in both the neurogenic and nephrogenic types. Moreover, the treatment of nephrogenic diabetes insipidus appears to be enhanced by the administration of abundant quantities of water at short intervals and feedings containing limited electrolytes and minimum but nutritionally adequate amounts of protein.

Chlorpropamide (Diabinese) has been found to have an antidiuretic effect through its augmentation of endogenous ADH. It may be tried in cases with a partial deficiency in doses of 100–250 mg once or twice a day. Maximal effects may take 1–2 weeks. Hypotension and hypoglycemia are uncommon side-effects.

B. X-Ray Therapy: X-ray therapy is used for some cases of tumor (eg, reticuloendotheliosis).

Prognosis

In the absence of associated defects, life expectancy should be normal (if severe dehydration in infancy is avoided). Hydronephrosis and hydroureter are not uncommon sequelae of prolonged polyuria; patients should also be observed carefully for urinary tract infection.

Bode HH, Crawford JD: Nephrogenic diabetes insipidus in North America: The Hopewell hypothesis. New England J Med 280:750–754, 1969.

Ehrlich RM, Kooh SW: The use of chlorpropamide in diabetes insipidus in children. Pediatrics 45:236–245, 1970.

Kleeman CP, Marshall FB: The clinical physiology of water metabolism. New England J Med 277:1300–1307, 1967.

Richards MA, Sloper JC: Diabetes insipidus: The complexity of the syndrome. Acta endocrinol 62:627–646, 1969.

PINEAL

The pineal gland is made up of parenchymal cells (pinealocytes) and is often assigned an endocrine function. The pineal may be involved in regulation of somatic growth, sexual maturation, body pigmentation, blood sugar regulation, and a day/night-sensitive neuroendocrine regulatory function. Tumors destroying the pineal may be associated with sexual precocity in males, possibly either through loss of an inhibitor hormone produced by the pineal or by extension into the hypothalamus. Cases of gonadotropin-secreting chorioepitheliomas of the pineal with secondary Leydig cell activation and resultant sexual precocity have been reported. Inasmuch as other space-occupying lesions in the same region (eg, cysts, teratomas, and hamartomas) have been associated with sexual precocity (and, at times, retarded sexual maturation), probably as a result of pressure changes upon the hypothalamus and without associated destruction of the pineal gland, a definite endocrine effect cannot be assigned to the pineal at present. Intracranial calcification may be associated with disturbances of the pineal but may be of questionable significance in the older individual since calcification is noted in 70% of normal persons by the sixth decade.

Quay WB: Diagnosis of destructive lesions of the pineal. Lancet 2:42, 1970.

Relkin R: Relative efficacy of pinealectomy: Hypothalamic and amygdaloid lesions in advancing puberty. Endocrinology 88:415, 1971.

OVARY

The ovary produces 2 types of hormones: estrogens and progesterone. At least 3 natural estrogens have been isolated: estrone, estriol, and estradiol-17β (most potent). Estrogens stimulate the growth of the uterus, vagina, and breasts. Small amounts of estrogens are elaborated throughout childhood, with a marked increase at puberty, but it is not clear whether the prepubertal production is derived from the ovary or from the adrenal cortex.

Richardson GS: Ovarian physiology. New England J Med 274:1121, 1966.

OVARIAN TUMORS

Ovarian tumors are not rare in children and account for approximately 1% of cases of female sexual precocity. They may occur at any age; are usually large, benign, and unilateral; and may be estrogen-producing. The most common estrogen-producing tumor is the granulosa cell tumor (see below), but thecomas, luteomas, mixed types, and theca-lutein and follicular cysts have all been described in association with sexual precocity. Sexual development may be complete, with advanced skeletal development and sexual hair, nipple pigmentation, and menstrual bleeding; in other cases, sexual hair may be conspicuously absent. In most instances, the tumor is palpable abdominally or rectally by the time sexual development has occurred, but there are notable exceptions to this rule.

Urinary estrogens are elevated, and the vaginal smear is positive for estrogen effect. Urinary gonadotropins are usually normal or decreased for the age.

Other ovarian tumors (teratomas, chorioepitheliomas, and dysgerminomas) have been reported in association with sexual precocity.

Treatment is surgical removal, and recurrences are uncommon.

Abell MR: Nature and classification of ovarian neoplasms. Canad MAJ 94:1102–1124, 1966.
Lippe BM & others: Pelvic pneumography in the diagnosis of endocrine and gynecologic disorders in children. J Pediat 78:779, 1971.

TESTIS

The testes contain 3 types of cells: interstitial (Leydig) cells, germinal epithelium of the seminiferous tubules, and Sertoli cells. The Leydig cells produce the testicular androgens androstenedione and testosterone, both of which contribute to the urinary ketosteroid pattern. Testosterone is far more potent, and changes in its secretory rate may produce obvious masculinization without contributing significantly to the total urinary 17-ketosteroid fraction. (The other major ketosteroid precursors are produced by the adrenal cortex.) Testicular androgens, produced under the stimulation of anterior pituitary luteinizing hormone (LH, ICSH), appear in boys in appreciable amounts at about 11–12 years of age and are responsible, wholly or in part, for the growth of the penis and the development of secondary sexual characteristics, including pubic, axillary, and facial hair. FSH stimulates the development of germinal epithelium. The production of testicular androgens contributes to the maturation of testicular germinal epithelium and thus promotes spermatogenesis. Androgens induce nitrogen retention, accelerate bone growth, and determine the closure of epiphyseal junctions.

The Sertoli cells activate the germinal epithelium and may produce a hormone that depresses the formation of follicle-stimulating hormone (FSH) of the anterior pituitary. In addition, the Sertoli cells have the function of affording mechanical support for the germinal epithelium.

It is improbable that the testes have any major significant endocrine function before puberty.

Gonadal deficiency may be the result of absence or destruction of testicular tissue, or atrophy following pituitary insufficiency; it may be due to either a disturbed tubular or a disturbed Leydig cell function, but usually involves both.

Primary deficiency of testicular tissue or function may be due to a genetic or embryologic defect; hormone excess affecting the fetus in utero; inflammation and destruction following infection (mumps, syphilis, tuberculosis); trauma, irradiation, or tumor; or surgical castration. Secondary hypogonadism may result from pituitary insufficiency (destructive lesions in or near the anterior pituitary, irradiation of the pituitary, or starvation), diabetes mellitus, or dysfunction of either the thyroid or adrenals.

Degenhart HJ: Excretion and production of testosterone in normal children: Adrenogenital syndrome and sexual precocity. Pediat Res 4:309, 1970.
Pal SB: Urinary excretion of testosterone and epitestosterone in men, women and children in health and disease. Clin chim acta 33:215–227, 1971.

CRYPTORCHIDISM

Cryptorchidism (undescended testes) is a common disorder in children. It may be unilateral or bilateral and may be classified as ectopic, total, or incomplete.

Approximately 3% of term male newborns and 20% of premature males have undescended testes at birth. In over 1/2 of these cases, the testes will descend by the second month; by age 1 year, 80% of all undescended testes are in the scrotum. Further descent may occur through puberty, the latter perhaps stimulated by endogenous gonadotropin. If cryptorchidism persists into adult life, failure of spermatogenesis may occur but testicular androgen production usually remains intact.

The incidence of malignancy (usually seminoma) is appreciably greater in those testes which remain in the abdomen after puberty.

Cryptorchidism may merely represent delayed descent of the testes or may be due to prevention of normal descent by some mechanical lesion such as adhesions, short spermatic cord, fibrous bands, or endocrine disorders causing hypogonadism (uncommon). It is probable that many abdominal testes are congenitally abnormal and that this abnormality in itself prevents descent.

A causal relationship between failure of spermatogenesis and an abdominal location after puberty is assumed by many, but this relationship has not been established. The normally descended testis of a male with unilateral cryptorchidism may not have normal spermatogenesis; cases have been described in which persistent intra-abdominal testes have been associated with normal spermatogenesis. The apparent abnormality of an abdominal testis may be reversible (even if the testes are histologically abnormal at the time they are placed in the scrotum) since they may later manifest normal histology and function.

Treatment

The best age for medical or surgical treatment has not been determined. Although there is a difference of opinion about whether lack of descent until puberty will cause damage to the testes, in general, delaying treatment for 5–10 years (or even longer) undoubtedly involves no greater risk of sterility than early surgical correction (with the hazard of surgical injury to the testis). Surgical repair is indicated for cryptorchidism persisting beyond puberty since the incidence of malignancy is appreciably greater in those glands which remain in the abdomen beyond the second decade of life.

A. Unilateral: Most cases are due to local mechanical lesions or a defective testis on the involved side. If pseudocryptorchidism (see below) has been ruled out and if descent has not occurred by mid-puberty, surgical exploration and relocation should be attempted by a surgeon skilled in this procedure. Surgical intervention may be delayed until serum or urine gonadotropin have been at pubescent levels for 6–12 months.

Testes with short spermatic cords should be relocated at the abdominal wall and later to a scrotal site (if possible) after "stretching" has increased spermatic cord length.

Gonadotropin therapy (chorionic gonadotropins, 500 units IM 2–3 times a week for 5–8 weeks) is recommended by many before surgery and may be of value if surgery is carried out prior to puberty. When surgery is postponed until mid-puberty, it is doubtful that exogenous gonadotropins are more effective than the gonadotropin produced endogenously.

B. Bilateral: The child with bilaterally undescended testes should be evaluated for sex chromosome abnormalities and genetic sex determined by buccal smear or chromosome analysis as early as possible—preferably in the newborn period. The male child with bilateral cryptorchidism in whom pseudocryptorchidism has been ruled out should be managed in the same way as the child with unilateral cryptorchidism (see above).

Androgen treatment (eg, testosterone, methyltestosterone) is indicated only as replacement therapy in the male beyond the normal age of pubarche who has been shown to lack functional testes.

C. Pseudocryptorchidism: This disorder consists of retractile testes that are normally located extraabdominally but not found in the scrotum at the time of examination.

In palpating the scrotum for the testes, the cremasteric reflex may be elicited, with a resultant ascent of the testes into the inguinal canal or abdomen. To prevent this, the fingers first should be placed across the upper portion of the inguinal canal, obstructing ascent. Examination while the child is in a warm bath is also helpful.

No treatment is necessary, and the prognosis for testicular competence is excellent.

Abeyaratne MR, Aherne WA, Scott JES: The vanishing testis. Lancet 2:822–824, 1969.

Dykes JRW: Histometric assessment of human testicular biopsies. J Path 97:429–440, 1969.

Kirschner MA, Jacobs JB, Fraley EE: Bilateral anorchia with persistent testosterone production. New England J Med 282:240–244, 1970.

PRECOCIOUS SEXUAL DEVELOPMENT

Sexual development may be considered precocious if it develops before the age of 10 years in boys or 8½ years in girls. The causes are outlined in Table 24–8. True (complete) precocious puberty refers to sexual maturation in which the hypothalamic-pituitary mechanism initiates sexual development; in pseudoprecocity, the process is initiated elsewhere. True precocious puberty is always isosexual and may be associated with the production of mature sperm or ova. In pseudoprecocity, sex characteristics may be isosexual or heterosexual; secondary sexual characteristics develop, but the gonads do not mature and the patient is infertile. In the pseudosexual variety, gonadal development and fertility may occur at the normal time.

Constitutional Precocious Puberty

Precocious puberty is 9 times more common in girls than in boys. It may have its onset at any age. In constitutional precocious puberty, no etiologic factor can be found. The overwhelming majority of cases of true precocious puberty in females are of this type; in males, an appreciable proportion of those with precocious puberty have some abnormality. Sexual and genital maturation and body growth tend to proceed along the normal pattern but are accelerated. (The earliest recorded pregnancy occurred at age 5 years 7 months.) In males, a positive family history is often present. Breast development is usually the first sign in females, but the pattern of development may be variable; the interval between breast development and menstruation may be less than 1 year or more than 8 years. Psychologic development tends to be consistent with chronologic age. In contrast to male pseudoprecocious puberty, where the penis enlarges but the testes do not, the constitutional form in boys manifests enlargement of testes as well as the penis. However, enlargement of the testes may not be commensurate with that of the penis since tubular elements may not be stimulated to the same extent as in normal puberty. Children are usually tall in childhood but may be short as adults since osseous maturation ("bone age") is usually more advanced than height age.

When sensitive assays for pituitary gonadotropins are employed, pubertal elevations are demonstrable; however, bio-assay methods may not detect elevations since they lack sufficient sensitivity. 17-Ketosteroids

TABLE 24–8. Causes of precocious sexual development.

True (complete) precocious puberty
Constitutional (functional, idiopathic)
Tumors producing destruction of the pineal (principally in males)
Polyostotic fibrous dysplasia (McCune-Albright syndrome) (principally in females; often incomplete; usually infertile)
Hypothalamic lesions (hamartomas, hyperplasia, congenital malformations, tumors)
Tumors in vicinity of the third ventricle
Internal hydrocephalus
Cerebral and meningocerebral infections (postencephalitis, postmeningitis, toxoplasmosis)
Degenerative, possibly congenital encephalopathy
Tuberous sclerosis
Von Recklinghausen's disease
Cystic arachnoiditis
Therapeutic administration of gonadotropin
 	
Pseudoprecocious (incomplete) puberty
Adrenogenital syndrome
    Adrenocortical hyperplasia
    Adrenocortical tumors
Gonadal tumors
    Tumors of the ovary–Granulosa cell tumor (most common), theca cell tumor, teratoma, chorioepithelioma, dysgerminoma, luteoma
	Tumors of the testes–Interstitial (Leydig) cell tumor, teratoma
	Hyperplastic ectopic adrenal tissue
	Cushing's syndrome
	Premature pubarche (premature adrenarche) (both sexes)
	    Without cerebral disease (constitutional?)
	    With cerebral disease
	Premature thelarche (premature gynarche) (females)
	    Without cerebral disease (constitutional?)
	    With cerebral disease
	Drug-induced sexual precocity
	
	Unclassified causes
	With elevated gonadotropins
	    Associated with hypothyroidism
	    Presacral teratoma
	    Primary liver cell tumors (hepatoma)
	    Choriocarcinoma and seminoma of the testes
	Others
	    Primary liver cell tumors (hepatoma) (males only)
	    Hyperinsulinism
	    Primordial dwarfism
	    Silver's syndrome (short stature, congenital asymmetry, and variations in the pattern of sexual development)
	    Thyrotropin releasing factor excess

may be elevated to the pubertal range. Despite an absence of neurologic findings, the EEG may be abnormal. Luteal cysts of the ovaries are frequently found and probably reflect only gonadotropin activity, although an etiologic role has been inferred by some.

Treatment is seldom necessary. In girls, the administration of medroxyprogesterone acetate (Depo-Provera), 100–150 mg IM every 10 days, may arrest and reverse the condition either by inhibiting gonadotropin production or by a direct effect on the ovary, but treatment may be associated with increased acceleration of bone age and hypertension. Psychologic management of the patient and family is important.

Early menarche may be associated with late menopause.

Females with sexual precocity should have a thorough abdominal and rectal examination every 4–6 months for the presence of a possible ovarian neoplasm since evidence of precocious sexual development may precede the finding of a palpable abdominal mass by several months.

In males, observe carefully for tumors of the testes and adrenals.

Since certain cases of precocious puberty resulting from organic brain lesions may produce no clinical manifestations for prolonged periods, children should be examined periodically for evidence of increased intracranial pressure or other CNS disturbances (skull x-ray, eye examination, visual fields, EEG).

Benedict PH: Endocrine features in Albright's syndrome (fibrous dysplasia of bone). Metabolism 11:30–39, 1962.

Conly PW, Sandberg DH, Cleveland WW: Steroid metabolism in premature pubarche and virilizing adrenal hyperplasia. J Pediat 71:506, 1967.

Donovan BT, Van der Werff ten Bosch JJ: *Physiology of Puberty*. Arnold, 1965.

Grossman H, New M: Precocious sexual development: Roentgenographic aspects. Am J Roentgenol 100:48–62, 1967.

Kenny FM & others: Radioimmunoassayable serum LH and FSH in girls with sexual precocity, premature thelarche and adrenarche. J Clin Endocrinol 29:1272–1275, 1969.

Silver HK: Premature thelarche. Am J Dis Child 108:523, 1964.

DIABETES MELLITUS

(By Donough O'Brien, MD, FRCPE)

Essentials of Diagnosis

- Hyperglycemia and glycosuria, with or without ketonuria.
- Weight loss, polyuria, polydipsia, and abdominal or leg cramps.
- Enuresis, mild appetite loss, emotional disturbances, lassitude.

- 40–70% of cases present in coma or pre-coma.
- Diminished glucose tolerance.

General Considerations

Diabetes mellitus is a common disease in childhood. Its incidence in a clinically overt form may be as high as 0.4%. It was regarded primarily as an expression of insulin deficiency until technical advances in the ability to measure plasma insulin levels showed that this was not always the case.

In most cases of juvenile diabetes—if observed early—there is insulin in the circulating blood, and some investigators have observed hypertrophy of the islet tissue. However, this hypertrophic stage is short-lived, and early and progressive degenerative changes of the beta cells lead to the complete disappearance of insulin from the pancreases of young juvenile diabetics within 2 years after onset. These pancreatic changes are in striking contrast with the absent or mild ones noted in the maturity onset type of diabetes. Juvenile diabetics, with rare exceptions, are insulin-dependent, since endogenous insulin is insufficient and rapidly disappears completely.

It seems probable that the phenomenon of diabetes mellitus will ultimately be explained in terms of a number of causes. In some cases, based on evidence of increased concordance of the disease in monozygous as opposed to dizygous twins, there is evidence of an inherited factor. The exact nature of the gene defect has yet to be defined, although evidence now exists that the insulin molecule itself is abnormal in diabetes. These conjectures began with the observations that the rate of destruction of serum insulin by a crude rat insulinase preparation was much slower in diabetic than in normal serum, and that highly purified diabetic insulin showed a diminished ability to enhance the incorporation of ^{14}C-labeled glucose into rat diaphragm glycogen after intraperitoneal injection.

It is also possible that diabetes may represent a family of insulinopathies with such entities as the Prader-Willi syndrome, lipo-atrophic diabetes, and myotonic dystrophy, representing different steric arrangements.

Whether or not an altered insulin molecule is fundamentally responsible for diabetes, the basic biochemical lesion is that insulin no longer stimulates protein synthesis at the ribosomal level or effectively bonds hexokinase to the electron transport chain on the mitochondrial surface. The latter leads to diminished availability of oxaloacetate. To replace these lessened energy resources from glucose, increased breakdown of fat and protein to acetyl-coenzyme A occurs. Peripheral utilization of fatty acids and amino acids, however, is incomplete, and both are converted to ketone bodies in the liver.

Present evidence is that pro-insulin, the single chain precursor molecule of insulin, constitutes up to 15% of circulating insulin, but that it is not of importance in the causation of diabetes.

Clinical Findings

A. Symptoms and Signs:

1. Severe diabetes—In most affected children, diabetes is first recognized during the initial rapid deterioration in carbohydrate metabolism, with 40–70% of patients being actually in or near coma when first seen. Largely in retrospect, the characteristic symptoms of loss of weight, polyuria, polydipsia, and abdominal or leg cramps are recognized.

Evanescent diabetic states may occur with severe infections such as pneumonia, meningitis, or encephalitis, or as a complication of corticosteroid therapy.

2. Mild diabetes—In a minority of children, the disease may present in a more benign fashion. A few will be detected before overt symptoms appear, being accidentally discovered on urinalysis; others are the ketosis-resistant cases, with enuresis as evidence of polyuria, with moderate weight loss, or with mild problems of poor appetite and lassitude or emotional disturbances. It should be borne in mind also that diabetes may be seen in the newborn infant, either permanently established or as the transient "pseudo-diabetes mellitus." Very rarely, diabetes may present as a delayed overcompensation to a glucose load, with hypoglycemia 2 hours or so after a glucose load, or as nonketotic (hyperosmolar) coma. In children, there are usually no specific signs suggestive of diabetes other than dehydration, exhaled acetone, or coma. "Adult onset" diabetes is occasionally seen in an obese teenager. This can be managed by diet restriction with or without sulfonylureas. By extending screening programs to young people, more such cases might be identified.

Well controlled diabetics show no abnormal physical signs.

3. Prediabetes and pseudodiabetes—Prediabetes is a condition in which there is an abnormal response to a glucose load but no clinical evidence of diabetes mellitus. Criteria for diagnosis are as follows: (1) Two values above the 97th percentile at 60 and 120 minutes and one below the 50th percentile at 180 minutes, or one value at or above the 97th percentile at 60 or 120 minutes and one below the 10th percentile at 180 minutes. These reflect a delayed insulin response to the glucose load. (2) Three values above the 97th percentile at 60, 120, and 180 minutes. Either criterion must be met in 2 tests. (3) Two fasting levels > 110 mg/100 ml or one value at 30 minutes > 200 mg/100 ml. There is much argument about whether these children should be treated; on balance, the authors here do not recommend treatment.

Pseudodiabetes is a transient diabetic state occurring in the newborn or occasionally in older children with infections. It may require brief treatment with regular insulin.

4. Hyperosmolar nonketotic coma—This is characterized by severe hyperglycemia, hyperosmolality, and dehydration without ketoacidosis. It is usually seen in adult onset diabetes; it is not uncommon in children. Restoration of extracellular water is a primary goal of treatment.

B. Laboratory Findings:

1. Glycosuria—Glycosuria may be identified by glucose oxidase tapes, eg, Tes-Tape and Clinistix, which are very sensitive tests and thus not always suitable for routine urine testing in treatment despite their convenience. Clinitest tablets are less sensitive; 5 drops of urine plus 10 drops of water placed on a tablet elicits a colored precipitate which can be compared to a color chart to indicate glucose concentrations between 0.25 and 2%. Eight drops of urine placed in 5 ml of Benedict's solution and boiled will give comparable changes from translucent blue to a brown-red precipitate according to the degree of reduction.

2. Hyperglycemia—A fasting blood sugar of over 120 mg/100 ml is almost certainly indicative of diabetes mellitus; the upper limit of normal is usually regarded as 100 mg/100 ml, using a true glucose determination.

3. Glucose tolerance tests—Glucose tolerance tests, although a traditional confirmatory test for diabetes, are not usually necessary in childhood. The oral test is to take fasting 30, 60, 90, and 120 minute blood samples for serum glucose determination following an oral dose of glucose of 70 gm/sq m. (See surface area nomograms, Figs 38–1 and 38–2.) The glucose should be given as flavored corn syrup (Glucola). A level of over 120 mg/100 ml at 2 hours is considered evidence of diabetes. (Glucose solutions may be used instead but may produce nausea and vomiting.)

4. Serum insulin levels—Serum insulin levels may be normal or moderately elevated at the onset of juvenile diabetes. A delayed insulin response to glucose is indicative of prediabetes.

Differential Diagnosis

The differential diagnosis of diabetes mellitus is not difficult since this is virtually the only condition which gives rise to glycosuria and hyperglycemia with ketosis. Very occasionally, of course, hypophyseal tumors with clinical Cushing's syndrome or acromegaly will lead to hyperglycemia with glycosuria, but the particular association of physical signs will emphasize the differential diagnosis. The same is true of hyperthyroidism and other rare causes of hyperglycemia, eg, tumors secreting the pressor amine metabolites. Renal glycosuria is not associated with hyperglycemia.

Treatment

A. Management of Ketosis and Coma:

1. General—Treatment of the initial and subsequent episodes of ketosis must be prompt and based on fundamental principles. Thus, insulin is given to restore carbohydrate metabolism. The serum pH is corrected, not only for homeostatic reasons but specifically to permit effective insulin action. Extracellular volume must be restored to replace the water and salt loss which accompanies the considerable osmotic load of unmetabolized glucose on the kidney. Though a less urgent requirement, the intracellular stores of glycogen, potassium, fat, and protein must be restored.

If infection is present, it must be vigorously treated with antibiotics.

2. Insulin—A routine initial dose of crystalline insulin is 1.5 units/kg. Half should be given intravenously to rapidly saturate vacant acceptor sites in the cells, and the other 1/2 given intramuscularly. Higher doses should not be given at first, for there is a definite risk of hypoglycemia from overdosage.

3. Intravenous fluids—Restoration of normal plasma and extracellular volume and correction of acidosis must be started immediately. For the first 4 hours, these need not contain a greater amount of glucose than 5% in intravenous fluids or potassium. Table 24–9 gives a suggested treatment program.

In the remaining 20 hours of the first 24, the aim should be to restore the bulk of extracellular water loss, to satisfy insensible water requirements, and to replace glucose and the lost potassium. Intravenous fluids are not usually required after this period, although further restoration toward normal pH and additional potassium may occasionally be required.

4. Ketosis—Quantitative or semiquantitative measurement of the content of acetone in serum and urine provides a useful ancillary guide to the progress of resuscitation from coma. It should be remembered, however, that quite severe lactic acidosis which is not accompanied by ketoacidosis may occasionally occur in diabetic children being treated with biguanides. Conversely, with insulin doses > 1.5 units/kg, other children may become hypoglycemic in the presence of ketosis if sufficient glucose has not been administered.

Recovery from the initial coma is usually rapid and uneventful, although severe CNS complications rarely occur that are unrelated to any obvious error in fluid replacement. It is important to remember that the acidosis may have been precipitated by extraneous circumstances, notably by infection.

5. Continuing management of the ketotic patient—After the first period of adjustment, there is seldom any need to give insulin more than once a day. On the first convenient morning after admission, the patient should be started on a mixture of equal parts of ultra- and semilente insulin in a single dose consisting of 1/4 of the total required during the resuscitation period. One part of regular insulin to 2 parts of lente is also satisfactory. Other mixtures of soluble, NPH, protamine zinc, and lente insulins can be devised; the duration of action of these preparations is shown in Table 24–10. In general, the ultralente/semilente mixture is best, offering greater stability of insulin release and a smaller chance of subcutaneous fat necrosis and injection tumors. Most children seem to require a more nearly 50:50 proportion of the relatively short-acting semilente and ultralente than exists in the lente preparation (30:70 ratio of semi to ultra). Protamine zinc insulin is seldom used in children.

In the following days, the patient should be encouraged to return to full activity and a normal diet, while the insulin dosage is adjusted on the basis of serum and urine glucose levels and urine acetone along the lines suggested below for long-term management.

TABLE 24–9. A program for insulin and fluid and electrolyte management of diabetic acidosis.

Time From Onset of Treatment	Insulin Dosage	Mild and Moderate Acidosis	Severe Acidosis
0–4 hours	Crystalline: 0.75 units/kg IV stat 0.75 units/kg IM stat	(1) If serum HCO_3^- is below 10 mEq/liter, give $NaHCO_3$, 149 mEq/liter.* Otherwise, give 1/6 M sodium lactate in a dosage of ($[25-HCO_3^-$ in mEq/liter] × 2) ml/kg. (2) Lactated Ringer's injection,† 30 ml/kg IV less volume of lactate or bicarbonate already administered under (1) above. Total intravenous load in first 4 hours to be limited to 30 ml/kg.	(1) Give lactated Ringer's injection,† 20 ml/kg over 1 hour or less. (2) If serum HCO_3^- is below 10 mEq/liter, give $NaHCO_3$, 149 mEq/liter.* Otherwise, give 1/6 M sodium lactate in a dosage of ($[25-HCO_3^-$ in mEq/liter] × 2) ml/kg. (3) Continue lactated Ringer's injection to a total of 50 ml/kg IV in this period.
4–24 hours	Crystalline (subcut): 1.5 units/kg × $$\frac{\text{4-hour glucose in mg/100 ml} - 200}{\text{Initial glucose} - \text{4-hour glucose}}$$ Then at 8 and 16 hours give crystalline insulin subcut as 0.3 units/kg for each gm/100 ml of glucose in freshly passed urine.§**	Give evenly over this whole period the following fluids, intravenously: (1) Any residual lactate or bicarbonate to correct acidosis, within the limits set above. (2) 100 ml/kg (in moderate cases) and 120 mEq/kg (in severe cases) of a polyelectrolyte solution‡ containing the following: Na^+, 40 mEq/liter; K^+, 30 mEq/liter; Cl^-, 50 mEq/liter; bicarbonate, 10 mEq/liter; and phosphate, 10 mEq/liter.	
24 hours on	Equal amounts of semi- and ultralente in a total dose of 25% of all insulin given in initial regulatory period. Thereafter, adjust in relation to glycosuria and serum glucose level.	Normal unweighed exchange diet. Further intravenous therapy is not required.	

*$NaHCO_3$, 149 mEq/liter, is made up by adding 50 ml (44.6 mEq) sodium bicarbonate solution (Abbott) to 250 ml of 5% dextrose in water.

†Lactated Ringer's injection (Baxter) contains Na^+, 130 mEq/liter; K^+, 4 mEq/liter; Ca^{++}, 3 mEq/liter; Cl^-, 109 mEq/liter; and lactate, 28 mEq/liter.

‡Polyelectrolyte solution: From a 1000 ml bottle of 5% dextrose in water, remove and discard 30 ml, and replace with the following solutions: NaCl, 3 mEq/ml (Baxter), 10 ml; $NaHCO_3$, 44.6 mEq/50 ml (Abbott), 11.2 ml; KCl, 2 mEq/liter (Baxter), 10 ml; and potassium phosphate, 4 mEq/ml (Abbott), 2.5 ml.

§In mild and moderate cases and depending on the time of admission, it would be usual to omit the 16-hour regular insulin dose and to substitute the first dose of long-acting insulin on the morning following admission. In severe cases, regular insulin is continued in this dosage every 8 hours until the second morning.

**Clinitest: + = 0.5 gm/100 ml; ++ = 0.75 mg/100 ml; +++ = 1 gm/100 ml; ++++ = 2 gm/100 ml.

TABLE 24–10. Duration of action of various insulins.

Insulin	Duration of Maximum Effect (hours)	Total Duration of Effect (hours)
Regular	4–6	6–8
Actrapid pork	2–7	8–9
Globin	6–10	12–18
NPH	8–12	12–18
Crystal II beef	5–18	13–23
Protamine zinc (PZI)	14–20	24–36
Semilente	4–6	12–16
Lente 30% semi	8–12	18–24
70% ultra	8–12	18–24
Ultralente	16–18	24–36

At this stage, education of the patient and family must begin. After the nature and prospects of the disease have been explained, they must be shown the technics of giving insulin and of testing the urine for acetone and sugar. It is important to go over these routines repeatedly, especially in the early months of the disease. A good clinic nurse, especially one who can make home visits, can be invaluable in helping families to understand and manage diabetes in a child.

B. Management of Children Without Acidosis: Less than 1/2 of cases of juvenile diabetes present without acidosis. With these children, the initial phase of treatment can be conducted on an outpatient basis if the family and physician can assign sufficient time for the purpose. However, it is usually better to confirm the diagnosis, establish insulin treatment, and start patient education, both generally (about the disease) and specifically (in terms of insulin administration, diet management, and urine testing), while the child is an inpatient.

Patients without acidosis should be started on 0.5 units/kg/day of a mixture of equal parts of semi- and ultralente insulin. This should be given once a day 30 minutes before breakfast. A preliminary regimen involving 2 or more doses of regular insulin should not be necessary. The insulin is gradually increased until hyperglycemia and glycosuria are controlled. The patient should be ambulatory and active even in the hospital.

In all new cases, regardless of the severity of onset, it is wise to have the patient experience a controlled episode of hypoglycemia. This can be achieved by delaying breakfast after the morning insulin dose. This gives the patient an opportunity to recognize the symptoms of hypoglycemia and to demonstrate how these can be offset by glucose in the form of hard candy, lump sugar, orange juice, or glucose syrup.

C. Long-Term Management of All Patients: The objective of long-term management is to achieve "control." In children, this can be defined as a high level of physical and emotional health, continuing normal growth with freedom from hypoglycemic reactions, no acetone in the urine, and glycosuria that seldom exceeds 750 mg/100 ml in early morning, pre-lunch, pre-supper, or late evening urine specimens. The following are important factors in achieving this:

1. Patient follow-up and continuing education— Continued observation of the child with diabetes is most important. Initially, this should be weekly or at any time the need should arise; telephone contacts should be encouraged. During this period, if patients will keep careful records of urine glucose and acetone, it is usually possible to anticipate the fluctuations in insulin need which are characteristic of the early years of juvenile onset diabetes. Later on, supervision can be much less close and will depend primarily on the patient's and the family's confidence in managing diet and insulin dosage. Puberty is often a period of instability in carbohydrate metabolism, but more frequently the problems at this age are, again, the emotional ones which may stem from feelings of being different or apart from the group as a result of the diabetes. The patient must be encouraged to participate in all activities, even the strenuous ones, care being taken to avoid hypoglycemia. It is important, particularly in the early months, constantly to renew and augment the patient's and family's understanding of diabetes in both general terms and in the specific practical matters of giving the injections, diet management, activity, care of the feet, and immediate treatment of infections.

2. Insulin—Mixtures of equal parts of semilente and ultralente insulin, or regular and NPH or semilente insulin in the proportion of 1:2, are most often given for routine once a day use. Cases that are difficult to control can occasionally be improved by 2 doses of regular insulin, one each before breakfast and before supper. Insulin resistance is rare in children, but patients requiring over 2 units/kg/day may be helped

by using pure pork insulin, sulfated insulin, or dalanated insulin. Insulin should normally be administered subcutaneously, if possible by the patient, 30 minutes before breakfast. The anterior and lateral aspects of the thighs are easiest for self-administration, and the exact site should be changed daily so that a given site is used no oftener than once or twice a month. Some children are helped by "body maps," but in general it is very desirable to handle the disease with minimum attention to being different from the normal.

Initially, insulin requirements will increase to around 1 unit/kg/day, but in most new diabetics, after 3–4 months, the requirement will be reduced to the point at which the total dose may be < 5 units a day. (See oral hypoglycemic agents, below.)

Insulin dosage should be readjusted from time to time on the basis of glycosuria. Parents and patients should be encouraged to acquire confidence in making small adjustments in insulin dosage in response to gradual changes with growth and short-term increases with infection. Ready access to the pediatrician for advice is important. Ideally, daily physical exercise should be kept constant, but this is often difficult, especially for boys. Physical exertion diminishes insulin requirements.

3. Oral hypoglycemic agents—These drugs play a minimal role in the management of juvenile diabetes. They are helpful in the occasional case of maturity onset diabetes in young persons. It may also be possible to manage juvenile diabetics on oral hypoglycemic agents during the period 2–4 months after onset, when insulin requirements may be minimal. The sulfonylureas, which have an initial primary effect as stimulators of insulin secretion, are at least therapeutically warrantable. The biguanides, which appear to act primarily by interfering with the complete breakdown of glucose, would not only seem to have very little physiologic justification but may lead to marked lactic acidosis. In any case, all but a very small percentage of young diabetics eventually have to return to a regimen of injected insulin. It is poor management to raise false hopes of continued oral control at a time when the physician should be concentrating on educating the family about the care of the child.

4. Diet—Effective control can nearly always be achieved without a strict dietary regimen. The rather equivocal advantage, in terms of protracted cardiovascular complications, that is claimed for rigid dietary control is offset in children by the practical and emotional problems that accompany the restrictions required.

In the great majority of cases it is sufficient to establish, with the help of a dietitian, that the family diet offers a conventional assembly of calories (100 calories × age in year + 1000), of which about 15–20% are from proteins, 35–40% from fat, and 45–55% from carbohydrates. Thereafter, control can be sustained on an unweighed diet which follows the "exchange" system in the American Diabetes Association exchange list (Table 24–11).

TABLE 24–11. The food exchange system (American Diabetes Association).

In this system, the common foods used by diabetics are divided into 6 groups according to composition. In each of these groups, the quantities of various foods providing approximately the same values of carbohydrate, protein, fat, and calories are listed. Since the foods contained in any one group have approximately the same nutritive value in the quantities shown, they are freely exchangeable. Admittedly, food composition varies according to source, time, conditions of harvesting, storage, preparation, etc, but variations in bodily requirements vary even more.

The word "exchange" as used in the diabetic diet means the following:

   (1) Within each list of foods, any food in the stated amount may be traded or exchanged for any other food in the **same** list.

   (2) **Do not** exchange from one list to another.

   (3) **Do not** exchange from one meal to another.

The amount of food given in each of the 6 food groups is the amount allowed for **one exchange**. If ½ exchange is allowed, use ½ the amount of food. If 2 exchanges are allowed from one group, either double the amount for the food desired or use 2 different foods in the same list.

Composition of Food Groups

List	Food	Measures	gm	CHO	Prot	Fat	Cal
1	Milk exchanges	½ pint	240	12	8	10	170
2a	Vegetable exchanges as desired	-	-	-	-	-	-
2b	Vegetable exchanges	½ cup	100	7	2	-	36
3	Fruit exchanges	Varies	-	10	-	-	40
4	Bread exchanges	Varies	-	15	2	-	68
5	Meat exchanges	1 oz	30	-	7	5	73
6	Fat exchanges	1 tsp	5	-	-	5	45

List 1. Milk Exchanges

	Amount to Use
Whole milk (plain or homogenized)	1 cup
Skim milk*	1 cup
Evaporated milk	½ cup
Powdered whole milk	¼ cup
Powdered skim milk (nonfat dried)*	¼ cup
Buttermilk (made from whole milk)	1 cup
Buttermilk (made from skim milk)*	1 cup
Plain yogurt (made from whole milk)	1 cup
Plain yogurt (made from skim milk)†	1 cup

*If the meal plan allows whole milk and the patient desires a type of milk which is (*) starred, he should also have one additional fat exchange for each ½ cup milk allowed in the meal plan.

†If the patient uses this in place of whole milk, add one additional fat exchange for each 1 cup milk allowed in the meal plan.

Vegetable Exchanges

All vegetables contain natural sugar, but some have more natural sugar than others. The vegetables have been divided into groups according to the amount of natural sugar they contain. List A vegetables have the smallest amount of sugar. List B vegetables have more sugar.

List 2a. Vegetable Exchanges A

	Cooked	Raw
Asparagus	1 cup	...
Broccoli	1 cup	...
Brussels sprouts	1 cup	...
Cabbage	1 cup	Any amount
Celery	1 cup	Any amount
Chicory	...	Any amount
Cucumbers	...	Any amount
Escarole	...	Any amount
Eggplant	1 cup	...
Greens		
Beet	1 cup	...
Chard	1 cup	...
Collard	1 cup	...
Dandelion	1 cup	...
Kale	...	Any amount
Mustard	1 cup	...
Spinach	1 cup	Any amount
Turnip	1 cup	...
Lettuce	...	Any amount
Mushrooms	1 cup	...
Okra	1 cup	...
Green peppers	1 cup	Any amount
Radishes	...	Any amount
Sauerkraut	1 cup	Any amount
String beans, young	1 cup	...
Summer squash	1 cup	...
Tomatoes	1 cup	1 cup
Watercress	...	Any amount
Zucchini squash	1 cup	...

List 2b. Vegetable Exchanges B

	Cooked	Raw
Beets	½ cup	...
Carrots	½ cup	½ cup
Onions	½ cup	½ cup
Peas, green	½ cup	...
Pumpkin	½ cup	...
Rutabagas	½ cup	...
Squash, winter	½ cup	...
Turnips	½ cup	...

TABLE 24-11 (cont'd). The food exchange system (American Diabetes Association).

List 3. Fruit Exchanges

Each exchange of fruit shown below contains about the same amount of sugar. The size of serving varies for each fruit because the amount of natural sugar varies from one fruit to another. The patient may use fresh, dried, cooked, canned, or frozen fruit as long as no sugar has been added.

Apple, fresh (2 inch diameter)	1 small
Apple juice	1/3 cup
Applesauce, canned, without sugar	½ cup
Apricots, fresh or canned, without sugar	2 medium
Apricots, dried	4 halves
Apricot juice	1/3 cup
Banana	½ small
Blackberries, fresh frozen, without sugar	1 cup
Blueberries, fresh frozen, without sugar	2/3 cup
Blended juice	½ cup
Cantaloupe (6 inch diameter, no rind)*	¼
Cherries, fresh or canned, without sugar	10 large
Cranberry juice, regular sweetened	1/3 cup
Dates	2
Figs, fresh	2 large
Figs, dried	1 small
Fruit cocktail, canned, without sugar	½ cup
Grapefruit*	½ small
Grapefruit juice*	½ cup
Grapes, Tokay or American	12
Grape juice	¼ cup
Honeydew melon (7 inch diameter, no rind)	1/8
Mango	½ small
Nectarines	1 medium
Orange, with rind*	1 small
Orange juice*	½ cup
Papaya	1/3 medium
Peach, fresh or canned, without sugar	1 small
Peach nectar	1/3 cup
Pear, fresh or canned, without sugar	1 small
Pear nectar	1/3 cup
Pineapple, fresh or canned, without sugar	½ cup
Pineapple juice	1/3 cup
Plums, fresh or canned, without sugar	2 medium
Prunes, dried	2 medium
Prune juice, unsweetened	¼ cup
Raisins	2 tbsp
Raspberries, fresh frozen, without sugar	1 cup
Strawberries, fresh frozen, without sugar*	1 cup
Tangerine*	1 large
Tomato juice*	1 cup
Watermelon, no rind (3 × 1½ inches)	1 cup

*These foods are rich sources of vitamin C. Try to use one of these in your diet each day.

List 4. Bread Exchanges

Bread, whole wheat, white, rye	1 slice
Biscuit, roll (2 inch diameter)	1
Plain muffin (2 inch diameter)	1
Cornbread (1½ inch cube)	1
Cereals: Cooked	½ cup
Cereals: Dry, flake, and puff types	¾ cup
(not sugar-coated)	
Grapenuts	3 tbsp
Rice, grits, cooked	½ cup
Spaghetti, noodles, macaroni, cooked	½ cup

Crackers	
Graham (2½ inch square)	2
Oyster (½ cup)	20
Saltines (2 inch square)	5
Soda (2½ inch square)	3
Round, thin (1½ inches)	6
Melba toast	4 slices
Ry-Krisp	3 wafers
Zwieback	2 slices
Cornstarch and flour	2½ tbsp
Vegetables	
Mixed vegetables	½ cup
Beans and peas, dried, cooked	½ cup
(lima, navy, split pea, cowpeas, etc),	
baked beans, no pork	¼ cup
Corn	1/3 cup
Corn on the cob	½ ear
Popcorn	1 cup
Parsnips	2/3 cup
Potatoes, white	1 small
Potatoes, white, mashed	½ cup
Potatoes, sweet, or yams	¼ cup
Tortilla (about 6 inch diameter)	1

List 5. Meat Exchanges

The meat should be baked, boiled, broiled, roasted, or pan broiled.

The following can be used for 3 meat exchanges: 2 pork chops (medium sized), 2 meat balls, 2 chicken legs, or 2 lamb chops (medium sized). A 3 oz serving of cooked meat is about equal to ¼ lb (4 oz) of raw meat.

Meat and poultry: Lean, cooked, no bone	1 oz
3 × 2 × 1/8 inch—beef, veal, lamb,	
pork, liver, chicken, turkey, etc	
Cold cuts (4½ × 1/8 inch)	1 slice
salami, minced ham, bologna	
liverwurst, luncheon loaf	
Frankfurter (8–9/lb)	1
Fish: Canned and drained	¼ cup
salmon, tuna, crab, lobster	
Fish: Fresh or frozen (2 × 2 × 1 inch)	1 oz
Shrimp, clams, oysters, etc	5 small
Sardines	3 medium
Egg	1
Cheese: American, Swiss, or cheddar	1 oz
Cottage cheese	¼ cup
Peanut butter*	2 tbsp

*Limit peanut butter to one exchange per day.

List 6. Fat Exchanges

The fat planned for the diet may be used in preparing meats and vegetables or eaten at mealtime as butter or margarine on a slice of bread.

Butter or margarine	1 tsp
Bacon, crisp	1 slice
Cream, light	2 tbsp
Cream, heavy	1 tbsp
Cream cheese	1 tbsp
Avocado (4 inch diameter)	1/8
French dressing	1 tbsp
Mayonnaise	1 tsp
Oil or cooking fat	1 tsp
Nuts	6 small
Olives	5 small
Gravy	2 tbsp
Sour cream	2 tbsp

TABLE 24–11 (cont'd). The food exchange system (American Diabetes Association).

Free Foods	Miscellaneous Exchange Items
Foods that the patient does not need to measure and that he may use often include the following:	Some common foods and how the patient can count them into his exchanges.

Free Foods		Miscellaneous Exchange Items
Coffee	Cranberries, fresh and	1 cup cream soup = 1 bread exchange + 1 meat exchange
Tea	unsweetened	1 cup rice or noodle soup with chicken or beef = 1 bread exchange
Decaffeinated coffee	Rhubarb, fresh and	1 cup vegetable soup = 1 B vegetable exchange
such as Sanka	unsweetened	1 hamburger or hot dog bun = 2 bread exchanges
Clear broth	Noncalorie or artificial	15 potato chips (2 inch diameter) or 1/3 cup Fritos = 1 bread exchange + 2 fat exchanges
Bouillon cubes	sweeteners	10 pieces French fried potatoes = 1½ bread exchanges + 2 fat exchanges
Unsweetened gelatin,	Salt, pepper, and other spices	1½ inch cube sponge or angel cake = 1 bread exchange
plain or flavored	Herbs, mustard, vinegar, and	1/3 cup regular sweetened, flavored gelatin = 1 bread exchange
Lemon wedge	other seasonings	¼ cup sherbet = 1 bread exchange (use no more than once a week)
Unsweetened dill or	One calorie soft drinks	½ cup plain vanilla ice cream = 1 bread exchange + 2 fat exchanges (use no more than once a week)
sour pickles	Low-calorie salad dressings	1 pancake or waffle (4 inch diameter) = 1 bread exchange
		1 cup macaroni and cheese = 2 meat exchanges + 2 bread exchanges + 2 fat exchanges
		1/10 of a 12 inch pizza (meat or cheese topping) = 1 bread exchange + 1 meat exchange

5. Managing hypoglycemia—It is wise for the patient to carry hard candy in case hypoglycemic symptoms are experienced. This is especially likely following unanticipated strenuous physical exertion. In certain cases, it is also advisable for the parents to be instructed in the use of glucagon to counteract hypoglycemia by giving 1 mg IM. If glucagon is used, the child must be given some easily absorbed carbohydrate as soon as possible to restore the liver glycogen.

6. Urine testing—Patients should be told to use the early morning urine as it is voided when making estimations of urine sugar. With other specimens, the bladder should first be emptied and a second specimen, voided 15–30 minutes later, used for the actual test. In cases where control is poor, it may be helpful to take serial blood sugars over a single day as a guide to insulin adjustment and to collect a number of 24-hour urine specimens for total sugar output. Urine sugar may be estimated with sufficient accuracy for clinical purposes with Clinitest tablets (trace, 250 mg/100 ml; +, 500 mg/100 ml; ++, 750 mg/100 ml; +++, 1 gm/100 ml; ++++, 2 gm/100 ml) and should not exceed 8 gm/sq m/24 hours. Twenty-four hour collections should not be asked for on a school day unless this can be arranged unobtrusively with the aid of the school nurse. Glucose oxidase tapes such as Tes-Tape or Clinistix are rather sensitive albeit convenient in juvenile diabetes.

Urine samples should also be tested for acetone using Acetest papers. It is usually sufficient to do this in the evenings only except during periods of poor control.

7. Blood sugar estimations—Isolated blood sugar estimations are of limited value in day-to-day management. However, in cases that are difficult to control, it may be very helpful to obtain blood glucose samples every 3 hours 1 hour before and 2 hours after each meal (6 hours between meals) as well as overnight for a single 24-hour period.

Complications

Complications during the course of diabetes in children are not common. During presenting coma, extensive neurologic signs may develop, but the outlook is good. Hypoglycemia, which is also rarely a presenting symptom, may be frequent and severe enough to cause brain damage. Urinary tract infections and tuberculosis are modest special risks. Degenerative vascular disease, peripheral neuritis, and exudative retinopathy may occasionally be seen in childhood. Poorly controlled diabetes in young children over a long period may lead to a syndrome of hepatomegaly and dwarfism (Mauriac's syndrome). Emotional disturbances are common, especially in the early teen years, and may require psychiatric help.

Perhaps one of the commonest iatrogenic sequels is the Somogyi phenomenon, which comes from sequential overdosage of insulin as a response to occult hypoglycemia, followed by pressor amine-induced hyperglycemia spuriously interpreted as due to insufficient insulin. Treatment in this instance consists of reduction of the insulin dosage.

Prognosis

Parents will want to know in what ways the overall expectancy of life may be altered for their diabetic children. In this respect, there is now a mean expectancy of some 20 years after the onset of the disease before the onset of major complications. Evidence shows, however, that the prepubertal years do not contribute to the anticipated time of onset of these complications.

The continuing management of the diabetic may present 2 outstanding difficulties. The first and most frequent is environmental. Poor family understanding of the diabetic, ranging from overprotection to neglect, often results in personal anxieties. This is often particularly evident in the teen-age girl who feels "different" from others in her age group because she is diabetic. Not only does this difficulty lead to carelessness in diet and insulin administration, but the stress itself has metabolic consequences of increased ketoacidosis, related probably to epinephrine secretion with diminished peripheral glucose utilization.

The second difficulty is intrinsic instability of carbohydrate management. Present evidence is that in children this is rarely due to insulin antibodies, though there have been occasional reports of the successful use of pure pork, sulfated, or dalanated insulins—or even

corticosteroids—in cases of resistance to beef insulin. One of the most common factors is overdosage of insulin. Glucagon, growth hormone, and corticosteroid output are also increased in hypoglycemia, and any of these factors could play a role in rebound hyperglycemia.

Camerini-Davalos RA, Cole HS: *Early Diabetes*. Academic Press, 1970.
Drash A: Diabetes mellitus in childhood. J Pediat 78:919, 1971.
O'Brien D: Childhood diabetes. Clin Pediat 5:21, 1966.
Schwarz R: Diabetic acidosis and coma. Pediatrics 47:902, 1971.

PRADER-WILLI SYNDROME

These children show obesity, short stature, and mental retardation with amyotonia in the newborn period. The males show hypogonadism. There is a tendency to develop diabetes in later childhood.

Dunn MG: The Prader-Labhart-Willi syndrome. Acta paediat scandinav, Suppl 186, 1968.

●　●　●

General References

Barnett HL: *Pediatrics*. Appleton-Century-Crofts, 1968.
Danowski TS: *Clinical Endocrinology*. Vols 1–4. Williams & Wilkins, 1962.
Gardner LI: *Endocrine and Genetic Diseases of Childhood*. Saunders, 1969.

Stanbury JB, Wyngaarden JB, Fredrickson DS (editors): *The Metabolic Basis of Inherited Disease*, 2nd ed. McGraw-Hill, 1966.
Williams RH: *Textbook of Endocrinology*, 4th ed. Saunders, 1968.

25 . . .
Disorders of Nutrition

Donough O'Brien, MD, FRCP, & H. Peter Chase, MD

DISEASES OF GENERALIZED UNDERNUTRITION

Undernutrition has long been recognized as the single most important problem in child health the world over. It was considered to be rare in the USA, although recent investigations have shown that this is regrettably far from true. Subclinical nutrition is not uncommon among the poor and usually takes the form of iron-deficiency anemia. Vitamin A deficiency may be seen in special groups such as children of migrant farm workers; and vitamin C deficiency is common in children of American Indians. Severe malnutrition usually occurs as a complex product of want and ignorance, with some element of the battered child syndrome. There is increasing evidence that severe maternal malnutrition in the last trimester or nutritional deprivation in the first year of life results in irrevocable impairment of normal intellectual development. The morbidity for infections is greatly increased in undernourished children, as is overall childhood mortality as well.

Chase HP, Martin HP: Undernutrition and child development. New England J Med 282:933–939, 1970.
National Nutrition Survey: *Nutrition and Human Needs.* Part 3. US Government Printing Office, Washington, DC, 1969.
Sandstead HH: Nutritional deficiencies in disadvantaged children. Am J Dis Child 121:455, 1971.

INFANTILE CALORIC UNDERNUTRITION
(Marasmus)

Marasmus is a syndrome of generalized undernutrition in infancy secondary to inadequate caloric intake. The term should be applied to children weighing less than 60% of the expected mean weight (Table 2–4) for age who have no edema. The causes are many and include underfeeding of breast milk, which in turn may be due to severe undernutrition in the mother or to various social, emotional, or economic causes. Inadequate intake of cow's milk in areas where prolonged breast feeding is not practiced is also an important cause. Again, the basic operative factors may be ignorance or poverty. Other precipitating causes are

prematurity with difficulty in feeding, infections, obstructive diseases of the oropharynx and upper gastrointestinal tract, disease of the mouth, malabsorption syndromes, inborn errors of metabolism, any serious organic disease, and maternal anxiety and insecurity. In the USA over half of the children hospitalized for "failure to thrive" in infancy are the victims of inadequate feeding.

Clinical Findings

A. Symptoms and Signs: The clinical picture depends to some extent on the causes as well as the severity and duration of undernutrition. Loss of subcutaneous fat (which can be quantitated with calipers) is striking and may be confused with dehydration, particularly if diarrhea complicates the history. Muscle wasting, particularly over the buttocks and in the extremities, is usually quite evident. The infant loses interest and acquires a pinched appearance, with sunken eyes. The abdomen may be somewhat distended, usually because of an enlarged liver which contains increased fat stores. Characteristically, there is no detectable edema, hair changes, or dermatosis.

B. Laboratory Findings: The diagnosis is a clinical one, although many laboratory tests are altered and can be followed as a general index to recovery. The total serum protein and albumin should be checked as these may be low, even though the child is not edematous. The serum BUN level (< 9 mg/100 ml) and amylase activity (< 5 units/100 ml) are often low and will rise with rehabilitation. The hemoglobin (< 10 gm/100 ml) may be low as a result of associated poor iron intake. It is important to follow the stool pH since disaccharidase deficiency is present in over half of cases and will lead to further problems. (See also Table 4–3.)

Treatment

Treatment consists of providing for adequate nutrition and treating the primary cause if there is one. Initial therapy should be aimed at intravenous restoration of adequate blood volume if the child is dehydrated. The milk formula should initially be lactose-free even if diarrhea is not present, since many of these children develop diarrhea when given a large lactose load. Disaccharidase intolerance may last for several months after rehabilitation, although it usually disappears in the first month. Vitamins should be given during recovery because of the body's increased needs during rapid growth. It is frequently necessary to gradually increase the caloric intake to 150–200 calories/kg body weight before weight gain finally starts. If possible, the child should not be exposed to other children with infections during early rehabilitation because of the increased morbidity and mortality that results.

Prognosis

Severely affected infants have a poor prognosis and frequently acquire secondary infections and adapt slowly to nutritional therapy. The ultimate height, weight, and head circumference is related to the timing, severity, and duration of the malnutrition. Low head circumference relates to poor brain growth and is important in estimating adult intellectual capacity.

Bouré MO, Barbezat GO, Hansen JOL: Carbohydrate absorption in malnourished children. Am J Clin Nutr 20:89–97, 1967.

Rutishauser IHE, McLance RA: Caloric requirements for growth after severe undernutrition. Arch Dis Childhood 43:252, 1968.

Scrimshaw NS: Synergism of malnutrition and infection. JAMA 212:1685, 1970.

PROTEIN MALNUTRITION
(Kwashiorkor)

Kwashiorkor is a multiple deficiency disease due mainly to inadequate protein intake in the presence of an adequate or even high carbohydrate intake. The diagnosis specifically denotes children who are 60–80% of the expected mean weight for age and who also have edema. The frequent occurrence of caloric undernutrition with protein deficiency has resulted in the term "marasmic kwashiorkor," which applies to children who are less than the 60% of the expected mean weight for age and who have edema. As with infantile malnutrition, there may be a variety of underlying causes other than simple nonavailability of adequate protein. Moreover, in the early years of life, a balanced but calorie-deficient diet is less of a threat to life than an unbalanced but calorically sufficient diet.

A great variety of metabolic aberrations occur in kwashiorkor. There is fatty infiltration of the liver; glucose is not readily mobilizable by epinephrine; and hypoglycemia is common. The ratio of essential to nonessential amino acids in the plasma is decreased, and generalized aminoaciduria is frequently present. It has been shown that total body water is not increased but that there is a definite shift of intracellular water toward the extracellular space. Muscle biopsies consistently demonstrate increased sodium and decreased potassium content. A malabsorption pattern is often seen, with morphologic small bowel changes and deficient disaccharidase enzymes.

Kwashiorkor usually occurs in children 1–5 years of age. This coincides with weaning from breast milk, which provides sufficient proteins and calories. Kwashiorkor can occur anywhere in the world—isolated cases have been reported in the USA—but almost all cases occur in the underdeveloped tropical world where the staples are incomplete protein foods (rice, maize, cassaba, etc).

Clinical Findings

The principal manifestations of kwashiorkor are growth failure; edema, which is usually peripheral but which may involve the rest of the body; wasted muscles and persistence of subcutaneous fat; lethargy, lack of interest in the environment, and poor appetite; and sparse, silky hair, unusually light in color. Other common symptoms and signs include anemia, loose, foamy stools, hepatomegaly, and skin manifestations. The dermatologic expression of the disease includes dark-colored patches on a background of relatively normal skin and striae over areas of stretched skin. The patches are most often seen on the backs of the thighs, on the buttocks, and in moist skin areas, leaving areas of depigmentation when they peel off. Small skin ulcers are often present, especially over pressure points.

Prevention & Treatment

Kwashiorkor can be prevented by making sure that cheap proteins such as whole dried fish meal, protein concentrates from soy, cottonseed, and peanut flours, lysine-fortified flour, and dried milk are available to deprived populations. Population control and improved agriculture are likewise important.

Therapy consists initially of treating severe electrolyte imbalance and anemia. Blood and plasma in small amounts so as not to precipitate congestive heart failure are often beneficial. Antibiotics should be used as indicated for infections. Hypoglycemia may be severe and, when it occurs in association with hypothermia and coma, is a poor prognostic sign. The cause of the encephalopathy that occasionally is seen is not known, but it is apparently more frequent with too rapid rehabilitation.

Liquids are usually necessary for initial oral feedings, and, because of the multiple intestinal and pancreatic enzyme deficiencies, should consist of as simple a formula as possible. A lactose-free formula should always be used, and, when available, hydrolyzed proteins are probably better than whole protein. A protein of high biologic value (with high content of all essential amino acids) such as casein is essential. The protein should be reintroduced gradually, or the patient's condition may actually worsen. Formulas containing medium-chain triglycerides (MCT) may reduce the steatorrhea, as lipase enzymes are not necessary for MCT absorption. Vitamin supplementation is also important.

Prognosis

The overall mortality in good hospitals is between 15 and 30%, and is even higher in severe cases. Hypothermia and encephalopathy are signs of a poor outcome. Congestive heart failure due to cardiac myopathy and rapid shifts of water and electrolytes during initial therapy may be fatal. Hypoglycemia is also considered by some to be a frequent cause of death.

The eventual height, weight, and intellectual attainment depends, as with marasmus, on the timing, severity, and duration of undernutrition. The brain is not apparently as severely affected by undernutrition after the first year of life as during the first year, when it is growing very rapidly.

Balmer S, Howells G, Wharton B: The acute encephalopathy of kwashiorkor. Develop Med Child Neurol 10:766–771, 1968.

Brinkman GG & others: Body weight composition in kwashiorkor. Pediatrics 36:94–103, 1965.

Gomez F & others: Malnutrition in infancy and childhood, with special reference to kwashiorkor. Advances Pediat 7:131–169, 1955.

Wharton B: Hypoglycemia in children with kwashiorkor. Lancet 1:171–173, 1970.

Whiteheard RG, Dean RFA: Serum amino acids in kwashiorkor. Am J Clin Nutr 14:313–330, 1964.

FAILURE TO THRIVE

The term "failure to thrive" is commonly applied to infants who, for a variety of reasons, show a striking lag in somatic growth. By far the most common cause is nutritional deprivation, and a meticulous nutritional history will elicit this. Nutritional problems in turn may reflect ignorance, poverty, or emotional conflicts over the child.

Organic causes for failure to thrive must also be considered. The list given in Table 24–1 for short stature can be used as a diagnostic guide.

VITAMIN DEFICIENCIES, DEPENDENCIES, & INTOXICATIONS

Vitamins are necessary organic substances which cannot be made in sufficient quantities by the body. Vitamins A, D, E, and K make up the fat-soluble vitamins, and, with vitamin C, are the most frequent causes of vitamin deficiency in the USA. The fat-soluble vitamins are stored in the body tissues, in contrast to the water-soluble vitamins which are minimally stored and which are readily excreted in the urine. Toxicity from fat-soluble vitamins is more common than with water-soluble vitamins, and food supplementation has in consequence been more restricted. Deficiency states for fat-soluble vitamins are

thus also more common. In addition, in any medical condition associated with fat malabsorption (undernutrition, celiac disease, sprue, cystic fibrosis), the fat-soluble vitamins are poorly absorbed.

1. FAT-SOLUBLE VITAMINS

VITAMIN A

Vitamin A is a fat-soluble alcohol derived in the animal body from certain of the carotenoid plant pigments, of which β-carotene is the most important. β-Carotene has a unique and specialized role in the photochemical basis of vision. The photosensitive pigment rhodopsin is formed from vitamin A and a protein called opsin. The general effect of vitamin A on cellular function is to reduce the stability of lysosomes; it has some influence also on sulfur metabolism by activating sulfate in mucopolysaccharide formation, and on steroid hormone production. It is considered important in the maintenance of epithelial membranes in the body.

Vitamin A is present in food primarily as the palmitate ester and is hydrolyzed to its free alcohol, retinol, in the intestine. Within intestinal cells, retinol is reesterified, primarily to palmitate, incorporated into the chylomicrons of the mucosa, and absorbed into the lymphatic system.

1. VITAMIN A DEFICIENCY

Clinical Findings

A. Symptoms and Signs: Night blindness and loss of visual acuity in poor light are early eye symptoms, followed by squamous metaplasia that produces dryness of the conjunctivas, xerophthalmia, and, very often, typical small gray-white patches called Bitot spots on the bulbar conjunctivas. As metaplasia progresses, the cornea becomes cloudy and soft (keratomalacia) and, eventually, secondarily infected and ulcerated, at which point corneal damage and loss of vision are irreversible except for the possibility of corneal transplant. Hypertrophy or atrophy of tongue papillae occurs early in vitamin A deficiency. Follicular hyperkeratosis on the buttocks and extensor surfaces of the extremities is common, as are skin and upper respiratory tract infections also.

Vitamin A deficiency (serum level $<$ 20 μg/100 ml) has been shown to be present in 2% of preschool children in the USA. In high-risk populations such as Mexican-Americans, 1/3 of preschool children have been shown to have levels under 20 μg/100 ml and over 1/2 have levels under 30 $\mu g/100$ ml. Vitamin A deficiency is common in children with kwashiorkor. Vitamin A levels are lower in sera of children born of mothers who have not received prenatal vitamin supplementation.

B. Laboratory Findings: The normal plasma vitamin A level in childhood has been suggested to be > 20 $\mu g/100$ ml or more prior to age 6 months and > 30 $\mu g/100$ ml or more thereafter. The mean value in preschool children in the USA has been determined to be $33 \pm 7.6 \ \mu g/100$ ml.

Serum carotene determination is a helpful test in cases of nutritional vitamin A deficiency or fat malabsorption. The normal levels are approximately 70 $\mu g/100$ ml at birth, rising to approximately 340 $\mu g/100$ ml at age 1. The levels fall to about 150 $\mu g/100$ ml at age 3½; thereafter, they are between 100 and 150 $\mu g/100$ ml. Since β-carotene is carried attached to β-lipoproteins, conditions in which β-lipoproteins are elevated, such as hypothyroidism, will be associated with high circulating levels of β-carotene.

Prevention & Treatment

Ideally, the patient should receive a diet with adequate amounts of vitamin A. Vitamin A is found primarily in liver and in yellow vegetables. The content of vitamin A in some common foods is shown in Table 25–1.

The minimum requirement of vitamin A varies with age but is in the range of 1000 IU (330 μg)/day in the child under age 6 years, 2000 IU/day between ages 6 and 10 years, and 3000 IU/day thereafter. Vitamin A has approximately equal concentrations in breast and cow's milk (53 and 34 $\mu g/100$ ml, respectively). The recommended daily dose of vitamin A in cases of vitamin A deficiency is 25,000 IU for 1–2 weeks in conjunction with a high-protein diet. Prophylactic doses are then continued. It is usually necessary to replenish liver stores of vitamin A before the serum levels increase, which may take several weeks. It is also possible to treat deficiency with single massive doses. In cases of malabsorption, a water-miscible vitamin A preparation is given in twice the recommended amount (5000–10,000 IU) as a minimum requirement.

Prognosis

When xerophthalmia is part of a malabsorption syndrome and treatment is early, effective, and sustained, the progress is good. If vitamin A deficiency is associated with general malnutrition, scarring and

secondary infection of the cornea have occurred and subsequent blindness is common.

Chase HP: Nutritional status of preschool Mexican-American migrant farm children. Am J Dis Child 122:316–324, 1971.

McLaren DS & others: Xerophthalmia in Jordan. Am J Clin Nutr 17:117–130, 1960.

Olson JA: Metabolism and function of vitamin A. Fed Proc 28:1670–1677, 1969.

Sandstead HH & others: Nutritional deficiencies in disadvantaged preschool children. Am J Dis Child 121:455, 1971.

Strikantia SG, Reddy V: Effect of a single massive dose of vitamin A on serum and liver levels of the vitamin. Am J Clin Nutr 23:114–118, 1970.

2. VITAMIN A TOXICITY

The availability without prescription of high-potency vitamin A preparations, which have come to be rather extensively prescribed for acne, has led to an increase in vitamin A toxicity. Patients may show peeling of the skin, particularly over the fingers and hands. Long bone pain is marked over the distal extremities, and the child may refuse to walk. Loss of appetite, hypertrophy and hyperemia of gums, skin pigmentation, and alopecia are also found. Signs and symptoms of pseudotumor cerebri occur and can last for several months after vitamin A is discontinued. Radiologically, there is evidence of subperiosteal new bone formation.

The only treatment is discontinuation of excessive doses of vitamin A. Clinical improvement begins within a few days, but a return of the bones to normal may not occur for several months.

Committees on Drugs and on Nutrition, American Academy of Pediatrics: The use and abuse of vitamin A. Pediatrics 48:655–656, 1971.

Lascari AD, Bell WE: Pseudotumor cerebri due to hypervitaminosis A: Toxic consequences of self medication for acne in an adolescent girl. Clin Pediat 9:627, 1970.

VITAMIN D

Vitamin D is absorbed by the intestine in solution in triglyceride particles. It is then carried on an a_2 globulin to the liver, where it is converted to the more active forms 25-hydroxycholecalciferol (25-HCC) and 25-hydroxyergocalciferol. These forms are essential to normal bone physiology and to the maintenance of adequate concentrations of calcium and phosphorus within the extracellular fluid. They also appear to enhance the enzymatic processes necessary for the calcification of the bone matrix. In the presence of parathormone, vitamin D promotes the reabsorption of

TABLE 25–1. Vitamin A content in some common foods.

Liver (2 oz fried)	37,000 IU
Carrots (1 large or 2 small)	11,000 IU
Sweet potato (1 small)	8,100 IU
Spinach (1/2 cup cooked)	7,300 IU
Cantaloupe (1/2 cup)	4,100 IU
Milk (1 cup, whole fresh)	340 IU

phosphate by kidney tubules and may increase the tubular reabsorption of amino acids. Sunlight promotes the endogenous synthesis of vitamin D.

The kidney is now known to form 1:25 dihydroxy HCC, a derivative of 25-HCC which is specifically active in promoting the synthesis of the calcium transport protein in the intestinal villus, a discovery that facilitates the understanding of the mechanisms of rickets in chronic renal disease (see p 461).

Rickets is a disorder of the deposition of hydroxyapatite in bone matrix and in preosseous cartilage at the zone of provisional calcification. By definition, it is conditional on active growth. Although first recognized in relation to vitamin D deficiency, rickets can also result from disorders of phosphate transport and of the bone matrix itself. The classification shown in Table 25–2 is appropriate in the light of present knowledge.

De Luca M: Role of kidney tissue in metabolism of vitamin D. New England J Med 284:554, 1971.

1. VITAMIN D DEFICIENCY

Essentials of Diagnosis

- History of insufficient dietary intake of vitamin D or of malabsorption.
- Listlessness, hypotonicity, and retarded motor development.
- Bony deformities clinically and on x-ray.
- Normal serum calcium, low serum phosphorus, elevated serum alkaline phosphatase.

General Considerations

Vitamin D deficiency rickets continues to be a significant problem in those parts of North America where there is little direct sunlight and where the milk supply is not fortified with vitamin D. Minor degrees

TABLE 25–2. A classification of rickets.

Essential calcium deficiency
  Responsive to normal doses of vitamin D_3 or 25-HCC
    Vitamin D deficiency
  Responsive to high doses of vitamin D_3 or 25-HCC
    Fat malabsorption syndrome
    Chronic renal disease
    Vitamin D dependency
Essential phosphorus deficiency
  The renal tubular dystrophies (See Table 18–3.)
  Phosphate depletion from overuse of aluminum hydroxide gels
Essential matrix abnormalities
  Metaphyseal dysostosis
  Hypophosphatasia and pseudohypophosphatasia

of clinical rickets are common in underprivileged groups such as migrant farm workers, especially those with pigmented skins, and in bedridden children in institutions.

Clinical Findings

A. Symptoms and Signs: Clinical findings include beading of the ribs; widening of the wrists, knees, and ankles; frontal bossing, craniotabes, the development of Harrison's sulcus in the chest wall, and, very rarely, pathologic fractures. In addition there may be lethargy, hypotonicity, muscle pain, hyperextensibility of joints, and motor retardation followed, as the severity increases, by convulsions and tetany. A history of poor vitamin D intake or of exclusion from sunlight is usual.

B. Laboratory Findings: These include variable hypocalcemia and hypophosphatemia. Alkaline phosphatase levels are usually elevated except in generally malnourished children. Generalized aminoaciduria and some impairment of tubular hydrion excretion may also be present, as may minimal glucosuria.

C. X-Ray Findings: Cupping, fraying, and flaring are seen at the ends of the bones. Bony trabeculae lose their sharp definition, which accounts for the general decrease in skeletal radiodensity.

Differential Diagnosis

The history should provide a clear differentiation from cases that are secondary to malabsorption of vitamin D. The vitamin D dependency syndrome presents in an identical clinical fashion; however, there may be a history of a normal vitamin D intake and a family history suggestive of an autosomal recessive condition. Vitamin D dependency will only respond to doses of the order of 40,000 IU daily. In hypophosphatasia and pseudohypophosphatasia, the bone changes are similar to those observed in rickets, serum calcium levels may be elevated, there is vitamin D resistance and phosphoethanolaminuria, and serum alkaline phosphatase levels are low or normal. In hereditary metaphyseal dysostosis, the bone changes are also similar, but there are no biochemical changes, no response to vitamin D even in large doses, and the children are essentially healthy, albeit stocky and bowlegged. This last condition is also sometimes associated with neutropenia, hair hypoplasia, and pancreatic insufficiency.

Prevention

The addition of vitamin D to fluid milk, evaporated milk, and to special milk products and substitutes has helped eradicate vitamin D deficiency rickets in the USA. It is important to remember, however, that 400 IU of vitamin D will only prevent rickets if the intakes of calcium and phosphorus are adequate and there is no absorption defect.

Treatment

Vitamin D deficiency rickets is cured by vitamin D, 5000 IU orally every day for 4–5 weeks. Evidence of cure is rapid. Radiologic and biochemical signs of improvement appear after the first week of therapy. It has occasionally been noted that in 3 weeks' time the radiologic evidence of rickets has completely disappeared.

The disturbance of calcium absorption in malabsorption syndromes is secondary to enteric losses of vitamin D with stool fat. For this reason, doubling the recommended prophylactic dose of vitamin D is usually sufficient; however, in certain cases of hepatobiliary disease, a true resistance to vitamin D has been described.

Daeschner CW & others: Metaphyseal dysostosis. J Pediat 57:844, 1960.
Fraser D: Hypophosphatasia. Am J Med 22:730, 1957.
Lewin PK & others: Iatrogenic rickets in low birth weight infants. J Pediat 78:207, 1971.
Lux SE & others: Chronic neutropenia and abnormal cellular immunity in cartilage-hair hypoplasia. New England J Med 282:231, 1970.
Scriver CR, Cameron D: Pseudohypophosphatasia. New England J Med 281:604, 1969.

2. VITAMIN D DEPENDENCY

Vitamin D dependency rickets has recently been differentiated as a form of vitamin D resistant disease which is probably due to a disorder in the formation or activity of the intestinally active polar form of 25-HCC, 1:25 dihydroxy HCC. The clinical features appear in the first year of life and mimic closely those of vitamin D deficient rickets. In this condition, other siblings may be affected and there is usually a history of normal vitamin D ingestion. There is a prompt response with administration of about 40,000 IU of vitamin D per day, but none to normal daily requirements. The presence of hyperaminoacidemia and renal tubular acidosis distinguishes the condition from X-linked hypophosphatemic vitamin D resistant rickets. Differentiation from the complex Fanconi type renal tubular dystrophy is, however, more difficult; vitamin D dependency will respond to vitamin D alone, whereas the former requires phosphate supplementation as well.

Arnaud C & others: Vitamin D dependency. Pediatrics 46:870, 1970.
Scriver CR: Vitamin D dependency. Pediatrics 46:361, 1970.

3. VITAMIN D INTOXICATION

Two forms of vitamin D intoxication are recognized. In the first, relatively small daily ingestion of vitamin D, ie, 5000 IU/day or less from oversupplemented foods, appears to have led to idiopathic hypercalcemia (see p 615) in sensitized children. The outbreaks occurred primarily in Britain, and the condition is now very uncommon in infancy.

In persons not resistant to vitamin D, ingestion of doses of the order of 1000–3000 IU/kg/day may lead to hypercalcemia together with nausea, anorexia, constipation, polyuria, and transient nitrogen retention. Later, nephrocalcinosis and irreversible renal failure can occur.

Treatment consists of immediate discontinuance of vitamin D.

Committee on Nutrition, American Academy of Pediatrics: The prophylactic requirement and toxicity of vitamin D. Pediatrics 31:512, 1963.

VITAMIN E DEFICIENCY

Vitamin E is believed to be important in stabilizing biologic membranes. Deficiency in laboratory animals results in decreased reproductive ability, muscular dystrophy, and anemia. Vitamin E is widely distributed in foods eaten by man, particularly vegetable fats, plant seeds, nuts, egg yolk, and leafy vegetables.

Lack of vitamin E through absolute dietary deficiency or secondary to steatorrhea has been shown to result in hemolytic anemia in premature infants. Although reduced virility has not been described in humans, focal necrosis of striated muscle occurs in deficient individuals.

The low levels in some premature infants apparently result both from low storage at birth, with little adipose tissue, and inadequate dietary intake. Ten to 15 mg of vitamin E per day orally prevents deficiency in the young infant.

Oski FA, Barness LA: Vitamin E deficiency: A previously unrecognized cause of hemolytic anemia in the premature infant. J Pediat 70:211, 1967.
Symposium: Hematologic aspects of vitamin E. Am J Clin Nutr 21:1–56, 1968.
Symposium: Tocopherol. Lipids 6:238–253, 281–306, 1971.

VITAMIN K

Vitamin K affects the rate of hepatic synthesis of prothrombin (factor II) and of factors VII, IX, and X. A large number of dietary components have biologic vitamin K activity, including green vegetables, soybeans, and fish. Intestinal bacteria also produce considerable quantities of vitamin K for human absorption.

1. VITAMIN K DEFICIENCY

Vitamin K deficiency is most frequently found in newborn infants, particularly when breast-fed, since human milk contains only 1/4 the amount of vitamin K found in cow's milk. The incidence of severe bleeding in newborn infants given vitamin K is 0.3%, compared to 2–5% for infants not given vitamin K.

Diarrhea, oral antibiotics, fat malabsorption, some special formulas, and—since bile salts are important in vitamin K absorption—obstructive jaundice may lead to vitamin K deficiency. Bacterial colonization of the infant's intestine is frequently inadequate at age 24 hours, when maternal prothrombin disappears from the newborn infant's blood.

Newborn infants are usually given 1 mg of the water-soluble form of vitamin K (eg, AquaMephyton) IM in the first day of life, which lessens the incidence of neonatal hemorrhage.

Committee on Nutrition, American Academy of Pediatrics: Vitamin K supplementation. Pediatrics 48:483, 1971.

2. VITAMIN K TOXICITY

Excessive administration of vitamin K, or administration of the fat-soluble forms, can result in hemolytic anemia. This may accentuate hyperbilirubinemia in the newborn infant.

2. WATER-SOLUBLE VITAMINS

Deficiencies of water-soluble vitamins are much less frequent in the USA because of the frequent fortification, particularly with B vitamins, of many foods. Most bread and wheat products are now routinely fortified with B vitamins, including rolls, crackers, cookies, and other bakery goods.

There is less danger of toxicity from water-soluble vitamins because excesses can be excreted in the urine. However, deficiency states can also develop more quickly than with the fat-soluble vitamins because of the limited stores of water-soluble vitamins.

THIAMINE DEFICIENCY

Thiamine (vitamin B_1) is an essential cofactor in the oxidative decarboxylation of pyruvic acid to acetyl-coenzyme A and of other α-keto acids. With magnesium, it activates transketolase in the regeneration of fructose-6-phosphate from ribulose-5-phosphate in the hexose monophosphate shunt. The vitamin is water-soluble and easily destroyed by heat; nevertheless, overt deficiency states are exceedingly rare in North America. Where deficiency does occur, the impact is predominantly on the heart and peripheral nerves. The myocardium shows fatty degeneration, and there is edema of the heart and interstitial tissues. Myelin and axonal degeneration is found in the peripheral nerves. Low red cell transketolase in 20% of underprivileged children in the USA offers some evidence of subclinical involvement in this group.

Clinical Findings

A. Symptoms and Signs: Symptoms are most likely to appear in early infancy, especially if the mother is providing thiamine-deficient breast milk. The infant becomes restless, has attacks of crying as though from abdominal pain, and may vomit breast milk. The vomiting may increase and be accompanied by abdominal distention, flatulence, constipation, and insomnia.

In the acute cardiac forms, there is tachycardia, gallop rhythm, dyspnea, cyanosis, cardiomegaly, hepatomegaly, and pulmonary edema. The condition is rapidly fatal unless treated. In endemic deficiency areas, cardiac failure of unknown etiology should always be treated with thiamine. Less dramatic (but equally serious) is the meningitic form which starts with a bulging fontanel, head retraction, and dilated pupils and may go on to convulsions and coma.

In older infants a chronic form is common in which the symptoms are anorexia, weight loss, weakness, diarrhea, constipation, and edema. Peripheral palsies, which may include vocal cord paralysis, may be seen, and the stretch reflexes are usually absent. Ataxia is a common finding.

B. Laboratory Findings: A blood thiamine level under 4 μg/100 ml (normal: 10 ± 5 μg) is suggestive of thiamine deficiency, but perhaps the most helpful test is to show a level of thiamine in the milk of < 7 μg/100 ml. Normal pasteurized cow's milk contains about 40 μg/100 ml.

Differential Diagnosis

The initial symptoms must be differentiated from pyloric stenosis and other high obstructions. The cardiac forms may be confused with fibroelastosis, congenital heart disease, Pompe's disease, and severe pneumonitis. A sterile CSF culture excludes pyogenic meningitis. Chronic thiamine deficiency must be distinguished from lead poisoning.

Prevention & Treatment

The disease can be prevented by a normal diet containing at least 0.4 mg of thiamine daily. In acute deficiency states, 25 mg of thiamine should be given IV, followed by 20 mg IM twice daily for 3 days and 10 mg orally daily for 6 weeks.

Prognosis

Complete recovery is expected provided an adequate thiamine intake can be assured.

Field CE: Infantile beriberi. Chap 8, pp 194–199, in: *Diseases of Children in the Subtropics and Tropics.* Trowell HC, Jelliffe DB. Arnold, 1958.

Sandstead HH & others: Nutritional deficiencies in disadvantaged preschool children. Am J Dis Child 121:455, 1971.

THIAMINE DEPENDENCY SYNDROMES

Anomalies of the branched chain keto acid decarboxylase system (see p 878) are known to present as a number of traits. One of these is thiamine dependent and responds to 10 mg/day of the hydrochloride.

Thiamine dependency has also been reported in a syndrome with optic atrophy and intermittent ataxia, lactic acidosis, and hyperalaninemia due to pyruvate decarboxylase deficiency.

Lonsdale D & others: Ataxia, hyperpyruvic acidemia, hyperalaninemia, hyperalaninuria. Pediatrics 43:1025, 1969.

Scriver CR & others: Thiamine-responsive maple syrup urine disease. Lancet 1:310, 1971.

RIBOFLAVIN DEFICIENCY

Riboflavin (vitamin B_2) is a constituent of a number of flavoprotein enzymes involved in intermediary metabolism. As riboflavin phosphate, it is incorporated into Warburg yellow enzyme, cytochrome c reductase, and D-amino acid dehydrogenase. As the flavin adenine nucleotide it is the prosthetic group in glycine oxidase, xanthine oxidase, and diaphorase. Riboflavin is water-soluble and is a constituent of both animal and vegetable protein foods (eggs, meat, fish, beans, etc), and for this reason riboflavin deficiency often accompanies protein malnutrition.

Breast milk and cow's milk provide adequate amounts of riboflavin, so that the disorder appears only in children on restricted protein intakes or in those with protein malabsorption. The characteristic triad of signs is sore red lips, seborrheic skin lesions with fissuring of the nasolabial folds and extending from the angle of the mouth, and a purplish-red smooth tongue with enlarged papillae. Corneal injection may also occur at the limbus, with eye pain, tearing, photophobia, and ultimately interstitial keratitis. Excretion of less than 125 μg of riboflavin per gram of creatinine in a random urine sample is suggestive of riboflavin deficiency.

The deficiency state can be prevented by a diet containing 0.6 mg riboflavin/1000 calories. Treatment consists of giving riboflavin, 2 mg IM daily for 2 days, followed by 10 mg IM daily for 3 weeks. Thereafter, a diet containing adequate amounts of riboflavin must be maintained.

NICOTINIC ACID DEFICIENCY
(Pellagra)

Nicotinic acid (niacin) may be ingested from natural food sources or derived endogenously as one of the end products of the kynurenine pathway of tryptophan breakdown. The molecule is a component of nicotinamide adenine dinucleotide (NAD) and nicotinamide adenine dinucleotide phosphate (NADP), which act as hydrogen and electron transfer agents by reversible oxidation and reduction. Nicotinic acid is plentiful in most protein foods and in grains. The only critical diet is one in which there is a substantial content of highly milled maize, which also has a relatively low tryptophan content.

Pellagra tends to be associated with a state of chronic, difficult to define ill health. The most typical lesions are found on the exposed parts of the skin and are aggravated by sunlight and sometimes confused with sunburn. The lesions start as an erythema which then becomes darkly pigmented and progresses to a rough, sharply demarcated, fissured, scaly dermatosis with little tendency to desquamate. The mouth and tongue become red and painful and there is widespread gastrointestinal inflammation with dysphagia, nausea, vomiting, and attacks of diarrhea. Apathy is seen in childhood, but not the more severe psychoses that occur in adult pellagra.

The skin lesions may be confused with those of kwashiorkor. In kwashiorkor, however, the lesions tend not to be on the exposed extremities but around pressure sites in the groin and trunk. The diarrhea must be differentiated from that due to parasitic diseases (including amebiasis) and other infections.

Prevention & Treatment

The condition may be prevented by ensuring a nicotinamide intake of 6–10 mg/day orally, depending on age. Treatment consists of giving 10–25 mg of nicotinamide 3 times daily for 2 weeks, followed by a continuing adequate diet containing sufficient B complex vitamins.

PYRIDOXINE DEFICIENCY

Pyridoxine (vitamin B_6) deficiency was first produced artificially in 2 retarded infants. One developed a marked hypochromic anemia and the other, more characteristically, severe convulsions. Both infants responded promptly to intravenous pyridoxine and were ultimately stabilized on 150 µg/day orally. Shortly afterward, a group of infants given a proprietary liquid milk formula were observed to become hyperirritable between 6 weeks and 4 months of age. Generalized seizures followed which were treated successfully with oral pyridoxine or with a formula containing normal amounts of pyridoxine. A similar history was given by a mother whose breast milk was shown to contain unusually low amounts of pyridoxine. These infants all had normal interictal EEGs, showed no familial incidence of convulsions, and developed unexceptionally on a proper diet. Xanthurenic aciduria was apparent on tryptophan loading; the correction of this abnormality was notable in that greater amounts of pyridoxine were required for its correction than for control of the convulsions. Although pyridoxal phosphate is a coenzyme in a wide range of reactions, the key pyridoxal-dependent reaction in causing convulsions is thought to be that of the formation of gamma-aminobutyric acid from glutamic acid by glutamic acid decarboxylase.

For practical purposes, pyridoxine deficiency occurs only in infancy. It should be considered when convulsions or anemia is otherwise unexplained.

Complete recovery may be expected after the administration of 5 mg of pyridoxine IM followed by 0.5 mg daily by mouth for 2 weeks together with a normal dietary intake.

Coursin DB: Vitamin B_6 metabolism in infants and children. Vitamins Hormones 22:756, 1964.

THE PYRIDOXINE (VITAMIN B_6) DEPENDENCY SYNDROMES

In the neonatal period, affected infants show hyperirritability and generalized convulsions. In some instances the seizures have certain additional characteristics, such as blinking and a startled expression. There is definite familial bias, and the interictal EEG is abnormal. The convulsive tendency is completely resolved by administration of pyridoxine, 2–10 mg/day orally, but withdrawal even after long periods may lead to resumption of seizures. These cases show no abnormality of kynureninase activity nor any other readily accessible pyridoxine-dependent enzyme.

The prompt response to pyridoxine makes it clear that there is no delay in conversion of the coenzyme to pyridoxal phosphate. The key enzyme involved is thought to be glutamic acid decarboxylase, which converts glutamic acid to gamma-aminobutyric acid, an important substrate for cerebral energy metabolism.

Another group of these related syndromes are those associated with an abnormality of kynureninase. In the first category were 2 mentally defective young women with no history of convulsions and no abnormal physical findings. There was a kynureninase defect, as judged by xanthurenic aciduria, and an abnormally high hydroxykynurenine/hydroxyanthranilic acid ratio of 6/0 in the urine of both cases (normal: < 2/0). These abnormalities reverted to normal after administration of 100 mg of pyridoxine IV or orally for several days. The prompt response to intravenous pyridoxine and the normal excretion of 4-pyridoxic acid seem to rule out relative vitamin B_6 deficiencies due to a defect of pyridoxal kinase or excessive conversion of pyridoxine to 4-pyridoxic acid, but these observations do not exclude excessive renal loss of pyridoxal or pyridoxamine.

These syndromes are analogous to homocystinuria and cystathioninuria, in which there are defects of the cystathionine synthetase and cleavage enzymes which can be overcome by large doses of pyridoxine. Also in this group are some cases of infantile spasm. These patients develop massive myoclonic jerks at age 2–12 months and usually become severely retarded. Changes in kynurenine metabolism are the same as reported above, and these may, again, be restored by pyridoxine in doses of about 1 mg/kg IV. Although the biochemical abnormality may be corrected in this manner, only about 1/3 of cases show any clinical response to oral pyridoxine in doses of 4–10 mg/kg/day. All of these groups probably represent defects in the coenzyme binding site of kynureninase; the nature of the cerebral disorder is not known.

Finally, there is a recent report of an 11-year-old girl who suffered from severe stomatitis and reddening of the buttocks in infancy, "failed to thrive," was anemic, and showed a number of bony abnormalities, including defects of the lower dorsal and first lumbar vertebrae, ribs, and short and long bones and delayed ossification of the right femoral epiphyses. Vitamin B supplements were given, but she made slow progress and was considered to be retarded at age 8 with an IQ of 78. On tryptophan loading she was shown to have a virtual absence of kynureninase activity, with a massive xanthurenic aciduria, hydroxykynureninuria, and no hydroxyanthranilic acid in the urine. N^1 Methylnicotinamide and its pyridone derivative were not measured, but the child improved in growth and intellectual function on a regimen consisting of 10 mg nicotinic acid daily. This defect might be interpreted as one of the substrate binding sites on the apoenzyme kynureninase.

In practical terms, diagnosis can easily become unprofitably cumbersome. In typical infantile pyridoxine dependency, pyridoxine, 100 mg IM, followed by 10 mg/day orally, immediately and completely abates convulsions. The forms in which kynureninase activity is affected can only be diagnosed by the measurement of urinary tryptophan metabolites before and after pyridoxine administration. This is overelaborate for general use, and it is probably expedient simply to administer pyridoxine, 100 mg/day orally for at least 3 months, and to observe for clinical improvement.

Infantile pyridoxine dependency responds promptly and well to continued pyridoxine therapy. Myoclonic epilepsy with a kynureninase defect responds variably, and the other types show little, if any, response.

French JM & others: Pyridoxine and infantile myoclonic seizures. Neurology 15:101–113, 1965.

Gentz J & others: Vitamin B$_6$ metabolism in pyridoxine dependency with seizures. Acta paediat scandinav 56:17–26, 1967.

VITAMIN C DEFICIENCY

Essentials of Diagnosis

- Dietary history of an infant 6–12 months of age fed cow's milk and no citrus fruits or green vegetables.
- Fretfulness, anorexia, weight loss, and tenderness of the lower extremities. Legs held in the "frogleg" position.
- Hemorrhages in the gums, skin, or mucous membranes.

General Considerations

Scurvy is rare today. Social and economic factors determining dietary habits have a lot to do with its development.

Structurally, ascorbic acid resembles monosaccharide sugars. Most animal species can synthesize ascorbic acid and thus have no dietary requirement for this vitamin. However, man, the other primates, and guinea pigs cannot metabolize glucose to ascorbic acid because of the absence of the enzyme L-gulonolactone oxidase.

Ascorbic acid has many metabolic roles. Because of its reversible oxidation-reduction capacity, it is active in microsomal electron transport. It is important in preventing depolymerization of collagen and in maintaining the integrity of ground substance. Ascorbic acid presumably has an effect on hematopoiesis since anemia usually accompanies scurvy.

By protecting the enzyme parahydroxyphenylpyruvic acid oxidase from inhibition by its substrate, tyrosine, vitamin C plays an essential role in the metabolism of tyrosine in the newborn period.

Clinical Findings

Populations where breast feeding is in disfavor and where most newborns are fed cow's milk have a higher incidence of symptomatic scurvy. A history of a poor intake of fruits and vegetables is also suggestive. The time required for the development of scurvy after a grossly deficient diet is instituted is about 4–7 months. Certain groups such as the Navajo Indians are especially susceptible.

A. Symptoms and Signs: Nonspecific symptoms appear before any physical changes are evident. Irritability, weakness, anorexia, weight loss, and tenderness of the extremities, particularly of the legs, are common. In more advanced stages of the disease, the affected infant lies quietly in the frogleg position and may exhibit pseudoparalysis because the slightest motion causes severe pain. Small or large hemorrhages may occur anywhere in the body but are most frequent under the periosteum of the long bones, particularly the lower end of the femur and the proximal end of the tibia; this may not be detectable on x-ray until healing has begun with superficial calcification. Gastrointestinal, genitourinary, and meningeal bleeding have been reported occasionally in advanced stages. Hemorrhaging under the mucous membranes of the gums is common if teeth have erupted or are about to erupt. Conjunctival and tongue hemorrhagic lesions are also common. Costochondral beading, which differs from the rachitic rosary by its sharpness ("bayonet" deformity), often occurs.

B. Laboratory Findings: A fasting serum ascorbic acid level of < 0.1 mg/100 ml suggests scurvy. Levels in the 0.1–0.19 mg/100 ml range are considered "low." Samples must be assayed within 48 hours of collection. A more satisfactory procedure is to perform a tolerance test by giving ascorbic acid, 20 mg/kg IV as a 4% solution in normal saline. A 4-hour urine sample containing > 1.5 mg/100 ml rules out scurvy.

C. X-Ray Findings: The earliest x-ray changes appear at the sites of most active growth, eg, the knees, and are characterized by thickening and irregularity at the epiphyseal lines with a subepiphyseal zone of rarefaction. There is thinning of bone cortices and atrophy of the trabecular structure, causing increased transparency ("ground glass" appearance). Shadows of the subperiosteal hemorrhages give the affected long bones a club shape; they become more clearly outlined after several days of treatment, when bone formation is initiated in the periphery.

Differential Diagnosis

If there are no gum hemorrhages, the signs may resemble those of acute pyogenic arthritis. However, the radiologic evidence is distinctive.

Prevention & Treatment

Breast-fed infants usually ingest 20–50 mg/day of ascorbic acid unless the mother's diet is very inadequate. Cow's milk contains insignificant amounts of vitamin C. Attempts at adding vitamin C to proprietary formulas have been successful despite the fact that vitamin C is extremely susceptible to oxidation and heat.

The therapeutic dose of ascorbic acid is 100 mg 3 times a day for infants and children. Infants should receive—in formula, citrus fruit juice, or green vegetables—50 mg of ascorbic acid daily.

Prognosis

Dramatic clinical improvement occurs within 24 hours after therapy with vitamin C is started. X-ray signs show some degree of amelioration within 10 days of the onset of therapy.

Brailsford JF: Some radiographic manifestations of early scurvy. Arch Dis Childhood 28:81–86, 1953.

3. TRACE ELEMENTS

Nutritional disease may result from deficiencies of essential trace elements other than iron and iodine. The extent and importance of such deficiencies is not known, but new analytic technics are resulting in a rapid increase in knowledge of the biologic roles of these elements.

Copper Deficiency

Hypocupremia is a known sequel of hypoproteinemia. Prolonged hypocupremia secondary to a severe malabsorption state may be associated with anemia, neutropenia, and skeletal lesions.

Zinc Deficiency

Zinc deficiency in adolescence, which is endemic in the Middle East, has been correlated with clinical features of retarded growth and delayed sexual maturation. It responds promptly to dietary zinc supplementation.

Chromium Deficiency

Dietary deficiency of chromium can result in impaired glucose tolerance and is an environmental factor to be considered in diabetes mellitus. Chromium deficiency may also be a factor in both the impaired glucose tolerance and the hypoglycemia associated with protein-calorie malnutrition.

Cordano A, Graham GC: Copper deficiency complicating severe chronic intestinal malabsorption. Pediatrics 38:596–604, 1966.

Hopkins L, Masas A: Improvement of CHO metabolism of malnourished infants by administration of chromium. Fed Proc 25:303, 1966.

Mertz W: Biological role of chromium. Fed Proc 26:186, 1967.

Prasad A: Nutritional metabolic role of zinc. Fed Proc 26:172–185, 1967.

Sandstead HH & others: Current concepts on trace minerals: Clinical considerations. M Clin North America 54:1509, 1970.

Cadmium Intoxication

Bone pain, osteomalacia, aminoaciduria, and glycosuria with multiple fractures have been reported as possible sequelae of cadmium intoxication.

Cadmium pollution and itai-itai disease. Lancet 1:382, 1971.

•   •   •

General References

Barness L: Nutritional disorders. Pages 164–185 in: *Textbook of Pediatrics,* 9th ed. Nelson W, Vaughan VC, McKay RJ (editors). Saunders, 1969.

Consultation on Human Testing of Protein-Rich Foods. World Health Organization, 1970.

Davidson S: *Human Nutrition and Dietetics,* 4th ed. Williams & Wilkins, 1969.

Fomon SJ: *Infant Nutrition.* Saunders, 1967.

International Conference on Prevention of Malnutrition in the Preschool Child: *Preschool Child Malnutrition: Primary Deterrent to Human Progress.* National Research Council, 1966.

Metcoff T & others: Biomolecular studies of fetal malnutrition in maternal leukocytes. Pediatrics 47:180, 1971.

O'Neal RM, Johnson DC, Schaeffer AE: Guidelines for classification and interpretation of group blood and urine data collected as part of the National Nutrition Survey. Ped Res 4:103, 1970.

Scrimshaw NS, Gordon JE: *Malnutrition, Learning and Behaviour.* MIT Press, 1967.

White House Conference on Food, Nutrition and Health: *Final Report.* US Government Printing Office, Washington, DC, 1970.

26...

Infections: Viral & Rickettsial

Vincent A. Fulginiti, MD

I. VIRAL INFECTIONS*

Laboratory Diagnosis

The specific etiologic diagnosis of viral infections is seldom possible on clinical grounds alone. Apart from exanthems such as measles and chickenpox and certain CNS infections (paralytic poliomyelitis and rabies), the clinical syndromes caused by different viruses frequently resemble one another. Therefore, laboratory tests are required for specific diagnosis.

The proper collection, shipping, and identification of specimens are essential to adequate diagnosis. In the discussions of specific viral diseases which follow are listed the specimens to be submitted, special procedures in handling and shipping such specimens (where applicable), and what information the physician can expect from the viral diagnostic laboratory.

General considerations which apply to the diagnosis of viral diseases are as follows:

(1) Viral diagnosis usually depends upon isolation of the offending agent or demonstration of the host response on the basis of a rising titer of specific serum antibody (or both).

(2) Specimens for isolation of viruses consist of appropriate body fluids, secretions, or tissue. An adequate sample can usually be obtained by swabbing the appropriate orifice or mucous membrane and immersing the swab immediately in media designed to protect the agent during shipping and handling—usually a mixture of salts and protein which can be supplied by the laboratory. (Veal infusion broth with 0.5% albumin or Hank's balanced salt solution is adequate.) It is almost always necessary to freeze the specimen immediately and keep it frozen until it reaches the laboratory. (Respiratory syncytial virus and cytomegalovirus may be destroyed by freezing and must be kept on ordinary ice during transport.)

(3) Viral antibody titration depends upon the collection of paired sera—a first ("acute") specimen collected as early as possible in the course of the illness and a second ("convalescent") serum collected usually 2–4 weeks later. Accurate serologic diagnosis depends upon aseptic direct venipuncture, careful separation of serum to avoid hemolysis, and maintenance in the frozen state until receipt in the laboratory.

(4) "Quick" diagnostic technics are available for some viral infections, eg, fluorescent antibody diagnosis of rabies, inclusion body identification in herpetic, vaccinal, and varicella infections. In general, these are presumptive tests which require confirmation by means of more elaborate technics.

Horstmann DM, Hsiung GD: Principles of diagnostic virology. In: *Viral and Rickettsial Infections of Man,* 4th ed. Horsfall FL, Tamm I. Lippincott, 1965.

Lennette EH, Schmidt NJ: *Diagnostic Procedures for Viral and Rickettsial Diseases,* 4th ed. American Public Health Association, Inc, 1969.

POXVIRUSES

VARIOLA
(Smallpox)

Essentials of Diagnosis

- History of contact with smallpox patient within past 2 weeks.
- Severe prodrome with high fever, severe backache, and prostration.
- Occasionally a "swimming trunk" rash, centrifugal in distribution, that lasts 3 days.
- Secondary rise in temperature.
- Typical rash appears on third to fifth days, beginning on the face and distal extremities and spreading centrally. Macules progress rapidly to papules, vesicles, umbilication, pustules, and crusts in 3 weeks.
- Early hemorrhagic form may only have prodrome and purpura (no rash).

General Considerations

All ages are susceptible. Immunity following vaccination varies with the interval from last successful vaccination. Vaccination confers virtually complete protection for 1 year, but protection diminishes progressively to nil by 20 years.

A minor form of the disease with lessened mortality is noted in some parts of the world (variola minor,

*For prevention, see Chapter 5.

649

alastrim), although the virus causing this type is indistinguishable from that of smallpox.

Clinical Findings

A. History: A history of prior contact and vaccination status is essential. The incubation period is usually 11–12 days, but it can vary from 7–21 days. No illness is usually apparent until the prodrome, but a nonspecific flu-like "illness of contact" is rarely noted shortly after exposure. Reported "successful" vaccination should be corroborated by observation of a scar.

B. Symptoms and Signs:

1. Prodrome–The onset of the illness is abrupt, with a sudden rise in temperature to 40–40.6° C (104–105° F), severe backache, and extreme prostration. This prodromal period lasts 2–4 days. A morbilliform eruption may occur in the groin and lower abdomen (swimming trunk rash) during the prodrome.

2. Rash–The typical rash heralding the disease appears on the third to fifth day. It begins on the face, wrists, and ankles and spreads over the extremities. At first, erythematous macules appear, each of which become a papule, then a vesicle, and finally a pustule, often with umbilication. The course in a given patient may vary, but the rash usually·progresses for 7–14 days after its first appearance. Encrustation occurs, and a scar results, particularly with secondary bacterial infection. Mucosal lesions are seen at the time of appearance of the skin rash. Corneal infection may occur.

The more fulminant forms of the disease are associated with a confluent rash; the less severe forms with discrete or even minimal rash.

3. Hemorrhagic smallpox–Hemorrhage may appear in the prodrome in "early" hemorrhagic disease, and death occurs before the pocks appear. A "late" hemorrhagic form is recognized in which hemorrhage occurs into established typical smallpox lesions.

C. Laboratory Findings: Leukopenia occurs early, but leukocytosis is more common by the time the disease is recognizable. Other hematologic abnormalities may be expected, with bleeding, bacterial superinfection, and electrolyte imbalance.

Hemorrhagic disease (early) is associated with accelerator globulin deficiency, depression of prothrombin, and marked thrombocytopenia. Late hemorrhagic disease is accompanied by thrombocytopenia.

Virus may be isolated in relatively high titer from the blood and papules early in the disease. In hemorrhagic forms, viremia is persistent until death.

Rapid diagnosis may be accomplished by light microscopic identification of elementary bodies (Gutstein stain), electron microscopic visualization of virus, fluorescent antibody staining of virus antigen in infected cells, and by identification of virus by precipitation with antisera in agar or by fixation of complement. The best source of material for all of these tests is scrapings from the base of a papule collected with a sharp No. 11 scalpel blade after light cleansing with alcohol. The scrapings and swabs (collected simultaneously) may be shipped dry to the laboratory or, where available, in appropriate virologic material (veal infusion broth or Hank's balanced salt solution with added antibiotics). Freezing during transit is desirable but not essential.

Appropriate bacterial cultures should be obtained.

D. X-Ray Findings: Radiologic examination of the chest and bones may help in the diagnosis of pneumonia and osteomyelitis.

Differential Diagnosis

The prodrome is frequently confused with dengue, enterovirus infections, and almost any febrile illness. The prodromal rash may be confused with that of measles. A history of contact and isolation of virus from the blood establish the diagnosis.

Hemorrhagic smallpox must be distinguished from meningococcemia, coagulation disorders, typhus, and other acute hemorrhagic exanthems.

Eruptive smallpox is most frequently mistaken for varicella. In smallpox, the rash has a centrifugal distribution, all lesions are in the same stage of development, and there is a history of a severe, febrile 3-day prodrome and of contact with a case of smallpox within the past 3 weeks.

Complications & Sequelae

Virus multiplication in tissues other than skin results in keratitis and blindness, laryngeal ulceration and edema, encephalitis, pneumonia, and osteomyelitis. Acute psychoses and orchitis have been reported also.

Secondary bacterial infection of the skin, abscess formation, and septicemia are common. Bronchial pneumonia is common later in the course.

Prevention

Routine smallpox vaccination is no longer recommended. Prevention of the disease in exposed susceptibles can be achieved with methisazone (Marboran) given during the incubation period (see p 957).

Treatment

Give supportive care, with attention to shock, blood replacement, and fluid and electrolyte balance. Appropriate antibacterial therapy should be employed when bacterial superinfection occurs.

Prognosis

The overall mortality in smallpox is 25%, but this is because fulminating and hemorrhagic diseases are almost universally fatal, whereas discrete smallpox is rarely fatal (1% or less). Recovery is usually complete in survivors, although postencephalitic symptoms and osteomyelitis may prolong convalescence.

Dixon CW: *Smallpox.* Churchill, 1962.

Kempe CH: Smallpox. In: *The Biologic Basis of Pediatric Practice.* Cooke R (editor). McGraw-Hill, 1969.

Rao AR, Prahlad I, Swaminathan M: A study of 1000 cases of smallpox. J Indian MA 35:296, 1960.

COMPLICATIONS OF
SMALLPOX VACCINATION

Essentials of Diagnosis

- History of recent vaccination.
- Typical vaccinial vesicles in sites other than vaccination area.
- Lack of healing of primary vaccination site after 15 days.
- Rash, corneal ulceration, and CNS symptoms following vaccination.
- Personal or family history of serious infections or hematologic or immunologic disease.

General Considerations

In most individuals, dermal vaccination results in a predictable, benign, local skin infection beginning on the third postinoculation day as a papule, progressing to vesiculation, forming a pustule, scabbing, and ultimately scarring during the next 3 weeks. In a few patients, untoward reactions occur which can be classified as shown in Table 26–1. As can be seen, most complications are infections, and many occur because of poor selection of vaccinees (immunologic deficiency states, malignancies, eczema, etc) or poor or ill-advised local care of the vaccination site.

Clinical Findings

Findings vary with specific complications. Important elements are the history of recent vaccination, excessive trauma in the preparation of the vaccination site, bathing during the "take," manipulation or irritation of the site, the prior presence of a bacterial respiratory or skin infection, allergic conjunctivitis and prior or concurrent inflammatory skin lesions (eczema, burns, pyoderma, exanthems, etc).

A. Symptoms and Signs of Specific Complications:

1. Noninfectious rashes—Macular, maculopapular, or vesicular rashes of presumed "allergic" or "hypersensitivity" origin have been noted at the height of the primary take (7–14 days). The rash may be localized or generalized, and is usually intensely erythematous and associated with a marked degree of erythema and induration surrounding the normal-appearing primary site. Pruritus and excoriation may be present. This is not an infective complication, and virus is not recoverable from the rash. No complications are observed.

2. Bacterial superinfection—This usually occurs in a child with recurrent or concurrent streptococcal respiratory infection. It may also be associated with skin infections (streptococcal or staphylococcal) elsewhere on the body. Manipulation of the primary vaccination causes seeding of the bacteria. Examination reveals an impetiginous vaccination site, and lifting a corner of the scab allows a thin, serous exudate to escape which on bacteriologic examination with Gram's stain is seen to contain many cocci and which

TABLE 26–1. Complications of vaccination.

Major Category	Specific Syndromes	Comment
Noninfectious rashes	"Erythema multiforme," macular ("toxic eruption"), maculopapular	
	Vesicular, urticarial	Differentiate from generalized
Bacterial superinfection	Streptococcal, staphylococcal, mixed	Often hyperkeratotic
	Tetanus, syphilis	Of historical interest in USA
Vaccination by abnormal route	Intramuscular, oral, etc	
Accidental inoculation (may occur in vaccinated individual or be acquired by contact with vaccinated individual)	Into normal skin, but more often into abnormal skin—eg, burns, pyoderma, exanthem, eczema; other dermatitides—eg, varicella, herpes	
	Mucosal (usually oral or conjunctival)	
	Corneal (keratitis)	
Congenital vaccinia	Disseminated infection	Acquired in utero
Generalized vaccinia	Benign or progressive ("malignant")	
Progressive vaccinia	In hypogammaglobulinemic (congenital x-linked, thymic alymphoplasia) In dysgammaglobulinemia With malignancies (chronic lymphatic leukemia, Hodgkin's, lymphoma, etc)	
Encephalitis	Postvaccinial	
Unusual	Hemolytic anemia, arthritis and osteomyelitis, laboratory infections, pericarditis and myocarditis	

on culture yields a profuse growth of streptococci or staphylococci (or both). Secondary lesions may be noted near the primary site or elsewhere.

3. Accidental inoculation—"Secondary" lesions may occur anywhere on the body at the time of or shortly after the vesiculopustular stage of vaccination, but are most frequent on exposed surfaces (nares, face, periorbital regions, extremities). If the child has been bathed, the diaper area may be involved. The individual lesions resemble a primary vaccination, and virus may be recovered from them.

Significant areas may become involved if the skin was previously abnormal. Thus, life-threatening vaccinia virus spread occurs in eczema (exczema vaccinatum), severe burns, and extensive dermatitides. The secondary lesions resemble primary vaccinations, but they are modified by the underlying disease and their atypical appearance may cause a delay in diagnosis. A history of contact with a recently vaccinated individual may lead to rapid diagnosis. Fever may be marked, and secondary bacterial infection with purulent drainage may occur. Virus is recoverable from the skin, and failure to detect serum antibody 1 week or more after onset is a grave prognostic sign.

Accidental inoculation of the conjunctivas is manifest by intense inflammation characterized by increased vascularity, pannus formation, and occasionally by a purulent exudate. If keratitis occurs, cloudiness of the cornea, severe photophobia and pain, and a fluorescein-stainable ulcer are noted.

4. Congenital vaccinia—This rare complication may occur following vaccination of a pregnant woman or contact of a pregnant woman with a vaccinated individual. Death in utero or massive, generalized infection of the infant with multiple cutaneous lesions may occur and may be fatal.

5. Generalized vaccinia—Blood-borne spread of vaccinia virus results in typical "pocks" on normal skin in an individual with a normal-appearing primary "take." The vaccination response is generally at its height (6–8 days). Virus can be recovered from the secondary lesions, and serum antibody, although it may be delayed, is produced in normal amounts.

6. Progressive vaccinia (vaccinia necrosa or gangrenosa)—Failure of the primary vaccination site to heal after 2 weeks establishes the diagnosis of progressive vaccinia. Bacterial infection must be ruled out, but the diagnosis should not be unduly delayed. The primary lesion fails to resolve normally, and slow progression at the margin with a "soft" vesicular border is observed. Central necrosis may be pronounced. Small "satellite" lesions may appear in uninoculated skin surrounding the primary site or at a distance from it. They resemble a primary take at first, but each progresses as does the primary. With delayed diagnosis, large areas of skin become involved and extensive peripheral spread is noted. The child usually remains well, with little fever or systemic signs. Secondary bacterial infection, usually due to gram-negative organisms, occurs late.

Virus is recovered in high titer from all skin lesions. Serum antibody is usually absent. No skin reaction at 24–48 hours is noted following intradermal injection of killed vaccinia virus. Other findings include those of the underlying disease (decreased serum globulins in hypogammaglobulinemia, abnormal peripheral blood and bone marrow in leukemia, etc).

7. Postvaccinial encephalitis—Following primary vaccination by 10–13 days, headache, vomiting, and drowsiness may herald encephalitis. Physical findings include cranial nerve palsies, coma, spastic paralysis, and occasionally nuchal rigidity. CSF pleocytosis (lymphocytic) and increased CSF protein are usually observed. Virus is usually not recoverable from CSF or autopsy material.

B. Laboratory Findings: Definitive diagnosis of the infectious complications depends upon isolation or other identification of vaccinia virus (complement fixing, hemagglutinating, precipitating antigens) from skin lesions. This is best accomplished by scrapings or swab specimens from the base of a scalpel-denuded papular or vesicular lesion. Identification of virus in blood can be accomplished in progressive vaccinia.

Determination of the immune response of the host is also important in the diagnosis. Intradermal injection of 0.1 ml of heat-inactivated vaccinia virus produces a delayed type skin response in normal vaccinees. This reaction is absent in patients with progressive vaccinia.

Serum neutralizing antibody can almost never be detected in progressive vaccinia nor in overwhelming eczema vaccinatum.

Underlying diseases such as hypogammaglobulinemia, leukemia, etc should be investigated by appropriate laboratory tests. Bacterial infections are identified by standard bacteriologic technics utilizing material from pustules, blood specimens, or other appropriate materials.

Prevention

Smallpox vaccination is no longer recommended for children. (See Chapter 5.)

Treatment

A. Hypersensitivity Reactions: Use of antihistamines, starch baths, and sedation aid in control of severe pruritus.

B. Bacterial Superinfection: Appropriate antibiotic therapy based upon bacteriologic findings is indicated.

C. Accidental Inoculation: Most cases require no therapy. With lesions around the eyes or in areas exposed to trauma and moisture, the use of vaccinia immune globulin (VIG), 0.3–0.6 ml/kg body weight, may result in more rapid healing.

Eczema vaccinatum or any extensive infection of skin in patients with no immunologic defect may respond to VIG, 0.6–1 ml/kg. With lack of serum antibody and overwhelming infection, higher doses of VIG (up to 10 ml/kg), methisazone (see Progressive Vaccinia, below), or exchange transfusion may be helpful.

D. Congenital Vaccinia: If the pregnant woman has been vaccinated, VIG is indicated to help prevent viremic spread to the fetus.

E. Generalized Vaccinia: No therapy is usually necessary.

F. Progressive Vaccinia: Because of the slowly progressive nature of this illness and because the mortality rate without treatment is 100%, all patients should be treated in centers experienced with this complication. Massive amounts of VIG may be necessary. Experiments have shown that methisazone (Marboran) in a dosage of 200 mg/kg orally stat followed by 200 mg/kg/day in 4 divided doses for 3 days is of value in 50% of cases. Repeated exchange transfusions with blood from a recently vaccinated donor may be beneficial.

Prognosis

If recovery occurs, it is usually complete. This is especially true of those complications that do not constitute a threat to life. In progressive vaccinia, the mortality rate is 100% without therapy and 30% or less with current therapy. Eczema vaccinatum is occasionally fatal despite therapy.

The mortality in postvaccinial encephalitis is 30–40%; residual neurologic damage is frequent in survivors.

Sequelae include blindness (keratitis), neurologic handicap (encephalitis), scarring (bacterial infection), and osteomyelitis (progressive vaccinia).

Fulginiti VA, Kempe CH: Poxvirus diseases. Chap 25, pp 1–27, in: *Practice of Pediatrics.* Vol 2. Brennemann-Kelley. Prior, 1970.

Kempe CH: Studies on smallpox and complication of smallpox vaccination. Pediatrics 26:176, 1960.

Neff JM & others: Complications of smallpox vaccination, U.S., 1963. Pediatrics 39:916, 1967.

MOLLUSCUM CONTAGIOSUM

The typical lesions of this uncommon viral infection are white to pink, pearly, hard, rapidly maturing asymptomatic papules which umbilicate and extrude a central core of friable exudate. The most common sites are the face, back, arms, and buttocks. The incubation period is believed to be 2 weeks.

A history of contact is not usually present in sporadic cases, but outbreaks have been observed in schools or institutions. The histologic picture is diagnostic. Prickle cells of the epithelium undergo degeneration, and round hyaline cytoplasmic masses are seen (molluscum bodies, or Henderson-Paterson inclusions). Virus isolation is possible but not readily available.

Molluscum contagiosum is rarely confused with other lesions. Solitary lesions must be distinguished from malignancies.

Surgical excision is rarely necessary. Incision or cautery, usually chemical—or both incision and cautery—is successful in eradicating lesions. Podophyllum, silver nitrate, trichloroacetic acid, and phenol have all been used successfully.

Molluscum contagiosum is usually a self-limited, benign disease. Autoinoculation (rare) results in hundreds of lesions and a chronic course.

Barefoot SW: Molluscum contagiosum: Its incidence and further experiences in treatment with resins of podophyllum. South MJ 49:1270, 1956.

Overfield TK, Brody JA: An epidemiological study of molluscum contagiosum. J Pediat 69:640, 1966.

MYXOVIRUSES

INFLUENZA

Except in major epidemics, clinical identification of influenzal infection may be impossible. Influenza is mimicked by other respiratory viral infections. "Flu" syndrome as identified in adults is uncommon in children.

Virus isolation is both possible and desirable. Increase in serum antibody is valuable in identifying epidemics.

Influenza viruses cause sporadic clinical illness in infants and children in nonepidemic infections which account for 5–10% of all serious respiratory infections. Most frequent is the upper respiratory infection (URI) syndrome, although croup, bronchiolitis, and pneumonia also occur. During epidemics, a sudden onset of fever and "toxic" symptoms may accompany respiratory manifestations.

Clinical Findings

A. History: The history is compatible with various types of respiratory infections of "viral" nature. A history of the same illness in other members of the family or school group, or more severe illness in younger siblings, can often be obtained.

B. Symptoms and Signs: There are no distinguishing clinical characteristics except the abrupt onset of high fever and "toxic" symptoms which are in contrast to most other respiratory viruses. Influenza C virus has been associated with the croup syndrome in infants.

C. Laboratory Findings: The usual laboratory tests are of little help. Specific diagnosis depends upon isolation of virus from respiratory secretions. A swab of nasopharyngeal or throat secretions should be sent in appropriate media to the laboratory. Paired sera obtained early in the course of the illness and after 2–3 weeks are of value in retrospective diagnosis. Early identification of virus type is important in control of epidemics by immunization.

D. X-Ray Findings: Chest x-rays may reveal extensive bronchial pneumonia or simply hyperaeration.

Differential Diagnosis

This is primarily an etiologic differential diagnosis since many viruses produce the same syndrome. With croup, it is important to differentiate from *Hemophilus influenzae* epiglottitis (cherry-red epiglottis, severe systemic illness, positive throat and blood cultures) and spasmodic or allergic croup (history of early respiratory symptoms or fever, x-ray demonstration of foreign body or its effects).

Complications & Sequelae

Pneumonia may be followed by bacterial superinfections (particularly staphylococcal), with empyema, pyopneumothorax, etc. Croup may be associated with drying of the tracheal mucous membranes (with subsequent encrustation and obstruction), cardiac arrest, subcutaneous or mediastinal emphysema, and pneumothorax.

Prevention

Amantadine (Symmetrel), may reduce the risk of influenza due to type A_2 if administered prior to infection. The dosage is as follows: 1–9 years: 4–9 mg/kg/day (do not exceed 150 mg/day) in 2 or 3 doses. 9–12 years: 200 mg/day in 2 doses (total dose).

Influenza vaccine is discussed in Chapter 5.

Treatment

Supportive measures are critical, especially in croup. Support of the airway, judicial tracheostomy, and attention to hydration and nutrition and to peripheral cardiovascular integrity may be lifesaving. (Croup is discussed further in Chapter 12.)

Prognosis

In general, complete recovery is the rule. Children—particularly young infants with croup—may die from cardiac arrest or other complications. Tracheostomy may prolong convalescence and require care beyond the period of acute infection.

Chanock RM, Parrott RH: Acute respiratory disease in infancy and childhood: Present understanding and prospect for prevention. Pediatrics 36:21, 1965.

Clark PS & others: An influenza B epidemic within a remote Alaska community. JAMA 214:507, 1970.

Lindsay MI & others: Hong Kong influenza. JAMA 214:1825, 1970.

Parrott RH & others: Clinical syndromes among children. Am Rev Resp Dis 88:73, 1963.

PARAINFLUENZA

The parainfluenza viruses are among the more important respiratory viruses in childhood because they cause croup and upper respiratory illness. Parainfluenza type 3 is most important very early in life, as most 1-year-old infants have been infected. The his-

tory, differential diagnosis, complications, and treatment are as for influenza (see above).

Although it is difficult to distinguish parainfluenza infections from other respiratory viral illness, the presence of hoarseness suggests this etiology. This is particularly true if one member of the family has croup and the others upper respiratory infection with hoarseness. Viral diagnosis is feasible, and identification of group and type is possible by laboratory examination of secretions and by antibody titration.

Recovery is the rule. Reinfection is common, but second infections tend to be less severe and with less fever.

MUMPS

Essentials of Diagnosis

- History of exposure 14–21 days previously.
- Unilateral or bilateral parotid gland swelling.
- Aseptic meningitis with or without parotitis.
- Pancreatitis, orchitis, oophoritis (or combination).

General Considerations

Mumps is a common childhood infection which is asymptomatic in 30–40% of cases. Most children are infected, and lifetime immunity results. A few remain susceptible throughout adolescence and adult life, when parotitis with orchitis may occur.

Clinical Findings

A. History: Contact results in infection 14–21 days later. Only 60–70% of cases develop symptoms, and bilateral (or unilateral) painful swelling of the parotid glands is usually the only manifestation of the disease. Parotitis may be accompanied by mild respiratory symptoms. Occasionally, CNS symptoms appear prior to or in the absence of parotid gland involvement. Abdominal pain is a frequent complaint and may represent pancreatic involvement.

B. Symptoms and Signs:

1. Parotitis or salivary gland form—Smooth, tender enlargement of the affected salivary gland or glands is the most common finding. Lymphedema of the face is frequently present also and makes the swelling indistinct at its margins. Obliteration of the angle of the mandible is a useful diagnostic sign, as is the alignment of the fusiform swelling with the line formed by the long axis of the ear and the ramus of the mandible. Upward and lateral displacement of the earlobe is noted. The opening of Stensen's duct may be pointed and reddened.

Submaxillary or sublingual gland involvement produces swelling in the lateral and anterior aspects of the neck, respectively. Both are palpated just beneath the mandible and may appear to be fused with it as a result of surrounding lymphedema.

Systemic symptoms may consist of high fever and headache or mild respiratory symptoms, or may be absent.

2. Meningoencephalitis—Mumps virus is the most common cause of aseptic meningitis in childhood. CSF pleocytosis is said to occur in 10–50% of all cases of mumps, although overt clinical symptoms are less common.

Aseptic meningitis may be accompanied by, may precede, or may occur in the absence of parotitis. Fever and headache increase, nuchal rigidity is noted, and gastrointestinal symptoms (nausea and vomiting) may occur. CNS irritability is uncommon, and convulsions are rare. Recovery is rapid, with symptoms subsiding in 3–10 days, almost always without sequelae.

3. Pancreatitis—Mild to moderate abdominal pain may be present in the parotitic form of mumps. When severe epigastric pain occurs in association with nausea, persistent vomiting, high fever, chills, and severe prostration, pancreatitis should be suspected.

4. Orchitis or oophoritis—The gonads may be involved in postpubertal individuals with sudden onset of fever, chills, systemic symptoms, and testicular (males) or lower abdominal pain (females). Testicular swelling and extreme pain occur. Symptoms subside in 3–14 days, with abdominal tenderness being most persistent.

5. Other glandular involvement—Rarely, overt inflammation of the thyroid, Bartholin's glands, and breasts may be seen.

6. Endocardial fibroelastosis and subacute thyroiditis have recently been said to be due to mumps virus infection, but the association has not been proved.

C. Laboratory Findings: In almost 75% of patients, serum amylase levels rise in proportion to the glandular swelling. Return to normal values occurs in 2–3 weeks. CSF pleocytosis with lymphocytosis (often 500–1000 cells/cu mm) is associated with elevated CSF protein and normal CSF glucose values.

Mumps virus may be isolated from saliva, the pharynx, or urine and, in cases of aseptic meningitis, from the CSF. A 4-fold rise in serum antibody titer is diagnostic, and is particularly useful in the diagnosis of nonsalivary gland forms of the disease. Serum should be collected as early as possible in the clinical course and again in 2 weeks.

Differential Diagnosis

The glandular forms of the disease must be distinguished from other acute causes of swelling in the neck: cervical lymphadenitis (location; coexistence of pharyngeal, tonsillar, or skin infection; leukocytosis with shift to the left; discreteness, absence of serum amylase elevation), acute suppurative parotitis (local inflammation, unilateral involvement, leukocytosis, purulent secretion from salivary duct), acute obstructive parotitis (visualization of calculus in the duct, history of previous episodes), other viral parotitides (coxsackievirus and lymphocytic choriomeningitis

virus infections, distinguishable by virologic methods), acute lymphoma or lymphosarcoma (painless enlargement, involvement of lymph nodes, bone marrow findings), and acute episodes of recurrent parotitis (history of previous episodes; sialography reveals sialectasia).

Pancreatitis and oophoritis may be confused with other causes of acute abdominal pain such as a ruptured viscus, acute appendicitis (especially in females with right-sided oophoritis), peptic ulcer, etc. A history of exposure to mumps, a high degree of suspicion, and serum amylase elevation all contribute to accurate diagnosis.

Meningoencephalitis occurring in the absence of parotitis must be distinguished from all other causes. This can usually be done by means of laboratory evaluation.

Complications

Rare sequelae of meningoencephalitis include deafness (auditory nerve damage), postinfectious encephalitis syndrome or myelitis, and facial neuritis.

Contrary to common belief, mumps orchitis and oophoritis do not result in sterility. Most often it is unilateral, and even with bilateral infection total atrophy of the gonads is unlikely.

Mumps myocarditis, arthritis, and hepatitis are rare.

Treatment

Control of fever, pain, and discomfort is occasionally necessary. Orchitis is best treated by conservative management, with rest, testicular support, and analgesics, although some physicians favor systemic corticosteroid therapy, which may result in more rapid subsidence of testicular swelling. Surgical intervention and hormonal therapy appear to offer no advantages. To prevent orchitis, administration of mumps hyperimmune gamma globulin appears to be effective in reducing the incidence by 75%. Several commercial preparations are available.

Prognosis

Mumps is usually a self-limited infection lasting approximately 1 week in all forms. Recovery is spontaneous and complete, and sequelae are rare. Immunity is lifelong. Recurrent episodes of parotitis are due to other causes.

Azimi PH & others: Mumps meningoencephalitis in children. JAMA 207:509–512, 1969.

Blitz D: The clinical evaluation of mumps in an orphanage. New York J Med 51:2765, 1951.

Bruyn HB, Sexton HM, Brainerd HD: Mumps meningoencephalitis: A clinical review of 119 cases. California Med 86:153, 1957.

Gellis SS, McGuiness AC, Peters M: A study on the prevention of mumps orchitis with γ-globulin. Am J Med Sc 210:661, 1945.

Levitt LP & others: Mumps in a general population. Am J Dis Child 120:134–138, 1970.

RESPIRATORY SYNCYTIAL VIRUS (RSV) DISEASE

Essentials of Diagnosis

- Bronchiolitis in very young infants is probably due to RSV.
- Illnesses are indistinguishable from other respiratory viral diseases (see Influenza).

General Considerations

RSV is the single most important cause of viral respiratory disease in infants and children, accounting for nearly 40% of all serious respiratory illnesses and for almost 70% of all cases of bronchiolitis. Children are infected early in life, and by age 1 most have acquired antibody. RSV infection appears to occur even when serum neutralizing antibody is present, and reinfection is common.

Clinical Findings

A. History: (See also Influenza.) A history of preceding upper respiratory symptoms is frequent in RSV infections, which then progress to lower tract disease. Fever is a more frequent finding in RSV infection than in other myxovirus diseases.

B. Symptoms and Signs:

1. Upper respiratory infections—Nonspecific symptoms of rhinitis, nasal stuffiness, and bronchitis. Cough and fever may be more frequent with RSV infections.

2. Bronchiolitis—Dyspnea and, frequently, severe respiratory distress, usually associated with copious, occasionally thick nasal and pharyngeal secretions, are the principal manifestations. Hyperaeration of lungs occurs, with fine rales and marked expiratory wheezing. Fever may be high. Retractions may be evident, and severe respiratory effort is a frequent finding.

3. Bronchial pneumonia—Dyspnea and tachypnea are evident. Rales may or may not be present. Expiratory wheezing is not part of the picture of bronchial pneumonia.

C. Laboratory Findings: Virologic diagnosis depends upon isolation of RSV or demonstration of 4-fold antibody rise in paired sera. Throat or nasopharyngeal swabs placed in appropriate media and kept cold but not frozen are essential. Freezing may destroy the virus.

D. X-Ray Findings: In bronchiolitis, generalized hyperaeration is often quite marked, with depression of the diaphragm, precardiac and retrosternal hyperaerated lungs, and diminished respiratory excursion on fluoroscopy. Pneumonia results in a similar pattern to a less marked degree. Patchy, diffuse peripheral infiltrates may be seen with both but are more prominent in pneumonia.

Differential Diagnosis

The differentiation between RSV and other respiratory viral infections can only be made by laboratory identification of the virus. Clues to RSV infection include wheezing, fever, and cough, which are prominent in RSV infection but may occur with other types of infection also. Bronchiolitis must be distinguished from pneumonia (lack of expiratory wheezing, prominence of pulmonary infiltrates) and allergic asthma (history of recurrence, family history, other signs or symptoms of atopy). Aspiration of a foreign body is characterized by a history of unilateral emphysema and endoscopic visualization; cystic fibrosis is diagnosed on the basis of sweat chloride determination, family history, and a history of meconium ileus or gastrointestinal symptoms.

Complications

Secondary bacterial infection may occur. Cardiac failure is a rare complication.

Treatment

Maintenance of airway and oxygenation is critical, and may be lifesaving in bronchiolitis. Cold vapor produced by bubbling oxygen through water should be administered by means of a croup tent. Hydration—usually by administration of intravenous fluids, since patients handle feedings poorly and may aspirate oral liquids—is essential. Expectorants have been used but seem less satisfactory than moist oxygen. If cardiac failure develops, administer digitalis.

Less well documented therapeutic attempts include administration of epinephrine (0.1 ml of 1:1000 solution subcut) or aminophylline (5 mg/kg IV every 6 hours), intravenous administration of hydrocortisone (25 mg every 6 hours), tracheostomy, and intermittent positive pressure breathing. Controlled trials have not shown these methods of therapy to be superior to good nursing care with attention to oxygenation and moist air.

Antibiotics have also been advocated, but there is no rationale for their use.

Prognosis

Bronchiolitis is rarely fatal, and recovery is usually complete. Respiratory symptoms and signs, cough, and wheezing may persist or may recur with subsequent respiratory infections whether or not they are due to RSV. There is some evidence linking RSV bronchiolitis to subsequent asthma.

Beem M, Oehms M: Observations on the etiology of acute bronchiolitis in infants. J Pediat 61:864, 1962.

Chanock RM & others: Respiratory syncytial virus. Am J Pub Health 52:918, 1962.

Glezen WP & others: Epidemiologic patterns of acute lower respiratory disease of children in a pediatric group practice. J Pediat 78:397–406, 1971.

MEASLES
(Rubeola)

Essentials of Diagnosis

- History of exposure 9–14 days previously.

- Three-day prodrome consisting of fever, conjunctivitis, coryza, and cough.
- Koplik's spots–pathognomonic small whitish specks on a red base on buccal mucous membranes–appear 1–2 days before rash.
- Maculopapular, confluent rash begins at hairline and spreads downward over the face and body in 3 days.
- Leukopenia. Multinucleated giant cells (Warthin-Finkeldey cells) in oral and nasal scrapings.

General Considerations

Measles is an acute, highly contagious disease usually affecting preschool children. Over 95% of persons are infected prior to age 15. Immunity is solid and lifelong.

Clinical Findings

A. History: A history of contact can usually be elicited and is particularly important in sporadic episodes. During epidemics, contact may be frequent and usually is with another member of the family.

B. Symptoms and Signs: After an incubation period of 9–14 days, the illness begins with high fever and lassitude, which persist and are accompanied in the next 3 days by increasing cough, coryza, and conjunctivitis. The cough is barking and harsh, and more noticeable at night. Severe conjunctival inflammation may be present, and photophobia is common. Preceding or accompanying the rash, Koplik's spots appear as small white specks on an intensely red base. Koplik's spots may be absent, but when present are pathognomonic of measles. They may be few in number or may involve the entire buccal mucous membrane, and occasionally are seen on the nasal mucous membranes also. The rash begins near the hairline as faint macules and papules and rapidly progresses to involve the face, trunk, and arms. When the rash appears on the lower extremities, it begins to fade on the face, and then gradually disappears over a 3–6 day interval. The lesions begin as discrete macules and papules and rapidly coalesce, involving large areas of skin. Fine desquamation may accompany healing. The coryzal symptoms reach their peak during the first 4–5 days and are accompanied by a harsh "barking" cough which persists throughout the illness, which lasts 9–10 days, and may be manifest after all other symptoms have subsided.

The general appearance (the "measly" look) of a child with florid measles is characteristic. The patient is red-eyed, with puffy eyelids and a swollen bridge of the nose, a distressed look, and copious, thin nasal secretions. The child with measles sits listlessly in bed, his apathy punctuated by violent harsh coughing. Combined with a confluent red rash, the clinical picture is one of extreme (though temporary) distress.

C. Laboratory Findings: Marked leukopenia is present early in the course. White counts as low as 1500–3000/cu mm are not uncommon, and lymphocytosis is marked. If bacterial superinfection occurs, abrupt leukocytosis with a shift to the left may be evident.

In doubtful prodromal cases, examination of nasal secretions or oral scrapings may reveal the characteristic Warthin-Finkeldey giant cells (large multinucleated cells).

Measles virus can be recovered from the blood or nasal and oropharyngeal secretions during the prodrome and early part of the rash. However, this is seldom necessary to establish the diagnosis. A 4-fold rise in serum antibody can be demonstrated in paired sera.

D. X-Ray Findings: In typical, uncomplicated measles, chest x-rays may reveal patchy pneumonic infiltrates or the typical "hilar pneumonia" pattern. Overaeration is frequent, and in the presence of bacterial pneumonia the x-ray may reveal lobular or lobar consolidation. With staphylococcal or, less commonly, pneumococcal pneumonia, empyema or pyopneumothorax may be evident.

Differential Diagnosis

Measles must be differentiated from other common exanthematous diseases of childhood. Table 26–2 lists the principal distinguishing features.

Abdominal pain (see below) in measles may be due to appendicitis or may result from gastrointestinal infection without appendicitis.

Acute prodromal measles with CNS manifestations must be differentiated from other causes of fever and convulsions. The presence of conjunctivitis and cough is helpful, as is the finding of giant cells in nasal scrapings or the presence of Koplik's spots.

Complications & Sequelae

A. Upper and Lower Respiratory Tract: Bacterial infection occurs in 5–15% of all cases of measles; otitis media and pneumonia are the most common forms. Sinusitis, mastoiditis, tonsillopharyngitis, and cervical adenitis also occur.

Viral complications include severe bronchial pneumonia and a peculiar viral pneumonia known as Hecht's giant cell pneumonia. The latter occurs frequently without rash and may be fatal.

B. Encephalitis: Occurring in 1:1000 instances of measles, this illness begins with fever, CNS signs (coma, convulsions, bizarre behavior, etc), and vomiting 3–8 days after the onset of rash. Sixty percent of patients recover completely; 25% have severe sequelae; and the remainder die.

Diagnosis can be suspected clinically and confirmed by the finding of CSF pleocytosis (lymphocytosis) and an elevated CSF protein, with normal or slightly elevated CSF glucose content.

C. Hemorrhagic Measles: Rarely, a fulminating form of measles is seen, with hemorrhage into the gastrointestinal tract, mucous membranes, and CNS. Fever and toxicity are pronounced, and the rash is purpuric and typically morbilliform. CNS symptoms (coma, convulsions, etc) may be prominent.

TABLE 26–2. Differential diagnosis of exanthematous diseases.

Disease	Incubation Period	Prodrome	Exanthem	Enanthem	Other Diagnostic Features
Measles	9–14 days	3 days. Cough, coryza, conjunctivitis.	Red, maculopapular, confluent, face to feet, lasts 7–10 days, may desquamate.	Koplik's spots	Cough prominent.
Rubella	16–18 days	Usually none	Pink, maculopapular, discrete, spreads rapidly, lasts 3–5 days.	None or faint	Lymphadenopathy may be prominent.
Roseola infection	10–14 days	3 days fever; "well" child.	Rose, macular, discrete, fleeting.	None	Child remains well. Occasional febrile convulsion with first rise in temperature.
Fifth disease (erythema infectiosum)	About 7–14 days	None	"Slapped cheek," lace-like rash on extremities, may reappear, lasts 7–14 days.	Variable	Rash is characteristic. May appear when extremity is warmed (bathing, clothing, etc).
Scarlet fever	2–5 days	1–2 days. Fever, vomiting, sore throat.	Red, punctate, sandpaper feel, confluent blush, lasts 7 days, desquamation.	Red pharynx, tonsillitis, palatal petechiae, strawberry tongue.	Circumoral pallor, increased rash in skin folds, "toxic" child.
Enterovirus infection	Variable (usually short)	Variable	May resemble any of above. Echo, petechial; coxsackie, vesicular.	Variable	Concurrent familial illness, gastroenteritis, epidemic locally.

D. Thrombocytopenia: Following the onset of the rash, or days later, bleeding may occur into the rash. This is usually associated with a decrease in the platelet count.

E. Gastrointestinal Complications: These are uncommon in the USA but are a leading cause of death elsewhere. True appendicitis, diarrhea, and vomiting may be observed, often with a progressive course and fatal outcome.

F. Eyes: Secondary bacterial conjunctivitis is common. Corneal ulceration, gangrenous meibomianitis, membranous conjunctivitis, and optic nerve damage are rare complications of measles.

G. Cardiac Complications: Myocarditis and cardiac failure occur occasionally.

H. Effect on Other Diseases and Conditions: Measles during pregnancy may result in stillbirth, abortion, or premature delivery. Tuberculosis is exacerbated by intercurrent measles, and transient anergy to tuberculin is frequent. Nephrosis, asthma, and eczema may temporarily abate during measles virus infection.

Treatment

Good nursing care is essential, with attention to relief of cough, maintenance of clear nasal passages, reduction of fever, and cleansing of the conjunctivas.

Bacterial complications should be specifically diagnosed and effective antimicrobial therapy employed. Streptococcal infections are common.

Antimicrobial prophylaxis should not be used since it may result in bacterial infections with resistant organisms.

Prognosis

Measles is usually a self-limited disease lasting 7–10 days. Most often it is without permanent sequelae, although it is a severe infection.

The most serious complication, encephalitis, may result in permanent disability or death in 40% of cases.

Rarely, a progressive degenerative CNS disease, ending in death, occurs as a late sequel (years after infection) of measles. This disease has had various eponyms attached to it but is currently termed subacute sclerosing panencephalitis (SSPE).

Jabbour JI & others: Subacute sclerosing panencephalitis. JAMA 207:2248–2254, 1969.

Kempe CH, Fulginiti VA: The pathogenesis of measles virus infection. Arch Virusforsch 16:103, 1965.

Robbins F: Measles: Clinical features. Am J Dis Child 103:266, 1962.

PICORNAVIRUS INFECTIONS

...roviruses
...and the

...in size,
...aracteris-
...a large
...s can be
...we will
...hen refer
...e groups.

A. Fever ...ses
A. Fever alone: ... may be ...mpanied
...

B. Respiratory Illness. Undifferentiated upper
...

C. Gastrointestinal Illness. Nausea ...ting, and
diarrhea have been associated with enteroviral infec-
...

D. Exanthematous Illness: A variety of rashes
has been reported, including scarlatiniform, morbilliform, rubelliform, petechial, and vesicular varieties.

E. **Combinations of Above:** Illnesses in which all
or some of the above symptoms occur together have
been recorded. This is particularly true for the echovirus group.

F. **CNS Infections:**

1. Aseptic meningitis—Fever, gastrointestinal
symptoms associated with nuchal rigidity, headache,
lethargy, and CSF pleocytosis can result from infection
with any of the enteroviruses.

2. Encephalitis—Cortical symptoms, including
disturbances of sensorium, convulsions, and coma,
have been noted.

3. Paralytic illness—Although occasionally due to
the echoviruses or coxsackieviruses, this syndrome is
almost exclusively produced by polioviruses and will
be considered separately below.

G. **Isolated Myocarditis:** Inflammation of the
myocardium with attendant precordial chest pain,
dyspnea, cough, tachycardia, cyanosis, and fulminant
congestive heart failure has been attributed to poliovirus and coxsackievirus infection.

1. PARALYTIC POLIOMYELITIS

Essentials of Diagnosis
- Muscle weakness, headache, stiff neck, fever,
nausea, vomiting, sore throat.

- Lower motor neuron lesion (flaccid paralysis) with decreased deep tendon reflexes
and muscle wasting.
- CSF shows excess cells. Lymphocytes predominate; rarely more than 500/cu mm.
- No history of immunization.

Clinical Findings

A. **Symptoms and Signs:** Following (or blending
with) an undifferentiated illness (fever, lassitude,
gastrointestinal symptoms), the onset of paralysis is
heralded by nuchal rigidity and stiffness of the back.
Varying degrees of CNS depression or excitability may
be observed, followed by pain and tenderness in the
affected muscles, a brief period of hypertonicity and
spasm with transient hyperactive reflexes, asymmetric
flaccid paralysis, and loss of superficial and deep
reflexes but maintenance of sensation. Deviations from
the above pattern are common, especially in very
young infants.

Involvement of the cervical spinal cord segments
and the brain stem may lead to respiratory muscle
paralysis and cranial nerve involvement with palatal,
facial, and laryngeal paralysis. Severe involvement
results in loss of function of the respiratory and circulatory centers with irregular respirations, apnea, and
peripheral vascular collapse.

Paralysis generally extends during the first week,
reaching its limits as the fever subsides. No progression
or improvement is noted for days or weeks; if spontaneous recovery is to occur, muscle strength and function and reflexes begin to improve at this time. The
ultimate extent of paralysis should not be judged until
12−18 months have passed without continuing
improvement.

B. **Laboratory Findings:** Poliovirus may be isolated from the throat or the stools. Fecal excretion
may persist for weeks beyond the acute phase. Specific
viral etiology can be detected by serum antibody
increase in paired sera.

CSF findings are those of aseptic meningitis.
There may be mild early pleocytosis with polymorphonuclear leukocytosis rapidly shifting to lymphocytosis.
Protein concentration is normal initially, but during
the second to third weeks of illness it rises roughly in
parallel with the paralysis.

Differential Diagnosis

Aseptic meningitis due to any cause may be confused with poliovirus infection. However, paralysis is
usually due to poliovirus infection and must be differentiated from Guillain-Barré syndrome or infective
polyneuritis (sensory loss frequently present, symmetric paralysis, CSF shows albuminocytologic dissociation, ie, high protein concentration, little or no
increase in leukocytes), other infective polyneuritides
(history of preceding illness, mumps, diphtheria, etc),
and paralysis or pseudoparalysis due to other causes
(signs of scurvy, syphilis, fractures, arthritides, infection of bone, etc).

Complications & Sequelae

Bulbar poliomyelitis may result in respiratory arrest, muscular or central in origin, requiring assisted ventilation and tracheostomy.

Paralysis may remain and result in loss of function necessitating relearning, bracing, wheelchair ambulation, etc.

Hypertension is usually brief in duration but may persist.

Immobilization in a respirator may result in stasis pneumonia, decubitus ulcers, renal calculi, and disuse atrophy of nonparalyzed muscles. Careful attention to skin care, exercising, and coughing will help to prevent these complications.

Treatment

Complete bed rest is essential. The immediate disability must be accurately assessed so that difficulties can be anticipated and treated promptly rather than as an emergency. Special attention must be given to neurologic evaluation to detect beginning respiratory paralysis.

The Kenny method (heat packs) reduces spasm and tenderness and makes possible early rehabilitation to avoid disease atrophy and reeducate involved muscle groups.

A clear airway should be maintained, preferably without the use of intubation, either endotracheal or transtracheal. If necessary, tracheostomy should be anticipated and performed electively in an operating suite with experts in attendance under optimal conditions. The use of oxygen, assisted ventilation, and humid respirators may be necessary.

Prognosis

The mortality rate in paralytic disease varies from 5–10%, and permanent incapacitating paralysis occurs in 15% of cases. Mild paralysis may occur in as many as 30% of cases. In general, pregnant women and other adults are more severely affected than infants and children.

Abramson H, Greenberg M: Acute poliomyelitis in infants under one year of age. Pediatrics 16:478, 1955.

Chin TD, Marine WM: The changing pattern of poliomyelitis observed in two urban epidemics. Pub Health Rep 76:553, 1961.

WHO Expert Committee on Poliomyelitis: *First, Second, & Third Reports.* WHO Technical Report Series Nos. 81, 145, 203. World Health Organization, 1954, 1958, 1960.

2. HERPANGINA
(Coxsackie Group A, Types 2–6, 8, and 10)

There are usually no prodromal symptoms. Similar illnesses may be observed in the community, or other forms of coxsackievirus infection may be noted.

Herpangina is characterized by fever, sore throat and painful swallowing, anorexia, and vomiting, which occur with abrupt onset in association with tiny vesicles (which rapidly ulcerate) on the anterior fauces and elsewhere in the posterior pharynx. The ulcers are often arrayed linearly on the anterior fauces, lending a characteristic (diagnostic) appearance to the throat. Fever may be prominent, particularly in the young. Convulsions may occur with the first rise in temperature. Symptoms and signs persist for 2–6 days.

Virus can be isolated from throat swab and stool specimens. Serologic diagnosis is of aid only in epidemics, where the specific virus type has been isolated.

Herpangina in its classic form is seldom confused with other illnesses. Oral ulceration associated with fever is seen in primary herpetic gingivostomatitis (ulcers over most of the oral mucosa, lack of epidemic pattern). Distinguish also from aphthous ulceration (usually no fever; lesions may be anterior), ulcerative pharyngitis associated with leukemia or its treatment (lymphadenopathy, splenomegaly, etc; characteristic peripheral blood and bone marrow changes), and other viral exanthems (history of contact, exanthem, course of disease).

Parotitis or vaginal ulceration may occur, but recovery is complete.

The disease is self-limited, and only symptomatic therapy is required.

Huebner RJ & others: The importance of coxsackie viruses in human disease, particularly herpangina and epidemic pleurodynia. New England J Med 247:249, 1952.

Parrott RH: The clinical importance of group A coxsackie viruses. Ann New York Acad Sc 67:230, 1957.

3. PLEURODYNIA
(Coxsackie B Viruses; Epidemic Myalgia; Bornholm Disease)

Pleurodynia may begin with vague prodromal symptoms of malaise, anorexia, headache, and muscle aches, but the onset is usually unheralded and abrupt. Other coxsackievirus infections may be observed in the community. Pleurodynia may be epidemic.

Pleurodynia characteristically begins with severe, usually unilateral chest pain which frequently is paroxysmal and pleuritic and therefore is aggravated by respiratory movements. The patient is asymptomatic between episodes. The pain is severe and dramatically described by the patient as crushing or vise-like (hence the name "devil's grip"). Headache, fever, malaise, apprehension, abdominal pain, hiccups, vomiting, diarrhea, and stiff neck have all been noted. The illness may last as long as a week but is quite variable. Mild forms are also seen. Physical signs include apprehension, fever, limitation of respiratory excursions, muscle tenderness, normal breath sounds, and an ipsilateral pleural friction rub in 1/4 of cases. Mild to moderate nuchal rigidity may be present.

Virus can be recovered from the stools or from throat swabs. Serologic diagnosis may be possible since coxsackievirus B3 and B5 are the most common offenders, but any of the group B coxsackieviruses can produce the disease.

Any cause of sudden pleurisy must be distinguished from pleurodynia. Thus, bacterial pneumonia (leukocytosis, empyema, productive cough, bacteriologic findings), tuberculosis (history of exposure, positive tuberculin test, identification of mycobacteria), and other infectious and noninfectious causes of pleuritis must be differentiated. Abdominal or muscular pain may suggest acute surgical conditions (appendicitis, ulcer, perforation, etc). The superficial nature of the tenderness, the associated fever and pulmonary findings, and epidemiologic evidence may suggest the diagnosis of pleurodynia.

Almost all patients recover completely without complications. A few cases have been reported associated with aseptic meningitis, orchitis, pericarditis, and pneumonia.

Analgesics, splinting of the chest, and other supportive measures to relieve pain and discomfort are indicated.

See Huebner reference, above.

4. GENERALIZED NEONATAL INFECTION
(Coxsackie B Viruses)

Sudden onset of fever associated with acute heart failure occurring in more than one infant should arouse the suspicion of generalized neonatal infection. Sick infants are usually in nurseries or recently discharged. Case-finding is important, and may lead to the correct diagnosis. A history of mild gastrointestinal symptoms 1–2 days before the major illness is common. The mother may have had an upper respiratory tract infection just prior to delivery. Cyanosis, tachycardia, and increasing size of the liver and heart are all observed. Pneumonic symptoms may predominate early, and cough, dyspnea, and vomiting are prominent manifestations. In more than 1/2 of cases, the disease progresses rapidly to death in circulatory collapse. Cardiac murmurs are not heard. Despite the preponderance of cardiac signs and symptoms, the infection is a generalized one, and encephalitis, pancreatitis, focal hepatitis, and myositis are all observed at autopsy. ECG changes are those of severe myocardial damage. Chest x-ray reveals a large heart.

In general, the illness is produced by coxsackievirus groups B3 and B4. Virus can be recovered from the feces before death and from the myocardium and other tissues postmortem. Serologic confirmation is possible in surviving infants.

Other causes of acute congestive heart failure in neonates must be considered, but the epidemic nature and findings of coxsackievirus infection should be diagnostic.

Intensive supportive measures, including oxygenation, support of ventilation and circulation, and digitalization, are mandatory.

Reported mortality rates are variable, but approach or exceed 50%. If the patient survives, recovery is rapid and complete.

Gear J: Coxsackie virus infections. Yale J Biol Med 34:289, 1961–1962.

5. ISOLATED MYOCARDITIS & PERICARDITIS
(Coxsackie B Viruses)

Myocardial or pericardial infection with coxsackieviruses occurs in humans and in several other animal species. The clinical findings are similar to those observed in myocarditis or pericarditis due to other causes. Severity ranges from very mild clinical disease to fulminant fatal infections. The diagnosis is suggested by the clinical findings and substantiated by virus isolation from the stools or pericardial fluid during life, from the myocardium postmortem, or by a rise in serum antibody in paired sera in survivors.

Myocarditis is treated as outlined above for generalized neonatal infection. Pericardial aspiration is indicated for pericarditis.

Burch GE & others: Interstitial and coxsackie B myocarditis in infants and children. JAMA:203:55–62, 1968.
Lewes D, Lane WF: Acute benign pericarditis due to coxsackie virus, group B. Lancet 2:1385, 1961.

6. ACUTE LYMPHONODULAR PHARYNGITIS
(Coxsackie A10)

Papular whitish-yellow lesions of the uvula, anterior pillars, and pharynx in association with sore throat, fever, and headache have been observed in a single outbreak of coxsackievirus A10 infection. The illness lasted for 1–2 weeks and was uncomplicated. The papules did not vesiculate, which differentiates this disease from herpangina.

Treatment is symptomatic.

Steigman AJ, Lipton MM, Braspenickx H: Acute lymphonodular pharyngitis: A newly described condition due to coxsackie A virus. J Pediat 61:331, 1962.

7. VESICULAR EXANTHEM
(Hand-Foot-Mouth Disease; Coxsackie A5, A10, & A16)

Several epidemics of a vesicular exanthem which in its complete form involves the oral mucosa, tongue, and interdigital and digital surfaces of both the upper and lower extremities (hence the term hand-foot-mouth disease) have occurred due to infection with coxsackievirus A16. Incomplete forms are also seen, and coxsackievirus A16 may cause nonvesicular disease in the community at the same time.

Diagnosis is by virologic isolation and serology.

Treatment is symptomatic.

Adler JA & others: Epidemiologic investigation of hand, foot, and mouth disease. Am J Dis Child 120:309–313, 1970.

Robinson CR, Doane FW, Rhodes AJ: Report of an outbreak of febrile illness with pharyngeal lesions and exanthema: Lorento, summer 1957: Isolation of group A coxsackie virus. Canad MAJ 79:615, 1958.

8. ECHOVIRUS EXANTHEMATOUS DISEASE

Echovirus types 4, 9, and 16 have been definitely associated with epidemics of exanthematous illness; 10 other echovirus types have also been related to such illnesses. Other clinical findings have also been noted, including the aseptic meningitis syndrome.

Echovirus types 4 and 9 cause a usually maculopapular but sometimes petechial rash, and vesicular rashes, even with crusting, have occasionally been noted. Association with aseptic meningitis and lymphadenitis has been observed. The rash is usually present for just a few days but may persist for 10 days.

In echovirus type 16 disease (Boston exanthem), the rash appears during or shortly after defervescence, thus simulating roseola infantum. A punched-out ulcerative exanthem may be seen. Aseptic meningitis due to echovirus 16 usually occurs without rash. The rash lasts 1–5 days and may be associated with pharyngitis and cervical, suboccipital, and postauricular lymphadenopathy, but there are no appreciable respiratory symptoms.

Cherry J: Newer viral exanthems. Advances Pediat 16:233–286, 1969.

Lerner AM & others: New viral exanthems. New England J Med 269:678, 1963.

RHINOVIRUSES

A large group of viruses with properties similar to those of the enteroviruses have recently been shown to cause the common cold in adults. Their role in the production of disease in infants and children is not completely understood at present. They have been isolated from the nose and throat in a wide range of upper respiratory illnesses in children and less frequently in lower tract diseases.

HERPESVIRUSES

HERPES SIMPLEX

Essentials of Diagnosis

- Recurrent small grouped vesicles on an erythematous base, especially around oral and genital areas.
- May follow minor infections, trauma, stress, or sun exposure.
- Regional lymph nodes may be swollen and tender.

General Considerations

Primary herpesvirus infection is asymptomatic in most individuals. When manifestations occur, they usually take the form of gingivostomatitis in children under 4 or 5 years of age. Secondary or recurrent herpes occurs far more frequently even in the absence of a history of primary infection; thus, the virus is felt to remain hidden or "latent" following first infection. Various excitants (fever, menses, trauma, severe infections, sunshine, etc) result in uncovering of the virus with a resulting "fever blister" or "cold sore" type of infection. Thus, immunity is imperfect despite demonstrable levels of circulating antibody.

Two types of herpesvirus have been identified. Type 1 is involved in lesions of the oral cavity, CNS, and skin. Type 2 is responsible for genital disease and probably accounts for all cases of congenital herpes infection. Type 2 has also been linked with carcinoma of the cervix.

Clinical Findings

A. History: In primary infections, no history of previous disease is elicited; in recurrent disease, a history of severe gingivostomatitis or vulvovaginitis in early childhood can sometimes be elicited. In recurrent herpes, a history of similar episodes following exposure to the same excitants is usually present.

B. Symptoms and Signs:

1. Herpetic gingivostomatitis—Fever, irritability, pain in the mouth and throat and upon attempted swallowing, and lassitude with disinterest in surroundings are seen in varying degrees. Examination reveals extensive shallow, yellowish ulcers of the buccal, gingival, tonsillar, and pharyngeal mucosa, frequently with crusting of the lips, a half-open mouth with drooling, foul breath odor, and cervical lymphadenopathy. The disease lasts 7–14 days.

2. Herpetic vulvovaginitis or urethritis—Manifestations are similar to those of gingivostomatitis (both may occur) except that they appear on the vulva and vagina. Urination may be painful or withheld, especially in males. Inguinal lymphadenopathy is frequently present.

3. Recurrent herpetic lesions—Sensory symptoms varying from vague discomfort to neuralgic pain may precede or accompany the appearance of erythematous papules on the mucocutaneous junction of the lips. Rapid vesiculation, pustulation, and crusting occur. Fever is usually absent unless it is the inciting factor. Regional lymphadenopathy and lymphadenitis occur infrequently. Lesions appear in groups and tend to involve the same area in recurrences. Severity is variable, and the illness often causes discomfort without being incapacitating.

4. Herpetic keratoconjunctivitis—A variety of forms of herpetic corneal infection have been described according to the depth and extent of the infection. Almost all forms are accompanied by conjunctival inflammation, often purulent in appearance. Cloudiness and ulceration of the cornea may be noted. Ulceration may be diagnosed by application of fluorescein to the eye, whereupon a dendritic (branched) pattern may be seen. Deeper forms include stromal edema and hypopyon with rupture of the globe. Ophthalmologic consultation is indicated for accurate diagnosis and treatment.

5. Herpetic encephalitis—This rare disease may take the form of aseptic meningitis (or mumps or enterovirus encephalitis) or may begin with cortical symptoms and cranial nerve palsies. Convulsions and coma are frequent, and death occurs in the second to third weeks of illness.

6. Neonatal herpetic infection—This form of infection occurs in infants of nonimmune parents, and a history of recent herpes infection in either parent may be obtained. The illness may be present at birth but usually manifests itself in the first week of life with generalized vesiculation of the skin, high or low temperature, jaundice, progressive hepatosplenomegaly, dyspnea, signs of cardiac failure, hemorrhage, and CNS manifestations. Death occurs following a 2–4 day course of illness. "Mild" neonatal herpes infections result in vesicular rash usually unassociated with overt CNS disease. The rash may recur repeatedly in the first months of life, and CNS function may ultimately be impaired.

7. Eczema herpeticum (Kaposi's varicelliform eruption)—The appearance of fever, prostration, and vesicular lesions in a patient with eczema should lead to a diagnosis of intercurrent herpesvirus or vaccinia virus infection. Although varying in severity, eczema herpeticum is frequently fulminant and fatal, especially when large areas of skin are involved.

C. Laboratory Findings: CSF pleocytosis (lymphocytosis) is present in aseptic meningitis. Virus can be recovered from vesicular fluid, skin and corneal scrapings, throat swabs, blood, CSF, and appropriate tissue specimens. Enrichment of collection media with protein enhances virus stability if a delay in handling specimens is unavoidable.

A 4-fold or greater rise in serum antibody is detectable in paired sera from patients with primary infection. This is of little aid in recurrent infection since titer rises do not occur. In lesions simulating herpes, a negative titer may help to rule out this diagnosis.

Smears taken from the bases of vesicles or ulcers suspected of being herpetic can be stained with hematoxylin and eosin to reveal the typical Cowdry type A intranuclear inclusion bodies. These consist of eosinophilic oval masses within the nucleus, which has marginal chromatin. Fixation produces a distinct halo around the inclusion. Giemsa stains of tissue best visualize the giant cells with their multinucleate or syncytial structure.

Electronmicroscopic examination of vesicular fluid may result in rapid identification of herpes simplex virus.

Differential Diagnosis

Herpetic gingivostomatitis must be differentiated from herpangina (posterior pharyngeal ulcers only, linear array on anterior pillars, isolation of coxsackie A viruses); aphthous ulceration (one or only a few ulcers, previous history, lack of systemic symptoms); ulcerative pharyngitis of agranulocytic disease (history, other physical findings, blood and bone marrow findings), and Stevens-Johnson syndrome (multiple mucosal involvement, "iris" lesions of skin, history of sulfonamide or other drug ingestion).

Recurrent herpes labialis can easily be differentiated from impetigo by the characteristic history and course of the former and bacterial isolation and response to treatment of the latter.

Herpetic keratoconjunctivitis must be differentiated from vaccinial keratoconjunctivitis (history or presence of recent vaccination or contact, isolation of virus) and from adenovirus keratoconjunctivitis (pain in adenovirus infection of cornea, epidemic nature, isolation of virus).

Meningoencephalitis can only be differentiated from other causes by laboratory studies.

Generalized neonatal infection is differentiated from similar illness due to coxsackie B viruses by lack of skin involvement, epidemic nature in nursery, and isolation of virus.

Eczema vaccinatum can be differentiated from eczema herpeticum by the history of exposure to smallpox vaccination, typical vacciniform lesions, and the fact that eczema vaccinatum lesions tend to be in the same stage. In some cases, differentiation is difficult and laboratory diagnosis is necessary.

Complications, Sequelae, & Prognosis

Primary skin and mucosal infections are usually self-limited, with complete and prompt recovery, although limited recurrences occur.

Herpetic keratoconjunctivitis can lead to blindness or perforation of the cornea with loss of the eye.

Encephalitis or neonatal generalized infection is frequently fatal.

Treatment

A. Specific Measures: Idoxuridine (IDU, Herplex, Stoxil, Dendrid) has been used successfully in superficial mucosal, corneal, and skin infections. It is of proved curative effect if used promptly in superficial ulcerative keratitis and possibly of ameliorative effect in skin infections. One to 2 drops are instilled onto the cornea every 1–2 hours around the clock for maximum effect. (Follow manufacturer's directions, as new formulations may appear.)

There is no specific therapy for other forms of herpes infection.

B. General Measures: In gingivostomatitis, considerable discomfort is experienced, with resultant lack of fluid and caloric intake. Since this is a 7–14 day illness, maintenance of fluid intake is vital. Dehydration can be avoided by hospitalization and intravenous administration of fluids and electrolytes. In less severe instances, discovering the optimal temperature of fluids tolerated (cool is usually best) can ensure intake. It is rarely necessary to use topical "caine" anesthetics, thus avoiding potential sensitization. Mild antiseptic mouthwashes are occasionally of benefit. There is no rationale to the use of local antibiotics. Systemic administration of analgesics occasionally is necessary and facilitates intake of food and fluids.

The treatment of encephalitis and neonatal infection is symptomatic and supportive.

Herpetic keratoconjunctivitis is best treated with idoxuridine (see above). The use of topical corticosteroids in the acute ulcerative disease is contraindicated. In instances of stromal edema or of persistent deep lesions, topical corticosteroids may be of aid but should be combined with idoxuridine and given only under an ophthalmologist's direction.

Eczema herpeticum is best treated as an extensive "burn" so that appropriate attention is directed to replacement of fluid and electrolytes and to protein nutrition. Prevention of secondary bacterial infection is accomplished by continuous bacteriologic guidance and antibacterial therapy.

In severe complications, the use of systemic corticosteroids is often advocated. There are theoretical objections to the use of such agents since experimental evidence indicates that they enhance viral spread. Pooled adult gamma globulin has been advocated, but there is no evidence that it has a beneficial effect.

Recurrent herpes labialis has been treated in a variety of ways, including injections of vitamin B_{12}, the use of reticulose (a supposed antiviral substance), and repeat smallpox vaccination. No evidence of a controlled nature is available to indicate that any of these or other forms of therapy are uniformly beneficial. Saline injections and no other treatment can result in "cure" of recurrent herpes. Smallpox vaccination has resulted in untoward effects in some patients and should be avoided.

Kauffman HE: Successful therapy of viral keratitis. Postgrad Med 35:518, 1964.

McNair Scott TF: Epidemiology of herpetic infections. Am J Ophth 43:134, 1957.

Nahmias AJ, Dowdle WR: Antigenic and biologic differences in herpes virus hominis. Progr Med Virol 10:110–159, 1968.

VARICELLA (Chickenpox) & HERPES ZOSTER (Shingles)

Essentials of Diagnosis

Varicella:

- History of exposure within 2–3 weeks; appearance of characteristic vesicles over a 2–5 day period, usually without prodrome.
- Lesions rapidly evolve from macules to papules to "dewdrop" superficial vesicles to encrustation in centripetal distribution. Macules, papules, vesicles, and crusts are all observable at any one time (pleomorphic).

Herpes Zoster:

- History of chickenpox.
- Preeruptive pain (infrequent in children) in region of rash.
- Clusters of confluent vesicles in unilateral dermatomal distribution. Successive crops may appear.
- Examination of early vesicular scrapings reveals Tszank giant cells or characteristic intranuclear inclusions (see Herpes Simplex, above).

General Considerations

Varicella and herpes zoster are caused by the same virus. Varicella is the primary infection and herpes zoster appears to be a recurrent infection. In the USA, varicella is primarily a disease of childhood; in large areas of the tropics, it is principally a disease of adults. No known animal reservoir exists, and the disease is transmitted from man to man in epidemics with a high degree of contagiousness (80–90% of exposed susceptibles are infected). Herpes zoster is sporadic and considerably less infectious, resulting in varicella in 15% of exposed susceptibles.

Clinical Findings

A. History: A history of contact 10–20 days (average, 12–13 days) prior to onset is typically obtained. There is usually no prodrome, but a mild febrile illness with rhinitis is occasionally noted for 1–3 days before the rash appears. A history of contact may be lacking in zoster, but the disease has occurred (in adults) following exposure to varicella. Severe pain along the nerve root distribution of the rash may precede the rash by several days.

B. Symptoms and Signs:

1. Varicella–In typical varicella, the onset is abrupt with the appearance of the rash. Systemic symptoms, if any, are mild. The rash appears in crops, with faint erythematous macules rapidly developing into papules and vesicles. The vesicles are characteristic; they are thin-walled, and superficially located on the skin with a distinct areola (dewdrop on a red base). They rupture easily, rapidly encrust, and frequently become impetiginized. Successive crops (usually 3) appear in the next 2–5 days, giving rise to the pleomorphic appearance of the rash: lesions in all stages can be seen at one time. The rash is heaviest on the trunk and sparse on the extremities. Barring bacterial infection, the crust falls off in 1–3 weeks, leaving no scars.

Deviations from the above pattern vary from very mild disease with just a few vesicles to as many as 5 successive crops with involvement of most of the skin. Rarely, hemorrhagic lesions occur and are associated with thrombocytopenia, particularly in children with leukemia receiving antimetabolites. Infrequently, a zoster-like cluster of lesions appears during the course of primary varicella. Bullous and gangrenous forms are recognized.

Systemic symptoms are usually absent or mild but may be severe, and generally parallel the extent of skin involvement.

An enanthem is recognizable which consists of shallow mucosal ulceration (the vesicle is rarely seen). When it involves the posterior pharynx or esophagus, swallowing may be painful and difficult.

2. Zoster—Herpes zoster is usually unilateral and limited to one or more adjacent dermatomes. Thoracic and lumbar forms are most common, although the ophthalmic division of the trigeminal nerve, cervical roots, and other divisions may be affected. Maculopapules appear in closely arrayed patches, rapidly vesiculate, and frequently coalesce; they follow the dermal distribution of the nerve root, and often end abruptly at the midline of the body. Concomitant or preceding pain, often very severe, occurs less frequently in children than in adults.

C. Laboratory Findings: The usual laboratory tests are of little aid. Sepsis may be accompanied by an abrupt increase in the white blood count with neutrophilia.

Although virus isolation and serologic tests are available, they are seldom necessary. Etiologic identification may be important in distinguishing varicella from smallpox or in the diagnosis of unusual and atypical forms of the disease.

Giant cells with multinucleate or syncytial structure may be found in vesicular scrapings, as may inclusion bodies of the eosinophilic intranuclear type (Cowdry type A) also.

D. X-Ray Findings: Chest films may reveal diffuse nodular pneumonia ("viral") and emphysema in varicella pneumonia.

Differential Diagnosis

Typical chickenpox is seldom confused with other illnesses. Severe forms must, in rare cases, be differentiated from smallpox (history of exposure, typical 3-day severe prodrome, lesions all in same stage of development, centrifugal distribution, hard, pearly, nodular, deep-seated lesions, absence of giant cells and intranuclear inclusions, isolation of the virus) and mild forms from the vesicular exanthem due to coxsackievirus infection (sparseness of rash, history of chickenpox, failure to form crusts, isolation of specific virus). Also to be distinguished are impetigo (lack of exposure

history, response to therapy), multiple insect bites or papular urticaria (history of bites, papular and excoriated but no vesicles), rickettsialpox (primary eschar, smaller lesions, lack of crusting, serologic diagnosis), and dermatitis herpetiformis (chronic course, symmetry of eruption, urticaria, residual pigmentation).

Complications & Sequelae

There are usually no complications. Secondary bacterial infection may occur if the lesions are manipulated. Septic sequelae may then ensue, including local abscesses, lymphangitis, septicemia, osteomyelitis, and others.

Varicella pneumonia is rare in children except in severe generalized forms of the disease such as occur in neonatal disease and disseminated forms associated with malignancy or immunosuppressive drug therapy. Its onset is in the first week of rash with fulminant pulmonary manifestations (cough, dyspnea and tachypnea, pain, cyanosis, rales, splinting). Chest films show characteristic diffuse pulmonary nodular infiltrates throughout both lung fields. The disease may be fatal, especially in adults and in disseminated forms.

Varicella in the neonate is often mild but may be fulminant, with extensive visceral infection and death.

Varicella occurring in patients with malignancies or receiving immunosuppressive therapy can be very severe and often fatal. Hemorrhagic forms of the disease and disseminated visceral lesions, including pneumonia, are common. The role of corticosteroid therapy is controversial, but most authorities feel that the underlying disease is more important in the development of severe infections than is administration of corticosteroids alone.

Patients receiving corticosteroids for illnesses not associated with immunologic suppression (eg, asthma, juvenile rheumatoid arthritis) require no adjustment in dose upon exposure. Those patients whose underlying illness predisposes to disseminated disease should have the dose of corticosteroids reduced as much as possible and zoster-immune globulin administered.

Varicella encephalitis occurs infrequently and is milder than measles encephalitis. Eighty percent fully recover; 15% have sequelae; and 5% die. The onset is insidious, usually in the first week of rash, and is followed by varying CNS signs and symptoms.

Fatal hypoglycemia has been reported in infants with varicella and is believed to be associated with decreased carbohydrate intake and concomitant salicylate therapy.

Rare complications include transverse myelitis, optic neuritis, hepatitis, and orchitis.

Treatment

Symptomatic measures include fluids, control of itching (sedative antihistamines, colloidal baths), attention to cleanliness (trimming of nails, handwashing, bathing), and antipyretics where indicated (avoid high or repeated doses of aspirin, especially in young infants). Antimicrobial agents should not be administered prophylactically, but infections should be treated as they occur. Topical therapy is often sufficient for mild skin infection, but systemic administration may be necessary.

Supportive and symptomatic treatment for the complications of varicella are indicated. In the disseminated forms of infection, massive amounts of passive antibody in the form of zoster-immune globulin or convalescent plasma from adults recently ill with zoster may be of aid. Recent evidence suggests that idoxuridine and probably cytosine arabinoside (cytarabine) may be useful.

Prognosis

Varicella is usually benign and self-limited. Complications in children are infrequent and fatalities rare.

Gordon JE: Chickenpox. Am J M Sc 244:362, 1962.

Ross AH: Modification of chickenpox in family contacts by administration of gamma globulin. New England J Med 267:369, 1962.

Winkelman RK, Perry HO: Herpes zoster in children. JAMA 171:376, 1959.

ARBOVIRUSES

Four clinical syndromes of importance in children are associated with arbovirus infection: encephalitis, dengue, yellow fever, and febrile illnesses such as Colorado tick fever. In general, a cycle of infection between an arthropod and nonhuman vertebrates is established in nature, and man is infected as a secondary host. Dengue and urban yellow fever are exceptions, as the mosquito transmits the viruses directly from human to human.

ENCEPHALITIS SYNDROMES

Essentials of Diagnosis

- High fever, severe headache, nuchal rigidity, stupor, coma, convulsions, and other CNS symptoms predominate.
- CSF pleocytosis and slight protein elevation (normal in St Louis encephalitis).
- Isolation of virus from blood, CSF, or postmortem specimens (brain, blood).
- Identification of serum antibody rise in paired specimens obtained 3–4 weeks apart.

General Considerations

In the USA the equine encephalitides—eastern equine encephalitis (EEE), western equine encephalitis (WEE), and St Louis encephalitis (SLE)—are the most important illnesses caused by arboviruses.

Clinical Findings

A. History: A history of encephalitic death in horses may precede human cases of EEE and WEE. The epidemic nature of the illness may alert the physician to new cases.

B. Symptoms and Signs: After an incubation period of 5–10 days (as long as 3 weeks in SLE), a sudden onset of high fever and headache heralds the illness. Signs of CNS irritability (convulsions, nausea and vomiting) and depression (coma, stupor, lethargy) appear in association with a stiff neck or back, increased deep tendon reflexes, tremors, muscle weakness, and occasionally paralysis. Mild or asymptomatic infections are observed in WEE and SLE but are uncommon with EEE.

The illness may be abortive, with rapid recovery, or may progress to severe illness and even death. In general, EEE tends to be the most severe.

C. Laboratory Findings: In EEE and WEE, CSF pleocytosis of moderate degree is noted (50–1000 cells/cu mm) and protein concentration may be slightly elevated. CSF glucose concentration remains normal.

Attempts at virus isolation should be made early in the course of an epidemic in order to alert physicians and to inform public health officials. Heparinized blood, CSF, and CNS tissue from fatal cases should be submitted to appropriate diagnostic laboratories. The USPHS maintains diagnostic facilities for this purpose. Serologic diagnosis can be accomplished by demonstration of a 4-fold or greater antibody rise between acute and convalescent sera (7–21 days apart).

Differential Diagnosis

Arbovirus encephalitis must be differentiated from other causes of encephalitis by appropriate laboratory means. Brain tumor, lead and other poisonings, and CNS injuries occurring during an epidemic of arbovirus encephalitis must also be differentiated. The history, appropriate neurologic and neurosurgical diagnostic procedures, and negative virologic studies aid in the differentiation.

The abortive forms must be distinguished from aseptic meningitis due to any cause and from enteroviral infections, particularly since the peak incidence of both illnesses often coincides. Only laboratory study can make the distinction, as the clinical syndromes may be identical. For this reason, throat and stool specimens as well as blood and CSF should be submitted to the virus diagnostic laboratory.

Complications & Sequelae

Infants may develop convulsions, hydrocephalus, mental retardation, and severe CNS damage.

Treatment

Control of convulsions by barbiturates is indicated. The unconscious patient requires continuous care, with attention to the airway, oxygenation, and support of the circulation.

Prognosis

Mortality from encephalitis is greatest with EEE and may exceed 50%, whereas the mortality rate in WEE and SLE is usually less than 25% (often 5–7%).

Hammon WM: The viral encephalitides in man. Ann New York Acad Sc 70:292, 1958.

McAllister RM: Viral encephalitis. Ann Rev Med 13:389, 1962.

DENGUE
(Group B Arboviruses)

Dengue in children usually occurs during the preschool or early school years. It is characterized by a sudden onset of fever, severe headache, and retro-ocular pain; severe pain in the extremities and back (thus the term breakbone fever), lymphadenopathy, and a maculopapular or petechial (hemorrhagic) rash.

The fever and course are often diphasic, with an "exacerbation" following temporary improvement. CNS and pneumonic symptoms may occur. Shock and peripheral vascular collapse may result in death in the first week of illness.

Leukopenia and thrombocytopenia may be marked. Hemorrhagic disease may be associated with prolonged bleeding time and maturation arrest of megakaryocytes. Virus may be recovered from the blood. Complications include hemorrhage, shock, and postinfectious asthenia. Fatality rates vary from epidemic to epidemic but are usually low.

Treatment consists of supportive measures for shock, blood replacement for severe hemorrhage, and, in severe cases, corticosteroids. Antipyretics and analgesics suffice for uncomplicated cases.

No sequelae have been observed in survivors. Fatality rates vary but are usually low.

Doherty RL: Clinical and epidemiological observations on dengue fever in Queensland. MJ Australia 1:753, 1957.

Hammon W & others: New hemorrhagic fevers of children in the Philippines and Thailand. Tr Ass Am Physicians 73:140, 1960.

YELLOW FEVER

The severity of yellow fever varies, and mild and inapparent infections occur. In the classic illness, 3 phases are seen following an incubation period of 3–7 days. The first is nonspecific, with abrupt onset, fever, headache, lassitude, nausea and vomiting, and vague muscle aching. A short period of remission is followed by the severe "toxic" phase with high fever associated with bradycardia (Faget's sign), severe jaundice, and gastrointestinal hemorrhage often progressing to shock and death. The disease may be fulminant, with no remissive period; or may be abortive, with only mild nonspecific symptoms. The disease is usually less severe in children.

Leukopenia is the rule. Proteinuria, azotemia, hyperbilirubinemia, elevated BUN, and disturbed liver function tests are observed. Virus can be isolated from the blood in the first 3–4 days of illness and irregularly thereafter. Serologic diagnosis is possible by examination of paired sera obtained 2–4 weeks apart. Midzonal hepatic cell necrosis with eosinophilic inclusions (Councilman bodies) and relative absence of inflammation are seen at postmortem examination and can be diagnostic.

Treatment is symptomatic and supportive, including fluid and blood replacement, antipyretics, and support of peripheral circulation.

Despite prolonged convalescence in some severely affected patients, no permanent sequelae are noted in survivors. Mortality rates vary, and may be conditioned by age, race, and the status of other arbovirus immunity.

Cahill KM: Yellow fever. New York J Med 63:2990, 1963.

Elton NW, Romero A, Trejos A: Clinical pathology of yellow fever. Am J Clin Path 25:135, 1955.

COLORADO TICK FEVER

Three to 6 days after the bite of an infected tick (*Dermacentor andersoni*), a sudden onset of high fever occurs with retro-ocular, back, and muscular pain. This phase lasts 2–3 days, and a remission of 2–3 days may follow, whereupon a second, usually more severe episode of fever, severe headache, and muscular pain occurs. Rarely, several such episodes occur. In 10–15% of patients, a generalized maculopapular or petechial rash may be present. Symptoms subside slowly, and recovery is usually complete within 10–14 days.

Marked leukopenia (often 1500–2000/cu mm), with a shift to the left occurring on the third to sixth day, is characteristic. In the hemorrhagic forms, thrombocytopenia may be present. Virus may be regularly isolated from the blood during the illness and occasionally from CSF. Serologic testing reveals an increase in antibody 4–6 weeks after onset.

Any cause of fever must be considered in the early phases, but the typical clinical course, leukopenia, and virus isolation serve to distinguish Colorado tick fever. The appearance of a rash may lead to confusion with other viral exanthems, meningococcemia, and various thrombocytopenic states. Bacteriologic and hematologic studies may be of aid in diagnosis.

Encephalitis and severe hemorrhages have been reported. Nuchal rigidity, stupor, headache, or signs of CNS irritability suggest meningoencephalitis and should prompt a lumbar puncture.

Hemorrhage (frequently severe) involving the skin, mucous membranes, gastrointestinal tract, and genitourinary tract may occur.

Treatment is symptomatic and supportive. Transfusion of whole blood may be necessary if hemorrhage occurs.

Most cases are uncomplicated and self-limiting.

Ecklund CM & others: The clinical and ecological aspects of Colorado tick fever. Proceedings of the Sixth International Congress of Tropical Medicine and Malaria, Libson 5:197, 1958.

Silver HK, Meiklejohn G, Kempe CH: Colorado tick fever. Am J Dis Child 101:30, 1961.

ADENOVIRUSES

There are more than 24 human types of adenoviruses, but relatively few produce illness in children. A carrier state involving one or more adenoviruses is common in young children. Immunity is type-specific.

Many forms of adenovirus disease are recognized:

(1) Pharyngoconjunctival fever: Fever, exudative pharyngitis, and follicular conjunctivitis.

(2) Follicular conjunctivitis: Sporadic illness with preauricular adenopathy and occasional corneal opacification.

(3) Epidemic keratoconjunctivitis: Epidemics of severe conjunctivitis and corneal infiltration traceable to some common source, eg, ophthalmologic examination.

In most of the respiratory infections caused by adenoviruses, the signs and symptoms are not unlike those produced by any of the respiratory viruses. Conjunctivitis and exudative pharyngitis are more commonly due to adenoviral infection than to other viruses and may provide an etiologic clue in local outbreaks.

Specific diagnosis can be made by virus isolation from stools, respiratory secretions, or conjunctival specimens and by identification of antibody responses. A 4-fold antibody rise in paired sera is essential to the diagnosis. Since these viruses may be "carried" in the pharynges of normal children, serologic evidence of infection should be sought; lack of evidence of other respiratory viral etiology supports the diagnosis.

Van Der Veen J: The role of adenoviruses in respiratory disease. Am Rev Resp Dis 88:1967, 1963.

MISCELLANEOUS VIRUSES

RUBELLA

Essentials of Diagnosis

- Variable clinical expression in childhood.

"Typical case":

- Maculopapular, discrete rash with rapid caudal progression (3 days).
- Lymphadenopathy preceding and outlasting rash.
- Minimal respiratory and systemic symptoms.

In congenital rubella (usually in combination):

- Thrombocytopenic purpura.
- Deafness.
- Cataract, glaucoma, retinopathy.
- Congenital heart defect.
- Psychomotor retardation.
- Growth retardation.
- Evidence for specific organ infection (hepatitis, osteomyelitis, etc).

General Considerations

It is now appreciated that rubella may be an asymptomatic illness or one associated solely with lymphadenopathy, although the typical illness in children consists principally of a 3-day exanthem. This virus is of major importance because of its proved teratogenic effects on the unborn fetus of a susceptible woman.

Clinical Findings

A. History: The incubation period is 14–21 days (usually 17 days), and in children there is no prodrome. (In adults and adolescents, fever, mild respiratory and constitutional symptoms, and lymphadenopathy may precede the eruption by 1–5 days.)

Maternal exposure to rubella, particularly during the first 12 weeks of gestation, may be associated with fetal disease whether or not a history of illness is elicited in the mother.

B. Symptoms and Signs: Lymphadenopathy may be the first sign of the illness, and is often present for several days prior to rash. Any nodes may be involved, but the suboccipital and postauricular groups are most frequently enlarged. (Lymph node enlargement is not pathognomonic of rubella.) The rash appears first about the face as a pinkish, discrete, macular eruption and rapidly spreads to the trunk and proximal extremities. Within 2 days it fades from the face and trunk and involves the distal extremities. Thereafter, it rapidly disappears and only rarely desquamates.

Fever and systemic symptoms are usually absent or are very mild. Rarely, in infancy, a severe rash and constitutional symptoms may be present. In the epidemic form in 1964, many children were observed with systemic symptoms, some so severe as to suggest rubeola.

Purpura and petechiae may occur in a small percentage of patients during an epidemic. Arthritis is not uncommon, particularly among adolescent girls and young women. The involved joints may be normal in appearance or may simulate acute rheumatoid arthritis.

An infant born following maternal rubella infection may be normal, or any or all of the following findings may be present: purpura, jaundice, bulging fontanel, hepatosplenomegaly, heart murmurs (rarely, cyanosis and congestive heart failure), pneumonia, microphthalmia with or without cataract, growth retardation (small for gestational age), abnormal dermatoglyphics (simian line, distal axial triradius), seborrheic dermatitis, intermittent skin mottling, excess sweating.

As these infants grow, the effects of congenital rubella may become apparent. Thus, deafness, cataract, congenital heart disease, and psychomotor and growth retardation may only become evident with the passage of time.

C. Laboratory Findings: Leukopenia or thrombocytopenia is seen in some patients. Virus may be recovered prior to the rash (up to 7 days) and as late as 2 weeks after onset. Throat specimens and urine are good sources, but blood must be examined before the onset of rash. Fecal specimens may also yield the virus.

A rise in rubella antibody may be detected between paired sera collected 2 or more weeks apart. Since antibody may be present early in the rash stage of rubella, it is important to collect specimens as early as possible.

In congenital rubella, the following may be detected:

1. Thrombocytopenia, frequently $< 10,000$ platelets/cu mm.

2. Hemolytic anemia, neuroblastemia, reticulocytosis, an erythroid hyperplastic marrow, and eventual decrease in hemoglobin.

3. Increased levels of direct-reacting bilirubin and evidence of hepatocellular dysfunction.

4. Virus may be removed from peripheral leukocytes, throat, stool, and urine for as long as 8 months after birth. Recovery of virus from the lens has occurred after even longer intervals.

5. High and persistent rubella antibody titer in the serum.

6. Abnormalities in immunoglobulin concentration (variable, but includes depression of IgA and IgG levels with increased IgM levels).

7. A defect in cellular immunity.

D. X-Ray Findings: Signs of pneumonia may be present in congenital rubella. Radiographic evidence of rubella osteomyelitis consists of alternating linear densities and translucent streaks in the metaphyses of the long bones.

Differential Diagnosis

Rubella must be differentiated from other acute viral exanthematous diseases (Table 26-2). In general, the 3-day course of the pinkish rash, prior lymphadenopathy, and minimal or absent prodromal symptoms serve as useful clinical criteria for diagnosis. However, in cases where the distinction is important (as in the pregnant female), virus isolation and serology are essential.

Arthritis or arthralgia raises the possibility of rheumatoid arthritis (fever, splenomegaly, history, multiple joint involvement), and the distinction may be blurred by a positive latex fixation test. The transient nature of rubella arthritis may aid in the differentiation.

Congenital rubella must be differentiated from other infections acquired in utero, including toxoplasmosis (by specific antibody studies), cytomegalovirus infection (by virus recovery and specific antibody studies), and congenital syphilis (by serologic study).

Complications & Sequelae

A. Encephalitis: Encephalitis occurs in no more than one out of 6000 cases of rubella. The manifestations are those of postinfectious encephalitis due to any cause, although rubella encephalitis tends to be mild, with less frequent sequelae and few fatalities.

B. Rubella During Pregnancy: Rubella in pregnant women is not unusually severe, but the potential risk to the fetus is great. The following generalizations may be made in the light of currently available evidence:

The risk to infants following maternal rubella is greatest in the first 3-4 months of pregnancy. In Cooper's study, only one out of 16 infants born to mothers infected after the fourth month were abnormal, whereas 243 out of 291 were abnormal if infection occurred before the end of the fourth month. The greatest risk in this series was in the first 2 months, when 75 out of 166 infants were abnormal, and least in the fourth month, with 22 out of 43 infants involved.

Gamma globulin adminstered to the exposed pregnant female probably has no effect in preventing fetal infection. However, the data are controversial and sometimes contradictory, and firm recommendations cannot be made until controlled trials with a standard gamma globulin are completed.

Treatment

A. Specific Measures: Despite the demonstration of antiviral activity of amantadine in vitro, no specific therapy for rubella is available.

B. General Measures: The usual case requires no therapy. Purpura is usually confined to the skin, and no treatment is necessary. It is conceivable that severe hemorrhage might occur, requiring transfusion of whole blood or platelets. Arthritis is controlled with aspirin and limitation of motion.

C. In Pregnancy: Therapeutic abortion is recommended in some pregnancies. This practice is tempered by local standards, religious beliefs, and law.

Prognosis

Rubella is almost always a self-limited, uncomplicated disease with complete recovery. Congenital rubella can result in death or prolonged handicap.

Bellanti JA: Congenital rubella. Am J Dis Child 110:464, 1965.

Cooper LZ & others: Rubella: Clinical manifestations and management. Am J Dis Child 118:18–29, 1969.

Green RH & others: Rubella: Studies in its etiology, epidemiology, clinical course and prevention. Tr Ass Am Physicians 77:420, 1964.

Heggie AD, Robbins FC: Natural rubella acquired after birth. Am J Dis Child 118:12–17, 1969.

Horstmann DM: Rubella and the rubella syndrome: New epidemiologic virologic observations. California Med 102:397, 1965.

Plotkin SA: Virologic assistance in the management of German measles in pregnancy. JAMA 190:105, 1964.

CYTOMEGALIC INCLUSION DISEASE
(Cytomegaloviruses)

Essentials of Diagnosis

- The syndrome of hepatosplenomegaly, microcephaly, and chorioretinitis occurring in a jaundiced infant with a petechial rash is classical.
- Variants occur with only part of the syndrome.
- Periventricular intracranial calcification.
- Inclusion bodies (owl's eye) in cells sedimented from freshly voided urine or in liver biopsy.
- Detection of virus in urine or saliva. (*Note:* Do not freeze specimens. Keep at 0–4° C.)

General Considerations

It was originally thought that the cytomegaloviruses produce only a characteristic fulminant, generalized neonatal infection, but it has recently been shown that in older children and adults they may cause pulmonary or gastrointestinal infections also. Patients receiving immunosuppressive therapy may develop clinical disease by unmasking of latent virus infection, usually in the lungs.

Many investigators believe that additional illnesses will be attributable to the cytomegaloviruses since they are ubiquitous and most individuals are infected (as shown by the finding of serum antibody and, occasionally, asymptomatic virus excretion).

Cytomegalovirus infection may result from infusion of blood containing the virus. An appreciable risk occurs in a susceptible patient receiving large quantities of whole blood (cardiac surgery, etc).

Clinical Findings

A. History: Since the maternal disease is asymptomatic, the history is of little value.

B. Symptoms and Signs: In full-blown neonatal disease, jaundice, massive hepatosplenomegaly associated with CNS signs (lethargy, convulsions, etc), and a petechial-purpuric rash are present. Milder forms of the disease are seen. Fewer infants have chorioretinitis and cerebral calcification, but almost all have some degree of microcephaly, occasionally striking. Surviving infants are usually severely mentally and physically handicapped, and hepatosplenomegaly and jaundice may persist. A syndrome resembling infectious mononucleosis may occur without accompanying heterophil antibody rise. Isolated hepatitis has been described.

C. Laboratory Findings: Anemia, thrombocytopenia, and hyperbilirubinemia are usually present. CSF pleocytosis and elevated protein with normal glucose concentration are found. Typical owl's eye intranuclear basophilic inclusions can be found in cells in freshly voided urine. Delay in examination may result in lack of visualization of the inclusions. Tissue from other organs can also be utilized; examination of liver biopsy material can establish the diagnosis.

Virus can regularly be isolated from the urine for many months and even years after birth. Salivary and fecal excretion of virus is also detectable, but for shorter periods.

Diagnosis by antibody determination is clouded by the widespread incidence of infection; more than 70% of all infants have antibody in their cord sera. Therefore, serologic diagnosis is less helpful than isolation of virus and histologic technics.

D. X-Ray Findings: Skull films may show typical periventricular calcification.

Differential Diagnosis

Cytomegalic inclusion disease must be differentiated from other causes of jaundice, hepatosplenomegaly, and petechial rash in the newborn, principally toxoplasmosis (diagnosed by elevated Feldman-Sabin dye test antibody titer and suggested by generalized instead of periventricular cerebral calcification); generalized herpetic neonatal infection (presence of vesicular skin lesions, lack of cerebral calcification, specific virologic tests); generalized coxsackievirus infection (myocarditis predominates, epidemic nature, isolation of virus); hemolytic disease of newborn (no microcephaly, positive Coombs tests, demonstration of incompatibility for rhesus or ABO antigens); bacterial sepsis, including syphilis (positive blood culture or serology, osseous changes, lack of microcephaly); and galactosemia (galactosuria and galactosemia, proteinuria, aminoaciduria, and absence of other signs of cytomegalovirus infection).

Pneumonia in older individuals must be differentiated from *Pneumocystis carinii* infection which is usually accomplished by identification of the parasite.

Complications & Sequelae

Residual cerebral damage frequently results in mental and physical retardation of marked degree. Institutionalization may be necessary for total care.

Treatment

There is no specific treatment. Symptomatic therapy may reduce immediate morbidity but usually does not influence the final outcome.

Floxuridine may be of benefit in severe cytomegalovirus infections in children with leukemia or other diseases associated with immunosuppression.

Prognosis

The exact mortality is difficult to estimate because of a broad base of asymptomatic infections. Fulminant forms of the disease are almost universally fatal in the neonatal period.

Medearis DN Jr: Cytomegalic inclusion disease: Analysis of clinical features based on literature and six additional cases. Pediatrics 19:467, 1957.

Weller TH, Hanshaw JB: Virologic and clinical observations on cytomegalic inclusion disease. New England J Med 266:1233, 1962.

Clemens HH: Exanthem subitum (roseola infantum): Report of 80 cases. J Pediat 26:66, 1945.

Kempe CH & others: Studies on the etiology of exanthem subitum (roseola infantum). J Pediat 37:561, 1950.

ROSEOLA INFANTUM
(Exanthem Subitum)

Roseola infantum is a usually benign, self-limited infection which has been transmitted by filtrates of blood. No specific virus has been isolated.

Clinical Findings

A. History: The typical clinical picture is 3 days of sustained high fever, often with a febrile convulsion at onset, in a child who otherwise appears well. Roseola occasionally occurs in epidemics, even in young adults.

B. Symptoms and Signs: A discrete pink rash is the most characteristic finding. It is often evanescent, and typically appears as the fever decreases or shortly thereafter. The rash is occasionally generalized and may coalesce. Any sustained fever in an infant or child under 3 years of age should therefore alert the physician and parents to look for a rash, which may be mild or transient. The temperature falls to lower than normal after defervescence. Edema of the eyelids has been said to be diagnostic, but this is not regularly observed and may not be specific.

C. Laboratory Findings: Leukocytosis with a shift to the left may be present at onset, but leukopenia is more common and may be marked at the time of rash.

Differential Diagnosis

The presence of high fever and the frequency of initial convulsions may suggest other causes of this combination, including bacterial meningitis and encephalitis. The age of the child, well-being following recovery from the seizure, and the typical course plus a normal CSF are helpful in the differentiation.

Complications & Sequelae

Some workers claim that encephalitis is common, but sequelae occur infrequently if at all.

Treatment

Fever can be controlled with supplemental fluids, gentle tepid water sponge baths, and aspirin. Convulsions are usually self-limited and single, requiring no therapy. Barbiturates are rarely required. With a history of prior "febrile" convulsions, administration of elixir of phenobarbital, 15 mg 3 times daily, should be considered. Antimicrobial agents are not indicated and are of no benefit.

Prognosis

Roseola is almost universally benign, and complete recovery is the rule.

ERYTHEMA INFECTIOSUM
(Fifth Disease)

This disease (of presumed viral origin) is characterized by an intensely erythematous, slightly raised, hot eruption of the cheeks ("slapped face") followed after 1 day by a maculopapular eruption on the extensor surfaces of the proximal extremities. With spread and continued evolution, the rash assumes a striking reticular or lacy pattern. The rash is frequently enhanced by a warm bath or by wrapping the arm in a towel. It lasts for a few days to several weeks, often clearing and reappearing. There are usually no other symptoms, and resolution is eventually complete.

There are no known complications or sequelae, and treatment is not necessary.

Gellis S, Finegold M (editors): Picture of the month. Am J Dis Child 110:543, 1965.

Greenwald P, Bashe WJ Jr: An epidemic of erythema infectiosum. Am J Dis Child 107:30, 1964.

INFECTIOUS MONONUCLEOSIS

Essentials of Diagnosis

- Fever, pharyngitis, lymphadenopathy, and splenomegaly.
- Lymphocytosis with atypical lymphocytes.
- Positive heterophil test.

General Considerations

Infectious mononucleosis is an acute, self-limiting infectious disease characterized by increased numbers of atypical lymphocytes and monocytes in the peripheral blood. The disease is presumed to be due to a virus (EB virus). The disorder can occur at any age but is seen most frequently in children and young adults. In the majority of patients the serum reveals an increased titer of agglutinins for sheep red cells (heterophil antibody test). However, in children under 5 years of age, the heterophil test is often negative.

Clinical Findings

A. Symptoms and Signs: Children with infectious mononucleosis often present with fever, sore throat, exudative tonsillitis, malaise, generalized lymphadenopathy, and splenomegaly. Other clinical features may be headache, epistaxis, jaundice, and abdominal pain. A morbilliform or maculopapular exanthem is not unusual. Almost any system may be involved; hepatitis, encephalitis, meningitis, polyradiculoneuritis, and carditis have all been reported. There is an increased susceptibility to rupture of the spleen.

B. Laboratory Findings:

1. Peripheral blood—The leukocyte count varies greatly; although the usual white count is 10–20 thousand/cu mm, a normal or low count may be present. A rather constant feature is the appearance of increased numbers of atypical lymphocytes and monocytes in the peripheral blood smear, ranging from 50–90% of the total differential count. The hemoglobin, hematocrit, and platelets are usually normal. Thrombocytopenia and autoimmune hemolytic anemia occasionally may be complicating factors.

2. Serology—The heterophil antibody (Paul-Bunnell) test is often positive in a titer above 1:112. Early in the course of the disease or in young children, this test may be negative. An attempt to make the heterophil test more reliable uses differential agglutination after absorption as follows:

Serum Source	Heterophil Agglutinins Present After Absorption By	
	Guinea Pig Kidney	Beef Cells
Infectious mononucleosis	+	–
Normal sera	–	+
Serum sickness	–	–

Differential Diagnosis

Differential diagnosis includes leukemia (usually with pancytopenia or circulating "blast" cells), acute infectious lymphocytosis (increase in small mature lymphocytes), viral exanthems (clinical course differs), infectious hepatitis (fewer atypical lymphocytes and absence of lymphadenopathy), and aseptic meningoencephalitis (absence of splenomegaly and lymphadenopathy). In addition, many young infants and children have a few atypical lymphocytes without evidence of illness.

Treatment

Treatment is symptomatic. Emphasis is on supportive care when the major systems (liver, heart, nervous system) are involved. In older children and adolescents the symptoms may be quite severe, and hospitalization and bed rest are often necessary.

Prognosis

The prognosis is good for complete recovery after a period of illness of 3–6 weeks or, with major system involvement, longer. Rupture of the spleen and secondary infection are the major complications.

Pejme J: Infectious mononucleosis. Acta med scandinav, Suppl 413, 1964.
Ragab AH, Vietti TJ: Infectious mononucleosis, lymphoblastic leukemia, and the EB virus. Cancer 24:261–265, 1969.

Schumacher HR, McFeely AE, Maugel TK: The mononucleosis cell. 3. Electron microscopy. Blood 33:833–842, 1969.
Smith CH: *Blood Diseases of Infancy and Childhood.* Mosby, 1960.

RABIES

Essentials of Diagnosis

- History of animal bite (wild, sick, or unidentified).
- Early hypesthesia or paresthesia in area of bite.
- Increasing irritability with clear sensorium.
- Hydrophobia—initially to drinking, later to sight of water.
- Progressive symptoms to death.
- Isolation of rabies virus from animal brain confirming Negri body visualization or fluorescent antibody identification.
- CSF may be normal, or there may be pleocytosis and slightly elevated protein.
- Mild to moderate peripheral leukocytosis.

General Considerations

Rabies is an almost unexceptionally fatal disease which is transmitted to humans by the bite of a rabid animal. The variable results following such bites are due to the presence or absence of virus in the animal's saliva, the extent and location of the wound, the promptness with which preventive measures are instituted, and the immune status of the bitten individual. Accurate diagnosis and correct therapy depend upon determination of the presence or absence of rabies. This requires knowledge about the prevalence of rabies in the community; the immunization status of the animal; and observation of the living animal for at least 10 days following the bite.

Clinical Findings

A. History:

1. The animal bite—In most instances, a clear-cut history of animal bite is obtained. The animal is usually a dog, but may be a wild skunk, fox, wolf, etc or unknown to the patient. Multiple bites may have occurred. If the animal was a pet, unusual behavior and an unprovoked bite should suggest rabies. Death of the animal complicates the history. With prolonged incubation periods, the history of animal bite, particularly in a young child or if the wound was slight, may be lacking.

Rabies may also be transmitted by bats; rarely, the bat's environment, particularly in caves, may serve as a means of transmission where no bite is involved.

2. The animal—Peculiar behavior of an animal during observation is noted. The dog, the usual offender, may become hyperirritable and begin to bite anything in its environment. Conversely, progressive lethargy and paralysis may be seen ("dumb" rabies). If the animal remains healthy for 10 days or more after the bite, the possibility of rabies is remote.

3. The patient—Following the bite, no symptoms occur for 10 days to many months. The duration of the incubation period is related to the site of the bite in relation to the brain and to the severity of the bite (and therefore to the amount of rabies virus inoculated). Very short incubation periods have been associated with direct intracranial bites and prolonged ones with slight trauma to the distal extremities.

B. Symptoms and Signs: The first symptom in the typical form of the disease relates to the region of the bite. Tingling or loss of sensation is reported. The patient then experiences increasing apprehension, anxiety, and hyperexcitability despite a clear sensorium. Episodes of convulsive movements, irrational behavior, or frank delirium may alternate with lethargy. Progressive aversion to water or the act of swallowing ensues, and drooling and spasmodic contraction of the muscles of deglutition follow.

The course is progressive and culminates in death. Increasing CNS depression, cardiovascular and respiratory instability, and fever end in death 5–7 days after onset.

C. Laboratory Findings: Rabies virus may be recovered from saliva during life or from CNS tissue or salivary glands after death. Virus identification rarely leads to premortem diagnosis because death occurs before laboratory studies can be completed. A presumptive diagnosis can be made on the basis of examination of the animal's brain, if available, for rabies virus content. Fluorescent antibody or Negri body identification should always be confirmed by virus isolation.

Examination of CSF is of little aid. Most often it is normal, although elevation of the white cell count and protein may occur. The presence of peripheral leukocytosis is of little diagnostic significance.

Differential Diagnosis

Differentiation from other forms of encephalitis is usually not difficult. The history of animal bite, an appropriate incubation period, and the characteristic clinical course should be sufficient. Adequate virologic diagnosis of other forms of encephalitis should be attempted.

Prevention*

Despite adequate support, almost all patients die. Therefore, treatment at the time of the animal bite is directed at preventing the clinical disease.

The World Health Organization has outlined its recommendations for the use of rabies hyperimmune serum and vaccines in the prophylactic treatment of animal bites. However, local conditions should modify these recommendations, particularly because the risk of bites by domestic animals in many areas is almost negligible as a result of absence of a convenient reservoir in the wild animal population or insufficient

*See also Chapter 5.

opportunities for contact between domestic and wild animals. The guidelines laid down by the California State Department of Public Health (see below and Chapter 5) can be made applicable to local conditions. Early and adequate local treatment of the wound, local epidemiologic factors, veterinary consultation, adequate field investigation, and the facts and circumstances associated with the bite may modify the physician's judgement with regard to the systemic treatment indicated in individual cases. The following is intended only as a guide.

A. Local Treatment of the Wound: If the animal is not overtly rabid and has been impounded, cleanse the wound carefully with bland soap and water and irrigate copiously with saline solution. Debride devitalized tissues. Give tetanus prophylaxis. If the animal is known to be rabid, or if the attack was unprovoked and the animal has been killed or has escaped, cauterize the wound with fuming nitric acid, irrigate copiously with saline, and cleanse with soap and water.

B. Antirabies Immunization:*

1. No lesion (indirect contact; licks of unabraded skin)—No treatment even if animal is overtly rabid.

2. Licks of abraded or scratched skin or mucosa— No treatment if animal remains healthy. Start vaccine at first sign of rabies in animal.

3. Bites other than multiple bites or face, head, or neck bites—

a. Start vaccine at first sign of rabies in animal.

b. Stop treatment on fifth day after exposure if the animal at first showed signs suggestive of rabies but is normal after 5 days.

c. Start vaccine immediately (see Chapter 5) if the animal is overtly rabid or if he has escaped, was killed, or cannot be identified.

4. Multiple bites or face, head, or neck bites—

a. Start serum immediately. Give no vaccine as long as the animal remains normal.

b. Start vaccine at first sign of rabies in animal.

c. Stop vaccine if animal is normal on fifth day after exposure.

d. Give serum immediately, followed by vaccine, if the animal is rabid, escaped, killed, or unknown; or for bites by a wild animal (especially a skunk or bat).

Treatment

Experience with 3 recent cases of rabies suggests that prolonged survival and, in one case, apparent recovery may occur if vigorous early supportive therapy is utilized. Early tracheostomy, careful attention to maintaining oxygenation, circulatory support, and ventilation are suggested.

Prognosis

Although rare instances of survival in suspected rabies have been reported, the disease is almost always

*Modified from recommendations of the California State Department of Public Health, May, 1960. Physicians in rabies-enzootic areas are advised to consult WHO Technical Report Series No. 121, 1957, prepared by the Expert Committee on Rabies of the World Health Organization.

fatal. Whether application of vigorous early supportive therapy will alter this prognosis cannot be stated at present.

Habel K: Rabies prophylaxis in man. Pediatrics 19:923, 1957.
Rabies Prophylaxis: Recommendations. California State Department of Public Health, May, 1960.
WHO Expert Committee on Rabies: *Third Report.* WHO Technical Report Series No. 121. World Health Organization, 1957.

II. RICKETTSIAL INFECTIONS (RICKETTSIOSES)

The rickettsiae are pleomorphic coccobacillary organisms which are intracellular parasites. They are now classified as true bacteria.

Characteristically, human infections occur as a result of arthropod contact. Only those diseases encountered in pediatrics will be considered here.

Common characteristics of rickettsiae and the infections they produce may be listed as follows:

(1) Asymptomatic multiplication in the arthropod host.

(2) Intracellular replication.

(3) Limited geographic and seasonal occurrence related to arthropod ecology.

(4) Local primary lesions (rickettsialpox, scrub typhus, tick typhus).

(5) Fever, rash, and respiratory symptoms predominate.

(6) Nonspecific (Weil-Felix reaction, H proteus agglutinins) and specific antibodies develop following human infection.

(7) Infections respond to the tetracyclines and chloramphenicol.

RICKETTSIALPOX

Rickettsialpox is an acute, self-limited disease caused by infection with *Rickettsia akari.* It is transmitted by mites from the common house mouse. Following an incubation period of 2 weeks, fever, chills, myalgia, headache and photophobia appear abruptly. At the site of the mite bite, a primary firm, red papule appears which vesiculates and becomes crusted with a black eschar. Two to 4 days after onset, a generalized papulovesicular eruption appears which evolves to crusting within 2 days. The crusts are shed in 1—2 weeks. The differential diagnosis includes varicella, variola, flea typhus, Rocky Mountain spotted fever, and scrub typhus. Leukopenia is frequent early in the illness, and complement-fixing antibodies appear during or after the second week of illness.

The drug of choice is tetracycline (see Chapter 39).

TICK TYPHUS
(Rocky Mountain Spotted Fever, Boutonneuse Fever, North Queensland Tick Typhus, Spotted Fevers, Etc)

The tick-borne rickettsioses have many features in common, and are all produced by rickettsiae which may be considered subspecies of *R rickettsii.* They differ in the locale of infection and bear regional names for the illnesses. All are transmitted by the hard ticks, including the genera Dermacentor, Haemaphysalis, Amblyomma, and Rhipicephalus. Animal hosts vary and include rodents, rabbits, and dogs.

1. ROCKY MOUNTAIN SPOTTED FEVER

The name of this disease is a misnomer since it is seen throughout the USA and is found with greater frequency in some eastern and southeastern states than in the Rocky Mountain region. The ixodid ticks serve as the vector for *Rickettsia rickettsii.* Most cases are seen in the late spring and early summer in children who frequent wooded and rural areas.

Following an incubation period of 3—7 days, chills, fever, and influenza-like symptoms appear suddenly. There may be associated headache, sore throat, retro-orbital pain, photophobia, nosebleed, myalgias, arthralgias, gastrointestinal symptoms, and abdominal pain. Severe CNS manifestations may occur, ie, coma, delirium, stupor, and profound lethargy. Physical findings initially include conjunctivitis, fever, splenomegaly (in 50% of cases), and, occasionally, cyanosis, hepatomegaly, and jaundice. Within 2—11 days (usually 3—5 days), a tiny red macular eruption appears on the wrists and ankles and spreads to involve the entire extremities and the trunk, usually sparing the face. The macules grow larger and become petechial within 2—3 days.

Laboratory findings may include proteinuria, bilirubinuria, and hematuria. The diagnosis may be established by isolation of the rickettsiae from blood by inoculation into guinea pigs or embryonated hens' eggs or by specific complement-fixing antibody increases in 2 weeks. Proteus OX-19 and OX-2 agglutinins become detectable during the second week (Weil-Felix reaction). The illness may be complicated by myocarditis, pneumonia, and cerebral infarction.

Before the availability of antimicrobial agents, the mortality rate was 25—75%. Specific therapy includes the tetracyclines or chloramphenicol (see Chapter 39).

For persons with a high exposure risk, a vaccine is available. The dose is 1 ml subcut for 3 doses at intervals of about 1 week.

2. OTHER FORMS OF TICK TYPHUS

African tick typhus is generally mild, usually terminating by rapid lysis in the second week. An abrupt onset is usual, with severe headache, constipation, insomnia, photophobia, myalgia, and arthralgia. Mental disturbances may occur but are not severe. In a varying proportion of cases, an eschar is already developed at onset, with painful enlargement of regional lymph nodes. The eschar may be anywhere on the body, at the site of the tick bite, but is usually on covered parts. The rash is similar to that of the American type, but is less often petechial and may be transitory or absent, especially outside the Mediterranean region. In the mildest cases, there may be no more than a few days of fever with headache, with or without an eschar and lymphadenopathy.

North Queensland tick typhus has been little studied. Fever lasts less than a week and may be intermittent. The rash is variable in character and may be fleeting.

EPIDEMIC TYPHUS
(Louse Typhus)

This disease is produced by infection with *R prowazeki* and is transmitted in the feces of the body of the louse. Following an incubation period of 8–12 days, during which malaise, cough, nausea, coryza, headache, and chest pain may occur, the disease begins with an abrupt rise in temperature accompanied by chills and severe prostration. Headache, nausea and vomiting, gastrointestinal symptoms, cough, nonpleu-ritic chest pain, stupor and delirium, and severe muscle aching may occur. Conjunctivitis, flushing, splenomegaly (1/3 of cases), rales, low blood pressure, and a rash may be seen. The rash is characteristic, beginning on the third to eighth day of illness with pink maculopapules that appear on the trunk and spread to the extremities. The rash usually spares the face, scalp, palms, and soles, and may become hemorrhagic.

Leukopenia may be present during the first week, and leukocytosis during the second. Proteinuria is common, and hematuria may occur. Although rickettsiae can be isolated, the diagnosis is usually made by the appearance of proteus OX-19 (and occasionally OX-2) agglutinins and specific complement-fixing antibody titers during or after the second week of illness.

The illness usually lasts 2–3 weeks, and convalescence may be prolonged. A recrudescent form of the disease is seen in adults (Brill's disease).

Therapy consists of tetracyclines or chloramphenicol (see Chapter 39).

ENDEMIC TYPHUS
(Murine Typhus)

Endemic typhus is caused by *R mooseri* and is usually transmitted by fleas from a rodent (house rat) reservoir. Body lice may become infected and transmit the agent in their feces.

The illness is gradual in onset. Although the symptoms resemble those of epidemic typhus, they are milder and shorter in duration. The prognosis is also better, and fatalities and complications are rarely seen. Proteus OX-19 agglutinins and specific complement-fixing antibody titers appear in the second week.

● ● ●

General References

Blanic H, Rake C: *Rickettsial Disease of the Skin, Eye and Mucous Membranes of Man.* Little, Brown, 1955.

Committee on Infectious Diseases: *Report,* 16th ed. American Academy of Pediatrics, 1970.

Cooke R (editor): *The Biologic Basis of Pediatric Practice.* McGraw-Hill, 1969.

Horsfall FM, Tamm I: *Viral and Rickettsial Infections of Man,* 4th ed. Lippincott, 1954.

Jawetz E, Melnick JL, Adelberg EA: *Review of Medical Microbiology,* 10th ed. Lange, 1972.

Krugman S, Ward R: *Infectious Diseases of Childhood,* 4th ed. Mosby, 1970.

Lennett EH, Schmidt NJ: *Diagnostic Procedures for Viral and Rickettsial Diseases,* 4th ed. American Public Health Association, Inc, 1969.

27...

Infections: Bacterial & Spirochetal

Jerry J. Eller, MD

BACTERIAL INFECTIONS

GROUP A BETA-HEMOLYTIC STREPTOCOCCAL INFECTIONS

Distinct clinical entities are seen in specific age groups.

(1) In early childhood, the disease is mild, with low-grade fever, serous nasal discharge, pallor, and failure to thrive.

(2) In middle childhood, an abrupt onset of fever, sore throat with exudate, and vomiting may be prominent symptoms. The eruption of scarlet fever is finely papular, erythematous, and in appearance much like a mild sunburn. The diagnosis is confirmed by a positive culture of group A beta-hemolytic streptococci from a throat swab.

(3) The adult type (after 10 years of age) has a more insidious onset with fewer toxic symptoms.

Streptococcal respiratory infections are caused by group A beta-hemolytic streptococci. Transmission is by inhalation of droplets from an infected individual. The average incubation period is 1–3 days. Outbreaks of group A streptococcal infections on maternity and newborn services have occurred. Raw and processed powdered milk and contaminated eggs are sources of organisms in food-borne epidemics, which are occasionally reported.

Streptococcal infections of the lungs, brain, and endocardium are life-threatening unless promptly treated.

Vaginal, skin, and respiratory tract infections are of concern principally because they may lead to the development of sensitizing antibodies which predispose to the later development of rheumatic fever or acute glomerulonephritis.

In scarlet fever, the host responds to the erythrogenic toxin of the streptococcus by development of an erythematous eruption, strawberry tongue, Pastia's lines, and other manifestations. Strain differences between streptococci causing infection without eruption and those causing scarlet fever have been demonstrated, and the difference in clinical response relates to the presence in the host of specific antibodies against the erythrogenic toxin.

Clinical Findings

A. Symptoms and Signs:

1. Respiratory infections—

a. Infancy and early types—The onset is insidious, with very mild constitutional symptoms, ie, failure to thrive, low-grade fever, chronic serous nasal discharge, chronic cervical adenitis, and pallor. Otitis media is common. Pharyngitis and exudate are rare in this age group.

b. Childhood type—Sudden onset with high fever —at least 39–40° C (102–104° F), with marked malaise and usually repeated vomiting. The pharynx is sore and edematous and the tonsillar area generally shows exudate. Anterior cervical lymph nodes are tender and enlarged. Small petechiae are frequently seen on the soft palate. Fine discrete petechiae on the upper abdomen and trunk may suggest meningococcemia, leukemia, idiopathic thrombocytopenic purpura, and subacute bacterial endocarditis. In scarlet fever, the skin is diffusely erythematous and appears like a sunburn. The rash is most intense in the axillas and groin and on the abdomen and trunk. It blanches on pressure except in the skin folds, which do not blanch and are pigmented (Pastia's sign). The rash usually appears 24 hours after the onset of fever and rapidly spreads over the next 1–2 days. Desquamation begins on the face at the end of the first week and becomes generalized by the third week. A retrospective diagnosis of scarlet fever may be made by observing desquamation of the fingers several weeks after a febrile disease. Early, the surface of the tongue is coated white, with the papillae enlarged and bright red ("white strawberry tongue"). Subsequently, desquamation occurs and the tongue appears beefy red ("red strawberry tongue"). The face generally shows circumoral pallor. Petechiae may be seen on all mucosal surfaces.

c. Adult type—The adult type is characterized by exudative or nonexudative tonsillitis with fewer systemic manifestations, lower fever, and no vomiting. Complications due to sensitization do occur. Scarlet fever is not common in this age group.

2. Impetigo—Streptococcal impetigo begins as a papule that vesiculates, leaving a denuded area covered by a honey-colored crust. A mixture of *Staphylococcus aureus* along with streptococci is isolated in about 66% of cases. The lesions spread readily and diffusely. Local lymph nodes often become swollen and inflamed. Such a child may develop high fever and be acutely ill.

3. Cellulitis—The portal of entry is often an insect bite or superficial abrasion on an extremity. There is a diffuse and rapidly spreading cellulitis which involves the subcutaneous tissues and extends along the lymphatic pathways with only minimal local suppuration. Local acute lymphadenitis occurs. The child is usually acutely ill, with fever and malaise. The involved area is swollen, warm, tender, and painful. The infection may extend rapidly from the lymphatics to the blood stream.

4. Necrotizing fasciitis—*(This is a medical and surgical emergency.)* Formerly called streptococcal gangrene, this is an uncommon but dangerous entity. Infection with group A beta-hemolytic streptococci after trauma to an extremity causes extensive necrosis of superficial fascia with undermining of surrounding tissue and extreme systemic toxicity. Initially, the skin overlying the infection is pale red without distinct borders, resembling subcutaneous cellulitis. Blisters or bullae may appear. The pale red skin progresses to a distinct purple color. The involved area may develop mild to massive edema.

5. Group A streptococcal infections in newborn nurseries—Group A beta-hemolytic streptococcal nursery epidemics are still of importance. The organism may be introduced into the nursery from the vaginal tract of a mother or from the throat or nose of a mother or a member of the staff. The organism then spreads from infant to infant. The umbilical stump is colonized while the infant is in the nursery. As is true also in staphylococcal infections, there may be no or few clinical manifestations while infants are still in the nursery; most often, a colonized infant develops a chronic, oozing omphalitis days later at home. The organism may spread from the infant to other family members. More serious and even fatal infections may develop, including sepsis, meningitis, empyema, septic arthritis, and peritonitis.

B. Laboratory Findings: Leukocytosis with a marked shift to the left is seen early. Eosinophilia regularly appears during convalescence and is a useful retrospective diagnostic sign.

Beta-hemolytic streptococci are cultured with ease from the throat. The organism may be cultured from the skin—and by needle aspiration from subcutaneous tissues and other involved sites—and from infected nodes. Occasionally, with overwhelming infections, blood cultures are positive. Group A streptococci may be identified most easily by demonstrable sensitivity on disks containing standardized concentrations of bacitracin. Few false-negatives are reported by this method. Grouping by fluorescent antibody technics is preferred and correlates best with the original precipitin reactions described by Lancefield. Grouping is dependent upon the presence of a specific "C carbohydrate substance" in the cell wall. Typing is dependent upon the presence of specific M precipitins or T agglutinins in the cell wall and is sufficiently cumbersome to perform to be reserved for epidemiologic surveys.

Antistreptolysin (ASO) titers rise above 150 units within 2 weeks after an acute infection.

"Pyoderma" strains (types 2, 49, and others) of group A beta-hemolytic streptococci are seldom associated with rheumatic fever but are associated with an increased incidence of acute glomerulonephritis. Elevated ASO and anti-DNase titers are useful in documenting prior throat infections in cases of acute rheumatic fever. On the other hand, elevated anti-DNase B and anti-hyaluronidase titers are most useful in associating pyoderma and acute glomerulonephritis. Elevation of 2 or more of these antibody titers in children 5–18 years of age with isolated Sydenham's chorea suggests a streptococcal etiology.

Confirmation of the presence of erythrogenic toxin in scarlet fever may be obtained during the first hours of the rash by a blanching reaction following the local intradermal injection of 0.1 ml of human gamma globulin. Blanching is best seen 8–14 hours after injection. This is best done on the lateral chest or abdominal wall.

The urine may show proteinuria, cylindruria, and minimal hematuria early. More commonly, true sensitizing poststreptococcal nephritis is seen 2–4 weeks after the respiratory infection.

Differential Diagnosis

Streptococcosis of the early childhood type must be differentiated from pneumococcosis and from adenovirus and other respiratory virus infections. Streptococcal pharyngitis must be differentiated from such virus infections as herpangina (coxsackievirus A), acute lymphonodular pharyngitis (coxsackievirus A-10), nonbacterial exudative pharyngitis (adenoviruses), herpes simplex stomatitis, and pharyngeal erythema associated with respiratory syncytial and parainfluenza viruses.

In diphtheria, systemic symptoms, vomiting, and fever are all less marked; the pseudomembrane is confluent and adherent; and the throat is less red.

Infectious mononucleosis causes more marked generalized adenopathy and splenomegaly and shows a typical blood picture and a positive heterophil test.

Pharyngeal tularemia causes white rather than yellow exudate. There is little erythema, and cultures for beta-hemolytic streptococci are negative. Response to specific antibiotic therapy is prompt. Leukemia and agranulocytosis may be diagnosed by bone marrow examination.

Scarlet fever must be differentiated from other exanthematous diseases, principally rubella. Erythema due to sunburn, drug reactions, fever, and the prodromal rashes of chickenpox and smallpox must at times be considered.

Complications

The most common complications of group A beta-hemolytic streptococcal infections are chronic purulent or serous rhinitis, sinusitis, otitis, mastoiditis, cervical lymphadenitis (which may be suppurative), pneumonia and empyema, septic arthritis, and meningitis. Spread of streptococcal infection from the throat to other sites, principally the skin (impetigo) and vagina, is common also and should be considered in every instance of chronic vaginal discharge or chronic skin infection such as that complicating childhood eczema.

Rheumatic fever occurs in 0.5–3% of untreated infections. The average latent period is about 3 weeks, but it may occur within the first week after infection. Rheumatic fever is still an important cause of death in children age 6–10 years. For unknown reasons, the incidence of primary rheumatic fever in certain areas of the USA is declining. On the other hand, recurrent attacks are a frequent complication of streptococcal infection.

Acute glomerulonephritis, caused principally by the nephrogenic type 12 group A beta-hemolytic streptococcus (less commonly by types 1, 4, 6, 24, and 49), is usually seen during the second to fourth week after infection. The incidence is about 3%, and the disease is benign in over 95% of cases.

Prevention of Complications

Penicillin G, 200,000 units orally twice daily, or benzathine penicillin G, 1.2 million units IM once a month (usually for life), prevents reinfection with the group A beta-hemolytic streptococcus in individuals with proved rheumatic fever and thus prevents recurrences. A similar approach to the prevention of recurrences of acute glomerulonephritis is debatable but probably worthwhile in childhood when there is any suspicion that repeated streptococcal infections coincide with flare-ups of acute glomerulonephritis.

Treatment

A. Specific Measures: Treatment is directed not only toward eradication of acute infection but also to the prevention of rheumatic fever and nephritis. This is best accomplished with penicillin. The use of sulfonamides in the treatment of streptococcal disease is to be discouraged because they do not prevent the development of sensitizing antibodies and therefore do not lower the incidence of rheumatic fever or nephritis.

1. Penicillin—In children, oral penicillin is adequate for most infections. Give penicillin G, 200–400 thousand units, or penicillin V, 125–250 mg every 6 hours between meals for 10 days. Parenteral therapy is indicated if there is vomiting or sepsis and other serious infections.

A single dose of benzathine penicillin G (Bicillin), 0.6–1.2 million units IM, is preferred for treatment of pharyngitis and impetigo. Mild cellulitis may be similarly treated. Cellulitis requiring hospitalization should be treated with aqueous penicillin G, 150,000 units/kg/day IV or IM in 4 divided doses until there is marked improvement. Procaine penicillin G, 25,000 units/kg/day IM in 2 doses, may then be given to complete a 7- to 10-day course. Acute cervical lymphadenitis may require incision and drainage. Treatment of necrotizing fasciitis requires emergency surgical debridement. Aqueous penicillin G should be given as 300,000 units/kg/day IV in 6 divided doses for 7 days

after surgery. Smaller doses may then be given intramuscularly until the patient is completely healed.

Ampicillin, nafcillin, cloxacillin, and dicloxacillin are also effective in the treatment of streptococcal infections. Penicillinase-producing staphylococci play a controversial role in penicillin treatment failures.

2. Other antibiotics—For serious, life-threatening infections in patients with known penicillin allergy, give cephalothin, 100–200 mg/kg/day in 4–6 divided doses. For milder infections, give erythromycin, 40 mg/kg/day orally in 4 divided doses.

Clindamycin and cephalexin are 2 new effective oral antibiotics. The dosage of clindamycin is 75 or 150 mg 3 times daily; for cephalexin, 25 mg/kg/day in 3 divided doses. Each of these drugs should be given for 10 days. Lincomycin may be effective. Tetracycline-resistant strains have been reported.

3. Reasons for treatment failure include the following:

a. Failure to take or absorb full course of antibiotics as prescribed.

b. Streptococci found after adequate treatment frequently are other than beta-hemolytic group A.

(1) Reported falsely as beta-hemolytic if human blood agar rather than sheep blood agar plate is used.

(2) Reported falsely as group A if the wrong concentration of bacitracin disk is used. (The laboratory should use 0.02 unit—not 0.1 unit—bacitracin disks.)

c. Reinfection by another family member—A sick child will spread organisms to about 40% of childhood siblings and to about 20% of adult members of the household. These family members then may reinfect the originally sick and treated child.

d. The creation in vivo of protoplasts no longer sensitive to penicillin, with later reversion to the parent pathogenic form, is another interesting but presently speculative cause of penicillin treatment failures.

e. Unknown reasons for failure.

4. Control of nursery epidemics—

a. Treat all infants with positive cultures with aqueous penicillin G, 100,000 units/kg/day IM in 2 doses for 10 days.

b. Apply bacitracin ointment every 8 hours to the umbilical stump of each infant until discharge from the nursery.

c. Treat all other infants prophylactically with a single IM dose of 150,000 units of benzathine penicillin G.

d. Continue prophylactic bacitracin ointment and benzathine penicillin G for 15 days or until the outbreak is controlled.

B. General Measures: Analgesic lozenges or gargles with 30% glucose or hot saline solution may be used for relief of sore throat. A soft, bland diet, including noncarbonated high-glucose drinks such as apple juice, grape juice, and pear juice, and iced milk or sherbet is helpful. Aspirin may be useful in reducing high temperatures.

With impetigo, crusts should first be soaked off; areas beneath the crusts should then be washed with 3% hexachlorophene 3 times daily.

C. Treatment of Complications: Acute complications are best treated with penicillin. Prevention of rheumatic fever and glomerulonephritis is best accomplished by early adequate penicillin treatment of the streptococcal infection (see above).

D. Treatment of Carriers: Carriers of group A beta-hemolytic streptococci are much less likely to spread the disease to contacts than acutely infected individuals. Carrier states are difficult to abolish, and it may be well to be certain that a group A hemolytic strain is involved before it is attempted.

Contacts should be cultured 2 days after initiating treatment in the index case, and all contacts with positive cultures should be treated. As an alternative plan, all family contacts may be treated. Treatment consists of a single dose of benzathine penicillin G, 1.2 million units IM, or therapeutic doses of oral penicillin G or V. Hemolytic streptococci found after adequate treatment frequently are other than group A.

Prognosis

Death is rare except in sepsis or pneumonia in infancy or early childhood. The febrile course is shortened and complications eliminated by early and adequate penicillin treatment.

Derrick CW, Dillon HC Jr: Further studies on the treatment of streptococcal skin infection. J Pediat 77:696–700, 1971.

Dillon HC Jr: Streptococcal skin infection and acute glomerulonephritis. Postgrad MJ 46:641–652, 1970.

Gill CC, Castle WK, Mortimer EA Jr: Group A streptococcal infections in newborn nurseries. Pediatrics 46:849–854, 1970.

Kaplan EL & others: Diagnosis of streptococcal pharyngitis: Differentiation of active infection from the carrier state in the symptomatic child. J Infect Dis 123:490–501, 1971.

Margileth AM, Mella GW, Zilvetti EE: Streptococci in children's respiratory infections: Diagnosis and treatment. Clin Pediat 10:69–77, 1971.

Sheehe PR, Feldman HA: Streptococcal epidemics in two populations of "normal" families. J Infect Dis 124:1–8, 1971.

Shrand HN: Rheumatic fever after streptococcal otitis media. New England J Med 284:221–228, 1971.

Wannamaker LW: Differences between streptococcal infections of the throat and of the skin. New England J Med 282:23–31, 78–85, 1970.

STREPTOCOCCAL INFECTIONS OTHER THAN GROUP A

Group B and group D (enterococcus) hemolytic streptococci are etiologic agents in sepsis and major infections in the newborn and are effectively treated using penicillin or ampicillin parenterally. Enterococcus is the second most common cause of urinary tract infections and can be treated with ampicillin. Viridans streptococci are the commonest cause of subacute bacterial endocarditis; and enterococci cause about 10% of cases.

Treatment of Subacute Bacterial Endocarditis (See

Chapter 13 for cardiovascular management.)

Subacute bacterial endocarditis is best treated with both penicillin and streptomycin. Endocarditis caused by a viridans streptococcus sensitive to 0.2 μg/ml or less of penicillin G may be successfully treated with penicillin V, 125 mg/kg/day orally in 6 divided doses every 4 hours for 3–4 weeks. An average serum killing level of 1:16 or higher should be maintained. Strains resistant to 0.2 μg/ml of penicillin G should be treated with aqueous penicillin G given intravenously. Streptomycin is also given in a dosage of 30 mg/kg/day IM in 2 divided doses.

For enterococcal endocarditis, give 300,000 units/kg/day of aqueous penicillin G by continuous IV infusion or in 6 divided doses IV for 6 weeks. Concurrently, streptomycin is given for 2 weeks in a dosage of 30 mg/kg/day IM in 2 divided doses and then 15 mg/kg/day for an additional 4 weeks. The maximum dose of streptomycin for adolescents is 2 gm/day. Two hours after an intramuscular injection of streptomycin, the serum killing level should be 1:8 or higher.

In case of penicillin allergy, treatment may be given after desensitization. Otherwise, vancomycin is given in a dosage of 40 mg/kg/day IV in 4 divided doses every 6 hours for 6 weeks, along with streptomycin. The maximum dose of vancomycin for adolescents is 2–3 gm/day.

Croxson MS, Altmann MM, O'Brien KB: Dental status and recurrence of streptococcus viridans endocarditis. Lancet 1:1205–1209, 1971.

Mandell GL & others: Enterococcal endocarditis: An analysis of 38 patients observed at the New York Hospital-Cornell Medical Center. Arch Int Med 125:258–264, 1970.

Rogers KB: Neonatal meningitis and pneumonia due to Lancefield group B streptococci. Arch Dis Childhood 45:147, 1970.

PNEUMOCOCCAL INFECTIONS

Essentials of Diagnosis

- Very high fever, with few other signs of illness in the early childhood form.
- Marked leukocytosis.
- Cough and diffuse rales (pneumonia).
- Bulging fontanels and neck stiffness (meningitis).
- Diagnosis confirmed by blood, sputum, or CSF culture.

General Considerations

Pneumococcal fever (with bacteremia), pneumococcal pharyngitis, sinusitis, otitis, pneumonitis, and occasionally pneumococcal meningitis, vaginitis, and peritonitis are all part of a spectrum of "pneumococcosis" that may occur at any time during childhood. The incubation period of pneumococcal fever is 1–7 days.

Eighty-two types of pneumococci have been identified. In patients of all age groups, types I–VIII are most invasive. In infants and young children, types XIV, VI, V, XIX, and I occur most frequently (in that order). Twenty to 50% of the population may carry virulent pneumococci in their nasopharynges.

In recent years, the incidence of pneumococcal pneumonia in children has dropped sharply. This may be due to the widespread use of antibiotics, but it may also be that viral studies are now available which establish a viral etiology for serious lower respiratory tract infections previously misdiagnosed as due to pneumococci.

The highest incidence of pneumococcal meningitis is during the first year of life, but the disease may occur at any age. The child with sickle cell disease appears unusually susceptible.

The pneumococcus is the most frequent bacteriologic agent isolated from middle ear aspirates (33%) in cases of acute otitis media. There is likely to be high fever, marked pain, and unilateral involvement.

Disseminated intravascular coagulation with or without Waterhouse-Friderichsen syndrome has been observed with pneumococcal bacteremia. In the reported cases, there is a high incidence of asplenia. The spleen seems to be important in the control of pneumococcal infection by clearing organisms from the blood and producing an opsonin which enhances phagocytosis. Autosplenectomy may explain why the older child with sickle cell disease is at increased risk of developing serious pneumococcal infections.

Clinical Findings

A. Symptoms and Signs: Fever usually appears abruptly, often accompanied by chills, in an otherwise well appearing child. There may be no respiratory symptoms, and in a child under 2 years of age a diagnosis of roseola infantum may be suspected because the child appears well otherwise. There may be some irritability; mild pharyngitis may be present, but exudate is not seen. Cervical adenopathy is uncommon. In pneumococcal sinusitis, mucopurulent discharge may occur. In infants and young children, cough and diffuse rales are found more often than the lobar distribution characteristic of adult forms of pneumococcal pneumonia. Respiratory distress is manifest by flaring of the alae nasi, chest retractions, and tachypnea. In older children, the adult form of pneumococcal pneumonia with signs of lobar consolidation may be found, but sputum is rarely bloody. Thoracic pain due to pleural involvement is sometimes present. With involvement of the right hemidiaphragm, pain may be referred to the right lower quadrant.

Vomiting is common at onset but seldom persists. Convulsions are relatively common at onset in infants. It is not unusual for the infant to have meningismus manifested by nuchal rigidity.

Meningitis. In infants, fever, irritability, and convulsions are common. Some neck stiffness may be detected. The most important sign is a tense, bulging anterior fontanel. In older children, fever, chills, head-

ache, and vomiting are common symptoms. Classical signs are nuchal rigidity associated with positive Brudzinski and Kernig signs. With progression of untreated disease, the child may develop opisthotonos, stupor, and coma.

B. Laboratory Findings: Leukocytosis is pronounced (20,000–45,000/cu mm), with 80–90% polymorphonuclear neutrophils. Bacteremia is more likely to be detected in infections with types I, III, and XIV. The presence of pneumococci in the nasopharynx is not diagnostic, whereas large numbers in endotracheal aspirates are much more confirmatory. Needle aspiration of the lung rarely is indicated. CSF usually shows an elevated white count of several thousand, chiefly PMNs, with decreased glucose and elevated protein levels. Gram-positive diplococci are often seen on stained smears of CSF sediment.

Differential Diagnosis

Roseola infantum is apparent when the diagnostic rash coincides with the disappearance of symptoms 3–4 days after onset. Leukopenia is present instead of leukocytosis.

Infants and young children with signs of upper respiratory tract infection who develop moderate respiratory distress and signs of lower respiratory disease are most likely to be infected with respiratory syncytial virus or parainfluenza virus types 1, 2, or 3. Hoarseness is often present, and there may be a marked bronchiolitic component. X-ray of the chest shows perihilar infiltrates and increased bronchovascular markings.

Staphylococcal pneumonia causes early cavity formation and empyema.

In primary pulmonary tuberculosis, x-rays show a primary focus associated with hilar adenopathy and often signs of pleurisy. Miliary tuberculosis presents a classical x-ray appearance.

The child with cystic fibrosis has patchy infiltrates, areas of emphysema and atelectasis, and a positive sweat test.

Pneumonia caused by *Mycoplasma pneumoniae* is rare under 5 years of age and is most likely to occur in "closed populations" such as institutions.

Pneumococcal meningitis is excluded or diagnosed by lumbar puncture.

Complications

Complications include otitis media, mastoiditis, and occasionally meningitis and sinusitis secondary to pneumococcal fever or pneumococcal pharyngitis, and empyema accompanying pneumonia. Peritonitis is often a complication of chronic glomerulonephritis and nephrosis. Both pneumococcal meningitis and peritonitis are more likely to occur independently without coexisting pneumonia.

Treatment

A. Specific Measures: Penicillin is the drug of choice, but erthromycin is also effective. In recent years there have been several reports of occasional pneumococcal strains (including type XIV) resistant to tetracyclines. For several reasons, tetracyclines are not the drugs of choice for children under 5 years of age (See Chapter 38.)

1. Pneumonia—For infants, give aqueous penicillin G, 50–100 thousand units/kg/day IM in 2 or 3 divided doses. Aqueous procaine penicillin G, 600,000 units IM daily for 7 days, is recommended for children. Pneumonia which is not severe may be treated with oral penicillin G, 400,000 units 4 times daily for 7–10 days. In case of penicillin allergy, give erythromycin, 40–50 mg/kg/day orally in 4 divided doses. Oral cephalexin or clindamycin may be used.

2. Otitis media—Treat with oral penicillin or ampicillin or a substitute as described above for 10–14 days.

3. Meningitis—Until pneumococcal meningitis is confirmed by culture, give ampicillin, 300 mg/kg/day IV in 6 divided doses. After bacteriologic confirmation, give aqueous penicillin G, 300,000 units/kg/day IV in 6 divided doses. Intrathecal penicillin is occasionally given at onset in small children and infants. Treatment must be continued until the patient has been afebrile for 5 days, the CSF white cell count is 30/cu mm or less, and CSF glucose and protein have returned to normal. This usually requires 10–14 days.

B. General Measures: Supportive and symptomatic care is required.

Prognosis

Case fatality rates of less than 1% should be achieved in pneumococcal disease other than meningitis, in which rates of 5–20% still prevail.

Austrian R: Current status of bacterial pneumonia with special reference to pneumococcal infection. J Clin Path 21 (Suppl 2):93–97, 1968.

Cronberg DS, Nilsson IM: Pneumococcal sepsis with generalized Shwartzman reaction. Acta med scandinav 188:293–299, 1970.

Dowling JN, Sheehe PR, Feldman HA: Pharyngeal pneumococcal acquisitions in "normal" families: A longitudinal study. J Infect Dis 124:9–17, 1971.

Grant MD, Horowitz HI: Waterhouse-Friderichsen syndrome induced by pneumococcemic shock. JAMA 212:1373–1374, 1970.

Hansman D & others: Increased resistance to penicillin of pneumococcus isolated from man. New England J Med 284:175–177, 1971.

Howle VM, Ploussard JH, Lester RL Jr: Otitis media: A clinical and bacteriological correlation. Pediatrics 45:29–35, 1970.

Lund E: Types of pneumococci found in blood, spinal fluid and pleural exudate during a period of 15 years. Acta path microbiol scandinav 78:333–336, 1970.

STAPHYLOCOCCAL INFECTIONS

Staphylococcal infections are an important cause of serious neonatal infections and lung diseases in early childhood. There are marked strain differences in pathogenicity. Penicillin has revolutionized the specific therapy of diseases caused by strains of staphylococci which are not penicillinase producers. More than 80% of strains causing hospital-acquired staphylococcal disease are resistant to penicillin. Resistance is due to inactivation of penicillin by penicillinase (β-lactamase), an enzyme which opens the beta-lactam ring of the penicillin molecule.

The incubation period of staphylococcal infection is 1–7 days. Coagulase production correlates well with virulence. Brain abscess occurs by extension or metastatically from such infected peripheral sites as chronic otitis media, sinusitis, infected skin lesions, and infected myelomeningoceles. Brain abscess also occurs in association with cyanotic congenital heart disease and pulmonary arteriovenous fistulas and after penetrating head wounds, including those inflicted by lead pencil points.

Cultures from brain abscesses most often reveal aerobic and anaerobic streptococci. *Staphylococcus aureus* is the second most frequently isolated pathogen. Isolates include a great variety of aerobic and anaerobic gram-positive and gram-negative bacteria and fungi.

The staphylococcal scalded-skin syndrome has been expanded to include several different dermatologic reactions all of which are probably produced by a toxin elaborated by infection with phage group II staphylococcus. Reactions in the skin include, in infants, generalized exfoliative (Ritter's) disease; in children, toxic epidermal necrolysis, generalized scarlatiniform erythema without exfoliation (staphylococcal scarlet fever), and localized bullous impetigo.

Septic (purulent) pericarditis without antecedent infection is rare. *S aureus* is the most common primary etiologic agent and is found in 40–50% of cases. The primary sites of infection in purulent pericarditis due to *S aureus* are the lungs and pleura in 20% of cases and the skin and wound and soft tissue abscesses in 30% of cases. Less commonly, the pericardium may become infected by *S aureus* from the upper respiratory tract, osteomyelitis, or meningitis. After *S aureus,* the most common organisms causing purulent pericarditis are the pneumococci, *Hemophilus influenzae,* and meningococci, followed by gram-negative coliforms. Bacteroides and anaerobic streptococci have rarely been reported as causes of purulent pericarditis.

Clinical Findings

A. Symptoms and Signs:

1. Pyoderma is seen as impetigo, primarily in the neonatal period; in older children, acute and chronic skin infections are often seen as part of a family infection. Impetigo caused purely by *S aureus* begins as a papule that becomes and remains bullous.

2. Osteomyelitis frequently follows trauma, primarily to the head or to the long bones, and is regularly accompanied by septicemia.

3. Staphylococcal pneumonia in infancy is characterized by abdominal distention, high fever, respiratory distress, and toxemia. It often occurs without predisposing factors or after minor skin infections. The organism is necrotizing, producing broncho-alveolar destruction. Pneumatoceles, pyopneumothorax, and empyema are frequently encountered. Rapid progression of disease is characteristic. Presenting symptoms may be typical of paralytic ileus, suggestive of an abdominal catastrophe. When this is suspected, the abdominal films should always be accompanied by a chest film to rule out the staphylococcal pneumonitis. Staphylococcal pneumonia is usually peribronchial and diffuse.

Staphylococcal pneumonia usually begins with a focal infiltrative lesion progressing to patchy consolidation. Most often only one lung is involved (80%), more often the right. Purulent pericarditis occurs by direct extension in about 10% of cases, with or without empyema.

4. The most common source of staphylococcal food poisoning produced by enterotoxin is poorly refrigerated and contaminated food. The disease is characterized by vomiting, prostration, and diarrhea occurring within 2–6 hours after ingestion of contaminated foods.

5. Brain abscess is characterized by fever, headache, irritability, focal neurologic signs, and signs of increased intracranial pressure. Percussion tenderness over the abscess is an important localizing sign. Skull films, serial EEGs, brain scans, and echoencephalograms are helpful in diagnosis. A definitive diagnosis prior to surgery is most frequently made by carotid arteriography or ventriculography.

6. Septic pericarditis is characterized by symptoms and signs of the primary infection and high spiking fever. A pericardial friction rub is audible in about 20% of cases. Clinical, x-ray, and ECG evidence of a pericardial effusion develops. Pus is commonly aspirated from the pericardial sac. On occasion, a large effusion will be coagulum-free but grow the organism.

B. Laboratory Findings: Moderate leukocytosis, (15,000–20,000/cu mm) with a shift to the left is usually found. The sedimentation rate is elevated. Cultures of pus from sites of infection prove the diagnosis. Cultures of tracheal aspirates and material from pleural taps are positive in pneumonia. Blood cultures are often sterile in pneumonia but positive in osteomyelitis. CSF culture is usually negative with brain abscess, but CSF pressure is usually elevated, with mild pleocytosis and elevated protein. Culturing large numbers of *S aureus* in suspected food suggests that the organism is responsible in cases of food poisoning.

Bacteriophage typing is extensively utilized for epidemiologic studies.

Differential Diagnosis

Klebsiella pneumoniae (Friedländer's) pneumonia is rare but tends to cause lobar consolidation with bulging fissures seen on x-ray. Rare nursery outbreaks have been reported. The organism is a secondary invader associated with antibiotic usage, debilitating states, and chronic respiratory conditions and rapidly forms abscesses or empyema.

Primary pneumonias caused by group A hemolytic streptococci and *H influenzae* may also cause pneumatoceles and empyema.

See pneumococcal diseases for further differential diagnosis of bacterial pneumonia.

Tracheo-esophageal fistulas in infancy may be demonstrated by careful x-ray examination. Such infants may develop aspiration pneumonia involving the upper lobes.

Staphylococcal osteomyelitis may be confused with conditions causing pain and limitation of motion of an extremity, including rheumatic fever, septic arthritis, cellulitis, and fractures and sprains.

Staphylococcal enterocolitis is associated with the suppression of normal intestinal flora and the presence of large numbers of the organisms on smears and cultures of the stool. Staphylococcal food poisoning as a separate entity is usually epidemic in nature and usually is not associated with fever. Shigellosis and salmonellosis must be distinguished. Brain abscess must be distinguished from viral encephalitis, meningitis, generalized sepsis, lead poisoning, brain tumors and other encephalopathies, and space-occupying lesions.

Purulent pericarditis must be distinguished from pericarditis with acute rheumatic fever, in which there are usually murmurs and manifestations of endocarditis. Collagen diseases (especially rheumatoid arthritis) with pericarditis must also be differentiated. Tuberculous pericarditis is usually painless and is associated with a friction rub lasting for weeks or months. The child usually has pulmonary tuberculosis. Viral pericarditis is associated with chest pain, a prominent friction rub, and pericardial effusion which is either serous, containing fibrin and a few lymphocytes, or serosanguineous. There is usually evidence of other infections in the community due to coxsackievirus B1–6, including pleurodynia, aseptic meningitis, or perhaps a nursery outbreak of encephalomyocarditis. Pericarditis associated with hemolytic anemia or uremia occasionally must be distinguished from purulent pericarditis.

Complications

Various infections of the skin (particularly in newborns and infants), including impetigo, paronychia, and cellulitis, may be followed by mastitis, omphalitis, pneumonia, meningitis, and brain abscess. Ritter's disease is a generalized bullous exfoliative dermatitis associated with phage types 3B/55/71. Epidemic strains in nurseries have included phage types 52A/79/80/81/71 and 77. Extension of the osteomyelitic process may lead to septic arthritis and subcutaneous abscesses. Chronic osteomyelitis still occurs in inadequately treated acute cases. Septic pericarditis leads to heart failure and fatal tamponade.

Treatment

A. Specific Measures:

1. **Pneumonia**–Prompt administration of a penicillinase-resistant penicillin, eg, methicillin, oxacillin, or nafcillin, is indicated until the sensitivity of the etiologic agent to penicillin G has been determined. The

---

Prevention of Cross-Infection in Hospitalized Patients

(1) Avoid unnecessary treatment with antibiotics.

(2) Observe strict aseptic technic in operating rooms. (Heart-lung machines have been found to be contaminated with staphylococci.)

(3) Observe strict isolation precautions for patients with infectious diseases.

(4) Maintain scrupulous cleanliness in the hospital to reduce dust-borne and other types of contamination from fomites.

(5) Care of patients with purulent discharges:

(a) Observe strict isolation, especially from patients with burns, eczema, etc.

(b) Use masks and gloves.

(c) Dispose of infectious material promptly in impermeable bags.

(d) Disinfect unit after patient is discharged.

(6) Choose antibiotics carefully by means of sensitivity tests. Monitor "serum killing powers" at intervals.

(7) Prevent contact between patients and staphylococcal infections or carrier states.

(8) Establish an infection committee to review nosocomial infections continuously and make recommendations.

---

dosage of methicillin is 200–300 mg/kg/day IV in 6 divided doses. The dosage of oxacillin is 100–200 mg/kg/day in 6 divided doses; of nafcillin, 50–100 mg/kg/day IV in 4 divided doses.

A few methicillin-resistant strains associated with serious illness have been reported in the USA, and more such reports have come from Europe. If the organism is penicillin-sensitive, penicillin G is preferred. Give 300,000 units/kg/day IV in 4 or 6 divided doses. Parenteral therapy is continued for 3 weeks or until there has been marked clinical improvement. Pyopneumothorax and empyema should be treated by placement of one or more chest tubes into the pleural space accompanied by massive systemic antibiotic therapy.

2. Newborn infections–(See also Chapter 3.) Methods available to stop a nursery epidemic include the following:

a. Prompt and adequate management of known infections.

b. Prevention of colonization of newborns with epidemic strains by the following means:

(1) Daily hexachlorophene (pHisoHex) baths.

(2) Removal and treatment of personnel carrying the epidemic strain.

(3) Segregation of infants according to age, and early discharge (within 3 days after birth).

(4) Complete cleansing and disinfection of nurseries after discharge of colonized and infected infants.

(5) Restriction of visitors to the nursery area.

(6) Elimination of breast feeding.

(7) Consideration of prophylactic antibiotics.

(8) Elective colonization of infants with a relatively nonvirulent strain of *S aureus* such as 502A. This procedure is still in the investigational stage but shows promise provided strict methodology is adhered to.

c. "Rooming-in" has definite psychologic benefits but probably is not so important in stopping an epidemic as once thought.

3. Skin infection–See Chapter 8.

4. Brain abscess–(See Chapter 21 for neurosurgical management.) An established abscess must be treated surgically. Some neurosurgeons prefer repeated aspirations; others prefer total excision of the abscess as an initial surgical maneuver. Broad spectrum antibiotic coverage should begin before the first surgical procedure, using penicillin G, 300,000 units/kg/day IV in 4 or 6 divided doses, and kanamycin, 15 mg/kg/day IM in 2 or 3 divided doses. In cases where the organism is identified by culture, drugs shown to be appropriate by sensitivity tests should be used. Although the value of topical antibiotics has not been determined, the abscess cavity may be irrigated with bacitracin solution, 500 units/ml, prior to surgical closure and for 1 or 2 days postoperatively. Systemic antibiotics should be continued for 3–4 weeks or until the abscess has healed.

5. Osteomyelitis–(See Chapter 19 for surgical management.) Some orthopedists believe that immediate surgical drainage of the metaphysis is the local treatment of choice in the early stage of metaphysitis. Antibiotic treatment should be started immediately with methicillin, 200–300 mg/kg/day IV in 6 divided doses. Penicillin G, 300,000 units/kg/day IV in 4–6 divided doses, should be given if the organism is penicillin-sensitive. It is mandatory that a serum killing power be determined at the time of the expected peak blood level of the antibiotic (about 10 minutes after an intravenous dose). The level of the drug should be maintained at a serum killing power of 1:32 or higher. If there is metaphysitis without x-ray changes, parenteral antibiotic therapy should be continued for 3 weeks. With x-ray changes of osteomyelitis, parenteral therapy should be continued in the hospital for 5 weeks. The serum killing power should be determined every other day for the first week and then weekly for the next 4 weeks. During the sixth week of hospitalization, a transition from parenteral to oral therapy may be made, maintaining a peak serum killing power of 1:32. Oral therapy should be continued for an additional 3 or 4 weeks. Dicloxacillin, 25–100 mg/kg/day orally in 4 divided doses, or penicillin V, 250–500 mg orally 4 times daily, may be used. Probenecid (Benemid), 10 mg/kg/dose given 4 times daily, with penicillin V may be required to give adequate penicillin blood levels.

Persistence of fever is due to (1) inadequate drainage, (2) multiple lesions, (3) metastatic lesions, (4) phlebitis (drug-induced), and (5) drug fever. Drug fever associated with methicillin most commonly occurs during the second or third week of treatment. In association with an elevated temperature, leukopenia, eosinophilia, and micro- or macroscropic hematuria are seen. These signs subside usually within 24 hours after the drug is stopped. Eosinophilia usually persists for a while.

6. Septic pericarditis—When pus is present in the pericardial sac, optimum treatment consists of maximim intravenous doses of antistaphylococcal antibiotics for 4 weeks plus surgical pericardiostomy, which permits constant drainage and prevents reaccumulation of fluid. The child should be digitalized preoperatively or immediately after surgical drainage.

B. General Measures: Moist heat applied to local infections will hasten localization and drainage. Oxygen, intravenous fluids, and other supportive care are indicated in staphylococcal pneumonia and other systemic infections. Blood transfusion may be indicated if the patient is severely anemic.

Prognosis

Septicemia, brain abscess, and widespread pneumonitis in infancy all have a serious prognosis. Infants who recover from serious staphylococcal pneumonia appear to have a good long-term prognosis without development of chronic respiratory disease. Osteomyelitis is now never fatal if promptly treated.

Even with optimal treatment, the mortality rate of septic pericarditis remains about 20%.

Breckinridge JC, Bergdoll MS: Outbreak of food-borne gastroenteritis due to a coagulase negative enterotoxin-producing staphylococcus. New England J Med 284:541—543, 1971.

Melish ME, Glasgow LA: The staphylococcal scalded-skin syndrome: Development of an experimental model. New England J Med 282:1114—1119, 1970.

Melish ME, Glasgow LA: Staphylococcal scalded-skin syndrome: The expanded clinical syndrome. J Pediat 78:958—967, 1971.

Richards F, McCall C, Cox C: Gentamicin treatment of staphylococcal infections. JAMA 215:1297—1300, 1971.

Ridley M & others: Antibiotic-resistant *Staphylococcus aureus* in hospital antibiotic policies. Lancet 1:230—233, 1970.

Shinefield HR, Ribble JC, Bons M: Bacterial interference between strains of *Staphylococcus aureus,* 1960—1970. Am J Dis Child 121:148—152, 1971.

MENINGOCOCCAL INFECTIONS

Essentials of Diagnosis

- Fever, headache, vomiting, convulsions.
- Petechial rash of skin and mucous membranes.
- Signs of meningitis.

General Considerations

Infection with *Neisseria meningitidis* is most commonly a subclinical nasopharyngitis or upper respiratory carrier state. Fewer than 1% of carriers develop serious illness via the blood stream with involvement of the meninges, joints, or other sites or with fulminating sepsis followed by rapid circulatory collapse and death. Group A strains cause epidemics every 10—20 years. Groups B and C now cause most sporadic cases and outbreaks. In recent years, over 95% of the strains submitted to the Center for Disease Control are in groups B and C. Sulfonamide resistance has been reported in all 3 groups but is 90% for group C. Disease among the military has accounted for about 10% of reported cases during the past 2 years. Children from ages 2—4 to age 12 develop progressive immunity by virtue of an asymptomatic carrier state. These children usually carry nontypable, nonpathogenic strains which nevertheless produce cross-reacting protective antibodies. Young adults carry a higher percentage of typable and pathogenic organisms. The meningococci are second only to *Hemophilus influenzae* type B as a cause of meningitis in children. The highest attack rate occurs within the first year of life.

Pathogenic strains differ in their virulence. Endotoxins may damage the walls of blood vessels directly and cause hemorrhage. Endotoxins may also induce disseminated intravascular coagulation, resulting in the production of damaging fibrin thrombi. Myocarditis is a significant factor in the fatal outcome of acute meningococcal infections. Pulmonary edema may result from the direct action of endotoxins on the CNS.

Clinical Findings

A. Symptoms and Signs: Disseminated meningococcal infection is generally one of 3 types: meningococcemia, meningitis, or fulminating sepsis.

1. Meningococcemia—There often is a prodrome of upper respiratory infection followed within 2 days by high fever, headache, nausea, and often diarrhea. A petechial rash on the skin and mucous membranes and occasionally bright pink tender macules or papules over the extremities and trunk are seen and may have hemorrhagic centers. Chronic meningococcemia is characterized by periodic bouts of fever, arthralgia or arthritis, and recurrent petechial lesions. Splenomegaly is often present. The patient may be fairly free of symptoms between bouts.

2. Meningitis—In most children, meningococcemia is followed within a few hours by the onset of a typical acute purulent meningitis with severe headache, stiff neck, nausea, vomiting, and stupor. The Kernig and Brudzinski signs are positive.

3. Fulminating sepsis—A most virulent and rapidly progressing form of meningococcemia (Waterhouse-Friderichsen syndrome) is seen in which massive skin and mucosal hemorrhages and shock occur. This syndrome may occur in other generalized bacterial infections, particularly those due to *H influenzae* or pneumococcosis. Characteristically, the blood pressure falls rapidly as massive bleeding into the skin and mucosal membranes occurs. Death occurs generally within 12 hours. In those who survive, marked renal impairment, extensive skin necrosis, and prolonged convalescence are usual. Meningitis may or may not be present.

B. Laboratory Findings: Leukocytosis is marked. If petechial or hemorrhagic lesions are present, meningococci can readily be demonstrated on smear by puncturing the lesions and expressing a drop of tissue fluid. Meningococci are also readily found in smears of buffy coat. The spinal fluid is generally cloudy and contains more than 1000 white cells per cu mm, with many polymorphonuclear cells containing gram-negative intracellular diplococci. A gram-stained smear of the CSF sediment may fail to show the organisms, however, even in the absence of previous antibiotic therapy. Meningococci can usually be cultured from the nasopharynx or blood by the use of chocolate agar incubated in an atmosphere of 5–10% CO_2. In the case of partially treated meningitis, nonviable organisms from the CSF may be identified as meningococci, using an immunofluorescent antibody technic. Examination of a stained blood smear for the presence of platelets will show whether significant thrombocytopenia is present. The combined findings of severe thrombocytopenia, markedly abnormal prothrombin time and partial thromboplastin time (PTT), and significant depletion of prothrombin, factor V, factor VIII, and fibrinogen indicate intravascular coagulation.

Differential Diagnosis

The petechial lesions of meningococcemia may be mistaken for the skin lesions seen in other disseminating infections due to *H influenzae* or pneumococci or caused by enteroviruses (echovirus types 6, 9, 16; coxsackievirus types A-2, 4, 9, and 16 and type B-4).

Eruptions seen in bacterial endocarditis, leptospirosis, Rocky Mountain spotted fever, and other rickettsial diseases as well as the prodrome of smallpox must also be differentiated.

Blood dyscrasias as a cause of petechial eruptions may be excluded by bone marrow examination.

Complications

Blood-borne infections may lead to arthritis, osteomyelitis, endocarditis, pericarditis, pneumonia, unilateral ophthalmia, and bilateral deafness. Meningitis may lead to chronic CNS damage manifested by convulsions, paralysis, and impairment of intellectual functions. Subdural collections of fluid and hydrocephalus are important complications.

Prevention

Chemoprophylaxis with sulfadiazine, 0.5 gm every 12 hours for 4 doses, will reduce the carrier rate and limit spread of the disease among contacts if strains are sulfonamide-sensitive. If the strain is resistant to sulfonamides, rifampin appears to be the drug of choice. It is given orally, 8 mg/kg/day for 4 days in single daily doses. A 40 kg child should receive one 300 mg capsule and an adult 2 capsules daily.

A group C meningococcal polysaccharide vaccine has been extensively tested among a large number of military recruit volunteers. The vaccine was found to be safe and effective. An 87% reduction in group C disease was statistically significant. Group C carrier acquisitions among vaccinated persons were also markedly reduced.

Treatment

A. Specific Measures: Give aqueous penicillin G, 400,000 units/kg/day IV in 6 divided doses. Treatment is continued until the patient has been afebrile for 5 days, the CSF count shows fewer than 30 white cells, and the CSF glucose and protein levels are normal. Patients allergic to penicillin should probably be treated with chloramphenicol or with penicillin G after rapid desensitization and concomitant corticosteroid administration.

B. General Measures: Fluid overload is a common cause of circulatory failure, and careful blood volume determinations are of great value in clinical management of seriously ill patients.

In some patients, decreased cardiac output associated with increased central venous pressure (CVP) has been observed. With heart failure, the CVP usually exceeds 16 cm water. With constant monitoring, 1–2 ml/kg of isotonic electrolyte solution, plasma, or blood are infused over a 10-minute period in order to treat hypovolemic shock. During the infusion, if the CVP increases by more than 5 cm water, the infusion is stopped. There should be a 10-minute waiting period before infusing more fluid. A rise of CVP of 2 cm water is acceptable. If, after 10 minutes, the CVP has risen more than 5 cm water, the patient should be treated for heart failure. If hypovolemic shock is present, intermittent infusions should be continued until the CVP is constant in a normal range of 5–8 cm water. With heart failure, the intravenous administration of a rapidly acting digitalis preparation is recommended with constant ECG monitoring. A continuous infusion of isoproterenol (Isuprel), 0.2–0.4 mg in 100 ml of isotonic solution, is given to patients who do not respond to digitalis alone.

In the presence of demonstrated brain edema, intravenous urea, 0.5 gm/kg every 12 hours, or mannitol, 2 gm/kg given in 30 minutes, may greatly improve the patient's vital signs.

The routine use of corticosteroids is not advised. The use of corticosteroids is safer *if preceded by heparinization. In serious disease with some evidence of shock, hydrocortisone sodium succinate (Solu-Cortef) is given intravenously in a dose of 125–250 mg followed every 8 hours by 125 mg for the next 48 hours. The dosage can then be tapered or changed to oral prednisone, 1 mg/kg/day, decreasing gradually over the next 7 days.

Heparinization is indicated if there is laboratory evidence of disseminated intravascular coagulation. An initial dose of 50 units/kg IV is given. One hundred units per kg are added to the infusion every 4 hours. The dosage should be titrated to give a clotting time of 20–30 minutes.

Prognosis

With prompt treatment, the prognosis is excellent, except in the fulminating form of the disease. Convalescence may require several weeks, especially if skin involvement is pronounced.

Artenstein MS & others: Prevention of meningococcal disease by group C polysaccharide vaccine. New England J Med 282:417–420, 1970.

Denmark TC, Knight EL: Cardiovascular and coagulation complications of group C meningococcal disease. Arch Int Med 127:238–240, 1971.

Dixon LM, Sanford HS: Meningococcal pericarditis in the antibiotic era. Mil Med 136:433–438, 1971.

Eickhoff TC: In-vitro and in-vivo studies of resistance to rifampin in meningococci. J Infect Dis 123:414–420, 1971.

Ellman L: Meningococcemia and consumption coagulopathy treated with heparin and dextran 70. Arch Int Med 127:124–126, 1971.

Hardman JM, Earle KM: Myocarditis in 200 fatal meningococcal infections. Arch Path 87:318–325, 1969.

Nielsen LT: Chronic meningococcemia. Arch Dermat 102:97–101, 1970.

GONOCOCCAL INFECTIONS*

Vaginitis in preadolescent girls has been shown to be commonly caused by other bacterial or parasitic pathogens than gonococci. In adolescence, however, gonorrheal infections of the adult type are becoming increasingly important in the USA. An increased resistance to penicillin has been observed in cases treated in Southeast Asia. This has now become a problem in the USA: Increased penicillin resistance of gonococcal strains recovered in 7 metropolitan cities in the USA has been observed.

Clinical Findings

A. Symptoms and Signs:

1. Vaginitis—Pruritus, discharge, and often dysuria are present. Ten to 15% of infected females may be entirely asymptomatic.

2. Urethritis—Adolescent males after sexual contact with infected partners develop a purulent discharge and burning on urination. There may be fever, although systemic symptoms are usually mild.

B. Laboratory Findings: Gram-negative intracellular diplococci may be demonstrated on smears taken from males. Smears are entirely unreliable taken from females, giving both false-negative and false-positive findings. Culture on enriched chocolate agar is usually reliable. Colonies can be identified after 48 hours of anaerobic incubation.

Differential Diagnosis

Gonococcal vaginitis must be distinguished from physiologic leukorrhea of adolescence and from vaginal

*Gonococcal ophthalmia neonatorum is discussed in Chapter 9.

discharge due to infectious pneumococci, streptococci, trichomonads, oxyuris, and herpesvirus and due to foreign bodies.

Urethritis in the adolescent male may be caused by trauma or mycoplasma infection.

Complications

Gonorrhea in the male may lead to epididymitis, prostatitis, arthritis, and endocarditis. In girls, salpingitis or pelvic peritonitis may occur.

Prevention

Prevention of gonorrhea is principally a problem of sex education.

Treatment

Check with the local Health Department regarding penicillin resistance of gonococcal strains. A single injection of 2.4 million units of procaine penicillin G IM is usually sufficient treatment for genitourinary infections in adolescence when the strain is penicillin sensitive. In children, 1.2 million units IM may be given. Ampicillin appears at present to be the drug of choice where there is relative penicillin resistance. Give 0.5 gm of ampicillin orally every 6 hours.

An asymptomatic female should be treated if there is a history of contact with a positive male. Follow-up culture should be taken when possible.

In all cases of gonorrhea, laboratory tests for syphilis should also be performed.

Prognosis

The prognosis is excellent with antibiotic therapy.

Allen ES: Identification of the asymptomatic female carrier of *N gonorrhoeae:* Treatment with ampicillin. Brit J Ven Dis 46:334–335, 1970.

Blumberg N: Penicillin resistant gonorrhea. J Urol 101:106, 1969.

Holmes KK & others: Recovery of *Neisseria gonorrhoeae* from "sterile" synovial fluid in gonococcal arthritis. New England J Med 284:318–320, 1971.

Kvale PA & others: Single oral dose ampicillin-probenecid treatment of gonorrhea in the male. JAMA 215:1449–1453, 1971.

Thatcher RW, Pettit TH: Gonorrheal conjunctivitis. JAMA 215:1494–1495, 1971.

ANTHRAX

Anthrax is a diseased caused by *Bacillis anthracis* and is transmitted to man through broken skin or mucosa or by inhalation or ingestion from a variety of domestic animals. The characteristic lesion of human anthrax is a necrotic cutaneous ulcer, the "malignant pustule." A degree of suspicion is necessary in making the diagnosis, especially if a potential source of contamination is present. Cases have occurred among children of industrial workers. A specific toxin affecting capillary permeability and leading to fluid loss has been identified.

Clinical Findings

A. Symptoms and Signs:

1. Cutaneous anthrax ("malignant pustule")—This form of the disease usually begins on an exposed body surface as a painless, mildly pruritic, erythematous papule which soon vesiculates. Within 1 day, ulceration leads to the formation of a black eschar. The ulcer may be surrounded by marked edema and swelling which is nontender and nonpitting. Mild tenderness and enlargement of regional lymph nodes is seen. Constitutional symptoms may be very mild despite extensive local changes. Septicemic spread may occur with extensive systemic manifestations, but this is uncommon.

2. Pulmonary anthrax (woolsorter's disease)—The pneumonic form of the disease is characterized by high fever, malaise, headache, cough, and evidence of widespread pneumonitis by auscultation and x-ray. Widening of the mediastinum is suggestive of the disease.

3. Gastrointestinal anthrax—A central necrotic ulcer of the stomach surrounded by edema may be accompanied by massive ascites.

B. Laboratory Findings: The exudate from a "malignant pustule" usually shows little cellular reaction, and the causative gram-positive bacilli are present in small numbers. The smear may also show contamination with staphylococci. Cultures of the skin exudate, blood, and sputum may be positive for *B anthracis*. A serologic test exists with which a diagnosis can be made in patients· who have been given antibiotics prior to collection of specimens for culture.

Differential Diagnosis

In scrub typhus, a cutaneous black eschar is associated with a generalized maculopapular eruption.

Pneumonitis associated with Q fever may need to be distinguished from pulmonary anthrax. Infection occurs by inhalation of contaminated products of infected sheep and cattle.

The pulmonary lesions may resemble those of tuberculosis, neoplasms, sarcoidosis, and fungal infections.

The cutaneous lesion may be mistaken for tuberculosis, pyoderma, carcinoma, and granulomas.

Treatment

Treatment consists of procaine penicillin G, 50,000 units/kg/day IM in 4 divided doses for 10–14 days. Streptomycin may be added if there is no clinical response within 24 hours. One of the tetracyclines may be given as an alternative to penicillin in a dosage of 25–50 mg/kg/day orally in 4 divided doses. Erythromycin or streptomycin may also be used.

Prognosis

Mortality approaches 20% in the untreated cutaneous form of the disease. Prognosis with early treatment is excellent. Pulmonary anthrax has a serious prognosis.

Brachman PS: Anthrax. Ann New York Acad Sc 174:577–582, 1970.

Dutz W, Saidi F, Kohout E: Gastric anthrax with massive ascites. Gut 11:352–354, 1970.

BOTULISM

Essentials of Diagnosis

- Nausea and vomiting.
- Diplopia.
- Difficulty in swallowing and speech occurring within 12–36 hours after ingestion of home-canned food.

General Considerations

Botulism is a serious food poisoning caused by the ingestion of preformed toxin of *Clostridium botulinum*. CNS symptoms characteristically develop and are due to prevention of release of acetylcholine by toxin from cranial nerve motor endplates. Man is affected with types A, B, E, and F. Most cases follow improperly prepared home-canned foods, the remnants of which are often fed to domestic animals such as chickens, causing their death and confirming the diagnosis. The immunologically distinct strain designated as type F was recognized in an outbreak caused by the ingestion of homemade liver paste on the Dutch island of Langeland in 1960. Type F subsequently was recovered from marine samples taken off the coasts of California and Oregon and from salmon in the Columbia River. An outbreak caused by type F occurred in California in 1966.

Clinical Findings

A. Symptoms and Signs: An abrupt onset occurs 12–36 hours after ingestion of food which may have had a rancid or putrid odor or taste. There is lassitude or fatigue, generally with headache. Double vision followed by photophobia and nystagmus occurs, and within a few hours, difficulty in swallowing and in speech. Pharyngeal paralysis occurs in serious cases, and food may be regurgitated through the nose and mouth. The sensorium is clear and the temperature normal. Death usually results from respiratory failure.

B. Laboratory Findings: Suspected food should be recovered and examined for the presence of toxin by injection into mice. Laboratory findings in the patient are usually normal. With the use of electrophysiologic technics, electrical abnormalities can be found. Early in the course, when the patient has marked clinical weakness, the rested muscle shows a depressed response to a single supramaximal stimulus applied to the nerve (normal, 6–12 mv). Later in the course, a marked augmentation of muscle action potential is seen after rapid repetitive stimulation (50/second) of the nerve. This finding is characteristic of neuromuscular block.

Differential Diagnosis

Spinonuchal rigidity and CSF pleocytosis distinguish bulbar poliomyelitis from botulism.

A symmetrical ascending motor paralysis associated with sensory findings and albumino-cytologic dissociation are seen in Guillain-Barré syndrome (infectious neuritis).

The history and related findings characterize post-diphtheritic polyneuritis.

In methyl chloride poisoning, pulmonary edema is associated with CNS depression.

In sodium fluoride poisoning, there is severe nausea, vomiting, and diarrhea in addition to CNS depression. Poisoning with methyl alcohol, organic phosphorus compounds, or atropine may have to be ruled out.

Tick paralysis is characterized by a flaccid ascending motor paralysis which begins in the legs.

Myasthenia gravis usually occurs in adolescent girls and is characterized by ocular and bulbar symptoms with normal pupils, fluctuating weakness, and the absence of other neurologic signs.

Complications

Difficulty in swallowing leads to aspiration pneumonia. Serious respiratory paralysis may be fatal.

Prevention

Proper sterilization of all canned foods is indicated. Energetic boiling for 10 minutes before eating home-canned food would prevent the disease. Cans with bulging lids or jars with leaking rings should be destroyed. Prophylactic antitoxin should be given to asymptomatic persons within 72 hours of ingesting an incriminated food. Vomiting should be induced, and purgatives and high enemas should be administered.

Treatment

A. Specific Measures: Botulinus antitoxin, trivalent (types A, B, and E), should be given intravenously as soon as the diagnosis is made or suspected after skin testing for horse serum sensitivity. The antitoxin as well as 24-hour diagnostic consultation, epidemic assistance, and laboratory testing services are available from the Center for Disease Control. The trivalent antitoxin contains 7500 IU of type A, 5500 IU of type B, and 8500 IU of type E per vial. It is recommended that 2 vials be given as initial therapy. This dose may be repeated within 2–4 hours. A small supply of quadrivalent antitoxin (types A, B, E, and F) is stored at the Center for Disease Control. Guanidine hydrochloride, 15–35 mg/kg/day orally in 3 doses, reverses the neuromuscular block and is a useful adjunct in the treatment of botulism.

B. General Measures: General and supportive therapy consists of absolute rest in bed, aspiration of the respiratory tract through a tracheostomy (if necessary), oxygen and assisted respiration for respiratory paralysis, fluid therapy, and administration of purgatives and high enemas. Treatment with penicillin will eliminate viable organisms continuing to produce toxin.

Prognosis

The mortality rate is 65% in the USA but much lower in Europe. In nonfatal cases, symptoms subside over 2–3 months and recovery is eventually complete.

Cherington M, Ginsberg S: Type B botulism neurophysiologic studies. Neurology 21:43–46, 1971.

Cherington M, Ryan DW: Treatment of botulism with guanidine: Early neurophysiologic studies. New England J Med 282:195–197, 1970.

Fusfeld RD: Electromyographic abnormalities in a case of botulism. Bull Los Angeles Neurol Soc 35:164–168, 1970.

Gangarosa EJ: Botulism in the US, 1899–1967. J Infect Dis 119:308–311, 1969.

Gangarosa EJ & others: Botulism in the United States, 1899–1969. Am J Epidem 93:93–101, 1971.

Stuart PF & others: Botulism among Cape Dorset Eskimos and suspected botulism at Frobisher Bay and Wakeham Bay. Canad J Public Health 61:509–517, 1970.

TETANUS

Essentials of Diagnosis

- History of puncture wound.
- Spasms of jaw muscles (trismus).
- Stiffness of neck and back muscles, with hyperirritability and hyperreflexia leading to fatal convulsions.

General Considerations

Clostridium tetani is an anaerobic, gram-positive organism which produces an acute CNS intoxication by fixation of a potent exotoxin. The organism enters the body by contamination of a wound which may be very minor. In many cases, no history of wound contamination can be obtained. In the newborn, infection frequently occurs through the umbilical cord. It may also occur after smallpox vaccination if an infected poultice is used. The incubation period ranges from 1–54 days (in nearly 90% of cases, within 14 days). In the USA there is an increased incidence of tetanus in the lower Mississippi Valley and in the Southeast. Wounds leading to tetanus usually have 2 things in common: (1) they have not been washed and kept clean, and (2) they often have scabbed over to allow a little pus to form beneath.

Clinical Findings

A. Symptoms and Signs: The first symptom is often minimal pain at the site of inoculation followed by hypertonicity and spasm of the regional muscles. Characteristically, difficulty in opening the mouth (trismus) is evident within 48 hours. The disease may then progress to extensive stiffness of the jaw and neck, increasing dysphagia and irritability, and generalized hyperreflexia with extreme rigidity and spasms of all muscles of the abdomen and back. There is no involvement of the sensorium, and the patient is conscious and lucid. Difficulty in swallowing and convulsions triggered by minimal stimuli such as sound, light, or movement may occur. Recurrent spasms are seen, as well as opisthotonos, clenching of the fists, and pain lasting 10–20 seconds. In most cases the temperature is only mildly elevated. A high or subnormal temperature is a bad prognostic sign. A profound circulatory disturbance associated with sympathetic overactivity may occur on the second to fourth day, which may contribute to the mortality. This is characterized by elevated blood pressure, increased cardiac output, tachycardia (> 120 beats/minute), and dysrhythmia.

B. Laboratory Findings: The diagnosis is made on clinical grounds. There is a mild polymorphonuclear leukocytosis. The CSF is normal with the exception of some elevation of pressure.

Differential Diagnosis

Poliomyelitis is characterized by asymmetric paralysis in an incompletely immunized child.

The history of a bite, absence of trismus, and pleocytosis of the spinal fluid distinguish rabies.

Local infections of the throat and jaw should be easily recognized.

In strychnine poisoning, spasms of the jaw muscles are not common, and periods of relaxation between spasms are more obvious.

Tetany is confirmed by finding hypocalcemia.

Complications

Malnutrition, pneumonitis, and respiratory obstruction are complications which can be prevented by skilled nursing care.

Prevention

A. Tetanus Toxoid: Active immunization with tetanus toxoid is routinely advised. Primary immunization of infants is completed after 4 injections. A booster is given upon entry into school. A diphtheria and tetanus (DT) booster is then required every 10 years. A serum antitoxin content of 0.01 unit/ml indicates that protection is adequate. A booster at the time of injury is practical if none has been given in the past 3 years, or if none has been given within 1 year in case of a heavily contaminated wound.

An attack does not confer immunity, and every patient who recovers from an attack should be given a complete course of active immunizations without delay.

B. Tetanus Antitoxin: Horse serum antitoxin was formerly used in nonimmunized individuals with soil-contaminated wounds, compound fractures, gunshot wounds, etc. Tetanus immune gamma globulin (human) should now be employed instead. Much lower doses are required than with horse serum, and the child does not require prior sensitivity testing or observation following its administration. For children under 5 years of age, give 125 units IM; for children 10 years of age or older, 250 units IM. After severe exposure or delayed therapy, 500 units may be required. Tetanus toxoid should be administered at the same time since

there is no apparent evidence for significant interference with immune response by the concomitantly administered immune globulin.

C. Treatment of Wounds: Proper surgical cleansing and debridement of possibly contaminated wounds will decrease the likelihood of tetanus.

Treatment

A. Specific Measures: Human tetanus antitoxin, 3000–6000 units IM, is preferred to horse serum (50,000–100,000 units IV) because it causes no sensitivity reactions and has a much longer half-life. Surgical exploration of wounds with excision of all necrotic tissue is indicated after effective relaxant therapy has been initiated. Local therapy with antitoxin is contraindicated. Penicillin G is given in a dosage of 150,000 units/kg/day IV for 14 days.

B. General Measures: The patient is kept in a quiet dark room with minimal stimulation. Diazepam (Valium) is given in a dosage of 0.6–1.2 mg/kg/day IV in 6 divided doses. In the newborn, the drug may be given in 2 or 3 divided doses. Large doses (up to 25 mg/kg/day) may occasionally be required for older children. Diazepam is given intravenously until muscular spasms become infrequent and the generalized muscular rigidity much less prominent. The drug may then be given in the same total daily dose orally in 3 divided doses. With continued improvement, the daily oral dose may be reduced after physical therapy is started and then finally discontinued.

A synthetic corticosteroid has been tried and has been associated with decreased mortality. The optimal dose of dexamethasone for children is 20–40 mg daily IM. The drug should be started as soon as the diagnosis is made and continued until there is marked clinical improvement.

Tracheostomy is generally desirable early in the course of the disease. Hyperbaric oxygen therapy is said to be of value but requires specialized equipment not generally available. Intravenous fluids are used as required to minimize the need for oral feeding.

Cardiovascular instability may be treated with propranolol (Inderal), beginning with 0.2 mg IV and guided by continuous monitoring of the ECG, heart-rate, and intra-atrial pressure. Further increments of 0.2 mg are given at 2–3 minute intervals until a normal sinus rhythm at a rate of 100/minute or less is reached. The total intravenous dose should not exceed 3 mg. The drug may then be given in a maintenance dosage of 0.5–0.8 mg/kg/day intragastrically in 4 divided doses until the patient has recovered sufficiently to reduce the oral dose of sedative. In some cases, hypertension associated with elevated systemic resistance may persist after the heart rate has been stabilized with propanolol. In such a case, bethanidine (Esbatal) or other hypotensive agent may be efficacious; bethanidine is given intragastrically every 2 hours for a total dose of 0.6–0.8 mg/kg/day.

Prognosis

The fatality rate in newborns is high (70–90%). A fatality rate of 20–40% can be expected in pediatric practice. Many deaths are due to pneumonia or respiratory embarrassment. If the patient lives, recovery is complete.

Mortality rates tend to increase when (1) the incubation time is short, (2) the site of infection is less accessible and closer to the CNS, (3) there is no acquired immunity, (4) spasms are more frequent and severe and associated with apnea, and (5) the temperature is under 36.7° C (98° F) or over 38.9° C (102° F).

Edsall G: The current status of tetanus immunization. Hosp Practice 6:57–88, July 1971.

Hardegree MC & others: Immunization against neonatal tetanus in New Guinea. 2. Duration of primary antitoxin responses to adjuvant tetanus toxoids, and comparison of booster responses to adjuvant and plain toxoids. Bull World Health Organ 43:439–451, 1970.

LaForce FM, Young LS, Bennett JV: Tetanus in the US (1965–1966): Epidemiologic and clinical features. New England J Med 280:569–574, 1969.

Murphy KJ: Fatal tetanus with brain stem involvement and myocarditis in an ex-serviceman. MJ Australia 2:542–544, 1970.

Peebles TC & others: Tetanus-toxoid emergency boosters: A reappraisal. New England J Med 280:575–581, 1969.

Prys-Roberts C & others: Treatment of sympathetic overactivity in tetanus. Lancet 1:542–545, 1969.

Sanders RKM: Tetanus: New treatment and prophylaxis. Lancet 2:526–527, 1970.

Sherman RT: Prevention and treatment of tetanus in the burn patient. S Clin North America 50:1277–1281, 1970.

GAS GANGRENE

Essentials of Diagnosis

- Massive edema, skin discoloration, and pain in an area of trauma with contamination.
- Serosanguineous exudate from wound.
- Crepitation of subcutaneous tissue.
- Clostridia cultured or smeared from exudate.

General Considerations

Gas gangrene (clostridial myositis) is an infection caused by one or more of several anaerobic gram-positive bacilli of the genus Clostridium *(Cl perfringens [Cl welchii], Cl novyi,* and *Cl septicum).* These are soil and fecal organisms usually placed in traumatized devitalized tissue. They produce potent toxins which are necrotizing to tissue and which, when produced massively, cause prostration, shock, and hemolysis. The spread of alpha toxin, in particular, is responsible for the clinical features. Alpha toxin production can be suppressed in broth cultures of *Cl perfringens* by increasing the partial pressure of oxygen in the broth to 250 mm Hg by exposure of cultures to a pressure of 3 atmospheres.

Clinical Findings

A. Symptoms and Signs: The onset is sudden, usually 1–5 days after a traumatic injury with an open wound which has been inadequately debrided or has been closed by suture after fairly heavy contamination. The skin around the wound becomes discolored, there is a serosanguineous exudate, and crepitation may be felt in the subcutaneous tissues. Pain and swelling are usually intense. If clostridial septicemia occurs, intravascular hemolysis and jaundice are the rule. Shock and renal failure are ominous signs of far-advanced disease.

B. Laboratory Findings: Isolation of the organism is accomplished by anaerobic culture. Smears may demonstrate morphologically characteristic clostridia.

C. X-Ray Findings: Although the diagnosis is generally made on clinical grounds, x-ray may demonstrate subcutaneous gas.

Differential Diagnosis

Gangrene caused by streptococci is associated with massive bullae. Crepitus in the subcutaneous tissues or x-ray evidence of gas is diagnostic of gas gangrene.

Treatment

A. Specific Measures: Give penicillin G, 150,000 units/kg/day IV in 4 divided doses, and continue until clinical remission occurs. Treatment may be supplemented with tetracyclines.

Polyvalent gas gangrene antitoxin is now rarely employed in pediatric practice because of the danger of horse serum sensitivity and the adequacy of other specific measures.

Tetanus toxoid with or without antitoxin should be given.

B. Surgical Measures: Where hyperbaric oxygen is used, surgery should be limited to incisions into the phlegmonous area in cases with massive necrosis; removal of necrotic tissue after clinical resolution; and reconstructive measures as necessary.

C. Hyperbaric Oxygen: Hyperbaric oxygen therapy has been shown to be dramatically effective. An environmental oxygen pressure of 2 atmospheres (30 psi) will produce a partial pressure of oxygen in gangrenous tissue of 250 mm Hg at a depth of 5 cm. A patient may be exposed to 2 atmospheres absolute (30 psi) in pure oxygen in a small "one-man chamber" for 2-hourly periods for as many sessions as necessary until there is clinical remission of disease. Hyperbaric oxygen therapy is usually continued for 2 or 3 sessions after clinical remission has occurred. Large chambers that can accommodate medical staff as well as the patient are unnecessary in the treatment of gas gangrene. Care must be taken to eliminate risks from pressure, 100% oxygen, and spark production.

Prognosis

Without adequate and early therapy, the prognosis is extremely poor.

Calwill MR, Maudsley RH: The management of gas gangrene with hyperbaric oxygen therapy. J Bone Joint Surg 50B:732–742, 1968.

Hoffman S, Katz JF, Jacobson JH: Salvage of a lower limb after gas gangrene. Bull New York Acad Med 47:40–49, 1971.

Mackay NNS & others: Primary *Clostridium welchii* meningitis. Brit MJ 1:591–592, 1971.

Nakamura M, Schulze JA: *Clostridium perfringens* food poisoning. Ann Rev Microbiol 24:359–372, 1970.

DIPHTHERIA

Essentials of Diagnosis

- A gray, adherent pseudomembrane, most often in the pharynx but also in the nasopharynx or trachea.
- Sore throat, serosanguineous nasal discharge, hoarseness, and fever in a nonimmunized child.
- Peripheral neuritis or myocarditis.
- Positive culture.

General Considerations

Diphtheria is an acute infection, usually of the throat or nose but also of the mucous membranes or skin, caused by a gram-positive pleomorphic rod, *Corynebacterium diphtheriae,* which produces a powerful exotoxin. Transmission is from the respiratory tract of the patient or carrier or from skin contact, particularly in the presence of existing skin lesions such as burns and wounds. Skin infections may be of major importance in the transmission of virulent organisms from person to person, eventually reaching the respiratory tract and causing clinical illness. The incubation period is 1–6 days. More serious damage by exotoxin involves the heart, causing early myocarditis. A late manifestation is polyneuritis.

Clinical Findings

A. Symptoms and Signs: A presumptive diagnosis of diphtheria is made on clinical grounds without waiting for laboratory confirmation and should result in immediate specific treatment.

1. Pharyngeal diphtheria—Early manifestations of diphtheritic pharyngitis are a mild sore throat, moderate fever, and malaise, fairly rapidly followed by severe prostration and circulatory collapse. The pulse is more rapid than the fever would seem to justify. A membrane forms in the throat and may spread into the nasopharynx or the trachea, producing respiratory obstruction. The membrane is tenacious and gray and is surrounded by a narrow zone of erythema and a broader zone of edema. Difficulty in swallowing is present, and noisy breathing becomes evident even without laryngeal obstruction. High fever and prostration are characteristic. Palatal paralysis may occur. A disturbed sensorium is seen. Hemorrhages from the mouth and nose are common. Petechiae may appear on the skin and mucous membranes. The cervical lymph nodes become swollen, and swelling is associated with brawny edema of the neck ("bull neck").

2. Nasal diphtheria—Primary nasal diphtheria occurs in about 2% of cases and is characterized by a serosanguineous nasal discharge and excoriation of the upper lip. Fever and constitutional manifestations may be absent.

3. Laryngeal diphtheria—In about 25% of cases, the larynx is invaded. Occasionally, it may be the only manifestation of the disease. Stridor is apparent. Progressive laryngeal obstruction can lead to cyanosis and suffocation.

4. Other forms—Cutaneous or vaginal diphtheria and wound diphtheria comprise fewer than 2% of cases and are characterized by ulcerative lesions with membrane formation. These may be particularly difficult to identify in the presence of burns or wounds thought to be necrotic on a nonspecific basis. Prompt diagnosis and treatment are essential.

B. Laboratory Findings: The white blood count is usually normal, but there may be a slight leukocytosis. The red cell count may show evidence of rapid destruction of erythrocytes and hemoglobin. Smear of the exudate with methylene blue shows rods with midpolar bars. Bacterial culture will confirm the diagnosis. Fluorescent antibody staining may permit early identification. Urinalysis frequently shows proteinuria of a transient nature. In postdiphtheritic neuritis, the CSF may show an albumino-cytologic dissociation. A positive Schick test indicates susceptibility to diphtheria. In this test, 0.1 ml of solution containing 1/50 MLD of diphtheria toxin is injected intracutaneously. A positive reaction is characterized by 10 mm or more of erythema and induration on the fourth to fifth day.

Differential Diagnosis

A foreign body in the nose can be seen with a nasal speculum.

Infants with "snuffles" have other signs of congenital syphilis.

Nasal discharge associated with respiratory viral infections is usually clear and not blood-tinged. Other family members often have symptoms.

The child with acute streptococcal pharyngitis has a sudden onset of high fever, sore throat, and appears acutely ill. Exudate is usually confined to the tonsils.

Exudative pharyngitis may be associated with adenovirus infections. Normal flora is obtained on throat culture. There is no clinical response to penicillin.

Infectious mononucleosis is differentiated by generalized lymphadenopathy, a characteristic blood picture, and a positive heterophil agglutination test.

Agranulocytosis and leukemia are diagnosed by bone marrow examination. (See streptococcal infections for a more complete differential diagnosis of pharyngitis.)

Acute epiglottitis caused by *Hemophilus influenzae* type B is identified by physical examination and culture.

Acute spasmodic croup is recurrent, worse at night, and may be of allergic origin.

Croup caused by the parainfluenza viruses is associated with symptoms of the common cold with or without fever. Many children in the community will have colds, with some degree of hoarseness. Unpredictably, the occasional child with a mild "croupy cough" will develop stridor and upper airway obstruction rapidly and require a tracheostomy.

Complications

A. Myocarditis: Diphtheritic myocarditis is characterized by a rapid, thready pulse, indistinct and poor heart sounds, cardiac arrhythmias, cardiac failure, hepatomegaly, and fluid retention. Cardiac failure most commonly occurs during the second week. ECG changes are characteristic of myocarditis. Conduction system disturbances are not uncommon. Left hemi-anterior block is frequent. Complete heart block signifies a poor prognosis.

B. Toxic Polyneuritis: This complication involves principally the nerves innervating the palate and pharyngeal muscles during the first or second week. Nasal speech and regurgitation of food through the nose are seen. Diplopia and strabismus associated with ocular palsy occur during the third week or later. Neuritis may also involve peripheral motor nerves supplying the intercostal muscles and diaphragm and other muscle groups. Generalized paralysis usually occurs after the fourth week.

C. Bronchopneumonia: Secondary pneumonia is common in fatal cases, especially in association with the laryngeal form.

D. Nephritis: Mild generalized edema, proteinuria, and hyaline casts associated with a decreased urine output are seen in 10–15% of cases.

Prevention

Immunizations with diphtheria toxoid combined with pertussis and tetanus toxoids (DPT) should be employed routinely for infants for a total of 4 injections. A booster is given at 4–6 years, and then an adult type of diphtheria and tetanus (DT) toxoids at 12–14 years. Thereafter, a DT booster is indicated every 10 years.

Care of exposed susceptibles. Children exposed to diphtheria should be examined for signs and symptoms of early diphtheria. If any are found, treat as for diphtheria. Asymptomatic individuals should receive diphtheria toxoid and either erythromycin orally or benzathine penicillin G intramuscularly and be observed daily.

1. Benzathine penicillin G–Age 1–5 years, 600,000 units IM as single dose; over 5 years, 1.2 million units IM as single dose.

2. Erythromycin–Up to 50 lb, 250 mg as estolate (syrup) twice daily for 7 days; 50–100 lb, 250 mg (capsule) 3 times daily for 7 days; over 100 lb, 250 mg (capsule) 4 times daily for 7 days. Failure to take the full course of prescribed drug means that the carrier state will not be eradicated. In epidemic situations where there are many exposed contacts, treatment with benzathine penicillin G is effective and assures

that the person is treated. A previously unimmunized, asymptomatic individual who cannot be observed daily should receive, in addition to the above, 10,000 units of diphtheria antitoxin IM.

Treatment

A. Specific Measures:

1. Diphtheria antitoxin must be given when the diagnosis is seriously entertained without waiting for laboratory confirmation. The intravenous route is preferable in all cases. Conjunctival and skin tests for horse serum sensitivity should be done and desensitization carried out if necessary. A single dose should suffice, and retreatment should never be necessary because of the serious risk of increasing sensitization to horse serum. Diphtheria antitoxin is administered on the basis of the following schedule: Mild pharyngeal diphtheria, 40,000 units; moderate pharyngeal diphtheria, 80,000 units; severe pharyngeal or laryngeal diphtheria, combined types, or late cases, 120,000 units. Diphtheria antitoxin is infused in 100–200 ml of isotonic saline over a 30-minute period.

2. Procaine penicillin G, 300–600 thousand units IM daily for 7 days, slightly speeds the disappearance of the organism from the throat. Penicillin is also intended for suppression of group A beta-hemolytic streptococcus invaders, which are commonly present.

3. Corticosteroids may be of use in acute laryngeal diphtheria. Give hydrocortisone sodium succinate (Solu-Cortef), 4.4 mg/kg/day IM or IV in 3 divided doses for 1 or 2 days. An equivalent dose of prednisone is then given orally when possible and gradually reduced over a 5–8 day period. In severe cases, prednisone, 1 mg/kg/day orally in 3 divided doses for 2 weeks, may lessen the incidence of myocarditis.

B. General Measures: A liquid or soft bland diet may be tolerated. During this period, the child should be fed, bathed, and allowed the least possible amount of voluntary activity. Frequent evaluation for appearance of complications is essential.

Discharge of patients is delayed until 2 consecutive daily pharyngeal cultures obtained no less than 24 hours after discontinuation of antibiotic therapy are negative for *C diphtheriae*. Most patients require 2 weeks of hospitalization. With evidence of myocarditis, total bed rest is required for at least 4 weeks and until the ECG is normal.

C. Treatment of Complications:

1. **Myocarditis**–No specific treatment exists. Oxygen and intravenous hypertonic glucose solution (10–20%) may be of value. Digitalis and quinidine are indicated if an arrhythmia with a rapid pulse rate supervenes. Digitalis should not be withheld in case of heart failure. Digitalis is probably contraindicated in case of any degree of heart block.

2. **Neuritis**–Nasal feeding should be administered early if paralysis of the soft palate exists. The presence of stridor, dyspnea, and cyanosis indicates upper airway obstruction. Examination by direct laryngoscopy and the use of a nasotracheal tube may provide an adequate airway. Tracheostomy is now considered to

be a safe and effective method of management. The procedure is best done before the child becomes exhausted. The mechanical respirator is of value in intercostal paralysis.

D. Treatment of Carriers: The elimination of virulent diphtheria organisms from asymptomatic individuals should be attempted by treatment with penicillin. Results may be disappointing. Tonsillectomy and adenoidectomy are occasionally required. Carriers should be isolated until virulent organisms are no longer demonstrated by culture.

Prognosis

Mortality rates vary from 3–25%, and are particularly high in the presence of early myocarditis. Neuritis is fatal only if an intact airway and adequate respiration cannot be maintained. Permanent damage due to myocarditis occurs rarely.

Death may occur as a result of respiratory obstruction or acute toxemia and circulatory collapse. The patient may succumb after a somewhat longer time as a result of cardiac damage or may recover after perhaps showing evidence of neurotoxic injury.

Bezjak V, Farsey SJ: *Corynebacterium diphtheriae* in skin lesions in Uganda children. Bull World Health Organ 43:643–650, 1970.

McCloskey RV & others: The 1970 epidemic of diphtheria in San Antonio. Ann Int Med. In press.

Morales AR & others: Pathological features of cardiac conduction disturbances in diphtheritic myocarditis. Arch Path 91:1–7, 1971.

Stewart JC: Analysis of diphtheria outbreak in Austin, Texas, 1967–1969. Pub Health Rep 85:949–954, 1970.

ESCHERICHIA COLI INFECTIONS

Essentials of Diagnosis

- Sudden onset of explosive watery stools with fever and vomiting in newborns or gradual onset of foul-smelling, green diarrheal stools in children under 2 years of age.
- Sick newborn with labile temperature, poor feeding, irritability, jaundice, irregular respirations.
- Child with symptoms of acute urinary tract infection.

General Considerations

Institutional epidemics of gastroenteritis are caused by *Escherichia coli,* including serotypes 026, 055, 086, 091, 0111, 0112, 0119, 0124, 0128, and 0142, which are spread to the infant from hospital personnel, mothers, or infected infants (who may be asymptomatic). Early diagnosis and treatment, including that of carriers in institutions, is essential to prevent widespread disease. Strains of *E coli* not necessarily associated with gastroenteritis can cause neonatal

sepsis, the diagnosis of which must be made on clinical grounds and prompt therapy started while awaiting results of blood cultures. Most acute urinary tract infections in children are due to *E coli* infection.

There is growing evidence that "nonbacterial" diarrhea in older children and adults may be due to strains of *E coli* which may or may not be recognized as being "enteropathogenic" in infants but may nevertheless produce a dysenteric syndrome ("colitis") either by intestinal epithelial penetration (as in shigellosis) or a salmonella-like illness (enteritis) by elaboration of an enterotoxin similar to that of cholera.

Clinical Findings

A. Symptoms and Signs:

1. Enteropathic *E coli* gastroenteritis—Usually there is a gradual onset of diarrhea which is not associated with high fever or vomiting in a child under 2 years of age. The stools are loose, slimy, foul-smelling, and green. In a nursery outbreak, the newborn may have fever and associated vomiting and rapidly develops dehydration and metabolic acidosis. In the latter case, weight loss may be spectacular. Within a period of 6–8 hours, 10% dehydration may occur.

2. Neonatal sepsis—Overt signs include jaundice, hepatosplenomegaly, fever, and anemia; subtle signs include listlessness, labile temperature control, apneic spells or irregular respiration, irritability, and failure to suck vigorously. Meningitis is associated with sepsis in 25–40% of cases. Other metastatic foci of infection may be present, including pneumonia and pyelonephritis. Sepsis may also lead to congestive heart failure, hyponatremia, tissue hypoxia, lactic acidemia, severe metabolic acidosis, circulatory collapse, disseminated intravascular coagulation, and death.

3. Neonatal meningitis—High fever, full or bulging fontanels, vomiting, coma, twitching or frank convulsions, pareses or paralyses (ocular, facial, limb), poor or absent Moro reflex, and opisthotonos; occasionally, hyper- or hypotonia and stiff neck. Sepsis coexists or precedes meningitis in a large number of cases. Thus, signs of sepsis often accompany those of meningitis. CSF shows a cell count of over 10/cu mm, usually several hundred or thousands, mostly PMNs. (More than a few PMNs almost always indicate meningitis.) Gram-stained smear of CSF may show organisms. CSF glucose concentration is low, usually less than 1/2 that of blood. CSF protein is elevated to 100 mg/100 ml in full-term newborns. CSF protein is normally elevated in prematures (mean, 180 mg/100 ml) even in the absence of meningitis. The diagnosis is established by a positive culture of CSF.

4. Acute urinary tract infection—Classical symptoms include dysuria, increased urinary frequency, and fever in the older child. Such nonspecific symptoms as anorexia, vomiting, irritability, failure to thrive, and unexplained fever are seen in children under 2 years of age. As many as 1% of girls of school age and 0.05% of boys have undiagnosed and asymptomatic but significant urinary tract infections.

B. Laboratory Findings: Culture of enteropathogenic *E coli* by repeated anal swab is routine, but for rapid diagnosis fluorescent antibody studies give an almost immediate answer which permits control measures to prevent epidemic spread in nurseries. Blood cultures are positive in neonatal sepsis. Cultures of spinal fluid, urine, and the umbilicus should also be obtained. A positive culture with a significant colony count (100,000 colonies per ml) from a bladder tap or a clean catch, midstream urine sample confirms the diagnosis of acute urinary tract infection.

Differential Diagnosis

The clinical picture of enteropathogenic *E coli* infection may resemble salmonellosis or shigellosis or certain enterovirus (echovirus 18, 9) and adenovirus infections. The diagnosis depends upon stool cultures.

Neonatal sepsis can be clearly differentiated only by blood culture identification.

Complications

Gastroenteritis frequently results in metabolic acidosis and dehydration, requiring vigorous corrective therapy. (See Chapter 37.) Neonatal sepsis may result in seeding of meninges, brain, bone, etc and the development of hemolytic anemia. Recurrent urinary tract infections associated with vesicoureteral reflux may lead to irreversible kidney damage and early death from uremia.

Treatment

A. Specific Measures:

1. *E coli* gastroenteritis–The drug of choice is neomycin, 100 mg/kg/day orally in 3 divided doses for 3–5 days. If the organism is neomycin-resistant, give colistin, 5–10 mg/kg/day orally in 2–3 doses. Good results have also been obtained with gentamicin, 25 mg/kg/day orally in 2 divided doses.

2. *E coli* sepsis, pneumonia, pyelonephritis–Give ampicillin, 100 mg/kg/day, or penicillin G, 50,000–100,000 units/kg/day, IV or IM in 2 or 3 divided doses. In addition, give kanamycin, 15 mg/kg/day IM in 2 divided doses. Since there is increasing resistance of *E coli* to kanamycin at some centers, be sure the *E coli* isolate is kanamycin-sensitive. Treatment should be continued for 10 days. In case of kanamycin resistance, substitute gentamicin, 3–5 mg/kg/day, or polymyxin B, 2–4 mg/kg/day, in 3 divided doses.

3. *E coli* meningitis–Give ampicillin, 100 mg/kg/day IV or IM in 3 divided doses, and gentamicin, 3–5 mg/kg/day IM in 3 doses. In addition, give gentamicin intrathecally daily for 5 days. The dose for a full-term infant is 1 mg intrathecally and that for a small premature is 0.5 mg intrathecally. Treat with parenteral antibiotics for 3 weeks. Stop treatment and then reevaluate sterility of CSF after 2–4 days of observation. Do not perform subdural taps unless a symptomatic subdural collection is suspected on the basis of bulging fontanels, enlarged head circumference, seizures, focal neurologic signs, or persistent or recurrent fever. In such a case, perform daily subdural taps with caution, removing a maximum of 10–15 ml daily from each side of the coronal suture for 2 weeks. In case of subdural empyema, continue parenteral antibiotics and introduce 0.5–1 mg of gentamicin into the infected subdural space at the time subdural taps are performed.

4. Acute urinary tract infection–Treat for 3–4 weeks with sulfisoxazole or triple sulfonamides, penicillin V or G, or with ampicillin, 125–250 mg orally 3 times daily. Cultures and sensitivity tests should be repeated while treatment is being given. Nalidixic acid, 55 mg/kg/day orally in 3–4 doses, or methenamine mandelate (Mandelamine), 250 mg/30 lb/day orally in 4 doses, may be given for long-term suppressive therapy when indicated. If methenamine mandelate is used, acidification of the urine to a pH below 5.5 with ascorbic acid is recommended.

B. General Measures: In gastroenteritis, early correction of metabolic acidosis and dehydration is indicated. The jaundice encountered in hemolytic *E coli* sepsis of the newborn often requires blood transfusion. Principles of importance in the management of urinary tract infection, in addition to specific treatment, include the following: (1) diagnosis of existing mechanical defects by intravenous urography, voiding cystourethrography, cinefluoroscopy, and cystoscopy; (2) surgical correction of defects; (3) frequent culture after an initial infection to detect significant asymptomatic bacteriuria before the onset of repeated clinical illness (every 3 months for the first year, then every 6–12 months for an indefinite period); and (4) long-term suppressive therapy (for years) in cases not controlled by the above means.

Prognosis

Gastroenteritis should no longer be of serious import provided general and specific therapy is given early. On the other hand, neonatal sepsis still carries a mortality of over 50%. As many as 20% of children with recurrent urinary tract infections may eventually succumb to the effects of the disease.

Brumfitt W & others: Antibiotic-resistant *Escherichia coli* causing urinary tract infections in general practice: Relation to fecal flora. Lancet 1:315–317, 1971.

DuPont HL & others: Pathogenesis of *Escherichia coli* diarrhea. New England J Med 285:1–9, 1971.

McCracken GH: Changing pattern of the antimicrobial susceptibilities of *Escherichia coli* in neonatal infections. J Pediat 78:942–947, 1971.

Orskov F, Orskov I: *Escherichia coli* serotypes and renal involvement in urinary tract infection. Lancet 1:1312–1314, 1971.

South MA: Enteropathogenic *Escherichia coli* disease: New developments and perspectives. J Pediat 79:1–11, 1971.

Valman HB, Wilmers MJ: Use of antibiotics in acute gastroenteritis among infants in hospital. Lancet 1:1122–1123, 1969.

PROTEUS & PSEUDOMONAS INFECTIONS

Essentials of Diagnosis

- Organisms tend to lodge in damaged or infected tissues in debilitated children.
- Occurs as a "superinfection" in patients treated for some other infection or receiving prophylactic chemotherapy.
- Positive cultures.

General Considerations

Members of the proteus and pseudomonas groups, although not hardily invasive, are becoming increasingly important as causes of infection in debilitated individuals or those receiving antibiotic therapy. Spread from local sites can occur in many locations, including the urinary and respiratory tracts, ears, mastoids, paranasal sinuses, eyes, and skin. Invasion of the meninges is occasionally seen. There is a tendency for infection to occur in debilitated patients or those with neoplastic disease or extensive burns. Pseudomonas can be isolated from the respiratory tract of a majority of patients with cystic fibrosis of the pancreas as the disease progresses. Pseudomonas produces a vasculitis affecting the media of small blood vessels which leads to infarction and gangrene. Pyoderma (ecthyma) gangrenosum is a term used to describe gangrenous involvement of the skin in association with pseudomonas sepsis. Nosocomial infections with *Pseudomonas aeruginosa* and *Proteus vulgaris* are spread by a variety of hospital equipment and solutions. Proteus is second only to *Escherichia coli* as a gram-negative rod associated with urinary tract infection.

Clinical Findings

The diagnosis is made by specific culture. Pseudomonas infection is frequently associated with a low white count and agranulocytosis.

Prevention

A. Burned Patients: Colonization of extensive second and third degree burns by pseudomonas can lead to fatal septicemias. Topical treatment with 0.5% silver nitrate solution, 10% mafenide (Sulfamylon) cream, or gentamicin ointment will greatly inhibit pseudomonas contamination of burns. Silver nitrate can lead to serious systemic depletion of sodium and chloride, so that children on silver nitrate therapy must have their serum electrolytes checked frequently. Mafenide (Sulfamylon) may cause pain, sensitization, and acidosis. Gentamicin is an excellent topical agent, but many centers discourage its topical use because of its potential for selecting out resistant organisms. Silver sulfadiazine is an experimental drug which is as effective as any of the above, although thorough clinical testing has not been completed. There is also a commercially available vaccine against pseudomonas that is injected in doses of 20 mg/kg at intervals of 4 days for the first 3 injections and then weekly therafter. This vaccine has not achieved widespread use.

No matter what topical agents or vaccines are used, the burns must be debrided frequently and kept clean or pseudomonas will colonize dead tissue beneath the eschar and invade the dermal vessels and lymphatics.

B. Nosocomial Infections: Faucet aerators, communal dispensers of green soap, improperly cleaned inhalation therapy equipment, infant isolettes, and numerous back rub solutions and lotions have all been associated with pseudomonas epidemics. Constant vigilance and frequent cultures are essential in order to minimize spread of pseudomonas between patients.

Treatment

A. Proteus: Some strains of *Proteus mirabilis* are relatively susceptible to penicillin V or to ampicillin, 100–300 mg/kg/day orally in 4 divided doses. Other strains are susceptible to the cephalosporins and kanamycin. Gentamicin, 3–5 mg/kg/day IM in 3 divided doses, is quite effective. Carbenicillin is a new semisynthetic penicillin which is active against indole-positive proteus and appears to be quite useful clinically, especially for urinary tract infections. The dose is 50–200 mg/kg/day IV or IM in 4 divided doses.

B. Pseudomonas: The drugs of choice for the treatment of systemic and local pseudomonas infections have been polymyxin B and colistin. Gentamicin is also effective in a dosage of 5–20 mg/kg/day orally or 1–3 mg/kg/day IM in 3 doses. For local therapy, polymyxin B, 0.1% solution or ointment, may be useful. Gentamicin may also be used as an ointment.

Synergy against pseudomonas has been reported with mixtures of carbenicillin and gentamicin. Thus, for serious, life-threatening infections, it is recommended that the 2 antibiotics be used together. In such cases, carbenicillin should not be used as the single agent. The dosage of carbenicillin is 350–400 mg/kg/day IV in 6 divided doses for 10–14 days.

Intrathecal administration of gentamicin, 1–3 mg daily, is now the preferred treatment for pseudomonas meningitis. Gentamicin should also be given IM in a dosage of 1–4 mg/kg/day.

Until recently, the intrathecal administration of polymyxin B (0.5–1 mg/ml) was the only specific treatment. If there is no clinical response and the CSF continues to grow pseudomonas after 5 days of intrathecal and intramuscular gentamicin treatment, intrathecal polymyxin B should be used. The dose for children under 2 years of age is 2 mg and for older children 5 mg given as a single daily intrathecal dose. When sepsis is associated with pseudomonas meningitis, polymyxin B may also be given in a dosage of 2.5 mg/kg/day IM in 4 divided doses.

The intrathecal administration of either gentamicin or polymyxin B is continued daily for 4 or 5 days and then every other day for 2–3 weeks after CSF culture is negative and CSF sugar is normal. The intrathecal administration of gentamicin should be supplemented by daily parenteral administrations.

Solutions for nebulizer inhalation should contain 2–10 mg of polymyxin B per ml. The dose for inhalation is 2 ml 4 or more times per day.

Prognosis

As debilitated patients are most frequently affected, the mortality rate is high. The disease may, however, have a protracted course.

Burke JP & others: *Proteus mirabilis* infections in a hospital nursery traced to a human carrier. New England J Med 284:115–121, 1971.

Cooke EM & others: Faecal carriage of *Pseudomonas aeruginosa* by newborn babies. Lancet 2:1045–1046, 1970.

Diaz F, Mosovich LL, Neter E: Serogroups of *Pseudomonas aeruginosa* and immune response of patients with cystic fibrosis. J Infect Dis 121:269–274, 1970.

Fox CL Jr, Rappole BW, Stanford W: Control of pseudomonas infection in burns by silver sulfadiazine. Surg Gynec Obst 128:1021–1026, 1969.

Grieble HG & others: Fine particle humidifiers. Source of *Pseudomonas aeruginosa* infections in a respiratory-disease unit. New England J Med 282:531–535, 1970.

Pseudomonas bronchopneumonia. Lancet 2:1110–1111, 1971.

Roe R, Jones RJ, Lowbury EJL: Transfer of antibiotic resistance between *Pseudomonas aeruginosa, Escherichia coli,* and other gram-negative bacilli in burns. Lancet 1:149–152, 1971.

Schemmer KE, Alexander JW, Fisher MW: Immunologic response of patients with severe burns to pseudomonas vaccination. 55th Clinical Congress of the American College of Surgeons, San Francisco, California, October 1969.

KLEBSIELLA-ENTEROBACTER INFECTIONS

The klebsiella-enterobacter organisms are encapsulated gram-negative bacilli found among the normal flora of the mouth, respiratory tract, and intestines. For historical reasons, organisms isolated from the respiratory tract have been called klebsiella and those from the genitourinary tract aerobacter (enterobacter). One-fourth to one-third of children with acute urinary tract infections have a recurrence of the infection within a year. Enterobacter is second only to *E coli* as a gram-negative rod associated with urinary tract infections and is more likely to be a cause of recurrent or chronic infections. Klebsiella causes a progressive, serious (sometimes fatal) bronchopneumonia which may lead to cavity formation. The organism is a secondary invader associated with antibiotic usage, debilitating states, and chronic respiratory conditions. Rare nursery outbreaks have occurred. Nosocomial colonization with kanamycin-resistant *Klebsiella pneumoniae* in nurseries is becoming an increasing problem.

Clinical Findings

A. Symptoms and Signs: *K pneumoniae* rapidly forms abscesses or empyema. The onset is usually sudden, with chills, fever, dyspnea, cyanosis, and profound toxicity. The sputum is often red ("currant jelly"), mucoid, sticky, and difficult to expectorate. Physical findings and white counts are variable. The disease may be fulminating and progress rapidly to a fatal outcome. In subacute forms, there is a tendency to necrosis of lung tissue and abscess formation. Lobar consolidation with bulging fissures is seen on x-ray.

B. Laboratory Findings: The diagnosis is established by culture of the sputum, pleural fluid, or blood and urine.

Differential Diagnosis

Staphylococcal pneumonia in the first 2 years of life is many times more common as a cause of pneumatoceles, cavity formation, and empyema.

Treatment

A. Specific Measures: Many of these infections are difficult to treat, and antibiotic sensitivity tests are desirable. At present, cephalothin, 75–100 mg/kg/day IV or IM in 4 divided doses, is the drug of choice for a *K pneumoniae* superinfection in the newborn. Treatment should be continued for 7–10 days. In older children, doses of 100–200 mg/kg/day IV may be used for serious infections. Other effective antibiotics include gentamicin, polymyxin B, colistin, kanamycin, cephaloridine, and cephalexin (oral preparation). Despite the historical aspects of nomenclature, the majority of isolates from the urinary tract are non-motile and belong to the Klebsiella genus. These latter organisms causing acute infections are susceptible to oral cephalexin given as 25 mg/kg/day in 3 divided doses for 14–21 days. However, isolates classed as Enterobacter species are usually motile and are resistant to cephalexin.

Recurrent urinary tract infections should be treated for 6 weeks to 3 months before stopping an effective antibiotic. (See under *E coli* infections for management of urinary tract infections.) Combinations of chloramphenicol or streptomycin and tetracyclines have also been used successfully.

B. General Measures: Causes of urinary tract obstruction should be investigated and surgically corrected. Oxygen and supportive therapy are required for klebsiella pneumonia. Intercostal tube drainage connected to a water seal is needed to manage empyema.

Prognosis

Klebsiella is usually a secondary invader, and, in the respiratory tract, progresses rapidly, causing abscesses, empyema, and necrosis. The mortality rate in untreated cases is upward of 80%. With vigorous, adequate treatment, this may be reduced to 40%.

Adler JL & others: Nosocomial colonization with kanamycin-resistant *Klebsiella pneumoniae,* types 2 and 11, in a premature nursery. J Pediat 77:376–385, 1970.

Price DJE, Sleigh JD: Control of infection due to *Klebsiella aerogenes* in a neurosurgical unit by withdrawal of all antibiotics. Lancet 2:1213–1215, 1970.

Russell JP: Antibiotic sensitivity of klebsiella-enterobacter. Am J Clin Path 51:384–389, 1969.

Seldon R & others: Nosocomial klebsiella infections: Intestinal colonization as a reservoir. Ann Int Med 74:657–664, 1971.

Steiner BE, Putnoky G: *Klebsiella pneumoniae* (Friedländer's bacillus) infections in infancy. Arch Dis Child 31:96–100, 1956.

SALMONELLA & GASTROENTERITIS & MENINGITIS

Essentials of Diagnosis

- Nausea, vomiting, headache.
- Fever and diarrhea.
- Abdominal pain.
- Meningismus.
- Culture of organism from stool, blood, or other specimens.

General Considerations

Salmonella enteral infections in childhood occur in 2 major forms: (1) gastroenteritis (including food poisoning), which may be very mild or severe and complicated by sepsis with or without focal suppurative complications; and (2) enteric fever (typhoid fever and paratyphoid fever). (See next section.) While the incidence of typhoid fever has decreased, the incidence of salmonella gastroenteritis caused by a variety of strains has greatly increased in the past 15 years in the USA. The highest attack rates occur in children under 6 years of age, with a peak in the age group from 6 months to 2 years old. Nursery epidemics have occurred, and infants under 6 months of age are susceptible.

The organisms are widespread in nature, infecting domestic animals (pets, including pet turtles, and fowl), rodents, and arthropods. Most nonhuman isolations of salmonellae are from poultry. Contaminated egg powder and frozen whole egg preparations used to make ice cream, custards, and mayonnaise are often responsible for outbreaks. Animal-to-man transmission occurs by ingestion of animal excreta, infected animal meat, and animal products. Transmission from man to man occurs by the fecal-oral route via contaminated food, water, and fomites.

Most cases of salmonella meningitis (80%) have occurred in infancy. About 25% of cases have occurred in nursery epidemics. In newborns, meningitis tends to run a rapid course, with diarrhea as a prominent manifestation.

Clinical Findings

A. Symptoms and Signs: The infant develops fever, vomiting, and diarrhea. The older child may complain of headache, nausea, and abdominal pain. Stools may be watery or may contain mucus and in some instances blood. Diarrhea may be mild to moderate, or profuse, suggestive of shigellosis. Drowsiness and disorientation may be associated with striking meningismus. Splenomegaly is occasionally noted. In the usual case, diarrhea is moderate and subsides after 4–5 days, but it may be protracted.

B. Laboratory Diagnosis: Diagnosis is made by isolation of the organism from the stools and blood and in some cases from the urine, CSF, or pus from a suppurative lesion. The white count usually shows a polymorphonuclear leukocytosis. Typing of the isolate is done with specific antisera.

Differential Diagnosis

In staphylococcal food poisoning, the incubation period is shorter (2–4 hours) than in salmonella food poisoning (12–24 hours). In shigellosis, pus cells are likely to be seen on a Wright-stained smear of stool, and there is more likely to be a shift to the left in the peripheral white count. In shigellosis as well as in enteropathogenic *E coli* enteritis and other diarrheal diseases, culture of the stools or other appropriate diagnostic laboratory tests will establish the diagnosis. Meningitis may need to be excluded by lumbar puncture.

Complications

Bacteremia can occur. Septicemia with focal manifestations occurs most commonly with *Salmonella choleraesuis* but also with *S enteritidis, S typhimurium,* and *S paratyphi* B and C. The organism may localize in any tissue, producing abscesses and causing arthritis, osteomyelitis, cholecystitis, endocarditis, meningitis, pericarditis, pneumonia, and pyelonephritis. In sickle cell anemia and other hemoglobinopathies, there is an unusual predilection for osteomyelitis to develop. Severe dehydration and shock are more likely to occur with bacillary dysentery but may occur with salmonella gastroenteritis.

Prevention

Measures for the prevention of salmonella infections include thorough cooking of foodstuffs derived from potentially infected sources; proper refrigeration during storage; and recognition and control of infection among domestic animals, combined with proper meat and poultry inspections. Adults with occupations involving care of young children should have negative stool cultures for 3 successive days.

Patients traveling to an endemic area should be vaccinated.

Treatment

A. Specific Measures: In the usual case of uncomplicated salmonella gastroenteritis not associated with sepsis, there is no evidence that antibiotic treatment shortens the course of the clinical illness or the length of time the organism is present in the gastrointestinal tract. In fact, there is evidence that antibiotic treatment prolongs the carrier state.

However, antibiotic treatment is indicated for newborns, young infants moderately or severely ill, and in cases of sepsis or where there are focal suppurative complications. Ampicillin, 100–150 mg/kg/day IM or orally in 4 divided doses for 5–7 days, is recommended. Longer treatment is indicated for specific complications. If clinical improvement does not follow and in vitro sensitivity tests indicate resistance to ampicillin, oral or parenteral colistin, gentamicin, or tetracyclines are alternative drugs which may be effective.

Salmonella meningitis is best treated with both chloramphenicol, 100 mg/kg/day IV, and ampicillin, 200–300 mg/kg/day IV, each given in 4 divided doses.

Chloramphenicol should be given for 2–3 weeks; ampicillin for 4–6 weeks. An average CSF killing level of 1:4–1:8 should be maintained. Selection of a multiple antibiotic-resistant strain is less likely to occur if both antibiotics are used to treat this serious disease.

Nursery or hospital epidemics. An outbreak may be stopped by treating hospitalized asymptomatic contacts with colistin, 10 mg/kg/day orally in 3 divided doses, until they can be discharged. Excretion of the organism in the stools will stop while the infants are taking oral colistin. The carrier state will occur as soon as the colistin is stopped. Sick infants should be treated with ampicillin as outlined above to prevent bacteremia and suppurative complications. They should then be treated with oral colistin until discharge from the hospital.

B. Treatment of the Carrier States: About 1/2 of patients are still infectious after 4 weeks. During the first year of life, particularly under 6 months, there is a greater tendency to remain a convalescent carrier. Antibiotic treatment of carriers is not indicated.

C. General: Careful attention must be given to maintaining fluid and electrolyte balance, especially in infants. Severe dehydration must be vigorously treated as outlined in the section on bacillary dysentery.

Prognosis

In gastroenteritis, the prognosis is good if adequate measures are used to control diarrhea. In sepsis with focal suppurative complications, the prognosis is more guarded.

The case fatality rate for salmonella meningitis is about 85% in infants. There is a strong tendency for relapse to occur if treatment is not prolonged.

Aaron E & others: Urban salmonellosis. Am J Pub Health 61:337–343, 1971.

Adler JL & others: A protracted hospital-associated outbreak of salmonellosis due to a multiple-antibiotic-resistant strain of *Salmonella indiana*. J Pediat 77:970–975, 1970.

Aserkoff B, Bennett JV: Effect of therapy in acute salmonellosis on salmonellae in feces. New England J Med 281:636–640, 1969.

Bergstrand CG, Nilsson K: Neonatal meningitis caused by *Salmonella thompson*. Acta paediat scandinav 59:427–431, 1970.

Spread of salmonellas. Lancet 1:744–745, 1971.

Wilner EC, Fenichel GM: Treatment of salmonella meningitis. Clin Proc Child Hosp DC 25–26:362–366, 1969–1970.

TYPHOID FEVER & PARATYPHOID FEVER

Essentials of Diagnosis

- Acute onset of headache, anorexia, vomiting, constipation or diarrhea, dehydration, and fairly high fever.
- Meningismus, splenomegaly, and rose spots with abdominal distention and tenderness.
- Leukopenia; positive blood, stool, and urine cultures.
- Elevated Widal agglutination titers.

General Considerations

Typhoid fever is caused by the gram-negative rod *Salmonella typhi;* paratyphoid fevers, which may be clinically indistinguishable, may be caused by a variety of strains but most frequently by *S paratyphi* A, B, and C. Children have a shorter incubation period than do adults (usually 5–8 days instead of 8–14 days). Symptoms of typhoid fever in children may vary from the mildest to the most severe, but in general, except for the very young, the disease is milder than in adults. The organism enters the body through the walls of the intestinal tract and multiplies in the reticuloendothelial cells of the liver and spleen. Reinfection of the intestinal tract occurs as organisms are excreted from the biliary tract. The onset of disease depends upon when a sufficient number of *S typhi* reach the blood stream and mesenteric lymph nodes. Symptoms appear to be due to the systemic effects of endotoxin and other bacterial products. Bacterial emboli in the capillaries of the skin produce the characteristic skin lesions.

Clinical Findings

A. Symptoms and Signs: In children, the onset is apt to be sudden rather than insidious, with malaise, headache, crampy abdominal pains and distention, and sometimes constipation followed within 48 hours by diarrhea, high fever, and considerable toxemia. Disturbances of the sensorium may be seen with irritability, confusion, delirium, and stupor. Vomiting and meningismus may be prominent in the young. The classic 3-stage disease seen in adult patients seems to be shortened in children. Thus, the prodrome may be shortened to only 2–4 days, whereas the fastigium, which is characterized by fever, diarrhea, and abdominal distention and mild to marked toxemia, may last only 2–3 days. The defervescence stage generally lasts 1–2 weeks. Relapse may occur 1–2 weeks after the temperature returns to normal.

During the prodromal stage, physical findings may be absent or there may merely be some abdominal distention and tenderness, meningismus, and minimal splenomegaly. The typical typhoidal rash (rose spots) tends to appear during the second week of the disease, and may erupt in crops for the succeeding 10–14 days. Rose spots are pink papules 2–3 mm in diameter which fade on pressure, are found principally on the trunk and chest, and generally disappear within 3–4 days.

B. Laboratory Findings: Blood, stool, and urine cultures may be positive at any time during the first week. During the second week of the disease, a rise in antibodies (Widal test) is noted either by a rise in titer in sera taken 1 week apart or by a single specimen showing a somatic (O) antibody titer of 1:160. Leukopenia is commonly encountered in the second week of the disease. However, total leukocyte counts above 10,000 are not unusual. Urinalysis generally reveals 1+

or 2+ protein. Mild anemia may be present unless massive bleeding occurs (see Complications, below). Disseminated intravascular coagulation has been reported in association with typhoid fever.

Elevated sedimentation rates and the presence of C-reactive proteins are seen during the febrile period.

Differential Diagnosis

Typhoid and paratyphoid fevers must be distinguished from other serious prolonged fevers associated with normal or low white counts. These include typhus, primary atypical pneumonia, brucellosis, tularemia, miliary tuberculosis, psittacosis, and lymphomas.

A positive diagnosis of typhoid fever is made by laboratory means.

Complications

The most important complication of typhoid fever is hemorrhage from the gastrointestinal tract. This generally occurs toward the end of the second week or during the third week of the disease. The clinical signs and symptoms are those of acute blood loss, including the appearance of gross blood in the stools and early evidence of shock. Epistaxis is the most common type of hemorrhage.

Intestinal perforation is a dangerous complication and one of the principal causes of death. The sites of perforation generally are the terminal ileum or the proximal part of the colon. The clinical manifestations are indistinguishable from those of acute appendicitis, with pain, tenderness, and rigidity in the right lower quadrant. The x-ray finding of free air in the peritoneal cavity is diagnostic.

Bacterial pneumonia, meningitis, septic arthritis, and osteomyelitis are uncommon complications, particularly if specific treatment is given promptly. Cardiovascular collapse and electrolyte disturbances may lead to death. Occasionally there are metastatic abscesses. Hepatic involvement with jaundice occurs occasionally. Acute cholecystitis associated with gallstones is rare. Infection of the urinary tract occurs in about 25% of cases.

Prevention

Paratyphoid A and B vaccines or triple vaccines should no longer be employed. Routine typhoid immunization is not recommended in the USA. Selective typhoid fever immunization is indicated in the following circumstances: (1) Intimate exposure to a known typhoid carrier, as would occur with continued household contact. (2) Community or institutional outbreaks of typhoid fever. (3) Foreign travel to areas where typhoid fever is endemic. There are no data to warrant continuing the practice of typhoid vaccination for persons attending summer camps or where flooding has occurred.

A. Primary Immunization: Children 6 months to 10 years, 0.25 ml subcutaneously on 2 occasions separated by 4 or more weeks; adults and children over 10 years, 0.5 ml subcut on 2 occasions separated by 4 or more weeks.

B. Booster: Under conditions of continued or repeated exposure, a booster dose should be given every 3 years. Even if more than 3 years have elapsed, a single booster injection should be sufficient. The booster dose, regardless of age, is 0.1 ml intradermally.

Treatment

A. Specific Measures: Chloramphenicol is the drug of choice in typhoid fever. Ampicillin is much less effective. The dose of chloramphenicol is 50–100 mg/kg/day orally given in 4 divided doses. For infants under 1 month of age, the daily dose should not exceed 25 mg/kg. Oral therapy is preferable to systemic therapy. Where vomiting is a problem it is well to supplement parenteral therapy with oral medication as soon as possible. Occasionally, drug administration through a gastric tube is required. Chloramphenicol palmitate, while well tolerated, is not advised because of the irregular absorption of this lipase-dependent compound. A suspension of the crystalline form from the capsule is to be preferred.

If chloramphenicol therapy is contraindicated (hematologic disorders, anemia, etc), give parenteral ampicillin in doses of 150 mg/kg stat followed by 150 mg/kg/day in 4 divided doses. Treatment should be continued for 14–21 days. Fever usually returns to normal within 3–5 days.

Hetacillin, a new synthetic derivative of 6-aminopenicillanic acid, has an antimicrobial spectrum similar to that of ampicillin. It is, however, more stable in acid medium, is better absorbed following oral administration, and achieves higher serum and urine concentrations. A recent report indicates that hetacillin and chloramphenicol have comparable efficacy in the treatment of typhoid fever in children. The dosage is 50 mg/kg/day orally in 3 divided doses, with a minimum daily dose of 1.5 gm. If the results of this report are confirmed by other workers, hetacillin may become the drug of choice.

B. General Measures: If toxicity is marked, a short course of corticosteroids may be indicated when antibiotics are begun. Prednisone, 1 mg/kg/day orally during the first 4 days of chloramphenicol therapy, generally results in marked improvement of the patient's condition.

General support of the patient is exceedingly important and includes rest, good oral hygiene, and careful observation with particular regard to evidence of internal bleeding or perforation. A high-caloric liquid diet should provide ample calories and at least 2 gm of protein per kg body weight. Potassium depletion should be corrected. Small transfusions with whole blood may be needed in the anemic patient even in the absence of frank hemorrhage.

Prognosis

A convalescent carrier stage in children often continues for 3–6 months after the acute infection. This does not require retreatment with antibiotics nor exclusion from school or other activities.

With specific antibiotic therapy, the prognosis is excellent.

Chawla V & others: A comparative trial of hetacillin and chloramphenicol in typhoid fever. J Pediat 77:471–473, 1970.

Hornick RB & others: Typhoid fever: Pathogenesis and immunologic control. New England J Med 283:686–691, 739–746, 1970.

Leffall LD Jr & others: Massive gastrointestinal hemorrhage due to specific infections. J Nat Med Ass 63:99–103, 1971.

Maloney CT: Surgical treatment of typhoid perforation of ileum. New York J Med 71:663–664, 1971.

Nourmand A, Ziai M: Typhoid and paratyphoid fever in children: Review of symptoms and therapy in 165 cases. Clin Pediat 8:235–238, 1969.

BACILLARY (SHIGELLA) DYSENTERY

Essentials of Diagnosis

- Cramps and bloody diarrhea.
- High fever, malaise, clouded sensorium, convulsions.
- Pus and mucus in diarrheal stools; isolation of shigella strain.

General Considerations

Shigellosis is a serious disease of children under 2 years of age with an appreciable mortality rate. Because of the variability of antibiotic sensitivity for strains of shigella now encountered, it remains an important therapeutic problem. In older children, the disease tends to be self-limited and milder.

The Flexner and Sonne strains of *Shigella dysenteriae* are responsible for most cases of shigella dysentery in the USA.

Clinical Findings

A. Symptoms and Signs: Onset is abrupt, with abdominal cramps, tenesmus, chills and fever, malaise, dairrhea, and often a cloudy sensorium suggesting encephalitis. In the most severe forms, blood and mucus are seen in the watery stool and convulsions may occur. In older children, the disease may be mild and the diagnosis therefore missed. In young children, a fever of 39.4–40° C (103–104° F) is common.

Respiratory symptoms of bronchitis are common. The anal sphincter shows lax tone. Rarely, there is rectal prolapse. In over 50% of cases, other family members will also have diarrhea.

B. Laboratory Findings: The white count is high, with a shift to the left. The appearance of more band forms than segmented neutrophils in the differential smear may be an important diagnostic clue. The stool shows blood, mucus, and pus and a positive culture for shigella. Hemoconcentration with a marked elevation in hematocrit is common shortly after onset.

Differential Diagnosis

Diarrhea due to echovirus infections tends to be seen in the summer months in outbreaks. Intestinal infections caused by salmonellae and enteropathogenic *Escherichia coli* are differentiated by culture. Amebic dysentery is diagnosed by microscopic examination of fresh stools. Intussusception is distinguished by an abdominal mass, currant jelly stools, and absence of fever. Epidemic outbreak and an incubation period of 6 hours or less characterize staphylococcal food poisoning.

Complications

Dehydration, acidosis, and shock occur in infancy. In some cases, a chronic form of dysentery occurs characterized by mucoid stools and poor nutrition. Otitis media, pneumonia, and nonsuppurative arthritis are occasional complications.

Treatment

A. Specific Measures: Ampicillin is the antibiotic of choice and is given IV, IM, or orally in a dosage of 100 mg/kg/day in 4 divided doses for 5–7 days. Therapeutic failure with ampicillin correlates closely with in vitro resistance. Tetracycline, 25 mg/kg/day orally in 4 divided doses, may be effective. Oral colistin or gentamicin and parenteral kanamycin are other alternative antibiotics if in vitro resistance to ampicillin is demonstrated.

B. General Measures: In severe cases, immediate rehydration by means of saline, glucose, and potassium is an emergency procedure, generally requiring a cutdown in a suitable vein. To combat circulatory collapse and shock, special nursing observation is required.

In milder cases, after initial rehydration with parenteral fluids, clear liquids may be required for 2 or 3 days followed by glucose-containing liquids such as grape juice, apple juice, liquid jello, or ginger ale. Subsequently, boiled skimmed milk or any 12 calorie/oz formula may be introduced, followed by return to a regular light diet somewhat low in fat.

A mild form of chronic malabsorption syndrome may supervene and require fairly prolonged dietary controls.

Prognosis

Except in the very young patient with septicemia, the prognosis is excellent if ampicillin is given early and vascular collapse is treated promptly by adequate fluid therapy.

Davies JR, Farrant WN, Uttley AHC: Antibiotic resistance of *Shigella sonnei.* Lancet 1:1157–1159, 1970.

DuPont HL & others: The response of man to virulent *Shigella flexneri* 2a. J Infect Dis 119:296–299, 1969.

Martin DG: Antibiotic sensitivities of shigella isolates in Vietnam, 1968–1969. Mil Med 135:560–562, 1970.

Nelson JD, Haltalin KC: Accuracy of diagnosis of bacterial diarrheal disease by clinical features. J Pediat 78:519–522, 1971.

CHOLERA

Essentials of Diagnosis

- Sudden onset of very severe diarrhea.
- Persistent vomiting without nausea.
- Extreme and rapid dehydration and electrolyte loss, with rapid development of vascular collapse.
- Contact with a case of cholera and the presence of a cholera epidemic in the community.
- Positive smears and culture.

General Considerations

Cholera is an acute diarrheal disease caused by *Vibrio cholerae* and transmitted by contaminated water or food in the endemic areas of the world. The incubation period is very short, 1–3 days, and the disease is generally so dramatic that in a frank case the diagnosis is obvious. Mild cases are important causes of infection in others. Young children may play an important role in transmission of the infection. Higher titers of vibriocidal antibody are seen with increasing age. Infection occurs in individuals with low titers. The age-specific attack rate is highest in the age group under 5 years and declines with age. Sanitation and personal hygiene may prevent cholera in areas where the vibrios persist in the environment. A protein enterotoxin produced by *V cholerae* has been shown to be highly active in inducing experimental cholera in animals. The enterotoxin elicits an increased vascular permeability of the skin and is probably responsible for the outpouring of fluid from the gut.

Clinical Findings

A. Symptoms and Signs: Sudden onset of massive, frequent, watery stools, generally light gray in color ("rice water") and containing some mucus but no pus. Vomiting may be projectile and is not accompanied by nausea. Within 2–3 hours, the tremendous loss of fluids has resulted in severe and life-threatening dehydration, hypochloremia, and loss of cellular potassium, with marked weakness and collapse. This is a medical emergency. Renal failure with uremia and irreversible peripheral vascular collapse will occur if fluid therapy is not administered.

B. Laboratory Findings: Markedly elevated hemoglobin (20 gm/100 ml), marked acidosis, hypochloremia, and hyponatremia are seen.

Using darkfield microscopy and Ogawa/Inaba specific antisera, a presumptive diagnosis can be made within a matter of minutes. This is based on the immobilization by specific antisera of the highly motile cholera vibrios. In the absence of such facilities, confirmation of a clinical diagnosis will take 16–18 hours for a presumptive diagnosis and 36–48 hours for a definitive bacteriologic diagnosis after the arrival of a specimen of stool or rectal swab at the laboratory.

Prevention

Cholera vaccine is given as 2 injections, 0.5 ml subcut, not less than 4 weeks apart, with boosters of 0.5 ml every 6 months while at risk. In endemic areas, all water and milk must be boiled, food protected from flies, and rigid sanitary precautions observed. All patients with cholera should be strictly isolated and their surroundings carefully decontaminated.

Chemoprophylaxis is indicated for household and other close contacts of cholera patients. Drug administration should be initiated as soon as possible after the onset of the disease in the index patient. One of the tetracyclines given as a single daily dose of 500 mg for 5 days is effective in preventing subsequent infection in children.

Treatment

Physiologic saline must be administered at once in large amounts to restore blood volume and urine output and to prevent irreversible shock. Potassium supplements are required. Sodium bicarbonate, 2–4% solution given intravenously, may also be needed initially to overcome profound acidosis. In general, children need more potassium and less sodium replacement than adults. Some hypotonic fluids should also be given intravenously in order to replace water lost in excess of electrolytes.

Recent reports indicate that moderate dehydration and severe acidosis can be corrected in 3–6 hours by oral therapy alone. Give 1000 ml/hour of warmed (45°C) oral solution during a 6-hour period. The composition of the solution (in mEq/liter) is as follows: Na^+, 120, HCO_3^-, 48, Cl^-, 87, and K^+, 25—together with 110 mM glucose per liter. Intravenous fluids should be given initially in cases with frank shock.

Treatment of children with one of the tetracyclines, 25 mg/kg/day orally in 4 divided doses for 5 days, modifies the clinical course of the disease and prevents clinical relapse.

Prognosis

With early and rapid replacement of fluids and electrolytes lost through the massive diarrhea, the case fatality rate should be less than 1%. If significant symptoms appear and no treatment is given, the mortality rate is over 50%.

Cash RA & others: Rapid correction of acidosis and dehydration of cholera with oral electrolyte and glucose solution. Lancet 2:549–550, 1970.

Change in Cholera Vaccination Requirement. Morbidity and Mortality Weekly Report. Center for Disease Control, Atlanta, Georgia, Dec 1970.

Gangarosa EJ, Foich GA: Cholera: Risk to American travelers. Ann Int Med 74:412–415, 1971.

Mahalanabis D & others: Water and electrolyte losses due to cholera in infants and children: A recovery balance study. Pediatrics 45:374–385, 1970.

MacKenzie DJM: Cholera: Its nature, management and prevention. South African MJ 45:3–7, 1971.

Nalin DR, Cash RA, Rahman M: Oral (or nasogastric) maintenance therapy for cholera patients in all age groups. Bull World Health Organ 43:361–363, 1970.

BRUCELLOSIS

Essentials of Diagnosis

- Intermittent fevers, primarily in the evenings or at night.
- Easy fatigability, arthralgia, anorexia, sweating, and irritability.
- Relative lymphocytosis, positive blood culture, agglutination titer of 1:160 or greater.

General Considerations

Brucella infections in man are caused by 3 species: *B abortus* (cattle), *B suis* (hogs), and *B melitensis* (goats). Infection usually occurs through ingestion of contaminated milk or milk products or by contact through minor skin or mucosal abrasions. The incubation period is 8–30 days. In the USA, the disease has been maintained by infection in swine.

Clinical Findings

A. Symptoms and Signs: The onset is insidious, with vague symptoms of weakness and exhaustion, intermittent night fevers, and sweating. In children, physical findings are generally absent, although splenomegaly is occasionally seen. Slight lymphadenopathy may be present.

B. Laboratory Findings: The white count is normal, with absolute lymphocytosis. The organism can be recovered from the blood and urine and, though rarely, from the CSF and other tissues. There is little difficulty in obtaining positive blood cultures from patients infected with *B melitensis* or *B suis.* However in *B abortus* infections there are fewer organisms circulating in the blood. In case of suspected *B abortus* infections, it is well to obtain about 0.5 ml/kg of venous blood and distribute it among a series of blood culture bottles. All blood cultures should be subcultured twice a week for at least 8 weeks before a negative result is reported. An elevated brucella agglutinin titer (1:160 or above) confirms the diagnosis.

Where there is a questionable or doubtful positive agglutination test, 2 additional serologic tests may be helpful. An agglutination test may be repeated after treating the serum with mercaptoethanol. A titer of 1:40 or higher is considered positive. If the serum fixes complement using brucella antigen at a titer of 1:10 or higher, it is considered positive.

In case of involvement of the CNS, the CSF may rarely show a growth of brucella in culture or be positive for agglutinins.

An intracutaneous test with brucella antigens may be performed and read at 48–72 hours. A positive test indicates prior exposure to the antigenic components of the organism. It does not indicate the current status of infection.

Four-fold rises in serum antibody may occur after performing a skin test. The skin test should not be used in routine diagnosis when serologic tests are available.

Differential Diagnosis

A variety of causes of fever without localization, including neoplastic and granulomatous diseases which may cause lymphadenopathy and hepatosplenomegaly, have to be distinguished. It is desirable to look for evidence of brucellosis in patients with arachnoiditis or meningomyelitis of obscure origin.

Complications

Following hematogenous spread, secondary foci of infection may lead to endocarditis, pyelonephritis, meningoencephalitis, and osteomyelitis. In older children, infection of the bile ducts results in jaundice. In the malignant form, hepatic necrosis may occur. Neurologic complications may appear at the onset of the illness or at any time during the clinical course, including convalescence, or long after acute symptoms have subsided. Leptomeningitis is an early feature and may lead to adhesive arachnoiditis in the cranium or in the spinal cord.

A psychiatric form of the disease is well known which is likely to be associated with a mild encephalitis.

Treatment

A. Specific Measures: One of the tetracyclines, 30 mg/kg/day orally in divided doses every 6 hours, is given for 21 days. In case of a relapse, treatment is repeated. Only in very severe cases of acute brucellosis or in suppurative brucellosis due to *B suis*, simultaneous administration of streptomycin, 15 mg/kg IM as a single daily dose for 1 week, is advised. During the second week, streptomycin is continued at the level of 7 mg/kg while tetracycline is continued orally for the full 21 days.

B. General Measures: Limited physical activity and bed rest are indicated while there is fever. Aspirin will relieve headache and somatic pains. Codeine sulfate, 30 mg orally every 12 hours, is occasionally required early in the course of antibiotic therapy.

Prognosis

With specific therapy, the prognosis is now excellent and the chance for prolonged invalidism markedly reduced.

Bergin WN, Bergin WC: Brucellosis in Hawaii. Hawaii MJ 29:628–632, 1970.

Boycott JA: Diagnosing brucellosis. Lancet 1:255–256, 1969.

Bradstreet CMP & others: Intradermal test and serological tests in suspected brucella infection in man. Lancet 2:653–656, 1970.

Foley BV, Clay MM, O'Sullivan DJ: A study of a brucellosis epidemic. Irish J Med Sc 3:457–462, 1970.

Hall WH, Manion RE: In vitro susceptibility of brucella to various antibiotics. Appl Microbiol 20:600–604, 1970.

TULAREMIA

Essentials of Diagnosis

- A cutaneous or mucous membrane lesion at the site of inoculation and regional lymph node enlargement.
- Sudden onset of fever, chills, and prostration.
- History of contact with infected animals, principally wild rabbits.
- Culture of mucocutaneous ulcer or regional lymph nodes confirms the diagnosis.

General Considerations

Tularemia is caused by *Pasteurella tularensis,* a gram-negative organism usually acquired from infected animals, principally wild rabbits, by ingestion of contaminated meat or infected water; by contamination of the skin or mucous membranes; by inhalation of infected material; and by bites of ticks or fleas or deerflies which have been in contact with infected animals. Strains of high virulence for man are usually associated with tick-borne tularemia of rabbits; those of lowered virulence are linked with the water-borne disease of rodents. The incubation period is short, usually 3–7 days.

Clinical Findings

A. Symptoms and Signs: Several clinical types are seen in children. Most infections start as a reddened papule which may be pruritic, quickly ulcerates, and is not very painful (ulceroglandular form). Shortly thereafter, there may be marked systemic manifestations, including high fever, chills, weakness, vomiting, and enlargement of the regional lymph nodes which are usually very tender and quickly become fluctuant. Drainage may occur. Pneumonitis occasionally is found clinically or by x-ray (pneumonic form). A detectable skin lesion is occasionally absent, and localized lymphoid enlargement exists alone (glandular form). Oculoglandular and oropharyngeal forms also occur in children. In the absence of any primary ulcer or localized lymphadenitis, a prolonged febrile disease reminiscent of typhoid fever can be seen (typhoidal form). Splenomegaly is common, and an evanescent maculopapular rash is often seen on the trunk and extremities.

B. Laboratory Findings: *P tularensis* can be recovered from ulcers or regional lymph nodes as well as from sputum in patients with the pneumonic form. An intradermal skin test is positive early in the disease; it resembles the tuberculin skin tests. The skin test does not result in a significant serologic response and may therefore be used in addition to serologic tests for diagnosis. The white blood count is not remarkable, and the ESR is usually normal. Agglutinins are present after the second week of illness, and in the absence of a positive culture their development confirms the diagnosis. An agglutination titer of 1:160 or higher is considered positive.

Differential Diagnosis

The typhoidal form of tularemia may mimic typhoid, brucellosis, miliary tuberculosis, Rocky Mountain spotted fever, and infectious mononucleosis. Pneumonic tularemia resembles atypical and mycotic pneumonitis and bacterial pneumonia. The ulceroglandular type of tularemia resembles pyoderma caused by staphylococci or streptococci, rat-bite fever, plague, anthrax, cat scratch fever, and rickettsialpox as well as accidental vaccinia inoculation. The oropharyngeal type must be distinguished from herpetic gingivostomatitis, herpangina, and lymphonodular pharyngitis due to coxsackievirus type A, nonspecific tonsillopharyngitis due to adenovirus, infectious mononucleosis, and blood dyscrasias.

Prevention

Reasonable attempts should be made to protect children from bites of insects, principally ticks, fleas, and deerflies, by the use of proper clothing and repellents. Drinking water from streams in endemic areas should be avoided. Children should be cautioned to stay away from wild game. If contact occurs, thorough washing with soap and water is indicated.

Treatment

A. Specific Measures: Give streptomycin, 30–40 mg/kg/day IM in 2 divided doses for 8–10 days. The maximum daily dose is 1 gm. The tetracyclines and chloramphenicol are also effective but are not advised as sole medication.

B. General Measures: Antipyretics and analgesics may be given as necessary. Skin lesions are best left open. Glandular lesions occasionally require incision and drainage.

Prognosis

With streptomycin treatment, the prognosis is excellent.

Anderson RA: Oculoglandular tularemia: A case report. J Iowa Med Soc 60:21–24, 1970.

Brooks GF, Buchanan TM: Tularemia in the United States: Epidemiologic aspects in the 1960's and follow-up of the outbreak of tularemia in Vermont. J Infect Dis 121:357–359, 1970.

Buchanan TM, Brooks GF, Brachman PS: The tularemia skin test–325 skin tests in 210 persons: Serologic correlation and review of the literature. Ann Int Med 74:336–343, 1971.

PLAGUE

Essentials of Diagnosis

- Sudden onset of fever, chills, and prostration.
- Regional lymphangitis and lymphadenitis with suppuration of nodes (bubonic form).

- Hemorrhages into skin and mucous membranes and shock (septicemia).
- Cough, dyspnea, cyanosis, and hemoptysis (pneumonic form).
- History of exposure to infected animals.

General Considerations

Plague is an extremely serious, acute infection caused by a gram-negative bacillus, *Pasteurella pestis.* It is a disease of rodents which is transmitted to man by the bites of fleas. Rodent plague in animals of the field and forest is called sylvatic plague; plague in rodents associated with man is called murine plague. Plague bacilli have been isolated from rodents in 15 of the western states in the USA. Cases associated with wild rodents occur sporadically.

Recent cases have occurred in "hippies" and other persons living in the open under primitive conditions in the southwestern USA.

Clinical Findings

A. Symptoms and Signs: The disease assumes several different clinical forms, the 2 most common being bubonic and pneumonic.

1. Bubonic plague—Bubonic plague begins with a sudden onset of high fever, chills, headache, vomiting, and marked delirium or clouding of consciousness. Although the flea bite is rarely seen, the regional lymph node is painful and tender, 1–5 cm in diameter, and usually suppurates and drains spontaneously after 1 week. The plague bacillus is known to produce an endotoxin which causes vascular necrosis. Bacilli may overwhelm regional lymph nodes and enter the circulation to produce septicemia. Severe vascular necrosis results in widely disseminated hemorrhages in skin, mucous membranes, liver, and spleen. The term "black death" was used during the Middle Ages because of the large, discolored hemorrhagic skin areas. Myocarditis and circulatory collapse may result from damage by the endotoxin.

Plague meningitis may occur secondarily following bacteremic spread from an infected lymph node, and suboptimal antibiotic therapy employing penicillin may permit multiplication of organisms in a protected site in the meninges.

2. Pneumonic plague—The pneumonic form occurs primarily during epidemics as a result of man-to-man airborne transmission. Lung necrosis results in abundant sputum that is initially watery but rapidly becomes bloody and loaded with organisms. Patients are toxic, cyanotic, and dyspneic.

B. Laboratory Findings: Aspiration of a bubo leads to visualization of bacilli on a stained smear. Pus, sputum, and blood all yield the organism, although laboratory infections are common enough to make isolation dangerous. Blood-agar cultures yield positive results in 24–48 hours. The white count is markedly elevated, with a shift to the left.

Differential Diagnosis

The febrile phase of the disease may be confused with such illnesses as typhoid fever and typhus. The bubonic form resembles tularemia, anthrax, cat scratch fever, streptococcal adenitis, and cellulitis. Skin lesions may suggest a rickettsial infection. Buboes in the groin need to be differentiated from chancroid, lymphogranuloma venereum, and incarcerated hernia. Primary gastroenteritis and appendicitis may have to be distinguished.

Prevention

Proper disposal of household and commercial wastes and chemical control of rats are basic measures for control of the reservoir of murine plague. Flea control is instituted and maintained with the liberal use of DDT and other insecticides. Children of vacationing parents in remote camping areas should be cautioned not to handle dead or dying animals.

Vaccination is recommended for persons traveling or living in an area of high incidence. (See Chapter 5 for details.)

Treatment

A. Specific Measures: Streptomycin and tetracyclines should both be used. The dose of streptomycin is 20–40 mg/kg IM in 2 divided doses for 5 days followed by one of the tetracyclines, 50 mg/kg/day IM in 3 divided doses. The total daily dose of streptomycin should not exceed 1 gm. Treatment should be continued until the patient has been afebrile for 4 or 5 days. In simple bubonic plague, sulfonamides are also effective.

In septicemia and pneumonic plague, treatment must be started in the first 15–24 hours of the disease if survival is to be expected. Treatment with streptomycin started 36–48 hours after onset of the disease may result in death due to liberation of plague toxin. The mechanism may be analogous to the Jarisch-Herxheimer reaction, with release of toxin from dead plague bacilli. Any case of painful bubo should be treated without delay.

Bubonic plague is not highly contagious. Every effort is made to effect resolution of buboes without resorting to surgery. Pus from draining lymph nodes should be handled with rubber gloves.

B. General Measures: Pneumonic plague is highly infectious, and rigid isolation is required. All contacts should receive sulfonamide prophylaxis given as 45 mg/kg/day orally in 3 divided doses for 7 days.

Prognosis

The mortality rate in untreated bubonic plague is about 50%; it is 90% in the septicemic form, and nearly 100% in the pneumonic form. The mortality rate of the septicemic form is reduced to 10% or less with early streptomycin treatment.

Expert Committee on Plague: *Fourth Report.* WHO Technical Report Series No. 44. World Health Organization, 1970.

Beasley P: Human plague in the United States. JAMA 208:1024–1025, 1969.

Henderson RJ: Summary of recent abstracts: VI. Plague. Trop Dis Bull 67:745–750, 1970.

Kadis S, Montie TC, Ajl SJ: Plague toxin. Sc Am 220:92–100, 1969.

Reed WP & others: Bubonic plague in the southwestern United States: A review of recent experience. Medicine 49:465–486, 1970.

Reiley CA, Kates ED: Clinical spectrum of plague in Vietnam. Arch Int Med 126:990–994, 1970.

HEMOPHILUS INFLUENZAE TYPE B INFECTIONS

Essentials of Diagnosis

- Purulent meningitis in children under age 2 years with direct smears of CSF showing long filamentous forms as well as gram-negative pleomorphic rods.
- Acute epiglottitis: High fever, dysphagia, and croup. White blood count > 20,000/cu mm.
- Otitis media: Low-grade fever, chronic nasal discharge, and bilaterally inflamed tympanic membranes with little pain.
- Septic arthritis: Fever, circumferential redness, swelling, local heat, and pain with active or passive motion of the involved joint.
- Orbital cellulitis: Sudden onset of pain, swelling of the orbital area, purple discoloration of involved skin, and bilateral haziness of maxillary and ethmoid sinuses.
- Insidious onset of pneumonia in an infant, with x-ray picture of lobar consolidation or patchy bronchopneumonia; empyema.
- High, spiking fever in an infant with meningitis or pneumonia, transient pericardial friction rub, ST segment and T wave ECG changes, clinical and x-ray evidence of pericardial effusion, and aspiration of pus from the pericardial sac.
- In all cases, a positive culture from the blood or from aspirated pus confirms the diagnosis.

General Considerations

Hemophilus influenzae type B is perhaps the most important bacterial pathogen in childhood. The organism is a cause of meningitis, acute epiglottitis (supraglottic croup), acute otitis media, acute septic arthritis, orbital cellulitis, pneumonia, and septic pericarditis. *H influenzae* type B infections occur most frequently in the age group from 6 months to 4 years (epiglottitis: 3–7 years). Indeed, with the exception of pneumonia and septic pericarditis, this organism is the leading cause of all these infections in this age range. This age distribution for infection was explained by the classic work of Fothergill and Wright almost 40 years ago. They demonstrated that 90% of the blood from neonates showed bactericidal antibody, presumably reflecting passive transfer of antibody from protected mothers. The age of distribution for *H influenzae* type B infections was explained by the loss of passive protection by 4–6 months and the progressive infection of susceptibles and acquisition of protective antibodies in early childhood. In the past decade, 2 important trends have been observed at various medical centers: (1) There has been a gradual increase in the frequency of infections due to *H influenzae* type B; and (2) a change in age distribution of infections has been observed. The frequency of distribution of infections is still highest in the age group from 6 months to 4 years. However, an increasing incidence of infection with this organism has been reported in newborns and older children and adults. Among the pediatric population at Fitzsimons Army Hospital (Denver) in the 10-year period from 1960–1969, the highest age-specific attack rate for hospitalized *H influenzae* type B meningitis occurred in the age group from 0–3 months. A recent study by Graber and his associates (see reference below) explains the occurrence of infections in neonates and adults. In this study of neonatal and maternal sera, bactericidal antibody to *H influenzae* type B was demonstrated in only 10% of newborn infants (cord blood) and in 25% of the mothers. An apparent increase in the frequency of *H influenzae* otitis media and sinusitis in older children and adults has been documented. There is no clear explanation of the increase in the number of illnesses due to this organism requiring hospitalization during the past 10–20 years.

Clinical Findings

A. Symptoms and Signs:

1. Meningitis—Findings may be very minimal. Nothing clinically distinguishes it from other forms, although petechiae are less common than in meningococcal meningitis and fever and generalized toxemia are apt to be very high. Characteristically, there is a history of upper respiratory infection in a young infant who subsequently frowns a good deal, becomes increasingly stuporous, and who may show nuchal rigidity. If the fontanel is open, evidence of increased intracranial pressure may be seen.

2. Acute epiglottitis—The most characteristic clinical aid in the early diagnosis of *H influenzae* croup is evidence of dysphagia characterized by a refusal to eat or swallow saliva even by very young children. This finding, plus the presence of a high fever in a toxic child—even in the absence of direct examination of the epiglottis (cherry-red epiglottis)—should strongly suggest the diagnosis and lead to prompt intubation. (See Chapter 12 for details.)

3. Otitis media, septic arthritis, orbital cellulitis, pneumonia, septic pericarditis—See Essentials of Diagnosis, above.

B. Laboratory Findings: Very high leukocytosis (> 20 thousand/cu mm) with a marked shift to the left is characteristic of *H influenzae* infections. Blood culture is almost always positive. Positive culture of aspirated pus or fluid from or near the involved site proves the diagnosis.

In meningitis (before treatment), spinal fluid smear reveals, in addition to the characteristic pleomorphic gram-negative rods, pathognomonic long filamentous forms.

C. X-Ray Findings: A lateral view of the neck should be taken in suspected acute epiglottitis. Haziness of maxillary and ethmoid sinuses occurs with orbital cellulitis; lung consolidation and pleural fluid with pneumonia; and a characteristically enlarged heart shadow with purulent pericarditis.

D. Electrocardiography: Elevated ST segments and flattened T waves and low voltage occur with purulent pericarditis.

Differential Diagnosis

A. Meningitis: Differentiate from head injury, brain abscess, tumor, lead encephalopathy, and other forms of meningoencephalitis due to viral, fungal, and bacterial agents, including tuberculous meningitis.

B. Acute Epiglottitis: In croup caused by viral agents (parainfluenza 1, 2, and 3, respiratory syncytial virus, influenza A, adenovirus), the child has more definite upper respiratory symptoms, slower progression of obstructive signs, and only low-grade fever. Spasmodic croup occurs typically at night in a child with the history of previous attacks; these attacks may be of allergic origin. A history of sudden onset of choking and paroxysmal coughing suggests aspiration of a foreign body. Occasionally, retropharyngeal abscess or laryngeal diphtheria may have to be differentiated from epiglottitis.

C. Septic Arthritis: Acute osteomyelitis, prepatellar bursitis, cellulitis, rheumatic fever, and fractures and sprains.

D. Orbital Cellulitis: Erysipelas, paranasal sinus disease without orbital cellulitis, allergic inflammatory disease of the lids, vaccinal or herpes simplex conjunctivitis, herpes zoster infection, metastatic neuroblastoma, and primary orbital tumors.

E. Pneumonia: See pp 265–267.

F. Septic Pericarditis: See p 321.

Complications

A. Meningitis: Subdural effusion, subdural empyema, involvement of cranial nerves, hydrocephalus; late intellectual sequelae include handicaps of perceptual and motor functioning and abstract thinking ability.

B. Acute Epiglottitis: Mediastinal emphysema, pneumothorax; rarely, bacteremic spread to meninges or joints.

C. Otitis Media: Sinusitis, mastoiditis, and occasionally bacteremic spread to other sites.

D. Septic Arthritis: May result in rapid destruction of cartilage and ankylosis if diagnosis and treatment are delayed.

E. Orbital Cellulitis: Cavernous sinus thrombosis is a rare sequel. With the onset of this complication, the child develops severe pain and general toxicity, papilledema, and decreased vision.

F. Pneumonia: Empyema; rarely, pneumatoceles and pneumothorax.

G. Septic Pericarditis: Myocardial abscesses and heart failure; cardiac tamponade.

Treatment

With the exception of acute otitis media, all of these diseases are potentially fatal and require immediate hospitalization and treatment. Each disease should be treated with ampicillin, 200–400 mg/kg/day IV in 6 divided doses until there is marked improvement; in some cases, the treatment course may then be completed with ampicillin given intramuscularly in 4 divided doses. Chloramphenicol, 100 mg/kg/day IV in 4 divided doses, is the drug of choice if there is a known allergy to ampicillin.

A. Meningitis: A repeat lumbar tap should be performed after 24–36 hours of treatment. The CSF should then be sterile. Treatment should be continued until the patient has been afebrile for 5 days, the CSF cell count is 30 cells or less, and the sugar and protein have returned to normal; this usually requires 10–14 days. It is preferable to give the entire course of antibiotic intravenously in 6 divided doses per day. There will be no treatment failures if a dosage of 300 mg/kg/day is used. The intravenous site should be rotated every 48–72 hours.

Most common causes for exacerbation of fever or persistence of fever beyond 6 days are the following: chemical phlebitis at injection site, drug fever, subdural effusions, acquisition of hospital-acquired viral or bacterial superinfection, and metastatic disease requiring drainage (eg, subdural empyema, septic pericarditis, arthritis).

In case of subdural effusion, a maximum of 15 ml are allowed to drip freely from each side of the anterior fontanel daily. If fluid is still present after 2 weeks neurosurgical consultation is advised.

Supportive therapy with intravenous fluids, oxygen, sedation, and tube feeding should be given as required.

B. Acute Epiglottitis: An immediate intravenous dose of 200–300 mg/kg of ampicillin is given, followed by 200 mg/kg/day IV in 6 divided doses. In most cases, establishment and maintenance of a free airway are most important considerations. Signs of increasing airway obstruction are a clear indication for tracheostomy, which should be done electively with the assistance of a skilled bronchoscopist. Antibiotic treatment should be continued for 10 days. In case of penicillin sensitivity, give chloramphenicol as an alternative drug.

High humidification and intravenous fluids are required. Improvement of cyanosis by placing the child in an oxygen atmosphere gives a false sense of security to the physician. The basic problem is upper airway obstruction, which may require tracheostomy.

C. Otitis Media: Give ampicillin orally in a dosage of 100 mg/kg/day in 4 divided doses for 14–21 days. There is some clinical evidence of an increased incidence of serous otitis following oral ampicillin treatment. Erythromycin, 40 mg/kg/day orally in 4 divided doses, is effective. Some physicians still prefer to use an oral penicillin-sulfonamide combination preparation.

Oral decongestants may be used but are now considered less important than once thought. Careful follow-up for the secondary occurrence of serous otitis and hearing loss should be made.

D. Septic Arthritis: Ampicillin is given in a dosage of 200–300 mg/kg/day IV in 6 divided doses until there is marked improvement. The same dose may then be given intramuscularly in 4 divided doses to complete a 3-week course of treatment. On admission, surgical incision and drainage are required whenever there is a significant collection of pus in the joint.

The joint should be immobilized. Give antipyretics and analgesics as required and maintain adequate hydration.

E. Orbital Cellulitis: Give ampicillin as for septic arthritis and supportive and symptomatic treatment as required. There is usually marked improvement after 72 hours of treatment. Antibiotics should be given for 7–10 days.

F. Pneumonia: Give ampicillin as for septic arthritis and oxygen, intravenous fluids, and other supportive care as required. Treat for 3 weeks. Empyema should be treated by placement of one or more chest tubes into the pleural space. When possible, a chest tube should be removed after 4 or 5 days.

G. Septic Pericarditis: Give ampicillin as for septic arthritis. Treat for 4 weeks. Pericardiocentesis may be lifesaving to prevent fatal tamponade. Open pericardiostomy should be performed to allow for continuous drainage of pus and to prevent reaccumulation.

Digitalis, oxygen, and intravenous fluids should be given as required.

Prognosis

The case fatality rate for *H influenzae* meningitis is 5–10%. Young infants have the highest mortality rate. Nuerologic sequelae should be watched for but are appreciably reduced with prompt antibiotic treatment.

The case fatality rate in acute epiglottitis is 15–20%; mortality is associated with bacteremia and the rapid development of airway obstruction.

With optimal medical and surgical drainage, the case fatality rate for septic pericarditis in infants still is 20%.

The prognosis for the other diseases requiring hospitalization is good with the institution of early and adequate antibiotic therapy.

Achtel RA: Recurrent bacteremia following ampicillin treatment of *Hemophilus influenzae* meningitis. Acta paediat scandinav 59:211–213, 1970.

Almquist EE: The changing epidemiology of septic arthritis in children. Clin Orthop 68:96–99, 1970.

Balagtas RC & others: Secondary and prolonged fevers in bacterial meningitis. J Pediat 77:957–964, 1970.

Graber CD & others: Changing pattern of neonatal susceptibility to *Hemophilus influenzae.* J Pediat 78:948–950, 1971.

Levine MS, Boxerbaum B, Heggie AD: Recrudescence of *H influenzae* meningitis after therapy with ampicillin. Clin Pediat 9:54–57, 1970.

McLinn SE, Nelson JD, Haltalin KC: Antimicrobial susceptibility of *Hemophilus influenzae.* Pediatrics 45:827–838, 1970.

Rapkin RH: Acute epiglottitis: Pitfalls in diagnosis and management. Clin Pediat 10:312–314, 1971.

Winkelstein JA: The influence of partial treatment with penicillin on the diagnosis of bacterial meningitis. J Pediat 77:619–624, 1970.

Wright L, Jimmerson S: Intellectual sequelae of *Hemophilus influenzae* meningitis. J Abnorm Psychol 77:181–183, 1971.

PERTUSSIS
(Whooping Cough)

Essentials of Diagnosis

- Staccato, paroxysmal expiratory cough ending with a high-pitched inspiratory "whoop."
- Prodromal catarrhal stage (1–3 weeks) characterized by cough, coryza, and occasionally vomiting.
- Leukocytosis with absolute lymphocytosis.
- Diagnosis confirmed by fluorescent stain or culture.

General Considerations

Pertussis is an acute communicable infection of the respiratory tract caused by *Bordetella (Hemophilus) pertussis.* It is of most serious import to children under 2 years of age. Transmission is through infected individuals, generally as a family contact. The incubation period is 7–14 days, and infectivity is greatest during the catarrhal and early paroxysmal cough stage (for about 4 weeks after onset). Half of cases occur before 4 years of age, and no deaths from whooping cough are reported after age 2 in the USA.

Clinical Findings

A. Symptoms and Signs: In children over 2 years of age, mild cases lasting 5–14 days occur, and symptoms may consist only of low-grade fever and irritating cough with mild paroxysms. In the younger child, symptoms of pertussis last about 8 weeks. The onset is insidious, with mild catarrhal upper respiratory tract symptoms (rhinitis, sneezing, and an irritating cough). Slight fever may be present. After about 2 weeks, cough becomes paroxysmal, with each cough followed by a sudden inspiratory whoop. Vomiting commonly occurs, and coughing through tenacious mucus may result in large bubbles at the nose and mough. Coughing is accompanied by sweating, prostration, and exhaustion. This stage lasts for 2–4 weeks, with gradual improvement. Cough suggestive of chronic bronchitis lasts for another 2–3 weeks and then usually fades away. Paroxysmal coughing may continue in the absence of any active infection for some months.

B. Laboratory Findings: White blood cell counts of 20–30 thousand/cu mm with 70–80% lymphocytes appear near the end of the catarrhal stage. The blood picture may resemble lymphocytic leukemia. Identification of *B pertussis* by fluorescent antibody technic or culture from nasopharyngeal swabs proves the diagnosis. The organism may be found in the respiratory tract in diminishing titers beginning in the catarrhal stage and ending about 2 weeks after the beginning of the paroxysmal stage. A Bradford wire swab specimen is obtained from the nasopharynx. Culture of the specimen is done on special media. The combination of culture and fluorescent antibody staining is the diagnostic method of choice. Sterilized Bordet-Gengou agar base should be stored in the refrigerator and liquefied just prior to use. Freshly withdrawn defibrinated sheep's blood is added to make a final concentration of 20% in pour plates. Plates used for culture should have been prepared within 72 hours. Serum agglutinins appear late in the infection and are of little value in diagnosis.

Differential Diagnosis

Cough in acute bacterial pneumonias in infants is usually associated with high fever, tachypnea, and chest retractions, often out of proportion to auscultatory findings. In viral respiratory infections, several members of a family usually have symptoms. The infant may develop stridor, wheezing, or signs of pneumonia. Pertussis is differentiated by the progressive course and characteristic "whoop." Children with cystic fibrosis of the pancreas have a positive sweat test, steatorrhea, and often a positive family history. A positive chest x-ray and tuberculin test distinguish the young child with tuberculosis. A foreign body aspirated into the tracheobronchial tree may be identified by proper x-ray and endoscopic technics. Parapertussis resembles mild pertussis and can be distinguished only by culture. A pertussis-like illness may be caused by at least 3 adenovirus types (2, 5, and 12).

Complications

Pneumonia may be widespread and may be the direct cause of death, particularly in an infant. Asphyxia in children having serious paroxysmal attacks may lead to brain damage with or without convulsions. Cerebral edema is a common postmortem finding. Cerebral hemorrhage and bleeding into the conjunctivas or from the nose may occur. Increased intrapulmonary pressure may also lead to interstitial or subcutaneous emphysema and pneumothorax.

Pertussis probably has been an important primary respiratory disease, leading to chronic bronchiectasis.

Diagnostic lumbar puncture is occasionally desirable to ascertain the presence of blood when subarachnoid hemorrhage is suspected on clinical grounds.

Prevention (See Chapter 5.)

Active immunization should be routinely administered with pertussis vaccine given in combination with diphtheria and tetanus toxoids (DPT). Little or no maternal immunity is passively transferred to the newborn.

Passive immunization of exposed susceptible contacts in the family—particularly those under 2 years of age—is accomplished by giving 2.5 ml of hyperimmune gamma globulin IM.

In exposed immunized children, a booster injection of pertussis vaccine should be given.

Treatment

A. Specific Measures: The elimination of *B pertussis* from patients can be accomplished with antimicrobial therapy. The patient should be considered noncontagious only after confirmation by negative culture and fluorescent antibody studies. Antibiotic treatment does not modify the clinical course. Give ampicillin, 150 mg/kg/day orally in equal doses at 6-hour intervals day and night for 7 days. When oral therapy is not possible, give 150 mg/kg/day IV in 4 divided doses.

In some geographic areas, the majority of strains are ampicillin-resistant. If the organism is resistant to ampicillin, give erythromycin, 50 mg/kg/day orally in 4 divided doses for 7 days.

In controlled studies, pertussis immune globulin has not been shown to be of benefit in the treatment of pertussis. Therefore, its use is no longer recommended.

B. General Measures: Nursing care to permit adequate nutritional support during the period of most exhausting paroxysms is one of the most important therapeutic considerations. Frequent small feedings, and refeeding if vomiting occurs, are recommended. Gavage tube feeding and parenteral fluid supplementation may be essential in serious cases in which the nutritional state is poor and continued weight loss cannot be prevented by other means. Gastrostomy feedings may be required.

Minimizing stimuli which trigger paroxysms is probably the best way of controlling cough. In general, cough mixtures are of little benefit.

C. Treatment of Complications: Respiratory insufficiency due to pneumonia or other pulmonary complications should be treated with oxygen and with high humidity. Control convulsions by means of oxygen and parenteral sodium phenobarbital.

Prognosis

The prognosis of pertussis is much improved in recent years because of adequate attention to nursing care. The disease is still of serious importance in infants under 1 year of age; about 70% of deaths due to pertussis occur in this age group. For unknown reasons, the mortality rate is higher among females.

Balagtas RC & others: Treatment of pertussis with pertussis immune globulin. J Pediat 79:203–208, 1971.

Bass JW & others: Antimicrobial treatment of pertussis. J Pediat 75:768–781, 1969.

Brooksaler FS: The pertussis syndrome. Texas Med 67:56–61, 1971.

Connor JD: Evidence for an etiologic role of adenoviral infection in pertussis syndrome. New England J Med 283:390–394, 1970.

Lone WC & others: What causes whooping-cough? Lancet 2:1142, 1970.

Nelson JD: Antibiotic treatment of pertussis. Pediatrics 44:474–476, 1969.

Wilkins J & others: Agglutinin response to pertussis vaccine. I. Effect of dosage interval. J Pediat 79:197, 1971.

TUBERCULOSIS

Essentials of Diagnosis

- All types: Positive tuberculin test, chest x-ray, history of contact, and demonstration of organism by stain and culture.
- Pulmonary: Fatigue, irritability, and undernutrition, with or without fever and cough.
- Glandular: Chronic cervical adenitis.
- Miliary: Classical "snowstorm" appearance of chest x-ray; choroidal tubercles.
- Meningitis: Fever and manifestations of meningeal irritation and increased intracranial pressure.

General Considerations

Tuberculosis is a chronic granulomatous disease caused by *Mycobacterium tuberculosis*. It remains a leading cause of death throughout the world, although in the USA human disease caused by the bovine type has been virtually eliminated by pasteurization of milk and control of disease in cattle. The case rate in children under 15 years of age showing a demonstrable lesion is 7 per 100,000 population. For every case of diagnosed disease there are about 80 asymptomatic infections manifested only by tuberculin skin test conversion. Children under 3 years of age are most susceptible, and lymphohematogenous dissemination through the lungs and spread to extrapulmonary sites, including the brain and meninges, eyes, bones and joints, lymph nodes, kidneys, intestines, larynx, and skin are more likely to occur in infants. Increased susceptibility occurs again in adolescence, particularly in girls within 2 years of menarche. Prolonged household contact with an active adolescent or adult case usually leads to infection of infants and children. This is a particularly serious problem among crowded urban populations. The case rate and death rate in nonwhite children are 2–5 times those in white children. The primary complex in infancy and childhood consists of a small parenchymal lesion in any area of the lung with caseation of regional nodes and healing by calcification. There is a strong tendency for lymphohematogenous spread early in primary infection, but chronic pulmonary disease is not common (see Chapter 12). Postprimary tuberculosis in adolescents and adults occurs in the apexes of the lungs and is likely to cause chronic, progressive cavitary pulmonary disease with no tendency for hematogenous dissemination.

Clinical Findings

A. Symptoms and Signs:

1. Pulmonary—See Chapter 12.

2. Miliary—Diagnosis is made on the basis of a classical snowstorm appearance of lung fields on x-ray. The majority also have a fresh primary complex and pleural effusion. Choroidal tubercles are seen in as many as 60% of cases. Other lesions may be present and may be associated with osteomyelitis, arthritis, meningitis, tuberculomas of the brain, enteritis, and infection of the kidneys.

3. Meningitis—Symptoms include fever, vomiting, headache, lethargy, and irritability, with signs of meningeal irritation and increased intracranial pressure, including cranial nerve palsies, convulsions, and coma. Choroidal tubercles are pathognomonic when associated with these signs and symptoms. Otorrhea or acute otitis media may be seen.

4. Glandular—The primary complex may be associated with a skin lesion drained by regional nodes or chronic cervical node enlargement and infection of the tonsils. Involved nodes may become tender, fixed to the overlying skin, and suppurative and may drain.

5. Enteritis—Chronic diarrhea, tenesmus, anemia, fever, and wasting are seen.

B. Laboratory Findings: The Mantoux test using intermediate strength PPD, 0.0001 mg (5 TU) or 0.0002 mg (10 TU), is read as positive at 48–72 hours if there are over 10 mm of induration. The tine test or Heaf test may be used in surveys, but positive responses should be verified by Mantoux testing. The white count is not helpful. The ESR is usually elevated. The CSF in tuberculous meningitis shows slight to moderate pleocytosis (50–300 white cells), decreased glucose, and increased protein.

The detection of mycobacteria in body fluids or discharges is now best done by examination of auramine O stained preparations with blue light (incandescent lamp) fluorescence microscopy, which is superior to the Ziehl-Neelsen method. Specimens are plated for isolation and direct susceptibility to primary drugs (INH, streptomycin, ethambutol, PAS) without reference to microscopic findings on specific culture media. A tentative bacteriologic diagnosis can usually be made within 6 weeks. Sensitivities of the organism should be checked at regular intervals.

C. X-Ray Findings: Chest x-ray shows a fresh primary complex or pleural effusion.

Differential Diagnosis

Pulmonary tuberculosis must be differentiated from sarcoidosis, fungal, parasitic, and bacterial pneumonias, lung abscess, foreign body aspiration, lipoid pneumonia, and mediastinal malignancy. Cervical lymphadenitis is most apt to be due to streptococcal, staphylococcal, or recurrent viral infections. Cat scratch fever and infection with atypical mycobacteria may need to be distinguished from tuberculosis also. Viral meningoencephalitis, head trauma (battered child), lead poisoning, brain abscess, acute bacterial meningitis, brain tumor, and disseminated fungal infections must be excluded in tuberculous meningitis.

Prevention

A. BCG Vaccine: BCG vaccination confers definite but only partial protection and is advised for tuberculin-negative children known to be exposed (limited contact) to adults with active or recently arrested disease. It is advisable to give BCG to newborn infants of tuberculous mothers. BCG is administered intracutaneously over the deltoid or triceps muscle. The dosage is 0.05 ml for newborns and 0.1 ml for older infants and children. The child should not remain in contact with the infected member of the family for at least 2 months afterwards. BCG should never be given to a tuberculin-positive individual; to one with definite or suspected agammaglobulinemia, thymic alymphoplasia, or dysplasia; or to one with skin infection or burns or a recent smallpox vaccination. Some authorities feel that BCG vaccination should be made compulsory for tuberculin-negative school children in slums (urban and rural) before they are admitted to school.

B. Isoniazid (INH) Chemoprophylaxis: Daily administration of INH in therapeutic doses is advised for children who cannot avoid intimate household contact with adolescents or adults with active disease. The dose of isoniazid is 10 mg/kg orally, not to exceed 300 mg daily. Isoniazid is continued throughout the period of exposure and for 6 months after the contact has been broken. BCG is not given during the period of isoniazid chemoprophylaxis.

C. Other Measures: The source contact (index case) should be identified, isolated, and treated to prevent other secondary cases. Exposed tuberculin-negative children should be skin tested every 2 months for 6 months after contact has been terminated. Tuberculin skin testing is advised annually for preschool children and every 2–3 years through adolescence.

Among very malnourished and very ill children with overwhelming infection with bacteriologically proved tuberculosis, it is very common (30%) to find no reaction to intermediate strength PPD. Usually (but not always) the second strength test will be positive. About 20% of patients with recently acquired active disease which is not an overwhelming infection will have negative intermediate strength PPD reactions shortly after admission to a diagnostic ward. After a few weeks, about 98% of these latter cases will have positive intermediate tuberculin reactions.

Certain viral infections, including measles, influenza, varicella, mumps, and probably others; some viral vaccines (measles, influenza, rubella); and administration of corticosteroids and other immunosuppressants may depress or suppress tuberculin reactivity for 2–6 weeks. Malnutrition may have a similar effect.

Treatment

A. Specific Measures: Most patients in the USA are hospitalized at the beginning of treatment but receive most of the prolonged drug course as outpatients. Treatment failure is usually due to the inability of patients (and parents) to cooperate in the long program of therapy.

1. Isoniazid (INH)—INH is given alone to any child without a demonstrable lesion who is tuberculin-positive (with Mantoux reaction measuring less than 18 mm) and is (1) under 6 years of age, (2) adolescent, (3) known to have converted within 1 year, or (4) receiving corticosteroids, antimetabolites, or ionizing irradiation. The dosage is 10–20 mg/kg orally once a day (or intravenously or intramuscularly if the drug causes vomiting) for 12 months.

2. Ethambutol (Myambutol)—This drug has replaced aminosalicylic acid (PAS) in the primary drug regimen used at Fitzsimons General Hospital and at the National Jewish Hospital, Denver. This substitution has been made because of the relatively high incidence of PAS intolerance and because ethambutol is both effective and well tolerated. In children, the dosage is 15–20 mg/kg/day orally in 2 divided doses. Retrobulbar neuritis is an uncommon complication of ethambutol treatment in adults, but routine visual acuity testing is recommended when the drug is being given.

3. Aminosalicylic acid (PAS)—Since children have a better tolerance for PAS than do adults, there is still a role for PAS in the primary drug regimen for the treatment of tuberculosis in children. Sodium or potassium PAS, 250–300 mg/kg/day orally in 3 or 4 divided doses, is given in addition to INH for 18–24 months in the following conditions: cervical or hilar lymphadenitis; segmental lung shadow or pleural effusion; tuberculin conversion within the year where there is a demonstrable or "suspicious" lesion; tuberculin-positive reaction measuring 18–23 mm; or tuberculin-positive girl with a reaction measuring 12 mm or more whose menarche has occurred or will occur within 2 years. If the organism is suspected or shown to be resistant in vitro to INH, ethambutol, and PAS, the dosage of INH is increased to 30 mg/kg/day, and ethionamide (Trecator), 15–20 mg/kg/day orally in 3–4 divided doses, is substituted for ethambutol or PAS. A new drug, rifampin, has been shown in European studies to be as effective as INH alone. It is likely that triple therapy in a primary drug regimen will soon consist of INH, rifampin, and ethambutol. The dosage of rifampin is 10–20 mg/kg/day given orally as a single daily dose, either 1 hour before or 2 hours after a meal.

4. Streptomycin or kanamycin—In serious or progressive forms, including meningeal, miliary, renal, osseous, cavitary, and chronic pulmonary tuberculosis, give streptomycin, 20–30 mg/kg/day IM in 1 or 2 doses, for 2–4 months in addition to 2 oral drugs. In case of streptomycin resistance, kanamycin, 15 mg/kg/day IM, is given for 1–3 months. Periodic audiometric tests are advisable when either drug is used.

B. General Measures:

1. Corticosteroids—These drugs are useful for suppressing inflammatory reactions in meningeal, pleural, and pericardial tuberculosis and for the relief of bronchial obstruction due to hilar adenopathy. Prednisone is given orally, 1 mg/kg/day for 6–8 weeks, with gradual withdrawal at the end of that time.

2. Bed rest—Rest in bed is only indicated while the child feels ill. Isolation is necessary only for children with draining lesions or renal disease and those with chronic pulmonary tuberculosis. Otherwise, children receiving INH or INH plus ethambutol or PAS are noninfectious and may attend school.

Prognosis

If bacteria are sensitive and treatment is completed, most patients make lasting recovery. Retreatment is more difficult and less successful. With antituberculosis chemotherapy (especially isoniazid), there should now be nearly 100% recovery in miliary tuberculosis. Without treatment, there is nearly a 100% mortality in both miliary tuberculosis and tuberculous meningitis. In the latter form, about 2/3 of treated cases survive with treatment. There may be a high incidence of neurologic abnormalities among survivors if treatment is started late.

Bivibo NO: Tuberculosis of the cervical lymph nodes: Clinical studies of children in East Africa. Clin Pediat 9:733–735, 1970.

Darney PD, Clenny ND: Tuberculosis outbreak in an Alabama high school. JAMA 216:2117–2118, 1971.

Ehrlich RM, Lattimer JK: Urogenital tuberculosis in children. J Urol 105:461–465, 1971.

Kendig EL: The place of BCG vaccine in the management of infants born of tuberculous mothers. New England J Med 281:520–523, 1969.

Mitchell RS: Control of tuberculosis up-to-date. New England J Med 284:1380–1381, 1971.

Newman R & others: Rifampin in initial treatment of pulmonary tuberculosis. A United States Public Health Service trial. Am Rev Resp Dis 103:461–476, 1971.

Smith DT: Which children in the United States should receive BCG vaccination? Clin Pediat 9:632–634, 1970.

Smith MHD: Tuberculosis in adolescents: Characteristics, recognition, management. Clin Pediat 6:9–15, 1967.

Stegen G, Jones K, Kaplan P: Criteria for guidance in the diagnosis of tuberculosis. Pediatrics 43:260–263, 1969.

Steiner M & others: Primary drug-resistant tuberculosis: Report of an outbreak. New England J Med 283:1353–1358, 1970.

Vall-Spinosa A & others: Rifampin in the treatment of drug-resistant *Mycobacterium tuberculosis* infections. New England J Med 283:616–621, 1970.

INFECTIONS WITH ATYPICAL MYCOBACTERIA

Essentials of Diagnosis

- Chronic unilateral cervical lymphadenitis.
- Granulomas of the skin.
- Chronic bone lesion with draining sinus (chronic osteomyelitis).
- Reaction to PPD-S (standard) of 5–8 mm, negative chest x-ray, and history of contact with tuberculosis.
- Positive skin reaction to a specific atypical antigen.

General Considerations

Various species of acid-fast mycobacteria other than *Mycobacterium tuberculosis* are now known to cause asymptomatic subclinical infections in wide segments of the population with occasional manifest clinical disease closely simulating tuberculosis. Strain cross-reactivity with *M tuberculosis* can be demonstrated by simultaneous skin testing (Mantoux) with PPD-S (standard) and PPD prepared from one of the atypical antigens. The larger skin reaction represents infection with the homologous strain.

The Runyon classification of mycobacteria now used includes the following:

Group I—Photochromogens (PPD-Y): Yellow color develops upon exposure to light in previously white colony grown 2–4 weeks in the dark. Group includes *M kansasii* and *M balnei* and tends to be more prevalent in the midwestern USA.

Group II—Scotochromogens (PPD-G): Colony is definitely yellow-orange after incubation in the dark. Organisms may be found in small numbers in the normal flora of some human saliva and gastric contents. Subclinical infection is widespread in the USA, but clinical disease appears rarely. Group includes *M scrofulaceum.*

Group III—Nonphotochromogens (PPD-B): "Battey-avian-swine group" grows as small white colonies after incubation in the dark with no significant development of pigment upon exposure to light. Infection with *M intracellulare* ("Battey bacillus") is prevalent in the south and southeastern USA and probably in the New England states. Infection with avian strains is prevalent in Great Britain.

Group IV—"Rapid growers": *M fortuitum* is the recognized pathogen. Within 1 week after inoculation, forms a colony closely resembling *M tuberculosis* morphologically.

Clinical Findings

A. Symptoms and Signs:

1. Pulmonary disease—*M kansasii* accounts for 60% and *M intracellulare* for 30% of pulmonary tuberculosis due to organisms other than *M tuberculosis.* Clinical features and x-ray appearance can be identical to disease caused by *M tuberculosis.*

2. Cervical lymphadenitis—Due to *M intracellulare, M kansasii,* and *M scrofulaceum.* The submandibular or anterior cervical (tonsillar) node is enlarged on one side and persists as a troublesome lump which is discovered fortuitously. There is no response to treatment with penicillin. Such a child might show evidence of pulmonary infection on x-ray (uncommonly) or evidence of disseminated disease (rarely).

3. Granulomas of the skin—Due to *M balnei.* Outbreaks have been shown to be associated with infected water in swimming pools.

4. Chronic osteomyelitis—Due to *M kansasii* and *M scrofulaceum.* The child has swelling and pain over a distal extremity, radiolucent defects in bone, fever, and clinical and x-ray evidence of bronchopneumonia. Such cases are rare.

5. Meningitis—Due to *M kansasii*. Disease may be indistinguishable from tuberculous meningitis.

B. Laboratory Findings: In most cases there is a small reaction (< 10 mm) when Mantoux testing is done with PPD-S. The chest x-ray is negative, and there is no history of contact with tuberculosis. Biopsy of the lesion shows a granulomatous reaction with caseation. Acid-fast bacilli are demonstrated in stained biopsy material. Tuberculosis may be suspected and treatment started with antituberculosis drugs. With these findings, including a Mantoux reaction of < 10 mm, disease due to one of the atypical mycobacteria should be suspected. Simultaneous tuberculin testing with the infecting atypical antigen (PPD-Y, G, or B) will usually give a reaction 2—5 mm greater than the reaction to PPD-S.

Definitive diagnosis is made by isolating the causative agent from clinical material on a medium as described for the isolation of *M tuberculosis.*

Differential Diagnosis

See section on differential diagnosis in the discussion of tuberculosis above and in Chapter 12.

Treatment

A. Specific Measures: Treatment should be individualized, based on in vitro drug sensitivity studies. Photochromogens and scotochromogens may or may not be susceptible to isoniazid, aminosalicylic acid, streptomycin, ethambutol, capreomycin, and kanamycin. Battey strains are often resistant to most of the antituberculosis agents. Complete surgical excision of involved cervical nodes (regardless of the type of antibiotic coverage) usually results in uneventful recovery and is the treatment of choice. In case of pulmonary and disseminated disease where in vitro resistance appears complete, a combination of isoniazid (30 mg/kg/day orally in divided doses), aminosalicylic acid, and streptomycin may be effective. Rifampin may become the drug of choice.

B. General Measures: Isolation of the patient is not usually necessary. General supportive care is indicated for the child with disseminated disease.

Prognosis

The prognosis is good, though fatalities have occurred.

Dawson DJ: Potential pathogens among strains of mycobacteria isolated from house dusts. MJ Australia 1:679—681, 1971.

Gruhl VR, Reese MH: Disseminated atypical mycobacterial disease presenting as "leukemia." Am J Clin Path 5:206—211, 1971.

Kubica GP: Known clinical mycobacterial organisms. Ann New York Acad Sc 174:840—846, 1970.

Salyer KE, Votteler TP, Dorman GW: Cervical adenitis in children due to atypical mycobacteria. Plast Reconstr Surg 47:47—53, 1971.

Wiant JR: Mycobacterial diseases. Arizona Med 28:96—100, 1971.

LEPROSY

Essentials of Diagnosis

- Pale, anesthetic macular—or nodular and erythematous—skin lesions.
- Superficial nerve thickening with associated sensory changes.
- History of residence in endemic area.
- Acid-fast bacilli in skin lesions or nasal scrapings, or characteristic histologic nerve changes.

General Considerations

Leprosy is a mildly contagious chronic infectious disease caused by the acid-fast rod *Mycobacterium leprae.* The mode of transmission is unknown, and attempts to infect human volunteers have been unsuccessful. Susceptibility to leprosy may involve a hereditary factor.

Clinical Findings

The onset of leprosy is insidious. The lesions involve the cooler tissues of the body: skin, superficial nerves, nose, pharynx, larynx, eyes, and testicles. The skin lesions may occur as pale, anesthetic macular lesions 1—10 cm in diameter; diffuse or discrete erythematous, infiltrated nodules 1—5 cm in diameter; or as a diffuse skin infiltration. Neurologic disturbances are manifested by nerve infiltration and thickening, with resultant anesthesia, neuritis, paresthesia, trophic ulcers, and bone resorption and shortening of digits. The disfiguration due to the skin infiltration and nerve involvement in untreated cases may be extreme.

The disease is divided clinically and by laboratory tests into 2 distinct types: lepromatous and tuberculoid. In the lepromatous type the course is progressive and malign, with nodular skin lesions; slow, symmetric nerve involvement; abundant acid-fast bacilli in the skin lesions, and a negative lepromin skin test. In the tuberculoid type, the course is benign and nonprogressive, with macular skin lesions, severe asymmetric nerve involvement of sudden onset with no bacilli present in the lesions, and a positive lepromin skin test. In the lepromatous type an acute febrile episode with evanescent skin lesions may occur and may last for weeks. Eye involvement (keratitis and iridocyclitis), nasal ulcers, and epistaxis may occur in both types but are most common in the lepromatous type.

Systemic manifestations of anemia and lymphadenopathy may also occur.

Histologic nerve changes are usually characteristic.

Differential Diagnosis

The skin lesions of leprosy must often be distinguished from those of lupus erythematosus, sarcoidosis, syphilis, erythema nodosum, erythema multiforme, and vitiligo; nerve involvement, sensory dissociation, and resulting deformity may require differentiation from syringomyelia and scleroderma.

Complications

Intercurrent tuberculosis is common in the lepromatous type. Amyloidosis may occur with long-standing disease.

Treatment

Drug therapy must be given during periods of exacerbation of the disease. Drugs should be given cautiously, with slowly increasing doses, and must be withheld when they show signs of producing an induced exacerbation with leprotic fever; progressive anemia with or without leukopenia; severe gastrointestinal symptoms, allergic dermatitis, hepatitis, or mental disturbances; or erythema nodosum. It is important, therefore, to observe temperature, blood counts, and biopsy changes in lesions at regular intervals. The duration of treatment must be guided by progress, preferably as judged by biopsy. Treatment must be continued for several years but often indefinitely because recrudescence may occur after cessation of therapy.

A. Dapsone (Avlosulfon, DDS) is given orally to a maximum of 300 mg a week (occasionally up to 600 mg/week, the full adult dose). Start with 25 mg twice weekly and increase to the maximum by 25 mg increments every week, by which time the dose of 300 mg weekly may be spread in daily or other fractions. Selected cases may be treated as outpatients. Children tolerate all the sulfones well in doses proportionate to age (eg, 300 mg/week for a child of 12). If the lepra reaction occurs, stop treatment until recovery is complete and then start again at the beginning or change to another sulfone. (Although all sulfones apparently act in the body in the same way as DDS, some produce fewer reactions.)

B. Solapsone (Sulphetrone), a complex substituted derivative of DDS, may be given orally or parenterally. The adult oral dose is 0.5 gm 3 times daily initially, increasing gradually until a total daily dose of 6–10 gm is being given. The parenteral preparation (50% aqueous solution) is given deeply subcutaneously or intramuscularly in doses beginning with 0.1 ml twice a week and doubling each 2 weeks to a maximum of 3 ml/week in divided doses.

C. Diphenylthiourea (DPT) is given orally in divided doses, beginning with 250 mg/day and increasing to a maximum of 2 gm/day. This drug is indicated if intolerance develops to the above drugs. It may be continued for about 3 years before resistance develops.

D. Sulfoxone sodium (Diasone) is given orally, 300 mg daily Monday through Friday for 1 week and 600 mg daily Monday through Friday thereafter.

E. Surgical care of the extremities (hands and feet) requires careful consideration.

F. BCG vaccination is being studied and shows promise as a means of immunizing children. Both dapsone and BCG are being tested for their prophylactic value for family contacts of patients with lepromatous leprosy.

G. Rifampin: A recent small clinical trial showed that rifampin was just as effective in the treatment of lepromatous leprosy as standard treatment with dapsone. Rifampin is a bactericidal agent, whereas all other conventional antileprosy drugs are bacteriostatic. If these clinical findings are confirmed in larger trials, rifampin could become the drug of choice.

Prognosis

Untreated lepromatous leprosy is progressive and fatal in 10–20 years. In the tuberculoid type, spontaneous recovery usually occurs in 1–3 years; it may, however, produce crippling deformities.

With treatment, the lepromatous type regresses slowly (over a period of 3–8 years), and recovery from the tuberculoid type is more rapid. Recrudescences are always possible and it may be safe to assume that the bacilli are never eradicated. Deformities persist, however, after complete recovery, and may markedly interfere with function and appearance.

Bechelli LM, Guinto RS: Some recent laboratory findings on *Mycobacterium leprae*: Implications for therapy, epidemiology and control of leprosy. Bull World Health Organ 43:559–569, 1970.

Pearson JMH, Weddell G: Changes in sensory acuity following radial nerve biopsy in patients with leprosy. Brain 94:43–50, 1971.

Quagliato R, Bechelli LM, Marques RM: Bacterial negativity and reactivation (relapse) of lepromatous outpatients under sulfone treatment. Internat J Leprosy 38:250–263, 1970.

Rees RJW, Pearson JMH, Waters MFR: Experimental and clinical studies on rifampicin in treatment of leprosy. Brit MJ 1:89–92, 1970.

Sabin TB: Preservation of sensation in a cutaneous vascular malformation in lepromatous leprosy. New England J Med 282:1084–1085, 1970.

Sehgal VN & others: Inoculation leprosy subsequent to smallpox vaccination. Dermatologica 141:393–396, 1970.

Slem G: Clinical studies of ocular leprosy. Am J Ophth 71:431–434, 1971.

Warren G: Facets of leprosy of orthopaedic interest. Australian New Zealand J Surg 40:296–298, 1971.

BARTONELLOSIS
(Oroya Fever, Carrión's Disease)

Bartonellosis is an acute or chronic infection caused by *Bartonella bacilliformis,* a gram-negative, pleomorphic microorganism occurring in certain mountainous areas of South America. It is transmitted to man by the sandfly *Phlebotomus verrucarum.* The acute and noneruptive phase (Oroya fever) is characterized by mild or severe fever occurring 2–6 weeks after infection. There may be malaise, headaches, bone and joint pains, and moderate to severe anemia which is of the macrocytic, hypochromic type. Hepatospleno-megaly and lymphadenopathy are common. Super-infection with bacterial pathogens, especially salmonel-lae, is common at this stage. The acute phase lasts 2–6 weeks. In the severe form of the acute disease, mortality has been 90–95%. In those who survive, the eruptive phase (verruga peruana) begins 2–6 weeks later and lasts from a few weeks to 2 years. Hemangioma-like lesions (verrugas) 1–3 mm in size appear in the skin. There are also subcutaneous lesions, but the miliary skin lesions are more widespread and may become secondarily infected. No scars form unless infections are not treated. In Oroya fever the orga-nisms are seen in the peripheral blood smear by Giemsa stain or by blood culture. Skin lesions may also reveal the organisms. Leukocytosis is rare, but hyperbili-rubinemia, reticulocytosis, and megaloblasts and normoblasts are commonly seen.

Chloramphenicol is the drug of choice, especially because of its effect on salmonella superinfection. Penicillin, streptomycin, and the tetracyclines in large doses have all been used effectively. Blood transfusion is often required.

Reyes del Pozo E: Bartonellosis or Peruvian verruca. J Am Med Wom Ass 24:422–423, 1969.
Schultz MG: A history of bartonellosis (Carrión's disease). Am J Trop Med 17:503–515, 1968.
Wernsdoyer G: Possible human bartonellosis in the Sudan: Clini-cal and microbiological observations. Acta trop 26:216–234, 1969.

PSITTACOSIS
(Ornithosis)

Essentials of Diagnosis

- Fever, cough, malaise, chills.
- Rales all over chest; no consolidation.
- Long-lasting x-ray findings of broncho-pneumonia.
- Isolation of bedsonia or rising titer of com-plement-fixing antibodies.
- Exposure to infected birds.

General Considerations

Psittacosis is due to *Chlamydia psittaci,* a rela-tively large organism of the psittacosis-LGV-trachoma group acquired from contact with birds (parrots, para-keets, pigeons, chickens, ducks, and many others). Human-to-human spread is rare. The incubation period is 7–15 days.

Clinical Findings

A. Symptoms and Signs: The onset is usually rapid, with fever, chills, headache, backache, malaise, myalgia, epistaxis, dry cough, and prostration. Signs include those of pneumonitis, alteration of percussion note and breath sounds, and rales. Pulmonary findings may be absent early. Rose spots, splenomegaly, and meningismus are occasionally seen. Delirium, constipa-tion or diarrhea, and abdominal distress may occur. Dyspnea and cyanosis may occur later.

B. Laboratory Findings: The white count is nor-mal or decreased, often with a shift to the left. Pro-teinuria is frequently present. The organism may be isolated from the blood and sputum by mouse inocula-tion. Complement-fixing antibodies appear during or after the second week. The rise in titer may be mini-mized or delayed by early chemotherapy.

C. X-Ray Findings: The x-ray findings in psittaco-sis are those of central pneumonia which later becomes widespread or migratory. Psittacosis is indistin-guishable from viral pneumonias by x-ray.

Differential Diagnosis

This disease can be differentiated from acute viral pneumonias only by the history of contact with poten-tially infected birds. Rose spots and leukopenia suggest typhoid fever.

Complications

Myocarditis, pericarditis, hepatitis, and secondary bacterial pneumonia.

Treatment

Give tetracyclines in full doses for 14 days. Supportive oxygen is often needed. The patient should be kept in strict isolation.

Coli R, Horner I: Cardiac involvement in psittacosis. Brit MJ 4:35–36, 1967.
Cornog JL Jr, Hanson CW: Psittacosis as a cause of miliary infiltrates of the lung and hepatic granulomas. Am Rev Resp Dis 98:1033–1036, 1968.
Cunningham AI, Walker WJ: Psittacosis in Hamilton: A case report and epidemiological study. Canad MAJ 102:69–73, 1970.
Meyer KF: The present status of psittacosis-ornithosis. Arch Envir Health 19:461–466, 1969.
Schaffner W & others: The clinical spectrum of endemic psittacosis. Arch Int Med 119:433–443, 1966.
Timberger RJ, Armstrong D: Ornithosis without direct bird exposure: Response to erythromycin. Am Rev Resp Dis 99:936–939, 1969.
Wisnieroski HJ, Piraino FF: Review of virus respiratory infec-tions in the Milwaukee area, 1955–1965. Pub Health Rep 84:175–181, 1969.

CAT SCRATCH DISEASE

Essentials of Diagnosis

- History of a cat scratch or contact (95%).
- Healing primary lesion (papule, pustule, con-junctivitis) at site of inoculation.
- Regional lymphadenopathy.

- Aspiration of sterile pus from a node.
- Negative laboratory studies excluding other causes.
- Positive skin test.
- Biopsy of enlarged node showing histopathology consistent with cat scratch disease.

General Considerations

Cat scratch disease is a nonfatal infectious disease of uncertain cause, although the agent is now believed to belong to the chlamydia group, which includes also the agents of psittacosis, lymphogranuloma venereum, and trachoma. Stained sections of primary skin lesions and involved lymph nodes show large numbers of intracellular and extracellular granule-like elementary bodies similar to those seen in psittacosis. Herpes-like virus particles have been seen in cell cytoplasm in tissue taken from infected people. These viruses may be passengers and not etiologic agents. It is possible that more than one agent produces cat scratch disease.

The cat or kitten is merely the healthy carrier of the agent. Also implicated as the source of the scratch or bite are dogs, monkeys, thorns, codfish bones, and wooden splinters. The clinical picture is that of a regional lymphadenitis associated with a distal skin lesion without intervening lymphangitis. The disease occurs worldwide and is more common in the fall and winter.

Clinical Findings

A. Symptoms and Signs: About 50% of patients develop a primary lesion at the site of the scratch or inoculation. The lesion usually is a papule or pustule and is located most often on the arm or hand (50%), head or leg (30%), or trunk or neck (10%). The lesion may be conjunctival (10%). Symptoms are usually not manifest until regional lymphadenopathy accompanied by malaise, lassitude, headache, and fever develop, 10–30 days after the original inoculation. At that time there is some exacerbation of redness and swelling of the primary lesion, which is healing. Axillary, cervical, submental, preauricular, epitrochlear, inguinal, and femoral nodes are commonly involved. Multiple site involvement is seen in about 10% of cases. Involved nodes may be hard or soft and 1–6 cm in diameter. They are usually tender. About 25% of involved nodes suppurate. Overlying skin may or may not be inflamed. Lymphadenopathy may persist for 2 weeks to 8 months but usually lasts about 2 months.

Unusual clinical manifestations include exanthem with nonpruritic maculopapular rash, erythema multiforme or nodosum, or purpura; conjunctivitis with syndrome of Parinaud, parotid swelling, pneumonia, chronic sinus drainage, osteolytic lesions, mesenteric and mediastinal adenitis, and compression peripheral neuritis.

Encephalopathy, believed to represent a delayed hypersensitivity reaction, is unusual but may occur within 1–6 weeks of the onset of adenopathy. Manifestations include coma or convulsions, involvement of cord and nerve roots, lethargy or confusion, choreoathetosis, behavior disorders, and optic neuritis.

B. Laboratory Findings: Skin test antigens are prepared from materials aspirated from nodes of infected individuals. Antigens should be shown to be sterile. Lack of chemical standardization and antigenic variation among different lots of test material are obvious disadvantages. The test is performed by the intracutaneous injection of 0.1 ml of antigen. A positive reaction consists of 5 mm or more of induration or any degree of erythema at the injection site 48–72 hours later. A positive reaction indicates prior contact with the etiologic agent and is not necessarily diagnostic of the present illness. The skin test should be repeated in 1 month in a case where cat scratch disease is clinically suspected but the initial skin test is negative.

Histopathologic examination shows characteristic changes. The lymph node architecture is displaced by multiple areas of central necrosis showing acidophilic staining and surrounded by foci of epithelioid cells and scattered giant cells of the Langhans type. There is usually some elevation in the sedimentation rate. In cases with CNS involvement, the CSF is usually normal but may show a slight pleocytosis and modest elevation of protein.

Differential Diagnosis

Cat scratch disease must be distinguished from pyogenic adenitis, tuberculosis (typical and atypical), tularemia, plague, brucellosis, Hodgkin's disease, lymphoma, rat-bite fever, acquired toxoplasmosis, infectious mononucleosis, lymphogranuloma venereum, and fungal infections.

In the atypical forms of cat scratch disease such as encephalitis, rash, Parinaud's syndrome, parotid swelling, or purpura, the differential diagnosis includes the common causes of these manifestations.

Treatment

The best therapy is reassurance that the adenopathy is benign and will subside spontaneously within 4–8 weeks in most cases. Aspirin may be given for pain. In case of suppuration, node aspiration under local anesthesia with an 18 or 19 gauge needle relieves painful adenopathy within 24–48 hours. In the rare instance of compression peripheral neuritis, excision of the involved node is indicated. In encephalitis, corticotropin gel, 0.8 units/kg/day IM in divided doses every 12 hours for 2–3 weeks, is recommended in addition to supportive therapy.

Prognosis

The prognosis is uniformly good.

Carithers HA: Cat-scratch disease: Notes on its history. Am J Dis Child 119:200–203, 1970.

Hughes JH: Cat scratch disease: Report of a case presenting as an intra-oral mass. Ohio Med J 67:139–140, 1971.

Kalter SS, Kim CS, Heberling RL: Herpes-like virus particles associated with cat scratch disease. Nature 224:190, 1969.

Margileth AM: Cat scratch disease: Non-bacterial regional lymphadenitis. The study of 145 patients and a review of the literature. Pediatrics 42:803–818, 1968.

Sweeney VP, Drance SM: Optic neuritis and compressive neuropathy associated with cat scratch disease. Canad MAJ 103:1380–1381, 1970.

SPIROCHETAL INFECTIONS

SYPHILIS

Essentials of Diagnosis

- *Congenital:* In all types, there will be a history of untreated maternal syphilis, a positive serologic test, and positive darkfield examination.
- *Newborn:* Hepatosplenomegaly, characteristic x-ray bone changes, anemia, increased nucleated red cells, thrombocytopenia, abnormal spinal fluid, jaundice, edema.
- *Young infant (3–12 weeks):* Snuffles, maculopapular skin rash, mucocutaneous lesions, pseudoparalysis (in addition to x-ray bone changes).
- *Childhood:* Stigmas of early congenital syphilis (saddle nose, Hutchinson's teeth, etc), interstitial keratitis, saber shins, gummas of nose and palate.
- *Acquired:* Chancre of genitalia, lip, or anus in child or adolescent. History of sexual contact.

General Considerations

Syphilis is a chronic, generalized infectious disease caused by a slender spirochete, *Treponema pallidum.* In the acquired form, the disease is transmitted by sexual contact. Primary syphilis is characterized by the presence of an indurated chancre. A secondary eruption involving the skin and mucous membranes appears in 4–6 weeks. After a long latency period, late lesions of tertiary syphilis involve the eye, skin, bone, viscera, CNS, and cardiovascular system.

After a precipitous decline in incidence between 1947 and 1957, a great increase has been reported in adults, adolescents, and even young children.

Congenital syphilis results from transplacental infection after the fourth month of gestation and may result in stillbirth or manifest illness in the newborn, in early infancy, or later in childhood. Syphilis occurring in the newborn and young infant is comparable to secondary disease in the adult but is more severe and life-threatening. Late congenital syphilis (developing in childhood) is comparable to tertiary disease.

Clinical Findings

A. Symptoms and Signs:

1. Congenital syphilis—

a. Newborn—Jaundice, anemia with or without thrombocytopenia, increase in nucleated red blood cells, hepatosplenomegaly, and edema are seen. There may be overt signs of meningitis (bulging fontanel, opisthotonos), but CSF is more likely to be abnormal (increased protein, modest increase in cells). The majority of affected newborns show x-ray changes in the long bones.

b. Young infant (3–12 weeks)—The infant may appear normal for the first few weeks of life only to develop "snuffles," a syphilitic skin eruption, mucocutaneous lesions, and pseudoparalysis of the arms or legs. Shotty lymphadenopathy may sometimes be felt in addition to organomegaly. Other signs of disease seen in the newborn may be present. "Snuffles" (rhinitis) almost always appears and is characterized by a profuse mucopurulent discharge which excoriates the upper lip. A syphilitic rash is common on the palms and soles but may occur anywhere on the body; it consists of bright red, raised maculopapular lesions which gradually fade. Moist lesions occur at mucocutaneous junctions (nose, mouth, anus, genitalia) and lead to fissuring and bleeding.

Syphilis in the young infant may lead to stigmas recognizable in later childhood. Thus, such a child may have rhagades or scars around the mouth or nose, a "saddle" nose, and a high forehead (secondary to mild hydrocephalus associated with low-grade meningitis and frontal periostitis). The permanent upper central incisors may be peg-shaped with a central notch (Hutchinson's teeth), and the cusps of the sixth-year molars may have a lobulated mulberry appearance.

c. Childhood—Bilateral interstitial keratitis (6–12 years) is characterized by photophobia, increased lacrimation, and vascularization of the cornea associated with exudation. Chorioretinitis and optic atrophy may also be seen. Meningovascular syphilis (2–10 years) is usually slowly progressive, with mental retardation, spasticity, abnormal pupil response, speech defects, and abnormal spinal fluid. Deafness sometimes occurs. Thickening of the periosteum of the anterior tibias produces saber shins. A bilateral effusion into the knee joints (Clutton's joints) may occur but is not associated with sequelae. Gummas may develop in the nasal septum, palate, long bones, and subcutaneous tissues.

2. Acquired syphilis—The primary chancre of the genitals, mouth, or anus may occur as a result of intimate sexual contact. If the chancre is missed, signs of secondary syphilis may be the first manifestation of the disease.

B. Laboratory Diagnosis:

1. Darkfield microscopy—Treponemes can be seen in scrapings from a chancre and from moist lesions.

2. Serologic tests for syphilis (STS)—Routine tests include the following: quantitative VDRL (Venereal Disease Research Laboratory), quantitative Kolmer, etc, and the RPCF (Reiter's protein complement fixation). Infected newborns may have negative or low titers at birth. High cord blood titers may reflect passive transfer of antibodies. Elevated IgM (> 20 mg/100 ml) or IgA (> 10 mg/100 ml) strongly suggests prenatal infection. Rising titers usually occur within 4 months in infected infants. The VDRL or FTA-ABS test should be employed to screen umbilical cord or neonatal serum for serologic evidence of congenital syphilis, and the IgM FTA-ABS test is especially useful when production of intrauterine IgM antibody has already begun but VDRL and routine FTA-ABS antibody levels have not reached a sufficient magnitude in relation to maternal values to be of diagnostic significance.

C. X-Ray Findings: Osteochondritis and periostitis involve the long bones. Occasionally the phalanges and metatarsals are involved. Periostitis of the skull is seen. Bilateral symmetrical osteomyelitis with pathologic fractures of the medial tibial metaphyses (Wimberger's sign) is almost pathognomonic.

Differential Diagnosis

Syphilis is known as the "great imitator" among diseases and must be considered in the differential diagnosis of a wide variety of disorders.

Prevention

A serologic test for syphilis should be performed at the initiation of prenatal care and repeated once during pregnancy. Adequate treatment of mothers with secondary syphilis before the last month of the pregnancy will reduce the incidence of congenital syphilis from 90% to less than 2%. The serology of the father and siblings should also be checked.

Treatment

A. Specific Measures: Penicillin is the drug of choice against *T pallidum.* If the patient is allergic to penicillin, erythromycin or one of the tetracyclines may be used.

1. Congenital—Prompt treatment of the infant with penicillin is indicated if there is clinical or x-ray evidence of disease or the cord blood serology is positive and the mother has not been adequately treated. With equivocal findings, the infant may be given protective treatment or followed at monthly intervals with quantitative serologic tests and physical examinations. Rising titers or clinical signs usually occur within 4 months in infants with infection.

Newborns and infants should be treated with procaine penicillin G in a dosage of at least 100,000 units/kg/day IM for 8–10 days. Procaine penicillin G may be given once daily IM for 10 consecutive days: 150,000 units/day for children under 2 years of age, and 300,000 units/day for older children. Benzathine penicillin G may be given as a single IM dose of 100,000 units/kg. It may be necessary to repeat this dose in 1–2 weeks.

For interstitial keratitis, a topical corticosteroid (drops or ointment) should be applied to the affected eye at 2-hour intervals. Herpetic keratitis must be excluded before using topical corticosteroids. The pupil should be kept dilated with a mydriatic.

2. Acquired—1.2 million units of benzathine penicillin G is given IM in each buttock (total dose of 2.4 million units).

B. General Measures: Care should be given to the maintenance of adequate nutrition. Treatment of anemia with transfusion may be necessary before penicillin treatment to prevent a severe Herxheimer reaction.

Prognosis

Severe disease, if unexpected, may be fatal in the newborn. Complete cure can be expected if the young infant is treated with penicillin. Serologic reversal will usually occur within 1 year. Treatment of primary syphilis with penicillin is curative. Permanent neurologic sequelae may be seen with meningovascular syphilis.

Alford CA Jr & others: IgM-fluorescent treponemal antibody in the diagnosis of congenital syphilis. New England J Med 280:1086–1091, 1969.

Al-Salihi FL, Curran JP, Shteir OA: Occurrence of fetal syphilis after a nonreactive early gestational serologic test. J Pediat 78:121–123, 1971.

Bernfeld WK: Hutchinson's teeth and early treatment of congenital syphilis. Brit J Ven Dis 47:54–56, 1971.

Drucker MG, Mankin HJ: Congenital syphilis in 1970: A case report. Bull Hosp Joint Dis 31:132–140, 1970.

Fiumara NJ, Lessell S: Manifestations of late congenital syphilis. An analysis of 271 patients. Arch Dermat 102:78–83, 1970.

Kraus SJ, Haserick JR, Lantz MA: Fluorescent treponemal antibody-absorption test reactions in lupus erythematosis: Atypical beading pattern and probable false-positive reactions. New England J Med 282:1287–1290, 1970.

Lee RV, Thornton GF, Conn HO: Liver disease associated with secondary syphilis. New England J Med 284:1423–1425, 1971.

Naeye RL: Fetal growth with congenital syphilis: A quantitative study. Am J Clin Path 55:228–231, 1971.

Sparling PF: Diagnosis and treatment of syphilis. New England J Med 284:642–653, 1971.

Wilkinson RH, Heller RM: Congenital syphilis: Resurgence of an old problem. Pediatrics 47:27–30, 1971.

ENDEMIC SYPHILIS
(Bejel, Skerljevo, Etc)

Endemic syphilis is an acute and chronic infection caused by an organism morphologically indistinguishable from *Treponema pallidum;* it is distinguished from sporadic syphilis by its occurrence in children in crowded, poor households in particular localities, by virtual absence of primary lesions, and the predilection of secondary lesions for oral and nasopharyngeal mucosa as well (in places) as the soles (plantar hyperkeratosis). It is distinguished from yaws by its occurrence in areas in which yaws is not endemic and by the absence of primary lesions and the presence of buccal lesions. It may be confused with angular stomatitis due to vitamin deficiency. It has been reported in a number of countries, including Latin America, often with local names: bejel in Syria and Iraq; skerljevo in Bosnia; dichuchwa, njovera, and siti in Africa. Each has local distinctive characteristics.

Secondary oral lesions are the most common manifestations. Generalized lymphadenopathy and secondary and tertiary bone lesions are common in bejel. Secondary lesions tend to heal in about a year.

Laboratory findings and treatment are the same as for primary syphilis.

Guthe T, Luger A: The control of endemic syphilis of childhood. Dermat Int 5:179–199, 1966.

International work in endemic treponematoses and venereal infections, 1948–1963: Endemic treponematoses of childhood. WHO Chronicle 18:403–417, 1964.

PINTA
(Carate)

Pinta is a nonvenereal spirochetal infection caused by *Treponema carateum.* It occurs endemically in rural areas of Latin America, especially in Mexico, Colombia, and Cuba; the Philippines; and some areas of the Pacific. A nonulcerative, erythematous primary papule spreads slowly into a papulosquamous plaque showing a variety of color changes (slate, lilac, black). Secondary lesions resemble the primary one and appear within a year after it. These appear successively, new lesions together with older ones. They are commonest on the extremities, but may cover most of the body. Mild local lymphadenopathy is common. Atrophy and depigmentation occur later. Some cases show pigment changes and atrophic patches on the soles and palms, with or without hyperkeratosis, which are indistinguishable from "crab yaws."

Diagnosis and treatment are the same as for primary syphilis.

Kuhn VSG & others: Inoculation pinta in chimpanzees. Brit J Ven Dis 46:311–312, 1970.

Mikhail GR, Tanay A: Pinta or pinta-like syphiloderm? Dermat Trop 3:131–135, 1964.

Padillia-Goncalves A: Immunologic aspects of pinta. Dermatologica 135:199–204, 1967.

Pardo-Castello V: Dermatoses of the Americas. Dermat Trop 2:232–237, 1963.

Rodriguez HA & others: Langerhans' cells in late pinta: Ultrastructural observations in one case. Arch Path 91:302–306, 1971.

YAWS
(Pian, Frambesia)

Yaws is a contagious disease largely limited to tropical regions which is produced by *Treponema pertenue.* It is characterized by granulomatous lesions of the skin, mucous membranes, and bone. Yaws is rarely fatal, although if untreated it may lead to chronic disability and disfigurement. Yaws is acquired by direct nonvenereal contact. The disease is usually acquired in childhood, although it may occur at any age. The "mother yaw," a painless papule which later ulcerates, appears 3–4 weeks after exposure. There is usually associated regional lymphadenopathy. Six to 12 weeks later, similar secondary lesions appear and last for several months or years. Late gummatous lesions may follow, with associated tissue destruction and alterations involving large areas of skin and subcutaneous tissues. The late effects of yaws, with bone change, shortening of digits, and contractions, may be confused with similar changes occurring in leprosy. CNS, cardiac, or other visceral involvement is rare. The Wassermann and flocculation tests are positive, and the spirochetes may be demonstrated by darkfield examination.

Cleanliness of lesions is very important in treatment. Specific measures consist of giving one of the following: (1) procaine penicillin G, 300,000 units IM daily for 7–10 days; (2) one of the tetracyclines, 0.5 gm orally every 6 hours for 10 days; or (3) dichlorophenarsine (Chlorarsen), 40 mg IV weekly for 3–6 weeks.

Browne SG: Contractures of the fingers associated with framboesial palmar hyperkeratosis. Dermat Int 7:104–108, 1968.

Cahill KM: Tropical medicine for temperate climates: Treponematosis and rickettsiosis. New York J Med 64:647–650, 1964.

Fluker JL, Hewitt AB: Late yaws. Brit J Ven Dis 46:264, 1970.

Garner MF, Blackhouse JL, Tibbs GJ: Yaws in an isolated Australian aboriginal population. Bull World Health Organ 43:603–606, 1970.

Taneja BL: Yaws: Clinical manifestations and criteria for diagnosis. Internat J Med Res 56:100–113, 1968.

RELAPSING FEVER

Relapsing fever is the name of a group of clinically similar acute infectious diseases caused by several different species of spirochetes of the genus Borrelia. The disease is transmitted to man by insect vectors (head and body lice and ticks). The insect is infected by feeding on human acute cases (lice) or the animal reservoir (ticks), and transmits the disease to humans when insect feces or crushed insects are rubbed into the bite puncture wound, excoriated areas of skin, or the eyes. The disease is endemic in various parts of the world, including western USA. The incubation period is 2–15 days (average about 7 days).

Clinical Findings

A. Symptoms and Signs: The disease is characterized by relapses occurring at intervals of 1–2 weeks after the preceding episode with an interim asymptomatic period. The relapses duplicate the initial attack but become progressively less severe. Recovery occurs after 2–10 relapses.

The attack is of sudden onset with fever, chills, tachycardia, nausea and vomiting, myalgia, arthralgia, bronchitis, and a dry, nonproductive cough. Hepatomegaly and splenomegaly appear later. Jaundice may be present. An erythematous rash appears early in the course of the disease over the trunk and extremities, followed later by rose-colored spots in the same area. Petechiae may also be present. In severe cases, neurologic and psychic manifestations are present. After 3–10 days, the fever falls by crisis. Jaundice, iritis, conjunctivitis, cranial nerve lesions, and uterine hemorrhage are more common in the relapses.

B. Laboratory Findings: During the acute episodes, the urine shows protein, casts, and occasionally erythrocytes; the blood shows a marked polymorphonuclear leukocytosis and, in about 1/4 of cases, a false-positive serologic test for syphilis. During the paroxysm, spirochetes may be found in the patient's blood on darkfield examination or on a blood smear stained with Wright's or Giemsa's stain; or the blood may be injected into a rat and the spirochetes found 3–5 days later in the tail blood. The Weil-Felix test may be positive in a titer of 1:80 or more.

Differential Diagnosis

The late manifestations of relapsing fever may be confused with those of malaria, leptospirosis, dengue, yellow fever, and typhus.

Complications

Facial paralysis, eye diseases such as iridocyclitis, vitreous opacities, and optic atrophy, and possibly hypochromic anemia.

Treatment

Treatment either with (1) tetracycline drugs, 0.5 gm orally every 6 hours for 7 days; or (2) aqueous penicillin, 50,000 units IM every 3 hours, or procaine penicillin G, 300,000 units IM daily for 10 days. Chloramphenicol is often of value.

The more severely ill patients should be hospitalized and should receive intensive care during and after reaction to treatment. Antibiotic treatment should be started at the beginning of a paroxysm or after the fever has dropped in order to avoid a "Jarisch-Herxheimer" reaction, which can be dramatic and even fatal. This reaction is probably due to released endogenous pyrogen. Some severely ill patients have died within hours of an intravenous dose of tetracycline or penicillin.

Prognosis

The overall mortality rate is usually about 5%. Fatalities are most common in debilitated or very young children. With treatment, the initial attack is shortened and relapses largely prevented.

Bryceson ADM & others: Louse-borne relapsing fever: A clinical and laboratory study of 62 cases in Ethiopia and a reconsideration of the literature. Quart J Med 39:129–170, 1970.

Goodman RL, Arndt KA, Steigbigel NH: Borrelia in Boston. JAMA 210:722–724, 1969.

Parry EHO & others: Some effects of louse-borne relapsing fever on the function of the heart. Am J Med 49:472–479, 1970.

Smith L, Brown TG: Relapsing fever: A case history. California Med 110:322–324, 1969.

Thompson RS & others: Outbreak of tick-borne relapsing fever in Spokane County, Washington. JAMA 210:1045–1050, 1969.

RAT-BITE FEVER
(Sodoku)

Rat-bite fever is an acute infectious disease caused by *Spirillum minus* and transmitted to man by the bite of a rat. The organism gains entry into the rat's oral cavity from the drainage of a primary eye infection. The incubation period is 5–28 days.

Clinical Findings

A. Symptoms and Signs: The original rat bite, unless infected by other organisms, heals promptly, only to be followed after the incubation period by a flare-up at the original site. The area of the rat bite then becomes swollen, indurated, and painful, assumes a dusky purplish hue, and may ulcerate. Regional lymphangitis and lymphadenitis, fever, chills, malaise, myalgia, arthralgia, and headache are present. Splenomegaly may occur. A dusky red, sparse maculopapular rash appears on the trunk and extremities.

After a few days, both the local and systemic symptoms subside, only to reappear again in a few days. This relapsing pattern of fever of 24–48 hours alternating with an equal afebrile period becomes established and may persist for weeks. The local and systemic findings, however—including the rash—usually recur only during the first few relapses.

B. Laboratory Findings: Leukocytosis is often present, and a blood STS may be falsely positive. The organism may be identified by darkfield examination of the ulcer exudate or aspirated lymph node material or by animal inoculation of exudate or blood. The organism cannot be cultured in artificial media.

Differential Diagnosis

In case of a rat bite, the chief problem is distinguishing between infection with *S minus* and *Streptobacillus moniliformis*. *S moniliformis* is characterized by a short incubation period (usually less than 10 days), lack of flare-up of the primary lesion at the onset of systemic symptoms, a high incidence of arthritis (50%), and a low incidence of false-positive STS (15%). This organism can usually be isolated from blood, joint fluid, or pus. Agglutinins against the organism develop during the second or third week of illness. A prolonged incubation period, relapsing instead of sustained fever, and few or no manifestations of arthritis suggest *S minus* infection.

Rat-bite fever may also need to be distinguished from tularemia, relapsing fever, malaria, and chronic meningococcemia.

Treatment

Treat with aqueous penicillin, 100,000 units every 3 hours IM; procaine penicillin G, 300,000 units IM every 12 hours; or tetracycline drugs, 0.5 gm orally every 6 hours for 7 days. Give supportive and symptomatic measures as indicated.

Prognosis

The reported mortality rate is about 10%, but this should be markedly reduced by prompt diagnosis and treatment.

Arkless HA: Rat-bite fever at Albert Einstein's Medical Center. Penn Med 73:49, 1970.

Cale JS, Stell RW, Bulger RJ: Rat-bite fever: Report of three cases. Ann Int Med 71:979–981, 1969.

Farquahar JW, Edmunds PN, Tilley JB: Sodoku in a child. Lancet 2:1211, 1958.

Pardo-Castello V: Dermatoses of the Americas. Dermat Trop 2:232–237, 1963.

LEPTOSPIROSIS

Essentials of Diagnosis

- Biphasic course lasting 2 or 3 weeks.
- Initial phase characterized by high fever, headache, myalgia, and conjunctival injection.
- Apparent recovery for a few days.
- Return of fever associated with meningitis.
- Jaundice, hemorrhages, and renal insufficiency (severe cases).
- Culture of organism from blood and CSF (early) and from urine (later).
- Positive leptospiral agglutination test during convalescence.

General Considerations

Leptospirosis is due to *Leptospira icterohaemorrhagiae*. The rat is the principal host. At present, about 130 known serotypes have been reported. Infection occurs in a variety of wild mammals in addition to rodents, and domestic animals are an important source for the spread of infection. Infected animals (particu-larly rodents) are rarely symptomatic, but shed leptospira localized in the convoluted tubules of the kidney into the urine for months or years. The organism remains viable in damp soil or water for as long as 6 weeks. It usually enters the human body through abraded skin and intact mucous membranes, particularly the conjunctivas.

Human infection is widespread in the USA, occurring principally as sporadic cases but occasionally in outbreaks. Serologic surveys suggest that inapparent infection may not be uncommon. Many of the reported cases are relatively mild and anicteric. The most important serotypes are *L icterohaemorrhagiae, L canicola,* and *L pomona.* Infection with *L icterohaemorrhagiae* often occurs after immersion in water contaminated with rat urine. *L canicola* infections more commonly occur in the home and are associated with exposure to dogs. *L pomona* infections occur on the farm in association with cattle and swine. The incubation period is 7–12 days. Cases have been reported in young children, but the disease is more common among teenagers.

Clinical Findings

A. Symptoms and Signs:

1. Initial phase—Chills, fever, headache, myalgia, and conjunctivitis (episcleral injection) occur commonly. This phase lasts for a few days up to 1 week.

2. Phase of apparent recovery—Symptoms typically subside for 2–3 days, but this does not always occur.

3. Systemic phase—Fever reappears, completing the "saddleback" temperature curve, and is associated with muscular pain and tenderness in the abdomen and back, nausea and vomiting, and headache. Signs of lung, heart, and joint involvement are occasionally seen.

a. CNS—The CNS is the organ system most commonly involved. Mild nuchal rigidity is usual, but delirium, coma, and focal neurologic signs may be seen.

b. Renal and hepatic—In about 50% of cases, either or both organs become involved early in the illness. Gross hematuria and oliguria or anuria are sometimes seen. Dysuria is not prominent. Jaundice may be associated with an enlarged and tender liver.

c. Hemorrhage—Petechiae, ecchymoses, and gastrointestinal bleeding may be severe.

B. Laboratory Findings: Leptospires may be grown from the blood and CSF early in the illness on Fletcher's semisolid medium. Identification by dark-field examination is not reliable. Organisms are present in the urine beginning in the second week. The white count may be normal but is more likely to show leukocytosis with liver involvement. Serum bilirubin levels, when elevated, usually remain below 20 mg/100 ml but may go higher. Other liver function tests may be abnormal, although the SGOT usually shows only slight elevation. CSF shows a moderate elevation of cells ($<$ 500) and protein (50–100 mg/100 ml), but CSF glucose is normal. Urine often shows microscopic pyuria, hematuria, and, less often, proteinuria (++ or greater). BUN is usually below 100 mg/100 ml. The ESR is usually markedly elevated. With lung involvement, chest x-ray may show pneumonitis. EEG and ECG occasionally show abnormal tracings.

Microscopic and macroscopic agglutination tests are the most basic and widely used serologic tests for the diagnosis of leptospiral disease. Titers become elevated during the second or third week of illness.

Differential Diagnosis

Fever and myalgia associated with the characteristic conjunctival (episcleral) injection should suggest leptospirosis early in the illness. During the prodrome, causes of fever and general myalgia such as malaria, typhoid fever, typhus, rheumatoid arthritis, brucellosis, and influenza may be suspected. Depending upon the organ systems involved, a variety of other diseases need to be distinguished, including aseptic meningitis of viral or tuberculous origin, encephalitis, poliomyelitis, polyneuritis, viral hepatitis, glomerulonephritis, viral or bacterial pneumonia, rheumatic fever, and acute surgical abdomen.

Prevention

Preventive measures include avoidance and treatment of contaminated water and soil, rodent control, vaccination of dogs and other domestic animals, and good sanitation.

With known exposure, give procaine penicillin G, 50,000 units/kg/day IM for 7 days.

Treatment

A. Specific Measures: The efficacy of specific antibiotic treatment has not been clearly established. Treatment within the first 4 days of illness (prodrome) reduces the severity of the disease but has little effect if started later. Give procaine penicillin G, 50,000 units/kg/day IM in 4 divided doses. Continue treatment for 7–10 days. A predictable increase in fever and other signs and symptoms occurs in the majority of patients after the initiation of penicillin treatment.

Tetracyclines may be used as an alternative to penicillin. Give 20 mg/kg/day orally in 4 divided doses.

B. General Measures: Symptomatic and supportive care is indicated, particularly for renal and hepatic failure and hemorrhage.

Prognosis

In the vast majority of cases, leptospirosis is anicteric and recovery is complete. The disease usually lasts 1–3 weeks, but the course may be prolonged. Relapse may occur.

There are usually no permanent sequelae associated with CNS infection. The mortality rate may reach 20% or more in patients who have severe kidney and hepatic involvement.

Allen GL, Weber DR, Russell PK: The clinical picture of leptospirosis in American soldiers in Vietnam. Mil Med 133:275–280, 1968.

Hubbert WT, Humphrey GL: Epidemiology of leptospirosis in California: A cause of aseptic meningitis. California Med 108:113–117, 1968.

Poh SC, Soh CS: Lung manifestations in leptospirosis. Thorax 25:751–755, 1970.

Problems in leptospirosis. WHO Chronicle 22:159–160, 1968.

Turner LH: Leptospirosis. Brit MJ 1:231–235, 1969.

Zack MD, Barr AB, Sinally NP: Leptospirosis in city slum: Clinical and epidemiologic aspects. New York J Med 71:880–883, 1971.

● ● ●

General References

Committee on Infectious Diseases: *Report,* 16th ed. American Academy of Pediatrics, 1970.

Eickhoff TC: Surveillance of nosocomial infections in community hospitals. J Infect Dis 120:305, 1969.

Gotoff SP, Behrman RE: Neonatal septicemia. J Pediat 76:142, 1970.

Jawetz E, Melnick JL, Adelberg EA: *Review of Medical Microbiology,* 10th ed. Lange, 1972.

Krugman S, Ward R: *Infectious Diseases of Children,* 4th ed. Mosby, 1968.

28...

Infections: Parasitic

Jacob T. John, MD

PROTOZOAL INFECTIONS

MALARIA

Essentials of Diagnosis

- Fever—often, but not always, paroxysmal and with chills, rigors, and sweating.
- Splenomegaly and anemia, especially in chronic stage.
- Severe headache, delirium, coma, convulsions, gastrointestinal disorders, and jaundice.
- Malarial parasites in blood smears (extremely rare in newborn babies of mothers from endemic areas).

General Considerations

Despite all eradication campaigns, approximately 25 million people a year still contract malaria. Malaria is the leading cause of death in childhood where it is still prevalent.

Four species of parasites infect man: *Plasmodium vivax, P falciparum, P malariae,* and *P ovale* (in declining order of frequency). Various species of female anopheline mosquitoes act as vectors. Male and female gametocytes ingested by the mosquito fertilize and develop into sporozoites which are injected into fresh hosts. They develop in the reticuloendothelial cells of the liver (pre-erythrocytic cycle), resulting in the release of merozoites into the circulation. Those that escape phagocytization infect red blood cells, mature, and divide into merozoites which are released when the erythrocytes rupture (erythrocytic cycle, schizogony). These merozoites may infect fresh red cells and repeat the erythrocytic cycle, or they may infect and develop in liver cells (exo-erythrocytic cycle). A few merozoites develop into gametocytes. In time the erythrocytic cycles dwindle and disappear, and the exo-erythrocytic cycle forms the source for new erythrocytic cycles, causing relapses.

Because falciparum malaria has no exo-erythrocytic cycle, relapses after long intervals do not occur.

Malarial infections constitute an intense form of antigenic stimulation leading to the production of antimalarial antibodies detectable by various technics. Susceptibility to malarial infection varies in different populations, and some individual genes confer some degree of natural immunity (eg, hemoglobin S, hemoglobin F, glucose-6-phosphate dehydrogenase deficiency, thalassemia). Natural immunity is easily overcome by the sporozoites, but clinical manifestation of the disease is delayed and modified until acquired immunity is achieved.

Active infection results in partial immunity involving primarily cellular rather than humoral defenses. Passive immunity is possibly acquired by the newborn via placental antibody transfer. Congenital malaria is relatively common in babies born to nonimmune but infected mothers but is rare in babies of immune mothers despite heavy placental infestations with *P falciparum.*

Transfusion malaria must be considered in nonmalarial areas when the clinical syndrome with fever occurs in a patient who has received blood.

Clinical Findings

A. Symptoms and Signs: The clinical manifestations vary to some degree according to the species of parasite. Minor variations also occur between strains of the same species. On first exposure, the incubation period is 2 weeks for vivax, falciparum, and ovale malaria and about 3—5 weeks for quartan (malariae) malaria. Initially, intermittent or continuous fever occurs and lasts for a variable period. The fever may disappear, only to appear in further episodes. Periodicity characteristic of the species may become established in first or subsequent attacks. In vivax (benign tertian), falciparum (malignant tertian), or ovale malaria, fever occurs on alternate days. In the quartan type, the day of fever is followed by 2 afebrile days. Fever that occurs every day is called quotidian. Considerable variation in the above periodicities occurs as a result of "broods" of the same species or mixed infection. Each paroxysm consists of chills lasting up to 1 hour accompanied by headache, back and muscle pains, and nausea and vomiting; rapid elevation of temperature lasting for several hours accompanied by prostration; and then remission with intense perspiration. These paroxysms coincide with the periodicity of the erythrocytic cycle of the parasites, which for unknown reasons develops a curious synchrony. Thus, in its classical form, malaria is manifested as remissions and relapses of paroxysmal fever.

Between attacks, the child may feel well or ill. The spleen gradually becomes palpable and continues to enlarge. Rapid splenic enlargement may cause pain.

Herpetic lesions may appear on the lips. Anemia and slight jaundice may become manifest. In the absence of reinfections and complications, the relapses die down in less than a year for falciparum malaria and in a few years for vivax. Quartan malaria may remain dormant or "cryptic" for years or decades and then reappear.

B. Laboratory Findings: The most important part of the investigation is thick and thin blood smears, the former for screening and the latter for detailed study. The parasites seen in blood smears are trophozoites, schizonts, and gametocytes.

Serologic methods, including complement fixation and flocculation tests, are occasionally used but are of limited value.

Other laboratory findings include low red and white cell counts, increased unconjugated blood bilirubin, and increased serum gamma globulin.

Differential Diagnosis

Malaria must often be differentiated from tuberculosis, typhoid, and other febrile illnesses, especially recurrent ones such as brucellosis, rat-bite fever, relapsing fever, febrile episodes of lymphoreticular diseases, urinary tract infections, and periodic fevers. Malaria may coexist with other diseases or may be present in unusual circumstances such as undiagnosed postoperative fever. The various complications of *P falciparum* infection are a diagnostic challenge.

Complications & Sequelae

Apart from malignant tertian malaria, the other forms of malaria are relatively free from complications. Chronic malaria may result in anemia and debility. An enlarged spleen may rupture on trivial trauma. Red cells infected with *P falciparum* trophozoites have a tendency to adhere to blood vessels, and in certain viscera infected red cells and the population of parasites increase in a vicious cycle, causing obstruction and anoxic necrosis which may result in enteritis with gastrointestinal bleeding, interstitial pneumonia, and "encephalitis" (commonly called cerebral malaria).

Severe intravascular hemolysis resulting in hemoglobinuria and shock (blackwater fever) occurs rarely in falciparum malaria. The mortality rate is very high in cerebral malaria and in blackwater fever. Blackwater fever was very common in the past when quinine was widely used as a therapeutic agent.

Severe hemolytic reactions, which may be fatal, occur in Negro patients who have erythrocyte deficiency of glucose-6-phosphate dehydrogenase and are given full doses of primaquine. Where the condition is suspected, 1/8 of the recommended dose is given to start and very gradually increased.

The nephrotic syndrome is seen as a complication of *P malariae.* Massive splenomegaly may lead to hypersplenism with anemia. Serologic tests for syphilis may be falsely positive.

Heavy placental infection with the malarial parasite in the pregnant woman interferes with the growth of the fetus and is a common cause of low birth weight.

Prevention

Widespread prophylaxis may not be justified in malarial areas with immune populations of children because later withdrawal of prophylaxis leaves the child highly susceptible to severe disease. However, for nonimmune children living in endemic areas and therefore constantly at risk of infection or reinfection, the best procedure is prophylaxis. Since true prophylaxis (prevention of infection by the destruction of sporozoites) is unavailable, a drug is given that suppresses schizogony and clinical symptoms. The most commonly used suppressive drug is chloroquine, given as follows (dosage expressed as portions of a 250 mg tablet): up to age 1 year, ¼ tablet per week; age 1–3 years, ½ tablet per week; age 7–10 years, ¾ tablet per week; age 11–16 years, 1 tablet per week; over age 16 years, 2 tablets per week. Other suppressive drugs include chloroguanide (proguanil, Paludrine), 2–3 mg/kg/day; amodiaquine (Camoquin), 7.5 mg/kg/week; and pyrimethamine (Daraprim), 0.5 mg/kg/week. If the suppressive drug is taken for about 4–6 weeks after a person leaves the endemic area, falciparum malaria usually does not become manifest but the others may because of the uncontrolled exoerythrocytic cycle. To avoid this, a course of primaquine may be given as described below.

Because malaria parasites may become resistant to all the suppressive drugs, it is recommended that chloroquine be reserved for treatment and not used for suppression. A new drug, cycloguanil pamoate (Camolar), given intramuscularly, protects for up to a year. If initial results are authenticated and the drug is found to be suitable for wide use, it holds great promise.

Since most malarial vectors are night biters, the use of mosquito nets to sleep in and mosquito repellents are important preventive measures. However, prevention of malaria ultimately depends upon mosquito control.

Treatment

Any fever of high and intermittent nature in a malaria-endemic area must be presumed to be malaria until proved otherwise and treated as such.

A. Specific Measures: In a child with malaria, the first aim of treatment is to terminate the paroxysms with drugs that act on the erythrocytic cycle, ie, chloroquine (Aralen) or quinine. Primaquine may also be used in conjunction with chloroquine to prevent relapses in vivax infections.

1. Chloroquine diphosphate (Aralen)—Given once daily orally for 4 days, this is the drug of choice for *P vivax* and *P falciparum* infections, which it completely eradicates. Toxic symptoms include nausea, vomiting, and diarrhea. The dosage is as follows:

a. Give 10 mg/kg as initial dose, followed by 5 mg/kg twice daily for 2 days.

b. If oral therapy is not possible, give chloroquine hydrochloride, 2 mg/kg IM or IV stat and the same dosage once each day.

2. Quinine—In chloroquine-resistant falciparum infection, fever persists over 48 hours. Change treatment to quinine.

a. Quinine sulfate, 0.6 gm 3 times daily orally for 5–7 days.

b. Quinine dihydrochloride, 0.5 gm IV diluted in 100 ml or more of physiologic saline solution. Give slowly. Use only for patients unable to take oral medication. Follow with oral medication. *Caution:* A very dangerous drug.

3. Primaquine phosphate—A drug used in combination with chloroquine in *P vivax* infections only. It is reported to eradicate the infection and prevent relapses. *Caution:* Primaquine is a toxic drug and must be used with careful laboratory follow-up. Never use in Negroes. If anemia, leukopenia, or methemoglobinemia appears, discontinue drug immediately. Never use with quinacrine or within 5 days of quinacrine therapy.

Give orally once daily for 14 days as follows: up to 15 lb, 2 mg; 15–40 lb, 4 mg; 40–80 lb, 6 mg; 80–120 lb, 10 mg; over 120 lb, 20 mg.

B. General Measures: Fluid therapy is most important. Urge oral intake and, if not satisfactory, give parenteral fluids. Control high fever and treat anemia with iron.

Prognosis

In the majority of cases, the prognosis with proper therapy is excellent. In small infants and in the presence of malnutrition or chronic debilitating disease, the prognosis is more guarded.

Collins WE & others: Fluorescent antibody studies in human and Simian malaria. Am J Trop Med 15:11, 1966.

Gilles HM, Hendrickse RG: Nephrosis in Nigerian children: Role of *Plasmodium malariae* and effect of antimalarial treatment. Brit MJ 2:27, 1963.

Kruatrachue M, Klongrumnuanhara K, Harinasuta C: Infection rates of malarial parasites in red blood cells with normal and deficient glucose-6-phosphate dehydrogenase. Lancet 1:404, 1966.

Powell RD, Brewer GJ: Glucose-6-phosphate dehydrogenase deficiency and falciparum malaria. Am J Trop Med 14:358, 1965.

Shute PG: Some observations on malaria in children returning from holidays in the tropics. Lancet 2:1232, 1965.

WHO Expert Committee on Malaria: *Twelfth Report.* Pages 21–27. Technical Report Series No. 324. World Health Organization, 1965.

Ziai M & others: Malaria prophylaxis and treatment in G-6-PD deficiency: An observation on the toxicity of primaquine and chloroquine. Clin Pediat 6:243, 1967.

AMEBIASIS

Essentials of Diagnosis

- Acute dysentery: Evidence of colitis, ie, diarrhea with blood and mucus, pain, and tenderness.

- Chronic dysentery: Recurrent symptoms of diarrhea and abdominal pain.
- Hepatic amebiasis: Enlarged and tender liver.
- Amebic abscess: Reddish-brown pus.
- Amebas or cysts in stools or abscesses.

General Considerations

Amebiasis in children is a common and serious problem in some tropical countries but is rare where sanitation is good. Infants and children of all ages may be infected, and the younger the patient the greater the chance that infection has been acquired within the family.

The trophozoites (vegetative forms of *Entamoeba histolytica*) invade tissues, and the cysts survive outside the host and infect others. Infection occurs by ingestion of the cysts. The question of pathogenicity of strain variants and other species of amebas is controversial. *Entamoeba coli* is nonpathogenic.

Infection by *E histolytica* does not always cause disease. Asymptomatic carriers often pass cysts and, rarely, vegetative forms.

Clinical Findings

A. Symptoms and Signs: The symptoms of amebic dysentery vary greatly .in severity. Typically there is diarrhea with several small stools, not too foul-smelling, with clear mucus and a variable amount of blood. The onset may or may not be sudden. Fever is variable and not usually high. Older children may complain of abdominal pain, either localized over the cecum or sigmoid or generalized. In severe cases, dehydration and prostration may supervene.

Symptoms in chronic intestinal amebiasis also vary greatly in severity. Recurrent complaints of changing bowel habits, abdominal pain, and tenderness over the colon are usual. Chronic dysentery may or may not be preceded by an acute attack. Amebomas are rare in children.

B. Laboratory Findings: The most important investigation is that of satisfactory stool specimens. In acute dysentery, a fresh fecal sample is mounted in warm saline on a warm slide and examined under the microscope. The trophozoites are distinguished by their ameboid movement, size (50–60 μm), a clear ectoplasm, and ingested red cells. In acute dysentery in children, sigmoidoscopy is not usually recommended. It may be done, however, for obtaining ulcer scrapings to look for amebas. Characteristically, the mucosa looks inflamed, with shallow ulcers scattered over otherwise intact mucosa.

In suspected chronic amebiasis, stools are examined for cysts. They are round or oval, with a diameter 1–2½ times that of a red cell. Immature cysts contain 1–2 nuclei, and often 2 chromatoid bodies. More mature cysts contain 4 nuclei and no chromatoid bodies. Staining with Lugol's iodine brings the above features into prominence. If necessary, the stools may be collected after a saline purge.

Other laboratory technics such as cultivation of amebas and serology (complement fixation, hemagglutination, ameba immobilization, and gel diffusion tests) are of limited value at present. Barium enema helps in the differentiation of chronic dysentery from other colonic lesions.

Moderate leukocytosis may be present.

Differential Diagnosis

Acute bacillary dysentery has a more explosive onset and foul-smelling diarrhea, often with blood and mucus. Fever and leukocytosis are often high. A smear of feces reveals the presence of large numbers of pus cells and bacteria. The final proof is the cultural demonstration of pathogenic bacteria and the absence of amebas.

Other causes of bloody stools such as polyps, anaphylactoid purpura, and nonspecific ulcerative colitis must be differentiated from amebiasis. Schistosomiasis, balantidiasis, regional enteritis, and tuberculous enteritis must be distinguished from acute or chronic amebiasis.

Other causes of chronic and recurrent diarrhea also need to be considered, eg, sprue and malabsorption syndromes.

Complications & Sequelae

Complications may be generally classified as alimentary or extra-alimentary. Acute dysentery may result in perforation of the bowel and peritonitis. Granulomatous proliferations (ameboma) are extremely rare in children.

Amebic hepatitis following amebic colitis consists of hepatic enlargement and tenderness in the absence of demonstrable abscesses. Liver function tests may be slightly abnormal.

Amebic liver abscess is usually solitary and in the right lobe. Fever, chills, hepatic enlargement, and tenderness are usually present, but may be absent in debilitated children. Rarely, such abscesses rupture into the peritoneum, pleura, lungs, or pericardium. Metastatic abscesses may occur in the lungs, brain, or spleen. Cutaneous and genital lesions are extremely rare.

Treatment

A. Medical Treatment: Several antiamebic drugs are available, and no one drug can be expected to eradicate all infections. The choice of drugs varies with the severity, chronicity, and site of infection.

1. Amebic dysentery—In severe amebic dysentery, emetine hydrochloride (1 mg/kg/day or as follows: up to 3 years, 10 mg/day; 3–6 years, 20 mg/day) is given by deep subcutaneous or intramuscular injection for 3–5 days. Dehydroemetine, 1 mg/kg/day IM for 5–8 days, appears to be less toxic and therefore preferable. The relapse rate is often high, and so treatment with emetine should be followed by a course of diloxanide (Entamide) furoate, 20 mg/kg orally for 10 days. Metronidazole (Flagyl) is also now established as a useful amebicidal drug.

Tetracyclines, erythromycin, or paromomycin (Humatin) in pediatric doses may be given for 7–10 days, starting with or following emetine or dehydroemetine. Paromomycin may be given in a dosage of 25 mg/kg orally in 3 divided daily doses. Combined therapy effectively controls the acute symptoms.

After the acute symptoms are controlled, diiodohydroxyquin (Diodoquin) for 3 weeks or glycobiarsol (Milibis) or carbarsone for 7–10 days should be given to ensure the eradication of infection. Diiodohydroxyquin, 40 mg/kg, or carbarsone, 10 mg/kg, may be given orally in 2–3 divided doses each day. Children under 6 years of age may be given 250 mg and older children 500 mg of glycobiarsol orally each day.

2. Amebic hepatitis—In amebic hepatitis (and suspected liver abscess), emetine or preferably dehydroemetine should be given as described above, accompanied by chloroquine phosphate (Aralen), 10 mg/kg orally twice daily for 2 days and then once daily for 19 days. Abscesses threatening to rupture should be aspirated with a needle. The liver may be needled with suitable precautions to confirm a diagnosis of abscess. Opinions vary regarding aspiration as a therapeutic measure in all liver abscesses. It is advisable to treat as outlined above to eradicate chronic infection.

3. Chronic amebiasis—Chronic intestinal infection is occasionally difficult to eradicate. Diiodohydroxyquin (Diodoquin), glycobiarsol (Milibis), or carbarsone may be given as described above. Diloxanide furoate (Furamide), 15–20 mg/kg orally for 10 days, may suffice to eradicate infection. However, it is better to combine 2 drugs for higher cure rates.

In cases of extra-abdominal amebiasis with pus, vigorous antiamebic therapy combined with surgical drainage may be required.

B. Follow-Up Care: A diligent examination of several (at least 3) samples of feces should be done to make sure that infection has been eradicated in all treated cases.

Prognosis

With prompt diagnosis and adequate treatment, if complications can be avoided, the prognosis is good. In ruptured liver abscesses and in brain abscesses, the prognosis is poor.

Ninochiri E: Observations on childhood amoebiasis in urban family units in Nigeria. J Trop Med 68:231–236, 1965.

Olatunbosum DA: Amoebiasis and its complications in Nigerian children (a necropsy survey). Tr Roy Soc Trop Med Hyg 59:72–79, 1965.

Salem HH, Abd-Rabbo H: Dehydroemetine in acute amoebiasis. Tr Roy Soc Trop Med Hyg 58:539–544, 1964.

Scragg J: Amoebic liver abscess in African children. Arch Dis Childhood 35:171–176, 1960.

WHO Expert Committee: *Amoebiasis Report.* Pages 1–52. Technical Report Series No. 421. World Health Organization, 1969.

GIARDIASIS

Most infections with *Giardia lamblia* are asymptomatic or cause only mild symptoms. Diarrhea of insidious onset is the most common manifestation. In some children, steatorrhea with large frothy stools may occur. Vague abdominal pain and tenderness occasionally occur, with few constitutional symptoms.

The organisms usually reside in the duodenum and jejunum. The diagnostic feature is the presence of the organisms in fresh stools: vegetative forms in diarrheic stools and cysts in formed stools. The trophozoites are pear-shaped, with 4–5 pairs of notable flagella. There are 2 nuclei with central karyosomes and 2 parabasal bodies, altogether resembling the caricature of a face. They are 12–15 μm in diameter. The cysts are elliptical, with a clear wall and 4 nuclei with karyosomes. Excretion of the cysts is responsible for spread of infection.

Giardiasis must be differentiated from tuberculous enteritis, steatorrhea due to other causes, and chronic amebiasis. Giardiasis may coexist with any of these diseases, and a therapeutic trial may help to clarify the role of giardia in the total clinical picture.

Quinacrine (mepacrine, Atabrine), 8 mg/kg/day in 3 doses for 5 days, will usually clear the infection. Chloroquine (Aralen) is also effective. (For dosage, see Amebiasis.) Metranidazole (Flagyl) has also been reported to be effective.

Moore GT & others: Epidemic giardiasis at a ski resort. New England J Med 281:402–407, 1969.
Ninochiri E, Lantum D: Giardiasis, a cause of recurrent enteritis in Nigerian outpatients. J Trop Med 68:47–49, 1965.
Yardley JH, Takano J, Hendrix TR: Epithelial and other mucosal lesions of the jejunum in giardiasis: Jejunal biopsy studies. Bull Johns Hopkins Hosp 115:389–406, 1965.

BALANTIDIASIS

Dysentery due to *Balantidium coli* infection is far less common than amebiasis. The·clinical picture may mimic that of amebic dysentery. It is believed that pigs are the main source of infection. Ingested cysts result in colonic infection by trophozoites. *B coli* may live free in the lumen of the intestine or cause ulceration in the colon. In severe infection, the entire lower bowel may be affected.

There may be no symptoms, or symptoms essentially similar to those of acute amebiasis may occur, ie, diarrhea with or without blood and mucus. Slight leukocytosis may be present, and some degree of eosinophilia is not uncommon.

Examination of fresh feces reveals motile trophozoites, ciliated ovoid bodies approximately 100 × 50 μm with a reniform macronucleus, a micronucleus, and several vacuoles. The cysts are about 40 × 60 μm, containing most of the internal features of the trophozoite.

Intestinal perforation is the major complication. Liver lesions do not occur.

Treatment is with tetracyclines, 20–50 mg/kg/ day orally in divided doses for a week, or carbarsone (as for amebiasis).

Woody NC, Woody HB: Balantidiasis in infancy. J Pediat 56:485–489, 1960.

TOXOPLASMOSIS

Essentials of Diagnosis

- Congenital toxoplasmosis: Fever, rash, hepatosplenomegaly, chorioretinitis, hydrocephalus or microcephaly, and mental retardation (in various combinations).

- Acquired toxoplasmosis: Fever, rash, lymphadenopathy, chorioretinitis, encephalitis, and myocarditis (in various combinations). Chronic infection may be afebrile and associated only with lymphocytosis.

- In both cases, the demonstration of *Toxoplasma gondii* or serologic evidence of infection is required for confirmation.

General Considerations

Toxoplasma gondii is a protozoal parasite of various animals and man. Widespread occurrence of asymptomatic infection in man has been demonstrated by serology. The organism is crescentic and 4–7 μm long. It has a single nucleus. In tissues the parasites appear intracellularly, often in clusters forming "pseudocysts."

Toxoplasmosis may be congenital or acquired. Congenital toxoplasmosis is acquired in utero from the mother. Most acquired infections, including those of gravid women, remain clinically unrecognized.

The mode of transmission remains unclear. The organisms may persist in tissues for long periods.

Clinical Findings

A. Congenital Toxoplasmosis: The infected newborn may manifest skin rash (hemorrhagic or otherwise), hepatosplenomegaly, and jaundice. Thrombocytopenia is common. Some infants exhibit CNS disease during the first several weeks of life. Hydrocephalus, microcephaly, CSF pleocytosis and elevated protein, intracranial calcifications, and mental retardation occur in various combinations. Chorioretinitis is common. The systemic manifestations may occur alone or be accompanied or followed by the encephalitic features.

The organisms may be visualized in or isolated (usually in mice) from infected tissues or CSF. High levels of antibodies (demonstrated by the Sabin-Feldman dye test or hemagglutination test) are present both in the mother and the baby. The demonstration of IgM (19 S) antibodies in the baby is further proof of infection.

B. Acquired Toxoplasmosis: Symptomatic acquired infection, though rare, may occur at any age. The clinical manifestations include fever and the following features in varying combinations: generalized lymphadenopathy, muscular pain, maculopapular rash, hepatosplenomegaly, encephalitis, usually unilateral chorioretinitis, pneumonia, and myocarditis. The course may be short or may extend over several weeks. The diagnosis may be confirmed by the demonstration of the organisms or by serology.

The toxoplasmin skin test is of only limited diagnostic value. Some clinicians feel that the skin test may aggravate acquired toxoplasmic chorioretinitis.

Differential Diagnosis

Congenital toxoplasmosis may be mistaken for hepatitis due to other causes, septicemia, cytomegalovirus infection, and maternal rubella syndrome. The acquired form must be differentiated from viral encephalitis, viral myocarditis, infectious mononucleosis, and lymphoreticular and lymphoproliferative diseases. Because of the lymphoid proliferation, it may be difficult to differentiate lymphoid toxoplasmosis from lymphosarcoma even on biopsy.

Treatment

A combination of pyrimethamine (Daraprim) and a sulfonamide (sulfadiazine or trisulfapyrimidines) is recommended for 3–4 weeks in suspected or proved cases. Pyrimethamine is given orally in doses of 0.5 mg/kg twice daily in infants and once daily in older children. Sulfadiazine or trisulfapyrimidines are given orally in a dosage of 100 mg/kg daily in 4 divided doses for 2 weeks. Both of these drugs may cause gastrointestinal upsets which may necessitate interruption of treatment. Pyrimethamine may cause leukopenia, thrombocytopenia, and, very rarely, agranulocytosis; frequent blood counts should be performed and the drug stopped if the counts fall very low. Folic acid, 10 mg/day orally, may be given to combat the drug toxicity.

The neurologic damage that occurs in congenital toxoplasmosis does not subside after treatment. In acquired toxoplasmosis, in the absence of encephalitis and myocarditis, one must use discretion in instituting potentially dangerous therapy. The infection is usually self-limited.

In chorioretinitis, especially in the acquired form, a course of corticosteroids should be given along with antitoxoplasmosis drugs, eg, prednisone, 1 mg/kg orally initially and then reduced gradually. The corticosteroid may be stopped in 3–4 weeks and anti-infective therapy continued until the activity of the eye lesion abates. For recurrence of eye lesions, corticosteroids may be given alone.

Feldman HA: Toxoplasmosis. Pediatrics 22:559–574, 1958.

Fleck DG: Toxoplasmosis. Public Health 83:131–135, 1969.

Hogan MJ, Kimura SJ, O'Connor GR: Ocular toxoplasmosis. Arch Ophth 72:592–600, 1964.

Jones TC, Kean BH, Kimball AC: Toxoplasmic lymphadenitis. JAMA 192:1–5, 1965.

Jones TC: Acquired toxoplasmosis. New York J Med 69:2237–2242, 1969.

Stern H: Microbial causes of mental retardation: The role of prenatal infections with cytomegalovirus, rubella virus and toxoplasma. Lancet 2:443–449, 1969.

LEISHMANIASIS

1. VISCERAL LEISHMANIASIS
(Kala-Azar)

Essentials of Diagnosis

- High fever, remittent or intermittent—occasionally hectic.
- Splenomegaly and hepatomegaly; often lymphadenitis.
- Progressive anemia, leukopenia, and wasting.
- Demonstration of *Leishmania donovani* in smears of bone marrow or in splenic or lymph node aspirate.
- Positive formol-gel test, complement-fixation test, or immunofluorescence test.

General Considerations

Leishmania donovani is a protozoal parasite transmitted by the sandfly from man to man (India) or from dogs and rodents to man (Mediterranean regions). Infantile kala-azar is common in the Mediterranean area; in India, older children are more susceptible; and in other parts of the world, leishmaniasis is primarily an adult disease.

The parasites infect and multiply in the reticulo-endothelial cells of the spleen, liver, bone marrow, and lymph nodes. In the human body they exist as ovoid bodies, 2–4 μm in diameter. With Leishman's stain they exhibit a round nucleus and a rod-shaped rhizoplast enclosed in faintly bluish cytoplasm. Appropriate smears show these organisms intracellularly or extracellularly. In the sandfly as well as in artificial (NNN) medium, the parasites exist in a flagellated form.

Clinical Findings

A. Symptoms and Signs: In infants and children, the onset is usually acute, with high fever and gastrointestinal upsets. The spleen enlarges rapidly. There may also be enlargement of the liver (though to a lesser degree) and lymphadenopathy.

In older children, the illness is usually less severe and more prolonged. They remain febrile over long periods, develop hyperpigmentation, lose weight, and become progressively anemic and wasted.

Hypopigmented patches and nodular lesions may occur on the face, forearms, and thighs in patients who have been treated for visceral leishmaniasis. This condition, called dermal leishmanoid and post-kala-azar leishmaniasis, has been reported in India and Africa. The nodular lesions harbor the parasites.

B. Laboratory Findings: The diagnosis is confirmed by the presence of *L donovani* in smears of bone marrow or splenic or lymph node aspirate. Rarely, blood smears may reveal the organisms. Blood or bone marrow may be cultured on NNN medium to prove the diagnosis. In chronic cases, a drop of commercial formalin coagulates about 1 ml of serum at room temperature (aldehyde or formol-gel test). A complement-fixation test and an immunofluorescence test are also available.

Leukopenia is common, and often quite marked. Thrombocytopenia (with skin hemorrhages) also is common. Anemia and markedly elevated serum gamma globulins are also characteristic.

Differential Diagnosis

Febrile illnesses associated with splenomegaly such as bacterial endocarditis, typhoid fever, brucellosis, lymphoproliferative and lymphoreticular diseases, trypanosomiasis, schistosomiasis, and malaria must be differentiated from kala-azar. Dermal leishmanoid simulates leprosy, yaws, or lupus vulgaris.

Treatment

Correction of nutritional deficiencies (including anemia) and treatment of complicating infections should be done along with specific therapy.

The drugs used in kala-azar are ethylstibamine (Neostibosan), urea stibamine, and sodium antimony gluconate (pentavalent antimony compounds), and pentamidine isethionate (Lomidine).

Indian leishmaniasis is easily controlled by treatment, but in Africa the response to specific treatment has been less satisfactory.

The antimony compounds may be given intramuscularly or by slow intravenous injection. Ethylstibamine is given on alternate days in doses of 25 mg in infants less than age 1 and 50 mg in older children for 5 or 6 injections. If parasitism persists after about 2 months, treatment should be repeated. Urea stibamine is given in doses of 10–50 mg on alternate days for a total of 150–750 mg. Sodium antimony gluconate is given in doses of 0.1 ml/kg (20 mg antimony per ml) for 6 injections on alternate days. Antimony compounds may cause vomiting, diarrhea, and muscle cramps; temporary interruption of therapy may be necessary.

Pentamidine may be given intramuscularly in doses of 3 mg/kg of the base daily for 10 days. This drug is useful where the disease is resistant to antimony compounds.

For the nodular type of dermal leishmanoid, a course of a pentavalent antimony compound must be given.

Prognosis

In untreated cases, death usually occurs as a result of bacterial complications such as pneumonia.

Manson-Bahr PEC, Southgate BA: Recent research in kala-azar in East Africa. J Trop Med 67:79–84, 1964.

2. CUTANEOUS LEISHMANIASIS
(Oriental Sore)

Leishmania tropica is morphologically identical with *L donovani*. The vector is the sandfly. Cutaneous leishmaniasis has been reported from all inhabited continents. Endemic foci are mostly in India, the Asian countries west of India, and North Africa. Russian investigators recognize 2 forms: the dry type, in urban areas, spread from man to man; and the moist type, in rural areas, transmitted from animals to man.

The lesions develop at the sites of sandfly bites after an incubation period of weeks to months. They begin as itchy papules and develop into granulomatous ulcers with scabs. The ulcers gradually extend, and satellite lesions occasionally appear. These lesions occur mostly on the face and limbs, especially in children. The lesions occasionally remain atypical with no ulceration. The onset may or may not be accompanied by fever. After several months, the lesions heal slowly, leaving behind depressed and deforming scars.

In endemic areas the diagnosis is suspected on clinical grounds and confirmed by demonstration of the causative organisms in smears of fluid aspirated from the base of the lesions. Such specimens may also be cultured on NNN medium.

The leishmanin skin test is positive in all cases.

Discrete ulcers may be cleaned and treated with local or systemic antibacterial therapy and allowed to heal, assuring immunity and avoiding potentially toxic drugs. Mild chemical cauterization is recommended by some investigators. In instances of multiple or extensive ulceration and lesions on the face, antibacterial therapy should be accompanied by specific therapy with pentavalent antimony compounds as for visceral leishmaniasis. Stibophen (Fuadin), supplied in 5 ml ampules of 6.3% solution, is an alternative drug. It is given intramuscularly as follows: 0.5 ml on the first day; 1 ml on the second day; third day onward, 1 ml for children weighing less than 15 kg, or 1 ml/15 kg on alternate days for 9 injections.

Prognosis

The prognosis is good except for deforming scars which can be minimized by early treatment.

Chavarria AP, Kotcher E, Lizano C: Preliminary evaluation of cycloguanil pamoate in dermal leishmaniasis. JAMA 194:1142–1144, 1965.
Fraser WM & others: Cutaneous leishmaniasis. JAMA 186:155–157, 1963.

3. MUCOCUTANEOUS LEISHMANIASIS

Except for a few reports, especially from North America, most cases of leishmania infection are reported from South America. Several different species are now recognized: *L braziliensis* causes espundia; *L mexicana* causes chiclero's ulcer in Mexico, Guatemala, and Honduras; *L peruviana* causes uta in British and French Guiana and Peru; *L americana* has been recently described in Venezuela. *L braziliensis* is morphologically identical with *L donovani*. It is presumed to be transmitted by sandflies. The chronic ulcerative lesions may be indistinguishable from those of oriental sore, or they may develop into destructive mucocutaneous lesions over the naso-oral regions. Healing is slow, and in untreated cases heavy scarring occurs. Lesions similar to oriental sore or punched-out ulcers may occur on the face or limbs.

The diagnosis is confirmed by demonstration of *L braziliensis* at the base of the ulcer. The leishmanin test is usually positive.

Treatment is similar to that of oriental sore, with pentavalent antimonials and antibacterial therapy. Cycloguanil pamoate has recently been reported to be curative. The dose (given in one injection) is 140 mg of the base for infants; 280 mg for children 1–5 years of age; and 350 mg for older children. Pyrimethamine (Daraprim) given orally has been found useful. It is given in 3 ten-day courses of 50 mg/day orally with a rest period of 1 week between courses.

AFRICAN TRYPANOSOMIASIS
(Sleeping Sickness)

Essentials of Diagnosis

- Trypanosome chancre and erythematous nodule at the site of fly bite.
- Fever, progressive anemia and debility, splenomegaly, lymphadenitis, skin rash.
- Changes in personality, disturbances of speech and gait, progressive apathy and somnolence, involuntary movements, and coma.
- Detection of trypanosomes in a wet blood film in rhodesiense infections and by lymph node puncture in gambiense infections.

General Considerations

Trypanosomiasis occurs in parts of tropical Africa. The more virulent Rhodesian form, caused by *Trypansoma rhodesiense,* occurs chiefly in East Africa, but the Gambian form, caused by *T gambiense*, is more widespread. Both species are transmitted by the bites of tsetse flies (glossina). In human blood the 2 are morphologically similar—actively motile, slender, wavy, spindle-like bodies with a central nucleus and a prominent flagellum.

Gambian trypanosomiasis occurs more commonly in children than the Rhodesian form, except in epidemics of the latter.

Clinical Findings

A. Signs and Symptoms:

1. Rhodesian trypanosomiasis—During the first week, an erythematous, pruritic, and occasionally painful nodule appears at the site of fly bite and subsides in a few days. Some patients do not develop this reaction. Fever appears by the second week. It varies in intensity but occurs intermittently or continuously, accompanied by headache, muscular pain, tenderness, and transient skin rashes. Progressive splenomegaly and, to a lesser degree, hepatomegaly are common. Cervical, femoral, or axillary lymph nodes may become palpable. In a few months, weakness, lassitude, emaciation, personality changes, disturbances of speech and gait, and involuntary movements appear. Death may occur before the onset of the classical somnolence.

2. Gambian trypanosomiasis—The early and intermediate stages are similar to those of the Rhodesian form but the progression is slow. Lymphadenitis is more prominent, especially of the posterior cervical glands (Winterbottom's sign). CNS involvement sets in after several months to years. The child becomes very lethargic and sleeps most of the time. Severe emaciation and edema are common. Terminally, coma is followed by death.

B. Laboratory Findings: A wet or stained thick blood smear should be examined for trypanosomes. Repeated examinations are sometimes necessary. Bone marrow aspirate or, preferably, a lymph node aspirate is more likely to be positive in the early and intermediate stages. In the late stages, CSF, especially after centrifugation, may exhibit the organisms. CSF pleocytosis and elevated protein are usually found. Even in the absence of gross CNS symptoms and signs, pleocytosis and elevated protein are evidences of CNS invasion.

Anemia, elevated erythrocyte sedimentation rate and serum gamma globulins, and hypoproteinemia are some of the accompanying nonspecific features.

Differential Diagnosis

Malaria is not usually difficult to distinguish, but kala-azar may at times be mistaken for trypanosomiasis. Fever, splenomegaly, and lymphadenitis may occur also in lymphoreticular and lymphoproliferative diseases and should be differentiated from trypanosomiasis in endemic areas. Meningitis, especially tuberculous and cryptococcal, and intracranial neoplasms may mimic the CNS manifestations of this disease.

Treatment

A. Specific Measures:

1. Suramin (Antrypol, etc), an organic urea compound, is the drug of choice in the early and intermediate stages without CNS involvement in both the Rhodesian and Gambian forms. Give fresh 10% aqueous solution intravenously in the following dosage: Give a test dose of 20–50 mg with facilities for resuscitation in the event of severe reaction. Continue with 5 doses of 20 mg/kg on days 1, 3, 7, 14, and 21. The appearance of heavy and persistent proteinuria or dermatitis is an indication for discontinuing therapy.

2. Pentamidine isethionate (Lomidine) is an alternative drug which may be given in doses of 3–4 mg/kg IM daily for 10 days. It may induce hypotension or hypoglycemia. It is less effective in the Rhodesian form than the Gambian form.

Suramin and pentamidine do not penetrate the CNS, so that when the brain is involved, treatment with arsenicals is necessary.

3. Melarsoprol (Mel B), an arsenical, is the drug of choice in stages with CNS involvement, especially in patients with average nutrition and little renal or hepatic damage. It is given IV as 3.6% solution in propylene glycol, 3.6 mg/kg on alternate days for 3 injections. In severe CNS disease, the course may be repeated after 3 weeks. Any evidence of arsenical toxicity such as mental confusion, encephalopathy, or peripheral neuritis should immediately be treated with dimercaprol (BAL). Headache, vomiting, and proteinuria are indications for discontinuing therapy.

A closely related drug, Mel W, is water-soluble and may be given intramuscularly or subcutaneously. Give fresh 5% aqueous solution in doses of 1, 2, 2, and 4 mg/kg on successive days. In advanced late cases, repeat after 2 weeks. It is less toxic than melarsoprol but is also less effective in Rhodesian trypanosomiasis.

4. Tryparsamide, another arsenical, is less toxic than melarsoprol but may cause optic atrophy. It is more effective against *T gambiense* in CNS than against *T rhodesiense.* The dose is 20–40 mg/kg IV given at weekly intervals for 10 injections. Treatment should be stopped at the appearance of the slightest symptom related to the eyes. In severe and late cases, the course may be repeated after a month.

During the treatment of CNS disease, suramin or pentamidine also should be given to eradicate parasites from the blood and reticuloendothelial system.

B. General Measures: When facilities are available, patients should be hospitalized for therapy. Concurrent infections and nutritional deficiencies should be adequately treated.

Prognosis

Spontaneous recovery occurs occasionally in early cases, and early and intermediate cases do well with treatment. After the CNS has been invaded, the prognosis is less favorable. Untreated cases have an extremely high mortality rate, ie, death occurs within 1 year in Rhodesian and within 10 years in Gambian forms.

Robertson DHH: Chemotherapy of African trypanosomiasis. Practitioner 188:80–83, 1962.

Weinman D: Problems of diagnosis of trypanosomiasis. Bull WHO 28:731–743, 1963.

AMERICAN TRYPANOSOMIASIS
(Chagas' Disease)

Essentials of Diagnosis

- Chagoma—an erythematous, painful nodule at the site of primary cutaneous infection.
- Unilateral conjunctivitis and palpebral and facial edema—"Romaña's sign."
- Fever, lymphadenitis, myocarditis, occasionally meningoencephalitis.
- Mega-esophagus, megacolon.
- *Trypanosoma cruzi* in blood, bone marrow, or aspirates of lymph nodes or spleen.

General Considerations

Chagas' disease is confined to South and Central America, with the highest incidence in Brazil and Argentina. The causative agent, *Trypanosoma cruzi,* infects man and various animals. It is transmitted through the feces of reduviid bugs—by rubbing feces in skin abrasions or the eye. The organisms multiply locally and invade blood and other tissues.

Clinical Findings

A. Symptoms and Signs: Infants and children are frequently infected in endemic areas. In most cases, a transient lesion (chagoma) develops at the site of primary infection, characterized by an erythematous painful nodule. It is soon followed by local lymphadenitis, unilateral palpebral and facial edema, conjunctivitis, intermittent or continuous fever, generalized lymphadenitis, hepatosplenomegaly, and myocarditis (tachycardia, cardiomegaly, arrhythmias, and cardiac failure). Occasionally meningoencephalitis may occur.

In chronic cases, especially in older children and young children who survive the early stages, the main abnormality is myocardial damage. Damage to the myenteric nerve plexuses may result in mega-esophagus and megacolon.

B. Laboratory Findings: In acute Chagas' disease, wet and stained thick blood smears should be examined for *T cruzi.* If they are negative, bone marrow and lymph node or splenic aspirate should be examined. Blood or other specimens may be inoculated into mice, rats, or guinea pigs or cultured in NNN medium. Another method is to feed laboratory-grown bugs on patients and to look for the organisms in the bugs' feces after 3–8 weeks. A complement fixation test is also available.

In the acute phase, there is often high leukocytosis, mostly due to mononuclear cells. Cases with myocarditis have x-ray and ECG abnormalities.

Differential Diagnosis

Trichinosis, kala-azar, and bacterial sepsis should be differentiated. In endemic areas, nonpathogenic trypanosomes (*T rangeli*) may be found in blood.

Treatment

There is no specific therapy. Bed rest, good nutrition, and management of myocarditis and cardiac failure are indicated.

Prognosis

Acute infection may prove fatal to infants and children. Mortality is particularly high in meningoencephalitis. Chronic disease with myocardial damage carries a poor prognosis.

Laranja FS & others: Chagas' disease: A clinical, epidemiologic and pathologic study. Circulation 14:1035–1060, 1956.

METAZOAL INFECTIONS

1. NEMATODAL INFECTIONS

HOOKWORM DISEASE

Essentials of Diagnosis

- Weakness and pallor, with a hypochromic, microcytic anemia.
- Abdominal discomfort, weight loss.
- Occult blood in stool.
- Ova in fecal smears.

General Considerations

The hookworms that commonly infect man are *Ancylostoma duodenale* and *Necator americanus.* Their life cycles are identical, and both occur widely in the tropical and subtropical regions of the world.

The adult worms reside mostly in the jejunum. They feed on blood, and it has been found that about 20 worms remove 1 ml of blood per day. Ova are deposited in the bowel and expelled in feces. In suitable damp, shaded soil the eggs hatch and develop into infective larvae. On contact with human skin (walking bare-footed or handling soil), they penetrate and enter the blood stream, reach the lungs, exit into the alveoli, migrate toward the pharynx, and are swallowed. In the upper intestine, they develop into adults.

In some communities where no organized drainage and sanitation are available, over 90% of individuals may be infected.

Another species, *A braziliense,* is a rare human parasite. The infective larvae cause cutaneous larva migrans. This condition has been reported mainly from the American continents.

Clinical Findings

A. Symptoms and Signs: At the skin sites where large numbers of larvae penetrate, especially on and between the toes, intense itching ("ground itch") may occur, particularly in rainy seasons. In cutaneous larva migrans, the larvae penetrate the skin and wander under it, causing irritation, redness, and a slowly creeping eruption.

Small numbers of worms cause no symptoms, and symptoms directly related to the presence of these parasites are never notable. Abdominal pain, discomfort, and distention and changes in bowel habits occasionally occur with heavy infection.

B. Laboratory Findings: Diagnosis is made by identification of ova in fecal smears. They are oval, about 60 X 40 μm, with a segmented egg cell or coiled embryo visible through the thin eggshell.

Tests for occult blood in feces are usually positive if there are a sufficient number of worms. Mild to moderate eosinophilia is common.

Complications & Sequelae

By causing a continuous loss of blood, hookworm aggravates nutritional deficiencies. Thus, a progressive iron deficiency anemia is produced in people who are on a low iron intake. Supplemental iron prevents hookworm anemia. In patients with borderline folic acid intake, megaloblastic anemia may be produced. The anemia is so insidious that patients may seek medical attention only after cardiac decompensation has occurred. In addition to cardiac failure, hypoalbuminemia may also exist and contribute to anasarca.

Prevention

Prevention is achieved by avoiding fecal contamination of soil and skin contact with contaminated soil.

Treatment

A. Specific Measures:

1. Bephenium hydroxynaphthoate (Alcopara) is the drug of choice, particularly for *A duodenale* infection. It is also effective against roundworms (ascaris) and can be administered very cautiously in mixed infections. It is given in a single dose, on an empty stomach, 2.5 gm for children under 20 kg and 5 gm for those above. Food should be withheld for 2 hours after administration, but no purgation is necessary. Because of its bitter taste, it is best mixed with fruit juice, flavored liquid, or milk. It may provoke nausea and vomiting, but other side-effects are few. Treatment may be repeated after an interval of 3–4 weeks.

2. Tetrachloroethylene is equally effective and widely used, especially for North Americans. It is given orally in a single dose of 0.1–0.12 ml/kg to a maximum of 5 ml on an empty stomach. No purgation is necessary, but a light supper with no fat on the previous night is recommended to prevent absorption of the fat-soluble drug. In severely anemic or debilitated children, treatment for anemia should precede the above therapy. Since it may stimulate roundworms into activity and migration, tetrachloroethylene is better avoided in mixed infection or only given after piperazine therapy. The drug may cause abdominal discomfort and nausea and vomiting. It deteriorates unless kept in a cool place in dark air-tight containers.

3. Cutaneous larva migrans may be arrested by repeated ethyl chloride sprays to kill the larvae, which are eventually resorbed. Diethylcarbamazine (discussed under filariasis) and thiabendazole have been claimed to be effective.

B. General Measures: In many anemic children, oral iron therapy is of greater value than anthelmintics. Exchange blood transfusions may be lifesaving in severely anemic children in cardiac failure. In less severe cases, parenteral iron therapy is of value.

Prognosis

Except in severely anemic children, the prognosis is good.

CCTA-WHO: *African Conference on Ancylostomiasis.* Brazzaville, 1961. WHO Technical Report Series No. 255. World Health Organization, 1963.

Gilles HM, Williams EJW, Ball PAJ: Hookworm infection and anemia: An epidemiological, clinical and laboratory study. Quart J Med 33:1–24, 1964.

Goodwin LG, Jayewardene LG, Standen OD: Clinical trials with bephenium hydroxynaphthoate against hookworm in Ceylon. Brit MJ 2:1572–1576, 1958.

Pitchomoni CS & others: Hookworm disease, malabsorption and malnutrition. Am J Clin Nutr 22:813–816, 1969.

ASCARIASIS

Essentials of Diagnosis

- Abdominal discomfort and colic.
- The passage of roundworms in feces or the demonstration of ascaris ova.

General Considerations

The roundworm, *Ascaris lumbricoides,* is a cosmopolitan human parasite. Where indiscriminate defecation by children is allowed, the ova are spread widely in the soil where they remain viable for long periods. The ova contaminate food, fingers, toys, etc and are swallowed, to hatch in the upper small intestine. The escaping larvae penetrate the gut wall and, through the portal circulation and the right side of the heart, reach the pulmonary capillaries. They penetrate into the alveoli, are coughed up and swallowed, and mature in the small intestine. Males and females mate, and the female lays thousands of eggs each day.

Clinical Findings

A. Symptoms and Signs: In the great majority of instances, the infection remains silent. However, abdominal pain, anorexia, gastrointestinal upsets, loss of weight, irritability, and short febrile episodes have been attributed to the presence of these worms. Occasionally the worms are excreted in feces or ascend to the stomach and are vomited out.

Large numbers of the larvae migrating through the lungs may cause an acute and often transient "pneumonia" accompanied by eosinophilia (Löffler's syndrome). This syndrome seems to be rare in India. In pediatric practice, large numbers of worms in the gut lumen can cause symptoms of intestinal obstruction.

B. Laboratory Findings: Except when a history of passing roundworms is obtained, the diagnosis is made by the detection of ova in fecal smears. They are approximately 45 X 60 μm with a brown (bile-stained) mamillated outer coat, a thick middle, and a delicate inner coat covering a densely granular egg cell.

Complications

Large numbers of worms occasionally cause intestinal obstruction, which may be precipitated by treatment in cases of massive infection.

Worms may penetrate the gut wall and cause peritonitis; block the appendiceal lumen, causing acute appendicitis; or block the common bile duct and cause acute obstructive jaundice.

Treatment

In asymptomatic infections, especially in older children, there is no urgency for treatment. The infection is self-limited unless reinfection occurs.

Piperazine compounds (citrate, adipate, hydrate, or phosphate) are the drugs of choice. They are available as tablets or syrup. Dosage is usually calculated in terms of the hydrous base, piperazine hexahydrate. Piperazine citrate (Antepar) is widely used as a single dose of 100 mg/kg taken orally after breakfast. The maximum recommended dose is 3 gm for children over 30 kg body weight. No purge is required, and treatment can be repeated after a week if necessary. Little or no toxicity is encountered.

Other suitable drugs include bephenium hydroxynaphthoate (Alcopara) and hexylresorcinol (Crystoids Anthelmintic). The dosage of bephenium hydroxynaphthoate is discussed under hookworm (above) and that of hexylresorcinol under trichuriasis (below).

In massive infection, treatment may result in intestinal obstruction by masses of paralyzed worms.

In the presence of surgical complications, enterotomy with evacuation is perhaps the safest procedure. The administration of a piperazine drug is recommended after about 2 weeks.

Prognosis

The prognosis is good except when massive infection results in bowel gangrene or perforation and peritonitis; in these instances, death may result.

Fernando N: Surgical ascariasis in children (a review of 50 cases). J Trop Pediat 4:61–70, 1958.

Goodwin LG, Standen OD: Treatment of ascariasis with various salts of piperazine. Brit MJ 1:131–133, 1958.

Myalvaganam C & others: Extra-intestinal ascaris granuloma. J Trop Med 72:98–100, 1969.

ENTEROBIASIS
(Oxyuriasis, Pinworm or Seatworm Infection)

Essentials of Diagnosis

- Pruritus ani, especially at night.
- Worms in stool; ova on perianal skin.

General Considerations

Enterobiasis occurs all over the world. Infection is caused by the pinworm or seatworm, *Enterobius (Oxyuris) vermicularis.* The adult worms reside in the cecum and colon. The gravid females crawl out and deposit thousands of eggs in the skin folds of the anus, especially at night, causing intense itching. When the child scratches, the ova stick to the fingertips and under the nails and eventually get to the mouth and are swallowed, resulting in auto-infection. Contamination of clothes and the environment leads to the infection of fresh hosts; it is not unusual for several members of the same household to harbor pinworms.

Clinical Findings

A. Symptoms and Signs: The commonest manifestation is pruritus ani, especially at night. In young girls, vaginitis and pruritus vulvae may occur. Rarely, the worms may fill the appendiceal lumen and cause acute appendicitis.

B. Laboratory Findings: The diagnosis is confirmed by the detection of ova on the perianal skin. A transparent adhesive tape held tight over the bottom of a test tube with the sticky surface outward is applied to the anus and perianal skin; this is preferably done in the morning, before defecation or washing. The tape is then mounted over a drop of toluene on a glass slide and examined under the microscope. Occasionally, ova and even adult worms may be seen in stools.

The ova measure about 50–60 X 20–30 μm and are oval with one flat surface. The coiled larva is usually visible through the translucent shell.

Differential Diagnosis

All instances of pruritus ani or vulvae are not caused by enterobiasis, though in the absence of other demonstrable causes a therapeutic trial is justifiable.

Treatment

A. Specific Measures: To prevent intrafamilial cross-infection, it is worthwhile treating all infected individuals in a household simultaneously.

1. Piperazine compounds (citrate, adipate, hydrate, or phosphate) are nontoxic in therapeutic dosage and are widely used in syrup form. The dosage is 50 mg/kg to a maximum of 2 gm daily in the evenings for 7 days. The course may be repeated after 1 week. The cure rate is high.

2. Pyrvinium pamoate (Povan) in syrup, single dose of 5 mg/kg body weight (maximum of 0.25 gm), repeated after 2 weeks. It may cause nausea and vomiting, and turns the stools red.

3. Stilbazium iodide (Monopar), single dose of 10–15 mg base/kg body weight, in enteric-coated capsules. The stools become colored red.

4. Dithiazanine iodide (see under strongyloidiasis and trichuriasis) is also effective against enterobiasis.

B. General Measures: Strict personal hygiene helps prevent auto-infection. Infected children should wear undergarments even while sleeping so that direct contact of fingers with perianal skin can be avoided. The nails should be kept short and clean. Bedclothes and undergarments of infected children should be removed without shaking (to prevent dispersal of ova) and laundered frequently.

Leuin MB: Night cries in little girls. Pediatrics 44:125–126, 1969.

Mathias AW Jr: *Enterobius vermicularis* infection: Certain effects of host-parasite relationship. Am J Dis Child 101:174–177, 1961.

TRICHURIASIS
(Trichocephaliasis, Whipworm)

The whipworm, *Trichuris trichiura,* is a worldwide human and animal parasite. The adult worms reside in the cecum and colon, and ova are passed in feces. The ova reach the human alimentary canal in contaminated soil, vegetables, toys, etc and hatch in the upper small intestine. There are usually no symptoms except when infection is heavy, causing abdominal pain especially in the right iliac fossa, abdominal distention, and diarrhea. Massive colonic infection may cause dysentery clinically similar to amebic dysentery. The diagnosis is based on demonstrations of ova in fecal smears. They are about 50 X 20 μm, brown, and oval, with 2 polar plugs in the shell. Proctoscopy may reveal grayish-white worms with narrow anterior and broad posterior portions attached to hyperemic mucosa. The whole worm measures 3–5 cm.

Mild to moderate eosinophilia is usually present.

Asymptomatic and mild infections may be left untreated. The drugs of proved efficacy include dithiazanine iodide and hexylresorcinol. Dithiazanine iodide (no longer available in the USA) may cause anorexia, nausea, vomiting, and abdominal cramps. These side-effects may be minimized if the drug is given after meals. The dose is 10 mg/kg (to a maximum of 300 mg) in 3 divided doses on the first day followed by double the dose for the next 4 days. The course may be repeated after 2 weeks. The drug should be discontinued if it causes severe gastrointestinal symptoms.

Hexylresorcinol (Crystoids Anthelmintic) is a local irritant to skin and mucosa but causes little systemic toxicity in therapeutic doses. It may be given either orally, as enteric-coated tablets, or rectally as a 0.1% or 0.2% retention enema. The oral dose is 1 tablet (100 mg) per year of age, to be given on empty stomach on the morning following a light nonresidue supper. In children with no diarrhea, a saline cathartic may be given after 2 hours. *Caution:* Tablets of hexylresorcinol should not be chewed. The retention enema should be given with petroleum jelly to protect perianal skin. The enema should be retained for 15 minutes.

Jung RC, Beaver PC: Clinical observations on *Trichocephalus trichiuris* (whipworm) infestation in children. Pediatrics 8:548–557, 1951.

Paine DHD, Lower ES, Cooper TV: Treatment of trichuriasis with dithiazanine in a hospital for mental defectives. Brit MJ 1:770–774, 1960.

STRONGYLOIDIASIS

Essentials of Diagnosis

- Productive cough, blood-streaked sputum.
- Abdominal pain, distention, diarrhea.
- Progressive nutritional deficiencies, eosinophilia.
- Larvae in stool or duodenal aspirate.

General Considerations

Unlike the other helminths considered in this chapter, *Strongyloides stercoralis* has parasitic and free-living forms. As a human parasite, it has been found in many tropical and subtropical regions of the world. The adult worms live in the submucous tissue and the mucosal folds of the duodenum and occasionally occupy the entire length of the intestines. Ova are deposited in the lumen of the bowel and hatch rapidly. Therefore, both in feces and in duodenal aspirates, the larvae are found commonly but the ova rarely.

In suitable soil, the larvae undergo various stages of development and become infective. Contact with human skin (walking bare-footed or handling soil) facilitates the penetration of skin by the larvae, which reach the pulmonary capillaries through the blood stream. They escape into alveoli, traverse up the bronchial tree, and enter the alimentary canal. In the duodenum, they mature into adults.

Older children and adults are more often affected than young children. Even in areas where the general incidence of strongyloidiasis is low, an occasional patient presents with massive parasitization.

Clinical Findings

A. Symptoms and Signs: The site of skin penetration may go unnoticed, or a transient pruritic papular eruption may occur. After heavy exposure, respiratory signs and symptoms may be caused by the migrating larvae. Cough, often productive, with streaks of blood in the sputum may occur. Abdominal pain, distention, vomiting, and diarrhea with large and pale stools, often with mucus, are the common features.

B. Laboratory Findings: The diagnosis is confirmed by the presence of larvae in feces and duodenal aspirates. They are about 225 μm long, with a double-bulb esophagus which is almost 1/2 the length of the larva.

Larvae can sometimes be seen in sputum. A mild to moderate eosinophilia may be present.

C. X-Ray Findings: There may be patchy areas of infiltration on chest x-ray. A barium meal may reveal evidence of duodenitis, including coarse mucosal folds, a widened lumen, and clumping of barium. In severe cases, a pipe-like appearance may occur in duodenum and elsewhere. These findings simulate those of sprue, regional enteritis, and occasionally ulcerative colitis.

Differential Diagnosis

Symptomatic strongyloidiasis must be differentiated from sprue, other causes of malabsorption, regional enteritis, tuberculous enteritis, and hookworm disease.

Complications & Sequelae

In heavy infection with strongyloides, chronic diarrhea eventually leads to severe nutritional deficiencies and debility. Paralytic ileus has been known to occur. Several workers have reported fatal cases of strongyloidiasis.

Treatment

A. Specific Measures: The treatment of choice has been dithiazanine iodide (Abminthic, Delvex, Telmid), 10 mg/kg/day in 3 divided doses orally for 14–21 days. This drug has now been withdrawn from the market in the USA. In Britain, it is available for use only in hospitals. (The side-effects are discussed under trichuriasis.) Close follow-up of treated patients is recommended, as relapses are common. In such instances, specific therapy should be repeated.

Alternative drugs and dosages are as follows: (1) thiabendazole (Thibenzole, Mintezol), 25 mg/kg/day for 2 days; or (2) pyrvinium pamoate (Povan), 5 mg/kg as a single dose. (*Note:* Pyrvinium colors the stools red.)

B. General Measures: In serious infections, attention to the nutritional and fluid and electrolyte needs is urgent. In many fatal cases, death appears to be due to the severe nutritional defects or to paralytic ileus.

Prognosis

The prognosis is good in mild infection but poor in symptomatic heavy infections with complications.

Bras G & others: Infection with *Strongyloides stercoralis* in Jamaica. Lancet 2:1257–1260, 1964.

Huchton P, Horn R: Strongyloidiasis. J Pediat 55:602–608, 1959.

Swartzwelder JC & others: Dithiazanine, an effective broad spectrum anthelmintic: Results of therapy of trichuriasis, strongyloidiasis, enterobiasis, ascariasis and hookworm infection. JAMA 165:2063–2067, 1957.

TRICHINOSIS

Trichinella spiralis parasitizes the alimentary canal of man and several species of animals, especially the pig. The adult females secrete larvae which penetrate the mucosa and enter the blood stream. The larvae reach the skeletal muscles, where they encapsulate between muscle fibers. Man becomes infected by eating raw or undercooked pork containing the larvae. Even the use of a contaminated knife to cut other meats may lead to infection.

Trichinosis is more common in North America and Europe than elsewhere. Infants and young children are seldom affected.

Among pork-eating people, subclinical infection is common and may be recognized only at autopsy.

Heavy exposure may be followed by gastroenteritis (due to intestinal parasitization) after about 5–7 days.

The next stage of symptoms consists of fever, periobital edema, muscular pains in the neck, chest, and limbs, swellings in the limbs, and skin eruptions in varying combinations. Meningitic and encephalitic symptoms may occur. Myocarditis and splenomegaly are not uncommon. Marked eosinophilia is present in almost all cases.

A history of exposure is helpful in diagnosis. An intradermal test and serologic tests are available. The diagnosis can be confirmed by the demonstration of young larvae in muscle biopsy (gastrocnemius, deltoid, or biceps).

The larvae eventually die and become calcified, when they can be demonstrated by radiography.

Cholera, typhoid fever, collagen diseases, and many other diseases may be mimicked by trichinosis.

The importance of prevention of parasites in pigs and the need for adequate cooking of pork to kill the larvae cannot be overemphasized. Freezing also kills the larvae.

There is no specific treatment against the larvae. Thiabendazole may prove to be of use. If exposure is suspected, saline purgation might help in the elimination of the developing parasites.

Supportive symptomatic measures are the mainstay of therapy. Some workers have reported rapid relief on giving corticosteroids.

Heavy infection may result in death in a few weeks. Recovery is the rule in mild to moderate infections.

Gould SE & others: Diagnostic patterns: *Trichinella spiralis.* Am J Clin Path 40:197–208, 1963.
Maynard JE, Kagan IG: Trichinosis. Practitioner 191:622–629, 1963.

DRACUNCULOSIS
(Dracontiasis, Guinea Worm Infection)

Dracunculus medinensis (guinea worm) is a common parasite of man and animals in some parts of India, West Asia, and Africa. Infection results from drinking water containing small crustaceans (cyclops) harboring mature larvae. The larvae penetrate the intestinal mucosa and migrate to the subcutaneous tissues of the lower extremities or back. They may also reach various other tissues and die, causing few or no symptoms.

Larvae are discharged through the skin ulcer caused by the female adult worm, especially when the skin is in contact with water. Thus, farm workers and water carriers who wade into steep wells both suffer from and perpetuate dracunculosis.

There have been few reports on dracunculosis in children, though pediatric infection is known to occur in India.

The symptoms mostly refer to the blister or ulcer caused by the worm. The lesion is usually on the lower limb, and discharges a milky fluid that shows the white worm. Fever and urticaria may occur prior to or during the blister formation. In cryptic infection, eosinophilia may be the sole evidence, although intense pruritus occasionally occurs. Calcified worms can be seen on x-rays and may be palpable. The ulcer may become bacterially infected. Premature death of worms in the subcutaneous tissues may result in inflammatory lesions and sometimes in a sterile abscess. A filarial skin test is available which is seldom needed for diagnosis.

In ulcerated dracunculosis, a moist antiseptic dressing (eg, acriflavine) accelerates the discharge of larvae and the death of the worm. Afterward the worm can be pulled out gradually, about 2–3 cm a day, using a suitable instrument such as a clean match stick on which it can be wound. If more rapid withdrawal is attempted, the worm might rupture and cause a severe cellulitis.

A neomycin-bacitracin cream or systemic antibiotics should be given when bacterial infection is evident.

Diethylcarbamazine (Hetrazan) has been reported to be effective against immature forms and in maximal doses even against adult forms.

Hodgson C, Barrett DF: Chronic dracunculosis. Brit J Dermat 76:211–217, 1964.

VISCERAL LARVA MIGRANS
(Toxocariasis)

Essentials of Diagnosis
- Marked eosinophilia and hepatomegaly in children with pica.
- The demonstration of larvae in liver biopsy.

General Considerations
Visceral larva migrans is a recently described condition in young children infected with the larvae of the dog or cat roundworm, *Toxocara canis* or *T cati.* Most of the reported cases are from North America and the British Isles. A history of pica is helpful in diagnosis. The presence of worm-infested dogs in the environment leads to the ingestion of ova.

The life cycle and transmission of dog and cat roundworms are quite similar to those in man. When the ova are ingested in large numbers by children, they hatch in the intestines and the larvae migrate through the blood stream and are caught up in granulomatous inflammatory lesions in the liver, occasionally in the lungs, and rarely in other tissues.

A similar syndrome can also be caused by the rodent whipworm, *Capillaria hepatica.*

Clinical Findings

A. Symptoms and Signs: The common presenting symptoms are anorexia, fever, and pallor. Abdominal distention and cough occur occasionally. Hepatomegaly is common, and splenomegaly is not unusual. Cutaneous hemorrhagic lesions have been reported in a few instances. Blindness and epileptiform convulsions may be atypical forms of presentation.

B. Laboratory Findings: Anemia is usually present and may be the reason for the pica. High leukocytosis, mainly due to eosinophilia (30–90%), is almost a constant feature. The diagnosis may be confirmed by finding nematode larvae in a liver biopsy specimen, preferably performed by the open method. The larvae may be seen in secretions in granulomatous lesions or in crushed or papain digested specimens. In fatal cases, larvae have been demonstrated in muscle and brain also.

C. X-Ray Findings: Infiltrations can often be seen on chest x-ray.

Differential Diagnosis

Pallor and pica in children with other symptoms may be associated with lead poisoning. These 2 conditions have been reported to occur simultaneously. Transient eosinophilia (less than 3 weeks) may occur during the migration of ascaris larvae. More prolonged eosinophilia may occur in strongyloidiasis and trichinosis. Other helminths do not usually cause eosinophilia to a comparable degree.

Tropical eosinophilia may occur in infants and toddlers, especially in India. Pulmonary signs and symptoms are common, and hepatomegaly and fever may occur. Pica is not a feature.

Eosinophilia may be prominent in schistosomiasis and hydatid disease in association with hepatomegaly. Collagen diseases with eosinophilia and eosinophilic leukemia also should be differentiated.

Complications & Sequelae

Myocarditis, convulsive disorders, encephalitis, and ocular involvement such as retinal mass and endophthalmitis may occur due to the presence of larvae in these tissues. The ocular complications may be mistaken for retinoblastoma.

Treatment

A. Specific Measures: Diethylcarbamazine (Hetrazan) is the only drug with some action against the larvae. The dosage is 10–30 gm/kg/day orally in 3 divided doses for 2 weeks. Medical treatment is especially indicated when pulmonary symptoms are prominent.

B. General Measures: In most cases, the prevention of reinfection is all that is required since the condition disappears without treatment. Removal of the source of toxocara ova is important. The treatment of anemia with iron may be of value in stopping pica.

For endophthalmitis or for severe cases, especially with massive pulmonary infiltrates, corticosteroids have been recommended.

Prognosis

Some severe cases have been fatal. Endophthalmitis leads to blindness. The majority of patients recover if continued infection is avoided.

Shrand H: Visceral larva migrans: *Toxocara canis* infection. Lancet 1:1357–1359, 1964.
Synder CH: Visceral larva migrans: Ten years' experience. Pediatrics 28:85–91, 1961.

ONCHOCERCIASIS

Essentials of Diagnosis

- Localized or generalized pruritus.
- Subcutaneous nodules (adult worms).
- Superficial punctate keratitis.
- Late iridocyclitis.
- Eosinophilia.
- Biopsy evidence of *Onchocerca volvulus*.

General Considerations

Onchocerca volvulus is a filarial nematode found in Africa, Central and South America, and southern Mexico. It is transmitted by Simulium black flies in the larval form. The larvae develop slowly in subcutaneous tissue. Microfilariae may be found in locally infested areas of the body (skin and eyes) but do not invade the blood.

Clinical Findings

A. Symptoms and Signs: Almost 1/2 of infected patients develop localized areas of nodularity associated with itching and resulting in excoriation and chronic pigmentary and morphologic skin changes. Common sites include the bony prominences of the trunk, extremities, and head. Few patients develop more than 3–6 nodules.

Ocular infestation results in an early superficial punctate keratitis. Iridocyclitis may ultimately occur and is a serious complication which may lead to glaucoma, cataracts, and blindness.

B. Laboratory Findings: Eosinophilia of 15–50% is common. Aspiration of nodules will usually reveal eggs and microfilariae, and adult worms may be demonstrated in excised nodules. Microfilariae are not found in the blood but can be identified in skin or conjunctival snips or in skin shavings. The snip is performed by tenting the skin with a needle and cutting off a bit of skin above the needle tip. A blood-free shaving may be cut with a razor blade from the top of a ridge of skin firmly pressed between thumb and forefinger. Cocaine improves rather than detracts from the value of conjunctival snips. The snip or shaving is examined in a drop of saline under a coverslip on a slide. Shavings or snips should be taken from several sites over bony prominences of the scapular region, hips, and thighs. In ocular onchocerciasis, slit lamp examination will usually reveal many microfilariae in the anterior chamber. Complement-fixation and skin tests are of doubtful value because of high false-positive reaction rates.

Treatment
A. Specific Measures:
1. Diethylcarbamazine citrate (Hetrazan, Banocide) is almost nontoxic and fairly effective. Give 2–3 mg/kg orally 3 times daily for 14–21 days. To prevent severe allergic symptoms, which may be provoked early in therapy as microfilariae are rapidly killed, start treatment with small doses and increase the dosage over 3–4 days. When the eyes are involved, particular caution is necessary, starting with a single daily dose of 0.25 mg/kg. Use antihistamines to control allergic symptoms.

One course of diethylcarbamazine will eradicate the infection in about 40% of patients and halt progression in the remainder. Two or 3 courses will cure almost all cases.

2. Suramin sodium (Antrypol, Naphuride) is more effective than diethylcarbamazine in eradicating infection in a single course, but it has the disadvantage of potential renal toxicity (proteinuria, casts, red cells). Renal disease is a contraindication. For adults, give 1 gm as a 10% solution in distilled water IV every 4–7 days to a total dose of 5–10 gm. Start treatment with a test dose of 0.2 gm.

B. Surgical Measures:
Surgical removal of nodules is not curative but removes many adult worms and is particularly justifiable when nodules are located close to the eyes. Nodulectomy may also be indicated for cosmetic reasons.

Prognosis
With chemotherapy, progression of all forms of the disease usually can be checked. The prognosis is unfavorable only for patients seen for the first time with already far-advanced ocular onchocerciasis.

Duke BOL: Onchocerciasis. Brit MJ 1:301–304, 1968.
Woodruff AW & others: Papers and discussion on onchocerciasis. Tr Roy Soc Trop Med Hyg 60:695–734, 1966.

FILARIASIS

Essentials of Diagnosis
- Lymphangitis of the legs and genitals; obstructive lymphatic disease.
- Recurrent episodes lacking in periodicity.
- Characteristic microfilariae in blood.
- Leukocytosis with marked eosinophilia.
- Positive skin test to dirofilaria antigen.
- Positive complement-fixation, hemagglutinating, or flocculating antibody tests.

General Considerations
Filariasis is caused by infection with worms of the superfamily Filarioidea. They parasitize the blood and lymphatic systems and involve muscles, serous cavities, and connective tissues. The 2 principal human pathogens are *Wucheria bancrofti* and *Brugia malayi*. Both are transmitted by mosquitoes (*W bancrofti* by Culex and Aedes and *B malayi* by Anopheles and Mansonia). *W bancrofti* infection is widely prevalent in the tropics and subtropics throughout the world; *B malayi* is found mostly in India, Ceylon, and Southern Asia. Microfilariae are ingested by the mosquito vector and migrate to the thoracic muscles; larvae are deposited onto the skin of humans close to the bite of the mosquito. The larvae migrate into the puncture wound and pass to the lymphatics, where they reside for approximately 1 year, reaching maturity in the interval. Adults reside in the lymphatics of the extremities and genitals, where they give rise to microfilariae which reach the circulation. Microfilariae of *W bancrofti* are in the blood at night (an exception is a non-nocturnal variety in the South Pacific). *B malayi* may demonstrate nocturnal periodicity but can be semiperiodic (present at all times but more plentiful at night).

Man is the only definitive host for both filariae. *B malayi* tends to occur in regions along coastlines dotted with multiple ponds bearing water plants of the genus Pistia.

Other species of filarial worms infect man but are of little consequence clinically. These include *Tetrapetalonema perstans* (African and South American tropics), *Mansonella ozzardi* (West Indies and Central and South America), and worms of the genus Dirofilaria (Southern USA, especially Florida).

Clinical Findings
A. Symptoms and Signs:
Three clinical forms are apparent in children: the asymptomatic, the inflammatory, and the obstructive stages.

Asymptomatic infection is observed with both *W bancrofti* and *B malayi*. Children are exposed early in life and may exhibit microfilariasis in the blood without symptoms. By age 6, most children will be affected in endemic regions. Physical examination may reveal moderate lymphadenopathy, commonly of the inguinal nodes but not limited to this group. With death of the adult worms, the disease is "cured" and microfilariae disappear.

Inflammatory disease is probably related to hypersensitivity to antigens or products of the living and dead adult worms. Localized areas of lymphangitis involving the lower extremities and episodes of epididymitis, orchitis, and funiculitis are common. Systemic manifestations include fever, chills, vomiting, malaise, and achiness lasting for days or weeks. Abscesses occasionally occur in areas where adult worms have died. A chronic proliferative fibroblastic reaction eventually results in signs of obstructive lymphatic disease.

The obstructive stage develops in only a portion of those infected with filariae. Obstructive filariasis is a slow, chronic, progressive state resulting in edema of the affected parts. Elephantiasis results from multiple channel obstruction and can terminate in gross distortion of the extremities and genitalia. Recurrent inflammatory episodes may punctuate the progressive obstructive signs. Lymphatic rupture can result in the extrusion of lymph into serous cavities or organs (chyluria, chylous ascites, hydrocele).

B. Laboratory Findings: Eosinophilia in children may vary between 5–25% early in the disease. With progression and reduction of inflammatory episodes, the eosinophil count falls.

Microfilariae may be found in night blood specimens in the asymptomatic form of the disease as well as in the inflammatory form, but decrease as the obstructive phase progresses. Differentiation of *W bancrofti* and *B malayi* from nonpathogenic microfilariae may be difficult and requires an experienced observer. Adult worms can be identified in biopsy specimens, but biopsies should be performed judiciously to avoid further damage to lymphatic drainage channels.

Antibody determinations may be useful when microfilariae cannot be identified. The skin test employs dirofilaria antigen and has a 10% false-positive response.

Differential Diagnosis

During the inflammatory stage, diagnosis may be difficult, and many common childhood infections must be considered. In endemic areas or with a history of a stay in such areas, the presence of fever, lymphangitis, and lymphadenitis associated with eosinophilia should suggest filariasis. Various inflammatory lesions of the genitalia (gonorrhea, mumps orchitis, epididymitis) must be differentiated. Elephantiasis is strongly suggestive of filariasis but must be differentiated from hernia or hydrocele, Milroy's disease, venous thrombosis, or lesions resulting in anasarca or dependent edema (congestive heart failure, nephrosis, hepatic disease).

Prevention

Control of mosquitoes and human sources is necessary. Insecticide control of mosquitoes and attempts to reduce breeding areas are useful. Diethylcarbamazine therapy in humans results in a diminishing reservoir for mosquito infestation.

Treatment

A. General Measures: Rest and relocation in a cooler climate appear to aid in alleviation of inflammatory episodes. All secondary infections—particularly those affecting the lymphatics, such as streptococcal infections—should be diagnosed promptly and treated vigorously. Inflammatory genital lesions in the male are relieved by suspension of the affected part.

B. Surgical Measures: Plastic surgical correction of the involved genitalia may be accomplished with good results. Surgical treatment of limbs is unsatisfactory. Drainage of chyle, when it results in discomfort or reduced function, may be useful on a temporary basis.

C. Specific Treatment: Diethylcarbamazine citrate (Hetrazan, Banocide) is the drug of choice. The dose is 2 mg/kg orally 3 times daily for 14–21 days. Allergic reactions are minimized by reducing each dose in relation to the occurrence and severity of prior reactions. The drug kills microfilariae but has little effect on the adult worms. Relapses can occur 3–12 months after a course of therapy, and retreatment over a period of 1–2 years is often necessary. Obstructive filariasis is not benefited by drug therapy.

Prognosis

In asymptomatic disease, the prognosis is excellent in young children. With progression, relocation can result in improvement provided the disease is in its early stages and is mild. Severe elephantiasis requires surgical correction, which may have a satisfactory result in the genital region but a poor result if extremities are involved.

Wijetunge HPA: Clinical manifestations of early bancroftian filariasis. J Trop Med 70:90–94, 1967.

Wilson T: Filariasis in Malaya: A general review. Tr Roy Soc Trop Med Hyg 55:107–129, 1961.

2. CESTODAL INFECTIONS

TAENIASIS & CYSTICERCOSIS

Essentials of Diagnosis

- Abdominal discomfort, pain, or diarrhea (taeniasis).
- Passage of segments (proglottids) or ova of tapeworm per rectum (taeniasis).
- Demonstration of cysticerci in tissue biopsy specimens or on x-ray (cysticercosis).

General Considerations

Taeniasis may be caused by the beef tapeworm (*Taenia saginata*) or pork tapeworm (*T solium*). The adult worms reside in the alimentary canal of man. The mature segments passed per rectum discharge ova in feces and soil which are then ingested by cattle and pigs. The hatched larvae develop into encysted forms mainly in the skeletal muscles (cysticercosis). When man consumes raw or undercooked meat, the larvae are liberated and develop into adults in the small intestine. The worm attaches itself to the mucosa by its head.

Human cysticercosis is usually caused by the larvae of *T solium* but may rarely be caused by larvae of *T saginata*. It occurs as a result of ingestion of ova, which hatch in the intestines; from the intestines the larvae migrate into muscle and other tissues. It may be that ova produced by the worm already in the intestine can hatch and cause cysticercosis.

Both of these disorders are worldwide in distribution. They are more prevalent in areas where control over the quality of meat is inadequate.

Clinical Findings

A. Symptoms and Signs: In the majority of tapeworm infections there are no symptoms other than the passage of segments per rectum. The worms are often passed in feces, and are seen as white motile bodies about 1–2 cm long and 5 mm thick. Occasionally, the proglottid moves out of the rectum and crawls on the skin of the thigh.

Infants are not infected since they are not exposed. Toddlers and older children may harbor the infection for years. Abdominal pain, diarrhea, excessive appetite, failure to gain weight, abdominal distention, and anorexia may occur. Symptoms may be related to the number of worms present.

Most cases of cysticercosis go undiagnosed since there are few or no symptoms. The development of subcutaneous or muscle nodules is often the sole manifestation. After several years the cysticerci calcify and appear as opacities on x-ray. Cysticerci in the brain may remain silent or may cause symptoms and signs of epilepsy, brain tumor, hydrocephalus, and basal meningitis. In the eye they may cause uveitis, retinal detachment, and hemorrhage. The diagnosis is difficult to confirm except when nodules are available for biopsy or are visible in radiographs. The presence of *T solium* in the gut is of diagnostic significance.

B. Laboratory Findings: The diagnosis is confirmed by the demonstration of the proglottids or ova. Ova may be seen in fecal smears or may be detected on the perianal skin by the method used in the diagnosis of enterobiasis (see above). They are globular, 30–60 μm in diameter, with a double wall showing radial striations and an embryo with 6 hooklets.

If a proglottid is compressed between 2 glass slides, the main lateral branches of the uterus may be examined. *T saginata* has more than 15 and *T solium* fewer than 14 such branches to each side.

Eosinophilia is mild or absent in most cases.

Treatment

A. Taeniasis: Until recently, quinacrine was the best drug available though not completely satisfactory. Aspidium oleoresin (extract of male fern) is more effective but more toxic and not recommended for children. The duodenal introduction of warm hypertonic salt solutions has been successfully used but is too cumbersome for general use. Dichlorophen (Anthiphen) is a promising drug if preliminary results are confirmed.

Niclosamide (Yomesan) now appears to be the best available drug. Toxicity is slight or absent in therapeutic doses. It is given orally in doses of 1 gm for children 2–8 years of age, 1.5 gm for children over 8, and 2 gm for adults—on an empty stomach on the morning following a light nonresidue supper. A saline cathartic is recommended after 2 hours only in *T solium* infection to prevent spillage of ova into the intestines, which may lead to cysticercosis.

If niclosamide is not available, give quinacrine (mepacrine, Atabrine) in doses of 10–15 mg/kg orally up to a maximum of 800 mg, either as a single dose or in 2 divided doses 1 hour apart on an empty stomach in the morning as in niclosamide therapy. The purpose of dividing the dose is to prevent vomiting, but antiemetics may be given prior to administration or sodium bicarbonate (200 mg) may be given with the drug. A saline cathartic is recommended in both types of taeniasis.

If segments are not passed per rectum for at least 3 months, that is sufficient evidence of complete expulsion of the worms.

B. Cysticercosis: There is no specific treatment for cysticercosis. Operative removal of cysticerci is of value when individual lesions cause symptoms.

Prognosis

The prognosis is good in taeniasis. In cerebral cysticercosis, the prognosis is unpredictable. Symptoms may disappear after a variable interval. In heavy infections, death may follow.

Dixon HBF, Hargreaves WH: Cysticercosis (*T solium*). Quart J Med 13:107–121, 1944.

Nieto D: Cysticercosis of the nervous system: Diagnosis by means of the spinal fluid complement fixation test. Neurology 6:725–738, 1956.

HYMENOLEPIASIS

Hymenolepis nana infects children commonly and *H dimínuta* rarely. *H diminuta* is a rat tapeworm with cysticercus stages in fleas and insects. Children acquire the infection by eating contaminated grains. *H nana* occurs in South and Southeast Asia, North Africa, southern Europe, South America, and the southern United States. It is primarily a human parasite and requires no intermediate host. The ova may hatch inside the intestinal lumen and perpetuate infection. Fecal-oral contamination is necessary for infection of fresh hosts.

Unlike other tapeworms, *H nana* is very small (1 cm), and numerous worms may be present in the intestines. Infection is usually asymptomatic, but diarrhea and abdominal pain may occur. The diagnosis is confirmed by detecting ova in feces. They appear oval or globular, 40–60 μm, and double-walled without radial striations; the embryo has 6 hooklets.

Quinacrine (mepacrine, Atabrine) is the usually recommended drug, but it is only moderately effective. (For dosage, see Taeniasis.) Hexylresorcinol may be tried if quinacrine fails (see Trichuriasis). Tetrachloroethylene may be of value in some cases (see Hookworm Disease).

Niclosamide (Yomesan) has been used recently with success, but experience with this drug in the treatment of hymenolepiasis is small (see Taeniasis).

Since these drugs do not kill the ova, a second course of therapy should be administered after an interval of 10 days to eliminate the newly developing worms.

Beaver PC, Sodeman WA: Treatment of *Hymenolepis nana* (dwarf tapeworm) infection with quinacrine hydrochloride (Atebrin). J Trop Med 55:97–99, 1952.

DIPHYLLOBOTHRIASIS

Human infection with the fish tapeworm, *Diphyllobothrium latum,* occurs in the Scandinavian, Baltic, and Mediterranean regions, in Japan, and around the Great Lakes region of the USA and Canada. One or more adult worms live inside the human intestine, attached to the mucosa by its head. Adults and children are infected.

The ova develop in crustaceans, which are eaten by fish. The larvae develop further and encyst in the muscle and connective tissues of the fish. Pike, salmon, trout, and barbels may become infected. Man acquires the infection by consuming raw caviar or raw or undercooked fish. Smoking or ordinary kippering does not destroy the larvae.

In many cases the infection remains silent. No segments (proglottids) are passed per rectum. Abdominal pain, vomiting, diarrhea, and nutritional deficiency occur occasionally.

The diagnosis is made by the detection of ova in stools. They are oval, operculated, 45 × 70 μm, with a brownish shell enclosing several granulated, tightly packed yolk cells.

In fewer than 1% of cases, progressive macrocytic, megaloblastic anemia occurs as a result of vitamin B_{12} deficiency. The megaloblastic anemia may be complicated by spinal cord lesions.

Quinacrine, hexylresorcinol, and tetrachloroethylene are moderately effective against this worm (see Hymenolepiasis). Niclosamide (Yomesan; see Taeniasis), dichlorophen (Anthiphen), or bithionol (Actamer, Bitin) may, if preliminary studies are confirmed, replace the conventional drugs.

In the majority of instances of megaloblastic anemia, the expulsion of the worms results in a hematologic remission. In severe cases, cyanocobalamin (vitamin B_{12}) may be given parenterally in a single dose of 15–30 μg by deep subcutaneous or IM injection. Oral cyanocobalamin is of little value until after the expulsion of the worms.

Nagahana M & others: Treatment of *Taenia saginata* and *Diphyllobothrium latum* infections with bithionol. Am J Trop Med 15:351–354, 1966.

Von Bonsdorff B & others: Vitamin B_{12} deficiency in carriers of the fish tapeworm, *Diphyllobothrium latum.* Acta haemat 24:15–19, 1960.

ECHINOCOCCOSIS

Essentials of Diagnosis

- Cystic tumor of liver or lung; rarely, of kidney, bone, brain, and other organs.
- Urticaria and pruritus secondary to rupture of cyst.
- Eosinophilia.
- Protoscoleces, brood capsules, or daughter cysts in lesion.
- Elevated titers on indirect hemagglutination (> 1:400) or bentonite flocculation (> 1:5) tests.
- Positive skin test (Casoni).

General Considerations

Echinococcus granulosus is a tapeworm that infects dogs and some cats and other carnivores. The adult worm lives in the intestines, and eggs are excreted in dog feces. Man serves as an intermediate host. After eggs are ingested, the embryonic worm passes into intestinal lymphatics, reaching various parts of the body via the circulation. A cyst develops in organs where the embryonic worms settle. There is a predilection for the liver (60–70%) and the lung (20–25%). A unilocular spherical cyst is the most common form of the disease. It grows over a period of years and may reach 10 inches in diameter, although most are between ½ and 3 inches. A well defined structure exists in the cyst. Infection with *E multilocularis* results in cysts which are multilocular or alveolar.

Clinical Findings

A. Symptoms and Signs: Clinical findings are dependent upon several phenomena: pressure by the enlarging cysts, erosion of blood vessels, and circulation of sensitizing parts of the cyst or worm. Cysts in the liver present as slowly growing tumors. Jaundice may be present if biliary obstruction occurs. Most cysts are in the right lobe, extending downward into the abdomen; ¼ are on the upper surface and may go undetected for many years.

Hemorrhage may result from erosion. Omental torsion is also observed.

Pulmonary cysts rarely produce pressure symptoms but may erode into a bronchus, resulting in cough and atelectasis.

Rupture of a cyst and discharge of its contents may result in sudden episodes of coughing if in the lung. Asthma, urticaria, and pruritus may be observed. The sputum is blood-tinged and frothy and contains bits of the cyst and worm. Common signs in pulmonary cyst rupture are coughing, dyspnea, hemoptysis, chest pain, and increase in pulse and respiratory rates.

Cysts of the brain may produce focal neurologic signs and convulsions; of the kidney, hematuria and pain; of bone, pain.

B. Laboratory Findings: In suspected cases of echinococcosis with allergic manifestations, a search for protoscoleces, brood capsules, or daughter cysts should be made. Specimens for examination will depend on the site of the cyst but include sputum or bronchoscopic aspirates, urine, ascitic fluid or pleural fluid, and CSF.

Eosinophilia occurs irregularly and to a variable extent.

Serologic tests include indirect hemagglutination (titer of > 1:400 positive) and bentonite flocculation (titer of > 1:5). In liver disease, 80–85% have positive serologic results; in lung disease, only 30–50% are positive. A complement-fixation test is available and is positive in 80–90%. Complement-fixation titers decrease with removal of the cyst. The Casoni test is positive in 85% of patients with echinococcosis but has a high false-positive rate (18%). Positive reactions persist for years after surgical removal or death of the worm.

C. X-Ray Findings: X-ray of the chest may reveal the cyst. Special studies of the CNS may reveal evidence of an intracranial mass and increased pressure. Calcified cysts in any organ may be noted; destruction of bony structure is visible in osseous lesions.

Differential Diagnosis

Hydatid cysts in any site may be mistaken for a variety of malignant and nonmalignant tumors or for abscesses, both bacterial and amebic. In the lung, a cyst may be confused with an advanced tubercular lesion. Syphilis may also be confused with echinococcosis. Allergic symptoms arising from cyst leakage may resemble those associated with many other diseases.

Complications

Sudden rupture of a cyst leading to anaphylaxis and sometimes death is the most important complication of echinococcosis. If the patient survives the rupture, he still faces the danger of multiple secondary cyst infections arising from seeding of daughter cysts. Segmental lung collapse, secondary infections of cysts, secondary effects of increased intracranial pressure, and severe renal damage due to kidney cysts are other potential complications.

Treatment

The only definitive treatment is surgical removal of the intact cysts, preferably preceded by inoculation into the cyst of hydrogen peroxide, Lugol's iodine, glycerin, or formalin. Often, however, the presence of a cyst is only recognized when it begins to leak or when it ruptures. Such an event calls for vigorous treatment of allergic symptoms or emergency management of anaphylactic shock. There is no treatment for alveolar cysts in the liver.

Bunamidine derivatives have been reported to be effective (see Nature 206:408–409, 1965) and should be tested further.

Prognosis

Patients may live for years with relatively large hydatid cysts before their condition is diagnosed. Liver and lung cysts often can be removed surgically without great difficulty, but for cysts in sites less accessible to surgery the prognosis is less favorable. The prognosis is always grave in secondary echinococcosis and with alveolar cysts. About 15% of patients with echinococcosis may eventually die because of the disease or its complications.

Bonakdarpour A: Echinococcocus disease: A report of 112 cases from Iran and a review of all cases from the United States. Am J Roentgenol 99:660–667, 1967.

Hutchison, WF: Serodiagnosis of echinococcus infection. Am J Trop Med 17:752–755, 1968.

Webster GA, Cameron TWM: Epidemiology and diagnosis of echinococcosis in Canada. Canad MAJ 96:600–607, 1967.

3. TREMATODAL INFECTIONS

PARAGONIMIASIS, CLONORCHIASIS, FASCIOLIASIS, & FASCIOLOPSIASIS

Paragonimiasis, caused by the lung fluke *Paragonimus westermani,* occurs in East and Southeast Asia, parts of Africa, and in northern South America. Man and carnivorous animals acquire the infection by consuming uncooked shellfish, the intermediate hosts carrying encysted larvae.

Clonorchiasis and fascioliasis are caused by the liver flukes *Clonorchis sinensis* and *Fasciola hepatica.* The former occurs in East and Southeast Asia and the latter in Central America and the Caribbean. Ingestion of raw fish containing encysted clonorchis larvae or fresh aquatic plants with attached encysted fasciola larvae results in infections.

Fasciolopis buski, the intestinal fluke, causes fasciolopsiasis, found in East and Southeast Asia. The encysted larvae remain attached to water plants as in the case of fasciola.

Clinical Findings

A. Paragonimiasis: The lung fluke larvae migrate from the intestines to the lungs, where they mature and form cystic lesions with fibrous walls. Fibrous nodules also appear around eggs. The usual symptoms are cough with copious brownish sputum and frequent hemoptysis. In heavy infections the worms are also found in various abdominal viscera and even in the brain. In such instances, abdominal pain, dysentery, and convulsive and paralytic disease may occur. X-ray changes in the lungs and clubbing of the fingers are common. The diagnosis depends on the demonstration of ova in sputum or feces.

B. Clonorchiasis and Fascioliasis: The larvae of these liver flukes migrate and mature in the liver tissues. Most infections remain asymptomatic. Fever, upper abdominal pain, hepatomegaly, jaundice, urticaria, and eosinophilia in varying combinations are the early features in heavy and continued infections, especially in older children. Cholangitis, cholecystitis, and cholelithiasis may occur in episodes. Cirrhosis of the liver is a late complication. The diagnosis is confirmed by the demonstration of ova in feces or duodenal aspirate.

C. Fasciolopsiasis: The flukes inhabit the duodenum and the jejunum. The usual symptoms are abdominal pain and diarrhea. Gradually, progressive malnutrition, ascites, and generalized edema appear. Severe and untreated infections may cause death. The diagnosis is confirmed by the presence of ova in feces.

Treatment

A. Paragonimiasis, Clonorchiasis, and Fascioliasis: There are no specific effective drugs against lung and liver flukes. Emetine hydrochloride, 1 mg/kg/day IM for 5–7 days, is the usually recommended therapy, especially for paragonimiasis and fascioliasis. An alternative drug is chloroquine, 10 mg/kg orally daily for 3 weeks, especially for paragonimiasis and clonorchiasis. It may be advisable to give one course each of both drugs. Gentian violet is also useful in clonorchiasis.

Bithionol (Bitin), given in a dose of 5 mg/kg orally in 3 divided doses on alternate days, has been found useful in paragonimiasis.

B. Fasciolopsiasis: Intestinal fluke infection may be treated either with oral hexylresorcinol (Crystoids Anthelmintic) or tetrachloroethylene. These drugs are discussed under trichuriasis and hookworm disease, respectively.

Brown HW & others: The treatment of *Fasciolopsis buski* infections with dithiazanine iodide, 1-bromo-naphthol-(2)ascaridol, piperazine and tetrachloroethylene. J Formosan Med A 58:792–797, 1959.

Ehrenworth L, Daniels RA: Clonorchiasis sinensis: Clinical manifestations and diagnosis. Ann Int Med 49:419–427, 1958.

Neghime A, Ossandon M: Ectopic and hepatic fascioliasis. Am J Trop Med 23:545–550, 1943.

Nwokolo C: Paragonimiasis in eastern Nigeria. J Trop Med 67:1–4, 1964.

SCHISTOSOMIASIS
(Bilharziasis)

Essentials of Diagnosis

- A transient itchy papular rash following exposure to fresh water.
- Fever, urticaria, joint pain, cough, lymphadenitis, eosinophilia.
- Anorexia, loss of weight, diarrhea or dysentery.
- Hematuria (usually terminal), painful micturition.
- Demonstration of ova in stools, urine, or rectal biopsy specimen.

General Considerations

Schistosomiasis is caused by the blood flukes, *Schistosoma haematobium, S japonicum,* or *S mansoni. S haematobium* is prevalent in tropical and subtropical Africa and some parts of western Asia. *S japonicum* occurs in East and Southeast Asia. *S mansoni* is common in tropical Africa and South America.

The infective larvae are found in fresh water. When in contact with human skin, they penetrate, invade the blood vessels, and migrate to certain sites. Respectively, the preferential sites of *S haematobium, S japonicum,* and *S mansoni* are the vesical venous plexus, the draining veins of the small intestine, and those of the large bowel. They mature at these sites, mate, and the females lay eggs. The eggs escape into the perivascular tissues, cause inflammatory lesions, and exude into the lumen of the bladder and bowel. This is accompanied by extravasation of blood.

The ova that escape in urine and feces hatch in fresh water and the larvae enter and develop in the intermediate host, the snail. At a later stage, the infective larvae live free in water.

Clinical Findings

In highly endemic areas, large proportions of the population may be infected with many showing no symptoms but discharging ova. Symptoms follow heavy and continued exposure. The diagnosis is readily suspected in endemic areas. Otherwise, a history of residence in endemic areas is of great value in alerting the pediatrician.

A. Symptoms and Signs: Irritation of the skin may rarely occur at sites of larval entry with a transient itchy papular rash. During the migration of the larvae, fever and urticaria may occur. The larvae may escape into the alveoli, causing cough and hemoptysis. Liver and spleen gradually enlarge and become tender. After lodgement of the flukes in their favorite venous plexuses, fever and toxemia occur and last for several days to weeks. In bladder infection, painful and frequent micturition and hematuria are common. Bladder stones and incontinence of urine may follow. Secondary pyelonephritis, ureterovesical reflux, and anatomic changes in the ureters demonstrable by intravenous urograms are common. In the intestinal types, abdominal pain, diarrhea (often bloody), and progressive abdominal enlargement due to increasing splenomegaly and ascites occur.

B. Laboratory Findings: The diagnosis is usually confirmed by the demonstration of schistosome ova in feces or urine. *S japonicum* ova are seen only in feces. *S mansoni* ova are frequently seen in feces and occasionally in urine. If there are no ova in feces and urine, rectal biopsy specimen may reveal *S mansoni* eggs. *S haematobium* ova are frequently seen in urine and occasionally in feces.

The ova of *S mansoni* and *S hematobium* measure about 140 × 60 μm and those of *S japonicum* about 90 × 70 μm. *S haematobium* ova have a terminal spine, whereas the ova of *S mansoni* and *S japonicum* have a lateral hook or spine.

An intradermal test is available and is of value especially in *S japonicum* infection.

Marked eosinophilia is common.

Complications & Sequelae

The complications and sequelae of *S hematobium* infection are anemia, renal calculi, ascending bacterial infection of the urinary tract, strictures and fistulas, lymphedema of the genitalia, uremia, hypertension, and malignancy of the bladder. Schistosomal granulomas in the female genital tract or in the spinal cord (with paraplegia) have been described.

Anemia, cirrhosis of the liver, portal hypertension, and bleeding from esophageal varices may occur in alimentary forms of schistosomiasis. Pulmonary hypertension and cor pulmonale may occur late in *S mansoni* infections.

Severe nutritional deficiencies and death are not uncommon in unchecked and heavy infections.

Prevention

In endemic areas, prevention of infection by avoiding skin contact with contaminated fresh water (bathing, wading) is of paramount public health importance.

Treatment

A. General Measures: It is important to look for and treat intercurrent bacterial or parasitic infections and nutritional deficiencies. For fibrotic and calcified lesions in the older child, especially of the urinary tract, corrective surgery should be done to relieve symptoms or arrest the progression of renal damage. Splenectomy and portacaval shunt are palliative measures in advanced alimentary schistosomiasis.

B. Specific Measures:

1. Antimony compounds—Antimony potassium or sodium tartrate (tartar emetic) is recommended only for *S japonicum* infections. It is given intravenously as a freshly prepared 0.5% solution. Injections are given on alternate days, starting with 4 ml on the first day and increasing by 2 ml on alternate days up to 14 ml, and continued at this level (ie, 14 ml on alternate days) until 200–250 ml have been given to children under 40 kg and 300 ml for those over 40 kg. It must be given very slowly, avoiding leakage into perivascular tissue. The patient must rest in bed during the injection and for several hours afterward. When intravenous therapy is difficult, stibophen (see below) may be given intramuscularly as for *S haematobium* or *S mansoni* infections.

One of the following antimonials given intramuscularly is recommended in *S haematobium* and *S mansoni* infections.

Antimony sodium dimercaptosuccinate is given for *S haematobium* and *S mansoni* in total doses of 40–60 mg/kg for children under 20 kg and 30–50 mg/kg for older children in 5 or 6 IM injections, 1–2 injections per week. Persistent rash or fever and excessive vomiting are indications for a temporary suspension of therapy.

Stibophen (Fuadin) is given IM as a 6.3% aqueous solution in doses of 1 ml/15 kg, not exceeding 5 ml per injection. A test dose of 0.5 or 1 ml is given first and the dose increased in 2–3 steps. A short course consists of 8 injections and a long course consists of 5 injections per week for 4 weeks. Recurrent vomiting, the appearance of proteinuria, and joint pains call for cessation of therapy.

Antimony lithium thiomalate (Anthiomaline) is given IM on alternate days to a total of 40–45 ml for children under 15 years. The first dose is 0.5 ml; thereafter, give 2 ml for children under 10 and 2.5–3 ml for those above.

2. Niridazole (Ambilhar)—This drug has given cure rates equal to or better than those achieved with antimonials. The results are best with *S haematobium*, and *S japonicum* is least responsive. The daily dose is 25 mg/kg (maximum, 1.5 gm) in 2 divided doses daily for 7 days.

3. Lucanthone hydrochloride—Lucanthone (Miracil D, Nilodin) has the advantage of oral administration. It is given in doses of 5 mg/kg 2–3 times daily up to a total of 100 mg/kg. Anorexia, nausea, and vomiting occur frequently. Children tolerate this drug better than adults, who may experience circulatory disturbances, psychoses, and convulsions.

Prognosis

The prognosis is good in mild infections and in heavy, symptomatic infections treated early. Otherwise, the prognosis is poor, especially with involvement of the lungs, liver, spleen, and urinary tract.

Fernandez A, Steigmann F, Villa F: Schistosomiasis: Mimicry of gastrointestinal diseases. Am J Gastroenterol 40:482–486, 1963.

Forsyth DM, MacDonald G: Urological complications of endemic schistosomiasis in school children. Part I. Usagara School. Tr Roy Soc Trop Med Hyg 50:171–178, 1965.

Forsyth DM: Treatment of urinary schistosomiasis: Practice and therapy. Lancet 2:354–358, 1965.

• • •

General References

Adams ARD, Maegraith BG: *Clinical Tropical Diseases,* 4th ed. Blackwell, 1966.

Brown HW, Belding DL: *Basic Clinical Parasitology,* 2nd ed. Appleton-Century-Crofts, 1964.

Faust EC, Russell PF: *Craig and Faust's Clinical Parasitology,* 7th ed. Lea & Febiger, 1964.

Jawetz E, Melnick JL, Adelberg EA: *Review of Medical Microbiology,* 10th ed. Lange, 1972.

Manson-Bahr P, Walters JH: *The Chemotherapy of Tropical Diseases.* Thomas, 1961.

Manson-Bahr P: *Manson's Tropical Diseases,* 16th ed. Tindall & Cassell, 1966.

Meyers FH, Jawetz E, Goldfien A: *Review of Medical Pharmacology,* 3rd ed. Lange, 1972.

Trowell HC, Jelliffe DB: *Diseases of Children in the Subtropics and Tropics.* Arnold, 1958.

29 . . .

Infections: Mycotic

Vincent A. Fulginiti, MD

ACTINOMYCOSIS

Essentials of Diagnosis

- Chronic suppurative lesions of the skin, with sinus tract formation.
- "Sulfur granules"—actinomyces colonies 1–2 mm in diameter—found in pus from lesion.
- Gram-positive hyphae.
- Association with gram-negative bacteria.
- Isolation of organism from sulfur granule or pus.

General Considerations

Human actinomycosis is almost always caused by *Actinomyces israelii.* Many investigators feel that the presence of gram-negative bacilli is necessary before infection can occur, and it is true that gram-negative bacilli are found almost invariably in association with *A israelii.* The organism is a frequent oral and dental saprophyte, and infection is endogenous.

Actinomycosis is characteristically a chronic, slowly progressive disease. There is no consistent occupational association.

Clinical Findings

A. Symptoms and Signs: Three forms of the disease are recognized: cervicofacial, thoracic, and abdominal.

1. Cervicofacial actinomycosis (lumpy jaw)— Granulomas appear in the mandible or maxilla and are of dental or oral origin. These break down and suppurate, and may seal over but do not heal. Sinus tracts form and reform, and without treatment the disease has a chronic unremitting course.

2. Thoracic actinomycosis—This form is heralded by fever (often of septic nature), pleural pain, cough, and weight loss. Mucopurulent or sanguineous sputum or sinus tract drainage may be present. Dullness to percussion and signs of consolidation may be present, and sinus tracts communicating with the skin may form.

3. Abdominal actinomycosis—Abdominal actinomycosis usually begins with inflammation of the appendix and weight loss. Fever, chills, and vomiting over a protracted course are associated with painful, palpable masses.

B. Laboratory Findings: Identification of typical sulfur granules and gram-positive hyphae in secretions should lead to culture of *A israelii,* which establishes the diagnosis.

C. X-Ray Findings: With bony involvement, periostitis and osteomyelitis are visible on x-ray examination. Heavy hilar and basilar infiltration is characteristic of pulmonary actinomycosis.

Differential Diagnosis

Actinomycosis must be distinguished from similar fungal diseases (culture); pulmonary, intestinal, or lymphatic tuberculosis (PPD, isolation of mycobacteria, response to therapy); and lymphomas (biopsy, absence of sinuses, blood or bone marrow changes). Bacterial infection of the cervical lymph nodes, bones, chest, or abdomen can usually be differentiated on the basis of culture, acuteness, and response to therapy.

Complications

Extension of the infection from the primary site to contiguous structures (irrespective of anatomic limits) results in osteomyelitis, brain abscess, hepatic or renal involvement, and skin abscesses and sinus tracts.

Treatment

A. Specific Treatment: Penicillin is the drug of choice. Daily doses ranging up to 2 million units in infants and up to 20 million units in older children are necessary. Initial intravenous therapy followed by intramuscular and then by oral administration must usually be continued for as long as 1–1½ years. Broad spectrum antibiotics and sulfadiazine are useful adjuncts but should not be used alone.

B. General Measures: Surgical excision is frequently necessary, particularly with chronic, multiple sinus tracts. Preoperative therapy with penicillin is always indicated.

Prognosis

Penicillin therapy has greatly improved the prognosis. Unless the course has been prolonged and complications such as brain abscess or meningitis have appeared, recovery is the rule. Convalescence may be prolonged.

Coodley EL: Actinomycosis: Clinical diagnosis and management. Postgrad Med 46:73–78, 1969.

Harvey TC & others: Actinomycosis: Its recognition and treatment. Ann Int Med 46:868–885, 1957.

Peabody JW, Seabury JH: Actinomycosis and nocardiosis. Am J Med 28:99–115, 1960.

ASPERGILLOSIS

Opportunistic infection due to *Aspergillus fumigatus* and other species of this genus is rare in childhood. These organisms are found commonly in nature, particularly in decaying vegetation. A number of cases have occurred in children receiving corticosteroids or immunosuppressive drugs; other predisposing causes include chronic bronchopulmonary disease, tuberculosis, and morphologic abnormalities of the respiratory tract.

A chronic course is characteristic, and a history of long-standing symptoms may be elicited. Fever, productive cough, and increasing lassitude often precede cavitary pulmonary changes. Pulmonary infection may become disseminated to other viscera, often with a fatal outcome. Mucopurulent sputum or hemoptysis is frequently present. Chronic otomycosis is manifested by obstruction of the auditory canal with a plug composed of fungus, wax, and epithelial debris. In the absence of bacterial infection, the canal is dry. There are no laboratory aids to the diagnosis save for culture of the fungus or identification of hyphae in sodium hydroxide preparations from specimens of sputum, pus, or ear curettage.

There is no specific therapy. Iodides, amphotericin B (Fungizone), and vaccine therapy have all been employed with variable success.

International symposium on opportunistic fungus infection. Lab Invest 11:1017–1241, 1962.

Khoo TK & others: Disseminated aspergillosis. Case report and review of world literature. Am J Clin Path 45:697–703, 1966.

Wahner HW & others: Pulmonary aspergillosis. Ann Int Med 58:472–485, 1963.

Young RC: Aspergillus lobar pneumonia. JAMA 208:1156–1162, 1969.

NORTH AMERICAN BLASTOMYCOSIS

Blastomyces dermatitidis, a budding yeast form in human infection, is present in soil, but its exact mode of transmission is not known. The disease is widely distributed in North and Central America, with a high prevalence in the Mississippi Valley. Childhood illness is uncommon.

There are 2 basic forms—pulmonary and cutaneous—and a disseminated form that may arise from either and is characterized by chronic suppurative bronchopulmonary disease with insidious and often prolonged (months) early symptoms of cough, fever, weight loss, increasing chest pain, and hoarseness. Purulent or bloody sputum may be present. With dissemination, cutaneous lesions, bone pain, chills, and sweats become apparent. CNS symptoms are heralded by severe headache, and focal neurologic signs, particularly paralysis, are common.

Cutaneous lesions are usually single, beginning as a nodular papule on an exposed surface and gradually ulcerating and failing to heal. Multiple sites may be present and are all associated with pulmonary disease. Spread is believed to be via the blood stream. The individual lesion has a raised border with a multiply abscessed crater. Purplish discoloration is frequent, and small abscesses can be found in the border.

Dissemination results in involvement of the brain, kidneys, bones, skin, and subcutaneous tissues. Symptoms referable to these tissues in a patient with chronic pulmonary infection should lead one to suspect blastomycosis.

Pus from sputum or cutaneous lesions should be examined in a sodium hydroxide preparation. A thick-walled, broad-based, budding spherical fungus (8–15 μm in diameter) is almost diagnostic but should be confirmed by isolation of a characteristic white, dry mold on Sabouraud's medium. Since infection in laboratory personnel is a risk, material for culture should be carefully handled and culture plates or slants sealed and maintained for more than 30 days. A positive blastomycin skin test reaction indicates contact with the organism. A rise in complement fixation titer occurs in paired sera.

Iodides and diamidines have been employed with variable success. Amphotericin B (Fungizone) by intravenous infusion may be helpful (see Chapter 39). Surgical drainage and excisional therapy are of limited benefit but may be useful in selected cases and as an adjunct to antifungal therapy.

Mild forms of the pulmonary disease may exist, but the usual clinically apparent case, if untreated, usually disseminates, leading to death.

Baum GL, Schwarz J: North American blastomycosis. Am J M Sc 238:661–683, 1959.

Kunkel WM & others: North American blastomycosis. Surg Gynec Obst 99:1, 1954.

Parker JD & others: A decade of experience with blastomycosis and its treatment with amphotericin B. Am Rev Resp Dis 99:895–902, 1969.

Pfister AK & others: Pulmonary blastomycosis. South MJ 59:1441–1447, 1966.

CANDIDIASIS

Essentials of Diagnosis

- Plaque-like and ulcerative lesions of the oral mucosa.

- Vulvovaginitis, skin fold infections, paronychia; pulmonary, CNS, and disseminated disease.
- A compatible clinical picture, a susceptible host, and the repeated finding of oval, budding yeasts in clinical specimens should establish the diagnosis.

General Considerations

Candida albicans is the major human pathogen of the genus. It is a ubiquitous, dimorphic fungus which usually reproduces by budding. The yeast forms are vegetative; in most human tissue infections, the mycelial form is observed. Although many host defense factors have been described, no consistent relationship to infection or disease has been established. Delayed hypersensitivity to candida appears to be important in that clinically significant disease states are almost always associated with a lack of skin test reactivity.

C albicans exists as a normal inhabitant of the gastrointestinal flora, and its growth is held in check by the presence of other members of the flora. With the exceptions of thrush in neonates and vaginitis in pregnant women, it seldom produces disease in healthy individuals. Reduction in host defenses or a significant change in the indigenous flora results in overgrowth of candida and can lead to local and systemic disease. Thus, lymphopenic immunologic deficiencies, the use of corticosteroids or other immunosuppressive therapy, and the administration of antibiotics all may result in systemic candidiasis. Candidiasis is also commonly associated with diabetes mellitus, but the important pathogenetic factors are obscure. Topical candidiasis may occur in areas of the skin macerated or exposed to excessive moisture (eg, the diaper area).

Other species of candida may also produce disease in humans. Specific identification rests with an experienced bacteriologist.

Clinical Findings

A. Symptoms and Signs:

1. Oral candidiasis—White patches with superficial mucosal ulceration appear on the entire oral and pharyngeal mucosa and frequently result in loss of appetite, difficulty in swallowing, and even respiratory distress. Individual lesions are surrounded by intensely red areolas; occasionally, in severe forms, coalescence occurs. The illness may be seen in neonates or even 1–2 weeks later.

2. Skin infection—Diaper dermatitis is common, with an intensely red, "scorched" appearance extending to the perianal and anterior abdominal areas. Sharp demarcation is sometimes evident. Scaling, weeping lesions, vesicles, pustules, and papules are occasionally present. Satellite lesions are frequent.

Vulvovaginitis may present with the above changes plus a thick, often yellowish exudate associated with itching (often intense).

3. Pulmonary infection—*C albicans* pneumonia (uncommon) tends to occur only in diseases associated with deficiency or abnormalities of lymphocyte function. On the other hand, candida is commonly isolated from sputum or on autopsy, and it is sometimes difficult to determine what etiologic role candida played in the pneumonia. This is especially true if antibiotics or corticosteroids have been administered. Symptoms consistent with candidal pneumonia include low-grade fever, chronic cough, and mucoid or mucosanguineous sputum. Rales, signs of pleuritis, and effusion may be present. A bronchopulmonary or bronchial form is also recognized.

4. Other forms—CNS infection of the meningitic type may occur. Endocarditis, pyelonephritis, and candidemia are also seen, with attendant symptoms. All of these forms are rare in childhood and limited to patients who are rendered susceptible by therapy with antibiotics, corticosteroids or other immunosuppressive agents, or underlying disease.

A chronic progressive granulomatous skin lesion, occasionally associated with oral candidiasis, is characterized by horny excrescences.

Paronychia and onychia due to candida are observed in children as part of the clinical illness characterized by hypoadrenalism, hypoparathyroidism, pernicious anemia, and steatorrhea. Candidiasis usually precedes the other manifestations, but all combinations are seen.

B. Laboratory Findings: Direct examination of scrapings, pus, or sputum will reveal ovoid, budding yeast cells in large numbers. With tissue invasion, typical mycelial elements may be found.

The organism is readily cultured on the usual laboratory media or on Sabouraud's medium.

A skin test is available, but the ubiquitousness of the fungus and the large number of positive reactions precludes its clinical usefulness. Furthermore, lymphopenic states associated with a high incidence of candidiasis are frequently characterized by anergy to candida extract injected intradermally.

Serology is of little use in diagnosis.

Differential Diagnosis

Characteristic mucosal or skin lesions, isolation of the fungus, and response to therapy should establish the diagnosis in most cases. To be differentiated are agranulocytic mucosal lesions, herpes simplex, herpangina, contact or allergic dermatitis, avitaminosis, bacterial infections, and toxic or drug eruptions of the skin.

Complications

Dissemination from oral and skin infection is the most serious complication. The severity of candidal infection is directly related to the type of underlying disease and the amount of therapy with antibiotics, corticosteroids, or immunosuppressive agents.

Treatment

Mild candidiasis is usually a benign disease that is easily treated with a single course of topical gentian violet or nystatin (Mycostatin) (see Chapter 39). Sodium caprylate, various propionates, and potassium permanganate have also been used for skin lesions. The diaper area should be kept dry and open to the air if possible. Bland powder should be applied to prevent accumulation of moisture.

The visceral, systemic, and chronic forms of candidiasis are more difficult to treat because of the underlying disease process or because it is necessary to continue antibiotic, corticosteroid, or immunosuppressive therapy for other reasons. In these forms of candidiasis, amphotericin B (Fungizone) may have to be employed adjunctively (see Chapter 39). Whenever possible, modification or elimination of predisposing causes should be attempted.

Prognosis

Most superficial forms are self-limited and, with topical therapy, curable. In some cases, only suppression is achieved, and the disease recurs upon discontinuing antifungal therapy.

The prognosis is usually grave in systemic or visceral forms of the disease.

Appleyard WJ & others: Candida septicemia. Brit MJ 1:577, 1969.

Curtis GH: Systemic moniliasis. Arch Dermat 99:121–123, 1969,

Newcomer VD & others: Candida granuloma. Arch Dermat 93:149–161, 1966.

Seelig MS: The role of antibiotics in the pathogenesis of Candida infections. Am J M Sc 40:887–917, 1966.

Sheft D, Shrago G: Esophageal moniliasis. JAMA 213:1859, 1970.

Toala P & others: Candida at Boston City Hospital. Arch Int Med 126:983, 1970.

Winner HI, Horley R: *Candida Albicans.* Little, Brown, 1964.

COCCIDIOIDOMYCOSIS

Essentials of Diagnosis

- Primary pulmonary form: Fever, pleuritis, productive cough, anorexia, weight loss, and (in 10%) generalized macular skin rash.
- Erythema nodosum and multiforme with arthralgia ("desert rheumatism").
- Extrapulmonary form: Traumatic site, indurated ulcer 1–3 weeks later, regional adenopathy.
- Disseminated lesions in skin, bones, viscera, and meninges.
- Sporangia (30–60 μm) in pus, sputum, CSF, etc.
- Gray, cottony growth on Sabouraud's medium.
- Delayed type skin test reaction (induration more than 5 mm) to coccidioidin.
- Precipitin (early, 1–4 weeks) and complement-fixing (late, 6–12 weeks) antibodies develop.

General Considerations

Coccidioidomycosis is caused by the dimorphic fungus *Coccidioides immitis.* The infective forms (arthrospores) are found in soil in the lower sonoran life zone, and the disease is endemic in parts of California, Arizona, New Mexico, Texas, Mexico, and South America. Infection is acquired by inhalation or skin inoculation. Many rodents are naturally infected. The human disease is not contagious, but laboratory infections can occur from cultured coccidioides.

Almost 2/3 of infections are asymptomatic; of the remainder, less than 0.5% will disseminate.

Clinical Findings

A history of residence or travel in an endemic area is essential to the diagnosis. The incubation period of 7–28 days seems to be directly related to the intensity of exposure; brief and minimal exposure is associated with a longer interval. Children in agricultural communities are at risk.

A. Symptoms and Signs: The primary forms of coccidioidomycosis are usually pulmonary and rarely dermal. Severity varies from a mild upper respiratory illness to a severe influenza-like syndrome. In the latter, fever is prominent and may be prolonged. Associated symptoms include pleural pain, myalgia, headache, severe lassitude and malaise, anorexia with weight loss; cough, which may be productive of clear to purulent sputum; and arthralgia ("desert rheumatism"). Milder forms of the disease are associated with milder symptoms of brief duration. Skin rashes may be prominent, with 10% of patients exhibiting a generalized erythematous macular eruption early in the illness. A few patients will develop tender, indurated nodules on the lower extremities (erythema nodosum), and a more generalized pleomorphic rash (erythema multiforme).

Apart from fever and skin eruptions, physical findings are usually few and limited to the lungs. Rales, signs of consolidation, and a pleural friction rub may be noted.

An indolent indurated ulcer at the site of skin trauma is observed in primary dermal coccidioidomycosis. Regional lymphadenopathy is usually present.

Chronic pulmonary coccidioidomycosis may be asymptomatic. Some patients complain of chest pain and cough, and a few produce sputum, which may be bloody. The pulmonary lesion is cavitary and may elicit signs of consolidation or, if it is subpleural, may rupture and cause empyema or pneumothorax.

Dissemination may be heralded by a biphasic course with recurrence and extension of symptoms following initial improvement. However, dissemination may occur rapidly in the primary illness. Symptoms are similar to the primary illness but more severe and persistent. Also, signs referable to the organs involved will appear (eg, meningitic signs in CNS involvement).

B. Laboratory Findings: Direct examination of pus, CSF, sputum, or other clinical specimens treated with sodium hydroxide may reveal the characteristic sporangia (30–60 μm). India ink may be useful for contrast, but staining is of no value. The fungus can be cultured on Sabouraud's agar, but the slants should be sealed and never opened to avoid laboratory infections. *C immitis* grows rapidly, and gray, cottony colonies appear in a few days. Occasionally, mouse inoculation will aid in diagnosis.

Precipitating antibodies appear in the first to third weeks of infection and disappear by 4–6 weeks. Complement-fixing antibodies develop much later, if at all. Mild and asymptomatic illness is associated with no complement-fixing antibodies; moderate to severe illness is associated with a complement-fixing antibody rise which disappears in 6–8 months; and disseminated illness is associated with a persistent and high titer of complement-fixing antibodies. The presence of complement-fixing antibody in CSF is diagnostic of meningitis.

A skin test with coccidioidin results in an area of induration more than 5 mm in diameter within 2–21 days after onset. In patients with allergic manifestations (erythema nodosum), extreme skin sensitivity is present and the coccidioidin should be diluted 10–100 times before testing. Reactivity may persist for years in convalescence but may decrease or disappear with dissemination.

The sedimentation rate is elevated during the acute phase. An intense eosinophilia has been described just prior to dissemination.

C. X-Ray Findings: Roentgenologic evidence of pneumonia, pleural effusion, granuloma, or cavitation may be present at various stages of the pulmonary disease. Osteomyelitis may be noted.

Differential Diagnosis

Coccidioidomycosis must be distinguished from acute viral and bacterial pneumonias and acute tuberculosis. The chronic pulmonary lesion must be distinguished from chronic tuberculosis and malignancy. The disseminated forms will resemble diseases with manifestations in the organs involved (osteomyelitis, meningitis, etc).

Complications

These are primarily pulmonary, with pleural effusion, empyema, pneumothorax, or combinations occurring in association with a subpleural cavity.

Treatment

A. Specific Measures: There is no universally effective drug. Amphotericin B (Fungizone) may be of value in individual cases, particularly with dissemination. (See Chapter 39.) In the meningitic form, systemic amphotericin B alone is of little benefit. Intracisternal administration of amphotericin B, initially on a daily basis and subsequently at intervals of 1–6 weeks, may result in prolonged survival.

B. General Measures: Bed rest is mandatory until fever and pulmonary findings resolve. The sedimentation rate should be normal before ambulation is permitted.

C. Surgical Measures: Surgery may be indicated in cavitary lesions or with chronic draining sinuses.

Amphotericin B should be administered prior to and for 4 weeks following excisional surgery.

Prognosis

Complete recovery is the rule for all but a very few patients. Those with disseminated disease are at greatest risk, and as many as 50% died prior to the availability of amphotericin B. Negroes and Filipinos appear to be at greater risk of dissemination (10 times the rate for Caucasians) and, therefore, mortality. Meningitis and diffuse disseminated disease carry the worst prognosis. An increasing complement-fixing antibody titer and a decrease or reversion of a positive skin test are unfavorable prognostic signs.

Richardson HB, Anderson JA, McKay BM: Acute pulmonary coccidioidomycosis in children. J Pediat 70:376–382, 1967.

Winn WA: Long term study of 300 patients with cavitary-abscess lesions of the lung of coccidioidal origin. Dis Chest 54:268, 1968.

Zierina WH, Rockas HR: Coccidioidomycosis: Long-term treatment with amphotericin B. Am J Dis Child 108:454–459, 1964.

CRYPTOCOCCOSIS

Cryptococcus neoformans is a spherical fungus found worldwide in soil and in the old excreta of pigeons. It is an opportunistic organism that is frequently associated with seriously altered host mechanisms, eg, leukemia. It is commonly found at autopsy. Man is probably infected by inhalation.

Systemic cryptococcosis may result in widespread infection. Particular sites of localization include the CNS, eyes, skin, and bone. Skin lesions vary from papules to ulcerative abscesses. Bony lesions are indurated and painful and result in extensive local destruction, although periosteal proliferation is minimal or absent.

Several forms of the disease exist. Most commonly observed is the insidious cryptococcal meningitis. Recurrent or progressive headache, changes in personality and ambition, dizziness, and vomiting herald the onset of meningeal infection. The patient may have mild fever, slight nuchal rigidity, and alteration in lower extremity reflexes. Signs of progressive increase in intracranial pressure follow, with papilledema, cranial nerve paresis, and optic atrophy. The symptoms usually progress slowly over a period of several months, but chronic forms may last for years.

Sporadic cases of acute pulmonary cryptococcosis are seen and asymptomatic granulomas are frequently detected at necropsy. Thus, it is likely that the lungs are the portal of entry for the fungus.

Clinical laboratory specimens are usually very mucoid owing to the capsule of the fungus. Direct visualization of the 5–20 μm fungi is enhanced by India ink contrast. Any specimen containing cellular debris should be digested with 10% sodium hydroxide. Culture from pus, sputum, or CSF is possible. When CSF is inoculated, care must be taken to use sufficient volume. As much as 2–20 ml should be inoculated into a single culture, as the fungus cell content may be quite low.

Chest x-rays may reveal solitary or multiple lesions; bone films may show areas of osteolysis.

Amphotericin B (Fungizone) (see Chapter 39) is the only therapeutic agent of proved value, and its use (intravenously or intrathecally) may result in complete cure. Surgical excision may be of adjunctive value.

The disease process may be relatively acute or may progress slowly over a period of several years. In the chronic forms, remissions and exacerbations are frequent. The disseminated and meningeal forms are frequently fatal.

Campbell GD: Primary pulmonary cryptococcosis. Am Rev Resp Dis 94:236–243, 1966.

Gordon MA, Vedder DK: Serologic tests in diagnosis and prognosis of cryptococcosis. JAMA 197:961–967, 1966.

Littman ML, Walter J: Cryptococcosis: Current status. Am J Med 45:922–932, 1968.

Watkins JS & others: Two cases of cryptococcal meningitis, one treated with 5-fluorocytosine. Brit MJ 3:29–31, 1969.

HISTOPLASMOSIS

Essentials of Diagnosis

- History of residence in or travel to endemic areas.
- Pulmonary calcification.
- Hepatosplenomegaly, anemia, leukopenia.
- Positive skin test.
- Isolation of organism or identification in smears (2–4 μm oval budding yeasts with narrow neck).

General Considerations

Histoplasmosis is caused by the dimorphic fungus *Histoplasma capsulatum.* Its tissue form is a budding oval yeast, 2–4 μm in diameter. Benign histoplasmosis was first noted in tuberculin-negative individuals with pulmonary calcifications. Such individuals were histoplasmin reactive (positive). The endemic areas include central and eastern USA. The fungus is found in soil, especially when enriched by bat feces. It is believed that infection is acquired by inhalation, and over 65% of children acquire asymptomatic infections in the endemic areas.

Clinical Findings

A history of residence or travel to the endemic areas is essential. Heavy contact with potentially infected soil or excreta (bat feces) may provide an etiologic clue.

A. Symptoms and Signs: Three forms of infection are recognized: asymptomatic benign infection, pneumonia, and disseminated disease.

1. Asymptomatic infection–The diagnosis is made by observation of pulmonary calcifications in the absence of delayed hypersensitivity to other antigens and a positive histoplasmin skin test.

2. Histoplasmal pneumonia–This form of the disease is manifested by nonproductive cough, chest pain, hemoptysis, and dyspnea. Cyanosis and hoarseness may also be noted. Influenza-like symptoms may also occur, with fever, muscle and joint pains, and malaise. Night sweats and weight loss may simulate tuberculosis. Physical signs may be absent, or typical findings of pneumonia (rales, bronchial breathing, etc) may be observed. A chronic pulmonary disease may be seen in adults but almost never in children.

3. Disseminated histoplasmosis–The disseminated form of the disease has all of the pulmonary features plus signs and symptoms referable to the lymphatic system. Thus, hepatosplenomegaly, severe wasting, and generalized lymphadenopathy occur. Ulceration of the gastrointestinal and respiratory tracts occurs occasionally. Pallor may be a prominent finding.

B. Laboratory Findings: Anemia and leukopenia, often profound, occur in the disseminated form. Isolation of the fungus provides a specific diagnosis. This usually is unrewarding in the benign infection, although rarely the organism may be found in the urine. Examination of sputum, urine, biopsy material, bone marrow, or blood may yield the organism in the disseminated form. Morphologically, *H capsulatum* appears as 2–4 μm oval cells on a smear stained with Giemsa's or Wright's stain. A large vacuole and crescent-shaped eosinophilic masses of cytoplasm may be visible in the larger end of the ovoid. If budding is observed, the neck is seen to be narrow and may appear as a separate ovoid. Such cells are identified within monocytes or macrophages but often are found free. Upon culture (with agar at 20–30° C), the organism may be isolated and specifically identified. Mouse inoculation is an extremely sensitive method for isolation of histoplasma. Complement fixation and precipitin antibody tests are available. Both are positive in the first few weeks after infection and remain elevated only with dissemination.

C. X-Ray Findings: Pulmonary calcifications, solitary or multiple, may be noted in an asymptomatic child. In acute pulmonic disease, bilateral bronchial pneumonia is the rule. Miliary distribution occasionally occurs.

Differential Diagnosis

Pulmonary histoplasmosis with or without symptoms must be differentiated from tuberculosis. The use of skin tests and serologic and isolation technics permits differentiation. The disseminated form of the disease mimics miliary tuberculosis and leukemia. Differentiation is based upon isolation of the organism. Serology may be helpful if the disease is not fulminant.

Complications

Benign and mild symptomatic infections require no specific therapy, and recovery is the rule. With concomitant disease (lymphatic malignancies, tuberculosis) or with immunosuppressive therapy, dissemination may occur.

Treatment

Benign or mild forms require no treatment. Selective extirpative surgical therapy may be of benefit in localized pulmonary disease. Amphotericin B (Fungizone) appears to be effective. (See Chapter 39.)

Prognosis

In benign or mild forms, the prognosis is excellent for recovery and complete healing. Chronic infection may result from more marked pulmonary disease. Disseminated histoplasmosis has a variable course and severity. Fulminant histoplasmosis, histoplasmosis associated with concomitant tuberculosis or malignancy, or histoplasmosis occurring in a patient receiving immunosuppressive therapy has a very poor prognosis.

Comparison of treated and untreated severe histoplasmosis. JAMA 183:823–829, 1963.

Crawford SE: Histoplasmosis in infants and children. GP 30:78–85, Jan 1964.

Holland P, Holland NH: Histoplasmosis in early infancy. Am J Dis Child 112:412–421, 1966.

Tesh RB & others: Histoplasmosis in children. Pediatrics 33:894–903, 1964.

NOCARDIOSIS

Nocardiosis is infrequent in childhood. It is caused by *Nocardia asteroides,* an aerobic, gram-positive, partially acid-fast actinomycete. Pulmonary infection is common and may lead to chronic pneumonia or dissemination to the meninges or brain. Typical gram-positive, short-branching rods or coccal forms are seen which are also acid-fast. Culture establishes the diagnosis.

The sulfonamides are the drugs of choice (see Chapter 39).

Ballenger CN, Goldring D: Nocardiosis in childhood. J Pediat 50:145–169, 1957.

Murray JF & others: The changing spectrum of nocardiosis. Am Rev Resp Dis 83:315–330, 1961.

SPOROTRICHOSIS

Sporotrichosis is caused by *Sporotrichum schenckii.* Localized lymphatic sporotrichosis may follow a prick with a thorn or splinter which results in an ulcer or nodule followed by others along the route of lymphatic return from the injured part. Dissemination to the skin and mucosa can occur, but the viscera are usually spared. Diagnosis is best accomplished by culture of aspirates or drainage from local lesions or nodes.

Potassium iodide is said to be effective, although some cases may require amphotericin B (Fungizone) (see Chapter 39). Potassium iodide can be administered orally as the saturated solution. The dose is variable. Initially, give 3–5 drops 3 times daily after meals. Increase the dose to 40 drops 3 times daily by adding 1 drop per dose. Continue therapy for 2 weeks or until signs of disease activity have disappeared. Then reduce the dose by 1 drop per dose until 5 drops is reached, at which time therapy is discontinued. *Note:* If signs of iodism appear, the dosage must be reduced. Potassium iodide is indicated only in sporotrichosis and not in other fungal diseases.

Hanrahan JB, Erickson ER: Sporotrichosis in western Pennsylvania. JAMA 197:814–816, 1966.

Scott SM & others: Pulmonary sporotrichosis. New England J Med 265:453–457, 1961.

•   •   •

General References

Conant NF & others: *Manual of Clinical Mycology.* Saunders, 1954.

Dalldorf G (editor): *Fungi and Fungous Diseases.* Thomas, 1962.

Dubos RJ, Hirsch JG: *Bacterial and Mycotic Infections of Man,* 4th ed. Lippincott, 1965.

Emmons CW & others: *Medical Mycology.* Lea & Febiger, 1963.

Fetter BF & others: *Mycoses of the Central Nervous System.* Williams & Wilkins, 1967.

Halde C: Systemic mycoses. Chap 23 in: *Current Medical References,* 6th ed. Chatton MJ, Sanazaro PJ (editors). Lange, 1970.

Hildick-Smith G & others: *Fungus Diseases and Their Therapy.* Little, Brown, 1964.

Lewis GM & others: *An Introduction to Medical Mycology.* Year Book, 1958.

Salvin SB: Immunologic aspects of the mycoses. Progr Allergy 7:213–331, 1963.

Sweany HC (editor): *Histoplasmosis.* Thomas, 1960.

Wilson JW, Plunkett OA: *The Fungous Diseases of Man.* Univ of California Press, 1965.

30...

Emergencies & Accidents

John D. Burrington, MD

INITIAL EMERGENCY EXAMINATION & MANAGEMENT

Initial Management

A. Emergency Measures:

1. Relieve asphyxia—

a. Clear the upper air passages. Pull the tongue forward and insert an airway. Draw the chin forward with the patient supine by inserting the second and third fingers behind the angles of the mandibles. Suction mucus or blood. If indicated, insert an open type of endotracheal tube or perform tracheostomy.

b. Close sucking wounds of thorax.

c. Institute artificial respiration if necessary.

d. Administer oxygen if necessary.

2. Cardiac resuscitation if necessary.

3. Stop hemorrhage with pressure or tourniquet— Examine for concealed hemorrhage into the thorax, abdomen, gastrointestinal tract, or soft tissues.

4. Treat shock promptly.

5. Avoid spinal cord damage in any patient suspected of back injury. Maintain normal alignment of the vertebrae both in examination and transportation.

B. Follow-Up Measures: If indicated, arrange for administration of plasma, plasma substitutes, or blood. Splint fractures before moving patient.

Insert a 14 gauge plastic intravenous catheter at once. Meticulously cleanse the site of insertion; insert the needle; take measures to prevent catheter embolus; and apply antibiotic ointment. Change to the other arm at least every 48 hours.

Relieve pain. However, narcotics and sedatives may mask pain of diagnostic importance. Use narcotics cautiously in the presence of shock because of the danger of sudden absorption of multiple doses on recovery.

Initial Rapid Survery Examination

Record initial and serial findings. Diagnosis often depends on changing signs. Record fluid intake and urinary output. Explain to and reassure friends or family.

A. History: (From the patient himself or from relatives, friends, bystanders, police, ambulance drivers, previous charts, other patients, other physicians.)

---

*Other medical emergencies are discussed in appropriate chapters elsewhere in this book. Poisoning, including snakebite, spider bite, scorpion bite, and insect stings, is discussed in Chapter 31.

1. **Present illness**—Prodrome, onset, recent illness, progression of symptoms, environment, medicines, syringes, etc. In case of injury, elicit exact details.

2. **Past history**—Previous attacks, chronic illness, habits, medications, occupation (student, part-time employment, etc). Examine patient's personal effects (diabetic or epileptic identification card, prescription labels, etc).

B. **Physical Examination:**

1. **General Observations**—Note position of body and extremities, evidence of external or internal bleeding, skin color, rate and quality of pulse and respiration, temperature, blood pressure (both arms), state of consciousness, and unusual odors. Note neck vein distention; check pulsation in major arteries, paradoxic pulse.

2. **Head, neck, and eyes**—Injuries of skull and face, neck rigidity, breath aroma, appearance of pupils and reaction to light, ophthalmoscopic examination in coma, fluid or blood from ears or nose, mucous membranes of mouth, position of trachea, crepitation in the neck.

3. **Chest**—Note pattern of breathing, retraction, paradoxic motion, bruising, sucking sounds. Test chest wall stability with gentle anteroposterior and lateral compression. Check trachea for mediastinal shift. Listen and percuss for breath sounds, dullness, mediastinal crunch, murmurs, or increased cardiac dullness.

4. **Abdomen**—External evidence of injury, distention, presence of rigidity or tenderness, bowel sounds. Percuss bladder and other palpable or percussable organs.

5. **Back**—Examine for injuries. Maintain normal alignment of vertebrae.

6. **Extremities**—Note position, deformity, color, and pulses in extremities. Check active and passive motion. Compress wings of ilium; palpate symphysis pubis and examine perineum for hematoma, genital injury, or extravasated urine.

7. **Neurologic examination**—Deep and superficial reflexes, flaccidity or rigidity; response to pinprick or noxious stimuli. Elicit cranial nerve abnormalities when possible.

CARDIAC ARREST

Irreversible CNS damage will occur within 4 minutes after cardiac arrest. Valuable time should not be lost by auscultation or taking an ECG. Whether the arrest is secondary to ventricular fibrillation or standstill (asystole) is of no immediate consequence. Initial resuscitative measures are identical in both circumstances.

Treatment

Initial treatment is directed at restoring circulation and oxygenation of tissues.

A. **Heart Massage:**

1. Begin closed chest cardiac massage immediately. (See Technic, below, and Fig 30–1.)

2. Open heart massage is indicated only in the operating room if closed chest massage is unsuccessful.

B. **Pulmonary Ventilation:** Must be initiated immediately. (See Technic, below, and Fig 30–2.)

1. Patients often aspirate vomitus or secretions before cardiac arrest. Using mechanical suction if available, clear the throat and trachea before beginning positive pressure breathing.

2. Mouth-to-mouth breathing is the most efficient of the commonly available methods of administering immediate artificial respiration. The mask and bag method is also an efficient method (Fig 30–4).

3. Endotracheal intubation and 100% oxygen therapy should be initiated as soon as equipment is available.

C. **Intravenous Fluids:** Introduce an 18 gauge or larger plastic cannula into a vein. A central venous catheter can be introduced via the basilic vein at the elbow or via the external jugular. Begin lactated Ringer's injection and add plasma or blood as indicated. If arrest has occurred, give 0.9 M sodium bicarbonate according to the following formula:

Weight (in kg) $\times$ 0.3 $\times$ 10 = ml of 0.9 M sodium bicarbonate

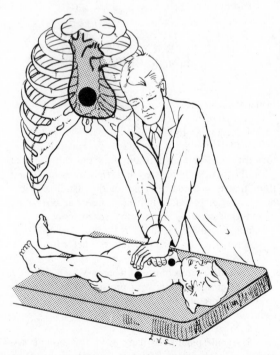

FIG 30–1. Technic of closed chest cardiac massage. (Heavy circle in heart drawing shows area of application of force. Circles on supine figure show points of application of electrodes for defibrillation.)

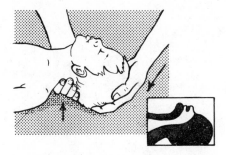

The operator takes his position at the patient's head.

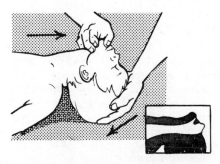

With the right thumb and index finger he displaces the mandible forward by pressing at its central portion, at the same time lifting the neck and tilting the head as far back as possible.

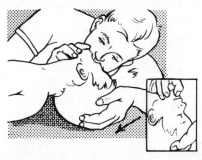

After taking a deep breath, the operator immediately seals his mouth around the mouth (or nose) of the victim and exhales until the chest of the victim rises.

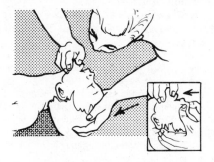

The victim's mouth is opened by downward and forward traction on the lower jaw or by pulling down the lower lip.

FIG 30–2. Technic of mouth-to-mouth insufflation.

This assumes a base deficit of 10 and should be repeated every 3–5 minutes during resuscitation. All other measures will fail if acidosis is not corrected.

D. Electrocardiogram: Determine by ECG whether the heart is in ventricular fibrillation or asystole.

E. Management of Fibrillation: (See Technic, below, and Fig 30–1.) Use of a defibrillator is indicated.

F. Management of Asystole:

1. Correct acidosis with 0.9 M sodium bicarbonate as above.

2. Strike the chest shraply with the fist 2 or 3 times.

3. Ensure adequate ventilation.

4. Single electric shocks from a defibrillator may initiate contraction.

5. Calcium has an inotropic action and should be used if asystole continues. Give 1 ml of 10% calcium gluconate by direct intracardiac injection or through a central venous catheter.

6. For persistent asystole, epinephrine, 1–3 ml of 1:10,000 solution by direct intracardiac injection, may restore the heartbeat.

7. Once a regular heartbeat and palpable peripheral pulses have been established, determine arterial pH, P_{O_2}, P_{CO_2}, and base deficit. Repeat these determinations at least hourly until the patient's condition has stabilized since resuscitation may wash metabolic acids out of tissues and lead to profound acidosis.

8. Plan on endotracheal intubation and assisted or controlled ventilation for at least several hours after resuscitation from cardiac arrest.

9. Watch carefully for cardiac tamponade and pneumothorax if direct intracardiac medications have been given.

Prognosis

The reversibility of the arrest depends on the cause. Patients who arrest during an acute hypoxic episode can often be resuscitated. Cardiac arrest following prolonged shock is not easily reversible, and the results are often disappointing.

Technics of Cardiac Massage, Pulmonary Ventilation, & External Defibrillation

A. External Cardiac Massage: (Fig 30–1.)

1. The back must be on a firm surface. A "resuscitation board," placed between the patient's back and the bed, provides a satisfactory surface. In small infants, one hand can be used to support the back while external massage is given with the other.

2. The heel of one hand is placed over the junction of the middle and lower 1/3 of the sternum; the second hand is placed on the dorsum of the first hand to reinforce pressure.

3. The sternum is pressed downward 2 cm in an infant or 3–5 cm in an older child, 60 times a minute. The compression phase is very fast (about 0.4 second). This is followed by a rapid release and then a delay period of about 0.6 seconds. The tendency is to mas-

sage too rapidly and not allow adequate time for cardiac filling.

4. The criterion of good technic is a palpable femoral or carotid pulse.

5. If only one physician is available, he should interrupt cardiac massage every 30 seconds and inflate the lungs several times by the mouth-to-mouth technic.

B. Pulmonary Ventilation:

1. The mouth-to-mouth technic is the most efficient of the commonly available means of achieving immediate ventilation.

a. Position the patient flat on his back and extend his neck.

b. Clear the oropharynx and pull the tongue forward.

c. If there is evidence of aspiration and suction is immediately available, aspirate both mainstem bronchi.

d. Occlude the nostrils.

e. Cup the patient's lips and exhale into the patient's mouth.

f. Continue a rate of 40 breaths per minute in newborns or 20 breaths per minute in older children.

2. Hand pulmonators (Fig 30–4) are advantageous because the physician can more easily observe the patient's response and because 100% oxygen can be delivered. The manual resuscitator consists of a pliable bag, nonrebreathing valve, and face mask. Effective positive pressure ventilation can be achieved by applying the mask firmly over the nose and mouth and squeezing the bag, which recoils promptly to the full position when released. Oxygen can be administered if desired by attaching the oxygen tubing to the air intake valve at the end of the bag. The manual resuscitator should be available in ambulances, coronary care and intensive care units, and wherever there might be victims of heart attack, cardiac arrest, suffocation, drowning, etc.

3. Wherever oxygen and an AMBU (self-inflating) bag are available, there should be a laryngoscope and an assortment of endotracheal tubes.

4. The criteria of adequate ventilation are chest excursion and breath sounds, improvement in nail bed and skin color, and serial determinations showing normal arterial blood gases and pH.

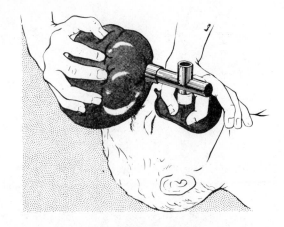

(1) Lift the victim's neck with one hand.

(2) Tilt head backward into maximum neck extension. Remove secretions and debris from mouth and throat, and pull the tongue and mandible forward as required to clear the airway.

(3) Hold the mask snugly over the nose and mouth, holding the chin forward and the neck in extension as shown in diagram.

(4) Squeeze the bag, noting inflation of the lungs by the rise of the chest wall.

(5) Release the bag, which will expand spontaneously. The patient will exhale and the chest will fall.

(6) Repeat steps 4 and 5 approximately 12 times per minute.

FIG 30–4. Portable manual resuscitator.

C. External Defibrillation:

1. Place one electrode in the second intercostal space of the right sternal border and a second electrode in the 4th intercostal space of the left midaxillary line (Fig 30–1). Be sure that adequate electrode paste has been applied and that no personnel are touching the patient at the time of defibrillation.

2. Begin in the low ranges of 50 watt-seconds and increase in increments of 25 watt-seconds (values are for DC defibrillators).

3. If single shocks are ineffective, attempt paired shocks at intervals as short as the defibrillation machine will allow.

Emergency Resuscitation Team Manual: A Hospital Plan. American Heart Association, 1968.

Lefer AM: Role of corticosteroids in the treatment of circulatory response. Clin Pharmacol Therap 11:630–655, 1970.

Resnekov L: Electroconversion of cardiac dysrhythmias. Am Heart J 78:581–586, 1970.

Riker WL: Cardiac arrest in infants and children. P Clin North America 16:661–669, 1969.

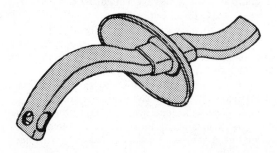

FIG 30–3. Airway for use in mouth-to-mouth insufflation. The larger airway is for adults. The guard is flexible and may be inverted from the position shown for use with infants and children.

SHOCK

Shock is a clinical syndrome characterized by prostration and hypotension resulting from a profound depression of vital cell functions associated with or secondary to poor tissue perfusion. If cellular function is not improved, shock becomes irreversible and death will ensue even though the initiating cause of the shock is corrected.

Clinical Findings

Early signs of shock are pallor, agitation, confusion, and thirst. As shock progresses, the patient will become less and less responsive and eventually comatose.

The skin is pale, mottled, and cold. The nail beds are cyanotic, and local and peripheral edema may occur. Poor capillary filling and decreased skin turgor can be demonstrated. Tachycardia and tachypnea are present.

Newborns in shock appear lethargic, pale, and slightly gray. Late shock may be manifested by a decrease in skin temperature, particularly of the extremities.

Immediate Treatment of Shock

(1) Lay the patient flat. Elevation of the legs is helpful except in instances of respiratory distress, when it is contraindicated.

(2) Establish a patent upper airway and administer oxygen by mask or nasal catheter. If the clinical condition deteriorates, consider the use of an endotracheal tube and intermittent positive pressure breathing.

(3) Establish an intravenous site with a large bore catheter (No. 18 or larger).

(4) Initiate fluid therapy with lactated Ringer's injection or isotonic saline solution at a rate calculated for daily maintenance plus correction of existing dehydration. (See Chapter 37.)

(5) Establish a central venous pressure monitor in all cases of shock that are not easily reversible.

(6) Consider an arterial catheter as a useful guide to monitoring pressure and as a source of specimens for blood gases and arterial pH.

Treatment of Specific Types of Shock

A. Hypovolemic (Hemorrhagic) Shock: This is defined as a reduction in the size of the vascular compartment, with a falling blood pressure, poor capillary filling, and a low central venous pressure. Treatment consists of preventing further fluid loss and volume replacement of existing losses. Vasopressors should not be used. The choice of fluid used as a volume expander depends on the cause of the hypovolemia.

1. Blood Loss—Whole blood is the replacement fluid of choice for shock due to hemorrhage. Type-specific blood is strongly recommended; however, unmatched type O Rh-negative blood has been used without causing serious transfusion reactions in emergency situations. The rate of blood replacement is judged by the rate of blood loss, the patient's response, and a rising central venous pressure. Hemorrhagic shock is usually accompanied by marked metabolic acidosis, which must be corrected.

2. Plasma loss—Dextran is a good temporary volume expander which is most useful when large amounts of plasma have been lost. Twenty ml/kg can be given in 30 minutes as a 6% w/v solution in normal saline. More may be administered according to the estimated amount and rate of blood loss. Burn cases respond well; however, the use of low molecular weight dextran in actively bleeding patients is not recommended since it has the property of coating and suspending platelets and thus inhibiting normal platelet agglutination. It may also interfere with blood crossmatch, so the specimen should be obtained prior to dextran infusion. Dextran is excreted in the urine and leads to very high urine specific gravity.

3. Dehydration—Isotonic salt solutions are indicated in all instances of dehydration, including hypertonic dehydration, when there is an absolute depletion of body salt and fluid even though there is a relative hypertonicity. Lactated Ringer's injection or 0.5 N saline solution with added sodium bicarbonate (30 mEq of $NaHCO_3$ per 500 ml bottle) should be started at a rate of 25—35 ml/kg/hour IV until skin turgor improves and electrolyte values can be obtained.

4. Burns and Infection—Albumin and plasma are good volume expanders which are particularly useful in cases of burns or massive infection, where protein loss is significant.

B. Cardiogenic Shock: This is defined as shock resulting from decreased cardiac output, eg, due to cardiac tamponade, myocarditis, abnormal rates and rhythm, and biochemical abnormalities.

1. Cardiac tamponade is usually secondary to fluid collection in the pericardial space, but it can also occur secondary to constrictive pericarditis. The only effective treatment is to relieve the tamponade by evacuating the pericardial space or surgically excising the pericardium. Temporary treatment can be achieved by increasing the venous pressure with a transfusion of blood or blood substitutes. Vasodilators cause a drop in venous pressure and are contraindicated.

2. Myocarditis results from viral infections and toxins secondary to bacterial infections.

3. Abnormal heart rate and rhythm results in decreased cardiac output.

a. Marked sinus bradycardia can occur during anesthesia, particularly when associated with surgery of the neck and thorax. Sinus bradycardia can be blocked with atropine, 0.01 mg/kg as a single IM dose. The minimum dose for newborns is 0.15 mg regardless of weight. The maximum dose for older children is 0.6 mg.

b. Atrioventricular block may occur secondary to inflammatory disease, surgical trauma, or ischemic injury to the conduction system. Prednisolone, 1 mg/kg/day IV or IM in 4 equally divided doses, may be useful in such conditions. If slowing persists, the ventricular rate can often be increased with isoproterenol, 3–5 μg/kg/minute by IV drip. The infusion is then adjusted according to the pulse response.

c. Ventricular arrhythmias may be secondary to hypoxia, acidosis, or myocarditis. Procainamide (Pronestyl), 50 mg/kg/day IV, is useful in controlling premature ventricular contractions. (For discussion of defibrillation, see Cardiac Arrest, above.)

4. Biochemical disturbances can result in decreased cardiac output. These include acidosis, hypoxia, and hyperkalemia. (See Chapter 37.)

C. Bacteremic (Endotoxin, Septic) Shock: This type of shock occurs when overwhelming sepsis and circulating bacterial toxins result in peripheral vascular collapse. Clinical recognition depends on the toxic appearance of the patient, often in association with purpura, splinter hemorrhages, hepatosplenomegaly, and jaundice. Adequate treatment of bacterial shock depends on proper antibiotic therapy of the primary infection. In addition to anti-infective agents, several other procedures are useful in supporting the patient with bacterial shock.

1. Crystalloid and colloid should be administered to keep central venous pressure within the range of 10–14 mm Hg.

2. When bacteremic shock is due to gram-negative organisms, corticosteroids should be used early. Give prednisolone, 2–4 mg/kg/day IV, or hydrocortisone, 10–40 mg/kg/day IV.

3. Hypotention often persists in spite of a high central venous pressure. However, tissue perfusion is more important than arterial pressure per se. Isoproterenol (Isuprel), 1 mg in 500 ml of saline solution by IV drip, will often give adequate peripheral perfusion even though the arterial pressure is as much as 20 mm Hg below normal systolic pressure. Levarterenol (Levophed) is rarely used in treating shock since it elevates central arterial pressure partly by inducing profound vasoconstriction.

4. Heparin is of value when bacterial infections are complicated by intravascular coagulation.

D. Anaphylactic Shock: This is an extreme form of allergy or hypersensitivity to a foreign substance which results in circulatory and respiratory distress. The diagnosis is established by a history of exposure to an antigen and by clinical signs of respiratory distress and circulatory collapse. Urticaria and angioneurotic edema are often present. The pathophysiologic mechanisms are the release of histamine, serotonin, and bradykinins and their effects on various body tissues. The net effect of these compounds is to cause arteriolar dilatation, venular constriction, increased capillary permeability, and bronchial constriction. Such physiologic changes cause marked hypovolemia and respiratory distress.

1. If shock is precipitated by a drug given intramuscularly, apply a tourniquet proximal to the site of injection tight enough to restrict venous return but not to interrupt arterial flow.

2. Give epinephrine, 1:1000 aqueous solution, 0.1 ml/kg IM stat. Follow with 0.1 ml/kg IV and repeat in 20 minutes if the response is not satisfactory. (If cardiac arrest occurs, treat as outlined above.)

3. Give antihistamines, eg, diphenhydramine (Benadryl), 5 mg/kg/day in 4–6 divided doses by IV push over a 5–10 minute interval.

4. Give prednisolone, 2 mg/kg/day IV in 4–6 divided doses.

5. For treatment of respiratory distress or wheezing, give aminophylline, 12 mg/kg/day by IV drip in 4 divided doses every 6 hours.

6. Secretions should be suctioned and may require repeated bronchoscopy. Laryngeal edema may necessitate intubation followed by tracheostomy.

7. Hypovolemia should be treated vigorously with isotonic saline solution at rates of 25 ml/kg/hour until the patient voids or the central venous pressure monitor indicates a rise to normal values.

E. Neurogenic Shock: This includes all forms of shock in which interruption of the normal neuronal control results in decreased cardiac output and vascular tone. There is usually a history of exposure to anesthetic agents, spinal cord injuries, or ingestion of barbiturates, narcotics, or tranquilizers. Examination reveals abnormal reflexes and muscle tone, tachycardia and tachypnea, and low blood pressure. The pathophysiologic mechanism is loss of vessel tone with subsequent expansion of the vascular compartment, resulting in relative hypovolemia. Many anesthetic agents have a direct effect on the myocardium which causes a decrease in cardiac output.

1. Fluids—Neurogenic shock responds well to volume therapy. Give isotonic saline solution, 25 ml/kg/hour IV, until peripheral circulation and skin turgor improve.

2. Vasopressors—Vascular tone can be improved by several drugs which have a primary effect on vessels and little or no effect on the myocardium. They should be administered only if fluid therapy is not successful. Give either of the following:

a. Methoxamine (Vasoxyl), 0.25 mg/kg IM as a single dose, or 0.08 mg/kg IV given over a 10–15 minute interval.

b. Phenylephrine (Neo-Synephrine), 0.1 mg/kg IM as a single dose.

3. Isoproterenol (Isuprel), 1 mg in 500 ml of saline solution by IV drip, markedly improves perfusion but does not elevate blood pressure.

F. Shock Due to Miscellaneous Causes:

1. Following pulmonary embolism—Shock secondary to pulmonary emboli is rare in pediatrics, but the possibility should be considered if there is a fracture or significant soft tissue injury followed by symptoms of chest pain, dyspnea, cyanosis, and signs of right heart failure. Treatment is supportive, with oxygen and analgesics. If hypotension occurs, isoproterenol (Isuprel) is the drug of choice since it provides a bronchodilator effect. If right heart failure develops, a rapid-acting digitalis preparation such as digoxin should be given. The digitalizing dose of digoxin is 0.05 mg/kg IV or IM. The maintenance dose is about 1/5 the digitalizing dose.

2. Respiratory disease—Respiratory disease due to any cause can result in sufficient hypoxia to cause shock. Shock of this nature is reversible only to the extent that the lung disease is reversible, and treatment should be directed toward the primary pulmonary disorder. Oxygen and alkali therapy will only temporarily improve the patient's condition.

3. Metabolic shock—Shock may be secondary to a number of metabolic conditions, such as adrenocortical insufficiency and diabetic acidosis.

Prognosis

With prompt and effective emergency care for both the shock itself and the underlying condition, the immediate prognosis is excellent.

Hardaway RM & others: Intensive study and treatment of shock in man. JAMA 199:779–790, 115–126, 1967.

Johnson DG: Surgical pediatrics. P Clin North America 16:621–635, 1969.

Lillehei RC & others: Modern treatment of shock based on physiologic principles. Clin Pharmacol Therap 5:63, 1964.

Sonnenschein H: Endotoxin shock. Clin Pediat 10:240, 1971.

Weil MH, Shubin H: *Diagnosis and Treatment of Shock.* Williams & Wilkins, 1967.

PULMONARY EMBOLISM

Pulmonary embolism is rare in children. Major thrombi may originate in the right side of the heart or in the deep veins of the leg and pelvis. Thromboembolic disease is not uncommon in disseminated lupus erythematosus.

Small emboli do not usually give rise to respiratory distress unless there is already existing respiratory or cardiac disease. Large emboli cause severe dyspnea, substernal or generalized chest pain, sweating, cyanosis, anxiety, and sometimes convulsions. P_2 is loud, neck veins are distended, and the right border of the heart may be percussible beyond the right sternal border.

Thrombophlebitis should be treated with anticoagulants to prevent pulmonary embolism.

The patient should be placed in a sitting position and given oxygen. Narcotics may be required if the pain is severe, and antitussives should be given for cough. Heparin, 100 units/kg IV, should be given every 4 hours; or continuous administration can be given via an indwelling intravenous catheter with a heparin lock. Pleural effusions may need tapping, and it may be necessary to sustain blood pressure with levarterenol (Levophed), 0.12 mg/kg/24 hours by slow IV drip.

Embolectomy may have to be considered.

TRAUMA

FIRST AID

General Principles

(1) Determine the extent of injury quickly but thoroughly.

(2) Treat immediately such life-endangering conditions as cardiac arrest, airway obstruction by blood or vomitus, arrhythmias or serious bleeding, and shock.

(3) Improvise dressings, splints, and transportation, and arrange for prompt definitive treatment.

Evaluation of the Patient

A. History: Take a sufficient history to ascertain the degree and type of damage and any serious underlying medical problems, eg, cardiac disease or diabetes mellitus.

B. Physical Examination: Examine the patient thoroughly after major trauma.

1. External wounds—Control bleeding promptly (see below).

2. Respiratory distress—Stridor and suprasternal or intercostal retraction indicate airway obstruction. Shortness of breath may be due to chest injury or shock. Respiratory depression may occur in head injury or in severe shock. Cyanosis is due to poor oxygenation from any cause. Check the position of the trachea; a shift indicates either collapse of one lung or tension pneumothorax in contralateral thorax.

3. Shock—Typical signs are faintness, pallor; cool, moist skin; thirst, air hunger; and a weak, usually rapid pulse. Distinguish neurogenic from oligemic shock.

4. Fractures and dislocations—Palpate carefully from head to foot. Move all joints cautiously, and exert gentle pressure on the spine, chest, and pelvis. Pain, swelling, ecchymosis, deformity, and limitation of motion are classical signs of fracture and dislocation. Few or none of these may be apparent immediately after injury.

5. Brain and spinal cord damage—Assess CNS injury by noting state of consciousness, gross skin sensation, and ability to move extremities actively.

6. Internal injury—Overt localizing signs are often minimal. Hypovolemic shock in the absence of external bleeding or extensive soft tissue trauma suggests internal hemorrhage. Chest pain with respiratory distress and abdominal pain with signs of peritoneal irritation point to visceral injury.

Management of External Bleeding

A. Major Arterial Bleeding: Serious bleeding is usually due to the laceration of a major artery. Speed is essential.

1. Direct pressure on the wound will reduce or stop the flow.

2. Compression of the major artery proximal to the wound may make local pressure effective, permit

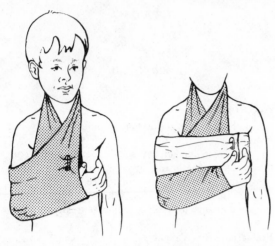

FIG 30—5. Method of application of sling and swathe.

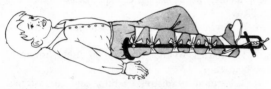

FIG 30—6. Keller-Blake half-ring splint for transportation of patient with fracture of thigh or leg. Spanish windlass on a Collins hitch.

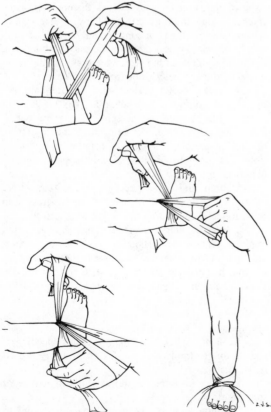

FIG 30—7. Method of tying Collins hitch.

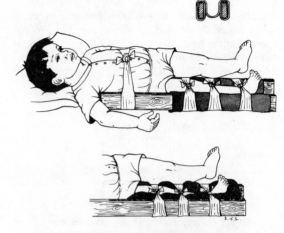

FIG 30—8. Padded board splints for transportation of patient with fracture of thigh and leg. Outer board extends to axilla.

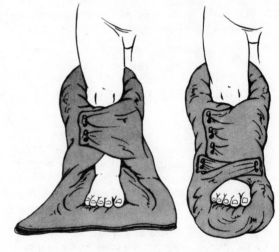

FIG 30—9. Method of application of pillow splints.

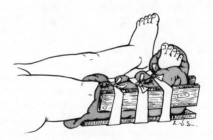

FIG 30—10. Reinforcement of pillow splint for transportation of patient with injury of ankle and foot.

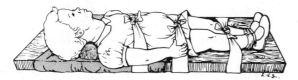

FIG 30–11. **Board or door used for transportation of patient with injured spine.**

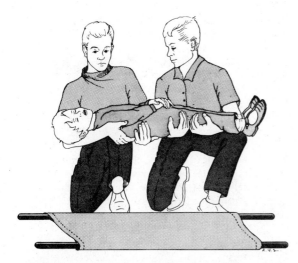

FIG 30–12. **Method of lifting injured patient onto stretcher.**

grasping of a bleeder with a hemostat, or allow time for fashioning a tourniquet.

3. A tourniquet is necessary when other methods fail. Do not use a tourniquet when direct pressure on the wound will control bleeding. *Caution:* Faulty use of a tourniquet may cause irreparable vascular or neurologic damage. Tourniquets can be made from rubber tubing, rope, neckties, belts, handkerchiefs, stockings, or strips of cloth. Keep the tourniquet exposed and release it briefly at least every 30 minutes.

B. Venous and Minor Arterial Bleeding: These can be controlled by direct pressure on the wound with sterile gauze or a clean cloth and elevation of the part.

Management of Respiratory Distress

A. When Due to Airway Obstruction:

1. Remove secretions and foreign material from the mouth and throat. Use suction if available.

2. Hold up the patient's chin or pull out his tongue when relaxation of the tongue and jaw obstruct the hypopharynx, as in comatose patients.

3. Tracheostomy may be necessary if a foreign body or edema obstructs the larynx.

B. When Due to Other Causes: Maintain a clear airway, treat the underlying cause, and administer oxygen if available.

C. In Respiratory Arrest: Clear the airway and institute artificial respiration by mouth-to-mouth

insufflation. Intubate the trachea and control ventilation when possible.

Management of Shock

Anticipate and prevent shock by the measures outlined above.

(1) Control hemorrhage and such contributing causes as exposure and pain.

(2) Keep the patient comfortably warm in the recumbent, slightly head-down position. Avoid rapid position changes.

(3) Splint fractures and apply traction if necessary to relieve pain. Pneumatic splints are compact and light. When inflated to 35–40 mm Hg, they immobilize the fracture and control local edema. Check peripheral circulation frequently.

(4) Transport as gently and as quickly as possible to a hospital.

(5) If profound or progressive shock develops, give blood, plasma, or a plasma substitute as soon as possible.

Control of Pain

Distinguish fear and excitement from real pain. Severe injuries frequently cause surprisingly little discomfort. Immobilization of injured parts often relieves distress. *Note:* Narcotics are contraindicated in coma, head injuries, and respiratory depression. Morphine sulfate, 1 mg/10 lb IM, will relieve pain and anxiety. The intravenous route is quick and sure; peripheral vasoconstriction may delay absorption of a subcutaneous or intramuscular injection, and will lead to overdosage if multiple injections are later absorbed at the same time. Inform other attendants that the patient has received morphine, and record the time and dosage on a note or tag affixed to his wrist or ankle.

Care of Open Wounds

(1) Remove gross foreign debris; apply a dry, sterile dressing or a clean cloth and secure it firmly in place.

(2) Do not place antiseptic solutions or antibacterial powders in the wound. It is not necessary to cleanse the skin around the wound with soap or antiseptic.

(3) Arrange for the earliest possible cleansing, debridement, and closure under aseptic conditions.

Transportation of Injured Patients

Improper methods of moving patients can increase injuries. Lift severely injured patients with care (see above), and improvise stretchers from blankets, boards, and doors when necessary. (See accompanying illustrations.) Transport the following types of cases in the recumbent position, on a stretcher, preferably in an ambulance: head and internal injuries; fractures of the spine, pelvis, and long bones of the lower extremities; shock; and major wounds in general. The physician administering first aid is morally and in some areas legally responsible for ensuring the safe transfer of the patient to a medical facility or to another physician.

EMERGENCY ROOM WORK-UP

Examine accident victims promptly and thoroughly. Record history and findings in accurate detail. Obtain the following information in cases of acute injury.

Identification

Obtain as much of this as possible from the family or from adults accompanying the child.

(1) Patient's name, address, phone number, age, sex, and race.

(2) Date and exact time brought to emergency room.

(3) Brought to emergency room by (give name and address).

(4) Referring physician (name and address).

(5) Next of kin (name and address).

(6) If injured at school, record the name, address, and phone number of the school and the name of the school's insurance carrier.

History of Injury

(1) Date and exact time of accident.

(2) Where and how it occurred.

(3) Accurate description of the mechanism of injury, including symptoms, subsequent course, and treatment given.

(4) Note and record exact medications and doses that have been administered.

(5) In major injuries, take a complete general history.

Physical Examination

(1) In minor injuries, describe accurately the local findings. Line drawings are frequently helpful in showing the location and configuration of wounds.

(2) Severe trauma commonly causes multiple injuries, and symptoms may not become manifest for many hours. Palpate such patients carefully and completely in order not to overlook occult fractures and visceral damage.

Laboratory Examination

(1) In major injuries determine the hematocrit, hemoglobin, white blood count, and differential count, and perform a urinalysis.

(2) Group and cross-match for blood transfusion as required.

(3) Obtain appropriate x-rays. All sites of suspected fracture should be x-rayed as soon as the patient's condition permits.

(4) Special laboratory tests as indicated.

Diagnostic Impression & Differential Diagnosis

Signature of examiner

Date and hour of examination

Disposition

(1) Discharge; date of return visit.

(2) Referral (name and address of physician).

(3) Hospital admission.

ABDOMINAL INJURIES

Nonpenetrating Abdominal Injuries

May be accompanied by varying degrees of shock, hemorrhage, or peritonitis. The nature and direction of injury should be ascertained. Serial examinations are imperative. Pass a nasogastric tube and aspirate the stomach contents. Test for blood. Leave on suction. Measure abdominal girth at the navel. After initial x-rays, tap the abdomen in either or both lower quadrants if indicated by the clinical findings.

A. Liver Rupture: Manifestations are due to hemorrhage, shock, and possible bile peritonitis. Liver rupture is characterized by a history of injury followed immediately or after a few hours by right upper quadrant pain, tenderness, and signs of hemorrhage. Shock and rapid exsanguination may occur.

B. Splenic Rupture: Manifestations are due to hemorrhage and shock. Splenic rupture is characterized by a history of injury followed immediately or after days (subcapsular hemorrhage) by left upper quadrant and shoulder pain, rebound tenderness, muscle rigidity, signs of bleeding (including shifting dullness), a mass in the left upper quadrant, and shock. Spontaneous rupture may occur with malaria, leukemia, or infectious mononucleosis.

C. Intestinal Rupture: Manifestations are due to localized peritonitis or to gangrene of the bowel following a mesenteric tear with impairment of blood supply. Characterized by history of injury followed by symptoms due to peritonitis, anemia, or gangrene of bowel. Upright x-rays of the abdomen or chest show free air under the diaphragm, ileus, and free fluid in the abdomen.

D. Kidney Rupture: Manifestations are due to perirenal bleeding and urinary extravasation or intrarenal bleeding. Characterized by a history of injury followed by flank pain, hematuria, local costovertebral angle tenderness, swelling, muscle spasm, a palpable mass, nonshifting flank dullness, shock, and ecchymosis. An intravenous urogram is valuable for confirmation and to determine the extent of injury.

E. Bladder Rupture: Manifestations are due to local injury with intra-or extraperitoneal extravasation of urine or blood. Rupture is caused by trauma to a full bladder or by a pelvic fracture. Characterized by history of injury to the lower abdomen, followed by persistent pain, suprapubic tenderness, muscle spasm, and hematuria. Signs of free fluid in the peritoneal cavity may be present. A boggy suprapubic mass may be felt or percussed. X-rays of the pelvis should be taken to determine if fracture has occurred. A simple procedure is to empty the bladder, instill 300 ml of sterile saline solution, and measure the return. A cystogram is the most dependable test for bladder injury: instill sterile radiopaque contrast fluid and take anteroposterior and oblique views. (The capacity of the bladder in a 1-year-old child is 75–100 ml; in an adult, 250–300 ml.)

F. Urethral Rupture: Manifestations depend upon the segment of urethra involved; extravasation of urine or blood may be around the bladder, in the anterior abdominal wall, periprostatic, or perineal. An abdominal or perineal injury is followed by pain, blood at the urethral meatus, difficulty in voiding, and signs of extravasation (see above). Urethrograms (5–20 ml radiopaque material instilled into urethra by catheter) should be taken to confirm and localize the site of rupture. A catheter may not pass the area of urethral injury.

Penetrating Abdominal Injuries

All penetrating abdominal injuries must be explored. A minute entry wound may mask extensive internal damage. Penetrating abdominal wounds always require exploratory laparotomy. The patient should be stripped and carefully examined for entry and exit wounds and for evidence of associated injuries or bleeding contributing to shock. Symptoms, signs, and laboratory evidence of severe hemorrhage must be evaluated promptly so that lifesaving surgery may be done—in spite of shock, if necessary.

The status of the patient depends upon (1) the organs involved, as suggested by the type and direction of the injury and specific symptoms and signs; (2) the severity of hemorrhage, shock, and peritonitis; (3) the time elapsed since injury; and (4) treatment already administered.

Symptoms and signs of specific organ involvement are reviewed above. Manifestations of hemorrhage and shock are reviewed on p 755.

PERINEAL INJURIES

Perineal injuries most often result from falls on a bicycle seat, falls in a bath tub, or sexual assault.

Injuries to the labia often cause bruising, edema, and urinary retention. Have the child attempt to urinate while sitting in a tub of warm water. Catheterization is rarely necessary.

Vaginal injuries require thorough examination under sedation or anesthesia. If associated with fever, abdominal pain, lower abdominal tenderness, or free air in the abdomen, the abdomen must be explored. Otherwise, lacerations can be sutured loosely and the patient begun on sitz baths.

Urethral injuries are rare if the pelvis is not fractured or the symphysis pubis disrupted.

Testicular pain following trauma should suggest torsion of the testes or rupture of the tunica albuginea. Persistence of pain for 1–2 hours after trauma is indication for exploration of the testes. In torsion of the

testis, the testis is tense and tender and the cord may be thick and shortened. Torsion of appendix testis may follow trauma or activities such as bicycle or horseback riding. The earliest sign is a tender, firm, palpable nodule. Later, the entire testis becomes larger because of effusion into the tunica vaginalis. The scrotum is often red on the involved side. Surgery reduces morbidity and shortens convalescence, but the disease is self-limited.

CHEST INJURIES

External evidence of injury may not be present.

Rib Fracture

Localized pleuritic pain (sharp pain with breathing), localized severe pain with pressure at the fracture site, or pain with compression of sternum or lateral chest. Pleural friction rub may be present. Examine for fluid (hemothorax) and pneumothorax.

Flail Chest

Multiple rib fractures may result in separation of an area of chest wall which then functions independently of the rib cage proper. With inspiration, the segment is sucked in, limiting expansion of the lung on the involved side. Flail chest is characterized by pain, dyspnea, cyanosis, and paradoxic motion of the involved segment. Immediate immobilization is required. This may require endotracheal intubation and support with a positive pressure ventilator.

Pneumothorax

Pneumothorax is classically characterized by dyspnea and cyanosis, chest lag, absence of fremitus, hyperresonance, and absence of breath and voice sounds on the involved side. Upright chest x-ray will confirm the diagnosis. The classical picture varies greatly with the amount of air. If fluid is also present, findings of pneumothorax predominate. There are 4 types: spontaneous, traumatic, tension, and open.

A. Spontaneous Pneumothorax: Usually in older children; rupture of bleb with leakage of air into the pleural cavity; source of leak seals spontaneously. Characterized by a sudden onset of dyspnea, pleuritic pain, respiratory lag, hyperresonance, and absent breath and voice sounds on the involved side. Symptoms and signs do not progress.

B. Tension Pneumothorax: Failure of the lung leak to seal results in an increasing amount of air in the pleural space with each breath. This causes mediastinal shift, rapidly progressive dyspnea and cyanosis, and physical findings as noted above. Marked intrathoracic pressure may prevent hyperresonance. Tension pneumothorax may result from lung trauma (penetrating wounds) or may occur with spontaneous pneumothorax. Immediate measures must be taken to aspirate air and to allow continued escape of trapped air.

C. Open Pneumothorax: Characterized by the presence of an open wound, severe respiratory distress with cyanosis, audible sucking sounds, and ingress or egress of frothy, blood-tinged fluid with each breath. The opening must be closed **at once** with an airtight bandage and the patient placed on the injured side. Vasoline gauze covered with a bulky bandage will usually suffice.

Hemothorax

Signs of pleural fluid as evidenced by absent fremitus, loss of resonance, absent breath and voice sounds, and tracheal shift to the opposite side, together with general symptoms of hemorrhage following chest injury; may be associated with pneumothorax. Physical findings of pneumothorax may obscure those of hemothorax. Confirm by needle aspiration after upright chest x-ray.

Penetrating Wounds of Chest

May be closed or open.

A. Closed Wounds: A minute point of entry may be associated with extensive intrathoracic damage. Check for rib fracture, pneumothorax, hemothorax, subcutaneous (palpation) or mediastinal emphysema (crunching sound with each heartbeat), and cardiac contusion.

B. Open Wounds: Open wounds inevitably produce critical pneumothorax; see above.

Cardiac Injury

May consist of simple contusion, a penetrating wound, valve rupture, or cardiac tamponade. Contusion may be associated with arrhythmia or nonspecific ECG findings. Rupture occurs most commonly in the aortic valve and is manifested by a loud, "cooing" diastolic murmur; signs of acute left heart failure may be present.

Cardiac tamponade due to blood in the pericardial sac progresses to limitation of diastolic filling of the heart with resultant progressive narrowing of pulse pressure, increase in pulse rate, paradoxic pulse, engorged neck veins, and eventually critically low cardiac output. Pericardial paracentesis may be lifesaving.

Pulmonary Contusion

Chest trauma is often associated with hemorrhage into contused areas of lung. This appears as floccular or large densities on x-ray. The patient becomes progressively cyanotic and agitated. Blood may be present in the tracheal aspirate. Increased pulmonary shunting leads to a progressive rise in P_{CO_2} and a fall in P_{O_2}. Administration of oxygen by mask or nasal catheter may help, but the patient often requires endotracheal intubation and positive pressure ventilation. Oxygen concentration should be just adequate to maintain an arterial P_{O_2} of 60–80 mm Hg. Prolonged exposure to high concentrations of oxygen can lead to permanent lung damage. Treat the patient with salt-poor albumin, salt restriction, furosemide (Lasix), 1 mg/2.5 kg IV,

and maintenance fluids. Pulmonary contusion is completely reversible.

Ruptured Bronchus

Persistent pneumothorax after placement of a chest tube, air in the mediastinum, and hemoptysis should suggest traumatic rupture of a bronchus. In children, this can occur without rib fracture. Bronchoscopy is indicated as soon as possible if this diagnosis is suspected.

ARTERIAL OCCLUSION

Traumatic

A cold, pale, pulseless extremity following trauma to an extremity suggests arterial occlusion. This may be from direct penetration or division, from local pressure, or from entrapment in a fracture site. Once the patient is stable and the fractured extremity has been placed in traction, persistent signs and symptoms demand immediate arteriography to demonstrate the site of occlusion. Corrective surgery within 4 hours can save the limb.

Neonatal

Arterial occlusion can occur in the newborn. Emboli from the occluding ductus arteriosus or umbilical arteries are the usual cause, although iatrogenic complications of umbilical artery catheterization may occur. The limb appears pale at first, and then cyanotic or mottled. Pulses are absent below the occlusion. The extremity may swell. Immediate therapy consists of heparin, 100 units/kg body weight IV every 4 hours, to maintain a clotting time 3–4 times normal. If symptoms progress, embolectomy must be attempted and can be successful in the neonate.

FRACTURES*

General Features

Clinical manifestations of fracture include pain, local tenderness, ecchymosis, deformity due to swelling and bone displacement, impaired function, abnormal motion, and crepitus at the site of fracture. In some instances, only pain is present. Simple inspection is often diagnostic. X-ray confirmation is mandatory. Evaluate sensory changes and voluntary motion of joints distal to the fracture for evidence of nerve damage. Check distal portion of extremity for evidence of impaired blood supply.

Spinal Injuries

Vertebral fractures and spinal cord injuries are suggested by the nature of the injury, back pain, and

*See also Chapter 19.

abnormal position or mobility of the neck, back, or extremities. All unconscious patients or those who complain of back or neck pain should be treated as potential spinal cord injury cases. Every effort should be made to maintain the normal alignment of the spine both in examination and transportation. Never transport such patients in a sitting or semireclining position; use a flat stretcher without a pillow. By asking the patient to move his toes, legs, and hands, one can roughly determine the presence of significant cord injury and its approximate location. Loss of sensation to pain will further identify the level of the cord injury.

LACERATIONS

All lacerations sufficiently deep to penetrate the skin must be thoroughly explored. When possible, place the extremity in about the same position it was in when injury incurred. This may reveal more extensive injury than previously suspected.

Aqueous benzalkonium chloride (Zephiran) makes an excellent cleansing solution. Clean the skin thoroughly about the laceration. Then inject sufficient 0.5% procaine or lidocaine (Xylocaine) to achieve good anesthesia before cleansing the depths of the wound. All clots and debris must be removed.

Remove all dead fat, muscle, and fascia with sharp scissors or scalpel. Debride the edges of the wound if they are ragged, crushed, or heavily impregnated with grease or dirt. The edges should be straight, clean, and bleeding freely.

Interrupted sutures of fine silk or nylon give the best cosmetic results. They should be evenly placed and should approximate the edges accurately. Sutures should not be tighter than necessary to give skin edge approximation.

Give a tetanus toxoid booster as indicated.

Lacerations heal faster and with less scarring if the extremity is at rest. Use splints, slings, and bed rest as necessary.

See patient in 24 hours. Check the edges of the wound for erythema, drainage, or undue tenderness. Warn the parents what to look for.

The face is very vascular and rarely under tension. Remove ½ of the stitches on the third day and the rest on the 5th day. Support with Steri-Tapes if in doubt. The hands, arms, and neck usually heal in 7 days. The feet, knees, pretibial areas, and shoulder require 10–14 days to heal.

EXTREMITY AMPUTATION

Stop major bleeding by pressure around the ends of the stump. Retrieve the extremity if feasible for possible reimplantation. First attention must always be paid to the patient; he may be neglected in the haste of retrieving the limb.

Treat blood loss and associated injuries.

FINGER INJURIES

Door Injuries

Car doors and metal cabinet doors may partially amputate a fingertip. The terminal phalanx is usually fractured and the nail bed is usually avulsed.

Cleanse the area thoroughly, realign all viable tissue, and approximate skin loosely with 3 or 4 sutures. Splint the digit.

These injuries often become infected and must be checked frequently. If infection develops, remove sutures near the site of infection and begin frequent soaks. Use antibiotics as indicated by cultures.

Finger Amputations

Amputated fingers should not be sewed on if more than just skin is lost. The amputated part can supply skin for a skin graft. Clean the amputation site thoroughly. Remove crushed tissue and bone fragments before approximating the skin loosely over the fingertip.

EMERGENCIES DUE TO LOCAL INFECTIONS & INFLAMMATION

PARONYCHIA

Paronychia is a staphylococcal infection around the base or side of a fingernail. There is usually a history of nailbiting. Drain under digital block using 0.5% lidocaine (Xylocaine) or procaine anesthesia. Soak the hand twice daily in warm water till healing occurs.

FELON

This consists of an infection, usually staphylococcal, in the pulp space of a finger. It often follows sliver or thorn injury to the finger pad. It is very painful and can progress to ischemic necrosis of the terminal phalanx.

Treatment consists of drainage by lateral incision deep into the pulp space after adequate digital block.

TESTICULAR PAIN

If the diagnosis of the cause of persistent testicular pain is in doubt, explore the testes as soon as possible because of the high incidence of torsion of the testes (see p 761).

Orchitis may be secondary to mumps. Check the history and draw acute phase serum for antibody titer determination. Treat with bed rest, fluids, and analgesics as necessary.

Epididymitis is uncommon in children who have no urinary tract infection or catheter. The epididymis can often be felt and is tense and tender. Treat urinary infection as indicated and check the prostate for prostatitis.

Abscesses

A. Cervical Abscesses: These usually follow cervical adenitis following tonsillitis, oral trauma, or dental operations. The lymph nodes are tender and the child febrile.

Treatment consists of a 10-day course of penicillin or other antibiotic as indicated by throat culture. If no response is obvious in 10 days, stop antibiotics and wait for the nodes to suppurate. Surgical drainage is indicated only when a node is clearly fluctuant.

B. Groin Abscesses: Adenopathy below the groin crease is usually secondary to sepsis in the foot or leg. Adenopathy above groin crease is usually secondary to diaper rash or vulval lesions. Enlargement of nodes above the groin crease may be confused with incarcerated hernia or hydrocele of the cord.

If the diagnosis is not clear, exploration of the groin is indicated. If the swelling is clearly a lymph node enlargement, treat for 10 days with penicillin and drain only when fluctuant.

URINARY RETENTION

Urinary retention is rare in children. The most common cause is chronic constipation, resulting in a large fecal concretion that presses on the bladder neck. Tumors (rhabdomyosarcoma of the prostate or cystosarcoma phyllodes) can cause retention.

Catheterization is rarely necessary except in cases of tumor.

BATTERED CHILD SYNDROME (CHILD ABUSE)

Essentials of Diagnosis
- Unexplained or inadequately explained signs of trauma.

- Multiple fractures at different stages of healing.
- Failure to thrive that responds to nutritional therapy alone.
- Isolated, depressed, immature parent without emotional support.

General Considerations

Child abuse can be defined as a lack of reasonable care and protection of children by their parents, guardians, or relatives. The incidence of child abuse is generally 6/1000 live births. Half of these children are physically abused; 1/2 are nutritionally deprived. The prevalence of child abuse is approximately 300 cases per million population per year. Therefore, in a city of 100,000 people, about 30 new cases can be detected per year.

The abused child is often an infant. Young children are at greater risk because they are demanding, defenseless, and nonverbal. Estimates of the usual age for child abuse are that 1/3 occur under 1 year of age, 1/3 from ages 1–3, and 1/3 over age 3.

The laws on child abuse are clear. In every state of the USA, reporting of suspected cases of child abuse by the physician is mandatory, and penalities exist for failing to report. The laws also protect the physician from liability suits regarding release of confidential information. Despite these laws, physicians sometimes go to great lengths to avoid diagnosing child abuse. They often fear that detection and reporting of child abuse will require them to personally treat this complex psychosocial problem. The responsibility for proper treatment rests with the child welfare facilities in the community—not with the physician.

Classification

A. Physical Abuse: Approximately 10% of accidents are due to physical abuse. These injuries can occur in several ways.

1. Injury in anger—Misbehavior makes parents angry. Some parents hit the child before they can control themselves.

2. Harsh punishment—Some parents attempt to discipline children in painful ways. This type of discipline is not acceptable to society when it results in an injury that requires medical attention or when it is employed frequently.

3. Accidents due to neglect—When children are not adequately supervised, accidents increase in number. Accident repeaters generally need reporting after the third accident—or after the second accident if the injury is major.

4. Deliberate assault or murder—This occurs rarely. Such parents are usually psychotic.

B. Nutritional Abuse: Caloric deprivation is the most common cause of failure to thrive. Over 30% of cases of failure to thrive are due to this cause. Many of these children also have developmental delays due to emotional deprivation. Older children who are emotionally deprived occasionally develop deprivational dwarfism (see Chapter 24).

C. Sexual Abuse (Incest): Incest often remains undiagnosed unless the physician looks carefully at the reasons behind unexplained urinary tract infections or vaginitis or running away by a young girl. A stepfather or a mother's boy-friend living in the home is more likely than a natural father to be involved in this kind of problem. Incest requires reporting to child welfare and separation from the offending adult.

D. Emotional Abuse: Emotional abuse concerns the continual scapegoating, terrorizing, and rejection of a specific child. Such treatment mutilates the developing personality. Proving this type of child abuse is nearly impossible. Perhaps it is fortunate that these children are eventually physically abused, abandoned, or imprisoned in their room. At this point, the child can be legally removed from his destructive environment.

Etiology

Most parents who abuse their children were also abused as children. They are often lonely, immature, isolated, unloved, depressed, and angry people. The parent who batters his child has poor impulse control; the parent who starves his child has relatively good impulse control but can deny the needs of his child. An overlap between caloric deprivation and physical abuse can occur.

Parents who abuse children come from all racial, religious, geographic, socioeconomic, and educational backgrounds. Either parent can be responsible, although the father is more likely to be the offender when multiple children are harmed. In cases of failure to thrive, the mother is almost always responsible.

Clinical Findings

Child abuse should be considered in any of the following medical problems: skin bruises, soft tissue swellings, fractures, dislocations, tender extremities, burns, head injuries, subdural hematomas, unexplained seizures, unexplained comas, undernutrition problems, or "crib deaths." Poisoning and lacerations are uncommon.

A. Symptoms: The diagnosis of child abuse is usually confirmed by the presence of several of the following suggestive data:

1. The injury is completely unexplained.
2. The described accident is vague, bizarre, or variable.
3. There is a discrepancy between the type of accident and the baby's developmental age.
4. There is a discrepancy between the accident and the physical findings.
5. Accidents have been repeated.
6. The parents have delayed in seeking medical care.
7. The parents disappear during admission; they rarely visit; or they don't ask about discharge.
8. Medical care has been neglected (eg, no immunizations, previous illnesses without medical attention).

9. A history of anorexia, recurrent vomiting, or recurrent diarrhea is not confirmed in the hospital setting (especially in the case of infants who fail to thrive).

B. Signs:
1. Pathognomonic skin lesions include lash marks, cigarette burns, grab marks, cord loop marks, belt buckle marks, human bites, tie marks.
2. An injury that could not have been self-inflicted (eg, a dunking burn).
3. Multiple old and new signs of trauma.
4. Retinal hemorrhages mean severe shaking if they are present without a fracture or scalp bruise.
5. Obvious fear of a parent.
6. Failure to thrive.
7. Signs of neglect (eg, cradle cap, long nails, diaper rash, unwashed).
8. Signs of emotional deprivation (eg, blank face, no speech, no curiosity, no complaint on venipuncture).

C. X-Ray Findings: Radiographic evidence of multiple fractures at different stages of healing is diagnostic of physical abuse. If a single injury is present, abuse can be suspected when metaphyseal chip fractures or exuberant periosteal reactions are found: When the initial film is normal, a follow-up film 2 weeks later will often confirm the suspicion of a non-displaced epiphyseal fracture by demonstrating metaphyseal fragmentation and callus formation. Any case in which a child is brought in dead on arrival is an indication for total body x-rays in addition to autopsy.

D. Diagnostic Trial of Caloric Rehabilitation: The diagnosis of failure to thrive secondary to nutritional deprivation is confirmed by rapid weight gain on unlimited feedings in the hospital. The same milk that was used at home is preferred. The infant usually responds within 2 weeks. The same personnel should feed the child to the extent that that is possible.

E. Consultations: The child with a developmental delay may need a baseline developmental quotient assessed by a developmental pediatrician or a psychologist.

F. Family Assessment: Certain psychosocial factors are usually present in child abuse families. In any case where child abuse is suspected, these factors should be assessed. A psychiatrist, social worker, or specially trained pediatrician can gather this information. Even when the child's injury is explained and plausible, this assessment should be done if (1) the child is under 6 months of age, (2) the injury was major and required hospitalization, or (3) the child is an accident repeater. The inquiry should establish the following:

1. The parents' stability—How is the mother doing? (Depressed, overwhelmed, etc?) Does either parent have a temper problem?

2. The mother-child relationship—Can the parent say anything positive about the child? Is there a bond of love with the child?

3. Discipline—What does the parent expect of the child? Does the child cause problems—eg, crying, eating, sleeping? What discipline is necessary?

4. Crisis—Was there a family crisis at the time of the accident—eg, moving, sick baby, absent husband, new pregnancy?

5. Rescue source—Does the parent have someone to talk to? Does the parent have someone to count on? (This is unlikely if there are marital problems or no extended family.)

Differential Diagnosis

Rare bone disorders may resemble nonaccidental trauma (eg, osteogenesis imperfecta, scurvy, syphilis), but a skilled radiologist can easily differentiate these entities. In children who fail to thrive, laboratory tests for rare malabsorptive disorders (eg, celiac disease) should be withheld until after an adequate trial of feeding.

Treatment

A. General Measures: The following 11 steps are recommended when a physician sees a child whom he suspects has been abused:

1. Hospitalize the child—The purpose of hospitalization is to protect the child until the safety of his home can be evaluated. The reason given to the parents for hospitalization is that, "His injuries need to be watched." It is not helpful to mention to the parents the possibility of nonaccidental trauma at this time. If the parents refuse hospitalization, a court order can be obtained. This is rarely needed and should not be a routine procedure.

2. Treat the child's injuries—Once the child is in the hospital, the medical and surgical problems should be cared for in the usual manner. Orthopedic consultation is commonly needed. Ophthalmologists, neurologists, neurosurgeons, and plastic surgeons are occasionally consulted.

3. Obtain necessary laboratory tests—Every suspected case should receive a skeletal survey. Avoid using incriminating terms (eg, "rule out battering") on requisitions. The x-ray findings may establish a definite diagnosis of nonaccidental trauma. If there are bruises or a history of "easy bruising," one should obtain a "routine clot screen." If there are visible physical findings, photographs should be taken. These require a parental consent form or a court order.

4. Maintain a helping approach to the parents—This is the hardest step. It is natural to feel angry with these parents, but expressing anger is very damaging to parent cooperation. Confrontation, accusation, and interrogation must be avoided. The primary physician must see or phone these parents daily. They become suspicious quite easily if communication is not optimal. If the child is brought in dead or with multiple life-threatening injuries, the parent must receive an emergency psychiatric evaluation because he may be psychotic or suicidal.

5. Report to Child Welfare by phone within 24 hours—Tell the parents the diagnosis and the need to report it before doing so. Tell them, "This is an unexplained injury," or, "Your explanation of the injury is insufficient." Then add, "I am obligated by law to report any injury to any child that is hard to explain." The physician must also tell the parents of the subsequent visit by a child welfare worker. He can add that the police will not be involved, that the matter will be kept confidential, and that everyone's goal is to help them find better ways of dealing with their child.

This call goes to the agency charged with child welfare in the patient's county of residence.

6. Report to Child Welfare in writing within 72 hours—The official report should be written by a physician and should contain the following data:

a. Description of the injury from the history, physical findings, and x-rays.

b. The alleged cause of the injury.

c. Past medical history of other injuries.

d. Concluding statement about why this represents nonaccidental trauma.

7. Obtain psychiatric consultation and social service consultation within 72 hours: Psychiatric consultation should be obtained as soon as practicable. The psychiatrist determines how safe the home is, how disturbed the parents are, and how likely they are to accept therapy. The social worker evaluates the marital relationship and the total family problems. The pediatrician is not usually able to do this. Child Welfare usually carries out their evaluation concurrently. The evaluations by the hospital social worker and psychiatrist should be typed and submitted to Child Welfare.

8. Attend disposition meeting—The psychiatrist, social worker, pediatrician, consultants, house staff, and child welfare worker should meet within 3 work days of admission. All evaluations should have been completed. All possible suspects (including babysitters, neighbor's children, boy-friends) should have been interviewed. The meeting should decide upon the best long range plan for the patient. The hospital social worker will convey these recommendations to Child Welfare and any other agencies involved if their representatives have not been able to attend.

9. Discharge the patient when Child Welfare authorizes it—Child Welfare should first decide whether the child will have a dependency hearing and whether they will seek placement of the child in a foster home if dependency filing is sustained. The pediatrician is obligated to keep the child in a protected environment until Child Welfare decides on the best course of action. If this takes too long, Child Welfare can be asked to place the child temporarily in a foster home.

10. Follow-up of physical status by the pediatrician—The battered child needs more frequent well child care than the average child. He should be seen once a week for a while. He needs follow-up to detect any recurrence of physical abuse. If he has sustained head injury, he needs follow-up for mental retardation, spasticity, and subdural hematomas. If he has experienced nutritional neglect, he needs careful monitoring of weight gain. If the parents come from a great distance, the pediatric follow-up should be requested of a physician in that community. If the child is reinjured and the injury itself does not warrant hospitalization,

Child Welfare should be called to decide what protective services should be provided.

11. Follow-up and treatment of psychosocial problems by Child Welfare—The pediatrician should not feel responsible for restoration of these families to emotional health. Child Welfare is primarily responsible for provision of psychotherapy, for home visits, and for finding the patient who becomes "lost to follow-up." The pediatrician can contribute to the therapeutic process by giving the parent his telephone number to call "if things get rough." It is best if the parent has several helping people available as lifelines. After the parent calls, Child Welfare should be notified that the parent is upset and urgently needs help.

B. Psychotherapy: The parents in child abuse cases usually do not accept interpretive psychotherapy and respond better to therapists who can reach out. Home visits are often necessary. Professional therapists are not always required. Laymen have been trained as mothering aides or homeworkers. Other battering parents have been helped by group therapy. Day care centers are very important in giving the mother a part of her day free from her child.

C. Legal Aspects of Management:

1. Dependency hearing—A dependency petition is a legal instrument that permits Child Welfare to request temporary protective custody of an abused child. If the petition is sustained by the court, the child becomes a ward of the state. The court can then insist that psychotherapy, marital counseling, or certain changes in the home be carried out. The parents cannot legally remove their child from the state during this period of time.

2. Placement—If the home is considered dangerous for the child, he should be placed in a foster home. However, the ultimate goal is to reunite the family. In 90% of cases in one large state where this problem has been extensively studied, the children are returned to their own homes after the court has observed improvement in the parents. Only 10% of cases require termination of parental rights and permanent placement. Danger signals that strongly suggest the need for placement are (1) a parent who does not want help; (2) a parent with no emotional support currently available; (3) a delusional or depressed psychotic, or aggressive psychopathic parent; (4) signs of neglect in addition to trauma; (5) injuries in the name of discipline; or (6) a severe injury in an infant. Occasionally, the physician must insist that placement be considered because of his special knowledge of the family.

3. Police intervention—Police are rarely needed in child abuse cases except to provide court holds at night or on weekends. Arrests, interrogations, or public incriminations by the police are detrimental to helping these parents. These cases should be managed by the juvenile court system and the Protective Services Division of Child Welfare.

Prognosis

The main objective in child abuse is to prevent repeated injuries to the child. In cases of child abuse

where the child is returned to his parents without any intervention, 5% are killed and 35% suffer permanent physical damage from repeated abuse. The untreated survivors also have emotional problems. Physically abused children often relate violently to the world when they grow up; emotionally deprived children often relate only shallowly to people. Early detection and intervention are mandatory in the syndrome known as the battered child.

Helfer RE, Pollock CB: The battered child syndrome. Page 9 in: *Advances in Pediatrics.* Vol 15. Levine SZ (editor). Year Book, 1968.

Helfer RE, Kempe CH (editors). *The Battered Child.* Univ of Chicago Press, 1968.

Holter JC, Friedman SB: Child abuse: Early casefinding in the emergency department. Pediatrics 42:128, 1968.

Kempe CH & others: The battered child syndrome. JAMA 181:17, 1962.

Kempe CH: The battered child and the hospital. Hosp Practice 4:44, 1969.

Kempe CH: Pediatric implications of the battered baby syndrome. Arch Dis Childhood 46:28, 1971.

Kempe CH, Helfer RE (editors): *Helping the Battered Child and His Family.* Lippincott, 1971.

EMERGENCIES DUE TO PHYSICAL AGENTS

BURNS

A second degree burn of 10% or more of the body surface in a child under 1 year of age or of 15% of the body surface in an older child is a serious injury and requires hospitalization for proper treatment. Initial management is the most important factor in survival.

Classification & Characteristics of Burn Wounds

A. First Degree: Involves superficial epidermis (partial thickness burn). The skin area is pink or red in appearance, blanches with pressure, and is painful to touch. Causes include sunburn, scalds, and distant flash fires.

B. Second Degree: Involves entire epidermis (partial thickness). The skin is red, blistered, or moist with exudate, and painful to pinprick or touch. Causes include scalds and flash fires.

C. Third Degree: Involves dermis or underlying fat, muscle, or bone (full thickness). The skin is white, dry or charred, and painless. Causes include scalds from live steam, open flame burns, or contact with chemicals or electric current.

Treatment of Minor Burns

First degree burns and second degree burns of less than 10% of the body surface that do not involve the hands, the feet, the perineum, or the face can be treated on an outpatient basis with plain petrolatum or antibiotic-impregnated gauze and clean dressings, which should be changed every 48–72 hours. All children with burns of the hands and most children with burns of the feet should be hospitalized so that proper splinting of the extremity and careful local wound care can be performed. Burns of the face need close observation for airway obstruction and careful local wound care to avoid infection so near the CNS.

Treatment of Major Burns

Major burns are second degree burns involving more than 10% of the body surface and any third degree burns.

A. Emergency Measures:

1. Cool the burned area immediately by running cool water over it or by immersing the patient in salt water (2 tsp of salt per quart of water) kept cool to 15° C (59° F) with ice cubes.

2. Transport the child to a hospital wrapped in a clean sheet.

3. If analgesia is needed, give meperidine, 2 mg/kg subcut, or morphine, 0.1 mg/kg subcut, and make certain that a written record of the amount given stays with the patient when he is transported to the hospital.

4. Begin fluid replacement if hospitalization will be delayed for several hours after injury.

B. Definitive Measures:

1. **Treatment of burned area–**

a. Using sterile technic (with gown, gloves, cap, and mask), remove burned clothing and carefully examine the patient for other injuries. Determine his general condition.

b. In facial burns, verify the patency of the airway and evaluate the need for tracheostomy.

c. Clean the wound of all grease and ointments and uncover blisters if topical antibiotics are to be used (see below).

d. Record areas of second and third degree burn as percentage of total body area, using the chart as adapted from Lund & Browder (Fig 30–13). (The "rule of nines," so useful in adult burns, does not apply to children.)

2. **Fluid administration–**

a. Place a large bore catheter in a vein. If a central catheter can be placed via the external jugular, subclavian, or cephalic vein, it can be used to obtain central venous pressure readings.

b. Place a catheter in the bladder and record hourly urine output.

c. Type and cross-match blood. Do a complete blood count and determine serum electrolytes.

d. Calculate fluid requirements (see Chapter 37) and begin fluid replacement.

3. **Prevention of infection–**

a. Administer tetanus toxoid or hyperimmune serum if not immunized.

b. Culture burn wound and nose and throat secretions.

c. Begin antibiotics (penicillin G and oxacillin) for control of streptococcal and staphylococcal infections.

Infant Less Than One Year of Age

Name _____ Age _____ Ward _____

1st degree erythema not to be included

2nd degree

3rd degree

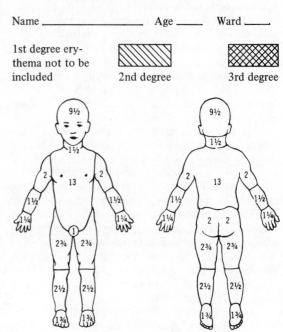

Variations from Adult Distribution in Infants and Children (in Percent).

	Newborn	1 Year	5 Years	10 Years
Head	19	17	13	11
Both thighs	11	13	16	17
Both lower legs	10	10	11	12
Neck	2			
Anterior trunk	13			
Posterior trunk	13			
Both upper arms	8	These percentages		
Both lower arms	6	remain constant at		
Both hands	5	all ages.		
Both buttocks	5			
Both feet	7			
Genitals	1			
	100			

FIG 30–13. Lund and Browder modification of Berkow's scale for estimating extent of burns. (The table under the illustration is after Berkow.)

d. Apply topical antibiotics (see below).

4. **Topical burn therapy–**Survival in major burns has been improved by the use of topical agents such as 0.5% silver nitrate, mafenide (Sulfamylon), and gentamicin (Garamycin). To be most effective, these drugs should be applied as soon as possible before the burn wound becomes heavily infected. Mafenide (Sulfamylon) cream is easily applied but tends to sting for a while after its application and may produce a metabolic acidosis secondary to inhibition of carbonic anhydrase by the absorbed and metabolized drug. In

addition, hyperchloremia occurs as the chloride salt is absorbed. If acidosis and hyperchloremia are a problem, use of the cream may be discontinued for 24–48 hours without decreasing the bacteriostatic effect.

Silver nitrate (0.5% by weight) for topical use is very hypotonic and can cause severe sodium and chloride deficits. Therefore, in the initial treatment period, serum electrolytes must be determined 2 or 3 times a day and appropriate sodium chloride replacement given. Silver nitrate, 1%, is toxic to new epithelium, whereas 0.1% is not bactericidal; therefore, the bulky dressings must be kept wet with 0.5% silver nitrate at all times to protect regenerating skin, maintain the correct concentration of the drug, and retard water evaporation with its concomitant energy losses.

C. General Measures: Give nothing by mouth for 24–48 hours, since ileus and gastric dilatation occur frequently in burns of children. Admit the patient to a ward where special burn nursing care is available.

Haynes BW Jr, Gayle WE Jr, Madge GE: Sulfamylon therapy in severe burns. Ann Surg 170:696–704, 1969.

Lund CC, Browder NC: The estimation of areas of burns. Surg Gynec Obst 79:352, 1944.

Moncrief JA & others: The use of topical sulfanilamide in the control of burn wound sepsis. J Trauma 6:407, 1966.

Moyer CA & others: Treatment of large human burns with 0.5% silver nitrate solution. Arch Surg 90:812, 1965.

Symposium on burns. S Clin North America 50:1191–1495, 1970.

Wilde JN: A comparison of silver nitrate treatment with other techniques in the treatment of burns. Plast Reconstr Surg 40:271–276, 1967.

HEAT STROKE

Heat stroke is rare in children but may occur with prolonged exposure to high ambient temperatures which result in failure of the thermoregulatory mechanism. In temperate climates, newborn infants, especially the sick and premature, have suffered from heat stroke when placed in cots next to radiators that have suddenly been turned on.

Symptoms and signs include headache, dizziness, nausea, visual disturbances, convulsions, and loss of consciousness. Rectal temperature may exceed 42° C (107.6° F); the pulse is rapid, irregular, and weak; and the skin is hot, flushed, dry, and incapable of sweating. Plasma and extracellular water volume and composition are normal.

Treatment

Place the child in a cool place and remove all clothing. Bring the rectal temperature down to 39° C (102.2° F) by fanning after sprinkling with water, by ice packs, or by immersion in cold water. Do not bring the temperature below 39° C. When that temperature is reached, discontinue antipyretic therapy.

Massage all 4 extremities to maintain peripheral circulation.

Avoid sedation. Give maintenance fluids, electrolytes, and calories intravenously.

Treat shock if present.

Avoid reexposure to similar conditions. If possible, a child who has suffered an episode of heat stroke should be moved to a temperate climate.

Eichler AC: Heat stroke. Am J Surg 118:855–863, 1969.

Sohar E: Heatstroke caused by dehydration and physical effort. Arch Int Med 122:159, 1969.

HEAT EXHAUSTION

Heat exhaustion is due to excessive depletion of plasma and extracellular volume as a result of sweating profusely in a high ambient temperature. Chloride losses are more critical than water losses, which explains the high risk of this condition in patients with cystic fibrosis in hot weather.

Headache and muscle cramps are common, especially in the calves. Perspiration is profuse, and there is weakness, dizziness, and stupor. The skin is pale and cool, and the temperature is normal or low. The tongue is dry, the eyes may be sunken, and the subcutaneous tissues have an inelastic quality due to loss of extracellular water. Oliguria is present, and sometimes hypotension. The condition is liable to occur in children with unusual salt losses, eg, those with cystic fibrosis or salt-losing renal diseases. It may also occur in healthy active children who replace sweat losses with water and not salt. Therefore children undergoing strenuous physical exertion in hot weather should satisfy thirst with water containing 1/4 tsp of salt to the pint. Certain proprietary drinks are pleasantly flavored, eg, Gatorade.

Treatment

Extracellular fluid volume should be restored intravenously and maintenance fluid and electrolytes given according to the principles outlined in Chapter 37. In severe heat exhaustion, a volume of isotonic lactated Ringer's injection equal to 8% of the body weight should be given intravenously over 24 hours, with 2/3 administered in the first 6 hours. Maintenance water should be 600 ml/sq m/24 hours and maintenance sodium 6 mEq/kg/24 hours until hydration is normal.

Varga C: *Handbook of Pediatric Medical Emergencies.* Mosby, 1968.

COLD INJURY
(Frostbite)

The severity of a frostbite injury depends on several factors: (1) The intensity of the cold exposure (a function of both temperature and wind velocity*) as well as increased rate of heat loss from the tissues due to contact with water or metal and restrictive or tight clothing proximal to the involved area. (2) Duration of exposure to cold is important in the progression of frostbite from superficial to deep involvement. (3) The rate of rewarming. Severe tissue damage will occur if the area is warmed too slowly or warmed and then refrozen. Thawing should not be attempted until facilities are available to properly rewarm the frostbitten tissue.

Clinical Findings & Classification

Cold injury is characterized by loss of sensation of affected parts and white, cold skin over affected areas in a child with a history of cold exposure.

A. First Degree (Frost Nip): Erythema of the skin and edema of the part but without blister formation. No significant tissue damage.

B. Second Degree: Blister and bulla formation.

C. Third Degree: Necrosis of the thick layers and subcutaneous tissues without loss of the part.

D. Fourth Degree: Complete necrosis with gangrene and loss of the affected part.

Complications

Complications include necrosis of the affected area and bacterial infection through broken skin. Late sequelae involving frostbitten areas and lasting months to years have included persistent pain, hyperhidrosis, skin tenderness, cold sensitivity, and retarded epiphyseal growth.

Treatment

A. Frost Nip: Treat by local warming.

B. Superficial and Deep Frostbite:

1. Loosen any garments which restrict blood flow.

2. Remove any wet garments which are in contact with the skin.

3. Cover the involved area with dry bulky garments.

4. Elevate the affected area.

5. Protect the part from trauma. Do not rub frostbitten tissue, for this macerates the area and causes further damage.

6. Rewarming—Transport the patient to a warm environment and rewarm the frostbitten area by immersion in a large volume of water preheated to 37.8–40.6° C (100–105° F) for about 20 minutes.

---

*Eg, 15° F when there is no wind has a "cooling power" of 15°; with winds of 25 mph, the cooling power would be −22° F at the same thermometer reading.

a. Rewarming with an oven, fire, or other source of dry heat should not be attempted, since unequal exposure with result in tissue burns.

b. Analgesics may be required during the rewarming period.

c. Low molecular weight dextran given during the rewarming phase prevents red cell and platelet agglutination and promotes tissue perfusion. An adequate dose is 1 gm/kg given once as a 5–10% solution IV.

7. Place the patient at bed rest with the part elevated.

8. Maintain local hygiene by whirlpool baths twice a day for 20 minutes at body temperature.

9. Avoid all surgical procedures on cold-injured skin. Do not remove or puncture bullae or blisters.

10. Sympathectomy and paravertebral block are of little value.

11. Amputation of a necrotic limb should be postponed 2–3 months until optimal healing has occurred. If uncontrolled infection supervenes, early amputation may be required.

Prognosis

With proper therapy, full recovery is the rule. Complications of infections are unusual in frostbite cases.

Jarrett JR & others: Cold injury. Missouri Med 67:169–173, 1970.

Knize DM & others: Use of antisludging agents in experimental cold injuries. Surg Gynec Obst 129:1019–1026, 1969.

Lapp N, Juergens JL: Frostbite. Mayo Clin Proc 40:932–948, 1965.

Vellar ID: Four cases of pedal cryopathy. MJ Australia 1:64–67, 1970.

ELECTRIC SHOCK & ELECTRIC BURNS

The danger of injury from electric shock depends upon the voltage and the frequency. Alternating current is more dangerous than direct current. At a frequency of 25–300 cycles, voltages below 230 volts can produce ventricular fibrillation. High voltages (which may be encountered in television circuits) produce respiratory failure. Faulty wiring of home appliances may lead to electric shock. In homes with young children, it is advisable to install occlusive safety outlets in the play area.

Electric Shock

Consciousness is rapidly lost. If the current continues, death from asphyxia due to ventricular fibrillation or respiratory arrest occurs within a few minutes.

Interrupt the power source or knock wire away from the skin with a dry piece of wood or other nonconducting material and institute external cardiac massage or mouth-to-mouth respiration, depending on whether asphyxia is cardiac or respiratory. Supply oxygen if available and institute treatment for shock.

Electric Burns

Momentary contact, particularly with a high-voltage outlet, will lead to localized, sharply demarcated, painless gray areas without associated inflammation of the skin. The examiner should search for a second area of grayness where the current has left the body. Sloughing occurs after a few weeks. With simple burns, the skin should be cleansed and a dry dressing applied. Deeper burns should be treated conservatively with mafenide (Sulfamylon) cream, or with gentamicin (Garamycin) under an occlusive dressing. Management is the same as for other types of burns. Infection occurs less often with electric burns, but reconstructive surgery for scarring after healing may be required.

Baxter CR: Present concepts in the management of major electrical injury. S Clin North America 50:1401–1418, 1970.

Lee WR: The nature and management of electric shock. Brit J Anaesth 36:572–580, 1964.

Lievens JB: Electrical accidents. Comm Health 2:88–194, 1970.

Robinson DW & others: Electrical burns: A review and analysis of 33 cases. Surgery 57:385–390, 1965.

Thomson GH, Juckes AW, Farmer AW: Electrical burns to the mouth in children. Plast Reconstr Surg 35:466–477, 1965.

DROWNING

Various forms of drowning are described:

(1) **Drowning without inhalation of water**: Water enters the mouth in large quantities and is swallowed. The clinical picture is that of asphyxia, and these patients have the best chance of survival. They may subsequently develop cerebral and pulmonary edema.

(2) **Drowning with inhalation of water**: The amount of water inhaled and the degree of pollution determine the severity. Asphyxia, cardiac failure, and cerebral edema may occur. There is marked loss of protein from the blood into the alveoli, producing frothy foam in the lung.

(3) **Secondary drowning**: Secondary drowning may occur in as many as 25% of all cases of drawning. Consciousness is recovered after the initial episode, but increasing respiratory distress occurs hours or days later.

(4) **Immersion syndrome**: Sudden death occurs on immersion, usually in cold water.

The results of experimental work in animals may be misleading in the clinical management of humans. It is said that in sea water drowning (sea water is hypertonic relative to blood) intravascular water enters the alveoli. Sodium, magnesium, and chloride in the sea water enter the blood, and protein is rapidly transferred into the alveoli. Hemoconcentration occurs and there is an increasing load on the heart. Pulmonary edema occurs in 4–5 minutes. In the case of fresh water drowning, water is immediately absorbed into the circulation, resulting in hemodilution and hemolysis of red blood cells, with release of potassium. Circulatory failure and ventricular fibrillation occur.

In man, no significant evidence of electrolyte imbalance, hemodilution, or hemoconcentration occurs. Hemoglobinuria, hemoglobinemia, and renal complications have rarely been reported. Clinically, no difference is seen between fresh water and salt water drowning.

Clinical Findings

A. Symptoms and Signs: Near drowning causes variable degrees of unconsciousness, trismus, motor hyperactivity, convulsions, fear and headache, pyrexia, cyanosis, apnea or tachypnea, chest pain, and bronchospasm. Pink, frothy sputum from the nose and mouth is indicative of pulmonary edema. Cardiovascular manifestations include tachycardia, arrhythmias, cardiac arrest, and hypotension, with pallor and sweating. Vomiting may be a prominent symptom.

B. Laboratory Findings: Urinalysis shows acetonuria, proteinuria, and hemoglobinuria. Other laboratory findings include hemoglobinemia and leukocytosis, which may be as high as 40,000/cu mm. The blood volume is usually normal or low. Arterial oxygen tension is decreased. CO_2 tension is increased or decreased. A base deficit develops, indicating a metabolic acidosis.

C. X-Ray Findings: Pneumonitis or pulmonary edema may be observed on chest films.

Complications

The complications of near drowning include respiratory failure (pneumonitis and secondary infection), cardiac failure, and arrhythmias.

Treatment

It is important to consider drowning from the purely clinical point of view and not from the theoretical standpoint. The treatment is similar for both fresh and salt water drowning.

A. Emergency Treatment: Ventilation and an adequate circulation must be restored as soon as possible. Regardless of the patient's status after resuscitation, he should be admitted to the hospital. On the way to the hospital, the patient may require ventilatory and cardiac support and oxygen.

B. Hospital Treatment: If the patient is unconscious or semiconscious, an adequate airway should be established and aspiration prevented by intubating the patient and passing a nasogastric tube. The pulse, ECG, blood pressure, and temperature should be monitored. An accurate account of fluid intake and output should be made and the central venous pressure monitored as necessary.

If shock develops, volume expanders (plasma) should be used. Cerebral edema can be treated with osmotic diuretics (mannitol), corticosteroids, and hypothermia. If pulmonary involvement is obvious, serial blood gases are essential in management. If the arterial oxygen tension continues to fall despite increasing inspired oxygen concentration, assisted ventilation may be necessary.

Bronchospasm is treated with bronchodilators. Aspiration pneumonitis may be treated with postural drainage and steroids.

Prognosis

If the patient can be kept alive for 24 hours, there is a good chance he will make a complete recovery. If coma returns after initial resuscitation, the prognosis is poor.

Giammona ST: Drowning: Pathophysiology and management. Curr Probl Pediat 1:7, 1971.

Miles S: Drowning. Brit MJ 3:597, 1968.

Redding JS: Resuscitation and treatment following drowning. Pediatrics 37:666–668, 1966.

Rivers JF & others: Drowning: Its clinical sequelae and management. Brit MJ 2:157, 1970.

IRRADIATION REACTIONS

The effects of radiation may develop during or after the course of therapeutic x-ray or radium administration or after any exposure to ionizing radiation (eg, x-rays, neutrons, gamma rays, alpha or beta particles). The harmful effects of radiation are determined by the degree of exposure, which in turn depends not only upon the quantity of radiation delivered to the body but also the type of radiation, which tissues of the body are exposed, and the duration of exposure. Three hundred to 500 R (400–600 rads) of x-ray or gamma radiation applied to the entire body at one time would probably be fatal. (For purposes of comparison, a routine chest x-ray delivers about 0.3 R.) Tolerance to radiation is difficult to define, and there is no firm basis for evaluating radiation effects for all types and levels of irradiation.

ACUTE (IMMEDIATE) RADIATION EFFECTS ON NORMAL TISSUES

Diagnosis

A. Injury to Skin and Mucous Membranes: Irradiation causes erythema, depilation, destruction of fingernails, or epidermolysis, depending upon the dose.

B. Injury to Deep Structures:

1. Hematopoietic tissues—Injury to the bone marrow may cause diminished production of blood elements. Lymphocytes are most sensitive, polymorphonuclear leukocytes next most sensitive, and erythrocytes least sensitive. Damage to the blood-forming organs may vary from transient depression of one or more blood elements to complete destruction.

2. Blood vessels—Smaller vessels (the capillaries and arterioles) are more readily damaged than larger blood vessels. If injury is mild, recovery occurs.

3. Gonads—In males, small single doses of radiation (200–300 R) cause temporary aspermatogenesis and larger doses (600–800 R) may cause sterility. In females, single doses of 200 R may cause temporary cessation of menses and 500–800 R may cause permanent infertility. Moderate to heavy radiation of the embryo in utero results in injury to the fetus or to embryonic death and abortion.

4. Lungs—High or repeated moderate doses of radiation may cause pneumonitis.

5. Salivary glands—The salivary glands may be depressed by radiation, but relatively large doses may be required.

6. Stomach—Gastric secretion may be temporarily (occasionally permanently) inhibited by moderately high doses of radiation.

7. Intestines—Inflammation and ulceration may follow moderately large doses of radiation.

8. CNS—The brain and spinal cord may be damaged by high doses of radiation because of impaired blood supply.

9. Resistant Structures—The normal thyroid, pituitary, liver, pancreas, adrenals, and bladder are relatively resistant to radiation. Peripheral and autonomic nerves are highly resistant to radiation.

C. Systemic Reaction (Radiation Sickness): The basic mechanisms of radiation sickness are not known. Anorexia, nausea, vomiting, weakness, exhaustion, lassitude, and in some cases prostration may occur, singly or in combination. Radiation sickness associated with x-ray therapy is most likely to occur when the therapy is given in large dosage to large areas over the abdomen, less often when given over the thorax, and rarely when therapy is given over the extremities. With protracted therapy, this complication is rarely significant. The patient's emotional reaction to his illness or to the treatment plays an important role in aggravating or minimizing such effect.

Prevention

Persons handling radiation sources can minimize exposure to radiation by recognizing the importance of time, distance, and shielding. Areas housing x-ray and nuclear materials must be properly shielded. Untrained or poorly trained personnel should not be permitted to work with x-ray and nuclear radiation. Any unnecessary exposures, diagnostic or therapeutic, should be avoided. X-ray equipment should be periodically checked for reliability of output, and proper filters should be employed. When feasible, it is advisable to shield the gonads, especially of young persons. Fluoroscopic examination should be performed as rapidly as possible, using an optimal combination of beam characteristics and filtration; the tube-to-table distance should be at least 18 inches, and the beam size should be kept to a minimum required by the examination. Special protective clothing may be necessary to protect against contamination with radioisotopes. In the event of accidental contamination, removal of all clothing and vigorous bathing with soap and water should be followed by careful instrument (Geiger counter) check for localization of ionizing radiation.

Treatment

There is no specific treatment for the biologic effects of ionizing radiation. The success of treatment of local radiation effects will depend upon the extent, degree, and location of tissue injury. Treatment is supportive and symptomatic.

A systemic radiation reaction following radiation therapy (radiation sickness) is preferably prevented, but when it does occur it is treated symptomatically and supportively. The antinauseant drugs, eg, dimenhydrinate (Dramamine), 100 mg 1 hour before and 1 hour and 4 hours after radiation therapy, may be of value. Whole blood transfusions may be necessary if anemia is present. Transfusion of marrow cells has been employed recently. Disturbances of fluid or electrolyte balance require appropriate treatment. Antibiotics may be of use in the event of secondary infection.

DELAYED (CHRONIC) EFFECTS OF EXCESSIVE DOSES OF IONIZING RADIATION

Diagnosis

A. Somatic Effects:

1. Skin scarring, atrophy, and telangiectases, obliterative endarteritis, pulmonary fibrosis, intestinal stenosis, and other late effects may occur.

2. Cataracts may occur following irradiation of the lens.

3. Leukemia may occur, perhaps only in susceptible individuals, many years following radiation.

4. The incidence of neoplastic disease is increased in persons exposed to large amounts of radiation, particularly in areas of heavy damage.

5. Microcephaly and other congenital abnormalities may occur in children exposed in utero, especially if the fetus was exposed during the first 4 months of pregnancy.

B. Genetic Effects: Alteration of the sex ratio at birth (fewer males than females) suggests genetic damage. The incidence of congenital abnormalities, stillbirths, and neonatal deaths when conception occurs after termination of radiation exposure is apparently not increased.

Treatment

See treatment of acute radiation reactions.

BITES

ANIMAL BITES

Animal bites are important as potential sources of pyogenic and anaerobic infections. In these cases, wounds should be treated by conventional surgical cleansing and debridement as necessary. A special problem, present largely in the minds of parents, is the possibility of rabies. Even though only 1–2 cases of rabies occur each year in the USA, about 30,000 individuals receive antirabies treatment each year. The decision to use rabies vaccine or hyperimmune serum is a difficult one. These products have been associated with numerous side reactions, and some cases of disability and death have resulted from their use. For further discussion, see Chapter 26.

Treatment

Wash and irrigate animal bite wounds with soap and water and then with a quaternary ammonium solution, eg, Cetab. Bites should be debrided but not immediately sutured. Systemic broad spectrum antibiotics are indicated. If the patient has been immunized against tetanus, give a tetanus toxoid booster (0.5 ml subcut). If the child has not been immunized, give human tetanus immune globulin, 4 units/kg subcut.

Specific antirabies treatment should be given after careful individual consideration. See Chapter 26 for details.

Chambers GH & others: Treatment of dog-bite wounds. Minnesota Med 52:427–430, 1969.

Paton BC: Bites: Human, dog, spider, and snake. S Clin North America 43:537, 1963.

HUMAN BITES

Most human bites inflicted by children on playmates are superficial and require only local hygiene for prompt healing.

Deep bites extending below subcutaneous tissue levels should be treated vigorously since a wide variety of pathogenic organisms are present in the human mouth. Most are sensitive to penicillin G.

Swabbings should be collected for culture.

Treatment

A. Local Measures:

1. Cleanse the wound with soap and water and irrigate vigorously. For deep wounds, force large quantities of sterile water into the wound with a syringe.

2. Surgically debride the wound as indicated.

3. Do not suture skin over a bite wound.

B. Specific Measures for Deep Wounds: Give full doses of broad spectrum antibiotics. Combinations of penicillin, kanamycin, and colistin provide a wide coverage for most organisms. After the results of cultures have been received, specific antibiotic therapy can be instituted.

Paton BC: Bites: Human, dog, spider, and snake. S Clin North America 43:537, 1963.

•   •   •

General References

Abramson H (editor): *Resuscitation of the Newborn Infant and Related Emergency Procedures: Principles and Practice,* 2nd ed. Mosby, 1966.

Gans SL (editor): Symposium on surgical pediatrics. P Clin North America 16:529–669, 1969.

Hill LF (editor): Symposium on medical emergencies. P Clin North America 9:1–309, 1962.

Varga C & others: *Handbook of Pediatric Medical Emergencies,* 4th ed. Mosby, 1968.

31 . . .

Poisoning

John E. Ott, MD

Poisonings, the fourth most common cause of death in children, are the result of a complex interaction of the agent, the child, and family environment. Most victims are between 18 and 24 months of age. Accidents occur most frequently in children under 5 years of age as a result of insecure storage of drugs, household chemicals, etc. Repeated poisonings are more likely to occur in a family under emotional stress. Older children and adolescents often become poisoned while experimenting with drugs or while attempting suicide or making suicidal gestures.

The best treatment for poisoning is prevention. Parents must be taught to identify potentially toxic household items and store them safely. Children should be taught not to taste unfamiliar substances unless they are provided by a responsible adult. Flavored medicines should not be called candy; dangerous drugs should not be flavored; and taking medicine should not be made a game. One ounce of ipecac syrup should be presented by the pediatrician to each family with young children with instructions to keep it in the medicine chest for emergencies. In case of poisoning, parents should call their family doctor, local poison control center, or the emergency department of the nearest hospital for instructions before giving ipecac.

Physicians can also decrease the number of serious poisonings by labeling all prescriptions and requesting that potentially dangerous drugs be dispensed in strip packs or Palm-N-Turn safety containers. The routine use of safety containers could decrease the accidental drug poisoning rate by over 80%. Although dispensing prescriptions in safety containers is the most important step in reducing the number of accidental ingestions, fewer than 1% of prescriptions are being dispensed in this manner.

The following suggestions will significantly decrease the number of accidental ingestions:

(1) Keep medicines and poisons in locked cabinets, separate from foodstuffs.

(2) All poison containers should be properly labeled and read before using.

(3) Do not transfer poisons from their original containers to drinking glasses or soft drink bottles.

(4) Unused medications and poisons should be discarded by flushing down a toilet. (Clean out the medicine cabinet annually.)

(5) Household chemicals such as polishes, kerosene, and lye should not be stored under the sink or in other accessible places.

(6) Household chemicals in aerosol spray cans or bottles with very small openings are less toxic because less of the chemical is likely to be accidentally ingested.

(7) Poisonous ornamental plants should be kept out of the home.

Treatment of Acute Poisoning

The treatment of acute poisoning may be divided into 3 stages: emergency care, evaluation of the patient, and definitive care.

A. Emergency Care: The physician usually first hears of a poisoning by a telephone call from a distraught mother. He must determine quickly whether or not the child's life is in imminent danger by ascertaining the presence of shock, respiratory arrest, cardiac failure, seizures, or severe bleeding. Telephone numbers of the fire and rescue squad and ambulance service should be immediately available so that, if the patient's life is in danger or the mother's hysteria makes evaluation impossible, emergency personnel rather than the mother can bring the child to the office or hospital. Mothers often are not calm enough or knowledgeable enough to render necessary first aid. For greater details on emergency treatment, see below.

B. Initial Evaluation of the Patient: If the patient's life is not in immediate danger, the following information should be obtained:

(1) Name, address, and telephone number.

(2) Age and weight of the child.

(3) Name of the suspected poison. (If the product is not labeled, find out the name of the manufacturer, pharmacist, etc.)

(4) Estimate the amount ingested and the interval between probable ingestion and discovery.

Since most childhood poisonings are acute and self-limited, this information will usually provide a basis for treatment or reassurance. If there is no contraindication to emetic therapy (eg, ingestion of a caustic agent or hydrocarbon), syrup of ipecac, 15−20 ml, should be given, followed by 2 or 3 glasses of water. Ipecac should be administered even though several hours have elapsed since ingestion, especially if tablets have been taken, because many drugs delay gastric emptying time. Ipecac is more effective if the patient remains ambulatory. If the first dose is ineffective, it may be repeated once. Given this way, ipecac produces vomiting 97% of the time. If ipecac is not available, the flat handle of a spoon can be used to produce gagging by touching the posterior pharynx. However, most traditional methods of inducing vomiting are ineffective.

All suspected products or drugs should be brought to the hospital or office with the patient. Collecting vomitus in a plastic bag may help with precise diagnosis. While the patient is being transported to the physician, he can contact the poison control center for further information. The telephone number of the nearest poison control center can be obtained from the local medical society and should be kept on file. If the local poison control center does not provide 24-hour service, the following regional centers may be contacted:

Athens, Georgia	404-543-4311, Ext 223
	(Night: 543–5304)
Chicago	312-738-4411, Ext 2267
Denver	303-758-0430
Kansas City	816-471-5250, Ext 213
	(Night: Ext 220)
Los Angeles	213-664-2121
Memphis	901-525-6541, Ext 281
	(Night: Ext 241)
New Orleans	504-899-3409
New York	212-340-4495
San Francisco	415-221-1200, Ext 764

Toxic ingredients in commercial products should be listed on the label. If ingredients are not listed, call the manufacturer collect. For information about a drug, call the office of the pharmaceutical company's medical director collect. Medications can frequently be identified by comparing their shape, color, and identifying markings with the product identification section in *Physicians' Desk Reference.*

Selected toxicology references should be available in every physician's office. (See list at end of this chapter.)

C. Definitive Care: Patients who have ingested a single drug will usually present with typical physical findings. Paradoxical responses occasionally occur **which** confuse clinical evaluation. When multiple drugs with different actions are taken, a clinical diagnosis may be impossible. Initial clinical evaluation of the patient should emphasize the circulatory, respiratory, and central nervous symptoms. Arousable patients with intact reflexes are likely to recover rapidly. More deeply comatose patients should be admitted to an intensive care unit.

State of Activity

The severity of hyperactivity, restlessness, seizures, and psychosis seen in some poisoned patients can be evaluated by using the hyperactivity scale shown in Table 31–1.

The degree of coma in an unconscious patient can be estimated by using the scale shown in Table 31–2.

Emergency Treatment

The combined use of specific therapeutic procedures in addition to meticulous conservative manage-

TABLE 31–1. Clinical classification of hyperactivity.

Symptoms	Severity
Restlessness, irritability, insomnia, tremor, hyperreflexia, sweating, flushing	+
Hyperactivity, confusion, hypertension, tachypnea, tachycardia, mild fever, sweating	++
Delirium, mania, self-injury, marked hypertension, tachycardia, arrhythmia, hyperpyrexia	+++
Above plus: Convulsions and coma, circulatory collapse, and death	++++

ment of the poisoned patient should result in a 98% survival rate. Particular attention must be focused on measures that will prevent the 3 most common causes of death: aspiration, hypoxia, and cerebral edema.

The 2 major goals in treating an acutely poisoned patient are to maintain vital functions and eliminate the toxin.

A. Respiratory Care: Failure to maintain adequate air exchange is the most common cause of death in poisoning. An adequate airway must be established after debris has been removed from the mouth. An oral airway is not adequate. If there is respiratory failure or difficulty in aspirating bronchial secretions, an endotracheal tube should be inserted. A nasogastric tube with suction should be used in a comatose patient after an endotracheal tube is inserted.

B. Induced Vomiting: Induced vomiting is more efficient than gastric lavage. Give syrup of ipecac unless contraindicated by the presence of coma, seizures, or the ingestion of caustics. There are conflicting opinions regarding the use of syrup of ipecac in hydrocarbon ingestion, but it is probably justified in cases of high exposure. (*Caution:* Fluidextract of ipecac should never be used to induce vomiting.)

Apomorphine may be utilized to induce vomiting, but only by physicians acquainted with its pharmacology since it may produce respiratory and cardiac depression, especially in small children. Give 0.06

TABLE 31–2. Clinical classification of coma.

Symptoms	Class
Asleep, but can be aroused and can answer questions.	0
Comatose, does not withdraw from painful stimuli, reflexes intact.	1
Comatose, does not withdraw from painful stimuli, no respiratory or circulatory depression, most reflexes intact.	2
Comatose, most or all reflexes absent but without depression of respiration or circulation.	3
Comatose, reflexes absent, respiratory depression with cyanosis, and circulatory failure or shock (or both).	4

mg/kg IM and follow with nalorphine (Nalline), 0.15 mg/kg IV, within 10 minutes to counteract respiratory depression. Vomiting will occur within minutes. Apomorphine must be stored in a dark, tightly stoppered bottle and should be checked for discoloration every 3–4 weeks.

C. Gastric Lavage: Gastric lavage should be limited to situations in which emetic therapy is contraindicated. If the patient is comatose or has a depressed gag reflex, a cuffed nasotracheal or oral endotracheal tube must be inserted. The patient should be lying head down on his left side. A large-bore nasogastric tube is inserted. Lavage is continued until the return fluid is clear. Aspiration of stomach contents must be prevented, or aspiration pneumonia will result. If aspiration pneumonia develops, treatment with antibiotics and corticosteroids is probably worthwhile. Early bronchoscopy may be required to assure a clear airway.

D. Charcoal: The use of activated charcoal is commonly neglected, but it is very useful, especially when treating ingestions of multiple medications. Activated charcoal must be stored in a tightly sealed container to maintain its potency. Charcoal adsorbs the following compounds particularly well: atropine, barbiturates, chloroquine, chlorpromazine (Thorazine), mercurials, phenol, propoxyphene hydrochloride (Darvon), salicylates, sulfonamides, and strychnine. It is not useful in the treatment of poisoning with alcohols, cyanide, strong acids or bases, and most pesticides. "Universal antidote," consisting of burnt toast, tannic acid, and magnesium oxide, is worthless.

A charcoal slurry is made by adding 1 rounded tsp of charcoal to 2 oz of water. The amount of charcoal used should be 5–10 times the estimated weight of drugs ingested. It can be used prior to apomorphine or gastric lavage but should not be used with ipecac since ipecac is efficiently adsorbed by charcoal.

E. Cathartics: Cathartics may reduce the gastrointestinal tract absorption of toxins, especially if sustained-release preparations have been ingested. Saline cathartics should be used because they are fast, predictable in their action, and have a relatively short duration of action. Fleet's Phospho-Soda, 15–30 ml diluted 1:4, or sodium sulfate, 150–200 mg/kg diluted 1:2, or magnesium sulfate (Epsom salts), 250 mg/kg/dose, will usually be sufficient.

F. Analeptics: Analeptic drugs such as doxapram (Dopram), ethamivan (Emivan), amphetamines, pentylenetetrazol (Metrazol), and methylphenidate (Ritalin) are contraindicated as they increase rather than decrease mortality rates. Analeptic drugs can cause adverse effects such as nausea, vomiting, laryngospasm, hypertension, hyperpyrexia, arrhythmia, and convulsions which formerly were attributed to the original toxic agent.

G. Clearing Noxious Gases: Blood or tissue levels of toxic gases usually fall rapidly when the patient is removed from a contaminated atmosphere. Oxygen therapy and suctioning are usually the only measures necessary. Bronchospasm and bronchorrhea may be caused by caustic gases such as chlorine. Corticosteroid therapy, hydration, intermittent positive pressure breathing, and bronchidilators may be required.

H. Skin Decontamination: Skin decontamination is essential following exposure to substances that penetrate or burn the skin (eg, caustics, alkalies, acids, hydrocarbons, pesticides, and cyanides). Immediate thorough washing of the exposed area, including a shampoo and nail cleansing, with tincture of green soap and copious amounts of warm water is necessary. If tincture of green soap is not available and contamination with pesticides or hydrocarbons has occurred or is suspected, the skin should be cleaned with alcohol as well as with soap and water since hydrocarbons are more soluble in alcohol than in water. Care should be taken not to abrade the skin since this increases absorption. Vinegar, lemon juice, and olive oil or other oily or greasy substances should not be used following contamination with any of these agents because they may interfere with the treatment of resulting burns.

I. Eye Decontamination: Substances accidentally splashed into the eye may be removed by copious irrigation with warm saline solution or water while the lids are held apart. Continue irrigation for at least 5 minutes if contact with an acid has occurred and for 20 minutes if contact with an alkali has occurred. Chemical antidotes should not be used. Topical anesthetics, miotics, and mydriatics should not be administered until an ophthalmologist has evaluated possible corneal damage.

J. Specific Antidotes: Some poisons described in more detail elsewhere in this chapter have relatively specific antidotes:

    Amphetamines: Chlorpromazine
    Belladonna alkaloids: Physostigmine
    Carbon monoxide: Oxygen
    Cyanide: Thiosulphate
    Heavy metals
        Arsenic: BAL
        Iron: Deferoxamine
        Lead: EDTA and BAL
        Mercury: BAL
    Narcotics: Nalorphine (Nalline) or naloxone (Narcan)
    Nitrites and nitrates: Methylene blue
    Phenothiazines: Diphenhydramine (Benadryl)
    Phosphate ester insecticides: Protopam (2-PAM) and atropine

Hospital Management

A. General: Over 98% of hospitalized poisoned patients can be treated effectively by means of conservative medical and nursing care. Meticulous attention must be paid to cardiorespiratory problems (airway obstruction, aspiration, and cardiac failure), correction of metabolic deficiencies (acid-base balance, electrolytes, hypoglycemia), and renal failure. The comatose patient should be turned regularly and given passive exercises. Since analeptics (see above) lower the seizure threshold and do not increase the drug's metabolism or excretion, they should not be used. If the vital functions can be stabilized, the body will gradually metabolize and excrete the offending substance until it falls below toxic levels.

B. Consultative Services: Consultative services are available from several sources. Toxicologists are sometimes available in medical examiners' offices. The local offices of the Department of Agriculture frequently have lists of commonly used products in a given area. A Physicians' Poison Consultation Service may be available at a nearby medical center. Consultation services for any critically ill patient may be arranged by calling the American Academy of Clinical Toxicology in Houston (713–524–7547). Rapid laboratory determinations are available 7 days a week from Poisonlab, 1469 South Holly Street, Denver 80222.

(Call 303-758-0430 to arrange air freight pick-up service.)

C. Special Procedures: Specialized treatments such as forced diuresis, hemodialysis, exchange transfusion, or peritoneal dialysis (Table 31–3) should be used in combination with conservative management, not in place of it. Meticulous conservative therapy at all stages of the illness coupled with specialized technics should markedly increase the likelihood of survival in even the most seriously poisoned patient.

1. Forced diuresis–(Table 31–3.) Forced diuresis is indicated in serious poisonings involving long-acting barbiturates, amphetamines, alcohols, salicylates, strychnine, isoniazid, bromides, and other drugs excreted primarily by the kidneys. Forcing diuresis means increasing the amounts of fluid and imposing an

---

TABLE 31–3. Drugs and toxic substances for which dialysis or forced diuresis is indicated, may be indicated, or is contraindicated.*

Immediate Dialysis Indicated Regardless of Clinical Condition	Potassium
Amanita phalloides (mushroom) ingestion	Quinidine
Antifreezes (glycol type)	Quinine·
Heavy metals in soluble compounds	Salicylates (in combination with forced alkaline
Heavy metals, after acute therapy with chelating	diuresis)
agents	Strychnine
Methanol	Thiocyanates
Dialysis Indicated on Basis of Condition of Patient	**Dialysis Not Indicated; Therapy Consists of Intensive Conservative Care**
Alcohols (other than methanol)	Antidepressants including tricyclic compounds
Ammonia	and MAO inhibitors
Amphetamines (forced acid diuresis is indicated)	Antihistamines
Anilines	Chlordiazepoxide (Librium)
Antibiotics	Propoxyphene (Darvon)
Barbiturates	Diazepam (Valium)
Boric acid	Digitalis and related drugs
Bromides	Diphenoxylate (Lomotil)
Calcium	Glutethimide (Doriden)†
Chloral hydrate	Hallucinogens
Diphenylhydantoin (Dilantin)	Heroin and other opiates‡
Ethchlorvynol (Placidyl)§	Methaqualone (Quaalude)
Fluorides	Methyprylon (Noludar)
Iodides	Oxazepam (Serax)
Isoniazid	Phenothiazines
Meprobamate (Equanil, Miltown)	Synthetic anticholinergics and belladonna com-
Paraldehyde	pounds**

*Authorities do not always agree on the drugs which can be dialyzed. For another opinion, consult Schreiner G: Dialysis of poisons and drugs: Annual review. Tr Am Soc Artific Int Organs 16:544–568, 1970.

†Hemodialysis for glutethimide (Doriden) intoxication has not been shown to reduce coma or other manifestations of toxicity to a significant degree. A recent review of cases in several hospitals suggests that patients who are dialyzed do no better than patients who are not dialyzed. Therefore, dialysis is probably not indicated in glutethimide intoxication.

‡These drugs are antagonized effectively by nalorphine (Nalline) or other narcotic antagonists. Although they are well cleared by hemodialysis, antagonists are the treatment of choice.

§Hemodialysis for this drug has not significantly reduced the morbidity or mortality. Although a significant quantity of drug is demonstrable in the dialysis fluid, this cannot be related to the clinical situation of the patient.

**Anticholinergic compounds produce a syndrome of central stimulation, confusion, and then coma combined with peripheral muscarinic signs. All of these may be reversed by administration of physostigmine salicylate, 1–2 mg IV every 1–2 hours as needed.

osmotic load that will increase the proximal tubular excretion of drugs. Sufficient fluids should be given to maintain a urine output of 5–7 liters/sq m/24 hours, or 2–4 times normal excretion. Fluid loading in small children can be followed most closely by the use of a sensitive bed scale. A 25% solution of mannitol (0.5 gm/kg) should be given IV every 4–6 hours or whenever the urine specific gravity falls below 1.025. Sodium bicarbonate may be used to alkalinize the urine in the diuresis of weakly acidic drugs such as phenobarbital or salicylates. Acidification of the urine by intravenous ascorbic acid or arginine monohydrochloride (Argivene), or with ammonium chloride orally or intravenously, is useful in treating poisoning due to basic drugs such as amphetamines or strychnine. Large fluid volumes may be sufficient to produce an acid urine in young people. Serum electrolytes must be evaluated frequently to avoid hyponatremia or hypokalemia, which are the most common complications of prolonged forced diuresis. Calcium and magnesium should also be monitored if the urine is alkalinized.

2. Peritoneal dialysis–(Table 31–3.) Although peritoneal dialysis is less efficient than hemodialysis, it is useful in small children when technical problems prevent hemodialysis. Peritoneal dialysis requires a minimum of equipment and can be used in the smallest hospitals. It is not useful for drugs which are highly tissue-bound, such as most antidepressants, tranquilizers, antihistamines, and hallucinogens.

Peritoneal dialysis fluid varies in osmolar concentration and potassium content. The precise composition of the fluid employed must be determined by the patient's electrolytes, acid-base balance, and blood gases. Five percent albumin added to the dialysis fluid will increase the clearance of highly protein-bound drugs.

3. Hemodialysis–(Table 31–3.) Indications for hemodialysis have become stricter in recent years. They include the following:

a. Poisons excreted primarily by the kidneys.

b. Stage 3 or 4 coma or hyperactivity caused by a dialyzable drug which cannot be treated by conservative means.

c. Hypotension threatening renal or hepatic function which cannot be corrected by adjusting circulating blood volume.

d. Apnea in a patient who cannot be adequately ventilated by a mechanical respirator.

e. Marked hyperosmolality which is not due to easily corrected fluid problems.

f. Severe acid-base disturbance requiring rapid correction and not responding to conventional therapy.

g. Severe electrolyte disturbance which cannot be readily corrected by conventional means.

h. Marked hypothermia or hyperthermia.

4. Exchange transfusion–Exchange transfusion has been used most often with small children who have ingested drugs which are highly protein-bound, remain in the circulation for a long time, or form toxic metabolites which accumulate in the blood. It is helpful in massive poisoning. Exchange transfusion can now be accomplished efficiently and safely in patients of any size and age by the use of the isovolumetric technic. Electrolytes, acid-base balance, and vital functions must be carefully monitored. All blood should be administered at body temperature to minimize heat loss. This complex procedure must be done by an experienced physician.

LABORATORY EVALUATIONS

Drug screening or quantitative determinations should be done by the laboratory to identify or confirm the presence of a toxin in seriously ill patients thought to have a toxicologic problem. As many biologic fluids as possible (preferably blood, urine, and gastric fluid) should be obtained so that the best specimen will be available for a given determination. For most studies, blood should be collected in a heparinized fluoride or oxalated tube. If the laboratory determinations cannot be done promptly, it is usually best to refrigerate (not freeze) the specimens until they can be sent to the laboratory. It is better to prepare the specimens and then not do the analysis than to wish in retrospect that appropriate specimens had been obtained.

Any history or physical findings which suggest or rule out certain drugs or groups of drugs should be relayed to the laboratory so that the analyst can organize his sequence of procedures to confirm or disprove this information in the shortest possible time.

If there is no clue to the drug or drugs ingested, it may be useful to request a screening test based on the predominating clinical findings such as a coma, heavy metal, drug of abuse, or narcotics screen. The laboratory can then use a variety of methods, such as thin-layer chromatography and gas-liquid chromatography, which will identify a number of causes of poisoning in that group. The exact procedures and therefore the drugs identified can be varied somewhat depending upon the drugs which are the most common toxins at a specific time.

The following lists include drugs which are commonly identified in screening tests.

(1) Coma screen: Alcohols, barbiturates, glutethimide (Doriden), meprobamate (Miltown, Equanil), methyprylon (Noludar), chlordiazepoxide (Librium), diazepam (Valium), promazine (Sparine), chlorpromazine (Thorazine), trifluoperazine (Stelazine), morphine, codeine, methadone, propoxyphine (Darvon), imipramine (Tofranil), paracetamol, phenactin, salicylates, chlorinated hydrocarbons. **Blood and urine required**: Flurazepam (Dalmane), methaqualone (Quaalude), oxazepam (Serax), chloral hydrate, ethchlorvynol (Placidyl), belladonna alkaloids.

(2) Narcotics screen: Heroin, morphine, meperidine, codeine, propoxyphene (Darvon), oxymorphone (Numorphan), etc can be identified in urine.

(3) Heavy metal screen: Lead, arsenic, mercury, bismuth, antimony, selenium, silver, and tellurium. (Blood and urine are required and should be collected in acid-washed containers.)

(4) Drugs of abuse: Amphetamines, mescaline, narcotics, belladonna alkaloids, and cocaine can be identified in urine. Tranquilizers, antidepressants, and sedatives can usually be identified in urine or blood. Marihuana, LSD, and related compounds cannot be identified in biologic fluids but can be isolated from the raw material if it is available.

The information from screening procedures is often qualitative or semiquantitative in nature. Naturally occurring substances in the body occasionally mimic the behavior of drugs in the analytical procedures used. If the laboratory findings do not correlate well with the clinical findings, a definitive procedure such as quantitative specific drug determinations, mass spectrophotometry, or infrared spectrophotometry should be used to identify the substance in question. A negative drug screen does not necessarily mean the patient did not take a drug in this group. The biologic fluid examined may not have been appropriate; some drugs can be identified in urine but not blood, and vice versa. The test may not have been sensitive enough to identify small amounts of the drug, or the drug ingested may be a less frequently used one which is not identified by the analytical procedures used.

Intelligent use of the toxicology laboratory can be quite rewarding, but it is unreasonable to ask the analyst to identify a drug without giving him any clues to what drugs are to be considered. In many instances qualitative determinations will be sufficient; in others, specific quantitative drug determinations will be necessary. The analyst and clinical toxicologist, functioning as consultants, can help the physician make the best possible use of the laboratory. The laboratory results must always be considered in relation to the clinical findings in a given patient.

Arena JM: *Poisoning: Diagnosis–Symptoms–Treatment,* 2nd ed. Thomas, 1970.

Dreisbach RH: *Handbook of Poisoning: Diagnosis & Treatment,* 7th ed. Lange, 1971.

Gleason MN, Gosselin RE, Hodge HC: *Clinical Toxicology of Commercial Products,* 3rd ed. Williams & Wilkins, 1969.

Goodman LS, Gilman A: *The Pharmacological Basis of Therapeutics,* 4th ed. Macmillan, 1970.

Maher JF, Schreiner G: The dialysis of poison and drugs. Tr Am Soc Artific Int Organs 14:440–453, 1968.

Matthew H, Lawson AA: *Treatment of Common Acute Poisonings,* 2nd ed. Livingstone, 1970.

Poisoning in children. P Clin North America 17:471–754, 1970.

Stracener CE, Scherz RG, Crone RI: Results of testing a child-resistant medicine container. Pediatrics 40:286–288, 1967.

Teitelbaum DT: Initial management of poisoning. Emergency Med 2:32, 1970.

Thienes CH, Haley TJ: *Clinical Toxicology,* 5th ed. Lea & Febiger, 1971.

MANAGEMENT OF SPECIFIC COMMON POISONS

Unless otherwise directed, syrup of ipecac or apomorphine should be given to all conscious patients poisoned by the substances listed in the following section. Gastric lavage is usually indicated for comatose patients after an endotracheal tube is inserted.

ACIDS
(Hydrochloric, Nitric, & Sulfuric Acids)

Strong acids are commonly found in metal and toilet bowl cleaners, batteries, etc. Sulfuric acid is the most toxic and hydrochloric acid is the least toxic of these 3 substances. However, even a few drops can be fatal if aspirated into the trachea.

Painful swallowing, mucous membrane burns, bloody emesis, abdominal pain, respiratory distress due to edema of the epiglottis, thirst, shock, and renal failure can occur. Coma and convulsions sometimes are seen terminally. Residual lesions include esophageal, gastric, and pyloric strictures as well as scars of the cornea, skin, and oropharynx.

Treatment

Emetics and lavage are contraindicated. Water or milk is the ideal substance to dilute the ingestant because a heat-producing chemical reaction does not occur. Alkalies should not be used. The use of gas-forming carbonates is contraindicated since they increase the likelihood of perforating an already weakened stomach wall. Burned areas of the skin, mucous membranes, or eyes should be washed with copious amounts of warm water. Olive oil should not be applied to denuded areas unless the surgeon concurs. Opiates for pain and antibiotics may be needed. Treatment of shock is often necessary. An endotracheal tube may be required to alleviate laryngeal edema. Esophagoscopy should be performed promptly. If this procedure is not done, it must be assumed that the patient has esophageal burns. Corticosteroids in high doses (eg, prednisone, 2 mg/kg/24 hours orally) should be given for 3 weeks if there is evidence of esophageal burns. Surgical repair of a gastric perforation may be necessary.

Cameron JL: Aspiration pneumonia: Results of treatment by positive-pressure ventilation in dogs. J Surg Res 8:447–457, 1968.

Cho KJ: Management of acid intoxication. J Laryng 81:533–549, 1967.

ALCOHOL, ETHYL
(Ethanol)

Alcoholic beverages, tinctures, cosmetics, and rubbing alcohol are commonly overlooked causes of poisoning in children. Concomitant use of other depressant drugs increases the seriousness of the intoxication. Barbiturates decrease the rate of metabolism by alcohol dehydrogenase. Symptoms correlate well with blood levels, though the clinical effects are more pronounced when concentrations are rising than when they are falling. A potentially lethal dose in small children is approximately 3 mg/kg. (Blood levels cited are for adults; comparable figures for children are not available. In most states, alcohol levels of 50–80 mg/100 ml are considered compatible with impaired faculties, and levels of 80–150 mg/100 ml are considered evidence of intoxication.)

50–150 mg/100 ml: Incoordination, slow reaction time, and blurred vision.

150–300 mg/100 ml: Visual impairment, staggering, and slurred speech. Marked hypoglycemia may be present. (Legal intoxication in some jurisdictions. In others it is much lower.)

300–500 mg/100 ml: Marked incoordination, stupor, hypoglycemia, and convulsions.

> 500 mg/100 ml: Coma and death.

The urinary alcohol level is approximately 130% of the blood level. Complete absorption of alcohol by the stomach and small bowel requires 30 minutes to 6 hours depending upon the volume, the presence of food, the time spent in consuming the alcohol, etc. The rate of metabolic degradation is constant (about 20 ml of 100 proof alcohol per hour in an adult). Less than 10% is excreted in the urine.

Treatment

Supportive treatment, including aggressive management of hypoglycemia and acidosis, are usually the only measures required. Glucagon does not correct the hypoglycemia because hepatic glycogen stores are reduced. If the patient is conscious, vomiting should be induced with syrup of ipecac. Apomorphine should not be used without nalorphine (Nalline) or other narcotic antagonists because it is also a respiratory depressant. Although forced diuresis will increase the clearance rate of ethanol somewhat, it is not usually indicated as it increases the likelihood of cerebral edema. If a short-acting diuretic is used, ethacrynic acid (Edecrin) should probably not be used since it is thought to inhibit alcohol dehydrogenase. Monitoring of blood gases and oxygen administration are indicated in serious overdoses because death is usually caused by respiratory failure. Cerebral edema should be treated prophylactically with dexamethasone, 0.1 mg/kg IV or IM every 4–6 hours. Peritoneal dialysis and hemodialysis are indicated in life-threatening ethanol intoxication.

Beard JD: Fluid and electrolyte abnormalities in alcoholism. Psychosomatics 11:502–503, 1970.

Mendelson JH: Effects of alcohol on the central nervous system. New England J Med 284:104–105, 1971.

Nichols MM: Acute alcohol withdrawal syndrome in a newborn. Am J Dis Child 113:714–715, 1967.

ALCOHOL, METHYL
(Methanol)

Nausea, vomiting, muscle cramps and pain, and blurred vision may be present. Blindness may be partially reversible if treatment is given promptly. Toxic signs usually develop 8–36 hours after ingestion and are primarily related to (1) the severe metabolic acidosis caused by formic acid, (2) specific toxicity of these metabolites for retinal cells, and (3) CNS depression.

As little as 10 ml of methyl alcohol, a common constituent of paints, varnishes, paint removers, antifreeze, and Sterno, may be toxic in an adult. Methyl alcohol is commonly used to denature ethyl alcohol. The poisoning may be aggravated by absorption of methyl alcohol through the skin. The metabolic products formed in the conversion of methyl alcohol to formaldehyde and formic acid cause the toxic reactions. The rate of degradation of methyl alcohol is constant (less than 2 ml/hour). Laboratory analysis by gas-liquid chromatography is necessary to differentiate methanol from ethanol.

Treatment

Vomiting should be induced if the patient is conscious. Hemodialysis should be started as soon as the diagnosis is made—if the blood level of methanol exceeds 20 mg/100 ml, preferably before the onset of symptoms. If hemodialysis is not available, peritoneal dialysis and forced diuresis as well as bicarbonate and ethyl alcohol loading should be started. Ethyl alcohol, 100 proof, should be given every 4 hours IV in a dosage of 0.75 ml/kg because it competitively inhibits the oxidation of methyl alcohol, reducing methyl alcohol toxicity. The blood level of ethyl alcohol should be about 0.1%. Acidosis must be treated aggressively with sodium bicarbonate. Marked hypokalemia can occur. Folic acid may increase the biotransformation of methanol.

Kane RL & others: A methanol poisoning outbreak in Kentucky. Arch Envir Health 17:119–128, 1968.

AMINOPHYLLINE

Irritability, agitation, anxiety, tremors, delirium, coma, convulsions, nausea, vomiting, dehydration, shock, fever, respiratory distress, proteinuria, headache, vertigo, and vision disorders suggest aminophylline toxicity. Nausea and vomiting, the most constant sign, is due primarily to medullary stimulation. Severe dehydration may be associated with respiratory alkalosis. Early toxic signs are frequently attributed to the disease being treated rather than the aminophylline.

Although idiosyncratic reactions do occur, most intoxications are the result of overdosage. The dose should not exceed 3.5 mg/kg IV or IM, 5 mg/kg orally, or 7 mg/kg rectally, nor should a dose be given more often than every 6–12 hours. Peak drug levels occur within minutes following intramuscular or intravenous administration, within 1 hour after ingestion of uncoated tablets, and within 3–5 hours after rectal administration. Rectal absorption is unpredictable. Chronic administration of the drug and other bronchodilators increases the drug's effects. Concomitant antihistamine administration with aminophylline may increase the risk of seizures. Rapid intravenous administration of aminophylline may cause a cardiac arrhythmia and cardiovascular collapse. Warming the solution to body temperature may help prevent the arrhythmia.

Treatment

Induce emesis unless hyperreflexia is present. Oxygen and other antishock measures should be given as indicated. Anticonvulsants may be needed to control seizures. Fluid and electrolyte balance must be restored and maintained. Allopurinol (Zyloprim), 3–4 mg/kg orally 3 times daily, may be useful in the treatment of aminophylline intoxication since it is closely related structurally to xanthine and uric acid.

Dworetzky M: The dangers of therapeutic agents used in the treatment of asthma. South MJ 62:649–654, 1969.
Takaori M: Ventricular arrhythmias induced by aminophylline during halothane anaesthesia in dogs. Canad Anaesth Soc J 14:79, 1967.

AMPHETAMINES

Acute poisoning. Amphetamine poisoning is common because of the widespread availability of "diet pills" and the use of "speed" by adolescents. Symptoms include CNS stimulation, anxiety, hyperactivity, hyperpyrexia, hypertension, abdominal cramps, nausea and vomiting and inability to void urine. A toxic psychosis indistinguishable from paranoid schizophrenia may occur.

Chronic toxicity. Amphetamines are common causes of dependency and perhaps addiction. Chronic users develop such a high tolerance that more than 1500 mg of intravenous methamphetamine can be used daily. Hyperactivity, disorganization, and euphoria are followed by exhaustion, depression, and coma lasting 2–3 days. Upon awakening, the patient is ravenously hungry. Heavy users, taking more than 100 mg a day, have restlessness, incoordination of thought, insomnia, nervousness, irritability, and visual hallucinations. Psychosis may be precipitated when amphetamines are withdrawn. Depression, weakness, tremors, gastrointestinal complaints, and suicidal thoughts occur frequently.

Treatment

Because chlorpromazine (Thorazine) (0.5–1 mg/kg every 30 minutes as needed) brings about dramatic decreases in hyperactivity in intoxication, it should replace barbiturates in the management of intoxication with these drugs. When combinations of amphetamines and barbiturates (diet pills) are used, the action of the amphetamines begins first, followed by a rebound depression caused by the barbiturates. In these cases, particularly, treatment with additional barbiturates is contraindicated because of the risk of respiratory failure. Cathartics should be used to decrease the absorption of sustained-action medications. Amphetamines are excreted by the kidney most efficiently at an acid pH (4.5–5.5). Forced diuresis and mannitol may be sufficient to produce an acid urine. If necessary, mandelic acid or ammonium chloride can be used to acidify the urine. Vomiting should be induced. Peritoneal dialysis and hemodialysis are both effective in severe cases.

Chronic users may be withdrawn rapidly from amphetamines. If amphetamine-barbiturate or amphetamine-phenothiazine combination tablets have been used, the barbiturates or phenothiazines must be withdrawn gradually to prevent withdrawal seizures. Psychiatric treatment should be considered.

Espelin DE, Done AK: Amphetamine poisoning. New England J Med 278:1361–1365, 1968.

ANESTHETICS, LOCAL

Intoxication caused by local anesthetics may be associated with CNS stimulation, anxiety, delirium, shock, convulsions, and death. Some of the newer local anesthetics, such as prilocaine (Citanest), cause methemoglobinemia, which should be treated if levels in the blood exceed 40% or if blood levels are unavailable.

Accidental injection of mepivacaine (Carbocaine) into the unborn baby's head during caudal anesthesia has caused neonatal asphyxia, cyanosis, apnea, bradycardia, convulsions, and death.

Treatment

If ingested, activated charcoal should be followed by induced vomiting. Any contaminated mucous membranes should be carefully cleansed. Oxygen administration, with assisted ventilation if necessary, is indicated. Methemoglobinemia is treated with methylene blue, 1%, 0.2 ml/kg IV over 5–10 minutes; this should dramatically relieve the cyanosis. Exchange transfusion is indicated in a newborn with mepivacaine toxicity. Continuous gastric suctioning may also be of value.

Sinclair J: Intoxication of the fetus by a local anesthetic. New England J Med 273:1173–1177, 1965.

ANTIHISTAMINES

Although antihistamines typically cause CNS depression, children often react paradoxically with excitement, hallucinations, delirium, tremors, and convulsions followed by CNS depression, respiratory failure, or cardiovascular collapse. Anticholinergic effects, such as dry mouth, fixed dilated pupils, flushed face, and fever may be prominent.

Antihistamines are common causes of childhood poisonings because they are widely available in the home, in allergy, cold, and antiemetic preparations as well as in over-the-counter sedatives. Many antihistamines are supplied in enteric-coated or sustained-release forms, which increases the likelihood of dangerous overdoses. They are rapidly absorbed, and metabolized by the liver, lungs, and kidneys. A potentially fatal dose of most antihistamines is 25–50 mg/kg, or 20–30 tablets of the most commonly used antihistamines.

Treatment

Activated charcoal should be used to delay drug absorption. Emetics may be ineffective if the antihistamine is structurally related to phenothiazines. A saline cathartic is indicated for sustained-release preparations. Physostigmine, 0.5–3 mg IV, dramatically reverses the central and peripheral anticholinergic effects of antihistamines. Diazepam (Valium), 1–2 mg/kg IV, can be used to control seizures. Forced diuresis is not helpful. Exchange transfusion with 5% albumin should be considered in very severe intoxications, since most antihistamines are highly protein-bound and are concentrated in the serum.

Schipior PG: An unusual case of antihistamine intoxication. J Pediat 71:589–591, 1967.
Slovis TL & others: Physostigmine therapy in acute tricyclic antidepressant poisoning. Clin Toxicol 4:451–460, 1971.

ARSENIC

Acute poisoning. Abdominal pain, vomiting, watery and bloody diarrhea, cardiovascular collapse, paresthesias, difficulty in walking, and exfoliative dermatitis occur. Convulsions, coma, and anuria are later signs. Inhalation may cause pulmonary edema. Death is the result of cardiovascular collapse.

Chronic poisoning. Anorexia, generalized weakness, giddiness, colic, abdominal pain, polyneuritis, dermatitis, nail changes, alopecia, and anemia often develop.

Arsenic is commonly used in insecticides, rodenticides, weed killers, and wallpaper. It is well absorbed primarily through the gastrointestinal and respiratory tracts, but skin absorption may occur. Arsenic can be found in the urine, hair, and nails by laboratory testing. A potentially fatal dose of arsenic is 1–2 mg/kg.

Treatment

In acute poisoning, give dimercaprol (BAL), 2.5 mg/kg IM, immediately and follow with 2 mg/kg IM every 4 hours. After 4–8 injections, dimercaprol should be administered twice daily for 5–10 days. If possible, hemodialysis should be started as soon as dimercaprol is begun. The dimercaprol-arsenic complex is dialyzable.

Dimercaprol is not effective in the treatment of arsine gas intoxication, which should be treated by hemodialysis or exchange transfusion. Vomiting should always be induced.

Chronic arsenic intoxication should be treated by intermittent (5–10 day) courses of dimercaprol with measurement of urinary arsenic excretion between courses.

Lugo G, Cassady, G, Palmisano P: Acute maternal arsenic intoxication with neonatal death. Am J Dis Child 117:328–330, 1969.
Teitelbaum DT, Kier LC: Arsine poisoning. Arch Envir Health 19:133–143, 1969.

BARBITURATES

A patient who has ingested barbiturates in toxic amounts can present with a variety of findings including confusion, poor coordination, coma, miotic or fixed dilated pupils, increased or (more commonly) decreased respiratory effort, etc. Respiratory acidosis is commonly associated with pulmonary atelectasis, and hypotension frequently occurs in severely poisoned patients. Ingestion of more than 6 mg/kg of either long- or short-acting barbiturates is usually toxic; however, chronic users of barbiturates can tolerate levels up to 25 mg/100 ml.

Bullous lesions of the skin, which have been ascribed to barbiturates or glutethimide ingestion, may be seen in any patient in prolonged coma with respiratory depression and shock. They are the result of pressure and usually occur over bony prominences, suggesting that the patient has been deeply comatose for at least 12 hours.

Treatment

If the patient is awake, activated charcoal and induced vomiting is indicated. Careful conservative management with emphasis on maintaining a clear airway, adequate ventilation, and control of hypotension is critical in cases of coma due to barbiturate poisoning. Since phenobarbital is excreted unchanged by the kidney, forced alkaline diuresis is useful and often eliminates the need for dialysis. If the patient develops increasing respiratory acidosis after initial improvement during forced alkaline diuresis, pulmonary edema ("shock lung") is suggested and constitutes a probable indication for dialysis. If this or other clinical indications are present and the short-acting barbiturate level is higher than 3.5 mg/100 ml—or if the long-acting barbiturate (phenobarbital) level is higher than 8–9 mg/100 ml—hemodialysis or peritoneal dialysis should be done. Forced alkaline diuresis is not of significant help in the treatment of poisoning with short-acting barbiturates.

Analeptics are not helpful and actually increase morbidity and mortality rates.

Bloomer HA: A critical evaluation of diuresis in the treatment of barbiturate intoxication. J Lab Clin Med 67:898–905, 1966.
Hadden J & others: Acute barbiturate intoxication. JAMA 209:893–900, 1969.
Gröschel D, Gerstein A, Rosenbaum J: Skin lesions as a diagnostic aid in barbiturate poisoning. New England J Med 283:409–410, 1970.

BELLADONNA ALKALOIDS
(Atropine, Scopolamine, Stramonium, Asthmador, Jimsonweed, & Potato Leaves)

Patients with atropinism have been characterized as "red as a beet, dry as a bone, and mad as a hatter." Common complaints include dry mouth, thirst, decreased sweating associated with hot, dry, red skin, high fever, and tachycardia which may be preceded by bradycardia. The pupils are dilated and vision is blurred. Speech and swallowing may be impaired. Hallucinations, delirium, and coma are common. Leukocytosis may occur, confusing the diagnosis.

The onset of symptoms is quite rapid, but symptoms usually last only 3–4 hours unless large overdoses have been taken. Atropinism has been caused by normal doses of atropine or homatropine eyedrops, especially in children with Down's syndrome. Many common plants and over-the-counter sleeping medications contain belladonna alkaloids.

Treatment

Activated charcoal and cathartics are indicated. Vomiting should be induced with apomorphine, since syrup of ipecac is well adsorbed by charcoal. Physostigmine, 0.5–3 mg IV (repeated once or twice as needed), dramatically reverses the central and peripheral signs of atropinism. Neostigmine is ineffective because it does not enter the CNS. High fever must be

controlled. Catheterization may be needed if the patient cannot void. Short-acting barbiturates are preferable to sedation with phenothiazines because the latter may have a synergistic effect with belladonna alkaloids.

Bernstein S, Leff R: Toxic psychosis from sleeping medicine containing scopolamine. New England J Med 277:638–639, 1967.
Duvoisin RC, Katz R: Reversal of central anticholinergic syndrome in man by physostigmine. JAMA 206:1963–1966, 1968.

BORIC ACID

Boric acid is a worthless antiseptic which has been commonly used to treat diaper rash and burns. It is rapidly absorbed through broken skin and is potentially toxic to all organs, especially the CNS, kidneys, and pancreas. About 1/2 of the ingested dose will be excreted in the first 24 hours. The estimated lethal dose in children is 5–6 gm. The amount of boric acid present in baby powder is safe under normal conditions, but all other boric acid preparations should be removed from pediatric areas to minimize the possibility of ingestion.

Anorexia, weight loss, and mild diarrhea are the most common initial findings. Later, the "boiled lobster" skin, a characteristic erythematous exfoliating rash which desquamates in 1–2 days, is seen. Fever, vomiting, dehydration, anuria, and convulsions are commonly associated with the rash. CNS signs (irritability, high-pitched cry, exaggerated startle reflex, and opisthotonos) are common in children.

Treatment

Unless contraindicated, induced vomiting followed by catharsis should be used to remove ingested boric acid. If boric acid is being absorbed through the skin or mucous membranes, it should be removed with water and its use discontinued. Ten percent glucose in water given intravenously will induce diuresis. Anticonvulsants may be needed. Peritoneal dialysis and hemodialysis are more effective than exchange transfusion in severe boric acid poisoning.

Levin S: Diapers. South African MJ 44:256–263, 1970.
Skipworth GB: Boric acid intoxication from medicated talcum powder. Arch Dermat 95:83–88, 1967.

CARBON MONOXIDE

The degree of toxicity correlates well with the carboxyhemoglobin level. Symptoms are more severe if the patient has exercised, taken alcohol, or lives at a high altitude. Normal blood may contain up to 5% carboxyhemoglobin. The patient is often asymptomatic with levels up to 20%. Between 20–30%, nausea, vomiting, dizziness, decreased visual acuity, confusion, and headache develop. Over 50%, severe symptoms occur, including hallucinations, severe ataxia, respiratory collapse coma, thready pulse, and a pink discoloration of the skin. (This discoloration is not a regular or reliable sign. Many victims have pallor or cyanosis.) Death occurs rapidly if the carboxyhemoglobin level is more than 80%.

Proteinuria, glycosuria, elevated serum transaminase levels, or ECG changes (including S–T segment and T-wave abnormalities, atrial fibrillation, and interventricular block) may be present in the acute phase. Myocardial infarction most commonly occurs about a week after an acute serious exposure. Permanent cardiac, liver, renal, or CNS damage occasionally occurs. Even in extremely severe poisoning, CNS damage may be completely reversible, although months may be required for total recovery.

Treatment

Remove the patient from the contaminated area and administer oxygen. (Carboxyhemoglobin concentrations will drop 50% in 3–4 hours if the patient is exposed to air, or in 20–40 minutes if exposed to 100% oxygen.) The addition of CO_2 is more hazardous than beneficial. A hyperbaric chamber at 2–2.5 atmospheres of oxygen is the ideal treatment. Hypothermia appears to be a useful adjunct to therapy. Dexamethasone, 0.1 mg/kg IV or IM every 4–6 hours, should be started to combat cerebral edema. Although the mechanism of action is unknown, a slow continuous intravenous infusion of procaine is helpful in arousing the patient if he remains comatose after carboxyhemoglobin levels have returned to normal.

The patient should be closely observed for at least a week following a severe acute poisoning because myocardial infarction, pulmonary edema, and myoglobinuria may occur during convalescence.

Anderson TB: Natural gas: Unnatural causes. Lancet 1:466, 1970.

Garrel S & others: Neuro-psychiatric syndrome following carbon monoxide poisoning. Electroenceph Clin Neurophysiol 29:534, 1970.

Gore I: Treatment of carbon-monoxide poisoning. Lancet 1:468–469, 1970.

Lzdungham IM: Hyperbaric oxygen in shock. Internat Anesth Clin 7:819–839, 1969.

CAUSTICS
(Clorox, Purex, Sani-Clor, Drano, Liquid-Plumr, Clinitest Tablets)

Alkalies produce more severe injuries than acids do. Some substances, such as Clinitest Tablets or Drano, are quite toxic, while the chlorinated bleaches (3–6% solutions of sodium hypochlorite) are not as toxic as formerly thought. When sodium hypochlorite comes in contact with the acid pH of the stomach, hypochlorous acid, which is very irritating to the mucous membrane and skin, is formed. However, the rapid inactivation of this substance prevents systemic toxicity from developing. If a chlorinated bleach is mixed with a strong acid such as a toilet bowl cleaner, chloramine, which is extremely irritating to the eyes and respiratory tract, is produced.

Alkalies can cause burns of the skin, mucous membranes, and eyes. Respiratory distress may be due to edema of the epiglottis, pulmonary edema resulting from inhalation of fumes, or pneumonia. Mediastinitis or other intercurrent infections or shock can occur. Perforation of the esophagus or stomach is rare.

Treatment

The skin and mucous membranes should be cleansed with copious amounts of water. A local anesthetic can be instilled in the eye if necessary to alleviate blepharospasm. The eye should be irrigated for at least 20–30 minutes. Ingestions should be treated with sodium thiosulfate (5–10 gm orally in 200 ml of water), which rapidly reduces the hypochlorite ion to a nontoxic substance. However, 300–500 ml of water is also effective. Routine esophagoscopy is no longer indicated to rule out burns of the esophagus due to chlorinated bleaches unless an unusually large amount has been ingested; however, it is indicated if the patient continues to complain of dysphagia or pain. The absence of oral lesions does not rule out the possibility of oropharyngeal burns. A 3-week course of corticosteroids in high doses (prednisone, 2 mg/kg/24 hours orally) is indicated for the treatment of esophageal burns. Bougienage is not used as often as previously but may be helpful in selected cases. Antibiotics may be needed.

Egan RS: Corrosive esophagitis: A review of therapy. Northwest Med 68:1007–1009, 1969.

Kinnman JE: Management of severe lye corrosions of the esophagus. J Laryng 83:899–910, 1969.

Leape L & others: Hazard to health: Liquid lye. New England J Med 284:578–581, 1971.

Yarlongton C: The experimental causticity of sodium hypochlorite in the esophagus. Ann Otol Rhin Laryng 79:895–899, 1970.

CONTRACEPTIVE PILLS

The only known toxic effects following acute ingestion of oral contraceptive agents are nausea, vomiting, and vaginal bleeding in girls.

COSMETICS & RELATED PRODUCTS

The relative toxicities of commonly ingested products in this group are listed in Table 31–4.

Permanent wave neutralizers may contain bromates, peroxides, or perborates. Bromates have been removed from most products because they can cause nausea, vomiting, abdominal pain, methemoglobinemia, shock, hemolysis, renal failure, and convulsions. Four gm of bromate salts are potentially lethal. Poisoning is treated by induced emesis or gastric lavage with 1% sodium thiosulfate followed by demulcents to relieve gastric irritation. Sodium thiosulfate, 1%, 100–500 ml, can be given IV, but methylene blue should not be used to treat methemoglobinemia in this situation because it increases the toxicity of bromates. Dialysis is indicated in severe bromate poisoning. Perborate can cause boric acid poisoning.

Finergnail polish removers usually contain toluene or aliphatic acetates which produce CNS irritation and depression. Treatment is supportive.

Cobalt, copper, cadmium, iron, lead, nickel, silver, bismuth, and tin are sometimes found in metallic hair dyes. In large amounts, they can cause skin sensitization, urticaria, dermatitis, eye damage, vertigo, hypertension, asthma, methemoglobinemia, tremors, convulsions, and coma. Treatment for ingestions is to administer demulcents and the appropriate antidote for the heavy metal involved.

Home permanent wave lotions, hair straighteners, and hair removers usually contain thioglycollic acid salts which cause irritation and perhaps hypoglycemia.

Shaving lotion, hair tonic, hair straighteners, cologne, and toilet water contain denatured alcohol which can cause CNS depression and hypoglycemia.

Deodorants usually consist of an antibacterial agent in a cream base. Antiperspirants are aluminum salts which frequently cause skin sensitization. Zirconium oxide can cause granulomas in the axilla.

Chronic inhalation of hair sprays containing synthetic and natural resins has reportedly caused

TABLE 31–4. Relative toxicities of cosmetics and similar products.

High toxicity	Low toxicity
Permanent wave neutralizers	Perfume
Fingernail polish remover	Hair removers
	Deodorants
	Bath salts
Moderate toxicity	
Fingernail polish	**No toxicity**
Metallic hair dyes	Liquid make-up
Home permanent wave lotion	Vegetable hair dye
Bath oil	Cleansing cream
Shaving lotion	Hair dressing (non-alcoholic)
Hair tonic (alcoholic)	Hand lotion or cream
Cologne, toilet water	Lipstick

thesaurosis (hilar lymphadenopathy and diffuse pulmonary infiltration) as well as ocular irritation and keratitis.

Arena JM: Pages 422–427 in: *Poisoning: Toxicology–Symptoms–Treatments*, 2nd ed. Thomas, 1970.

COUGH MEDICATIONS

Cough mixtures often contain ephedrine-like compounds, antihistamines, and cough depressants such as codeine or dextromethorphan. The latter 2 can produce respiratory depression, excitement, coma, and seizures.

Nalorphine (Nalline) is a pharmacologic antagonist to codeine, but its value in dextromethorphan poisoning is not established. (See Antihistamines and Narcotics.)

Induce vomiting.

Bass M: Sudden sniffing death. JAMA 212:2075–2079, 1970.
Hanison AJ: A case history of drug addiction and a T.L.C. system for the separation and identification of some drugs of addiction in sub-microgram amounts. J Forensic Sc Soc 9:165–167, 1969.

CYANIDE

Cyanide poisoning may cause a bitter, burning taste with an odor of bitter almonds on the breath, salivation, nausea (usually without vomiting), anxiety, confusion, vertigo, giddiness, stiffness of the lower jaw, coma, convulsions, opisthotonos, paralysis, dilated pupils, cardiac irregularities, and transient respiratory stimulation followed by respiratory failure. A prolonged expiratory phase is characteristic.

Cyanide is commonly used in rodenticides, metal polishes (especially silver), electroplating, and photographic solutions as well as in fumigation products. Aqueous solutions are readily absorbed through the skin, mucous membranes, and lungs, but alkali salts are toxic only when ingested. Lethal doses vary greatly with the individual, but death has usually been associated with ingestion of 200–300 mg of the sodium or potassium salt, or blood cyanide levels of 0.26–3 mg/100 ml. Death usually occurs within minutes following inhalation and within an hour following ingestion.

Treatment

If the patient is apneic or has gasping respirations, artificial respiration must be started immediately. The patient should inhale amyl nitrite for 15–30 seconds of every minute while a sodium nitrite solution is being prepared for intravenous injection. Amyl nitrite alone is not adequate treatment because the maximum methemoglobin level obtainable in this way is about 5%. Cyanide kits (Lilly Stock No. M76) which contain instructions *(for use in adults)* should be carried in all emergency vehicles. Intravenous sodium nitrite is given first followed immediately by sodium thiosulfate. Adult doses are 10 ml of 3% sodium nitrite IV (2–5 ml/min), followed by 50 ml of 25% sodium thiosulfate IV at the same rate. The amount of sodium nitrite required to raise the methemoglobin level to the ideal level of 40% in a child with a hemoglobin of 12 gm/100 ml is approximately 15 mg/kg. It should be safe to administer 10 mg/kg of sodium nitrite while the hemoglobin is being determined. Children weighing more than 25 kg who are not anemic should receive adult doses of both sodium nitrite and sodium thiosulfate. If marked hypotension occurs during treatment, epinephrine or ephedrine can be given. Oxygen increases the effects of nitrites and thiosulfates but is not adequate treatment by itself. It should be continued after the thiosulfate is given because methemoglobinemia decreases the ability of blood to carry oxygen. Exchange transfusion or infusion of whole blood is indicated if methemoglobin levels rise over 50%.

Activated charcoal is not useful in cyanide poisoning, and lavage is not usually helpful because cyanide is absorbed very rapidly. Contaminated clothing must be removed and affected skin areas washed carefully with soap and water. As long as the heart is beating, prompt and vigorous treatment is likely to be successful.

The patient should be observed for 24–48 hours since evidence of toxicity may reappear. If a relapse occurs, the patient should be retreated using 1/2 of the above doses of sodium nitrite and sodium thiosulfate.

Bain JTB: Successful treatment of cyanide poisoning. Brit MJ 2:763, 1967.
Berlin C: The treatment of cyanide poisoning in children. Pediatrics 46:793–796, 1970.

DIGITALIS & OTHER CARDIAC GLYCOSIDES

Manifestations include nausea, vomiting, diarrhea, headache, delirium, confusion, and occasionally coma. Cardiac irregularities such as atrial fibrillation, paroxysmal atrial tachycardia, and atrial flutter often occur. Death usually is the result of ventricular fibrillation.

Toxic reactions occur with doses of digitoxin greater than 0.07 mg/kg. The long duration of action of digitoxin makes its use undesirable in children.

Transplacental intoxication by digitalis has been reported. An accurate radioimmune assay for digitalis is now available.

Treatment
Induce vomiting. Withdrawal of the digitalis and administration of potassium is the treatment of choice.

If renal function is adequate, up to 5 mEq/kg of potassium chloride may be given daily IV. Intravenous solutions containing more than 40 mEq/liter should be avoided. The patient must be monitored carefully for ECG evidence of hyperkalemia. The correction of acidosis will better demonstrate the degree of potassium deficiency present. In some cases, diphenylhydantoin (Dilantin), beta-adrenergic blocking agents such as propranolol (Inderal), or procainamide (Pronestyl) are necessary to correct arrhythmias. The intravenous administration of sodium or dipotassium (not calcium) edetate produces a hypocalcemia that rapidly counteracts the toxic symptoms of digitalis.

It has recently been noted that digitoxin has an enterohepatic circulation.

The use of oral binding agents such as cholestyramine resin (Cuemid, Questran) has been suggested in massive digitalis overdoses.

Dreifus LS & others: Current status of diphenylhydantoin. Am Heart J 80:709–713, 1970.
Selzer A, Cohn KE: Production, recognition, and treatment of digitalis intoxication. California Med 113:1–7, Oct 1970.

DIPHENOXYLATE HYDROCHLORIDE
(Lomotil)

Lomotil is a combination of diphenoxylate hydrochloride, a synthetic narcotic, and atropine sulfate. Early signs of Lomotil intoxication are due to its anticholinergic effect and consist of fever, facial flush, tachypnea, and lethargy. However, the miotic effect of the narcotic predominates. Later, hypothermia, increasing CNS depression, and loss of the facial flush occur. Seizures are probably secondary to hypoxia. Small amounts of Lomotil are potentially lethal when ingested by children, and the use of this drug in pediatrics should be discouraged.

Treatment
After an adequate airway has been established with an endotracheal tube, gastric lavage may be useful because of the prolonged delay in gastric emptying time. Narcotics are not adsorbed by activated charcoal, but atropine is. Nalorphine (Nalline), 0.1–0.2, mg/kg/dose IM or IV, or naloxone (Narcan), 0.01 mg/kg IV, should be given. A transient improvement in respiratory status may be followed by respiratory depression because the duration of action of diphenoxylate is considerably longer than that of the antagonists. The anticholinergic effects can be reversed temporarily by the use of physostigmine, 0.5–3 mg IV.

Ament ME: Diphenoxylate poisoning in children. J Pediat 74:462, 1969.

Bargman G: Near fatality in an infant following Lomotil poisoning. Pediatrics 44:770–771, 1969.

Ginsburg CM, Angle CR: Diphenoxylate-atropine (Lomotil) poisoning. Clin Toxicol 2:377–382, 1969.

DISINFECTANTS & DEODORIZERS

1. NAPHTHALENE

Naphthalene is commonly found in moth balls as well as in disinfectants and deodorizers commonly used in bathrooms, toilets, and garbage cans.

Naphthalene's toxicity is often not fully appreciated. It is absorbed not only when ingested but also through the skin and lungs. Naphthalene is very soluble in oil and relatively insoluble in water. It is potentially hazardous to store baby clothes in naphthalene because baby oil is an excellent solvent which increases absorption of the drug through the skin.

Metabolic products of naphthalene cause a severe hemolytic anemia similar to that due to primaquine toxicity 3–7 days after ingestion. Other physical findings include nausea, vomiting, diarrhea, jaundice, oliguria, anuria, coma, and convulsions. The urine may contain hemoglobin, protein, and casts.

Treatment

Induced vomiting should be followed by a saline cathartic. Forced alkaline diuresis prevents blocking of the renal tubules by acid hematin crystals. Repeated small blood transfusions may be necessary to bring the hemoglobin level up to 60–80% of normal. Corticosteroids are said to be useful in minimizing naphthalene hemolysis. Anuria may persist for 1–2 weeks and still be completely reversible.

2. *p*-DICHLOROBENZENE, SODIUM BISULFATE, & PHENOLIC ACIDS

Disinfectants and deodorizers containing *p*-dichlorobenzene or sodium bisulfate are much less toxic than those containing naphthalene. Disinfectants containing phenolic acids are highly toxic, especially if they contain a borate ion. Phenol precipitates proteins and causes respiratory alkalosis followed by metabolic acidosis. Some phenols cause methemoglobinemia.

Local gangrene occurs after prolonged contact with tissue. Phenol is readily absorbed from the gastrointestinal tract, causing diffuse capillary damage and, in some cases, methemoglobinemia. Pentachlorophenol, which has been used in terminal rinsing of diapers, has caused infant fatalities.

The toxicity of alkalies, quaternary ammonium compounds, pine oil, and halogenated disinfectants

varies with the concentration of active ingredients. Wick deodorizers are usually of moderate toxicity. Iodophor disinfectants are the safest. Spray deodorizers are not usually toxic because a child is not likely to swallow a very large dose.

Manifestations of acute ingestion include diaphoresis, thirst, nausea, vomiting, diarrhea, cyanosis, hyperactivity, coma, convulsions, hypotension, abdominal pain, and pulmonary edema. Acute liver or renal failure may develop later.

Treatment

Activated charcoal should be used prior to emesis or gastric lavage. Castor oil dissolves phenol and retards its absorption. Mineral oil and alcohol are contraindicated because they increase the gastric absorption of phenol. A saline cathartic should follow the castor oil. The metabolic acidosis must be carefully managed. Anticonvulsants or measures to treat shock may be needed.

Because phenols are absorbed through the skin, exposed areas should be irrigated copiously with water.

Arena J: Pages 144–145, 364–365 in: *Poisoning: Toxicity–Symptoms–Treatments,* 2nd ed. Thomas, 1970.

George JM & others: Heinz body hemolytic anemias. New York J Med 70:2574–2582, 1970.

GLUTETHIMIDE
(Doriden)

Although no clinical signs are specific for glutethimide poisoning, affected patients may have nystagmus, mydriasis, dry mouth, ileus, and CNS depression manifested by absent deep tendon reflexes, coma, and either hypothermia or hyperpyrexia. Respiratory depression with normal respiratory rates, sudden apnea, and alternating levels of consciousness occur. The anticholinergic effects of glutethimide often predominate in children.

There is a narrow range between therapeutic and toxic blood levels. Doses exceeding 25–50 mg/kg are toxic in children. Blood levels greater than 3 mg/100 ml are generally associated with coma and serious illness. Glutethimide levels usually fall at a rate of 1.5–2 mg/100 ml/day. As in any other sedative poisoning, coma often is prolonged and varies in depths from moment to moment, but patients usually awake when blood levels decline to 1.5 mg/100 ml.

Treatment

Meticulous conservative management is the most successful approach. Induced emesis with apomorphine is preferable to lavage in a conscious patient since glutethimide is very insoluble in water. Because glutethimide is well dissolved in castor oil, it should be used for gastric lavage. An endotracheal tube must be inserted before gastric lavage is undertaken. Glutethimide is well adsorbed by activated charcoal.

Forced diuresis, peritoneal dialysis, and hemodialysis (including lipid dialysis) have not been helpful in reducing the duration of coma, morbidity, or mortality rate, although enhanced excretion of inert metabolites of the drug has been demonstrated. Fluids should be used cautiously because there is an increased likelihood of pulmonary or cerebral edema.

Chazan JA, Garella S: Acute glutethimide intoxication: A prospective study of 70 cases treated without hemodialysis. Clin Toxicol. In press.

Comstock EG: Glutethimide intoxication. JAMA 215:1668, 1971.

Wright N, Roscoe P: Acute glutethimide poisoning: Conservative management of 31 patients. JAMA 214:1704–1706, 1970.

HYDROCARBONS
(Petroleum Distillates, Kerosene, Benzene, Charcoal Lighter Fluid, Gasoline, etc)

Ingestion causes irritation of mucous membranes, vomiting, blood-tinged diarrhea, respiratory distress, cyanosis, tachycardia, and fever. Although 10 ml are potentially fatal, patients have survived ingestion of several ounces of petroleum distillates. The more aromatic and the lower the viscosity rating of a hydrocarbon, the more toxic it is. Benzene, gasoline, kerosene, and red seal oil furniture polish are the most dangerous. A dose exceeding 1 ml/kg is likely to cause CNS depression. A history of coughing or choking, as well as vomiting, suggests aspiration with resulting hydrocarbon pneumonia, an acute hemorrhagic necrotizing disease which usually develops within 24 hours of the ingestion and resolves without sequelae in 3–5 days. However, several weeks may be required for resolution of a hydrocarbon pneumonia. Pneumonia may be caused by a few drops of petroleum distillate being aspirated into the lung or by absorption from the circulatory system. Pulmonary edema and hemorrhage, cardiac dilatation and arrhythmias, hepatosplenomegaly, proteinuria, and hematuria can occur following large overdoses. Hypoglycemia is occasionally present. A chest film may reveal pneumonia shortly after the ingestion. An abnormal urinalysis in a child with a previously normal urinary tract suggests a large overdose.

Treatment

Both emetics and lavage should be avoided if only a small amount has been ingested. It is impossible to do a "cautious gastric lavage" unless a cuffed endotracheal tube is inserted. Under these circumstances, gastric lavage may be done using saline or 3% sodium bicarbonate solution. Following lavage, mineral oil and sodium sulfate should be left in the stomach. (Mineral oil itself is capable of causing a low-grade lipoid pneumonia.)

Emetics are probably preferable to gastric lavage if massive ingestion has occurred. Epinephrine should not be used since it may affect an already sensitized myocardium. Analeptic drugs are contraindicated. The usefulness of prophylactic antibiotics is debated. Corticosteroids (at least 100 mg or equivalent of cortisone) appear helpful in reducing pulmonary inflammation. Prophylactic use of corticosteroids for 48 hours is also advisable and will not affect the patient's endocrine status. Oxygen and mist are helpful.

Lazner J: Summer poison hazards for young children. MJ Australia 2:1098, 1970.

INSECTICIDES

Insecticides are common causes of poisoning. The petroleum distillates or other organic solvents used in these products are often as toxic as the pesticide. Unless otherwise indicated, induced vomiting or gastric lavage is warranted after insertion of an endotracheal tube.

DePalma AE, Kwalich DS, Zukerberg N: Pesticide poisoning in children. JAMA 211:1979–1981, 1970.

Hayes WJ: *Clinical Handbook on Economic Poisons*. US Department of Health, Education, and Welfare, 1963.

1. CHLORINATED HYDROCARBONS
(Aldrin, Carbinol, Chlordane, DDT, Dieldrin, Endrin, Heptachlor, Lindane, Toxaphene, Etc)

Common signs of intoxication include salivation, gastrointestinal irritability, abdominal pain, nausea, vomiting, diarrhea, CNS depression, and convulsions. Inhalation exposure causes irritation of the eyes, nose, and throat, blurred vision, cough, and pulmonary edema.

Chlorinated hydrocarbons are absorbed through the skin, respiratory tract, and gastrointestinal tract. These compounds or their metabolic products are chronically stored in fat. Decontamination of skin (tincture of green soap) and evacuation of the stomach contents are critical. All contaminated clothing should be removed. Castor oil, milk, and other substances containing fats or oils should not be left in the stomach as they increase absorption of the chlorinated hydrocarbons. Convulsions should be treated with sodium phenobarbital, 6 mg/kg IV, diazepam (Valium), 2 mg/kg IV, or paraldehyde, 0.15 ml/kg IM. Epinephrine should not be used as it may cause cardiac arrhythmias.

2. ORGANIC PHOSPHATE
(CHOLINESTERASE INHIBITING) INSECTICIDES
(Chlorthion, Co-Ral, DFP, Diazinon, Malathion, Para-oxon, Parathion, Phosdrin, TEPP, Thio-TEPP, Etc)

Dizziness, headache, blurred vision, miosis, tearing, salivation, nausea, vomiting, diarrhea, hypoglycemia, cyanosis, sense of constriction of the chest, dyspnea, sweating, weakness, muscular twitching, convulsions, loss of reflexes and sphincter control, and coma can occur.

The clinical findings are the result of cholinesterase inhibition, which causes an accumulation of large amounts of acetylcholine. Serum or red cell cholinesterase levels are helpful, especially if preexposure values are available. (Some normal individuals have a low cholinesterase level.) Normal values vary in different laboratories. A screening test apparatus for cholinesterase levels (Unopette #5820, Becton, Dickinson & Co, Rutherford, N.J. 07070) should be available in every hospital emergency room. In general, a decrease of 40% in red cell cholinesterase indicates significant exposure to organophosphate insecticides.

Repeated low-grade exposures may result in sudden, acute toxic reactions. This syndrome usually occurs after repeated household spraying rather than agricultural exposure.

Treatment

Atropine plus a cholinesterase reactivator, pralidoxime (Protopam), are chemical antidotes for organophosphate insecticide poisoning. After establishing a clear airway and eliminating any cyanosis, large doses of atropine should be given and repeated every few minutes until signs of atropinism are present. An appropriate starting dose of atropine in an adult is 2–4 mg IV (approximately 10 times the normal dose). As much as 50 mg per 24 hours of atropine may be needed in an adult.

Because atropine antagonizes the parasympathetic effects of the organophosphates but does not alter the muscular weakness, pralidoxime should also be given immediately in more severe cases and repeated every 8–12 hours as needed (1 gm IV for older children and 250 mg IV for infants at a rate of no more than 500 mg/minute). Pralidoxime should be used in addition to—not in place of—atropine; however, smaller doses of atropine will probably be needed if the 2 drugs are used concomitantly. Pralidoxime is probably not useful later than 36 hours after the exposure. Artificial ventilation equipment must be available and the heart should be monitored, since anticholinesterases may cause heart block. Morphine, theophylline, aminophylline, succinylcholine, and tranquilizers of the reserpine and phenothiazine types should be avoided.

Decontamination of the skin (including nails and hair) and clothing with tincture of green soap is extremely important. Decontamination of the skin must be done carefully to avoid abrasions which increase organophosphate absorption significantly.

Melby TH: Prevention and management of organophosphate poisoning. JAMA 216:2131–2133, 1971.

3. CARBAMATES
(Carbaryl, Sevin, Zectran, Etc)

Carbamate insecticides are reversible inhibitors of cholinesterase. The reversal is often so rapid that measurements of blood cholinesterases are near normal, whereas β-naphthol, a metabolite, is present in significant amounts. The signs and symptoms of intoxication are similar to those associated with organophosphate poisoning but are generally less severe. Atropine in large doses is sufficient treatment. Pralidoxime may be harmful because it causes such a rapid reversible inhibition of cholinesterase levels.

4. BOTANICAL INSECTICIDES
(Raid, Black Flag Bug Killer, Black Leaf CPR Insect Killer, Flit Aerosol House and Garden Insect Killer, French's Flea Powder, Etc)

Pyrethrins, allethrin, ryania, and rotenone do not commonly cause signs of toxicity. Antihistamines, short-acting barbiturates, and atropine are helpful when needed.

INSECT STINGS
(Bee, Wasp, & Hornet)

Insect stings are painful but not usually dangerous; however, these insects cause more deaths in the USA than snakes do. Deaths from insect stings are usually due to severe allergic reactions. Bee venom, for example, has hemolytic, neurotoxic, and histamine-like activities which can on rare occasions cause hemoglobinuria and severe anaphylactoid reactions. If possible, a tourniquet should be applied above the bite and the stinger removed, being careful not to squeeze the venom sac. Epinephrine, 0.01 ml/kg of 1:1000 solution, should be administered IV or subcut above the site of the sting. Three to 4 whiffs from an isoproterenol (Isuprel) aerosol inhaler may be given at 3–4 minute intervals as needed. Corticosteroids (hydrocortisone, 100 mg IV) or diphenhydramine (Benadryl), 1.5 mg/kg IV, are useful ancillary drugs but have no immediate effect. Ephedrine or antihistamines may be used for 2 or 3 days to prevent recurrence of symptoms.

A patient who has had a potentially life-threatening insect sting should be desensitized against the hymenoptera group since the honey bee, wasp, hornet, and yellow jacket have common antigens in their venom.

For the more usual stings, cold compresses, aspirin, and diphenhydramine (Benadryl), 1 mg/kg orally, are useful.

IRON

Four stages of intoxication occur following iron intoxication: (1) Hemorrhagic gastroenteritis, which usually occurs 30–60 minutes after ingestion and may be associated with shock, acidosis, coagulation defects, and coma. This phase usually lasts 4–6 hours and is commonly followed by a 6–24 hour asymptomatic period. (2) Delayed shock may occur 24–48 hours after ingestion and is usually associated with a serum iron level greater than 500 mg/100 ml. Metabolic acidosis, fever, leukocytosis, and coma may also be present. (3) Liver damage with hepatic failure. (4) Residual pyloric stenosis, which usually develops at least 4 weeks after the ingestion.

Ferrous sulfate is 20% elemental iron. The average lethal dose is about 200–250 mg of iron/kg but deaths in small children have been caused by as little as 600 mg of iron. Although the correlation between serum iron and clinical symptoms is not good, it appears that serum iron levels greater than the total serum iron-binding capacity (300–500 μg/100 ml) are necessary to produce severe symptoms.

Once iron is absorbed from the gastrointestinal tract, it is not normally eliminated in feces or urine. Iron found in feces represents iron that was unabsorbed. A reddish discoloration of the urine suggests a serum iron level greater than 350 μg/100 ml. Abdominal x-ray will show radiopaque tablets remaining in the gastrointestinal tract, but finely dispersed iron will often not be identified.

Treatment

Shock must be treated in the usual manner. After inducing vomiting, leave sodium bicarbonate or Fleet's Phospho-Soda (15–30 ml diluted 1:2 with water) in the stomach to decrease iron absorption. A saline cathartic is indicated since most iron preparations are enteric-coated. Deferoxamine (Desferal) has replaced edathamil as the chelating agent of choice in severe iron intoxication. It is a useful adjunct but does not replace careful conservative management. Deferoxamine is a specific chelating agent for iron and does not chelate other heavy metals. Very little is absorbed when given orally. When given parenterally, it forms a soluble complex which is excreted largely in the urine. It is contraindicated in patients with renal failure.

Deferoxamine should not be delayed in serious cases of poisoning until serum iron levels are available, but it should not be used in all patients with iron poisoning. Some authorities suggest that 5–10 gm of deferoxamine be given orally to complex iron remaining in the gastrointestinal tract. Because of its bitter taste, administration by a nasogastric tube is usually necessary. Intravenous administration is indicated *only* if the patient is in shock, in which case 1 gm may be given at a rate not to exceed 15 mg/kg/hour. Rapid intravenous administration causes hypotension, facial flushing, urticaria, tachycardia, and shock. The dose may be repeated every 4–12 hours if clinically indicated. Deferoxamine, 1–2 gm IM every 3–12 hours, may be given if clinically indicated. Blood levels of deferoxamine given intramuscularly and intravenously are about equal in 15 minutes if the patient is not in shock.

Hemodialysis, peritoneal dialysis, or exchange transfusion can be used to increase the excretion of the dialyzable complex, if necessary. Urine output should be monitored and urine sediment examined for evidence of renal tubular damage. Initial laboratory studies should include blood typing and cross-match, total protein, serum iron, total iron-binding capacity, serum sodium, potassium, chloride, CO_2, pH, and liver function tests. Serum iron levels fall rapidly even if deferoxamine is not given.

After the acute episode, liver function studies and an upper gastrointestinal series are indicated to rule out residual damage.

The mortality rate following iron ingestion is much less than previously reported.

Helfer RE, Rodgerson DO: The effect of deferoxamine on the determination of serum iron and iron binding capacity. J Pediat 68:804–810, 1966.

James JA: Acute iron poisoning: Assessment of severity and prognosis. J Pediat 77:117–119, 1970.

Leiken S, Vossough P, Mochir-Fatemi F: Chelation therapy in acute iron poisoning. J Pediat 71:425–430, 1967.

Soots M & others: Reaction to iron sorbitol injection. Brit MJ 4:54, 1970.

Whitten CF, Chen Y, Gibson GW: Studies in acute iron poisoning. Pediatrics 38:102–110, 1966.

LEAD

Clinical Findings

Lead poisoning causes weakness, irritability, weight loss, vomiting, personality changes, ataxia, constipation, headache, transient abdominal pain, and a "lead line" on the gums. Late manifestations consist of retarded development, convulsions, and coma associated with increased intracranial pressure. The latter is a medical emergency.

Plumbism usually occurs insidiously in children under 5 years of age. The most likely sources of lead include pica involving flaking leaded paint, artist's paints, fruit tree sprays, leaded gasoline, solder, brass alloys, home-glazed pottery, and fumes from burning batteries. Only paint containing < 1% lead is safe for interior use (furniture, toys, etc). Repetitive ingestions of small amounts of lead are far more serious than a single massive exposure.

Toxic reactions are likely to occur if more than 0.5 mg of lead per day is absorbed, but fatality usually does not occur unless more than 0.5 gm/day is absorbed. Only uncombined lead is removed by deleading agents. Children under 2 years of age have a poor prognosis, whereas children who develop peripheral neuritis without evidence of mental retardation or encephalitis usually recover completely.

Many laboratory tests are helpful in establishing a diagnosis of plumbism. Urinary δ-aminolevulinic acid determination is probably the best screening test; with levels > 6 mg/liter, some symptoms appear, and levels > 19 mg/liter are associated with definite symptoms of plumbism. Twenty-four-hour urinary lead level exceeds 80 μg/day without treatment and should increase to > 1.5 mg/day on any one of the first 3 days on calcium edathamil therapy. Dehydration and acidosis may falsely lower urinary lead levels. Glycosuria, proteinuria, hematuria, and aminoaciduria occur frequently. Blood lead levels should exceed 80 μg/100 ml in symptomatic patients. Abnormal blood and urinary lead levels should be repeated because the determinations are technically difficult to do. Specimens must be meticulously obtained in acid-washed containers. A normocytic, slightly hypochromic anemia with basophilic stippling of the red cells and reticulocytosis is usually present in plumbism. Stippling of red blood cells is absent in cases of sudden massive ingestion. Fecal excretion of > 125 μg of lead in a given stool is a more sensitive indication of lead ingestion than is the blood lead level.

Increased density of the metaphyseal lines of the wrists and knees as well as radiopaque densities in the gastrointestinal tract can be seen. The CSF protein is moderately to markedly elevated, and the CSF white cell count is usually less than 100 cells/ml. CSF pressure is usually elevated. Lumbar punctures must be performed very cautiously to prevent herniation of the brain stem in patients with encephalopathy.

Treatment

Induced vomiting followed by a saline cathartic is indicated. Using the combination of dimercaprol (BAL), 4 mg/kg/dose every 4 hours IM, and calcium disodium edathamil, 12.5 mg/kg/dose (maximum dose 75 mg/kg/day) IV or IM starting with the second dose of dimercaprol, should reduce the mortality of acute lead encephalopathy to < 5%. This treatment is indicated for a symptomatic patient or one with a blood lead level of 100 μg/100 ml. It should be started as soon as urine flow is initiated. Unless the patient is severely affected, 50 mg/kg/day of calcium disodium edathamil (EDTA) is an adequate dose which is less likely to damage the kidneys or cause hypercalcemia. Elevated lead levels will usually return to normal in 3–5 days when the combination method is used; this is rarely true when calcium disodium edathamil is used alone. After a 2-day pause, another course of treatment can be given if desired. Dimercaprol can be used

with complete renal shutdown but not in patients with severe hepatic insufficiency. Dimercaprol (but not calcium disodium edathamil) increases the fecal excretion of lead. The development of lacrimation, blepharospasm, paresthesias, nausea, tachycardia, and hypertension suggests a toxic reaction to dimercaprol. Iron should not be given to patients being treated for plumbism since it forms a toxic substance with dimercaprol. Dimercaprol is usually used instead of penicillamine (Cuprimine) because it results in a greater excretion of lead than penicillamine.

If the blood lead level is 80–100 μg/100 ml, calcium disodium edathamil and dimercaprol can be given for 2 days and then replaced with penicillamine orally for 5 days if there is no lead in the gut, or calcium disodium edathamil can be given alone for 5 days or dimercaprol and calcium disodium edathamil can be given concomitantly for 3 days.

A brief course of edathamil or a longer course of penicillamine is indicated for lead levels of 60–80 μg/100 ml. Chelation therapy is not indicated for lead levels below 60 μg/100 ml unless there is additional evidence of toxicity.

Fifty mg/kg/day of the hydrochloride salt of penicillamine given orally on an empty stomach is an investigational method of treating milder forms of lead poisoning. Doses up to 100 mg/day have been given for up to 7 days without serious adverse effects, but doses larger than 40 mg/kg/day of the free base or 50 mg/kg/day of the hydrochloride salt should not be used for chronic therapy. Excessive doses cause the nephrotic syndrome, bleeding phenomena, leukopenia, and neutropenia.

Anticonvulsants may be needed. Mannitol or corticosteroids are indicated in patients with encephalopathy. Fluid intake should be restricted. One expert investigator feels that surgical decompression is contraindicated, but others disagree. Hypothermia and corticosteroid therapy have not altered mortality rates significantly. A high-calcium, high-phosphorus diet and large doses of vitamin D remove lead from the blood by depositing it in the bones.

Daily urinalysis, serum calcium and phosphorus, and BUN should be done every 2 days. Calcium gluconate given intravenously as a 10% solution is helpful in controlling the colic which sometimes occurs.

A public health team should evaluate the source of the lead. Necessary corrections should be completed before the child is returned home.

Chisolm J: Treatment of acute lead intoxication: Choice of chelating agents and supportive therapeutic measures. Clin Toxicol 3:527–540, 1970.

Chisolm J, Kaplan E: Lead poisoning in childhood: Comprehensive management and prevention. J Pediat 73:942–950, 1968.

Klein M: Earthenware containers as a source of fatal lead poisoning. New England J Med 283:669–672, 1970.

MATCHES

Potassium chlorate has replaced yellow phosphorus in matches (330 mg in 20 wooden kitchen matches or 180–270 mg in 20 book matches). Five gm of potassium chlorate are considered a toxic amount, but ingestion of as little as 1 gm has caused death. If large numbers of matches have been ingested, induced vomiting should be followed by a saline cathartic.

Red phosphorus, which (unlike yellow* or white phosphorous) is relatively nonabsorbable and nontoxic, and antimony sulfide, which is also insoluble and relatively inert, are commonly used in the striking surface of the box. Red phosphorus may be contaminated with up to 0.6% white phosphorus.

Treatment

If large numbers of matches have been ingested, induce vomiting and follow with a saline cathartic.

MEPROBAMATE
(Miltown, Equanil)

Respiratory depression, coma, cardiac arrhythmias, and occasional convulsions associated with hyperexcitability occur. Death is the result of cardiac or respiratory failure.

Meprobamate is a general depressant, anticonvulsant, and muscle relaxant which causes habituation and a withdrawal syndrome. In addition to being detoxified in the CNS and liver by an acetylation process, meprobamate is excreted unchanged in the urine. There are genetic variations in the rate of acetylation which are of great significance in patients who have taken massive overdoses of meprobamate. People who are rapid acetylators tolerate higher serum levels without toxicity. Serum meprobamate levels of 10–20 mg/100 ml are usually associated with severe toxicity. However, toxicity may occur at much lower levels in patients who are slow acetylators.

Treatment

Gastric lavage is not very effective because meprobamate is highly insoluble in water. Delayed gastric emptying is common, and the drug is absorbed slowly from the gastrointestinal tract. Induced vomiting is indicated if the patient is awake and should be followed by a saline cathartic. Patients who show an initial improvement may relapse and die as a result of delayed absorption from concretions of meprobamate in the stomach.

Treatment in mild intoxications is supportive. If the patient deteriorates rapidly or develops deep coma with seizures or cardiac arrhythmias, hemodialysis, peritoneal dialysis, or forced diuresis is indicated.

*See Phosphorus, below, for toxicity due to fireworks.

Jenis EH, Payne RJ, Goldbaum LR: Acute meprobamate poisoning. JAMA 207:361–362, 1969.

MERCURY

Mercury poisoning is manifested by a metallic taste, thirst, severe vomiting, bloody diarrhea, cough, pharyngeal and abdominal pain, dyspnea, pulmonary embolization, dermatitis, corneal ulcers, nephrosis, renal failure, hepatic damage, ulcerative colitis, and shock. Acrodynia occurs in children after chronic exposure to small amounts of mercury in diaper rash ointments and teething lotions.

Chronic inorganic mercury poisoning causes salivation, loosening of teeth, bad oral odor, gingivitis, mouth ulcerations, dermatitis, fatigue, loss of memory, irritability, apprehension, tremors, decreased visual acuity and night vision, and staggering and slurred speech ("mad hatter syndrome"). Both organic and inorganic mercury poisoning can cause similar physical signs, although organic mercury intoxication characteristically causes dysarthria, ataxia, and constricted visual fields.

Elevated mercury levels have recently been noted in tuna and swordfish, and human mercury poisoning has been attributed to eating large amounts of contaminated swordfish. Mercury is a possible constituent of antiseptics, cathartics, diuretics, fumigants, and fungicides. All forms of mercury are potentially poisonous, but organic mercurials are generally less toxic than inorganic mercurials because they are poorly absorbed. A small amount of metallic mercury from a thermometer is nontoxic under normal circumstances because it is not well absorbed.

Treatment

Activated charcoal should be followed by induced vomiting and a saline cathartic. Dimercaprol (BAL) as for lead poisoning (see above) is often used. (Edathamil is contraindicated.) Penicillamine is also effective and has the advantage of being given orally. N-Acetylpenicillamine has also been used successfully in a few patients but is still considered an experimental drug. Demulcents and analgesics are indicated, as well as correction of fluid and electrolyte imbalances. Hemodialysis may be indicated for renal failure but not for removal of mercury.

Eyl TB: Alkylmercury contamination of foods. JAMA 215:287–288, 1971.

Javett SN, Kaplan B: Acrodynia treated with D-penicillamine. Am J Dis Child 115:71–73, 1968.

Kark RAP & others: Mercury poisoning and its treatment with N-acetyl-D,L-penicillamine. New England J Med 285:1–16, 1971.

Teitelbaum DT, Ott JE: Elemental mercury self-poisoning. Clin Toxicol 2:243–248, 1969.

MUSHROOMS

Many toxic species of mushrooms are difficult to separate from edible varieties. Symptoms vary with the species ingested, the time of year, the stage of maturity, the quantity eaten, the method of preparation, and the interval since ingestion. A mushroom that is toxic to one individual may not be toxic for another. Drinking alcohol and eating mushrooms may cause a reaction similar to that seen with disulfiram (Antabuse) and alcohol. Cooking destroys some toxins but not the deadly one produced by *Amanita phalloides,* which is responsible for 90% of deaths due to mushroom poisoning. Mushroom toxins are absorbed relatively slowly. Onset of symptoms within 2 hours of ingestion suggests muscarinic toxin, whereas a delay of symptoms for 6–48 hours after ingestion strongly suggests Amanita poisoning. Patients who have ingested *A phalloides* may relapse and die of hepatic or renal failure following initial improvement.

Mushroom poisoning may be manifested by muscarinic symptoms (salivation, vomiting, diarrhea, cramping abdominal pain, tenesmus, miosis, and dyspnea), coma, convulsions, hallucinations, hemolysis, and hepatic and renal failure.

Treatment

Induce vomiting and follow with activated charcoal and a saline cathartic. If the patient has muscarinic signs, give atropine, 0.025 mg/kg IM (0.02 mg/kg in toddlers) and repeat as needed (usually every 30 minutes) to keep the patient atropinized. Large doses of atropine are required. Hypoglycemia is most likely to occur in patients with delayed onset of symptoms. If the patient is deteriorating clinically or if *A phalloides* is identified or suspected, prompt dialysis is lifesaving and should minimize the danger to the liver and kidneys. If the specific mushroom is unknown and the patient is toxic, dialysis is indicated. Blood transfusions may be necessary to compensate for the hemolytic anemia which is sometimes seen.

Beargie RA: Beware of mushroom poisoning. Consultant, pp 44–47, April 1967.
Harrison DC: Mushroom poisoning in five patients. Am J Med 38:787–792, 1965.

NARCOTICS & SYNTHETIC CONGENERS*
(Heroin, Morphine, Codeine, Propoxyphene)

Physicians may be called upon to treat various narcotic problems, including drug addiction, withdrawal in a newborn infant, and accidental overdoses. Accidental ingestions of propoxyphene (Darvon) and

*Diphenoxylate (Lomotil) poisoning is discussed above in alphabetic sequence.

diphenoxylate (in Lomotil) are becoming increasingly more frequent. A detailed discussion of this complex subject is not possible in this short presentation, but the following information should be kept in mind.

Narcotics are often administered parenterally because their absorption in the gastrointestinal tract is variable. Unlike other narcotics, methadone is readily absorbed from the gastrointestinal tract. Drug abusers often use the intravenous route of administration. Most narcotics, including heroin, methadone, meperidine, morphine, and codeine, are excreted in the urine within 24 hours and can be readily detected in the urine.

The treatment of a narcotic addict–who usually is a demanding, manipulating, and irritating patient–is often quite difficult. If an addict seeks medical help, the physician must decide whether to treat the patient himself or refer him to another physician.

Narcotic addicts often have other medical problems, including cellulitis, abscesses, thrombophlebitis, tetanus, bacterial endocarditis, tuberculosis, hepatitis, malaria, foreign body emboli, thrombosis of pulmonary arterioles, diabetes mellitus, obstetric complications, and peptic ulcer.

Treatment of Overdosage

Children receiving an overdose of narcotics can develop respiratory depression, stridor, coma, increased oropharyngeal secretions, sinus bradycardia, and urinary retention. Methadone is less likely to cause miosis than other narcotics. Pulmonary edema rarely occurs in children; deaths usually result from respiratory arrest and cerebral edema.

The treatment of choice appears to be naloxone hydrochloride (Narcan), 0.01/mg/kg IV, which rapidly produces a marked improvement without causing respiratory depression. The dose can be repeated as needed. If naloxone is not available, nalorphine (Nalline), 0.1 mg/kg IM or IV, is indicated. Nalorphine may increase respiratory depression if the diagnosis is incorrect, especially if the respiratory depression is due to barbiturates; therefore, it should not be repeated if the diagnosis is in question and there is no dramatic response. An improvement in respiratory status may be followed by respiratory depression since the depressant action of narcotics may last 24–48 hours while the narcotic antagonist's duration of action is only 2–3 hours. Intravenous fluids should be given cautiously, as narcotics exert an antidiuretic effect and may precipitate cerebral or pulmonary edema.

Withdrawal in the Addict

The severity of narcotic withdrawal signs in an addict can be evaluated by observing and scoring the following physical findings on a 0–2 point basis: yawning, dilated pupils, restlessness, lacrimation, gooseflesh, muscle cramps, insomnia, hyperactive bowel sounds, diarrhea and tachycardia or systemic hypertension. A score of 1–5 indicates mild, 6–10 moderate, and 11–15 severe withdrawal from narcotics. A seizure indicates a severe withdrawal pattern regardless of the score.

Diazepam (Valium), 10 mg every 6 hours orally, has been recommended for the treatment of mild narcotic withdrawal in ambulatory adolescents. Ambulatory or hospitalized patients with moderate or severe withdrawal signs can be given the same dose of diazepam intramuscularly. Diazepam is recommended because it is nonhepatotoxic, nonmutagenic, does not affect the fetus when given to pregnant women, and is a good anticonvulsant. Diazepam therapy can be discontinued when the withdrawal score falls below 2. Diphenoxylate (Lomotil) is used to treat severe diarrhea and abdominal cramps. Chloral hydrate is the drug of choice for insomnia; barbiturates should not be used.

Methadone maintenance is not usually recommended for adolescents, although it may be used for withdrawal purposes. One method of administration is to give methadone orally every 12 hours, starting with a 25 mg dose and decreasing the amount by 5 mg every 12 hours. When the dose of methadone is 10 mg, add 3 tablets of diphenoxylate with atropine (Lomotil) 3 times daily for 1 day followed by 2 tablets 3 times daily for 2 days. If signs of withdrawal recur, 10 mg of methadone orally or diazepam (orally or IM) are given.

The abrupt discontinuation of narcotics (cold turkey method) is not recommended and may cause severe physical withdrawal signs.

Withdrawal in the Newborn

A newborn infant in narcotic withdrawal is small for his gestational age and demonstrates yawning, sneezing, decreased Moro reflex, hunger but uncoordinated sucking action, jitteriness, tremor, constant movement, a shrill, protracted cry, increased tendon reflexes, convulsions, vomiting, fever, watery diarrhea, cyanosis, dehydration, vasomotor instability, and collapse. The onset of symptoms commonly begins in the first 48 hours but may be delayed as long as 8 days depending upon the timing of the mother's last fix and her predelivery medication. The diagnosis can be easily confirmed by identifying the narcotic in the urine of the mother and baby.

Several methods of treatment have been suggested for narcotic withdrawal in the newborn. Chlorpromazine (Thorazine), 1 mg/kg/day in 4 doses IM or orally for the first 4 days and gradually reduced as signs abate, can be given for 10–21 days. Phenobarbital, 8 mg/kg/day IM or orally in 4 doses for 4 days and then reduced by 1/3 every 2 days as signs decrease, may be continued for as long as 3 weeks. Paregoric is given in gradually increasing doses until a clinical response is seen—2–4 drops/kg orally every 4–6 hours, increasing to as high as 20–40 drops/kg/day if necessary—and then lowered gradually as the signs diminish. Methadone, 0.1–0.5 mg/kg/day orally in 4 doses for 4 days, has also been recommended, but the side-affects of this drug in neonates are not well understood. The dose is gradually tapered.

It is not clear whether prophylactic treatment with these drugs decreases the complication rate. The mortality rate of untreated narcotic withdrawal in the newborn may be as high as 45%.

Dole VP & others: Methadone poisoning. New York J Med 71:541, 1971.

Gary NE & others: Acute propoxyphene hydrochloride intoxication. Arch Int Med 121:453–457, 1968.

Harries JT, Rossiter M: Fatal Lomotil poisoning. Lancet 1:150, 1969.

Ingall D, Zucherstatter M: Diagnosis and treatment of the passively addicted newborn. Hosp Practice 5:101, 1970.

Kahn E, Neumann L, Polk G: The course of heroin withdrawal syndrome in newborn infants treated with phenobarbital and chlorpromazine. J Pediat 75:495, 1969.

Litt I, Colli A, Cohen M: Diazepam in the management of heroin withdrawal in adolescents: Preliminary report. J Pediat 78:692–696, 1971.

Sey MJ, Rubenstein D, Smith D: Accidental methadone intoxication in a child. Pediatrics 48:294–296, 1971.

NITRITES & NITRATES

Nausea, vertigo, vomiting, cyanosis (methemoglobinemia), cramping abdominal pain, tachycardia, cardiovascular collapse, tachypnea, coma, shock, convulsions, and death are possible manifestations of nitrite or nitrate poisoning.

Nitrite and nitrate compounds found in the home include amyl nitrite, glyceryl trinitrate (nitroglycerin), pentaerythritol tetranitrate (Peritrate), sodium nitrite, and spirits of nitre. High concentrations of nitrites in water or spinach have been the most common cause of nitrite-induced methemoglobinemia. Symptoms do not usually occur until 40–50% of the hemoglobin has been converted to methemoglobin.

Treatment

After administering activated charcoal, induce vomiting and follow by a saline cathartic. Decontaminate any affected skin with soap and water. Oxygen and artificial respiration may be needed. If the blood methemoglobin level exceeds 40% or if levels can not be obtained, give 0.2 ml/kg of a 1% solution of methylene blue IV over 5–10 minutes. Avoid perivascular infiltration since it causes necrosis of the skin and subcutaneous tissues. A dramatic change in the degree of cyanosis should occur. Transfusion is occasionally necessary. Epinephrine and other vasoconstrictors are contraindicated. If reflex bradycardia occurs, atropine can be used to block it.

Bakshi SP, Fahey JL, Pierce LE: Sausage cyanosis: Acquired methemoglobinemic nitrite poisoning. New England J Med 277:1072, 1967.

Carlson DJ & others: Methemoglobinemia from well water nitrates: A complication of home dialysis. Ann Int Med 73:757–759, 1970.

TABLE 31—5. Poisoning due to plants.

	Symptoms and Signs	Treatment
Autumn crocus (colchicum)	Abdominal cramps, severe diarrhea, CNS depression, and circulatory collapse. Occasionally, oliguria and renal shutdown. Delirium or convulsions occur terminally.	Fluid and electrolyte monitoring. Abdominal cramps may be relieved with meperidine or atropine.
Caladium (arum family) Dieffenbachia, calla lily, dumbcane	Burning of mucous membranes and airway obstruction secondary to edema caused by calcium oxalate crystals.	Accessible areas should be thoroughly washed. Corticosteroids relieve airway obstruction. Apply cold packs to affected mucous membranes.
Castor bean plant	Mucous membrane irritation, nausea, vomiting, bloody diarrhea, blurred vision, circulatory collapse, acute hemolytic anemia, convulsions, uremia.	Fluid and electrolyte monitoring. Saline cathartic. Forced alkaline diuresis will prevent complications due to hemagglutination and hemolysis.
Foxglove and cardiac glycosides*	Nausea, diarrhea, visual disturbances, and cardiac irregularities (eg, heart block).	If ECG is normal, treat symptomatically. If abnormal, give potassium chloride to protect against irritability of cardiac muscle. (Do not use potassium if renal function is impaired.) Quinidine, procainamide, or calcium disodium edathamil may be useful in treating marked arrhythmias. Epinephrine may precipitate ventricular tachycardia.
Jimsonweed: See Belladonna Alkaloids, p 784.		
Larkspur (Delphinium)	Nausea and vomiting, irritability, muscular paralysis, and CNS depression.	Symptomatic. Atropine may be helpful.
Monkshood (Aconitum)	Numbness of mucous membranes, visual disturbances, tingling, dizziness, tinnitus, hypotension, bradycardia, and convulsions.	Activated charcoal, oxygen. Atropine is probably helpful.
Oleander (dogbane family)	Nausea, bloody diarrhea, respiratory depression, tachycardia, and muscle paralysis.	Symptomatic. Atropine may be helpful. Dipotassium edathamil chelates calcium, decreasing cardiac toxicity of oleandrin.
Poison hemlock	Mydriasis, trembling, dizziness, bradycardia, CNS depression, muscular paralysis, and convulsions. Death is due to respiratory paralysis.	Symptomatic. Oxygen and cardiac monitoring equipment are desirable. Assisted respiration is often necessary. Give anticonvulsants if needed.
Rhododendron	Abdominal cramps, vomiting, severe diarrhea, muscular paralysis, CNS and circulatory depression. Hypertension with very large doses.	Atropine can prevent bradycardia. Epinephrine is contraindicated. Antihypertensives may be needed.
Rosary pea (jequirity bean)	Nausea, vomiting, abdominal and muscle cramps, hemolysis and hemagglutination, circulatory failure, respiratory failure, and renal and liver failure.	Symptomatic. Renal failure can be prevented by alkalinizing the urine. Gastric lavage or emetics are contraindicated because the toxin is necrotizing. Saline cathartics are indicated.
Yellow jessamine (active ingredient related to strychnine)	Restlessness, convulsions, muscular paralysis, and respiratory depression.	Symptomatic. Because of the relation to strychnine, forced acid diuresis and diazepam (Valium) for seizures would be worth trying.

*See also Digitalis, p 787.

PHENOTHIAZINES
(Chlorpromazine [Thorazine], Prochlorperazine [Compazine], Trifluoperazine [Stelazine], Etc)

Extrapyramidal crisis. Episodes characterized by torticollis, stiffening of the body, spasticity, poor speech, catatonia, and inability to communicate although conscious are typical manifestations. These episodes usually last a few seconds to a few minutes but have rarely caused death. Extrapyramidal crises may represent idiosyncratic reactions and are aggravated by dehydration. The signs and symptoms occur most often in children who have received prochlorperazine (Compazine). They are commonly mistaken for psychotic episodes.

Overdose. Lethargy and deep prolonged coma commonly occur. Promazine, chlorpromazine, and prochlorperazine are the drugs most likely to cause respiratory depression and precipitous drops in blood pressure. Occasionally, paradoxical hyperactivity and extrapyramidal signs as well as hyperglycemia and acetonemia are present. Seizures are uncommon.

Phenothiazines are rapidly absorbed by the gastrointestinal tract and bound to tissue. They are principally conjugated with glucuramic acid and are then excreted in the urine.

Treatment

Extrapyramidal signs are dramatically alleviated within minutes by the slow intravenous administration of 1–5 mg/kg of diphenhydramine (Benadryl). No other treatment is usually indicated. Dialysis is contraindicated.

Patients with overdoses should be treated conservatively. An attempt should be made to induce vomiting with apomorphine after administration of activated charcoal. Charcoal adsorbs chlorpromazine and probably other phenothiazines very well. Emetics are often unsuccessful in this situation because phenothiazines are potent antiemetics; gastric lavage, therefore, may be the only practical way to remove gastric contents. A large amount of intravenous fluid without vasopressor agents is the preferred method of treating tranquilizer-induced neurogenic hypotension. If a pressor agent is required, norepinephrine (levarterenol) should be used. Epinephrine should *not* be used because phenothiazines reverse epinephrine's effects.

Patients rarely die if properly managed.

Alexander CS, Nino A: Cardiovascular complications in young patients taking psychotropic drugs. Am Heart J 78:757–769, 1969.

Davies DM: Treatment of drug-induced dystanesias. Lancet 1:567–568, 1970.

Moser RH: Reactions to phenothiazine and related drugs. Clin Pharmacol Therap 7:683–684, 1966.

Thomas J: Fatal case of agramulocytosis due to chlorpromazine. Lancet 1:44–45, 1970.

PHOSPHORUS
(Yellow Phosphorus)

Yellow phosphorus, used in fertilizers, pesticides, and fireworks, is extremely toxic. Ingestion of 0.1 mg/sq m can cause severe toxicity. Nausea, vomiting, diarrhea, and a garlic odor of the breath and feces, followed by cardiac failure, hepatic, and renal damage can occur. The onset of symptoms is 1–2 hours after ingestion. Abdominal pain, gastrointestinal bleeding, hypoglycemia, hypocalcemia, jaundice, shock, convulsions, and coma are late signs. Patients may initially improve and then relapse.

Alterations in carbohydrate, fat, and protein metabolism occur. Glycogen deposition is inhibited, as is bone formation also.

Yellow phosphorus on the skin causes a second or third degree burn which is slow to heal, but usually no systemic signs.

Red phosphorus, which is used in matches and match book striking surfaces, is not absorbed and is generally nontoxic unless contaminated with yellow phosphorus.

Treatment

Treatment is nonspecific. Induced vomiting or gastric lavage with an oxidizing substance such as potassium permanganate (1:5000 solution) or 2% hydrogen peroxide is indicated and should be followed by a saline cathartic. Fluids containing large amounts of carbohydrate are indicated. Calcium administration may be needed.

Fluids and electrolytes must be carefully monitored. Vitamin K should be given if the prothrombin level is decreased.

The skin should be washed with water for at least 15 minutes if it was contaminated with yellow phosphorus.

Marin GA & others: Evaluation of corticosteroid and exchange transfusion treatment of acute yellow-phosphorus intoxication. New England J Med 284:125–128, 1971.

Rodriguez-Iturbe B: Acute yellow phosphorous poisoning. New England J Med 284:157, 1971.

PLANTS

Many common ornamental, garden, and wild plants are potentially toxic. Small amounts of a plant may cause severe illness or death. These effects usually involve the cardiovascular, gastrointestinal, and central nervous systems and the skin. Table 31–5 lists the most toxic plants, symptoms and signs of poisoning, and treatment.

TABLE 31−6. Commonly abused drugs.

Type and Name of Drug (and Slang Terms)*			How Taken	Clinical Findings	Duration of Action
Stimulants					
Amphetamines			Swallowed or injected	Agitation, talkativeness, insomnia, anorexia, diarrhea. May develop weight loss, hypertension, toxic psychosis resembling paranoid schizophrenia, exhaustion, etc. Psychologic dependence can occur. Physiologic dependence probably does not occur.	Single dose commonly lasts 4−8 hours
Beans	Dexies	Splivins			
Bennies	Eye-openers	Truck drivers			
Black beauties	Footballs	Ups			
Bombita	Greenies	Uppers			
Browns	Hearts	Wake-ups			
Cartwheels	Jolly beans	Whites			
Chicken powder	Lid poppers				
Coast-to-coasts	L-A turnabouts	**Intravenous:**			
Co-pilots	Oranges	Bombido			
Crank	Peaches	Crack			
Crink	Pep pills	Crystal			
Cris	Purple hearts	Drivers			
Christmas trees	Roses	Meth			
Christina	Splash	Speed			
Crystal	Speed				
Cocaine			Sniffed, swallowed, or injected	CNS stimulation, euphoria, pupillary dilatation, vasoconstriction, loss of sense of time, hyperactive reflexes, vertigo, confusion, exhaustion, convulsions, hallucinations, tachycardia, vomiting. Psychologic dependence occurs.	A few minutes to 4 hours
Bernice	Charlie	Gold dust			
Bernice's flakes	Cholly	Joy powder			
Big bloke	Coke	Leaper			
Blow	Dream	Nose candy			
"C"	Dust	Snow			
Carrie cecil	Girl	Stardust			
Sedatives					
Barbiturates			Swallowed or injected	Slurred speech, staggering, confusion, and mood shifts. See also discussion of barbiturates in this chapter.	4−8 hours
Barbs	Goof balls	Seccy			
Bluebirds	Peanuts	Seggy			
Blue devils	Rainbows	Sleeping pills			
Blue heavens	Red birds	Stoppers			
Blues	Red and blues	Yellow jackets			
Candy	Red devils	Yellows			
Double trouble	Reds				
Codeine			Swallowed	Drowsiness, difficulty in concentration, dulled perceptions. Psychologic and physiologic dependence can occur.	4 hours
Cough syrup					
Number 4's					
Schoolboy					
Heroin			Injected or sniffed	Euphoria, drowsiness, and confusion (see also narcotics), constipation, malnutrition, respiratory arrest, infections common. Psychologic and physiologic dependence occur.	4−8 hours
Blow horse	Harry	Skid			
Dujie	Horse	Smack			
Foolish powder	Noise	TNT			
"H"	Pee	White junk			
Marihuana			Smoked, sniffed, or swallowed	Euphoria, mood swings, loss of inhibitions, distortion of time and space sense. Depressant effect more prominent than hallucinatory effect. "Dropout syndrome." Psychologic dependence occurs.	2−4 hours
Acapulco gold	Indian bay	Pod			
Ace	Indian hay	Pot			
Bhang	Jive	Stick			
Bobo bush	Jive sticks	Reefer			
Cannabis	Loco weed	Roaches			
Fine stuff	Log	Rope			
"FU"	Love weed	Sativa			
Gage	Mary Jane	Splim			
Grass	Mary Warner	Sweet Lucey			
Griefo	Mezz	Tea			
Joint	Mootos	Texas tea			
Hay	Moragrifa	Viper's weed			
Hemp	Muggles	Weed			
Hot sticks	Mutah				

*Slang terms vary in different localities and may even designate different drugs.

TABLE 31−6 (cont'd). Commonly abused drugs.

Type and Name of Drug (and Slang Terms)*			How Taken	Clinical Findings	Duration of Action
Sedatives					
Morphine			Swallowed or injected	Euphoria, difficulty in concentration, depressant effect. Respiratory depression and arrest, constipation. Psychologic and physiologic dependence.	4−8 hours
Cube juice	Miss Emma	White			
Emsel	Morph	merchandise			
Hard stuff	Morphie	White stuff			
Hocus	Morpho				
"M"	Unkie				
Hallucinogens					
Dimethoxymethylamphetamine (STP)			Swallowed	Euphoria, confusion, hallucinations, violence, respiratory arrest. Chromosomal damage not proved. Psychologic damage occurs.	3−14 days
Serenity, tranquility, and peace					
Lysergic acid diethylamide (LSD)			Swallowed or injected	Euphoria, rapid mood shifts, depersonalization, toxic psychosis. Chromosomal damage not proved. Psychologic dependence occurs.	8−10 hours
Acid	Grape parfait	Purple haze			
Blue heaven	Hawaiian sun-	Purple ozoline			
California sun-	shine	Smears			
shine	Micro dots	Squirrels			
Chocolate chips	Orange wedges	Strawberry			
The cube	Owsley's acid	field			
"D"	Peace	Wedges			
Domes	Peace tablets	White lightning			
Flats	Purple barrels	Yellow dimples			
Mescaline (peyote)			Swallowed, injected, or sniffed	Nausea, vomiting, anxiety, hallucinations, drug psychosis. May be confused with appendicitis, but blood counts and temperature are normal. Psychologic dependence occurs.	Up to 12 hours
Cactus	Berkeley grape	White light			
Big chief	(orange or green)				
Phencyclidine (veterinary anesthetic)			Swallowed	Depersonalization, hallucinations.	6−8 hours on 25 mg
Angel dust	DOA	Peace pill			
Dead on arrival	Dust of angels				
Psilocybin			Swallowed	Nausea, vomiting, headaches, hallucinations, drug psychosis.	6−8 hours
Mushrooms					
Tryptamine derivatives (DET, DMT)			Swallowed, injected, smoked	Exhilaration, hallucinations. Chromosomal damage not proved. Psychologic dependence occurs.	30 minutes to 4 hours
Businessman's lunch					

Combination drugs (see previous discussions for Clinical Findings, etc).

Heroin and cocaine: Speedball, dynamite, whiz-bang

Heroin, amphetamine, and Tuinal (amobarbital and neobarbital): Bombita

Oxycodone (Percodan) and methamphetamine (Methedrine): Speedball

LSD and methamphetamine: Speedball

Scrap iron: Bootleg drug made with alcohol, mothballs, and a hypochlorite solution.

Mix 'em or match 'em: A variety of pills are pooled. Then each person eats a handful. The pills can be all similar in appearance (match 'em) or a wide variety (mix 'em, or "fruit salad").

Hardin JW, Arena JM: *Human Poisoning From Native and Cultivated Plants.* Duke Univ Press, 1969.

Kozma JJ: *Killer Plants: A Poisonous Plant Guide.* Milestone Publishing Co., 1969.

PSYCHOTROPIC DRUGS

Psychotropic drugs consist of 4 general classes: stimulants (amphetamines), depressants (narcotics, barbiturates, etc), antidepressants and tranquilizers, and hallucinogens (LSD, etc).

The following clinical findings are commonly seen in patients abusing drugs:

Stimulants. Agitation, euphoria, grandiose feelings, tachycardia, fever, abdominal cramps, visual and auditory hallucinations, mydriasis, coma, convulsions, and respiratory depression.

Depressants. Emotional lability, ataxia, diplopia, nystagmus, vertigo, poor accommodation, respiratory depression, coma, apnea, and convulsions. Dilatation of conjunctival blood vessels suggests marihuana ingestion. Narcotics cause miotic pupils and occasionally pulmonary edema.

Antidepressants and tranquilizers. Hypotension, lethargy, respiratory depression, coma, and extrapyramidal reactions.

Hallucinogens and psychoactive drugs. Belladonna alkaloids cause mydriasis, dry mouth, nausea, vomiting, urinary retention, confusion, disorientation, paranoid delusions, visual and auditory hallucinations, fever, hypotension, aggressive behavior, convulsions, and coma. **Psychoactive drugs** such as LSD cause mydriasis, unexplained bizarre behavior, hallucinations, and generalized undifferentiated psychotic behavior.

See Table 31−6 for a list of commonly abused drugs and their synonyms, the clinical findings associated with their use, and their durations of action. See also other entries discussed in alphabetical sequence in this chapter (narcotics, barbiturates, belladonna alkaloids, etc).

Management of the Patient Who Abuses Drugs

Only a small percentage of the persons using drugs come to the attention of physicians; those who do are usually suffering from adverse reactions such as panic states, drug psychoses, homicidal or suicidal thoughts, and respiratory depression which could not be satisfactorily managed by their friends.

Even with cooperative patients, an accurate history is difficult to obtain. The user often does not really know either the dose or the specific drug or drugs he has been taking. "Street drugs" are almost always adulterated with one or more other compounds. Multiple drugs are often taken together ("fruit salad"), making it impossible to clinically define the type of drug. Friends may be a useful source of information. A drug history is most easily obtained in a quiet spot by a gentle, nonthreatening, honest examiner.

The general appearance, skin, lymphatics, cardiorespiratory status, gastrointestinal tract, and CNS should be stressed during the physical examination since they often provide clues suggesting drug abuse. A drug history should not be taken from an adolescent in the presence of his parents.

Although it is desirable to know the specific drug taken, it is often impossible to obtain this information. Hallucinogens are not life-threatening unless the patient is frankly homicidal or suicidal. A specific diagnosis is usually not necessary to manage the patient; instead, the presenting signs and symptoms are treated. Does the patient appear intoxicated? Does he seem to be in withdrawal? Is he having a "flashback" experience? Does he have some illness or injury (eg, head trauma) that is being masked by a drug? (Remember that an obvious "hippie" who is a known drug user may still be hallucinating because he has meningoencephalitis.)

The signs and symptoms in a given patient are a function not only of the drug and the dose but also the level of acquired tolerance, the "setting," the patient's physical condition and personality traits, the potentiating effects of other drugs, and many other factors.

The most common drug problem in most hospital emergency rooms is the "bad trip," which is usually a panic reaction. This is best managed by "talking the patient down" and minimizing auditory and visual stimuli. It is helpful to communicate a light mood and join with the patient in his trip while trying to focus on realities. If a negative response occurs, quickly change the subject. The physician should not attempt to use "street language" unless he is comfortable with it. A friend of the patient can often help by sitting with him. Trips may last 8 hours or more. The physician's job is not to end the trip but to help the patient over the bad sensations he is experiencing.

Drugs are often unnecessary and may complicate the clinical course of a patient with a panic reaction. Although phenothiazines have been commonly used to treat "bad trips," they should be avoided if the specific drug is not known since they may cause a precipitous drop in blood pressure if STP has been taken or paradoxical hyperactivity which makes management difficult. Diazepam (Valium), 20 mg orally every 30 minutes as necessary, is the drug of choice if a sedative is required. Physical restraints are rarely if ever indicated and usually increase the patient's panic reaction.

For treatment of life-threatening drug abuse, consult the section on the specific drug elsewhere in this chapter and the section on general management at the beginning of the chapter.

After the acute episode, the physician must decide whether psychiatric referral is indicated; in general, patients who have made suicidal gestures or attempts and adolescents who are not communicating with their families should be referred. On the other hand, adolescents who are "experimenting" with drugs often do not need psychiatric referral.

Pillard R: Marijuana. New England J Med 283:294–301, 1970.

Teitelbaum DT: Poisoning with psychoactive drugs. P Clin North America 17:557–567, 1970.

Tjio J, Pahnke W, Kurland A: LSD and chromosomes: A controlled experiment. JAMA 210:849–856, 1969.

Weil A, Zinberg N, Nelson J: Clinical and psychological effects of marihuana in man. Science 162:1234–1242, 1968.

RIOT CONTROL CHEMICALS

Every physician should know what chemicals are most likely to be used as riot control compounds in his area. This information can be obtained from local law enforcement officials.

Most currently used riot control chemicals produce burning and irritation of the eyes, profuse tearing, conjunctivitis, and irritation of the skin. Corneal damage is usually limited to the epithelium unless the chemical is discharged at close range, which may result in greater penetration of the epithelium, corneal opacification, and cataracts. A burning sensation or feeling of tightness in the chest, associated with cough, can occur after the use of Pepper Fog. Other chemicals can cause disorientation, second degree burns, and hyperpigmentation as well as nausea and vomiting. Repeated exposure to these chemicals may cause allergic conjunctivitis, blepharitis, and dermatitis. The estimated lethal dose for each chemical is more than 100 times the incapacitating dose.

Chloroacetophenone (tear gas, CN). This is the most commonly used riot control chemical and is the usual constituent of tear gas pen guns. It is now usually sold in a pressurized aerosol can containing a hydrocarbon solvent which prolongs the exposure to the skin, resulting in more second degree burns. Severe damage to the eyes, including burns, glaucoma, cataracts, hemorrhage, etc, has occurred after firing the weapon at close range. Permanent anesthesia of the hands and fingers has been reported.

Chloroacetophenone with kerosene and methyl chloroform (Mace, Peacemaker, Streamer). This is sprayed in a stream of tiny droplets which are converted to a gas which envelops the subject. Recommended firing distance from the victim is 12–15 feet. Its effect lasts approximately 30 minutes. Second degree burns and hyperpigmentation of the skin develop when the firing distance is too short. Skin sensitization, corneal scarring, and hypertension have also been reported.

Other forms of chloroacetophenone; chloropicrin. Chloroacetophenone is also marketed in combination with chloroform (CNC) and with benzene and carbon tetrachloride (CNB); chloropicrin is combined with chloroform (CNS). CNS produces vomiting and choking in addition to the more common symptoms. Its effects are longer lasting because of the chloropicrin.

Bromobenzyl cyanide (BBC). This compound has the odor of sour fruit but is otherwise similar to other riot control agents.

Orthochlorobenzylmalononitrile (CS, Pepper Fog). This agent is contained in a hand grenade which causes a vapor cloud that smells like pepper.

Gum cambogia (gamboge). This resin, also present in water colors, causes severe vomiting, diarrhea, cardiovascular collapse, and death. It should not be used for riot control.

Treatment

Management of exposure to the commonly used riot control chemicals is similar. Removing the patient from the contaminated atmosphere will aid greatly in removing the volatile tear gas. Exposed areas, including the nails and hair, should be washed with soap and water to remove dirt and oils which entrap the irritant. The area should then be flushed with copious amounts of cool water. Clothes must also be decontaminated by washing well in soap and water.

Copious irrigation of the eyes with water or saline is indicated. Topical anesthesia and ophthalmic ointments should not be used because they can retard healing and may concentrate the offending agent. Prevention of secondary infection and treatment of complications, such as iritis and glaucoma, are the only definitive treatment.

Anon: A little more about CS. Lancet 2:788, 1969.

Leopold IH, Lieberman TW: Chemical injuries of the cornea. Fed Proc 30:92–95, 1971.

Penneys NS: Contact dermatitis to chloroacetophenone. Fed Proc 30:96–99, 1971.

Pinkus JL: Chemical mace. New England J Med 281:1431–1432, 1969.

SCORPION BITES

Scorpion bites are common in arid areas of the southwestern USA. Scorpion venom is more toxic than most snake venoms, but only minute amounts are injected. Although neurologic manifestations of the bite may last a week, most clinical signs subside within 24–48 hours.

Bites by less toxic scorpion species cause local pain, redness, and swelling. Bites by more toxic species cause tingling or burning paresthesias at the site of the bite which tend to progress up the extremity, plus throat spasm, a feeling of a thickening of the tongue, restlessness, muscular fibrillation, abdominal cramps, convulsions, urinary incontinence, and respiratory failure.

A specific antiserum for scorpion bites is available from Laboratories "MYN," S.A., Av. Coyoacan 1707, Mexico 12, D.F. In addition, calcium gluconate, 10% solution, 5–20 ml IV, relieves muscular cramps. Hot compresses of sodium bicarbonate will soothe the bitten area. Sedation and corticosteroids may be indicated.

The prognosis for life is good except in infants and young children.

Bartholomew C: Acute scorpion pancreatitis in Trinidad. Brit MJ 1:666–668, 1970.

Gueron M & others: Cardiovascular manifestations of severe scorpion sting: Clinicopathologic correlations. Chest 57:156–162, 1970.

Zlotkin E & others: Recent studies on the mode of action of scorpion neurotoxins: A review. Toxicon 7:217–221, 1969.

SNAKEBITE

Considering the lethal potential of venomous snakes, human morbidity and mortality are surprisingly low. The outcome depends on the size of the child, the site of the bite, the degree of envenomization, and the effectiveness of treatment.

Poisonous snakebites are most common and most severe in the early spring. Children in snake-infested areas should wear boots and long trousers, should not walk barefoot, and should be cautioned not to explore under ledges or in holes where a snake might be hiding.

Being bitten by a poisonous snake does not always cause envenomization.

Ninety-eight percent of poisonous snakebites in the USA are caused by pit vipers (rattlesnakes, water moccasins, and copperheads) or elapids (coral snakes). Snake venom is a complex mixture of noxious components which may have predominantly cytotoxic, neurotoxic, hemotoxic, or cardiotoxic effects but other effects as well. The snake does not use all its venom in a single bite. Thirty percent of bites by pit vipers do not result in venom injection.

Pit viper venom is predominantly cytotoxic and hemotoxic, causing a severe local reaction with pain, discoloration, and edema, as well as hemorrhagic effects. Peripheral and central neurologic abnormalities can also occur. Convulsions are not uncommon in children. Coral snakes, found in southern USA, usually cause little local reaction but marked neurotoxic signs, including euphoria or dysphoria, salivation, ptosis, dysphagia, and bulbar paralysis. Convulsions often occur within an hour of envenomization and death in the first 24 hours.

Organic signs of systemic poisoning rarely appear within 30 minutes of the bite. Local pain is not helpful in the diagnosis because it may occur without systemic poisoning and may also be due to bites by non-poisonous snakes.

Pit viper envenomization can be ruled out if local swelling has not occurred a few minutes after the bite. Early systemic signs of pit viper envenomization may include blood-stained spit, abnormal blood clotting, and disseminated intravascular coagulation. Viper envenomization is considered severe if swelling is present above the elbow or knee within 2 hours or if shock and hemorrhagic signs other than hemoptysis are present.

Coral snake envenomization causes little local pain, swelling, or necrosis, and systemic reactions are often delayed for 10 hours, although children may convulse within 1 hour after being bitten. The early signs of coral snake envenomization include bulbar paralysis, dysphagia, and dysphoria; these may appear in 5–10 hours and may be followed by total peripheral paralysis and death in 24 hours.

Treatment

The treatment of snake bite envenomization is controversial, but the following approach seems most useful.

A. Emergency (First Aid) Treatment: The most important first aid measure is reassurance. If possible, clean the wound with a germicidal preparation. Splint the affected extremity and minimize the patient's motion. If systemic signs are present or if a significant delay cannot be avoided before definitive care can be provided, a tourniquet completely occluding the blood supply is indicated. *Caution:* The tourniquet should **not** be released until the patient has been adequately treated with antivenin. The extremity may have to be sacrificed to save a life. Release of the tourniquet before sufficient antivenin has been given may result in sudden shock and death.

Incision and suction are useful if done within a few minutes after the envenomization. The incision should not be more than 1/4 inch in length and should cut only through the skin. Multiple incisions following the line of progressive edema do not increase the amount of venom recovered. Incision and suction are contraindicated if the venom is primarily neurotoxic and is not helpful if there is little local effect.

B. Definitive Medical Management: Blood should be drawn for typing and cross-match, hematocrit, clotting time and platelet function, and serum electrolyte determinations. Close monitoring of the hematocrit and electrolytes is indicated. The venom may make it difficult to do blood typing and cross-matching. The massive destruction of red cells may be associated with hyperkalemia. Establish 2 secure intravenous sites for the administration of antivenin, blood, and other medications.

Specific antivenin is indicated only when definite signs of envenomization are present. Polyvalent pit viper antivenin and coral snake antivenin are available from Wyeth Laboratories, Box 8299, Philadelphia 19104. Coral snake antivenin can also be obtained from Charity Hospital, New Orleans, or from the National Center for Disease Control, Atlanta, Georgia, telephone (404) 633-3311.

After horse serum sensitivity tests (see Chapter 5) are negative, antivenin should be given intravenously and can be given at any desired concentration or rate. Ten to 100 ml may be required. (Antivenin should not be given intramuscularly or subcutaneously because it is slow-acting, inefficient, and impossible to control if adverse reactions occur. Antivenin injected into the bite site has little effect.) If anaphylaxis occurs despite negative skin tests, it will occur at the onset of treatment. Epinephrine, 0.3 ml of 1:1000 solution, should be drawn up in a syringe before antivenin is administered. Horse serum sensitivity must be reevaluated if another course of antivenin is required over 36 hours after the first. The hemorrhagic tendency, pain, and shock are rapidly improved by adequate amounts of antivenin.

Injection of edathamil into the bite site probably decreases the amount of local hemorrhage and necrosis. Heparinization (initial dose of 100 units/kg IV followed by a maintenance dose of 50 units/kg every 4 hours) is indicated for disseminated intravascular coagulation. Codeine, 1–1.5 mg/kg/dose orally, or meperidine (Demerol), 0.6–1.5 mg/kg/dose orally or IM, is occasionally necessary to control pain during the first 24 hours. Cryotherapy is contraindicated since it commonly causes tissue damage severe enough to necessitate amputation. Early physiotherapy minimizes contractions. In rare cases fascial splitting procedures to relieve pressure are required to save the function of a hand or foot. Corticosteroids (hydrocortisone, 1–2 gm IV every 4–6 hours) are useful in the treatment of serum sickness or anaphylactic shock. Ampicillin (200 mg/kg/day orally) is given to treat gram-negative infections which are often associated with snake bite.

A fluid tetanus toxoid booster is adequate if the patient was previously immunized against tetanus. If the patient has not completed his primary immunizations, 250 units of tetanus immune globulin (human) should be given IM. Tetanus antitoxin is not given if tetanus immune globulin is available.

Glass TG: Snakebite. Hosp Med 7:31–55, July 1971.

Lonjo MF: Review of current management of snakebites. J Louisiana Med Soc 123:9–12, 1971.

McCollough NC, Gennaro JF: Treatment of venomous snakebite in the United States. Clin Toxicol 3:483–500, 1970.

Reid HA: The principles of snakebite treatment. Clin Toxicol 3:473–482, 1970.

Sadan N, Soroker B: Observations on the effects of the bite of a venomous snake on children and adults. J Pediat 76:711, 1970.

SOAPS, HEXACHLOROPHENE, & DETERGENTS

1. SOAPS

Soap is made from salts of fatty acids. Some toilet soap bars contain both soap and detergent. Ingestion of soap bars may cause vomiting and diarrhea, but they have a low toxicity.

Dilute with milk or water. Induced emesis is unnecessary.

2. HEXACHLOROPHENE

Hexachlorophene is an antibacterial agent which is found in soaps, detergents, creams, etc. It is also dispensed as a 3% solution (pHisoHex). Cleansing of extensive areas of burned or abraded skin with pHisoHex and the application of pHisoHex wet dressings has resulted in a significant degree of absorption, CNS irritation, and convulsions. pHisoHex should be thoroughly cleaned off with water or saline to minimize its absorption.

pHisoHex placed in a cup or glass has also been confused with milk of magnesia and formula, resulting in ingestion, absorption of large amounts of the agent, and deaths. Nausea, vomiting, diarrhea, abdominal cramps, convulsions, dehydration, and shock have occurred following ingestion of pHisoHex.

Induce vomiting and carefully monitor fluid and electrolyte balance. Anticonvulsants, vasoconstrictors, and sedatives may be needed.

3. DETERGENTS

Detergents are nonsoap synthetic products used for cleaning purposes because of their surfactant properties. Commercial products include granules, powders, and liquids. Electric dishwasher detergent granules are very alkaline and can cause hypocalcemia, shock, and cyanosis. Low concentrations of bleaching and antibacterial agents as well as enzymes are found in many preparations. Although these pure compounds are moderately toxic, the concentration used is too small to significantly alter the product's toxicity although occasional primary or allergic irritative phenomena have been noted in housewives and in employees manufacturing these products.

There are 3 general types of detergents: cationic, anionic, and nonionic.

Cationic Detergents (Zephiran, Diaperene, Ceepryn, Phemerol)

Nausea, vomiting, collapse, coma, and convulsions may occur. The estimated fatal dose is approximately 1 gm of pure product/sq m of body area. Death is most likely in the first 4 hours, as cationic detergents are rapidly inactivated by tissues and ordinary soap.

Induce vomiting and follow with a saline cathartic. Ordinary soap is an effective antidote for unabsorbed cationic detergents. Anticonvulsants may be needed. Analeptics are likely to aggravate seizures and should not be used.

Anionic Detergents

Most common household detergents are anionic—Tide, Cheer, etc. Laundry compounds (All, etc) have water softener (sodium phosphate) added, which acts as a corrosive and may reduce ionized calcium. Anionic detergents irritate the skin by removing natural oils. Although ingestion causes diarrhea, intestinal distention, and vomiting, no fatalities have been reported. The LD_{50} in animals ranges from 1–5 gm/kg.

The only treatment usually required is to discontinue use if skin irritation occurs. Induced vomiting is not indicated following ingestion of electric dishwasher detergent because of its strong alkalinity. Dilute with water or milk. Give 5 ml of 10% calcium gluconate IV if the patient has hypocalcemia.

Nonionic Detergents (Tritons X-45, X-100, X-102, X-114 and Brij products)

These compounds include lauryl, stearyl, and oleyl alcohols and octyl phenol. They have a minimal irritating effect on the skin and are nontoxic when swallowed.

Anon: Enzyme detergents. Brit MJ 1:518, 1970.

Calandra JC & Faucher OE: *Cleaning Products and Their Accidental Ingestion.* The Soap and Detergent Association (New York), 1969.

Jeven JE: Severe dermatitis and "biological" detergents. Brit MJ 1:299, 1970.

Newhouse ML & others: An epidemiological study of workers producing enzyme washing powders. Lancet 1:689–693, 1970.

SPIDER BITES

At least 50 species of spiders have been implicated in human spider bites, but most toxic reactions in the USA are caused by the black widow spider (*Latrodectus mactans*) and the North American brown recluse (violin) spider (*Loxosceles reclusus*). Many spider venoms have common chemical and pharmacologic properties. Positive identification of the spider is helpful since many spider bites may mimic those of the brown recluse spider.

Black Widow Spider

The black widow spider, which is endemic to nearly all areas of the USA, causes most of the deaths due to spider bites. The initial bite may be hemorrhagic and associated with a sharp fleeting pain. Local and systemic muscular cramping, abdominal pain, nausea and vomiting, and shock can occur. Convulsions are more commonly seen in small children. Systemic signs of black widow spider bite are often confused with other causes of acute abdomen. Although paresthesias, nervousness, and transient muscle spasms may persist for months in survivors, recovery from the acute phase is generally complete within 3 days.

Following negative intradermal or conjunctival skin tests for horse serum sensitivity (see Chapter 5), 2.5 ml of restored Lyovac antivenin (Merck Sharp & Dohme) should be given IM. If sensitivity tests for horse serum are positive, antivenin should not be given

unless essential to save life. Symptoms usually subside in 1–3 hours, but a second dose of antivenin is occasionally required. Give 5–20 ml of 10% calcium gluconate IV to relieve muscle cramps. Hydrocortisone, 25–100 mg IV, or methocarbamol (Robaxin), 15 mg/kg/dose IV every 6 hours at a rate not to exceed 3 ml/minute, may be useful. Morphine or barbiturates may occasionally be needed for control of pain or restlessness, but they increase the possibility of respiratory depression.

Local treatment of the bite is not helpful.

Brown Recluse Spider (Violin Spider)

The North American brown recluse spider is most commonly seen in the central and midwestern areas of the USA. Its bite characteristically produces a localized reaction with progressively severe pain within 8 hours. The initial bleb on an erythematous ischemic base is replaced by a black eschar within a week. This eschar separates in 2–5 weeks, leaving a poorly healing ulcer which may result in keloid formation. Systemic signs include cyanosis, morbilliform rash, fever, chills, malaise, weakness, nausea and vomiting, joint pains, hemolytic reactions with hemoglobinuria, jaundice, and delirium. Fatalities are rare.

There is no specific antivenin. Local infiltration with phentolamine (Regitine) has been tried because the venin contains norepinephrine, but this procedure is not recommended because of the potential serious systemic reactions that may occur. Hydrocortisone sodium succinate (Solu Cortef), 1 gm/24 hours IV, is specifically indicated for systemic complications. Hydroxyzine (Atarax, Vistaril), 1 mg/kg/day IM, is reportedly useful because of its muscle relaxant, antihistaminic, and tranquilizing effects. The advisibility of total excision of the lesion at the fascial level to minimize necrosis is debatable.

Arena JM: Pages 454–458 in: *Poisoning,* 2nd ed. Thomas, 1970.

Bolton M: The brown spider bite. J Kansas Med Soc 71:197–201, 1970.

Frazier CA: *Insect Allergy: Allergic and Toxic Reactions to Insects and Other Arthropods.* Warren Green, 1969.

Gorham JR, Rheney TB: Envenomation by the spiders *Chiracanthium inclusum* and *Argiope aurantia.* JAMA 206:1958–1962, 1968.

Russell FE, Waldron WG: Spider bites, tick bites. California Med 106:247–148, 1967.

STRYCHNINE

Strychnine poisoning is characterized by restlessness, apprehension, perceptual difficulties, and simultaneous contraction of all muscles, resulting in opisthitonos, respiratory depression, cyanosis, and a characteristic tetanic contraction of the face (risus sardonicus). The patient is conscious throughout the convulsion and is in great pain. Complete muscle relaxation frequently occurs between convulsions. The onset of symptoms is 10–20 minutes after exposure.

Strychnine can be found in household products such as rodenticides, tonics, and cathartics. It is also occasionally added to hallucinogenic drugs. Deaths have been reported after ingestion of as little as 15 mg.

Treatment

If the patient is seen before the onset of symptoms, vomiting should be induced after administration of activated charcoal, which is a very efficient adsorber of strychnine. Apomorphine should be used to induce vomiting since ipecac is also adsorbed by activated charcoal. Convulsions can be controlled with diazepam (Valium), 1–2 mg/kg IV, short-acting barbiturates, or mephenesin (Tolserol), 2% solution, 1–3 ml/kg slowly IV. External stimulation should be minimized. Forced acid diuresis and peritoneal dialysis are very helpful since strychnine is not significantly protein-bound and is present in large concentration in the serum. It is rapidly cleared in the urine. The hyperacute nature of strychnine intoxication makes hemodialysis impractical.

Maron BJ, Krupp JR, Tane B: Strychnine poisoning successfully treated with diazepam. J Pediat 78:697–699, 1971.
Teitelbaum DT, Ott JE: Management of strychnine intoxication. Clin Toxicol 3:267–273, 1970.

THYROID PREPARATIONS
(Desiccated Thyroid, Sodium Levothyroxine [Synthroid])

Ingestion of the equivalent of 50–150 gr of desiccated thyroid can cause signs of hyperthyroidism, including irritability, mydriasis, hyperpyrexia, tachycardia, and diarrhea. Maximal clinical effect occurs about 9 days after ingestion—several days after the PBI has fallen dramatically.

Induce vomiting. Chlorpromazine (Thorazine) is useful if the patient develops clinical signs of toxicity because of its adrenergic and anticholinergic activity.

Funderburk SJ, Spaulding JS: Sodium levothyroxine (Synthroid) intoxication in a child. Pediatrics 45:298–301, 1970.

TURPENTINE

Turpentine is used as a solvent in oil-base paints, polishes, and varnishes. Children have died after ingesting 15 ml of it. Nausea, vomiting, abdominal pain, and diarrhea are common early signs in intoxicated patients. CNS stimulation followed by depression and respiratory arrest occur later. Reversible renal damage may occur, but renal failure is rare. The urine has an odor of violets due to the turpentine-glycuronate complex in the urine.

Induce vomiting and then give milk or other demulcent to reduce gastric irritation. Oxygen and artificial respiration may be required. If pulmonary and renal function are satisfactory, forced diuresis should be done. If symptoms were due to inhalation, the patient should be removed from the contaminated atmosphere.

Sperling F: In vivo and in vitro toxicology of turpentine. Clin Toxicol 2:21–35, 1969.
Wahlberg P: Turpentine and thrombocytopenic purpura. Lancet 2:215–216, 1969.

VITAMINS

Accidental ingestion of excessive amounts of vitamins rarely causes significant problems. Occasional cases of hypervitaminosis A and D do occur, however, particularly in patients with poor hepatic or renal function. The fluoride contained in many multivitamin preparations is not a realistic hazard since a 2 or 3 year old child could eat 100 tablets, containing 1 mg of sodium fluoride per tablet, without producing serious symptoms.

Moncrieff MW: Nephrotoxic effect of vitamin D therapy in vitamin D refractory rickets. Arch Dis Child 44:571–579, 1969.
Morrice G: Papilledema and hypervitaminosis A. JAMA 213:1344, 1970.
Seelig MS: Vitamin D and cardiovascular, renal, and brain damage in infancy and childhood. Ann New York Acad Sc 147:539–582, 1969.

WARFARIN

Warfarin is used as a pesticide. It causes hypoprothrombinemia and capillary injury. It is readily absorbed from the gastrointestinal tract but is absorbed poorly through the skin. One to 2 mg/kg/day (or 0.5 kg of rat bait at one ingestion) are required to cause severe toxic effects in humans. Warfarin is more toxic to dogs. A prothrombin time is helpful in establishing the severity of the poisoning. Chloral hydrate potentiates the hypoprothrombinemic effect of warfarin.

Treatment consists of induced vomiting followed by a saline cathartic. If bleeding occurs or the prothrombin time is prolonged, give 10–50 mg of vitamin K IV.

Monro P: Iatrogenic encephalopathy. Postgrad MJ 46:327–329, 1970.
Sellers EM: Potentiation of warfarin-induced hypoprothrombinemia by chloral hydrate. New England J Med 283:827–831, 1970.

●   ●   ●

General References

A Directory of Information Resources in the United States: General Toxicology. Library of Congress, US Government Printing Office, 1969.

Browning E: *Toxicity and Metabolism of Industrial Solvents.* Elsevier, 1965.

Browning E: *Toxicity of Industrial Metals,* 2nd ed. Butterworth, 1969.

Dreisbach RH: *Handbook of Poisoning: Diagnosis & Treatment,* 7th ed. Lange, 1971.

Gleason MN, Gosselin RE, Hodge HC: *Clinical Toxicology of Commercial Products,* 3rd ed. Williams & Wilkins, 1969.

Goodman LS, Gilman A: *The Pharmacological Basis of Therapeutics,* 4th ed. Macmillan, 1970.

Hardin JW, Arena JM: *Human Poisoning From Native and Cultivated Plants.* Duke Univ Press, 1969.

Hayes WJ: *Clinical Handbook on Economic Poisons.* US Department of Health, Education, & Welfare, 1963. [Available through most state health departments.]

Kozma JJ: *Killer Plants: A Poisonous Plant Guide.* Milestone Publishing Co., 1969. [Available from the author, Director, Poison Control Center, Passavant Memorial Area Hospital, Jacksonville, Ill.]

Matthew H, Lawson AA: *Treatment of Common Acute Poisonings.* Livingstone, 1967.

Meyer L, Herxhamer A: *Side Effects of Drugs.* Williams & Wilkins, 1968.

Moeschlin S: *Poisoning: Diagnosis and Treatment.* Grune & Stratton, 1965.

Polson CJ, Tattersall RN: *Clinical Toxicology.* Lippincott, 1969.

32 . . .

Neoplastic Diseases

Charlene P. Holton, MD

Cancer is the most common fatal disease of American children past the age of 1 year. Leukemias represent 40% of these cases, and various solid tumors constitute the remaining 60%. Survival rates are increasing, in part because of an increased awareness on the part of physicians that children may be born with or can develop cancer. Neoplastic diseases may masquerade as many other pediatric diseases and may present with almost any symptomatology. They should be kept in mind as diagnostic possibilities even in an apparently healthy child.

If malignancy is suspected or diagnosed, the determination of its cell type has assumed more importance with the development of multimodal therapy, incorporating surgery, radiation therapy, and chemotherapy early in treatment as indicated. In many hospitals, it has been estimated that approximately 30% of childhood cancers are either misdiagnosed or undiagnosed. The likelihood of diagnosis is increased through the use of special stains, tissue culture technics, biochemical studies, and electron microscopy.

Referral of children with neoplastic diseases should be made to regional cancer centers or universities that have multidisciplinary teams capable of developing a plan of therapy and follow-up using the latest combinations of anticancer drugs, supervoltage radiation therapy, surgery, and optimal supportive care. The primary physician has an important role in the multidisciplinary team approach to childhood cancer as a diagnostician in early case detection, as the on-site cancer therapist in the child's home community, and as a counselor to families with children who have cancer.

The causes of cancer in man are not known, although viral infection has been implicated in a few cases. Genetic disorders may predispose to certain types of neoplasia, and the role of environmental influences such as radiation or certain chemicals may be significant. A great number of childhood solid tumors are of embryonal origin and may be seen in the newborn nursery; the role of intrauterine environment in the causation of cancer needs further investigation.

LEUKEMIA

Essentials of Diagnosis

- Pallor, petechiae, fatigue, fever, bone pain.
- Lymph node enlargement, hepatosplenomegaly.
- Thrombocytopenia; low, normal, or elevated white count; normal or low hemoglobin.
- Diagnosis confirmed by bone marrow examination.

General Considerations

The acute leukemias of childhood constitute the major form of childhood neoplasia. Ninety percent are stem cell, undifferentiated, or lymphoblastic types, followed in frequency by myeloblastic leukemia. Chronic myelocytic leukemia makes up about 2.5% of cases and may be of the adult variety, with the Philadelphia chromosome present, or the juvenile form, which is not associated with a chromosomal abnormality and is more difficult to treat.

In acute leukemia, the median age at onset is 4 years, but the disease may be present at birth. When the disease presents in adolescence, it is often more difficult to control. Males are affected more frequently than females. Black children appear to respond less well to all forms of treatment.

In recent years the survival rate has increased 6-fold, and children are now enjoying longer periods of disease-free life. The advent of aggressive combination chemotherapy, advances in supportive care with blood component therapy, newer antibiotics to combat the infectious complications, and the recognition that foci of disease in the CNS and genitourinary tract must also be controlled have increased the rate of remissions and their duration.

Clinical Findings

A. Symptoms and Signs: The variable presenting complaints of children with acute leukemia are referable to marrow replacement with immature blast cells that crowd out normal elements of the marrow and to organ infiltration. The lack of red cell precursors leads to anemia, which may make the child pale, listless, irritable, and chronically tired. The lack of mature granulocytes makes the child more susceptible to infection, and a history of repeated infections prior to definitive diagnosis of leukemia is not unusual. The thrombocytopenia predisposes to bleeding episodes: epistaxis, petechiae, hematomas, or life-threatening hemorrhage. Organs may be infiltrated by disease and not function properly, may cause discomfort because of their large size, or may cause symptoms due to pressure on other structures. It is important to assess renal and liver function before chemotherapy is started so that drug toxicity will not occur if these organs are malfunctioning.

B. Laboratory Findings: Many patients present with elevated, normal, or low white blood counts, some degree of anemia, and thrombocytopenia. "Blasts" may predominate or may be absent on the peripheral blood smear. The diagnosis is confirmed by marrow examination, which shows a homogeneous infiltration of blast cells replacing the normal precursor cells. Special stains may be helpful in classifying the various types of acute leukemia. An elevated serum lactic acid dehydrogenase, sedimentation rate, and serum uric acid are nonspecific findings that support the diagnosis of leukemia.

Diagnostic Work-Up

Accurate evaluation of the child is essential in planning for therapy. The patients may present acutely ill with hemorrhage, infections, fluid and electrolyte imbalance, and malnutrition. In 5% of cases, CNS involvement is present at the time of diagnosis.

Prior to initiation of therapy, the following studies should be obtained:

A. Complete History and Physical Examination: Important features of the history are a family history of cancer, drugs used, radiation exposure, immunizations, and infectious diseases. A baseline photograph is often helpful to assess nutritional status and growth.

B. Laboratory Studies:

1. Complete blood count, phase platelet count, reticulocyte count, prothrombin time, and bone marrow aspiration or biopsy (or both).

2. Lumbar puncture with study of a Wright-stained smear of sediment for blast cells; sugar and protein determinations.

3. BUN, serum uric acid, bilirubin, SGOT, alkaline phosphatase, proteins, sodium, potassium, and lactic acid dehydrogenase.

4. Urinalysis.

5. Cultures and smears of mouth, throat, blood, bone marrow, skin lesions, urine, CSF, and stool should be taken immediately when infection is suspected. Fungal and viral cultures and serology should also be obtained when needed.

6. PPD intermediate strength skin test and endemic fungal skin tests.

C. ECG and X-Ray Studies: Electrocardiogram, intravenous urogram, chest x-ray, and skeletal survey.

D. Psychiatric Evaluation: A psychosocial inventory is often helpful as a baseline for future management of difficult emotional problems that might occur.

Differential Diagnosis

Early in the course of the disease, leukemia may mimic rheumatic fever, rheumatoid arthritis, viral diseases such as infectious mononucleosis or hepatitis, or other neoplastic diseases such as neuroblastoma or Letterer-Siwe disease.

Specific Treatment

The goal of therapy is to prolong useful life and disease-free status.

A. Acute Lymphocytic and Stem Cell Leukemia: The theoretical aim of antileukemic chemotherapy is the elimination of blasts from the body; an average 30 kg child might present with 1 kg of blast cells at the time of diagnosis. This leukemic blast population doubles in number approximately every 4 days.

The average duration of induction therapy to achieve complete remission (absence of measurable signs of disease) is about 4–6 weeks. The use of vincristine (Oncovin), 1.5 mg/sq m in an IV push weekly for 4–6 weeks, and prednisone, 40 mg/sq m orally daily in 3 divided doses for 4–6 weeks, has induced complete remission in 85–95% of children with acute lymphocytic leukemia with little toxicity.

Patients in complete remission with improved clinical status can then tolerate high-dosage intensive combinations of chemotherapy aimed at further reduction of residual leukemia cells. An intensive course of therapy is given daily for 1 week with large intravenous doses of methotrexate, mercaptopurine, and cyclophosphamide.

The child is then maintained on oral combination chemotherapy for 3–5 years depending upon response and toxicity. More often, the dosage of chemotherapeutic agents is tailored to the patient's biologic response to therapy rather than administered in calculated set dosages, ie, the physician attempts to keep the child's white blood count somewhere between 2000–3500/cu mm without oral ulceration, severe vomiting, diarrhea, hematuria, or repeated intercurrent infections. The average tolerated dosage schedule is as follows: mercaptopurine, 50 mg/sq m/day orally; one weekly dose of methotrexate, 20 mg/sq m orally; and cyclophosphamide, 200 mg/sq m orally.

Some centers are attempting periodic reinductions as "pulse" therapy every 3 months with vincristine and prednisone to attack cells that may manifest resistance to drugs used during the maintenance phase.

B. Central Nervous System Leukemia: The problem of CNS involvement with leukemia has been recognized in up to 50% of cases of acute lymphocytic leukemia at some time in the course of the disease. Symptoms include headache, vomiting, cranial nerve palsies, photophobia, lethargy, meningismus, hyperphagia, polydipsia, polyuria, and weight gain. The diagnosis may be suspected if ophthalmoscopic examination reveals blurred optic disks or if x-ray shows a spreading of cranial sutures in younger children. A lumbar puncture with examination of a Wright-stained smear of the centrifugate from a 2–5 ml sample of spinal fluid may reveal lymphoblasts. This complication may be treated with methotrexate, 12 mg/sq m intrathecally (diluted with sterile water without preservatives) weekly until the fluid is clear. Cranial or cranial and spinal radiation is being studied as a means of preventing this problem, and may be used therapeutically if resistance to methotrexate develops.

If a child relapses in spite of the above measures, reinduction with vincristine and prednisone may result in 40–70% second and third induction rates. Should induction fail, newer experimental agents such as adriamycin or L-asparaginase may be considered if the child can be carefully monitored by physicians trained in chemotherapy.

C. Acute Myeloblastic Leukemia: The treatment of acute myeloblastic leukemia has also improved with the advent of combination therapy; 50–60% of patients achieve initial remission. Combination chemotherapy consists of mercaptopurine, 75 mg/sq m orally for 28–42 days, plus vincristine, 1.5 mg/sq m IV weekly, and prednisone, 40 mg/sq m orally daily in 3 divided doses. Arabinosyl cytosine (cytarabine), 150 mg/sq m IV or IM weekly, and mercaptopurine, 50 mg/sq m orally daily, is suggested maintenance. Cyclophosphamide, 300 mg/sq m orally or IV, is also used by some experts in combination with the above.

D. Chronic Myelocytic Leukemia: Chronic myelocytic leukemia in the adult form that demonstrates the Philadelphia (Ph) chromosome is treated with busulfan (Myleran) beginning with 10–12 mg/day orally and reducing the dosage to 2–4 mg/day when the white blood count reaches 15,000/cu mm. The white count should remain between 5000–10,000/cu mm, and the dosage is adjusted as necessary to achieve this response.

The juvenile non-Philadelphia chromosome (Ph-negative) form of chronic myelocytic leukemia is seen in younger children. Bleeding secondary to thrombocytopenia, organomegaly, and repeated infections makes this form of disease difficult to control clinically. Attempts at various forms of chemotherapy have not been successful. Transient relief of pressure symptoms has been accomplished by splenic irradiation with [60]Co. Splenectomy has improved survival in few patients.

E. Erythroleukemia: Erythroleukemia and monocytic leukemia are extremely rare. The drugs used in the treatment of acute myeloblastic leukemia may be used.

Supportive & Adjunctive Treatment

A. Massive Tumor Tissue: In the presence of leukemic leukocytosis, massive splenomegaly, nephromegaly, thymomegaly, or initial hyperuricemia, initiate the following regimen and continue it during the period of maximum tumor catabolism (3–7 days).

1. Give allopurinol (Zyloprim), 100–150 mg/sq m orally twice daily.

2. Provide liquids, 2–3 liters/sq m orally or IV (or both). Avoid potassium-containing parenteral solutions during tumor catabolism.

3. Give sodium bicarbonate, 3–4 gm/sq m/day orally in 4–6 divided doses, to maintain a urine pH of 6.5–7.0.

4. Record liquid intake and urinary output.

5. Determine urine pH (at bedside) at each voiding, to determine whether urine pH is 6.5–7.0.

6. Perform urinalysis and determine BUN, serum uric acid, and serum potassium daily for 3 days or until values are normal.

7. Prescribe a regular diet for age with no salt added.

B. Nephromegaly: If there is considerable nephromegaly as manifested by palpable kidneys or by calyceal abnormalities on urography—or if there is evidence of renal dysfunction—the following measures are suggested:

1. Start chemotherapy using only prednisone, 20 mg/sq m/day orally in 2 divided doses.

2. Deliver radiotherapy to the kidneys in a total dosage of 100–300 rads over several days.

3. When renal function appears to be normal, prednisone and vincristine in full doses should be initiated cautiously.

C. Hepatic Dysfunction: If there is evidence of hepatic dysfunction (not hepatomegaly only) as manifested by such signs as elevation of serum bilirubin, SGOT, and alkaline phosphatase and prolonged prothrombin time, vincristine should be used cautiously.

D. Infection: Cultures of blood and bone marrow and smears and cultures of the pharynx, nasopharynx (if no bleeding), rectal swabs, and urine should be taken on admission and repeated as necessary. Gram-stained smears of infected lesions and body orifices should be examined immediately. Full doses of appropriate bactericidal antibiotics should be used as soon as infection is suspected. If paronychia or other skin infections occur, 0.3 ml saline should be injected and aspirated for smear and culture. Do not wait for "pointing." Urinary tract infections may exist without pyuria in the granulocytopenic child. Do not delay antibiotic chemotherapy. Suspect *Escherichia coli,* klebsiella-enterobacter, or staphylococcal infection if the child has been on penicillin. Suspect pseudomonas or candida infection if the child has been receiving broad spectrum antibiotics. Antibiotic therapy should be narrow spectrum whenever possible, pinpointing the target bacteria. Intravenous administration is recommended.

Prolonged antibiotic therapy should be avoided. It is better to risk some recurrences than to upset the child's flora more than absolutely necessary.

Unusual infections such as *Pneumocystis carinii* pneumonia may be treated with pentamidine given cautiously intravenously. Fungal infections require prolonged treatment with amphotericin B given intravenously. The patient is often plagued by his own flora, which, in the debilitated state that occurs during relapse, may lead to sepsis with *E coli,* pseudomonas, or staphylococci.

The classical symptoms of infection may be masked by immunosuppressive chemotherapy. Children may have life-threatening infections with rubeola and varicella. The parents need to be educated regarding notification of the physician when the child shows symptoms of infection or has been exposed to contagious diseases. No live virus vaccines should be given to leukemic children.

E. Persistent Leukemic Organomegaly: Local radiotherapy should be given for leukemic organomegaly persisting at day 28 of induction therapy. Chemotherapy should not be interrupted.

F. Additional Precautions:

1. A "no salt added" diet is prescribed when the patient is on prednisone.

2. Avoid deep venipunctures, intramuscular injections, and instrumentation with catheters, laryngoscopes, and the like in children with bleeding tendencies. Avoid tight clothing.

3. Avoid administration of barium sulfate during vincristine therapy. Give the child fruit, fruit juice, and plenty of liquids to help prevent constipation due to vincristine. Peri-Colace may be tried.

4. For nausea and vomiting, give antiemetics orally or as suppositories and fluids if needed.

5. Good nutrition and well balanced meals are essential. Providing extra fluids on the day before and the day of cyclophosphamide therapy helps decrease bladder toxicity.

G. Psychologic Support of Patient and Family: The emotional impact of the diagnosis of leukemia is often overwhelming and affects the entire family. A thorough discussion with the parents regarding diagnosis, prognosis, plan of therapy, toxicities of treatment, and their own role in the care of the child is mandatory initially and throughout the course of the disease.

What to tell the patient depends upon the maturity of the child and the judgment of physicians and family about the problems at hand. The author recommends a frank discussion of the disease with the adolescent patient. The discussion should be factual and honest, emphasizing the hopeful aspects and offering reassurance that progress is being made.

At times, psychologic guidance may be needed for siblings, parents, and patient, and appropriate professional consultation should be obtained.

Prognosis

In the past, the average survival in acute leukemia was 3–6 months and the leading cause of death was hemorrhage. The leading cause of death is now infection and resistant disease. Centers are now reporting mean survival rates (6-year leukemia-free intervals) of 17% when modern combination chemotherapy, radiation, and supportive care are used. Physicians must realize that advances in treatment have been made and are available for their patients.

Aur RJA & others: Central nervous system therapy and combination chemotherapy of childhood lymphocytic leukemia. Blood 37:272, 1971.

Crowther D & others: Combination chemotherapy using L-asparaginase, daunorubicin, and cytosine arabinoside in adults with acute myelogenous leukemia. Brit MJ 4:513, 1970.

George P & others: A study of "total therapy" of acute lymphocytic leukemia in children. J Pediat 72:399, 1968.

Holton CP, Johnson WW: Chronic myelocytic leukemia in infant siblings. J Pediat 72:377, 1968.

Pinkel D & others: Drug dosage and remission duration in childhood lymphocytic leukemia. Cancer 27:247, 1971.

LYMPHOMAS

1. HODGKIN'S DISEASE

Essentials of Diagnosis

- Fever, night sweats, pruritus.
- Fatigue and weight loss.
- Hepatomegaly, splenomegaly, lymphadenopathy.
- Cold intolerance..

General Considerations

The clinical course of Hodgkin's disease has been favorably altered by advances in diagnostic and therapeutic technics introduced in the past several years. The obsolete view that Hodgkin's disease was invariably fatal has been challenged by modern concepts of diagnostic evaluation and therapy such as lymphangiography, laparotomy, splenectomy, and optimal treatment with intensive extended-field megavoltage radiation therapy and combination chemotherapy.

The disease occurs twice as frequently in men as in women, with its peak incidence in the third decade. It has been reported in children as young as 3 years of age. The cause is not known.

The histologic classification of Hodgkin's disease has been modified from the classical Jackson & Parker description as shown in Table 32–1.

Clinical staging has also been modified. The proposed Stanford Classification of 1970 is shown in Table 32–2.

The subclassification of (A) absence or (B) presence of systemic symptoms (fever, night sweats, pruritus, and a 10% weight loss) is also of prognostic value in staging.

Clinical Findings

A. Symptoms and Signs: The occurrence of anorexia, weight loss, fatigue, weakness, fever, malaise, pruritus, night sweats, and pain on ingestion of alcohol are variable in degree. The most common site of nodal involvement is the cervical region. Involved nodes are usually firm and nontender and may produce pressure symptoms depending upon their location, which may be anywhere. Hepatosplenomegaly and extranodal disease in any organ may be present.

TABLE 32–1. Histologic classification of Hodgkin's disease.

Jackson & Parker	Rye, 1965	Distinctive Features	Relative Frequency
Paragranuloma	Lymphocyte predominance	Abundant stroma of mature lymphocytes, histiocytes, or both; no necrosis; Reed-Sternberg cells may be sparse.	10–15%
	Nodular sclerosis	Nodules of lymphoid tissue, partially or completely separated by bands of doubly refractile collagen of variable width; atypical Reed-Sternberg cells in clear spaces ("lacunae") in the lymphoid nodules.	20–50%
Granuloma	Mixed cellularity	Usually numerous Reed-Sternberg and atypical mononuclear cells with a pleomorphic admixture of plasma cells, eosinophils, lymphocytes, and fibroblasts; foci of necrosis commonly seen.	20–40%
Sarcoma	Lymphocyte depletion	Reed-Sternberg and malignant mononuclear cells usually, though not always, numerous; marked paucity of lymphocytes; diffuse fibrosis and necrosis may be present.	5–15%

B. Laboratory Findings: Hematologic findings may be normal or may show anemia, leukocytosis, leukopenia, thrombocytosis, thrombocytopenia, eosinophilia, or elevated sedimentation rate. Kidney and liver function tests or scans may reflect abnormalities if involved with disease.

Immunologic defects as a reflection of abnormalities of the cell-mediated immune responses may be seen in abnormal delayed hypersensitivity to PPD, candidal extract, and streptokinase-streptodornase skin test antigens. Hemolytic anemia and abnormal levels of immunoglobulins may also occur.

The diagnosis is confirmed by biopsy of the involved node followed by bone marrow biopsy, clinical staging, and laparotomy with multiple abdominal node biopsies, liver biopsy, and splenectomy.

C. X-Ray Findings: Chest x-ray may show parenchymal or mediastinal nodal disease. Skeletal survey may show bone involvement. The intravenous urogram may show diversion of the ureter or bladder; a lateral view is often helpful to show anterior displacement. Lymphangiography may reveal a "foamy" enlarged node which implies tumor filling the node.

Complications

Patients with Hodgkin's disease are more susceptible to herpes zoster, tuberculosis, and fungal infections. Side-effects of treatment such as nausea, vomiting, anorexia, neurotoxicity, alopecia, bladder toxicity, and marrow depression should be monitored closely and medication adjusted. Radiation pneumonitis, growth changes, skin changes, and marrow depression secondary to radiation therapy may also occur.

The psychologic effects of this diagnosis and its treatment occurring in the adolescent age group commonly require good rapport between the patient and physician.

Treatment

After the patient is properly staged, he should receive the optimum benefits of megavoltage extended-field radiation by a radiation therapist skilled in the treatment of the growing child to minimize the side-effects of radiation.

Combination chemotherapy is superior to single drug therapy, as shown by a 50% response rate in patients receiving 4-drug therapy versus a 15% response rate in patients treated with mechlorethamine alone. Agents commonly used in combination are vincristine plus cyclophosphamide, prednisone, and procarbazine. The dosage, schedule, and duration of therapy are dependent on the stage of the disease and the patient's tolerance. Experimental drugs such as BCNU (bis-chlor-nitrosourea) and streptonigrin are under study.

A. Stages I and I-E:

1. Induction phase–

a. Radiation therapy–Supervoltage radiation to begin as soon as possible after diagnosis. Deliver 3500 rad tumor dose to the involved area and a similar dose to contiguous lymph node areas.

TABLE 32–2. Clinical staging of Hodgkin's disease.

Stage I	Involvement of a single lymph node region (I) or of a single extralymphatic organ or site (I-E).
Stage II	Involvement of 2 or more lymph node regions on the same side of the diaphragm (II), or solitary involvement of an extralymphatic organ or site and of one or more lymph node regions on the same side of the diaphragm (II-E).
Stage III	Involvement of lymph node regions on both sides of the diaphragm (III), which may also be accompanied by involvement of the spleen (III-S) or by solitary involvement of an extralymphatic organ or site (III-E), or both (III-SE).
Stage IV	Multiple or disseminated foci of involvement of one or more extralymphatic organs or tissues, with or without associated lymph node involvement.

b. Rest period—For 4 weeks after completion of radiation therapy.

c. Chemotherapy—Begin after rest period if white count is above 3000/cu mm. Give cyclophosphamide, 3–5 mg/kg/day orally for 6 weeks, and vincristine, 1.5 mg/sq m/week IV for 6 weeks. (Top dosage level is 2 mg.)

2. Continuation phase—None.

B. Stage II:

1. Induction phase—

a. Radiation therapy—Supervoltage radiation to begin as soon as possible after diagnosis. Deliver 3500 rad tumor dose to extended fields well beyond the limits of the known nodal involvement.

b. Rest period—For 3 weeks after completion of radiation therapy.

c. Chemotherapy—Begin after rest period if white count is above 3000/cu mm. Give cyclophosphamide, 3–5 mg/kg/day orally for 6 weeks, and vincristine, 1.5 mg/sq m/week IV for 6 weeks.

2. Continuation phase—Cyclophosphamide, 3–5 mg/kg/day orally for 2 years, and vincristine, 1.5 mg/sq m every 2 weeks IV for 2 years.

C. Stages II-E and III:

1. Induction phase—

a. Radiation therapy—Deliver 3500 rad tumor dose to extended fields if tolerated.

b. Rest period—For 4 weeks following completion of radiotherapy.

c. Chemotherapy—Give one dose on first day of radiotherapy of vincristine, 1.5 mg/sq m IV, and cyclophosphamide, 300 mg/sq m IV. Give prednisone, 40 mg/sq m orally for 6 weeks, and then taper and discontinue.

2. Continuation phase—Vincristine, 1.5 mg/sq m IV every 2 weeks, and cyclophosphamide, 3–5 mg/kg/day orally for 2 years.

D. Stages III-S, III-E, III-SE, and IV:

1. Induction phase—

a. Radiation therapy—Give radiation therapy immediately in life-threatening disease; otherwise, withhold until completion of induction phase chemotherapy. Give radiation therapy to residual tumor masses after induction chemotherapy. Radiation therapy may be increased to 400 rads in adolescents at the discretion of the radiation therapist.

b. Chemotherapy—Give cyclophosphamide, 3–5 mg/kg/day orally for 6 weeks; vincristine, 1.5 mg/sq m/week IV for 6 weeks; procarbazine, 100 mg/sq m/day orally for 6 weeks; and prednisone, 40 mg/sq m/day orally for 6 weeks, and then taper and discontinue.

2. Continuation phase—Cyclophosphamide, 3–5 mg/kg/day orally for 2 years, and vincristine, 1.5 mg/sq m every 2 weeks IV for 2 years.

3. Pulse phase—Procarbazine pulse every 4 months: 100 mg/sq m/day orally for 3 weeks and then discontinue; prednisone pulse every 4 months: 40 mg/sq m/day orally for 3 weeks and then taper and discontinue.

Prognosis

The prognosis in adequately irradiated patients who have been staged with laparotomy has been greatly improved. In stages I and II, 5-year survival rates range from 85–90%; in stage III-A, the average survival rate is 70%; and in stage III-B it is 40–50%. Duration of symptom-free life is also being lengthened by chemotherapy in stage IV disease.

Glatstein E & others: The value of laparotomy and splenectomy in the staging of Hodgkin's disease. Cancer 24:709, 1969.

Kadin M, Glatstein E, Dorfman R: Clinicopathologic studies of 117 untreated patients subjected to laparotomy for the staging of Hodgkin's disease. Cancer 27:1277, 1971.

Rosenberg S, Kaplan H: Hodgkin's disease and other malignant lymphomas. California Med 113:23, Oct 1970.

NONHODGKIN'S LYMPHOMA

A new classification of this diverse group of lymphomas proposed by Gall & Rapport is based on the architecture of the node, whether the disease is nodular or diffuse, and the cytologic differentiation of lymphocytes and histiocytes. This group includes the former "lymphosarcomas"—reticulum cell sarcomas or tumors with giant follicular cell patterns.

Burkitt's tumor (African lymphoma) is a special type of childhood lymphoma found principally in Africa. A few cases have been reported in the USA. This tumor is responsible for 1/2 of all cancer deaths in children in Uganda and Central Africa. A viral etiology has been assumed, and Epstein-Barr virus is under scrutiny. The tumor is characterized by (1) primary involvement of abdominal nodes and viscera, (2) predilection for the facial bones and mandible, and (3) massive proliferation of primitive lymphoreticular cells and phagocytosis on histologic examination.

Clinical Findings

A. Symptoms and Signs: The primary site of involvement differs from that of Hodgkin's disease in the mode of presentation. The gastrointestinal tract in the region of the terminal ileum, cecum, appendix, ascending colon, and mesenteric nodes is the most common site. Boys outnumber girls 9:1. Acute abdominal pain, intussusception, gastrointestinal tract perforation, and hemorrhage may occur. Involvement of the tonsillar region, cervical nodes, and nasopharynx may be diagnosed by the presence of a mass or compression symptoms. The mediastinum and retroperitoneal nodes may be involved as well as any superficial nodal chain. The incidence of children developing marrow involvement with a leukemia-like picture is 20–50% of cases; this is most frequently seen when the mediastinum is involved. The CNS may also be involved; a lumbar puncture or brain scan may be helpful in confirming this diagnosis.

B. Laboratory Findings: These patients should be studied as Hodgkin's patients with the exception of routine exploratory laparotomy and splenectomy. Laboratory findings depend on organ, nodal, or marrow involvement.

Treatment

Surgical resection of extranodal disease, when possible, is advocated, followed by megavoltage radiation therapy to the tumor bed or regional nodes. Combination chemotherapy should be started as soon as possible and continued for 2–3 years. The drugs most commonly used are vincristine, 1.5 mg/sq m IV weekly for 6 weeks and then every 2 weeks; prednisone, 40 mg/sq m orally daily in 3 divided doses; cyclophosphamide, 300 mg/sq m IV weekly for 6 weeks and then every 2 weeks; and procarbazine, 100 mg/sq m IV weekly for 6 weeks and then every 2 weeks. Mercaptopurine and methotrexate are occasionally used.

Prognosis

The prognosis in non-Hodgkin's lymphoma is not as good as in Hodgkin's disease, and many children die with a conversion to a leukemic phase.

Jenkins T, Sonley M: The management of malignant lymphoma in childhood. Pages 305–320 in: *Neoplasia in Childhood.* Year Book, 1969.

Rosenberg S, Kaplan H: Hodgkin's disease and other malignant lymphomas. California Med 113:23, Oct 1970.

NEUROBLASTOMA

Essentials of Diagnosis

- Asymptomatic abdominal mass, subcutaneous nodules, posterior mediastinal mass, and organomegaly.
- Fever, anemia, weakness, "black eyes," proptosis, opsoclonia, and diarrhea.
- Bone pain, paraplegia, and ataxia.

General Considerations

Neuroblastoma is a tumor arising from cells in the sympathetic ganglia and adrenal medulla. It is the third most frequent pediatric neoplasm. Clinically, the survival rates are much better in children under 2 years of age, in children with extra-adrenal tumor, and in those with localized disease. These tumors may spontaneously regress in 5–10% of cases. In routine autopsies of infants under 3 months of age dying of other causes, neuroblastoma in situ in the adrenal is seen 40 times more frequently than expected.

Immunologic factors may be very significant in the understanding of the biology of neuroblastoma. Many tumors show infiltration with lymphocytes and plasma cells. The colony inhibition test (Hellstrom) has shown the lymphocytes of neuroblastoma patients and, in some cases, of their mothers to be lethal in reacting against tumor cells in tissue culture.

Clinical staging of extent of disease is the basis of therapeutic planning. Several staging systems are advocated in the USA. The system used at The Children's Hospital of Denver, Colorado, and at St. Jude's Children's Research Hospital in Memphis, Tennessee, is as follows:

Stage I: Local, completely resected.
Stage II: Regional.
        A. Partially resected.
        B. Not resected.
Stage III: Systemic.
        A. Without involvement of bone marrow.
        B. With involvement of bone marrow.

Clinical Findings

A. Symptoms and Signs: The child most commonly presents at about age 2 with a palpable abdominal mass. The symptomatology depends upon the extent of disease at the time of diagnosis. Bone pain, weight loss, and fever may be the presenting complaints. Newborn infants may present with subcutaneous nodules and adrenal masses with marrow involvement. A high index of suspicion is needed for early diagnosis of this disease.

B. Laboratory Findings: Anemia and thrombocytopenia may be present secondary to marrow replacement by neuroblasts which may mimic leukemia.

The VMA spot test is a useful screening test for catecholamine excretion; a 24-hour excretion study of catecholamines preoperatively may be helpful as a baseline in following the patient if catecholamines are elevated initially. If the levels increase during follow-up, a recurrence may be suspected and reevaluation is advised. Urinary cystathionine is also present in 50% of children with neuroblastoma; it is independent of VMA excretion and may offer additional diagnostic help if the VMA is normal.

C. X-Ray Findings: Chest x-ray, skeletal survey, and intravenous urography aid in preoperative staging of the disease. Angiography may aid the surgeon in identifying the extent of the tumor and its blood supply; the tumor may be extremely vascular.

Treatment

Total surgical removal followed by megavoltage radiation to the tumor bed or area of regional spread, followed by vincristine and cyclophosphamide, is advocated in all stages. The duration and dosage of radiation therapy and chemotherapy are dependent on the age of the patient and the stage of the disease. Inoperable tumors often become amenable to surgery after radiation therapy and chemotherapy. Experimental agents under study in this disease are CCNU (chloroethyl-cyclohexyl-nitrosourea), daunomycin, adriamycin, and streptozotocin.

A. Stage I:

1. Surgical resection.
2. Radiotherapy (1800–3000 rads).

3. Chemotherapy—Vincristine, 1.5 mg/sq m IV, and cyclophosphamide, 300 mg/sq m IV, concurrently weekly for 6 weeks.

B. Stages II-A and II-B:

1. Radiotherapy (1800—3500 rads).

2. Chemotherapy—Vincristine, 1.5 mg/sq m IV, and cyclophosphamide, 300 mg/sq m IV, concurrently weekly for 6 weeks and then every other week for 46 weeks. Continue chemotherapy if evidence of disease persists at 46 weeks.

3. Surgical resection if and when it becomes possible.

C. Stages III-A and III-B:

1. Chemotherapy—Vincristine, 1.5 mg/sq m IV, and cyclophosphamide, 300 mg/sq m IV, concurrently weekly for 6 weeks and then every other week for 46 weeks. Continue chemotherapy if evidence of disease persists at 46 weeks.

2. Radiotherapy to local tumor masses; dosage and port must be individualized.

3. Surgical resection if and when only a local residual tumor persists.

Prognosis

The major problem in control of this disease is the fact that 75% of patients who present with symptoms related to metastatic spread are over age 2. Until physicians become more conscious of the cancer problem in children, the progress that has been made in treatment cannot be utilized to its fullest extent.

Pinkel D & others: Survival of children treated with combination chemotherapy. J Pediat 73:928—931, 1968.

Rubin P & others: Cancer of the urogenital tract: Wilms's tumor and neuroblastoma. JAMA 205:153—166, 1968.

Thurman W, Donaldson M: Current concepts in the management of neuroblastoma. Page 175 in: *Neoplasia in Childhood.* Year Book, 1969.

RENAL TUMORS

1. WILMS'S TUMOR

Essentials of Diagnosis

- Asymptomatic abdominal mass or abdominal pain.
- Hematuria, genitourinary anomalies, aniridia.
- Hypertension, fever.

General Considerations

Wilms's tumor follows neuroblastoma in frequency of occurrence of pediatric solid tumors. It is believed to be embryonal in origin, develops within the kidney parenchyma, and enlarges with distortion and invasion of the adjacent renal tissue. This tumor may be associated with congenital anomalies, and patients should be evaluated for Wilms's tumor if the following entities occur: hemihypertrophy, aniridia, ambiguous genitalia, hypospadias, undescended testes, duplications of the ureters or kidneys, horseshoe kidney, or Beckwith's syndrome.

Wilms's tumor more commonly presents as an abdominal mass—in contrast to renal tumors in adults, which usually present with hematuria. The incidence of bilateral Wilms's tumor is 2%. Metastases to the liver and lungs are present in 25% of patients under 2 years of age at the time of diagnosis; in children over 2 years of age, 50% show spread of disease at diagnosis.

Several systems of tumor staging exist for Wilms's tumor. The system used at The Children's Hospital in Denver, Colorado, and the University of Colorado Medical Center is as follows:

Stage I: Tumor confined to kidney.

    A. Tumor limited to kidney and less than 6 cm in size without renal capsule involvement.

    B. Tumor limited to kidney and greater than 6 cm in size with extension to renal capsule.

Stage II: Tumor confined to renal fossa.

    A. Local extension beyond renal capsule but no invasion of adjacent viscera or metastasis.

    B. Tumor in renal vessels.

    C. Positive lymph nodes at renal hilus.

Stage III: Tumor confined to abdomen.

    A. Invasion of adjacent viscera by direct extension only (ie, diaphragm, spleen, colon, stomach, pancreas, liver).

    B. Metastases confined to abdomen only. Tumor ruptured at time of surgery with peritoneal dissemination. Primary tumor not resectable.

    C. Involvement by tumor of vena cava; bilateral Wilms's tumor.

Stage IV: Disseminated tumor.

    Distant metastases outside abdomen (ie, lungs, bone, bone marrow, etc).

Clinical Findings

A. Symptoms and Signs: Children with Wilms's tumor may be asymptomatic, and a mass may be felt by the parent while dressing or washing the child or by a physician on a routine well baby examination. Occasionally, a tumor may be ruptured by a fall or trauma to the abdomen, and symptoms of an acute surgical abdomen occur.

The work-up of a child with an abdominal mass should be accomplished within 24 hours, and palpation of the abdomen should be gentle and infrequent.

B. Laboratory Findings: Complete blood count, reticulocyte count, platelet count, and bone marrow examination are needed as baselines for staging and for following therapy. Wilms's tumor rarely metastasizes to bone marrow, whereas neuroblastoma does so frequently. Urinalysis and urine culture may reveal hematuria or infection. BUN, serum creatinine, uric acid, bilirubin, alkaline phosphatase, lactic acid dehydrogenase, and SGOT are other baseline studies of importance for following treatment. Erythropoietin levels are followed in some centers and may aid in detecting tumor activity.

C. X-Ray Findings: Posterior-anterior, lateral, and oblique views of the chest should be taken to rule out pulmonary metastases. Intravenous urograms to define the tumor mass and an inferior venacavagram to rule out vascular invasion are suggested. In right-sided Wilms's tumor, a liver scan is helpful to rule out hepatic metastases.

Treatment

In 1956, a 47% cure rate with total excision of Wilms's tumor was reported. It is now proper to use a transabdominal approach to allow early ligation of the renal vessels, to avoid manipulation of the tumor, and to examine the abdominal viscera, nodes, and the opposite kidney for staging.

Radiation therapy to the renal fossa postoperatively has increased survival rate in some cases to 60%. Therapy with megavoltage equipment is begun following surgery. Dosages of 2000–3500 rads are given, depending on the age of the patient and the stage of the tumor. If the tumor is ruptured, the entire abdomen should be treated using lead shields to protect the remaining kidney.

In 1966, survival rates of 89% were reported when chemotherapy with dactinomycin was added to surgery and radiation therapy in 53 patients with operable tumors; 53% survival rates were reported in 15 children presenting with metastases. Chemotherapy with vincristine and dactinomycin in courses of 6–12 weeks has been effective and has tolerable toxicity. Radiation and chemotherapy are given concurrently; wound healing and adequate nutrition are important factors in following patients postoperatively. Chest films, complete blood counts, and renal function studies should be monitored during therapy. The duration of therapy depends on the patient's age and the extent of the disease.

The following treatment methods are those in use at The Children's Oncology Center and the University of Colorado Medical Center. Postoperative treatment (based on staging), radiation therapy, and chemotherapy are begun as soon as possible after recovery from surgery or when the diagnosis is established —usually within 72 hours.

A. Stage I-A:

1. **Chemotherapy**—Give the following concurrently for 6 weeks and then discontinue: vincristine, 1.5 mg/sq m IV weekly, and dactinomycin, 0.4 mg/sq m IV weekly.

2. **Radiation therapy**—None.

B. Stage I-B:

1. **Chemotherapy**—As above.

2. **Radiation therapy**—Deliver 2000–3000 rads (1000 rads/week) to the renal fossa with supervoltage radiation therapy equipment.

C. Stages II-A and II-B:

1. **Chemotherapy**—Give the following concurrently for 6 weeks: vincristine, 1.5 mg/sq m IV weekly, and dactinomycin, 0.4 mg/sq m weekly. Discontinue the dactinomycin and continue the vincristine for weeks 8, 10, and 12. Repeat this schedule every 3 months for 1 year and then discontinue if there is no recurrence.

2. **Radiation therapy**—Deliver 2000–3500 rads to the renal fossa with a 2–4 cm margin included in ports.

D. Stage II-C:

1. **Chemotherapy**—Same as for stages II-A and II-B for 1 year.

2. **Radiation therapy**—Deliver 2000–3500 rads to the entire abdomen with shielding of the remaining kidney after 1500 rads.

E. Stage III:

1. **Chemotherapy**—Same as in stages II-A and II-B, but extend every 3-month schedule for 2 years and discontinue.

2. **Radiation therapy**—Deliver 2000–3500 rads to the entire abdomen with the remaining kidney shielded. With bilateral tumors and involvement of the vena cava, dosage and ports must be individualized.

F. Stage IV:

1. **Chemotherapy**—Same as in stages II-A and II-B for 2 years; then reevaluate for further therapy.

2. **Radiation therapy**—Must be individually considered because of varied anatomic locations and age.

a. Pulmonary metastases—Both lungs are treated regardless of the number and location of metastases. The port is from the clavicle to the level of L1. The shoulders are shielded. The dosage is 1400 rads.

b. Liver metastases—In nonresectable lesions, deliver radiation to the involved part of the liver. If the entire organ is involved, the dosage is 3000 rads in 3½–4 weeks. The right kidney should be shielded if uninvolved.

c. Other—Bony lesions should have a 3 cm margin in any direction. In the case of cerebral metastases, treat the entire ipsilateral hemisphere with a minimum dosage as in liver metastases.

Prognosis

The 2-year survival rate continues to improve and is better in children under 2 years of age with localized disease. A National Wilms's Tumor Study is currently under way, various modalities of therapy are being tested, and new data will be generated for this disease, which now has a better outlook than in the past.

Farber S: Chemotherapy in the treatment of leukemia and Wilms's tumor. JAMA 198:826, 1966.

Fleming I, Johnson W: Clinical and pathologic staging as a guide in the management of Wilms's tumor. Cancer 26:660–665, 1970.

Martin RG: Multimodal treatment for Wilms's tumor. Pages 165–173 in: *Neoplasia in Childhood.* Year Book, 1969.

Rubin P & others: Cancer of the urogenital tract: Wilms's tumor and neuroblastoma. JAMA 205:153–166, 1968.

Schneider B & others: Wilms's tumor: The evaluation of a treatment program. Am J Roentgenol 108:92–97, 1970.

2. HYPERNEPHROMA

Hypernephroma, or clear cell carcinoma, rarely occurs in children. It presents with hematuria, abdominal pain, fever, and a palpable mass. Treatment consists of nephrectomy; the tumor is relatively resistant to radiation therapy. Chemotherapy in children with this disease has not been studied to any significant extent. The prognosis is good.

Edwardsen KF: Bilateral primary hypernephroma. Brit J Urol 39:746, 1967.

3. RENAL TUMORS IN THE NEONATAL PERIOD

Mesenchymal tumors of the kidney are rarely manifest in the first month of life, though common renal neoplasms are of nephroblastic origin. They should be differentiated from the malignant Wilms's tumor so that children are not overtreated with radiation and chemotherapy. These tumors are benign and may represent fibromyomas or fibromyomatous hamartomas.

Surgical removal is curative. The prognosis is good.

Favara B, Johnson W, Ito J: Renal tumors in the neonatal period. Cancer 22:845–854, 1968.

SOFT TISSUE TUMORS

Tumors arising in tissues of mesodermal origin may be malignant or benign. Histologically, they are of connective, fatty, or muscle tissue origin. The most common clinical complaint is of a painless lump that may arise at any site. These lumps should not be "watched" for long periods of time; surgical consultation with excisional biopsy is warranted. These tumors are too often diagnosed by means of incisional biopsy, which may disseminate the tumor and make a potentially curable lesion a widespread disease.

Classification

A. Malignant:
1. Rhabdomyosarcoma.
2. Malignant mesenchymoma.
3. Fibrosarcoma.

B. Benign:
1. Juvenile fibromatosis.
2. Lipomas.
3. Epulis.
4. Giant cell tumor.

1. RHABDOMYOSARCOMA

Rhabdomyosarcoma is the most common type of sarcoma in the somatic soft tissues of children. It is most commonly found in the first 2 decades of life and is an embryonal tumor. The 4 histologic types (with definite overlapping) are embryonal, alveolar, botryoid, and pleomorphic. Common sites of occurrence are the head and neck, extremities, orbits, and pelvic regions. The histologic pattern is variable and may be related to the site, ie, if arising in a luminal structure such as the bladder or nasopharynx where there is poor support, the tumor may assume a gelatinous or botryoid "grape-like" appearance—in contrast to the fleshy sarcomatous tumor within the body of a muscle bundle in an extremity, where a more alveolar pattern with cross-striations may be noted. This tumor is often misdiagnosed as neuroblastoma; special electron microscopic studies are needed for clarification and show primitive Z bands in the myofibrils.

The work-up should include chest x-ray, intravenous urograms, and bone marrow examination. Rhabdomyoblasts may appear in the marrow as primitive "tadpole" cells. Creatinine phosphokinase and lactic acid dehydrogenase may show some changes; renal and liver function studies should be obtained as baselines.

Treatment must be coordinated with staging:

Stage I: Localized disease, completely resectable.
Stage II: Regional disease.
    A. Completely resectable.
    B. Nonresectable or partially resectable, ie, pelvic lymph node involvement from sarcoma botryoides, infiltration of base of skull from a primary nasopharyngeal tumor.
Stage III: Generalized disease.
    A. Distant metastases with normal bone marrow.
    B. Distant metastases with positive bone marrow.

Cures are rare when single therapeutic modalities are used because of early infiltration of blood and lymphatics by tumor.

Surgery with wide margins is advocated, followed by radiation with ^{60}Co or electron beam therapy using the betatron with energies up to 25 meV at dosage levels of 4000–6000 rads. Ports should extend beyond the confines of the tumor, and treatment should be given over a period of 5–8 weeks. Chemotherapy with intravenous vincristine, dactinomycin, and cyclophosphamide is given for 1 year in stages I and II-A. Stages II-B, III-A, and III-B receive chemotherapy for 2 years.

The prognosis is improving when this tumor is treated early and aggressively.

Treatment

A. Stages I and II-A:

1. **Surgery**—Radical excision if possible.

2. **Radiation therapy**—Deliver 4000–6000 rads to the tumor bed if feasible.

3. **Chemotherapy**—Total therapy is 364 days. Follow phase I and II schedule (see below), then repeat phases I and II.

B. Stage II-B:

1. **Surgery**—Partial excision when possible.

2. **Radiation therapy**—Deliver 4000–6000 rads to the tumor bed if possible, depending upon location.

3. **Chemotherapy**—Total therapy is 728 days. Follow phase I and II schedule (see below), then repeat phases I and II 3 times each.

C. Stages III-A and III-B:

1. **Surgery**—None.

2. **Radiation therapy**—Deliver 4000–6000 rads to local tumors for palliation.

3. **Chemotherapy**—Total therapy is 728 days. Follow phase I and II schedule (see below), then repeat phases I and II 3 times each.

D. Chemotherapy Schedules:

1. **Phase I—**

a. Vincristine, 1.5 mg/sq m IV on days 1, 8, 15, 22, 29, 36, 50, 64, and 78.

b. Dactinomycin, 0.4 mg/sq m IV on days 1, 8, 15, 22, 29, and 36.

c. Cyclophosphamide, 300 mg/sq m IV on days 1, 8, 15, 22, 29, 36, 50, 64, and 78.

2. **Phase II—**

a. Vincristine, 1.5 mg/sq m IV on days 85, 99, 113, 127, 141, 155, and 169.

b. Dactinomycin, 0.4 mg/sq m IV on days 85, 92, 99, 106, 113, and 120.

c. Cyclophosphamide, 300 mg/sq m IV on days 85, 99, 113, 127, 141, 155, and 169.

Burrington JP: Rhabdomyosarcoma of the paratesticular tissues in children: A report of 8 cases. J Pediat Surg 4:503, 1969.

Pratt C: Response of childhood rhabdomyosarcoma to combination chemotherapy. Pediatrics 74:791–794, 1967.

Pratt C, Fleming I, Hustu HO: Multimodal therapy of childhood rhabdomyosarcoma. Proc Am A Cancer Res 103:29, 1971.

Sutow W & others: Prognosis in childhood rhabdomyosarcoma. Cancer 25:1384–1390, 1970.

2. MALIGNANT MESENCHYMOMA

This tumor consists of 2 or more anaplastic mesenchymal elements. It follows rhabdomyosarcoma in frequency. It may be found in any superficial soft tissue as well as in viscera.

Since the most common differentiated element in this tumor is the rhabdomyosarcoma, treatment is as above.

Kauffman S, Stowt A: Congenital mesenchymal tumors. Cancer 18:460–475, 1965.

3. FIBROSARCOMA

Fibrosarcoma may be found as a nodule of varying size which invades locally and may metastasize to the lung. It may be present at birth but more commonly is noted in the first year of life. A variant arising in the nerve sheath called neurilemmoma may be seen in Recklinghausen's disease.

Surgical excision is the treatment of choice. The prognosis is good.

4. JUVENILE FIBROMATOSIS

This includes a diverse group of relatively benign fibrous tumors such as dermoid fibromatosis, plantar and palmar fibromas, and keloids. Histologically, these tumors are often difficult to distinguish from fibrosarcomas. Another form of fibromatosis involves the sternocleidomastoid muscle in infancy; this may result from trauma at birth.

Surgical resection is the treatment of choice. The prognosis is good.

5. LIPOMAS

Lipomas tend to be soft, circumscribed subcutaneous masses. Generalized lipomatosis is rare, but it may occur in childhood or even as a congenital lesion.

Surgical removal is the treatment of choice. The prognosis is good.

6. EPULIS

This is a term applied to any pedunculated or sessile growth of the gums. It consists of multinucleated giant cells containing fibrous tissue.

Treatment consists of surgical removal. Recurrence is uncommon, and metastases do not occur.

TABLE 32–3. Antineoplastic agents commercially available in common use.

Agent	Dosage and Route	Spectra	Toxicity
Arabinosyl cytosine (cytarabine, Cytosar)	100–150 mg/sq m/week IV or IM; 5–50 mg/sq m once or twice weekly intrathecally for CNS leukemia until CSF clears.	Acute myeloblastic and acute lymphocytic leukemia.	Nausea, vomiting, anorexia, bone marrow depression, hepatotoxicity.
Cyclophosphamide (Cytoxan)	75–100 mg/sq m/day orally or 300 mg/sq m/week IV.	Leukemia, Hodgkin's lymphoma, neuroblastoma, sarcomas, retinoblastoma, hepatoma, rhabdomyosarcoma, Ewing's sarcoma.	Nausea, vomiting, anorexia, alopecia, bone marrow depression, hemorrhagic cystitis.
Dactinomycin (Cosmegen)	0.4 mg/sq m/week IV in 6 doses in phases with varying rest periods.	Wilms's tumor, sarcomas, rhabdomyosarcoma.	Nausea, vomiting, anorexia, bone marrow depression, alopecia, chemical dermatitis if leakage at intravenous site, tanning of skin if used with radiation therapy.
Fluorouracil (Efudex)	300–360 mg/sq m IV. Dosage should be scheduled based upon the specific disease stage. Maximum dose: 800 mg/day.	Hepatoma, gastrointestinal carcinoma.	Nausea, vomiting, oral ulceration, bone marrow depression, gastroenteritis, alopecia, anorexia.
Mercaptopurine (Purinethol)	50–100 mg/sq m/day orally.	Acute myeloblastic and acute lymphocytic leukemias.	Nausea, vomiting, rare oral ulcerations, bone marrow depression.
Methotrexate	15–20 mg/sq m orally or IV twice a week until relapse. Give 12 mg/sq m/week intrathecally for CNS leukemia until CSF clears.	Acute lymphocytic leukemia, CNS leukemia, lymphomas, choriocarcinoma, brain tumors, Hodgkin's disease.	Oral ulcers, gastrointestinal irritation, bone marrow depression, hepatotoxicity. Do not use in presence of impaired renal function.
Prednisone	40 mg/sq m/day orally in 3 divided doses for 4–6 weeks.	Acute myeloblastic and lymphocytic leukemia, lymphoma, Hodgkin's disease, bone pain from metastatic disease, CNS tumors.	Increased appetite, sodium retention, hypertension, provocation of latent diabetes or tuberculosis, osteoporosis.
Procarbazine (Matulane)	100–125 mg/sq m/day orally for 4–6 weeks depending on schedule.	Hodgkin's disease, lymphomas.	Nausea, vomiting, anorexia, bone marrow depression (3-week delay). Do not give with narcotics or sedatives; has "Antabuse effect." Monitor liver and renal function.
Vincristine (Oncovin)	1.5 mg/sq m/week IV for 4–6 weeks, then every 2 weeks. Maximum dose: 2 mg.	Acute lymphocytic and myeloblastic leukemia, lymphoma (Hodgkin's), rhabdomyosarcoma, Wilms's tumor, neuroblastoma, Ewing's sarcoma, retinoblastoma, hepatoma, sarcomas.	Alopecia, constipation, abdominal cramps, jaw pain, paresthesia, myalgia and muscle weakness, neurotoxicity, decrease in deep tendon reflexes, chemical dermatitis. Do not use in presence of severe liver impairment.

7. GIANT CELL TUMOR

The giant cell tumor arises in the tendon sheath and may show considerable lipid, hemosiderin, and multinucleated giant cells. Cellular hyperchromatism may be of sufficient degree to be confused with malignant features. However, the presence of foam and giant cells identifies this lesion as benign.

Surgery is the treatment of choice. The prognosis is good.

TERATOMAS & HAMARTOMAS

Teratoma is a neoplasm that contains many types of tissue, including tissues not normally present at the site of origin. These tumors often contain all 3 types of embryonic tissue, ie, ectodermal (skin, teeth, nerve), mesodermal (connective tissue, vascular), and endodermal (respiratory or intestinal tract). Teratomas tend to arise in the midline of the body and produce signs and symptoms by pressure on vital areas or by metastases if they become malignant. The usual sites of teratomas in children are the pineal gland, nose, palate, base of skull, thyroid, mediastinum, retroperitoneal area, ovary, testes, and sacrococcygeal area. The usual treatment is complete surgical excision.

Hamartomas consist of normal tissues which produce tumor-like deformities due to excessive growth of certain tissue elements, eg, angioma. They differ from embryomas (Wilms's tumor) and teratomas in that they are not neoplastic in the pathologic sense and are governed by the general mechanisms of growth. Adenomas of the liver and rhabdomyomas of the heart are examples of this group of tumors.

Emery JL: Teratomas. P Clin North America 6:573–581, 1959.

Woolley MW & others: Teratomas in infancy and childhood: Review of clinical experience at Children's Hospital of Los Angeles. Z Kinderchir 4:289, 1967.

.　　.　　.

PRINCIPLES OF TREATMENT OF CANCER IN CHILDREN

The use of multimodal anticancer therapy in children requires careful monitoring of blood counts, nutritional status, and liver and kidney function and prompt attention to suspected infectious complications as susceptibility to infection is increased.

Table 32–3 shows the commercially available drugs in common use. Dosages and schedules depend upon the disease being treated and must be modified when the drugs are used in combination with other agents. Consultation is recommended for dosage, scheduling, and duration of therapy based on the age of the patient and the stage of the disease at diagnosis.

New drugs being investigated are L-asparaginase, daunomycin, adriamycin, BCNU (bis-chlor-nitrosourea), CCNU (chloroethyl-cyclohexyl-nitrosourea), streptozotocin, and cycloleucine. Some of these agents show activity when these diseases become resistant to conventional drugs and may offer hope for the future.

Cancer research efforts in all aspects of pediatric neoplasia make it important that good case reporting to cancer registries be done so that epidemiologic, familial, and environmental factors may be studied. The work of tumor immunologists and cancer virologists also offers hope for the possibilities of immunotherapy and vaccines.

●　　●　　●

General References

Anderson Hospital: *Neoplasia in Childhood.* Year Book, 1967.

Anderson Hospital: *Tumors of Bone and Soft Tissue.* Year Book, 1963.

Cline MJ: *Cancer Chemotherapy.* Saunders, 1971.

Dargeon HW: *Reticuloendothelioses in Childhood.* Thomas, 1966.

Easson WM: *The Dying Child: The Management of the Child or Adolescent Who is Dying.* Thomas, 1970.

Marsden HB, Steward JK: *Tumours in Children.* Springer-Verlag, 1968.

National Cancer Institute: *Human Tumor Cell Kinetics.* Monograph No. 30. US Department of Health, Education, and Welfare, 1969.

33...

Allergic Disorders

David Pearlman, MD, & Winona G. Campbell, MD

Allergic disorders include a variety of local and systemic manifestations all of which are ultimate expressions of the union between antigen and antibody. Although this union triggers the chain of events that culminates in the clinical allergic reaction, nonimmunologic factors are important in modifying this chain of events. In some instances, nonimmunologic factors can be completely responsible for clinical reactions indistinguishable from immunologically induced reactions (eg, urticaria caused by histamine-releasing drugs such as codeine and polymyxin B).

Allergic reactivity is normal. The reaction that results from the transfusion of mismatched blood is an allergic reaction; the repeated injection of antitoxin in the form of foreign serum often leads to the development of serum sickness; and contact with poison ivy frequently causes an allergic dermatitis. Some forms of allergic reactivity, however, occur only in certain members of the population. These disorders (which include allergic rhinitis, asthma, and atopic dermatitis) are called **atopic disorders**, signifying an unusual form of reactivity for which there is some unknown predisposition.

GENERAL PRINCIPLES OF DIAGNOSIS

By definition, allergic reactions stem from an antigen-antibody interaction; identification of these participants is of prime importance both in the diagnosis and in the therapy of allergic disorders. It is often difficult to identify the antigens (allergens) responsible for a particular clinical disorder, but the most helpful procedure by far is a thorough and detailed history. Tests for the presence of a specific antibody which will implicate specific allergens are helpful but are never a substitute for a thorough history.

Antibodies differ in their biologic activities. Since certain types of antibodies are involved in some disorders and others in different disorders, it is essential to select the appropriate immunologic test for the disorder being investigated. In atopic disorders, reaginic or skin-sensitizing antibody is important.* The usual

immunologic test for this type of antibody is the scratch or intradermal skin test. In this test, the union of skin-sensitizing antibody with antigen is responsible for the liberation of histamine, which in turn induces local vasodilatation and edema with consequent wheal and erythema ("hive") formation. As with all immunologic tests, the presence of antibody does not itself signify its clinical importance since antibody can often be identified in the absence of any clinical symptoms. When correlated with the history, however, the results of skin tests for this type of antibody can be highly informative.

Skin-sensitizing antibody plays no significant role in contact dermatitis. In this type of disorder, cell-bound antibody or delayed hypersensitivity characteristic of the tuberculin reaction is responsible. Unlike the wheal and erythema response, delayed hypersensitivity reactions are characterized by infiltration around the allergen of a variety of cells, including sensitized lymphoid cells, which cause tissue destruction by other mechanisms. In contact dermatitis, "patch testing" (placing the suspected allergen in direct contact with the skin for 24–48 hours under cover of a "patch") is used to detect the offending antibody and thus implicate the specific allergen.

The presence of a particular antibody does not always identify the cause of a given allergic disorder, ie, the presence of antibody is necessary but not in itself sufficient to produce allergic symptoms. The suspicion of the clinical importance of an allergen, however, may be confirmed by the use of a "provocative test," ie, challenging a given individual with the suspected allergen and observing the response. In a sense, "patch testing" in contact dermatitis is a provocative test since this is both the route of sensitization and the point of reaction. Inhalation of pollens and molds by patients with asthma or hay fever and the feeding of milk to patients with suspected milk allergy are other examples of provocative tests. However, since allergic sensitivity can be inordinately great, provocative testing is potentially dangerous and should not be used routinely. Provocative tests may prove a relationship between the provoking substance and a clinical reaction, but they do not necessarily establish that the reaction is allergic. For example, in children with lactase deficiency, milk may elicit gastrointestinal symptoms similar to those of milk allergy.

*The major portion of reaginic antibody activity appears to reside in the IgE fraction, and IgE levels are often elevated in atopic disorders. This is not a practical diagnostic tool, however.

GENERAL PRINCIPLES OF TREATMENT

Environmental Control of Exposure

Since the clinical allergic reaction stems from the union of antigen with antibody, avoidance of the offending antigen is the most effective means of therapy of all allergic disorders. In many instances, complete avoidance of identified allergens is impossible, but it is frequently feasible to reduce the incidence and severity of reactions by minimizing the contact. Many nonimmunologic factors can precipitate or aggravate atopic disorders (eg, irritational smoke, or cold air in asthma) and avoidance of such known or suspected irritants is also of prime importance in the therapy of allergic disorders.

Sample directions for environmental control of common allergens. The following refers mainly to the patient's bedroom, but the principles are applicable to the rest of the house as well.

(1) House dust is a common offender. The accumulation of dust may be minimized by the avoidance of dust catchers and dust producers such as wool (in rugs, blankets), flannel (in bedding, pajamas), mattresses, furniture, and toys stuffed with plant or animal products, chenille (bedspreads, drapes, and rugs), cotton quilts, stuffed cotton pads, and venetian blinds.

(2) Rooms should be dusted daily with a damp or oiled cloth. The room should be cleaned thoroughly at least once a week—never with the patient present.

(3) All forced air ducts, which frequently contain dust and molds and tend to stir up room dust, should be sealed off. An electric radiator may be substituted as a source of heat, if necessary. If pollenosis is a problem, windows should be kept closed during the pollen seasons. Air cleaners (electronic precipitators) and refrigerated air conditioners may be usefully employed. Automatic humidifiers with provision for humidity not to exceed 40% can be helpful in dry climates and winter time heating systems.

(4) Plant products (kapok, cotton) and animal products (feathers, horse and cow hairs) commonly used for pillows, stuffing of furniture, toys, bedding, and hair pads for rugs should be eliminated. Alternatively, all mattresses, box springs, and pillows in the bedroom should be completely enclosed in impermeable plastic or rubber casings. Inexpensive casings may be obtained from department stores; better quality encasings may be obtained from Allergy-Free Products for the Home, 1162 West Lynn, Springfield, Missouri 65892, or 224 Livingston Street, Brooklyn, NY 11201; or from Allergen-Proof Encasings, Inc, 4046 E Superior Ave, Cleveland, Ohio 44103. Especially if plastic casings are used, they should be checked periodically for tears or punctures. Furniture, bedding, and clothes stuffed solely with synthetic products (eg, Dacron pillows or rubber) are permissible; the latter, however, may harbor molds. Toys stuffed with old nylon stockings or synthetic foam, with plain nonfuzzy cotton or synthetic coverings, are very satisfactory.

(5) Cleaning equipment, wool, and fur coats should not be kept in or near the child's room or closet.

(6) Basements and attics, particularly if unfinished, are forbidden territory for an atopic child.

(7) Sensitization to animals develops so frequently in atopic individuals that close contact with animals of any sort should be avoided. If there is any reason to suspect already existing sensitivity, it is important to rid the environment completely of animals.

Hyposensitization

If avoidance of offensive allergens is not possible, specific hyposensitization is sometimes attempted. The value of hyposensitization is limited mainly to atopic disorders and to severe insect allergy. There are a variety of hyposensitization procedures, but the same general principle applies to all: Extremely small amounts of allergen are injected subcutaneously at frequent intervals and in increasing amounts until a "top dose" is reached; this is usually the highest tolerated dose of a given allergen extract, or that amount which induces a state of clinical hyporeactivity to the allergen as demonstrated after natural contact. When perennial therapy is adopted, the top tolerated dose is used as a maintenance dose, with carefully regulated lengthening of intervals (by not more than an additional week at a time) up to 6 weeks, as tolerated.

Most allergists agree that the majority of well selected patients with pollen asthma (or hay fever) are significantly improved after 3–4 years of therapy on a "perennial" injection regimen of aqueous antigens, and there is evidence to substantiate the beneficial effects of hyposensitization even in perennial asthma. The effectiveness of therapy is dose-related. Repository therapy using pyridine-extracted, alum-precipitated extracts (Allpyral) are useful mainly in increasing the antigen dosage in individuals who are extremely sensitive to small amounts of aqueous antigen. Theoretically, fewer injections of alum-precipitated material are required to reach a maintenance dose of antigen, and maintenance injections need to be given less frequently. However, information on the efficacy of this form of therapy is not as complete as that relating to aqueous therapy. Mold hyposensitization therapy is believed by some to offer significant protection, but the extent or importance of various individual molds (involving innumerable species) in the production of asthma is not known. Certainly the value of mold hyposensitization is questionable. The value of hyposensitization against house dusts is not well substantiated; it may be beneficial but is no substitute for good environmental control. The efficacy of bacterial extracts is extremely controversial; its usefulness in allergic disorders is based mainly on testimonial evidence, and its effectiveness has been brought into question by the results of well controlled studies.

Drug Therapy (Table 33–1.)

A variety of drugs are effective in the treatment of allergic disorders. However, inappropriate use of

TABLE 33–1. Preparations and dosages of drugs commonly used in allergic disorders.

	Dosage
Adrenergic Agents*	
Epinephrine aqueous, 1:1000 (V, B)	0.1–0.3 ml subcut or IM. (May repeat at 20-minute intervals.)
Sus-Phrine 1:200 (V, B)	0.1–0.2 ml subcut every 8–12 hours. (Shake well before administering.)
Ephedrine sulfate (V, B)	3 mg/kg/day orally in 4–6 doses.
Phenylephrine hydrochloride (V) (Neo-Synephrine)	3–10 mg 3 times daily orally; 0.1–0.2 mg/kg subcut or IM.
Ophthalmic preparation, 0.125%	1–2 drops in each eye as necessary.
Pseudoephedrine hydrochloride (V, B) (Sudafed)	5 mg/kg/day orally in 4–6 doses.
Isoproterenol sulfate (B) aerosol (Medihaler-Iso) (Duo-Medihaler) with phenylephrine	1–2 inhalations as necessary.
Isoproterenol hydrochloride (B) (Norisodrine, Isuprel)	1–2 inhalations as necessary.
Naphazoline ophthalmic solution (0.1%)	1–2 drops in each eye as necessary.
Metaraminol (V) (Aramine) in 1 ml and 10 ml vials, (10 mg/ml)	15–100 mg (1.5–10 ml) in 500 ml 5% dextrose in water or isotonic NaCl. Adjust rate of infusion to maintain blood pressure.
Levarterenol (V) (Levophed) 0.2% solution in 4 ml ampules	1 ampule (4 ml) in 1000 ml 5% dextrose in water. Adjust rate of infusion to maintain blood pressure.

*V = Induces vasoconstriction. B = Induces bronchodilatation.

Drugs With Antihistaminic Activity	
Chlorpheniramine maleate (Chlor-Trimeton)	0.35 mg/kg/day orally in 4–6 doses.
(Teldrin)	0.35 mg/kg/day orally in 2 doses.
Injectable	4–8 mg IV (slowly) or IM (10 mg/ml in 1 ml vials; 100 mg/ml in 2 ml vials).
Diphenhydramine hydrochloride (Benadryl)	5 mg/kg/day orally in 4–6 doses.
Injectable	25 mg IV (slowly) or IM (ampules, 50 mg/ml; vials, 10 mg/ml).
Brompheniramine maleate (Dimetane)	0.35 mg/kg/day orally in 4 doses.
Tripelennamine hydrochloride (Pyribenzamine)	5 mg/kg/day orally in 4–6 doses.
Hydroxyzine (Atarax, Vistaril)	2 mg/kg/day orally in 4 doses.

Combination Drugs for Allergic Rhinitis, Allergic Serous Otitis Media, and Urticaria	
Phenylephrine and chlorpheniramine (Novahistine)	Elixir: ½–1 tsp every 4 hours. Forte capsules: 1 capsule every 8 hours (older children).
Phenylephrine and chlorpheniramine (Demazin)	Syrup: ½–2 tsp every 6 hours depending on age. Repetabs: 1–2 twice daily depending on age.
Pseudoephedrine and triprolidine (Actifed)	Syrup: ½–2 tsp 3 times daily depending on age. Tablets: ½–1 tab 3 times daily depending on age.

Combination Drugs for Asthma

Each Tablet Contains	Tedral	Quadrinal	Verequad	Marax
Ephedrine	24 mg	24 mg	24 mg	25 mg
Phenobarbital	8 mg	24 mg	8 mg	10 mg*
Theophylline†	130 mg	130 mg	130 mg	130 mg
Potassium iodide	. . .	320 mg	. . .	. . .
Glyceryl guaiacolate	. . .	. . .	100 mg	. . .

*Contains hydroxyzine instead of phenobarbital.
†As the anhydrous base.
Each tsp of syrup = ½ tablet (except for Marax, which = ¼ tablet).
Dosage: ½ tsp up to 1 tablet every 4–6 hours depending on weight.

Sedatives	
Chloral hydrate	15 mg/kg orally or rectally every 6–8 hours (maximum 1 gm/dose).

TABLE 33–1 (cont'd). Preparations and dosages of drugs commonly used in allergic disorders.

	Dosage
Expectorants	
Syrup of hydriodic acid	1.5 ml/year of age (to age 15) orally 3 times daily.
Potassium iodide, saturated solution (= 1 gm KI/ml)	25 mg/kg/day orally in 3–4 doses.
Glyceryl guaiacolate (Robitussin)	1 tsp every 4–6 hours.
Xanthines	
Aminophylline, theophylline	IV: 4 mg/kg every 6 hours (infuse over 20–30 minute period).
	Oral: 5 mg/kg every 6 hours.
	Rectal: Suppositories, 5–7 mg/kg every 8 hours.
	Enema, 4–6 mg/kg every 6 hours.

Adrenal Glucocorticoids

Most rapid therapeutic effect follows intravenous or oral administration, but there may be no perceptible effect for hours. In acute situations, high doses of corticosteroids (eg, 100–400 mg hydrocortisone in 2 or 4 divided doses) are generally employed the first day and the dose tapered as rapidly as possible to maintenance levels or withdrawn completely.

Approximate equivalents of activity: 100 mg hydrocortisone = 4 mg dexamethasone = 25 mg prednisolone = 20 mg methylprednisolone.

Intravenous preparations	
Hydrocortisone sodium succinate (Solu-Cortef)	100 mg vials.
Dexamethasone-21-phosphate (Decadron)	Each ml contains 4 mg dexamethasone-21-phosphate (in 1 ml and 5 ml vials).
Methylprednisolone (Solu-Medrol)	40 mg/ml in 1 ml vials.
Prednisolone-21-phosphate (Hydeltrasol)	20 mg/ml in 2 and 5 ml vials.
Dermatologic preparations	
Fluocinolone acetonide (Synalar)	0.025% cream or ointment and 0.01% cream.
Flurandrenolone (Cordran)	0.05% and 0.025%.
Cort-Dome cream	1/8% up to 2% hydrocortisone in Acid Mantle base.

drugs may aggravate the reaction, and a thorough understanding of the pharmacologic actions of these drugs is essential. The principal groups include adrenergic agents, antihistamines, methyl xanthines, expectorants, oxygen, and adrenal corticosteroids. The selection of drugs obviously depends upon the pathologic processes involved.

A. Adrenergic Agents: As a group, adrenergic agents exhibit many pharmacologic effects. Their usefulness in allergic disorders depends mainly on their ability to constrict blood vessels and relax other smooth muscle. The manifestations of many allergic reactions are due, at least in part, to chemical mediators such as histamine and acetylcholine which produce varying degrees of vasodilatation, edema, and smooth muscle spasm. Adrenergic agents are the principal pharmacologic antagonists of these chemical mediators, and at times may even reverse their effects completely. However, the pharmacologic properties of adrenergic drugs as a group are not shared uniformly by all members of the group, and these drugs cannot be used interchangeably to produce a given effect. In urticaria, for example, phenylephrine, an effective vasoconstrictor but a poor smooth muscle dilator, would be especially useful. Isoproterenol, on the other hand, although devoid of vasoconstrictor action, is the most effective bronchodilator of the group and is useful in asthma. In asthma, and in anaphylaxis—in which vasodilatation, edema, and asthma may all be a problem—epinephrine, which is a potent antagonist of all of these effects, is the drug of choice.

Adrenergic drugs are not always effective in a given disorder and are not without undesirable effects. Epinephrine resistance may occur in severe asthma, for example, and its use in such cases may actually aggravate the disorder by increasing the patient's anxiety and contributing to venous congestion and mucus plugging. The injection of epinephrine in the face of severe hypoxemia and acidosis may produce cardiac arrhythmia or arrest. Isoproterenol in inhalant form, although frequently effective in asthma even in epinephrine-resistant cases, may also severely aggravate asthma if used excessively. Aerosols containing adrenergic drugs should be used cautiously and only as adjuncts to other appropriate pharmacologic management of asthmatic patients.

B. Antihistamines: The antihistamines act through competition with histamine for receptor sites, thereby preventing histamine from exerting its activity. Antihistamines are particularly useful in urticaria, anaphylaxis, and allergic rhinitis; for reasons not well understood, they may not be effective (and may be harmful) in certain other syndromes such as asthma and atopic dermatitis in which vascular reactions are certainly involved. Although antihistamines may be very useful in severe allergic disorders, they are not the drug of first choice in medical emergencies due to allergic reactions but may be administered after epinephrine has been given. Antihistamines have antipruritic properties, however, and are useful in atopic dermatitis and in contact dermatitis, in which histamine does not appear to play a major role. The sedation which occurs as a side-effect, although undesirable in many instances, may be an advantage in others.

The transition between the antihistamines and the anticholinergic group of drugs is a subtle one, and many agents classified as one have both actions. For example, antihistamines in general have a notable atropine-like drying effect; and many antipsychotic tranquilizers, particularly the phenothiazines and hydroxyzine (Atarax), are especially good antihistamines. Because of their antihistaminic actions, these tranquilizers have been found useful in some conditions in which antihistamines are helpful (eg, urticaria) and should be used cautiously in those in which antihistamines may be harmful (eg, asthma).

C. Methyl Xanthines: Theophylline and its ethylenediamine derivative, aminophylline, are effective bronchodilators which appear to act at a different point but in the same pathway through which epinephrine exerts its smooth muscle dilating effect. The improper use of these agents has been associated with severe toxic reactions, in some cases resulting in death. Overdosage frequently occurs following the use of rectal suppositories and as a result of failure to appreciate the variability of rate and extent of absorption with different routes of administration. Toxic reactions include headache, palpitation, dizziness, stomach ache, nausea and vomiting, excessive thirst, and hypotension. (Nausea and stomach ache are common complaints, particularly with the initial use of oral methyl xanthines, and are not necessarily indicative of overdosage.) The diuretic action of theophylline or aminophylline should always be kept in mind when calculating fluids needs, particularly since dehydration may be part of the clinical problem in an asthmatic attack. When used properly, theophylline and aminophylline are valuable drugs with a bronchodilating effect equal to that of any of the adrenergic agents. Prolonged administration of appropriate amounts of these drugs causes few side-effects.

Rectal administration of theophylline in fluid form usually results in prompt and efficient absorption of the drug which may be almost as efficient as intravenous administration. Absorption from rectal suppositories tends to be slow and erratic. Absorption following oral administration is also somewhat erratic, but effective drug levels can be achieved by this route, and the oral route is the route of choice for chronic administration of methyl xanthines.

D. Expectorants: Expectorants such as iodides and glyceryl guaiacolate are used mainly in bronchial asthma to liquefy thick, tenacious mucus, but it is not clear whether the therapeutic effectiveness of these agents is in fact due to their expectorant action. Iodides seem more effective than guaiacolate and are relatively nontoxic, but (especially with prolonged use) goiter, salivary gland inflammation, gastric irritation, skin eruptions, and acne may occur. Acne is rarely provoked before adolescence. *Note:* It is important to keep in mind that adequate hydration is essential to effective expectoration. Expectorant preparations containing narcotics are contraindicated in asthma.

E. Corticosteroids: Adrenal glucorticoids have been used in the treatment of all of the allergic disorders. Their effectiveness is apparently due to their "anti-inflammatory" actions. They are most useful in disorders of delayed hypersensitivity (such as contact dermatitis) and in asthma. They appear to be least effective in urticarial disorders. The untoward side-effects of prolonged corticosteroid administration (eg, growth suppression, myopathy, Cushing's syndrome, hypertension, peptic ulcer, diabetes, and electrolyte imbalance) limit their use mainly to those conditions which are refractory to other measures or are life-threatening. Even then, however, their slow onset of action (even when given intravenously) precludes first-choice administration of these drugs in acute allergic emergencies. Most allergic syndromes are amenable to other forms of therapy, and the systemic use of the corticosteroids is rarely necessary. When chronic use is necessary, alternate-day corticosteroid therapy with a short-acting preparation (eg, prednisone) in the early morning every other day should be attempted. There are virtually no advantages to the use of corticotropin over the glucocorticoids themselves when glucocorticoid action is deemed necessary in the treatment of allergic disorders.

The main indications for the use of systemic corticosteroids are severe, acute life-threatening asthma and control of chronic severe disorders such as asthma and atopic dermatitis which are refractory to other appropriate therapy. In some instances, administration of a short course of corticosteroids for self-limiting allergic disorders (eg, serum sickness) may be warranted.

Topical corticosteroids are extremely effective anti-inflammatory agents in the control of allergic dermatitis—mainly contact dermatitis and atopic dermatitis. Topical application is the preferred route of administration in such disorders.

F. Sedatives: Sedatives have been grossly misused in asthma and have been responsible for the deaths of some asthmatics. Although the psyche undoubtedly exerts a significant influence on asthma and other allergic disorders, the anxiety associated with extreme asthma is more often a reflection of the severity of the respiratory distress than the main cause of it. Sedatives which suppress the respiratory center (as the barbiturates do) should not be used in the therapy of severe asthma. If sedatives are necessary, chloral hydrate may be used (Table 33−1).

G. Oxygen: Oxygen is extremely important in the treatment of severe asthma. Hypoxemia usually occurs early in the course of moderately severe or severe asthma, much in advance of any detectable cyanosis. Oxygen is potentially very drying and should be humidified when administered. Excessively high concentrations of oxygen should be avoided since they can lead to atelectasis.

H. Antibiotics: There are no special indications for the use of antibiotics in allergic disorders. Antibiotics should, of course, be used when evidence of bacterial infection exists. However, their excessive use in children with allergic disorders when no clear indication does exist has led to the frequent sensitization of children to penicillin and other antibiotic and chemotherapeutic agents.

Erythromycin seems to be one of the least sensitizing antibiotics, and offers good coverage against many respiratory pathogens.

I. Cromolyn Sodium (Intal): This drug is a promising adjunct for the treatment of severe asthma and, possibly, allergic rhinitis. It is currently under intensive study and may become commercially available in the USA in the near future.

Deamer WC: Injection therapy in asthma and allergic rhinitis. P Clin North America 16:243–255, 1969.

Falliers CJ: Cromolyn sodium (disodium cromoglycate). J Allergy 47:298–305, 1971.

Ferrara A: Environmental control: Conferences with parents. P Clin North America 16:67–83, 1969.

Norman PS: A rational approach to desensitization. J Allergy 44:129–145, 1969.

Sadan N & others: Immunotherapy of pollinosis in children. New England J Med 280:623–627, 1969.

Siegel SC: Corticosteroids and ACTH in the management of the atopic child. P Clin North America 16:287–304, 1969.

Tempero KF, Hunninghake DB: Antihistamines. Postgrad Med 48:149–154, 1970.

MEDICAL EMERGENCIES DUE TO ALLERGIC REACTIONS

Skin testing, hyposensitization with allergen extracts, drugs, vaccines, toxoids, sera, blood transfusions, and insect bites and stings are the most common causes of severe allergic reactions. Anaphylactic shock, angioedema, and bronchial obstruction, alone or in combination, are the principal life-threatening manifestations of severe allergic reactions. Lightheadedness, paresthesias, sweating, flushing, palpitations, and urticaria may precede or accompany severe reactions.

Prevention

Prevention consists mainly of avoiding allergens known or believed to be responsible for allergic reactions. A history suggestive of a reaction to a given drug is an indication for the selection of an alternative and unrelated drug for therapeutic use. Skin tests should be performed before foreign serum is administered.

Treatment

A. Emergency Measures: Immediate treatment is essential for successful management of these reactions.

1. Epinephrine, 1:1000, 0.2–0.4 ml, should be injected IM without delay. This may be repeated at 15–20 minute intervals as necessary. If the reaction is due to the recent injection of a drug, serum, or other substance, a tourniquet should be applied proximal to the injection. If the offending substance has been injected intradermally or subcutaneously, absorption of the material may be delayed further by injecting epinephrine, 0.2 ml subcut near the site of injection. Subsequent therapy depends partly upon the response.

2. Antihistamines (Table 33–1) should be given intramuscularly or intravenously. When intravenous infusions are used, they should be given over a 5–10 minute period since untoward reactions, particularly hypotension, have been induced by too rapid administration.

3. Aminophylline is useful when bronchospasm occurs. Further treatment of bronchial obstruction is discussed under Asthma.

4. Tracheostomy may be lifesaving in cases of profound laryngeal edema.

5. Fluids—Since anaphylactic shock is in part produced by hypovolemia secondary to massive exudation of intravascular fluid, maintenance of a proper volume by intravenous fluids (5% dextrose in water) is particularly important.

B. Follow-Up Measures:

1. Adrenal corticosteroids have little place in the treatment of acute reactions but may be employed with persistent severe reactions. The onset of action of these drugs is slow (hours, even by intravenous administration). If used, they should be given only after epinephrine and antihistamines have been administered.

2. Mild sedation may also be indicated.

C. Hyposensitization for Insect Bites: Individuals who have experienced serious reactions following an insect sting should be hyposensitized. A polyvalent vaccine consisting of bee, wasp, yellow jacket, hornet, and mosquito antigens is commercially available and is recommended over species-specific antigen. Hypersensitivity to insect allergens is often so great, however, that testing and therapy are best left to physicians experienced in dealing with insect allergy. Treatment kits for anaphylactic reactions should be available for immediate use in individuals with insect hypersensitivity and should be kept in the home or taken along by a responsible person when the sensitive person travels in an area likely to be infested with the offensive insects.

Barr SE: Allergy to hymenoptera stings: Review of the world literature, 1953–1970. Ann Allergy 29:49–66, 1971.

Heimlich EM, Siegel SC: Anaphylaxis. Chap 66 in: *Brenneman's Practice of Pediatrics.* Vol 2. Harper, 1968.

ATOPIC DISORDERS

Certain individuals are predisposed to allergic rhinitis, asthma, or atopic dermatitis. The incidence tends to be familial, but little is known about the constitutional factors responsible. Sensitization is usually to substances considered to be innocuous for other people. Animal danders, feathers, kapok (used as stuffing in mattresses and toys), and house dusts are the most common perennial allergens. Accruing evidence indicates that the emanations of house dust mites (high in mattress flock) and of cockroaches (abundant in poor housing situations) may be important factors contributing to the allergenicity of house dust. Many varieties of trees, grass and weed pollens, and molds cause atopic disorders in a more or less seasonal incidence. Foods and a number of other substances may contribute to perennial or seasonal problems. Atopic individuals commonly become sensitized to one or more of these sensitizing substances, and "environmental control" (see above) is therefore recommended for any child with an atopic syndrome. Particular emphasis is placed on the bedroom.

Diagnosis

The diagnosis of atopic disease is based primarily on the clinical findings. Laboratory procedures (including skin testing) can be very helpful but should be interpreted in the light of the history and physical findings. To arrive at a diagnosis of any or all atopic diseases, a detailed history and complete physical examination are essential. More than one atopic disease (precipitated in many instances by the same allergens) may be present, and a history of familial atopic disorders or of other past or present atopic symptoms is especially useful. The following is a guideline for the overall history and physical examination. Indicated laboratory procedures will be included under individual atopic diseases.

    A. History:

    1. Chief complaint of patient.

    2. Specific allergens or any atopic disease in other family members, past or present (asthma, allergic rhinitis, atopic dermatitis).

    3. Details of development of first episode (eg, infection), change in environment (family move, acquisition of pets or toys, different household furnishings), season of year, ingestion of "new" food, special occasions, emotional and social upheavals.

    4. Circumstances of subsequent and most recent episodes (as above).

    5. Associated atopic or other allergic diseases (past or present), especially allergic rhinitis, bronchial asthma, "allergic cough," atopic dermatitis, food intolerance, "allergic rashes," angioedema.

    6. History of pneumonia, bronchiolitis, "croup," recurrent ear infections, sinusitis, removal of tonsils and adenoids.

    7. Food-related symptoms, eg, vomiting, colic, diarrhea, abnormal stools, abdominal pain, skin rashes, headache.

    8. Presence of "continuity symptoms," eg, itchy or stuffy nose, night cough, breathlessness, cough or wheezing (with exercise, laughter, crying, "frustration"), fatigue, irritability.

    9. Wheezing, cough, rashes, or nose, ear, or eye symptoms following contact with the following:

    a. Animals, especially house pets and household furnishings or clothing of animal origin (feather pillows, hair rug pads, mohair [goat], felt [rabbit and cow hair], wool).

    b. Seasonal agents—In winter, predominantly house dust and respiratory infections; in spring, trees; in late spring to early summer, grasses; in late summer to early fall, weeds.

    c. Seasonal sources of pollen, eg, flowers, grass mowing, harvesting, play or work in weed patches.

    d. Mold, eg, outside seasonal molds (wet, warm periods), moldly foods, mildew, old storage areas (attics, damp basements).

    e. Cosmetics, eg, bubble bath, hair spray, facial cosmetics, shampoos, soaps, enzyme detergents.

    10. Emotional and social factors and habits— Family structure, general attitudes and behavior; family, school, and social adjustments; temper tantrums, enuresis.

    B. Physical Examination: A complete physical examination is essential. The following signs deserve special emphasis:

    1. General appearance for state of nourishment and physical development, including weight and height; degree of activity; signs of fatigue; sneezing; cough and its character; dyspnea.

    2. Attitudes, responses, and relationships of patient to parents, physician, nurses, etc; general level of intelligence.

    3. Vital signs—Blood pressure, temperature, pulse rate, and character of respirations.

    4. Skin—Rashes, pallor, cyanosis, temperature changes, sweating, degree of dryness.

    5. Eyes—"Allergic pleats" (lower lid edema, eyeshadowing), conjunctival injection, blebs, itching, cataracts (in severe, long-standing atopic dermatitis), blepharitis (from chronic rubbing), tearing.

    6. Nose—Itching ("allergic salute," "bunny nose," nasal crease), excoriation of nares, hyperemia, mucosal edema, polypoid changes, purplish pallor, excessive serous or mucoid discharge.

    7. Ears—With allergic rhinitis, retraction of drums; with recurrent serous otitis media, hearing loss, changes in drum (distortion, retraction, fullness, opacity, narrow and "chalky" malleus), evidence of fluid in middle ear; discharge in canal uncommon.

    8. Mouth—For palatal malformations, character of speech, "canker sores," changes in tongue (geographism, grooving).

    9. Throat—Presence and appearance of tonsils and pharyngeal lymphoid tissue, appearance of mucosal epithelium (anterior pillars, soft palate, pharyngeal wall), nasopharyngeal secretions.

    10. Chest—Configuration ("barrel chest," "pigeon breast," prominent Harrison's grooves—all may be present in long-standing asthma), evidence of hyper-

inflation, pattern of breathing, development and use of muscles for accessory respiration (eg, hypertrophy of pectorals, trapezii, sternocleidomastoids), retractions (especially in infants).

11. Lungs–Relationship to inspiratory-expiratory cycle of gross or auscultatory wheezes (including after exercise and forced expiration), rhonchi and their pitch, rales, degree and equality of air exchange; degree of resonance and level and movement of diaphragm.

12. Heart–Tachycardia, size, accentuation of pulmonic second sound (for evidence of pulmonary hypertension in asthma).

13. External genitalia–Vulvitis (girls in pollen season), meatal ulcer (boys with contact dermatitis).

14. Signs of associated infections–Pyoderma, purulent nasal or ear discharge, purulent bronchial secretions, significant adenopathy.

C. Supplementary Diagnostic Procedures:

1. Skin tests–In all atopic disorders, skin testing for the presence of reaginic antibody is a potentially useful procedure in identifying allergens. As a general rule, atopic individuals have reaginic antibody to many antigens, and the finding of multiple positive skin tests tends to confirm a suspicion of atopy. Scratch testing should be done first since it is less likely than intradermal testing to cause severe reactions in very sensitive individuals. Intradermal testing is about 100 times more sensitive than scratch testing. The tests are read at the peak of the urticarial reaction, which is usually within 15–20 minutes. If scratch tests are negative, intradermal tests may be used. Skin testing is a potentially dangerous procedure in highly sensitive individuals, and epinephrine and a tourniquet should always be at hand.

A positive skin test reaction consists of an immediate erythema, wheal, and flare (triple response) to "scratch" or intracutaneously injected allergens. In interpreting the skin tests and assessing their clinical significance, the following should be kept in mind: (1) A negative control of diluent should always be used for comparison. (2) Infants may react predominantly with flaring; older children, with wheal reactions. (3) Mild reactions (1–2+) are less likely to be clinically significant than more strongly positive (pseudopodic wheal) reactions. Also, a positive reaction elicited by scratch or puncture testing is more likely to be clinically significant than a positive test which can be elicited only by intradermal testing. (4) When a skin test does correlate with clinical sensitivity, the size of the reaction cannot be taken as an index of the severity of the clinical syndrome. (5) False-positive and false-negative reactions to foods are especially common, particularly in older children. (6) A definitely positive skin test means only that reaginic antibody is present in the skin. It may reflect a past, present, or potential clinical hypersensitivity manifest as one or more of the atopic diseases; on the other hand, the patient may never develop an atopic disease due to the specific allergen. (7) Up to 10% of nonatopic individuals may have positive skin reactions to a few allergens, especially house dust.

2. The Prausnitz-Küstner reaction–Passive transfer of antibody by injecting serum from a sensitized individual into the skin of a nonsensitized individual, followed by local challenge of the transfer site with the suspected allergen, is occasionally employed when skin testing is not feasible.

3. Conjunctival tests are infrequently used and appear to offer little advantage in testing.

4. Provocative testing may be employed, but is not recommended as a routine procedure for any potentially severe disorder such as asthma. Provocative tests are most valuable in determining clinical sensitivity to foods. Elimination and subsequent challenge with the following may be especially revealing: (1) Foods eaten more or less daily (unless there is a history of vomiting or angioedema involving the mouth and throat immediately following ingestion), eg, cow's milk, legumes, cereal grains, potatoes, chocolate, eggs. (2) Foods eaten less often, eg, nuts, peanuts, fish or seafood, sunflower seeds, and melons–if vomiting and angioedema have not occurred. In most cases, the parent or patient is already aware of the relationship between allergen and reaction if severe asthma or angioedema has immediately followed ingestion.

Procedure for provocative testing. After environmental factors are stabilized, withhold all suspected foods for at least 3 weeks; then challenge with a single food in at least twice the quantity usually ingested. Repeated offerings for a few days may be necessary to establish a hypersensitivity reaction.

Direct provocative inhalant testing is potentially hazardous and should be performed in a hospital setting. The "natural" casual contacts of the patient with the inhalant allergens is not only very helpful in a definitive diagnosis, but usually bears permissible risk.

5. Eosinophilia–Increased numbers of eosinophils in the blood or bodily secretions (nasal, gastrointestinal) are frequently present in a variety of allergic conditions, especially in atopic disorders, and the presence of eosinophilia may strengthen a suspicion of allergic diatheses. Nasal eosinophilia is practically diagnostic of allergic rhinitis, but eosinophilia itself is by no means pathognomonic of other clinical allergies. Conversely, the absence of eosinophilia does not rule out allergy, particularly since a variety of factors (eg, concurrent infection) may suppress eosinophils. Nasal eosinophilia in infants up to 3 months of age is considered normal.

6. Other tests–Numerous other tests (leukocyte histamine release in vitro, in vitro basophil degranulation test, the induction of blast transformation or peripheral blood lymphocytes by antigen in vitro, skin window test) have been employed in attempts to identify allergens which may be responsible for particular allergic reactions. In some cases (eg, the induction of blast transformation in lymphocytes), the validity of the test for implicating allergens is questionable; others are more promising and may aid in the identification of problem allergens. For various reasons, however, their use on a general basis is impractical at this time, and these procedures can be considered chiefly to be research tools.

Bronsky EA, Ellis EF: Inhalation bronchial challenge testing in asthmatic children. P Clin North America 16:85–94, 1969.

Eisen AN: The role of infection in allergic disease. P Clin North America 16:67–83, 1969.

Hannaway PJ, Hyde JS: Scratch and intradermal skin testing: A comparative study in 250 atopic children. Ann Allergy 28:413–419, 1970.

Johnstone DE, Dutton AM: Dietary prophylaxis of allergic disease in children. New England J Med 274:715–719, 1966.

Lecks HI, Kravis LP: The allergist and the eosinophil. P Clin North America 16:125–148, 1969.

Levy DA: Studies of histamine release from human leukocytes. Ann Allergy 27:511–518, 1969.

Norman PS: Antigens that cause atopic disease. Chap 44 in: *Immunological Diseases*, 2nd ed. Samter M (editor). Little, Brown, 1971.

BRONCHIAL ASTHMA

Essentials of Diagnosis

- Paroxysmal or chronically exacerbating dyspnea characterized by bilateral wheezing, prolongation of expiration, "air trapping," and hyperinflation of lungs.
- Restoration of abnormal pulmonary function to (or significantly toward) normal by injection of epinephrine, inhalation of isoproterenol (1:200 dilution), or other therapeutic measures.
- Eosinophilia of sputum and blood (common).
- Positive immediate skin test reactions to provoking allergens (supportive only).
- Provocation of attacks of dyspnea and wheezing on contact with specific allergens, infectious agents, irritants, or emotional upsets.

General Considerations

Bronchial asthma is a reversible obstructive process predominantly of the lower pulmonary tract caused by mucosal edema, increased and unusually viscid secretions, and bronchiolar constriction. Especially in protracted asthmatic episodes, the obstructive pathologic changes may cause not only hypoxemia but retention of CO_2 and respiratory acidosis.

The incidence of asthma has been reported to be less than 10% of the total population but to constitute 26–63% of all atopic diseases. Before adolescence, boys are affected twice as frequently as girls. Onset is rare in the first year of life, but asthma is not uncommon by the second year. In the majority of cases in childhood, the onset is by the seventh year.

In up to 40% of patients, offensive allergens cannot be definitely identified by history or suggested by skin testing. The most common allergens causing asthma in children are inhalants: house dust and its usual ingredients of old kapok, cotton linters, indoor molds, insects, epidermals (especially feathers and the hair and danders of cats, dogs, horses, cattle, rabbits, and sheep), and airborne pollens (trees, grasses, weeds), and out-of-doors seasonal molds. Foods occasionally provoke asthma, especially in infants, but this is less common in later childhood. The most common food allergens are egg whites, cow's milk, fish, and foods of seed origin, eg, nuts, legumes, chocolate, and wheat and other cereal grains. It is probable that foods act as allergens in fewer than 10% of cases. The same allergens that cause asthma frequently cause allergic rhinitis in the same patient; many children with initial hay fever develop asthma, but there are divergent opinions regarding the number who do so (eg, 7% versus 60% in 2 different series.)

In addition to allergic reactions, numerous factors trigger or aggravate asthma, principally upper and lower respiratory tract infections. The specific role of bacterial organisms and their products in the production of asthma is a disputed question. Other triggering factors are rapid changes in temperature or barometric pressure, the common air pollutants in cities, cooking odors, smoke, paint fumes, and emotional upheavals. Psychologic factors appear to be important in some cases but are seldom the sole cause.

Clinical Findings

A. History: Onset may be in the early weeks of life, but in most cases the onset is between 3–8 years. In infancy, the first attack usually follows a respiratory infection, and there is frequently a history of allergic rhinitis. As age increases, there is a progressively greater tendency for initial and subsequent episodes to be associated with inhalants, pollens, and molds.

A history of atopic dermatitis or allergic rhinitis is often obtainable. A family history of atopic diseases (especially allergic rhinitis and bronchial asthma) is often present.

B. Progressive Symptoms and Signs: (During an acute severe attack or if an attack is prolonged.)

1. Flushed, moist skin; pallid cyanosis; dry mucous membranes.

2. Restlessness, apprehension, fatigue, drowsiness, coma.

3. Distressing cough, dyspnea, increasing prolongation of expiration, high-pitched rhonchi and wheezes throughout the chest (diminishing in intensity as the obstruction becomes more severe), secretions (variable but decreasing in amount with ensuing dehydration), hyperinflation of the chest, poor air exchange to areas of imperceptible air exchange. Worse at night.

4. Increasing tachycardia; initially, there may be mild hypertension; ultimately, hypotension; and, rarely, signs of cardiac failure.

5. Initially good and prompt response to epinephrine or other adrenergic drugs or methyl xanthines. If the attack is very prolonged, the response to the above drugs may be poor—especially the response to epinephrine ("epinephrine fastness").

C. Special Clinical Findings:

1. Episodes of asthma in association with infections are frequently insidious in onset and prolonged;

those due to specific identifiable allergens tend to be acute in onset and brief if the causative agent is removed.

2. Bronchial asthma in infants (under 2 years of age) deserves special comment. The first attack usually follows by a few days the onset of a respiratory infection; some degree of wheezing persists for prolonged periods and becomes worse with subsequent "colds."

3. In infants under 1 year of age, the predominant symptoms may be dyspnea, excessive secretions, noisy and rattly breathing, cough, and, in many cases, some intercostal and suprasternal retractions—rather than the typical pronounced expiratory wheezes that occur in older children. Initial and repeated diagnoses of these episodes are apt to be "croup," "bronchiolitis," "pneumonia," and "whooping cough." Definite clinical and epidemiologic evidence of infection is often present. A high percentage of these infants have positive skin tests to egg white, and this in combination with atopic dermatitis increases the likelihood of chronic disease.

D. Laboratory Findings: Eosinophil accumulations (eg, clumps of eosinophils in a nasal or sputum smear) and peripheral eosinophilia are commonly found but are often absent in infection or if corticosteroids or antihistamines are being given.

Hematocrit is elevated with dehydration, prolonged attacks, or severe, chronic disease. In severe asthma, the first sign is hypoxemia without CO_2 retention. Acidosis and increased CO_2 tension may ensue. (Moderately severe hypoxemia may occur with low CO_2 tension due to a combination of hyperventilation and ventilation-perfusion disturbances.)

E. X-Ray Findings: Bilateral hyperinflation; bronchial thickening and peribronchial infiltration; and areas of densities (patchy atelectasis or associated bronchopneumonia) may be present. (Patchy atelectasis is a common finding and is often misread as pneumonitis.) The pulmonary arteries may also appear prominent.

F. Pulmonary Function Studies: (See Chapter 12.) Increased airway resistance with a decrease in the 1-second forced expiratory volume (FEV_1) and maximum flow rates, decreased vital capacity (VC), and increased functional residual capacity (FRC) and residual volume (RV). The first 3 may be normal in asymptomatic intervals.

G. Skin Testing: Positive skin reactions (immediate wheal and flare reactions) to "scratch" or intracutaneously injected allergens are usually present. (Supportive evidence only.)

H. Provocative Tests:

1. Food—Positive clinical reactions usually occur within hours after ingestion. Foods causing low-grade hypersensitivity reactions may not induce a reaction for a few days and are very difficult to document.

2. Inhalants—A positive clinical reaction usually occurs immediately after inhalation but may not occur until a few hours after challenge. Asthma may occasionally be provoked by skin testing with the appropriate allergens.

Differential Diagnosis*

Bronchial asthma may be confused with middle and lower respiratory tract infections (eg, laryngotracheobronchitis, acute bronchiolitis, bronchopneumonia, and pertussis), especially in the very young.

Nasal "wheezes" may be transmitted to the chest (especially in infants) from upper airway edema, increased secretions, or other obstructing factors such as allergic rhinitis, upper respiratory tract infections, adenoidal hypertrophy, foreign body, choanal stenosis, and nasal polyps (incidence high in cystic fibrosis).

Congenital laryngeal stridor is usually associated with other anomalies.

In tracheal or bronchial foreign body, dyspnea or wheezing is usually of sudden onset; on auscultation, the wheezes are usually but not always unilateral. X-ray findings are characteristic.

The differentiation between bronchial asthma and cystic fibrosis is made on the basis of high sweat chloride, a history (often present) of serious pulmonary infections since birth, a personal and family history of associated intestinal disturbances with profuse, bulky stools, and pancreatic enzyme deficiency.

Tracheal or bronchial compression by extramural forces may resemble asthma and may be due to a foreign body in the esophagus, aortic ring, anomalous vessels or inflammatory or neoplastic lymphadenopathy.

Complications & Sequelae

Chronic recurrent bronchial asthma may lead to invalidism, both organic and psychologic, barrel chest, and perhaps emphysema (presumably as a result of complicating infections); atelectasis and massive pulmonary collapse, mediastinal emphysema and pneumothorax, and death due to respiratory insufficiency or improper medication (oversedation, misuse of aerosols, theophylline, tranquilizers, narcotics). Sudden death may occur as a result of unknown causes other than respiratory insufficiency.

Treatment of Mild & Moderate Asthma

As is true of all atopic diseases, bronchial asthma can be controlled but not cured.

A. Specific Measures: Insofar as possible, the patient should avoid contact with proved or suspected irritants and allergens in the environment. (See Environmental Control of Exposure, above.) **Hyposensitization therapy** is generally believed to be justified for patients whose allergens cannot be avoided, eg, pollens, seasonal molds, and house dusts.

B. General Measures: General management should be directed in a comprehensive fashion to include the measures listed below. Depending upon the frequency and severity of asthma in a given child, some or all of these measures may be used, mainly with the onset of an asthmatic attack or as a constant regimen—especially during the times of year when asthma is most severe.

---

*See also Other Allergic Pulmonary Disorders, p 843.

1. **Education**—The patient must be educated to live optimally with his chronic problem. Complete understanding of all recommendations made is essential.

2. **Liquefaction and expectoration of mucus**—Maintain adequate hydration by encouraging oral fluid intake, or give intravenous fluids if necessary. Warm humidification (not cold or steam) and expectorants may be used as necessary. Isoproterenol (Isuprel) inhalations may be used twice daily (followed by postural drainage) or every 2–6 hours, depending upon the severity of asthma and the tolerance of the patient.

3. **Relief of mucosal edema**—Give vasoconstrictive adrenergic drugs (epinephrine, phenylephrine, ephedrine).

4. **Bronchodilatation**—Bronchodilating adrenergic drugs (epinephrine, isoproterenol, and ephedrine), aminophylline, theophylline.

5. **Correction of metabolic acidosis**, if present, by providing an adequate energy source to diminish ketosis (eg, 5% dextrose IV), food if tolerated, and bicarbonate (see below).

6. **Corticosteroids**—In severe acute asthma or in chronic asthma unresponsive to other measures, adrenal glucocorticoids may be indicated (see below).

7. **Antibiotics**—With evidence of bacterial infection, appropriate antibiotics should be given. However, leukocytosis up to 15,000/cu mm is common in severe asthma without any evidence of bacterial infection. Patchy atelectasis must not be confused with pneumonitis on x-ray.

8. In children with chronic or recurrent asthma, breathing and fitness exercises under the guidance of a well oriented physical therapist may assist the patient in aborting some attacks of asthma and improving muscular functions of the thoracic cage.

9. Children with frequent overt asthma attacks (eg, 1 or 2 per week) and evidence of more or less constant pulmonary obstruction should be on constant pharmacologic therapy including a daily regimen stimulating coughing and encouraging expectoration (eg, postural drainage at least twice a day).

Treatment of Severe Asthma (Status Asthmaticus, Intractable Asthma)

This is a medical emergency!

A. Emergency Care: Epinephrine (1:1000 aqueous solution, 0.1–0.3 ml subcut) is the drug of first choice. It may be repeated at 20-minute intervals for a total of 3 doses. If the response to epinephrine is good but relatively short-lived, a longer acting epinephrine preparation (eg, Sus-Phrine) may then be employed. If a response to epinephrine is not apparent by the second or third injection, discontinue the drug since excessive use of epinephrine, particularly in the face of "epinephrine resistance," may actually aggravate asthma. Relative or apparently complete lack of responsiveness to epinephrine ("epinephrine fastness") may be due to hypoxemia and acidosis, bronchial obstruction with thick mucus plugs, pneumothorax, or simply severe asthma. Epinephrine sensitivity may improve after initiation of other therapy.

B. Hospital Care: If signs are relatively early, an overnight ward may suffice.

1. With the first evidence of resistance to epinephrine, with poor fluid intake or vomiting or signs of dehydration, provide warm humidification (not cold or steam) and give 5% dextrose solution with 0.2% saline intravenously. (Use 1½ times maintenance fluid requirements.)

2. Give moisturized oxygen (by mask or nasal prongs—not by tent) in a concentration of about 40%.

3. Give aminophylline, 4 mg/kg, in intravenous tubing over a 20–30 minute period (if not used in previous 4 hours); may repeat every 6 hours.

4. Take an arterial or venous blood sample for pH and an arterial sample for P_{CO_2} and P_{O_2}. (Determination of gases or pH on capillary blood is unreliable.)

5. Correction of acidosis (pH 7.3 or below) with sodium bicarbonate should be attempted. The appropriate dosage may be calculated by means of the following formula:

$$\text{mEq bicarbonate needed} = \text{negative base excess} \times 0.3 \times \text{body weight in kg}$$

The bicarbonate can be given rapidly by the intravenous route.* Arterial or venous pH should be redetermined 5–10 minutes later, and further correction of acidosis, using bicarbonate, should be considered at that time if necessary. In respiratory failure, in the absence of a pH determination, 2 mEq/kg body weight may be infused initially.

6. Give isoproterenol (Isuprel), 1:200, by inhalation (2–3 good "whiffs") followed by postural drainage every 2–4 hours as tolerated.

7. **Corticosteroids**—If the patient is already receiving corticosteroids, do not withdraw but increase the dose temporarily. If he is not receiving corticosteroids, they should be withheld for about 2–4 hours in most cases to ascertain the benefits of the measures listed above. Corticosteroids should be added initially when the asthma is of sufficient severity to be life-threatening or the patient has been on prolonged daily corticosteroid therapy (at least 2 weeks) in the past year. If it is decided that corticosteroids are to be used, one of the following should be given intravenously in the following initial doses every 6 hours around the clock: (1) Hydrocortisone sodium succinate (Solu-Cortef), 100 mg. (2) Prednisolone sodium phosphate (Hydeltrasol), 20 mg. (3) Dexamethasone sodium phosphate (Decadron), 4 mg.

With amelioration of symptoms, the dose should be decreased as rapidly as possible. (If the patient has not been on prolonged corticosteroid therapy within the past year, the corticosteroids can be discontinued abruptly rather than tapered. It is frequently feasible to use high doses of corticosteroids for 48 hours or less.)

8. Give antibiotics as indicated.

*Sodium bicarbonate for injection may be obtained in ampules or multidose vials which contain approximately 1 mEq/ml.

9. Chloral hydrate, 15 mg/kg rectally, may be given for restlessness or apprehension.

10. In respiratory failure unresponsive to the above therapy, assisted ventilation by a mechanical respirator may be required.

C. Precautions in Therapy: Note the following "don'ts":

1. Don't use antihistamines or antihistaminic tranquilizers. (They may dry secretions.)

2. Don't use narcotics or barbiturates. (They depress the respiratory center. Tranquilizers may do the same in the presence of severe hypoxemia.)

3. Don't use epinephrine excessively. (The patient has probably already had too much; it tends to dry secretions, depletes glycogen stores, and increases apprehension.)

4. Don't use 100% oxygen. (It may cause respiratory arrest and atelectasis and is very drying.)

5. Don't use isoproterenol aerosols excessively—they may aggravate asthma. Discontinue if responsiveness to aerosol therapy is not apparent.

D. Follow-up Therapy:

1. Fluids—When the patient is improved and is able to take fluids and oral medications, continue humidification and give oral fluids in the form of fruit juices with added sugar, eg, grape, apple, pineapple, Kool-Aid, carbonated drinks (but not caffeine and chocolate containing colas). Give no milk or iced drinks.

2. The following medications are of value at this stage:

a. Isoproterenol (Isuprel) inhalations, 1:200, every 3–6 hours, followed by postural drainage for 20 minutes.

b. Ephedrine-theophylline combination (eg, Marax, Quadrinal, Tedral, or Verequad) every 6 hours (dosage according to weight).

c. Saturated solution of potassium iodide, 25 mg/kg/day.

d. If corticosteroids have been started, withdraw after 48 hours or taper gradually and discontinue as soon as possible.

Prognosis

There is no evidence that bronchial asthma can be cured, and the old adage still holds: "Once an asthmatic, always an asthmatic." However, the prognosis for symptom-free control in childhood asthma is fairly good. The largest series of cases with the longest follow-up in children with onset under 13 years of age (420 for at least 20 years) was reported by Rackemann in 1959. Thirty percent were completely free of symptoms, 20% were asymptomatic unless in contact with the offending agent, and 21% were free of asthma but still had hay fever—giving a total of 71% who had "done well." Fifteen percent still had mild symptoms, largely with provocation of wheezing by occasional respiratory infections; 11% had significant symptoms, but only 2 patients required hospitalization for asthma; and 2.4% (11 patients) had died, but only 4 deaths were known to be due to asthma.

Recent reports indicate that in the past 25 years the morbidity and mortality rates in asthma may have increased, but it is not clear whether this increase is due to the diagnosis of more cases of "infectious" or "intrinsic" asthma, increased air pollution, the use of isoproterenol aerosols, or corticosteroid therapy. Mortality statistics indicate that a high percentage of deaths have been due to indiscriminate use of sedatives, narcotics, and aminophylline. In the pediatric age group, the highest mortality rates have been reported in infants with onset of asthma under 2 years of age.

In general, the earlier the onset of asthma, the more serious the disease. "Continuity" symptoms of night cough, breathlessness, and provocation of wheezing with exercise or stress are usually indicative of more serious disease than the occasional, spontaneous, and brief attacks due to recognizable allergens (eg, epidermals, kapok, pollens) with symptom-free periods in between.

Johnstone DE, Dutton AM: The value of hyposensitization therapy for bronchial asthma in children: A 14-year study. Pediatrics 42:793–802, 1968.

Rackemann FM: The prognosis of asthma in children. P Clin North America 6:725–729, 1959.

Reisman RE: Asthma induced by adrenergic aerosols. J Allergy 46:162–177, 1970.

Richards W, Siegel SC: Status asthmaticus. P Clin North America 16:9–29, 1969.

Strick L: Breathing and physical fitness exercises for asthmatic children. P Clin North America 16:31–42, 1969.

ALLERGIC RHINITIS

Essentials of Diagnosis

- Chronic or recurrent nasal obstruction; itching and sneezing (frequently paroxysmal) with seromucoid discharge. There may be accompanying conjunctival injection and itching, with or without tearing. Bilateral "vacuum" headaches often present.

- Mucosal hyperemia to purplish pallor and edema of nasal mucous membranes; polypoid changes of turbinates may occur.

- Eosinophilia of nasal secretions when symptomatic. (May be absent with infections, or possibly with corticosteroid therapy.)

- Positive immediate skin test reactions to provoking allergens (supportive evidence only).

General Considerations

Allergic rhinitis is the most common atopic disease, perhaps because the nose is anatomically and physiologically vulnerable to inhalant allergens. The pathologic changes are chiefly hyperemia, edema, goblet cell and connective cell proliferation, cellular infiltration (especially with eosinophils and lymphocytes), and exudation of serous and mucoid secretions, all of which lead to variable degrees of nasal obstruction, rhinorrhea, and pruritus. Inhalant allergens are principally responsible for causation of symptoms, but food allergens on occasion may provoke rhinitis.

Classification

Allergic rhinitis may be classified as perennial or seasonal (hay fever), but these 2 entities frequently occur concomitantly. Children with allergic rhinitis seem to be more susceptible to upper respiratory infections, which in turn intensify the symptoms of existing allergic rhinitis.

A. Perennial Allergic Rhinitis: Perennial allergic rhinitis occurs to some degree all year long but is usually more severe in winter. Characteristically, it "blows up" when forced air heating systems are turned on in the fall, causing increased exposure to house dusts. Nasal stuffiness, frequent sniffing, or constant rhinorrhea with evidence of mild to moderate itching (frequent nose rubbing) are often the dominant symptoms, although more severe symptoms, including paroxysmal sneezing, may occur. Sneezing is often most pronounced in the morning shortly after waking. Symptoms may be related to periods of shedding of hair of house pets (early fall and early spring), redecoration procedures, and changes in home furnishings. Greater exposure to house dust during the winter months is due to increased indoor activities, the use of winter blankets and wool or hairy clothing, dry air and heating systems which raise, disperse, and circulate dust, and indoor housing of pets.

This disease frequently begins before the second year of life. It often accompanies bronchial asthma and may be provoked by the same allergens. Dental abnormalities and disturbances in dental arch growth and malocclusion have been attributed to longstanding perennial allergic rhinitis.

B. Seasonal Allergic Rhinitis (Hay Fever): Hay fever occurs seasonally as a result of exposure to specific wind-borne pollens. The major important pollen groups in the temperate zones are trees (late winter, early spring), grasses (spring to early summer), and weeds (late summer to early fall). Seasons may vary significantly in different parts of the country. Mold spores may also be a significant cause of seasonal allergic rhinitis, principally in the summer and fall.

The age at onset is generally later than for perennial allergic rhinitis. Hay fever is rare before age 1; in most cases it begins after 3 years of age. Worsening or extension of pollen sensitivities over a period of several years after onset can be expected.

Clinical Findings

A. Symptoms and Signs: Nasal obstruction is manifested by mouth breathing, snoring, difficulty in nursing or eating, nasal speech, and inability to clear the nose with blowing. Nasal seromucoid secretions are increased, with anterior drainage, sniffling, "nasal stuffiness," postnasal drip, and loose cough. Nasal itching leads to nose rubbing ("allergic salute," "bunny nose"), nose-picking, epistaxis, and sneezing. Eye manifestations consist of itching, unilateral or bilateral tearing, conjunctival injection, lid edema, "allergic pleats," and eye shadows. There may be headache or a feeling of fullness. Palatal and pharyngeal itching may occur.

The symptoms and signs of perennial allergic rhinitis and hay fever differ little except for seasonal incidence and, in hay fever, severe intense itching, coryza, and sneezing. Examination shows decreased or absent patency of nasal airways, increased seromucoid discharge anteriorly and posteriorly (usually more serous in seasonal rhinitis), and excoriation of the nares. The mucous membranes (especially over the turbinates) are pale blue to purplish, swollen, and boggy, with dimpling in the turbinates or pedunculated polyps. Bleeding points or ulceration may be seen on the anterior nasal septum. A horizontal crease may be seen extending across the lower third of the nose due to frequent upward rubbing of the nose. Malocclusion (overbite), presumably due to excess pressure of digit sucking to relieve palatal itching, may be seen in longstanding cases.

The florid conjunctival injection, coryza, intense itching of the eyes and nose, and violent sneezing experienced by older children and adults are not so commonly seen in young children. Paroxysmal sneezing, however, is a frequent symptom even in young children.

B. Laboratory Findings: Eosinophilia can be demonstrated on smears of nasal secretions or blood (usually higher in seasonal than perennial rhinitis.) The technic of examination of nasal secretions is as follows:

1. Obtain nasal secretions by having the patient blow onto a piece of wax paper or by nasal swab; spread on a microscope slide and allow to dry.

2. Cover the slide with Hansel's stain for 1−2 minutes.

3. Add enough distilled water to take up staining solution and allow to stand 1 minute.

4. Wash with distilled water.

5. Flood with 95% ethanol and drain off immediately; allow to dry.

6. Examine under the oil immersion objective. (Look for greater than 4% eosinophils, or accumulations [clumps] of eosinophils.)

C. Skin Testing: Positive immediate reactions to scratch or intradermal tests with offending allergens.

D. Provocative Tests: Positive on ingestion or inhalation of offending allergens.

E. X-Ray of Head Sinuses: Allergic sinusitis may accompany allergic rhinitis and is frequently demonstrable on x-ray (mucosal thickening, fluid levels, or complete opacification of sinuses).

Differential Diagnosis

These disorders must be differentiated from the common cold, other infectious diseases (eg, purulent rhinitis and sinusitis, nasal diphtheria, congenital syphilis), adenoidal hypertrophy, foreign bodies (usually unilateral), nasal polyposis with cystic fibrosis, choanal stenosis, nasopharyngeal neoplasms, palatal malformations (eg, congenitally high arch, cleft palate), "vasomotor rhinitis," and nasal polyps with prolapse of nasal mucous membranes (unusual in children).

Treatment

A. Specific Measures: Avoid exposure to proved allergens insofar as is reasonably possible. (See Environmental Control of Exposure, above.)

1. Perennial allergic rhinitis–Hyposensitization should not be considered unless symptoms are severe and all other measures have failed; unless the disease is definitely associated with recurrent serous otitis media and hearing loss; or unless it is accompanied by significant seasonal allergic rhinitis. The only allergen for which hyposensitization might be of benefit in perennial allergic rhinitis is house dust. However, the efficacy of hyposensitization therapy specifically with house dust is not clearly established and the trauma of prolonged injection therapy should be seriously weighed against the questionable benefit.

2. Hay fever–Hyposensitization may be beneficial in seasonal rhinitis due to specific allergens identified by clinical history and skin tests. It should be reserved for cases which have become progressively worse and cannot be controlled by antihistamines or adrenergic drugs (or both), or those which are accompanied by asthma. There is evidence that hyposensitization for hay fever may prevent the onset of asthma; some allergists therefore favor hyposensitization therapy in all children with hay fever in whom an inciting allergen can be identified.

B. General Measures:

1. Give antihistamines with or without vasoconstricting adrenergic drugs by mouth. (Table 33–1.)

2. Treat associated infections.

3. Avoid all nasal topical drugs except for minimal use of decongestants (eg, phenylephrine) for severe episodes. Corticosteroids should be used only for short periods in polypoid states or acute severe nasal obstruction not controllable by other means.

4. Surgical removal of nasal polyps is indicated if other measures fail.

Prognosis

A. Perennial Allergic Rhinitis: Unless specific allergens can be identified and eliminated from the environment or diet (unusual cases), this atopic disease tends to be very protracted. As the child grows older—presumably because of increasing caliber of the nasal airway and if polypoid growths do not appear—nasal obstruction becomes less troublesome.

B. Seasonal Allergic Rhinitis: Hay fever patients tend to repeat their seasonal symptoms if exposure to offending allergens is high. On moving to a region devoid of specific allergens, they may be free of seasonal allergic rhinitis for 1–3 years but frequently acquire new pollen hypersensitivities from airborne pollens in the areas to which they move. (*Example:* On moving to the Rocky Mountain region from mid-eastern USA, patients usually become less symptomatic to ragweed because of low exposure but acquire hypersensitivity to tumbleweeds and sages.)

About 70% of patients seem to improve significantly on hyposensitization therapy over a 2–4 year period. About 25% of boys seem to improve spontaneously during adolescence; girls often get worse during these years (and may also develop seasonal rhinitis for the first time during adolescence). Continued hyposensitization with prolongation of intervals between infections (if possible) or resumption of a previous injection program may be necessary in some patients.

Norman PS, Lichtenstein LM: Allergic rhinitis: Clinical course and treatment. Chap 47 in: *Immunological Diseases,* 2nd ed. Samter M (editor). Little, Brown, 1971.

Norman PS, Winkenwerder WL, Lichtenstein LM: Maintenance immunotherapy in ragweed hay fever. J Allergy 47:273–282, 1971.

Sadan N & others: Immunotherapy of pollenosis in children. New England J Med 280:623–627, 1969.

RECURRENT ALLERGIC SEROUS OTITIS MEDIA ("Glue Ear")

Essentials of Diagnosis

- Recurrent or protracted nonpurulent otitis media characterized by episodes of mild to moderate hearing loss with or without earaches.
- Presence of viscid secretions within the middle ear; distortion of tympanic membranes.
- Nasal eosinophilia (common).
- Positive immediate skin test reaction to offending allergens (supportive only).
- Provocation of symptoms with inhalation or ingestion of provoking allergens.

General Considerations

Recurrent serous otitis media is probably a misnomer since the secretions within the middle ear are more mucoid than serous. In most cases, this entity is thought to be an extension of the pathologic changes of allergic rhinitis (edema and increased secretory activity of the mucosa) involving the eustachian tubes and the epithelial lining of the middle ear. The result is episodic obstruction of the eustachian tubes, metaplastic mucosal changes, accumulation of viscid secretions within the middle ear, fullness or retraction of the tympani, hearing loss, often earache and ear plugging, and, sometimes, rupture of the tympani. Hearing loss and frequent "colds" are common complaints.

This entity is most common in small children and is seldom seen after 8 years of age. Many cases previously believed to be due to inadequately treated acute or subacute otitis media of infectious origin or primary hypertrophy of adenoid tissues are now thought to be part of an allergic diathesis. The atopic young child seems to be particularly prone to the development of serous otitis media. In one study of 512 allergic infants and children with this syndrome, 98% had concurrent allergic rhinitis, 34% a history of asthma, and 25% a history of eczema. Major allergy was present in at least one member of the immediate family in 81% of cases and a bilateral family history occurred in 50%. In the vast majority of patients, repeated myringotomies and multiple courses of antibiotics had failed before the institution of allergy management. Nasal eosinophilia (about 10%) was present in 88%. Fluctuating hearing loss was found in 51%. On the basis of the history and skin testing, inhalants (eg, dust, epidermals, molds, and pollens) appeared to be the major allergens. Skin testing for commonly eaten food allergens, however, has been of little assistance in implicating specific allergens, and the importance of their role in this entity remains controversial and undetermined. Although thought to be contributory to the disease in many instances, they are rarely identified as the sole cause.

Intercurrent ear infections are common in this disorder and tend to complicate the underlying problem. Although allergic factors appear to be important in many cases of serous otitis media, other causes must be considered.

Clinical Findings

A. Symptoms and Signs: A history of allergic rhinitis appears common. The incidence of recurrent episodes of infectious otitis media is high. Recurrent episodes of ear plugging and earaches since infancy are frequently reported; there may be complaints of "popping" sounds in the ears. Rupture of the drum and discharge of mucoid secretions in the ear canal are uncommon.

Hearing impairment is recurrent and variable (usually mild to moderate); audiographic changes are usually variable and for the most part reversible. Difficulties in social and school adjustment due to hearing loss are often encountered.

Vertigo seems to be rare.

The tympani may be scarred, distorted, full, very retracted, opaque, and amber to bluish in color, and movement of the tympanic membrane may be limited. Chalky appearance and narrowing of the malleus are prominent signs. Tympanic bleb formation is sometimes present. A fluid level or "bubbles" behind the tympani may be observed. Occasionally, the ears may appear normal.

B. Laboratory Findings: Eosinophilia of nasal secretions (see Allergic Rhinitis, above) is often present. Smears of middle ear secretions are usually negative for eosinophils and other cells.

C. Audiometry: A bilateral hearing loss of up to 10–40 db in all frequencies (usually reversible with treatment) may be seen.

D. Skin Testing: Positive immediate skin reactions to provoking allergens is supportive evidence for allergic etiology.

E. Provocative Tests: Symptoms subside with elimination of offending allergens and recur with inhalation or ingestion of offending allergens.

Differential Diagnosis

This entity must be differentiated from viral otitis media, inadequately treated bacterial otitis media, anomalies of the eustachian tube and nasopharynx, hypertrophy of adenoidal tissue due to nonallergic causes, growths in the nasopharynx (eg, nasal polyps, carcinoma), or otosclerosis in later childhood.

Complications & Sequelae

Complications include permanent hearing loss, recurrent and chronic infectious otitis media and its sequelae, and problems of learning and social adjustment.

Treatment

The treatment of recurrent serous otitis media in which an allergic etiology is suspected is as outlined for allergic rhinitis (see above), with the following additional considerations: (1) ENT consultation as required, eg, when the question of intubation and drainage of the middle ear arises. (2) Special schools may be necessary in cases of hearing loss. (3) Elimination of identified causative allergens and daily use of antihistamines coupled with decongestants. (4) Prompt treatment of bacterial infections of ears and nose. (5) Hyposensitization with proved inhalant allergens must be considered if elimination of allergens and drug therapy are of little benefit. (6) Provision of adequate and controlled humidification (40%).

Adenoidectomy gives poor results. Temporary improvement is reported with myringotomy or intubation.

Prognosis

The problem of recurrent serous otitis media appears to diminish with age. Recent reports indicate that, in those patients in whom an allergic diathesis is recognized and appropriately treated, the overall prognosis is good.

The benefit of hyposensitization against inhalant allergens is questionable, and there is no substantial evidence for the value of hyposensitization with microbial antigens.

McGovern JP, Haywood TJ, Fernandez AA: Allergy and secretory otitis media: An analysis of 512 cases. JAMA 200:134–138, 1967.

Miller GF: Influence of an oral decongestant on eustachian tube function in infants. J Allergy 45:187–193, 1970.

Murray AB & others: A survey of hearing loss in Vancouver school children. Part 2. The association between secretory otitis media and enlarged adenoids, infections, and nasal allergy. Canad MAJ 98:995–1001, 1968.

Sale CS: Control of allergy and humidity in secretory otitis media of children. South MJ 63:1042–1046, 1970.

ATOPIC DERMATITIS

Essentials of Diagnosis

- Appearance of the lesions: from erythematous and papular to scaling, vesicular, and tous and papular to scaling, vesicular, and oozing; in more chronic forms, lichenification.

- Predilection for cheeks and flexural creases.
- Pruritus, frequently intense.
- Family history of atopy or presence of other atopic disorder in the same patient (frequent).

General Considerations

Atopic dermatitis is a confusing disorder with a poorly understood pathophysiology. It is generally accepted as an atopic disorder largely because of its frequent association with other atopic disorders and because skin-sensitizing antibodies are often demonstrable. It is frequently difficult to implicate specific allergens, however, and it is by no means certain that allergic mechanisms are always involved.

Individuals with atopic dermatitis exhibit certain physiologic or pharmacologic peculiarities: (1) "White dermographism"–a white line instead of the usual erythematous line in response to firm stroking of the skin–can be elicited in most patients. (2) A "delayed blanch" reaction, which occurs a few minutes after the intradermal injection of acetylcholine or methacholine (see below), has been demonstrated in 70% or more of patients (mostly adults) with atopic dermatitis. (3) Patients with atopic dermatitis exhibit unusually sensitive alterations in blood flow in response to changes in temperature. (4) The skin of patients with atopic dermatitis has been shown to release twice as much histamine, to harbor 15 times as much acetylcholine, and to bind greater amounts of norepinephrine than that of normal subjects.

When specific allergens can be established, foods appear to be a particularly common offender in early life; inhalants and contactants may also play a role and are the most important antigens in later childhood. Atopic dermatitis has been reported to occur more commonly in infants fed cow's milk than breast milk or a soybean preparation for the first few months of life. Intense heating of cow's milk lessens its antigenicity, and the use of heat-processed evaporated or powdered milk formulas may account for an apparent decrease in incidence of this disorder in young infants in recent years. Egg white, a commonly incriminated allergen, has been reported to elicit a positive skin test in 76% of infants with atopic dermatitis. However, only about 50% of these children were found to be clinically sensitive to egg white. Conversely, an occasional infant with a negative skin response to egg white can be found to react clinically to ingestion of this antigen. Follow-up observations of infants with atopic dermatitis show that 30–80% develop at least one respiratory allergy later in childhood.

Children with atopic dermatitis behave as if they have generally "itchy skin." The pruritus is aggravated and frank dermatitis provoked by a variety of factors in addition to allergic and psychic mechanisms. The trauma of scratching plays a major role in the occurrence and progression of dermatitis. Local infection is a frequent aggravating factor. Autosensitization is believed by some authorities to be a significant factor in the development of the lesions.

Decreased sweating, possibly due to increased absorption factors by a relatively defatted hydrophilic keratin content in the epidermis, may account for the abnormally high pH of the skin of patients with atopic dermatitis. The abnormal dryness of skin seen in these patients is thought to be due to diminished surface secretions of both sweat and sebaceous material, but a heritable (autosomal dominant) form of ichthyosis may also be present in these children. Seborrheic dermatitis, which often accompanies atopic dermatitis in early infancy, differs in its predilection for the scalp and the postauricular and axillary creases and its coarse, scaling, nonpruritic lesions which may appear the first few days of life. If unaccompanied by atopic dermatitis, the areas of unaffected skin appear normal.

Clinical Findings

A. Symptoms and Signs: The infantile forms typically appear at 3–6 months of age but may occur earlier. Lesions appear first on the cheeks and forehead and then spread in a patchy or generalized distribution over the extremities and trunk and eventually involve the flexural creases (antecubital, popliteal, neck). In late infancy, or in middle or late childhood, the rash usually appears first in flexural creases and subsequently in areas easily accessible to scratching as well as areas predisposed to friction and contact irritation (extensor surfaces), which become equally involved.

A rare but severe form of atopic dermatitis which may occur in the first few weeks of life, *atopic erythroderma,* is characterized by diffuse dermatitis, marked generalized lymphadenopathy, and cold, blue extremities. It usually responds poorly to any form of treatment. Severe infection of the skin may be important in prolonging the disease.

The parent or the patient often complains of unusual dryness and itchiness of the skin and intolerance to extreme heat or cold at all ages. Pruritus, evidenced by signs of scratching, may occur as early as 2 months of age.

Recurrent florid pyoderma is common (50% in the experience of one author). In these cases, repeated upper respiratory infections, impetigo, acne, or poor general hygiene in the patient or other family members are common. Low-grade inflammatory reactions are the rule in areas of frequent scratching.

Occasionally, in infantile atopic dermatitis, the first appearance of rash follows soon after the introduction of a "new" food, eg, a prepared cow's milk supplement to breast feeding, dairy milk, egg, or wheat. In these cases, coincident colic, vomiting, nasal symptoms, or wheezing may also occur, suggesting a single food allergen. Citrus fruits and tomatoes commonly aggravate this disorder in infants–particularly the facial lesions. In the authors' experience, foods rarely provoke atopic dermatitis in older children, the exception being an occasional urticarial response to egg or an infrequently eaten food such as walnuts, peanuts, shellfish, trout, or chocolate. When this occurs, it is sometimes followed by exacerbation of the existent atopic dermatitis.

In older infants and in children, the onset of atopic dermatitis can sometimes be related to the increased contacts in the child's environment, eg, the creeping infant on a wool carpet, house pets, feather pillow, outside play in the spring (tree or grass pollen), or play in a weed patch (weed pollen) or dusty basement (house dust). Whether such agents provoke atopic dermatitis by inhalation, by absorption through the skin, or by direct contact on the surface of the epidermis is disputable.

Atopic dermatitis in older children is usually an extension of the dermatitis developed initially in infancy.

Chemicals, dyes, and rough or wool clothing commonly exacerbate an existent dermatitis, particularly in areas of direct contact. The sudden appearance of a generalized vesicular rash should suggest a new laundry soap, detergent (particularly those with enzymes), bleach, water softener, crease-resistant treated fabrics, or bubble bath; involvement of the extensor surfaces of the legs suggests that the cause may be friction-producing trousers or repeated contact with some particular object in that area. Worsening of flexural crease lesions usually occurs during such episodes.

The history of use (and effect) of previously used local or systemic medications is helpful in making a specific diagnosis, in evaluating the severity of disease, and in assessing the effects of a specific drug on the patient—all of which are invaluable in outlining a plan of management.

The acute stage of dermatitis is characterized by an intensely pruritic, erythematous, papular to vesicular rash in various stages of eruption and disruption of skin with exudation of serum and crusting. The rash shows a predilection for the cheeks and flexural creases and may be generalized or distributed patchily in areas of greatest friction or sweating. Evidence of scratching (excoriation) is often present.

Subacute or chronic stages are characterized by various degrees of fading erythema, dryness, cracking of the skin in areas of greatest involvement, and patchy plaques of thickening and lichenification, especially in flexural creases.

Areas of normal skin often show unusual dryness; itching and scratching may be provoked on touch. The skin is often generally pale. The skin of the extremities may be cool. Purplish discoloration of the palms and soles is occasionally seen.

B. Laboratory Findings: A "delayed blanch" frequently occurs in areas of normal or involved skin in response to the intradermal administration of acetylcholine, 1:10,000, or methacholine (Mecholyl), 1:5000. (This test is rarely used and seldom necessary.) Blood eosinophilia is frequently seen.

C. Allergic Testing: Positive immediate skin test reactions are common but do not necessarily identify the causative agents.

Differential Diagnosis

Seborrheic dermatitis often accompanies atopic dermatitis but may be distinguished by lack of significant pruritus, its predilection for the scalp ("cradle cap"), the skin behind the ears, and the axilla; the coarse "potato chip" scales; and orange and yellow nonvesicular lesions occurring in plaques with intervening normal skin.

Candidiasis occurs predominantly in the diaper region and is characteristically intensely red, with satellite lesions. Denudation and weeping occur in creases. Cultures and smears for *Candida albicans* are positive.

Contact dermatitis is chiefly distinguished by the distribution of lesions (extensor and exposed areas).

Nummular eczema is characterized by large, coin-shaped, thick denuding plaques and easy bleeding. Pruritus is minimal at times but may be intense at night.

Scabies is characterized by a papulovesicular, relatively nonerythematous eruption, chiefly in interdigital and waistline distribution. Itching occurs mostly at night. Mites may be seen with a magnifying glass.

Aldrich's syndrome is a sex-linked recessive disorder of male infants characterized by melena, thrombocytopenia, absence of heterologous isohemagglutinins, severe recurrent infections (particularly otitis media), and early death. Eczematous lesions frequently occur and may be indistinguishable from those of atopic dermatitis.

Children with phenylpyruvic oligophrenia (phenylketonuria) may have a rash simulating atopic dermatitis in infancy. This disorder is characterized by an odorous urine containing an excess of phenylpyruvic acid, elevated serum phenylalanine levels, and, in untreated cases, mental retardation, convulsions, and an abnormal EEG pattern.

Leiner's disease (erythrodérma desquamativum) is a rare disease with onset of 1–3 months of age. It is characterized by thick, yellow scaling and crusting scalp lesions; generalized desquamation of skin in large, opaque scales, leaving an erythematous base; nail deformities; blotchy red hands and feet; vesiculation; associated gastrointestinal symptoms; malnutrition; absence of pruritus; and lymphadenopathy. It is thought to be a form of seborrheic dermatitis. If the patient survives (the mortality rate is about 30%), recovery is complete in 3 months and there are no allergic sequelae.

Ritter's disease (dermatitis exfoliativa neonatorum) is an unusual disorder which occurs as a manifestation of infection, usually streptococcal or staphylococcal, of the skin in newborns. Vesicles, bullae, and denuding lesions over the body are usually heralded by peripherally spreading erythematous patches originating around the mouth. Widespread exfoliation may occur. Nikolsky's sign (removal of epidermis by slight rubbing) and cultures for the appropriate bacterial agent are positive.

Complications & Sequelae

Bacterial skin infections, particularly staphylococcal and streptococcal, may occur. Viral infections include Kaposi's varicelliform eruption (eczema herpeticum) and eczema vaccinatum due to vaccinia virus, most often acquired from recently vaccinated siblings but sometimes from the patient's own vaccination site.

Nutritional disturbances may result from too vigorous restrictions in diet imposed by the physician or parents.

Cataracts in late childhood or adulthood may occur in very severe, protracted cases.

Emotional disturbances may occur in severe cases as a result of feelings of disfigurement, imposed restrictions, and unhealthy attitudes of parents toward a child with this disease.

Prevention of Serious Complicating Infections

Smallpox, chickenpox, herpes simplex, and staphylococcal and streptococcal infections should be prevented if possible. No child with atopic dermatitis or eczematoid lesions of any kind should be vaccinated with live vaccinia virus or have direct contact with individuals so vaccinated. In the event of smallpox vaccination of other family members, either the patient or the vaccinated individual should be removed from the home until the vaccinia lesion is healed.

If the patient with active atopic dermatitis has not had chickenpox, avoidance of systemic corticosteroid therapy and contact with chickenpox is especially important. Patients with atopic dermatitis should not have direct contact with individuals with overt lesions of herpes simplex, impetigo, or florid acne.

Treatment

A. Specific Measures: Elimination of proved food and environmental allergens is the only specific treatment available. Hyposensitization is of doubtful value.

B. General Measures: The patient and the parents must be educated to live optimally with a chronic problem characterized by periodic exacerbations. A nutritionally adequate diet must be provided and undue physical limitations avoided. In the authors' experience, good general skin care and vigorous specific local treatment are the most important aspects of treatment of atopic dermatitis.

C. General Skin Care:

1. Provide generous lubrication, eg, with hypoallergenic bath oils (Lubath, Alpha-Keri, Domol) in bath water and with lotions (Lubriderm, Alpha-Keri, Domol lotion) after washing. Bath oils should be added to the bath only after allowing the skin to be hydrated by water in the bath (it is usually sufficient to add the oil half way through the bath). Hypoallergenic soaps (Basis, Lowila) or detergents (pHisoHex) may be used. Excessive use of the latter may be especially drying, and, if applied vigorously over widely denuded areas, sufficient absorption of hexachlorophene can occur to cause toxic symptoms, eg, convulsions and coma.

2. Use only mild detergents in washing clothes and rinse *thoroughly* 3 times in the laundry. Detergents with added enzymes and bleaches should be avoided.

3. Avoid direct contact of skin with irritants and dyes (eg, wool, chemicals, harsh soaps). Wash new clothing before wearing. Use light cotton pajamas–not silk or flannel. Minimize scratching by keeping the fingernails short and clean. Provide good coverage of the body with light clothing. (Avoid direct contact of skin with silk, wool, or flannel.) Swathing and restraints should be avoided if possible but may be necessary in infants in severe cases.

4. For itching, give oatmeal-starch baths (eg, Aveeno). Burow's solution is also an effective antipruritic, especially when used on weeping skin.

D. Specific Treatment of Dermatitis: Care should be taken not to apply any ointment or cream thickly enough to occlude sweat glands or to cover encrusted infected areas. Do not use creams or ointments in the weeping stage unless an antibiotic cream is selected for infection, in which case it should be used sparingly.

1. **Acute weeping stage–**

a. Burow's solution (aluminum subacetate) soaks are made up as a 1:20 solution using 1 Domeboro tablet or packet per pint of water. Apply for 20 minutes as often as every 3 hours.

b. Treat any evidence of infection–(1) Substitute for Burow's solution, benzalkonium chloride (Zephiran) solution, 1:5000, or potassium permanganate, 1:6000 (one 0.3 gm tablet in 2 quarts of water). (2) Topical antibiotics (Bactracin Solvets, 500 units/ml as soaks; bacitracin ointment, 500 units/gm, or neomycin ointment) may be used twice daily if infection is confined to the skin. Infection due to group A beta-hemolytic streptococci, however, should be treated systemically. Remove crusts with soaks before applying antibiotic. (Because topical medications are particularly sensitizing, systemic antibiotics are preferred by the authors.)

c. Pruritus–Diphenhydramine (Benadryl), tripelennamine (Pyribenzamine), trimeprazine (Temaril), and hydroxyzine (Atarax) are the preferred drugs for pruritus. They are especially useful at night, when itching may be most intense.

2. **Healing or subacute stage**–Corticosteroid creams are particularly effective at this stage in diminishing inflammation, pruritus, and further trauma secondary to pruritus. Hydrocortisone (0.5–1%) or one of the more potent fluorinated steroids, eg, fluocinolone acetonide (Synalar), 0.025 or 0.01%, are useful. Other effective, less expensive compounds:

a. Lassar's paste–Zinc oxide, 1 part; corn starch, 1 part; white petrolatum, 2 parts.

b. 1-2-3 ointment (Rosen and Glaser)–Burow's solution, 1:20, 1 part; Hydro-Sorb (fatty acid esters of diethanolamine in petrolatum), 2 parts; Lassar's paste, 3 parts. If infection is still present, benzalkonium chloride (Zephiran), 17%, may be added to the above mixture to a final concentration of 1/600 parts. A prescription may be compounded as follows:

R	Burow's solution, 1:20	10.0
	Hydro-Sorb	20.0
	Lassar's paste	30.0
	Benzalkonium chloride, 17%	0.6

c. Plain Acid Mantle cream with buffered aluminum acetate in a water-miscible base, pH 4.2.

Although reported experience is limited, the use of topical heparin (100 mg/30 gm cream base) holds promise as an important adjunct in local skin therapy.

3. Chronic stage—Apply coal tar solution, 2–5% in acid mantle cream, Lassar's paste, or vanishing cream base. Corticosteroid creams and ointments are effective, particularly in lichenified lesions, and may be used alone or in combination with coal tar. A good combination in the latter case is hydrocortisone, 0.5%; coal tar solution, 2%; and iodochlorhydroxyquin, 1%, in acid mantle vehicle (Cor-Tar-Quin, 0.5%). Because of their photosensitizing qualities, coal tar products should be discontinued with extended exposure to direct sunlight. In the presence of seborrheic dermatitis, use iodochlorhydroxyquin (Vioform) cream cut to 1–2% with acid mantle cream.

Systemic corticosteroids should be used only in the most refractory cases and for the shortest period of time possible.

Optimal lubrication of the skin of patients with atopic dermatitis during quiescent periods tends to decrease the frequency and severity of episodes of frank dermatitis. For this purpose, continued use of lubricating bath oils and lubricating after-bath creams are recommended. An inexpensive means of encouraging good skin lubrication, particularly over areas of skin which characteristically become affected by the dermatitic process, is to apply a thin layer of white petrolatum over the wet skin at night. (After bathing at night, do not dry skin completely, and coat with petrolatum.)

Prognosis

Most cases of simple atopic dermatitis clear by 2½–3 years of age with reasonably good skin and general pediatric care and elimination of offending allergens. (Atopic dermatitis may also disappear without known definitive therapy.) However, persistent dermatitis may extend through adult life. Many patients, especially those in whom the onset is in middle or late childhood, benefit only slightly from specific "anti-allergic" or other means of therapy. Emotional problems may become paramount and require special consideration.

Dockhorn RJ: Topical heparin treatment of eczema. Ann Allergy 28:573–579, 1970.

Holt LE Jr (editor): Conference on infantile eczema. J Pediat 66:153–274, 1965.

Sulzberger MB, Frick OL: Atopic dermatitis. Pages 680–697 in: *Dermatology in General Medicine*. Fitzpatrick TB & others (editors). McGraw-Hill, 1971.

FOOD ALLERGY

Allergic reactions can be provoked by food antigens in virtually any tissue of the body containing blood vessels, smooth muscle, or mucous and secretory epithelium. A wide variety of signs and symptoms are encountered, many of which may appear extremely vague. Significant serious reactions include anaphylaxis, acute angioedema of the upper airway, and severe bronchial asthma provoked especially by eggs, shellfish, trout, cow's milk (see Chapter 16), walnuts, peanuts, pork, melons, and certain seeds (sesame, sunflower). Such reactions usually occur within 1–2 hours. Other symptom complexes of lesser consequence can also occur in response to a variety of common foods. These are more likely to appear after several hours.

Classification

"Syndromes" which may be induced by hypersensitivity to foods include the following:

A. Angioedema: (Often accompanied by urticaria.) In mild cases, periorbital and lip edema, a few hives, mild arthralgia, malaise; in severe cases, tongue, pharyngeal and laryngotracheal edema and joint swelling. Death may occur from asphyxia. (See Medical Emergencies Due to Allergic Reactions.)

B. Anaphylaxis: Immediate reaction with lightheadedness to syncope, flushing to pallor, paresthesias, generalized itching—especially palms and soles, palpitation and tachycardia; symptoms and signs of pulmonary edema, bronchial asthma and vascular collapse. (See Medical Emergencies Due to Allergic Reactions.)

C. Gastrointestinal Intolerance: In milder cases, nausea, diarrhea, flatulence, bloating, and abdominal discomfort; in severe cases, forceful vomiting, severe colic, bloody and mucoid diarrhea, and dehydration. Prolonged episodes of food gastrointestinal intolerance can result in malnutrition and growth retardation. A curious syndrome of melon and banana sensitivity coincident with ragweed pollinosis has been recently reported. The predominant manifestations of the former are oral pruritus and gastrointestinal and mouth symptoms, including swelling of the lips.

D. Perennial Allergic Rhinitis, Bronchial Asthma, Atopic Dermatitis, Urticaria: See elsewhere in this chapter.

E. Tension-Fatigue Syndrome: A combination of fatigue, lassitude, irritability, sleeplessness, disturbed behavior, disinterest, pallor, "shadowy" eyes with "allergic pleats," "run-down feeling," and sometimes generalized headache with vague abdominal complaints has been reported. This syndrome may be associated with other atopic or allergic disorders. It may be related to inhalant allergens but frequently seems to be provoked by food antigens commonly and abundantly eaten, eg, cow's milk, cereal grains, chocolate, eggs, pork. The diagnosis of this syndrome is frequently difficult, and, in the authors' opinion, one of exclusion of many other mild and chronic disease states, particularly in a patient who has no other evidence of allergic disease.

F. Migraine: In addition to other causes, certain foods may precipitate a migrainous episode. A true hypersensitivity reaction is questioned. Certain foods such as chocolate, strong cheeses (cheddar), and some wines and beers in which significant amounts of tyramine has been found have been demonstrated to precipitate migraine.

Clinical Findings

A. History; Symptoms and Signs: See above; the section on history in the discussion of atopic disorders; and individual disorders.

B. Laboratory Findings:

1. Eosinophilia of stool mucus may be present in cases of gastrointestinal intolerance but may be a normal finding in the first 3 months of life; blood eosinophilia may occur.

2. Skin testing for food hypersensitivity is generally of little value; however, positive reactions may give leads to possible allergens, especially those provoking a sudden onset, eg, angioedema, anaphylaxis, and severe gastrointestinal symptoms. Use scratch tests only.

3. Provocative food tests are important in the less serious entities. Elimination, challenge, and rechallenge must be relied upon for definitive diagnosis. In immediate or very serious reactions such as angioedema, anaphylaxis, and bronchial asthma, the causative food is usually known by the patient or parents or can be identified by the physician with aid of a history. Food challenges and food skin testing would be hazardous in these situations. In the less serious and more obscure symptom entities, the likely food is a common one (eg, milk, cereal, chocolate); the suspected food should be withdrawn for a minimum of 3 weeks before challenge.

Differential Diagnosis of Important Symptoms

A. Gastrointestinal Intolerance: Differentiate from cystic fibrosis, pyloric stenosis, celiac disease, acute or chronic intestinal infections, gastrointestinal malformations, and carbohydrate enzyme deficiencies (eg, lactase).

B. Angioedema of the Upper Airway: Differentiate from acute epiglottitis and foreign body in upper airway.

C. Tension-Fatigue Syndrome: Because the symptomatology is often vague, the differential diagnosis is often not specific. Connective tissue disorders (early phase), low-grade chronic infections, nutritional and metabolic disorders, leukemia (early), chronic poisonings, and hypochondriasis must be considered.

Treatment

Treatment consists of elimination of the offending food or foods, but with specific advice for ensuring the nutritional adequacy of the diet. If milk or a comparable milk substitute is withdrawn from the diet for over 1 month in infants or over 2 months in older children, the daily maintenance requirement of calcium should be administered (see Chapter 4). *Note:* To be condemned—especially in the growing child—is the unnecessary and unjustified restriction of many foods over an indefinite period because they might be involved or happened to give a positive skin test reaction.

Treat specific signs or symptoms as indicated.

Prognosis

The prognosis is good if the offending food can be identified. In some of the vague chronic syndromes this may not be possible, in which case the patient will remain symptomatic. In the severe syndromes, the responsible food is usually known and can be avoided.

Feeney MC: Nutritional and dietary management of food allergy in children. Am J Clin Nutr 22:103–111, 1969.

Fries JH: Factors influencing clinical evaluation of food allergy. P Clin North America 6:867–880, 1969.

Goldstein GB, Heiner DC: Clinical and immunologic perspectives in food hypersensitivity: A review. J Allergy 46:270–299, 1970.

Unger L, Cristol JL: Allergic migraine. Ann Allergy 28:106–109, 1970.

CONTACT DERMATITIS

Essentials of Diagnosis

- Erythematous, papular eruption which may progress to include vesiculation, bulla formation, and denudation.
- Mild to intense pruritus.
- Eruption confined more or less to areas of direct skin contact with allergen.

General Considerations

Contact dermatitis is a delayed hypersensitivity reaction of the epidermis. The allergen is believed to conjugate locally with skin tissue elements. Sensitization after initial contact requires at least a few days and frequently takes much longer, but an already sensitized individual may react to contact with the allergen in as little as 24 hours. Fur, leather and fabric dyes, formalin, dye intermediates, soaps, enzymes in detergents, rubber compounds and impurities, insecticides and fungicides, cosmetics, topical antibiotics and other drugs, vegetable oleoresins and mineral oils, weeds, flowers, foods, wool, silk, rayon, and plastics are among the most common offenders in contact dermatitis.

Clinical Findings

A. History: A history of contact with possible allergens appropriate to the distribution of the lesions, in conjunction with the appearance of the lesions, may be sufficient for the diagnosis or may serve only as a starting point for further investigation. Itching is the rule, is frequently intense, and may precede the onset of observable lesions.

B. Physical Examination: The appearance and distribution of the lesions are the main criteria for diagnosis. The eruption may be confined to areas of contact with the offending allergen, and the inflammation sharply demarcated from normal skin. With more severe and chronic eruptions, however, dissemination may occur as a result of scratching and repeated contact with the allergen. If the eruption is mild, only erythema with some papulation may be present; more intense reactions include vesiculation with denudation of skin and frank weeping. Exfoliative dermatitis and secondary infection can also occur. There may be evidence of excoriation reflecting the pruritic nature of these lesions. With chronic dermatitis, skin thickening may be present.

C. Patch Testing: Patch testing with suspected allergens can be used to identify the contactants involved. In general, patch testing should not be performed when the dermatitis is active since this procedure may exacerbate the dermatitis. Patch testing kits of common contact allergens can be obtained from a variety of firms dealing with allergenic materials. The patch testing procedure is briefly as follows:

1. Material is applied to a gauze patch and secured to a nonhairy portion of the skin with adhesive tape (or an adhesive substitute in tape-sensitive persons).

2. The patch is removed after 48 hours—or sooner if itching, pain, or burning develops. The patch should be kept dry and remain securely fastened to the skin during the contact period.

3. The test is read 24–48 hours after removal of the patch. A positive test is one in which there is definite evidence of dermatitis which persists 24 hours or more. (A hand lens is helpful in interpreting mild or questionable reactions.) A control patch test should be employed. Be certain that the testing material is not itself a primary irritant. Solutions and oils can be soaked into the gauze; ointments and creams are merely smeared on the gauze.

Differential Diagnosis

Seborrheic dermatitis, atopic dermatitis, scabies, papular urticaria, nummular eczema, dermatophytoses, and candidiasis may at times be confused with contact dermititis.

Prevention

Sensitizing substances should be avoided to the extent possible. Inflamed skin is more susceptible to sensitization than normal skin, and one must regard virtually any substance applied to the skin as potentially sensitizing; a test application of a "new" topical agent to a very limited area is advised before more extensive use.

Hyposensitization is not generally successful and presents a number of problems. Moreover, the striking beneficial effects of a brief course of local or systemic corticosteroid treatment virtually nullify justification for hyposensitization at the present time.

Treatment

A. Early Treatment:

1. Terminate exposure to the contactant.

2. Burow's solution (Domeboro powder or tablet, 1 package or tablet to 1–2 pints of water), or potassium permanganate, 1:6000 (0.3 gm tablet plus 2 quarts of water), soaks may be used in the early stage, especially if oozing is present, to diminish itching.

B. Mild Dermatitis: Zinc oxide paste or calamine lotion may be used.

C. Severe Dermatitis: Creams containing corticosteroids—particularly the fluorinated corticosteroids—are helpful. These should be applied liberally and frequently so as to keep the inflamed areas covered at all times. In unusual circumstances, when the dermatitis is extremely severe and extensive, systemic corticosteroids should be considered. A short course of systemic corticosteroids followed by topical corticosteroid administration is frequently helpful in controlling acute severe contact dermatitis (eg, poison ivy dermatitis). In severe cases, a course of 3–4 weeks may be necessary. Pastes, ointments, and creams should not be applied to weeping skin.

D. General Measures:

1. Avoid all secondary irritants to the skin, eg, wool, detergents.

2. Treat infection, if present. Early, potassium permanganate solution may be employed instead of Burow's solution. Topical treatment may be sufficient, but with extensive lesions systemic antibiotic therapy must be used.

3. Give antihistamines for pruritus. Colloidal soaks, such as starch baths, may be employed with extensive dermatitis.

DeWeck AL: Contact eczematous dermatitis. Pages 669–680 in: *Dermatology in General Medicine.* Fitzpatrick TB & others (editors). McGraw-Hill, 1971.

Waldbott CL: *Contact Dermatitis.* Thomas, 1953.

SERUM SICKNESS

Essentials of Diagnosis

- Fever, malaise.
- Skin rash (usually urticarial).
- Local or generalized lymphadenopathy, polyarthralgia, or polyarthritis is frequent.
- History of recent administration of foreign serum or drug.

General Considerations

Antibiotics—particularly penicillin—have largely replaced foreign serum as the principal cause of serum sickness. In addition to antibiotics and foreign sera, vaccines, toxoids, and virtually any injectable foreign substance may cause this disorder. It may occur after the first encounter with a substance, usually requiring 7–10 days for sufficient sensitization to occur. Reexposure to the antigen in an already sensitized individual may result in symptoms as early as 1–4 days later. In unusually sensitive individuals, exposure to antigen may result in anaphylactic shock. Administration of antigen or, in atopic individuals, natural exposure (eg, to horse allergens) may sensitize an individual to the antigen without inducing clinically apparent symptoms.

Clinical Findings

A. Symptoms and Signs: This disorder usually begins with a low-grade fever and malaise which are followed to a variable extent by skin rash, lymphadenopathy, polyarthritis, and neurologic symptoms. Skin rashes occur in over 90% of cases. Most commonly, the skin rash is urticarial with an accompanying severe pruritus (which may precede the urticaria), but other erythematous eruptions may occur. Development of a localized erythematous or frankly urticarial reaction may first occur at the injection site. Lymphadenopathy may be localized to an area which drains the injection site or it may be generalized. Neurologic lesions, when they occur, are most commonly those of peripheral neuritis, but there may be CNS involvement as well. Gastrointestinal symptoms sometimes occur.

B. Laboratory Findings: Leukopenia may occur early, followed later by leukocytosis. Eosinophilia is not common but does occur. Proteinuria and microscopic hematuria may be seen.

Prevention

The patient should always be questioned about a history of previous reactions before the administration of drugs, sera, or other injectable foreign substances. (In atopic individuals, a history of respiratory allergy induced by contact with an animal from which the serum to be administered has been derived is strongly suggestive that the patient may react adversely.)

Since foreign sera are highly sensitizing, skin tests with the serum should be performed if a history of previous contact or suspected allergy is obtained. Caution is required, since anaphylactic reactions after skin tests have been known to occur. Scratch testing should be done first, followed by intradermal testing with a 1:20 dilution of the scratch test material. Unfortunately, the reliability of the skin test in predicting clinical sensitivity is much less than desired; both false-positive and false-negative reactions occur. Conjunctival tests are also unreliable.

Treatment

Treatment consists mainly of the discontinuance of the drug or other offending agent, the use of antihistamines with or without adrenergic drugs, and, in more severe and prolonged cases, administration of adrenal corticosteroids. When angioneurotic edema, bronchial constriction, and vascular collapse occur, epinephrine and theophylline may be lifesaving. (See Medical Emergencies Due to Allergic Reactions, above.) Joint pain, pruritus, and high fever may be amenable to treatment with aspirin. Sedation may also be in order.

Prognosis

In most cases serum sickness subsides in less than a week, but on occasion it may be more prolonged. The symptoms usually abate with the clearance of offending antigen from the circulation; persistence, therefore, suggests continued exposure.

Arbesman CE, Reisman RE: Serum sickness and human anaphylaxis. Chap 20 in: *Immunological Diseases,* 2nd ed. Samter M (editor). Little, Brown, 1971.

DRUG ALLERGY

Drugs are so widely used that drug reactions of one sort or another are commonplace. **Toxic drug reactions** are due to the inherent pharmacologic properties of the drug and are most frequently encountered after drug overdosage. Some individuals exhibit inordinate sensitivity to the recognized pharmacologic effects of a drug, however, and may therefore develop toxicity after administration of usually nontoxic amounts. **Drug idiosyncrasy** refers to an unusual response to the pharmacologic action of the drug (eg, hyperactivity rather than sedation following the administration of phenobarbital). This paradoxical reaction to barbiturates is not uncommon in patients with atopy. **Allergic reactions to drugs,** on the other hand, are independent of the drug's pharmacologic action and, as is true of all allergic reactions, are the result of antigen-antibody interaction. The allergen may not be the drug administered but a metabolic derivative of it produced in the body. Although the immunologic reaction is highly specific, cross-reactions with chemically related drugs are not infrequent. Allergy to one sulfonamide, for example, is often associated with allergy to many other sulfonamides, and there is potential cross-reactivity among the various kinds of penicillins.

The manifestations of drug allergy are extremely varied, and virtually all allergic syndromes can be produced by drugs. The most common manifestations are skin eruptions (see Chapter 8) and fever.

Although any drug is a potential sensitizer, some are more often associated with allergic reactions than others, particularly penicillin and the sulfonamides. The likelihood of sensitization is increased by repeated exposure. It is also probable that parenteral administration is more sensitizing than oral administration. Topical administration of drugs, especially over inflamed skin, is particularly sensitizing.

Exposure to sunlight may activate skin reactions to photosensitizing drugs such as sulfonamides, tetracycline antibiotics, and topically applied coal tar products.

In questioning a patient about drug reactions, it should be remembered that certain drugs such as benzathine penicillin G remain in the body for a long time. Reactions to a single depot injection of penicillin have been known to last for months.

With the exception of patch testing in contact dermatitis, skin testing has usually been a disappointing procedure in identifying or predicting drug allergy. The reasons are many, and in some cases at least the allergic reaction is due to a metabolically altered form of the drug. In the case of penicillin, some of the offensive metabolic derivatives have been identified; when these substances are used in skin testing, prediction of allergic reactions on the basis of a skin test reaction is more successful. However, these reagents are not readily available and until the exact allergens are identified and preparations containing the appropriate allergens become available, skin testing for drug allergy cannot be considered a reliable procedure.

The history of previous reactions to drugs remains the best means of diagnosing drug sensitivity. This is often difficult, however, and in any instance in which a reaction to a drug is questionable an alternative drug should be used (if possible) and the patient advised to avoid the drug even though a definite drug allergy has not been established.

Treatment

Regardless of the manifestation, the treatment of drug allergy includes discontinuance of the offending drug at the first sign of an allergic reaction and making certain that further contact with the drug is avoided. Small amounts of drugs to which a patient may be sensitive may be found in vaccines, foods, and other substances. Individuals with extreme hypersensitivity to a given drug should be warned, therefore, of other hidden sources of contact with the drug. Although desensitization has been used successfully, it is not recommended, and the physician is better advised to substitute a chemically unrelated drug for the offending drug.

Symptomatic treatment offers relief for manifestation of the drug reactions.

Prognosis

The prognosis is good, especially with early identification.

Adkinson NF Jr & others: Routine use of penicillin skin testing on an impatient service. New England J Med 285:22–24, 1971.
Alexander HC: *Reactions with Drug Therapy.* Saunders, 1955.
Kasik JE, Thompson JS: Allergic reactions to antibiotics. M Clin North America 54:59–73, 1970.
Levine BB, Zolov DM: Prediction of penicillin allergy by immunological tests. J Allergy 43:231–244, 1969.

URTICARIA

Essentials of Diagnosis

- Multiple (occasionally single) macular lesions, consisting of localized edema (wheal) with surrounding erythema.
- Pruritus, frequently intense.

General Considerations

Urticaria is a vascular reaction of the upper dermis consisting mainly of vasodilatation and perivascular transudation resulting in the classical "hive" or wheal and flare. Lesions are characteristically pruritic. Ordinarily, this vascular reaction is due to the liberation of histamine, but acetylcholine and other mediators also may be involved.

Urticarial reactions are usually very transient (hours) but have been known to persist for months or more. They may be the sole allergic manifestation or may represent only a part of the clinical picture, as in serum sickness. Emotional tension may be a precipitating factor. **Angioedema** is essentially an urticarial reaction of the lower parts of the dermis, resulting in the production of a more diffuse edema.

Hereditary angioneurotic edema is a rare syndrome characterized by periodic bouts of angioedema frequently involving one or more extremities but other anatomic areas as well. It is inherited as an autosomal dominant trait and appears to be related to a deficiency of a dual Cl esterase and kinin inhibitor. There is no good evidence that an allergic mechanism is involved.

Cholinergic urticaria, which is uncommon, seems to occur in some individuals during and following exercise, increased environmental heat, and emotional stress. Characteristically, the lesions appear as extremely small wheals accompanied by a large bright red flare. Abdominal cramps, diarrhea, increased sweating, and headache may also occur.

Clinical Findings

A. History: The history is of prime importance in ascertaining the possible cause. The most common causes of urticaria include the following:

1. Drugs, hyposensitization extracts, vaccines, toxoids, and hormone preparations.

2. Infections—Bacterial (especially group A beta-hemolytic streptococci), parasitic and, rarely, viral. (**Note:** An urticarial reaction following administration of anthelmintics may represent sudden destruction of the parasites and liberation of antigens rather than an allergic reaction to the drug used.)

3. Foods (especially eggs, milk, wheat, chocolate, pork, shellfish, fresh water fish, berries, cheese, and nuts).

4. Inhalants, pollens, molds.

5. Insect bites—Papular urticaria is a term given to a syndrome characterized by multiple papules resembling insect bites, found especially on the extremities. It is thought to be due to hypersensitivity to the bites of fleas, mites, mosquitoes, lice, or bedbugs.

6. Psychologic factors.

7. Physical factors (cold, heat), histamine liberators, and dermographism should be considered.

B. Symptoms and Signs: Urticarial lesions characteristically appear as erythematous areas with a pale center and usually occur in large numbers. Pruritus is the rule and is frequently intense; it may precede the appearance of the lesions. Pruritus is not so characteristic of angioneurotic edema (giant hives), however, which occurs most often as a solitary lesion or in conjunction with multiple urticaria. When urticaria involves the laryngeal area, it may be a threat to life.

Dermatographism may be symptomatic and occurs in approximately 10% of allergic patients.

In addition to the history, diagnostic procedures may include drug elimination, dietary elimination of suspected foods and their challenge, and a thorough search for a focus of infection. Skin testing more often than not is of little value in urticaria.

Differential Diagnosis

Urticaria is a prominent feature of mastocytosis (urticaria pigmentosa) and may occur in systemic diseases such as lupus erythematosus.

Treatment

Treatment consists mainly of the detection and elimination of the appropriate allergens, when possible, and psychotherapy if indicated. Antihistamines are usually the most useful therapeutic agents in urticarial disorders, but adrenergic agents with vasoconstrictor properties are frequently a useful adjunct. Epinephrine is especially effective when rapid relief is needed. Hydroxyzine (Atarax, Vistaril) has been reported to be effective in some instances in which antihistamines are not, eg, chronic urticaria and dermatographism. Mild sedation may also be indicated.

Adrenal corticosteroids are sometimes used in the more chronic form of urticaria, but their effectiveness is questionable. There is little place for these agents in the management of acute urticaria or angioneurotic edema.

Topical medications do not appear to be effective.

Prognosis

Except for life-threatening laryngeal edema, the prognosis is good. Identification of the offending agent is most important.

Collins-Williams C: Urticaria and angioedema. Chap 65 in: *Brenneman's Practice of Pediatrics.* Vol 2. Harper & Row, 1968.

Grolnick M: Evaluation of dermatographism. Ann Allergy 28:395–404, 1970.

Thompson JS: Urticaria and angioedema. Ann Int Med 69:361–380, 1968.

OTHER ALLERGIC PULMONARY DISORDERS

A variety of pulmonary disorders either known or thought to stem from an allergic reaction to inhaled or ingested antigens have been described. In some instances, evidence implicating an allergic mechanism in the pathogenesis of the disease is substantial; in others, the role of allergic mechanisms is mainly conjectural.

A syndrome thought to be related to **cow's milk hypersensitivity** has been described which consists of recurrent pulmonary infiltrates, wheezing, chronic cough, chronic or frequent otitis media and rhinorrhea, and iron deficiency anemia related to excessive gastrointestinal blood loss. Gastrointestinal symptoms (diarrhea, vomiting) and poor weight gain are also features of this disorder which is seen in children chiefly in the first 2 years of life. Some of these children have evidence of pulmonary hemosiderosis, and blood eosin-

ophilia is sometimes seen. Multiple precipitins to cow's milk can be demonstrated, but the significance of this finding is controversial. Dietary elimination of cow's milk antigens is followed by improvement of the disorder, although symptoms also have been reported to subside spontaneously.

Extrinsic allergic alveolitis (hypersensitivity pneumonitis) is an inflammatory reaction involving principally the alveoli and characterized clinically by malaise, fever, chills, cough, and dyspnea. Tissue damage stems from a hypersensitivity reaction to any of a variety of inhaled organic dusts or of fungi which may or may not also be infective. The disease is seen predominantly in adults as a result of occupational exposure to large concentrations of certain antigens (eg, proteinaceous material from bird droppings in bird fancier's lung; thermophilic actinomycetes from hay in farmer's lung or from contaminated air conditioners), but it can occur at any age. Pulmonary allergic aspergillosis, with or without tissue invasion by the organism, is seen with some frequency in Great Britain but is rare in the USA. These diseases occur principally in adults but have been reported in children also. The onset may be insidious or acute. Symptoms—particularly in the acute onset form—typically occur 4–8 hours after exposure to the offending antigen, reflecting, presumably, the nature of the specific allergic mechanism involved (a type III or immune complex mechanism). In asthmatic individuals, wheezing also may be a part of the picture, with involvement of reagin-mediated mechanisms as well. Rales may be heard, but physical findings referable to the lungs may be minimal. Chest x-ray reveals a variable pattern, with mottled densities or infiltrates early in the disease and a picture of interstitial fibrosis in more chronic cases. Pulmonary function studies reveal a restrictive defect with diminished diffusing capacity (Pa_{O_2} may be decreased, but Pa_{CO_2} is usually normal). Treatment consists mainly of avoiding the offensive inhalants. Glucocorticoids may be extremely helpful in minimizing the hypersensitivity reaction early in the disease. Accompanying fungal infection must also be treated (eg, amphotericin in aspergillosis). If recognized early, lesions are largely reversible and the prognosis is excellent. With chronic severe disease, pulmonary fibrosis may result, leading to severe respiratory insufficiency and death.

An association between **tissue and blood eosinophilia and pulmonary infiltrates** has been observed in various disorders (eg, asthma, pulmonary allergic aspergillosis, connective tissue diseases) and is thought to reflect an allergic pathogenesis in these disorders. Pulmonary infiltrates with eosinophilia (PIE) sometimes occur as an apparently distinct clinical entity characterized by mild (mainly cough) to absent clinical symptoms and fleeting pulmonary infiltrates which, on x-ray, appear to migrate from one area of the lungs to another over a few days (often called Löffler's syndrome). A number of drugs (especially sulfonamides and nitrofurantoin), parasites (eg, ascaris), and other antigens have been implicated at times in the production of this syndrome, but frequently no cause can be found. The disorder is generally self-limited, lasting less than a month; but more severe forms may be seen (eg, in many cases of so-called tropical eosinophilia associated with filariasis), and the tissue reaction may proceed to pulmonary fibrosis. Corticosteroids may be extremely beneficial, particularly early in the reaction, and should be used when the severity of the disorder warrants.

Banaszak EF, Thiede WH, Fink JN: Hypersensitivity pneumonitis due to contamination of an air conditioner. New England J Med 283:271–276, 1970.

Heiner DC, Wilson JF, Lahey MD: Sensitivity to cow's milk. JAMA 189:563–567, 1964.

Lecks HI, Kravis LP: The allergist and the eosinophil. P Clin North America 16:125–148, 1969.

Salvaggio JE, Buechner HA: Pulmonary hypersensitivity diseases associated with actinomycetes and fungi. Chap 1 in: *Management of Fungus Diseases of the Lungs.* Buechner HA (editor). Thomas, 1971.

TRANSFUSION REACTIONS

Essentials of Diagnosis
- Fever and chills during or after transfusion.
- Urticarial reaction with or without lymphadenopathy, joint pains, fever, hypotension, asthma.

General Considerations

The incidence of transfusion reactions is high—estimates ranging up to 20%. A common form is a febrile reaction which may be related to contamination with bacterial or other pyrogenic products or which may accompany hemolytic reactions or reactions in which transfused leukocytes are destroyed by antileukocyte antibodies present in the recipient. Urticarial reactions have been reported to occur in 1–3% of transfusions and are said to be more common in atopic individuals. Citrate toxicity, manifested largely as tetany and vascular collapse progressing at times to death, is an unusual complication of transfusion therapy. The transmission of serum hepatitis is also a potential problem, but careful screening of donors has helped to reduce the incidence of transmission.

Allergic transfusion reactions may be due to the transfusion of mismatched blood, resulting in symptoms and signs consequent to intravascular or extravascular hemolysis; or may result either from passive sensitization of the recipient through blood from a donor who is sensitive to foods, drugs inhalants, or other allergens, or from the infusion of allergen present in donor's plasma to which the recipient is sensitive. Hemolytic reactions are among the most severe transfusion reactions and are associated with a high mortality rate.

Clinical Findings

A. Symptoms and Signs: Chills and fever are particularly common and may be associated with septice-

mia, hemolytic reactions, or reactions due to the presence of leuko-agglutinins, especially if the patient has received multiple transfusions. Symptoms of hemolytic reactions may also include headache, nausea and vomiting, apprehension and anxiety, facial flushing, a feeling of warmth along the vein into which blood is being transfused, and abdominal or chest pains. Hypotension, oliguria, and frank renal failure with anuria may result.

Urticarial reactions with accompanying pruritus frequently occur without other symptoms but may also occur in conjunction with anaphylactic and hemolytic reactions. Anaphylactic reactions, which may include bronchial obstruction, hypotension, or laryngeal edema, are seen rarely. With allergic reactions, eosinophilia is sometimes noted.

B. Laboratory Findings: With hemolytic reactions, free hemoglobin is usually present in detectable amounts in the serum almost immediately and may also be found in the urine; serum bilirubin levels may become elevated within hours, as may methemoglobin levels also. The white blood count may be high or low. A Coombs test (direct and indirect) performed on post-transfusion recipient's blood should reveal the presence of antibody reactive with cells of the recipient or donor. In addition, red cell agglutinates can sometimes be seen in a sample of the recipient's blood.

Prevention

Antihistamines (Table 33–1) given 1 hour before the blood transfusion may be used prophylactically to decrease the incidence and severity of allergic reactions. This procedure has reportedly been very effective, but it would seem to make more sense to administer antihistamines only to those patients who develop allergic symptoms rather than to use the drug routinely. Used prophylactically, *antihistamines do not completely eliminate the possibility of a severe transfusion reaction.* Problems consequent to the administration of hemolyzed blood can largely be avoided with proper inspection of the blood and equipment prior to transfusion.

Treatment

Treatment consists chiefly of immediate discontinuation of the transfusion and maintenance of adequate blood volume and pressure by means of intravenous fluids and pressor amines. Other ancillary measures depend upon the degree and nature of the reaction.

Urticaria with pruritus unaccompanied by other signs or symptoms does not necessarily contraindicate continuing the transfusion, as is the case with mild febrile reactions.

The treatment of urticarial reactions, angioedema, laryngeal edema, asthma, serum sickness, and anaphylactic shock has been described elsewhere.

Epinephrine, 1:1000, 0.2–0.4 ml IM, remains the most important single drug early in the treatment of severe acute allergic reactions. Antihistamines may also be given intravenously. Corticosteroids have also been recommended for the treatment of allergic and hemolytic transfusion reactions, but their efficacy in acute reactions is questionable.

For citrate toxicity, the discontinuation of the transfusion and *slow* administration of chloride (5%) or gluconate (10%), 5–20 ml IV, is the treatment of choice.

With hemolytic reactions, recipient and donor blood should be retyped and cross-matched and recipient blood cross-matched against other possible donors. If the hemolytic reaction is severe–and in the absence of cardiac failure, severe dehydration, or intracranial bleeding–mannitol, 0.3 gm/kg of 20% solution IV over 10–15 minutes, should be given in addition to intravenous fluids in order to ensure adequate urine flow. This may be repeated once in 2 hours if adequate urine flow is not attained in this time.

Plasma expanders may be necessary to treat hypotension due to hypovolemia.

Corticosteroids–eg, hydrocortisone sodium succinate (Solu-Cortef), 4 mg/kg–should be added to intravenous fluids and infused over a 4- to 6-hour period.

Prognosis

The prognosis depends on the nature and degree of the reaction. Hemolytic reactions must be kept in mind since they are associated with a high fatality rate.

Baker RJ & others: Transfusion reaction: A reappraisal of surgical incidence and significance. Ann Surg 169:684–693, 1969.

Baker RJ, Nyhus LM: Diagnosis and treatment of immediate transfusion reaction. Surg Gynec Obst 130:665–672, 1970.

● ● ●

General References

Samter M (editor): *Immunological Diseases,* 2nd ed. Little, Brown, 1971.

Samter M, Durham OC: *Regional Allergy of the United States, Canada, Mexico, and Cuba.* Thomas, 1955.

Sheldon JM, Lovell RG, Matthews KP: *A Manual of Clinical Allergy,* 2nd ed. Saunders, 1967.

Sherman WB: *Hypersensitivity: Mechanisms and Management.* Saunders, 1968.

Speer F (editor): *The Allergic Child.* Harper, 1963.

Van Der Wert PJ: *Mold Fungi and Bronchial Asthma.* Thomas, 1958.

34 . . .

Genetic & Chromosomal Disorders

Arthur Robinson, MD

Recent developments in the science of genetics have greatly increased our understanding of the basic processes of heredity. Genetics is an essential discipline for an understanding of human biology; it helps to unify the physician's concept of disease and has great relevance to his clinical experience.

THE CELL

The central structure of any living cell is its complement of genes (located on the chromosomes) within the cell nucleus and consisting of a molecule whose 3-dimensional structure is that of a double helix. This molecule, deoxyribonucleic acid (DNA), is the chief constituent of the gene, which has a dual function: (1) to replicate itself (the central act of biologic reproduction); and (2) to be responsible, through the enzymes, for specific aspects of the cell's metabolism.

The information residing within a specific gene is necessary to permit synthesis of the polypeptide, a linear array of amino acids, which forms a segment of a protein. The enzymes, which are proteins, are necessary as catalysts for chemical reactions in the cell. This is in accord with the Beadle-Tatum "one gene, one enzyme" hypothesis.

A series of consecutive triplet pyrimidine and purine base pairs in the linear DNA chain code for, and are colinear with, the series of consecutive amino acids in the polypeptide chain. Many of the details of how this information is transcribed and translated have been worked out; and protein synthesis has even been observed in vitro in a cell-free system.

The majority of the genes are probably not "structural," ie, not responsible for the production of specific proteins, but are regulatory. These latter genes permit the cell to respond sensitively to its environment and to differentiate into the various kinds of cells within the organism. This has been shown in bacteria and is probably true in man, although this has yet to be proved.

CELL DIVISION

The cell cycle can be roughly divided into 4 periods (Fig 34–1): (1) S, the period of DNA replication; (2) M, the period of cell division; and (3) G1 and

(4) G2, the periods separating S and M in which protein synthesis may occur.

Cell division is of 2 types: meiosis, a form of cell division limited to those cells (germ cells or gametes) which participate in sexual reproduction; and mitosis, a form of asexual division occurring in somatic cells.

Meiosis occurs during gametogenesis (Fig 34–2). During the first meiotic division, homologous chromosomes are arranged in pairs (synapsis) along the equatorial plate, permitting genetic recombination, a process essential to human variability and evolution. The 2 homologues then separate and move to opposite poles (disjunction). Unlike the situation which exists in mitosis, described below, division occurs between (not through) the centromeres. As a result, the daughter cells have one member of each chromosome pair (haploid). Following the first meiotic (reduction) division, a second division, mitotic in character, occurs. Hence the mature germ cells, both sperm and ova, have the haploid number of 23 chromosomes. After fertilization, the fertilized egg (zygote) has the full diploid chromosome complement of somatic cells, 46.

It is worth stressing that, during the first meiotic division, chance alone determines which member of a

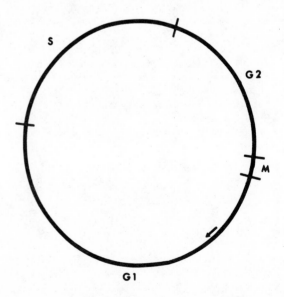

FIG 34–1. Diagram of the life cycle of a mammalian cell.

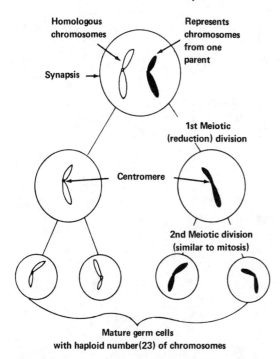

Since the chromosomes can only be delineated during mitosis, it is important to examine human material containing many cells in a dividing state. The only tissue in the body where this condition exists to any degree is the bone marrow. Because bone marrow is not readily available for routine biopsy, it becomes necessary to utilize tissue culture technics to stimulate rapid in vitro growth, so that many cells in mitosis may be examined. The period of culture varies with the tissues sampled. The lymphocytes of the blood, being most readily available, are most commonly cultured, requiring 3 days of growth in the presence of phytohemagglutinin (PHA), a mitogenic agent.

Chromosomes prepared from cultures consist of 2 arms separated by a light-staining centromere by which they are normally attached to the spindle. Because the DNA has already replicated (in the S period), each arm consists of 2 identical chromatids. Chromosomes may be designated, according to the position of the centromere, as metacentric, submetacentric, and acrocentric (nearly terminal centromere). The 10 acrocentrics are satellited.

The human somatic cell has 22 pairs of autosomes and 2 sex chromosomes. The female, being the homogametic sex, has 2 X chromosomes; the heterogametic male has one X and one Y (Figs 34–4 and 34–5).

The system for numbering and ordering the chromosomes adopted in 1960 by an international study group meeting in Denver is now used throughout the world. Although there is some difficulty in clearly distinguishing individual pairs within a given grouping, especially in suboptimal preparations, the "Denver system" has greatly simplified communication among cytogenetic laboratories in all countries. The finding, with the help of autoradiography, that chromosome replication in the S period occurs in a definite order has helped in the identification of specific chromosomes.

FIG 34–2. Diagrammatic representation of meiosis, demonstrating the conversion from the diploid somatic cell to the haploid gamete.

chromosome pair, the maternally or paternally derived one, will migrate to a given pole. This permits 2^{23} different combinations of chromosomes in the gametes and, in addition to the process of recombination, is responsible for the major part of human genetic variability. No 2 humans, with the exception of monozygotic twins, have ever been genetically identical.

During **mitosis**, the DNA coils up tightly so that the chromosomes become short and thick, which explains why they are only visible during this relatively brief segment of the cell cycle. During metaphase (Fig 34–3), the shortened chromosomes arrange themselves on the spindle; the centromere undergoes longitudinal division; and the separated chromosomal halves disjoin to opposite poles before the cell divides into 2 daughter cells. This permits the 2 daughter cells to have the identical genetic material that was present in the parent cell.

THE HUMAN CHROMOSOMES

A new era in cytogenetics began in 1956 with the discovery, by Tjio and Levan, that the human chromosomal number was 46. Since then, this field has advanced with explosive rapidity. Its importance to medicine may be judged by the fact that grossly abnormal karyotypes occur in about 1% of human live births.

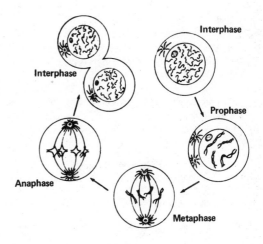

FIG 34–3. Diagram demonstrating the various stages of the mitotic cycle.

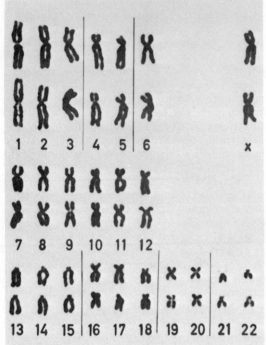

FIG 34—4. Female human chromosomes.

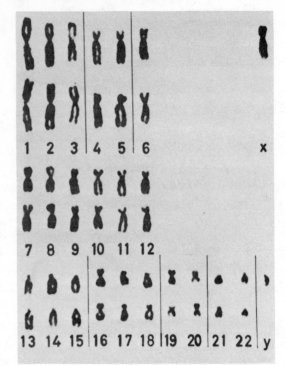

FIG 34—5. Male human chromosomes.

Very recently, 2 new staining technics make it possible easily and unequivocally to identify all the chromosomes in the karyotype and to arrange them in homologous pairs. The first of these utilizes the differential affinity of the various chromosomes and parts of chromosomes for the fluorescent dye, quinacrine mustard. Segments of chromosomes which take up the dye fluoresce brightly under ultraviolet microscopy whereas the other segments do not. This gives the individual pairs of chromosomes unique and characteristic banding patterns. The long arm of the Y chromosome fluoresces particularly intensely. The other staining method produces a very similar banding pattern on the chromosomes when they are stained with a very alkaline Giemsa stain.

Carter CO: Chromosomes and chromosome mutations. Lancet 1:1041, 1969.

Caspersson T & others: Identification of human chromosomes by DNA-binding fluorescent agents. Chromosoma 30:215, 1970.

Patil S, Merrick S, Lubs H: Identification of each human chromosome with a modified Giemsa stain. Science 173:821, 1971.

Puck TT: *The Mammalian Cell.* Holden-Day, 1971.

CHROMOSOMAL ABERRATIONS

With current technics, the cytogeneticist is able to recognize 2 classes of abnormality: numerical and morphologic. **Numerical abnormalities** are due to nondisjunction, ie, the failure of the chromosomes to divide equally between the 2 daughter cells. This may occur either during meiosis or mitosis, ie, during gametogenesis or as a postzygotic phenomenon. In the former eventuality, 2 types of gametes will be formed: those which lack a chromosome and those with an extra chromosome. If either of these gametes unites with a normal germ cell, the resulting conceptus will be either monosomic or trisomic for the involved chromosome rather than having the normal pair.

When the nondisjunction is postzygotic, the resulting individual may be a mosaic, ie, he may have 2 or more cell populations which differ in their chromosomal number. Mosaicism may also be due to chromosome lag, the failure of a chromosome to migrate to one pole of the dividing cell and its subsequent loss from one of the daughter cells. The phenotype of the mosaic individual will then depend upon when in development the nondisjunction occurred and which anlage had the aneuploid cells.

Morphologic aberration is the result of the breakage of chromosomes and the rejoining of the damaged ends in new ways. When such a rearrangement occurs between 2 nonhomologous chromosomes (reciprocal translocation) without significant loss of chromatin material (Fig 34—6), this is a balanced translocation and the individual is phenotypically normal. However, if duplication or loss of chromatin material (deletion) occurs, the somatic effects are frequently severe—even lethal. A break may occur at the centromere, with rehealing to form a metacentric structure known as an

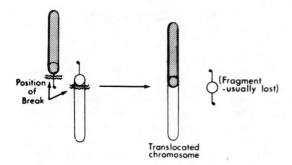

FIG 34–6. Reciprocal translocation between 2 non-homologous satellited chromosomes.

isochromosome, both arms of which originate from the chromatids of a single arm of the original chromosome. Hence the isochromosome will lack the genes on the other arm.

CAUSE OF CHROMOSOMAL ABERRATIONS

As many as 0.5% of human live births and 25–50% of spontaneous abortions are aneuploid, a fact which marks nondisjunction as one of the major causes of human disease whose origin requires investigation.

Nondisjunction has been observed to increase with maternal age and hence with the age of the maternal ova. An explanation of this "maternal age effect" may be that the ovary contains a full complement of oocytes at birth, at which time meiotic prophase has already begun. These oocytes remain in prophase until ovulation, which may occur 40 years later. It may well be that the completion of oogenesis in these older cells is attended by an increased risk of nondisjunction.

Another possible cause of nondisjunction is ionizing irradiation. At least 2 retrospective studies suggest that the mothers of children with Down's syndrome (which results from nondisjunction involving chromosome 21) have a history of significantly higher exposure to ionizing irradiation than do control groups.

Patients with a variety of aneuploid conditions, especially those with Down's syndrome, have been found to have elevated serum titers of thyroid autoantibodies. This has also been true of their close relatives, in whom there may be an increased incidence of so-called autoimmune disease. In view of the fact that several epidemiologic studies have revealed that aneuploidy tends to occur in clusters both in time and space in a manner suggestive of viral epidemics, some have suggested that nondisjunction may occur more frequently as a result of a specific viral insult in those genetically predisposed to autoimmune disease.

Recent studies on the occurrence of nondisjunction of the X chromosome have thus far provided presumptive evidence that nonrandom environmental

causes of nondisjunction exist, and that some of these are influenced by socioeconomic status and possibly by viral infection.

Viral infections, both in vivo and in vitro, have been shown to cause chromosomal breaks with or without abnormal rehealing. In 3 diseases—congenital aplastic anemia (Fanconi), Bloom's dwarfism, and ataxia-telangiectasia—an increased incidence of chromosomal breakage has been found. Whether viral infections are involved in the etiology of these breaks is unknown.

Finally, a variety of chemical agents, especially drugs, have been implicated as causes of chromosomal breakage. In many cases, especially in the case of LSD, the data are conflicting and a final conclusion has not yet been reached. If these drugs do, in fact, break chromosomes, their influence on the production of congenital malformations is also not yet known.

Carr DH: Chromosome studies in selected spontaneous abortions: Polyploidy in man. JM Genet 8:164, 1971.

Cohen MM, Hirschhorn K, Frosch WA: Cytogenetic effects of tranquilizing drugs in vivo and in vitro. JAMA 207:2425, 1969.

Hungerford DA & others: Cytogenetic effects of LSD 25 therapy in man. JAMA 206:2287, 1968.

Robinson A & others: Studies on chromosomal non-disjunction in man. Am J Human Genet 21:466, 1969.

CHROMOSOMAL DISEASES

Numerical abnormalities may involve either the sex chromosomes or the autosomes, predominantly the former. Gross autosomal imbalances produce severe phenotypic disturbances and, particularly when they involve loss of chromosomal material, are usually incompatible with life.

DERMATOGLYPHICS

In persons with a variety of congenital malformations, and especially in those with chromosomal disease, the dermatoglyphic patterns, ie, the fingerprints, palm prints, and foot prints, deviate from the normal (Fig 34–7).

Since the fine dermal ridges on the hands and feet begin to develop in their characteristic patterns between the second and fourth months of embryogenesis, deviations from normal embryonic development during this period may be reflected in abnormalities of the dermatoglyphic pattern. As a result, the presence of abnormal dermatoglyphics in a patient suggests some developmental trauma during the second to fourth months of pregnancy and should prompt a careful examination of the patient for associated, less obvious, congenital malformations.

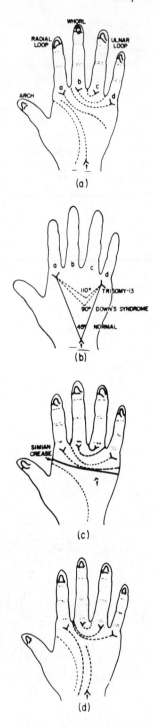

(a)

(b)

(c)

(d)

FIG 34–7. **Abnormal palm prints.** Schematic representation of **(a)** normal hand; **(b)** atd angle in normal person and in patients with Down's and trisomy 13–15 (D) syndrome; **(c)** dermatoglyphic pattern in a patient with Down's syndrome; **(d)** dermatoglyphic pattern in a patient with trisomy 18 syndrome. (Reproduced from Porter IH: *Heredity and Disease.* McGraw-Hill, 1968. Copyright © 1968. Used with permission of McGraw-Hill Book Company.)

THE SEX CHROMOSOMES

Unlike Drosophila, in which the fly with the XO pattern is the male, in the human the Y chromosome is necessary (but not sufficient) for maleness. The Y chromosome presumably contains few genes other than those necessary to produce "maleness." The X chromosome, on the other hand, carries many sex-linked (more correctly, "X-linked") genes.

The X chromosome has some unique characteristics that have thrown light on some fundamental properties of mammalian cells and have been of great importance to medicine. The first indication of this was the demonstration by Moore & Barr of a sexual dimorphism in the somatic cells of man which consisted of a deeply staining chromatin body in some cells of the normal female and its absence in the male (Fig 34–8). Subsequent studies revealed that humans may have 0–4 chromatin (Barr) bodies and that the number of such bodies is one less than the number of X chromosomes in the individual's karyotype (the "nuclear sex rule").

A hypothesis was proposed by Lyon and Russell (independently) to account both for the above phenomenon and for the "dosage compensation" effect—the fact that the amount of protein produced by a given X-linked gene such as the one for antihemophilic globulin is independent of the number of X chromosomes the individual has (eg, the female with 2 X chromosomes does not produce twice as much antihemophilic globulin as the male with only one). They suggested that only one X chromosome in any cell is fully active and that all others are genetically inactive during the major part of the cell's life cycle. Moreover,

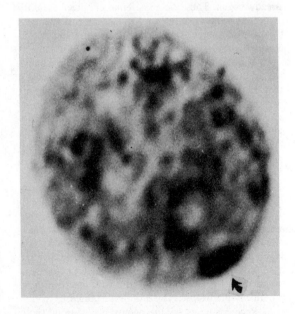

FIG 34–8. **Nucleus of cell obtained from the buccal mucosa, demonstrating the densely staining chromatin body.** Arrow points to chromatin body.

the hypothesis suggests that, early in embryogenesis (about the tenth to twelfth day in man), a random choice is made by each somatic cell about which X will remain active. Thereafter, the same X will remain active for all future progeny of a given cell. The normal female would then constitute a mosaic of clones with respect to the identity of the active X chromosome.

Much evidence has been accumulated to support the basic validity of the Lyon-Russell hypothesis. At present, it is thought that the Barr body represents the genetically inactive (or, more probably, the partially genetically inactive) X chromosome. Autoradiography has demonstrated that the various chromosome pairs have specific patterns of replication. The X chromosomes are remarkable for the degree of asynchrony they show in their patterns of replication, one of them being the last chromosome to replicate its DNA during the S period of the cell cycle. Whenever X polysomy (an increased number of X chromosomes) exists, all but one of the X chromosomes replicates late; and whenever one of the 2 X chromosomes has a morphologic abnormality, it, too, is late in replicating. The Barr body, then, is thought to represent the genetically inactive, late-replicating X chromosome. When one of the X chromosomes is morphologically abnormal and

hence late-replicating, the corresponding chromatin body may be abnormal in size.

The Lyon-Russell hypothesis provides an explanation for the observation that abnormalities of X chromosomal constitution are more likely to be compatible with life and to be associated with less severe phenotypic defects than those of autosomes.

A second type of sexual dimorphism which has the same significance as the Barr body is the "drumstick" on the nucleus of polymorphonuclear leukocytes (Fig 34–9). The presence of at least 6 of these in 500 polymorphonuclear leukocytes reflects chromatin positivity in the blood. A discrepancy between the "drumstick" condition and the sex chromatin status as determined by buccal smear reflects mosaicism.

The Barr test has become an effective means of screening patients for sex chromosomal abnormalities. The test may be performed rapidly by means of a buccal smear. Normal males have less than 3% positive cells in their buccal smears, whereas normal females have 25–50% positive cells. Intermediate counts suggest mosaicism. Recently, the amniotic membrane stripped from the placenta has been utilized to great advantage in screening populations of newborns for abnormalities of the X chromosomes.

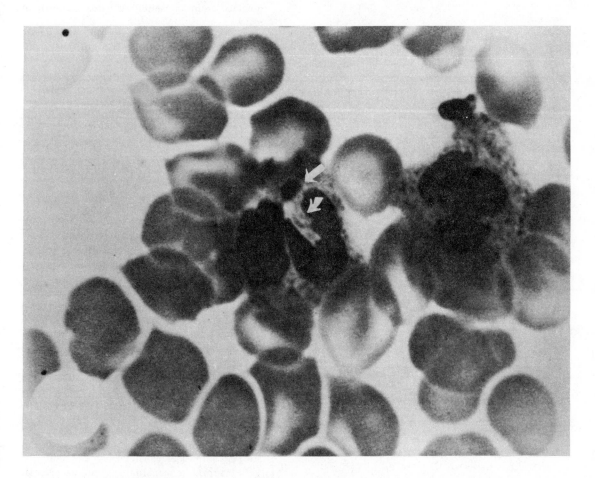

FIG 34–9. Nucleus of polymorphonuclear leukocyte. Arrows point to "drumstick."

The affinity of the long arm of the Y chromosome for fluorescent dyes is also being used in screening newborns for abnormalities of the Y chromosome by looking for the "Y body" in interphase cells (Fig 34–10).

Carr DH: Chromosomal abnormalities in clinical medicine. Chap 1 in: *Progress in Medical Genetics.* Vol 6. Steinberg AG, Bearn AG (editors). Grune & Stratton, 1969.

Greensher A & others: Screening of newborn infants for abnormalities of the Y chromosome. J Pediat 79:305, 1971.

DISEASES OF THE SEX CHROMOSOMES
(See Table 34–1.)

At least 0.25% of all live infants born at term and about 1% of the inmates of institutions for the retarded have sex chromosomal anomalies. Examination of the chromatin status can identify most of them.

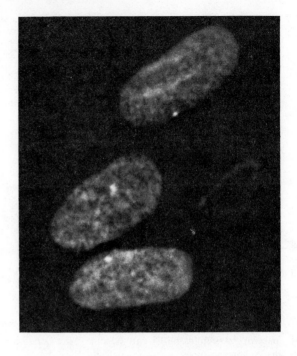

FIG 34–10. Fluorescent Y bodies in nuclei cells obtained from the umbilical cords of newborn males.

TABLE 34–1. Other diseases involving sex differentiation.

Lesion and Disease	Chromosome Number	Symptoms
XX male, possibly due to a chromosomal interchange between X and Y during meiosis in the male. Sex chromatin positive.	46	Like Klinefelter's or partial feminization, as in true hermaphrodite.
45,X/46,XY male pseudohermaphrodite, "mixed gonadal dysgenesis." Sex chromatin negative.	45/46	A variable degree of Turner's phenotype with infantile female secondary sex characters and a variable amount of masculinization of the genitals. Tendency to develop gonadoblastomas.
"Pure" gonadal dysgenesis, 46,XY male pseudohermaphrodite. Sex chromatin negative.	46	Tall female with underdeveloped secondary sex characteristics, streak gonads, primary amenorrhea, and sterility. Tendency to develop gonadal tumors.
Testicular feminizing syndrome, male pseudohermaphroditism, 46,XY. Sex chromatin negative.	46	Tall, well feminized, sterile female with testes. Probably an "end organ" insensitivity to androgens. May be suspected in sterile adult females with primary amenorrhea and in girls with bilateral inguinal hernias. Probably inherited as a sex-limited autosomal dominant disease. Tendency to develop gonadal tumors.
True hermaphrodite, 46,XX; 46,XY or 46,XX/46,XY (the latter possibly due to an ovum being fertilized by 2 sperms).	46	Varying degrees of abnormal phenotypic sexual indeterminacy. May have ovum on one side, testis on the other (lateral hermaphrodite) or ovotestis on one (unilateral) or both sides (bilateral hermaphrodite). In lateral hermaphrodites, internal genitals usually conform to gonad on that side. External genitals may vary widely.

Indications for Examining the Sex Chromatin

An incidence of sex chromosomal anomalies of 0.14% has been found in a survey of 27,000 newborns born in 2 Denver hospitals. Since most of the abnormal cases would not have been diagnosed by physical examination alone, it may be desirable for obstetrical services to establish the chromatin status of all newborns at birth by routine examination of the amniotic membranes.

Sex chromatin examination is especially indicated in the following cases:

(1) All individuals, including newborns, with any abnormalities of the external genitalia, including micro-orchidism.

(2) All those with mental retardation.

(3) All sterile individuals.

(4) All females with primary amenorrhea.

(5) All female newborns with somatic abnormalities suggestive of Turner's syndrome, eg, lymphedema of the dorsa of the feet, cubitus valgus, coarctation of the aorta, webbing of the neck.

(6) Older girls with hypoplastic nipples, short stature, facies suggestive of Turner's syndrome, and inguinal or femoral hernia.

Eller E & others: Prognosis of newborns with X-chromosomal abnormalities. Pediatrics 47:681, 1971.

Harris JS, Robinson A: X chromosome abnormalities and the obstetrician: The value of routine nuclear sexing of newborn infants. Am J Obst Gynec 109:574, 1971.

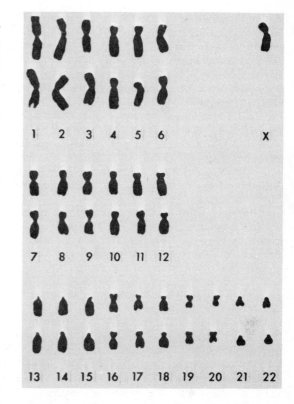

FIG 34–11. 45,X karyotype of girl with Turner's syndrome.

TURNER'S SYNDROME
(Gonadal Dysgenesis)

Essentials of Diagnosis

- Short stature, primary amenorrhea, and sexual infantilism in adults.
- "Streaked" gonads and partial or complete X-chromosomal monosomy (Fig 34–11) are found at all ages.

General Considerations

Turner's syndrome has an incidence of about 1/3000 live births, but the "45,X anomaly" may be 40 times as common in spontaneous abortions. The occurrence of some of the somatic stigmas of the disease varies greatly from case to case. Most cases are chromatin-negative.

Clinical Findings

The family history is noncontributory except that an increased incidence of twinning has been reported in families with gonadal dysgenesis. Birth weight tends to be low (especially for those with webbed neck and coarctation of the aorta). Newborns often display lymphedema, especially of the lower parts of the legs and the distal arms.

A. Symptoms and Signs: The characteristic findings are sexual infantilism and primary amenorrhea in a postpubertal female, shortness of stature, low birth weight, congenital lymphedema, cubitus valgus, a small "turned down" mouth, low hair line, retrognathia or micrognathia, webbing of the neck, and short neck. Other abnormalities may include coarctation of the aorta, pigmented nevi, deep-set nail beds, and hypoplastic nails. The IQ is usually normal, although many of these patients have perceptual difficulties and space blindness or have trouble with numbers (dyscalculia). Congenital malformations of the urinary tract are common, especially horseshoe kidneys and double ureter and pelvis. In addition, there may be "shield chest" combined with widely spaced nipples, abnormalities of the spine (epiphysitis), retardation of bone age, and osteoporosis. The growth rate throughout childhood is slow, and the ultimate height is usually 52–59 inches. Occasional patients have been reported who menstruate and have normal height; these are probably chromosomal mosaics.

B. Laboratory Findings: Sex chromatin is usually negative. 45,X/46,XX mosaicism is not uncommon; in these cases there may be some chromatin-positive cells but a lower percentage (< 20%) than one would normally expect to find. Occasionally the buccal smear is chromatin-positive but the bodies look particularly large; this suggests that the patient has an X-isochromosome of the long arm of the X (XX_{qi})* sex chromosomal constitution. If, on the other hand, the chromatin bodies look small, the patient may have an X-deletion X or X-isochromosome of the small arm (XX_{pi})* constitution.

In the typical case the karyotype reveals a 45,X condition. Mosaicism (45,X/46,XX or 45,X/46,XX/47,XXX)* is not rare. In these cases the phenotype may be modified so that many of the characteristic clinical findings are absent. Even mosaics, however, are likely to have "streak" gonads and primary amenorrhea.

Patients with 46,XX_{qi} usually have typical Turner's phenotypes. In addition, they have an increased incidence of Hashimoto's thyroiditis. When a deletion of part or all of the long arm of one X chromosome occurs, many of the characteristic signs and symptoms, including shortness of stature, are absent, but amenorrhea and the sterility which results from dysgenetic gonads persists.

Urinary FSH excretion is elevated by the 13th to 14th year. Prior to this, FSH may be higher than normal for the age.

The gonads appear as long, slender white "streaks" in the broad ligaments. They are composed of wavy connective tissue without any germinal epithelium.

C. X-Ray Findings: X-ray studies often reveal rarefaction of the bones, especially in the hands, feet, and spine, where epiphysitis may also be present. Bone age is only slightly retarded. Intravenous urography will often reveal urinary tract anomalies.

Differential Diagnosis

Turner's syndrome must be ruled out in all cases of females with shortness of stature, amenorrhea, webbing of the neck, or coarctation of the aorta. The diagnosis depends on the buccal smear and the chromosomal analysis. Patients with pseudohypoparathyroidism may have many of the stigmas of gonadal dysgenesis.

Complications & Sequelae

These relate primarily to the dangers of coarctation of the aorta when that is present. Rarely, the dysgenetic gonads may become neoplastic (gonadoblastoma). Sexual infantilism and the perceptual motor difficulties to which these patients are prone may have concomitant psychologic hazards.

Treatment

Treatment consists principally of identifying and treating perceptual problems before they become established. Cyclic hormone therapy should be started at 13–14 years of age to develop secondary sex characteristics and permit normal menstrual periods. This is psychologically most important. Teen-age patients

*Terminology adopted by Chicago Conference on the Human Chromosomes (1966).

need careful counseling so that they will have no doubt about their femininity. The need for hormone therapy should be carefully explained.

Prognosis

The prognosis for life is good, limited only by complications such as coarctation of the aorta. Sterility is permanent.

De la Chapelle A: Cytogenetical and clinical observations in female gonadal dysgenesis. Acta endocrinol 40 (Suppl 65), 1962.

POLYSOMY X SYNDROME
(XXX & XXXX)

The incidence of this syndrome in newborns is about 0.12% (significantly higher among retardates). These patients are phenotypic females with 2 or more sex chromatin bodies. In an as yet undetermined proportion of cases, there is underdevelopment of secondary sex characteristics, primary or secondary amenorrhea, and mild mental retardation. Occasional patients have epicanthus, transverse palmar lines, and curved little fingers.

All phenotypic females with mild mental retardation, epicanthic folds, transverse palmar lines, or primary or secondary amenorrhea should have buccal smears.

Treatment is supportive. Cyclic hormone therapy is indicated for older girls with underdeveloped secondary sex characteristics and amenorrhea.

TABLE 34–2. Sex chromatin in polysomy X.

Sex Chromatin	Karyotype
Two bodies	47,XXX
Three bodies	48,XXXX
Four bodies	49,XXXXX
Few double bodies	46,XX/47,XXX; 45,X/47,XXX
Few triple bodies	45,X/48,XXXX

When the syndrome is diagnosed in the newborn, the prognosis for mental development and fertility must be guarded.

The offspring of women with polysomy X have thus far had normal sex chromosomal constitutions, although there have been several children with Down's syndrome among the offspring of women with the tetra-X condition.

Court Brown WM & others: Abnormalities of the sex chromosome complement in man. Medical Research Council Special Report Series 305. Her Majesty's Stationery Office, London, 1964.

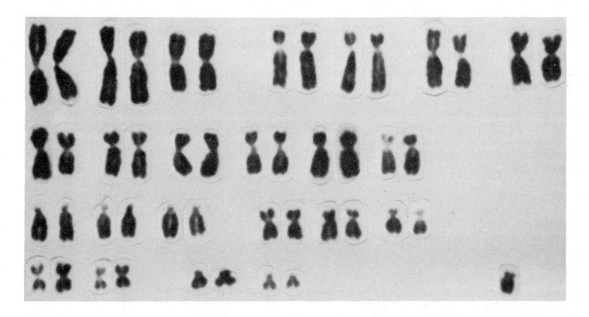

FIG 34–12. 47,XXY karyotype of man with Klinefelter's syndrome.

KLINEFELTER'S SYNDROME

Essentials of Diagnosis

- Micro-orchidism due to prepubertal testicular atrophy, azoospermia, and sterility in the adult (about 4 patients with this syndrome are said to have been fertile).
- Elevated urinary gonadotropins in puberty. 47,XXY chromosomal constitution (Fig 34–12).
- Chromosomal variants are occasionally seen.

General Considerations

The incidence in the newborn population is roughly 1/500, but it is about 1% in groups of male retardates and 3% in males seen at infertility clinics. The maternal age at birth is often advanced. The diagnosis is rarely made before puberty except as a result of screening tests for sex chromatin. Unlike gonadal dysgenesis, this lesion is rarely found in spontaneous abortions.

Clinical Findings

A. Symptoms and Signs: The findings are characteristic only in the postpubertal period. Micro-orchidism associated with otherwise normal external genitalia, azoospermia, and sterility are almost invariable in diagnosed cases. Gynecomastia, subnormal IQ, diminished facial hair, lack of libido and potency, and a tall, eunuchoid build are frequent. In chromosomal variants with 3 and 4 X chromosomes, mental retardation is severe and radio-ulnar synostosis may be present as well as anomalies of the external genitalia and cryptorchidism. In the XXXXY cases, these findings are especially prominent, as well as microcephaly, hypertelorism, epicanthus, prognathism, and incurved fifth fingers.

The adult XXYY patient tends to be taller and more retarded than the average XXY patient.

In general, the physical and mental abnormalities in Klinefelter's syndrome increase with the number of sex chromosomes.

B. Laboratory Findings: Sex chromatin is positive. Twenty to 40% of the cells of the buccal mucous membrane usually have one Barr body, although 2 and 3 Barr bodies may be found in individuals having one of the rare variants of Klinefelter's syndrome with more than 2 X chromosomes.

The majority of cases have a 47,XXY constitution. However, rare variants may have 48,XXXY, 49,XXXXY, 49,XXXYY, and 48,XXYY. A variety of mosaics containing combinations of the above and including 46,XY/47,XXY mosaicism have been reported. Some of these latter have been fertile and not mentally defective.

Urinary excretion of gonadotropins is high in adults, the levels being comparable to those found in postmenopausal women.

Histology of the testis in the adult is characterized by hyalinization and atrophy of the majority of seminiferous tubules, with large clumps of abnormal Leydig cells in between. A marked deficiency of germ cells (spermatogonia) has been found also in prepubertal patients (even in a 10-month-old child).

Differential Diagnosis

Chromatin-positive Klinefelter's syndrome must be differentiated from 2 chromatin-negative varieties: postpubertal testicular atrophy and germ cell aplasia. In both cases the diagnosis can be made by buccal smear for sex chromatin and testicular biopsy.

Adolescent obesity with delayed puberty and Prader-Willi syndrome may be confused with Klinefelter's syndrome. In both cases, the sex chromatin determination, absence of a eunuchoid build, and absence of true testicular atrophy should rule out Klinefelter's syndrome.

Complications & Sequelae

These patients may be more prone to a variety of conditions, including antisocial personality (especially sex crimes), schizophrenia, male breast cancer, asthma, and thyroid disease.

Treatment

Treatment consists of supportive care for the psychologic stresses of the disease and, occasionally, plastic surgery for the gynecomastia.

Prognosis

The prognosis is good for life but poor for fertility and normal IQ. It is not known what percentage of these patients will have normal intelligence, but undoubtedly some do.

XYY SYNDROME

The incidence of the 47,XYY karyotype in the newborn population is as yet unknown, although current estimates are that it is at least as frequent as the 47,XXY karyotype (about 1:500). It is worth stressing that these newborns in general are perfectly normal and do **not** have the "XYY syndrome," which may be present in 10% of tall men (over 6 feet) who come into conflict with the law because of their grossly defective, aggressive personalities.

These individuals may exhibit an abnormal behavior pattern from early childhood and are often slightly retarded. Fertility is normal. They are chromatin-negative except for an occasional chromatin-positive individual with a 48,XXYY karyotype. Hence, these patients are not identified by examination of the sex chromatin. However, they can be identified by a buccal smear stained for the fluorescent "Y body."

There is no treatment, and the long-term prognosis is not known.

Court Brown WM: Males with an XYY chromosome complement. JM Genet 5:341–359, 1968.

Marinello MJ & others: A study of the XYY syndrome in tall men and juvenile delinquents. JAMA 208:321, 1969.

AUTOSOMAL DISEASES
(See Table 34–3.)

Man is even more susceptible to autosomal disorders than to abnormalities of the sex chromosomes.

TABLE 34–3. Other diseases of the autosomes.

Lesion and Disease	Chromosome Number	Symptoms
Deletion of short arm of 17–18.	46	Microcephaly, epicanthic folds, rounded facies, hypotonia, short stature, severe psychomotor retardation.
Partial deletion of long arm of 17–18.	46	Mental and growth retardation, atresia of ear canals and deafness, high palate, microcephaly, retraction of middle part of face, receding chin, prominent antihelix, spindle-shaped fingers. IgA is often absent.
Deletion of long arm of chromosome 22–the Ph[1] chromosome.	46	Chronic granulocytic leukemia. The chromosomal abnormality is present in the bone marrow in 90% of cases. Less often, it is also present in cells cultured from the peripheral blood.
Bloom's dwarfism: multiple chromosome breaks, quadriradial figures, occasionally "pulverization" of chromosomes.	46	Dwarfism, chronic erythematous rash, tendency to malignancy, especially leukemia. Probably inherited as a single gene autosomal recessive. Increased chromosomal breaks may be seen in close relatives.
Congenital aplastic (Fanconi's) anemia: increased number of chromosomal breaks; chromosomes probably more susceptible to breakage by virus.	46	Skeletal (especially upper extremities) and hematopoietic abnormalities, increased hemoglobin F. Anemia often does not appear until 6–10 years of age. Hyperpigmentation, sexual and mental retardation, and microcephaly may also be present. Autosomal recessive inheritance.

Uniform autosomal monosomy is not compatible with life and has been observed only in spontaneously aborted fetuses. Similarly, only trisomy of the small autosomes (13, 18, and 21 [G group]) occur in living individuals and then only in the presence of serious disease. The belief that many abnormalities of the chromosomes do not permit the birth of a viable infant is strengthened by the finding of gross chromosomal aberrations in 20–50% of cases of spontaneous abortion.

Indications for Chromosomal Analysis

(1) Whenever the phenotypic and the chromatin sex do not agree.

(2) Whenever the chromatin examination suggests sex chromosome mosaicism.

(3) Whenever the Barr body is morphologically abnormal.

(4) Whenever the clinical condition suggests one of the autosomal syndromes, or the patient has gross structural anomalies involving a variety of systems and is retarded.

(5) Whenever there is an abnormal number of "Y bodies."

Polani PE: Autosomal imbalance and its syndromes, excluding Down's. Brit M Bull 25:81, 1969.

Stenchever MA & others: Testicular feminization syndrome: Chromosomal, histologic, and genetic studies in a large kindred. Obst Gynec 33:649, 1969.

DOWN'S SYNDROME

Essentials of Diagnosis

- Slow development, characteristic facies, short stature, abnormal dermatoglyphics.
- Trisomy 21 or chromosomal translocation.

General Considerations

The term Down's syndrome is preferred to mongolism since the latter term is descriptively inaccurate and is offensive to some. The most constant characteristic of the disease is mental retardation. IQ's may vary between 20 and 80, with the great majority being between 45 and 55. The incidence of Down's syndrome is about 1/600 in the general population, being roughly the same in various parts of the world and in all races. The patient's mother's age at the time of conception as well as the nature of the chromosomal malformation are important in genetic counseling.

Clinical Findings

A. Symptoms and Signs: The principal findings are a small, brachycephalic head, expressionless facies, flat nasal bridge, ruddy cheeks, dry lips, large protruding "scrotal" tongue, small ears, oblique palpebral fissures which narrow laterally, epicanthic folds, occasional Brushfield spots, and a short fleshy neck. Irregular development of teeth is common; in about 1/3 of cases, the upper lateral permanent incisors are missing.

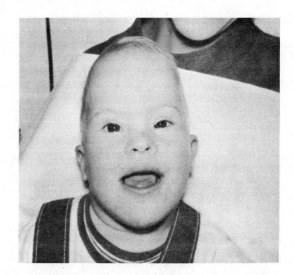

FIG 34–13. Facies of a child with Down's syndrome.

or defective. About 1/3 have congenital heart disease, most often an endocardial cushion defect or other septal defect. Patients tend to have short, stubby, spade-like hands with transverse palmar ("simian") lines and abnormal dermatoglyphics (see below). Generalized hypotonia is often present, as well as umbilical hernia. There is often a cleft between the big toe and second toe. Sexual development is retarded. The affected newborn is prone to have a third fontanel, prolonged physiologic jaundice, polycythemia, and a transient leukemoid reaction. "Cutis marmorata" is often present.

Patients with Down's syndrome display an increased sensitivity to the mydriatic effects of atropine when instilled into the conjunctiva.

Dermatoglyphic patterns are characteristic. In general, the dermal ridges are poorly formed, and the frequencies of arches, radial and ulnar loops on the various fingers, the distal location of the axial triradius on the palm, and the hallucal pattern on the sole of the foot differ from normals. Ford-Walker has combined frequency data on dermatoglyphic patterns on the fingers, palms, and soles into a "dermal index" which delineates 3 ranges—"Mongol," "normal," and "overlap." A single flexion crease on the fifth finger is often found.

B. Laboratory Findings: The chromosomal abnormalities are pathognomonic. The great majority of cases (95%) have 47 chromosomes with trisomy of 21 (Fig 34–14). However, about 4% of sporadic cases have 46 chromosomes, including an abnormal translocated chromosome formed as a result of centric fusion between 2 acrocentric chromosomes,* one of which is chromosome 21 (Fig 34–15). On the other hand, about 1/3 of the familial cases have a translocation. Ten percent of patients whose mothers are younger will have these "interchange" lesions, whereas this is true in only 3% of those with older mothers.

*Fusion between 2 centromere regions—a translocation.

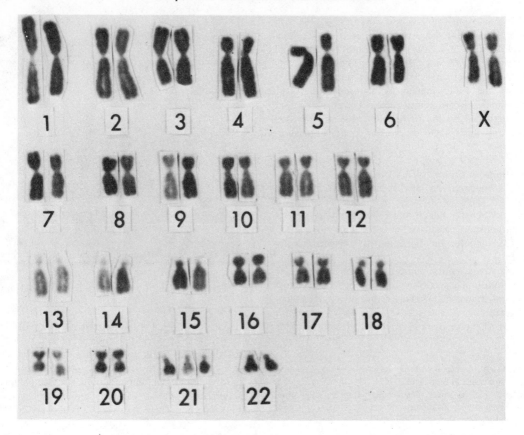

FIG 34–14. Karyotype of Down's syndrome: 47,XX,21⁺.

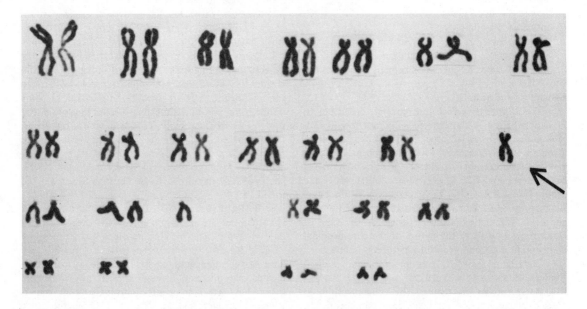

FIG 34–15. Karyotype of Down's syndrome: 46,XX,t D/G. The arrow points to an abnormal chromosome formed by a translocation between chromosome 21 and a chromosome of the 13–15 group (probably 14).

Mosaicism of the 46/47 type can also occur in persons with Down's syndrome. This may result in milder symptoms, especially in higher than expected IQ. Apparently normal mothers of affected children have occasionally been mosaics.

Although increased levels of leukocyte alkaline phosphatase have been reported, there has been a marked overlap in the distribution of patients and controls. This and increased levels of other enzymes (galactose-1-phosphate uridyl transferase and glucose-6-phosphate dehydrogenase) are probably nonspecific effects of a variation in the metabolism of leukocytes which occurs in association with Down's syndrome.

Total serum proteins are usually in the low normal range. Serum albumin is low but gamma globulin is often elevated.

Decreased urinary excretion of xanthurenic and indoleacetic acids after a tryptophan load is indicative of some abnormality of tryptophan metabolism.

C. X-Ray Findings: X-rays of the pelvic bones of affected infants reveal flattening of the inner edges of the ileum and widening of the iliac wings. The "iliac index" is 1/2 the sum of both acetabular and iliac angles. This index is low (below 65) in about 80–90% of infants under 9 months of age with Down's syndrome (over 80 in the controls).

Skull x-rays often reveal brachycephaly, with flattening of the occiput. The sinuses may be absent or poorly developed. X-rays of the hand show shortening of the metacarpal bones and phalanges. The second phalanx of the little finger, in particular, is often abnormally small.

Differential Diagnosis

Most of the individual signs and symptoms of Down's syndrome also occur in the normal population, and the diagnosis is based on the presence of a **combination** of symptoms. Other autosomal trisomies, and occasionally girls with the triple X syndrome, may have many similar findings. The dermatoglyphics, sex chromatin status, and chromosomal analysis will differentiate the latter from Down's syndrome.

Complications

Leukemia (not the transient leukemoid reaction of the newborn) is 20 times more common than normal in individuals with Down's syndrome. These patients are very susceptible to intercurrent infections and are subject to the complications of congenital heart disease when they have it.

Prevention

In general, Down's syndrome is not familial and the risk of having an affected child in a sibship varies with maternal age (1/2000 for mothers under 25; 1/200 for mothers over 35; 1/75 for mothers over 40). These figures are fairly accurate for families with trisomy 21 but much too low when one of the parents is a balanced translocation carrier.

In counseling parents who have produced one child with Down's syndrome about the risk of having a

repeat, the prognostic accuracy can be improved by studying the karyotypes of the affected child and his parents. Several different situations may be present:

A. Child Has Trisomy 21, Parents Have Normal Karyotypes: The risk is only slightly greater than for parents in the general population. In general, it is said to be 4 times the risk for a mother of the same age who has not had an affected child. For mothers less than 30 years old, it is 1–2%.

B. Trisomic Child, One Parent Mosaic: The risk will depend upon the degree of gonadal mosaicism of the affected parent. A rough estimate will be 1/2 of the proportion of abnormal cells in fibroblast cultures of the cells obtained from the parent.

C. Child Has 14/21 (D/G) Translocation, Parents Have Normal Karyotypes: The risks are similar to those under (A).

D. Child Has 14/21 Translocation, One Parent a Balanced Translocation Carrier:

1. When the mother is the carrier, about 15% of the children will be affected, 1/3 will be carriers, and 1/3 completely normal.

2. When the father is the carrier, there is a 1:20 chance of having another affected child and 1/2 of the apparently unaffected children may be carriers.

E. Child Has a 21/22 (G/G) Translocation:

1. **Both parents have normal karyotypes**—The prognosis is roughly the same as under (A), although there is some evidence that advancing paternal age may increase this risk slightly.

2. **One parent carries the translocation**—If it is an isochromosome of 21 (21/21), the risk is 100%. If it is a 21/22 translocation, the risk is as in (D).

Treatment

No form of medical treatment has been shown to have significant merit. Therapy is directed toward specific problems, eg, cardiac surgery or digitalis for heart problems, antibiotics for infections, special education and occupational training, etc. These children should be helped to make the most of their limited abilities. For this reason, in general, early institutionalization is not recommended. Support of the parents is important.

Chemke J, Robinson A: The third fontanelle. J Pediat 75:617, 1969.

Mikkelsen M, Stene J: Genetic counselling in Down's syndrome. Human Heredity 20:457, 1970.

Penrose LS: The causes of Down's syndrome. Advances Teratology 1:9–21, 1966.

Penrose LS, Smith GF: *Down's Anomaly.* Little, Brown, 1966.

TRISOMY 18 SYNDROME
(E₁ Trisomy)

Essentials of Diagnosis

- Mental retardation, failure to thrive, hypertonicity.

- Abnormal dermatoglyphics.
- Trisomy of chromosome 18 or, occasionally, an unbalanced translocation involving chromosome 18.

General Considerations

This disease has an incidence of about 1 in 4500 live births, and there is an approximately 1:3 sex ratio (male:female). The mean maternal age is advanced. Affected individuals usually die in early infancy, although occasional patients survive into childhood.

Clinical Findings

A. Symptoms and Signs: Trisomy 18 is characterized by failure to thrive, low birth weight, mental retardation, hypertonicity, prominent occiput, low-set, malformed ears, micrognathia, abnormal flexion of the fingers (index over third), equinovarus or "rocker bottom" feet, short sternum and narrow pelvis, congenital heart disease (often ventricular septal defect or patent ductus arteriosus), and inguinal or umbilical hernias. There is an increased occurrence of single umbilical arteries.

Dermatoglyphics show simple arches on fingers, a single flexion crease on the fifth finger, and transverse palmar lines.

B. Laboratory Findings: In place of uniform trisomy 18, chromosomal analysis occasionally reveals mosaicism for trisomy 18 or an unbalanced translocation involving a third number 18 and a chromosome of the 13–15 group. Rarely, double trisomies have been found in which X-trisomy or 21-trisomy is present in addition to 18-trisomy.

C. X-Ray Findings: X-ray often reveals gross retardation of osseous maturation, eventration of the diaphragm, and kidney abnormalities.

Differential Diagnosis

Trisomy 18 is differentiated from trisomy 13, in which failure to thrive, congenital heart disease, and retardation are also present. In the latter condition, the shape of the head; eye, ear, and palatal anomalies; dermatoglyphics; and the occurrence of apneic spells are all different. Other causes of failure to thrive must be considered.

Complications

Complications are related to associated lesions. Death is often due to heart failure or pneumonia.

Treatment

There is no treatment other than general supportive care.

Prognosis

Death usually occurs in infancy, although occasional patients have lived into early childhood.

Taylor AI: Autosomal trisomy syndromes: A detailed study of 27 cases of Edwards' syndrome and 27 cases of Patau's syndrome. JM Genet 5:227–252, 1968.

TRISOMY 13
(D Trisomy)

The incidence of this disorder is about 1 in 14,500 live births, and 60% of the patients are female. The mean maternal age is elevated. Death usually occurs by the second year of life, usually as a result of heart failure or infection.

The symptoms and signs consist of failure to thrive, mental retardation, arhinencephaly, sloping forehead, eye deformities (anophthalmia, colobomas), low-set ears, cleft lip and palate, capillary hemangiomas, deafness, apneic spells, seizures, polydactyly or syndactyly, and congenital heart disease (usually ventricular septal defect). Other abnormal findings may include hyperconvex, narrow fingernails, flexed and overlapping fingers, "rocker bottom" feet, retroflexible thumbs, urinary tract anomalies, umbilical hernia, and cryptorchidism or bicornuate uterus.

Although most patients have 13 trisomy (D trisomy), occasional patients are mosaic, and there are rare cases of an unbalanced (D/D) translocation with one of the parents carrying a similar translocation in the balanced state. Multiple projections and abnormal lobulation of the neutrophils are often present. Grossly elevated fetal hemoglobin and the presence of embryonic Gower's hemoglobin often occur.

Trisomy 18 patients are more hypertonic than these infants, and the head shape is different. The diagnosis of trisomy 13 should be considered in all

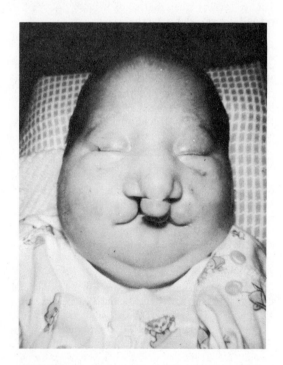

FIG 34–16. Facies of an infant with trisomy 13.

cases of failure to thrive associated with retardation and palatal anomalies.

Other forms of the first arch syndrome are differentiated by the absence of a sloping forehead and the usual absence of other generalized malformations.

Treatment is supportive. Prevention in the form of genetic counseling is indicated when one of the parents carries a balanced translocation, in which case the risks for future affected children are elevated (as in the analogous situation in Down's syndrome).

Taylor AI: Autosomal trisomy syndromes: A detailed study of 27 cases of Edwards' syndrome and 27 cases of Patau's syndrome. JM Genet 5:227–252, 1968.

CRI DU CHAT ("CAT CRY") SYNDROME

The incidence of this syndrome is not known. It occurs more commonly among females. Life expectancy is not seriously curtailed. The dimensions of the deleted chromosomal fragment are variable, which explains the variations observed in the phenotype.

Symptoms and signs consist of severe mental retardation, low birth weight, failure to thrive, microcephaly, hypertelorism, obliquity of palpebral fissures, epicanthic folds, low-set ears, a broad, flattened nasal bridge, "moon-like" facies, and micrognathia. The cry in the newborn and infant has a unique mewling quality like that of a kitten. It has a sharp timbre and plaintive tonality when emitted on expiration. It is due to small, flaccid, and somewhat rudimentary laryngeal structures, and becomes less typical as the child gets older.

These patients often have repeated respiratory infections and persistent feeding problems. Breathing may be difficult. Hypospadias, cryptorchidism, and curved little fingers have been reported.

Chromosomal analysis shows deletion of part of the short arm of chromosome No. 5. This is occasionally replaced by a "ring" chromosome No. 5 or by a translocation.

Dermatoglyphics are often abnormal, with distal axial triradii. Transverse palmar lines are frequently present.

Because of the lack of specificity of many of the symptoms associated with abnormalities of the autosomes, all children with severe mental retardation, microcephaly, and failure to thrive enter into the differential diagnosis.

Newborn infants with various kinds of weak cry and laryngeal stridor may be differentiated by the fact that the "cat cry" is an expiratory sound and that an affected baby has the associated malformations.

Few cases have been familial. However, when one parent carries a balanced translocation involving chromosome No. 5 with deletion of the short arm, the risks are increased as in the analogous situation in Down's syndrome.

Supportive care is all that can be given.

THE GENE

The genes, which occur in pairs in somatic cells, occur at similar sites on the homologous chromosomes. The members of a pair, although they encode for the same function, are not always the same but may constitute alternate forms (alleles). When the homologues are the same, the individual is said to be "homozygous" for the gene; if they are different, he is "heterozygous." Since the male has only one X chromosome, he is said to be "hemizygous" for X-linked genes.

GENE EXPRESSION

Most of what is currently known about a gene stems from how it expresses itself—its phenotype.

The phenotypic expression of a gene is the result of an interaction between the gene and its environment. The latter, in addition to the surrounding nucleoplasm and cytoplasm, includes the rest of the genome* which may have a modifying effect on a particular gene. It is this interaction that results in the variable severity of genetic diseases (expressivity) and occasionally completely prevents the expression of a defective gene (penetrance). The primary gene product, a protein, is least affected by environmental conditions. Hence, one of the criteria for determining that a gene product is primary is complete penetrance and little variation in expressivity. This would be true, for example, of hemoglobin S, a protein which is the direct result of a single mutation in the gene which produces the beta polypeptide chain of hemoglobin. An important point in clinical genetics is that the defective gene which is not expressed at all (nonpenetrant) can still be passed on to offspring, where it may be expressed.

Carr DH: Chromosomal errors and development. Am J Obst Gynec 104:327, 1969.

SINGLE GENE DEFECTS

Diseases which are due to defects in a single gene are said to be "autosomal" or "sex-linked" depending on whether the defective gene is located on an autosome or X chromosome. If the disease is present when the defective gene is present either in the heterozygous or in the homozygous state, it is a dominantly inherited disease. If, however, it is present only when the gene involved is in the homozygous state, it is a recessively inherited disease.

*Genetic complement.

TABLE 34–4. Some dominantly inherited diseases (autosomal).

Achondroplasia	Intestinal polyposis
Isolated cleft palate (when due to a genetic defect)	Marfan's syndrome
Ehlers-Danlos syndrome	Muscular dystrophy (facio-scapulohumeral type)
Epidermolysis dystrophica hereditaria	Neurofibromatosis
Gardner's syndrome	Osteogenesis imperfecta
Hereditary spherocytosis	Porphyria, hepatic form
Hidrotic ectodermal dysplasia	Retinoblastoma
Huntington's chorea	Treacher-Collins syndrome
	Tuberous sclerosis

AUTOSOMAL DOMINANT INHERITANCE

Some characteristics of dominantly inherited diseases (Table 34–4) are as follows:

(1) One of the parents of the propositus will have the disease. An exception to this is a mutation occurring in the parent's germ cell (see below) or when the disease in the parent was either not penetrant or of a greatly diminished expressivity.

(2) There is a 50% risk of involvement in each sibling of an affected individual.

(3) The disease is usually not so serious as a recessively inherited disease.

(4) Either sex may be affected.

(5) The pedigree tends to be "vertical," ie, there are affected individuals in several generations.

AUTOSOMAL RECESSIVE INHERITANCE

Some characteristics of recessively inherited diseases (Table 34–5) are as follows:

(1) The disease tends to be rare and more severe than many dominantly inherited conditions.

(2) Affected individuals tend to be in the same generation.

(3) Normal parents are carriers.

(4) The rarer the trait, the greater the incidence of consanguinity in the parents.

(5) There is a 25% risk of involvement of the sibs of an affected individual.

(6) Either sex may be affected.

(7) The pedigree is usually "horizontal," ie, affected individuals are in the same generation.

SEX-LINKED (X-LINKED) DISEASE

When a gene is located on the X chromosome, it is said to be sex-linked (X-linked). A disease due to a single gene defect, which is inherited in an X-linked fashion, may be inherited either as an X-linked dominant or X-linked recessive.

X-linked dominant traits are rare (Table 34–6). They have the following characteristics:

(1) The hemizygous male will exhibit the full disease. None of his sons will be involved. All of his daughters will be involved, but will show a milder form of the disease. There will be a 50% risk of involvement in each of his daughter's children.

(2) The homozygous female will have severe disease, and all of her children will be involved.

(3) The heterozygous female will have a milder form of disease, and there will be a 50% chance in all of her children, regardless of sex, of their being involved.

The X-linked recessive form of disease (Table 34–7) will have the following characteristics:

(1) Affected individuals are nearly always males.

(2) The mother is usually a carrier. She transmits the disease to half of her sons, ie, there is a 50% chance that each of her sons will be involved.

(3) One-half of a carrier mother's daughters will be carriers. All of an affected father's daughters will be carriers.

(4) The uninvolved sons do not transmit the disease.

(5) There is no father-son transmission.

TABLE 34–5. Some recessively inherited diseases (autosomal).

Albinism	Hurler's syndrome
Chondroectodermal dysplasia	Ichthyosis congenita
Congenital afibrinogenemia	Maple syrup urine disease
Cystic fibrosis of the pancreas	Microcephaly
Endemic goitrous cretinism	Morquio's syndrome
Epidermolysis bullosa dystrophica (severe recessive form)	Niemann-Pick disease
	Phenylketonuria
Familial amaurotic idiocy	Sickle cell anemia
Familial nonhemolytic jaundice with kernicterus	Thalassemia
Galactosemia	Virilizing adrenal hyperplasia
Gaucher's disease	Wilson's disease
Glycogen storage disease	Xeroderma pigmentosa

TABLE 34–6. X-linked dominant inheritance.

Hereditary hematuria: some types
Vitamin D-resistant rickets: some types
Xg(a) blood group

MUTATION

The word mutation means a sudden change in genotype. In the case of a gene, this is a point mutation to distinguish it from more gross changes in chromosomal structure. A mutation occurring in a germ cell will result in a child who differs at the given genetic locus from his parents. This mutant gene, however, will be passed on to the descendants of the individual having the mutation in the same manner as any other gene. It is obvious that mutations can only be recognized when the trait exhibits itself in the heterozygous condition—in other words, is dominantly inherited.

The causes of mutation are not completely known, although some factors, particularly high-energy radiation, which increase the rate of mutation are recognized.

SPORADIC OCCURRENCE OF DISEASE

It is especially important to investigate sporadic cases of disease occurring in a family when it is known that the disease is usually due to a single gene defect. The following causes should be considered:

(1) Mutation occurring in one of the parents. If this is true, then the disease should be dominantly inherited in the offspring of the affected individual; and, since the mutant event was a point mutation occurring in one germ cell, the parents of the affected individual are not at an increased risk that further affected children will result from conceptions involving other, nonmutated germ cells.

TABLE 34–7. X-linked recessively inherited diseases.

Aldrich's syndrome
Color blindness
Glucose-6-phosphate dehydrogenase deficiency
Hemophilia A
Hemophilia B
Hereditary anhidrotic ectodermal dysplasia
Lesch-Nyhan syndrome
Lowe's oculocerebrorenal syndrome
Microcephaly (some types)
Pseudohypertrophic muscular dystrophy (Duchenne)
Agammaglobulinemia

(2) The disease is a rare recessive. Both parents are healthy carriers, and any future children that the parents have will run the usual 25% risk of being involved.

(3) The disease is a phenocopy, ie, a predominantly environmentally determined disease which mimics a genetic disease. An example of this would be the microcephaly occurring as part of the rubella syndrome versus genetically determined microcephaly.

(4) The disease is dominantly inherited but has low penetrance, and has for this reason skipped the previous generation. It is possible that if one were to examine the parents by very sensitive technics, some abnormal manifestation might be found to show that they were, in fact, involved.

(5) One must always consider the possibility in sporadic cases of genetic diseases that there may be illegitimacy and that one of the supposed parents is not really the parent.

SEX-LIMITED DISEASE

A sex-limited disease is one which is actually autosomally inherited but which, because of factors in the environment such as the presence of certain sex hormones, is expressed only in one sex. An example of this is baldness, which is inherited as an autosomal dominant but occurs predominantly in the male.

POLYGENIC DISEASE

In addition to those traits which are due to the inheritance of a single gene, there are many traits and genetically determined diseases which are multifactorial in origin. Many of these traits occurring in the general population do not sharply divide the population up into those who have and those who do not have the trait but exhibit a continuous variability representing a varying interaction between a genotype of a certain composition and an environment. The inheritance of certain characteristics such as blood pressure, intelligence, and height is multifactorial. Unfortunately for the practical application of genetics to medicine, the more common diseases tend to be etiologically heterogeneous and due to many genetic and environmental factors. As a result, genetic counseling for these conditions is not as simple as it is for the aforementioned diseases in which simple types of inheritance occur.

TABLE 34–8. Empiric risks for some congenital diseases.

Mental deficiency of unknown etiology: Incidence 3:100
  Risks among siblings
      Both parents normal, 15% defective
      One parent defective, 35% defective
      Both parents defective, 85% defective

Anencephaly and spina bifida: Incidence 1:1000
  Male:female = 1:3. Incidence increases with maternal age and parity, and also in firstborn of very young mothers.
  Risk of repeat = about 3%. Risk of abnormal child or abortion = 25%.

Hydrocephalus: Incidence 1:2000 newborns
  Occasional X-linked recessive
  Often associated with meningocele or spina bifida
  May be nongenetic (toxoplasmosis, aminopterin, x-ray)
  Chance of repeat of some CNS anomaly = 3%
  Chance of repeat of hydrocephalus = 1%

CNS malformations in general: Incidence 29:10,000
  Siblings 6 times more likely to have CNS malformation
  Stillborn and abortion rates increased

	Cleft lip ± cleft palate	Cleft palate
Incidence	0.1%	0.04%
Negative family history	4.0%	2.0%
Normal parents; relatives involved	4.0%	7.0%
2 affected children	9.0%	1.0%
1 affected parent; no affected children	4.0%	6.0%
1 affected parent; 1 affected child	17.0%	15.0%

Congenital heart disease: Incidence 2:1000
  Neither parent involved, 1.4–1.8% risk of repeat*
  One parent involved, 5% risk of repeat*

Diabetes: Incidence 5:100
  One parent involved, 15% risk of repeat*
  Both parents involved, 25–75% risk of repeat*

Pyloric stenosis
  Male index patients:
      Brothers   3.2% ⎫
      Sons   6.8% ⎭   10 times greater than normal risk
      Sisters   3.0% ⎫
      Daughters   1.2% ⎭   20 times greater than normal risk

  Female index patients:
      Brothers   13.2% ⎫
      Sons   20.5% ⎭   35 times greater than normal risk
      Sisters   2.5% ⎫
      Daughters   11.1% ⎭   70 times greater than normal risk

Clubfoot: Incidence 1:1000 (male:female = 2.1)
  Sibling risk = 3–8%

Congenital dislocated hip: Incidence 1:1000
  Siblings of index case, 40 times greater than normal risk
  Aunts, uncles, nephews, nieces (of index case), 4 times greater than normal risk

*Many exceptions.

EMPIRIC RISK FIGURES

Where the pattern of inheritance is obscure, as in diseases in which a number of genes interacting with the environment seem to be responsible, it becomes difficult to provide accurate risk rates. In this case so-called empiric risk figures must be used. These are obtained by perusing the literature and finding pooled data on a large number of families with the disease. Because of the many variables involved, it is important to remember that these figures represent averages which may have little meaning in a specific case. However, they are the best available. It is also well to remember, in counseling, that where the pattern of inheritance is not clear a risk of a repeat is generally about one in 20, a figure much lower than the risks which must be quoted when single gene defects are involved (Table 34–8).

INBORN ERRORS OF METABOLISM
(See also Chapter 35.)

The concept of the inborn error was first suggested by Sir Archibald Garrod in 1908. This was greatly strengthened in 1926 when Beadle and Tatum presented their theory that one gene is responsible for the formation of one enzyme. At present, at least 80 of these inborn errors have been discovered, and there are undoubtedly many more. Fig 34–17 illustrates the different mechanisms by which an enzymatic block can produce clinically detectable disease: (1) Failure of production of a normal end product, eg, albinism. (2) Failure of production of a biologically active protein, eg, agammaglobulinemia. (3) The piling up of an abnormal and toxic metabolite, eg, phenylketonuria, galactosemia.

A list of commonly known inborn errors of metabolism is given in Table 34–9. Most of these dis-

TABLE 34–9. List of some inborn errors.

Phenylketonuria	Cystic fibrosis of the
Galactosemia	pancreas
Wilson's disease	Glycogen storage disease
Goitrous cretinism	Orotic aciduria
Adrenogenital syndrome	Gaucher's disease
Albinism	Cystathioninuria
Hemophilia	Maple syrup urine disease
Afibrinogenemia	Homocystinuria
Agammaglobulinemia	

eases are inherited as autosomal recessives. They tend to be rare, but frequently are serious life-threatening diseases which cause severe mental retardation. Many of them, such as phenylketonuria and galactosemia, have achieved an importance greater than their incidence would seem to warrant because by early diagnosis and appropriate treatment the serious forms of mental retardation can be prevented. In an increasing number of these inborn errors of metabolism, it has become possible for the alert physician to make a diagnosis of the enzymatic defect in the newborn baby. By circumventing the enzymatic block, usually by a dietary change, he can then prevent the serious aftermath of the disease. The identification of the carrier state, ie, the normal individual who is a heterozygote for this recessive trait, is of the utmost importance in genetic counseling. This has been achieved for galactosemia and, at least for this inborn error of metabolism, it is now possible to tell a married couple whether or not both members are carriers of this defect, which would then give them a 25% risk of having affected offspring. One of the major efforts in human genetics today is to develop technics for recognizing the carrier state in all of the inborn errors of metabolism.

Hsia DY & others: Metabolic disorders associated with mental retardation. P Clin North America 15:889, 1968.

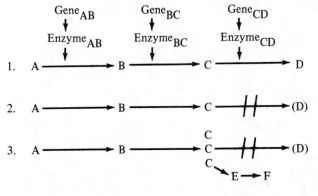

FIG 34–17. Mechanisms by which an enzymatic block in a metabolic pathway (A→B→C→D) can produce disease.

GENETIC COUNSELING

The most direct application of the advances in our understanding of basic genetic mechanisms is in the provision of genetic advice or genetic counseling. The advice usually stems from an inquiry about whether a given disease is likely to recur in the family.

The prime requisite for giving advice is the possession of all available facts about the patient and the disease. In order to give genetic advice, the physician must ask himself the following questions:

(1) What is the disease in the propositus? This requires the most accurate diagnosis available.

(2) Is the disease hereditary or is it a phenocopy, eg, is the cleft palate due to abortifacients? Is the mental deficiency due to a birth injury? Is the pseudohermaphroditism due to the use of oral progestins?

FAMILY HISTORY

History taking is a fundamental tool in every physician's armamentarium. In genetic counseling, however, there are points in the family history which should be stressed in order to pinpoint the genetic factors involved:

(1) **Parental age:** Mention has already been made of the maternal age effect, ie, the increasing risk of nondisjunction and the increasing risk of other congenital malformations with increasing parental age.

(2) **Siblings:** Their age, sex, and state of health is important. The larger the number of unaffected sibs, the less likely the condition is to be due to a single segregating gene.

(3) **Consanguinity:** The chance of both parents carrying the same rare recessive gene is greater if they are related. The likelihood of the patient's disease being recessively inherited is thus increased in the presence of consanguinity. Consanguinity rates in the general population have been decreasing throughout the world, being about 0.05% in the USA. Among the parents of children with albinism, however, there is a consanguinity rate of about 20%. This fact should be borne in mind when one is asked, "Should I marry my cousin?"

(4) **Radiation history:** The deleterious effect of x-irradiation on the embryo has been well documented. In addition, there occur genetic effects of irradiation such as point mutations, chromosomal breaks with abnormal healing, and increased incidence of nondisjunction. These effects are likely to occur prior to conception during gametogenesis. For this reason a history of radiation exposure to the gonads of either parent prior to conception is important. Because of the nature of gametogenesis in the female, inquiries should be made concerning exposure of the mother to x-ray at a time when she herself was an embryo.

(5) **History of exposure to drugs and virus infections early in pregnancy:** A positive history of exposure to a known teratogen may help in determining whether genetic or environmental factors were etiologically important in the child's disease.

(6) **History of previous pregnancies in the family:** Many abortions in the family may suggest the carrier state of a translocating chromosome, which should then be looked for in the patient. Similarly, diabetes or "prediabetes" should be ruled out.

(7) **Construction of a pedigree:** The diagrammatic representation of the family history helps one decide whether a disease is familial and, if so, whether it follows one of the single gene patterns of inheritance, ie, the vertical patterns of dominant inheritance, the horizontal pattern of recessive inheritance, or the oblique pattern of X-linked recessive inheritance. The larger the pedigree, the more typical the pattern (Fig 34–18).

PHYSICAL EXAMINATION

In addition to the physical examination that is performed on the affected patient for diagnostic pur-

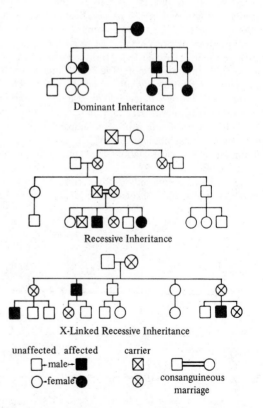

FIG 34–18. Pedigrees demonstrating various types of single gene inheritance.

poses, it is frequently desirable to examine the parents and the unaffected siblings of the patient in order to pick up cases where expressivity is diminished. This is important in determining whether a gene mutation has occurred in a parental germ cell, a fact which changes risk figures greatly. Sometimes a laboratory test on the parents, such as a blood phosphorus level when the patient has vitamin D-resistant rickets, will bring to light an expression of a previously unrecognized defective gene in a seemingly normal parent.

Finally, the literature on a specific disease should be carefully reviewed in order to determine the usual type of transmission and, if this is not clear, to estimate the empiric risks. This is particularly helpful if the patient's pedigree data are not too complete.

NATURE OF ADVICE

Counseling should be given with both parents present. If the mother is pregnant, the counseling should, in general, be deferred until after delivery unless an abortion or amniocentesis may be indicated.

Advice should never be given in a cold, impersonal way. Knowledge of the cultural, religious, and educational background of the family is helpful. Advantage should be taken of the opportunity for a thorough discussion of the nature of the disease in order to dispel the store of misinformation, anxiety, and guilt that is often present.

It is often helpful to remind the patient of the 5% chance in every pregnancy of a congenital abnormality. The risk resulting from the defect in question will frequently not add significantly to this figure.

When the patients are fully informed about the nature of the disease, and when the risks they will incur in future pregnancies are carefully explained, the actual decision about their future action is left up to them. The physician should be ready, however, to offer information on alternatives to normal reproduction such as sterilization, artificial insemination, contraception, and adoption.

Genetic counseling may be postconceptional as well as preconceptional. In the former case, the question to be answered is, "Should pregnancy be interrupted?" In most cases the investigative procedure is similar to what has been discussed above, and the patient is told the probability that the unborn child is affected, which may be anything from 1% to 50%. On the basis of this figure, one must decide whether there is a valid genetic indication for interrupting pregnancy, and pregnancy may be interrupted even though the fetus is actually more likely to be unaffected.

Intrauterine diagnosis usually converts the probability to a certainty, so that one knows that the fetus is or is not affected.

The procedure of amniocentesis has made possible intrauterine diagnosis for some diseases—in particular the cytogenetic diseases and those biochemical diseases that can be diagnosed by assaying for a specific enzyme on cultured fetal cells obtained from amniotic fluid (Table 34–10). The procedure consists of the suprapubic insertion of a needle into the uterine cavity at about 16 weeks of pregnancy and the aspiration of 5–10 ml of sterile amniotic fluid. Thus far, the complications have been negligible—certainly much less than 1%. For this reason, it seems reasonable to perform the procedure when the risk of diagnosable fetal disease is greater than 1%.

The indications for amniocentesis are as follows:

(1) Either parent is a carrier of a balanced translocation. The risk of an affected child is about 3–10% depending upon which parent is the carrier.

(2) A previous child with trisomy 21. The risk of a repeat may be as high as 2%, especially for mothers under 30.

(3) Parents are carriers of an autosomal recessively inherited disease that can be diagnosed in utero (Table 34–10).

(4) Mother is a carrier of an X-linked recessively inherited disease which cannot be diagnosed in utero (eg, muscular dystrophy, hemophilia A). However, the risk of being affected is 50% if the fetus is a male and close to zero if a female.

(5) Maternal age over 35 years (in some clinics, the indication is maternal age over 40 years). In the USA, the 10% of pregnant women who are over 35 years old are responsible for the birth of 50% of children with Down's syndrome.

Intrauterine diagnosis may well be one of the great advances in medicine in the second half of the 20th century.

Milunsky A & others: Pre-natal genetic diagnosis. New England J Med 283:1370, 1441, 1497, 1970.

Nadler HL: Prenatal detection of genetic defects. J Pediat 74:132, 1969.

TABLE 34–10. Some biochemical disorders which can be diagnosed antenatally.

Argininosuccinic acid	Juvenile GM_1 gangliosidosis
Branched chain ketoaciduria	
Cystathionine synthase deficiency	Ketotic hyperglycinemia
	Krabbe's syndrome
Cystinosis	Lesch-Nyhan syndrome and variants
Fabry's disease	
Fucosidosis	Mannosidosis
Galactokinase deficiency	Metachromatic leukodystrophy
Galactosemia	
Gaucher's disease (infantile)	Methylmalonic aciduria
Generalized gangliosidosis	Niemann-Pick disease
Hunter's and Hurler's syndromes	Orotic aciduria
	Pompe's disease
Hypervalinemia	Refsum's disease
I-cell disease	Sandhoff's disease
Isovaleric acidemia	San Filippo disease
	Tay-Sachs disease

GLOSSARY OF
GENETIC TERMS

Alleles: Genes that occupy homologous loci on homologous chromosomes. An individual can never have more than 2 allelic genes at a given locus.

Aneuploid: This refers to the chromosomal number of a cell population which is not an integral multiple of the haploid number.

Autosomes: All of the chromosomes other than the 2 sex chromosomes.

Chromatids: The 2 halves resulting from the longitudinal division of a chromosome through the centromere, each consisting of a double helix of DNA. Pictures of metaphase chromosomes will usually show sister chromatids on each side of the centromere and joined together at the centromere.

Consanguinity: The blood relationship of 2 individuals. It usually refers to a married couple.

Crossing-over: The physical process of exchange between chromatids in synapsis, which permits the process of recombination. This has the result that genes lying in one chromosome are not always passed on together to the descendants.

Diploid: The double set of chromosomes in the somatic cells of the organism. The diploid number in man is 46.

Gametes: The mature germ cells which have the haploid set of chromosomes.

Genotype: The genetic constitution of an organism.

Haploid: One-half of the diploid complement of chromosomes, in which only one chromosome of each homologous pair is present. The haploid number in man is 23.

Isochromosome: A morphologically abnormal chromosome which results from an abnormal "horizontal" division of the centromere, instead of its normally vertical division, during mitosis. The result is that the chromosome is metacentric, with the centromere in the center. The 2 arms of the chromosome arise from 2 homologous chromatids. Such a chromosome would possess a double set of genes from the arm of the parent chromosome which supplied the chromatids, and would be lacking the genes normally provided by the other arm of the parent chromosome.

Karyotype: The chromosomal constitution of an individual, as typified by the systematized array of the chromosomes of a single cell prepared by photography.

Meiosis: A form of cell division in which the haploid gametes are produced from diploid cells.

Monosomy: Having only one chromosome of a particular homologous pair, instead of 2.

Mosaic: An individual whose tissues are of two or more genetically different kinds, usually of different chromosomal constitution.

Phenocopy: A nongenetic condition which mimics that produced by a certain genotype.

Phenotype: The manifest constitution of an individual as determined by careful examination. This is the result of an interaction between his genetic makeup and the environment.

Proband or propositus: The index case, or starting case, from which a genetic investigation is undertaken.

Satellite: These are small deeply staining bodies situated at the end of the short arm of an acrocentric chromosome and separated from it by a short distance.

Trisomy: The presence of any single chromosome in 3 homologous forms, rather than the usual 2.

●   ●   ●

General References

Carr DH: Chromosomal abnormalities in clinical medicine. Chap 1 in: *Progress in Medical Genetics*. Vol 6. Steinberg AG, Bearn AG (editors). Grune & Stratton, 1969.

Holt SB: *The Genetics of Dermal Ridges*. Thomas, 1968.

McKusick V: *Mendelian Inheritance in Man*. Johns Hopkins Press, 1966.

Moore K: *The Sex Chromatin*. Saunders, 1966.

Penrose LS, Smith GF: *Down's Anomaly*. Little, Brown, 1966.

Porter IH: *Heredity and Disease*. McGraw-Hill, 1968.

Reisman LE, Matheny AP Jr: *Genetics and Counseling in Medical Practice*. Mosby, 1969.

Thompson J, Thompson M: *Genetics in Medicine*. Saunders, 1966.

Yunis JJ (editor): *Human Chromosome Methodology*. Academic Press, 1965.

35...

Inborn Errors of Metabolism

Donough O'Brien, MD, FRCP

In his Croonian Lecture to the Royal College of Physicians of London in 1908, Sir Archibald Garrod described 4 diseases—alkaptonuria, cystinuria, albinism, and pentosuria—at the same time coining the term inborn errors of metabolism. Since then, and particularly in the last few years, there has been a prodigious increase in our understanding of the molecular mechanisms of genetic misinformation. Technical developments in fields such as gas chromatography and mass spectroscopy have also extended diagnostic possibilities to other areas of intermediary metabolism than amino acids and lipids.

Most of these conditions are rare autosomal recessive traits. However, the development of inexpensive screening procedures and the increased potential for confirmatory identification and treatment as well as the wider acceptance of termination of pregnancy following antenatal diagnosis have made them an important group of pediatric diseases. Some of the better known and more common syndromes are described below or in Tables 35–4 to 35–6. Others are described elsewhere in this book—eg, the hyperbilirubinemias in Chapter 18, glucose-6-phosphate deficiency and the hemoglobinopathies in Chapter 14, and the immune globulin disorders in Chapter 15.

Bergsma D (editor): Intrauterine diagnosis: A symposium. Birth Defects 7(5), April 1971.
Hsia DYY: Use of white blood cells and cultured somatic cells in clinical genetic disorders. Clin Genet 1:5, 1970.

DISORDERS OF CARBOHYDRATE METABOLISM

GALACTOSEMIA

Galactosemia now refers to a group of conditions characterized by galactose intolerance in which the enzymatic block varies in both site and severity. These can be divided into the galactose-1-phosphate uridyl transferase deficiencies and galactokinase deficiency.

1. GALACTOSE-1-PHOSPHATE URIDYL TRANSFERASE DEFICIENCY

In the severe form of this disease the galactose-1-phosphate uridyl transferase activity in red blood cells and in liver is negligible. Several variants have been described, indicating the heterogeneity of the disease, including the Negro, Kelly, Rennes, unstable, and Duarte types. The latter is by far the commonest; homozygotes are asymptomatic and have about 50% of the enzyme activity of the normal person. All are autosomal recessive traits.

The liver shows extensive fatty infiltration, occasional giant cells, pericellular cirrhosis, and, later, advanced cirrhosis. Autopsy evidence from untreated cases is scanty, but there are occasional reports showing a small brain with narrow gyri and evidence of a gliotic encephalomyelopathy. In the kidneys, the epithelial cells of proximal and distal convoluted tubules are usually swollen, with perinuclear vacuolation.

The cataracts that usually develop are due to osmotic damage from accumulation of unmetabolized galactitol, a reduction product of galactose.

Clinical Findings

A. Symptoms and Signs: In the severe form of the disease the onset is with vomiting and diarrhea in the newborn period after a milk feeding. The infant becomes jaundiced and develops hepatomegaly. Without treatment, death frequently occurs in a few days. Cataracts usually develop within 2 months in untreated cases and may be visible much earlier.

Not all cases are severe, as shown by the occasional identification of a patient with galactosemia in mental institution surveys. Mental retardation occurs unless treatment is given and seems to be irreversible. Clinical and laboratory evidence of the disease abates promptly with effective treatment.

B. Laboratory Findings: Laboratory findings in infancy include galactosuria, hypergalactosemia, proteinuria, and aminoaciduria. The simplest way to make the diagnosis is by the detection of reducing substances in the urine followed by one-dimensional paper chromatography to confirm the presence of excess galactose. This may not be entirely satisfactory if the infant is sick and on a low milk intake. Elevated serum galactose levels, especially after a galactose load, help to confirm the diagnosis but are technically hard to

TABLE 35–1. The glycogen storage diseases.*

Type	Enzyme Deficiency	Clinical Description	Ancillary Laboratory Tests	Definitive Laboratory Tests
I	Glucose-6-phosphatase	Onset may be in neonatal period; marked hepatomegaly; tendency to fasting hypoglycemia.	High serum uric acid, cholesterol, total lipids; flat serum glucose response to epinephrine, glucagon, intravenous fructose and galactose; low alkaline phosphatase.	Glucose-6-phosphatase on liver biopsy ($<$ 5 μM/minute/gm wet tissue)
II	Acid maltase	Usually striking cardiomegaly with poor muscle tone; pseudohypertrophic macroglossia; normal mentally; early death.	Granular (not vacuolar) appearing liver cells; periodic acid-Schiff positive glomeruli and tubules.	Acid maltase on liver biopsy. No activity. (Normal, $>$ 10 μM/minute/gm wet tissue.)
III	Amylo-1,6-glucosidase; debranching enzyme	Hepatomegaly, growth retardation, tendency to hypoglycemia with attendant complications; also called limit dextrinosis.	Diminished but significant rise in serum glucose after epinephrine and glucagon; hyperglycemia after intravenous fructose and galactose; very high red cell glycogen.	Amylo-1,6-glucosidase assay on liver biopsy and leukocytes ($<$ 1 μM/minute/gm wet tissue)
IV	Amylo-1,4:1,6-transglucosidase; branching enzyme	Failure to thrive, hepatomegaly, and hypotonia. May treat with a-glucosidase.	Coincidental evidence of chronic liver disease; characteristically flat iodine spectrum and high degradation by β-amylase.	Amylo-1,4:1,6-transglucosidase assay in leukocytes.
V	Muscle phosphorylase	Easy fatigability in childhood; later, weakness with muscle pain and stiffness on minimal exertion; transient myoglobinuria.	Work capacity increased by glucose infusion; venous blood lactate falls during exercise.	Muscle phosphorylase assay ($<$ 80 μM/minute/gm)
VI	Liver phosphorylase	Consanguinity of parents; liver enlargement sometimes in early infancy; growth retardation; tendency to hypoglycemia with convulsions.	Diminished but significant rise in serum glucose after epinephrine and glucagon; hyperglycemia following intravenous fructose or galactose.	Liver phosphorylase assay ($<$ 20 μM/minute/gm)
VII	Phosphoglucomutase	Hepatomegaly without splenomegaly; extensive glycogen deposition in liver.	Single case only; unlikely to be defined except by elaborate enzymic investigation.	Phosphoglucomutase assay
VIII	Phosphofructokinase	Easy fatigability, weakness, muscle stiffness on exertion in children of consanguineous parents.	Failure of venous blood lactate to rise on exertion.	Phosphofructokinase assay
IX	Phosphorylase kinase	Onset at birth with marked hepatomegaly but normal muscles.	As for type VI.	Specific enzymic assay.
X	Glycogen synthetase	Mental retardation; hypoglycemia with convulsions after overnight fast; no hepatosplenomegaly.	Rise in serum glucose with glucagon after meal but not fasting; reduced catecholamine response to hypoglycemia.	UDPG-glycogen-1, 4-transglucosylase assay
Mauriac's syndrome	None	Obesity, hepatosplenomegaly, and dwarfism in badly controlled diabetic children, usually males.	High liver glycogen, hypersensitivity to insulin.	None

*Modified and reproduced, with permission, from O'Brien, Ibbott, & Rodgerson: *Laboratory Manual of Pediatric Microbiochemical Techniques,* 4th ed. Hoeber, 1968.

perform. Moreover, galactose loading may lead to severe hypoglycemia and is not advised. Specific confirmation of defective red cell galactose-1-phosphate uridyl transferase activity must always be carried out; both screening and quantitative methods are available. Normal levels are $\geqslant 300$ international milliunits (ImU)/ gm hemoglobin; in galactosemia, they are < 8 ImU/gm hemoglobin.

Treatment

A galactose-free diet should be instituted as soon as the diagnosis is made. In the USA, regimens based on hydrolysates such as Nutramigen with added Dextri-Maltose have proved satisfactory. For the detailed implementation of such a regimen, the reader should consult the references given below.

The efficacy of the diet should be monitored by measuring red cell galactose-1-phosphate concentration, which should not exceed 2 mg/100 ml packed red cell lysate. However, results must be corroborated with dietary history as in certain conditions galactose-1-phosphate can be produced endogenously from UDP-galactase. Avoidance of galactose should be lifelong in severe cases, although there is some increased tolerance with age. Mothers of identified cases are advised to take a galactose-free diet during subsequent pregnancies.

Prognosis

With prompt institution of a galactose-free diet, the prognosis for life is excellent. Long-term follow-up still suggests, however, that the majority of severely affected individuals suffer some intellectual impairment.

California State Department of Public Health. *Galactose-Free Diet for Professional Use and Parent's Guide for the Galactose-Free Diet.* [Available from the department office at 2151 Berkeley Way, Berkeley, California 94704.]

Chacho CM & others: Unstable galactose-1-phosphate uridyl transferase: A new variant of galactosemia. J Pediat 78:454, 1971.

Hsia DYY (editor): *Galactosemia.* Thomas, 1969.

Komrower GM & others: Long term follow-up of galactosemia. Arch Dis Child 45:367, 1970.

O'Brien D: *Galactosemia: A Reference Bibliography,* 2nd ed. US Department of Health, Education, & Welfare, 1972.

2. GALACTOKINASE DEFICIENCY

A few cases of hypergalactosemia and galactosuria due to galactokinase deficiency have been reported. These patients showed no evidence of hepatic or renal complications, but all developed severe cataracts in childhood. Heterozygotes have mild galactose intolerance and an increased incidence of cataracts.

Monteleone JA & others: Cataracts, galactosuria, and hypergalactosemia due to galactokinase deficiency. Am J Med 50:403, 1971.

FRUCTOSE INTOLERANCE

In this autosomal recessive disease there is a reduced ability to split fructose-1-phosphate into glyceraldehyde and dihydroxyacetone phosphate. The ill effects of this disorder are, however, those of hypoglycemia, for which 3 explanations have been offered. The first is that fructose-1-phosphate inhibits phosphoglucomutase and thus the release of glycogen from the liver. The second is that sequestration of phosphorus as fructose-1-phosphate may reduce hepatic glucose-1-phosphate formation from glycogen. The third hypothesis is that rapid fructose phosphorylation may reduce available hepatic ATP, which is needed for gluconeogenesis. A similar syndrome occurs with hepatic fructose-1,6-diphosphatase deficiency.

Infants and children with this disease are free of symptoms except after the ingestion of fructose. If the relation to particular foodstuffs is not recognized, the infant will fail to thrive and will have repeated episodes of vomiting, with the development of jaundice, hepatomegaly, and evidence of liver damage. Hypoglycemia with convulsions and loss of consciousness occurs, and there is fructosuria, proteinuria, and aminoaciduria. As survivors grow up, they recognize the association of nausea and vomiting with fructose-containing foods and learn to avoid them.

The typical history can be confirmed by detecting fructose in the urine after a fructose load. Fructosuria is, of course, also seen in benign fructosuria due to fructokinase deficiency. Hypoglycemia and hypophosphatemia following fructose loading (24 gm/sq m) is diagnostic; low serum aldolase levels are suggestive; and greatly reduced hepatic 1-phosphofructoaldolase activity on liver biopsy is confirmatory.

Treatment consists of the avoidance of cane sugar in the diet. If the disorder is recognized early enough, the prospects for normal intellectual and somatic development are good.

Köhlin P, Melin K: Hereditary fructose intolerance in four Swedish families. Acta paediat scandinav 57:24, 1968.

Levin B & others: Fructosaemia. Am J Med 45:826, 1968.

Rennert OM, Greer M: Hereditary fructosemia. Neurology 20:421, 1970.

GLYCOGEN STORAGE DISEASES

Glycogen is a branched chain polysaccharide which is stored in liver and muscle. The usual end-to-end linkage in the molecule, which may contain about

10,000 glucosyl residues, is between carbon atoms 1 and 4. The branching links, however, are formed by a-1,6-glucosidic bonds. About 1/2 of the bulk of the molecule is made up of free-end chains which are 7—10 glucosyl units long.

In the synthesis of glycogen, glucose is phosphorylated first in the 6 and then in the 1 position. Uridine diphosphoglucose is then formed by the enzyme UDPG pyrophosphorylase. In the next step, activated by glycogen synthetase, a glucosyl unit is added to the growing chain in a 1:4 bond. At the same time, the branching enzyme amylo-1,4:1,6-transglucosidase dislodges appropriate terminal chain segments and reattaches them in the 1,6 position. In the breakdown of glycogen, a small amount of glucose is liberated by the action of the debranching enzyme amylo-1,6-glucosidase; however, the bulk of the molecule is broken down to glucose-1-phosphate by phosphorylase. The activity of the latter enzyme is subject to a complex control mechanism initiated by glucagon and epinephrine and dependent on cyclic AMP.

The various types of glycogenoses are represented by different specific enzymatic defects in the above pathway. The more common types are described briefly below, and a guide to their laboratory diagnosis is given in Table 35—1.

Type I: Glucose-6-Phosphatase Deficiency

The clinical course of this condition is quite variable. It usually presents in early infancy with hepatomegaly. Symptoms are predominantly due to hypoglycemia, with episodes of drowsiness, vomiting, convulsions, and coma. There may also be a hemorrhagic diathesis. The mobilization of fat for energy leads to acidosis, ketonuria, hyperglycemia, and xanthomas. Excess glycogen is deposited in the kidneys and glycogen and fat in the liver. Blood lactate levels are elevated, as are those of uric acid also, which may ultimately lead to gout in geriatric patients. Serum glycerides and cholesterol are elevated, and phosphorus is low.

The diagnosis can be surmised in a young person who shows hepatomegaly with normal liver function tests and, on administration of glucagon, shows a rise in lactate levels but not in serum glucose. (Type VII is as severe clinically but shows some response to glucagon postprandially.)

The diagnosis must be confirmed by the specific enzyme assay.

Galactose and fructose restriction, frequent high-protein feedings, and glucagon, corticosteroid, or thyroid administration may be helpful in treatment.

Type II: Acid Maltase Deficiency (Pompe's Disease)

In this variant there is excessive glycogen deposition in both liver and muscle, with cardiac muscle especially involved. The symptoms are those of cardiac failure with marked muscle weakness as well as vomiting, anorexia, and failure to grow. These patients generally do not survive infancy. The large tongue may sometimes give rise to an erroneous diagnosis of Down's syndrome or cretinism. Radiologically, there is a greatly enlarged globular cardiac outline. Glucose tolerance tests are normal, and the final differentiation from other nonanatomic causes of cardiomegaly (eg, fibroelastosis) is on the basis of absent a-glucosidase or increased glycogen assay in the white blood cells.

Dietary and glucagon therapy may be of some help.

Dancis J & others: Absence of acid maltase in glycogenosis type 2 (Pompe's disease) in tissue culture. Am J Dis Child 117:108, 1969.
Hug G & others: Type II glycogenosis. Pediat Res 5:107, 1971.

Type III: Debranching Enzyme Deficiency

Symptomatology is similar to that of type I although—like types IV, VI, VII, and X—this type is more benign. Laboratory evaluation shows a partial reduction in the blood sugar response to epinephrine and glucagon and a normal rise in serum glucose after a galactose or fructose load. The red cell glycogen content is strikingly elevated.

Conventional treatment with frequent high-protein, low-starch feedings and glucagon may reduce hepatomegaly. In some cases described recently, portacaval diversions have been strikingly successful.

Esmann V & others: Heredity of leukocyte phosphorylase and amylo-1,6-glucosidase deficiency. J Pediat 74:96, 1969.
Fernandez J & others: Hexose and protein tolerance tests in children with liver glycogenosis caused by a deficiency of the debranching enzyme system. Pediatrics 41:935, 1968.
Justice P & others: Amylo-1,6-glucosidase in human fibroblasts. Biochem Biophys Res Comm 39:301, 1970.
Starzl TE & others: Portal diversion in glycogen storage disease. Surgery 65:504, 1969.

Type V: Muscle Phosphorylase Deficiency (McArdle's Syndrome)

Patients with this disease and with phosphofructokinase deficiency present with pain, weakness, and spasm of muscles after exercise. In the resting state, there are no abnormal neurologic or electromyographic changes and no fasciculations or fibrillations. Symptoms are relieved by rest. Responses to glucagon are normal, but the affected muscle is overloaded with normal glycogen. Specific diagnosis rests on a precise enzymatic determination.

Treatment consists of restricting exercise to tolerable limits and administering glucose during enforced activity.

Schmid R: Syndrome of muscular dystrophy with myoglobinuria. J Clin Invest 38:1040, 1959.

Type VI: Liver Phosphorylase Deficiency

Signs and symptoms of this disease are mild, although hepatomegaly may be present from birth. There is some elevation of serum glucose after glucagon, and fructose and galactose loading lead to hyperglycemia. Phosphorylase kinase deficiency can only be distinguished by specific enzymic assay.

Simple dietary evasion of hypoglycemia is all the treatment necessary.

Hug G: Liver phosphorylase. Am J Med 42:139, 1967.

THE HYPOGLYCEMIAS

Impaired ability to sustain normal serum glucose levels is a common metabolic problem in infancy and childhood. Precise definitions are difficult, so that diagnosis and treatment are designed to detect and treat hyperinsulinism on the one hand and disorders of glycolysis and gluconeogenesis on the other.

Table 35–2 sets out many of the recognized forms of infantile hypoglycemia and summarizes the differential diagnosis. The special importance of this group of disorders is worth repeated emphasis, namely, that failure to diagnose and treat correctly can lead to significant permanent cerebral damage.

Clinical Findings

A. Symptoms and Signs: Symptoms of hypoglycemia are quite variable. In the newborn, especially, there may be none, or the infant may show difficulty in feeding, apathy, hypothermia, pallor, cyanosis, a weak cry, and, later, episodes of tremors, eye rolling, or actual convulsions. The fontanel is sometimes distended, and there may be cardiomegaly in severe cases. In older children, the usual symptoms are those of faintness, headache, sweating, and feeling hungry. Patients may look pale and complain of muscle pains and paresthesia; they may become irritable and drowsy and ultimately develop convulsions. Clinical response to restoration of normal serum glucose levels is usually rapid at all ages unless neurologic involvement is marked.

B. Laboratory Findings:* Hypoglycemia is usually defined as a serum glucose level of $\leqslant$ 20 mg/100 ml in the premature and $\leqslant$ 30 mg/100 ml in newborn or older infants. The possibility of this diagnosis always warrants complete laboratory evaluation, which can usually be done as an elective procedure. Where toxic or other specific cause is indicated, the diagnosis is that of the supposed underlying condition. In other cases, the following procedure is suggested:

1. After 3 days of a high-carbohydrate diet, the child is admitted to the hospital and, after an overnight fast, is given a standard glucose test lasting 4 hours. This is followed immediately after the last sample by a glucagon tolerance test. An abrupt fall in blood sugar between 30 minutes and 60 minutes is indicative of hyperinsulinism, including leucine sensitivity: late hypoglycemia at 3–4 hours suggests the delayed hyperinsulinemia of prediabetes. A flat curve may suggest malnutrition. A normal glucagon tolerance test

indicates adequate hepatic glycogen and serves also as a screening test for normal glycolytic mechanisms.

2. On the second day, an insulin/glucose tolerance test should be given to evaluate the homeostatic responses to induced hypoglycemia. This test is safer than the insulin sensitivity test since it is less likely to induce severe hypoglycemia. Even so, it should only be done with an intravenous drip of 0.5 N saline set up so that 50% dextrose can be administered promptly if required. A positive test indicates failure of normal glycolysis or gluconeogenesis. The previous glucagon tolerance test will differentiate between the 2 processes.

3. Special tests—

a. Tests for galactosemia, glycogen storage disease, fructose intolerance, and fructose-1,6-diphosphatase deficiency should be performed as indicated by the clinical history.

b. Leucine loading test for leucine sensitivity when the history suggests that hypoglycemia follows protein loading. Hyperinsulinism with reactive hypoglycemia during an oral GTT may be seen.

c. Start a ketogenic diet (Colle E, Ulstrom J: J Pediat 64:632, 1964) if the patient is small for gestational age at birth and the history suggests a relationship between hypoglycemia and ketosis. Oral administration of medium chain triglycerides may also produce symptoms.

Complications

Uncontrolled hypoglycemic episodes may lead to progressive cerebral damage, with epilepsy and developmental retardation. In cases where a pancreatectomy has been performed, diabetes is an occasional complication.

Treatment

Treatment is directed at counteracting the imbalance in glucose homeostasis; it is not necessarily specific to the nature of the imbalance. The following program can be used as a guide.

A. Toxic Causes: Discontinue drug, provide high carbohydrate intake.

B. Newborn: Treat initially with 5 or 10% dextrose infusion. This sometimes does not prevent hypoglycemia and may occasionally provoke hypoglycemia if suddenly discontinued. Prednisone, 5 mg/day orally, glucagon, 15 μg/kg every 4 hours IM, or epinephrine, 1:200 (Sus-Phrine), 0.005 ml/kg IM, may sometimes be required for a few days in addition to a glucose infusion. Fructose can be used instead of glucose in equimolar amounts. It is less likely to cause reactive hypoglycemia if temporarily discontinued.

C. Idiopathic Hypoglycemia of Infancy: Treat acute episodes with glucagon, 15 μg/kg IM, repeated, if necessary, in 30 minutes. At the same time, give 10% dextrose in 0.5 N saline at a rate of 100 ml/kg/24 hours.

For long-term therapy, a high-protein intake with frequent small high-carbohydrate feedings may be successful. If this fails, prednisone, 1–2 mg/kg/day orally

*See Chapter 40 for details of the tests discussed in this section.

TABLE 35–2. **Guide to the diagnosis of hypoglycemic states.**

Causes and Types	Diagnosis
Newborn period (See General References.)	
Infants of diabetic mothers	Clinical history and serum glucose determination. Increased K_t (see p 838) following intravenous glucose may predict severe cases.
Prematurity	
Placental insufficiency	
Intracranial injury	
Sepsis	
Erythroblastosis fetalis	
Neonatal cold injury	
Cessation of intravenous glucose	
Metabolic disorders in older infants and children	
Disorders of glycolysis	
Glycogen storage diseases (see p 871)	
Glucagon deficiency	
Glucagon resistant ketotic hypoglycemia	Hypoglycemia with ketonuria. Hypoglycemia induced by ketosis. Small for gestational age infants. Some respond to diazoxide (Hyperstat).
Hypopituitarism	Clinical history and supportive laboratory evidence.
Hypoadrenocorticism	Clinical history and supportive laboratory evidence.
Primary liver disease	Poor response to glucagon and epinephrine.
Malnutrition	Rarely < 20 mg/100 ml, but serious if associated with hypothermia, coma, and bacterial or parasitic infection.
Catechol insufficiency (Zetterstrom type)	Defective catechol response to hypoglycemia. Technically hard to define.
Other disorders of hexose metabolism	
Galactosemia (see p 869)	Screen for red cell UDPgal transferase deficiency.
Fructose intolerance (see p 871)	Hypoglycemia after fructose load. Test for specific aldolase deficiency.
Fructose-1,6-diphosphatase deficiency	Acidosis and hypoglycemia on fasting; glycerol and fructose provoke hypoglycemia.
Lactose induced	Flat oral GTT. Hypoglycemic response to lactose.
Disorders of gluconeogenesis	
Idiopathic spontaneous hypoglycemia	Increased insulin sensitivity as shown by insulin/glucose tolerance test.
Hyperinsulinism	Often but not always an excessive insulin response to a glucagon, tolbutamide, or epinephrine tolerance test. Prompt and exaggerated hypoglycemic response to glucose loading.
Islet cell hyperplasia	Increased K_t on intravenous glucose tolerance test.
Islet cell adenoma or adenocarcinoma	Irregular hyperinsulinemia after a glucose load. May have paradoxical response to diazoxide (Hyperstat). May only be diagnosed at exploratory laparotomy.
Some extrapancreatic tumors	
Beckwith's syndrome	Associated with macroglossia, microcephaly, hepatomegaly, somatic gigantism, omphalocele.
Prediabetes	Delayed hypoglycemia following oral glucose tolerance test; later, glucose intolerance.
Leucine sensitivity	Positive leucine sensitivity test.
Maple syrup urine disease	Presence of typical smell, neurologic symptoms, acidosis, branched chain ketoaciduria.
Miscellaneous disorders	
Hypothyroidism	Clinical history, serum glucose levels.
Primary neurologic disorders	Clinical history, serum glucose levels.
Reye's syndrome	Clinical picture of encephalopathy, hepatomegaly, and acidosis.
Chronic diarrhea	Especially with enteric infection.
L-Asparaginase	In therapy for leukemia.
Methylmalonic aciduria	Specific organic aciduria.
Toxic	
Salicylates	Positive ferric chloride test, elevated blood salicylates.
EDTA	
Sulfonylureas	History of diabetes in the mother.
Manganese	Has been used in treatment of diabetes.
Biotin deficiency	

in 2 or 3 divided doses, may be helpful. Finally, diazoxide (Hyperstat), 6–12 mg/kg/day orally in 2 doses, may be given. If all these measures fail, subtotal pancreatectomy should be considered.

D. Leucine Sensitivity: Restrict protein intake to < 1.5 gm/kg/day (provided growth is adequate) and give frequent high-carbohydrate feedings. Diazoxide (Hyperstat) or prednisone may also be helpful.

E. Ketotic Hypoglycemia: Test urine routinely, using nitroprusside (Acetest) papers for acetone, and treat incipient ketosis with frequent high-carbohydrate feedings and snacks. In infection, administer glucose intravenously and, as in other cases, have glucagon available in the home should severe hypoglycemia develop.

F. Hyperinsulinism: The delayed inappropriate hyperinsulinism of early diabetes should be treated by carbohydrate restriction in the diet. Pancreatic or extrapancreatic insulin-secreting tumors should be removed. In the case of simple hyperplasia, 85% of the pancreas should be removed.

G. Failure of Glycogenolysis: In glycogen storage disease, give frequent carbohydrate feedings. Surgical shunting procedures may help (see Glycogen Storage Diseases, above).

H. Galactosemia, Fructose-1,6-diphosphatase Deficiency, Fructose Intolerance: Avoid appropriate monosaccharide in diet.

I. Deficient Pressor Amine Response: Apply measures as under C (above), but also try ephedrine, 0.5–1 mg/kg orally 3 times a day.

Prognosis

Treatment may be complex but is usually successful. Symptoms of hypoglycemia may persist into adult life.

Cornblath M, Schwartz R: Page 82 in: *Disorders of Carbohydrate Metabolism in Infancy.* Saunders, 1967.

Greenberg RE, Christiansen RD: The critically ill child: Hypoglycemia. Pediatrics 46:915, 1970.

Knoblock H & others: Prognostic and etiologic factors in hypoglycemia. J Pediat 70:876, 1967.

Kogut MD & others: Idiopathic hypoglycemia. J Pediat 74:853, 1969.

Mereu TR & others: Diazoxide in the treatment of infantile hypoglycemia. New England J Med 275:1455, 1966.

INBORN ERRORS OF AMINO ACID METABOLISM

The development of column chromatographic technics for the detection and quantitation of amino acids in biologic fluids has enormously expanded the possibilities of laboratory diagnosis and treatment of one rare but important group of inborn errors of metabolism, ie, those involving the amino acids. Most of these disorders are summarized briefly in Tables 35–4 to 35–6. A few of special interest or importance are described in the following paragraphs.*

PHENYLKETONURIA & THE HYPERPHENYLALANINEMIAS

Essentials of Diagnosis

- Serum phenylalanine levels persistently in excess of 20 mg/100 ml after the first few days of life with low serum tyrosine levels.
- Phenylalanine levels can only be lowered by a special low-phenylalanine formula.
- Tolerance to phenylalanine is very poor, and serum levels rise rapidly with any increase in intake. Tolerance is unchanged with increasing age.
- Untreated cases excrete phenylpyruvic and o-hydroxyphenylacetic acid in the urine and show a positive ferric chloride test.

General Considerations

In 1934, the Norwegian physician Følling described 10 children who excreted phenylpyruvic acid in their urines and were severely mentally retarded. Subsequently, it was shown that these children had virtually no phenylalanine hydroxylase activity and therefore were unable to convert phenylalanine to tyrosine. Treatment of these children on a low phenylalanine diet for the first few years of life was logical and has generally been successful in preventing retardation.

Routine testing for hyperphenylalaninemia in the newborn period shows that relatively large numbers of infants have phenylalanine levels ≥ 4 mg/100 ml in the first week of life. The great majority of these are associated with elevated serum tyrosine levels and are due to a transient deficiency of p-hydroxyphenylpyruvic acid oxidase activity. A small number of others are due to other mutant phenylalanine hydroxylases which have limited activity.

It is important to recognize these other possibilities so that parents may initially be reassured, when a high serum phenylalanine is detected, that it by no means necessarily implies a diagnosis of phenylketonuria. Transient p-hydroxyphenylpyruvic acid oxidase deficiency usually responds promptly to vitamin C or to a short-term lowering of protein intake. The other hyperphenylalaninemias respond to a conventional low-protein formula, and a definite attempt should be made to keep fasting serum phenylalanine levels below 10 mg/100 ml for the first 4–6 years of life.

O'Brien D: *Rare Inborn Errors of Metabolism in Children With Mental Retardation,* 2nd ed. Children's Bureau, 1971.

Phenylketonuria is a traditional example of an inborn error of metabolism associated with mental deficiency. Like most of these diseases, it is an autosomal recessive condition in which there is impaired conversion of phenylalanine to tyrosine due to a defect in phenylalanine hydroxylase. The incidence in the USA averages 1:10,000 births, but much higher incidences are reported in Yemenite Jews and people of Celtic origin. It is uncommon in Negroes and Orientals.

The biochemical abnormality leads to an accumulation of phenylalanine in all body fluids and to the excessive urinary excretion of normal derivatives such as phenylpyruvic acid, phenyllactic acid, o-hydroxyphenylacetic acid, and phenylacetylglutamine. It is still not clear, however, why the great majority of these children are severely mentally retarded. Phenylalanine in excess is known to interfere with pyruvate kinase and cerebroside sulfokinase, and phenylpyruvic acid with pyruvate decarboxylase. This prevents normal myelination, and has been clearly demonstrated in laboratory animals. The rate of myelination in man decreases rapidly in the first few months after birth and is maximal during the third trimester. This explains why heterozygous children of phenylketonuric mothers are retarded and why it is of great importance to institute early dietary therapy.

Clinical Findings

In infants, one of the earliest manifestations of phenylketonuria is vomiting. Another is a "mouse-like" odor of the urine and sweat, which contains excessive amounts of phenylacetic, phenyllactic, and phenylpyruvic acids. By 1 year of age, the untreated phenylketonuric infant is often quite obese. The excessive accumulation of phenylalanine also impairs melanin production: thus, the untreated phenylketonuric individual is often lighter complexioned than his unaffected relatives. For example, Negroes, Orientals, and Spanish individuals have been noted to have brown hair; eczema is also common. Neurologic impairment is usual but not universal. Most are mentally retarded and hypertonic and have hyperactive reflexes. Seizures and tremors may be noted. Some have autistic or psychotic manifestations. Because this is an inherited disorder, a family history of phenylketonuria or of some of the above manifestations may also be helpful.

Differential Diagnosis of a Positive Blood Phenylketonuria Screening Test

With increased understanding of the heterogeneity of phenylalanine hydroxylase, it has become increasingly important to differentiate the various types of hyperphenylalaninemia. These are summarized below.

A. Classical: Persistent elevation of serum phenylalanine levels > 20 mg/100 ml. Continuing intolerance to phenylalanine and phenylketonuria after the first few weeks of life. Boys are more commonly affected than girls. Treatment is indicated.

B. Other Isozymic Variants: These cannot be accurately differentiated at the present time but have been reported to include (1) a "modified" form with serum phenylalanine levels in the 10–25 mg/100 ml range, occasionally needing phenylalanine restriction; (2) a "benign" form with serum levels of < 10 mg/100 ml, not needing treatment; and (3) an "occult" form where abnormal levels may not be present in the first few months of life but later reach 25–30 mg/100 ml with phenylketonuria; phenylalanine restriction is indicated depending on the level.

C. Hydroxylase Immaturity: Marked early rise in serum pheylalanine with serum levels of > 20 mg/100 ml but increasing tolerance with age. May show phenylketonuria in early life but not later. Treatment may involve some limitation of protein initially.

D. p-Hydroxyphenylpyruvic Acid Oxidase Deficiency: This is especially frequent in the premature and is the most common cause of neonatal hyperphenylalaninemia. Tyrosine levels are also elevated (see next section).

E. Other Causes and Types:

1. Prematurity.

2. Heterozygotes, mixed homozygotes (phenylketonuria/hyperphenylalaninemia), or maternal phenylketonuria.

3. Phenylalanine transaminase deficiency.

4. Postmalnutrition protein loading.

5. Oasthouse syndrome.

6. Phenylketonuria with cystathioninuria.

Differential Diagnosis

Established phenylketonuria in a severely retarded older child with typical biochemical and physical characteristics is a straightforward diagnosis. In the newborn period, especially when there is no family history, the condition must be differentiated from other forms of hyperphenylalaninemia. The low tyrosine level will distinguish transient p-hydroxyphenylpyruvic acid oxidase deficiency. The true phenylketonuric will show a rapid rise in serum phenylalanine to over 20 mg/100 ml, and only a sustained low-phenylalanine diet will lower it. The parents show a typical heterozygote response to a phenylalanine load. Phenylalanine intolerance remains unchanged with age but should be briefly confirmed at 6 and 12 months.

Prevention

Prevention consists of early detection in infancy so that treatment can be instituted before intellectual impairment occurs. Genetic counseling of phenylketonuric women is advised so that heterozygous offspring can be protected by dietary management if pregnancy occurs.

Treatment

Treatment is aimed at limiting the intake of the essential amino acid phenylalanine to facilitate normal growth and development without producing neurologic impairment. This is generally possible through the use of a milk substitute (Lofenalac) and natural foods. Since excessive restriction of phenylalanine may produce bone changes, anemia, and retardation of growth and development, it is essential to monitor the treatment closely through serial serum phenylalanine determinations as well as ascertainment of general health, growth, development, and nutritional intake. Such coordination of care is frequently best done at clinics where specialists in each of these areas are in attendance. Although dietary treatment is most effective when initiated during the first few months of life, it is sometimes beneficial in reversing maladaptive behavior such as hyperactivity and excessive lethargy when started later in life.

The diet is calculated to assure adequate protein, caloric, and fluid intake as well as other nutrients. Various methods of diet calculation have been described. The phenylalanine, protein, caloric, and fluid requirements are first established. The phenylalanine requirement approximates 60 mg/kg/24 hours at 9 years of age. One must determine the extent to which Lofenalac meets these requirements. Other foods such as milk, cereals, vegetables, and fruits are also given in measured amounts or exchanges (since most contain phenylalanine) to meet all of the child's nutritional requirements.

Since the first few months and years of life are the most critical, the treatment is closely monitored during this time. The mother records diet histories daily during the first 6 months, weekly for the next 6 months, and once a month thereafter. Blood tests for phenylalanine determinations are performed weekly during the first year and once a month thereafter. These should be maintained between 5–10 mg/100 ml. Clinic evaluations are performed once a month during the first year and less frequently thereafter. As the child grows, his dietary needs change; thus, the treatment and progress of the child must be closely monitored.

Prognosis

Children treated promptly after birth and properly managed in terms of phenylalanine and tyrosine homeostasis develop well physically and have a good but less than normal expectation for intellectual development.

In general, dietary restrictions can be eased after the fifth year—although opinion differs on this matter.

Auerbach V, DiGeorge AM, Carpenter GG: Phenylalaninemia. Page 11 in: *Amino Acid Metabolism and Genetic Variation.* Nyhan WL (editor). McGraw-Hill, 1967.

Bickel H, Hudson FP, Woolf LI: *Phenylketonuria and Some Other Inborn Errors of Amino Acid Metabolism.* Thieme Verlag, Stuttgart, 1971.

Frankenburg WK: *PKU Diet Manual.* Univ of Colorado Medical Center Press, 1971.

Frankenburg WK: Maternal phenylketonuric implications for growth and development. J Pediat 73:560, 1968.

Koch R & others: Conference on sex ratio in phenylketonuria. J Pediat 78:157, 1971.

O'Brien D: *Phenylketonuria: A Comprehensive Bibliography.* US Department of Health, Education, & Welfare, 1972.

TYROSINOSIS
(Tyrosinemia)

Until quite recently, tyrosinosis was considered to be a single exceedingly rare abnormality of metabolism. With the advent of widespread screening programs for phenylketonuria and of more limited screening programs in the newborn which appraise a number of serum amino acids, it has become apparent that transient tyrosinosis is a common aberration of amino acid metabolism in the newborn infant.

Studies have now defined more clearly the relationship of the various clinical forms of tyrosyluria.

In the normal pathway for tyrosine metabolism, tyrosine is transaminated to p-hydroxyphenylpyruvic acid (pHPPA) and thence, after further oxidation and breaking of the ring, to fumarate and acetoacetate. The syndromes listed below represent transient and permanent inhibitions or abnormalities of pHPPA oxidase activity. In consequence, there is always an increased urinary content not only of pHPPA but also of p-hydroxyphenyllactic acid (pHPLA) and p-hydroxyphenylacetic acid (pHPAA). The proportions of these phenolic acids vary in different patient groups.

Serum tyrosine levels exceed 15 mg/100 ml.

As is the case with hyperphenylalaninemia, there are variants of pHPPA oxidase deficiency which may relate both to rates of maturation of activity and to stearic variants of the enzyme. These may be listed as follows:

(1) Transient pHPPA oxidase deficiency in the newborn. This condition is accentuated by vitamin C deficiency and by a high protein intake. In breast-fed infants, the overall incidence of tyrosinosis (ie, serum levels > 5 mg/100 ml) is around 1.5%; in artificially fed infants, it may be as high as 5%. However, figures are much higher for the premature (30% or more). Recovery of pHPPA activity is abrupt and may take place at any time between a few days and 3 months. The prognosis is good.

(2) Transient pHPPA oxidase deficiency and heterozygosity for phenylketonuria. Some of these are full-term infants with a modest hyperphenylalaninemia and thus are detected on screening. Again, the ultimate prognosis appears to be good, although symptoms occasionally occur.

(3) There is a single report of a 4-month-old child with vomiting, diarrhea, failure to thrive, and convulsions. Because of a positive ferric chloride test, the child was treated with and improved on a low phenylalanine diet. Tyrosinosis was inferred later on the basis of a normal serum phenylalanine level and increased urinary phenolic acids.

(4) Fulminating "neonatal cirrhosis" with tyrosinosis and fructosuria. The outcome is usually fatal.

(5) A syndrome presenting in infancy and childhood characterized by cirrhosis of the liver, multiple renal tubular dystrophies, vitamin D resistant rickets, hypertyrosinemia, and tyrosyluria. These may respond well to a low tyrosine and phenylalanine intake, indicating a partial pHPPA deficiency.

(6) The original case of Medes in a 49-year-old man with myasthenia gravis.

(7) Tyrosine transaminase deficiency with multiple congenital malformations.

The transient conditions in the newborn will be detected either as evanescent high serum phenylalanine levels or as a result of screening with technics such as one-dimensional paper chromatography. Confirmation can be obtained by column chromatography or special fluorescent technics. Phenolic acids can be examined by paper or gas chromatography.

Treatment

At present there is only tentative evidence that transient pHPPA deficiency in the newborn leads to any neurologic impairment. However, there have been animal studies which show an effect of tyrosinosis on myelination. It seems reasonable, therefore, to use a low-protein formula until enzyme activity is restored and to ensure an adequate vitamin C supplement.

In the groups with liver damage, control with a low-phenylalanine and low-tyrosine diet (50 mg of each per kg/24 hours) now seems mandatory.

Conference on hereditary tyrosinemia. Canad MAJ 97: 1045–1100, 1967.

Rizzardini M, Abeliuk P: Tyrosinemia and tyrosinuria in low birth weight infants. Am J Dis Child 121:182, 1971.

MAPLE SYRUP URINE DISEASE
(Branched Chain Ketoaciduria)

Maple syrup urine disease is due to a failure of decarboxylation of branched chain keto acids. The defect is seen in both liver and white blood cells. Mild, intermittent, and thiamine-dependent forms are also seen. The exact cause of the characteristic odor of the urine is not known.

In the severe form, the patients are normal at birth but in a few days become lethargic and refuse feedings. They may become comatose and convulse, and many die in the first month of life, usually from an intercurrent pneumonitis. The maple syrup urine odor is usually noticed at the end of the first week. Neurologic damage occurs. In the mild form, there may be transient episodes with neurologic signs.

Laboratory findings consist of elevation of the branched chain amino acids leucine, isoleucine, and valine in the serum. Excess urinary keto acids give a positive ferric chloride test.

If the characteristic odor is not noticed, these children may be thought to have an infection or intracranial damage. Once considered, the diagnosis can be quickly made by paper chromatography and confirmed by column chromatography. In the mild form, the diagnosis between attacks can only be made by assaying the enzyme in the white blood cells. Other forms should be considered in children who are retarded or fail to thrive.

Dietary Management (Severe Form)

Treatment initially consists of a largely synthetic formula comprised of a vitamin:mineral mixture and a Dextri-Maltose:corn oil powder with added amino acids (Table 35–3). Some branched chain amino acids (eg, about 80 mg/kg/24 hours of leucine, 50 mg/kg/24 hours of isoleucine, and 60 mg/24 hours of valine), given either alone or in milk or gelatin, must be added to sustain growth. Achieving normal growth while avoiding toxic levels of branched chain amino acids requires constant supervision in a center with a well equipped laboratory. Leucine is the most critical amino acid to control, although it appears that levels up to 3 times the upper limit of normal are not harmful.

A 30-day supply of powdered formula (Table 35–3) is mixed on a roller mixer and stored in the refrigerator in a polyethylene container. Liquid formula is then made up as follows: 237 gm of powdered formula are mixed with 600 ml of boiling water in a blender and water added to a total volume of 1000 ml. This should be stored in the refrigerator in 3 separate clean glass bottles. Each day, 330 ml of the above mixture are added to 100–200 ml of 2% butterfat cow's milk and sufficient boiled water is added to give a total daily formula volume of around 100 ml/kg in the first month, 150–200 ml/kg in the second and third months, and 120 ml/kg thereafter. To the daily formula, 5 gm of gelatin and 5 gm of yeast should be added—or these may be given mixed with puréed vegetables or fruits beginning in the second or third month. The formula is distributed in bottles and given in the usual way.

TABLE 35–3. Diet in branched chain ketoaciduria.

Amino Acid Mixture	24-Hour Requirement (gm)	30-Day Supply (gm)
Alanine	0.7	21
Aspartic acid	1.6	48
Glutamic acid	4.5	135
Cystine	1	30
Histidine	0.7	21
Proline	1.6	48
Phenylalanine	1	30
Tyrosine	1	30
Serine	1.1	33
Threonine	1.1	33
Arginine	0.9	27
Lysine HCl	1.3	39
Tryptophan	0.4	12
Methionine	0.5	15
Glycine	0.6	18
Total amino acid mixture (Ajinomoto Co.)	18	540
Mineral: vitamin base Z598 (Mead Johnson)	0.13	3.9
Dextri-Maltose: corn oil base Z618 (Mead Johnson)	60.7	1820

The amount of gelatin and cow's milk added is varied in relation to the serum levels of the branched chain amino acids—leucine, isoleucine, and valine.

Exclusive of additional amounts provided by the cow's milk, this formula contains the following amounts of vitamins, with added calcium gluconate, monobasic potassium phosphate, dibasic potassium phosphate, calcium hydroxide, potassium chloride, magnesium oxide, and ferrous sulfate:

Vitamin A palmitate, 1570 USP units
Vitamin D (calciferol), 419 USP units
Vitamin E, 5 IU
Ascorbic acid, 31 mg
Thiamine hydrochloride, 0.48 mg
Riboflavin, 1.8 mg
Niacinamide, 4.2 mg
Pyridoxine hydrochloride, 0.52 mg
Calcium pantothenate, 3.3 mg
Vitamin B_{12}, 4.8 μg
Biotin, 0.03 mg
Choline chloride, 157 mg

The mild and intermittent forms are treated by protein restriction; the thiamine-dependent form with 10 mg thiamine daily orally.

Dancis J, Hutzler J, Rokhones T: Intermittent branched chain ketonuria. New England J Med 267:84–89, 1967.
Goodman SI & others: The treatment of maple syrup urine disease. J Pediat 74:485, 1969.
Schulman JD & others: A new variant of maple syrup urine disease. Am J Med 49:118, 1970.
Scriver CR & others: Thiamine responsive maple syrup urine disease. Lancet 1:310, 1971.

HOMOCYSTINURIA

Homocystinuria is a condition associated with a marked decrease in hepatic cystathionine synthetase activity. At present, there are few tangible links between the biochemical abnormality and the multiple clinical manifestations. There is evidence that homocystine can enhance platelet adhesiveness, causing the thromboembolic phenomena, and there also appears to be an intrinsic abnormality of the platelets corrected by vitamin B_6. Methionine can, like phenylalanine, impair myelination in animals, so that hypermethioninemia could account for the mental retardation. The rather eccentric incidence of retardation may relate to actual methionine levels in the early months of life. Certainly there is heterogeneity, notably in relation to vitamin B_6 responsiveness. Transient neonatal hypermethioninemia with uneventful recovery has also been reported. Homocystinuria has also been reported with methylmalonic aciduria in cases with abnormal vitamin B_{12} metabolism.

In the original descriptions, it was thought that the clinical pattern was highly distinctive, ie, all patients were thought to be mentally retarded. This has been shown not to be true, as a survey of homocystinuric persons with ectopia lentis attending eye clinics showed most to be normal intellectually. Ectopia lentis itself is certainly common, but was not seen in 3 Spanish-American patients. The hair is usually fine and friable but not necessarily fair. There are a variety of bony deformities, including kyphoscoliosis, pes planus, genu valgum, and pectus carinatum, which may lead to an abnormal gait. Vascular manifestations include a malar flush, livedo reticularis, and a tendency to thromboembolic phenomena, supposedly due to increased platelet adhesiveness.

Laboratory findings consist of high serum methionine levels and an increased urinary excretion of homocystine. The cyanide-nitroprusside test for homocystine in the urine is positive. In this test, 5 ml of fresh urine are mixed with 0.5 ml of 1 N hydrochloric acid to which is added 2 ml of fresh 5% sodium cyanide. With the addition of 1 ml of 0.5% sodium nitroprusside, a positive test is shown by a distinctive purple color.

The bone and eye changes may be confused with those of Marfan's syndrome. However, if the clinical picture is suggestive, biochemical confirmation is simple. Children with cystinuria also have a positive cyanide-nitroprusside test but do not have elevated methionine levels on paper or column chromatography.

Treatment

It is uncertain whether dietary treatment is necessary since it is unlikely to influence the physical changes caused by the disease. There is some evidence that affected children with retarded older siblings will develop normally on a low-methionine diet. The indications for treatment in infancy would thus include a retarded sibling or a thromboembolic episode at any age.

Serum methionine levels may be lowered in 50% of cases by large oral doses (500 mg/day) of pyridoxine; serum homocystine is also lowered, but more strikingly, in responsive cases. Low-methionine diets are successful and nutritionally satisfactory. In infancy, the diet should be based on a Sobee formula supplemented with 100 mg/cystine/kg/24 hours and with iron, calcium, and B complex vitamins. Exchange lists of puréed vegetables and fruits and other foods for the older patient are now available.

Prognosis

Normal intellectual development can be expected on a low-methionine diet, and the regimen is not hazardous nutritionally. In at least one case, lenticular dislocation has occurred despite dietary and pyridoxine treatment from birth.

Control observations are not yet available.

Barber GW, Spaeth GL: The successful treatment of homocystinuria with pyridoxine. J Pediat 75:463, 1969.
Chase HP, Goodman SI, O'Brien D: Treatment of homocystinuria. Arch Dis Child 42:514–520, 1967.

TABLE 35–4. Syndromes associated with inborn errors of metabolism.
I. Disorders of amino acid metabolism.

	Amino Acids or Organic Acids Increased in Plasma	Amino Acids or Organic Acids Increased in Urine	Biochemistry	Clinical Features & Treatment
Sulfur-containing Amino Acid				
Cystathioninuria	. . .	Cystathionine	Cystathionine cleavage enzyme deficiency; homoserine dehydratase deficiency.	Mental retardation; congenital malformations; talipes, deafness, abnormal ears and sensation. One case with high phenylalanine, one with thrombocytopenia and renal calculi. Treat with large doses of pyridoxine.
Homocystinuria	Methionine	Homocystine, homolanthionine	Cystathionine synthetase deficiency. 50% are pyridoxine dependent. May have folate deficiency.	Mental retardation, spastic paraplegia, occasional convulsions, cataracts, lenticular dislocation, friable hair, malar flush, thromboembolic disease, bone changes. Treat with low-methionine, cystine-supplemented diet or with pyridoxine.
Cystinuria	. . .	Cystine, lysine, arginine, ornithine	Transport abnormality in renal tubules and bowel mucosa.	Somatic and occasional mental retardation; renal calculi with their complications. Treat with penicillamine, high water intake, alkalies, and sometimes low-methionine diet. Renal transplantation in severe renal failure.
Methionine malabsorption syndrome	. . .	a-Hydroxybutyric acid (also in feces)	Methionine, leucine, isoleucine, and valine: rejected by bowel wall; may be same as oasthouse syndrome.	Convulsions, episodic diarrhea, hyperventilation, mental retardation; smell as in oasthouse syndrome.
β-Mercapto-lactate cysteine disulfiduria	. . .	β-Mercapto-lactate cysteine disulfide	Unknown.	Severe retardation; increased tone in lower limbs; persisting suck reflex.
Sulfite oxidase deficiency	. . .	S-Sulfo-cysteine; also sulfite and thiosulfate	Sulfite oxidase deficiency.	Spastic quadriplegia; blindness; subluxation of lenses.
Urea Synthesis Cycle				
Argininosuccinic-aciduria	. . .	Argininosuccinic acid, citrulline	Argininosuccinate lyase deficiency.	Mental retardation, ataxia, convulsions, friable hair, rough skin, coma (due to ammonia intoxication). Treat with low-protein diet.
Ornithine transcarbamylase deficiency	. . .	Generalized aminoaciduria	Ornithine carbamoyl transferase deficiency.	Episodes of vomiting, restlessness, ataxia, coma in early life (from ammonia intoxication). Treat with low-protein diet.
Citrullinuria	Citrulline, methionine	Citrulline, alanine, aspartic acid, glycine, glutamic acid, histidine, N-acetylcitrulline	Argininosuccinate synthetase deficiency.	Mental retardation; episodes of severe vomiting and coma (due to ammonia intoxication). Treat with low-protein diet.
Carbamyl phosphate synthetase deficiency	Glycine; also ammonia	Glycine	Carbamyl phosphate synthetase deficiency.	Severe vomiting, hypotonia, lethargy, and dehydration in infancy. Responds to low-protein intake.
Hyperornithinemia	Ornithine, lysine; ammonia	Homocitrulline	Unknown.	Irritable, failure to thrive, intention tremors and myoclonic seizures.
Tryptophan Metabolism				
Congenital tryptophanuria	Tryptophan after oral load	Tryptophan	Possible tryptophan oxygenase deficiency.	Mental retardation, photosensitivity, rough hyperpigmented skin, telangiectasias of conjunctivas. Treat with nicotinic acid.

TABLE 35–4 (cont'd). Syndromes associated with inborn errors of metabolism.
I. Disorders of amino acid metabolism.

	Amino Acids or Organic Acids Increased in Plasma	Amino Acids or Organic Acids Increased in Urine	Biochemistry	Clinical Features & Treatment
Hartnup disease	. . .	Alanine, serine, glutamine, valine, leucine, isoleucine, phenylalanine, tyrosine, tryptophan, histidine; basic amino acids low	Tryptophan rejection by bowel and renal tubular epithelium.	Mental retardation in some cases, pellagra-like skin rash, ataxia and other cerebellar signs. Treat with nicotinic acid and low-protein diet.
Indolylacroyl glycine excretion	. . .	Indolylacroyl glycine	Possible malabsorption defect.	Mental retardation.
Hyperserotoninemia	Serotonin	. . .	Unknown.	Flushing episodes, ataxia, seizures.
Kynureninase deficiency	. . .	Kynurenine, hydroxykynurenine; xanthurenic acid.	Kynureninase deficiency. May be B_6-dependent.	Infantile spasms. May respond rapidly or slowly to vitamin B_6.
Imino Acid Metabolism				
Hyperprolinemia Type A	Proline	Proline, hydroxyproline, glycine	Proline oxidase deficiency.	Familial nephritis, deafness, renal hypoplasia, epilepsy, abnormal EEG.
Type B	Proline	Not recorded	Δ'-Pyrroline-5-carboxylic acid dehydrogenase.	Convulsions, coma, mental retardation.
Hydroxyprolinemia	Hydroxyproline	Hydroxyproline, 1-methylhistidine	Hydroxyproline oxidase deficiency.	Mental retardation, moderate hematuria and pyuria.
Joseph's syndrome	. . .	Proline, hydroxyproline, iminodipeptiduria		Convulsions, raised CSF protein, mental retardation.
Iminopeptiduria	. . .	Imino-C-terminal peptides	Unknown.	Mental retardation, splenomegaly; exophthalmos, unusual facies.
Histidine Metabolism				
Histidinemia	Histidine	Histidine, alanine, threonine	Histidine ammonia lyase.	Slurred, inarticulate speech. Variable incidence of mental retardation. Low-histidine diet has been reported; results questionable.
Formiminoglutamic-aciduria Type A	. . .	FIGLU after histidine load	Formiminotransferase deficiency.	Somatic and intellectual retardation, round face, obesity, hypersegmentation of polymorphonuclear leukocytes.
Type B	. . .	FIGLU before and after histidine load	(?) Folic acid transport defect.	Ataxia, megaloblastic anemia, mental retardation, convulsions.
Imidazole aminoaciduria in amaurotic idiocy	. . .	Anserine, carnosine; also histidine and 1-methylhistidine	Unknown.	Retardation, obesity, inactive, blind; later, increased muscle tone and decerebrate state.
Cyclohydrolase deficiency	Folic acid	No excess FIGLU	Cyclohydrolase.	Microcephaly, optic atrophy, hypsarythmia.
Carnosinemia	Carnosine	Carnosine	Carnosinase.	Grand mal seizures, myoclonic epilepsy.
Phenylalanine and Tyrosine Metabolism				
Phenylketonuria	Phenylalanine	Phenylalanine, *o*-hydroxyphenylacetic acid. Phenylpyruvic acid	Phenylalanine hydroxylase deficiency.	Usually (but not always) severe mental retardation. Convulsions, eczema, fair hair and complexion. Treat with low-phenylalanine diet.
Hyperphenylalaninemia	Phenylalanine	. . .	Not precisely known; phenylalanine transaminase in some cases.	May be normal; depends on type. Treat if level of serum phenylalanine > 20 mg/100 ml.

TABLE 35–4 (cont'd). Syndromes associated with inborn errors of metabolism.
I. Disorders of amino acid metabolism.

	Amino Acids or Organic Acids Increased in Plasma	Amino Acids or Organic Acids Increased in Urine	Biochemistry	Clinical Features & Treatment
Tyrosinosis (several clinical types)	Phenylalanine, tyrosine	Normal for age	Transient p-hydroxy-phenylpyruvic acid oxidase deficiency.	General failure to thrive, convulsions. Temporarily responds to low-phenylalanine diet.
Oasthouse syndrome	Not reported	Phenylalanine, methionine, tyrosine, (?) leucine and isoleucine, a-hydroxybutyric acid	Unknown.	Infantile spasms with interim flaccidity and unresponsiveness, sparse hair, retardation, general unawareness.
Branched Chain Amino Acid Metabolism				
Branched chain ketoaciduria	Isoleucine, valine, leucine, allo-isoleucine	Leucine, isoleucine, valine	Branched chain keto acid decarboxylase. Partial and intermittent forms described.	Neonatal difficulty in feeding, anorexia, convulsions, and other CNS signs. Mild, intermittent, and thiamine-dependent forms are seen.
Hypervalinemia	Valine	Valine	Not identified.	Failure to thrive, vomiting, nystagmus.
Isovaleric acidemia	Isovaleric acid, especially after valine load	Isovaleric acid, isovalerylglycine	Isovaleric dehydrogenase.	Mental and motor retardation. Smell of sweat in skin and urine.
Hydroxylysinuria	Hydroxylysine (slight increase)	Hydroxylysine and N-acetyl hydroxylysine increased	Defect in breakdown of hydroxylysine.	Mental and physical retardation.
β-Hydroxy-isovaleric acidemia	No abnormality detected	β-Hydroxy-isovaleric acid, β-methylcrotonyl-glycine	β-Methylcrotonyl carboxylase deficiency	Progressive hypotonia and muscular atrophy. Possibility a biotin dependency.
Methylhydroxy-butyric aciduria	. . .	a-Methyl-β-hydroxybutyric acid, a-methyl-acetoacetate	β-Hydroxy acyl dehydrogenase	Intermittment severe metabolic acidosis, macrocephaly, retardation.
Methylmalonic aciduria	Methylmalonic acid	Glycine, lysine, methylmalonic acid	Methylmalonyl-Co A isomerase. May also be error in B_{12} metabolism.	Acute episodes of vomiting and acidosis. Failure to thrive. B_{12} therapy should be attempted (500 μg daily IM initially).
Propionyl-Co A carboxylase deficiency				
Type A	Propionic acid	Propionic acid	Propionyl-Co A carboxylase.	Neonatal severe acidosis.
Type B	Glycine ++; also serine, alanine, glutamic acid	Glycine	Propionyl-Co A carboxylase.	Neonatal vomiting, ketosis, neutropenia, thrombocytopenia, osteoporosis.
Dibasic Amino Acid Metabolism				
Argininuria	. . .	Arginine	Unknown.	Convulsions, hepatomegaly, dry brittle hair.
Hyperlysinemia	Lysine; also ammonia	Lysine, N-acetyl lysine, homoarginine	Lysine acylase, lysine dehydrogenase, or lysine ketoglutarate reductase.	Convulsions and coma related to protein feeding.
Saccharopinuria	Lysine	Saccharopine, lysine, histidine, homocitrulline	Saccharopine cleavage enzyme.	Short stature, retardation.
Hyperdibasic aminoaciduria	Lysine, arginine, ornithine, homocitrulline	Dibasics are normal or low	Renal and enteric transport defect.	Mental and physical retardation, failure to thrive.

TABLE 35–4 (cont'd). Syndromes associated with inborn errors of metabolism.
I. Disorders of amino acid metabolism.

	Amino Acids or Organic Acids Increased in Plasma	Amino Acids or Organic Acids Increased in Urine	Biochemistry	Clinical Features & Treatment
Miscellaneous				
Aspartylglucos-aminuria	...	Aspartylglucos-amine	Unknown.	Coarse facies, retardation.
Hyperglycinemia	Glycine, serine, alanine, glutamic acid	Glycine, valine, leucine; taurine, serine may be low	Glycine-formyl FH_4 transferase deficiency.	Episodes of vomiting with severe dehydration, acidosis, ketosis, repeated infection, somatic and mental retardation.
Glutamicaciduria	Glutamic acid	Slight generalized increase in total amino nitrogen	Unknown.	Sparse, coarse, unpigmented hair, mental retardation, failure to thrive, other congenital malformations.
Raised CSF glutamic acid	Proline; also, perhaps, glutamic acid, leucine	Slight generalized increase in total amino nitrogen	Unknown.	Hypertonia, hyperreflexia, failure to thrive, mental retardation.
Sarcosinemia	Sarcosine (methyl-glycine)	Sarcosine (methyl-glycine)	Sarcosine oxidase deficiency.	Hypotonia; sometimes mental and physical retardation. Limb muscle contractures also reported.
Hyperalaninemia Type A	Alanine, lactic acid, pyruvic acid	Alanine, pyruvate, lactate	Pyruvate decarboxylase.	Severe acidosis, development retardation, ataxic convulsions. Treat with thiamine, 5 mg IM daily.
Type B	...	...	Pyruvate carboxylase	Mental retardation.
β-Aminoisobutyric aciduria	...	BAIB	Physiologic variant.	None.
β-Alaninemia	β-Alanine	β-Alanine, BAIB, taurine, GABA	Possibly β-alanine a-ketoglutarate transaminase.	Lethargy, somnolence, hypotonia, hyporeflexis, grand mal seizures.
Infantile keto-acidosis	Ketones	Lysine, glycine, phenylalanine, ketones	Muscle pyruvate kinase.	Severe ketosis with protein feeding.
Glutathionuria	Glutathione	Glutathione	Serum γ-glutamyl transpeptidase deficiency.	Moderate mental retardation.

Goodman SI & others: Homocystinuria with methylmalonic aciduria. Biochem Med 4:500, 1970.

Shih VE, Efron ML: Pyridoxine unresponsive homocystinuria. New England J Med 283:1206, 1970.

THE HYPERAMMONEMIAS & RELATED SYNDROMES

This is a group of diseases which involve the several enzymatic steps in the Krebs-Henseleit urea cycle and in lysine breakdown. They usually present in infancy with episodes of vomiting and neurologic signs, including coma. If untreated, the mortality rate is high and retardation is a common sequel. Hyperammonemia is usual, but individual enzyme assays are required for a specific diagnosis. They are important to recognize because affected patients respond well on a protein intake of < 1 gm/kg/24 hours. Argininosuccinic aciduria may later be associated with dry, friable hair, and both this condition and citrullinemia have been observed in otherwise normal persons.

Carton D & others: Argininosuccinic aciduria. Acta paediat scandinav 58:528, 1969.

Corbeel LM & others: Periodic attacks of lethargy in a baby with ammonia intoxication. Arch Dis Child 44:681, 1969.

Dancis J & others: Familial hyperlysinemia. J Clin Invest 48:1447, 1969.

Hommes FA & others: Carbamylphosphate synthetase deficiency. Arch Dis Child 44:688, 1969.

Morrow G & others: Citrullinuria with defective urea production. Pediatrics 40:465, 1967.

O'Brien D, Goodman SI: The critically ill child: Acute metabolic disease. Pediatrics 46:620, 1970.

TABLE 35–5. Syndromes associated with inborn errors of metabolism.
II. Lysosomal disorders of carbohydrate metabolism. (See also Table 37–8.)

Disease	Biochemistry	Enzyme Defect	Clinical Features
Hurler's (type 1)	Chondroitin sulfate B and heparitin sulfate in urine.	β-Galactosidase	Clouding of corneas; skeletal changes, hepatosplenomegaly.
Hunter's (type 2)	Chondroitin sulfate B and heparitin sulfate in urine.	β-Galactosidase	As above, without corneal clouding; milder course.
Sanfilippo (type 3)	Heparitin sulfate elevated in the urine.	β-Galactosidase	Minimal somatic changes; severe retardation.
Morquio's (type 4a)	Keratosulfate elevated in urine.	Not yet identified	Severe bone changes; may be retarded; corneas cloudy; aortic regurgitation.
Morquio-Ullrich (type 4b)	Keratosulfate and chondroitin sulfate B in urine.	Not yet identified	Bone changes, retardation, deafness.
Scheie's (type 5)	Chondroitin sulfate B elevated in urine.	Not yet identified	Stiff joints, coarse facies, cloudy corneas; may be retarded.
Generalized gangliosidoses	Accumulation in brain, liver, spleen, kidney, histiocytes of GM_1 ganglioside and galactose mucopolysaccharides.	β-Galactosidase	Progressive cerebral degeneration, bone changes.
Xylosidase deficiency	β-Xylosidase activity in cultured lymphocytes < 10% of normal. β-Galactosidase normal.	β-Xylosidase	Seizures, choreo-athetosis, episodes of vomiting, cortical atrophy, hypsarhythmia.
Farber's	Acid mucopolysaccharide excess in brain, liver, and spleen.	a-Mannosidase	Progressive neurologic disease, retardation, spasticity.
Fucosidosis	Accumulation of fucose containing ceramide, free and in vacuoles in liver cells.	a-Fucosidase	Progressive spasticity and mental retardation.
I-Cell disease		Multiple lysosomal enzyme defect	Similar to Hurler's disease.
β-Glucuronidase deficiency	Chondroitin sulfate A in urine.	β-Glucuronidase	Similar to Hurler's disease. No retardation.

TABLE 35–6. Syndromes associated with inborn errors of metabolism.
III. Miscellaneous.

Disease	Biochemistry	Enzyme Defect	Clinical Features
Hyperuricemia	Hyperuricemia, hyperuricuria. Basic defect is lack of intracellular nucleotides.	Hypoxanthine: guanine phosphoribosyl transferase	Cerebral palsy, choreo-athetosis, lip and nail biting. Treat with allopurinol and glutamate.
Methemoglobinemia	Methemoglobinemia.	Diaphorase	Cyanosis; cerebellar, pyramidal, and speech disorders. Give ascorbic acid, up to 500 mg daily orally.
Stale fish syndrome	Trimethycaminuria.	TMA oxidase	Similar to Turner's syndrome. Abnormalities in white blood cells.
Hypercalcemia	Probably an inborn error of sterol metabolism with excess production of vitamin D-like compounds.	Unknown	Unusual facies, renal failure, subaortic stenosis. Treat with corticosteroids.
Hyperoxaluria	Type 1, glycolic aciduria; type 2, L-glyceric aciduria.	Type 1, 2-oxoglutarate glyoxylate carboligase; type 2, D-glycerate dehydrogenase	Renal calculi and renal failure. Treat with calcium carbimide orally, 1 mg/kg/day; pyridoxine, 100 mg daily orally; and magnesium oxide, 10 mg/kg daily orally.
Goitrous cretinism	Defect in iodination of tyrosyl residues.	. . .	Congenital, familial, recessive condition with thyroid enlargement and hypothyroidism.
Acid phosphatase deficiency	. . .	Acid phosphatase	Early progressive neurologic signs, lethargy, and vomiting.
Lactic acidosis	Serum lactate elevated.	Not known	Hypotonia, convulsions, mental retardation.

LESCH-NYHAN SYNDROME

In this syndrome, patients are severely retarded and show choreoathetosis, limb spasticity, and compulsive lip and finger biting. The condition is thought to be the consequence of a deficiency of hypoxanthine/guanine phosphoribosyl transferase deficiency. This enzyme catalyzes the product of purine nucleotides from hypoxanthine and guanine. The deficiency results in uric acidemia and uricosuria: It is inherited as an X-linked recessive. Antenatal detection is possible on amniotic cells.

Allopurinol (Zyloprim), 8 mg/kg/24 hours, reduces uric acid formation; probenecid (Benemid), 80 mg/kg/24 hours, enhances excretion. Neither drug affects the neurologic changes in a major way. Adenine, 10 mg/kg/24 hours, orotic acid, and uracil are ineffective; but glutamine, 400 mg/kg/24 hours may be useful. Antipruritic drugs may be as helpful as anything.

Boyle JA & others: Lesch-Nyhan syndrome: Preventive control by prenatal diagnosis. Science 169:688, 1970.
Ghadimi H & others: The significance of the deficiency state in Lesch-Nyhan disease. Acta paediat scandinav 59:223, 1970.
Partington MW: The Lesch-Nyhan syndrome. Develop Med Child Neurol 9:563, 1967.

THE STORAGE LIPIDOSES

The storage lipidoses are rare conditions which have been recognized clinically for many years but have become of greater interest now that modern technics in lipid analyses have uncovered the basic biochemical defects. They are now classified as lysosomal disorders.

Desnick RJ & others: Diagnosis of glycosphingo-lipidoses by urinary sediment analysis. New England J Med 284:739, 1971.
O'Brien JS: Ganglioside storage diseases. New England J Med 284:893, 1971.

GAUCHER'S DISEASE

This condition may occur in an acute infantile or chronic adult form. The former is characterized by hepatosplenomegaly and by progressive bulbar signs which lead to death in the first year of life. In the latter, there is splenic and hepatic enlargement as well as involvement of the bone marrow, with anemia, frac-

tures, and joint swelling. Excess intracellular glucocerebroside is found primarily in the liver, spleen, and bone marrow. In the infantile form, large multinucleate macrophages with characteristically wrinkled cytoplasm are a more prominent finding. These reflect the excessive intracellular accumulation of glucocerebrosides, which was recently shown to be due to a defect in glucocerebroside cleaving enzyme. Fibroblasts and leukocytes can be used to identify heterozygotes.

Chang-ho M: Gaucher's disease. Am J Med Sc 254:303, 1967.
Drukker A & others: The infantile form of Gaucher's disease. Pediatrics 45:1017, 1970.

METACHROMATIC LEUKODYSTROPHY

This is a relatively common form of the demyelinating leukodystrophies. The onset is in childhood, with ataxia, dementia, disturbances of gait, and, later, grand mal seizures and pyramidal signs. The duration of the disease is 3–4 years. There is some evidence now that arylsulfatase A activity is low in brain, liver, and kidney tissue in children with metachromatic leukodystrophy. This is the enzyme that splits the sulfate radical from galactocerebroside. The diagnosis can be made by finding a diminished urinary sulfatase and increased urinary sulfatide. High urinary sulfatide levels may also be found in certain other progressive and nonprogressive neurologic disorders, as well as in the first months of life. Both low sulfatase and high sulfatide levels in the urine can be used in diagnosis.

Austin J & others: Metachromatic forms of diffuse cerebral sclerosis. Arch Neurol 14:259–269, 1966.

TAY-SACHS DISEASE

This disease is primarily an affliction of Ashkenazi Jews. It characteristically begins in infancy at around 6 months of age. Progressive loss of vision occurs, along with regression of motor development. In the ensuing months, the child becomes progressively more listless and hypotonic and totally blind. Optic atrophy is seen and, characteristically, a cherry-red spot at the macula. In the final stages, the child becomes decerebrate, spastic, and hyperreflexic.

The brain at autopsy is small and characteristically firm. There is a considerable deposition of lipid within the neurons.

Clinical findings in **Sandhoff's disease** are essentially the same. Here the enzyme defect also leads to some accumulation of visceral globoside. In juvenile GM$_2$ gangliosidosis, there is a progressive neurologic disorder starting usually at age 1–2 years but even as late as 5 years. A cherry-red spot is not always seen.

Brady RO: Tay-Sachs disease. New England J Med 281:1243, 1969.

O'Brien JS: Five gangliosidoses. Lancet 2:805, 1969.

O'Brien JS: Juvenile GM$_2$ gangliosidosis. J Pediat 77:1063, 1970.

NIEMANN-PICK DISEASE

The clinical picture in Niemann-Pick disease is extremely variable, both in the time and rate of onset as well as in the proportionate involvement of liver, spleen, and bone marrow vis-à-vis the CNS. Splenomegaly is common, and hepatomegaly to a lesser extent. Foam cells are present in the bone marrow. CNS involvement may include motor signs, a progressive paresis and dementia, macular degeneration, and blindness.

The lipid deposits are sphingomyelin, and it has now been shown that there is a defect in sphingomyelin cleavage enzyme although this has not yet been precisely defined.

Kamoshita S & others: Infantile Niemann-Pick disease. Am J Dis Child 117:379, 1969.

Reticuloendotheliosis: Niemann-Pick disease. J Pediat 72:291, 1968.

FABRY'S DISEASE

Fabry's disease is a condition where there is abnormal lipid storage in the ganglion cells, spleen, adrenals, lymph nodes, and striated musculature.

Characteristically, it starts at around 6 years of age, with fever, pains in the limbs, joints, and abdomen, paresthesias and corneal opacities. The classical skin lesions occur on and around the buttocks as red to purple macules 0.1–3 mm in diameter. Proteinuria and hematuria are present and may progress to chronic renal failure.

Skin lesions are not always present. The abnormal stored lipid is now known to be digalacto-gluco-ceramide (Gal-Gal-Glu-Cer). The derivation of the lipid is unknown, but it may well represent an accumulation of a normal degradation product of the GM$_2$ ganglioside.

Clark JTR & others: Ceramide trihexosidosis (Fabry's disease) without skin lesions. New England J Med 284:233–235, 1971.

REFSUM'S DISEASE

This is a rare autosomal recessive disorder characterized by peripheral neuritis with motor and sensory involvement, retinitis pigmentosa, ataxia, deafness, visual field restriction, cerebellar ataxia, and ichthyotic skin lesions.

There is a defect in the oxidation of exogenous phytanic acid (3,7,11,15-tetramethylhexadecenoic acid), which accumulates in the blood and tissues. Dietary restriction of phytanic acid is helpful.

Steinberg D & others: Studies on the metabolic error in Refsum's disease. J Clin Invest 46:313–322, 1967.

Steinberg D & others: Phytanic acid in patients with Refsum's syndrome and response to dietary treatment. Arch Int Med 125:75, 1970.

WOLMAN'S DISEASE

This uncommon condition is characterized by failure to thrive, vomiting, diarrhea, organomegaly, and adrenal calcification. There is visceral accumulation of triglycerides due to acid lipase and acid esterase deficiency.

Young EP: Wolman's disease. Arch Dis Child 45:664, 1970.

.   .   .

DISORDERS OF THE PLASMA LIPOPROTEINS

The intravascular transport of lipids is mediated via 2 protein-binding systems: one for free fatty acids and one involving lipoproteins. Free or unesterified fatty acids are the main currency of energy in the body during the postabsorptive state. They circulate as an albumin-fatty acid complex and are derived in part from enteric absorption of fatty acids with less than 12 carbons, but mainly from the triglyceride stores from which they are released by a series of complex homeostatic mechanisms. Primary disorders of this system (eg, green acyl dehydrogenase deficiency) are very rare and are not further discussed in this section.

Other lipids—primarily glycerides but also phospholipids, cholesterol, and the fat-soluble vitamins—are transported in the plasma in lipoprotein complexes. There are 4 main subdivisions of these lipoproteins characterized by their basic apoprotein, electrophoretic mobility, density, molecular size, and composition as shown in Table 35–7.

Exogenous glycerides are derived from the intestine. Ingested triglyceride is broken down by pan-

TABLE 35-7. Percentage composition of plasma lipoproteins.*

	Apoprotein	Protein	Cholesterol	Phospholipid	Glyceride	Electro-phoresis
Chylomicrons (exogenous glyceride)	A,B	1	4	5	90	chylo
Low density or beta lipoproteins	B	25	40	25	10	β
Very low density or prebeta lipoproteins (endogenous glyceride)	B	5	20	20	55	pre β
High density or alpha lipoproteins	A	50	20	25	5	α

*For normal values, see Chapter 40.

creatic lipase to micelles of monoglyceride and fatty acid. The short chain fatty acids move directly across the mucosal cell to the portal vein. The longer chain fatty acids and monoglycerides also enter the mucosal cell, where hydrolysis is completed and where triglycerides are resynthesized. The latter pass into the blood stream via the thoracic duct and are carried as chylomicrons to adipose tissue, liver, heart, and other organs, where they are immediately hydrolyzed as they enter the cells. In fasting plasma, the glyceride content is derived primarily from the liver.

Transport of cholesterol within the body is quantitatively much less than free fatty acids or glycerol. Exogenous cholesterol moves to the liver in the chylomicrons. From then on, transport of endogenous and exogenous cholesterol is on the alpha or beta lipoproteins. The phospholipids—mainly phosphatidyl choline and sphingomyelin—are also carried on the alpha and beta lipoproteins. Their biologic role is unclear but they are believed to stabilize the lipoprotein:plasma water interface.

The protein components of the alpha and beta lipoproteins are called A and B proteins. They are important in relation to conditions where there is an inborn deficiency of these proteins.

THE LIPOPROTEIN DEFICIENCY SYNDROMES

Familial Alpha Lipoprotein Deficiency (Tangier Disease)

This rare inherited condition was first identified in a kindred from Tangier Island in Chesapeake Bay. The most characteristic clinical features are the large lobulated tonsils with their red, orange, or yellowish banding. Hepatosplenomegaly and lymphadenopathy are common. Neurologic complications, including loss of pain and temperature sensation and peripheral neuropathy, are reported.

Plasma cholesterol levels are abnormally low, and alpha and prebeta lipoprotein bands are about 8% of normal on electrophoresis; levels in the parents are about 50% of normal. Serum triglycerides are normal or modestly elevated. The diagnosis can be confirmed by finding typical foam cells in the bone marrow or rectal mucosa. The appearance of the tonsils, together with hypo-alphaproteinemia, is unique except for LCAT deficiency (see below).

Tonsillectomy may be required because of their size. Treatment is not otherwise indicated, although, in time, CNS complications may constitute a significant handicap.

Koler RS & others: Familial α-lipoprotein deficiency (Tangier disease) with neurological abnormalities. Lancet 1:1341, 1967.

Lecithin: Cholesterol Acyltransferase (LCAT) Deficiency

LCAT deficiency is a rare inborn error of metabolism characterized by hypertriglyceridemia and hypercholesterolemia with lipid deposits in the corneas, proteinuria, and normochromic anemias. There is an almost complete absence of the normal alpha and prebeta lipoprotein bands on electrophoresis.

Serum phospholipids (especially lecithin) are increased to a greater extent than cholesterol. Only 3–4% of cholesterol is esterified; this is due to the absence of the enzyme transferring the acyl group from lecithin to cholesterol to form lysolecithin.

Norum VR & others: Familial plasma lecithin:cholesterol acyl transferase deficiency. Acta med scandinav 188:323, 1970.

Abetalipoproteinemia

This rare autosomal recessive condition is manifested in early infancy with failure to thrive and steatorrhea. Later in life, neurologic deficits include weakness, nystagmus, and posterior column, pyramidal tract, and cerebellar signs. Retinitis pigmentosa is also described.

Cholesterol and phospholipid levels are all extremely low, and chylomicrons are not formed after fat ingestion. Fasting glyceride levels are also abnormally low. Lipoprotein electrophoresis shows no chylomicron band and no beta or prebeta bands. Characteristically, the red blood cells demonstrate acanthocytosis.

Low cholesterol levels with steatorrhea are also found in celiac disease but without acanthocytosis, neurologic findings, or the typical lipoprotein pattern. In cystic fibrosis, there are respiratory symptoms and an elevated sweat chloride. In IgA deficiency, the immunoglobulin change can be measured.

The patient should be given a low-fat diet, but medium chain triglycerides are helpful as an additional source of calories. Supplements of water-soluble vitamin A (5000 IU/day) and vitamin D (500 IU/day) should be given.

Neurologic complications shorten normal life expectancy.

Fredrickson DS: Disorders of lipid metabolism. Page 979 in: *The Biologic Basis of Pediatric Practice.* Cooke RE (editor). McGraw-Hill, 1968.
Gotto AM & others: On the protein defect in abetalipoproteinemia. New England J Med 284:813, 1971.

Hypobetalipoproteinemia

A small number of patients have been reported with reduction of serum beta lipoprotein concentrations to 10–50% of normal with decreased serum levels of cholesterol, phospholipids, and glycerides. Acanthocytosis and neurologic symptoms may be seen. The condition must be differentiated from hypobetalipoproteinemias secondary to the celiac syndrome or the thalassemia trait.

A syndrome has also been described with low α- and β-lipoprotein, raised cholesterol and triglycerides, retardation, and hepatomegaly.

Van Buchem FS & others: Congenital β-lipoprotein deficiency. Am J Med 40:794, 1966.

THE FAMILIAL HYPERLIPOPROTEINEMIAS

The hyperlipoproteinemias can be characterized either in general etiologic terms or by physical characteristics. The primary lipoproteinemias are a group of heritable disorders of serum lipoprotein components; the secondary hyperlipoproteinemias are a reflection of a number of disorders such as nephrosis, hypothyroidism, and obstructive liver disease. Whether primary or secondary, the hyperlipoproteinemias can also be defined by certain biochemical parameters, the most important of which are serum total lipids, serum cholesterol, serum phospholipid, and the lipoprotein electrophoresis pattern.

Dietschy JM, Wilson JD: Regulation of cholesterol metabolism. New England J Med 282:1128, 1179, 1241, 1970.
Fredrickson DS, Levy RI, Lees RS: Fat transport in lipoproteins: An integrated approach to mechanisms and disorders. New England J Med 276:34, 94, 148, 215, 273, 1967.

Type I. Familial Hyperchylomicronemia (Lipoprotein Lipase Deficiency)

The onset is usually early in life, with bouts of abdominal pain. Later, moderate hepatosplenomegaly is noted and the retinal vessels are seen to be especially pale. Small cutaneous xanthomas are common.

The serum is characteristically lactescent, and on standing the chylomicrons rise to the top as a creamy layer on the plasma. Serum protein electrophoresis shows a great increase in the chylomicron band and a decrease in the alpha and beta bands. Postheparin lipoprotein lipase activity is reduced from the normal range of 240–600 nEq/ml of free fatty acids to 20–40 nEq/ml. The test is carried out following administration of 0.1 mg/kg of heparin IV by taking 15-minute samples from 0–90 minutes for lipoprotein lipase activity determination. Activity is maximal at 15 minutes.

Hyperglycemia and glycosuria have been reported but are not common (as in type IV; see below).

Hyperchylomicronemia quickly resolves on a low-fat diet (< 0.2 gm/kg/day). The alpha and beta lipoprotein bands will increase somewhat and the prebeta band which carries endogenous triglyceride will increase further. Caloric intake can be supplemented on a low-triglyceride diet (< 0.5 gm/kg/day) by giving medium chain triglycerides, either as a milk formula (Portagen) or as a special diet using MCT oil.

Episodes of abdominal pain, which may be accompanied by pancreatitis, can be controlled on this regimen, and so can the hepatosplenomegaly. Recent evidence is that there is no increased risk of atherosclerosis. The diagnosis is consistent with a normal life.

Ford S & others: Familial hyperchylomicronemia. Am J Med 50:536, 1971.
Schotz MC & others: A rapid assay for lipoprotein lipase. J Lipid Research 11:68, 1970.

Type II. Familial Hyperbetalipoproteinemia; Essential Familial Hypercholesterolemia

Familial hyperbetalipoproteinemia is the commonest lipoprotein disorder of childhood and is inherited as an autosomal dominant. Thus, evidence of hypercholesterolemia in at least one parent is essential to the diagnosis. The most striking clinical manifestations are the xanthomatous deposits which occur in tendons (particularly the Achilles tendon), over the extensor surfaces of the knees, hands, and elbows, and in pressure or trauma areas such as the buttocks. Xanthomas of the eyelids (xanthelasma) and corneal arcus are also common. Coronary atherosclerosis may be an early and life-threatening complication.

Hypercholesterolemia is striking; it has been reported elevated in cord blood, and levels over 500 mg/100 ml have been seen at 3 months of age. As with the appearance of xanthomas, the age at which hypercholesterolemia develops varies considerably, the more fulminating cases being seen in association with inheritance of the gene from both parents. Total cholesterol levels in childhood vary with age, but any level > 240 mg/100 ml should be considered abnormal. Serum phospholipid is moderately elevated but not to the same extent as cholesterol, and in some cases there may be a modest elevation of endogenous prebeta glycerides. Lipoprotein electrophoresis shows a characteristic intense increase in the beta band, with lipoprotein cholesterol exceeding 210 mg/100 ml. Hypercarotenemia is also seen due to the increased beta lipoprotein.

Hyperbetalipoproteinemia is reported in hypothyroidism, in obstructive liver disease, and in nephrosis. Florid xanthomatosis is, however, very rare in children with these conditions, and the differential diagnosis in the light of other evidence of thyroid, liver, or renal disease is easy to make. Type III hyperbetalipoproteinemia is an autosomal recessive condition which has not been described in childhood; in late adolescence, it would be distinguished by the small papular xanthomas on palm creases and fingertips, the tuberoeruptive lesions at the elbows, and, in the laboratory, by the opalescent serum with increased cholesterol and glyceride. Lipoprotein electrophoresis shows an intense conjoined broad beta and prebeta band.

Treatment of this condition in children is discouraging. However, because of the high risk of advancing coronary atherosclerosis, the following approaches should be tried:

A. Dietary Management: With the overall proviso that the diet should be palatable and contain adequate protein and calories, it is justifiable to limit the fat intake to 20% of calories, depending primarily on vegetable or polyunsaturated fats. Egg yolks and lean meat should be restricted. Obesity, if present, should be controlled, recognizing the difficulties of accomplishing this in young persons.

B. Drug Therapy:

1. Cholestyramine (Cuemid, Questran) is a resin which bonds bile acids, prevents their reabsorption, and, in turn, enhances the hepatic conversion of cholesterol to more bile acids. The dose is 0.7 gm/kg/day orally, but the drug is unpleasant to take and may cause steatorrhea. In some cases, the effect is to remove feedback inhibition of endogenous cholesterol synthesis, and levels rise.

2. D-Thyroxine (Choloxin) in a dose of 0.15 mg/kg/day orally sometimes lowers cholesterol levels.

3. Clofibrate (Atromid-S) inhibits the synthesis of mevalonic acid from acetate in the cholesterol synthesis pathway. The initial dose is 1 gm/sq m/24 hours orally in 3 or 4 divided doses; it may be justified to increase this to the limit of tolerance. Complications include leukopenia, mild hepatic damage, polyphagia, weakness, and muscle cramps. The drug is variably effective in type II disease in children.

4. Aminosalicylic acid (PAS), 0.2 gm/kg/day orally, has been reported to cause a modest lowering of cholesterol levels.

5. Nicotinic acid, 0.15 mg/kg/day orally, may lower cholesterol levels. The mechanism is not understood.

Type IV. Familial Hyperprebetalipoproteinemia

This is a common form of hyperlipoproteinemia in adults but is rare in childhood. It is characterized by turbid plasma and an increase in endogenous glyceride with a marked increase in the prebeta band on serum lipoprotein electrophoresis and a decrease in the alpha and beta bands. There are no chylomicrons on a low-fat diet. Hyperuricemia is common, and in most cases the lipemia is carbohydrate induced. The condition may be secondary to diabetes, type I glycogen storage disease, idiopathic hypercalcemia, hypoparathyroidism, and nephrosis.

Treatment consists of providing 40% of calories as fat, primarily polyunsaturated, and restricting carbohydrate sufficiently to reduce endogenous hyperlipemia. Nicotinic acid and clofibrate (Atromid-S) may also be helpful (see under type II, above).

Type V. Familial Hyperprebetalipoproteinemia With Hyperchylomicronemia

This condition is usually not seen until adult life, but it has been reported in the late teens. Clinically, patients tend to be obese and to have a family history of diabetes. There are widespread xanthomas with lipemia retinalis, hepatosplenomegaly, and foam cells in the bone marrow. On lipoprotein electrophoresis, there is an increase in both endogenous and exogenous glyceride, with cholesterol levels also elevated. Lipoprotein lipase activity is normal.

Treatment consists of reducing weight by caloric restriction. Clofibrate (Atromid-S) and nicotinic acid may also be helpful.

Correction of hyperlipoproteinemia. Lancet 1:276, 1971.

Lees RS, Wilson D: The treatment of hyperlipidemia. New England J Med 284:186, 1971.

• • •

General References

Cooke RE (editor): *The Biologic Basis of Pediatric Practice.* McGraw-Hill, 1968.

Hsia DYY: *Inborn Errors of Metabolism,* 2nd ed. *Part I. Clinical Aspects. Part II. Laboratory Methods.* Year Book, 1966.

Nyhan WL (editor): *Amino Acid Metabolism and Genetic Variation.* McGraw-Hill, 1967.

O'Brien D, Goodman SI: The critically ill child: Life-threatening metabolic disease in infancy. Pediatrics 45:620, 1970.

O'Brien D: *Rare Inborn Errors of Metabolism in Children With Mental Retardation,* 2nd ed. Children's Bureau, 1971.

Stanbury JB, Wyngaarden JB, Fredrickson DS (editors): *The Metabolic Basis of Inherited Disease,* 2nd ed. McGraw-Hill, 1966.

Symposium on treatment of amino acid disorders. Am J Dis Child 113:1 ff, 1967.

36 . . .

Diagnostic & Therapeutic Procedures

Ronald W. Gotlin, MD, & Henry K. Silver, MD

The care of children optimally does not end with diagnosis and treatment but includes an understanding of the specific procedures referable to this age group.

This chapter records those methods which have proved to be useful and effective. No claim is made of originality, and all possible pediatric procedures have not been included.

We recognize what may appear to be a lack of sufficient emphasis regarding the comfort and feelings of our pediatric patient and his parents. Were it not for limited space, we would continually reiterate the importance of patience and understanding when conducting procedures in children.

PREPARATION OF THE PATIENT & ORIENTATION OF THE PROCEDURE TEAM

With any diagnostic or treatment procedure, proper positioning and restraint are of greatest importance.

In the majority of cases, failure to complete a procedure is directly related to undue haste in preparing the patient. Young patients often have levels of apprehension and fear that do not lend themselves to "classic" adult physician-patient understanding; competence needs to be developed to balance reassurance and determination to carry out a procedure. This should be done by individualizing the approach for each patient.

Patience and adequate preparation are also necessary when dealing with understandably anxious parents. A few words of explanation to concerned family members will be most reassuring. In general, procedures go more smoothly when parents are not in the procedure room. However, in the event that a parent wants to be present, forcible ejection from the scene may be associated with harmful effects both to the patient and to the procedure team and it is usually advisable to allow the parent to remain under these circumstances. If parents are allowed to remain in the room, they should not be asked to become part of the procedure team or to play an active part in restraining the patient.

RESTRAINT & POSITIONING

The physician should acquaint himself with various methods of properly restraining and posi-

tioning a patient. It is usually very difficult and sometimes dangerous to attempt any procedure on an unrestrained young patient. Before actually starting a procedure, the physician should be certain that all necessary items of equipment are available and arranged for immediate use.

The commonly employed methods of restraint and immobilization are shown in the accompanying illustrations. (Figs 36–1, 36–2, 36–3.) Following immobilization of any extremity, the fingers or toes should be examined for adequate circulation by noting the temperature, color, and capillary pressure in the nail bed.

When total body restraint is necessary, the physician must be certain before and during the procedure that cardiorespiratory function has not been impaired. To assist in doing this a stethescope may be taped to the anterior chest of the patient to permit frequent evaluation.

Local subcutaneous infiltration with procaine or lidocaine (Xylocaine) before performing a lumbar puncture, bone marrow aspiration, or thoracic, pericardial, or peritoneal aspiration is frequently necessary and advisable. Whenever drugs are employed, a history of previous reactions to the drugs should be ascertained and equipment (suction apparatus, oral airway or endotracheal intubation device, laryngoscope, tourniquet, and epinephrine, 1:1000 solution) should be readily available to manage the rare but dangerous untoward reaction that may occur.

Following any procedure, the physician should personally observe the child long enough to be certain that he has not developed any untoward reaction.

DIAGNOSTIC PROCEDURES

COLLECTION & PROCESSING OF BLOOD SAMPLES

1. VENIPUNCTURE

The antecubital, femoral, and external or internal jugular veins are used most frequently for venipuncture and withdrawal of blood, but the sagittal sinus may be used if necessary. In older children, the scalp, wrist, hand, foot (Fig 36–4), and other veins of the extrem-

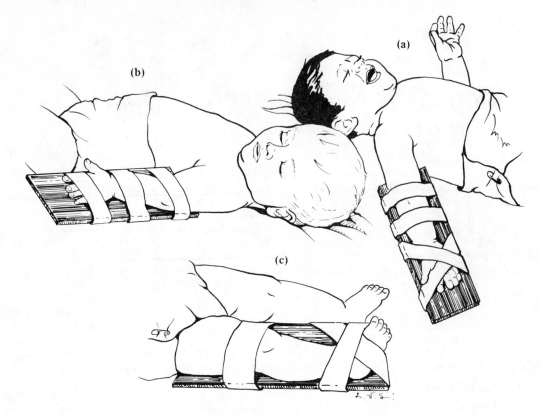

FIG 36–1. Restraining the extremities. (a) Upper extremity. **(b)** Hand. **(c)** Lower extremity.

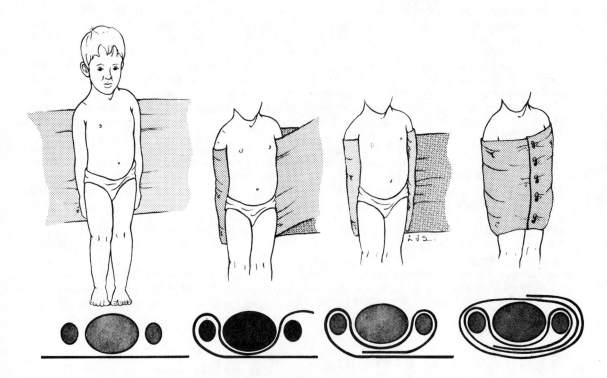

FIG 36–2. Body restraint.

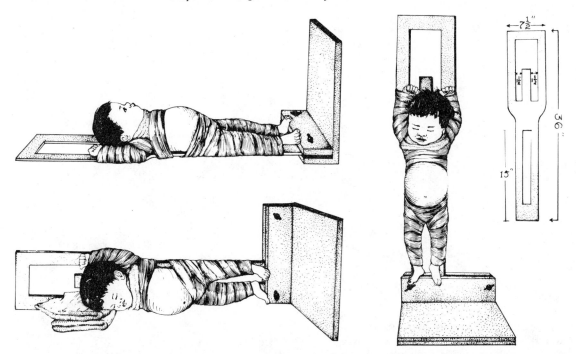

FIG 36—3. Immobilization board with various positions. Dimensions are shown at top right.

ities may be used, but they are usually too small in infants. In some instances, blood may be withdrawn from other veins in the extremities.

Large, accessible veins are best for purposes of injection. ***Caution:*** Do not inject materials into internal jugular, sagittal sinus, or other deep veins.

The skin should be cleansed thoroughly and a disinfectant (eg, an iodinated organic compound or isopropyl alcohol) applied. Iodinated solutions should not be used when blood is to be tested for various iodinated compounds (PBI, etc).

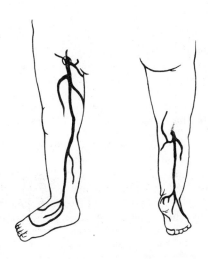

FIG 36—4. Veins of leg and foot.

Antecubital Vein Puncture

If available, the antecubital vein should be used for venipuncture in larger infants and children; frequently it may be entered readily in small infants.

A soft elastic tourniquet is applied proximal (cephalad) to the vein and the venous pattern observed. Dilatation of a vein may be facilitated by local warming; the wearing of red-tinted goggles by the operator may make the venous pattern more readily visible.

A short, sharp-beveled, 20 or 22 gauge needle applied firmly to an appropriate-sized syringe is used. The use of disposable syringes and needles is recommended.

The skin is entered with the needle at an approximately 10—30° angle with the bevel up. If gentle suction is applied to the syringe barrel, blood will be aspirated as the vessel is entered. Blood should be withdrawn gently and rapidly to avoid clotting and hemolysis. When the required quantity of blood has been obtained, the tourniquet is released and the needle withdrawn quickly. After the needle is removed, a dry sterile cotton ball is applied with pressure over the puncture site and held for approximately 3 minutes or until any evidence of bleeding has subsided. To avoid excessive hemolysis, the needle should be removed from the syringe prior to expelling the blood from the syringe into the specimen tube.

Femoral Vein Puncture (See Fig 36—5.)

Place the child on a flat, firm table. Abduct the leg so as to expose the inguinal region. Locate the femoral artery by its pulsation. The vein lies immedi-

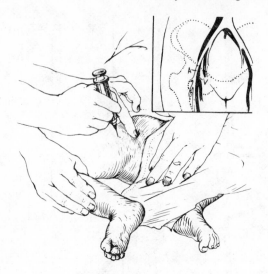

FIG 36–5. Femoral vein puncture.

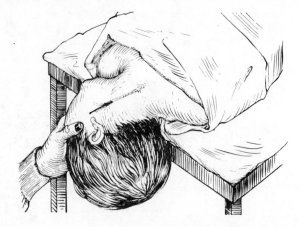

FIG 36–6. External jugular vein puncture.

ately medial to it. Be certain of the position of the femoral pulse at the time of puncture. Prepare the skin carefully with an antiseptic solution and carry out the procedure using strict sterile precautions. Insert a short-beveled needle, 20 or 21 gauge, into the vein (perpendicularly to the skin) about 3 cm below the inguinal ligament; use the artery as a guide. If blood does not enter the syringe immediately, withdraw the needle slowly, gently drawing on the barrel of the syringe; the needle sometimes passes through both walls of the vein, and blood is obtained only when the needle is being withdrawn. Use a large enough syringe to produce adequate suction to assist in withdrawing the blood.

After removing the needle, exert firm, steady pressure over the vein for 3–5 minutes. If the artery has been entered, check the limb periodically for several hours.

Dangers: Following femoral vein puncture, osteomyelitis of the femur and abscess of the hip may occur. Careful attention to aseptic technic is therefore mandatory. Arteriospasm which has resulted in serious vascular compromise of the extremity, particularly in the debilitated and dehydrated infant, has been reported secondary to arterial puncture or venipuncture. When arteriospasm occurs, it may be relieved by application of heat or by the subcutaneous administration of 2% procaine hydrochloride proximal to the site of puncture.

External Jugular Vein Puncture (See Fig 36–6.)

Wrap the child firmly so that arms and legs are adequately restrained. The wraps should not extend higher than the shoulder girdle. Place the child on a flat, firm table so that both shoulders are touching the table; the head is rotated fully to one side and extended partly over the end of the table so as to stretch the vein. Adequate immobilization is essential.

Use a very sharp No. 20 or 22 gauge needle for withdrawing blood. The child should be crying and the

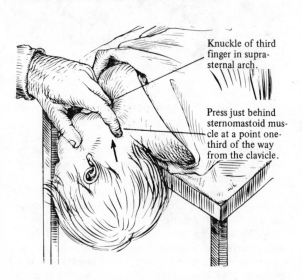

Knuckle of third finger in suprasternal arch.

Press just behind sternomastoid muscle at a point onethird of the way from the clavicle.

FIG 36–7. Direction of needle for internal jugular vein puncture.

vein distended when entered. First thrust the needle just under the skin; then enter the vein. Pull constantly on the barrel of the syringe and be certain that air is not drawn into the vein during aspiration.

After removing the needle, exert firm pressure over the vein for 3–5 minutes while the child is in a sitting position.

Internal Jugular Vein Puncture (See Fig 36–7.)

Prepare the child as for an external jugular vein puncture. Insert the needle beneath the sternocleidomastoid muscle at a point marking the junction of its lower and middle thirds. Aim at the suprasternal notch and advance the needle until the vein is entered. Avoid the trachea and the upper pleural space. Do not use this method in the presence of a hemorrhagic diathesis.

If no blood is obtained on inserting the needle, withdraw slowly and continue to pull gently on the barrel of the syringe. Not infrequently the needle passes through both walls of the vein and blood is obtained only when the needle is being withdrawn.

After completing the procedure, remove the needle and exert firm pressure over the area for 3–5 minutes with the child in a sitting position so as to reduce pressure in the vein.

Dangers: When properly performed, complications are rare. However, careless deep probing of the internal carotid vessel may result in injury to the trachea, vagus nerve, and pleura; the pleural cavity may be entered, and respiratory complications have been reported.

2. COLLECTION OF CAPILLARY BLOOD

The majority of determinations may be made on blood obtained from a finger and heel stick. An expertly performed heel stick (Fig 36–8) is much less traumatic for a small infant than is a femoral puncture and has the additional advantage that it may be repeated frequently and does not have the same risk of complications. The ear lobe is not a satisfactory site since puncture here may be associated with excessive bleeding which may be relatively difficult to control.

To ensure the formation of discrete drops of blood without hemolysis or clotting, the skin should first be wiped with ether. A free flow of blood without squeezing or "milking" is required. The small vein posterior to the medial malleolus is likely to bleed freely and should be used whenever possible. When blood is to be obtained from the heel, make a careful and deliberate puncture with a No. 11 Bard-Parker blade or a Hagedorn needle rather than a rapid stick as employed on the fingertip.

Collection of capillary blood may be difficult, and proficiency may be gained only after prolonged practice. In our laboratory the blood is collected in

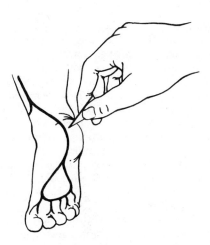

FIG 36–8. Heel puncture.

small glass tubes under a layer of mineral oil. The drop of blood may touch the top of the tube but at no time should the top of the collection tube come in contact with the skin since this is almost certain to produce hemolysis of the blood sample.

The flow of blood can be arrested by applying pressure with a sterile cotton ball. The site of puncture should be examined several times during the next 1–2 hours for evidence of oozing or ecchymoses.

3. ARTERIOPUNCTURE

Arteriopuncture is routinely employed in studying oxygen concentration, hemoglobin saturation, and in measuring arterial blood pressure. The femoral, brachial, radial, and temporal arteries are entered most readily; the umbilical artery may be employed in the newborn period. Oxygenated blood obtained by arteriopuncture is usually bright red in appearance.

Dangers: Firm pressure should be applied for at least 10–15 minutes after withdrawal of the blood specimen to avoid hematoma. Temporary or persistent arteriospasm with serious vascular compromise may occur. Distal obstruction of an artery due to the inadvertent injection of clots into the vessel during arteriopuncture has been reported. Arteriospasm may be relieved by the application of heat or by the subcutaneous administration of 2% procaine proximal to the site of puncture.

UMBILICAL VESSEL CATHETERIZATION

The use of an indwelling catheter in an umbilical artery or vein has become a common procedure in hospital nurseries. Catheterization of the artery generally provides a more useful source of diagnostic information and is safer than catheterization of the more frequently used umbilical vein.

Indications*
   A. Diagnostic Procedures:
   1. To obtain blood samples for analysis (particularly blood gas and pH analysis).
   2. To measure intravascular pressures (arterial and venous).
   3. Cardiac catheterization and angiocardiography.
   B. Therapeutic Procedures:
   1. Exchange transfusion.

*Because of the risks of serious complications, the use of peripheral veins is preferable to catheterization of umbilical vessels for routine blood withdrawal or infusion of therapeutic agents. However, when umbilical vessels are already catheterized for other reasons, use of the catheter obviates further peripheral vein puncture or capillary puncture.

2. Administration of fluids, blood, antibiotics, electrolytes, alkali (sodium bicarbonate, tromethamine), etc.

Procedure

The catheter should be made of flexible, nontoxic radiopaque material that will not kink when advanced through a vessel and will not collapse during blood withdrawal. Nonwettable material and a single, smooth-surfaced end hole reduce clot formation. A # 3.5 (Aloe Medical Corporation) catheter is used for infants weighing less than 1500 gm and a # 5 for larger infants. Dead space of the catheter system should be determined prior to catheterization.

The infant is loosely restrained, warmed (preferably under an overhead radiant heater), and the procedure carried out under sterile conditions.

In normal infants, arterial constriction may prevent catheterization after the first 15–30 minutes of life. (In the presence of hypoxia and acidosis, arterial constriction is usually diminished).

A standard cut-down tray is opened, and the wide end of the umbilical artery catheter is cut off so that the blunt needle adapter fits snugly into the catheter. Discarding the wide end and utilizing the needle adapter reduces the catheter capacity. A sterile syringe is filled with flushing fluid (eg, heparinized saline) and attached to a 3-way stopcock and, in turn, to the umbilical catheter. The entire system is filled with flushing fluid.

An assistant may elevate the umbilical cord by the cord clamp while the operator prepares the cord and adjacent skin with an iodine solution, which should then be removed with alcohol to prevent an iodine burn of the skin. The area is then draped. A purse-string suture (taking care not to puncture the umbilical vessels) or a loop of umbilical tape is placed at the base of the umbilical cord and tied loosely in order to control bleeding if necessary. The cord is then cut 1–1.5 cm above the skin with scissors or a scalpel blade.

The 2 thick-walled, round arteries and the single, thin-walled vein are identified. The rim of the cut vessel is grasped with a pointed forceps or mosquito clamp. The lumen of the vessel is then dilated with the tips of the forceps. Initially, the lumen may allow only one tip to enter. Both tips may then be inserted and allowed to spread, further dilating the vessel. The fluid-filled catheter is inserted into the lumen of the artery or vein and advanced. Any obstruction to advancement usually can be overcome by steady, gentle pressure. Forceful probing may lead to increased arteriospasm in the artery or perforation of the vein or artery. If the obstruction in one of the arteries cannot be overcome, the catheter should be removed and an attempt made to catheterize the other umbilical artery. If a similar obstruction occurs, the catheter should be removed and filled (0.1–0.2 ml) with 1–2% lidocaine (Xylocaine) in epinephrine. The catheter should be reinserted up to the obstruction and the lidocaine injected. This usually relaxes the arteriospasm after 1–2 minutes and allows the catheter to advance.

Frequent aspiration will demonstrate blood return. In arterial catheterization, the tip may be left at the bifurcation of the aorta (approximately at the level of the third lumbar vertebra on x-ray), but few complications occur when it is advanced so that the tip is above the level of the diaphragm (at the 12th thoracic vertebra—confirmed roentgenographically).

The catheter is tied in place by means of a purse-string suture at the base of the cord, securing the ends of the suture to the catheter, and the catheter taped to the infant's abdomen. An antibiotic ointment is applied to the stump and the stump examined frequently for signs of infection. Routine systemic antibiotics are not indicated.

Complications

The principal complications of this procedure are infection ("prophylactic" systemic antibiotics do not reduce the incidence of infection), hemorrhage, vasospasm (placement of the arterial catheter above the diaphram is not associated with this complication once placement is complete), and thrombosis and embolism. Thrombosis is rare in arterial catheterization above the diaphragm but is common (3–33%) in venous catheterization. Embolization occurs when air or clots are introduced, usually as a result of careless technic. Vascular perforation is a rare complication of portal vein catheterization. Vascular and tissue damage may occur secondary to the rapid infusion of hypertonic solutions.

Complications are exceedingly rare when the umbilical artery is employed and the catheter tip is placed in the abdominal aorta above the diaphragm.

Kitterman JA, Phibbs RH, Tooley WH: Catheterization of umbilical vessels in newborn infants. P Clin North America 17:895–912, 1970.

URINE COLLECTION

Midstream Catch (See Fig 36–9.)

Boehm and Haynes, utilizing a technic which they term "midstream catch," report minimal bacterial contamination. After feeding, and before the infant voids, the genital area is thoroughly cleansed with hexachlorophene detergent. The child is then held upside down. The spinal reflex of Perez is then elicited by stroking the back along the paravertebral muscles. Spontaneous voiding usually occurs within 5 minutes. The stream is directed into a sterile container.

The midstream specimen is the only one that is satisfactory for culture or bacterial count.

Attached Receptacle Method

A. Equipment: Pediatric Urine Collector (a Sterilon product), a plastic bag with a round opening surrounded by an adhesive surface to adhere to the skin, may be used. After application the diaper may be reapplied.

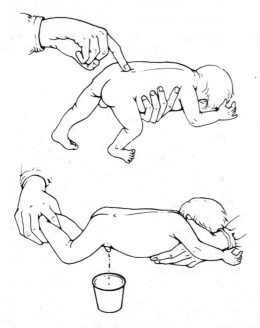

FIG 36–9. "Midstream catch" urine by the method of Boehm & Haynes. (Redrawn from Boehm JJ, Haynes JL: Bacteriology of "midstream catch" urines: Studies in newborn infants. Am J Dis Child 111:366, 1966.)

Urine may also be collected with a bird cup (for girls) or test tube (for boys) fitted in a specimen band.

B. Procedure: Remove diaper. Fit test tube or cup into band. Place child on his back and adjust band and container. Pin band tightly around child with safety pins. Prop up in bed in semi-Fowler position. Restrain arms and legs with diapers if necessary. Remove restraints and band as soon as specimen is obtained.

If a specimen is to be used for culture, the genitalia should first be cleansed thoroughly with soap and water and a mild disinfectant. Whenever possible a midstream specimen (see above) should be obtained. Catheterization is seldom necessary and should be avoided if possible.

For collection of a 24-hour specimen, the chamber of a plastic infusion set may be used. Cut the chamber and cover the rim with adhesive tape to prevent injury. Insert the penis into the tube and tape the tube against the pubic area. Prop the child in bed in the semi-Fowler position. This apparatus may be kept in place for several days without undue discomfort or irritation of the skin.

Clean Catch Method

The male prepuce and glans of the penis or the opening of the female urethra and external vaginal vestibule are cleansed by gentle scrubbing with hexachlorophene (pHisoHex). (In the event that the male is uncircumcised, the foreskin should first be retracted.) Benzalkonium chloride (Zephiran) sponges (1:750) are then employed for several more cleansings. If the patient is old enough, he is instructed to void into the sterile container; as soon as urine is passed, the container is sealed and sent immediately for laboratory analysis.

Metabolic Bed (See Fig 36–10.)

The metabolic bed is a crib in which the mattress has been replaced by a taut synthetic cloth mesh. The infant or young child is maintained without a diaper in the crib, and any urine that is passed flows through the mesh and onto a sloping surface beneath the crib. Children can usually tolerate the mesh for periods up to 24–48 hours without difficulty. This and similar devices have largely replaced the test tube and bird cup methods of urine collection in many hospitals.

Catheterization of the Urinary Bladder

Catheterization is seldom necessary. When it is used, sterile technic, including the use of sterile gloves and towels and adequate antiseptic preparation with hexachlorophene (pHisoHex) and benzalkonium chloride (Zephiran), should be employed.

If catheterization is necessary, catheters measuring 3–6 mm in diameter are usually satisfactory for most patients. Catheters made of inert Silastic or Teflon coated materials are preferred. They may be either straight or indwelling. The latter are double lumen tubes with an inflatable balloon near the distal opening. When inflated, removal is prevented until the bulb is deflated. This type of catheter is employed when continuous urine collection is necessary. If a retention catheter is employed, it should be changed at least every 2 days or replaced by a suprapubic cystocatheter. Acetic acid (0.25%) may be employed for bladder irrigation when a heavy urinary sediment is present. The urethral orifice and surrounding area should be cleaned at regular intervals and an appropriate antibiotic ointment (eg, polymyxin B-bacitracin-neomycin [Neosporin]) applied.

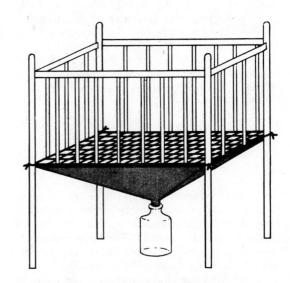

FIG 36–10. Metabolic bed (crib).

The patient is placed supine on a bed or table and immobilized and restrained when necessary. The skin is cleansed and the catheter is inserted into the external urethra. In the male, the penis is held initially at a right angle to the body, and in the female the labia majora and minora are widely separated. The female urethra is somewhat C-shaped and is more easily traversed than the relatively acute-angled male urethra. Trauma to the urethra or bladder can be minimized by using a catheter of the proper size and by gentle technic.

Suprapubic Percutaneous Bladder Aspiration

This method is particularly useful when a sterile urine sample is necessary (eg, suspected urinary tract infection). It is indicated in selected cases but does not lend itself to routine use.

The bladder *must* be full before the procedure is attempted. Cooperative patients should be urged to drink liberal quantities of fluid without voiding. In others, the bladder should be enlarged to palpation and percussion above the pubis before an attempt is made to aspirate urine. Local anesthesia may be used but is generally not necessary.

A. Procedure:

1. Prepare the skin carefully with an antiseptic solution, using strict sterile precautions. Remove hair if necessary.

2. Firmly introduce a sterile No. 21, long (4½ inch), spinal needle with obturator in place 1 or 2 cm above the pubis in the midline, with the needle perpendicular to the skin. After the skin and anterior wall have been penetrated, the tip of the needle will be lying against the bladder.

3. With a quick, firm motion, enter the bladder for a distance of 3–4 cm.

4. Remove the obturator and aspirate the urine with a sterile syringe.

5. After urine has been obtained, withdraw the needle with a single, swift motion.

6. Cover the area with a small sterile gauze dressing, and observe the patient carefully after the procedure.

B. Dangers: When the procedure is performed as outlined above, complications are uncommon. Failure to obtain urine usually indicates that the bladder was either not full or that the needle did not enter the bladder but passed to one side. The procedure may be repeated, but the patient must be fully hydrated and the bladder palpable.

COLLECTION OF NASOPHARYNGEAL FLUID

Nasopharyngeal secretions are frequently collected for culture in upper respiratory infections. In the newborn period, removal of fluid from the pharynx is frequently necessary after birth; passage of a nasopharyngeal tube is helpful in excluding choanal atresia.

Fluid is easily obtained with the use of an ordinary polyvinyl feeding tube to which a syringe has been attached for suction. The tube is introduced into either nostril or into the oral cavity and directed downward as necessary, applying gentle suction with the syringe.

GASTRIC ASPIRATION

Aspiration of the gastric contents of all newborn infants should be performed at the time of the initial examination; simultaneously, the possibility of choanal atresia may also be excluded and esophageal patency established. A positive culture of the gastric fluid or a finding of polymorphonuclear cells on stained smear may provide evidence of newborn sepsis. Intestinal distention may be temporarily relieved by this procedure.

Infants and children unable to cooperate are restrained in the supine position. A cooperative older child is best intubated in the sitting position, with neck and chin held forward without flexion or extension of the neck. When restraint is necessary, the patient is placed on his left side after insertion of the nasogastric tube, allowing the stomach to assume a dependent position. When the danger of pulmonary aspiration is present (ie, toxic ingestions), the patient should be placed with his head in a dependent position while gastric aspiration is being carried out.

The desired tube length is determined by measuring the distance from the patient's nose to the xiphoid process and adding 4 inches. This point is marked on the tube and another mark is made approximately 6 inches distal to that point for reference. The tube is lubricated and introduced into one nasal passage and directed posteriorly while the tip of the nose is held up (Fig 36–11). The tube is then advanced for a distance of 2–3 inches as the patient swallows. If the tube coils, it is best to remove it entirely and start over. To minimize coiling, the tube may be made stiff by prior cooling in ice. After passage of the tube, aspiration with a

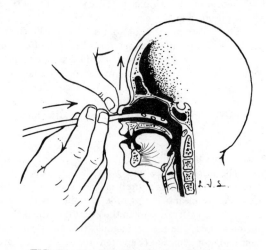

FIG 36–11. Inserting the nasogastric tube.

syringe is attempted. If gastric fluid is not obtained, air or sterile water is introduced while an assistant auscultates over the area of the stomach. A characteristic "gurgling" noise heard by the second observer will indicate that the stomach has been intubated properly; coughing indicates that the patient's respiratory tract has been intubated inadvertently.

The tube may have to be relocated by passing it farther or by withdrawing it 1–2 inches.

When prolonged intubation is necessary, the tube is secured to the cheekbone or forehead with nonirritating tape.

As an alternative, the oral route may be used, and is preferable in the newborn.

COLLECTION OF DUODENAL FLUID

Bile, duodenal, or pancreatic fluid may be needed for diagnostic analysis. The Miller-Abbott tube with weighted metal tip and double lumen is introduced as described above for gastric aspiration, and the gastric contents are aspirated with the patient placed on his right side. The tube is advanced approximately 6 inches and the patient asked to remain in that position for 30–60 minutes. In this position, the normal stomach will pass the tube beyond the gastric pylorus and into the duodenum. The appearance of bile and change in pH of the aspirated duodenal fluid or roentgenographic visualization of the metal tip verifies proper positioning of the tube.

OBTAINING SPINAL FLUID

The 4 procedures available for the collection of CSF are lumbar, subdural, cisternal, and ventricular punctures. Lumbar puncture is most frequently used for obtaining CSF for diagnostic purposes. It may be performed in either the lateral recumbent or sitting position.

Lumbar Puncture in Newborn & Small Infants

The sitting position is preferable in an infant and may be achieved by sitting the patient backward in a modified "infaseat" or "potty" chair. A small pillow or blanket between the abdomen and the back of the chair will increase the flexion of the back. When restraints are required, changes in cardiorespiratory activity should be monitored. When the lateral recumbent position is elected, the surface on which the child is placed should be firm and flat.

Lumbar Puncture in Children & Older Infants

Restrain the patient in the lateral recumbent position on a firm, flat table (Fig 36–12). Prepare the skin surrounding this area as for a surgical procedure with iodine and alcohol or other suitable antiseptic.

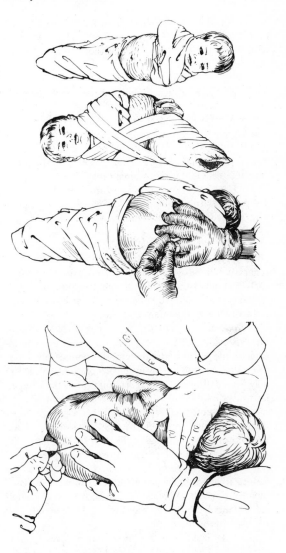

FIG 36–12. *Above:* Restraining the infant for lumbar puncture. *Below:* Lumbar puncture with assistance of nurse. (Drapes omitted to show positioning.)

Drape the area with sterile towels or a special drape. Infiltrate the skin and subcutaneous tissues with 1% procaine (not necessary in infants and young children).

Pertinent landmarks are the spinous processes and iliac crests. The line joining the tops of the iliac crests passes through the fourth spinous process. The space above (third) and 2 spaces below (fourth and fifth) are the sites of choice for puncture.

The operator sits with the puncture site at eye level and the light adjusted to shine over his operating hand. The needle and obturator are inserted into the chosen vertebral space in the exact midline and perpendicular to the plane of the body. The needle is directed slightly toward the head with the bevel facing the operator. In older children, a distinct "give" is usually felt when the dura is pierced; if in doubt, remove the stylet and examine the needle hub for the appearance of fluid. Gentle suction with a small syringe may be required in the small infant or in the case of purulent meningitis.

When fluid is obtained, the 3-way stopcock and manometer are attached and the stopcock opened. Pressure measurements are made before collection (opening pressure) and at the completion of collection (closing pressure). In addition, the presence of pressure changes with compression of the neck veins (Queckenstedt's test) is indicative of patency between the intracranial system and cerebrospinal canal.

After the closing pressure is obtained, the needle is removed with a quick deliberate movement and pressure applied for several minutes with a sterile sponge over the puncture site.

Note: When fluid is obtained in the infant or child for glucose determination, a concomitant blood sugar should be obtained as a comparison. Without such a comparison, a low CSF glucose may be meaningless since blood and spinal fluid sugar levels may be normally low in the infant and child.

Dangers: A "bloody tap" may occur without obvious cause and is most likely the result of penetration of the needle into the anterior venous plexus of the vertebral body. However, the presence of blood may be a pathologic finding. Herniation of the cerebellar tonsils may occur when increased intracranial pressure is present in the posterior fossa at the time of lumbar puncture; preoperative ophthalmoscopic examination of the retina may be helpful in indicating increased pressure. Increased intracranial pressure is not necessarily an absolute contraindication to the procedure if provision is made for neurosurgical management of possible complications. Introduction of chemical irritants and infectious agents should be avoided by the use of proper technic.

Postspinal headache is common when large amounts of CSF are removed rapidly or when leakage from the spinal canal into the subarachnoid space occurs. An analgesic may be required.

Cisternal Puncture

Whenever possible, the lumbar route is preferred, but cisternal puncture may be used to advantage for drainage and treatment when there is an obstruction of the spinal canal. Cisternal puncture is easier than lumbar puncture in the patient with marked opisthotonos, and there is less danger of medullary impaction when the intracranial pressure is high. However, the needle may pierce and damage vital centers in the medulla, and arterial damage with hemorrhage into the cistern or fourth ventricle may be fatal.

Hold the patient in the lateral recumbent position on a firm, flat table. Place a folded sheet or small firm pillow under his head to bring the cervical spine in line with the thoracic, with the whole spine horizontal. Use sterile precautions. Hold the patient very firmly if he is not fully cooperative, with the neck strongly flexed.

Insert a long 20 gauge lumbar puncture needle immediately below the suboccipital notch and stay in the sagittal plane, ie, parallel to the table surface, aiming toward a line drawn between the 2 external auditory meatuses. The forward progress of the needle must be under complete control by having one fingertip of the carrying hand resting firmly against the patient's neck or head. A distinct "give" will usually be felt and perhaps heard when the needle pierces the dura. Do not go any farther. If in doubt at any stage, withdraw the stylet and observe for the appearance of fluid. If none appears, withdraw the needle and make a fresh start. The assistance of a neurologist or neurosurgeon should be obtained if the operator has not had previous experience with a cisternal puncture.

Subdural Puncture (See Fig 36–13.)

Following CNS infection or trauma, bilateral subdural taps are frequently performed to determine the presence of, and remove, a subdural collection of fluid.

The anterior 2/3 of the scalp are shaved and sterile precautions are observed. The patient is restrained as shown.

Insert a short 19 or 20 gauge lumbar puncture needle with a very short bevel for a distance of 0.2–0.5 cm at the extreme lateral corner of the fontanel or farther out through the suture line, depending on the size of the fontanel. Piercing the tough dura is easily recognized. Normally, not more than a few drops (up to 1 ml) of clear fluid are obtained. If a subdural hematoma is present, the fluid will be grossly xanthochromic or bloody and more abundant. For children over age 2, a trephine opening usually is necessary.

Repeat the procedure on the other side. Do not remove more than 15–20 ml of fluid at any one time.

Remove the needle, exert firm pressure for a few minutes, and apply a sterile collodion dressing.

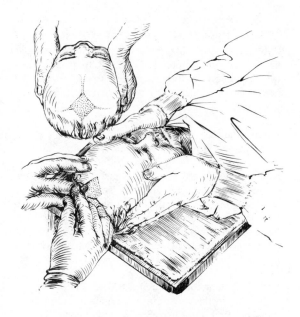

FIG 36–13. Subdural puncture.

Note: Hemorrhage may occur if the needle causes a laceration of a tiny vein communicating with the sagittal sinus. This may result in subsequent taps yeilding xanthochromic fluid from the blood introduced during the preceding procedures. Fistulous drainage is prevented by covering the orifice with a sterile collodion dressing.

BONE MARROW ASPIRATION

Bone marrow puncture is indicated in the diagnosis of blood dyscrasias, neuroblastoma, lipidosis, reticuloendotheliosis, lupus erythematosus, and to obtain culture material. The procedure should be performed with extreme caution when a defect of the clotting mechanism is suspected.

Sites for Punctures

The sites of choice for different age groups are listed in Table 36–1.

A. Iliac Crest: The site of choice for children is the posterior iliac crest. Restrain the child on his abdomen with a rolled sheet placed under his hips. Locate the iliac crest and enter at a spot approximately 1–2 cm posterior to the midaxillary line and approximately 1 cm below the crest.

B. Sternal Marrow: Seldom used in children.

C. Tibia: Between the tibial tubercle and the medial condyle over the anteromedial aspect. Recommended by some for infants.

D. Lumbar Spinous Process in the Midline.

Procedure

The patient should be adequately restrained. Sedation is often necessary for children. Prepare the skin surrounding the area as for a surgical procedure. Scrub and wear sterile gloves. Infiltrate with 1% procaine solution, through the skin and subcutaneous tissues to the periosteum.

Insert a short-beveled needle with stylet in place perpendicular to the skin, through the skin and tissues, down to the periosteum. (Use a 21 gauge lumbar puncture needle for infants, an 18 or 19 gauge special marrow needle with a short bevel for older children.) Push the needle through the cortex, using a screwing motion with firm, steady, and well controlled pressure. Some "give" is usually felt as the needle enters the marrow; the needle will then be firmly in place.

Immediately fit a dry syringe (20–50 ml) onto the needle and apply strong suction for a few seconds. A small amount of marrow will come up into the syringe; this should be smeared on glass coverslips or slides for subsequent staining and counting.

Remove the needle after withdrawing marrow, exert local pressure for 3–5 minutes or until all evidence of bleeding has ceased, and apply a dry dressing.

COLLECTION OF FLUID FROM BODY CAVITIES

Thoracentesis

Used for removing pleural fluid for diagnosis or treatment, to inject antibiotics in cases of empyema, or to induce or relieve pneumothorax.

A. Site: Locate the fluid or air by physical examination and by x-ray if necessary. If entering the base, locate the bottom of the uninvolved lung as a guide so that the puncture will not be below the pleural cavity.

B. Equipment: Use an 18 to 19 gauge needle with a very short bevel and a sharp point. The needle and a 10 or 20 ml syringe are attached to a 3-way stopcock (10 ml syringe is easier). If much fluid is to be removed, it can be pumped through a rubber tube attached to the sidearm of the stopcock, thereby avoiding leakage of air into the pleural space.

C. Procedure: When possible, the patient should be in a flexed position and lean forward against a chair back or bed stand. If too ill to sit up, he can lie on his uninvolved side on a firm, flat surface with a small pillow under his chest to widen the upper interspaces.

Use strict sterile precautions; scrub and wear sterile gloves. Prepare the skin surgically and use suitable drapes, preferably a large drape with a hole in the center. Infiltrate into the skin and down to the pleura with 1% procaine. A 3-way stopcock is attached to the aspiration needle, a section of rubber tubing is applied to the sidearm, and a 10 ml syringe is applied to the hub.

Insert the needle through an interspace, passing just above the edge of the rib. The intercostal vessels lie immediately below each rib. With gentle aspiration of the syringe, the needle is advanced slowly a few millimeters at a time until the pleural space is reached. It is usually not difficult to know when the pleura is pierced, but suction on the needle at any stage will show whether or not fluid has been reached. In cases of long-standing infection, the pleura may be thick and the fluid may be loculated, necessitating more than one puncture site. To prevent accidental penetration of the lung after the needle is in place, apply a surgical hemostat to the needle adjacent to the skin. Pleural

TABLE 36–1. Sites for bone marrow puncture.

Site	Age to Which Adaptable
Anterior iliac crest	Any age
Posterior iliac crest	Any age
Femur	Birth to 2 years
Spinous vertebral process	2 years and older
Sternum	6 years and older
Tibia	Birth to 2 years

*Reproduced, with permission, from Hughes WT: *Pediatric Procedures.* Saunders, 1964.

fluid is apt to coagulate unless it is frankly purulent, and an anticoagulant should be added after removal to facilitate examination. If a large amount of fluid is present, it should be removed slowly at intervals, 100–500 ml each time, depending on the size of the patient.

D. Dangers: Complications of this procedure include introduction of a new infection, pneumothorax or hemothorax from tearing of the lung, hemoptysis, syncope (pleuropulmonary reflex or air embolus), and pulmonary edema (from too rapid removal of large amounts of fluid). Careful sterile technic will decrease the risk of introducing infection. Hemodynamic imbalance is unlikely when only small quantities are removed slowly. Air embolism will not occur if the stopcock is closed, so that air cannot enter. Insertion of the needle into a blood vessel, heart, liver, and spleen can be prevented by proper selection and positioning of the puncture site. Pneumothorax should not occur if care is taken to avoid advancing the needle beyond the point where fluid should be present.

If the patient starts to cough, the needle should be removed.

Pericardiocentesis (See Fig 36–14.)

Pericardiocentesis is indicated for the diagnosis and treatment of purulent pericarditis or to relieve cardiac embarrassment due to collection of large amounts of blood or other fluid. The procedure is contraindicated if pericardial or myocardial adhesions are suspected.

A. Site: The puncture site is determined by physical or x-ray examination. The common site of aspiration is the fourth left interspace, 1–2 cm inside of the left outer border of percussion dullness or x-ray shadow. Other sites of entrance are just outside the apical pulsation; from below, in the chondroxiphoid angle; and occasionally from the back if a very large collection has collapsed the lung against the posterior chest wall.

B. Procedure: The patient sits forward at a 60° angle supported by bed or pillows. Using sterile technic, infiltrate the skin and subcutaneous tissues with 1% procaine. Connect a 50 ml syringe, 3-way stopcock, and 18 gauge needle. Insert the needle slowly at the lower border of the interspace just above the edge of the rib, directing it posteriorly and toward the spine. Aspirate, and then turn the stopcock to discharge fluid via the rubber tubing. When fluid is being aspirated with ease, attach a surgical clamp to the needle next to the skin to prevent the needle from slipping farther.

Continuous monitoring of the pulse and blood pressure is necessary during the removal of small increments of fluid. The needle is removed in one quick movement and pressure applied to the puncture site to ensure that air does not enter the pericardial or pleural space.

C. Dangers: Cardiac arrhythmias and penetration of the heart or coronary vessels have been reported to have resulted from pericardiocentesis.

Peritoneal Paracentesis

This procedure can be used as a therapeutic measure to remove excessive fluid in cases of nephrotic syndrome or hepatic cirrhosis or diagnostically for evidence of blood or intestinal contents. In cases of known or suspected trauma, a puncture in each of the 4 quadrants of the abdomen may be made ("4 quadrant tap") in search of blood or intestinal contents. Infrequently, peritoneal paracentesis may be used as a diagnostic measure to obtain bacteriologic specimens in peritonitis, but this involves the danger of puncturing the distended bowel, which frequently is adherent to the abdominal wall. Electrolyte solutions, albumin, blood, and antibiotics may be administered by the peritoneal route. Peritoneal dialysis may be of value for renal insufficiency and in the treatment of certain poisonings.

A. Procedure: Use an 18 or 19 gauge needle with a short bevel and a sharp point. The skin is cleansed and surgical safeguards employed to avoid peritoneal infection. A local anesthetic is injected and a small incision is made in the skin with a surgical knife. Enter at a level about ½ way between the symphysis and the umbilicus in the lower quadrant or in the midline. The needle should enter obliquely to avoid leakage afterward. Ascitic fluid will flow out readily. Pus may require aspiration.

B. Dangers: Perforation of the intestine has resulted when the intestines are distended or adhesions are present. Perforation of the bladder has resulted when the bladder is not empty. The removal of excessive amounts or excessively rapid removal of fluid may result in circulatory embarrassment. Peritonitis from the introduction of infectious agents has been ob-

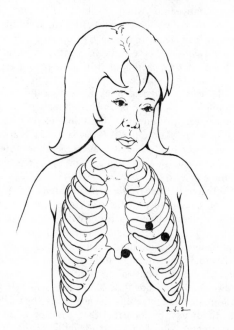

FIG 36–14. Sites of needle insertion for pericardiocentesis.

served; "prophylactic" antibiotics are no substitute for proper surgical technic and are usually not indicated.

THERAPEUTIC PROCEDURES

ADMINISTRATION OF FLUIDS

The administration of fluids may be necessary in a number of clinical situations. The available routes of administration are as follows: (1) Alimentary: Oral, gastric (gavage or gastrostomy), rectal. (2) Intravascular: Intravenous, intra-arterial. (3) Hypodermoclysis. (4) Intraosseous. (5) Intraperitoneal. (6) Intramuscular.

1. ALIMENTARY ROUTE

Oral

When available, the alimentary tract is the route of choice for the administration of all nutrients and fluids with the exception of blood. When the oral-gastric avenue is not competent, intubation of the stomach and duodenum is safe and easily accomplished.

Rectal

The rectal route may be used for diagnosis (culture or roentgenologic examination with barium), for cleansing (fecal impaction), or for therapy (administration of fluids, electrolytes, or drugs).

Because the vascular drainage of the rectum does not enter the portal system, the liver is bypassed and administered fluids and drugs that are absorbed can enter the systemic circulation directly without hepatic conjugation or detoxification. The portal bypass may be avoided by administering fluids into the colon by high enema or colonic flush.

A. Procedure: The older patient is placed either in the left lateral recumbent or the knee-chest position. The small infant may be placed on his back with his legs flexed and elevated. A rectal examination should be performed initially to rule out the presence of a foreign body. A rectal catheter of appropriate size is lubricated and introduced beyond the anal sphincter. Fluid (preferably warmed) is administered by the gravity method, holding or taping the buttocks together if necessary to prevent the loss of fluid.

B. Dangers: Rectal perforation, particularly in the small infant, is not rare but can be avoided with the use of a soft rubber catheter.

2. INTRAVENOUS ROUTE

Intravenous Therapy by the Gravity Method

For most infants and children a standard gravity apparatus or special equipment (Vacoset, to deliver fluids slowly, and Pedatrol, which permits controlled administration of fluid) should be used for giving large amounts of fluid slowly over a long period. Fluids are best administered through a 21 or 23 gauge needle.

A. Site: (Figs 36–15, 36–16, 36–17, 36–18.) For small infants, a scalp vein or one on the wrist, hand, foot, or arm will usually be most convenient. The superficial veins of the scalp do not have valves, and fluids may therefore be infused in either direction. Any accessible vein may be used in an older child. If a vein cannot be entered, blood may be given intraperitoneally in an emergency.

B. Equipment: A gravity apparatus is used with a closed drip bulb in the tubing not far below the container so that it will hang perpendicularly. The bulb should be 1/4–1/3 full and the connected tubing free of air. Flow is regulated by a screw clamp on the tubing.

C. Procedure: Use a Pediatric Scalp Vein Infusion Set (Cutter or Abbott) with a 21 gauge needle and rubber finger grip connected to plastic tubing or a short 21–24 gauge needle.

A syringe is attached to the catheter and the system is filled with saline. The skin over the area is prepared with an antiseptic and the tourniquet applied snugly but not tightly enough to impede arterial pressure. A warm sponge or gentle percussion over the vein will enhance distention of the vein. (The operator may wear red-colored glasses to facilitate visualization of the vessel.) The vein is stabilized by stretching the skin over it proximal to the puncture site. The needle is

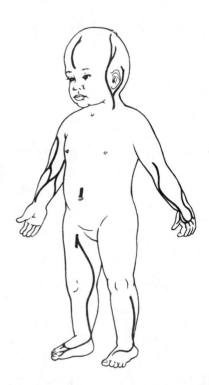

FIG 36–15. Superficial veins used most frequently for intravenous infusion.

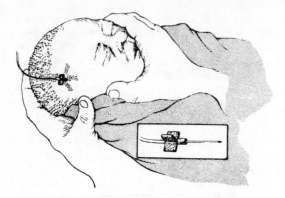

FIG 36—16. Intravenous fluids into scalp vein.

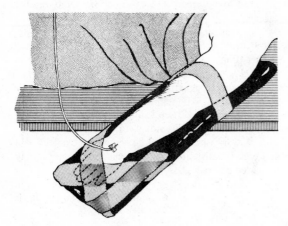

FIG 36—17. Intravenous fluids into wrist vein.

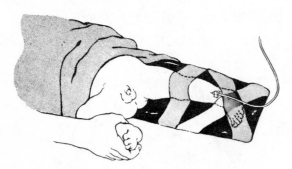

FIG 36—18. Intravenous fluids into ankle vein.

introduced bevel up and parallel to the long axis of the vein at a point just beneath the skin. A characteristic "give" is perceptible, and blood usually flows back into the catheter and syringe. The tourniquet is released and the winged tabs of the scalp vein set are held stable with the free hand. Very gentle pressure is applied to the syringe barrel to ensure patency of the system. If the syringe does not function easily, pressure should not be increased but merely maintained. Initial resistance is not uncommon and has been

attributed to "spasm" of the vessel. After a few seconds, the vein may open and saline will flow easily from the syringe.

The winged tabs are secured by taping; the syringe is removed and the scalp needle catheter is connected to an air-free gravity type infusion apparatus with a drip bulb. Final restraints are applied when necessary and the flow rate adjusted. Tape the needle firmly in place. Sandbags will be useful in securing the head, and sandbags or a padded board are employed to immobilize the hand and arm.

Superficial veins of the scalp of infants under the age of 2 years are easily visualized and can be distinguished from the superficial arteries of the scalp by palpation. When these veins are used, special care in cleansing the skin is mandatory since they communicate with the dural sinuses.

An ordinary rubber band will usually suffice as a tourniquet.

D. Rate: The rate can be calculated by counting the number of drops per minute delivered from the bottle. If a Pedatrol microdrop bulb is employed, drops/minute = ml/hour. When the adult set is used, drops/minute X 4 = ml/hour.

E. Precautions: *The rate of flow should be checked frequently.* An accurate record must be kept of the amount of fluid added. For small infants (particularly those who were prematurely born), never permit more than 1/3 of the daily fluid requirements to be in the container at any one time. It is advisable to remove the needle and change location each 48—72 hours to avoid phlebitis. If possible, avoid hypertonic solutions.

For the patient receiving fluids in an extremity, use foam rubber to maintain the limb in a position of comfort. Inspect the limb at regular intervals for evidence of undue pressure and circulatory embarrassment.

Intravenous Therapy by the Pump Method

In some infants, veins may be too small for the administration of fluids by the gravity method despite maximum elevation of reservoir bottle; in these cases, the solution can be pumped in slowly by syringe and a 3-way stopcock. With a needle and syringe on the terminal stopcock, one operator enters the vein and maintains the needle in the proper position. A second person "pumps" the solution in with a syringe on the second stopcock inserted farther up the tubing. If only one person is available, he can pump from the terminal stopcock. Twenty to 30 ml/kg body weight (except blood and plasma) may be administered slowly over the course of several minutes.

Percutaneous Catheterization

Catheterization of either a vein or an artery may be performed percutaneously by inserting a large bore, thin-walled needle into a relatively large vein and then threading a catheter through the needle and into the vein.

The needle is withdrawn and the catheter secured by taping to the skin. Leakage around the puncture site may occur but may be eliminated with the use of a Buffalo (Sterilon) needle. This device reverses the needle-catheter relationship, providing a needle within a catheter. As the needle is withdrawn, the puncture site is not reduced and leakage does not occur.

Cut-Down Intravenous

For small infants—or if fluids are urgently needed by a seriously ill older child and difficulty is encountered in entering a vein—expose a vein surgically and tie a piece of polyethylene tubing (or metal cannula if such tubing is not available) in place.

A. Site: The internal saphenous vein has been found to be the most satisfactory site. Its position is constant, running anterior to the medial malleolus of the tibia to the groove between the upper medial end of the tibia and the calf muscle. It can be entered at any point along its course. Hence, by starting at the ankle, the same vein can be used several times if necessary. The novice can easily identify it on his own leg first.

Other veins (small saphenous, median basilar, and cephalic) may also be used for "cut-downs," but their courses are more variable and difficult to define.

B. Equipment:

1. Sterile solution, container, tubing, drip bulb, and clamp are prepared as for continuous venoclysis.

2. Thin polyethylene tubing with the end cut on the slant is easiest to use and least irritating. A 19 gauge tubing is preferred, but tubing as small as 22 gauge may be used.

C. Procedure:

1. **Preparation**—Apply a tourniquet, cleanse the skin, and drape the leg as for a surgical procedure, using sterile precautions. The foot can be securely taped to a sandbag or board splint (Fig 36–19). Make a large wheal with 1 or 2% procaine solution in the skin over the vein.

2. **Incision**—With a scalpel, make an incision about 1 cm long just through the skin. The incision should be at a right angle to the direction of the vein. Using small, curved, sharp-pointed scissors or fine forceps, spread the incision widely.

3. **Identifying the vein**—The vein is usually seen lying on the fascia. Some dissection of subcutaneous fat may be necessary. Insert a curved clamp to the periosteum and bring the vein to the surface (Fig 36–20). Be certain it is a vein, not a nerve or tendon, by observing for the passage of blood. Using a small hook (eg, strabismus hook), dissect the vein free for a length of 1.5–2.5 cm. In small infants the vein is small and fragile, and great care must be taken in handling it.

4. **Placing ties**—Using No. 00 black silk, tie the vein off at the extreme distal (lower) end of the exposed portion. Leave the ends of the suture long so that they may be used later for traction. At the proximal end of the vein, loop a piece of suture loosely around the vein (Fig 36–21).

5. **Nicking the vein**—Using a fine-pointed scissors, sterile razor blade, or sharp-pointed scalpel blade, make a small incision through the wall of the vein a

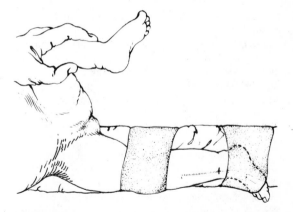

FIG 36–19. Position and taping of leg for cut-down incision.

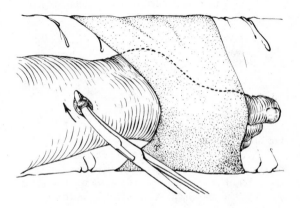

FIG 36–20. Isolation of vein for cut-down intravenous. (Drapes not shown.)

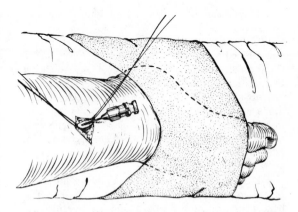

FIG 36–21. Cut-down intravenous with ligatures tied. (Drapes not shown.)

few millimeters above the lower ligature. Make certain that the lumen has been entered by lifting the vein on the handle of the hook or other instrument used so as to flatten it and draw it taut. Release tourniquet after tubing is in the vein.

6. Fixing the cannula—Insert the polyethylene tubing for a distance of at least 2 cm. Blood will usually drip from it; if not, note whether a small amount of the solution can be injected easily with a syringe and rubber adapter without producing a wheal or filling the incision site. Tie the upper proximal suture firmly around the vein and tubing to hold it in place. Connect the tubing from the reservoir of fluid to the polyethylene tubing in the vein with care to avoid pulling and tearing the vein.

7. Closing the wound—Close the wound with fine silk sutures which are removed in 3–4 days. The tubing must be firmly strapped in place. When using a needle or cannula, a pad of gauze under the hub will keep it in alignment with the vein. Cover the wound with gauze and roller bandage. Avoid restraint, which interferes with adequate circulation or causes pressure lesions.

The needle is withdrawn and the catheter secured by taping to the skin.

3. HYPODERMOCLYSIS

Use only isotonic solutions.

For Small Infants

A. Site: For small infants, hypodermoclysis may be given by syringe, using the subcutaneous tissues of the anterior and posterior axillary folds, the medial aspect of the mid-thigh, the upper back in the area of the inferior aspect of the scapula, or the lower abdominal wall. In most instances, the intravenous route is preferred since hypodermoclysis may be associated with erratic absorption or with a marked shift in body fluids.

B. Equipment: A 20 or 50 ml syringe and a 20 gauge needle.

C. Procedure: After aspirating to make certain that a blood vessel has not been entered, inject slowly; if the center of the injected area becomes pale, change the position of the needle point. Gentle massage will help to diffuse the fluid into the tissues. (Hyaluronidase may be used to facilitate spread and absorption.) In infants, up to 50 ml can be injected in each site at one time. Rigid aseptic precautions are necessary. The infant must be restrained to prevent bending or breaking the needle.

D. Dose: Thirty to 40 ml/kg body weight at one time. Larger amounts can be given over a longer period by a gravity apparatus with a Y-tube and 2 needles.

For Older Children

For older children, fluids by hypodermoclysis are best given slowly in the outer aspect of the mid-thigh by a gravity apparatus, using a Y-tube and 2 needles.

4. INTRAOSSEOUS THERAPY

Intraosseous (into the bone marrow) administration of fluids is a form of intravenous therapy. The effluent vessels of bone marrow provide a rapid and relatively complete drainage into the systemic circulation. However, the obvious consequences of infection preclude its general use.

5. INTRAPERITONEAL THERAPY

Isotonic fluids and blood may be administered by the intraperitoneal route, but the intravenous route is generally preferred.

6. INTRAMUSCULAR THERAPY

Intramuscular injections may be given into the upper outer quadrant of the gluteal area. With the child prone on a flat surface, locate the head of the greater trochanter of the femur and the posterior superior iliac spine. Direct the needle perpendicular to the table or bed in this space cephalad to the head of the trochanter.

Other satisfactory sites include (1) the anterolateral aspect of the thigh (use a 1 inch needle), with the needle directed downward at an oblique angle toward the bone; or (2) the ventral gluteal muscles, to the center of an area outlined by locating the anterior iliac tubercle, placing the index finger on the tubercle, and extending the middle fingertip along the crest of the ileum as far as possible, forming a triangle. The needle is directed slightly toward the iliac crest.

EXCHANGE TRANSFUSION FOR ERYTHROBLASTOSIS FETALIS

After an adequate preparation of the infant (respirations and temperature stabilized and maintained, gastric contents removed, proper restraint), drape the umbilical area. Cut off the cord about 1/2 inch or less from the skin. Control any bleeding. Identify the vein (the 2 arteries are white and cordlike; the single vein is larger and thin-walled). If the vein cannot be visualized in the cord stump, make a small transverse incision above the umbilicus. Cannulate the vein gently (usually to a distance of 6–8 cm) with a naked polyethylene tubing. Determine venous pressure and maintain below 10 cm with the child at rest.

Remove blood in 10–20 ml amounts and save the first aliquot for laboratory studies. Replace with an equivalent amount of fresh (less than 5 days old) type-specific or group O Rh-negative blood to which anti-A and anti-B soluble substances may be added. Heparinized blood is preferred. Give twice the blood volume (BV = about 85–100 ml/kg) for a "complete" exchange. When the infant is severely affected, a full exchange should not be attempted immediately after birth. Instead, small doses of sedimented erythrocytes should be given, alternating with slow withdrawal of the infant's blood until the venous pressure is less than 10 cm of water. Determine the pulse rate every 20–30 ml exchanged and the venous pressure every 100 ml exchanged; if venous pressure is elevated, gradually establish a deficit (10–100 ml). If hemorrhagic mani-festations, respiratory distress, yawning, pallor, or cyanosis develop, discontinue the exchange. Cardiac arrest occasionally occurs (see p 752 for treatment).

The administration of calcium gluconate has been suggested when ACD blood is employed. Administer calcium gluconate, 1–2 ml of 10% solution, slowly through the polyethylene tubing (rinsing tubing with saline solution before and after the drug is introduced). Do not give any further calcium if there is slowing of the pulse.

Give protamine sulfate, 0.5–1 mg IM, to terminate the heparin effect at the end of the exchange.

●   ●   ●

General References

Barnett HL: *Pediatrics,* 14th ed. Appleton-Century-Crofts, 1968.

DeSanctis AG, Varga C: *Handbook of Pediatric Medical Emergencies,* 4th ed. Mosby, 1968.

Gellis S, Kagan B: *Current Pediatric Therapy,* 3rd ed. Saunders, 1963.

Hughes W: *Pediatric Procedures.* Saunders, 1964.

Nelson WE, Vaughan VL, McKay RJ (editors): *Textbook of Pediatrics,* 9th ed. Saunders, 1969.

Shirkey HC: *Pediatric Therapy,* 3rd ed. Mosby, 1968.

Silver HK, Kempe CH, Bruyn HB: *Handbook of Pediatrics,* 9th ed. Lange, 1971.

37 . . .

Fluid & Electrolyte Therapy

John B. Moon, MD, & Donough O'Brien, MD, FRCP

PHYSIOLOGY OF THE FLUID SPACES IN CHILDHOOD

ELECTROLYTES

An electrolyte is any low molecular weight substance which, when dissolved in water, renders the solution capable of conducting an electric current. Conductivity is made possible because electrolytes in solution exist as ions and, therefore, have positive or negative charges. Positively charged ions are called cations (eg, Na^+, K^+, Ca^{++}), and negatively charged ions are called anions (eg, Cl^-, HCO_3^-). In any solution, the number of positive and negative charges is equal. Certain ions have more than one positive or negative charge, the number of charges per ion being the valence of the ion.

Molecular weight can be calculated as the sum of the weights of the individual atoms in a molecule. When expressed in grams, the value is known as a gram mol, and a solution containing 1 gram mol/liter is said to be 1 molar. If an ion has a valence of 2, then 1 mol of that ion can combine with 2 mols of any univalent reactant. The product of mols × valence gives equivalents. A solution containing 1 equivalent (Eq) per liter is said to be 1 normal. If the valence is 1, molarity equals normality. If the valence is 2, molarity is 1/2 of normality (0.5 N), etc. Electrolytes are customarily expressed as milliequivalents (mEq) per liter of solution, where 1 mEq is equal to 0.001 Eq.

In order to convert grams (gm), milligrams (mg), mols (M), or millimols (mM) to milliequivalents (mEq), the following formulas are used:

$$mEq = \frac{gm}{\text{Molecular weight}} \times valence \times 1000$$

$$mEq = \frac{mg}{\text{Molecular weight}} \times valence$$

$$mEq = Mols \times valence \times 1000$$

$$mEq = mM \times valence$$

BODY FLUIDS, MEMBRANES, & OSMOLALITY

Of the total water in the body (TBW), roughly 2/3 are intracellular (ICW) after early infancy, and the remainder is extracellular (ECW). Between the ECW and ICW lie all the cell membranes of the body, which may be considered as one large, aggregate membrane. This so-called cell membrane possesses 2 qualities of importance to clinicians: (1) It is water-permeable, and (2) it concentrates Na^+ into the ECW and K^+ into the ICW by virtue of a membrane-associated Na^+-K^+ "pump."

Water molecules cross the cell membrane constantly and equally in both directions; hence, the volumes of the ECW and ICW do not change. Particles dissolved in the water interfere with the movement of water molecules and thus lower the number which find "pores" in the membrane and cross to the opposite side. The number of dissolved particles per number of water molecules must therefore be equal on both sides of the cell membrane, or a net transfer of water or particles (or both) would result. If the membrane is impermeable to certain solute particles, addition of such particles to one side will lower the number of water molecules leaving that side and the number of water molecules entering from the opposite side will then be greater. A net transfer of water will occur until the ratio of particles to water molecules has again been equalized on both sides. The number of dissolved particles per number of water molecules is seldom computed as such, but a closely related value, osmolality, is employed. Osmolality is customarily expressed as mOsm/kg* of water.

The forces generated by separating solutions of differing osmolalities by a semipermeable membrane may be substantial, and will cause the transfer of water or particles or both. Much evidence exists that osmolality is the same throughout the TBW. Osmolality is often referred to as tonicity, and solutions which contain approximately 285 mOsm/kg are referred to as isosmolal, isotonic, or occasionally as normal. ("Normal" in this sense does not imply equivalents/liter.) Solutions containing less than or more than 285 mOsm/kg are spoken of as hypo- or hyperosmolal or

*mOsm = milliosmol = number of mM × number of particles formed when 1 molecule dissolves.

hypo- or hypertonic, respectively. Osmolality can be changed by selectively adding or taking away water, or by selectively adding or taking away solute particles. It is generally true that isosmolality (ie, 285 mOsm/kg) of the body fluids is optimal.

Some of the consequences of the cell membrane's ability to concentrate Na^+ into the extracellular fluid (ECF) and K^+ into the intracellular fluid (ICF) are shown in Fig 37–1.

EXTRACELLULAR FLUID

1. COMPONENTS

The components of the ECF are (1) plasma, (2) interstitial fluid, (3) connective tissue, cartilage, and bone fluids, and (4) transcellular fluids. (Table 37–2.)

Plasma

After early infancy, the plasma constitutes about 1/6 of the ECF volume, about 1/12 of the TBW, and about 1/20 of the weight of the patient (Table 37–1). It is separated from the interstitial fluid by the endothelial membranes lining the blood vessels. Endothelium allows the immediate passage of water and very rapid passage of ions but confines most of the albumin and globulin molecules to the intravascular compartment proper. This is presumably due to the large size of the protein molecules. The plasma proteins consist mostly of albumin of approximately

TABLE 37–1. Blood and plasma volume formulas.*

Boys

Blood volume in ml/kg = 7.57 − 0.114 × wt in kg

Blood volume in ml/sq m = 697 × surface area (in sq m) + 1312

Girls

Blood volume in ml/kg = 82.4 − 0.374 × wt in kg

Blood volume in ml/sq m = 360 × surface area (in sq m) + 1575

Plasma volume = blood volume × $\left(1 - \dfrac{0.93 \times hct}{100}\right)$

where Hct is a large vessel μ hematocrit.

*From Cropp JA: J Pediat 78:220, 1971.

60,000 mol wt and globulins ranging in mol wt from 180,000–1,000,000. The albumin molecules, though smaller, are much more numerous and contribute roughly 3/4 of the osmotic pressure attributable to the plasma proteins. This is frequently called colloid osmotic pressure. Compared to the osmotic pressure due to the more numerous low molecular weight electrolyte molecules of the plasma (eg, Na^+, K^+, Cl^-, HCO_3^-), the colloid osmotic pressure is negligible and constitutes only about 1 mOsm out of 285. Nevertheless, this difference plays a critical role in the maintenance of plasma volume.

Plasma is delivered to capillary beds under hydrostatic pressure. This pressure forces fluid out of the intravascular compartment into the interstitial fluid, concentrating the plasma proteins and raising the colloid osmotic pressure in the capillaries. As hydrostatic pressure falls and colloid osmotic pressure rises with further passage down the capillaries, a point is reached where the fluid, initially exuded, is reabsorbed back into the capillaries.

Interstitial Fluid (ISF)

The ISF may be regarded as an ultrafiltrate of plasma. Thus, the concentrations of Na^+, K^+, HCO_3^-, and Cl^- in ISF closely resemble those of plasma, and for all practical purposes plasma electrolyte analyses reflect interstitial fluid composition.

The ISF is the perfusate of the cells. Its composition is regulated chiefly by renal and pulmonary action on plasma. It represents a fluid "space" or "compartment" of considerable volume and therefore acts as a buffer against changes occurring in the much smaller plasma compartment. Excessive volume of ISF is manifested as edema. When ISF volume is diminished, the clinical signs include poor skin turgor, sunken eyes, depressed fontanels, and small tongue size. The ISF is thus an integral component of soft tissue structure.

Connective Tissue, Cartilage, & Bone Water

No particular symptoms are known to derive specifically from alterations in these fluids.

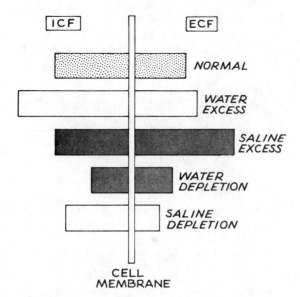

FIG 37–1. Changes in water distribution between ICF and ECF.

Transcellular Fluids

Transcellular fluids are body fluids which have been directly elaborated by cells. The fluids involved are spinal and ventricular fluid, bile, the humors of the eye, synovial fluid, and gastrointestinal fluids. Ordinarily, these fluids comprise less than 2% of TBW. The volume of gastrointestinal fluids, however, can expand enormously, creating a fluid pool of considerable size and importance.

2. CONTROL OF THE ECF

A wide variety of mechanisms play a role in the control of the composition and volume of the ECF. The most important ones are discussed below.

Thirst

Thirst is the perception of the need to drink, and control mechanisms operate with astonishing precision. ECF volume deficits evoke thirst, and the organism will use water to control volume at the expense of osmolality. Many fluid balance problems arise when thirst cannot be perceived, communicated, or satisfied.

Aldosterone

This potent adrenocortical hormone acts to enhance the tubular resorption of Na^+. Aldosterone secretion plays an important role in the control of ECF volume, as this depends mainly on the amount of Na^+ that it contains.

Antidiuretic Hormone (Vasopressin, ADH)

ADH acts to enhance renal resorption of water and thus allows formation of a concentrated urine of small volume. ADH is secreted from the posterior pituitary after synthesis in the anterior hypothalamus. ADH secretion, causing antidiuresis, is promoted by an increase in osmolality, a decrease in plasma (or ECF) volume, emotional stress (pain, fear, rage), exercise, and a number of drugs, including morphine, ether, barbiturates, nicotine, histamine, acetylcholine, and epinephrine. ADH secretion is inhibited, causing diuresis, by dilution of body fluids, distention of the left atrial wall, and alcohol.

INTRACELLULAR WATER

The bulk of the body water is intracellular, and for technical reasons quantitative assays are difficult, although it is sometimes of value to assay striated muscle biopsies for sodium, potassium, and magnesium content to give an approximation of their concentration in intracellular water.

It is clearly inappropriate to conceive of intracellular water as a simple homogeneous solution. As yet, however, there is no useful information about

regional differences in the volume and composition of intracellular water as between cytoplasm and organelles.

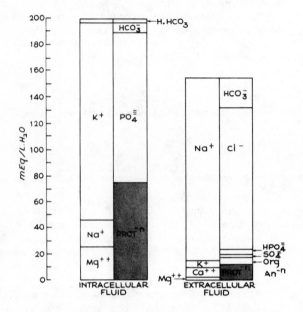

FIG 37–2. Electrolyte composition of intracellular and extracellular water.

DISTRIBUTION OF BODY WATER WITH AGE

An understanding of fluid and electrolyte problems requires an understanding of certain differences in ionic composition between extracellular and intracellular water (Fig 37–2), bearing in mind that the proportions of TBW in the various compartments vary with age (Table 37–2).

TABLE 37–2. Distribution of body water with age (in percentage of total body weight).

Age	Total (TBW)	Extra-cellular (ECW)	Intra-cellular (ICW)
0–11 days	77.8 (69–84)	42 (34–53)	34.5 (28–40)
11 days–6 months	72.4 (63–83)	34.6 (28–57)	38.8 (20–47)
6 months–2 years	59.8 (52–72)	26.6 (20–30)	34.8 (28–38)
2–7 years	63.4 (55–73)	25 (21–30)	40.4 (31–53)
7–16 years	58.2 (50–64)	20.5 (18–26)	46.7

MEASUREMENT OF BUFFER BASE
(The Metabolic Component)

Several different laboratory tests may be used to assess the metabolic (or "nonvolatile") component of the acid-base status. All in one way or another assess the concentration of buffer base in the blood.

The most important buffer base is HCO_3^- and the $[HCO_3^-]p$ is normally found by titration to be 22–24 mEq/liter.

Another laboratory test which gives similar values is the total CO_2, or CO_2 content of plasma. This value (which should not be confused with the PCO_2) is determined by volumetrically measuring all the gaseous CO_2 from a plasma sample by addition of strong acid. The total $CO_2 = HCO_3^- +$ dissolved CO_2. Average values for $[total\ CO_2]p$ are about 1–1.2 mEq/liter greater than $[HCO_3^-]p$. $[Total\ CO_2]p$ is usually used clinically to reflect the $[HCO_3^-]p$.

Unfortunately, the "metabolic indicators"– $[HCO_3^-]p$ and $[total\ CO_2]p$–are not independent of changes in the PCO_2. This is largely due to the presence of nonbicarbonate buffer bases, chiefly anionic groups on the plasma proteins and hemoglobin. Thus, a change in the PCO_2 (or $[H_2CO_3]$) produces a corresponding change in $[HCO_3^-]$ as indicated by the following equation:

$$H_2CO_3 + \boxed{Prot^-} = \boxed{HCO_3^-} + H\ Prot$$

Note, however, that a change in PCO_2 or $[H_2CO_3]$ produces changes in both $[Prot^-]$ and $[HCO_3^-]p$. These changes are precisely equal and in opposite directions, such that their **sum** does not change. Thus, the total buffer base concentration is independent* of the PCO_2 and can be used as an indicator of the metabolic component of the acid-base status. Normal values for total buffer base concentration range from 46–50 mEq/liter of whole blood.

The addition of strong, nonvolatile "metabolic" ·acid, on the other hand, generates no HCO_3^-. In fact, the total buffer base concentration will fall in direct proportion to the amount of nonvolatile acid added (see discussion of base excess, p 913).

ACID-BASE PHYSIOLOGY

Definitions
An acid is a substance which, when in solution, dissociates into hydrogen ions (H^+) and anions (A^-). Acids are, therefore, hydrogen ion donors, and a strong acid dissociates more completely than a weak acid. A base, when dissolved in solution, yields anions (A^-) capable of reacting with hydrogen ions, removing them from solution. Thus, a base is a hydrogen ion recipient.

A strong base has a greater affinity for H^+ than a weak base.

Buffers
A buffer is a mixture of a weak acid and its conjugate base. In the equilibrium $H_2CO_3 \rightleftharpoons HCO_3^- + H^+$, carbonic acid ($H_2CO_3$) is a weak acid and bicarbonate ion (HCO_3^-) is the conjugate base. In a buffer, or buffered solution, the weak acid is called a buffer acid and the weak base is called a buffer base.

Virtually all body fluids except gastric fluid are buffered, ie, they contain both buffer acids and buffer bases. The most significant buffer acid is carbonic acid. The most important buffer bases are bicarbonate ion, the anionic portions of plasma protein molecules and hemoglobin.

Acidity
Acidity refers to the concentration of hydrogen ions in a solution. The greater the $[H^+]$,* the greater the acidity. Alkalinity refers to the concentration of OH^- ions in solution; the greater the $[OH^-]$, the greater the alkalinity. Acidity and alkalinity are not independent of one another in that the product of $[H^+]$ X $[OH^-]$ is constant. Thus, a rise in $[H^+]$ (or acidity) is accompanied by an equivalent fall in $[OH^-]$ (or alkalinity) and vice versa.

The acidity of body fluids has come to be described not in terms of $[H^+]$ but by another term, pH, which is equal to $-log\ [H^+]$. This relationship may be rewritten as follows:

$$pH = log\ \frac{1}{[H^+]}$$

Hence, it can be seen that as acidity or $[H^+]$ rises, pH falls, and vice versa.

The pH of arterial blood is normally 7.40 ± 0.02.

When the pH of blood is 7.40, the $[H^+]$ is only 0.04 μEq/liter. At that pH, the buffer acids and buffer bases are present in milliequivalents per liter, making buffer acid and buffer base molecules many times more numerous than hydrogen ions. Fine control of $[H^+]$ (or pH) is accomplished by regulating buffer acid and buffer base concentrations, not hydrogen ions.

LABORATORY MEASUREMENT OF
ACID-BASE DISTURBANCES

The pH is governed by the concentrations of buffer acids and buffer bases by the following relationship:

$$pH = pK + log\ \frac{[Buffer\ base]}{[Buffer\ acid]}$$

*The use of brackets indicates concentration, eg, $[H^+]$ = hydrogen ion concentration; $[Na^+]_S$ = serum sodium concentration.

*Actually, this is strictly true only in vitro.

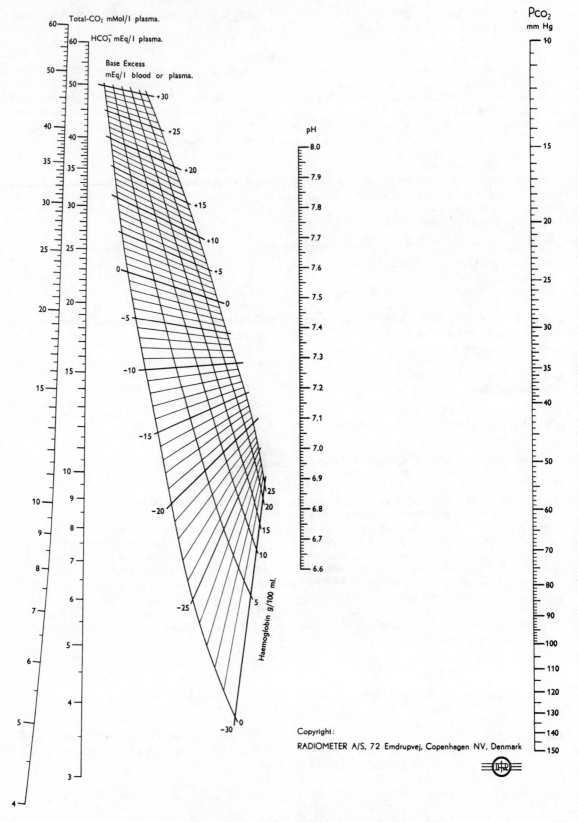

FIG 37–3. Siggaard-Andersen alignment nomogram.
(Reproduced by permission of the copyright holder, Radiometer A/S, Copenhagen.)

Accordingly, any adequate evaluation of acid-base status requires a knowledge of 3 variables, not just one. This in turn requires that at least 2 variables be measured in order that the third might be calculated.

Most modern laboratories are now equipped to measure blood pH. A variety of laboratory tests may be used to assess the other variables.

MEASUREMENT OF BUFFER ACID
(The Respiratory Component)

By far the most important (and the only conveniently measurable) buffer acid in the body is carbonic acid. This compound is formed by the hydration of metabolically produced CO_2 as shown in the equation $H_2O + CO_2 \rightleftharpoons H_2CO_3$. Most CO_2, however, is never hydrated but is carried in simple physical solution from the tissues where it is produced to the lungs where it is exhaled.

$[H_2CO_3]$ is not measured directly. Instead, the level of dissolved CO_2 is measured as the partial pressure of CO_2 (abbreviated P_{CO_2}). As the $[H_2CO_3] = 0.03 \times P_{CO_2}$, knowing the P_{CO_2} allows easy calculation of $[H_2CO_3]$.

The P_{CO_2} is an excellent index of the efficiency of ventilation and is directly proportional to the actual concentration of H_2CO_3. We can see that the $[H_2CO_3]$ is also dependent on the efficiency of ventilation. Hence, H_2CO_3 is called "volatile acid." All other buffer acids are "nonvolatile." Acid-base disturbances can thus be divided into 2 types: volatile or "respiratory" disturbances and nonvolatile or "metabolic" disturbances.

For example, if 10 mEq of strong, nonvolatile acid are added to 1 liter of blood originally containing a total buffer base concentration of 48 mEq/liter, the total buffer base concentration will fall to 38 mEq/liter. If H_2CO_3 (or CO_2) were added, no change would result.

The deviation of the total buffer base concentration from normal (in this case, −10 mEq/liter) is the basis for an extremely popular and useful laboratory measurement called the **base excess**. Like the total buffer base concentration (TBBC), the base excess is used to assess the "metabolic" component of the acid-base status of the blood. Normal values for base excess range from 0 to −4 mEq/liter of whole blood. Addition of strong nonvolatile acid causes the base excess to fall below 0 mEq/liter, thus acquiring negative values. Addition of buffer base causes the base excess to rise above 0 mEq/liter and take on positive values. Like the TBBC, the base excess changes very little with changes in the P_{CO_2}.

Fig 37−3 provides a means of relating pH, P_{CO_2}, $[HCO_3^-]p$, [total CO_2], and base excess. If any 2 values are determined experimentally, the remaining values may be calculated using a straight-edge.

GENERAL PRINCIPLES OF FLUID & ELECTROLYTE MANAGEMENT

All plans for the repair of fluid and electrolyte distortions are based on calculations first of maintenance requirements and then of volume and qualitative changes (correctional requirements).

MAINTENANCE REQUIREMENTS

Maintenance requirements are the fluids and electrolytes which must be given to maintain homeostasis for the next balance period (usually 24 hours). Predictions must be made for (1) sensible and insensible losses, (2) urinary output, (3) gastrointestinal (or other) losses, and (4) sufficient calories to prevent undue expenditure of the patient's own energy stores.

1. SENSIBLE & INSENSIBLE LOSSES

Table 37−3 lists approximate sensible and insensible losses. Both sweating and pulmonary losses must be considered.

Sweating

When planning ordinary sensible and insensible losses, no Na^+ is allocated, only free water, since most sweat Na^+ is normally reabsorbed within the duct.

When sweating becomes profuse, the duct's capacity to reabsorb Na^+ is saturated, and sweat is then produced which contains significant amounts of Na^+. Patients with cystic fibrosis have a limited capacity to reabsorb Na^+ in their excretory ducts and may require additional Na^+ to sustain body $[Na^+]$ in the presence of continued heavy sweating.

Patients with edema sweat very little. The same applies to patients with congenital absence of sweat glands, patients who are hypothermic, and to newborns. Sweating is minimal in cool mist but may be maximal in hot, humid environments.

Pulmonary Losses

Water loss through the lungs depends primarily upon tidal volume, respiratory rate, and the ambient humidity. Patients in mist thus lose significantly less water than those in dry air.

Sensible and insensible losses are obligatory and will continue whether provided for or not.

Zweymuller E, Preining O: The insensible water loss of the newborn infant. Acta paediat scandinav, Suppl 205, 1970.

TABLE 37–3. Estimated 24-hour requirements for infants and children on an intravenous regimen.
(All values except those for adults are in ml/kg.)

	Sensible and Insensible Losses (ml/kg)	Urinary Losses		
		Water (ml/kg)	Na⁺ (mEq/kg)	K⁺ (mEq/kg)
Prematures	20 (in mist) 30 (dry air)	30	3	0–2
Full-term–2 months	25 (in mist) 35 (normal) 45 (hypermetabolic)	40	3	1–3
2 months–10 kg	25	60	3	2–3
15 kg 30 kg 45 kg	400 ml/sq m/24 hours or 13 ml/kg/24 hours	750 ml/24 hours 1075 ml/24 hours 1500 ml/24 hours	25 mEq/24 hours 37 mEq/24 hours 50 mEq/24 hours	20 mEq/24 hours 30 mEq/24 hours 40 mEq/24 hours

2. URINARY OUTPUT

Table 37–3 lists estimated maintenance requirements for urinary output from infancy to adulthood. This table is intended for patients in whom no defect in concentrating ability exists. The previous day's urinary output should not be used in calculating maintenance requirements for urine production.

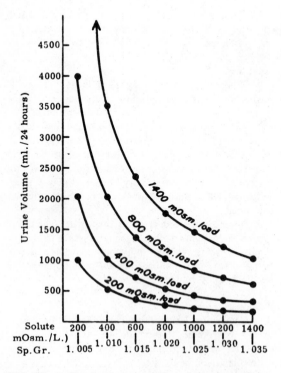

FIG 37–4. Total solute excretion and urine volume per given sp gr. (Redrawn and reproduced, with permission, from Bland JH: *Clinical Recognition and Management of Disturbances of Body Fluids.* Saunders, 1956.)

The normal newborn kidney can dilute effectively to about 50 mOsm/kg of urine water and can concentrate to approximately 600 mOsm/kg. A gradual increase in concentrating ability occurs until about 1 year of age, when roughly 1000–1200 mOsm/kg of urine may be excreted. If the kidney cannot concentrate effectively, an increased volume of urine must be excreted to clear the same milliosmolar load. If this volume is not provided, hyperosmolality may occur. Therefore, the maintenance requirements for urinary water may have to be raised somewhat if renal concentrating ability is impaired or if the patient is receiving a high solute load, eg, from a protein-rich diet. The same may apply if he is creating a high endogenous solute load from marked catabolism. If the solute load is low, as is often the case during intravenous therapy, water needs are minimal. The relation between urine volumes required to excrete varied milliosmolar loads is indicated in Fig 37–4.

Ziegler EE, Fomon SJ: Fluid intake, renal solute load, and water balance in infancy. J Pediat 78:561, 1971.

3. GASTROINTESTINAL & OTHER LOSSES

The most satisfactory guide for estimating anticipated gastrointestinal losses is the previous day's volume and trend. This requires that nasogastric fluid, biliary fistula fluid, etc be analyzed for electrolyte composition. However, adjustments always have to be made to adapt to the clinical situation.

For example, patients with ileus or pyloric obstruction may initially be estimated to lose gastric fluid at the rate of 20 ml/kg/24 hours until bowel activity returns. This fluid contains approximately 100 mEq/liter of NaCl and 10 mEq/liter of KCl.

Patients with gastroenteritis may lose large quantities of fluid and electrolytes in diarrheal stools. Nevertheless, the estimate of gastrointestinal losses may be zero, for as soon as patients are sustained intra-

TABLE 37–4. The approximate concentration of electrolytes (mEq/liter) in fluids obtained from the gastrointestinal tract.*

Fluid Type	Sodium	Potassium	Chloride	Total HCO$_3^-$
Stomach	20–120	5–25	90–160	0–5
Duodenal drainage	20–140	3–30	30–120	10–50
Biliary tract	120–160	3–12	70–130	30–50
Small intestine				
Initial drainage	100–140	4–40	60–100	30–100
Established	4–20	4–10	10–100	40–120
Pancreatic	110–160	4–15	30–80	70–130
Diarrheal stool	10–25	10–30	30–120	10–50

*Because of the wide range of normal values, specific analyses are suggested in long-term cases.

venously and given nothing by mouth, stooling usually ceases altogether.

Biliary fistulas, intra-abdominal drains, thoracic drains, and even CNS drains occasionally produce obligatory fluid loss that must be taken into account in calculating maintenance requirements.

4. CALORIES

If maintenance requirements are given as 5% glucose solutions, no additional source of calories need be added provided that such a regimen is not continued for longer than 3–4 days and the patient's caloric needs are not markedly increased, as in salicylate intoxication or the respiratory distress syndrome of prematurity. In these instances, 10% glucose in water may be substituted. Maintenance fluids given as 5% glucose solutions provide few calories, but they provide enough to prevent the patient from being hungry; they exert a substantial protein-sparing effect; and they prevent ketosis. Ordinarily, all intravenous fluids should contain at least 5% glucose. If water restriction is in force, however, insufficient protein-sparing calories will be administered if only 5% glucose is given. Fifteen to 20% glucose may then be used—if need be, with ethyl alcohol. Such solutions rapidly inflame veins and shorten the life of an intravenous site. If oral intake is allowed, cookies and candy may provide excellent therapy.

A special section of this chapter is devoted to the problem of prolonged intravenous alimentation.

Table 37–5 illustrates how 24-hour maintenance requirements are calculated for a 10 kg, 1-year-old child in normal fluid and electrolyte balance. (Data from Table 37–3.)

REPAIR OF EXISTING DEFICITS OR SURPLUSES

Calculations must be designed to correct both volume and qualitative distortions. In theory, adjustments should apply to all the body water compartments; however, knowledge of changes in the intracellular water in disease is limited because of the technical difficulties of measurement. From a practical viewpoint, therefore, correctional changes are applied as extracellular water, and there is experimental evidence that sodium may temporarily substitute for potassium as the main intracellular cation. Clinical response certainly justifies that approach. In making calculations, independent appraisals are made for (1) ECF volume changes and (2) qualitative changes in osmolality, acid-base balance, and electrolyte potassium balance.

1. EXTRACELLULAR FLUID DEPLETION

Clinical Features

Depletion of ECF, usually due to gastroenteritis, is one of the most common clinical problems in pediatrics. The symptoms and signs vary with the severity of fluid depletion. Skin turgor begins to be lost after 3–5% of the body weight is lost as isotonic ECF. The patient is thirsty, and urinary output is reduced. With a 10% loss of body weight, skin turgor becomes strikingly depressed, the eyes become sunken and soft, the fontanel, if present, is sunken, and the sutures in the skull may become prominent. Pulse rate is increased and pulse volume diminished. Orthostatic hypotension may occur in older children. Fever, oliguria, a dry mouth, diminished tearing, and lethargy are present. The skin, however, is pink, and the capillary refill time is prompt. The hematocrit is elevated. When over 10%

TABLE 37–5. Twenty-four hour maintenance requirements in a 1-year-old, 10 kg child.

	Fluid		Na$^+$		K$^+$		Cl$^-$	
	ml/kg	ml	mEq/kg	mEq	mEq/kg	mEq	mEq/kg	mEq
Estimated insensible losses	25	250	...	...	...	...	...	...
Estimated urinary losses	60	600	3	30	2	20	5	50
Totals	...	850	...	30	...	20		50

of the body weight is lost as ECF, the above signs become more prominent, but the hallmark of this end stage of acute ECF depletion is progressive cardiovascular collapse. Tachycardia increases, pulse volume decreases further, and the skin becomes cool and pale. A peculiar mottling of the skin occurs and is an ominous sign. Osmolality and $[Na^+]_S$ may remain normal up to the time of death.

Treatment

The treatment of ECF depletion is prompt restoration of a normal ECF volume. In severe cases, maintenance of the intravascular volume with plasma, isosmolal albumin solution, dextran, or any other suitable plasma expander takes first priority. Isotonic saline or lactated Ringer's injection may also be given as an interim measure to sustain peripheral circulation.

Once an adequate plasma volume is assured, the objectives of treatment are (1) to ensure a continuing adequate intake of calories, water, and electrolytes for maintenance or to compensate for other special losses. (2) to restore the remaining ECF deficit; and (3) to correct qualitative distortions of ECF homeostasis, such as acidosis and K^+ depletion (see below). The volume deficits may amount to 5–10% of the body weight. Where this is so, an ECF equivalent (eg, lactated Ringer's injection) should be given intravenously rapidly enough to halve the volume deficit in under 2 hours or until skin turgor, sunken eyes, and lethargy are substantially improved. In less severe cases, fluid restoration should be planned in such a way that the volume deficit is half-corrected during the first 8 hours and fully corrected by 24–48 hours.

In severe malnutrition, especially in infants, skin turgor may be markedly depressed in the absence of fluid depletion. Caution should be exercised lest such patients receive needless overexpansion of their ECF compartments.

In shigella dysentery, neurotoxins may cause dramatic lethargy, with eye rolling and stupor in the absence of correspondingly severe signs of ECF depletion. The sodium needs are obviously not determined solely by the state of consciousness.

In patients with cardiovascular disease and inadequate circulation, ECF replacement should be achieved more cautiously so as not to induce cardiac failure.

2. EXTRACELLULAR FLUID EXCESS

The accumulation of excess extracellular water, whether due to retention of water or salt and water or to a proportion shift between ECF and ICF, constitutes edema. The various forms are described below.

Systemic Edema

By the time edema has become manifest, significant ECF excess is already present. Rapid weight gain with no change in $[Na^+]$ indicates accumulation of ECF and may be the only sign available until edema

appears. Edema fluid is an ultrafiltrate of plasma, and its presence implies sodium excess.

Edema fluid is mobile and is distributed to the most dependent portions of the body. Children may have periorbital edema upon arising in the morning which disappears in a short time as the edema fluid is redistributed. Paroxysmal nocturnal dyspnea may occur when edema fluid within the legs is added to the circulation upon lying down, giving rise to acute episodes of pulmonary edema. Pulmonary edema is generally the most serious complication of systemic edema.

Edema of Hypoproteinemia

Significant hypoproteinemia (albumin concentration less than about 2 gm/100 ml) is usually accompanied by edema. This comes about in 2 ways. First, inadequate albumin concentrations cause the colloid osmotic pressure of plasma to fall below that necessary to reabsorb fluid filtered from capillaries under hydrostatic pressure. Second, the resulting decrease in plasma volume activates the renin-angiotensin-aldosterone system and increases the renal tubular reabsorption of sodium.

The "Third Space" Phenomenon

A special situation exists when edema fluid is sequestered in a particular location and can no longer readily exchange with the plasma. Such an accumulation of fluid is called a "third space." Examples include ascites, lymphedema, dermal sequestration in burns, and bowel edema in enterocolitis.

In all these instances, the third space must be allowed to form and sufficient isotonic saline or other ECF substitute made available. However, any third space may rapidly return its borrowed sodium to the circulation, as is frequently seen 3–4 days after a severe burn. The resulting volume distortion may be sufficient to cause pulmonary edema.

ICF to ECF Shifts

Occasionally in renal failure, a shift occurs in the distribution of water between extracellular and intracellular fluid, and children will become edematous without any change in total body water.

Treatment

The treatment of ECF excess depends upon whether the edema fluid is generalized or localized (third space) and whether or not serious hypoproteinemia exists (causing "obligate" edema).

Restriction of most dietary and all parenteral Na^+ is rational until evidence of generalized edema has disappeared. Edema fluid is an isotonic saline solution and contains nearly 150 mEq of Na^+ in each liter. Because of this, restriction of Na^+ should be accompanied by a proportionate restriction in water. If rapid correction of edema is desired, diuretics may be employed.

Neither sodium restriction nor diuretic therapy should be used in a patient in otherwise satisfactory fluid balance in order to alleviate a third space. In treating a third space, provide for it when it forms, beware of it when it resolves, and treat its cause whenever possible.

The treatment of edema due to hypoproteinemia usually consists of treatment of the primary disease. Administration of parenteral albumin is rational, but rapid administration is to be avoided lest the plasma volume be overexpanded by a sudden influx of interstitial fluid. Combinations of intravenous protein administration, diuretics (particularly furosemide), and sodium restriction are usually effective but seldom provide more than transient benefit unless protein can ultimately be retained in the plasma.

DISORDERS OF OSMOLALITY

1. HYPONATREMIA

Hyponatremia Due to Water Overload

Patients with normal renal function can ordinarily excrete a sudden water load with relative ease. However, many patients with impaired renal function and virtually all patients with acute renal failure or total obstructive uropathy are unable to tolerate water loading. Such patients are prone to develop hyponatremia with great rapidity and often make this fact known with an unexpected seizure. Treatment consists of water restriction, relief of urinary tract obstruction when present, and hypertonic saline only to control convulsions.

Hyponatremia With Normal ECW Volume

If a patient receives vasopressin (ADH) either iatrogenically or from inappropriate endogenous secretion, the urine output falls and the urine concentration increases. Thirst is unaffected, and the patient, if allowed access to water, will drink. As water is retained, the serum osmolality and serum sodium concentrations begin to fall. After 1–3 days, sufficient ECF volume expansion has occurred to inhibit aldosterone secretion, and a saline diuresis occurs which normalizes the ECF volume but leaves the osmolality and serum sodium concentration low. Administration of isotonic or hypertonic saline may result in transient rises of $[Na^+]_S$ but is quickly followed by brisk saline diuresis. Restriction of water can prevent this sequence from developing and will rectify the situation once it has developed.

The most common cause of this disorder is inappropriate secretion of vasopressin in the face of a normal ECF volume. Vasopressin is secreted in a variety of intracranial diseases, including tumors, head injuries, hydrocephalus, and meningitis. It also occurs with a variety of intrathoracic disorders varying from pneumonia to bronchogenic neoplasms. Drugs such as barbiturates, ether, morphine, and histamine may have

this effect, and strong emotional stress, rage, fear, and pain, as well as surgery, occasionally incite this inappropriate chain of events.

Hyponatremia is seldom associated with significant signs or symptoms until Na^+ concentrations fall below 120 mEq/liter. If hyponatremia develops gradually, anorexia, apathy, and mild nausea and vomiting may be the only symptoms. If it develops rapidly, headache, mental confusion, muscular twitching, eventual delirium, and, finally, convulsions occur. The signs and symptoms are related almost as much to the rate at which the hyponatremia developed as to the severity achieved. Extremely low Na^+ concentrations (90–110 mEq/liter) invariably cause CNS dysfunction but are not incompatible with either survival or recovery. CNS dysfunction due to rapid onset hypo-osmolality is sometimes called water intoxication.

Treatment consists of water restriction. Administration of isotonic or hypertonic saline solution results in overexpansion of the ECF. Hypertonic saline should be reserved for severe water intoxication with frank CNS disturbance. An occasional patient is helped by administration of ethanol, 7% solution, 20 ml/kg/24 hours, to inhibit ADH secretion.

Hyponatremia With Diminished ECW Volume

Depletion of the ECF in gastroenteritis, vomiting, adrenal insufficiency, renal salt-losing states, diabetic ketoacidosis, etc calls into play a number of mechanisms which act to protect plasma volume. Aldosterone conserves Na^+, thirst prompts the patient to drink, renin and catecholamines help to maintain blood pressure, and decreased glomerular filtration rate enhances both Na^+ and water resorption. In addition to the above, vasopressin is secreted, and as a result the organism will conserve water alone to maintain an adequate plasma volume at a lower than normal osmolality, if necessary. In the presence of a lowered ECF volume, renal clearance of free water (C_{H_2O}) is strikingly impaired. Thus, even though the organism is hypo-osmolal, excess water is now conserved. Rigid restriction of water will cause severe oliguria and will tend to normalize the osmolality, but it is poor treatment for the patient. If water alone is made available to the patient, he will drink water when sodium is needed.

The signs and symptoms are those typical of ECF depletion, ie, thirst, tenting skin, dehydrated appearance, dry mucous membranes, tachycardia, and oliguria.

Therapy is directed toward restoring a normal ECF volume by the administration of normal ECF-like fluids. This is usually associated with a water diuresis from the ICF compartment and rapid resolution of the hyponatremic state. If the hyponatremia is severe, correction of ECF depletion by saline may be combined with free water restriction.

Hyponatremia With Expanded ECW Volume

This type of hyponatremia is by far the most serious and most difficult to treat. The presence of hyponatremia in combination with edema implies that the osmoregulatory mechanisms have been reset at a lower level. Hyponatremia with edema usually occurs with severe heart failure, liver disease, or renal failure. If the underlying circulatory disturbance can be corrected, hyponatremia with edema usually resolves spontaneously. These patients may have gross edema and therefore a greater than normal total body Na^+ content.

The signs and symptoms are overshadowed by those of the underlying disease. Edema is obvious, and both the $[Na^+]_S$ and osmolality are low.

Vigorous water restriction should be instituted despite complaints of thirst. In many cases, this will amount to only enough fluid to allow the patient to swallow his food. The water allowance should be well below the estimated sensible and insensible water losses.

It is well known that hypo-osmolality impairs the ability of the kidney to manufacture a dilute urine. Thus, water restriction may be followed by slow improvement at first and by rapid improvement later. If this does not occur, the prognosis is usually grave.

Artifactual Hyponatremia

Plasma ordinarily contains about 93% water and 7% solids. The serum sodium concentration may be affected by the amount of solid present. Marked hyperproteinemia or hyperlipidemia may thus cause falsely low serum sodium concentrations. Osmolality, as determined by freezing point depression, is not significantly affected by this phenomenon. In children this is most common in diabetes and nephrotic syndrome.

2. HYPERNATREMIA

Hypernatremia always implies a deficit of water with respect to solute throughout the entire body. Therefore, it always indicates hyperosmolality. It may arise primarily from too little water or too much solute but is usually due to a combination of both. Hypernatremia is said to exist whenever the $[Na^+]_S$ exceeds 148 mEq/liter. Values over 160 mEq/liter are serious, yet patients have survived $[Na^+]_S$ in excess of 190 mEq/liter. Serious hypernatremia frequently causes intracerebral bleeding, brain damage, and subsequent mental retardation, convulsions, and death.

Hypernatremia Due to Primary Inability to Maintain Normal Body Water Content

A. Inadequate Water Intake: Patients who are denied access to water (or are unable to retain water, as in diabetes insipidus) are at risk of developing hypernatremia. Renal water conservation becomes extreme, but sensible and insensible water losses through the skin and lungs are unavoidable and, if continued, may cause hypernatremia. Unconscious patients and certain retardates are unable to communicate thirst and may develop water deficiency hypernatremia in spite of normal osmoregulatory capability.

B. Defective Osmoregulation: Tumors in or near the anterior hypothalamus, the third ventricle, the cerebral aqueduct, and certain other lesions associated with noncommunicating hydrocephalus may destroy the perception of thirst.

Patients with hypothalamic or hypophyseal (vasopressin-sensitive) diabetes insipidus, although generally thirst-perceptive, are at risk of developing hypernatremia if denied access to water.

Also at risk are patients with nephrogenic (vasopressin-resistant) diabetes insipidus and those with chronic hypercalciuria or chronic hypokalemia, both of which cause a vasopressin-resistant clinical picture similar to diabetes insipidus. In recovery from acute tubular necrosis, a water-losing state may exist.

C. Extrarenal Water Loss: Large sensible and insensible water losses occurring through the skin and lungs may predispose to hypernatremia. Patients with burns over large areas, prolonged high fevers, heat exhaustion (occasionally), hyperpnea due to diabetic ketoacidosis or salicylism, and patients with tracheostomies are all at risk.

Hypernatremia Due to Primary Salt Overloading

Salt overloading most commonly occurs when salt is accidentally used instead of sugar in making up the formula. In severe cases, the symptoms, signs, and treatment are the same as in hypertonic dehydration. If the mistake is detected early in an otherwise healthy infant, serum sodium levels may be restored by administration of chlorothiazide in a dose of 8 mg/kg/24 hours for 1 or 2 days. Peritoneal dialysis has been used effectively.

Hypernatremia Due to Water Loss in the Presence of Solute Gain

A. Hypernatremia Due to Infantile Diarrhea: This type of hypernatremia begins by lowering the ECF volume. The usual mechanisms of sodium and water conservation (thirst, vasopressin secretion, and aldosterone secretion) are called into play. If the patient is fed a high sodium load, hypernatremia may develop.

B. Hypernatremia Due to Large Solute Loads: The solute load required to produce hypernatremia need not be particularly rich in NaCl. Tube feeding of protein-rich foods to an unconscious patient or an infant creates a heavy solute load for renal excretion and results in an osmotic diuresis with the loss of much more water than salt. Hypernatremia may quickly follow if additional water is not provided. Chronic glycosuria in uncontrolled diabetes mellitus occasionally leads to hypernatremia in this fashion, as does overzealous therapy with mannitol or the absorption of the breakdown products of a gastrointestinal hemorrhage.

The signs and symptoms are referable to CNS dysfunction. Irritability, twitching, mental confusion, stupor, irregular respirations, frank convulsions, and eventually coma may occur. Thirst is severe, but the patient may be unable to swallow solid foods owing to the dryness of his mucosa. Weight loss may be severe, amounting to 20–25% of the body weight. There may be moderate fever, evidently due to lack of substrate with which to sweat.

Skin turgor may be normal, but the skin often feels "doughy" and inelastic. Subcutaneous fat may feel stiff or unusually firm. Pulse and blood pressure are usually normal. The hemoglobin tends to rise, MCV decreases, and the hematocrit changes little. BUN may be greatly elevated (> 100 mg/100 ml). Red cells, hyaline and granular casts, and protein appear in the urine.

Treatment consists of restoring deficits in ECW with isotonic solutions followed by slow, careful reduction of the $[Na^+]_S$ at a rate that should not exceed 15 mEq/24 hours. This is best accomplished by administering solutions which contain sodium concentrations about 60 mEq less than the patient's $[Na^+]_S$, with the rate of administration being governed by frequent laboratory determinations of $[Na^+]_S$. The $[Na^+]_S$ should never be lowered rapidly because doing so may precipitate convulsions. The administration of hypertonic saline solution may be helpful if convulsions do occur.

Patients with hypernatremia frequently have metabolic acidosis. Rapid alkalinization with sodium bicarbonate should not be attempted unless the acidemia is severe, since alkalinization enhances CNS irritability. Hypocalcemia commonly accompanies hypernatremia, although the reason for it is not clear. Therapy with calcium is, however, seldom necessary.

Lastly, not all patients with hyperosmolality have hypernatremia. The presence of large quantities of glucose may osmotically draw water into the plasma from the cells. The presence in the blood of 100 mg/100 ml of glucose is approximately equivalent to 2 mEq/liter added to the $[Na^+]_S$. A patient with a blood glucose concentration of 800 mg/100 ml and a $[Na^+]_S$ of 140 mEq/liter thus has about the same osmolality as a patient with a $[Na^+]_S$ of 156 mEq/liter. These changes are a complication of intravenous alimentation. Urea also contributes to osmolality, and uremia is frequently associated with a hyperosmolal state. However, because urea readily crosses cell membranes, shrinkage of the ICF volume does not occur.

POTASSIUM DISORDERS

Physiology

The total body potassium (TBK$^+$) of a 20 kg child is normally about 900 mEq. Roughly 20 mEq of this is in extracellular fluid; the remainder is intracellular. The $[TBK^+]$ has been measured by whole cadaver analysis and by counting the naturally occurring $^{40}K^+$ in whole body counters in "background-free" rooms. Ninety to 95% of the total body K$^+$ is more or less freely exchangeable, and this quantity, the "exchangeable K$^+$," may be assessed by following the 24- to 48-hour dilutional distribution of an injection of $^{40}K^+$ or $^{42}K^+$. Tissue $[K^+]$ may be investigated in muscle biopsy specimens, but such studies require rather broad inferences in their interpretation. $[K^+]_S$ is the only simple potassium determination available in most laboratories and is usually the only direct assessment of $[K^+]$ available to the physician. Red blood cell $[K^+]$ does not reflect total body or intracellular $[K^+]$.

The preponderance of K$^+$ lies within cells—about 60% of it specifically within skeletal muscle cells. Expressed as $[K^+]$/kg body weight, $[TBK^+]$ correlates well with total body water, lean body mass, and fat-free dry solid. The correlation of $[TBK^+]$ with weight falls off in obese patients and in those with malnutrition due to starvation or wasting illness. Postpubertal females tend to have less $[K^+]$/kg of body weight than postpubertal males, owing chiefly to differences in total body fat content. Neonates contain roughly 35–40 mEq/kg, a value which increases gradually to 50–55 mEq/kg in adult males and changes little throughout life in females.

Maintenance of normal $[K^+]_S$ is primarily dependent upon the Na$^+$-K$^+$ pump at the cell membrane. The normal skeletal muscle $[K^+]$ approximates 150–160 mEq/liter cell water. For comparison, in extracellular fluid the $[K^+]$ is normally only 4.5–5 mEq/liter.

The second most important regulator of $[K^+]$ is the kidney. The normal kidney is able to excrete a large load of K$^+$ but is poorly equipped to conserve K$^+$ on short notice. A massive crush injury which damages the integrity of large numbers of cell membranes and causes renal shutdown due to myoglobinuria and shock is, as might be expected, one of the quickest ways to dangerously elevate the $[K^+]_S$.

The distribution of K$^+$ between ICF and ECF is dependent upon ECF pH. Alkalemia promotes entry of K$^+$ into cells and lowers $[K^+]_S$. Acidemia, on the other hand, promotes exit of K$^+$ from cells and may raise $[K^+]_S$ if renal K$^+$ excretion lags behind. Nevertheless, the presence of symptoms or ECG changes (see below) which are referable to a potassium disturbance should always be taken seriously regardless of whether or not acid-base abnormalities are, in part, responsible.

When glycogen deposition occurs, K$^+$ enters cells and the serum level tends to fall. This is one of the factors explaining the low $[K^+]_S$ seen in diabetics following institution of insulin therapy. The Na$^+$-K$^+$ pump requires energy in the form of ATP. Uncoupling of oxidative phosphorylation, therefore, evokes rises in $[K^+]_S$.

$[K^+]_S$ may be raised artifactually in a number of ways. Hemolysis of red cells occurring between the time of sampling and centrifuging is well known and requires that blood drawn for $[K^+]_S$ determination be handled gently. Elevations of $[K^+]_S$ in patients with acute intravenous hemolysis are more difficult to evaluate. Storing of blood samples on ice (without freezing) is followed by rises in $[K^+]_S$. Blood with a grossly elevated leukocyte count (as in leukemia) may show artifactual elevations in $[K^+]_S$ due to damage of the leukocytes during clotting. Platelets are also rich in K$^+$, and thrombocythemic blood samples may show hyperkalemia if clotting is allowed to occur. The simple alternative is to do $[K^+]$ determinations on fresh plasma rather than serum.

Renal Aspects of $[K^+]$ Control

Under normal circumstances, the K$^+$ filtered by the glomerular membrane is mostly reabsorbed in the proximal tubule. Most of the potassium excreted is the product of distal tubular secretion. The quantity secreted by the distal tubular cells appears to result from an exchange with Na^+ from the distal tubular urine.

The amount of K^+ secreted also appears to depend on there being an adequate amount of Cl^- (or other directly reabsorbable anion) in the glomerular filtrate.

This may be more clearly understood by considering 2 glomerular filtrates: one contains 130, 105, and 25 mEq/liter of Na^+, Cl^-, and HCO_3^- respectively. The other contains only 85 mEq/liter of Cl^- plus 20 mEq/liter of nonreabsorbable anion (A^-). In the first filtrate, 105 mEq of Na^+ are resorbed by active transport and at the same time 105 mEq Cl^- are resorbed passively to maintain electroneutrality. Twenty-five mEq/liter of $NaHCO_3^-$ now remain. Twenty-five mEq/liter of H^+ are secreted in exchange for Na^+, the $[H^+] + [HCO_3^-] \rightarrow H_2CO_3 \rightarrow CO_2 + H_2O$. All the Na^+ has now been resorbed. In the second filtrate only 85 mEq of $NaCl$ may be resorbed, leaving 25 mEq of $NaHCO_3$ and 20 mEq of Na A^-. A 25 mEq/liter H^+ exchange for Na^+ occurs as before, but further H^+ secretion will now meet with an increasing H^+ gradient so that K^+ rather than H^+ will be exchanged for Na^+ across the inner tubule membrane.

Renal K^+ excretion may exceed 1000 mEq/1.73 sq m/24 hours. On the other hand, if dietary K^+ intake is totally curtailed, K^+ excretion will continue, decreasing only gradually for 2–3 weeks, by which time a significant negative K^+ balance will exist. The finding of a lowered urinary $[K^+]$ strongly implies that a K^+ depleted state exists and virtually excludes a renal K^+ wasting condition as the cause.

A number of factors enhance the renal secretion of K^+. Hypochloremia (eg, due to vomiting, prolonged nasogastric suction, $AgNO_3^-$ treatment of burns, chloridorrhea, or diuretic therapy) has been mentioned. Adrenal corticosteroids, by causing renal retention of Na^+, increase the quantity of Na^+ reaching the distal tubules and invoke wastage of K^+. If dietary Na^+ intake is minimized, corticosteroid-induced K^+ loss ceases. Diuretics of many types—in particular, thiazides, mercurials, and acetazolamide—effectively enhance the secretion of K^+.

Potassium Depletion

When 10–20% of the TBK^+ of the patient has been lost, symptoms of apathy and muscular weakness ensue. Paresthesias and tetany are occasionally seen. If the depletion worsens, the muscular weakness extends to a flaccid paralysis, eventually interfering with respiration. Extracellular replacement of K^+ may suffice to bring about dramatic but temporary relief from the muscular disability of K^+ depletion, but only as long as the K^+-containing infusion is running.

During serious K^+ depletion, typical ECG changes occur. These include T wave depression, the appearance of a U wave, and eventually ST segment depression. The Q–T interval may appear prolonged if a Q–U interval is mistakenly measured instead. A number of arrhythmias occur (Fig 37–5).

In the kidney, concentrating ability is impaired and a clinical picture similar to that of diabetes insipidus is produced which gives rise, occasionally, to hypernatremia. Tubular degeneration is seen on renal biopsy. Of the effects of hypokalemia, this is the slowest to resolve after proper therapy, and 2–3 weeks may be required for restoration of normal renal function. K^+ depletion also predisposes to digitalis intoxication, and a $[K^+]_S$ determination is always indicated when digitalis toxicity exists.

The treatment of K^+ depletion is to restore a $[K^+]_S$ sufficient to dispel any signs of muscular weakness or ECG abnormalities and to return the $[TBK^+]$ to normal. Such replacement may require several days.

Chronic K^+ depletion frequently complicates hypochloremic metabolic alkalosis. Until the Cl^- deficiency is corrected, administered K^+ continues to be wasted. The administration of KCl, therefore, corrects both the metabolic alkalosis and the K^+ depletion at the same time. The administration of K^+ with virtually any other anion (see above) effectively corrects neither. A variety of K^+-containing foods and juices provide excellent oral medication for this purpose (Table 37–6).

Changes in pH effect changes in the distribution of K^+ between intracellular and extracellular fluid. Acidemia causes K^+ to leave cells and enter the ECW, raising the $[K^+]_S$. Alkalemia causes the reverse. A normal $[K^+]_S$ in the presence of acidemia, therefore, suggests that K^+ depletion exists and that rapid correction of pH may be followed by a brisk fall in $[K^+]_S$. This is commonly seen during correction of diabetic ketoacidosis and acidosis which attends diarrhea. The deposition of glycogen also sequesters substantial amounts of K^+ in such instances.

Up to 5 mEq/kg/24 hours of additional KCl may be given to infants and small children as a correctional measure (in addition to maintenance K^+); 1–2 mEq/kg/24 hours may be given to older children. As K^+ depletion is corrected, the amount and especially the rate of administration should be lowered lest hyperkalemia occur. Actually, intravenous K^+ therapy in excess of that required for maintenance is not necessary to relieve symptoms of K^+ depletion; therefore, K^+ depletion should be treated without haste.

All intravenous K^+ should be evenly infused throughout the 24-hour balance period. If concentrations of K^+ greater than 40 mEq/liter are present in any bottle of intravenous solution, nurses should be given a maximum rate for the infusion. Concentrated K^+ solution must never be given by intravenous "push."

Hyperkalemia

The symptoms and signs of hyperkalemia are few. They include muscle weakness and, occasionally, tetany or paresthesias with ascending central paralysis. The major toxic symptoms and signs are cardiac in origin. ECG changes include tenting and then elevation of T waves, spreading of the QRS complex, atrial arrest, and, finally, a sine wave followed by ventricular

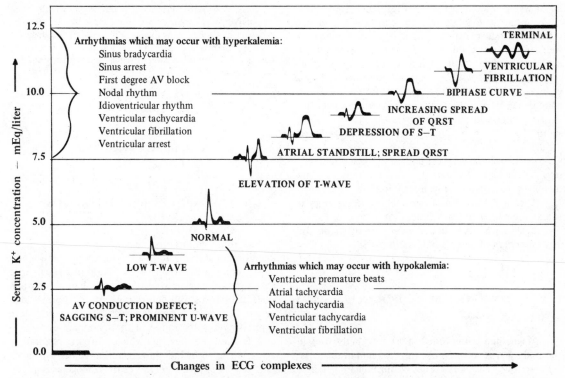

FIG 37–5. Rough correlation between $[K^+]_S$ and the ECG. (In hyperkalemia, the cardiotoxicity at a given $[K^+]_S$ becomes more marked by a decrease of $[Na^+]_S$. Thus, with severe hyponatremia, far-advanced cardiotoxicity may be seen with a $[K^+]_S$ of 7.5 mg/liter. (Reproduced, with permission, from Krupp MA, Chatton MJ: *Current Diagnosis & Treatment.* Lange, 1972.)

fibrillation and death. These changes, with their attendant arrhythmias, are shown in Fig 37–5.

The extent of treatment required depends upon the severity of the hyperkalemia, the ECG findings, the electrolyte profile of the serum, and the predicted behavior of the underlying disorder.

Ordinarily, $[K^+]_S$ values less than 6.5 mEq/liter require little more than curtailment of all K^+ intake. However, such levels might cause serious concern if, for example, QRS complex widening were noted, if the $[Na^+]_S$ were low, if alkalemia existed, if a previous value indicated a sharp rate of rise of $[K^+]_S$, if acute renal failure had occurred, or if digitalis toxicity were evident.

Serious hyperkalemia (levels greater than 8 mEq/liter) or serious ECG changes (widened QRS complexes, heart block, ventricular arrhythmias, etc) warrant vigorous measures. These are aimed at accomplishing 4 objectives: (1) counteracting the depolarization of cardiac muscle, (2) shifting K^+ from serum into cells, (3) ridding the body of excess K^+, and (4) preventing tissue catabolism.

Depolarization of cardiac muscle may be effectively counteracted for several minutes by administration of Ca^{++}. A slow intravenous infusion of 0.2–0.5 ml/kg of 10% calcium gluconate is given over 2–10 minutes. The infusion should be stopped at the first sign of bradycardia. It should be stressed that while Ca^{++} infusion may be lifesaving, it has no effect on $[K^+]_S$ and its cardiac effects are of brief duration.

K^+ may be shifted into cells by administration of sodium in high amounts, by raising the pH with HCO_3^-, and by promoting the deposition of intracellular glycogen with glucose. $NaHCO_3$ is usually marketed in hypertonic form in ampules which contain 44.6 mEq/50 ml. One to 3 ml/kg (at ampule strength) is given over a 5- to 20-minute time span by intravenous infusion. Ten to 20% glucose solutions may also be infused over 30–60 minutes at a dose of 1 gm/kg body weight. The effects of these measures may persist for several hours.

K^+ may be removed from the body by oral or rectal administration of ion exchange resins in their Na^+ or Ca^{++} cycles. For example, 0.2 gm/kg of sodium polystyrene sulfonate (Kayexalate) is mixed with 3–4

TABLE 37–6. Juices high in potassium.

	Approximate Content*	
	mEq	mg
Apple juice	3	100
Apricot juice	2.4	94
Pineapple juice	4	140
Grape juice	3	120
Grapefruit juice	4	150
Orange juice	5	190
Prune juice	7	260
Tomato juice	6	230

*1/2 cup quantities

ml of water or syrup per gram of resin and given orally or by intragastric tube; or 1 gm/kg of resin is mixed into a loose slurry with water and administered as a well mixed retention enema into the sigmoid or descending colon, where it is held for 4–8 hours and then flushed out with isotonic saline solution. In an emergency $[K^+]_S$ may be rapidly lowered by the administration of insulin, 0.25 unit/kg subcutaneously, or 0.1 unit/kg intravenously. Each unit of insulin should be covered by 3 gm of glucose given orally or intravenously.

Peritoneal dialysis–or, preferably, hemodialysis–may be used to rid the body of K^+ but only at some increased risk and a significant cost in time.

The administration of maximal calories is of great value in minimizing tissue catabolism.

Lastly, whenever hyperkalemia occurs, stop the administration of all oral and parenteral K^+.

MAGNESIUM DISORDERS

Magnesium is the fourth most abundant cation in the body and is second only to potassium in the intracellular water and soft tissues. Approximately 1/2 of the total body magnesium is contained in bone; the remainder exists primarily in the intracellular water of the soft tissues, where it acts as a cofactor in a wide spectrum of enzymic reactions.

Clinical Findings

Clinically, hypomagnesemia can present with muscular weakness and wasting, irritability, a positive Chvostek sign with a negative Trousseau sign, vertigo, tremors, and, in the newborn especially, convulsions. Hypomagnesemia (serum levels < 1 mEq/liter) are seen in the newborn as a familial condition or with hypoparathyroidism; in older infants and children, with malabsorption syndromes, protein-calorie malnutrition, chronic renal disease, and renal tubular dystrophies; and in diabetic acidosis and hyperparathyroidism.

Hypermagnesemia may be seen in the newborn if the mother has been given magnesium sulfate and in older children in renal failure. It is usually asymptomatic, but levels of over 6 mEq/liter may produce drowsiness and levels of over 10 mEq/liter may cause respiratory failure and heart block.

Treatment

Hypomagnesemia can be treated by administering magnesium intravenously as magnesium sulfate in amounts sufficient to restore the magnesium deficit in the extracellular water (Table 37–3). Magnesium sulfate may also be given orally in doses of 0.25 gm/kg/dose.

Hypermagnesemia only requires treatment in renal failure, where, in extreme cases, it would justify dialysis.

Friedman M & others: Primary hypomagnesaemia with secondary hypocalcaemia in an infant. Lancet 1:703, 1967.
Niklasson E: Familial early hypoparathyroidism associated with hypomagnesemia. Acta paediat scandinav 59:715, 1970.
Stromme JH: Familial hypomagnesemia. Acta paediat scandinav 58:433, 1969.

ACID-BASE DISORDERS

1. CHRONIC RESPIRATORY ACIDOSIS

Chronic respiratory acidosis involves a gradual impairment of the rate of CO_2 removal by the lungs, with a consequent trend to low blood pH. It can arise with normal lungs as a result of CNS damage or when skeletal or chest wall deformities prevent normal lung volume changes during the respiratory cycle. More typically, it results from primary pulmonary disease.

Disease entities in which chronic respiratory acidosis is seen include bulbar poliomyelitis, advanced muscular dystrophy, polymyositis, osteogenesis imperfecta, rickets, chronic severe asthma, and cystic fibrosis.

Clinically, the patient is dyspneic, shows peripheral cyanosis with clubbing of the fingernails, and may be uncooperative, disagreeable, depressed, and occasionally confused. Laboratory data typically show pH values only slightly below normal (7.27–7.35). The P_{CO_2} is, by definition, abnormally high, and base excess values are significantly elevated above normal (+3 to +15 mEq/liter). The elevated base excess values derive from augmented renal conservation of HCO_3^-, a so-called "compensatory mechanism" which acts to prevent dangerous depressions in pH.

Treatment

Treatment consists of correcting the ventilatory problem to the fullest possible degree, making sure that adequate oxygenation is achieved, and occasionally providing sufficient quantities of $NaHCO_3$ to effect near-complete compensation, ie, to normalize the pH in the presence of an abnormally high P_{CO_2}. Na^+ administration should be carefully controlled in the presence of cardiovascular complications.

2. ACUTE RESPIRATORY ACIDOSIS

Acute respiratory acidosis involves an abruptly developing retention of CO_2 and consequent H_2CO_3 elevation, as a result of which blood pH may fall abruptly. Acute respiratory acidosis can result from a variety of causes: perfusion failure (due to cardiac arrest, ventricular fibrillation), respiratory failure (due to CNS damage, poliomyelitis), upper airway obstruction (due to croup, epiglottitis, aspiration of foreign body), lower airway obstruction (due to asthma, aspiration of vomitus), and ventilation/perfusion disturbances (due to hyaline membrane disease).

Clinically, the patient is acutely air hungry; chest wall retraction may be evident; accessory muscles of respiration may be in use; and the patient is commonly dusky or frankly cyanotic.

Laboratory data include an elevated P_{CO_2}; a lowered arterial blood pH, occasionally to levels below 7.0; and a variable depression in base excess which usually ranges from −5 to −15 mEq/liter. The acidemia results directly from acute hypercapnia.

A greater hypobasemia is observed in premature and newborn infants with acute respiratory acidosis. This is chiefly because prematures have larger ISF volumes (on a percentage basis) than older children and adults.

Treatment

The management of acute respiratory acidosis depends upon the underlying cause. In cases due to acute upper airway obstruction, relief of the obstruction may be the only measure required. If it is impossible to correct the lesion, adequate ventilation should be provided by mouth-to-mouth resuscitation, mechanical ventilation, etc. If artificial ventilation is not feasible or advisable (as in most cases of hyaline membrane disease), therapy with buffer base may be started. The buffer base of choice is $NaHCO_3$, and whenever possible it is given until the blood pH has been restored to normal. This is frequently impossible when the P_{CO_2} has risen above about 70 mm Hg owing to the intolerably large Na^+ loads required. Most authorities feel that the hazards of rapid correction are significant and recommend several hours of $NaHCO_3$ infusion to alleviate acute acidemia of respiratory origin. $NaHCO_3$ should not be administered as it comes from ampules but diluted to near isosmolality (150 mEq/liter).

3. RESPIRATORY ALKALOSIS

Respiratory alkalosis is characterized by hyperventilation which lowers the P_{CO_2} below normal and thereby tends to raise the pH of blood above normal. The hyperventilation is nearly always the result of abnormal CNS stimulation and thus is usually seen in one of 3 clinical settings: hysterical hyperventilation, salicylate or salicylamide poisoning, or irritative CNS disorders such as meningitis and encephalitis.

Clinically, the patient may experience paresthesias about the fingers, toes, and lips. He may complain of dizziness, faintness, palpitations, heart pain, and even a band-like feeling about the chest. Hypocalcemic tetany is occasionally observed, and susceptible patients may have convulsions. Hyperventilation is usually apparent, and in salicylate intoxication this may mimic the Kussmaul respirations seen in diabetic ketoacidosis.

Laboratory data are helpful. The P_{CO_2} is depressed, occasionally to levels as low as 10 or 15 mm Hg. Arterial pH values above 7.65 are sometimes reported. Acutely, the base excess tends to be normal or slightly low. With greater chronicity (several days), base excess values as low as −15 mEq/liter may be observed. Whether such depressions in base excess derive from a compensatory process is not known, although hypocapnia stimulates red cells to produce abnormally large quantities of lactic acid.

Treatment

The management of respiratory alkalosis depends upon the disorder. If hysterical hyperventilation is the cause, simple rebreathing into a paper bag followed by administration of tranquilizers or psychotherapy (or both) usually suffices. If the disorder is caused by salicylate intoxication, management consists of suitable fluid and electrolyte administration to enhance excretion of the drug. If the patient is younger than about 4 years of age, metabolic acidosis with significant acidemia may soon supervene. Accordingly, zealous treatment of respiratory alkalosis due to salicylate intoxication is seldom practiced. Prolonged irritative CNS lesions may require administration of 2–4% CO_2. Apparatus designed to increase dead space or to allow partial rebreathing may be helpful. Careful laboratory monitoring of acid-base values is essential. The most effective therapy is usually directed at the underlying lesion.

4. METABOLIC ACIDOSIS

Metabolic acidosis is that primary pathophysiologic process which tends to lower the pH of blood by causing abnormal production or retention of strong nonvolatile acid, or by enhancing the loss of buffer base.

A wide variety of illnesses are associated with metabolic acidosis. Abnormal acid production is seen, eg, in diabetic or starvational ketoacidosis, lactic acidosis due to tissue hypoxia or metabolic poisoning, and ingestion of a large number of acidic or acidogenic products such as NH_4Cl, ethylene glycol, etc. Diminished acid excretion is seen in renal failure, primary renal tubular dystrophies of several kinds, and in renal hypoperfusion due to dehydration, shock, and other causes. Abnormal base loss causes metabolic acidosis in occasional diarrheal states (especially cholera) in which the stools are strongly alkaline. Biliary fistulas and certain HCO_3^- wasting nephropathies also produce metabolic acidosis by this route.

Regardless of the route, the clinical and laboratory pictures are similar. There is significant hypobasemia. Base excess values as low as −23 mEq/liter are occasionally encountered. There is usually a brisk compensatory hyperventilation, but compensation is seldom, if ever, complete. Arterial blood pH values lower than 7.0 are sometimes found.

Treatment

Management consists of the administration of $NaHCO_3$ and appropriate treatment of the underlying disorder. There is no advantage to using lactate, phosphate, citrate, or tromethamine instead of $NaHCO_3$. Once the pH approaches 7.25 or 7.30, then the rate of correction may be tapered. The compensatory hyperventilation which usually attends serious metabolic acidosis ordinarily requires 1–2 days to abate once hypobasemia has been resolved. If full correction of hypobasemia is undertaken in the first few hours of treatment, a transient (though seldom severe) respiratory alkalosis may occur. As usual, acid-base therapy is directed toward achieving a blood pH of 7.40 and then keeping the pH at that level.

In most cases, the objective is to correct the base excess in extracellular fluid within 24 hours. The dose of $NaHCO_3$ is calculated according to the following formula:

Dose of $NaHCO_3$ (mEq) = 0.3 × body weight (kg) × base excess. This formula usually provides a dose of bicarbonate that fully corrects the negative base excess.

When calculating the total daily requirement, equivalent amounts of sodium and chloride must be deducted from maintenance or replacement solutions.

5. METABOLIC ALKALOSIS

Metabolic alkalosis is caused by losses of excessive quantities of strong, nonvolatile acid or excessive gains of buffer base. The most frequent cause of metabolic alkalosis is loss of gastric fluid (HCl) via nasogastric tube or vomiting. Vomiting due to pyloric obstruction (eg, pyloric stenosis) is especially prone to cause metabolic alkalosis since the acidic emesis fluid is not contaminated with pancreatic (alkaline) fluid.

Any condition which selectively depletes the patient of Cl^- is prone to cause a metabolic acidosis in which hypokalemia, hypochloremia, hyperkaluria, and paradoxical aciduria are prominent features. Besides vomiting and nasogastric suction, diuretics, silver nitrate treatment of burns, and certain chronic diarrheas ("chloridorrheas") are well known causes.

Likewise, any condition which selectively conserves Na^+ without selectively conserving Cl^- results in the same syndrome, the only difference being a normal $[Cl^-]_S$. Examples include Calgagno's syndrome, adrenal 11β-hydroxylase deficiency, and certain juxtamedullary tumors of the kidney.

The laboratory picture is classical and consists of elevated blood pH, elevated base excess, and normal to very slightly elevated P_{CO_2}. Respiratory compensation appears to be limited, however, by oxygen need. A

common denominator underlies most cases of metabolic alkalosis, viz, a widened gap between $[Na^+]_S$ and $[Cl^-]_S$ (see p 920).

Treatment

The mainstay of management is the administration of Cl^-. A common misconception exists that K^+ is essential to treat the alkalosis. This is now known not to be so. Cl^-, as NaCl, KCl, or NH_4Cl, will correct the alkalosis. K^+ plus Cl^- is required to repair the K^+ depletion. Potassium gluconate, acetate, citrate, and bicarbonate have all been shown to be ineffective in treating either the K^+ depletion or the metabolic alkalosis.

PLANNING & ADMINISTRATION OF INTRAVENOUS FLUIDS

WRITING INTRAVENOUS FLUID ORDERS

Once maintenance and correctional requirements have been calculated and combined into 24-hour totals, intravenous fluid orders may be written. Some rounding-off of numbers is permissible in older children, but small infants should receive intravenous fluids almost exactly as calculated. Unless emergency considerations dictate otherwise, the 24-hour totals are evenly administered over a 24-hour balance period. The necessity for regular review of fluid orders in the light of clinical changes and ongoing laboratory data cannot be overestimated.

The sequence number and composition of each bottle should be stated in the orders and on the bottles themselves.

It is preferable that intravenous infusions for small children be constituted in a number of small bottles rather than a single large one. If 24-hour totals are mixed in a single bottle and then delivered to the patient by way of a smaller increment chamber (eg, Pedatrol or Metriset), then a hemostat should be placed between the large reservoir bottle and the increment chamber. As a general rule, quantities exceeding 150 ml should not be connected to children under 2 years of age, nor should quantities greater than 250 ml be connected to children under 5, nor quantities greater than 500 ml to children under 10.

All orders for intravenous fluids should contain specific instructions regarding the rate of infusion for each bottle. It is convenient to use a microdrop apparatus which delivers 60 drops/ml. When this is done, microdrops/minute equals ml/hour, and the rate of infusion may be readily calculated by dividing volume in ml by time in hours. Bottles containing K^+ should contain· instructions regarding the maximum rate of infusion lest a nurse fall behind schedule and try to catch up.

All orders for intravenous fluid therapy should be accompanied by orders to record careful daily weights and intake and output.

All output, whether gastric fluid or urine, should be saved and measured at the end of each therapy period. All empty or partly emptied intravenous fluid bottles should also be saved for the duration of each period.

ROUTES OF PARENTERAL FLUID ADMINISTRATION

A variety of routes other than the intravenous one are available for administration of parenteral fluids. These include hypodermoclysis, proctoclysis, and the intraperitoneal and intramedullary (bone marrow) routes. These are poor substitutes for intravenous infusion. Scalp vein needles have been perfected to such a degree that the above routes are seldom if ever indicated. If a vein cannot be found and it is important to use intravenous fluids, a venous cutdown should be performed.

HAZARDS IN THE ADMINISTRATION OF INTRAVENOUS FLUIDS

Infection is usually preventable with proper hygiene and rotation of sites. If an intravenous or cutdown site becomes infected, the site should be changed and appropriate therapy begun.

Sloughing can occur due to extravasation of hypertonic fluids, inadvertent administration into an artery, or pressure necrosis. Adequate padding is essential, especially beneath the heel when veins in the dorsum of the foot are used.

Rapid injection of certain substances may be fatal. K^+-induced ventricular fibrillation is a well known hazard. Rapid Ca^{++} infusion may cause cardiac arrest which is preceded by bradycardia. Ca^{++} infusions should never be given without monitoring the pulse. NH_4Cl or any NH_4^+-containing salt should never be given to patients with liver disease and should never be injected rapidly. A slow, even infusion over 24 hours, at a rate well below 0.1 mEq/kg/minute, does not exceed the normal hepatic clearance of NH_4^+. Sudden death may occur if given otherwise. Tromethamine (THAM-E) causes respiratory arrest if rapidly infused and offers no advantages over $NaHCO_3$.

KEEPING AN INTRAVENOUS INFUSION RUNNING

A variety of means may be employed to prolong the usable life of an intravenous site. Adequate immobilization of the site is extremely important, and so is nontraumatic insertion of the needle. This may sometimes be facilitated by warming the extremity around the vein and by the infiltration of small amounts of 1% lidocaine (Xylocaine).

Metal needles last longer than plastic catheters. Whichever is used, constant vigilance must be maintained for signs of phlebitis. Silastic (silicone rubber) tubing has been useful in larger veins.

Hypertonic solutions should be avoided.

The addition of 100 units of heparin and 1 mg of prednisolone to each liter of intravenous solution lengthens the life of a vein without causing significant systemic effects.

SOLUTIONS COMMERCIALLY AVAILABLE FOR PEDIATRIC INTRAVENOUS USE

Carrier Solutions

Dextrose, 2.5%, 250 ml
Dextrose, 5%, 250, 500, and 1000 ml
Dextrose, 10%, 500 ml
Dextrose, 20%, 500 ml
Dextrose, 50%, 50 and 500 ml
Water, 20, 250, and 500 ml

Straight Solutions

Lactated Ringer's injection, 500 ml (contains sodium, 130 mEq/liter, potassium, 4 mEq/liter, calcium, 3 mEq/liter, chloride, 109 mEq/liter, and lactate, 28 mEq/liter)
Dextrose, 2.5%, and sodium chloride, 0.45%, 250 and 500 ml
Dextrose, 5%, and sodium chloride, 0.45%, 250 and 500 ml
Dextrose, 5%, and sodium chloride, 0.9%, 250 and 500 ml
Dextrose, 10%, and sodium chloride, 0.9%, 500 ml
Sodium chloride, 0.9%, 250 and 500 ml
Sodium lactate, 1/6 M, 500 ml

Concentrated Electrolytes

(For Use in Carrier Solutions)
Sodium bicarbonate, 44.6 mEq in 50 ml
Ammonium chloride, 3 mEq/ml in 30 ml
Potassium chloride, 2 mEq/ml in 10 or 20 ml
Sodium chloride, 3 mEq/ml in 30 ml
Potassium phosphate, 3 mEq/ml in 10 ml

Special Solutions

Volume Expander: Dextran, 10% in 0.9% sodium chloride solution
Osmotic Diuretic: Mannitol, 15%, 150 and 500 ml
Hydrolysates:
(1) Casein, 5% (Travamin), dextrose, 5%, and ethanol 5%—Contains the following electrolytes (in mEq/liter) and amino acids (in

mg/100 ml): Na^+, 35; K^+, 18; Ca^{++}, 5; Mg^{++}, 2; Cl^-, 22; $PO_4^=$, 30; leucine, 410; valine, 310; lysine, 310; isoleucine, 260; phenylalanine, 200; threonine, 190; methionine, 130; histidine, 130; and tryptophan, 70.

(2) Casein hydrolysate, 5%, in 5% dextrose (eg, Travamin, Travenol); Hyprotigen is a 10% casein hydrolysate meant to be mixed in equal amounts with 5% dextrose.

For Peritoneal Dialysis: In mEq/liter: Na^+, 141; Ca^{++}, 3.5; Mg^{++}, 1.5; Cl^-, 101; lactate, 45. (Eg, Impersol.)

SPECIAL CLINICAL SITUATIONS

BURNS
(See also Chapter 30.)

One of the most difficult of all fluid balance problems is the treatment of the severely burned child, defined as any second or third degree burn involving more than 15% of the body surface area. Regional approximations of body surface area in children vary from adult norms but may be estimated from Table 37–7.

Fluid balance problems arise because large quantities of extracellular fluids, in particular plasma, are exuded onto the burned surface and into the burn itself. In addition, a poorly understood increased capillary "leakiness" allows transcapillary passage of plasma proteins—especially albumin—into the interstitial fluid. The burn acts as a third space, and hypovolemic shock may quickly ensue.

TABLE 37–7. Percentage of body surface area in infants and children. (After Berkow.)

	Newborn	1 year	5 years	10 years
Head	19	17	13	11
Both thighs	11	13	16	17
Both lower legs	10	10	11	12
Neck	2			
Anterior trunk	13			
Posterior trunk	13			
Both upper arms	8	These percentages		
Both lower arms	6	remain constant at		
Both hands	5	all ages.		
Both buttocks	5			
Both feet	7			
Genitals	1			
	100			

Burns of large areas cause significant immediate hemolysis. In addition, damaged red cells may continue to hemolyze over the next 24–48 hours. The usual danger from hemolysis is not anemia but acute tubular necrosis, which may occur when hemolysis is superimposed on hypovolemic shock. The principal need, therefore, is for expansion of the plasma volume rather than increase of red cell mass.

Early management is facilitated by (1) an indwelling urinary bladder catheter, (2) an indwelling central venous pressure apparatus, and (3) a large-bore catheter inserted via a venous cutdown. In the first 24 hours, establishment of an adequate urine output is vital, and urine volume should be determined hourly for the first 2 days. If prolonged severe shock can be avoided, significant oliguria due to acute tubular necrosis will also be avoided. A falling urinary output then becomes a sensitive indicator of hypovolemia. Central venous pressure measurement becomes mandatory if shock has been prolonged and significant renal damage is suspected. The urinary output should be 0.5 ml/kg/hour or more—preferably at least twice that much. Blood pressure is an insensitive criterion for assessing plasma volume. The hematocrit should be checked several times a day, since a rising hematocrit implies a need for plasma or saline. Serum proteins should also be followed. Rises imply the need for saline; falls may or may not imply a need for albumin.

Initially, an estimate of the needs for colloid (plasma or 5% albumin and saline) must be made. The following modified Brooke formula has been found suitable for children: (0.5 ml colloid + 1.5 ml ECF-like fluid) × % area burned (up to 50%) × body weight in kg = ml of fluid for first 24-hour correction needs. Half of this quantity is given in the first 8 hours and 1/2 in the next 16 hours. This formula is merely a starting point. Once begun, urine output must be sustained and elevations or depressions of central venous pressure prevented regardless of the formula. In addition, basic maintenance requirements for urine and insensible losses must be provided as outlined in Table 37–3 and the accompanying text. All K^+ is deleted from the administered fluids for at least the first 3 days.

During the second day, colloid needs usually fall sharply and colloid may often be discontinued or reduced by 50%, as can the third space ECW-like fluid also. On the second and third postburn days—and once urine output, venous pressure, and hematocrit have been stabilized—the minimum amount of fluid is given to sustain these signs. Usually on the third postburn day, the third space begins to resolve as the sequestered fluid returns to the circulation. Urinary output may increase or it may simply remain adequate. Colloid requirements typically fall to zero, and saline administration should be diminished or deleted as dictated by the needs of the patient. The respiratory rate and the auscultatory status of the lungs should be carefully monitored, along with central venous pressure. Failure to appreciate that a third space is resolving may result in serious ECF excess with pulmonary edema and death. Once the fluid and electrolyte status is secured, oral feeding should be employed.

ANURIA & OLIGURIA

The principles of conserving extracellular water homeostasis in renal failure are the same irrespective of etiology or duration. Careful attention to detail may sustain life for several weeks without the necessity of peritoneal or hemodialysis. Treatment of the primary condition, when possible, is implicit.

The first rule is to keep meticulous input and output records that are clear both to physicians and nursing staff. Reconciliation of these records must be made at regular intervals, never exceeding 24 hours. In difficult problems, calculations should be made on an 8-hour basis. Apart from reports of clinical changes, it is necessary to chart urine volume, patient's weight, and, if possible, plasma pH and levels of Na^+, K^+, Cl^-, and HCO_3^-. It may also be helpful to know the ionic composition of any urine, gastric fluid, etc.

The most difficult problem is to provide calories and to manipulate electrolyte distortions within a limited water intake. A suitable water allowance is 400 ml/sq m/24 hours; to this may be added the volume of passed urine in the previous calculation period plus the volume of any other extraneous losses. Water should be given as 20% dextrose. Electrolyte losses are replaced. Correction problems are dealt with as indicated elsewhere in this chapter. Hyperosmolality or hypernatremia is a considerable problem as it restricts alkali administration unless extracellular water is present in increased amounts. This is of no concern in the short term but may require dialysis if sustained. Hypo-osmolality requires treatment, but at the same time it affords an opportunity to counteract acidosis with parenteral bicarbonate administration. Hyperkalemia is usually satisfactorily managed by potassium restriction. Resins by enema will remove 1 mEq/gm. If necessary, dialysis may be used, and insulin, 0.1 unit/kg IV, may be given in an emergency. Low potassium levels are particularly likely to occur in the period immediately following recovery from acute tubular necrosis. Treatment consists of administering potassium in amounts necessary to restore extracellular levels to the normal range. Acidosis is treated with bicarbonate in the usual manner; it is more important to contain acidosis than normal extracellular water volume unless cardiac failure is present.

The indications for abandoning medical treatment for dialysis are a deteriorating clinical state and intractable acidosis or hyperkalemia.

Finally, it is essential not to neglect caloric intake. Where anuria is complete and due to acute tubular damage which promises to be relatively short-lived (ie, less than 2 weeks), it is advisable to depend entirely on the intravenous route for the first week. Thereafter, if good electrolyte control has been achieved or if some urine flow exists, hard candy and renal cookies can be allowed with some oral water intake.

SALICYLATE POISONING

Salicylate intoxication may occur as a chronic phenomenon in children treated for rheumatoid arthritis. It is seen principally in young children who have had access to a medicine cupboard or have been fed aspirin tablets by an older brother or sister. Occasionally it is the result of a suicide gesture by an older child.

It is important initially to make some judgment of the severity of salicylate poisoning based on the plasma level and of the degree of acidosis. In children under 5, the early phase of respiratory alkalosis is quickly superseded by metabolic acidosis. The physician should know which assay method the laboratory uses. The original ferric nitrate method does not measure salicyl conjugates such as salicylamide. The latter are not as toxic as aspirin itself but may nonetheless cause intoxication, so that a fluorimetric assay should be employed. Knowing whether or not a conjugated derivative was ingested will modify a judgment as to severity. (See Fig 37–6.)

Clinical Findings

Children with salicylate intoxication are hyperventilating, flushed, sweating, dehydrated, febrile, and often vomiting. Laboratory studies show serum salicylate levels over 40 mg/100 ml and abnormal blood-acid base values. Prolonged vomiting may lead to potassium depletion, with low serum levels. Hypoglycemia is occasionally seen. Disorientation, convulsions, and coma are frequent in severe intoxication.

Treatment

The objectives of treatment are to remove residual gastric salicylate content and facilitate urinary excretion by the administration of alkali and to restore normal intracellular potassium levels. In comatose patients, a urinary catheter should be inserted.

The following regimen achieves a half-life of the salicylate level of around 3 hours and, since it can be started immediately, obviates the necessity for more elaborate removal procedures such as exchange transfusion and dialysis. Salicylate levels are reduced 70% within 8 hours.

A. Immediately: Initiate vomiting or lavage to remove remaining salicylate. Give 3 mEq/kg sodium bicarbonate from an ampule containing 44.6 mEq in 50 ml. Repeat, giving 1.5 mEq/kg at intervals of 15, 30, and 45 minutes.

B. Over First 8 Hours: Give 200 mEq/sq m of potassium as potassium citrate orally if possible. Do not start until urine has been passed, and discontinue once urine pH reaches 7.0.

C. Over 24 Hours: Start up to 2000 ml/sq m in the first 8 hours and up to 4000 ml/sq m in the next 24 hours of a 5 or 10% dextrose solution containing 35 mEq/liter of KCl and 35 mEq/liter of $NaHCO_3$. The

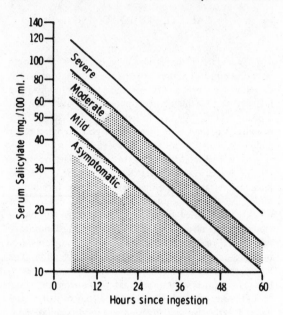

FIG 37–6. Nomogram relating serum salicylate concentration and expected severity of intoxication at varying intervals following ingestion of a single dose of salicylate. (Redrawn and reproduced, with permission, from Done AK: Salicylate intoxication. Pediatrics 26:800, 1960.)

KCl should only be added after urine flow is established. Hypoglycemia is averted by using dextrose solution. Coma may persist after salicylate levels have returned to normal. This is usually associated with cerebral edema and requires treatment with osmotic diuretics such as mannitol.

PREOPERATIVE & POSTOPERATIVE FLUID & ELECTROLYTE MANAGEMENT

Surgery in a child—especially in an infant—should be deferred until fluid and electrolyte balance has been achieved and his general nutritional status is optimal.

Special problems can be corrected according to instructions given elsewhere in this chapter. The following points should be considered.

(1) Complete volume replacements in plasma and ECF prior to surgery. Correct all electrolyte distortions.

(2) Arrange a planned review of fluid, electrolyte, and caloric balance for the operative and postoperative period.

(3) Except for minor procedures, use an intravenous infusion for at least 24 hours postoperatively.

(4) Maintenance fluid and electrolytes should be given evenly over the period of the operation. Whole blood is replaced in proportion to operative losses.

(5) The carrier vehicle for water and electrolytes should be 10% dextrose to provide minimum calories

until normal alimentation is restored. Prolonged parenteral feeding is discussed at the end of this chapter.

PYLORIC STENOSIS

The main problem in pyloric stenosis is that repeated vomiting of gastric contents without diarrhea leads to extracellular water depletion complicated by excessive potassium and chloride losses and metabolic alkalosis.

Consider the example of a typical case in a 3-week-old male infant weighing 3 kg and with the following serum values: Na^+, 140 mEq/liter; K^+, 3.5 mEq/liter; Cl^-, 85 mEq/liter; HCO_3^-, 44 mEq/liter; pH, 7.60; base excess, +19 mEq/liter; and P_{CO_2}, 45 mm Hg.

An infusion of isotonic NaCl is begun at once. Thirty minutes later, when 200 ml have been infused, his skin turgor is much improved and his listlessness diminished.

Basic maintenance and correctional requirements are now calculated (Tables 37–8 and 37–9).

The above case represents an example of severe saline depletion with hypokalemic, hypochloremic metabolic alkalosis due to vomiting from pyloric stenosis. The requirement was made up in 5% dextrose solution and mixed from ampules of electrolyte concentrate. The above totals were evenly administered over a period of 24 hours. On the following day, clinical dehydration had disappeared and all laboratory values were normal except the pH, which was 7.5; the base excess, which was +4 mEq/liter; and the [K^+], which was still slightly low at 4 mEq/liter. Basic maintenance requirements plus a KCl correctional allowance of 2 mEq/kg were given for an additional day, following which all values were normal and surgery was performed.

INTESTINAL OBSTRUCTIONS

In intestinal obstruction the bowel is distended with gas and accumulates substantial volumes of fluid. With continued vomiting there is a variable loss of sodium, potassium, chloride, and hydrogen, leading to reduced extracellular volume with changes in pH and ionic composition. These should be corrected according to the principles established elsewhere in the chapter, but the following guidelines should be observed.

(1) Maintain careful records of laboratory data, weight, etc and renew fluid and electrolyte balance at regular intervals.

(2) Delay surgery until these disturbances are corrected unless it is an emergency.

(3) Maintain continuous nasogastric suction, recording volume and, if necessary, ionic composition and pH of aspirated fluid. This will relieve distention.

TABLE 37–8. Basic maintenance requirements for the first 24 hours in the example (pyloric stenosis) cited above. (Data in part from Table 37–3.)

	ml/kg	ml	Na⁺/kg	Na⁺	K⁺/kg	K⁺	Cl⁻/kg	Cl⁻
Estimated insensible losses	25	75	...	...	...	...	...	...
Estimated urine output	40	120	3	9	3	9	6	18
Estimated gastrointestinal losses*	20	60	2	6	0.2	0.6	2.2	6.6
Maintenance totals		255		15		10		25

*Given only if vomiting continues. It usually does not continue once feedings are started unless there is a continuing gastritis.

TABLE 37–9. Correctional requirements in the example (pyloric stenosis) cited above.

	Volume 5% Dextrose	Na⁺	K⁺	Cl⁻	HCO₃⁻
Saline*	300	45	...	45	...
Acid-base	Will be self-correcting with administration of Cl⁻.				
K⁺ (2 mEq/kg)	...	...	6	6	...
Correctional total	300	45	6	51	...
Total 24-hour fluids	555	60	16	76	...

*200 ml were given initially and are included in this figure.

Give all fluids and calories intravenously until bowel sounds have returned postoperatively and the patient is free of distention and vomiting.

(4) Start alimentation as small frequent feedings, giving not more than 1/4 of the daily requirements by this route in the first 24 hours. Start with water or 0.225% saline in 10% dextrose, and then give fruit juices or milk before starting any solids.

ACUTE INFANTILE GASTROENTERITIS

This is perhaps the most common fluid and electrolyte problem in pediatric practice. The principles of management are illustrated by the following case.

A 1-year-old child is brought to the hospital with a history of profuse watery diarrhea of 2 days' duration. He has vomited virtually all oral intake. On physical examination, his rectal temperature is 39.4° C (103° F), pulse 160 but easily palpated, respiratory rate 56 and deep, weight 8 kg, and blood pressure 84/54. The fontanel is depressed, his eyes are sunken and frequently roll aimlessly, his oral mucosa is dry but not parched, his tongue is small, and his skin turgor is diminished but his skin is pink. Laboratory data are as follows: hematocrit, 45%; [Na⁺]$_S$, 138 mEq/liter; [K⁺]$_S$, 4 mEq/liter; [Cl⁻]$_S$, 106 mEq/liter; pH,

7.15; base excess, −20 mEq/liter; and P_{CO_2}, 24 mm Hg.

Fluid and electrolyte diagnoses are as follows:

(1) ECF depletion (severe), equal to approximately 10% of body weight.

(2) Metabolic acidosis (severe), with acidemia, hypobasemia, and compensatory hypocapnia.

(3) K⁺ depletion. (Note the low-normal [K⁺]$_S$ in the presence of a low pH.)

Fluid and electrolyte requirements are estimated as shown in Tables 37–10 and 37–11.

PROLONGED INTRAVENOUS ALIMENTATION IN INFANTS

Technical advances in major gastrointestinal surgery of young infants have necessitated comparable improvements in postoperative care. Although homeostasis of extracellular water has come to be rather well understood in recent years, data on intravenous nutrition are at present much more limited.

Ideally, a solution intended for intravenous feeding should be simple to prepare, sterile, not injurious to the venous intima, and capable of affording an adequate nutritional intake in a physiologic volume of water. Hypertonic solutions of glucose alone have been used in the past; they must be administered slowly into a large vein to avoid thrombosis, and sudden changes in flow rate may lead to hypoglycemia or hyperglycemia. Because of this, fructose and invert sugar—an equimolar mixture of fructose and glucose—have been extensively used as alternatives, and others such as xylitol are under consideration. To increase caloric intake in relation to volume, cottonseed oil emulsates were at one time popular. However, these led to occasional toxic reactions with a bleeding diathesis, fever, hepatosplenomegaly, and pigmentary deposits in the Kupffer cells. Soybean oil emulsates have now been reintroduced in Sweden. They appear to cause fewer complications, and as experience in their use grows they may become increasingly available in the USA. Intralipid is now approved for experimental use by the FDA.

TABLE 37–10. Basic maintenance requirements for the first 24 hours
in the example (acute infantile gastroenteritis) cited above.

	Fluid		Na^+		K^+		Cl^-	
	ml/kg	ml	mEq/kg	mEq	mEq/kg	mEq	mEq/kg	mEq
Estimated insensible losses	25	200	...	...	...	...	...	...
Estimated urinary output	60	480	3	24	2	16	5	40
Estimated gastro-intestinal losses	...	...	...	...	...	...	...	...
Totals	...	680	...	24	...	16	...	40

TABLE 37–11. Correctional requirements in the example (acute infantile gastroenteritis) cited above.

	Fluid	Na^+	K^+	Cl^-	HCO_3^-
ECW-like fluid (10% body weight)	800	72*	...	72	...
Potassium (2 mEq/kg/ 24 hours)	...	...	16	16	...
Acid-base (0.3 × body weight × base excess)	...	48*	...	...	48
24-hour totals (maintenance plus correction)	1480	144	32	128	48

*Note that part of the 120 mEq of Na^+ needed to make 800 ml of ECW-like fluid is given as NaCl and part as $NaHCO_3$ In actual practice, the above fluids should probably be given rapidly at first and the rate then tapered as clinical improvement is noted.

Most recent experience has been gained with a mixture of fibrin hydrolysate in hypertonic glucose with added minerals, vitamins, and electrolytes. The only nutritional omission is in unsaturated fatty acids, which should theoretically provide 2% of the calories. The incorporation of ethyl linoleate into the parenteral solution as an emulsate is being studied; in the meantime, however, essential fatty acids and trace mineral needs may be satisfied by giving 3 ml/kg of fresh frozen plasma IV every 4 days. For all the apparent simplicity of this program, it should only be undertaken where it is the only feasible means of nourishing the infant, and then only with good laboratory and pharmacy support together with a trained clinical team.

PREPARATION & COMPOSITION OF THE BASIC SOLUTION

The solution described here is one which can be easily dispensed in any well equipped hospital pharmacy. Ideally, it should be prepared in 48-hour batches since changes in sodium, potassium, and other contents may be required. A laminar air flow table should be used to preserve sterility. If such a unit is not available, solutions may be assembled with sterile disposable syringes with millipore filter attachments. The following materials and solutions are required to manufacture the base solution.

Equipment

(1) Laminar air flow table unit (Abbott).
(2) Swinnex-25 millipore filter units (0.22 μ).
(3) Sterile 250 ml vacuum bottles for intravenous use.
(4) Plexitron transfer sets for mixing sterile solution (Travenol).

Composition of Intravenous Solution Per 250 ml Bottle

Casein hydrolysate, 5%, in 5% dextrose with 3.5 mEq Na^+ and 1.8 mEq K^+ (Travamin, Travenol), 150 ml.

50% dextrose solution (Travenol), 100 ml

50% magnesium sulfate in 2 ml ampules (Abbott), 0.08 ml

20% calcium gluconate in 10 ml ampules (Endo), 2 ml

Potassium phosphate, 10 ml ampules (Travenol), 1 ml. (Contains 3 mEq K^+ and 65 mg P per ml.)

Sodium hydroxide in water for injection, 3 ml

Injectable vitamins (MVI), (USV Pharmaceutical Corporation) 1 ml

Sodium heparin, 1000 units/ml (Organon), 0.05 ml

Folvite folic acid solution, 10 ml ampules (Lederle), 0.01 ml. (Dilute 1:100 before use.)

Ducobee-1000, 1000 μg B_{12}/ml in 10 ml ampules (Breon), 0.4 ml

Astrafer injection, 20 mg Fe^{+++}/ml, 5 ml ampules (Astra), 50 μl. (Omit in infants below 3 months of age.)

Amigen and Hyprotigen are other commercial casein hydrolysates; the latter is supplied as a 10% solution. Products should be checked for electrolyte content.

If the above solution is administered at a rate of 125 ml/kg/24 hours, the infant will receive the corresponding amounts of nutrients, minerals, and vitamins shown in Table 37–12. The pH is approximately 7.3.

TABLE 37–12. Daily amounts of nutrients supplied by 125 ml/kg/24 hours of base solution.

Nutrient	Intravenous Administration/ 24 hours	Minimal Daily Requirement*
Total water (liter/sq m)	2.3	2–2.5
kcal/kg	126	100–120
Total amino nitrogen	476	290
(mg/100 kcal)		
Threonine (mg/kg)	118	45–87
Valine (mg/kg)	193	85–105
Methionine (mg/kg)	81	33–45
Isoleucine (mg/kg)	162	102–119
Leucine (mg/kg)	256	76–229
Phenylalanine (mg/kg)	124	47–90
Tryptophan† (mg/kg)	22	15–20
Lysine (mg/kg)	193	110–161
Histidine (mg/kg)	81	16–34
Linoleic acid (mg/100 kcal)		200
(ethyl linoleate)		
Sodium (mEq/kg)	2.7	1–3
Potassium (mEq/kg)	2.4	2–3
Magnesium (mEq/kg)	0.33	1.2
Calcium (mEq/kg)	0.9	2.5
Phosphorus (mg/100 kcal)	26	25
Iron (mg/100 kcal)	0.4	1
Copper (μg/100 kcal)	50	60
Iodine (μg/100 kcal)	< 1	10
Vitamin A (IU/100 kcal)	433	280
Ascorbic acid (mg/100 kcal)	22	8
Thiamine (B_1) (mg/100 kcal)	2.2	0.045
Riboflavin (B_2) (μg/100 kcal)	430	6
Pyridoxine (B_6) (μg/100 kcal)	67	200
Nicotinamide (mg/100 kcal)	4	0.8
Pantothenic acid (mg/100 kcal)	1.1	0.3
Vitamin D (IU/100 kcal)	43	40
Vitamin E (IU/100 kcal)	0.22	0.3
Folic acid (μg/100 kcal)	6	4
Vitamin B_{12} (μg/100 kcal)	174	150

*Figures for minimal daily requirement are based on those for oral feeding.

†Additional nicotinamide is derived from tryptophan in Aminosol.

MANAGEMENT

On the ward in preparation for intravenous alimentation, the following materials must be assembled:

(1) 250 ml bottles of solution described above.

(2) No. 2C0200 Plexitron solution administration set with filter (Travenol). Change every other day.

(3) Silastic tubing, 0.025 inches inner diameter, 0.047 inches outer diameter.

(4) Intramedic liver stub adaptors No. A1030/23, 23 gauge (Clay-Adams Inc).

The surgical staff should be requested to insert the catheter into the junction of the superior vena cava and the right atrium via the right external jugular vein.

The position should be confirmed by fluoroscopy. This should be done under sterile conditions and the catheter should then be passed through a subcutaneous tunnel from the right parietal area. The catheter opening on the skin should be sealed with polymyxin-bacitracin-neomycin (Neosporin) ointment and dressed with dry sterile gauze. The area should be cared for by the physician himself and inspected and redressed at least every 48 hours. The catheter itself should be changed every 48 hours. The solution should be administered at a rate of 125 mg/kg given evenly throughout the 24-hour period. Initially, however, a 1/2 strength solution in 5% dextrose should be used. The authors have not found it necessary to use a constant infusion pump. The system should not be used for drawing routine venous samples. Prophylactic antibiotics should not be given. Meticulous clinical, microbiologic, and biochemical monitoring is imperative, particularly in the first days of the regimen. Urine osmolality, glucose, serum osmolality, and levels of Na^+, K^+, Cl^-, HCO_3^-, Ca^{++}, Mg^{++}, and glucose should be monitored at least on alternate days until tolerance is stabilized. Body weight and total urine volume should be recorded daily.

COMPLICATIONS

Infection

The presence of an indwelling intravenous catheter carries a substantial risk of septicemia and bacterial endocarditis. Sepsis may not develop, however, until the catheter has been in place a week or more. It is wise to culture the flora of the skin, upper respiratory tract, bowel, and urine at weekly intervals. If there is clinical evidence of infection, it is important first to decide whether this is associated with the catheter or a separate event. In the latter case, specific treatment for the causative organism may be instituted. If there is no obvious basis for infection other than the catheter, the catheter should be removed, the tip cultured, and a new one inserted. The organisms most often involved are from the normal body flora, *Staphylococcus aureus, Streptococcus viridans,* proteus, klebsiella, and *Escherichia coli.* Saprophytes such as candida and aspergillus and weakly pathogenic organisms such as serratia may also be involved.

Pulmonary Embolism

Fronds of clot may develop from the external surface of the catheter around the tip. These may become infected or may detach to produce pulmonary emboli. Embolism is suggested by evidence of infection together with increased respiratory and pulse rates, cyanosis, and x-ray changes. The treatment is to heparinize the patient and to change the catheter. For major emboli, embolectomy is a possibility, but the likelihood of success is very small.

Control of Glucose Metabolism

Patients receiving intravenous nutrition frequently have been undernourished for a period of time, and glucose intolerance is a complication of undernutrition. It is usually necessary to increase the glucose concentrations in 2- to 4-day increments until the 23% concentration is tolerated.

Effective utilization of the glucose load can be enhanced by adding 1 unit of regular insulin to the infusate for each 5 gm of glucose and by giving up to 5 mEq of potassium per 100 kcal. The latter procedure requires that serum potassium be monitored. Serum and urine glucose levels must also be regularly checked to ensure that there is no osmotic overload.

Hypoglycemia is also a complication which is most liable to occur if the rate of glucose administration is allowed to fluctuate. Discontinuation of therapy must be done gradually. Under certain conditions, it may also be necessary to reduce amino acid concentration to keep up glucose levels, especially when Hyprotigen is used.

Amino Acids

The evidence so far is that, in the doses advocated, infants vary considerably in their ability to preserve normal levels of serum amino acids. Actual levels reflect the composition of the hydrolysate, eg, beef fibrin or casein. There has been no evidence of glutamate toxicity, but levels of branched chain amino acids and histidine tend to be low. The potential effects of infusing peptides are not now understood, but because of them it seems probable that hydrolysates will be replaced in time by simple amino acid mixtures such as Freamine.

Calcium & Vitamin Metabolism

The known actions of vitamin D are 2-fold: to enhance calcium absorption from the intestine and to mobilize calcium from bone. As the calcium is being given intravenously and it is not desired to mobilize bone calcium, it might be argued that vitamin D need not be given intravenously. It is apparent, however, that calcium may be precipitated by the phosphate buffer in the hydrolysate and that hypercalcemia may develop if other buffers are used. Until intravenous needs of calcium and vitamin D are more clearly understood they should be continued to be added to the solution.

Anemia

The constant infusion of a hypertonic solution may result in a mild hemolytic anemia. This should be monitored by weekly hemoglobin and hematocrit determinations and red cell counts. The appearance of anisocytosis and otherwise distorted red cells or serum haptoglobin saturation with hemoglobin are sensitive indications of hemolysis. Occasional transfusions of packed cells may be required.

Psychologic Problems

Older children and adults who have been encouraged to eat in order to maintain their nutritional status may become severely depressed at having failed when intravenous nutrition is initiated. Psychiatric help to allow them to ventilate their feelings is generally wise. Parents should be encouraged to hold infants receiving intravenous nutrition so that normal emotional attachments can develop.

Other Complications

Other reported complications include hypophosphatemia, intractable acidosis, copper depletion, and hepatic necrosis.

Filler RM & others: Long term total parenteral nutrition in infants. New England J Med 281:589, 1969.

Stegnik LD, Baker GL: Infusion of protein hydrolysates in the newborn infant: Plasma amino acid concentrations. J Pediat 78:595, 1971.

Wilmore DW & others: Total parenteral nutrition in infants with catastrophic gastrointestinal anomalies. J Pediat Surg 4:181, 1969.

● ● ●

General References

Cheek DB: Extracellular volume: Its structure and measurement and the influence of age and disease. J Pediat 58:103–125, 1961.

Christiansen HN: *Body Fluids and the Acid-Base Balance.* Saunders, 1964.

Darrow DC, Yannet H: The changes in the distribution of body water accompanying increase and decrease in extracellular electrolyte. J Clin Invest 14:266, 1935.

Gamble JL: *Chemical Anatomy, Physiology, and Pathology of Extracellular Fluid,* 7th ed. Harvard Univ Press, 1958.

Leaf A: The clinical and physiologic significance of the serum sodium concentration. New England J Med 267:24–30, 77–83, 1962.

Levinsky NG: Management of emergencies. VI. Hyperkalemia. New England J Med 274:1076–1077, 1966.

Moore FD & others: *The Body Cell Mass and Its Supporting Environment: Body Composition in Health and Disease.* Saunders, 1963.

Pitts RF: *Physiology of the Kidney and Body Fluids.* Year Book, 1968.

Schwartz EB, van Ypersele de Strihou C, Kassirer JP: The role of anions in metabolic alkalosis and potassium deficiency. New England J Med 279:630–639, 1968.

Siggaard-Andersen O: *The Acid-Base Status of the Blood.* Williams & Wilkins, 1964.

Talbot NB, Richie RH, Crawford JD: *Metabolic Homeostasis: A Syllabus for Those Concerned With the Care of Patients.* Harvard Univ Press, 1959.

Winters RW, Engel K, Dell RB: *Acid Base Physiology in Medicine.* A. Talbot Co (Canada), 1967.

38 ...

Drug Therapy

Henry K. Silver, MD

Precautions

Older children should never be given a dose greater than the adult dose. Adult dosages are given below to show limitation of dosage in older children when calculated on a weight basis. All drugs should be used with caution in children, and dosage should be individualized. In general, the smaller the child, the greater the metabolic rate; this may increase the dose needed. Dosage may also have to be adjusted for body temperature (metabolic rate is increased about 10% for each degree centigrade); for obesity (adipose tissue is relatively inert metabolically); for edema (depending on whether the drug is distributed primarily in extracellular fluid); for the type of illness (kidney and liver disease may impair metabolism of certain substances); and for individual tolerance (idiosyncrasy). The dosage recommendations on the following pages should be regarded only as estimates; careful clinical observations and the use of pertinent laboratory aids are necessary. Established drugs should be used in preference to newer and less familiar drugs.

Drugs should be used in early infancy only for significant disorders. In both full-term and premature infants, detoxifying enzymes may be deficient or absent; renal function relatively inefficient; and the blood-brain barrier and protein binding altered.

Dosages have not been determined as accurately for newborn infants as for older children.

At any age, oliguria requires a reduction of dosage of drugs excreted via the urine.

Whenever possible, reference should also be made to the printed literature supplied by the manufacturer or other recent authoritative sources, particularly for drugs that are used infrequently.

Determination of Drug Dosage*

Dosage rules based on proportions of the adult dose are not entirely satisfactory but may serve as a rough guide.

A. Surface Area: This is probably the most accurate method of estimating the dose for a child. (See Table 38–1 and Figs 38–1 and 38–2.)

$$\text{Child dose} = \frac{\text{Surface area of child in sq m} \times \text{adult dose}}{1.75}$$

or

Surface area in sq m $\times$ 60 = Percentage of adult dose.

B. Determination of Drug Dosage From Surface Area (Preferred Method): See Table 38–1.

Formula for calculating approximate surface area in children:

$$\text{Surface area (sq m)} = \frac{4W + 7}{W + 90}$$

where W is weight in kg.

C. Rule of Sixes Method:

$$\text{Child dose} = \frac{\text{Weight} \times \text{adult dose} \times \text{correction factor}}{70}$$

D. Clark's Rule: Based on weight, for children over 2 years.

$$\text{Child dose} = \frac{\text{Weight in lb} \times \text{adult dose}}{150}$$

E. Bastedo's Rule: Based on age.

$$\text{Child dose} = \frac{(\text{Age in years} \times \text{adult dose}) + 3}{30}$$

F. Cowling's Rule:

$$\text{Child dose} = \frac{\text{Age at next birthday} \times \text{adult dose}}{24}$$

G. Young's Rule: Based on age.

$$\text{Child dose} = \frac{\text{Age in years} \times \text{adult dose}}{\text{Age in years} + 12}$$

H. Dose in mg/kg if Adult Dose is 1 mg/kg (After Leach & Wood):

Age:	Adult	1
	12 years	1.25
	1–7 years	1.5
	2 weeks–1 year	2

*To convert dose in gm/kg to dose in gr/lb, multiply gm dosage by 7.

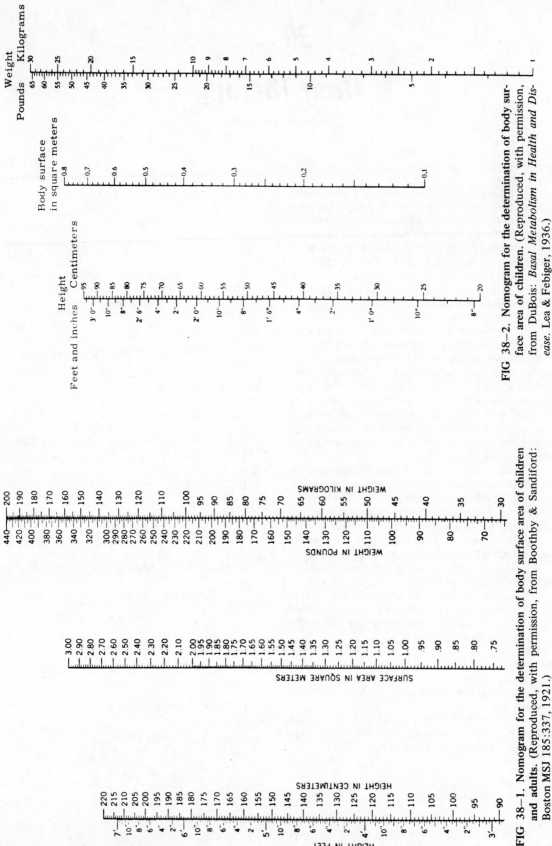

FIG 38–2. Nomogram for the determination of body surface area of children. (Reproduced, with permission, from DuBois: *Basal Metabolism in Health and Disease.* Lea & Febiger, 1936.)

FIG 38–1. Nomogram for the determination of body surface area of children and adults. (Reproduced, with permission, from Boothby & Sandiford: Boston MSJ 185:337, 1921.)

TABLE 38–1.

Weight		Approximate	Surface	% of
kg	lb	Age	Area (sq m)	Adult Dose
3	6.6	Newborn	0.2	12
6	13.2	3 months	0.3	18
10	22	1 year	0.45	28
20	44	5.5 years	0.8	48
30	66	9 years	1	60
40	88	12 years	1.3	78
50	110	14 years	1.5	90
65	143	Adult	1.7	102
70	154	Adult	1.76	103

*If adult dose is 1 mg/kg, dose for 3-month-old infant would be 2 mg/kg.

Administration of Drugs

A. Route of Administration:

1. Oral—Tablets may be crushed between spoons and given with chocolate, honey, jam, or maple or corn syrup. Many regularly prescribed drugs are commercially available in special pediatric preparations. The parent should be warned that the attractively flavored drug must be kept out of reach of children in the home.

a. Avoid administering drugs with important foods.

b. The powdered drug should be mixed in the vehicle and held between 2 layers, not floated on the top.

c. Attempt to administer the entire dose in 1 spoonful.

2. Parenteral—Parenteral administration of certain drugs may sometimes be necessary, especially in the hospital. Its use as a matter of convenience should be evaluated in the light of the psychic trauma which may result.

3. Rectal—Rectal administration is often very useful, especially for home use. (Rectal dosages are approximately twice the amount given orally.) The physician must make certain, however, that rectal absorption is adequate before depending upon this route for a specific drug. Drugs may be given rectally in corn starch (not more than 60 ml); they are best given through a tube, but an enema bulb may be used. Some drugs are prepared in suppository form.

B. Flavoring Agents for Drugs: Drugs for children should not be so flavorful that they are sought out as "candy." Syrups are more useful as flavoring agents than alcoholic elixirs, which have a burning taste.

Refusal of Medications

The administration of a drug to a child requires tact and skill. The parent or nurse should proceed as if she does not anticipate protest. Persuasion before it is necessary sets the stage for struggle. The child must understand that the drug will be given despite his protest, but great care should be exercised in a struggling child to avoid aspiration.

DRUG DOSAGES FOR CHILDREN

Acetaminophen (Tempra, Tylenol): 25 mg/kg/day in 4–6 doses orally. Under 1 year, 60 mg/dose; 1–3 years, 60–120 mg/dose; 3–6 years, 120 mg/dose; 6–12 years, 240 mg/dose. (Adult = 0.3–0.6 gm 3 times daily.)

Acetazolamide (Diamox): 5–30 mg/kg/day orally as single dose. (Adult = 5 mg/kg/day.) For hydrocephalus: 20–55 mg/kg/day orally in 2 or 3 divided doses. In salicylate intoxication: 5 mg/kg every 4 hours for 3 doses daily IM after diuresis is established. (For anticonvulsant use, see Table 21–2.)

ACTH: See p 623. Aqueous: 1.6 units/kg/day in 3 or 4 doses IV, IM, or subcut. Gel: 0.8 units/kg/day IM.

Actinomycin D: See Dactinomycin, Table 32–3.

Adrenalin: See Epinephrine.

Adroyd: See Oxymetholone.

Aerosporin: See Polymyxin B, Chapter 39.

Albumin, salt-poor: 0.5–1 gm/kg as 25 gm/100 ml solution (up to 100 ml) IV. (Adult = 50 mg/day IV.)

Aldactone: See Spironolactone.

Aldomet: See Methyldopa.

Aludrine: See Isoproterenol hydrochloride.

Aluminum hydroxide gel: 2–8 ml orally with meals. (Adult = 4–8 ml.)

Amantadine (Symmetrel): See p 937.

Amethopterin (methotrexate): (1) Orally or IM, 0.12 mg/day. (Adult = 5–10 mg/day.) (2) Intrathecally, 0.25–0.5 mg/kg/day. (3) IV, 3–5 mg/kg as single dose every other week. *Caution:* Toxic.

Aminophylline: (1) Orally, 2–5 mg/kg/dose. (Adult = 0.25 gm.) (2) IM or IV, 2–3.5 mg/kg/dose. (Adult = 0.25 gm.) (3) Rectally, 6 mg/kg/dose. (Adult = 0.5 gm.) Do not repeat in less than 6 hours. *Caution* in younger children.

Aminosalicylic acid (PAS): See Chapter 39.

Ammonium chloride: 75 mg/kg/day orally in 4 doses. For dysmenorrhea, 0.3–0.6 gm orally 3 times daily. (Adult = 0.6 gm 3 times daily.) Single expectorant dose, 0.06–0.3 gm orally/dose. (Adult = 0.3 gm.) As diuretic, 60–75 mg/kg/day orally. (Adult = 4 gm/day.)

Amobarbital sodium (Amytal): 3–12 mg/kg/dose IV (slowly) or IM. (Adult = 0.125–0.5 gm.) Use freshly prepared 10% solution and give slowly. Try smaller dose first. Orally, 6 mg/kg/day.

Amodiaquin: See Chapter 28.

Amphetamine sulfate (Benzedrine): 0.5 mg/kg/day in 3 doses orally or IM (not over 15 mg/day). (Adult = 5–15 mg.) The analeptic dose is 0.5 mg/kg IM or slowly IV. (For anticonvulsant use, see Table 21–2.)

Amphotericin B (Fungizone): See Chapter 39.

Ampicillin: See Chapter 39.

Amytal: See Amobarbital sodium.

Anadrol: See Oxymetholone.

Anhydrohydroxyprogesterone (ethisterone, Pranone, Progestoral, Lutocylol): 5–25 mg/day orally. (Same as adult dose.)

Ansolysen: See Pentolinium.

Antepar (piperazine): See pp 732 and 733.

Apomorphine: (1) Subcut, 0.06 mg/kg/dose. (2) Orally, 3–5 mg. (Adult = 5 mg.) May cause depression or excitability and potentiate the depressant action of CNS depressant drugs. May give levallorphan (see below) after vomiting is produced.

Apresoline: See Hydralazine.

Aralen: See Chloroquine.

Aramine: See Metaraminol.

Aristocort: See Triamcinolone.

Ascorbic acid (vitamin C): See Table 4–2 and p 647.

Asdrin: See Isoproterenol hydrochloride.

Aspirin: Analgesic, 65 mg/year of age/dose. (Adult = 0.3–0.65 gm.) For rheumatic fever, 65–130 mg/kg/day to maintain a blood level of 20–30 mg/100 ml. (Adult = 6–8 gm.) As antipyretic: up to 30–65 mg/kg/day. Try smaller dose first. Obtain blood levels for higher doses.

AT 10: See Dihydrotachysterol.

Atabrine: See Quinacrine.

Atarax: See Hydroxyzine.

Atropine methylnitrate (Eumydrin): 1:10,000 alcoholic solution. Initial dose: 0.05 mg; increase to 0.3 mg as necessary subcut. (Adult = 1–3 mg.)

Atropine sulfate: 0.005–0.02 mg/kg/dose subcut or orally. Maximum total dose: 0.4 mg. (Adult = 0.3–1 mg.) *Caution.*

Avertin: See Tribromoethanol.

Azathioprine (Imuran): 3–5 mg/kg/day orally.

Azulfidine: See Salicylazosulfapyridine.

Bacitracin: See Chapter 39.

BAL: See Dimercaprol.

Banthine: See Methantheline.

Belladonna tincture: 0.1 ml/kg/day orally in 3 divided doses. (Adult = 0.6 ml 3 times daily.) Do not give over 0.6 ml/dose or 3.5 ml/day.

Benadryl: See Diphenhydramine.

Benemid: See Probenecid.

Benodaine: See Piperoxan.

Bentyl: See Dicyclomine.

Benzedrine: See Amphetamine.

Betamethasone: See Table 24–7.

Bethanechol chloride (Urecholine Chloride): (1) Orally, 0.6 mg/kg/day in 3 divided doses. (Adult = 10–30 mg 3–4 times daily.) (2) Subcut, 0.15–0.2 mg/kg/day. (Adult = 2.5–5 mg.)

Bicillin (benzathine penicillin G): See Penicillins, Chapter 39.

Bisacodyl (Dulcolax): 0.3 mg/kg orally or rectally.

Bismuth glycolylarsanilate (Milibis): 20 mg/kg/day in 3 divided doses for 7 days. (Adult = 0.5 gm 3 times daily for 7 days.)

Blood: Packed erythrocytes, 15 ml/kg IV (not over 300 ml). Whole, 15–22 ml/kg IV as single transfusion. (Adult = 500 ml.)

Blood, whole: As a single transfusion, 15–22 ml/kg IV. (Adult = 500 ml.)

Bonine: See Meclizine.

Brewer's yeast (dried yeast tablets): 5–30 gm 3 times daily.

Bromides: See Table 21–2.

Brompheniramine (Dimetane): Children under 6 years: 0.1 mg/kg/day. Children over 6 years: 4 mg 3–4 times daily. (Adult = 4–8 mg 3–4 times daily.)

Busulfan (Myleran): 0.06 mg/kg/day orally. (Adult = 2 mg 1–3 times daily.)

Cafergot: See Ergotamine-caffeine, p 501.

Caffeine and sodium benzoate: (1) Subcut, IM, or IV, 6–10 mg/kg/dose. (Adult = 0.5 gm.) (2) Subcut or IM, 25% solution: 0.025–0.04 ml/kg/dose. This may be repeated. (Adult = 2 ml.)

Calciferol (ergocalciferol, vitamin D_2): 25–200 thousand units/day.

Calcium chloride (27% calcium): Newborn: 0.3 gm/kg/day orally as a 2–5% solution. Infants: 1–2 gm/day as dilute solution. Children, 2–4 gm/day. (Adult = 2–4 gm 3 times daily.) *Caution:* See p 86.

Calcium EDTA: See EDTA (edathamil).

Calcium gluconate (9% calcium): (1) Orally: Infants, 3–6 gm/day. Children, 6–10 gm/day in divided doses as a 5–10% solution. (Adult = 8 gm 3 times daily.) (2) IV, 0.1–0.2 gm/kg/dose (not over 2 gm) as a 10% solution. Inject slowly and stop if bradycardia occurs. (Adult = 5–10 ml.) *Caution.*

Calcium lactate (13% calcium): 0.5 gm/kg/day in divided doses orally in dilute solution. (Adult = 4–8 gm 3 times daily.)

Calcium mandelate: 2–8 gm daily orally, depending on age. (Adult = 3 gm 4 times daily.)

Caprokol: See Hexylresorcinol.

Carbacrylamine resins (Carbo-Resin): Over 5 years: 0.25 gm/kg/dose 3 times daily orally. (Adult = 8–16 gm 3 times daily.)

Carbamazepine (Tegretol): See Table 21–2.

Carbarsone: 10 mg/kg/day in divided doses.

Carbenicillin: See Chapter 39.

Carbo-Resin: See Carbacrylamine resins.

Carisoprodol (Soma): 25 mg/kg/day orally.

Cascara sagrada aromatic fluidextract: Infants, 1–2 ml/dose orally. Children, 2–8 ml/dose orally. (Adult = 4–8 ml orally.)

Castor oil: Infants, 1–5 ml/dose orally. Children, 5–15 ml/dose orally. (Adult = 15–60 ml orally.)

Cedilanid (lanatoside C): See p 284.

Celestone: See Betamethasone, Table 24–7.

Celontin: See Methsuximide, Table 21–2.

Cephaloridine: See Chapter 4.

Cephalothin (Keflin): See Chapter 39.

Chloral hydrate: (1) Orally or rectally: 12.5–50 mg/kg as single hypnotic dose (not over 1 gm). (Adult = 0.5–2 gm.) (2) Rectally or orally: 4–20 mg/kg as single sedative dose (not over 1 gm). (Adult = 0.25–1 gm.) May be repeated in 1 hour to obtain desired effect, and then may be repeated every 6–8 hours.

Chloramphenicol (Chloromycetin): See Chapter 39.

Chlorcyclizine (Perazil): 1.5 mg/kg/day orally.

Chlordiazepoxide (Librium): Over 6 years, 0.5 mg/kg/day orally in 3–4 doses.

Chloromycetin: See Chloramphenicol, Chapter 39.

Chloroquine (Aralen): 10 mg/kg/day orally.

Chlorothiazide (Diuril): 7–40 mg/kg/day in 2 divided doses orally. (Adult = 0.5–1 gm once or twice daily.)

Chlorpheniramine (Chlor-Trimeton, Teldrin): Infants, 1 mg 3–4 times daily. Children, 0.35 mg/kg/day in 4 doses orally or subcut. (Adult = 2–4 mg 3–4 times daily; long-acting, 8–12 mg 2–3 times daily.)

Chlorpromazine (Thorazine): (1) Orally, 0.5 mg/kg every 4–6 hours. (2) IM, up to 5 years: 0.5 mg/kg every 6–8 hours as necessary (not over 40 mg/day). 5–12 years: not over 75 mg/day. (3) Rectally, 2 mg/kg. (Adult = 10–50 mg.)

Chlorpropamide (Diabinese): Initially: 8 mg/kg/day in 3 divided doses. (Adult = 250 mg/day.) *Caution.*

Chlor-Trimeton: See Chlorpheniramine.

Cholestyramine (Cuemid, Questran): Children under 6 years: dose not yet established. Children over 6 years: initiate with 1/2 adult dose and adjust as necessary. (Adult = 4 gm 3–4 times daily.)

Citrovorum factor: 1–6 mg/day orally. (Adult = 3–10 mg.)

Codeine phosphate: (1) Orally, 0.8–1.5 mg/kg as a single sedative or analgesic dose; 3 mg/kg/day. (Adult = 8–60 mg.) (2) Subcut, 0.8 mg/kg. (Adult = 30 mg.) (3) For cough, 0.2 mg/kg/dose.

Colace: See Dioctyl sodium sulfosuccinate.

Colistimethate: See Colistin, Chapter 39.

Colistin (Coly-Mycin): See Chapter 39.

Coly-Mycin: See Colistin, Chapter 39.

Compazine: See Prochlorperazine.

Coramine: See Nikethamide.

Corticosteroids: See Table 24–7.

Corticotropin: See ACTH and p 623.

Cortisone: See Table 24–7.

Cosmegen: See Dactinomycin, Table 32–3.

Cotazym (pancreatic replacement): 0.3–0.6 mg with each feeding. (Adult = 3 capsules with meals.)

Cuemid: See Cholestyramine.

Curare: See Tubocurarine.

Cyclamycin: See Troleandomycin, p 950.

Cyclophosphamide (Cytoxan): See Table 32–3.

Cycloserine (Seromycin): 15–25 mg/kg/day orally. (Adult = 250 mg twice daily.)

Cyproheptadine (Periactin): 0.25 mg/kg/day orally in 3 or 4 doses. (Adult = 12–16 mg/day.)

Cytomel: See Triiodothyronine.

Cytoxan: See Cyclophosphamide, Table 32–3.

Dactinomycin (actinomycin D; Cosmegen): See Table 32–3.

Daraprim: See Pyrimethamine.

Darvon: See Propoxyphene.

Decadron: See Dexamethasone, Table 24–10.

Delalutin: See Hydroxyprogesterone caproate.

Delatestryl: See Testosterone enanthate.

Delestrogen: See Estradiol valerate.

Deltra: See Prednisone.

Demerol: See Meperidine.

Dendrid: See Idoxuridine, p 957.

Depo-Provera: See Medroxyprogesterone acetate.

Desoxycorticosterone: See Table 24–7.

Dexamethasone: See Table 24–7.

Dexedrine: See Dextroamphetamine, Table 21–2.

Dextroamphetamine (Dexedrine): See Table 21–2.

Dextromethorphan (Romilar): 1 mg/kg/day orally.

Dextropropoxyphene: See Propoxyphene.

Diamox: See Acetazolamide.

Dianabol: See Methandrostenolone.

Diazepam (Valium): See Table 21–2.

Dicodid: See Dihydrocodeinone bitartrate.

Dicyclomine (Bentyl): Infants: 5 mg as syrup 3 or 4 times daily. Children: 10 mg 3 or 4 times daily. (Adult = 10–20 mg 3 or 4 times daily.)

Diethylcarbamazine (Hetrazan): 15 mg/kg/day in a single dose for 4 days for ascariasis.

Diethylstilbestrol: See Stilbestrol.

Digitalis preparations: See p 284.

Dihydrocodeinone bitartrate (Dicodid): 0.6 mg/kg/day orally in 3–4 doses. (Adult = 5–10 mg.)

Dihydrotachysterol (AT 10): 1–4 ml (1.25 mg/ml) orally daily initially; 0.5–1 ml 3–5 times weekly as maintenance. (Adult = 4–10 ml initially and then 1–2 ml.)

Diiodohydroxyquin (Diodoquin): 40 mg/kg/day orally in 2–3 doses. (Adult = 0.2 gm/15 lb/day.)

Dilantin: See Diphenylhydantoin, Table 21–2.

Dimenhydrinate (Dramamine): 1–1.5 mg/kg/dose orally. (Adult = 50–100 mg.)

Dimercaprol (BAL): See p 792.

Dimetane: See Brompheniramine.

Dimocillin: See Penicillins, Chapter 39.

Dioctyl sodium sulfosuccinate (Colace, Doxinate): 3–5 mg/kg/day in 3 divided doses orally. (Adult = 60–480 mg daily.)

Diodoquin: See Diiodohydroxyquin.

Diodrast: See Iodopyracet.

Diphenhydramine (Benadryl): 4–6 mg/kg/day orally in 3–4 divided doses; 2 mg/kg IV over 5 minutes as an antidote for phenothiazine toxicity. (Adult = 100–200 mg/day orally.)

Diphenoxylate (in Lomotil): Children 3–6 months (*caution*): 3 mg/day and decrease dose as relieved. Older children: 2.5 mg 2 or 3 times daily and decrease dose as relieved. (Adult = 5 mg 3–4 times daily and reduce.)

Diphenylhydantoin (Dilantin): See Table 21–2.

Diuril: See Chlorothiazide.

Doxinate: See Dioctyl sodium sulfosuccinate.

Doxylamine succinate (Decapryn): 2 mg/kg/day orally.

Dramamine: See Dimenhydrinate.

Dropsprin: See Salicylamide.

Dulcolax: See Bisacodyl.

Durabolin: See Nandrolone.

Edathamil: See EDTA.

Edecrin: See Ethacrynic acid.

Edetate: See EDTA.

Edrophonium chloride (Tensilon): Test dose for infant: 0.2 mg/kg IV. Give only 1/5 of dose slowly initially; if tolerated, give remainder. (Adult = 5–10 mg IV.) Have atropine available as antidote.

EDTA (edathamil): 12.5 mg/kg IM (in solution containing procaine, 0.5–1.5%).

Emetine: 1 mg/kg once daily (not to exceed 0.06 gm per day) subcut or IM.

Emivan: See Ethamivan.

Ephedrine sulfate: 0.5–1 mg/kg/dose orally. May repeat every 4–6 hours. (Adult = 25 mg.) 0.2 mg/kg every 6 hours IM; 50 mg/1000 ml IV, adjusting drip rate to patient's response.

Epinephrine in oil injection, 1:500: For 1-year-old: 0.1 ml; 2-year-old: 0.15 ml; 5-year-old: 0.25 ml, IM. (Adult = 1 ml.)

Epinephrine solution, 1:1000 (aqueous): 0.01–0.025 ml/kg (maximum dose: 0.5 ml) subcut. (Adult = 0.5–1 ml.)

Epinephrine solution, 1:200 (aqueous) (Sus-Phrine): 0.05–0.1 ml subcut, 1 dose only. Use smallest effective dose.

Equanil: See Meprobamate.

Ergotamine-caffeine (Cafergot): See p 501.

Erythrocin (erythromycin): See Chapter 39.

Erythromycin (Erythrocin, Ilosone, Ilotycin, Pediamycin): See Chapter 39.

Esidrix: See Hydrochlorothiazide.

Estinyl: See Ethinyl estradiol.

Estradiol valerate (Delestrogen, Lastrogen): 10 mg/month IM for teenage girl. (Adult = 10–20 mg IM every 2–3 weeks.)

Etamon: See Tetraethylammonium chloride.

Ethacrynic acid (Edecrin): Children: Initial: 25 mg. Maintenance: increase by increments of 25 mg. *Caution.* (Adults: Initial: 50–100 mg. Maintenance: 50–200 mg on continuous or intermittent schedule.)

Ethambutol (Myambutol): See Chapter 39.

Ethamivan (Emivan): 1–2 mg/kg slowly IV. Titrate dose to patient. *Caution.*

Ethinyl estradiol (Estinyl): 0.02–0.05 mg/dose orally 1–3 times daily for teenage girl. (Adult = 0.05 mg 1–3 times daily.)

Ethosuximide (Zarontin): See Table 21–2.

Ethotoin (Peganone): See Table 21–2.

Eumydrin: See Atropine methylnitrate.

Ferrous salts: Medicinal iron. 4.5–6 mg/kg of elemental iron in 3 divided doses. See also Iron, Table 4–2 and p 330.

Fludrocortisone: See Table 24–7.

Fluorescein: 2 ml of 5% solution IV. (Adult = 3–4 ml of 20% solution.)

Fluorouracil: Adults: 15 mg/kg daily for 4 days, not to exceed 1 mg/day. If no toxicity occurs, give 7.5 mg/kg on 6th, 8th, 10th, and 12th days of treatment. Discontinue at end of 12th day even if no toxicity is apparent. May repeat in 6 weeks after last injection of previous course if no toxicity is reported.

Fluoxymesterone (Halotestin, Ultandren): Up to 0.15 mg/kg/day orally in 2 divided doses in prepuberal children and up to 0.1 mg/kg/day in puberal children. (Adult = 2–10 mg/day.)

Fluprednisolone: See Table 24–10.

Folic acid: 0.2–1 mg/day orally for maintenance. (Adult = 10–15 mg/day.)

Fulvicin: See Griseofulvin, Chapter 39.

Fumagillin (Fugillin, Fumidil): 0.5–1 mg/kg body weight in 3 doses for 10–14 days.

Fungicides: See Chapter 29.

Fungizone: See Amphotericin B, Chapter 39.

Furadantin: See Nitrofurantoin, Chapter 39.

Furazolidone (Furoxone): 5 mg/kg/day in 4 divided doses.

Furmethide: See Furtrethonium.

Furosemide (Lasix): Children: Contraindicated until safety is established. (Adults = Diuretic: 40–80 mg in a.m. Hypertension: 40 mg twice daily.)

Furoxone: See Furazolidone.

Furtrethonium (Furmethide): (1) Orally, up to 4 years: 2.5 mg; 4–9 years: 5 mg; 9–15 years: 5–20 mg 3 times daily. (Adult = 10–30 mg 2–3 times daily.) (2) Initial dose subcut: infants, 1 mg; young children, 2 mg; older children, 3 mg. May repeat in 30–60 minutes if necessary. (Adult = 5 mg.)

Gammacorten: See Dexamethasone, Table 24–7.

Gamma globulin: See pp 109, 115, and 417.

Gantrisin: See Sulfisoxazole, Chapter 39.

Garamycin: See Gentamicin, Chapter 39.

Gemonil: See Metharbital, Table 21–2.

Gentamicin (Garamycin): See Chapter 39.

Gentian violet (methylrosaniline chloride): 2 mg/kg/day orally in 3 divided doses. Not more than 30 mg should be given. (Adult = 65 mg.)

Glucagon: (1) Newborn, 0.025–0.1 mg/kg as single dose IV. Try smaller dose first. May repeat in 30 minutes. (2) Older child, 0.25–1 mg subcut, IM, or IV as single dose.

Gonadotropin, chorionic: 500–1000 units 2–3 times/week for 5–8 weeks IM.

Griseofulvin (Fulvicin): See Chapter 39.

Guanethidine (Ismelin): 0.2 mg/kg/day orally as single dose. Increase dose at weekly intervals by same amount. (Adult = 10 mg daily. Larger doses possible for hospitalized adults.) *Caution.*

Haldol: See Haloperidol.

Haloperidol (Haldol): Children: Contraindicated in children under 12 years of age; safety is not yet established. (Adults: No more than 15 mg/day. Initial: 1–2 mg 2 or 3 times daily. Maintenance: 1–2 mg 3–4 times daily.)

Halotestin: See Fluoxymesterone.

Heparin: (1) IV, 0.5 mg/kg/dose. This may be repeated every hour. One mg/kg every 4 hours is recommended for intravascular clotting. Control with clotting time. (Adult = 50 mg.) (2) Subcut, 4 mg/kg. Will prolong clotting time for 20–24 hours.

Herplex: See Idoxuridine, p 957.

Hetrazan: See Diethylcarbamazine.

Hexylresorcinol (Caprokol): 0.1 gm/year of age orally. Do not give over 1 gm. (Adult = 1 gm.)

Histadyl: See Methapyrilene.

Histamine: Provocative test: 0.02 mg/sq m IV. *Caution:* Phentolamine should be available.

HN2: See Mechlorethamine.

Hyaluronidase (Wydase): 500 viscosity units or 150 turbidity-reducing units in 1 ml sterile water or saline at site of fluid administration.

Hydralazine (Apresoline): (1) Orally, 0.15 mg/kg/dose 4 times daily. Increase to tolerance. (2) IM or IV with reserpine: 0.1–0.2 mg/kg every 6–24 hours. (3) IV or IM alone: 1.5–3.5 mg/kg/day in 4–6 divided doses. (Adult, initial parenteral dose = 20–40 mg; single oral dose = 100 mg.)

Hydriodic acid: 1–5 ml of 1.4% syrup every 4 hours in fruit juice.

Hydrochlorothiazide (Esidrix, HydroDiuril): 1/10 of chlorothiazide dose. (Adult = 25–200 mg/day.)

Hydrocortisone: See Table 24–10.

HydroDiuril: See Hydrochlorothiazide.

Hydroxyprogesterone caproate (Delalutin): 125 mg IM for teenage girl.

Hydroxyzine (Atarax): 1–2 mg/kg/day orally in 3 divided doses. Preoperatively, 1 mg/kg/day IM. (Adult = 25–50 mg 3 times daily.)

Hykinone: See Menadione sodium bisulfite.

Hyoscine: See Scopolamine.

Idoxuridine (Dendril, Herplex, Stoxil): See p 957.

Ilosone: See Erythromycin, Chapter 39.

Ilotycin: See Erythromycin, Chapter 39.

Imferon: See Iron-dextran complex, p 330.

Imipramine (Tofranil): Children: not generally recommended for children under 12 years. Adolescents: initial dose of 30–40 mg/day; may increase according to response and tolerance. Generally not more than 100 mg/day. (Adult = 75 mg initially, increased up to 150 mg daily.)

Imuran: See Azathioprine.

Inderal: See Propranolol.

Insulin: See Table 24–9.

Iodine solution, strong (Lugol's solution): 1–10 drops daily for 10–21 days.

Iodochlorhydroxyquin (Vioform): 0.25 gm orally 3 times daily for 14 days.

Iodopyracet (Diodrast): 35% for IV urography and retrograde aortography. 70% for IV angiocardiography. 7% in saline with hyaluronidase for subcut injection.

Ipecac syrup: 2–20 ml/dose orally. (Adult = 8–20 ml.) Repeat in 20 minutes if necessary. Recover dose (lavage) if not vomited. (Adult = 15 ml.) *Caution:* Never use fluidextract of ipecac as emetic.

Iron: See Table 4–2 and p 330. See also Ferrous salts, above.

Iron-dextran complex (Imferon): See p 330.

Ismelin: See Guanethidine.

Isoniazid: See Chapter 39.

Isonorin: See Isoproterenol.

Isoproterenol hydrochloride (Aludrine, Asdrin, Isonorin, Isuprel, Norisodrine, Proternol): 2–10 mg/dose sublingually 3 times daily for older children (not oftener than every 3–4 hours). Oral inhalation, 5–15 breaths of 1:200 solution (not more than 0.5 ml). (Adult = 15 mg sublingually 4 times daily.) Rectal, 5–15 mg 4 times daily. Subcut, 0.1–0.5 mg.

Isoproterenol sulfate (Isonorin, Norisodrine): 1:200 or 1:400, 1–2 inhalations.

Isuprel: See Isoproterenol hydrochloride.

Kanamycin (Kantrex): See Chapter 39.

Kantrex: See Kanamycin, Chapter 39.

Kaopectate: 3–6 years, 1–2 tbsp; 6–12 years, 2–4 tbsp.

Kayexalate: See Sodium polystyrene sulfonate.

Keflin: See Cephalothin, Chapter 39.

Kenacort: See Triamcinolone, Table 24–7.

Konakion: See Phytonadione.

Lanatoside C: See p 284.

Lasix: See Furosemide.

Lastrogen: See Estradiol valerate.

Latrodectus antivenin: 2.5 ml IM, repeated in 1 hour if symptoms have not markedly improved.

Leucovorin calcium: See Citrovorum factor.

Leukeran: See Chlorambucil, Table 32–3.

Levallorphan (Lorfan): 0.02–0.05 mg IV or IM for infant and repeat if necessary. (Adult = 1–2 mg.) May give levallorphan tartrate 1 minute after vomiting begins as result of administration of apomorphine for treatment of poisoning.

Levarterenol bitartrate (norepinephrine, Levophed): See pp 617 and 756.

Levophed: See Levarterenol, pp 617 and 756.

Levothyroxine sodium: Give orally. 100 mg desiccated thyroid = 0.1 mg sodium L-thyroxine = 25–30 µg triiodothyronine. (Adult = 0.3–0.6 mg.)

Lidocaine (Xylocaine): 1 mg/kg IV slowly for arrhythmia. Repeat as needed. (For anticonvulsant use, see Table 21–2.)

Lincocin: See Lincomycin, Chapter 39.

Lincomycin (Lincocin): See Chapter 39.

Liothyronine: See Triiodothyronine.

Liquid petrolatum, liquid paraffin: See Mineral oil.

Liquiprin: See Salicylamide.

Liver injection, crude: 2 ml/day IM. (Same as adult dose.)

Lomotil: See Diphenoxylate.

Lorfan: See Levallorphan.

Loridine: See Cephaloridine, Chapter 39.

Lugol's solution: See Iodine solution, strong.

Lypressin (lysine-8 vasopressin; Syntopressin): 30–55 units/day as a nasal spray.

Magnesium hydroxide: See Milk of magnesia.

Magnesium sulfate: (As anticonvulsant or for hypertension.) 0.1–0.4 ml/kg of 50% solution IM every 4–6 hours if renal function is adequate; or 10 ml (100 mg)/kg IV slowly as 1% solution. *Caution:* Check blood pressure carefully and have calcium gluconate available. As cathartic: 250 mg/kg/dose orally.

Mandelamine: See Methenamine mandelate, Chapter 39.

Mannitol (Osmitrol): Test dose for oliguria, 0.2 gm/kg IV. Edema, 1–2.5 gm/kg IV over 2–6 hours. Cerebral edema, 1–2.5 gm/kg over 30–60 minutes.

Marboran: See Methisazone, p 957.

Matulane: See Procarbazine hydrochloride.

Mebaral: See Mephobarbital, Table 21–2.

Mechlorethamine (HN2, Mustargen, nitrogen mustard): Inject slowly, diluted, 0.1 mg/kg/day for 4 days IV. (Same as adult dose.)

Mecholyl: See Methacholine chloride.

Meclizine (Bonine): 2 mg/kg every 6–12 hours orally. (Adult = 25–50 mg.)

Medrol: See Methylprednisolone, Table 24–7.

Medroxyprogesterone acetate (Depo-Provera): Children under 4 years, 100–150 mg per injection every 2 weeks. Children over 4 years, 150–200 mg per injection every 2 weeks.

Mellaril: See Thioridazine.

Menadiol sodium diphosphate (vitamin K analogue; Synkayvite): 1 mg IM. (Adult = 3–6 mg.)

Menadione sodium bisulfite (Hykinone): 1 mg IM. (Adult = 0.5–2 mg IM.)

Mepacrine: See Quinacrine hydrochloride.

Meperidine (Demerol): 0.6–1.5 mg/kg IM or orally as single analgesic dose; up to 6 mg/kg/day. (Adult = 50–100 mg.)

Mephenesin (Tolserol): (1) Orally, 40–130 mg/kg/day in 3–5 doses. (2) IV, 1–3 ml/kg as 2% solution slowly. (Adult = 1–3 gm 3 times daily.)

Mephentermine (Wyamine): 0.4 mg/kg orally, IM, or slowly IV as single dose. (Adult = 15–20 mg IM.)

Mephenytoin (Mesantoin): See Table 21–2.

Mephobarbital (Mebaral): See Table 21–2.

Meprobamate (Miltown, Equanil): Over 3 years: 7–30 mg/kg/day in 2–3 doses orally. (Adult = 400–800 mg 3 times daily.)

Meralluride (Mercuhydrin): See Mercurial diuretics.

Mercaptomerin sodium: See Mercurial diuretics.

Mercaptopurine (6-MP, Purinethol): See Table 32–3.

Mercuhydrin (meralluride): See Mercurial diuretics.

Mercurial diuretics (including mercaptomerin sodium and meralluride): Below 3 kg, 0.125 ml IM; 3–7 kg, 0.125–0.25 ml; 7–15 kg, 0.25–0.5 ml; 15–25 kg, 0.5–0.75 ml; 25–35 kg, 1 ml. Give daily to once weekly. (Adult = 1–2 ml.)

Mesantoin: See Mephenytoin, Table 21–2.

Mestinon: See Pyridostigmin.

Metaraminol (Aramine): 0.04–0.2 mg/kg subcut or IM; 0.3–2 mg/kg in 500 ml solution as IV infusion. (Titrate by effect or by blood pressure readings.) (Adult = 2–10 mg IM, 0.5–5 mg IV.)

Methacholine (Mecholyl): For arrhythmia in young child, 0.1–0.4 mg/kg subcut or IM. May be increased by 25% every 30 minutes. Oral starting dose: about 18 times greater.

Methacycline (Rondomycin): See Tetracycline, Chapter 39.

Methandrostenolone (Dianabol): 0.04 mg/kg/day orally. (Adult = 2.5–5 mg daily.)

Methantheline (Banthine): 4–8 mg/kg/day orally or IM in 4 divided doses. (Adult = 50–100 mg 3 times daily.)

Methapyrilene (Dozar, Histadyl, Thenylene): 0.2–0.3 mg/kg up to 5 times daily. (Adult = 50 mg/dose.)

Metharbital (Gemonil): See Table 22–2.

Methdilazine (Tacaryl): 0.3 mg/kg/day orally in 2 doses.

Methenamine mandelate (Mandelamine): See Chapter 39.

Methicillin: See Penicillins, Chapter 39.

Methimazole (Tapazole): 0.4 mg/kg/day in 3 divided doses. Maintenance, 1/2 initial dose. (See also p 607.) (Adult = 15–60 mg.)

Methionine: 250 mg/kg/day orally in 3–4 divided doses. (Adult dose to acidify urine: 12–15 gm/day orally.)

Methisazone (Marboran): See p 957.

Methocarbamol (Robaxin): 40–65 mg/kg/day orally in 4–6 divided doses. (Adult = 1.5–2 gm 3–4 times daily.)

Methotrexate: See Table 32–3.

Methoxamine (Vasoxyl): 0.25 mg/kg IM as single dose. (Adult = 15 mg IM.)

Methsuximide (Celontin): See Table 21–2.

Methylcellulose: 0.5 gm at bedtime.

Methyldopa (Aldomet): 2–4 mg/kg IV initially. Double dose in 4 hours if no effect. Dilute in 50–100 ml fluid and infuse over 30–60 minutes. Children: 10 mg/kg/day orally in divided doses every 6 hours, increasing at 2-day or greater intervals to 65 mg/kg/day. For crises, 20–40 mg/kg/day in divided doses every 6 hours, continuing with oral doses when controlled. *Caution.* (Adult = 250 mg 3 times daily initially; adjust at 2–7 day intervals.)

Methylene blue: 0.1–0.2 ml/kg/dose of 1% solution slowly IV. (Adult = 100–150 mg.)

Methylphenidate (Ritalin): 0.25–0.75 mg/kg/dose orally. (Adult = 10 mg 3 times daily.) *Caution.*

Methylphenylethylhydantoin: See Mephenytoin, Table 21–2.

Methylprednisolone: See Table 24–7.

Methylrosaniline chloride: See Gentian violet.

Methyltestosterone (Metandren, Oreton): 0.08–0.15 mg/kg/day sublingually. (Adult = 5–10 mg.)

Methysergide (Sansert): Children: Dosage has not been established. (Adult = 4–8 mg/day.) Do not continue for more than 6 months; interrupt for 3–4 weeks and begin again. Precede drug-free interval with dosage reduction.

Meticorten: See Prednisone, Table 24–7.

Milibis: See Bismuth glycolylarsanilate.

Milk of magnesia: 0.5–1 ml/kg/dose orally. (Adult = 30–60 ml.)

Milontin: See Phensuximide, Table 24–7.

Miltown: See Meprobamate.

Mineral oil: 0.5 ml/kg/dose orally. (Adult = 15–30 ml.)

Morphine sulfate: 0.12–0.2 mg/kg every 4 hours as necessary subcut (no more than 10 mg/dose). (Adult = 10–15 mg.) Infants, start with 1/2 the dose.

Mustargen: See Mechlorethamine.

Myambutol: See Ethambutol, Chapter 39.

Mycifradin: See Neomycin, Chapter 39.

Mycostatin: See Nystatin, Chapter 39.

Myleran: See Busulfan.

Mysoline: See Primidone, Table 21–2.

Nalidixic acid (NegGram): See Chapter 39.

Nalorphine (Nalline): 0.1–0.2 mg/kg/dose IV or IM. Repeat in 15 minutes if necessary. Use IV for shocky infant.

Nandrolone (Durabolin): Infants: 12.5 mg every 2–4 weeks IM. Children: 25 mg every 2–4 weeks IM.

NegGram: See Nalidixic acid, Chapter 39.

Nembutal: See Pentobarbital sodium.

Neo-Cultol: 4 ml at bedtime.

Neolin: See Penicillins, Chapter 39.

Neomycin (Mycifradin, Neobiotic): See Chapter 39.

Neostigmine (Prostigmin): (1) Orally, 0.25 mg/kg/dose. (Adult = 15 mg.) (2) IM, 0.025–0.045 mg/kg/dose. (Adult = 0.25–1 mg.) For myasthenia test, 0.04 mg/kg/dose IM. *Caution:* Atropine should be available.

Neo-Synephrine: See Phenylephrine.

Niacinamide (nicotinamide): See Table 4–1 and p 646.

Nicotinamide (niacinamide): See Table 4–1 and p 646.

Nikethamide (Coramine): 25 mg/kg/dose IV or IM.

Nilevar: See Norethandrolone.

Nitrofurantoin (Furadantin): See Chapter 38.

Nitrogen mustard: See Mechlorethamine.

Noctec: See Chloral hydrate.

Norepinephrine: See Levarterenol, pp 617 and 756.

Norethandrolone (Nilevar): 0.4–0.8 mg/kg/day orally. (Adult = 30–50 mg daily.)

Norisodrine: See Isoproterenol hydrochloride and sulfate.

Nystatin (Mycostatin): See Chapter 39.

Oleandomycin: See Troleandomycin, p 950.

Omnipen: See Penicillins, Chapter 39.

Oncovin: See Vincristine, Table 32–3.

Opium tincture, camphorated: See Paregoric.

Oreton: See Methyltestosterone.

Osmitrol: See Mannitol.

Ouabain (strophanthin): 0.01 mg/kg IV. Give 1/2 dose initially. Check ECG frequently.

Oxacillin: See Penicillins, Chapter 39.

Oxymetholone (Adroyd): 0.1–0.3 mg/kg/day orally. (2.5 mg for children weighing less than 20 kg and 3.75 mg for those over 20 kg.)

Pancreatin (pancreatic enzymes): 0.3–0.6 gm with each feeding. Increase as necessary. (Adult = 2.5 gm.)

Papaverine: 1–6 mg/kg/day orally, IV, or IM in 4 divided doses. (Adult = 0.1 gm.)

Paradione: See Paramethadione.

Paraldehyde: (1) Orally, 0.1–0.15 ml/kg/dose. (Adult = 4–16 ml.) (2) Rectally, 0.3–0.6 ml/kg/dose in 1 or 2 parts of vegetable oil. (Adult = 16–32 ml.) (3) IM, 0.1 ml/kg as single anticonvulsant dose (not over 10 ml). (Adult = 4–10 ml.) (4) IV, 0.02 ml/kg *very slowly.* (Adult = 1–2 ml.) *Caution:* IM administration may cause fat necrosis; IV administration may cause respiratory distress or pulmonary edema. Do not use plastic equipment.

Paramethadione (Paradione): See Table 21–2.

Paramethasone: See Table 24–7.

Parathyroid injection: 50–300 units subcut or IM, and then 20–40 units every 12 hours. (Adult = 20–100 units 3–5 times daily.)

Paregoric: 0.06 ml month of age up to 12 months. 5-year-old, 2 ml. May repeat every 3–4 hours if no drowsiness or respiratory depression. (Adult = 4 ml.) *Caution.*

PAS: See Aminosalicylic acid, Chapter 39.

Pediamycin: See Erythromycin, Chapter 39.

Peganone: See Ethotoin, Table 21–2.

Penbritin: See Penicillins, Chapter 39.

Penicillamine (Cuprimine): Infants over 6 months: 250 mg/day. Older children and adults: 1 gm/day in 4 doses orally. Increase as indicated. (Adult = 250–500 mg 3 times daily.)

Penicillins: See Chapter 39.

Pentobarbital (Nembutal): 1–1.5 mg/kg orally. Up to 3–5 mg/kg as single sedative dose. (Adult = 100 mg.)

Pentolinium (Ansolysen): (1) Orally, 1 mg/kg/day. (Adult = 20–200 mg 3 times daily.) (2) IM or subcut, 0.035–0.15 mg/kg dose. (Adult = 2.5–10 mg.) Start smaller dose and increase gradually.

Pentothal: See Thiopental.

Perazil: See Chlorcyclizine hydrochloride.

Periactin: See Cyproheptadine.

Permapen: See Penicillins, Chapter 39.

Pethidine hydrochloride: See Meperidine.

Phenacemide (Phenurone): See Table 21–2.

Phenergan: See Promethazine.

Phenobarbital: As sedative, 0.5–2 mg/kg as single dose orally every 4–6 hours. Anticonvulsant: 3–5 mg/kg/dose IM (IV only with extreme caution). **Epilepsy:** Starting doses: Under 3 years, 16 mg 3 times daily; 3–6 years, 32 mg twice daily; over 6 years, 32 mg 3 times daily. (Adult = 30 mg.) Hypnotic: 3–6 mg/kg/dose orally. (Adult = 100–200 mg.)

Phenobarbital sodium: (1) Subcut or IM, 4–10 mg/kg as anticonvulsant. (2) Orally, 1–5 mg/kg as single sedative dose. (Adult = 15–100 mg.) (3) IM or rectally, 1 mg/kg as single sedative dose. (Adult = 30 mg.) (4) Rectally, 3–5 mg/kg as anticonvulsant. Acts more rapidly than phenobarbital. (Adult = 0.3 gm.)

Phensuximide (Milontin): See Table 24–10.

Phentolamine (Regitine): (1) Test dose: 0.1 mg/kg IV. *Caution.* (2) Therapeutic, 5 mg/kg/day orally in 4 divided doses. (Adult = 5 mg IV.)

Phenurone: See Phenacemide, Table 21–2.

Phenylephrine (Neo-Synephrine): 3–10 mg orally for nasal vasoconstriction. (Adult = 10–25 mg.)

Phenoxymethyl penicillin: See Penicillins, Chapter 39.

Physostigmine: 1–2 drops of 0.25 or 0.5% solution or ointment several times daily.

Phytonadione (vitamin K$_1$, Mephyton, Aqua-Mephyton, Konakion): Prophylactic dose, 0.5–5 mg IM; therapeutic dose, 5–10 mg IM, IV, or orally. (Mephyton for oral use; others for parenteral use.)

Picrotoxin injection: 0.1–0.3 mg/kg every 20 minutes as necessary IM or IV. Not over 6 mg to a child. May repeat every 15 minutes with constant observation and IV barbiturate available. (Adult = 6–9 mg and repeat as necessary.)

Pilocarpine: 0.5, 1, and 2% as eyedrops.

Piperazine (Antepar): See pp 732 and 733.

Piperoxan (Benodaine) hydrochloride: Test dose, 0.25 mg/kg IV slowly. (Same as adult dose.)

Pitressin and Pitressin Tannate: See Vasopressin injection and Vasopressin tannate injection.

Pituitary, posterior, powder: Small pinch (approximately 40–50 mg) nasally 4 times daily as necessary. (Adult = 30–60 mg 2–3 times daily.)

Plasma: 10–15 ml/kg IV.

Polycillin: See Penicillins, Chapter 39.

Polymyxin B (Aerosporin): See Chapter 39.

Posterior pituitary: See Pituitary, posterior.

Potassium chloride: See pp 544 and 920 and Table 37–5.

Potassium iodide (saturated solution): 0.1–0.3 ml orally in cold milk or fruit juice. (Adult = 0.3 ml.)

Povan: See Pyrvinium pamoate.

Pralidoxime (Protopam): 25–50 mg/kg as 5% solution IV.

Pranone: See Anhydrohydroxyprogesterone.

Prednisolone: See Table 24–7.

Prednisone (Meticorten): See Table 24–7 and 32–3.

Primidone (Mysoline): See Table 21–2.

Priscoline: See Tolazoline.

Pro-Banthine: See Propantheline.

Probenecid (Benemid): Initial dose, 25 mg/kg, then 10 mg/kg every 6 hours orally. (Adult = 1–2 gm initially, then 0.5 gm every 6 hours.)

Procainamide (Pronestyl): (1) Orally, 8–15 mg/kg every 4–6 hours. (2) IM, 6 mg/kg every 4–6 hours. (3) IV, for emergency use only: 2 mg/kg, at a rate not to exceed 0.5–1 mg/kg/minute. Monitor by continuous ECG and blood pressure recording every minute.

Procarbazine (Matulane): 8 mg/kg orally as initial dose. *Caution.*

Prochlorperazine (Compazine): 0.25–0.375 mg/kg/day orally or rectally in 2–3 doses. (Adult = 25 mg rectally twice daily or 5 mg orally 3–4 times daily.) IM, 0.25 mg/kg/day. *Caution:* Avoid overdosage.

Progesterone: See Anhydrohydroxyprogesterone.

Progestoral: See Anhydrohydroxyprogesterone.

Promethazine (Phenergan): As antihistaminic, 0.5 mg/kg orally at bedtime; 0.1 mg/kg orally 3 times daily. For nausea and vomiting, 0.25–0.5 mg/kg rectally or IM. For sedation, 0.5–1 mg/kg IM.

Pronestyl: See Procainamide.

Propantheline (Pro-Banthine): 1–2 mg/kg/day orally in 4 divided doses after meals. (Adult = 15–30 mg 3–4 times daily.)

Propoxyphene (Darvon): 3 mg/kg/day orally. (Adult = 32–65 mg 3–4 times daily.)

Propranolol (Inderal): Adult: Arrhythmias, 10–30 mg 3–4 times daily, before meals and at bedtime. (Pediatric dosage has not been established.)

Propylthiouracil: 6–7 mg/kg/day in 3 divided doses at intervals of 8 hours. Maintenance: 1/3–1/2 initial dose. See also p 607.

Prostaphlin: See Penicillins, Chapter 39.

Prostigmin: See Neostigmine.

Protamine sulfate: 2.5–5 mg/kg, then 1–2.5 mg/kg IV. Newborn: 1–2.5 mg/kg IM or IV. (Adult = 50 mg every 4–6 hours IV.)

Protopam: See Pralidoxime.

Pseudoephedrine hydrochloride (Sudafed): 4 mg/kg/day in 4 doses.

Purinethol: See Mercaptopurine, Table 32–3.

Pyribenzamine: See Tripelennamine.

Pyridostigmin (Mestinon): 7 mg/kg/day orally in 6 doses. Increase as necessary by 5 mg. (Average adult dose = 600 mg/day.)

Pyrimethamine (Daraprim): 12.5 mg weekly (in syrup).

Pyronil: See Pyrrobutamine.

Pyrrobutamine (Pyronil): 0.6 mg/kg/day. (Adult = 15 mg 3–4 times daily.)

Pyrvinium pamoate (Povan): 5 mg/kg/day. (Same as adult dose.)

Questran: See Cholestyramine.

Quinacrine (mepacrine, Atabrine): Giardiasis, 8 mg/kg/day for 5 days in 3 doses orally. (Maximum, 300 mg/day.) Tapeworm, 15 mg/kg in 2 doses orally. (Maximum, 800 mg.)

Quinidine: Test dose: 2 mg/kg orally. If tolerated, give 3–6 mg/kg every 2–3 hours. (Adult = 200 mg.) Therapeutic dose: 30 mg/kg/day orally in 4–5 divided doses.

Quinine sulfate: 1 year: 0.13 gm orally 3 times daily. 5–10 years: 0.3–0.6 gm 3 times daily. (Adult = 0.6 gm 3 times daily for 5–7 days.)

Regitine: See Phentolamine.

Reserpine (Serpasil, etc): (1) Orally 0.005–0.03 mg/kg/day in 4 doses. (2) IM, 0.02–0.07 mg/kg every 12–24 hours. Initially, try smaller dose (except in life-threatening situations) and double in 4–6 hours if response is inadequate. May give with hydralazine (Apresoline). (Adult = 0.1–0.5 mg daily.)

Ritalin: See Methylphenidate.

Robaxin: See Methocarbamol.

Romilar: See Dextromethorphan.

Rondomycin (methacycline): See Tetracyclines, Chapter 39.

Salamide: See Salicylamide.

Salicylamide (Dropsprin, Liquiprin, Salamide, Salrin): 65 mg/year of age/dose orally 3 or 4 times daily. (Adult = 0.3–0.6 gm orally 3–4 times daily.)

Salicylazosulfapyridine (Azulfidine): 50–100 mg/kg/day orally at 4- to 6-hour intervals. (Adult = 1 gm 4–6 times daily.)

Salrin: See Salicylamide.

Sansert: See Methysergide.

Scopolamine: 0.006 mg/kg as single dose orally or subcut.

Secobarbital (Seconal): (1) Orally, 2–6 mg/kg as a single sedative or light hypnotic dose. (Adult = 100 mg.) (2) Rectally, 6 mg/kg as a minimal hypnotic dose. (Adult = 200 mg.)

Seconal: See Secobarbital.

Seromycin: See Cycloserine.

Serpasil: See Reserpine.

Sodium bicarbonate: See pp 63 and 923.

Sodium phosphate: 150–200 mg/kg/dose orally. (Adult = 4–8 gm.)

Sodium polystyrene sulfonate (Kayexalate): Children: 1 mEq potassium/gm resin. Calculate dose on basis of desired exchange. Instill rectally in 10% glucose. May be administered every 6 hours. (Adult = 15 gm orally 1–4 times daily in small amount of water or syrup; 3–4 ml/gm resin.)

Sodium salicylate: As a single analgesic or antipyretic dose, 65 mg/year of age orally. (Adult = 0.3–0.6 gm.) For rheumatic fever, 90–130 mg/kg/day orally to maintain a blood level of 20–30 mg/100 ml. (Adult = 0.3–4 gm.)

Sodium sulfate: 150–200 mg/kg/dose orally. Give as 50% solution. (Adult = 8–12 gm.)

Sodium thiosulfate: See p 787.

Spironolactone (Aldactone): (1) Diagnostic test: 0.5–1.5 gm/sq m/day in divided doses orally. (2) Edema and ascites: 1.7–3.3 mg/kg/day orally in divided doses. Start with smaller dose. *Caution.* (Adult = 25 mg 3–6 times daily orally.)

Stanozolol (Winstrol): 0.1 mg/kg/day orally.

Staphcillin: See Penicillins, Chapter 39.

Stilbestrol: 0.1–1 mg/day orally. (Adult = 0.5–1 mg.)

Stoxil: See Idoxuridine, p 957.

Streptomycin: See Chapter 39.

Strophanthin: See Ouabain.

Sudafed: See Pseudoephedrine hydrochloride.

Sulfisoxazole (Gantrisin): See Chapter 39.

Sulfonamides: See Chapter 39.

Sus-Phrine: See Epinephrine solution, 1:200.

Symmetrel: See Amantadine, p 957.

Synkayvite: See Manadiol sodium diphosphate.

Synthroid Sodium: See Levothyroxine sodium.

Tapazole: See Methimazole, p 607.

Tegretol: See Carbamazepine, Table 21–2.

Tempra: See Acetaminophen.

Tensilon: See Edrophonium chloride.

Testosterone: (1) Testosterone enanthate (Delatestryl): 200 mg IM every 4 weeks for teenage male. (2) Testosterone cyclopentylpropionate: 50–200 mg IM every 2–4 weeks for teenage male. (3) Testosterone propionate in oil: 10–50 mg 2–6 times a week IM for adult or teenage male. (4) Testosterone microcrystals in aqueous suspension: 100 mg IM every 2–3 weeks. (5) Testosterone pellets: 300 mg approximately every 3 months.

Tetrachloroethylene: (Do not give in presence of ascariasis; in mixed infections, treat ascariasis first.) Saline purge of 15–30 gm sodium sulfate on the night before therapy. Withhold all food. Give 0.2 ml per year of age as a single dose, in capsule form or as liquid with syrup, followed by bed rest for 24 hours. Two hours after therapy, repeat saline purge.

Tetracyclines: See Chapter 39.

Tetraethylammonium chloride (Etamon): Test dose, 250 mg/sq m IV. *Caution:* Phentolamine should be available. (Adult = 10–15 mg/kg IV or IM.)

Thiamine: See Table 4–2.

Thiopental (Pentothal): 10–20 mg/kg rectally *slowly* for basal anesthesia.

Thioridazine (Mellaril): Children 2–12 years: 0.5–3 mg/kg/day (maximum). Older children: 20–30 mg/day. Not for children under 2 years. (Adult = 20–200 mg/day. Psychosis: 200–800 mg/day.)

Thorazine: See Chlorpromazine.

Thyroid: See p 606.

L Thyroxine sodium: See Levothyroxine sodium.

Tigan: See Trimethobenzamide.

Tofranil: See Imipramine.

Tolazoline (Priscoline): Adult dosages = 25 mg orally 4–6 times daily; 25–75 mg subcut, IM, or IV 4 times daily. Pediatric dosages not established.

Tolserol: See Mephenesin.

Toluidine blue: Initial dose: 2.5–7.5 mg/kg/day IV. Subsequent dose: 2–5 mg/kg/day IV. (Adult = 6–8 mg/kg.)

Triacetyloleandomycin (Cyclamycin, TAO): See Troleandomycin, p 950.

Triamcinolone: See Table 24–7.

Tribromoethanol (Avertin): 65–100 mg/kg rectally. (Adult = 60 mg/kg.) Not over 8 gm should be given.

Trichlormethiazide: 0.03–0.1 mg/kg/day orally. (Adult = 2–8 mg daily.)

Tridione: See Trimethadione, Table 21–2.

Triethylenemelamine (TEM): Initial dose: 5 mg/day orally. Subsequent dose: 1 mg/day or 0.04 mg/kg orally. (Adult = 5 mg, then 2.5 mg.) *Caution.*

Triiodothyronine (liothyronine, Cytomel): 25–30 µg are equivalent to 100 mg thyroid USP or 0.1 mg levothyroxine sodium.

Trimethadione (Tridione): See Table 21–2.

Trimethobenzamide (Tigan): Children weighing less than 15 kg, 1/2 suppository (100 mg) 3 times daily. Children over 15 kg, 100 mg 3 times daily orally or 100–200 mg 3 times daily rectally.

Tripelennamine (Pyribenzamine): 3–5 mg/kg/day orally in 3–6 divided doses. (Adult = 50 mg 3–4 times daily.)

Troleandomycin: See Erythromycin, p 950.

Tubocurarine (curare): 0.2–0.4 mg/kg/day IM or subcut. *Caution.* (Adult = 6–9 mg.)

Tylenol: See Acetaminophen.

Unipen: See Penicillins, Chapter 39.

Urea: (1) 0.8 gm/kg/day in 3 divided doses orally. (Adult = 8 gm.) (2) 0.5–1 gm/kg IV over a period of 30–60 minutes. (Adult = 1–1.5 gm/kg.)

Urecholine Chloride: See Bethanechol chloride.

Valium: See Diazepam, Table 21–2.

Vancocin: See Vancomycin, Chapter 39.

Vancomycin (Vancocin): See Chapter 39.

Vasopressin (Pitressin) injection: 0.125–0.5 ml (20 units/ml) IM. Short duration. (Adult = 0.25–0.5 ml.)

Vasopressin (Pitressin) tannate injection: 0.2–2 ml (5 units/ml in oil) every 2–4 days as necessary IM. Start with smaller dose and increase. Effective 1–3 days. (Adult = 0.3–1 ml.)

Vasoxyl: See Methoxamine.

Velban: See Vinblastine, Table 32–3.

Versenate (edathamil): See EDTA.

Vinblastine (Velban): See Table 32–3.

Vincristine (Oncovin): See Table 32–3.

Vioform: See Iodochlorhydroxyquin.

Viokase (pancreatic replacement): 0.3–0.6 gm with each feeding. (Same as adult dose.)

Vitamins: See Table 4–2.

Vitamin A: See Table 4–2 and p 640.

Vitamin C: See Table 4–2 and p 647.

Vitamin D: See p 642.

Vitamin D_2 (Calciferol): 25–200 thousand units/day.

Vitamin K_1 (Mephyton): 0.5–5 mg orally, subcut, or IV. (Adult = 5 mg orally; in emergencies, 10–15 mg IV.)

Wyamine: See Mephentermine sulfate.

Wydase: See Hyaluronidase.

Xylocaine: See Lidocaine.

Zarontin: See Ethosuximide, Table 21–2.

•   •   •

General References

Gellis SS, Kagan BM: *Current Pediatric Therapy.* Saunders, 1970.

Physicians' Desk Reference, 26th ed, 1971. Medical Economics, Inc. 1972.

Shirkey C: *Pediatric Therapy.* Mosby, 1968.

Silver HK, Kempe CH, Bruyn HB: *Handbook of Pediatrics,* 9th ed. Lange, 1971.

Zaia M, Janeway A, Cooke RE: *Pediatrics.* Little, Brown, 1969.

39 . . .

Anti-infective Chemotherapeutic Agents & Antibiotic Drugs

C. Henry Kempe, MD, & Anne S. Yeager, MD

Antimicrobial therapy involves the use of chemotherapeutic agents for the treatment of an infectious disease by attack upon the etiologic agent. Maximum success in the use of these substances depends upon (1) identification of the pathogens to be eliminated, (2) selection of the therapeutic agent or agents most active against the pathogen, (3) selection of the appropriate route of administration in order to achieve maximum contact of the drug with the pathogen, and (4) administration of the appropriate amount of drug to reach and destroy the pathogen.

Methicillin, oxacillin, nafcillin, cloxacillin, and dicloxacillin are resistant to staphylococcal penicillinase and are used in the treatment of infections due to penicillin-resistant staphylococci. Parenteral nafcillin is as effective against pneumococci and streptococci as penicillin G. When used in proper dosage, drugs in this group are effective against penicillin-sensitive strains of staphylococci but are unnecessarily expensive; penicillin remains the drug of choice for penicillin-sensitive staphylococci. Gentamicin is a useful agent for topical and systemic treatment of pseudomonas and other resistant gram-negative infections. Carbenicillin is a useful adjunct in the therapy of pseudomonas infections but should generally be used with another drug and should be administered intravenously. Cephalexin is an improved oral drug which is similar in spectrum to cephalothin and achieves better blood levels than previously available oral cephalosporins. It should not be relied on for initiation of therapy in serious infections but is of use in urinary tract infections in which the organism is sensitive. Rifampin is an exceedingly effective drug against *Mycobacterium tuberculosis*. Because of fear of development of resistance with widespread use, it is recommended only for retreatment of refractory cases of tuberculosis and should be used only in combination with other drugs.

General Indications

Antibiotic and chemotherapeutic agents are indicated (1) for diseases in which a specific microbial etiologic agent has been identified by culture or serology, (2) for diseases in which the clinical picture implies a definite etiologic diagnosis, and (3) as a possible lifesaving measure for a desperately ill patient when an exact or complete etiologic diagnosis has not yet been made.

Development of Resistance

Resistance develops (1) if strains in the bacterial population which are by inheritance resistant to the agent being used become dominant by selection, or (2) if "spontaneous" mutation to a state of resistance should occur.

Adequate dosage and combined therapy prevent or slow down the development of resistant strains. Combined therapy is particularly important for treatment of tuberculosis.

Precautions in Newborns & Prematures

Especially in premature infants, newborn infants, and in oliguric children, great caution is necessary in preventing overdosage in order to avoid serious and permanent damage. Comments on dosage for newborn and premature infants are included in the text that follows.

Precautions in Oliguric Children

Regular drug dosages are too high for children with reduced renal function. Dosage and time schedules must be adjusted to renal output in the case of the more toxic agents (streptomycin, chloramphenicol, neomycin, kanamycin, bacitracin, polymyxin, colistin, novobiocin, and gentamicin). (See Table 39–1.)

PEDIATRIC ANTIMICROBIAL THERAPEUTIC AGENTS

Aminosalicylic Acid (PAS; PAS-C)
  Use: Tuberculosis.
  Dosage:
     Oral: PAS: 250–300 mg/kg/day in divided doses every 6 hours; PAS-C: 150 mg/kg/day in divided doses every 6 hours. **Adolescent:** 12 gm/day.
  Toxicity: Gastrointestinal symptoms, hypersensitivity (skin, fever, genital), renal irritation, goitrogenic, hematologic, hepatic.
  Comment: Avoid or reduce dosage by 1/2 when renal function is impaired. Stop drug at first sign of skin rash. PAS-C usually causes less gastric irritation than PAS.

TABLE 39–1. Use of antibiotics in patients with renal failure.*

Drug	Principal Mode of Excretion or Detoxification	Approximate Half-Life in Serum		Proposed Dosage Regimen† in Renal Failure‡	
		Normal	Renal Failure	Usual Initial Dose	Give Half the Initial Dose at Interval Of
Penicillin G	Tubular secretion	0.5 hours	10 hours	70,000 units/kg	8–12 hours
Ampicillin	Tubular secretion	0.5 hours	10 hours	50 mg/kg	8–12 hours
Methicillin	Tubular secretion	0.5 hours	10 hours	50 mg/kg	6–8 hours
Cephalothin	Tubular secretion	0.8 hours	15 hours	35 mg/kg	12 hours
Streptomycin	Glomerular filtration	2.5 hours	3–4 days	10 mg/kg	3–4 days
Kanamycin§	Glomerular filtration	3 hours	3–4 days	7.5 mg/kg	3–4 days
Gentamicin§	Glomerular filtration	2.5 hours	3–4 days	1.5 mg/kg	3–4 days
Vancomycin	Glomerular filtration	6 hours	8–9 days	10 mg/kg	8–10 days
Polymyxin B§	Glomerular filtration	5 hours	2–3 days	1.5 mg/kg	3–4 days
Colistimethate	Glomerular filtration	3 hours	2–3 days	2.5 mg/kg	3–4 days
Chloramphenicol	Liver and glomerular filtration	3 hours	4 hours	30 mg/kg	8 hours
Erythromycin	Liver and glomerular filtration	1.5 hours	5 hours	20 mg/kg (IV)	8 hours
Clindamycin	Glomerular filtration and liver (?)	4 hours	8 hours	5 mg/kg (orally)	8 hours

*This table should be used only as a guide. Serum killing power or μg/ml should be measured when possible, as well as minimal inhibitory concentration (MIC) of drug for specific organism.
†IV or IM unless otherwise specified.
‡Considered here to be marked by creatinine clearance of 10 ml/minute or less.
§See Kunin C: Antibiotic usage in patients with renal impairment. Hosp Practice 1:141, 1972.

Amphotericin B (Fungizone)

Use: Active against a variety of fungi (candida, cryptococcus, blastomyces, sporotrichum, coccidioides, histoplasma).

Dosage:

IV: 0.5–1 mg/kg/day or every other day, given over 4–6 hours.

Intrathecal: 0.5–1 mg in 10 ml spinal fluid every other day.

Incompatibility: Do not mix with penicillin G or tetracyclines.

Toxicity: Chills, fever, malaise. Significant renal, hepatic, and bone marrow damage. Thrombophlebitis, calcifications.

Comment: Indicated only in severe systemic fungal infections. Administration of corticosteroids before the daily dose is given may ameliorate side-effects. Blood levels should be followed (Am J Med 45:405, 1968).

Bacitracin

Use: Effective against gram-positive organisms; ineffective against gram-negatives.

Dosage:

Intrathecal, intraventricular: 500–5000 units/day (1000 units/ml).

Eye and skin: 500 units/ml.

Toxicity: Transient nephrotoxicity, nausea and vomiting. Topical or oral use harmless except for large denuded areas.

Comment: Superseded in other uses by the penicillinase-resistant penicillins.

Carbenicillin

Use: Covers only pseudomonas, indole-positive proteus, and some strains of serratia.

Dosage:

IM and orally: Do not use.

IV: 500–600 mg/kg/day in divided doses every 2–4 hours. **Newborn:** 300 mg/kg/day (not well established). **Adolescent:** Up to 30 gm/day.

Comment: Relatively high doses are required. It is of value in pseudomonas infections in patients with compromised renal function since toxicity is low. SGOT rises have been reported and may be due to muscle necrosis after intramuscular injection. Probably synergistic with gentamicin. Because of the rapid development of resistance, carbenicillin should be used only in combination with other drugs.

Cephalexin (Keflex)

Use: See Cephalothin.

Dosage:

Oral: 50–100 mg/kg/day (not well established). **Adult:** 1–2 gm/day.

Toxicity: Nausea, vomiting, diarrhea. Occasional SGOT rise, rash, pruritus.

Comment: The same precautions apply to the use of this drug in persons who are sensitive to penicillin as apply to cephalothin, cephaloridine, and cephaloglycin. The peak blood and urine levels are delayed when the drug is administered with food, but the absorption is still good. Bactericidal activity against sensitive organisms is not as rapid as with cephalothin and cephaloridine. Unit for unit, cephalexin is not quite as active as the latter 2 drugs against sensitive organisms. In general, blood levels are adequate for sensitive gram-positive organisms and for many gram-negative organisms, but the peak blood level achieved on a standard dose varies considerably from individual to individual. Cephalexin should not be relied on for initial therapy in seriously ill persons. 80–90% of the drug is excreted in the first 6 hours following a single dose. Because of rapid excretion, frequent doses of probenecid may be necessary if high blood levels must be maintained. Cephalexin is of use in the therapy of urinary tract infections caused by sensitive organisms. Blood levels are higher than those reached with cephaloglycin.

Cephaloglycin (Kafocin): See Cephalexin.

Cephaloridine (Loridine)

Use: Generally the same as for cephalothin (see below) except that it is less resistant to staphylococcal penicillinase, its efficacy in *Hemophilus influenzae* infections is somewhat uncertain, and it may penetrate tissue fluids (including the CSF) better.

Dosage:

    IV or IM: 30–50 mg/kg/day in divided doses every 4–6 hours given over 3–4 minutes or longer. **Newborn:** Do not use. **Adolescent:** Give no more than 4 gm/day. **Serious infections:** May be used in doses up to 100 mg/kg/day in divided doses every 4 hours, not to exceed 4 gm. Use the lowest effective dosage.

Toxicity: Definitely more toxic than cephalothin, with cases of oliguria and renal shutdown reported. Tends to build up after multiple injections, so that the 4-hour level is twice as high after multiple injections as after a single injection. Eosinophilia, leukopenia (rare). Impairment of free water clearance.

Comment: Less painful than cephalothin following intramuscular injection. May be associated with a higher rate of superinfections than cephalothin.

Cephalothin (Keflin)

Use: Equivalent to penicillin against gram-positive organisms except enterococcus (*Streptococcus faecalis*), which is relatively insensitive. Highly resistant to staphylococcal penicillinase. Effective against most *Escherichia coli,* indole-negative proteus, most klebsiella, and many strains of *Hemophilus influenzae.* Ineffective against pseudomonas, serratia, and most aerobacter (enterobacter). When used for gram-negative infections, individual sensitivities should be determined. This drug has been used successfully in penicillin-sensitive persons for treatment of meningococcal meningitis, but poor results have also been reported. Unusual prolongation of fever or lack of neurologic improvement should prompt reevaluation of the CSF and the choice of drug.

Dosage:

    Oral: Not absorbed.

    IM: 60–150 mg/kg/day in divided doses every 4–6 hours given into a large muscle.

    IV: 60–150 mg/kg/day in divided doses every 4–6 hours. **Newborn:** 50 mg/kg/day in divided doses every 6 hours. **Adolescent:** Up to 12 gm/day in the usual case. **Severe infections:** May be used in doses of 150–200 mg/kg/day in infections such as meningitis, with up to 24 gm being used in adults.

Incompatibility: Do not mix with polymyxin B, tetracyclines, erythromycin, calcium chloride, or calcium gluconate.

Toxicity: Pain at injection site; sterile abscesses, drug fever, positive direct Coombs test, anemia, thrombocytopenic purpura; brown-black precipitate in Benedict's test or Clinitest for glucose (when glucose is normal).

Comment: Cephalothin is of special use as a penicillin substitute in penicillin-sensitive persons. Anaphylaxis has been reported but is rare clinically, although the incidence of "sensitivity" to cephalothin as demonstrated by in vitro tests in penicillin-sensitive persons is high. The reason for this discrepancy is not known at present. The drug is relatively nontoxic to the kidneys. It causes a positive direct Coombs response in normal persons and, because of difficulty in cross-matching blood, should be avoided in persons who may require transfusion. In combination with methicillin or kanamycin, it may be beneficial in the treatment of methicillin-resistant staphylococcal infections. In combination with kanamycin, it may be synergistic in the treatment of resistant *Escherichia coli* infection.

Chloramphenicol (Chloromycetin)

Use: Bacteriostatic for a wide range of gram-positive and gram-negative organisms, rickettsiae, and chlamydiae. Drug of choice only for typhoid fever.

Dosage:

    Oral: 50–100 mg/kg/day (crystalline) in divided doses every 6 hours. Palmitate is poorly absorbed.

    IM: Should not be used since absorption is poor.

IV: Microcrystalline: 100–150 mg/kg/day in divided doses every 12 hours. Succinate: 100 mg/kg/day in divided doses every 6–8 hours. **Full-term newborn:** 25–50 mg/kg/day in divided doses every 6–12 hours. **Premature:** 25 mg/kg/day in divided doses every 6–12 hours. This drug should be avoided in premature infants. If used, serum levels should be followed to avoid toxicity initially and to avoid inadequate dosage as renal and liver function matures. An adequate blood level is 10–12 µg/100 ml. **Adolescent:** 100 mg/kg/day.

Incompatibility: Do not mix with polymyxin B, tetracyclines, vancomycin, hydrocortisone, B complex vitamins.

Toxicity: In newborns up to 4 months of age, vasomotor collapse (gray syndrome). Aplastic anemia and other hematopoietic toxicity. Gastrointestinal symptoms, stomatitis, candidal infections. Allergy, hepatitis, optic neuritis, and neurologic abnormalities occur rarely.

Comment: Should not be used when an equally effective drug is available. Mechanism of action is antagonistic to that of penicillin. Diffuses better than most penicillins (eyes, CSF). Uses include treatment of cases of hemophilus meningitis which fail to respond to ampicillin, meningococcal meningitis in penicillin-sensitive persons, bacteroides infections, typhoid fever, and peritonitis.

Clindamycin (Cleocin)

Use: Probably useful against common anaerobic organisms, including various species of Bacteroides and anaerobic streptococci.

Dosage:

Oral: 8–20 mg/kg/day in divided doses every 6–8 hours. **Adolescent:** 0.6–1.8 gm/day in divided doses every 6 hours.

Toxicity: Gastrointestinal disturbances (nausea, diarrhea, cramps). The incidence of rashes following the administration of clindamycin for the treatment of upper respiratory tract infections appears to be about 10%. Urticaria occurs rarely.

Colistin (Coly-Mycin S and Coly-Mycin C)

Use: *Pseudomonas aeruginosa;* some other gram-negatives. Not a good "broad spectrum" antibiotic. Proteus and gram-positive organisms are resistant.

Dosage:

Oral: Colistin sulfate: Not absorbed. 15 mg/kg/day in divided doses every 8 hours.

IM: Sodium colistimethate: 5–10 mg/kg/day in divided doses every 6–12 hours given deep into a muscle. **Newborn:** 1.5–5 mg/kg/day in divided doses every 12 hours (for the first week).

Toxicity: Proteinuria, cyclindruria, hematuria, increased BUN (reversible). Paresthesias, ataxia, drowsiness, confusion. Fever, rash, pain at injection site.

Comment: May be used orally for neomycin-resistant enteropathogenic *Escherichia coli* infections. Use with care if renal function is abnormal. Gains access to CSF only when used in doses greater than 10 mg/kg/day, so that other drugs should be used for CSF infection. Do not use intrathecally because the preparation contains dibucaine.

Erythromycin (Erythrocin, Ilotycin, Ilosone, Pediamycin)

Use: Gram-positive cocci, clostridia, *Hemophilus influenzae, H pertussis, Corynebacterium diphtheriae,* rickettsiae, brucella, some bacteroides. Resistance of some group A streptococci and some pneumococci has been reported, although this is rare at present. May be of use in chronic bronchitis, cystic fibrosis, and some urinary tract infections because of action against L forms. Probably as effective as tetracycline for symptomatic relief of mycoplasmal infections, although the organisms continue to be shed.

Dosage:

Oral: 30–50 mg/kg/day in divided doses every 6 hours.

IM: 10–20 mg/kg/day in divided doses every 6 hours.

IV: 40–70 mg/kg/day in divided doses every 6 hours given over a 20–60 minute period.

Full-term newborn and premature:

Oral: 20–40 mg/kg/day in divided doses every 12 hours.

IM, IV: 10 mg/kg/day in divided doses every 12 hours.

Adolescent: Up to 2 gm/day. Higher doses could be used in severe infections.

Toxicity: Painful injection, gastrointestinal symptoms, candidiasis, drug fever. Estolate (Ilosone) is associated with intrahepatic cholestatic jaundice when treatment is for more than 10 days.

Comment: Troleandomycin (triacetyloleandomycin, TAO) is similar to erythromycin in spectrum and activity. Do not use concomitantly with lincomycin.

Ethambutol (Myambutol)

Use: Tuberculosis.

Dosage: 15 mg/kg/day; retreatment, 25 mg/kg/day for 60 days, then 15 mg/kg/day.

Toxicity: Retrobulbar neuritis (3%). Patients should be routinely followed with monthly examination of visual acuity and color discrimination. Anaphylactoid reactions. Peripheral neuritis.

Comment: Experience in the pediatric age range is limited.

Gentamicin (Garamycin)

Use: Most gram-negatives, including pseudomonas and proteus. Of particular use in *Serratia marcescens* infections. Some activity against gram-positives, including activity against coagulase-positive staphylococci. Relatively inactive against pneumococci and streptococci.

Dosage:

Topical: Cream, 0.1% and ointment, 0.1%.

IM: 3–4 mg/kg/day in divided doses every 6–8 hours (may occasionally be used in higher dosage for brief periods).

IV: Little experience is available regarding intravenous use, and this route should be used only in the presence of a bleeding diathesis. Each dose should be given over a 2- to 4-hour period because of possible curare-like effect. The dose is the same as for IM administration. **Newborn:** 4 mg/kg/day (not well established).

Intraventricular: 4–8 mg/day (gives a CSF level of 3–5 μg/ml).

Toxicity: Irreversible vestibular damage has occurred, most often in uremic patients, and is related to excessive plasma levels. Transient proteinuria, elevated BUN, oliguria, azotemia, macular skin eruption, and elevated SGOT have been reported. If used in uremic patients, dosage schedule should be modified. Should be used with caution in patients receiving ototoxic drugs. Overall toxicity is probably the same as or less than that of kanamycin.

Comment: Parenteral therapy with this drug should be reserved for serious pseudomonas infections, hospital-acquired infections, and life-threatening infections of unknown but suspected gram-negative origin. If cultures later are positive for an organism sensitive to penicillin, methicillin, cephalothin, ampicillin, or kanamycin, therapy should be changed to one of these drugs. Every effort should be made to use this drug as little as possible so that drug resistance will not develop. Relative resistance has developed during therapy. Topical therapy with gentamicin for superficial infections of the skin and mucous membranes due to pseudomonas has been effective.

Griseofulvin (Fulvicin, Grifulvin, Grisactin)

Use: Tinea species, microsporum, trichophyton. Ineffective against candida, cryptococcus, blastomyces, histoplasma, and coccidioides.

Dosage:

Oral: Regular size: 20 mg/kg/day in divided doses every 6–12 hours. Microsize: 10 mg/kg/day in divided doses every 6–12 hours. Children 30–50 lb, 125–250 mg daily; over 50 lb, 250–500 mg daily.

Toxicity: Leukopenia and other blood dyscrasias, headache, incoordination and confusion, gastrointestinal disturbances, rash (allergic and photosensitivity), renal damage, lupus-like syndrome.

Comment: Do not use in patients with hepatocellular failure or porphyria.

Hetacillin (Versapen-K)

Use: See Ampicillin.

Dosage: For mild to moderate infections, 25–40 mg/kg/day orally, IM, or IV. The dosage for severe infections is not well established.

Toxicity: Probably similar to that of ampicillin.

Comment: Hetacillin is hydrolyzed in the body to ampicillin, which appears to be the active agent. Higher blood levels are achieved on oral administration if the drug is given in the fasting state. Peak blood levels following oral administration are in the range of 1 μg/ml, which is sufficient for sensitive gram-positive organisms but inadequate for systemic infections with common gram-negative organisms. Higher levels are achieved in urine, and (as with ampicillin) urinary tract infections due to sensitive gram-negative organisms may be treated with this drug. Hetacillin is more stable than ampicillin after reconstitution for intravenous use. Administration of hetacillin intravenously results in somewhat higher and more prolonged blood levels than the same dose of ampicillin.

Isoniazid (INH, Nydrazid)

Use: Tuberculosis.

Dosage:

Oral: 15–20 mg/kg/day in divided doses every 6–12 hours. Give no more than 600 mg/day.

IM: 10 mg/kg/day in divided doses every 12 hours. **Newborn:** Dosage is not well established, but there is some evidence that INH may compete with bilirubin for albumin-binding sites in newborns. BCG vaccination is a better alternative for the child of a tuberculous mother than INH prophylaxis.

Toxicity: Neurotoxic, due to pyridoxine deficiency (rare in children). Gastrointestinal symptoms, seizures, hypersensitivity. Reactions are rare, but more common in the elderly and the malnourished.

Kanamycin (Kantrex)

Use: Bactericidal for staphylococci, coliforms, proteus, some pseudomonas, mycobacteria.

Of use in special circumstances in some vibrio, salmonella, and shigella infections.

Dosage:

Oral: Not absorbed. Used for sterilization of bowel. 50–100 mg/kg/day in divided doses every 6 hours.

IM: 15 mg/kg/day in divided doses every 12 hours. **Full-term newborn:** 15 mg/kg/day. **Premature:** 10 mg/kg/day; avoid using IV. **Adolescent:** 1 gm/day in divided doses every 12 hours.

IV: 15–20 mg/kg/day in divided doses every 6–8 hours. (for serious infections only). **Adolescent:** In serious infections, 2 gm/day IV for a short time.

Intraventricular: 5 mg/day.

Aerosol: 1 mg 4 times daily (250 mg/ml).

Intrapleural and intra-articular: 2.5 mg/ml.

Toxicity: Limit use to 10 days. Irreversible deafness occurs after prolonged administration of high doses. (Cumulative ototoxicity with other ototoxic drugs occurs.) Nephrotoxicity is transient unless prior renal impairment was present. The safe total dose is 0.5 gm/kg.

Comment: Modify dosage and use with caution in oliguric patients.

Lincomycin (Lincocin)

Use: Gram-positive organisms except *Streptococcus faecalis.* Resistant pneumococci and group A streptococci have been reported but are rare at this time.

Dosage: Do not use in infants under 1 month of age.

Oral: 50–100 mg/kg/day in divided doses every 8 hours. **Adolescent:** 1.8–2.4 gm/day in divided doses every 6–8 hours.

IM: 10–20 mg/kg/day in divided doses every 12 hours.

IV: 10–20 mg/kg/day in divided doses every 8–12 hours.

Incompatibility: Do not mix with erythromycin or cyclamates.

Toxicity: Diarrhea, nausea, vomiting, rash, rectal irritation, vaginitis, urticaria. SGOT rise with or without jaundice. Neutropenia or leukopenia.

Comment: The evidence that this drug is as good as or better than penicillinase-resistant penicillins in osteomyelitis is scanty. It should only be used in cases in which the organism has been shown to be sensitive and when the serum levels can be followed.

Methacycline (Rondomycin). See Tetracyclines.

Methenamine Mandelate (Mandelamine)

Use: Genitourinary infections. Not effective against proteus.

Dosage: 100 mg/kg orally immediately and then 50 mg/kg/day in divided doses every 8 hours.

Comment: Urine should be kept acid.

Metronidazole (Flagyl)

Use: Trichomoniasis, giardiasis.

Dosage:

Oral: Adolescent: 250 mg every 8 hours.

Toxicity: Nausea, anorexia, and other gastrointestinal intolerance; glossitis and stomatitis; leukopenia; dizziness, vertigo, ataxia; urticaria, pruritus.

Comment: Has been used in the therapy of giardiasis infections and in the treatment of amebic dysentery in children in doses up to 50 mg/kg/day.

Nalidixic Acid (NegGram)

Use: Useful in gram-negative urinary tract infections with *Escherichia coli,* aerobacter (enterobacter), klebsiella, and proteus. Pseudomonas is generally resistant.

Dosage: 40–50 mg/kg orally in divided doses 4 times daily; may be reduced to 20–25 mg/kg/day for maintenance. **Adolescent:** 4 gm/day in divided doses every 6 hours; may be reduced to 2 gm/day for maintenance therapy.

Toxicity: Gastrointestinal symptoms, hypersensitivity (pruritus, rash, urticaria, eosinophilia), seizures.

Comment: Toxicity is low, and the drug may be used for months. Resistance may develop. Use cautiously in patients with liver disease or impaired renal function. Do not use in children under 1 month of age or for infections other than those of the urinary tract.

Neomycin (Mycifradin, Neobiotic)

Use: Bactericidal for gram-positive cocci, gram-negative bacilli, acid-fast bacilli, and actinomycetes.

Dosage:

Oral: Not absorbed. 100 mg/kg/day in divided doses every 6 hours. **Full-term newborn and premature:** 50 mg/kg/day in divided doses every 6 hours.

Toxicity: Nephrotoxic and ototoxic when used parenterally. Oral use causes diarrhea, reversible disaccharidase deficiency, malabsorption of carotene, glucose, and iron, and candidiasis. Topical use causes rashes and skin sensitization. Intrapleural or intraperitoneal use can lead to respiratory arrest (curare-like effect) which is potentiated by ether anesthesia and reversible by neostigmine. *Note:* Use with caution by all routes in patients with renal and hepatic disease, including the relatively oliguric newborn. Parenteral use is superseded by other drugs.

Nitrofurantoin (Furadantin)

Use: Many gram-negative organisms are susceptible to concentrations achieved in urine.

Dosage:

Oral: 5–7 mg/kg/day. Reduce dosage after 10–14 days. **Infant:** 1.5 mg/kg/day. **Adolescent:** 400 mg every day in divided doses every 6 hours.

Toxicity: Primiquine-sensitive hemolytic anemia, peripheral neuropathy, rash, chills, fever, myalgia-like syndrome, cholestatic jaundice.

Comment: Should only be used for urinary tract infections.

Nystatin (Mycostatin)

Use: *Candida albicans* and other yeasts.

Dosage:

Oral: Not absorbed. < 2 years, 400–800 thousand units/day. > 2 years, 1–2 million units/day in divided doses every 6–8 hours. **Full-term newborn and premature:** 200–400 thousand units/ day.

Eye and skin: 100,000 units/gm.

Toxicity: None.

Oleandomycin: See Erythromycin.

The Penicillins

Because of protein binding, serum killing power is the preferred test of bacterial sensitivity and efficacy of therapy.

All penicillins are cross-allergenic.

The mechanism of action of tetracyclines and chloramphenicol is antagonistic to that of the penicillins.

In serious infections, all penicillins should be given in divided doses so that a dose is given every 4 hours.

Until skin testing materials are commercially available, the following method may be used to desensitize the patient when penicillin must be used in the presence of possible penicillin sensitivity: (1) scratch test, 1000 units/ml; (2) scratch test, 10,000 units/ml; (3) intradermal injection, 0.1 ml of solution of 1000 units/ml; (4) if no reaction occurs, proceed with continuous intravenous therapy.

A. Penicillins Rendered Ineffective by Staphylococcal Penicillinase: (Ampicillin, penicillin G, procaine penicillin G, phenoxymethyl penicillin.)

1. Ampicillin (Polycillin, Penbritin, Omnipen)—

Use: 50–80% of *Escherichia coli,* some salmonellae, shigellae, proteus. Aerobacter (enterobacter) and klebsiella are usually resistant. Gram-positive cocci, nonpenicillinase-producing staphylococci, and *Hemophilus influenzae* are sensitive.

Dosage:

Oral: 50–150 mg/kg/day in divided doses every 6 hours.

IM, IV: 150–400 mg/kg/day in divided doses every 4 hours. Not stable in intravenous bottle. For meningitis, begin with > 200 mg/kg/day in divided doses every 4 hours. **Newborn:** 100 mg/kg/day in divided doses every 6–12 hours.

Toxicity: Low toxicity. Diarrhea, skin rash (especially in mononucleosis), drug fever. Superinfection.

Comment: Useful for genitourinary infections, some chronic salmonella carriers, and *Hemophilus influenzae* meningitis. A loading dose of 50 mg/kg is desirable in serious infections. Contains about 1.7 mEq Na^+ per 500 mg of drug. Ampicillin levels in the CSF drop after the third day in meningitis as the pleocytosis decreases. Although usually effective, one case of "relapse" of *Hemophilus influenzae* meningitis on intravenous therapy has been reported. The drug *must be given parenterally* for the entire course. Failure to improve, or increase in fever and irritability after initial improvement, should prompt repeat taps.

2. Penicillin G, potassium or sodium salt—

Use: Gram-positive and gram-negative cocci, gram-positive bacilli. In high doses, some gram-negative organisms.

Dosage:

Oral: 100–400 thousand units/dose in 5 doses 1/2 hour before meals.

IM: 20–50 thousand units/kg/day in divided doses every 4–6 hours.

IV: 20–500 thousand units/kg/day in divided doses every 4 hours. **Newborn:** 50,000 units/kg in divided doses every 8–12 hours. **Adolescent:** 20–60 million units.

Aerosol: 2 ml every 6 hours, 50,000 units/ml.

Intrapleural, intra-articular, intraperitoneal: 10–20 thousand units/ml.

Intrathecal, intraventricular: (Rare indications.) 5–10 ml/24 hours (1000 units/ml).

Incompatibility: Do not mix with amphotericin B, metaraminol, phenylephrine, tetracyclines, vancomycin, vitamin C.

Toxicity: Hypersensitivity (anaphylaxis, urticaria, rash, drug fever). Change in bowel flora, candidiasis, diarrhea, hemolytic anemia. Neurotoxic in very large doses.

Comment: High concentration in the urine makes this agent useful in treatment of some urinary tract infections with gram-negative rods. One million units of potassium penicillin G contain 1.7 mEq K^+. Avoid pushing large doses of potassium salt, as in initiating therapy for meningitis; use sodium salt instead.

3. Procaine penicillin G–

Dosage: 100–600 thousand units IM every 12–24 hours. **Newborn:** Do not use. Causes sterile abscesses. Also contains 120 mg procaine/300,000 in penicillin G, which may be toxic.

4. Benzathine penicillin G (Bicillin, Neolin, Permapen)–

Dosage: 0.6–1.2 million units IM every month.·

Comment: The preferred drug for rheumatic fever prophylaxis. Increasing the dose gives a more sustained rather than a higher blood level. In acute illness, the procaine penicillin in Bicillin C-R may be desirable.

5. Phenoxymethyl penicillin (V-Cillin, Pen-Vee, Compocillin V)–

Dosage:

Oral: 0.5–2 million units every 6 hours (125 mg = 200,000 units). **Newborn:** 90,000 mg/kg. **Adult** (serious infections): > 6 gm/day in divided doses every 4–6 hours.

B. Penicillins Resistant to Staphylococcal Penicillinase: (Methicillin, nafcillin, oxacillin, cloxacillin, dicloxacillin.)

1. Methicillin (Staphcillin, Dimocillin)–

Use: Penicillinase-producing staphylococci. Less effective than penicillin G for other gram-positive cocci.

Dosage:

IV, IM: 200–300 mg/kg/day in divided doses every 4 hours. Not stable in intravenous bottle. Deterioration in dextrose in water or normal saline solution is rapid and is prevented by adding $NaHCO_3$, 6 mEq/liter. **Full-term newborn:** 200–250 mg/kg in divided doses every 6–8 hours for the first 10 days and then every 4–6 hours.· **Premature:** 100 mg/kg in divided doses every 6–8 hours for the first 10 days and then every 6 hours.

Incompatibility: Do not mix with tetracyclines, kanamycin, neomycin.

Toxicity: Hypersensitivity, kidney damage, hematuria (thought to be a hypersensitivity phenomenon). Reversible bone marrow depression. Painful when given intramuscularly.

Comment: If therapy is initiated with methicillin because of suspected penicillin resistance, change to penicillin G when sensitivity to this agent is shown. One gram contains 2.5 mEq sodium.

2. Nafcillin (Unipen)–

Use: Penicillin-resistant staphylococci. Efficacy against pneumococci and streptococci, except enterococci, is similar to that of penicillin G.

Dosage: 50–150 mg/kg/day IM or IV in divided doses every 4–6 hours. **Adolescent:** 4–8 gm/day.

Incompatibility: Do not mix with B complex vitamins.

Toxicity: Similar to that of methicillin, but hematuria has not been reported.

Comment: Good choice for coverage of gram-positive cocci before sensitivity results are available.

3. Oxacillin–Nafcillin, cloxacillin, and dicloxacillin are preferred.

4. Cloxacillin (Tegopen)–

Use: Penicillinase-producing staphylococci.

Dosage: 50–100 mg/kg/day orally in divided doses every 6 hours given 1–2 hours before meals.

Toxicity: Probably similar to that of other penicillins.

Comment: Penicillinase-resistant. Dicloxacillin in equivalent dose is probably more active and better absorbed. For osteomyelitis, use a dosage of 100 mg/kg/day.

5. Dicloxacillin (Dynapen)–

Use: Penicillinase-producing staphylococci.

Dosage: 25–50 mg/kg/day. In serious infections, begin with 50 mg/kg/day and reduce dosage if serum killing power indicates this is possible.

Toxicity: Gastrointestinal irritation, which appears to be dose-related.

Polymyxin B (Aerosporin)

Use: Pseudomonas, some other gram-negative bacteria as determined by sensitivities on the specific organism. Not a good "broad spectrum" antibiotic for gram-negatives.

Dosage:

Oral: Not absorbed. 10–20 mg/kg/day in divided doses every 4–6 hours.

IM: 3.5–5 mg/kg/day in divided doses every 4–6 hours (not to exceed 200 mg/day). **Full-term newborn and premature:** 3.5–4 mg/kg/day in divided doses every 6 hours.

IV: 3.5–5 mg/kg/day in divided doses every 6–8 hours (not to exceed 200 mg/day). **Full-term newborn and premature:** 3.5–4 mg/kg/day in divided doses every 6 hours.

Intrathecal, intraventricular: 0.5–1 mg/ml. < 2 years: 2 mg/day or every other day. > 2 years: 5 mg/day or every other day.

Intra-articular, intraperitoneal: (Rare indications.) 1 mg/ml.

Incompatibility: Do not mix with cephalothin, chloramphenicol, heparin, tetracyclines.

Toxicity: Pain at injection site; neurotoxicity (paresthesias, ataxia, drowsiness); nephrotoxicity (cylindruria, hematuria, proteinuria, increased BUN); fever, rash.

Rifampin (Rifadin, Rimactane)

Use: Neisseria, mycobacterium, gram-positive cocci.

Dosage:

Oral: Not well established in children. **Adult:** 600 mg/day.

Toxicity: Hepatotoxic in animals but does not appear to have additive hepatotoxicity when used in various drug regimens for the therapy of tuberculosis. Appears to be well tolerated and relatively nontoxic.

Comment: The most striking contribution of rifampin has been to the care of patients infected with resistant strains of *Mycobacterium tuberculosis*. Although the results have been remarkably good, when used alone the development of resistance is rapid; therefore, the drug should always be used in combination with one or 2 drugs to which the organisms are sensitive. It should be reserved for patients in whom other drug regimens have failed. Early work has shown that it may have a place in the therapy of the carrier state of *Neisseria meningitidis.* It has also been used in the successful treatment of infections with *N gonorrhoeae* and staphylococci but offers no advantage over other drugs. Until more data are available, rifampin should be reserved for therapy of patients with infections due to *M tuberculosis* and *M leprae.*

Streptomycin Sulfate

Use: *Mycobacterium tuberculosis, Hemophilus influenzae,* some gram-negatives. Synergistic with penicillin against enterococci. Resistance develops quickly.

Dosage:

Oral: Not absorbed. 40 mg/kg/day in divided doses every 6 hours.

IM: 20–40 mg/kg/day in divided doses every 12–24 hours. **Newborn:** 10–20 mg/kg/day. Use with caution.

Aerosol: 2 ml every 6 hours (150 mg/ml).

Toxicity: Damage to vestibular apparatus. Fatal CNS and respiratory depression. Bone marrow depression, renal toxicity, hypersensitivity, superinfection.

Comment: Should never be used as the only drug. Dihydrostreptomycin is toxic to the eighth nerve and should not be used.

Sulfonamides: Sulfadiazine, Sulfisoxazole (Gantrisin), Sulfamethoxazole (Gantanol), Trisulfapyrimidines USP

Use: Bacteriostatic against gram-positive and gram-negative organisms. Approximately 80% of shigellae are resistant. Nocardia.

Dosage (for sulfadiazine, triple sulfas, and sulfisoxazole):

Oral: 120–150 mg/kg/day in divided doses every 6 hours.

IV: 120 mg/kg/day in divided doses every 6–12 hours; alkalinize urine. **Newborn:** Do not use.

Dosage (for sulfamethoxazole): 50 mg/kg/day orally in divided doses every 12 hours.

Toxicity: Crystalluria (mechanical urinary obstruction); keep fluid intake high. Hypersensitivity (fever, rash, hepatitis, lupus-like state, vasculitis). Do not use in kernicterus. Neutropenia, agranulocytosis, aplastic anemia, thrombocytopenia. Hemolytic anemia in individuals deficient in glucose-6-phosphate dehydrogenase. (There is a high correlation between G6PD deficiency and sickle cell anemia, so do not use in these patients.)

Comment: Useful in infections of the urinary tract and for rheumatic fever prophylaxis. (Should not be relied upon for treatment of group A streptococcal infections.) Long-acting preparations (Kynex, Madribon, sulfameter) are occasionally associated with serious reactions. Sulfadiazine is preferred for CNS infections since diffusion into the CSF is better. Sulfamethoxazole is intermediate-acting and causes a slightly higher incidence of urinary sediment abnormalities.

Tetracyclines (Many trade names.)

Use: Gram-positive and gram-negative bacteria, rickettsiae, bedsoniae, *Mycoplasma pneumoniae,* brucella, bacteroides. Many strains are resistant.

Dosage (for tetracycline, chlortetracycline, oxytetracycline):

Oral: 20–40 mg/kg/day in divided doses every 6 hours. Do not give with milk.

IM: 12 mg/kg/day in divided doses every 12 hours; achieves poor levels; painful.

IV: Do not use.

Aerosol: 1 ml every 12 hours (50 mg/ml in 75% propylene glycol).

Dosage (for demecycline [demethylchlortetracycline, Declomycin] and methacycline [Rondomycin]):

Oral: 12 mg/kg/day in divided doses every 6 hours. **Newborn:** Do not use.

Incompatibility: Do not mix with amphotericin B, cephalothin, chloramphenicol, heparin, hydrocortisone, methicillin, penicillin G, polymyxin B.

Toxicity: In children under 7 years of age, tetracyclines cause damage to teeth and bone. Deposition in teeth and bone of premature and newborn infants can result in enamel dysplasia and growth retardation. Outdated tetracyclines can produce Fanconi's syn-

TABLE 39–2. Choice of anti-infective agents. (Revised July 1972.)

Organism (and Gram Reaction)	Drug(s) of First Choice	Drug(s) of Second Choice
Actinomyces (+)	Penicillin	Tetracycline, sulfonamides
Bacillus anthracis (+)	Penicillin	Tetracyclines, erythromycin
Bacteroides (−)*	Chloramphenicol, clindamycin	Penicillin
Bedsoniae (agents of lymphogranu-loma venereum, psittacosis, and trachoma)	Tetracyclines	Chloramphenicol, sulfonamide
Bordetella pertussis (--)	Erythromycin	Ampicillin
Brucella (−)	Tetracyclines + streptomycin	Kanamycin
Candida albicans	Nystatin, amphotericin B	5-Fluorocytosine
Clostridia (+)	Antitoxin + penicillin	Erythromycin, kanamycin
Corynebacterium diphtheriae (+)	Antitoxin + penicillin	Erythromycin, lincomycin
Diplococcus pneumoniae (+)	Penicillin	Cephalothin, erythromycin, lincomycin
Enterobacter (Aerobacter) (−)*	Kanamycin, gentamicin	Polymyxin, colistin, tetracycline + streptomycin
Erysipelothrix (+)	Penicillin	Tetracyclines, erythromycin
Escherichia coli (−)*	Ampicillin, kanamycin, gentamicin, cephalexin, cephalothin	Tetracyclines, polymyxin, colistin, sulfonamides
Hemophilus influenzae (−)	Ampicillin	Chloramphenicol + streptomycin
Klebsiella pneumoniae (−)*	Kanamycin, cephalothin, cephalexin	Polymyxin, colistin, gentamicin, tetra-cycline + streptomycin
Leptospira icterohaemorrhagiae	Tetracyclines	Penicillin
Listeria monocytogenes	Ampicillin, tetracyclines	Penicillin, bacitracin
Mycobacterium leprae (+)	Sulfones	Solasulfone, sulfonamides, diphenyl-thiourea, sulfoxone, rifampin
M tuberculosis (+)*	Isoniazid + streptomycin + PAS or Isoniazid + streptomycin + ethambutol	Viomycin, cycloserine, ethionamide, pyrazinamide, rifampin
Mycoplasma pneumoniae (Eaton agent)	Tetracyclines, erythromycin	
Neisseria gonorrhoeae (−)	Penicillin + probenecid	Ampicillin + probencid, tetracyclines
N meningitidis (−)	Penicillin	Ampicillin, cephalothin, chloram-phenicol
Nocardia (+)*	Sulfonamides + cycloserine	Sulfonamides + agent chosen by sensi-tivity tests
Pasteurella pestis or *P tularensis* (−)	Streptomycin + tetracyclines	
Proteus mirabilis (−)*	Ampicillin, penicillin	Cephalothin, kanamycin
Proteus vulgaris, P morganii, *P rettgeri* (−)*	Kanamycin, gentamicin	Cephalothin, chloramphenicol
Pseudomonas aeruginosa (−)*	Gentamicin, carbenicillin	Kanamycin, tetracyclines, neomycin, polymyxin B, colistin
Rickettsiae (−)	Chloramphenicol (+ cortico-steroids for Rocky Mountain spotted fever)	Tetracyclines
Salmonella (−)*	Ampicillin	Chloramphenicol, cephalothin, tetra-cyclines, kanamycin
S typhi (−)*	Chloramphenicol, ampicillin	
Shigella (−)*	Ampicillin	Tetracyclines, cephalothin
Spirillum minus (−)	Penicillin	Tetracyclines
Staphylococcus (+)* if sensitive	Penicillin	Erythromycin, lincomycin, cephalothin
Staphylococcus (+) if resistant	Methicillin, nafcillin, dicloxacillin, cloxacillin	Cephalothin, erythromycin, lincomycin, kanamycin
Streptococcus (+)	Penicillin	Erythromycin, cephalothin, ampicillin
Str faecalis (+)*	Penicillin + streptomycin, ampicillin	Cephalothin
Treponema pallidum	Penicillin	Cephalothin, erythromycin

*Sensitivity tests usually indicated.

drome. Pseudotumor cerebri, bulging fontanels. Nausea, vomiting, diarrhea, stomatitis, glossitis, proctitis, candidiasis, and overgrowth of staphylococci in bowel. Disturbed hepatic and renal function. Drug fever, rash, photosensitivity.

Comment: Cross-resistance among the tetracyclines is complete.

Vancomycin (Vancocin)

Use: Staphylococci, other gram-positive cocci, clostridia, corynebacteria. Main use is in treatment of staphylococcal enterocolitis and methicillin-resistant staphylococcal infection.

Dosage:
Oral: Not absorbed. 2–4 gm/day in divided doses every 6 hours.
IV: 40 mg/kg/day. Adolescent: 2–3 gm/day in divided doses 4–6 hours.

Incompatibility: Do not mix with chloramphenicol, heparin, hydrocortisone, penicillin G.

Toxicity: Painful when given intramuscularly; do not use. Troublesome symptoms during intravenous administration include rash, chills, thrombophlebitis, and fever. Concomitant administration of corticosteroids may be necessary. Nephrotoxicity and irreversible ototoxicity have occurred. Does not interfere with the action of any known antibiotic.

Comment: Before the advent of the penicillinase-resistant antibiotics, vancomycin was used successfully in the treatment of subacute bacterial endocarditis, osteomyelitis, and serious soft tissue infections. High oral doses are exceedingly effective in staphylococcal enterocolitis.

ANTIVIRAL CHEMOTHERAPY

Few therapeutic agents are available for viral infections. The following drugs have limited usefulness.

Amantadine (Symmetrel)

Use: Limited to prophylactic administration during identified A_2 influenza virus epidemics. Of no therapeutic value. Does not appear to interfere with immunity induced by vaccination.

Dosage:
1–9 years: 2–4 mg/lb/day orally (do not exceed 150 mg/day) in 2 or 3 doses.
9–12 years: 200 mg/day orally in 2 doses (total dose).
Adult: 200 mg/day orally in 1 or 2 doses.

Toxicity: CNS irritability (nervousness, insomnia, dizziness, lightheadedness, drunken feelings, slurred speech, ataxia, inability to concentrate). Occasional depression and feelings of detachment; blurred vision (heightened with higher dosage, 300–400 mg/day, in elderly); less commonly, dry mouth, gastrointestinal upset, skin rash. Rarely, tremors, anorexia, pollakiuria, nocturia.

Idoxuridine (Dendrid, Herplex, Stoxil)

Use: At present, limited to acute superficial herpes simplex or vaccinia virus keratitis. Should be administered under an ophthalmologist's supervision. Some prefer concomitant local corticosteroid administration.

Dosage: Solution should be used initially; place 1 drop in each infected eye every hour while awake and every 2 hours. at night; with definite improvement, decrease to every 2 hours around the clock and continue treatment for 3–5 days after healing appears to be complete. Ointment: Instill 5 times a day (every 4 hours), with last dose at midnight.

Toxicity: Too frequent administration leads to small punctate defects in the cornea. Ingestion of 15 ml of solution or 20 mg of ointment is not known to be associated with poisoning.

Methisazone (Marboran)

Use: In the prophylaxis of smallpox if given in the first 9 days after exposure; in the therapy of complications of vaccination, especially eczema vaccinatum.

Dosage: Give a loading dose of 250 mg/kg/day orally followed by 50 mg/kg every 6 hours for 3 full days. An antiemetic should be given with the drug.

Toxicity: Vomiting, immediate gastric irritation, and late (5–6 hours) CNS stimulation. Short courses of therapy are not associated with other effects, but patients should be observed for hematologic and hepatic toxicity.

TABLE 39–3. Antibacterial spectrum of antimicrobial agents.

Mode of Action	Activity Principally Against		
	Gram-Positives	Broad Spectrum	Gram-Negatives
Bactericidal	Penicillins, bacitracin	Kanamycin, neomycin, cephalothin, ampicillin, penicillin*	Streptomycin, polymyxin B, colistin, gentamicin
Bacteriostatic	Erythromycin, troleandomycin, lincomycin, clindamycin	Tetracyclines, methacycline, sulfonamides, chloramphenicol	Nalidixic acid

*In very large doses, penicillin may be bactericidal against a number of gram-negatives.

• • •

General References

Baldwin DS: Renal failure and interstitial nephritis due to penicillin and methicillin. New England J Med 279:1245, 1968.

Bauer DJ & others: Prophylaxis of smallpox with methisazone. Am J Epidem 90:130–145, 1969.

Committee on Drugs, American Academy of Pediatrics: Infants of tuberculous mothers: Further thoughts. Pediatrics 42:393, 1968.

Cutler RE: Correlation of serum creatinine concentration and kanamycin half-life. JAMA 209:539, 1969.

Darrell JH: Carbenicillin resistance in *Pseudomonas aeruginosa* from clinical material. Brit MJ 3:141, 1969.

Drutz DJ: Treatment of disseminated mycotic infections. Am J Med 45:405, 1968.

Grossman ER: Tetracyclines and permanent teeth: The relation between dose and tooth color. Pediatrics 47:567, 1971.

International symposium on gentamicin. J Infect Dis 119:April-May 1969.

Kagan BM: *Antimicrobial Therapy.* Saunders, 1970.

Kunin CM: Limitations upon the use of antibiotics imposed by renal insufficiency. Mod Treat 7:355, 1970.

Lorber J: Treatment of ventriculitis with gentamicin and cloxacillin in infants born with spina bifida. Arch Dis Childhood 45:178, 1970.

Marsden HB: Gentamicin in childhood infections. Curr Ther Res 12:353, 1970.

Martin CM: Controlled trial of cephaloridine, lincomycin and nafcillin in severe gram-positive coccal infections. Antimicrob Agents Chemother 7:118, 1967.

McHenry MC: Gentamicin dosages for renal insufficiency. Ann Int Med 74:192, 1971.

Meyers BR: Cephalexin: Microbiological effects and pharmacologic parameters in man. Clin Pharmacol Therap 10:810, 1969.

Senra del Valle DA: Gentamicin in pediatric infections. J Infect Dis 119:453, 1969.

Southern P: Meningococcal meningitis. New England J Med 280:1163, 1969.

Summary of the Report of the Ad Hoc Advisory Committee on Isoniazid and Liver Disease. Morbidity and Mortality Weekly Report, July 3, 1971.

Vall-Spinosa A: Rifampin in the treatment of drug resistant *Mycobacterium tuberculosis* infections. New England J Med 283:616, 1970.

Yow MD: Ampicillin in the treatment of meningitis: An appraisal after 6 years of experience. J Pediat 74:848, 1969.

40 . . .

Interpretation of Biochemical Values*

Donough O'Brien, MD, FRCP, & Denis O. Rodgerson, PhD

SAMPLE COLLECTION

Blood

Laboratory personnel should be responsible for all sample collections, although this is not so important in older children in whom venipunctures are simple. Finger pricks are satisfactory in older infants, but heel pricks should always be used in newborns and young infants.

Materials and supplies taken to the bedside are as follows:

Ether and alcohol.

Hagedorn needles, 3 inches, one for each patient, each sterilized in a cotton-plugged test tube. (Disposable lancets have not been found satisfactory.)

Blood-collecting tubes containing heparin and a layer of mineral oil, capped with a rubber cap and labeled **H**. (If serum is required, the heparin is omitted and the tube labeled accordingly.)

Microhematocrit tubes, screw-cap vials containing 3 mg potassium oxalate.

The skin should be cleansed with ether and not alcohol, which will cause spreading and hemolysis; however, alcohol should be used for babies in incubators and the skin later dried with sterile cotton.

In order to prevent hemolysis of the sample and contamination with tissue fluid, it is essential to obtain a free flow of blood. This may require gentle "milking" but never squeezing. The small vein running posteriorly to the internal malleolus is likely to yield a free flow and should be used whenever it can be located. A careful and deliberate puncture should be made. The blood should drip into the collecting tube and fall at once through the mineral oil. It is permissible to touch the top of the tube against the drop, but the skin surface should never be in contact with the tube since hemolysis will occur. Directly after collection, a cotton ball is placed on the puncture site and pressure applied for a short time. When blood flow has ceased, a dressing is placed over the puncture site.

The tube of blood is covered with the rubber cap and the specimen is labeled appropriately.

On return to the laboratory, a Hagedorn needle is very gently passed circumferentially around the inner surface of the tube between the blood and the wall of the tube, the cap is replaced, and the sample is centrifuged for about 5 minutes.

Approximately 0.2 ml of whole blood should be allowed for each test described below, even though much less is required in many cases. For example, 0.23 ml of plasma will suffice for a combined plasma sodium, potassium, chloride, and CO_2 determination. Samples for sodium, potassium, urea by the urease method, calcium, and ammonia should be collected in heparin tubes. Samples requiring serum are collected in plain tubes.

Stools

Random stool samples should be sent directly to the laboratory. Twenty-four-hour or longer collections should be placed in polyethylene bags and stored in a special container in the freezer.

Urine

Random urine samples should be sent immediately to the laboratory. Several collections should be directly stored in a freezer or at 4° C after acidification with concentrated hydrochloric acid to pH 2.0 or less.

Cerebrospinal Fluid

Samples of CSF should always be sent immediately to the laboratory. At least 2 tubes are required—one for protein and glucose and one for cell count, differential count, culture, stained smear for bacteria, and animal inoculation. A third tube is required if a serologic test for syphilis or a colloidal gold curve is required.

SOURCES OF ERROR

Awareness of the possibility of error is important to the interpretation of laboratory data. All good laboratories have a reasonably accurate idea of the intrinsic error of their methods. Some typical ones are shown in Table 40–1.

---

*Normal values of most of the substances discussed in this chapter are given in Table 40–3 (alphabetically arranged).

Caraway WT: Accuracy in clinical chemistry. Clin Chem 17:63, 1971.

TABLE 40–1. Reproducibility of common micromethods. (95% confidence limits of a single estimation.)

	Mean and Variance	
Albumin (gm/100 ml)	4 (±5.2%)	
Total protein	6 (±2.2%)	
Alkaline phosphatase	50 IU/liter	±1.5 IU/liter (±2.9%)
Bicarbonate	20 mEq/liter	±0.4 mEq/liter (±2.2%)
Bilirubin (conjugated)	5 mg/100 ml	±0.12 mg/100 ml (±2.4%)
Bilirubin (unconjugated)	20 mg/100 ml	±1.3 mg/100 ml (±6.4%)
Calcium	5 mEq/liter	±0.3 mEq/liter (±6%)
Chloride	100 mEq/liter	±3 mEq/liter (±3%)
Cholesterol	200 mg/100 ml	±12 mg/100 ml (±6%)
Creatinine	1 mg/100 ml	±0.1 mg/100 ml (±11%)
Glucose	80 mg/100 ml	±3.7 mg/100 ml (±4.6%)
Hemoglobin	14 gm/100 ml	±0.1 gm/100 ml (±0.8%)
Magnesium	2 mEq/liter	±0.17 mEq/liter (±8.7%)
Phosphorus	5 mg/100 ml	±0.2 mg/100 ml (±4.2%)
Potassium	5 mEq/liter	±0.1 mEq/liter (±2%)
SGOT	50 IU/liter	±3.6 IU/liter (±7.3%)
SGPT	50 IU/liter	±14.7 IU/liter (±29.4%)
Sodium	140 mEq/liter	±2.1 mEq/liter (±1.5%)
Urea nitrogen (urease)	20 mg/100 ml	±1.2 mg/100 ml (±6%)
Uric acid	4 mg/100 ml	±0.4 mg/100 ml (±10.4%)
VMA	5 mg/liter	±0.5 mg/liter (±9.2%)

TESTS OF CARBOHYDRATE METABOLISM

Glucose in Serum, Plasma, & Cerebrospinal Fluid

A. Specimen and Test Requirements: 0.2 ml serum, CSF, or plasma. The patient should be fasted. Cells should be separated within 20 minutes. Plasma from heparinized blood must be precipitated at once.

B. Normal Values: Newborn, 10–80 mg/100 ml; older children, 60–105 mg/100 ml.

C. Interpretation: The most reliable methods are enzymatic, but their use is limited because they are only adaptable to discrete sampling systems for automation. Serum proteins are removed by precipitation with zinc hydroxide, and the glucose is converted to β-D-glucopyranose by the mutarotase present in all glucose oxidase preparations. The latter compound is then converted to gluconic acid and hydrogen peroxide by the glucose oxidase. o-Tolidine is present to give a blue color with hydrogen peroxide. The reaction can also be measured in terms of oxygen consumption.

Kadish AH: Determination of urine glucose by measurement of rate of oxygen consumption. Diabetes 18:467, 1969.

Oral Glucose Tolerance Test

A. Specimen and Test Requirements: Give 1.75 gm/kg of glucose as corn syrup or as a 20% solution with flavoring after 3 days of high-carbohydrate intake followed by an overnight fast. Children under 2 years of age should be given 2 gm/kg of glucose. Commercial products are available.

Take blood samples fasting and then at 30, 60, 90, 120, and 150 minutes for serum glucose determination. In cases of suspected carbohydrate-reactive hypoglycemia, post-fasting samples should be taken at 2, 3, 4, and 5 hours.

Collect urine prior to the test and after 1 and 2 hours to test for glycosuria. The criteria for the range of normal response are that the 30-minute level should be < 180 mg/100 ml and that fasting levels should be restored at 90–120 minutes.

Because the relatively large doses of glucose used in this test may lead to nausea and vomiting, corn syrup may be preferable. This could lead to error in the presence of a maltase deficiency. The glucose should be dissolved in ice cold water or soda water in a volume of 150 ml/sq m and flavoring added to make it palatable. Commercially prepared glucose solutions are available under various trade names.

B. Normal Values: The normal limits of glucose tolerance in children are shown in Fig 40–1.

C. Interpretation: Diminished glucose tolerance (elevated blood sugar values) is usually indicative of diabetes mellitus, but it may also be seen in states associated with excess anterior pituitary or adrenocortical hormones and with liver disease. An abrupt fall in serum glucose after the initial rise is sometimes seen with hyperinsulinism. Criteria for abnormality vary (see p 631), but 3 levels over the 97th percentile or a

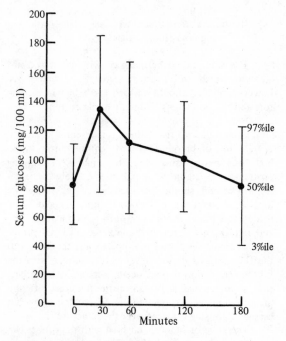

FIG 40–1. Serum glucose percentile levels after 1.75 gm/kg glucose orally.

sum of the fasting, 30, 60, and 120 minute levels > 625 would be considered positive.

Intravenous Glucose Tolerance Test

A. Specimen and Test Requirements: The patient should be fasted for 6 hours if under 6 months of age; otherwise, for about 12 hours.

Inject rapidly into a vein 0.66 ml 50% glucose solution per kg body weight. Collect blood every 4–5 minutes for 30–45 minutes for serum glucose measurement. From the calculation of glucose assimilation a constant (K) is determined as follows:

$$K = \frac{\log_{10} C_1 - \log_{10} C_2}{t_1 - t_2} \times 230.3$$

where C_1 and C_2 are serum glucose levels in mg/100 ml at times t_1 and t_2 in minutes, respectively.

B. Normal Values:

		Mean ± SD
6 months to 10 years		K = 2.8 ± 0.6
10–15 years	before puberty	K = 2.7 ± 0.8
	during puberty	K = 2.1 ± 0.7
	after puberty	K = 1.9 ± 0.4
Adult		K = 1.7 ± 0.3

C. Interpretation: The interpretation of diminished or increased glucose tolerance by the intravenous method is as for the oral test (above).

Loeb H: Variations in glucose tolerance during infancy and childhood. J Pediat 68:237, 1966.

Insulin Tolerance Test

A. Specimen and Test Requirements: Give 0.1 unit soluble insulin IV per kg body weight to the fasting patient.

Take serum samples for glucose fasting and at 20, 40, 60, 90, and 120 minutes. Safety precautions should be observed as in the insulin/glucose test (below), which is preferable.

B. Interpretation: Failure of the serum glucose to rise significantly after 20 minutes indicates pituitary or adrenal insufficiency.

Insulin/Glucose Tolerance Test

A. Specimen and Test Requirements: This test was developed as a somewhat safer means of detecting insulin sensitivity than the insulin tolerance test.

Administer 0.1 unit soluble insulin per kg body weight IV after an overnight fast. At 30 minutes, give 0.8 gram glucose per kg body weight orally in flavored aqueous solution. Collect samples for serum glucose fasting and after 30, 60, 90, 120, and 180 minutes. Glucagon and sterile 50% glucose should be on hand in case of a hypoglycemic reaction.

B. Interpretation: Failure of the serum glucose to rise after 30 minutes is indicative of insulin sensitivity.

Engel FL: The insulin glucose tolerance test. J Clin Invest 29:151, 1950.

Glucagon Tolerance Test

A. Specimen and Test Requirements: This is an overall test of glycogenolysis used in the diagnosis of various forms of glycogen storage disease and other liver diseases.

Administer 20 μg glucagon per kg of body weight IV to the fasting patient. Take samples for serum glucose determination fasting and at 10, 20, and 40 minutes.

B. Interpretation: Normal persons show a blood glucose rise of 50–100 mg/100 ml with a peak at 40 minutes and a return to normal by 2 hours.

Marks V: Glucagon test for insulinoma. S Clin Path 21:346, 1968.

Epinephrine Test

A. Specimen and Test Requirements: Inject epinephrine, 1:1000 solution subcut, to the fasting patient—0.03 ml/kg for infants and 0.01 ml/kg for children (maximum, 0.5 ml). Collect blood samples fasting and at 15, 30, and 60 minutes for serum glucose determination.

B. Interpretation: This is another test of glycogenolysis used in the evaluation of liver disease, in certain hypoglycemias, and in glycogen storage disease. In normal persons, blood sugar should rise significantly by 30 minutes.

Prednisone Glucose Tolerance Test

A. Specimen and Test Requirements: Perform a standard glucose tolerance test after giving 6 mg/sq m of prednisone orally 8½ and 2 hours before the first fasting sample.

B. Normal Values: As for Oral Glucose Tolerance Test.

C. Interpretation: This test is used in the detection of glucose intolerance in prediabetics among close relatives of known diabetics with a view to considering treatment with the sulfonylureas.

Rull JA & others: Levels of plasma insulin during cortisone glucose tolerance tests in "nondiabetic" relatives of diabetic patients. Diabetes 19:1, 1970.

Oral Tolbutamide Tolerance Test

A. Specimen and Test Requirements: Blood samples for glucose determinations are taken 20 minutes after an oral dose of 20 mg/kg tolbutamide with 1.2 gm/sq m of sodium bicarbonate to facilitate absorption. The tolbutamide may be given intravenously, but there is an increased risk of hypoglycemia.

B. Normal Values: Serum glucose levels should fall to between 20 and 40% of fasting in 20 minutes.

C. Interpretation: A fall of less than 15% at 20 minutes indicates insulin insufficiency. A fall greater than 50% by 20 minutes and to less than 70% of fasting at 90–120 minutes indicates hyperinsulinism. (See Fig 40–2.)

Cunningham GC: Tolbutamide tolerance test in hypoglycemic children. Am J Dis Child 107:714, 1966.

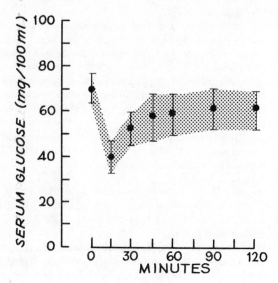

FIG 40–2. Serum glucose levels in children after 20 mg/kg of tolbutamide intravenously.

TESTS FOR FLUID & ELECTROLYTE & ACID-BASE DISORDERS

Bicarbonate or Total CO$_2$ in Plasma

A. Specimen: 0.03 ml heparinized plasma taken under oil.

B. Normal Values: 18–33 mM/liter.

C. Interpretation: (See Chapter 37.) Low values indicate metabolic acidosis or respiratory alkalosis. Elevated values indicate metabolic alkalosis or respiratory acidosis. It is usually advisable to have a simultaneous blood pH reading.

Various authors: Acta anaesth scandinav Suppl 37:10, 24, 27, 1970.

Blood & Plasma Volume

A. Specimen and Test Requirements: Evans blue dye or radioiodinated serum albumin (RISA) is injected intravenously, and samples of heparinized whole blood are drawn after allowing time for equilibration in the plasma volume. Technical details should be left to the laboratory.

B. Normal Values: See Table 40–3.

C. Method: The Evans blue dye and RISA methods are both simple dilution technics.

D. Interpretation: There is a definite role for the determination of blood volume in clinical work—particularly in judging the risk of transfusions in anemic patients and in assessing blood volume in diabetic acidosis, renal failure, severe burns, etc.

Cropp GJA: Changes in blood and plasma volumes during growth. J Pediat 78:220, 1971.

Body Water: Total, Extracellular, & Intracellular

A. Specimen and Test Requirements: For total body water, deuterium oxide (D$_2$O) is injected intravenously and allowed to equilibrate for 3 hours. Plasma water is distilled off under vacuum and the D$_2$O concentration measured by its specific infrared adsorbance. For extracellular water, a potassium bromide dilution technic is used. Bromide is measured polarographically.

B. Normal Values: See Table 40–3.

C. Interpretation: A measurement of total body water or extracellular water is occasionally of great value in renal failure and in other situations where an accurate appraisal of a severe fluid and electrolyte disturbance is important for therapy.

Cheek DB & others: Body water, height and weight during growth of normal children. Am J Dis Child 112:312, 1966.

Serum Calcium

A. Specimen: 0.1 ml serum, preferably fasting.

B. Normal Values: 4.4–5.3 mEq/liter.

C. Interpretation: Elevated values (between 6–9 mEq/liter) may be seen in idiopathic hypercalcemia, vitamin D intoxication, hyperparathyroidism, sarcoidosis, *Pneumocystis carinii* pneumonia, and in the blue diaper syndrome. Low levels are seen in hypoparathyroidism, pseudohypoparathyroidism, secondary to hypophosphatemia in chronic renal failure, in all forms of rickets, in postacidotic hypocalcemia, in hypoalbuminemia, in infantile tetany, and as a result of corticosteroid therapy.

Rodgerson DO: Measurement of serum calcium. Clin Chem 14:1207, 1968.

Serum Chloride

A. Specimen: 0.1 ml serum or plasma.

B. Normal Values: 97–104 mEq/liter.

C. Interpretation: The measurement of serum chloride, particularly in association with CO$_2$ content, offers in children a good index of acidosis, alkalosis, and the overall osmolality of the extracellular water provided excessive lipidemia is not present. Low values are found in pyloric stenosis and other instances of persistent vomiting; in overhydration, including states of inappropriate vasopressin secretion; and in rarer states where the intracellular tonicity has changed with a resultant migration of sodium and chloride into the cell. Somewhat high values normally occur in the thirsted infant at around the fourth day of life. High chloride values are also found in hyperchloremic renal acidosis, in hypertonic dehydration, and in some cases of diabetes insipidus. Salt retention may also occur in cerebral lesions, although it is more often associated with low serum chloride levels. Neurogenic hypochloremia may have a renal component. In some cases, end organ insensitivity to DOCA has been noted without other evidence of renal dysfunction.

Serum Magnesium

A. Specimen: 0.1 ml serum.

B. Normal Values: 1.2–1.6 mEq/liter.

C. Interpretation: Abnormally low levels may be found in gastroenteritis, the malabsorption syndromes, protein and calorie malnutrition, and in the renal tubular dystrophies or chronic renal disease. Low levels are occasionally seen in the newborn who is "twitchy" with or without hypocalcemia and also in diabetic acidosis and hyperparathyroidism. The associated clinical findings are muscular weakness and wasting, instability, tetany, vertigo, ataxia, tremors, and ultimately convulsions.

Elevated serum magnesium levels are most commonly encountered in chronic renal failure.

Tsang RC, Oh W: Serum magnesium levels in low birth weight infants. Am J Dis Child 120:44, 1970.

Osmotic Pressure

A. Specimen: 0.2 ml serum or urine.

B. Normal Values: 170–285 mOsm/liter serum.

C. Interpretation: Osmolality is measured in terms of freezing point depression. It is primarily a measure of the serum tonicity and parallels serum sodium.

pH of Whole Blood

A. Specimen: 0.03 ml heparinized whole blood.

B. Normal Values: 7.38–7.42 at 37° C.

C. Interpretation: A measure of acidemia or alkalemia (in conjunction with serum bicarbonate levels).

Sootarinen T: Acid base balance in the normal child. Acta anaesth scandinav Suppl 37:27, 1970.

Serum Phosphorus, Inorganic

A. Specimen: 0.1 ml serum, preferably fasting.

B. Method: Protein-free plasma is added to ammonium molybdate to form phosphomolybdate. This can be extracted by an isobutanol:petroleum ether solvent and reduced by stannous chloride to give a stable blue color.

C. Normal Values: 4.4–5.6 mg/100 ml.

D. Interpretation: Elevated plasma phosphorus levels are found in chronic renal disease, hypoparathyroidism, pseudohypoparathyroidism, and tetany of the newborn, where the elevation is caused by excessive phosphorus retention. The tetany found in infants of diabetic mothers is often normophosphatemic.

Low plasma phosphorus is encountered in rickets associated with malabsorption syndromes, in renal tubular dystrophies, postacidotic hypocalcemia, primary hyperparathyroidism, and in patients taking corticosteroids.

Kratiab AK, Forfar JO: Calcium, phosphorus and glucose levels in mother and newborn infant. Biol Neonat 15:26, 1970.

Serum Potassium

A. Specimen: 0.1 ml plasma or serum.

B. Normal Values: 4.1–5.6 mEq/liter.

C. Interpretation: High serum potassium levels occur in renal failure, respiratory distress syndrome, adynamia episodica hereditaria, and adrenal insufficiency. Low potassium is associated with congenital or acquired alkalosis and may result from persistent vomiting or diarrhea and from potassium-losing renal conditions.

Serum Sodium

A. Specimen: 0.1 ml plasma or serum.

B. Normal Values: 136–143 mEq/liter.

C. Interpretation: Serum sodium levels are obtained as a guide to serum osmolality. They are conspicuously low in adrenal insufficiency. The difference between the serum sodium level and the sum of the bicarbonate and chloride levels is an index of the degree of organic aciduria.

TESTS OF ENDOCRINE FUNCTION

ANTERIOR PITUITARY FUNCTION

The anterior pituitary gland is responsible for the elaboration of 7 tropic hormones: (1) follicle stimulating hormone (FSH), (2) luteinizing or interstitial cell stimulating hormone (LH, ICSH), (3) adrenocorticotropic hormone (ACTH, corticotropin), (4) thyrotropin (TSH), (5) somatotropin or human growth hormone (HGH), (6) luteotropic hormone or prolactin (LTH), and (7) melanocyte stimulating hormone (MSH). Methods of direct measurement of these hormones are being developed in many research laboratories employing both bioassay and radioimmunoassay methods, but at present these assays are rarely practical in clinical work. Pituitary gonadotropic activity (an estimation of both FSH and LH) may be helpful in the evaluation of premature sexual development and suspected cases of Turner's and Klinefelter's syndromes.

ACTH function and reserve may be assessed by the metyrapone (Metopirone) stimulation and dexamethasone suppression tests described briefly below.

Thyrotropic (TSH) and long-acting thyroid stimulating hormone (LATS) bioassays are now available in some university and commercial laboratories. *(Normal values:* TSH, up to 0.2 mU/ml serum; LATS, none detectable in normal serum.)

In clinical practice, a normal 4- or 24-hour uptake of ^{131}I is an index of a normally TSH-responsive thyroid and thus a guide to the level of endogenous TSH. In cases of suspected TSH excess, the T_3 (triiodothyronine) suppression of ^{131}I uptake by the thyroid gland is also useful.

Assays of growth hormone are being made more frequently, but there is substantial disagreement in the results reported by various investigators. In 2 groups, the mean plasma levels of HGH in fasting children and young adults were 1.5–5 ng/ml and 1.9 ± 0.2 ng/ml. Levels are usually at least double as a result of insulin hypoglycemia or the infusion of L-arginine; this is an important means of judging HGH secretive reserve.

Lazarus L, Young JD: Human growth hormone assay. J Clin Endocrinol 26:213, 1966.

ADRENAL FUNCTION

The basic measure of adrenal activity is the 24-hour urinary excretion of 17-hydroxycorticosteroids. Low levels are an absolute indication of hypoadrenalism, but normal values are obtained with low adrenal and pituitary reserve. Metyrapone (Metopirone) inhibits corticosteroid feedback control to the pituitary and leads to an increase in endogenous ACTH production and, secondarily, to increased levels of urinary hydroxycorticosteroids. If pituitary function is found to be normal, the corticotropin stimulation test can be used to detect suprarenal reserve. In some laboratories, serum levels of corticosteroids can be measured, and these can be used in lieu of 24-hour urine excretions, thus reducing the test time.

In cases of hyperadrenocorticism (Cushing's syndrome) and in the adrenogenital syndrome, the urinary corticosteroids are elevated and cannot usually be suppressed by small doses of dexamethasone (eg, 1.28 mg/sq m/24 hours for 3 days). Failure to suppress urinary corticosteroids with 3.75 mg/sq m/24 hours for 3 days is an indication of an autonomous adrenal adenoma, carcinoma, or pituitary neoplasm.

In cases of adrenogenital syndrome, 24-hour urine levels of 17-ketosteroids and pregnanetriol are substantially elevated.

Brief details of the corticotropin stimulation, metyrapone, and dexamethasone suppression tests are given below. In all cases, at least 2 preliminary 24-hour urine samples should be collected for baseline 17-hydroxycorticosteroid assays. No special precautions need to be taken other than to refrigerate samples pending the assays.

ACTH Stimulation Test
A. Specimen and Test Requirements: After 2 baseline 24-hour control collections, give 15 units corticotropin (USP) per sq m in 250–500 ml isotonic saline IV over a period of 8–12 hours, beginning at 8 a.m., or 20 mg/sq m corticotropin gel IM every 9–12 hours for 4 days. Collect 24-hour urine samples for 4 days following intravenous corticotropin or during intramuscular treatment, and measure 17-hydroxycorticosteroids.

B. Normal Values and Interpretation: Normally, ACTH stimulation produces a 3- to 5-fold increase over baseline levels in both plasma and urine. An abnormal response indicates hypoadrenocorticism, either primary or secondary to hypopituitarism. A normal response excludes primary hypoadrenocorticism.

Migeon CJ, Stempfel RS: Laboratory diagnosis in pediatric endocrinology. P Clin North America 4:959, 1957.

Metyrapone (Metopirone) Test
A. Specimen and Test Requirements: After 2 baseline 24-hour control collections, give metyrapone, 300 mg/sq m orally (never < 250 mg or > 750 mg) every 4 hours for 6 doses. Then collect two 24-hour urine samples following the last dose of the drug for 17-hydroxycorticosteroid assay.

B. Normal Values and Interpretation: The normal rise should be 3- to 5-fold, indicating normal pituitary and adrenal response. An abnormal test in the presence of a normal ACTH stimulation test indicates hypopituitarism.

Cushman P, Hilton JG: Metyrapone response in pituitary disease. J Endocrinol 43:377, 1969.

Dexamethasone Suppression Test
A. Specimen and Test Requirements: After 2 control collections have been made, give 1.25 mg/sq m/24 hours of dexamethasone orally in 4 divided doses for 3 days.

B. Normal Values: See Table 40–3 (17-hydroxycorticosteroids, 17-ketosteroids, and pregnanetriol).

C. Interpretation: If suppression of urinary hydroxycorticosteroids to a level of < 1.5 mg/24 hours or to < 50% of control values does not occur, increase the dose to 3.75 mg/sq m/24 hours and repeat the test. This is used to differentiate Cushing's syndrome (suppressible) from adrenal carcinoma, adenoma, or pituitary neoplasm (nonsuppressible).

Kendall JW, Sloop PR: Dexamethasone-suppressible adrenocortical tumor. New England J Med 279:532, 1968.

Plasma Hydrocortisone
Because there is considerable diurnal variation in plasma values of hydrocortisone (compound F), samples are always taken between 8 and 9 a.m., at which time 10–15 μg/100 ml is normal. The ACTH stimulation, metyrapone, and dexamethasone tests show the same proportionate changes for plasma as for urine.

THYROID FUNCTION

The laboratory appraisal of hypothyroidism and hyperthyroidism in children is primarily dependent on the triiodothyronine (T_3) uptake test, the T_4 test, and to a lesser extent (because of their technical difficulty) on butanol-extractable iodine (BEI) and protein-bound iodine (PBI) measurements. The radioiodine uptake test also has a complementary role.

In the precise evaluation of inborn errors of thyroxine metabolism, highly sophisticated procedures are required which are beyond the scope of this book. Some help may be obtained from noting the difference between the PBI, which measures tetra-, tri-, and diiodothyronine, and part of the monoiodothyronine, and the BEI, which measures only tri- and tetraiodothyronine.

Butanol-Extractable Iodine in Serum

A. Specimen: 0.5 ml serum.

B. Normal Values: $3-7$ μg/100 ml.

C. Interpretation: This test measures tri- and tetraiodothyronine but not iodinated tyrosyl residues. The results are high in thyrotoxicosis and low in hypothyroidism. The difference between PBI and BEI may indicate levels of mono- and diiodothyronine.

Protein-Bound Iodine in Serum

A. Specimen: 0.5 ml serum.

B. Normal Values: $4-8$ μg/100 ml.

C. Interpretation: As for BEI, above.

T$_3$ Uptake in Serum

A. Specimen: 0.5 ml serum.

B. Normal Values: $22-33\%$ (depends on laboratory).

C. Interpretation: The basis of the T$_3$ test is as follows. Plasma thyroid-binding globulin is normally partly saturated with T$_4$ and, to a very small extent, with T$_3$. The affinity for T$_4$, however, is greater than for T$_3$, so that if excess T$_3$ is added it does not displace the T$_4$. In the in vitro test, the added T$_3$ is labeled with ^{131}I and, after a period of equilibration, the residual unbound T$_3$ is adsorbed onto one of a variety of resins and the proportion of the original activity is measured.

In hypothyroidism, thyroid-binding globulin is relatively unsaturated and most of the labeled T$_3$ becomes attached to the protein. The converse is true in hyperthyroidism. Because of varying conditions, each laboratory should set up its own standards.

T$_4$ in Serum

A. Specimen: 0.5 ml serum.

B. Normal Values: $3.2-6.4$ μg/100 ml.

C. Interpretation: Serum is diluted and passed over an ion exchange column. The T$_4$ is eluted with acetic acid and the iodine measured with ceric sulfate. The test is specific. Elevated levels are seen in thyrotoxicosis and depressed levels in thyroid insufficiency.

Howarth PSN, Maclagan NF: Clinical applications of serum total thyroxin estimation. Lancet 1:224, 1969.

SCREENING & DIAGNOSTIC PROCEDURES FOR INBORN ERRORS OF METABOLISM

Amino Acids in Urine & Plasma

A. Specimens: 0.5 ml of a random urine acidified to pH 2.0; 0.1 ml serum.

B. Normal Values: See Table 40-2.

C. Interpretation: Disturbances of amino acid metabolism fall into 2 broad categories. In the first group, the changes in serum or urine amino acid levels are secondary to some other condition. Wilson's disease, galactosemia, chronic renal disease, rickets, scurvy, protein malnutrition, the renal tubular dystrophies, and heavy metal poisoning belong in this group. The increase in total urinary amino acid excretion may be striking, but the pattern of amino acids seen on paper chromatography usually reflects a generalized aminoaciduria and has little diagnostic value; measurement of total urinary amino acid nitrogen (expressed as μM/kg/24 hours) may be helpful.

In a second group, aminoaciduria or aminoacidemia reflects more precisely some inherited defect affecting the metabolism or transcellular movement of one or more amino acids. Improving technology for the precise measurement of amino acids and the increased use of screening technics in newborns and other special risk groups (institutionalized children, epileptics, psychotic children, etc) are now bringing to light new syndromes.

Scriver CR & others: Simple screening of plasma for aminoacidopathies. Lancet 1:230, 1964.

Chromatography of Sugars in Biologic Fluids

A. Specimens: 0.5 ml of a random urine acidified to pH 2.0; 0.1 ml serum.

B. Normal Values: Small amounts of hexoses and pentoses may be excreted by the normal person. For example, normal urine may contain up to 5 mg glucose/100 ml or 3 mg xylose/100 ml. Most tests for reducing sugars are insensitive to concentrations below 100 mg/100 ml, so that most pathologic melliturias require chromatography for their detection.

C. Interpretation:

1. Glycosuria—Diabetes, certain cerebral lesions, corticosteroid "diabetes," nephrosis, and primary and secondary renal tubular dystrophies.

2. Lactosuria—In milk-fed infants, up to 30 mg/100 ml; gastroenteritis, steatorrhea, and hepatitis.

3. Lactosuria, galactosuria, and fructosuria—Acute hepatitis, gastroenteritis, and rickets. It has been reported also in pyloric stenosis.

4. Fructosuria—Up to 20 mg/100 ml may normally be present in infants. Abnormal amounts may also be detected in diabetes, hepatitis, Wilson's disease, and mercury poisoning. Infantile fructosuria may also arise as a syndrome associated with vomiting, sweating,

TABLE 40–2. Normal values of amino acids and other ninhydrin-positive substances in plasma* and urine.†

	Newborn Plasma (Wk. 1)	Premature Plasma (Wk. 6)	Premature Urine (Wk. 6)	Full Term Plasma (Wk. 6)	Full Term Urine (Wk. 6)	Years 2–12 Plasma	Years 2–12 Urine	Adult Plasma	Adult Urine	% Tubular Reabsorption Infancy	% Tubular Reabsorption Childhood	% Tubular Reabsorption Adult
Phosphoethanol-amine	tr	...	...	...	...	...	.08–.28	...	...	...	...	...
Taurine	.01–.20	.05–.08	.03–.08	.02–.11	.01–.18	.06–.11	.76–1.9	.05–.08	0.4–1.3	96–98	93–95	72–95
Hydroxyproline	...	tr–.08	1.1–2.1	tr	0.7–2.6	...	0	0–tr	0	‡	...	...
Aspartic acid	tr–.02	.01–.02	tr–.04	.008–.02	tr–.32	.004–.02	tr–.07	.004–.01	.03–.09	§	92–99	85–98
Threonine	.04–.05	.15–.33	0.9–1.9	.17–.23	.67–1.4	.04–.10	.04–.17	.09–.14	.09–.14	71–91	92–99.5	97–99
Serine	.04–.30	.10–.16	0.8–1.3	.16–.20	1.1–2.3	.08–.11	.09–.34	.08–.11	.09–.31	54–86	92–99	97–99
Asparagine Glutamine	0.3–2.1	.40–.44	0.5–1.5	.36–.57	1.1–2.0	.06–.47	.04–.75	.4–.5	.17–.48	90–96	98–99.9	99+
Proline	.02–.43	.10–.31	0.6–1.7	.40–.48	0.7–5.4	.07–.15	tr–.04	.15–.25	0	53–94	99.5–100	99+
Glutamate	tr–.26	.08–.14	.02–.13	.06–.21	.04–.62	.02–.25	.01–.13	.05–.20	.008–.16	95–99	98.5–99.8	99+
Citrulline	...	.04–.07	.02–.17	tr–.04	tr–.04	...	tr–.03	tr–.03	0–tr	92–98	...	99+
Glycine	.05–.44	.12–.21	2.5–4.2	.18–.24	3.7–8.4	.12–.22	.33–1.5	.15–.24	.40–.90	15–63	93–99	94–99
Alanine	.04–.44	.20–.39	0.5–0.7	.46–.52	1.2–2.1	.14–.30	.04–.35	.35–.37	.09–.27	87–92	99–99.9	99+
α-Amino adipic	...	0	0.1–.23	0	.17–.23	...	...	0	0–.02	‡	...	‡
α-Amino butyric	tr–.07	0–tr	tr	tr–.02	0	...	tr–.06	.01–.03	.01–.04	‡	...	99
Valine	.03–.32	.12–.22	tr–0.2	.32–.35	.10–.16	.13–.28	tr–.08	.05–.08	tr–.05	98–99+	99.6–99.9	99+
Homocitrulline	...	tr	.13–.37	0	.12–.24	...	...	0	.02–.04	‡	‡	‡
1/2 Cystine	.02–.07	tr–.07	.04–.25	0	.14–.34	...	...	0	.02–.08	60–90	...	99+
Cystathionine	...	.005–.01	.09–.12	0–tr	.11–.17	...	...	0	.01–.02	35–65	...	‡
Methionine	tr–.08	.02–.04	.08–.14	.03–.05	.12–.14	.01–.02	.01–.04	.01–.04	.02–.04	85–97	98.3–99.7	98–99+
Isoleucine	.01–.09	.04–.08	.03–.07	.08–.12	.10–.16	.03–.08	.01–.07	.05–.08	.01–.04	96–99+	99.2–99.9	99+
Leucine	.01–.18	.1–.5	.04–.08	.14–.22	.15–.18	.06–.18	.02–.11	.10–.14	.02–.05	97–99+	99.6–99.9	99+
Tyrosine	.05–.30	.1–.4	.17–.60	.11–.21	.22–.38	.03–.07	.03–.12	.04–.07	.06–.10	93–99	98.2–99.3	98–99+
Phenylalanine	.02–.12	.05–.07	.08–.13	.06–.12	.11–.14	.03–.06	.01–.11	.04–.07	.04–.07	94–99	98.8–99.7	99+
β-Alanine	...	0	0	0	0	.02–.05	tr	0	0	...	...	...
BAIB	...	0	.09–.16	0	.17–.42	...	0–.19	0	.01–.09	...	...	...
Methylglycine	...	...	...	...	...	<.01	<.05	...	...	...	...	...
Hydroxylysine	...	0	.13–.27	0	.05–.11	...	...	0	0–.02	‡	...	...
GABA	tr–0.1	0	0–tr	0	0–tr	...	...	0	tr	...	...	‡
Ornithine	.01–.22	.08–.11	0–.08	.07–.10	.05–.08	.03–.09	.01–.03	.58–.90	tr	96–99+	99.5–99.8	99+
Lysine	.05–.35	.08–.15	0.2–0.6	.21–.34	0.7–1.4	.07–.15	.04–.21	.16–.18	.02–.20	81–96	98.5–99.8	99+
1-Methylhistidine	...	0	0	0	0–.03	...	...	0	.58–.90	...	...	...
Histidine	tr–.13	.05–.13	.34–.83	.05–.08	0.8–1.8	.02–.08	.11–1.0	.06–.07	.15–.53	30–80	90.3–98.4	92–98
3-Methylhistidine	...	0	0	0	0–.07	...	...	0	.08–.28	...	...	...
Arginine	tr–.12	tr–.07	0	.04–.10	tr–0.1	.02–.09	.01–.04	.03–.06	.02–.20	99+	99–99.9	99+

*Measured in $\mu M/ml$ (fasting).
†Measured in $\mu M/min/1.73$ sq m.
‡0–trace in plasma but significant amounts in urine.
§Detectable in plasma but not in urine except in traces.

hypoglycemia, and variable aminoaciduria, proteinuria, and hypophosphatemia.

5. **Galactosuria**—Up to 15 mg/100 ml may normally be present in small infants. Increased amounts may occur in children with galactosemia after galactose loads, although loading is not advised as a diagnostic test. Galactosuria may be present also in hepatitis.

6. **Sucrosuria**—Up to 15 mg/100 ml may be present in the urine of infants on alimentary loading. Sucrosuria is present also in pancreatic disease and has been described in a syndrome associated with hiatus hernia and mental retardation.

Wright SW & others: Studies on carbohydrates in body fluids. Am J Dis Child 93:173, 1957.

Screening Test for Galactosemia

A reliable screening test for galactosemia has been devised using 25 μl of heparinized blood. The test depends on the fluorescence formed when uridyl transferase converts galactose-1-phosphate to UDP galactose.

Beutler E, Baluda MC: Screening test for galactosemia. J Lab Clin Med 68:137, 1966.

Diagnostic Test for Galactosemia

A. Specimen: 1 ml heparinized blood cooled in ice water.

B. Normal Values: Galactose-1-phosphate uridyl transferase, 308–475 ImU/gm hemoglobin.

C. Interpretation: Homozygotes for galactosemia are < 8 ImU/gm hemoglobin. In Duarte variants and heterozygotes, the levels are 142–225 ImU/gm.

Tedesco TA, Mellman WJ: The UDPglu consumption assay for gal-1-P uridyl transferase. Page 66 in: *Galactosemia.* Hsia DYY (editor). Thomas 1969.

Mucopolysaccharides
A. Specimens: 5 ml of urine for screening test; a 24-hour urine sample for chromatographic test.
B. Normal Values: See Table 40–3.
C. Interpretation: In the last few years, a group of diseases have come to be identified which are now recognized to be associated with specific defects of lysosomal enzymes. Previously, they had been grouped together under the name of Hurler's syndrome, although they represented cases with a wide range of skeletal deformities, corneal clouding, hepatospleno-megaly, and intellectual impairment. As might be expected in an essentially connective tissue disorder, vascular and joint tissues may also be involved.

A satisfactory screening test for excess mucopoly-saccharides in urine is available which depends on a precipitate formed in the presence of a buffered acid-albumin reagent. More specific assay can be carried out using a saline gradient and column chromatography or urine. Specific enzyme assays will probably be increasingly used in the future.

Ferric Chloride Test for Phenylketonuria
A. Specimen: 5 ml urine.
B. Method: Add 10% ferric chloride solution, drop by drop, to 5 ml of urine in a test tube. Initially, a precipitate of ferric phosphate may form which may require filtering. A purple color is produced by both acetoacetic acid and salicylates, but the former color is heat-labile. A green color develops in the presence of phenylpyruvic acid. Other compounds reacting with ferric chloride are listed below.
C. Compounds Reacting in Ferric Chloride Test:
1. Metabolites—
   Phenylpyruvic acid: green
   p-Hydroxyphenylpyruvic acid: green fading rapidly
   a-Ketobutyric acid (oasthouse syndrome): purple going to brownish red
   3-Hydroxyanthranilic acid: brown
   Urocanic acid (histidinemia): green
   Homogentisic acid: very dark brown
   Xanthurenic acid (pyridoxine disorders): dark green going to brown
   Branched chain ketoacids (maple syrup urine): gray-green
   Pyruvic acid: yellow-brown
   Melanin: black
   Acetoacetic acid: red-brown, red
   Imidazole pyruvic acid (histidinemia): blue-green
   1-Methylhistidine: slow green

2. Drugs—
   Salicylates: purple
   Phenothiazines: purple
   Aminosalicylic acid: red-brown

Histidinuria Screening Test
A. Specimen: 1 ml random urine.
B. Interpretation: Excess histidine in urine will inhibit the formation of blue color given by bis-cyclohexane in the presence of copper. The screening test must be confirmed by a quantitative measurement of serum histidine.

Gerber MG: A simple screening test for histidinuria. Pediatrics 213:40, 1969.
Levy HL & others: A simple indirect method of detecting the enzyme defect in histidenemia. J Pediat 75:1056, 1969.

Methylmalonic Aciduria Screening Test
The following simple screening test for the presence of methylmalonic acid in urine is based on the formation of a green diazo derivative:

Fifty μl of urine are added to 0.75 ml of 0.1% *p*-nitroaniline in 0.16 N hydrochloric acid. Aqueous sodium nitrite, 0.5%, 0.25 ml, and 1 M sodium acetate buffer pH 4.3, 1 ml, are added, and the mixture is incubated for 1 minute in a boiling water bath. A green color appears at concentrations greater than 100 mg/100 ml of methylmalonic acid. This is sufficiently sensitive to detect cases of methylmalonate isomerase deficiency. Confirmation requires gas chromatography.

Giorgio AJ, Luhby AL: Rapid screening test for methyl malonic aciduria. J Clin Path 52:374, 1969.

Nitroprusside Cyanide Screening Test for Cystine & Homocystine in Urine
Acidify 5 ml of urine with 0.5 ml of 1 N hydro-chloric acid, add 2 ml of fresh 5% sodium cyanide solution, and let stand at room temperature for 30 minutes. Then add 1 ml of fresh 5.5% sodium nitro-prusside solution. A definite purple color indicates the presence of excess amounts of cystine, homocystine, or β-mercaptolactate cysteine disulfide. Faintly positive reactions may occur in older normal children, and more definite ones in small premature infants in the first trimester of life.

Orotic Aciduria Screening Test
A. Specimen: 0.5 ml random urine.
B. Method: Orotic acid is converted by bromine water and ascorbic acid to barbituric acid. The latter forms a yellow compound with Ehrlich's reagent. His-tidinuria may produce a false-positive test.
C. Interpretation: The test is valid for the detection of hereditary orotic aciduria and also as confirmation of hyperammonemia due to ornithine transcarbamylase deficiency.

Rogers LE, Porter FG: Hereditary orotic aciduria. II. A urinary screening test. Pediatrics 42:423, 1968.

TESTS OF LIVER FUNCTION

Alkaline Phosphatase

A. **Specimen:** 0.05 ml serum.

B. **Normal Values:** See Table 40–3.

C. **Interpretation:** Alkaline phosphatase is a lysosomal enzyme whose activity is found to be increased in 2 groups of diseases: those affecting liver function, and those in which there is involvement of osteoblastic activity in the bones. In hepatic disease, increased plasma alkaline phosphatase is generally accepted as an indication of biliary obstruction. In the second group, serum phosphatase activity is increased in primary hyperparathyroidism, in secondary hyperparathyroidism owing to chronic renal disease, in the various forms of rickets, and in osteitis deformans juvenilia—whether these be due to vitamin D deficiency, malabsorption, or renal tubular dystrophies. Levels may also be increased in Recklinghausen's disease with bone involvement and in a variety of malignant infiltrations of bone. Low values are found in hyperthyroidism and in the rare condition known as idiopathic hypophosphatasia, where it is associated with rickets and the excretion of excess phosphoethanolamine in the urine.

Derren JJ & others: Alkaline phosphatase. New England J Med 270:1277, 1969.

Acid Phosphatase

A. **Specimen:** 0.1 ml serum.

B. **Normal Values:** 8.6–13 IU/liter.

C. **Interpretation:** Serum acid phosphatase levels are elevated to about twice normal in Gaucher's disease. Elevations are also found in acute and chronic thrombocytopenic purpuras. Acid phosphatase activity is greatly reduced in a syndrome associated with early severe progressive neurologic disease.

Blood Ammonia

A. **Specimen:** 1 ml plasma collected in a heparinized tube in ice cold water.

B. **Normal Values:** 45–80 μg/100 ml.

C. **Interpretation:** Ammonia is produced by bacterial action in the bowel and absorbed into the portal circulation. It is also produced endogenously by the deamination of amino acids. Ammonia levels are of some value in gauging the severity or prognosis of liver failure, especially in Reye's syndrome, but are essential in the diagnosis of inborn errors in the Krebs-Henseleit urea cycle.

Conn HD: Sources and significance of blood ammonia. Yale J Biol Med 41:33, 1968.

Bilirubin in Serum

A. **Specimen:** 0.05 ml serum.

B. **Normal Values:** See Table 40–3.

C. **Interpretation:** Bilirubin is produced by the destruction of hemoglobin and is then converted in the liver to its diglucuronide for excretion in the bile. The unconjugated form is elevated in hemolytic diseases, in acute hepatitis, and in hereditary glucuronyl transferase deficiency. The conjugated form is elevated in acute and chronic hepatitis as well as in obstructive liver disease.

Robinson SH: The origins of bilirubin. New England J Med 279:143, 1968.

Bile Pigments in Urine & Feces & Associated Tests

A. **Hay's Test for Bile Salts:** Sprinkle a little dry, finely powdered sulfur onto the surface of about 10 ml of urine in a small beaker. The presence of bile salts is indicated by sinking of the sulfur particles, which can be very sensitively detected by examining the urine in reflected light.

B. **Fouchet's Test for Bilirubin in Urine:** Add 2 ml of 10% barium chloride to about 5 ml of urine, acidified if necessary with acetic acid. If there is no precipitate, add 1 or 2 drops of saturated ammonium sulfate solution. Mix and filter. Unfold filter paper and place it on another dry paper. Place 1 drop of Fouchet's reagent on the precipitate. The development of a green color denotes the presence of bilirubin.

C. **Fouchet's Test for Bilirubin in Feces:** Transfer a quantity of feces about the size of a pea to a 15 ml test tube containing 10 ml water. Cover tube with a square of Parafilm and shake vigorously to form a suspension. Place a few drops of this suspension on a white tile. Add (drop by drop) Fouchet's reagent (25 gm trichloracetic acid in 60 ml of water; 10 ml of 10% ferric chloride solution; water to make 100 ml).

D. **Urobilinogen and Porphobilinogen:** To 2 ml urine add 2 ml Ehrlich's reagent (dimethylaminobenzaldehyde, 7 gm; concentrated hydrochloric acid, 150 ml; water to make 250 ml), 4 ml saturated sodium acetate solution, and 3 ml chloroform. Mix and shake thoroughly for 5 seconds. A pink color in the chloroform layer indicates the presence of urobilinogen. Remove the aqueous layer and shake it with an equal volume of n-butanol; a pink color in the aqueous (lower) layer indicates porphobilinogen.

E. **Schlesinger's Test for Urobilin:** Add 3 drops 0.1 N iodine solution to 5 ml urine. Pour contents of this tube into another containing 5 ml absolute ethanol and 0.5 gm powdered zinc acetate. Mix thoroughly by repeated inversion and filter. A green fluorescence on looking down into the tube in a cross light indicates urobilin. Confirm by noting the characteristic band in the green/blue part of the spectrum.

F. **Stercobilin:** Place a quantity of feces about the size of a walnut in a large glass tube with 15 ml of a mixture of 1 ml concentrated hydrochloric acid to 100 ml of absolute ethanol. Mix thoroughly with a glass rod and let stand overnight. Filter.

The filtrate may be examined with a small hand spectroscope for the characteristic rather broad band at the juncture of the blue and the green part of the spectrum. Alternatively, the filtrate may be examined by fluorescence after neutralizing with sodium hydroxide, mixing with an equal quantity of alcoholic zinc acetate, and refiltering (see Schlesinger's Test, above).

G. Rothera's Test for Acetone and Acetoacetic Acid: Add 5 ml urine and 1 ml concentrated ammonia to approximately 1 gm of a powder containing 1 part sodium nitroprusside to 100 parts ammonium sulfate in a test tube. Cover tube with a Parafilm square and mix by inversion. The development of a permanganate color on standing indicates the presence of acetone or acetoacetic acid.

H. Bence Jones Protein: Filter the urine if it is not clear and make barely acid with dilute acetic acid. Put about 5 ml into each of 3 test tubes. To the second and third samples, add 1 and 2 drops of 33% acetic acid, respectively. Mix and place tubes in a water bath at room temperature. Place a thermometer in one of the tubes and gradually raise the temperature of the water bath. Bence Jones protein is precipitated between 40° and 60° C and dissolves on further heating. If albumin and globulin are present, boil and filter hot. Bence Jones protein will precipitate on cooling and may be redissolved by heating again.

More specific information can be obtained by electrophoresis of serum and urine proteins. The abnormal myeloma globulins show as dense, relatively narrow bands that lie in various positions in the β and γ areas.

I. Homogentisic Acid: If homogentisic acid is present, the urine will darken on standing, especially if alkaline. This process is greatly accelerated if strong base is added to the urine. Addition of 10% ferric chloride gives a transient blue or green color. Urine reduces Benedict's solution to give a brown precipitate.

The silver nitrate test for homogentisic acid is performed as follows: Add 5 ml 3% silver nitrate solution to 0.5 ml urine. Add a few drops of 10% ammonium hydroxide. A black color indicates the presence of homogentisic acid. Keep test tube out of direct sunlight.

Copper in Biologic Fluids

A. Specimens: 0.1 ml serum; 24-hour urine acidified to pH 2.0.

B. Normal Values: See Table 40–3.

C. Interpretation: Approximately 98% of circulating serum copper is bound to a blue alpha$_2$ globulin, ceruloplasmin. The remaining 2% exists in 2 forms: most is loosely bound to albumin, whereas the remainder exists as free ionic copper.

In Wilson's disease, urinary copper is increased and there is a decrease in serum copper and ceruloplasmin levels. In cirrhosis of the liver, urine copper is also elevated, but serum copper and ceruloplasmin (alpha$_2$ copper-binding protein) are increased. Serum copper oxidase assay is simple and specific since it relates closely to serum copper and ceruloplasmin levels, whose estimation is complex.

Wilson's disease should always be excluded as a cause of chronic liver disease in children. There is some recent evidence that, in a small number of cases of Wilson's disease, copper oxidase levels may be normal. Liver copper is the best index of Wilson's disease.

Slovis T & others: The varied manifestations of Wilson's disease. J Pediat 78:578, 1971.

Bromsulphalein Excretion Test

A. Specimen and Test Requirements: The patient should be fasting. Give 5 mg/kg Bromsulphalein in sterile 5% solution IV over a period of 1 minute. Draw a blood sample at 45 minutes. The test requires 0.1 ml serum. The method assumes a plasma volume of 50 ml/kg.

B. Normal Values: < 10% retention in children.

C. Interpretation: This is essentially a test of both the glutathione conjugating ability of the liver and the excretion of conjugates; outside of this specific role, it is a generally less useful test of liver function than enzyme assays and serum electrophoresis, especially in children. Bromsulphalein conjugates of glutamic acid and cysteine are also found in the bile.

Lindquist B, Paulson L: BSP elimination in infants and children. Acta paediat 48:223, 1959.

Serum Cholesterol

A. Specimen: 0.1 ml serum.

B. Normal Values: See Table 40–3.

C. Interpretation: Plasma cholesterol in the normal child varies within wide limits, and for this reason its estimation has a rather limited application. The level is elevated in diabetes, nephrosis, hypothyroidism, and biliary obstruction, as well as in idiopathic hypercholesterolemia and hyperlipidemia; it is depressed in hyperthyroidism, hepatitis, and sometimes in severe anemia or infection. In none of these instances does the measurement of serum cholesterol rank as more than a subsidiary test; in nephrosis, for example, serum protein electrophoresis provides a substantially more sensitive index of diagnosis and progress.

Rafstedt S: Serum lipids and lipoproteins in infancy and childhood. Acta paediat 44(Suppl 102):1, 1955.

Lactate Dehydrogenase, Serum & Cerebrospinal Fluid

A. Specimen: 0.1 ml serum or CSF.

B. Normal Values: 90–180 IU/liter.

C. Interpretation: Lactate dehydrogenase (LDH) is one of the increasing number of enzymes that can be separated into different protein fractions possessing the same substrate specificity. Each of the 5 common isozymes of LDH has been shown to be a tetramer comprised of combinations of 2 polypeptide chains, A and B. The enzyme shows an organ specificity, so that the predominant isozyme (60%) in heart muscle, type 1, appears in increased concentration in the serum following cardiac infarction, traveling in the neighborhood of albumin upon electrophoresis. On the other hand, the greatest serum LDH activity in hepatitis is in the slowest moving band, type 5. In myopathies, types 3, 4, and 5 are increased.

Levels of total serum LDH activity (2–5 times normal) have been reported in progressive forms of chronic hepatitis and hepatic cirrhosis. Abnormally high values have been detected in certain blood diseases, including sickle cell anemia, the hemolytic crisis in favism, acute acquired hemolytic anemia, and, particularly, in untreated pernicious anemia, in which levels more than 10 times normal are found. The serum LDH level is normal in anemias due to blood loss or iron deficiency.

LDH activity may be increased in the CSF following birth injury, results varying from 22–600 IU/liter in infants suspected of intracranial pathology.

Serum Leucine Aminopeptidase

A. **Specimen:** 0.1 ml serum.

B. **Normal Values:** 15–50 IU/liter.

C. **Interpretation:** Increases in the level of serum leucine aminopeptidase are associated (with the exception of pregnancy) almost exclusively with diseases of the liver, biliary tract, or pancreas. The determination has a special place in pediatric clinical chemistry in the differentiation of neonatal hepatitis and biliary atresia. In this respect, it ranks with rose bengal sodium I 131 as a diagnostic test. In neonatal hepatitis, values generally less than 120 IU/liter are recorded, but in atresia 90% are above this level.

Rutenburg AM & others: Serum leucine amino peptidates. Am J Dis Child 103:47, 1962.

Transaminase in Serum & Cerebrospinal Fluid

A. **Specimen:** 0.1 ml serum or CSF.

B. **Normal Values:** Up to 30 IU/liter.

C. **Interpretation:** The transaminases, as widely distributed intracellular enzymes, are raised in the serum in various kinds of tissue destruction, after major surgery, and in myopathies, but primarily in hepatitis and other forms of active liver disease. (The SGOT level in CSF following intracranial damage is 2.5–10.5 IU/liter.) High values are found in the newborn period; thereafter, values are remarkably uniform.

TESTS OF PANCREATIC & ENTERIC FUNCTION

Serum Amylase

A. **Specimen:** 0.1 ml serum or heparinized plasma.

B. **Normal Values:** 6–33 Close-Street units/100 ml.

C. **Interpretation:** Elevated levels of serum and urine amylase have been used as an index of pancreatitis following trauma or as a complication of mumps or infectious mononucleosis. In the above conditions, the serum amylase levels may initially exceed 250 Close-Street units. Levels may be increased in chronic pancreatic obstruction, in bowel obstruction, and in

peritonitis, but levels in serum do not exceed 120 units. Urine values are unsatisfactory due to interference from urinary citrate or concomitant impairment of renal function.

Disaccharidase in Jejunal Biopsy

A. **Specimen:** Assay requires 15–20 mg jejunal mucosa taken by biopsy.

B. **Normal Values:** (μM substrate split/minute/gram wet mucosal tissue.) Lactase, 0.2–19; maltase, 13–54; isomaltase, 4–13; sucrase, 6–17.

C. **Interpretation:** The enzymes are present in the brush border of the small intestine and in small amounts in the fluid within the lumen of the bowel. It will be apparent, therefore, that in conditions where the epithelium is itself damaged apparent disaccharidase deficiency will exist. This has been recorded during and after acute enteritis, in celiac syndrome (particularly with respect to lactase), and in cystic fibrosis. Less well documented accounts suggest similar deficiencies in regional ileitis, ulcerative colitis, peptic ulcer, abetalipoproteinemia, blind loop syndrome, and protein malnutrition.

Lactase deficiency alone is by far the most common of the heritable deficiencies. Congenital sucrase deficiency is theoretically possible, but the evidence to date is that it is rare and does not yet seem to have been reported with biopsy information. In the same way, isomaltase deficiency is possible and has now been recorded. Dahlqvist has shown that 75% of maltase activity is borne by isomaltase and invertase and the remainder by maltases II and III. In combined sucrase/isomaltase deficiency, this residual activity can hydrolyze an oral load of maltose. However, if starch is given and maltose is gradually released in passage down the intestine, intolerance may be shown.

These enteric enzyme deficiencies can also be measured by demonstrating a flat glucose tolerance test following an oral load of the appropriate disaccharide.

Duvois RS & others: Disaccharidase deficiency in children with immunologic deficits. J Pediat 76:377, 1970.

Absorption Tests for Lactase, Amylase, Maltase & Sucrase Activity

A. **Specimens and Test Requirements:** 0.1 ml serum at start of test and at 30 minutes for glucose assay. The oral loading dose of maltase and starch should be the same as that of glucose (see p 961). The dose for lactose and sucrose should be twice that amount. All carbohydrate is administered as a flavored 10% aqueous solution.

B. **Interpretation:** In normal children, there is a rise of over 50 mg/100 ml within 30 minutes. A rise of less than 20 mg/100 ml is suggestive of enzymatic defect.

Fat Absorption

A. **Specimen and Test Requirements:** The patient is placed on a normal diet containing 35% of calories as fat. On the third day, a 24-hour stool collection is made.

B. Normal Values: See Table 40–3.

C. Interpretation: About 40% of triglyceride is completely hydrolyzed in the small bowel: a further 40% is hydrolyzed to mono- and diglyceride, and about 20% is unhydrolyzed. Hydrolysis reflects the action of pancreatic lipase on emulsified triglyceride formed in the presence of bile salts, on fatty acids, and on mono- and diglycerides. Long chain fatty acids (> C-16) are absorbed in the free state or as monoglycerides into the mucosal cell, where they are resynthesized into triglyceride before passing into the lymph. Short chain fatty acids (< C-16, and especially < C-10) may be absorbed into mucosal cells in any form as mono-, di-, or triglyceride or in the free state. Within the cell, they may be resynthesized into triglyceride or become attached to albumin. In both ways they pass into the portal blood.

In children, excess stool fat is most commonly found in either cystic fibrosis of the pancreas or in the gluten-sensitive celiac syndrome. Other causes include obstructive liver disease which interferes with bile salt availability, chronic enteric infections, blind loop syndrome, small bowel resections, pancreatic achylias (including hereditary pancreatitis and absence of lipase), acrodermatitis enteropathica, abetalipoproteinemia, and hypoparathyroidism.

Anderson CM: Intestinal malabsorption in childhood. Arch Dis Child 41:571, 1966.

Free Fatty Acids in Plasma

A. Specimen: 0.1 ml plasma.

B. Normal Values: See Table 40–3.

C. Interpretation: The "free" fatty acids (FFA) of plasma represent metabolically active lipid in the process of being transported, albumin-bound, from the fat depots to the tissues. It is now clear that FFA form a readily available source of energy that can be metabolized by many tissues, notably cardiac and skeletal muscle. The respiratory quotient of newborn infants indicates that during the third to fifth days of life energy is derived from sources which are 80–90% fat. Although cord blood FFA levels are significantly lower than those of the mother at the time of delivery, the highest values achieved under normal conditions are found during the first day after birth. There ensues a gradual fall over the following year to levels slightly above normal adult levels. Infants born of diabetic mothers have cord blood levels which do not differ significantly from those of infants born of normal mothers.

The turnover rate of plasma FFA has been reported as 28% per minute, equivalent to about 250 μEq/liter/minute. During exercise, the turnover rate increases and the absolute level falls.

Elevated levels are found in hyperthyroidism, which is associated with an accelerated mobilization of fat. Fasting also results in an increased plasma FFA level, particularly in children up to age 10. A 19-hour period of fasting caused values higher than those following a 14-hour fast. While the same was true of adults, the levels found were considerably lower. The trauma experienced by an individual with burns is associated with raised FFA in plasma; the more pronounced the trauma, the greater and more prolonged the elevation. Four patients with nondetectable glucose-6-phosphatase levels had raised fasting FFA levels, presumably as a result of the hypoglycemic tendency typical of this glycogen storage disease. In the study of lipid levels of well controlled juvenile diabetics aged 2–13 years, no difference was found in the FFA levels when compared with normal children of the same age group. Twelve children age 13 months to 4 years suffering from kwashiorkor and a group with marasmus exhibited elevated levels of FFA in comparison with controls.

Lipase in Serum or Duodenal Secretion

A. Specimen: 0.1 ml serum or duodenal secretion.

B. Normal Values: 10–136 IU/liter (serum).

C. Interpretation: Traditionally, the assay of lipase in duodenal juice has been considered a diagnostic test for cystic fibrosis of the pancreas. However, it is apparent that pancreatic digestive secretions may be considerably diminished during and after any serious illness, whether enteric or not. There is also a rare condition of primary lipase deficiency.

Serum lipase levels are elevated in acute pancreatitis, a relatively common concomitant of mumps and glandular fever. In this condition, serum lipase levels tend to rise more slowly and, once elevated, to be more sustained than serum amylase levels. The difficulties and discomforts to the child of obtaining samples of duodenal juice, together with the effectiveness of the sweat chloride test, mean that this and similar enzyme tests are seldom now required in the diagnosis of fibrocystic disease.

Xylose Absorption

A. Specimen and Test Requirements: The test is performed as follows: The fasting child is given 10 ml/kg of a 5% solution of D-xylose and, subsequently, fasted and thirsted for 5 hours. Urine is collected over this period, and, after recording the total volume, an aliquot is preserved in the deep freeze. Blood samples are taken into fluoride-oxalate tubes before the test starts, at 30 minutes, and at 120 minutes.

B. Normal Values: See Table 40–3.

C. Interpretation: Xylose absorption is a technically simple, reliable, and informative gauge of upper small bowel absorption. This pentose is not digested in the bowel, but it is not clear whether it is absorbed in the small bowel solely by diffusion or by an active process involving phosphorylation or other specific enzymes. About 60% of absorbed xylose is metabolized via fructose-6-phosphate and through the Krebs cycle; the remainder is excreted within 5 hours in the urine. The test is primarily one of upper small bowel absorption.

Xylose absorption is normal in colitis, liver disease, and in primary pancreatic deficiencies. In children, it is abnormal in fibrocystic disease of the pancreas, indicating that the malabsorption in this state is not solely a reflection of deficient pancreatic enzymes.

Bunta H: Xylose test and its normal values in children. Kinderärztl Praxis 38:507, 1970.

BIOCHEMICAL TESTS FOR UNDERNUTRITION

The following tests are useful in the detection of undernutrition and in other situations which are outlined below. (See also Table 4–3 for levels indicating deficiencies.)

Ascorbic Acid

A. Specimens: 1 ml fresh plasma; 4 hour fresh urine collections.

B. Normal Values: See Table 40–3.

C. Interpretation: Ascorbic acid determinations may be useful when scurvy occurs with rickets and the typical radiologic picture is consequently obscured.

Estimates of ascorbic acid in fasting serum provide a rather crude assessment of the scorbutic state. Levels below 0.15 mg/100 ml are suggestive. A more satisfactory procedure is to perform a tolerance test by giving 20 mg/kg of ascorbic acid (IV or IM) as a 4% solution in sterile pyrogen-free saline. A 4-hour sample should show levels in excess of 1.5 mg/100 ml after the intravenous load and in excess of 0.6 mg/100 ml after the intramuscular load.

In scurvy, the urine level of ascorbic acid following an oral loading dose is < 1% in 24 hours.

Serum Proteins

A. Specimen: 0.1 ml plasma.

B. Normal Values: See Table 40–3.

C. Interpretation: Changes in serum protein levels occur in many childhood diseases. Albumin is depressed where there is proteinuria and in the exudative enteropathies. Alpha$_1$ proteins are elevated in acute and chronic infections and characteristically merge with the beta band in the acute stage of idiopathic nephrosis. Gamma globulins are increased in infection, in some immunodystrophies, and especially in disseminated lupus erythematosus and related diseases. The gamma globulins are diminished in the agammaglobulinemias.

Vitamin A & Carotene in Serum

A. Specimen: 0.1 ml serum.

B. Normal Values: See Table 40–3.

C. Interpretation: Vitamin A is fat-soluble, so that estimations of its level in plasma can be a measure of fat absorption. Low fasting levels are found in undernourished children and in those with malabsorption syndromes. Increased levels are noted in vitamin A intoxication and in some cases of idiopathic hypercalcemia of infancy. The absorption of vitamin A palmitate is a gauge of lipase function and chylomicron absorption, whereas vitamin A alcohol absorption is an index of chylomicron absorption only. Tolerance tests are a more sensitive index of malabsorption than fasting levels. They may also be used to demonstrate the augmented absorption often seen in idiopathic hypercalcemia, when values for vitamin A may rise from fasting values of 72–200 μg/100 ml to 4-hour levels of 360–1070 μg/100 ml.

β-Carotene occurs widely in leafy vegetables and in certain other fruits and roots. It is rather less well absorbed than vitamin A and more dependent on the presence of bile. Synthesis of vitamin A from β-carotene is thought to occur in the mucosa. Hypocarotenemia is found in malabsorption syndromes, and abnormally high levels may occur from a high intake of yellow vegetables and, occasionally, in diabetes and hypothyroidism.

Vitamin E in Serum

A. Specimen: 0.1 ml serum.

B. Normal Values: See Table 40–3.

C. Interpretation: The small premature infant fed evaporated milk unsupplemented by vitamin E may, by the second month of life, have a serum tocopherol level below that which is known to produce in vitro hemolysis of red blood cells. It has also been shown that children with cystic fibrosis of the pancreas may have hypovitaminosis E, often in association with ceroid deposits in the intestinal musculature.

Other Useful Laboratory Parameters Indicative of Malnutrition

Hemoglobin, < 10 gm/100 ml

Hematocrit, < 30%

Serum iron, < 30 μg/100 ml at 2 years to < 60 μg/100 ml at 12 years

Transferrin saturation, < 20%

Red cell folacin, < 140 ng/ml

Serum folacin, < 3 ng/ml

Urinary thiamine, < 120 (1–3 years), < 85 (4–6 years), < 60 (7–12 years) μg/gm creatinine

Urinary riboflavin, < 150 (1–3 years), < 100 (4–6 years), < 80 (7–15 years) μg/gm creatinine

Urinary iodine, < 25 μg/gm creatinine

Serum urea, < 8 mg/100 ml

Serum amylase, < 6 IU/100 ml

Chase MP & others: Nutritional status of migrant farm children. Am J Dis Child 122:316, 1971.

O'Neal RM & others: National Nutrition Survey 4:103, 1970.

TESTS OF RENAL FUNCTION

Urine Ammonia

A. Specimen and Test Requirements: Timed specimens should be acidified with concentrated hydrochloric acid to pH 3.0 as collected, and refrigerated. The assay is a simple colorimetric one using Nessler's reagent.

B. Normal Values: See Table 40–3.

C. Interpretation: The estimation of urine ammonia is one gauge of the renal tubular capacity to excrete hydrogen ion. Thus, in states of acidosis unaccompanied by renal impairment (eg, starvation and diabetic acidosis), there may be as much as a 5-fold increase in urine ammonia. Normal excretion is about 12 μEq/minute/sq m, but this varies with diet. The ammonium ion is derived from glutamine in the tubule cell, and in chronic renal disease the limitation of this mechanism is one of the causes of acidosis. As with all tests of renal function, the expanded capacity of remaining normal renal tissue conceals overall diminished performance until this is extensive.

Peonides A: The renal excretion of hydrogen ions in infants and children. Arch Dis Child 40:33, 1965.

Creatine & Creatinine in Plasma & Urine

A. Specimen: 0.1 ml serum, timed urine acidified to pH 2.0 and refrigerated.

B. Normal Values: See Table 40–3.

C. Interpretation: Serum creatinine is used as an index of glomerular failure, as is the creatinine clearance (urine concentration $\times$ urine volume per minute $\div$ plasma concentration). The latter value, which is generally less reliable than the inulin clearance, can also be used as a reference for calculating tubular reabsorption, eg, of amino acids or phosphorus. In muscular dystrophy, an increased urinary creatine coefficient and a decreased urinary creatinine coefficient may be diagnostically helpful. Creatinine excretion is not a reliable reference term in which to express the urinary content of other solutes.

Applegarth DA & others: Creatinine excretion in children. Clin Chem Acta 22:131, 1968.

Glomerular Filtration Rate (See also discussion in Chapter 18.)

A. Specimen: 0.1 ml fasting serum.

B. Normal Values: 45–95 ml/min/sq m.

Phosphorus, Tubular Reabsorption

A. Specimen: 0.1 ml serum; 1 ml urine.

B. Normal Values and Interpretation: The ratio of phosphorus and creatinine clearances can be used to calculate tubular reabsorption of phosphorus (TRP):

$$\% \text{ TRP} = 100\left[1 - \frac{(\text{Urine P} \times \text{Plasma creatinine})}{(\text{Plasma P} \times \text{Urine creatinine})}\right]$$

In normal subjects, the range is 78–97% reabsorption. This is greatly diminished in the phosphate-losing forms of vitamin D resistant rickets.

Nordin BEL, Fraser R: Assessment of urinary phosphate excretion. Lancet 1:947, 1960.

Blood Urea Nitrogen

A. Specimen: 0.1 ml heparinized whole blood.

B. Normal Values: See Table 40–3.

C. Interpretation: Urea is excreted by the glomeruli and reabsorbed by the tubules. Raised levels in the plasma offer only a rather crude index of renal failure since glomerular destruction must amount to about 80% before urea is retained. The same comment may be made about the urea clearance test. It is important to remember, however, that the blood urea may be raised up to 50 mg/100 ml or even more in small infants receiving a high dietary nitrogen load. In these circumstances, diminished urea clearance does not indicate renal disease.

Uric Acid in Plasma

A. Specimen: 0.2 ml plasma.

B. Normal Values: See Table 40–3.

C. Interpretation: Elevated in rheumatoid arthritis, in renal failure, in leukemia during treatment, and in the hyperuricemia/mental retardation syndromes.

SPECIAL TESTS FOR PHEOCHROMOCYTOMAS & NEUROBLASTOMAS

Pressor Amine Metabolites

A. Specimen: Timed or random urines, acidified to pH 2.0.

B. Normal and Abnormal Values:

Metanephrine

Normal children	0.02–0.16 μg/mg creatinine
Normal adults	0.1 μg/mg creatinine; 0.6 ± 0.3 mg/24 hours
Pheochromocytoma	0.2–3.5 μg/mg creatinine; 25 (3–113) mg/24 hours
Ganglioneuroma, neuroblastoma	Not strikingly increased.

Normetanephrine

Normal children	0.05–0.6 μg/mg creatinine
Normal adults	0.1 μg/mg creatinine
Pheochromocytoma	0.6–7 μg/mg creatinine
Ganglioneuroma, neuroblastoma	Some increase in the former; usually greatly increased in the latter.

Homovanillic acid (HVA)

Normal adults	2–4 μg/mg creatinine
Normal children	3–16 μg/mg creatinine

Pheochromocytoma,
    ganglioneuroma Some increase.
Neuroblastoma   Greatly increased.

3-Methoxy-4-hydroxymandelic acid (VMA)

Normal adults   1.5–3 μg/mg creatinine;
                   1–4 mg/24 hours
Normal children   2–12 μg/mg creatinine;
                   83 ± 26 μg/kg/24 hours
Pheochromocytoma
    (adults)   70–1200 μg/mg creatinine
Neuroblastoma
    (children)   86–14,000 μg/kg/24 hours

C. Interpretation: The estimation in urine of various pressor amine metabolites in children is of great importance in the diagnosis of pheochromocytomas, other sympathetic nervous system tumors, and perhaps also of dysautonomia. It is still true that clinical features are the main determinants in the diagnosis; the special value of biochemical data would seem to be in confirmation and in making some preoperative judgment on the extent and degree of malignancy of a tumor. Postoperatively, these measurements are likewise of value in judging the completeness of surgery as well as the establishment and growth of secondary deposits.

These estimations are probably most accurately made on 24-hour specimens of urine, although figures are now widely expressed in terms of creatinine despite the notorious variance of the latter from day to day in young persons.

The urinary excretion of a wide variety of phenolic metabolites in pheochromocytoma, ganglioneuroma, and neuroblastoma is now recorded. Fortunately, technics for the metanephrines, for 3-methoxy-4-hydroxymandelic acid (VMA), and for 3-methoxy-4-hydroxyphenylacetic acid or homovanillic acid (HVA) suffice for a very sophisticated appraisal. It is the metanephrines that are primarily increased in pheochromocytoma; VMA is usually elevated too, but HVA is not. In ganglioneuroma, it is primarily homovanillic acid which is increased. In neuroblastomas, normetanephrine may be strikingly elevated in the urine and metanephrine to a lesser extent, but VMA and HVA are uniformly greatly increased.

Technics are available for the estimation of urinary metanephrines and VMA. In practice, it is probably simpler to judge the HVA excretion from a chromatogram, although satisfactory and relatively simple technics for direct assay by column, thin layer chromatography, or spectrophotometry have now been developed.

An important ancillary assay is the urinary excretion of cystathionine and beta-aminoisobutyric acid (BAIB). These are not elevated in pheochromocytoma or in ganglioneuroma, but they are markedly increased in neuroblastoma, particularly in the more malignant growths and in those with extensive secondary deposits.

In dysautonomia, there is reported to be a change in the ratio of HVA/VMA in the urine from a normal value of 1.4 ± 0.55 to 4.7 ± 1.6. This is due to both a decrease in VMA and an increase in HVA. o-Tyrosine also appears to be much increased in urine.

Mention should also be made of the tyramine test for pheochromocytoma. A dose of approximately 580 μg/sq m of tyramine is given intravenously, which gives a mean rise of blood pressure in cases of pheochromocytomas of around 40 mm Hg as opposed to 3 mm Hg in normal subjects and 14 mm Hg in renal hypertensive patients. This appears to be an excellent test in adults, but few reports have been made in children. Glucagon produces a similar effect.

Gjessing LR: Studies of functional neural tumors. VI. Biochemical diagnosis. Scandinav J Clin Lab Invest 16:661, 1964.

TESTS FOR MUSCLE DISEASE*

Serum Aldolase

    A. Specimen: 0.2 ml serum.

    B. Normal Values: 4–10 IU/liter.

    C. Interpretation: Fructose diphosphate aldolase cleaves fructose-1:6-diphosphate to dihydroxyacetone phosphate and glyceraldehyde-3-phosphate. A second aldolase, predominantly in the liver, forms dihydroxyacetone phosphate and glyceraldehyde from fructose-1-phosphate.

Serum aldolase determinations are useful in differentiating primary diseases of muscle (eg, pseudohypertrophic muscular dystrophy) from disorders in which the lesion is neurogenic (eg, amyotonia). The activity of this enzyme is also increased in infective hepatitis, myocardial infarction, acute pancreatitis, and severe hemolytic anemia. Levels in portal cirrhosis and obstructive jaundice are within normal limits. Fructose-1-phosphate aldolase is absent in hereditary fructose intolerance and lowered in Tay-Sachs disease.

Niebroz-Dobosz I & others: Blood enzymes in Duchenne's progressive muscular dystrophy and their correlation with the clinical and histological pictures. Acta med pol 11:387, 1970.

Serum Creatine Kinase

    A. Specimen: 0.1 ml serum.

    B. Normal Values: 5–70 IU/liter.

    C. Interpretation: At present the most reliable laboratory confirmation of muscular dystrophy is provided by the serum creatine phosphokinase (CPK) level. This test has a further use in that it gives a moderately reliable indication of whether a young woman with affected male siblings is a carrier of the severe sex-linked form. The test is not helpful in identifying persons heterozygous for the mild X-linked and autosomal recessive forms.

*See also Lactate Dehydrogenase, p 969.

A refinement of this assay is provided by starch-gel electrophoresis of CPK isozymes: Muscular dystrophy patients show only the major and not the minor component. CPK activity is strikingly elevated in serum in hypothyroidism; it is diminished, but less obviously, in hyperthyroidism.

Cao A & others: Serum creatine phosphokinase isoenzymes in congenital hypoparathyroidism. J Pediat 78:134, 1971.

Katz RM, Liebman W: Creatine phosphokinase activity in central nervous systemic disorders and infections. Am J Dis Child 120:543, 1970.

TESTS FOR SALICYLISM & OTHER INTOXICATIONS

Serum Salicylate*

A. **Specimen:** 0.1 ml serum.

B. **Normal Values:** Therapeutic levels should be less than 30 mg/100 ml.

C. **Interpretation:** The estimation of plasma salicylate is no longer required to control therapy in rheumatic fever. It is, however, of great importance in the management and diagnosis of salicylism. The prognosis appears to be related to the initial salicylate load. In judging both appropriate treatment and prognosis, a single salicylate level must be related to time since ingestion. Done has suggested a formula—$\log S_O = \log S + 0.015\ T$—for calculation of the theoretical extrapolated zero-time salicylate level. S_O, which is based on measurements of salicylate half-life in the serum, is derived from the serum salicylate level (S) and the time (T) in hours since ingestion. Figures for S_O of 50 indicate no intoxication; 50–80, mild; 80–100, moderate; 100, severe; and 160, usually fatal. Because of delayed absorption, levels in the first hour to 6 hours after ingestion may not be maximal.

Conventional treatment of salicylism involves only the restoration of normal acid-base balance. In some instances, the additional use of acetazolamide may be justified. In severe toxicity, a slow exchange transfusion or peritoneal dialysis is an effective means of rapidly lowering tissue salicylate levels. Ready-made commercial solutions for dialysis are available (Peridial, Impersol). However, it has been shown that for peritoneal dialysis to be really effective the dialysate must contain albumin. A solution should therefore be made to contain 140 mEq Na^+/liter, 4 mEq K^+/liter, 4 mEq Ca^{++}/liter, 1.5 mEq Mg^{++}/liter, 103 mEq Cl^-/liter, 45 mEq lactate/liter, and 15 gm glucose/liter in 5% salt-free human albumin.

Done AK: Salicylate intoxication. Pediatrics 26:800, 1960.

Barbiturates

A. **Specimen:** 1 ml heparinized whole blood.

B. **Normal Values:** Therapeutic values of pentobarbital and secobarbital are 0.2–0.3 mg/100 ml; of phenobarbital (continuous treatment), 1–3 mg/100 ml. Lethal levels are in the region of 10 times the therapeutic ones.

Glutethimide

A. **Specimen:** 1 ml heparinized whole blood, serum, or plasma.

B. **Interpretation:** Using the method where the drug is extracted into chloroform and measured spectroscopically by its absorption in ultraviolet light at 235 nm, levels of 10 μg/ml are usually associated with coma. Lethal levels are in the range of 30–40 μg/ml.

Huttenlocher PR: Accidental glutethimide intoxication in children. New England J Med 269:38, 1968.

Screening Test for Phenothiazine Compounds

Add 1 ml of urine to 1 ml of a reagent containing 45 parts of 20% perchloric acid, 50 parts of 50% nitric acid, and 5 parts of 5% ferric chloride. The development of a pink to violet color within 5 minutes indicates increasing amounts of phenothiazines. Patients with phenylketonuria and those taking aminosalicylic acid may give false-positive results.

*See also discussion in Chapter 37.

TABLE 40–3. Normal values.

Acetylkynurenine (Urine)
1. 6–22.5 (mean, 9) μM/kg/7 hours after a tryptophan load.

Acid Maltase (Liver)
> 0.7 μM/minute/gm wet tissue.

Acid Phosphatase (Serum)
Newborn: 13.4 ± 3 IU/liter.
2–13 years: 10.8 ± 2.2 IU/liter.
Adults: Males, 0.5–11 IU/liter; females, 0.2–9.5 IU/liter.

Albumin: See Proteins in Serum, below.

Aldolase (Serum)
Adults: 1.8–4.9 IU/liter.
Newborns: 4 times adult value.
Children: Twice adult value.

Alkaline Phosphatase (Serum)
1–3 months: 73–226 IU/liter.
Thereafter: Steady fall to 57–151 IU/liter between ages 3–10. At puberty, values rise again, averaging 117 IU/liter but with a range between 57–258 IU/liter. This rise occurs at a slightly younger age in girls than in boys. After the pubertal rise there is a steady fall until the adult range of 18.8–38.4 IU/liter is reached at about age 16. Boys have slightly higher levels than girls.

Amino Acids (Plasma and Urine)
See Table 40–2.

Amino Nitrogen (Urine)
Older children: 129 μM/kg/24 hours (range, 66–204 μM/kg/24 hours).
Premature infants: Values are, on the average, 6 times as high.
Full-term newborns: About 3 times as high. Values are higher in breast-fed than in cow's milk fed babies.

Ammonia (Blood)
Newborns: 90–150 μg/100 ml; higher in premature and jaundiced infants.
Thereafter: 45–80 μg/100 ml.

Ammonia (Urine)
2–12 months: 11.8 (4.2–19.9) μEq/minute/sq m.
13 months–16 years: 12.1 (5.9–16.5) μEq/minute/sq m.

Amylase (Serum)
6–33 Close-Street units/100 ml.

Amylo-1,6-glucosidase (Liver)
1 μM/minute/gm wet tissue.

Ascorbic Acid
See Vitamin C, below.

Barbiturates (Blood)
Short-acting: 0.2–0.3 mg/100 ml.
Long-acting: 1–3 mg/100 ml.

Bicarbonate or Total CO_2 (Plasma)
18–33 mM/liter measured gasometrically with the Natelson apparatus.

Bilirubin (Serum)
Approximate maximal levels of total bilirubin:
Premature:
    Up to 24 hours: 8 mg/100 ml.
    Up to 48 hours: 12 mg/100 ml.
    Days 3–5: 24 mg/100 ml.
Full-term:
    Cord blood: 2.5 mg/100 ml.
    Up to 24 hours: 6 mg/100 ml.
    Up to 48 hours: 7.5 mg/100 ml.
    Days 3–5: 12 mg/100 ml.
After 1 month:
    Conjugated: 0–0.3 mg/100 ml.
    Unconjugated: 0.1–0.7 mg/100 ml.

Blood & Plasma Volume
Blood volume: 85.6 ml/kg (range, 69–112) at age 1. Similar values are found at birth, although they rise shortly after birth. The range in older children is 51–86 ml/kg (70 ± 8.3). In premature newborns, the mean is 98 ml/kg.
Plasma volume: 49.9 (39.1–76.9) ml/kg at birth, rising to 66 ml/kg at about 4 weeks and remaining at this level for the first year. The range in older children is 30–54 ml/kg.

Body Water
Values as percentage of body weight:
Total body water:
    0–11 days: 77.8 (69–84)%.
    11 days–6 months: 72.4 (63–83)%.
    2–7 years: (63.4 (55–73)%.
    7–16 years: 58.2 (50–64)%.
Extracellular water:
    0–11 days: 42 (34–53)%.
    11 days–6 months: 34.6 (28–57)%.
    2–7 years: 25 (21–30)%.
    7–16 years: 20.5 (18–26)%.
Intracellular water:
    0–11 days: 34.5 (28–40)%.
    11 days–6 months: 38.8 (20–47)%.
    2–7 years: 40.4 (31–53)%.
    7–16 years: 46.7%.

Bromsulphalein Test (Serum)
Newborn infants in respiratory distress: Up to 30% retention.
Normal newborn infants: Up to 15%.
Thereafter: < 10% retention.

TABLE 40–3 (cont'd). Normal values.

Calcium (Serum)	**Copper** (Serum)

Calcium (Serum)
4.4–5.3 mEq/liter by fluorometric assay.

Calcium (Urine)
40–80 mEq/24 hours during childhood (4–12 years).

Carbon Dioxide, Total (Serum)
18–23 mM/liter.

Carotene (Serum)
At birth: About 70 µg/100 ml, rising to about 340 µg/100 ml at age 1.
At age 3½: About 150 µg/100 ml.
Thereafter: 100–150 µg/100 ml.

Catecholamines, Total (Urine)
1 (0.4–2) µg/kg/24 hours.

Ceruloplasmin (Serum)
0.37 ± 0.06 absorbance units in 1-cm path cells. (Absorbance units × 87.5 = mg ceruloplasmin per 100 ml.)

Chloramphenicol (Serum)
Therapeutic levels are 15–30 µg/ml. Levels in excess of 50 µg/ml may be dangerous in the newborn.

Chloride
Serum: 97–104 mEq/liter.
Breast milk: 11 (2.5–30) mEq/liter.
Cow's milk: 37 (20–80) mEq/liter.
Muscle: 20–26 mEq/kg wet fat-free tissue.
Spinal fluid: 120–128 mEq/liter.
Sweat: 96% of children, up to 30 mEq/liter; in the remainder, up to 60 mEq/liter. (Adults: Up to 70 mEq/liter.)

Cholesterol (Serum)
Premature cord blood:
　Free: 23 (16–31) mg/100 ml.
　Ester: 44 (28–67) mg/100 ml.
　Total: 67 (47–98) mg/100 ml.
Full-term cord blood:
　Free: 24 (17–38) mg/100 ml.
　Ester: 43 (26–67) mg/100 ml.
　Total: 67 (45–98) mg/100 ml.
Full-term newborn (heel stick):
　Free: 31 (17–59) mg/100 ml.
　Ester: 54 (26–119) mg/100 ml.
　Total: 85 (45–167) mg/100 ml.
3 days–1 year:
　Free: 40 (26–66) mg/100 ml.
　Ester: 90 (51–132) mg/100 ml.
　Total: 130 (69–174) mg/100 ml.
2–14 years:
　Free: 54 (39–69) mg/100 ml.
　Ester: 134 (99–173) mg/100 ml.
　Total: 188 (138–242) mg/100 ml.

Copper (Serum)
Up to 6 months: < 70 µg/100 ml.
6 months–5 years: 27–153 µg/100 ml.
5–17 years: 94–234 µg/100 ml.
Adults: 70–118 µ/100 ml.

Copper (Urine)
Up to 30 µg/24 hours.

Copper Oxidase (Serum)
Same as Ceruloplasmin, above.

Creatine & Creatinine (Urine)
Creatinine coefficient:
　6–66 days (premature): 8.1–15 mg/kg/day.
　89–100 days (full-term): 10.4–19.7 mg/kg/day.
　1½–7 months: 10–15 mg/kg/day.
　7–15 years (males): 5.2–41 mg/kg/day.
　7–15 years: (females): 11.5–29.1 mg/kg/day.
Creatine coefficient:
　6–66 days (premature): 0–7.3 mg/kg/day.
　89–100 days (full-term): 5.4–18.2 mg/kg/day.
　1½–7 months: 5.4–13.7 mg/kg/day.
　7–15 years (males): Decrease from 5.7 to 1.5 mg/kg/day.
　7–15 years (females): Decrease from 6 to 1.2 mg/kg/day.

Creatine Kinase (Serum)
Males: 5–75 IU/liter.
Females: 6–50 IU/liter.

Creatinine (Serum)
0.4–1.2 mg/100 ml.

Cystine, Free (Urine)
45–485 µM/24 hours.

Epinephrine (Urine)
0.2 (0.02–0.7) µg/kg/24 hours.

Fats, Neutral (Serum)
10–350 mg/100 ml.

Fats (Fecal)
< 5 gm/24 hours.

Fatty Acids, "Free" (Serum)
Newborn: 905 ± 470 µEq/liter
4 months–10 years: 699 ± 199 µEq/liter (14-hour fast); 986 ± 235 µEq/liter (19-hour fast).
Adults: 448 ± 140 µEq/liter (14-hour fast); 560 ± 157 µEq/liter (19-hour fast).

Fibrinogen (Plasma)
200–500 mg/100 ml.

TABLE 40–3 (cont'd). Normal values.

Galactose   (Blood)
     Up to 20 mg/100 ml.

Galactose   (Urine)
     Up to 15 mg/100 ml on a milk diet.

Galactose-1-phosphate   (Red Cells)
     < 1 mg/100 ml packed erythrocyte lysate.

Galactose-1-phosphate Uridyl Transferase   (Red Cells)
     308–475 ImU/gm hemoglobin.

Glomerular Filtration Rate
     Older children and adults: 75 (45–95) ml/sq m.
         (These levels are reached by about 6
         months.)
     Newborns: About 50% of the above values.

Glucose   (Serum)
     Newborn: 20–80 mg/100 ml.
     Normal fasting level: 60–185 mg/100 ml.

Glucose   (Urine)
     Up to 5 mg/100 ml.

Glucose-6-phosphatase   (Liver)
     > 5 μM/minute/gm wet tissue.

Glucose-6-phosphate Dehydrogenase   (Red Cells)
     150–215 units/100 ml red cells.

Glycogen   (Red Cells)
     Cord blood: 123 (10–338) μg/gm hemoglobin.
     4½–19 hours: 150 (48–361) μg/gm hemoglobin.
     2–12 months: 78 (32–134) μg/gm hemoglobin.
     1–12 years: 66 (22–109) μg/gm hemoglobin.
     Adults: 57 (20–105) μg/gm hemoglobin.

Hematocrit
     Birth: 44–64%.
     14–90 days: 35–49%.
     6 months–1 year: 30–40%.
     4–10 years: 31–43%.

Hemoglobin   (Blood)
     Day 1: 19 (14–24) gm/100 ml.
     Day 2: 19 (15–23) gm/100 ml.
     Day 6: 18 (13–23) gm/100 ml.
     2 weeks: 16.5 (15–20) gm/100 ml.
     1 month: 14 (11–17) gm/100 ml.
     2 months: 12 (11–14) gm/100 ml.
     3 months: 11 (10–13) gm/100 ml.
     6 months: 11.5 (10.5–14.5) gm/100 ml.
     1 year: 12 (11–15) gm/100 ml.
     2 years: 13 (12–15) gm/100 ml.
     5 years: 13.5 (12.5–15) gm/100 ml.
     8–13 years: 14 (13–15.5) gm/100 ml.

Hemoglobin   (Plasma)
     No more than 3 mg/100 ml.
     A_2 hemoglobin: 2–3.5% of total hemoglobin.

Hemoglobin, Fetal   (Blood)
     Birth: 50–85% of total hemoglobin.
     1 year: < 15% of total.
     Up to 2 years: Up to 5% of total.
     Thereafter: < 2% of total.

Homovanillic Acid (See also p 973.)   (Urine)
     Children: 3–16 μg/mg urine creatinine.
     Adults: 2–4 μg/mg urine creatinine.

17-Hydroxycorticosteroids   (Serum)
     After 2 weeks: 10–15 μg/100 ml.

17-Hydroxycorticosteroids   (Urine)
     0–2 years: 2–4 mg/24 hours.
     2–6 years: 3–6 mg/24 hours.
     6–10 years: 6–8 mg/24 hours.
     10–14 years: 8–10 mg/24 hours.

5-Hydroxyindoleacetic Acid   (Urine)
     0.35 (0.11–0.61) μM/kg/7 hours. (Based on 15
         well nourished, apparently healthy mentally
         defective children on a tryptophan load.)

Hydroxyanthranilic Acid   (Urine)
     1.2–4.9 μM/kg/7 hours after a tryptophan load.

Hydroxykynurenine   (Urine)
     < 0.5–9.2 μM/kg/7 hours after a tryptophan
         load.

Hydroxyproline, Total   (Urine)
     5–14 years: 38–126 mg/24 hours.

Indole-3-acetic Acid   (Urine)
     3.1–8.1 mg/24 hours. (Based on 11 young adult
         normals.) Values for excretion after trypto-
         phan loading are not available.

Insulin   (Serum)
     Fasting: 5–40 μU/ml. (Varies with laboratory.)

Iodine, Butanol-Extractable   (Serum)
     Newborn: 3–13 μg/100 ml.
     6 weeks–16 years: 3–7 μg/100 ml.

Iodine, Protein-Bound   (Serum)
     4–8 μg/100 ml.

^{131}I-Labeled Triolein Absorption Test
     > 8% of ingested dose in total blood volume 4–6
         hours after ingestion.

TABLE 40–3 (cont'd). Normal values.

Iron (Serum)
190 ± 80 (2 SD) µg/100 ml at birth, falling in the first 4–6 months and then rising to 117 ± 58 (2 SD) µg/100 ml by age 3; by atomic absorption, 183 ± 96 (2 SD) µg/100 ml.

Iron-Binding Capacity (Serum)
Birth: 117 (59–175) µg/100 ml, rising steadily by age 1 to the levels of later childhood.
3–10 years: 350 (250–400) µg/100 ml.

17-Ketosteroids (Urine)
(Values in mg/24 hours.)
0–14 days: 0.5–2.5
2 weeks–2 years: 0–0.5
2–6 years: 0–2
6–8 years: 0–2.5
8–10 years: 0.7–4

	Boys	Girls
10–12 years:	0.7–6	0.7–5
12–14 years:	1.3–10	1.3–8.5
14–16 years:	2.5–13	2.5–11

Kynurenic Acid (Urine)
7.1 (3.4–20.6) µM/kg/7 hours after a tryptophan load.

Kynurenine (Urine)
15.6 (3.8–50.5) µM/kg/7 hours after a tryptophan load.

Lactate (Blood)
1–1.8 mM/liter after an overnight fast.

Lactate Dehydrogenase
Normal infants age 2½ hours–10 days:
Serum: 815 (308–1780) IU/liter.
CSF: 22.6 (2.3–84) IU/liter.
Adults:
Serum (males): 98–186 IU/liter.
Serum (females): 87–178 IU/liter.
CSF (both sexes): 6.3–30 IU/liter.

Lead (Blood)
< 50 µg/100 ml whole blood.

Leucine Aminopeptidase (Serum)
Newborn: 44 ± 15 IU/liter.
1 month–adult: 15–50 IU/liter.

Lipase
Serum: 20–136 IU/liter based on 4-hour incubation.
Duodenal juice: 8–35 IU/ml.

Lipoproteins (Serum)
Newborn:
Alpha: 134 ± 9 (71–176) mg/100 ml.
Beta: 103 ± 7.2 (51–158) mg/100 ml.

Omega: 77 ± 4.9 (48–106) mg/100 ml.
Total lipid: 314 ± 14 (170–440) mg/100 ml.
3–10 days:
Alpha: 194 ± 12 (116–266) mg/100 ml.
Beta: 277 ± 4.5 (215–320) mg/100 ml.
Omega: 138 ± 7.4 (84–190) mg/100 ml.
Total lipid: 609 ± 30 (430–760) mg/100 ml.
10 days–1 year:
Alpha: 169 (67–281) mg/100 ml.
Beta: 290 (122–450) mg/100 ml.
Omega: 124 (51–247) mg/100 ml.
Total lipid: 574 (240–800) mg/100 ml.
2–14 years:
Alpha: 251 ± 9.7 (147–327) mg/100 ml.
Beta: 412 ± 16 (225–541) mg/100 ml.
Omega: 176 ± 90 (98–268) mg/100 ml.
Total lipid: 839 ± 32 (490–1090) mg/100 ml.

Magnesium (Serum)
EDTA method: 1.2–1.8 mEq/liter.
Fluorometric method:
Children: 1.4 ± 0.18 mEq/liter.
Adults: 2.05 ± 0.22 mEq/liter.

Magnesium (Urine)
About 0.1 mEq/kg/24 hours by the fluorometric method.

Mercury (Urine)
< 50 µg/24 hours.

Metanephrine (See also p 973.) (Urine)
Children: 0.02–0.16 µg/mg urine creatinine.

Methemoglobin (Blood)
0–0.3 gm/100 ml.

3-Methoxy-4-hydroxymandelic Acid
See Vanilmandelic acid, below.

Methylnicotinamide (Urine)
Based on a group of 22 normal children without a tryptophan load: 0.85 (0.33–1.83) µM/kg/24 hours.
Based on a group of 15 well nourished, apparently healthy mentally defective children after a tryptophan load: 0.28 (0.12–0.44) µM/kg/7 hours.

Milliosmols (Plasma)
Same as Osmotic Pressure (see below).

Mucopolysaccharides (Urine)
(Values expressed as mg hexuronic acid/24 hours.)
2 years: 0–5 mg/24 hours.
4 years: 0–6 mg/24 hours.
6 years: 1–8 mg/24 hours.

TABLE 40–3 (cont'd). Normal values.

8 years: 1–9 mg/24 hours.
10 years: 1–10 mg/24 hours.
12 years: 1–11 mg/24 hours.
14 years: 2–12 mg/24 hours.
(Ratio of acid mucopolysaccharides to creatinine.)

1 year: 9/33	8 years: 4/21
2 years: 8/31	9 years: 3/20
3 years: 8/29	10 years: 2/18
4 years: 7/27	11 years: 2/15
5 years: 7/26	12 years: 1/14
6 years: 6/25	13 years: 0/13
7 years: 4/23	14 years: 0/12

Mucoproteins (Serum)
Mucoprotein carbohydrate: 21.8 ± 6.3 mg/100 ml.
Mucoprotein protein: 75.3 ± 28.5 mg/100 ml.
Mucoprotein tyrosine: 3.3 ± 1 mg/100 ml.

Nitrogen (Muscle)
29–34 gm/kg wet fat-free tissue.

Nonesterified Fatty Acids
See Fatty Acids, Free (above).

Norepinephrine (Urine)
0.8 (0.4–1.6) μg/kg/24 hours.

Normetanephrine (See also p 973.) (Urine)
Children: 0.05–0.6 μg/mg urine creatinine.

Osmotic Pressure (Plasma)
170–285 mOsm/liter plasma water.

Osmotic Pressure (Urine)
Infants: 50–600 mOsm/liter urine water.
Older children: 50–1400 mOsm/liter urine water.

Oxygen Capacity of Blood
1.34 ml/gm hemoglobin.

Oxygen Saturation of Venous Blood
Newborn: 30–80%
Thereafter: 65–85%

Packed Cell Volume
Birth: 44–64%.
14–90 days: 35–49%.
6 months–1 year: 30–40%.
4–10 years: 31–43%.

P$_{CO_2}$ (Blood)
40 mm Hg (at sea level).

pH (Whole Blood)
7.38–7.42 at 37° C.

Phenylalanine (Serum)
0.7–3.5 mg/100 ml on random specimens by fluorometric assay.

Phosphatase
See Acid Phosphatase and Alkaline Phosphatase, above.

Phospholipid (Serum)
Cord blood: 1.34 ± 0.36 μM/ml.
2–13 years: 2.67 ± 0.52 μM/ml.
3–20 years: 3.42 (2.49–4.36) μM/ml.

Phosphorus, Inorganic (Serum)
Premature:
Birth: 6.8 ± 0.6 mg/100 ml.
6–10 days: 8.9 ± 1.4 mg/100 ml.
Days 20–25: 8 ± 0.7 mg/100 ml.
Full-term:
Birth: 6.4 ± 0.7 mg/100 ml.
Day 3: 7.4 ± 0.8 mg/100 ml.
Days 6–12: 6.9 ± 1 mg/100 ml.
Childhood:
1 year: 5 ± 0.6 mg/100 ml.
10 years: 4.6 ± 0.5 mg/100 ml.
20 years: 4.1 ± 0.5 mg/100 ml.

Phosphorus, Inorganic (Muscle)
200–240 mg/kg wet fat-free tissue.

Plasma Volume
See Blood and Plasma Volume, above.

Porphyrins (Urine)
δ-Aminolevulinic acid:
Under 15 years: < 0.49 mg/100 ml.
Adults: 0.1–0.56 mg/100 ml.
Porphobilinogen:
Under 15 years: < 0.11 mg/100 ml.
Adults: < 0.2 mg/100 ml.
Coproporphyrin:
Adults: < 100 μg/24 hours. (Lower values are found in childhood, but the range is not yet known.)
Uroporphyrin:
Adults: 2.7–14.6 μg/liter. (Trace amounts only are present in children.)

Porphyrins, Total (Serum)
Adults: < 0.7 μg/100 ml. (Values for children are not available.)

Porphyrins (Red Cells)
Protoporphyrin (all ages): 15–100 μg/100 ml.
Coproporphyrin (all ages): 0.5–2 μg/100 ml.

Potassium
Serum: 4.1–5.6 mEq/liter.
Cow's milk: 20–45 mEq/liter.

TABLE 40–3 (cont'd). Normal values.

Breast milk: 12–17 mEq/liter.
Muscle: 160–180 mEq/kg wet fat-free tissue.

Pregnanetriol (Urine)
2 weeks–2 years: 0.02 (0–0.2) mg/24 hours.
2–16 years: 0.6 (0.3–1.1) mg/24 hours.

Pressor Amine Metabolites
See p 973.

Proline (Serum)
54 ± 20 (2 SD) μg/ml by colorimetric assay.

Protein (CSF)
Newborn: 40–120 mg/100 ml.
1 month: 20–70 mg/100 ml.
Thereafter: 15–40 mg/100 ml.

Proteins (Serum)
See accompanying chart.

Pyridoxic Acid (Urine)
2.3 (0.5–7.2) μg/kg/7 hours. (Based on results obtained from 21 apparently healthy, well nourished mentally defective children.)

Pyruvate (Blood)
55.3 ± 2.4 μM/liter. (Resting adult males; arterial samples.)

Pyruvate Kinase (Red Cells)
11 ± 3.7 (2 SD) units/gm hemoglobin.

Sodium
Serum: 136–143 mEq/liter.
Cow's milk: 22–26 mEq/liter.
Breast milk: 4.7–8.3 mEq/liter.
Muscle: 33–43 mEq/kg wet fat-free tissue.

Thymol Turbidity (Serum)
0–4 Maclagan units.

T_3 Uptake (Serum)
22–33% (varies with different laboratories).

T_4 (Serum)
3.2–6.4 μg/100 ml by column chromatography.

Transaminases (Serum)
Infants:
SGOT: Up to 67 IU/liter.

Proteins in Serum*
(gm/100 ml)

	First Week		4 Months	12 Months		4 Years
	Premature	Full-Term	Premature	Premature	Full-Term	and Over
Total						
5.29 (4.32–7.63) SD 0.72	5.97 (4.65–7.41) SD 0.8		5.76 (4.74–6.17) SD 0.8	6.47 (5.80–7.12) SD 0.47	6.41 (6.08–6.72) SD 0.40	6.79 (6.15–8.10) SD 0.43
Albumin						
3.38 (2.81–3.91) SD 0.35	4.17 (3.32–5.13) SD 0.65		3.90 (2.78–4.92) SD 0.53	3.76 (3.22–4.48) SD 0.37	4.48 (4.07–5.03) SD 0.28	4.58 (3.72–5.50) SD 0.40
Alpha$_1$						
0.21 (0.13–0.47) SD 0.08	0.17 (0.12–0.32) SD 0.04		0.23 (0.05–0.45) SD 0.08	0.35 (0.19–0.46) SD 0.09	0.22 (0.15–0.35) SD 0.06	0.22 (0.12–0.30) SD 0.06
Alpha$_2$						
0.39 (0.25–0.65) SD 0.12	0.38 (0.25–0.47) SD 0.04		0.57 (0.37–0.83) SD 0.13	0.77 (0.50–1.11) SD 0.18	0.54 (0.41–0.66) SD 0.13	0.57 (0.35–0.95) SD 0.11
Beta						
0.46 (0.31–1.16) SD 0.07	0.38 (0.17–0.61) SD 0.11		0.63 (0.41–1.13) SD 0.14	0.86 (0.64–1.08) SD 0.1	0.62 (0.52–0.83) SD 0.12	0.62 (0.47–0.92) SD 0.06
Gamma						
0.85 (0.48–1.56) SD 0.28	0.87 (0.40–1.41) SD 0.26		0.43 (0.12–0.67) SD 0.16	0.72 (0.33–1.20) SD 0.22	0.55 (0.45–0.66) SD 0.10	0.81 (0.53–1.20) SD 0.24

*Values are for paper electrophoresis. Using cellulose acetate, mean albumin levels increase by 0.3 gm/100 ml and gamma globulin decreases by 0.2 gm/100 ml.

TABLE 40–3 (cont'd). Normal values.

SGPT: In about 1/3 of infants the range is 27–54 IU/liter; in the remainder, the range is 0–27 IU/liter.
Older children:
SGOT: 3–27 IU/liter.
SGPT: 1–30 IU/liter.

Transaminases (CSF)
Infants:
GOT: 1–7 IU/liter.

Trypsin
Feces: Under age 1, dilution of feces of 1:100 or more digests gelatin.
Duodenal juice: 160–180 µg activated trypsin/ml. Dilution of 1:12.5 or more digests gelatin.

Tyrosine (Serum)
Normal newborn: 2.5 ± 2.3 (2 SD) mg/100 ml.
Adults: 1.1 ± 0.5 (2 SD) mg/100 ml.

Tubular Rejection Fraction Ratio
0.8–1.45

Urea Clearance
Premature: 2–10 ml/sq m/minute.
Newborn: 5–19 ml/sq m/minute.
2–12 months: 23–55 ml/sq m/minute.
2 years and over: 30 ml/sq m/minute.

Urea Nitrogen (Whole Blood)
1–2 years: 5–15 mg/100 ml.
Thereafter: 10–20 mg/100 ml.

Uric Acid (Serum)
2–5.5 mg/100 ml

Urobilinogen (Urine)
< 3 mg/24 hours.

Vanilmandelic Acid (VMA) (See also p 974.)   (Urine)
Children: 83 ± 26 µg/kg/24 hours, or 2–12 µg/mg urine creatinine.
Adults: 1–4 mg/24 hours, or 1.5–3 µg/mg urine creatinine.

Vitamin A (Serum)
Rises from 40 µg/100 ml at birth to 70 µg/100 ml at age 1, then falls slowly to 40 µg/100 ml by age 2.

Vitamin C
Plasma: 0.5–1 mg/100 ml.
Urine: > 5% of an oral 20 mg/kg loading dose in 24 hours; < 1% in scurvy.

Vitamin E (Serum)
Should exceed 0.5 mg/100 ml.

Xanthurenic Acid (Urine)
1.9 (0.8–5.6) µM/kg/7 hours after a tryptophan load.

Xylose (Urine)
Up to 3 mg/100 ml.

Xylose Absorption Test (Blood)
30–40 mg/100 ml 30 minutes after a xylose load.

Xylose Absorption Test (Urine)
(Mean 5-hour excretion expressed as percentage of ingested load.)
Under 6 months: 11–30%.
6–12 months: 20–32%.
1–3 years: 20–42%.
3–10 years: 25–45%.
Over 10 years: 25–50%.
Or: % excretion = > (0.2 × age in months) + 12.

Zinc (Serum)
107 ± 30 (2 SD) µg/100 ml by atomic absorption.

•   •   •

General References

O'Brien D, Ibbott FA, Rodgerson DO: *Laboratory Manual of Pediatric Micro-biochemical Techniques,* 4th ed. Hoeber, 1968.

Index